12TH EDITION

Maternity & Women's Health Care

DEITRA LEONARD LOWDERMILK

RNC-E, PhD, FAAN
Clinical Professor Emerita
School of Nursing
University of North Carolina at
    Chapel Hill
Chapel Hill, North Carolina

KATHRYN RHODES ALDEN

EdD, MSN, RN, IBCLC
Associate Professor, Retired
School of Nursing
University of North Carolina at
    Chapel Hill
Chapel Hill, North Carolina

SHANNON E. PERRY

RN, PhD, FAAN
Professor Emerita
School of Nursing
San Francisco State University
San Francisco, California

ELLEN F. OLSHANSKY

PhD, RN, WHNP-E, FAAN
Professor Emerita
Sue & Bill Gross School of Nursing
    and Founding Director
Program in Nursing Science
University of California Irvine
Irvine, California

KITTY CASHION

RN-BC, MSN
Clinical Nurse Specialist
Department of Obstetrics and
    Gynecology
Division of Maternal-Fetal Medicine
University of Tennessee Health
    Science Center
Memphis, Tennessee

ELSEVIER

3251 Riverport Lane
St. Louis, Missouri 63043

MATERNITY AND WOMEN'S HEALTH CARE, TWELFTH EDITION   ISBN: 978-0-323-55629-3

Notices

Knowledge and best practice in this field are constantly changing. As new research and experience broaden our understanding, changes in research methods, professional practices, or medical treatment may become necessary.

Practitioners and researchers must always rely on their own experience and knowledge in evaluating and using any information, methods, compounds, or experiments described herein. In using such information or methods they should be mindful of their own safety and the safety of others, including parties for whom they have a professional responsibility.

With respect to any drug or pharmaceutical products identified, readers are advised to check the most current information provided (i) on procedures featured or (ii) by the manufacturer of each product to be administered, to verify the recommended dose or formula, the method and duration of administration, and contraindications. It is the responsibility of practitioners, relying on their own experience and knowledge of their patients, to make diagnoses, to determine dosages and the best treatment for each individual patient, and to take all appropriate safety precautions.

To the fullest extent of the law, neither the Publisher nor the authors, contributors, or editors, assume any liability for any injury and/or damage to persons or property as a matter of products liability, negligence or otherwise, or from any use or operation of any methods, products, instructions, or ideas contained in the material herein.

Previous editions copyrighted 2016, 2012, 2007, 2004, 2000, 1997, 1993, 1989, 1985, 1981, and 1977.

Library of Congress Control Number: 2019934900

Senior Content Strategist: Sandra Clark
Content Development Specialist: Elizabeth Kilgore
Publishing Services Manager: Julie Eddy
Senior Project Manager: Rachel E. McMullen
Design Direction: Brian Salisbury

Printed in the United States of America

Last digit is the print number: 9   8   7   6   5   4   3   2   1

Working together to grow libraries in developing countries

www.elsevier.com • www.bookaid.org

DEITRA LEONARD LOWDERMILK

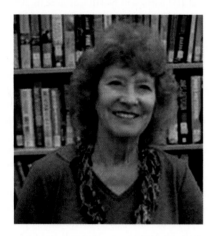

Deitra Leonard Lowdermilk is Clinical Professor Emerita, School of Nursing, University of North Carolina at Chapel Hill. She received her BSN from East Carolina University and her MEd and PhD in Education from UNC-CH. She is certified in In-Patient Obstetrics by the National Certification Corporation. She is a fellow in the American Academy of Nursing. In addition to being a nurse educator for more than 34 years, Dr. Lowdermilk has clinical experience as a public health nurse and as a staff nurse in labor and delivery, postpartum, and newborn units, and has worked in gynecologic surgery and cancer care units.

Dr. Lowdermilk has been recognized for her expertise in nursing education. She has repeatedly been selected as Classroom and Clinical Teacher of the Year by graduating seniors. She was a recipient of the Educator of the Year Award from both the District IV Association of Women's Health, Obstetric and Neonatal Nurses (AWHONN) and the North Carolina Nurses Association. She also received the 2005 AWHONN Excellence in Education Award.

She is active in AWHONN, having served as chair of the North Carolina Section of AWHONN and has served as chair and member of various committees in AWHONN at the national, district, state, and local levels. She has served as guest editor for the *Journal of Obstetric, Gynecologic and Neonatal Nursing* and served on editorial boards for other publications. Dr. Lowdermilk also is coauthor of *Maternity Nursing* (8th edition) and *Maternal Child Nursing Care* (5th edition).

Dr. Lowdermilk's most significant contribution to nursing has been to promote excellence in nursing practice and education in women's health through integration of knowledge into practice. In 2005 she received the first Distinguished Alumni Award from East Carolina University School of Nursing for her exemplary contributions to the nursing profession in the area of maternal-child care and the community. She was also Alumna of the Year for East Carolina University in 2005 and was selected as one of the 100 Incredible ECU Women in 2007 for Outstanding Leadership Among Women in the first 100 years of the university's founding.

In fall 2010, the East Carolina University College of Nursing named the Neonatal Intensive Care and Midwifery Laboratory in honor of Dr. Lowdermilk. In 2011 she was named one of the first 40 nurses inducted into the College of Nursing Hall of Fame.

SHANNON E. PERRY

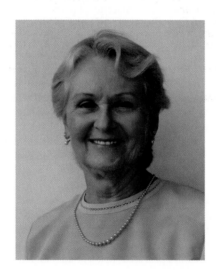

Shannon E. Perry is Professor Emerita, School of Nursing, San Francisco State University, San Francisco, California. She received her diploma in nursing from St. Joseph Hospital School of Nursing, Bloomington, Illinois; a baccalaureate in Nursing from Marquette University, an MSN from the University of Colorado Medical Center, and a PhD in Educational Psychology with a Specialization in Child Development from Arizona State University. She completed a 2-year postdoctoral fellowship in perinatal nursing at the University of California, San Francisco,

as a Robert Wood Johnson Clinical Nurse Scholar.

Dr. Perry has had clinical experience as a staff nurse, head nurse, and supervisor in surgical nursing, obstetrics, pediatrics, gynecology, and neonatal nursing. She has served as an expert witness and legal consultant. She has taught in schools of nursing in several states for more than 30 years and was interim director and director of the School of Nursing and director of a Child and Adolescent Development baccalaureate program at SFSU. She was Marquette University College of Nursing Alumna of the Year in 1999 and was the University of Colorado School of Nursing Distinguished Alumna of the Year in 2000. She received the San Francisco State University Alumni Association Emeritus Faculty Award in 2005 and the Excellence in Education Award from the Beta Upsilon chapter of Sigma Theta Tau International (STTI) in 2012.

She is coauthor of *Maternity Nursing* (8th edition), *Maternal Child Nursing Care* (5th edition), and *Clinical Companion for Maternity & Newborn Nursing* (2nd edition) and has authored numerous chapters and articles on maternal-newborn topics and the legal aspects of nursing. She is a fellow in the American Academy of Nursing, a member of AWHONN, Arizona Nurses Association (AzNA), and National League for Nursing (NLN), first vice president of the American Association for the History of Nursing (AAHN), and a member of the AAHN Communications Committee and the STTI Foundation Fellows Committee. Dr. Perry's experience in international nursing includes teaching international nursing courses in the United Kingdom, Ireland, Italy, Thailand, Ghana, and China and participating in health missions in Ghana, Kenya, and Honduras. She is participating in establishing a school of nursing in Kenya, has supported the establishment of the library, and has had a wing of a dormitory named after her. For her "exemplary contributions to nursing, public service, and selfless commitment and passion in shaping the future of international health," she received the President's Award from the Global Caring Nurses Foundation, Inc., in 2008. In January 2012, she and 47 other women climbed Mt. Kilimanjaro, the highest mountain in Africa, to raise awareness of human trafficking and to raise funds to support projects to combat human trafficking.

KITTY CASHION

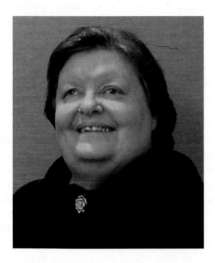

Kitty Cashion is a Clinical Nurse Specialist in the Maternal-Fetal Medicine Division, College of Medicine, Department of Obstetrics and Gynecology at the University of Tennessee Health Science Center in Memphis. She received her BSN from the University of Tennessee College of Nursing in Memphis and her MSN in Parent-Child Nursing from Vanderbilt University School of Nursing in Nashville, Tennessee. Ms. Cashion is certified as a high risk perinatal nurse through the American Nurses Credentialing Center (ANCC).

Ms. Cashion's job responsibilities at the University of Tennessee include providing education regarding low and high risk obstetrics to staff nurses in West Tennessee community hospitals. For more than 25 years Ms. Cashion has taught obstetric nursing in the clinical setting (mostly in Labor and Delivery) for students at Northwest Mississippi Community College in Senatobia, Mississippi, and Union University in Germantown, Tennessee.

Ms. Cashion has been an active AWHONN member, holding office at both the local and state levels. She also has served as an officer and board member of the Tennessee Perinatal Association and as an active volunteer for the Tennessee chapter, March of Dimes Birth Defects Foundation.

Ms. Cashion has contributed many chapters to maternity nursing textbooks over the years. She also coauthored a series of Virtual Clinical Excursions workbooks to accompany six obstetric nursing textbooks published by Elsevier. More recently she served as one of the authors for *Maternity & Women's Health Care* (10th and 11th editions), and *Clinical Companion for Maternity & Newborn Nursing* (2nd edition), and as an editor for *Maternal Child Nursing Care* (6th edition).

KATHRYN RHODES ALDEN

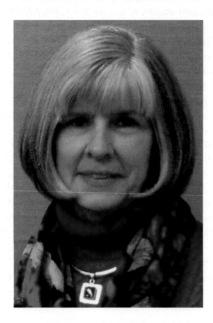

Kathryn Rhodes Alden is a retired Associate Professor, University of North Carolina at Chapel Hill School of Nursing. She received a BSN from the University of North Carolina at Charlotte, an MSN from the University of North Carolina at Chapel Hill, and a doctorate in adult education from North Carolina State University.

Dr. Alden has extensive experience as a nursing educator, having served on the faculty at the University of North Carolina at Charlotte and the University of North Carolina at Chapel Hill. Dr. Alden has clinical experience in pediatrics, pediatric intensive care, and neonatal intensive care. She is also experienced in home health care, having provided nursing care to pediatric and obstetric clients. She has worked as a nursing administrator and coordinator of quality improvement. As a certified lactation consultant, Dr. Alden has provided inpatient and outpatient care for breastfeeding mothers and infants and she has taught prenatal breastfeeding classes to expectant parents. She has taught continuing education courses on breastfeeding throughout North Carolina.

For nearly 30 years as an educator for baccalaureate nursing students at UNC-Chapel Hill School of Nursing, Dr. Alden has taught in maternal-newborn nursing courses, providing both classroom and clinical instruction. Dr. Alden coordinated and led the academic counseling program, providing assistance to students and to faculty. She was actively involved in the leadership of the undergraduate nursing program as member and former chair of the Baccalaureate Executive Committee.

She has received numerous awards for excellence in nursing education at UNC, being recognized for clinical and classroom teaching expertise as well as for academic counseling. Dr. Alden was selected for the Great 100 Nurses in North Carolina in 2008.

Dr. Alden was an early adopter of high-fidelity simulation and was instrumental in the use of this instructional strategy at UNC-Chapel Hill School of Nursing. She was actively involved in interprofessional collaboration with faculty from the UNC schools of Medicine and Pharmacy to offer obstetric and neonatal simulation learning activities to undergraduate nursing students, pharmacy students, and medical students in obstetrics and pediatrics. She has created numerous simulation scenarios including obstetric simulation cases for Elsevier. She has coauthored chapters on high-fidelity simulation and patient safety in publications by the Agency for Healthcare Research and Quality (AHRQ) and the NLN. Dr. Alden is an active member of AWHONN.

Dr. Alden has authored numerous chapters on a variety of topics in maternity texts for Elsevier. She is associate editor for *Maternal Child Nursing Care* (5th edition) and *Maternity Nursing* (8th edition).

ELLEN F. OLSHANSKY

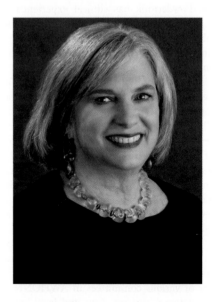

Ellen F. Olshansky is Professor Emerita in the Sue & Bill Gross School of Nursing at the University of California, Irvine (UCI) and Founding Director of the Program in Nursing Science at UCI. Dr. Olshansky earned a BA in Social Work from the University of California, Berkeley, and a BS, MS, and PhD from the University of California, San Francisco School of Nursing. She was previously a faculty member at the schools of nursing at the Oregon Health Sciences University, University of Washington, Duquesne University, and the University of Pittsburgh. She is a fellow in the American Academy of Nursing (the Academy) and served as co-chair and then chair of its Expert Panel on Women's Health and as a member of the Academy's Board of Directors. She is also a fellow in the Western Academy of Nursing.

Dr. Olshansky previously served as director of the Community Engagement Unit of the UC-Irvine Institute for Clinical and Translational Science, funded by a National Institutes of Health (NIH) Clinical Translational Science Award. Through this position she engaged community members in community-based participatory research, encouraging collaborative research between university faculty and community organizations. She has expertise in qualitative research and community-based participatory research.

Dr. Olshansky also served as Founding Chair of the Department of Nursing that was created as part of the Suzanne Dworak-Peck School of Social Work at the University of Southern California, and she continues an affiliation with USC as Distinguished Scholar in Nursing Science.

Dr. Olshansky is certified as an emeritus (lifetime) women's health nurse practitioner through the National Certification Corporation (NCC-Emeritus). Her research has focused on women's health across the life span, with a focus on reproductive health. Dr. Olshansky completed the Integrative Nurse Coach Certification Program through the International Nurse Coach Association. She is focused on working with people within their own communities to promote and maintain wellness. She is one of the founders of the Orange County Women's Health Project, which works to promote women's health and wellness in Orange County, California,

including holding annual women's health policy summits. She is also a member of the Board of Directors of MOMS of Orange County, a non-profit organization that served under-resourced pregnant and postpartum women.

She served for 10 years as editor of the *Journal of Professional Nursing,* the official journal of the American Association of Colleges of Nursing. She has published extensively in numerous nursing and other health-related journals as well as authored many book chapters, editorials, op-eds, and two books. She has authored many chapters in previous editions of Maternity and Women's Health Care and Maternal Child Nursing Care and served as associate editor for the 6th edition of Maternal Child Nursing Care, all published by Elsevier.

CONTRIBUTORS

Kathryn Rhodes Alden, EdD, MSN, RN, IBCLC
Associate Professor, Retired
School of Nursing
University of North Carolina at Chapel Hill
Chapel Hill, North Carolina

Jennifer T. Alderman, PhD, RNC-OB, CNL, CNE
Assistant Professor
School of Nursing
University of North Carolina at Chapel Hill
Chapel Hill, North Carolina

Rebecca Bagley, DNP, CNM, FACNM
Clinical Associate Professor
Director of Nurse-Midwifery Education
Advanced Practice Nursing & Education
College of Nursing
East Carolina University
Greenville, North Carolina

Deborah R. Bambini, PhD
Professor
Kirkhof College of Nursing
Grand Valley State University
Grand Rapids, Michigan

Melissa Schwartz Beck, PhD, RNC-OB, CHSE
Clinical Associate Professor
Department of Baccalaureate Education
College of Nursing
East Carolina University
Greenville, North Carolina

Beth Perry Black, PhD, RN, FAAN
Associate Professor
School of Nursing
University of North Carolina at Chapel Hill
Chapel Hill, North Carolina

Kitty Cashion, RN-BC, MSN
Clinical Nurse Specialist
Department of Obstetrics and Gynecology
Division of Maternal-Fetal Medicine
University of Tennessee Health Science
    Center
Memphis, Tennessee

Valerie Coleman, MSN, RN
Director of Lactation Services and Family
    Life Education
Department of Women's Health
VCU Health
Richmond, Virginia

Robin Webb Corbett, PhD, FNP-C, RNC
Associate Professor & Chair
Advanced Nursing Practice & Education
College of Nursing
East Carolina University
Greenville, North Carolina

Dusty Dix, MSN, RN
Assistant Professor
School of Nursing
University of North Carolina at Chapel Hill
Chapel Hill, North Carolina

Kelly Ellington, DNP, WHNP-BC, RNC-OB
Assistant Professor
School of Nursing
University of North Carolina at Wilmington
Wilmington, North Carolina

Lisa L. Ferguson, DNP, MSN, BSN
Clinical Assistant Professor
Department of Family, Community, and
    Health Systems Science
College of Nursing
University of Florida
Gainesville, Florida

Debbie Fraser, MN, RNC-NIC
Associate Professor
Faculty of Health Disciplines
Athabasca University
Athabasca, Alberta, Canada;
Neonatal Nurse Practitioner
NICU
St Boniface Hospital
Winnipeg, Manitoba, Canada

Pat Mahaffee Gingrich, MSN, WHNP-BC
Assistant Professor
School of Nursing
University of North Carolina at Chapel Hill
Chapel Hill, North Carolina

Nancy L. Havill, PhD, CNM, RN
Nurse Scientist
UNC Hospitals
Chapel Hill, North Carolina

Carol Ann King, DNP, FNP-BC
Clinical Professor
Assistant Director, Doctor of Nursing
    Practice Program
Department of Advanced Nursing Practice
    and Education
College of Nursing
East Carolina University
Greenville, North Carolina

Cheryl L. Kovar, PhD, RN, CNS
Assistant Professor
Advanced Nursing Practice & Education
College of Nursing
East Carolina University
Greenville, North Carolina

Rhonda K. Lanning, DNP, CNM, LCCE, IBCLC
Assistant Professor
School of Nursing
University of North Carolina at Chapel Hill;
Program Coordinator
Birth Partners Volunteer Doula Program
North Carolina Women's Hospital, UNC
    Healthcare
Chapel Hill, North Carolina

Nicole Lyn Letourneau, RN, BN, MN, PhD, FCAHS
Professor & ACHF Chair in Parent-Infant
    Mental Health & RESOLVE Alberta
    Director
Faculty of Nursing & Cumming School of
    Medicine (Pediatrics, Psychiatry &
    Community Health Sciences)
University of Calgary
Calgary, Alberta, Canada

Denise G. Link, PhD, WHNP-BC, CNE, FAAN, FAANP
Clinical Professor
College of Nursing & Health Innovation
Arizona State University
Phoenix, Arizona

Raquel Martinez-Campos, MSN, RN, FNP, WHNP-BC
Clinical Instructor
Sue and Bill Gross School of Nursing
UCI;
School Nurse
Health Services
Irvine Unified School District
Irvine, California

Kristen S. Montgomery, PhD, CNM
Adjunct Faculty
School of Nursing
Simmons University
Boston, Massachusetts

Amy Nichols, RN, MSN, EdD, CHSE
Clinical Professor
School of Nursing
Betty Irene Moore School of Nursing
Sacramento, California

Lecia Reardon, DNP, FNP-BC
Clinical Instructor
Advanced Nursing Practice & Education
College of Nursing
East Carolina University
Greenville, North Carolina

Christie W. Sawyer, MSN, APN, NNP-BC
Adjunct Faculty
School of Nursing
Vanderbilt University;
Neonatal Nurse Practitioner
Mednax Medical Group of Tennessee
Nashville, Tennessee

Ann Schreier, PhD, MSN, BSN
Professor
Nursing Science
College of Nursing
East Carolina University
Greenville, North Carolina

Patricia A. Scott, DNP, APRN, NNP-BC, C-NPT
TIPQC Infant Quality Improvement
    Specialist
Assistant Professor of Nursing—Neonatal
    and DNP Programs
Vanderbilt University School of Nursing;
Advanced Practitioner Coordinator
Mednax Medical Group of Tennessee
Nashville, Tennessee

Michelle Taylor Skipper, DNP, FNP-BC
Clinical Professor,
Director, Doctor of Nursing Practice
    Program
AGPCNP, FNP and PM APRN Specialties
Department of Advanced Nursing Practice
    and Education
College of Nursing
East Carolina University
Greenville, North Carolina

Renee Oakley Spain, DNP, MAED
Clinical Assistant Professor
Department of Advanced Nursing Practice
    and Education
College of Nursing
East Carolina University
Greenville, North Carolina

Genae Strong, PhD, APRN, CNM-BC, RNC-OB, IBCLC, RLC, CNE
Associate Professor
Loewenberg College of Nursing
University of Memphis
Memphis, Tennessee

Janet A. Tucker, PhD, MSN, RNC-OB
Assistant Professor
Loewenberg College of Nursing
University of Memphis
Memphis, Tennessee

Marcia Van Riper, PhD, RN, FAAN
Professor
School of Nursing
University of North Carolina at Chapel Hill
Chapel Hill, North Carolina

Jennie M. Wagner, EdD, RN, MBA, MSN, CNE, IBCLC
Assistant Professor
School of Nursing
University of North Carolina at Chapel Hill
Chapel Hill, North Carolina

LIST OF REVIEWERS

Women's health care encompasses reproductive health care and the unique physical, psychologic, and social needs of women throughout their life span. Maternity care includes care of the mother during the childbearing cycle and care of the normal and high-risk newborn. The specialties of women's health and maternity nursing offer challenges and opportunities. Nurses are challenged to assimilate knowledge and develop the technical and critical thinking skills needed to be reflective practitioners. Each woman, with her individual needs that must be identified and met, presents a challenge to nurses to provide optimal client-centered care. However, the opportunities are sufficiently extraordinary to make this one of the most fulfilling specialties of nursing practice.

The goal of nursing education is to prepare today's students to meet the challenges of tomorrow. This preparation must extend beyond mastery of facts and skills. Nurses must be able to provide safe, quality, client-centered care through the combination of clinical reasoning skills, technical competence, and compassionate caring. They must address the physiologic as well as the psychosocial needs of their clients. They must look beyond the condition and see the woman as an individual with distinctive needs. Yet they must consider her needs in the context of family-centered care and culture, realizing and acknowledging the influence and involvement of family members and significant others. Integral to family-centered care is awareness of and sensitivity to the needs of traditional and nontraditional families (e.g., same-sex couples). Above all, nurses must strive to improve practice on the basis of sound evidence-based information. Nurses can use evidence-based practice to produce measurable outcomes that can validate their unique and necessary role in the health care delivery system.

Maternity & Women's Health Care was designed to provide students with accurate and up-to-date information so that they can develop the knowledge and skills needed to become clinically competent, to think critically, and to attain the necessary sensitivity to become caring nurses. *Maternity & Women's Health Care* has been a leading maternity nursing text since it was first published in 1977. We are proud of the continued support this text has received. With this twelfth edition we have a responsibility to continue this leading tradition.

This edition has been revised and refined in response to comments and suggestions from educators, clinicians, and students. It includes the most accurate, current, and clinically relevant information available. We have had the assistance of expert faculty, nurse clinicians, and specialists from other health disciplines who authored, reviewed, and revised the text. Many exciting updates and additions will be noted throughout the book; they demonstrate the various dimensions of women's health care and areas of rapid and complex changes such as genetics, fetal assessment, and alternative therapies. However, we have retained the underlying philosophy that has been the strength of previous editions: our belief that pregnancy and birth and developmental changes in a woman's life are natural processes. We have also retained a base in physiology and a strong, integrated focus on the family and on evidence-based practice. There is new content related to needs and care of nontraditional families, recognizing that they often have unique concerns that nurses can address.

The text is also used as a reference for the practicing nurse. The most recent current recommendations and standards of practice based on evidence from research and clinical experts have been included from professional organizations such as the Association of Women's Health, Obstetric and Neonatal Nurses; the National Association of Neonatal Nurses; the American College of Obstetricians and Gynecologists; the American Academy of Pediatrics; the American Diabetes Association; the Centers for Disease Control and Prevention; and the U.S. Preventive Health Services Task Force. The text can be used to prepare for certification courses and for review in graduate programs of study. The text and its electronic resources are excellent references for the nursing unit.

APPROACH

Professional nursing practice continues to evolve and adapt to society's changing health priorities. The ever-changing health care delivery system offers new opportunities for nurses to alter the practice of maternity and women's health nursing and to improve the way care is given. Consumers of maternity and women's health care vary in age, ethnicity, culture, language, social status, marital status, sexual preference, and family configurations. They seek care from obstetricians, gynecologists, family practice physicians, certified nurse-midwives, nurse practitioners, nurses, and other health care providers in a variety of health care settings, including the home. Increasingly, many are self-treating, accessing web-based information, and using a variety of alternative and complementary therapies.

Nursing education must reflect these changes. Clinical education must be planned to offer students a variety of maternity and women's health care experiences in settings that include hospitals and birth centers, home health settings, clinics and private physician offices, shelters for the homeless or women in need of protection, prisons, and other community-based settings. Advances in nursing education include the increased use of simulation learning activities. Simulation laboratories have emerged in schools of nursing and in health care institutions to provide students and staff with opportunities to engage in care of clients in focused, challenging situations while in the safety of a controlled environment. Simulation experiences offer students in maternity and women's health courses opportunities that are otherwise unavailable due to shrinking opportunities for clinical placements, decreased clinical time, and increased numbers of students in clinical rotations. Within these laboratories, opportunities to engage in interprofessional simulations abound.

Today's prelicensure nursing students are challenged to learn more than ever and often in less time than their predecessors. Students are diverse. They may be new high school graduates, college students, or older adults with families. They may be male or female. They may have college degrees in other fields and be interested in changing careers. They may represent various cultures; English may not be their first language. Students may be enrolled in associate degree or diploma programs, in baccalaureate or accelerated baccalaureate nursing programs, or in entry-level master's programs. This twelfth edition, with its accompanying teaching and learning package, has been revised to meet these changing needs. Each chapter has been reviewed by a specialist and revised to improve readability and comprehension, especially by a diverse student population. Focused content is presented in a clearly written and easily read manner while retaining the comprehensiveness of previous editions. The text can be used by all levels of nursing education and in courses of varying lengths.

Health care today emphasizes *wellness* and *health promotion*. This focus is an integral part of our philosophy. Likewise, the developmental changes a woman experiences throughout her life are considered natural and normal. In women's health care, the goal is promotion of wellness for the woman through knowledge of her body and its normal functioning throughout her life span, while developing an awareness of conditions that require professional intervention. The unit on women's health care emphasizes the wellness aspects of care as well as social determinants of health and health care, while also including information about wellness aspects of care, and also includes information about common gynecologic problems and breast and gynecologic cancers. This unit has been placed before the units on pregnancy because many of the aspects of assessment and care can be applied to later chapters.

Pregnancy and birth are also part of a natural developmental process. We believe that students need to thoroughly understand and recognize the normal processes before they can identify complications and comprehend their implications for care. We present the entire normal childbearing cycle before discussing potential complications.

FEATURES

The twelfth edition features a contemporary design and spacious presentation. Students will find that the logical, easy-to-follow headings and attractive full-color design highlight important content and increase visual appeal. More than 450 color photographs (many of them new) and drawings throughout the text illustrate important concepts and techniques to further enhance comprehension. Each chapter begins with a list of *Learning Objectives* designed to focus students' attention on the important content to be mastered. *Key Terms* that alert students to new vocabulary are in blue, defined within the chapter, and included in a glossary at the end of the book. Each chapter ends with *Key Points* that summarize important content. *Community Activity* exercises are included in most chapters to provide opportunities for students to increase their knowledge of community and web-based resources to enhance client care. *Clinical Reasoning* case studies have been reconceptualized in this edition to help students prioritize client and family needs and concerns, recognizing that prioritization of care is essential for providing effective client-centered care. In addition, identification of the roles of the members of the interprofessional care team are integrated to guide students in applying their knowledge and increasing their ability to think and reflect critically about maternity and women's health care issues. References have been updated significantly, with most citations being less than 5 years old and all chapters having citations within 1 year of publication. An expanded table of contents and index make it easier for readers to locate exactly the information they are seeking. More of the additional outstanding features follow:

- *Care Management* is used as the consistent framework throughout nursing care chapters to discuss assessment, medical and surgical management, interprofessional care, and, more specifically, the nursing care related to each topic.
- *Nursing Care Plans* help students apply the nursing process in the clinical setting as they identify priority client problems or concerns, describe expected outcomes for client care, provide rationales for interventions, and include evaluation of care.
- *Teaching for Self-Management* boxes emphasize guidelines for the client to practice self-care and provide information to help students transfer learning from the hospital to the home setting.
- *Emergency* boxes alert students to the signs and symptoms of various emergency situations and provide interventions for immediate implementation.
- *Signs of Potential Complications* boxes alert students to signs and symptoms of potential problems and are included in chapters that cover uncomplicated pregnancy and birth.
- *Nursing Alert* and *Safety Alert* boxes and new *Medication Alert* boxes highlight critical information.
- *Evidence-Based Practice* is incorporated throughout in new boxes that integrate findings from several studies on selected clinical practices and changing practice. In addition, research findings

summarized in *The Cochrane Pregnancy and Childbirth Database* and other resources for evidence-based practices are integrated throughout the text.

- *Cultural Considerations* boxes describe beliefs and practices about pregnancy, labor and birth, newborn care and feeding, parenting, and women's health concerns, and emphasize the importance of understanding cultural variations and client preferences when providing care.
- *Legal Tips* are integrated throughout to provide students with relevant information to deal with these important areas in the context of maternity and women's health nursing.
- *Medication Guide* boxes include key information about medications used in maternity and women's health care, including their indications, adverse effects, and nursing considerations.

ORGANIZATION

The twelfth edition of *Maternity & Women's Health Care* comprises eight units organized to enhance understanding and learning and to facilitate easy retrieval of information.

Part 1, Introduction to Maternity & Women's Health Care, begins with an overview of contemporary issues in maternity and women's health nursing practice. Chapter 1 includes a section on historic milestones in maternity, women's health, and neonatal care and provides an overview of important therapies that can be used instead of or in addition to traditional techniques used in maternity and women's health care. Chapter 2 addresses the various forms of family as a unit of care and how family is related to culture and community. This chapter incorporates family theory, cultural aspects of care, and home care in relation to maternity and women's health nursing. Chapter 3 provides essential discussion about genetics in relation to maternity and women's health care.

Part 2, Women's Health, is a thoroughly revised unit on women's health. Eight chapters discuss health promotion, screening, and physical assessment, and then present common reproductive concerns. The chapter on assessment and health promotion incorporates normal anatomy and physiology of the female reproductive system and integrates health promotion for common women's health problems. There are separate chapters on reproductive problems and concerns, sexually transmitted infections and other infections, contraception and abortion, infertility, violence, problems of the breast, and structural disorders and neoplasms of the female reproductive system.

Part 3, Pregnancy, describes nursing care of the woman and her family from conception through preparation for birth. Nursing care during pregnancy includes both physiologic and psychologic aspects of care, as well as information on preparation for birth. A separate chapter on maternal and fetal nutrition emphasizes the important aspects of care, highlights cultural variations in diet, and stresses the importance of early recognition and management of nutritional problems.

Part 4, Labor and Birth, focuses on collaborative care among physicians, nurse-midwives, nurses, and women and their families during the processes of labor and birth. Separate chapters deal with the nurse's role in maximizing comfort during labor and birth and fetal monitoring, both of which have been updated significantly. All four chapters familiarize students with current labor and birth practices and focus on evidence-based interventions to support and educate the woman and her family.

Part 5, Postpartum, deals with a time of profound change for the entire family. Physiologic changes and nursing care based on the changes are addressed. The mother requires both physical and emotional support as she adjusts to her new role. The chapter on transition to parenthood discusses family dynamics in response to the birth of a child and describes ways nurses can facilitate parent–infant adjustment. Anticipatory guidance for the first few weeks at home and home follow-up care are addressed.

Part 6, The Newborn, has been updated and addresses physiologic adaptations of the newborn and assessment and care of the newborn. Information on the nutritional needs of the newborn and nursing care associated with breastfeeding and formula feeding are highlighted in a separate chapter.

Part 7, Complications of Pregnancy, discusses conditions that place the woman, fetus, infant, and family at risk. This unit has been revised and updated and includes a chapter on assessment of the high-risk pregnancy and eight other chapters covering specific pregnancy complications including hypertensive disorders, antepartal hemorrhagic disorders, endocrine and metabolic problems, medical-surgical problems, mental health problems and substance abuse, labor and birth complications, and postpartum complications.

Part 8, Newborn Complications, describes the nursing care for high-risk newborns, emphasizing the care of the preterm infant. There is enhanced content on care of late preterm infants in this edition. It addresses the most common acquired conditions of the neonate as well as hematologic disorders and congenital anomalies. All chapters have been revised and updated. A separate chapter on loss and grief discusses care of the family experiencing a fetal or neonatal loss.

TEACHING/LEARNING PACKAGE

Evolve, for Students: Evolve is an innovative website that provides a wealth of content, resources, and state-of-the-art information on maternity nursing. Learning resources for students include Case Studies, Content Updates, Printable Key Points, Nursing Skills, and NCLEX-Style Review Questions.

Simulation Learning System (SLS): The SLS is an online toolkit that helps instructors and facilitators effectively incorporate medium- to high-fidelity simulation into their nursing curriculum. Detailed client scenarios promote and enhance the clinical decision-making skills of students at all levels. The SLS provides detailed instructions for preparation and implementation of the simulation experience, debriefing questions that encourage critical thinking, and learning resources to reinforce student comprehension. Each scenario in the SLS complements the textbook content and helps bridge the gap between lectures and clinical practice. The SLS provides the perfect environment for students to practice what they are learning in the text for a true-to-life, hands-on learning experience.

Study Guide: This comprehensive and challenging study aid presents a variety of questions to enhance learning of key concepts and content from the text. Multiple-choice and matching questions are included, as well as Critical Reasoning Case Studies. Answers for all questions are included at the back of the study guide.

Virtual Clinical Excursions: Virtual Hospital and Workbook Companion: A Virtual Hospital and workbook package has been developed as a clinical experience to expand student opportunities for critical thinking. This package guides the student through a virtual clinical environment and helps the user apply textbook content to virtual clients in that environment. Case studies are presented that allow students to use this textbook as a reference to assess, diagnose, plan, implement, and evaluate "real" clients using clinical scenarios. The state-of-the-art technologies reflected in this virtual hospital demonstrate cutting-edge learning opportunities for students and facilitate knowledge retention of the information found in the textbook. The clinical simulations and workbook represent the next generation of research-based learning tools that promote critical thinking and meaningful learning.

Evolve, for Instructors includes these teaching resources:
- *Test Bank in ExamView format* contains more than 1000 NCLEX-style test items, including alternate-format questions. An answer key with page references to the text, rationales, and NCLEX-style coding is included.
- *TEACH for Nurses* includes teaching strategies; in-class case studies; and links to animations, nursing skills, and nursing curriculum standards such as BSN Essentials.
- *Image Collection,* containing more than 700 full-color illustrations and photographs from the text, helps instructors develop presentations and explain key concepts. Images can easily be inserted into *PowerPoint* presentations, thus helping make lectures more understandable and entertaining.
- *PowerPoint slides,* with lecture notes for each chapter of the text, assist in presenting materials in the classroom. *Case Studies* and *Audience Response Questions* for i-clicker are included.
- A *Curriculum Guide* that includes a proposed class schedule and reading assignments for courses of varying lengths is provided. This gives educators suggestions for using the text in the most essential manner or in a more comprehensive way.

ACKNOWLEDGMENTS

The twelfth edition of *Maternity & Women's Health Care* would not have been possible without the contributions of many people. First, we want to thank the many nurse educators, clinicians, and nursing students in the United States, Canada, Australia, and Taiwan whose comments and suggestions about the manuscript led to this collaborative effort by an outstanding group of contributors. A special thanks goes to these people, many of whom are new to this edition, whose names appear in the list of contributors. Their expertise and knowledge of current clinical practice and research have added to the relevancy and accuracy of the materials presented. We thank Jennifer Alderman for contributing to the Evidence-Based Practice boxes. We also thank Pat Gingrich for contributing to the Evidence-Based Practice boxes and Ed Lowdermilk, RPh for his assistance with Medication Guides and verification of other medication information. We are also appreciative of the critiques given by the reviewers, especially their attention to validating the accuracy of content and their challenge to present content differently and to include new ideas. These combined efforts have resulted in a revision that incorporates the most recent research and current information about the practice of maternity and women's health care.

We offer thanks for shared expertise and photographs to the staff of University of North Carolina Women's Hospital; University of North Carolina School of Nursing; Nurses Certificate Program in Interactive Imagery; Polly Perez at Cutting Edge Press; and Women's Birth & Wellness Center, Chapel Hill, North Carolina.

We also would like to thank the following photographers: Cheryl Briggs, RNC, Annapolis, MD; Michael S. Clement, MD, Mesa, AZ; Julie Perry Nelson, Loveland, CO; and Marjorie Pyle, RNC, Lifecircle, Costa Mesa, CA.

Thanks to the following individuals who allowed us to use their beautiful photos: Jennifer and Travis Alderman, Durham, NC; Freida Belding, Bird City, KS; Tiana Bennion, Gilbert, AZ; Jodi Brackett, Phoenix, AZ; Leona Cahill, Mesa, AZ; Racquel Martinez-Campos, Lake Forest, CA; David A. Clarke, Philadelphia, PA; Thomas and Christie Coghill, Clayton, NC; Christina and Eva Gardner, Memphis, TN; Amber and Zack Gaynor, Apex, NC; Kara and Casey George, Peoria, AZ; Regina Gomez-Vidal, Mesa, AZ; Patricia Hess, San Francisco, CA; Sharon Johnson, Petaluma, CA; Emily and Kevin Jones, Holly Springs, NC; Shannon Keller, CNM, Chapel Hill, NC; Carshawna Knighton, Memphis, TN; Sara Kossuth, Los Angeles, CA; Mahesh Kotwal, MD, Phoenix, AZ; Paul Vincent Kuntz, Houston, TX; Wendy and Marwood Larson-Harris, Roanoke, VA; Chelsea Lindblad, San Tan Valley, AZ; Lauren and Brian LiVecchi, Raleigh, NC; Ed Lowdermilk, Chapel Hill, NC; Barbra Manning, RN, MSN, Senatobia, MS; Ashley and Andrew Martin, Charlotte, NC; Shanika Mayfield, Joiner, AR; Norman L. Meyer, MD, PhD, Memphis, TN; Kim Molloy, Knoxville, IA; Amanda Politte, St. Louis, MO; Chris Rozales, San Francisco, CA; H. Gil Rushton, MD, Washington, DC; Brian and Mayannyn Sallee, Minot, ND; Shari Rivera Sharpe, Chapel Hill, NC; Mandi and Chase Steele, Millington, TN; Mark and Stephanie Stauder, Loveland, CO; Edward S. Tank, MD, Portland, OR; Danielle L. Tate, MD, Memphis, TN; Amy and Ken Turner, Cary, NC; Rebekah Vogel, Fort Collins, CO; Allison and Matthew Wyatt, Eagle, CO; Roni Wernik, Palo Alto, CA; and Randi and Jacob Wills, Clayton, NC.

Special words of gratitude are extended to Laurie Gower, Content Strategist; Elizabeth Kilgore, Senior Content Development Specialist; Julie Eddy, Publishing Services Manager; Rachel McMullen, Senior Project Manager; and Brian Salisbury, Book Designer, for their encouragement, inspiration, and assistance in preparing and producing this text. These talented and hardworking people helped change our manuscript into a beautiful book by editing the manuscript, designing an attractive format for our special features, and overseeing the production of the book from start to finish.

Deitra Leonard Lowdermilk
Shannon E. Perry
Kitty Cashion
Kathryn Rhodes Alden
Ellen F. Olshansky

CONTENTS

1

21st-Century Maternity and Women's Health Nursing

Nancy L. Havill

http://evolve.elsevier.com/Lowdermilk/MWHC/

LEARNING OBJECTIVES

- Describe the scope of maternity and women's health nursing.
- Evaluate contemporary issues and trends in maternity and women's health care.
- Examine social concerns in maternity nursing and women's health care.
- Integrate evidenced-based practice into care plans.

- Explain risk management and standards of practice in the delivery of maternity and women's health nursing care.
- Discuss legal and ethical issues in perinatal nursing.
- Examine *Healthy People 2020* goals related to maternal and infant care.

The chapter covers the **preconception** period, pregnancy (**prenatal** or **antepartum**), childbirth (**intrapartum**), and the first 6 weeks after birth (**postpartum**). The term **perinatal** is also used to describe all of these periods. Throughout the prenatal period, nurses, nurse midwives, and nurse practitioners provide care for women in many care settings, including clinics and private offices. Nurses teach classes to help families prepare for childbirth. Nurses provide care for women and their families during labor and birth in hospitals, freestanding birth centers (e.g., www.birthcenters.org), and women's homes. Highly trained nurses provide intensive care for high-risk neonates in special care units and for high-risk mothers in antepartum units, critical care obstetric units, or in the home. Maternity nurses teach about pregnancy; the process of labor, birth, and recovery; newborn care, and parenting skills. They provide continuity of care throughout the childbearing cycle.

Maternity nursing encompasses care of childbearing women, neonates, and their families through all stages of pregnancy, childbirth, and the first 6 weeks after birth.

Women's health care focuses on the physical, psychologic, and social needs of women throughout their lives. In the care of women, their overall experience is emphasized: general physical and psychologic well-being, childbearing functions, and diseases. Women's health nurses specialize in and investigate conditions unique to women (such as reproductive malignancies and menopause) and sociocultural and occupational factors that are related to women's health problems (such as poverty, rape, incest, family violence, and human trafficking), also referred to as social determinants of health. They also provide care for women and their families during the childbearing cycle.

Nurses caring for women have helped make the health care system more responsive to women's needs. They have been critically important in developing strategies to improve the well-being of women and their infants and have led efforts in quality improvement

by implementing clinical practice guidelines based on research evidence. Through professional associations, such as the Association of Women's Health, Obstetric, and Neonatal Nursing (AWHONN), nurses have a voice in setting standards and in influencing health policy by actively participating in the education of the public and state and federal legislators. In fact, nurses have a strong impact worldwide. Indeed, the World Health Organization (WHO) has declared 2020 as the year of the nurse and midwife (WHO, 2019).

CURRENT CONCERNS IN THE CARE OF WOMEN AND INFANTS

Although tremendous advances have taken place in the care of mothers and their infants during the past 150 years (Box 1.1), serious problems exist in the United States related to the health and health care of mothers and infants. Maternal mortality is increasing in the United States despite advances in health care and decreases in maternal mortality globally (WHO, 2018a, 2018b). Chronic medical conditions such as heart disease, diabetes, and obesity are likely contributory factors. Moreover, significant racial disparities exist: Black women face much greater risks of death related to childbirth than white women (Centers for Disease Control and Prevention [CDC], 2017). Lack of access to prepregnancy, pregnancy, and reproductive health services are major concerns. Sexually transmitted infections continue to affect reproduction adversely.

EFFORTS TO REDUCE HEALTH DISPARITIES

Racial and ethnic diversity is increasing within the United States, with trends toward a decrease in non-Hispanic Caucasians and an increase in other ethnic groups such that the current "majority" group will no longer be in the majority (Colby & Ortman, 2015).

BOX 1.1 Historic Overview of Milestones in the Care of Mothers and Infants in the Western World from 1847

1847—James Young Simpson in Edinburgh, Scotland, used ether for an internal podalic version and birth; the first reported use of obstetric anesthesia

1861—Ignaz Semmelweis wrote *The Cause, Concept and Prophylaxis of Childbed Fever*

1906—First U.S. program for prenatal nursing care established

1908—Childbirth classes started by the American Red Cross

1909—First White House Conference on Children convened

1911—First milk bank in the United States established in Boston

1912—U.S. Children's Bureau established

1915—Radical mastectomy determined to be effective treatment for breast cancer

1916—Margaret Sanger established first American birth control clinic in Brooklyn, New York

1918—Condoms became legal in the United States

1923—First U.S. hospital center for premature infant care established at Sarah Morris Hospital in Chicago, Illinois

1929—The modern tampon (with an applicator) invented and patented

1933—Sodium pentothal used as anesthesia for childbirth; *Natural Childbirth* published by Grantly Dick-Read

1934—Dionne quintuplets born in Ontario, Canada, and survive partly due to donated breast milk

1935—Sulfonamides introduced as cure for puerperal fever

1941—Penicillin used as a treatment for infection

1941—Papanicolaou (Pap) test introduced

1942—Premarin approved by the Food and Drug Administration (FDA) as treatment for menopausal symptoms

1953—Virginia Apgar, an anesthesiologist, published Apgar scoring system of neonatal assessment

1956—Oxygen determined to be a cause of retrolental fibroplasia (now known as retinopathy of prematurity)

1958—Edward Hon reported on the recording of the fetal electrocardiogram (ECG) from the maternal abdomen (first commercial electronic fetal monitor produced in the late 1960s)

1958—Ian Donald, a Glasgow physician, was first to report clinical use of ultrasound to examine the fetus

1959—*Thank You, Dr. Lamaze* published by Marjorie Karmel

1959—Cytologic studies demonstrated that Down syndrome is associated with a particular form of nondisjunction now known as trisomy 21

1960—American Society for Psychoprophylaxis in Obstetrics (ASPO/Lamaze) formed

1960—Birth control pill introduced in the United States

1960—International Childbirth Education Association founded

1962—Thalidomide found to cause birth defects

1963—Title V of the Social Security Act amended to include comprehensive maternity and infant care for women who were low income and high risk

1963—Testing for PKU begun

1965—Supreme Court ruled that married people have the right to use birth control

1967—First known helicopter transport under the nursing care of Sister M. Andre of a preterm infant from place of birth in Zion, IL to Peoria, IL for specialized care.

1967—Reva Rubin published article on maternal role attainment

1967—Rh$_o$(D) immune globulin produced for treatment of Rh incompatibility

1968—Rubella vaccine became available

1969—Nurses Association of the American College of Obstetricians and Gynecologists (NAACOG) founded; renamed Association of Women's Health, Obstetric and Neonatal Nurses (AWHONN) and incorporated as a 501(c)(3) organization in 1993

1969—Mammogram became available

1972—Special Supplemental Food Program for Women, Infants, and Children (WIC) started

1973—Abortion legalized in United States

1974—First standards for obstetric, gynecologic, and neonatal nursing published by NAACOG

1975—The Pregnant Patient's Bill of Rights published by the International Childbirth Education Association

1976—First home pregnancy kits approved by FDA

1978—Louise Brown, first test-tube baby, born

1987—Safe Motherhood initiative launched by World Health Organization and other international agencies

1991—Society for Advancement of Women's Health Research founded

1992—Office of Research on Women's Health authorized by U.S. Congress

1993—Family and Medical Leave Act enacted

1993—Female condom approved by FDA

1993—Human embryos cloned at George Washington University

1994—DNA sequences of *BRCA1* and *BRCA2* identified

1994—Zidovudine guidelines to reduce mother-to-fetus transmission of HIV published

1996—FDA mandated folic acid fortification in all breads and grains sold in United States

1998—Canadian Obstetric, Gynecologic, and Neonatal Nurses (COGNN) becomes AWHONN Canada

1998—Newborns' and Mothers' Health Act went into effect

1999—First emergency contraceptive pill for pregnancy prevention (Plan B) approved by FDA

2000—Working draft of sequence and analysis of human genome completed

2006—HPV vaccine available

2010—Centenary of the death of Florence Nightingale

2010—Patient Protection and Affordable Care Act signed into law by President Obama

2011—AWHONN Canada becomes the Canadian Association of Perinatal and Women's Health Nurses (CAPWHN)

2012—Scientists reported findings of the ENCODE (Encyclopedia of DNA Elements) project showing that 80% of the human genome is active

2012—U.S. Supreme Court upheld individual mandate but not the Medicaid expansion provisions of the Patient Protection and Affordable Care Act

2016—Zika virus discovered, spread by mosquitos, and sexually transmitted by sperm if a male is infected, affects the fetus/neonate (microcephaly)

HIV, Human immunodeficiency virus; *HPV*, human papillomavirus.

African Americans, Native Americans, Hispanics, Alaska Natives, Asian Americans, and Pacific Islanders experience significant disparities in morbidity and mortality rates compared to Caucasians. Shorter life expectancy, higher infant and maternal mortality rates, more birth defects, and more sexually transmitted infections are found among these ethnic and racial minority groups. The disparities are thought to result from a complex interaction among biologic factors, environment, socioeconomic factors, and health behaviors. Social determinants of health are those nonbiologic factors that have profound influences on health. Disparities in education and income are associated with differences in morbidity and mortality (Morbidity & Mortality Weekly, 2013).

In addition, people may have lifestyles, health needs, and health care preferences related to their ethnic or cultural backgrounds.

They may have dietary preferences and health practices that are not understood by caregivers. This presents a challenge for health care professionals to provide culturally sensitive care.

The Health Resources and Services Administration's (HRSA) Health Disparities Collaboratives are part of a national effort to eliminate disparities and improve delivery systems of health care for all people in the United States who are cared for in HRSA-supported health centers. The National Partnership for Action to End Health Disparities (NPA, 2016), sponsored by the Office of Minority Health, has developed priorities to address and end health disparities. The Institute for Healthcare Improvement (IHI, 2016) has implemented virtual training sessions on Advancing Safer Maternal and Newborn Care (www.ihi.org/education/WebTraining/Expeditions/AdvancingSafer-MaternalandNewbornCare/Pages/default.aspx). The National Institutes of Health (NIH) have a commitment to improve the health of minorities and provide funding for research and training of minority researchers (www.nih.gov). The National Institute of Nursing Research includes in its strategic plan support of research that promotes health equity and eliminates health disparities. The Black Mamas Matter Alliance (BMMA) has issued an important document that presents policy recommendations, framed through the lens of reproductive justice, to address the alarming disparities in pregnancy-related health among black women (BMMA, 2018).

The CDC publishes reports of recent trends and variations in health disparities and inequalities in some social and health indicators and provides data against which to measure progress in eliminating disparities. Topics specific to perinatal nursing that are addressed include infant deaths, preterm births, and adolescent pregnancy and childbirth. In 2015, the U.S. Department of Health and Human Services (USDHHS) released a progress report on its HHS Disparities Action Plan that provides a vision of eradication of disparities in health and health care in our nation (USDHHS, 2015). Through this plan, HHS will promote evidence-based programs, integrated approaches, and best practices to reduce disparities. The Action Plan complements the 2011 National Stakeholder Strategy for Achieving Health Equity prepared by the NPA. Since this strategy was developed, much progress has been made in addressing disparities and health equity through a comprehensive, community-driven approach to achieve health equity through collaboration and synergy (NPA, 2016). Through these initiatives, the United States is making a concerted effort to eliminate health disparities.

CONTEMPORARY ISSUES AND TRENDS

Healthy People 2020 Goals

Healthy People provides science-based 10-year national objectives for improving the health of all Americans. It has four overarching goals: (1) attaining high-quality, longer lives free of preventable disease, disability, injury, and premature death; (2) achieving health equity, eliminating disparities, and improving the health of all groups; (3) creating social and physical environments that promote good health for all; and (4) promoting quality of life, healthy development, and healthy behaviors across all life stages (www.healthypeople.gov/2020/about/default.aspx). The goals of *Healthy People 2020* are based on assessments of major risks to health and wellness, changes in public health priorities, and issues related to the health preparedness and prevention of our nation. Of the approximately 1200 objectives of *Healthy People 2020*, 33 are related to maternal, infant, and child health (Box 1.2). Objectives in this topic area include (1) reduce the rate of fetal and infant deaths, (2) reduce the rate of maternal mortality, (3) reduce preterm births, and (4) reduce cesarean births among low-risk women. (See https://www.healthypeople.gov/2020/topics-objectives/topic/maternal-infant-and-child-health/objectives for a complete list of objectives.)

Millennium Development Goals

The United Nations Millenium Development Goals (MDGs) are eight goals that were initially developed at the beginning of the millennium, adopted by 189 nations and signed by 147 heads of state and governments during the United Nations Millennium Summit in September 2000 (www.un.org/millenniumgoals). Goals 3 through 5 of the MDGs relate specifically to women and children (Box 1.3). Recently the U.N. has developed a new initiative, the U.N. Sustainable Development Goals for 2030, which consists of 17 broad goals that strive for peace and prosperity on the planet (https://sustainabledevelopment.un.org/?menu=1300).

Interprofessional Education and Care Management

Interprofessional education (IPE) incorporates collaborative education of various health professional students, including nursing, medicine, dentistry, pharmacy, social work, and public health. It is key in creating safe, high quality health care, where the client is the focus of care and the professionals work together by understanding the roles and responsibilities of each. This contributes to safer, higher quality health care. Teamwork and communication are critical aspects of this approach to care. Numerous organizations including the National League for Nursing (2019), the Interprofessional Education Collaborative (2019), the WHO, and many others have expressed support for IPE. IPE is identified as an important way to decrease medical errors and to prevent needless morbidities and mortalities due to such errors. The interprofessional collaborative practice competency domains include (1) values/ethics for interprofessional practice, (2) roles/responsibilities, (3) interprofessional communication, and (4) teams and teamwork.

Teamwork and communication are key aspects of IPE. Failure to communicate is a major cause of errors in health care. The Situation-Background-Assessment-Recommendation (SBAR) technique provides a specific framework for communication among health care providers about a client's condition, reducing the potential for errors. SBAR is an easy-to-remember, useful, concrete mechanism for communicating important information that requires a clinician's immediate attention (Kaiser Permanente of Colorado, 2014) (Table 1.1).

Problems With the U.S. Health Care System
Structure of the Health Care Delivery System

The U.S. health care delivery system is often fragmented and expensive and is inaccessible to many. Opportunities exist for nurses to alter nursing practice and improve the way care is delivered through managed care, integrated delivery systems, and redefined roles. Information about health and health care is readily available on the Internet (e-health). Consumers use this information to participate in their own care and consult health care providers with a knowledge base previously difficult to access.

Reducing Medical Errors

Medical errors are the third leading cause of death in the United States (Leapfrog Group, 2015; Makary & Daniel, 2016). Since the IOM released its report, *To Err Is Human: Building a Safer Health System* (Kohn, Corrigan, & Donaldson, 2000), a concerted effort has been under way to analyze causes of errors and develop strategies to prevent them. Hayes, Jackson, Davidson, and Power (2015) explored how nurses can decrease interruptions and distractions that contribute to medical errors. Recognizing the multifaceted causes of medical errors, the AHRQ prepared a fact sheet in 2000, *20 Tips to Help Prevent Medical Errors,* which was updated in 2014, for clients and the public. Clients are encouraged to be knowledgeable consumers of health care and ask questions of providers, including physicians, midwives, nurses, nurse practitioners, and pharmacists.

BOX 1.2 *Healthy People 2020* Maternal, Infant, and Child Health Objectives

- Reduce the rate of fetal and infant deaths.
- Reduce the 1-year mortality rate for infants with Down syndrome.
- Reduce the rate of child deaths.
- Reduce the rate of adolescent and young adult deaths.
- Reduce the rate of maternal mortality.
- Reduce maternal illness and complications due to pregnancy (complications during hospitalized labor and birth).
- Reduce cesarean births among low-risk (full-term, singleton, vertex presentation) women.
- Reduce low birth weight (LBW) and very low birth weight (VLBW).
- Reduce preterm births.
- Increase the proportion of pregnant women who receive early and adequate prenatal care.
- Increase abstinence from alcohol, cigarettes, and illicit drugs in pregnant women.
- Increase the proportion of mothers who achieve a recommended weight gain during their pregnancies.
- Increase the proportion of women of childbearing potential with intake of at least 400 mcg folic acid daily from fortified foods or dietary supplements.
- Reduce the proportion of women of childbearing potential who have lower (<25th percentile) red blood cell folate concentrations.
- Increase the proportion of women delivering a live birth who received preconception care services and practiced key recommended preconception health behaviors.
- Reduce the proportion of persons aged 18–44 years who have impaired fecundity (i.e., a physical barrier preventing pregnancy or carrying a pregnancy to term).
- Reduce postpartum relapse of smoking among women who quit smoking during pregnancy.
- Increase the proportion of women giving birth who attend a postpartum care visit with a health care worker.
- Increase the proportion of infants who are put to sleep on their backs.
- Increase the proportion of infants who are breastfed.
- Increase the proportion of employers that have worksite lactation support programs.
- Reduce the proportion of breastfed newborns who receive formula supplementation within the first 2 days of life.
- Increase the proportion of live births that occur in facilities that provide recommended care for lactating mothers and their babies.
- Reduce the occurrence of fetal alcohol syndrome (FAS).
- Reduce the proportion of children diagnosed with a disorder through newborn bloodspot screening who experience developmental delay requiring special education services.
- Reduce the proportion of children with cerebral palsy born LBW or VLBW.
- Reduce occurrence of neural tube defects.
- Increase the proportion of young children with autism spectrum disorder (ASD) and other developmental delays who are screened, evaluated, and enrolled in special services in a timely manner.
- Increase the proportion of children, including those with special health care needs, who have access to a medical home.
- Increase the proportion of children with special health care needs who receive their care in family-centered, comprehensive, and coordinated systems.
- Increase appropriate newborn bloodspot screening and follow-up testing.
- Increase the number of states, including the District of Columbia, that verify through linkage with vital records that all newborns are screened shortly after birth for conditions mandated by their state-sponsored screening program.
- Increase the proportion of screen-positive children who receive follow-up testing within the recommended time period.
- Increase the proportion of children with a diagnosed condition identified through newborn screening who have an annual assessment of services needed and received.
- Increase the proportion of VLBW infants born at level III hospitals or subspecialty perinatal centers.

Modified from HealthyPeople.gov. Maternal, infant, and child health. 2012. https://www.healthypeople.gov/2020/topics-objectives/topic/maternal-infant-and-child-health/objectives.

BOX 1.3 United Nations Millennium Development Goals

1. Eradicate extreme poverty and hunger.
2. Achieve universal primary education.
3. Promote gender equality and empower women.
4. Reduce child mortality.
5. Improve maternal health.
6. Combat HIV/AIDS, malaria, and other diseases.
7. Ensure environmental sustainability.
8. Develop a global partnership for development.

AIDS, Acquired immunodeficiency syndrome; *HIV,* human immunodeficiency virus.
Data from Millenium Development Goals and Beyond 2015. http://www.un.org/millenniumgoals/.

BOX 1.4 National Quality Forum Serious Reportable Events Pertaining to Maternal and Child Health

- Maternal death or serious injury associated with labor or birth in a low-risk pregnancy while being cared for in a healthcare setting
- Death or serious injury of a neonate associated with labor or birth in a low-risk pregnancy
- Artificial insemination with the wrong donor sperm or wrong egg
- Abduction of a client/resident of any age

Data from National Quality Forum (NQF). (2011). *Serious Reportable Events in Healthcare—2011 Update: A Consensus Report.* Washington, DC: NQF.

In 2002, the National Quality Forum (NQF) published a list of Serious Reportable Events in Healthcare. The list was most recently updated in 2011 (NQF, 2011), resulting in a total of 29 events. Of these 29 events, four pertain directly to maternity and newborn care (Box 1.4).

The NQF published *Safe Practices for Better Healthcare* in 2003 and updated it most recently in 2013 (http://www.hfap.org/pdf/patient_safety.pdf). The 34 safe practices included should be used in all applicable health care settings to reduce the risk for harm that results from processes, systems, and environments of care.

High Cost of Health Care

Health care is one of the fastest-growing sectors of the U.S. economy. Currently 17.5% of the gross domestic product is spent on health care (Centers for Medicare & Medicaid, 2015). These high costs are related to higher prices, readily accessible technology, and greater obesity. Most researchers agree that caring for the increased number of low–birth weight (LBW) infants in neonatal intensive care units (NICUs) contributes significantly to overall health care costs.

Nurse midwifery and advanced practice nursing care have helped contain some health care costs. However, not all insurance carriers reimburse nurse practitioners and clinical nurse specialists as direct care providers, nor do they reimburse for all services provided by nurse midwives, a situation that continues to be a problem. Nurses must become involved in the politics of cost containment because they, as knowledgeable experts, can provide solutions to many health care problems at a relatively low cost. Nurse practitioners are among the health care providers included in the Affordable Care Act (ACA). Despite this, only 21 states and the District of Columbia allow nurse practitioners to practice to their fullest potential without physician involvement (American Academy of Nurse Practitioners, 2015).

Limited Access to Care

Barriers to access must be removed so pregnancy outcomes and care of children can be improved. The most significant barrier to access is the inability to pay. Some improvement in ability to pay has been seen due to the ACA. The uninsured rate in 2014 was 10.4%, or 33 million people, which was lower than the rate of 13.3%, or 41.8 million people, in 2013 (Smith & Medalia, 2015). Lack of transportation and dependent child care are other barriers. In addition to a lack of insurance and high costs, a lack of providers for low-income women exists because many physicians either refuse to take Medicaid clients or take only a few such clients. This presents a serious problem because a significant proportion of births is to mothers who receive Medicaid.

Health Care Reform

In early 2010, President Obama signed into law the Patient Protection and ACA. The act aims to make insurance affordable, contain costs, strengthen and improve Medicare and Medicaid, and reform the insurance market. The act contained provisions to promote prevention and improve public health; improve the quality of care for all Americans; reduce waste, fraud, and abuse; and reform the health delivery system. In the early years of its implementation, the ACA gained ground on many of its goals, including the reduction in the number of uninsured Americans to fewer than 28 million by the end of 2016 (Henry J Kaiser Family Foundation). Professional associations such as The Association of Women's Health, Obstetric and Neonatal Nurses (AWHONN) and the American College of Nurse Midwives advocated successfully for the inclusion in the ACA of contraceptive methods, services, and counseling, without any out-of-pocket costs to clients; preventive services such as mammograms, well-woman visits, and screening for gestational diabetes; and providing breastfeeding equipment and counseling for pregnant and nursing women in new insurance plans. See Box 1.5 for resources for the ACA. Political forces rallying under a new administration seek to dismantle much of the Affordable Care Act.

Accountable Care Organizations

In 2011, the Centers for Medicare & Medicaid Services (CMS) finalized new rules under the ACA to help health care providers and hospitals better coordinate care for Medicare clients through Accountable Care Organizations (ACOs). An ACO is a group of health care providers and health care agencies that are accountable for improving the health of populations while containing costs. These groups of health care providers and hospitals voluntarily come together to coordinate high-quality care, eliminate duplication of services, and prevent medical errors, which results in savings of health care dollars.

Health Literacy

Health literacy involves a spectrum of abilities, ranging from reading an appointment slip to interpreting medication instructions. These skills must be assessed routinely to recognize a problem and accommodate clients with limited literacy skills. Most client education materials are written at too high a reading level for the average adult; e-health literacy has emerged as a concept. Individuals use the Internet for diagnosis, and more than half of these individuals seek the opinion of a medical professional rather than trying to care for themselves based on the information accessed.

The CDC (2018a) has a health literacy website (www.cdc.gov/healthliteracy) that highlights implementation of goals and strategies

---

TABLE 1.1   Sample SBAR Report to Physician or Midwife About a Critical Situation

S	Situation I am calling about Mary Smith. I have just assessed her and she saturated a peripad in the last hour. Her blood pressure is 112/62, pulse 86, and respirations 18. I think she is bleeding excessively.
B	Background Mrs. Smith is 12 hours postpartum after giving birth vaginally to a 9 lb, 12 oz term infant after an uncomplicated pregnancy. She had a rapid labor, just over 4 hours, and had no analgesia. She plans to bottle-feed this baby. She had an IV with 10 units of Pitocin but it was completed and discontinued about 2 hours ago. This is her sixth birth. All were uncomplicated and she had an uneventful recovery from them.
A	Assessment Her fundus becomes firm after massage but relaxes again. She has voided and her bladder feels empty. I think she might have retained placenta and she needs to be examined.
R	Recommendation I would like you to come and examine her immediately. Do you want her IV restarted? Do you want her to have a hemoglobin and hematocrit?

IV, Intravenous.
The SBAR tool was developed by Kaiser Permanente.

BOX 1.5   Resources for the Affordable Care Act

www.HealthCare.gov (CuidadDeSalud.gov) State-specific information
  www.medscape.org/viewarticle/782776
  CE module "What the Healthcare Marketplace Means for Practices and Patients"
  Marketplace.cms.gov

Downloadable Educational Materials
www.hhs.gov/healthcare/facts/bystate/statebystate.html Interactive map to show Americans how the ACA affects them; fact sheets

Social Media Resource
Facebook.com/HealthCare.gov (Facebook.com/CuidadoDeSalud.gov)
Twitter@HealthCareGov (Twitter@CuidadoDeSalud)
1-800-318-2596 (TTY: 1-855-889-4325)
Call center available 24/7 in 150 languages

BOX 1.6 Maternal/Infant Biostatistic Terminology

Abortus: An embryo or fetus that is removed or expelled from the uterus at 20 weeks of gestation or less, weighs 500 g or less, or measures 25 cm or less

Birth rate: Number of live births in 1 year per 1000 population

Fertility rate: Number of births per 1000 women between the ages of 15 and 44 years (inclusive), calculated on a yearly basis

Infant mortality rate: Number of deaths of infants younger than 1 year of age per 1000 live births

Maternal mortality rate: Number of maternal deaths from births and complications of pregnancy, childbirth, and puerperium (the first 42 days after end of the pregnancy) per 100,000 live births

Neonatal mortality rate: Number of deaths of infants younger than 28 days of age per 1000 live births

Perinatal mortality rate: Number of stillbirths and the number of neonatal deaths per 1000 live births

Stillbirth: An infant who, at birth, demonstrates no signs of life, such as breathing, heartbeat, or voluntary muscle movements

---

of the National Action Plan to Improve Health Literacy. Health literacy is part of the ACA.

As a result of the increasingly multicultural U.S. population, there is a more urgent need to address health literacy as a component of culturally and linguistically competent care. Older adults, racial or ethnic minorities, and those whose income is at or below the poverty level are most vulnerable. Lower health literacy is associated with adverse health outcomes (Dickens & Piano, 2013).

Health care providers contribute to health literacy by using simple common words, avoiding jargon, and assessing whether the client understands the discussion. Speaking slowly and clearly and focusing on what is important will increase understanding.

TRENDS IN FERTILITY AND BIRTH RATE

Fertility trends and birth rates reflect women's needs for health care. Box 1.6 defines biostatistical terminology useful in analyzing maternity health care. In 2017, the fertility rate, births per 1000 women from 15 to 44 years of age, was 60.3 (Martin, Hamilton, Osterman, et al., 2018). The birth rate for teens 15 to 19 years declined by 7% since 2016 to 18.8. Birth rates since 2016 decreased for women aged 20 to 30, while it increased for women in the early 40s. The cesarean birth rate increased slightly from 2016, when it was 31.9% to 32% in 2017 (Martin et al, 2018).

Low Birth Weight and Preterm Birth

The risks of morbidity and mortality increase for newborns weighing less than 2500 g (5 lb, 8 oz)—low–birth weight infants. In the United States in 2015, the LBW rate was 8.07 per 1000, a slight increase since 2012. Rates of LBW among non-Hispanic white women were stable at 9.93%. The rise in the overall LBW rates were due to increases in LBW births to non-Hispanic black women (13.35%) and Hispanic women (7.21%); non-Hispanic black infants are almost twice as likely as non-Hispanic white infants to be of LBW and to die in the first year of life (Martin et al., 2017).

The preterm birth rate also reversed trend for the first time since 2007 and showed a slight increase to 9.63% in 2015 (Martin et al., 2017). There was variation in the percentage according to race and Hispanic origin: 13.41% for non-Hispanic black births, 9.14% for Hispanic births, and 8.88% for non-Hispanic white births (Martin et al., 2017).

Multiple births contribute to the incidence of LBW and preterm birth. Increases in the rates of multiple births over the past few decades have been attributed to increased use of fertility drugs and older age at childbearing. Recent declines in this trend are linked to changes in medical procedures associated with assisted reproductive technologies (Martin et al., 2017). Overall multiple births accounted for 3.45% of births in 2015. The twin birth rate was 33.5 per 1000 in 2015. The downward trend in the birth rate of higher-order multiples (triplet, quadruplet, and greater) continued in 2015, with a rate of 103.6 per 100,000 (Martin et al., 2017).

Cigarette smoking is associated with LBW, prematurity, and intrauterine growth restriction. In 2010, 12.3% of pregnant women smoked, including 14.3% of non-Hispanic white women, 8.9% non-Hispanic black women, 3.4% of Hispanic women, 26% of American Indian/Alaska Native women, and 2.1% of Asian/Pacific Islander women (Tong et al., 2013).

Place of Delivery and Attendant

In 2015, 98.5% of births in the United States occurred in hospitals and were attended by nurse midwives (8.1%), medical doctors (84%), or doctors of osteopathy (7.1%). The remaining 61,000 births occurred either in women's homes (63.1%) or freestanding birth centers (30.9%) (Martin et al., 2017). Out-of-hospital births are attended primarily by certified nurse midwives, certified professional midwives, or certified midwives.

Infant Mortality in the United States

A common indicator of the adequacy of prenatal care and the health of a nation as a whole is the infant mortality rate. The U.S. infant mortality rate for 2015 was 5.9 deaths per 1000 live births (CDC, 2018b). The disparity in infant mortality rate between African American infants and non-Hispanic white infants has increased over time. The infant mortality rate continues to be higher for non-Hispanic black babies (11.3 per 1000) than for non-Hispanic whites (4.9 per 1000) and Hispanic (5.0 per 1000) babies (CDC, 2018b). Limited maternal education, young maternal age, unmarried status, poverty, lack of prenatal care, and smoking appear to be associated with higher infant mortality rates. Poor nutrition, alcohol use, and maternal conditions such as poor health or hypertension also are important contributors to infant mortality. To address the factors associated with infant mortality, a shift from the current emphasis on high-technology medical interventions to a focus on improving access to preventive care for low-income families must occur.

Congenital malformations are the leading causes of neonatal death. Other causes include: low birth weight, sudden infant death syndrome, maternal complications, unintentional injuries, cord and placental complications, newborn bacterial sepsis, newborn respiratory distress, circulatory system problems, and hemorrhage (Kochanek, Murphy, Xu, Arias, 2017). Racial differences in the infant mortality rates continue to challenge public health experts. Increased rates of survival during the neonatal period have resulted largely from high-quality prenatal care and the improvement in perinatal services, including technologic advances in neonatal intensive care and obstetrics.

Commitment at national, state, and local levels is required to reduce the infant mortality rate. More research is needed to identify the extent to which financial, educational, sociocultural, and behavioral factors individually and collectively affect perinatal morbidity and mortality. Barriers to care must be removed and perinatal services modified to meet contemporary health care needs.

International Infant Mortality Trends

Every day 7000 babies die within 28 days of birth (United Nations Inter-agency Group for Child Mortality Estimation, 2017), a rate that has increased since 2000. Half of all neonatal deaths occur in five countries: India (24%), Pakistan (10%), Nigeria (9%), the Democratic Republic of the Congo (4%), and Ethiopia (3%). In 2016, the infant mortality rate of Cuba (2.4/1000) was the lowest in the Americas, and that of the United States was (3.7/1000) (WHO). Decreases in the infant mortality rate in the United States do not keep pace with the rates of other industrialized countries. One reason for this is significant disparities in health which may result in the high rate of LBW infants in the United States in contrast with the rates in other countries.

Maternal Mortality Trends

The United Nations estimated that 303,000 women died of problems related to pregnancy or childbirth in 2015, a decline from approximately 358,000 in 2008 and 532,000 in 1990 (WHO, 2018). In the United States in 2014, the annual maternal mortality rate was 23.8 for 48 states and the District of Columbia (MacDorman, Declercq, Cabral, & Morton, 2016). The CDC began working with national and international groups in 2001 to develop and implement programs to promote safe motherhood. Although the overall number of maternal deaths in the United States is small (about 700 each year), maternal mortality remains a significant problem because a high proportion of deaths are preventable, primarily through improving the access to and use of prenatal care services. In the United States, there is significant racial disparity in the rates of maternal death: non-Hispanic black women (43.5), non-Hispanic white women (12.7), and women of other races (14.4) (CDC, 2017). Maternal mortality among black women is more than three times that of white women. Further data are needed to determine the maternal mortality rate of Hispanic women. The leading causes of maternal death attributable to pregnancy differ over the world. In general, three major causes have persisted for the past 50 years: hypertensive disorders, infection, and hemorrhage. The three leading causes of maternal mortality in the United States today are cardiovascular disease, noncardiovascular diseases, and infection/sepsis (CDC, 2017). Factors that are strongly related to maternal death include age (younger than 20 years and 35 years or older), lack of prenatal care, low educational attainment, unmarried status, and non-Caucasian race. The *Healthy People 2010* goal of 3.3 maternal deaths per 100,000 posed a significant challenge and was not achieved. The *Healthy People 2020* goal is 11.4 maternal deaths per 100,000 live births, which may also be difficult to achieve. Worldwide strategies to reduce maternal mortality rates include improving access to skilled attendants at birth, providing postabortion care, improving family planning services, and providing adolescents with better reproductive health services.

Maternal Morbidity

Although mortality is the traditional measure of maternal health and maternal health is often measured by neonatal outcomes, pregnancy complications are important. Currently no surveillance method is available to measure the incidence of maternal morbidity. This includes such conditions as acute renal failure, amniotic fluid embolism, cerebrovascular accident, eclampsia, pulmonary embolism, liver failure, obstetric shock, respiratory failure, septicemia, and complications of anesthesia (pulmonary, cardiac, central nervous system). Maternal morbidity results in a high-risk pregnancy. The diagnosis of high risk imposes a situational crisis on the family. The combined efforts of medical and nursing personnel are required to care for these clients, who often need the expertise of physicians and nurses trained in both critical care obstetrics and intensive care medicine or nursing.

Obesity

More than one third (38.3%) of women in the United States are obese (body mass index [BMI] of 30 or greater); in Canada less than one fourth (23.9%) of women are obese. Obesity in women demonstrates

significant racial disparities: in the United States 56.9% of non-Hispanic black women, 45.7% of Mexican-American women, and 35.5% of non-Hispanic white women ages 20 years and older are obese (Ogden, Carroll, Fryar, & Flegal, 2015). Approximately 52% of women in the United States have prepregnancy BMI in the overweight or obese categories. The two most frequently reported maternal medical risk factors are hypertension associated with pregnancy and diabetes, both of which are associated with obesity. Decreased fertility, congenital anomalies, miscarriage, and fetal death are associated with obesity. Obesity in pregnancy is associated with the use of increased health care services and longer hospital stays.

REGIONALIZATION OF PERINATAL HEALTH CARE SERVICES

Not all facilities can develop and maintain the full spectrum of services required for high-risk perinatal clients. A regionalized system focusing on integrated delivery of graded levels of hospital-based perinatal health care services is effective and results in improved outcomes for mothers and their newborns. This system of coordinated care can be extended to preconception and ambulatory prenatal care services. In 2015, the American College of Obstetricians and Gynecologists (ACOG) and the Society for Maternal-Fetal Medicine (SMFM) published a consensus statement on levels of maternal care (ACOG & SMFM, 2015).

Ambulatory Prenatal Care

Guidelines have been established regarding the level of care that can be expected at any given facility. In ambulatory settings, providers must distinguish themselves by the level of care they provide. *Basic care* is provided by obstetricians, family physicians, nurse midwives, and other advanced practice clinicians approved by local governance. Routine risk-oriented prenatal care, education, and support are provided. Providers offering *specialty care* are obstetricians who must provide fetal diagnostic testing and management of obstetric and medical complications in addition to basic care. *Subspecialty care* is provided by maternal-fetal medicine specialists and reproductive geneticists and includes the aforementioned in addition to genetic testing, advanced fetal therapies, and management of severe maternal and fetal complications. Collaboration among providers to meet the woman's needs is the key to reducing perinatal morbidity and mortality.

HIGH-TECHNOLOGY CARE

Advances in scientific knowledge and the large number of high-risk pregnancies have contributed to a health care system that emphasizes high-technology care. Maternity care has extended to preconception counseling, more and better scientific techniques to monitor the mother and fetus, more definitive tests for hypoxia and acidosis, and NICUs. The labors of virtually all women who give birth in hospitals are monitored electronically despite the lack of evidence of efficacy of such monitoring. The numbers of assisted labors and births are increasing. Internet-based information is available to the public that enhances interactions among health care providers, families, and community providers. Point-of-care testing is available. Personal data assistants are used to enhance comprehensive care; the medical record is increasingly in electronic form.

Strides are being made in identifying genetic codes, and genetic engineering is taking place. Women's health has expanded to emphasize care of older women, new cancer-screening techniques, advances in the diagnosis and treatment of breast cancer, and work on an AIDS vaccine. In general, high-technology care has flourished, whereas "health"

BOX 1.7   Principles for Social Networking and the Nurse

- Nurses must not transmit or place online individually identifiable client information.
- Nurses must observe ethically prescribed professional client-nurse boundaries.
- Nurses should understand that clients, colleagues, institutions, and employers may view postings.
- Nurses should take advantage of privacy settings and seek to separate personal and professional information online.
- Nurses should bring content that could harm a client's privacy, rights, or welfare to the attention of appropriate authorities.
- Nurses should participate in developing institutional policies governing online contact.

From American Nurses Association. (2011). *Principles for social networking and the nurse: Guidance for the registered nurse.* Washington, DC: Author.

care has become relatively neglected. Nurses must use caution and prospective planning and assess the effect of the emerging technology.

Telehealth is an umbrella term for the use of communication technologies and electronic information to provide or support health care when the participants are separated by distance. It permits specialists, including nurses, to provide health care and consultation when distance separates them from those needing care. This technology has the potential to save billions of dollars annually for health care, but these technologic advances have also contributed to higher health care costs.

Social Media

Social media uses Internet-based technologies to allow users to create their own content and participate in dialogue. The most common social media platforms are Facebook, Twitter, and LinkedIn, with others also gaining in popularity. Through use of these technologies, nurses can link with nurses with similar interests, share insights about client care, and advocate for clients (Casella, Mills, & Usher, 2014). However, there are pitfalls for nurses using this technology. Client privacy and confidentiality can be violated, and institutions and colleagues can be cast in unfavorable lights with negative consequences for those posting the information. Nursing students have been expelled from school, and nurses have been fired or reprimanded by a board of nursing for injudicious posts. To help make nurses aware of their responsibilities when using social media, the American Nurses Association (ANA) published six principles for social networking and the nurse (Box 1.7). In addition, the National Council of State Boards of Nursing (NCSBN) issued *White Paper: A Nurse's Guide to the Use of Social Media* (NCSBN, 2011). The paper details issues of confidentiality and privacy, possible consequences of inappropriate use of social media, common myths and misunderstandings of social media, and tips on how to avoid problems.

COMMUNITY-BASED CARE

A shift in settings, from acute care institutions to ambulatory settings including the home, has occurred (see Chapter 2). Even childbearing women at high risk are often cared for on an outpatient basis or in the home. Technology previously available only in the hospital is now found in the home. This has affected the organizational structure of care, the skills required in providing such care, and the costs to consumers.

Home health care also has a community focus. Nurses are involved in providing care for women and infants in homeless shelters and adolescents in school-based clinics and in promoting health at community sites, churches, and shopping malls. Nursing education curricula are increasingly community based.

CHILDBIRTH PRACTICES

Prenatal care can promote better pregnancy outcomes by providing early risk assessment and promoting healthy behaviors such as improved nutrition and smoking cessation. Prenatal care ideally begins before pregnancy because early decisions lay the foundation for the entire perinatal year. If at all possible, education continues in each trimester of pregnancy and extends through the early postpartum weeks. Some health care providers promote preconception care as an important component of perinatal services. Preconception or early pregnancy classes also emphasize health-promoting behavior as well as choices of care.

In the United States in 2012, 74.1% of all women received care in the first trimester. There is disparity in receiving prenatal care by race and ethnicity, with non-Hispanic black women and Hispanic women receiving significantly later prenatal care as compared to non-Hispanic whites. In spite of these statistics, substantial gains have been made in the use of prenatal care since the early 1990s, which are attributed to the expansion in the 1980s of Medicaid coverage for pregnant women.

Women can choose physicians or nurse midwives as primary care providers. In 2015, doctors of medicine attended 84% of all births, certified nurse midwives attended 8.1%, and doctors of osteopathy attended 7.1% (Martin et al., 2017). Women who choose nurse midwives as their primary providers participate more actively in childbirth decisions, receive fewer interventions during labor, and are less likely to give birth prematurely (Sandall, Soltani, Gates, et al., 2016). From 2014 to 2015, there was a decline in the rate of cesarean births from 32.2% to 32.0% (Martin et al.), although Thielking (2015) reported that the approximately one-third rate for cesarean births is too high for resulting benefits, as benefits usually plateau at about a 19% cesarean birth rate.

❓ CLINICAL REASONING CASE STUDY
Safety and Efficacy of Midwifery Care

A group of nurse midwives is setting up practice in your hometown. They are to collaborate with one of the groups of obstetricians in the same city. A letter to the editor appeared in the local newspaper stating that the presence of midwives will jeopardize the care of pregnant women in the community because midwives usually care for the poor and indigent, deliver babies at home, and therefore do not have the skills to work in hospitals and care for middle-class women who have insurance. The letter writer urged the community to boycott the midwives to ensure safe childbirth for women in the community.

1. What is the priority concern or client need in this situation?
2. List other client needs/problems in this case.
3. Identify any additional information needed by the nurse in addressing this situation.
4. Describe the roles/responsibilities of interprofessional health team members who may be involved in this situation.

With family-centered care, fathers, partners, grandparents, siblings, and friends may be present for labor and birth. Fathers or partners may be present for cesarean births and may participate in vaginal births by "catching the baby" or cutting the umbilical cord or both (Fig. 1.1). Doulas (i.e., trained and experienced female labor attendants) may be present to provide a continuous, one-on-one caring presence throughout the labor and birth. Ideally, newborns are placed skin-to-skin with the mother immediately after birth and are encouraged to breastfeed

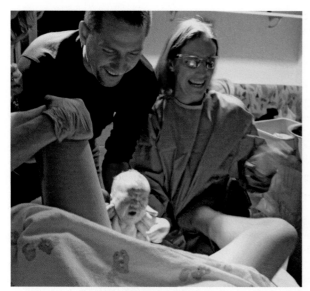

Fig. 1.1 Father "Catching" Newborn Daughter Who Cried Before Her Lower Body Emerged Following an Unmedicated Birth. (Courtesy Darren and Julie Nelson, Loveland, CO.)

as soon as possible. Neonates often remain in the room with their parents and may never transfer to a newborn nursery. Parents actively participate in newborn care on mother/baby units, in nurseries, and in NICUs.

Discharge of a mother and baby within 24 hours of birth has created a growing need for follow-up or home care. In some settings, discharge may occur as early as 6 hours after birth. Legislation has been enacted to ensure that mothers and babies are permitted to stay in the hospital for at least 48 hours after vaginal birth and 96 hours after cesarean birth, although they may choose to leave earlier. Focused and efficient teaching is necessary to enable the parents and infant to make the transition safely from the hospital to the home.

INVOLVING CONSUMERS AND PROMOTING SELF-MANAGEMENT

Self-management is appealing to clients as well as the health care system because of its potential to reduce health care costs. Maternity care is especially suited to self-management because childbearing is primarily health focused, women are usually well when they enter the system, and visits to health care providers can present the opportunity for health and illness interventions. Measures to improve health and reduce risks associated with poor pregnancy outcomes and illness can be addressed. Topics such as nutrition education, stress management, smoking cessation, alcohol and drug treatment, violence prevention, social support improvement, and parenting education are appropriate for such encounters.

INTERNATIONAL CONCERNS

High maternal and infant mortality is a serious problem in developing countries that have limited resources to address the problems. Two concerns that nurses in the United States and Canada might encounter are female genital mutilation and human trafficking.

Female genital mutilation, infibulation, and *circumcision* are terms used to describe procedures in which part or all of the female external genitalia is removed for cultural or nontherapeutic reasons (WHO, 2016). Worldwide, many women undergo such procedures. The International Council of Nurses and other health professionals have spoken out against procedures that result in mutilation as harmful to women's health. Although it is illegal in the United States to perform female genital mutilation on a person younger than 18 years of age, it is estimated that 513,000 women and girls in the United States have experienced or are at risk for female genital mutilation (Office of Women's Health, 2015).

Human trafficking is a serious crime, an illegal business that exists in the United States and internationally, in which mostly women and children are "trafficked," or forced into hard labor, sex work, and even organ donation (Budiani-Saberi, Raja, Findley, et al., 2014; United Nations Office on Drugs & Crime, 2016). Health care professionals may interact with victims who are in captivity. This provides an opportunity to identify victims, intervene to help them obtain necessary health services, and provide information about ways to escape from their situation (Fig. 1.2) (see Chapter 5). The National Human Trafficking Resource Center (1.888-373-7888) can provide assistance. AWHONN has published a position paper on nursing care of victims of human trafficking (AWHONN, 2016).

WOMEN'S HEALTH

Heart disease is the leading cause of death of women followed closely by malignant neoplasms, including breast cancer. Symptoms of a heart attack in women are different from symptoms in men. Nurses providing care for women have opportunities for client education to create awareness of these differences. Early detection of breast cancer through mammography can reduce the mortality rate resulting from this type of cancer. However, because of lack of information or lack of insurance and access, many women never have mammograms. Wide disparity exists between Caucasian women and women of other races and between older and younger women in their rates of mammography, detection, and treatment of breast cancer, and in their survival rates (see Chapter 10). Cancer genetic predisposition testing is increasingly available. Women may approach providers of women's health services to request such testing.

Various factors and conditions affect women's health. Race is a major factor: Caucasian women born in 2015 have a life expectancy at birth of 81.3 years, in contrast with 78.5 years for African American women (Arias, Heron, Jiaquan, 2017). The population has grown older: Approximately 50 million women are older than 50 years of age; 51 is the median age for menopause.

Violence is a major factor affecting women (see Chapter 5). Violence includes battery, rape or other sexual assaults, and attacks with various weapons. Rates of reported intimate partner violence have increased, possibly because of better assessment and reporting mechanisms. The incidence of battering increases during pregnancy. Violence is associated with complications of pregnancy such as bleeding. Alcoholism and substance abuse by the woman and her abuser are associated with violence and homelessness, which affect a growing number of women and children and place them at risk for a variety of health problems.

TRENDS IN NURSING PRACTICE

The increasing complexity of care for maternity and women's health clients has contributed to specialization of nurses working with these clients. This specialized knowledge is gained through experience, advanced degrees, and certification programs. Nurses

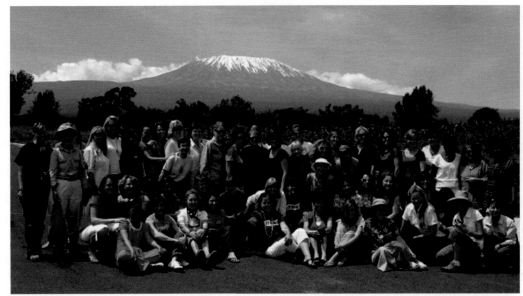

Fig. 1.2 In January 2012, a Group of 48 Women Participated in the Freedom Climb of Mt. Kilimanjaro, the Tallest Mountain in Africa. The women climbed to call attention to human trafficking and to raise funds to support projects to combat trafficking. The group raised more than $350,000, which went for projects such as prenatal care, education, safe houses, and micro loans for victims of trafficking in many countries served by Operation Mobilization (www.om.org). (Courtesy Shannon Perry, Phoenix, AZ.)

in advanced practice (e.g., nurse practitioners and nurse midwives) may provide primary care throughout a woman's life, including during the pregnancy cycle. In some settings the clinical nurse specialist and nurse practitioner roles are blended, and nurses deliver high-quality, comprehensive, and cost-effective care in a variety of settings. Lactation consultants provide services in the hospital setting, in clinics and primary care offices, and during home visits.

Nursing Interventions Classification

When the IOM proposed that all client records be computerized by the year 2000, a need for a common language to describe the contributions of nurses to client care became evident. Nurses from the University of Iowa developed a comprehensive standardized language that describes interventions that are performed by generalist or specialist nurses. This language is included in the Nursing Interventions Classification (NIC) (Bulachek, Butcher, Dochterman, & Wagner, 2013). Examples of interventions for childbearing care to assist in the preparation for childbirth before, during, and after the birth include breastfeeding assistance, childbirth preparation, circumcision care, electronic fetal monitoring, family planning, and kangaroo care.

Evidence-Based Practice

Evidence-based practice—providing care based on evidence gained through research and clinical trials—is increasingly emphasized. Although not all practice can be evidence based, practitioners must use the best available information on which to base their interventions. In 2013, AWHONN developed a draft document of quality measures for women's health and perinatal nursing, comparing NQF measures with AWHONN Nursing Care Quality measures (AWHONN, 2013). Discussion of nursing care and evidence-based practice boxes throughout this text provide examples of evidence-based practice in perinatal and women's health nursing (see Evidence-Based Practice box).

EVIDENCE-BASED PRACTICE

Seeking and Evaluating Evidence: A Necessary Competency for Quality and Safety

Evidence-Based Practice boxes are found throughout this textbook. These boxes provide examples of how any nurse, no matter how much experience he or she has, might conduct an inquiry into an identified practice question. Practice questions can emerge on any given shift. Curiosity and access to a virtual or real library are all the nurse needs to be confident that his or her practice has a sound foundation of evidence.

At the tertiary level professional organizations such as the AHRQ (www.ahrq.gov) or the National Guidelines Clearinghouse (NGC) (guideline.gov) may decide to address a broad practice question by sorting through all the available primary and secondary evidence and consulting experienced clinicians. After thoughtful review, the committee of experts in the organization crafts its consensus statement. These recommendations for best practice are derived from the work of the systematic analysts, who utilized the work of the primary researchers to create comprehensive systematic reviews.

Jennifer Taylor Alderman

Cochrane Pregnancy and Childbirth Database

The Cochrane Pregnancy and Childbirth Database was first planned in 1976 with a small grant from the WHO to Dr. Iain Chalmers and colleagues at Oxford. In 1993, the Cochrane Collaboration was formed, and the Oxford Database of Perinatal Trials became known as the Cochrane Pregnancy and Childbirth Database. The Cochrane Collaboration oversees up-to-date, systematic reviews of randomized controlled trials of health care and disseminates these reviews. The premise of the project is that these types of studies provide the most reliable evidence about the effects of care.

The evidence from these studies should encourage practitioners to implement useful measures and to abandon those that are useless or harmful. Studies are ranked in six categories:

1. Forms of care that are beneficial
2. Forms of care that are likely to be beneficial
3. Forms of care with a trade-off between beneficial and adverse effects
4. Forms of care with unknown effectiveness
5. Forms of care that are unlikely to be beneficial
6. Forms of care that are likely to be ineffective or harmful

Joanna Briggs Institute

Established in 1996 as an initiative of the Royal Adelaide Hospital and the University of Adelaide in Australia, the Joanna Briggs Institute (JBI) uses a collaborative approach for evaluating evidence from a range of sources (www.joannabriggs.edu.au). The JBI has formed collaborations with a variety of universities and hospitals around the world, including in the United States and Canada. The JBI uses the following grades of recommendation for evidence of feasibility, appropriateness, meaningfulness, and effectiveness: *A*, strong support that merits application; *B*, moderate support that warrants consideration of application; and *C*, not supported (JBI, 2013). The JBI provides another source for perinatal nurses to access information to support evidence-based practice.

Outcomes-Oriented Practice

Outcomes of care (that is, the effectiveness of interventions and quality of care) are receiving increased emphasis. Outcomes-oriented care measures effectiveness of care against benchmarks or standards. It is a measure of the value of nursing using quality indicators and answers the question, "Did the client benefit or not benefit from the care provided?" (Moorhead, Johnson, Maas, & Swanson, 2013). The Outcome and Assessment Information Set (OASIS) is an example of an outcomes system important for nursing. Its use is required by the CMS in all home health organizations that are Medicare accredited. The Nursing Outcomes Classification (NOC) (Moorhead, Johnson, Maas, Swanson, 2013) is an effort to identify outcomes and related measures that can be used for evaluation of care of individuals, families, and communities across the care continuum (Moorhead et al.); for example, the scale for *Breastfeeding Establishment: Infant* ranges from Not Adequate to Totally Adequate. Indicators include proper alignment and latching, proper areolar grasp and compression, correct suck and tongue placement, and audible swallowing. Through this assessment, the nurse can determine whether the infant met the desired outcome of ingesting adequate nutrition.

A Global Perspective

Advances in medicine and nursing have resulted in increased knowledge and understanding in the care of mothers and infants. Continued efforts at reducing mother-to-child transmission of HIV have had some success; antiretroviral treatment was accessed by three quarters of all pregnant women living with HIV in 2016, and the number of new cases of HIV infection among children aged 0 to 14 is declining (UNICEF, 2018). At the same time, new threats to fetal and neonatal health, such as the Zika virus, emerge requiring extensive resources to determine the cause, transmission, treatment, and prevention of such insults (Oduyobo, Polen, Walke, et al., 2017).

As the world becomes smaller because of travel and communication technologies, nurses and other health care providers are gaining a global perspective and participating in activities to improve the health and health care of people worldwide. Nurses participate in medical outreach, providing obstetric, surgical, ophthalmologic, orthopedic, or other services (Fig. 1.3); attend international meetings; conduct research; and provide international consultation. International student and faculty exchanges occur. More articles about health and health care in various countries are appearing in nursing journals. Several schools

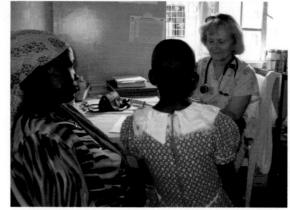

Fig. 1.3 Nurse Interviewing a Young Girl Accompanied by Her Mother in a Clinic in Rural Kenya. (Courtesy Shannon Perry, Phoenix, AZ.)

of nursing in the United States are World Health Organization Collaborating Centers.

STANDARDS OF PRACTICE AND LEGAL ISSUES IN PROVISION OF CARE

Nursing standards of practice in perinatal and women's health nursing have been described by several organizations, including the ANA, which publishes standards for maternal-child health nursing; AWHONN, which publishes standards of practice and education for perinatal nurses (Box 1.8); ACNM, which publishes standards of practice for nurse midwives; and the National Association of Neonatal Nurses (NANN), which publishes standards of practice for neonatal nurses. These standards reflect current knowledge, represent levels of practice agreed upon by leaders in the specialty, and can be used for clinical benchmarking.

In addition to these more formalized standards, agencies have their own policy and procedure books that outline standards to be followed in that setting. In legal terms, the standard of care is that level of practice that a reasonably prudent nurse would provide in the same or similar circumstances. In determining legal negligence, the care given is compared with the standard of care. If the standard was not met and harm resulted, negligence occurred. The number of legal suits in the perinatal area typically has been high. As a consequence, malpractice insurance costs are high for physicians, nurse midwives, and nurses who work in labor and birth settings.

LEGAL TIP
Standard of Care

When uncertain about how to perform a procedure, the nurse should consult the agency procedure book guidelines. These guidelines are the standard of care for that agency.

Risk Management

Risk management is an evolving process that identifies risks, establishes preventive practices, develops reporting mechanisms, and delineates procedures for managing lawsuits. Nurses should be familiar with concepts of risk management and their implications for nursing practice. These concepts can be viewed as systems of checks and balances that ensure high-quality client care from preconception until after birth. Effective risk management minimizes the risk of injury to clients

BOX 1.8   Standards of Care for Women and Newborns

Standards of Practice

Assessment
- Collects health data of the woman or newborn

Diagnosis
- Analyzes data to determine nursing diagnosis

Outcome Identification
- Identifies expected outcomes that are individualized

Planning
- Develops a plan of care

Implementation
- Performs interventions for the plan of care
  - (a) *Coordination of Care.* Coordinated care delivery within her/his scope of practice
  - (b) *Health Teaching and Health Promotion.* Employs teaching strategies to promote, maintain, or restore health

Evaluation
- Evaluates effectiveness of interventions in relation to expected outcomes

Standards of Professional Performance

Quality of Practice
- Systematically evaluates and implements measures to improve quality, safety, and effectiveness of nursing practice

Education
- Acquires and maintains knowledge and competencies that reflect current evidence-based practice

Professional Practice Evaluation
- Evaluates own practice in relation to current evidence-based information, standards and guidelines, statutes, rules and regulations

Ethics
- Decisions and actions determined in an ethical manner and guided by a sound ethical decision-making process

Collegiality
- Interacts with and contributes to professional development of peers, colleagues, and other health care providers

Collaboration and Communication
- Collaborates and communicates with women, families, health care providers, and the community in providing safe and effective care

Research
- Generates and/or integrates evidence to identify, examine, validate, and evaluate knowledge, theories, and approaches in providing care to clients

Resources and Technology
- Considers factors related to safety, effectiveness, technological advances, and costs in planning and delivering client care

Leadership
- Within appropriate roles, seeks to serve as a role model, change agent, consultant, and mentor to clients and other health care professionals

From Association of Women's Health, Obstetric, and Neonatal Nurses (AWHONN) (2019). Standards for professional nursing practice in the care of women and newborns. 8th ed. Washington, DC. Retrieved from: https://www.awhonn.org/store/ViewProduct.aspx?ID=12949365.

and the number of lawsuits against nurses, doctors, and hospitals. Each facility or site develops site-specific risk management procedures based on accepted standards and guidelines. The procedures and guidelines must be reviewed periodically.

Sentinel Events

The Joint Commission (2015) revised its definition of a sentinel event as any event that is not due to underlying conditions or natural courses of a client's condition that affects a client, resulting in death, permanent harm, or severe temporary harm. This refers to perinatal events, specifically the need for receiving 4 or more units of blood products and/or admission to the ICU. Kernicterus, a rare form of brain damage that can occur with jaundice, is an example of a sentinel event that may require four or more blood transfusions.

Failure to Rescue

Failure to rescue is the failure to recognize or act on early signs of distress. Key components of failure to rescue are (1) careful surveillance and identification of complications, and (2) quick action to initiate appropriate interventions and activate a team response. For the perinatal nurse, this involves careful surveillance, timely identification of complications, appropriate interventions, and activation of a team response to minimize client harm. Maternal complications that are appropriate for process measurement are placental abruption, postpartum hemorrhage, uterine rupture, eclampsia, and amniotic fluid embolism (Simpson, Knox, Martin, et al., 2011). Fetal complications

include nonreassuring fetal heart rate and pattern, prolapsed umbilical cord, shoulder dystocia, and uterine hyperstimulation (Simpson et al.).

Quality and Safety Education for Nurses

Quality and Safety Education for Nurses (QSEN) is an effort to provide nurses with the competencies to improve the quality and safety of the systems of health care in which they practice (QSEN, 2018). The competencies for nursing delineated by the IOM (2003) (Box 1.9) were adapted by QSEN faculty members and defined by describing essential features of a competent and respected nurse. They then developed knowledge, skills, and attitudes (KSAs) for each competency. Incorporation of these KSAs into prelicensure education for nurses helps faculty to plan learning experiences to prepare respected and qualified nurses.

ETHICAL ISSUES IN PERINATAL NURSING AND WOMEN'S HEALTH CARE

Ethical concerns and debates have multiplied with the increased use of technology and with scientific advances. For example, with reproductive technology, pregnancy is now possible in women who thought they would never bear children, including some who are menopausal or postmenopausal. Should scarce resources be devoted to achieving pregnancies in older women? Is giving birth to a child at an older age worth the risks involved? Should older parents be encouraged to conceive a baby when they may not live to see the child reach adulthood? Should a woman who is HIV positive have access to

BOX 1.9   Institute of Medicine Quality and Safety Education for Nurses Competencies for Nursing

Client-centered care
Teamwork
Collaboration
Evidence-based practice
Quality improvement
Safety
Informatics

Data from Institute of Medicine. (2003). *Health professions education: A bridge to quality*. Washington, DC: National Academies Press.

assisted reproduction services? Should third-party payers assume the costs of reproductive technology such as the use of induced ovulation and in vitro fertilizations? With induced ovulation and in vitro fertilization, multiple pregnancies occur, and multifetal pregnancy reduction (selectively terminating one or more fetuses) may be considered. Abortion is another controversial area in women's health, and taking care of women who choose abortion is part of nursing care.

Questions about informed consent and allocation of resources must be addressed with innovations such as intrauterine fetal surgery, fetoscopy, therapeutic insemination, genetic engineering, stem cell research, surrogate childbearing, surgery for infertility, assisted reproductive technology, fetal research, and treatment of very LBW (VLBW) babies.

The introduction of long-acting contraceptives has created moral choices and policy dilemmas for health care providers and legislators; that is, should some women (substance abusers, women with low incomes, or women who are HIV positive) be required to take these contraceptives? With the potential for great good that can come from fetal tissue transplantation, what research is ethical? What are the rights of the embryo? Should cloning of humans be permitted? Discussion and debate about these issues will continue for many years. Nurses and clients as well as scientists, physicians, attorneys, lawmakers, ethicists, and clergy must be involved in the discussions.

RESEARCH IN PERINATAL NURSING AND WOMEN'S HEALTH CARE

Research plays a vital role in establishing maternity and women's health science. It can validate that nursing care makes a difference. For example, although prenatal care is clearly associated with healthier infants, no one knows exactly which nursing interventions produce this outcome. The research into women's health must increase. In the past, medical researchers rarely included women in their studies, so more research in this area is crucial. Many possible areas of research exist in maternity and women's health care. The clinician can identify problems in the health and health care of women and infants. Through research, nurses can make a difference for these clients. Nurses should promote research funding and conduct research on maternity and women's health, especially concerning the effectiveness of nursing strategies for these clients.

Ethical Guidelines for Nursing Research

Research with perinatal clients may create ethical dilemmas for the nurse. For example, participating in research may cause additional stress to a woman concerned about outcomes of genetic testing or one who is waiting for an invasive procedure. Obtaining amniotic fluid samples or performing cordocentesis poses risks to the fetus. Nurses must protect the rights of human subjects (i.e., clients) in all of their research. For example, nurses can collect data on or care for clients who are participating in clinical trials. The nurse ensures that the participants are fully informed and aware of their rights as subjects. The nurse must also be knowledgeable about the need for Institutional Review Board (IRB) approval. The nurse can be involved in determining whether the benefits of research outweigh the risks to the mother and the fetus. Following the ANA ethical guidelines in the conduct, dissemination, and implementation of nursing research helps nurses ensure that research is conducted ethically.

KEY POINTS

- Maternity nursing focuses on women and their newborns and families during the childbearing cycle.
- Women's health nursing focuses on the special physical, psychologic, and social needs of women throughout their life spans.
- *Healthy People 2020* provides an update on goals for maternal and infant health.
- Nurses caring for women can play an active role in shaping health care systems to be responsive to the needs of contemporary women.
- A variety of factors, including race, age, violence, and human trafficking, affect women's health.
- Evidence-based practice and outcomes orientation are emphasized in current practice.
- Risk management and learning from sentinel events can improve quality of care.
- Research plays a vital role in establishing a scientific base for the care of women and infants.
- Ethical concerns have multiplied with the increasing use of technology and scientific advances.

REFERENCES

Agency for Healthcare Research and Quality. (2014). *20 tips to help prevent medical errors: Patient fact sheet*. December 2014, Rockville, MD. Retrieved from: http://archive.ahrq.gov/patients-consumers/care-planning/errors/20tips/index.html.

American Academy of Nurse Practitioners. (2015). *AANP voices support for senate bill empowering nurse practitioners in the veterans health administration*. Retrieved from: https://www.aanp.org/press-room/press-releases/166-press-room/2015-press-releases/1730-aanp-voices-support-for-senate-bill-empowering-nurse-practitioners-in-the-veterans-health-administration.

Arias, Heron, & Jiaquan. (2017). *United States Life Tables, 2014. National Vital Statistics Report*. Centers for Disease Control and Prevention. Retrieved from: https://www.cdc.gov/nchs/data/nvsr/nvsr66/nvsr66_04.pdf.

Association of Women's Health, Obstetric, and Neonatal Nurses (AWHONN). (2016). Human trafficking. *Journal of Obstetric, Gynecologic, and Neonatal Nursing*, 45, 458–460.

Association of Women's Health, Obstetric and Neonatal Nurses (AWHONN). (2013). *Women's health and perinatal nursing quality draft measures specifications*. Retrieved from: https://c.ymcdn.com/sites/www.awhonn.org/resource/resmgr/Downloadables/perinatalqualitymeasures.pdf.

Black Mamas Matter Alliance. (2018). Policy working group: Advancing holistic maternal care for black women through policy. Atlanta, GA.

Budiani-Saberi, D. A., Raja, K. R., Findley, K. C., Kerketta, P., & Anand, V. (2014). Human trafficking for organ removal in India: A victim-centered, evidence-based report. *Transplantation, 97*(4), 380–384.

Bulachek, B. M., Butcher, H. K., Dochterman, J. M., & Wagner, C. (2013). *Nursing interventions classification (NIC)* (6th ed.). St. Louis: Mosby.

Casella, E., Mills, J., & Usher, K. (2014). Social media and nursing practice: Changing the balance between the social and technical aspects of work. *Collegian, 21*(2), 121–126.

Centers for Disease Control and Prevention. (2017). *Leading causes of death in females, 2014.* Available at: https://www.cdc.gov/women/lcod/2014/race-ethnicity/index.htm.

Centers for Disease Control and Prevention. (2017). *Division of Reproductive Health, National Center for Chronic Disease Prevention and Health Promotion.* Pregnancy mortality surveillance system. Available at: https://www.cdc.gov/reproductivehealth/maternalinfanthealth/pmss.html.

Centers for Disease Control and Prevention. (2018a). *Health literacy.* Retrieved from: https://www.cdc.gov/healthliteracy/index.html.

Centers for Disease Control and Prevention. (2018b). National Center for Health Statistics. *National Vital Statistics Report, 67*(1).

Centers for Medicare and Medicaid. (2015). *NHE fact sheet.* Retrieved from: https://www.cms.gov/research-statistics-data-and-systems/statistics-trends-and-reports/nationalhealthexpenddata/nhe-fact-sheet.html.

Centers for Medicare & Medicaid Services (CMS). (2017). *National health expenditure projections 2017-2026: Forecast summary.* Available at: https://www.cms.gov/Research-Statistics-Data-and-Systems/Statistics-Trends-and-Reports/NationalHealthExpendData/Downloads/ForecastSummary.pdf.

Colby, S. L., & Ortman, J. (2015). *Projections of the size and composition of the US population: 2014-2016.* US Census Bureau. Retrieved from: https://www.census.gov/library/publications/2015/demo/p25-1143.html.

Dickens, C., & Piano, M. R. (2013). Health literacy and nursing: An update. *American Journal of Nursing, 113*(6), 52–57.

The Henry J. Kaiser Family Foundation. (2017). *Key facts about the uninsured population.* Available at: http://files.kff.org/attachment/Fact-Sheet-Key-Facts-about-the-Uninsured-Population.

Hayes, C., Jackson, D., Davidson, P. M., & Power, T. (2015). Medication errors in hospitals: A literature review of disruptions to nursing practice during medication administration. *Journal of Clinical Nursing, 24*(21–22), 3063–3076. (epub Aug 9, 2015).

Institute of Medicine. (2003). *Health professions education: A bridge to quality.* Washington, DC: National Academies Press.

Interprofessional Education Collaborative. (2019). What is professional education? Retrieved from: https//www.ipecollaborative.org/about-ipec.html.

The Joanna Briggs Institute. (2013). *JBI grading of recommendations.* Available at: http://joannabriggs.org/jbi-approach.html#tabbed-nav-Grades-of-Recommendation.

The Joint Commission. (2015). *Comprehensive accreditation manual for hospitals, Update 2. Sentinel events.* Retrieved from: http://www.jointcommission.org/assets/1/6/CAMH_24_SE_all_CURRENT.pdf.

Kaiser Permanente of Colorado. (2014). *SBAR technique for communication: A situational briefing model.* Available at: http://www.ihi.org/resources/Pages/Tools/SBARTechniqueforCommunicationASituationalBriefingModel.aspx.

Kochanek, K. D., Murphy, S. L., Xu, J., & Arias, E. (2017). *Mortality in the United States, 2016.* National Center for Health Statistics. Data Brief 293. Centers for Disease Control and Prevention. Retrieved from: https://www.cdc.gov/nchs/products/databriefs/db293.htm.

Kohn, L. T., Corrigan, J., & Donaldson, M. S. (2000). *To err is human: building a safer health system.* Washington, D.C.: National Academy Press.

Leapfrog Group. (2015). *Hospital errors are the third leading cause of death in the U.S., and new hospital safety scores show improvements are slow.* Washington, DC: Author. Retrieved from: http://www.hospitalsafetygrade.org/newsroom/display/hospitalerrors-thirdleading-causeofdeathinus-improvementstooslow.

MacDorman, M. F., Declercq, E., Cabral, H., & Morton, C. (2016). Recent increases in the U.S. maternal mortality rate: Disentangling trends from measurement issues. *Obstet Gynecol, 128,* 447–455. https://doi.org/10.1097/AOG.0000000000001556.

Makary, M. A., & Daniel, M. (2016). Medical error—The third leading cause of death in the United States. *British Medical Journal, 353,* i2139.

Martin, J. A., Hamilton, B. E, Osterman, M. J. K, et al. (2018). Births: Final data for 2017. *National Vital Statistics Reports, 67*(8). Hyattsville, MD: National Center for Health Statistics. Retrieved from: https://www.cdc.gov/nchs/data/nvsr/nvsr67/nvsr67_08-508.pdf.

Moorhead, S., Johnson, M., Maas, M., et al. (Eds.). (2013). *Nursing outcomes classification (NOC)* (5th ed.) St. Louis: Elsevier.

Morbidity and Mortality Weekly. (2013). *CDC health disparities and inequalities report.* Centers for Disease Control and Prevention. Atlanta, GA. Retrieved from: https://www.cdc.gov/mmwr/preview/ind2013_su.html#HealthDisparities2013.

National Council of State Boards of Nursing (NCSBN). (2011). *White paper: A nurse's guide to the use of social media.* Available at: www.ncsbn.org/Social_Media.pdf.

National League for Nursing. (2019). *Interprofessional education (IPE).* Washington, DC: National League for Nursing. Retrieved from: http://www.nln.org/professional-development-programs/teaching-resources/interprofessional-education-(ipe).

National Partnership for Action to End Health Disparities. (2016). *NPA background.* Rockville, MD: US Department of Health & Human Services, Office of Minority Health. Retrieved from: http://minorityhealth.hhs.gov/npa/templates/browse.aspx?1vl=1&1v1id=45.

National Quality Forum. (2011). Retrieved from: Serious reportable events in healthcare, 2011. https://www.qualityforum.org/Publications/2011/12/Serious_Reportable_Events_in_Healthcare_2011.aspx.

Oduyobo, T., Polen, K. D., Walke, H. T., et al. (2017). Update: Interim guidance for health care providers caring for pregnant women with possible Zika virus exposure – United States (including U.S. Territories). *Morbidity and Mortality Weekly Report, 66,* 781–793. https://doi.org/10.15585/mmwr.mm6629e1.

Office of Women's Health. (2015). *Female genital cutting.* Retrieved from: http://womenshealth.gov/publications/our-publications/fact-sheet/female-genital-cutting.html.

Ogden, C. L., Carroll, M. D., Fryar, C. D., & Flegal, K. M. (2015). Prevalence of obesity among adults and youth: United States, 2011–2014. *NCHS data brief.* (219). Hyattsville, MD: National Center for Health Statistics.

Quality and Safety Education for Nurses (QSEN). (2018). *QSEN Institute.* Retrieved from: http://qsen.org/.

Sandall, J., Soltani, H., Gates, S., Shennan, A., & Devane, D. (2016). Midwife-led continuity models versus other models of care for childbearing women. *Cochrane Database of Systematic Reviews, 2016*(4). Art. No.: CD004667. pub5. https://doi.org/10.1002/14651858.CD004667. Retrieved from: https://www.cochrane.org/CD004667/PREG_midwife-led-continuity-models-care-compared-other-models-care-women-during-pregnancy-birth-and-early.

Smith, J. C., & Medalia, C. (2015). *Health insurance coverage in the United States: 2014. Current Population Report.* US Census Bureau. 60–253. Washington, DC: US Government Printing Office Retrieved from: https://www.census.gov/content/dam/Census/library/publications/2015/demo/p60-253.pdf.

Thielking, M. (2015). *Sky-high C-section rates in the US don't translate to better birth outcomes. Stat.* Retrieved from: https://www.statnews.com/2015/12/01/cesarean-section-childbirth/.

UNICEF. (2017). *Children and AIDS: Statistical Update.* Available at: https://data.unicef.org/wp-content/uploads/2017/11/HIVAIDS-Statistical-Update-2017.pdf.

United Nations Inter-agency Group for Child Mortality Estimation (UN IGME). (2017). *Levels & trends in child mortality: report 2017, estimates developed by the UN inter-agency group for child mortality estimation.* New York: United Nations Children's Fund.

United Nations Development Programme. (2016). *Sustainable development goals.* Retrieved from: http://www.un.org/sustainabledevelopment/sustainable-development-goals/.

United Nations Office on Drugs and Crime. (2016). *Human trafficking.* Retrieved from: https://www.unodc.org/unodc/en/human-trafficking/what-is-human-trafficking.html.

U.S. Department of Health and Human Services. (2015). *HHS action plan to reduce racial and ethnic health disparities implementation progress report.* Washington, DC: Office of the Secretary, Office of the Assistant Secretary for Planning and Evaluation, and Office of Minority Health. Available at: https://minorityhealth.hhs.gov/assets/pdf/FINAL_HHS_Action_Plan_Progress_Report_11_2_2015.pdf.

U.S. Department of Health and Human Services. (2015). *National action plan to improve health literacy.* Washington, DC: Office of Disease Prevention and Health Promotion. Retrieved from: http://minorityhealth.hhs.gov/omh/browse.aspx?lvl=2&lvlid=10.

World Health Organization. (2018a). *Maternal and reproductive health.* Available at: http://www.who.int/gho/maternal_health/en/.

World Health Organization. (2018b). *Trends in maternal mortality.* Available at: http://www.who.int/gho/maternal_health/countries/usa.pdf?ua=1.

World Health Organization. (2019). *Executive board designated 2020 as The Year of the Nurse and Midwife.* Geneva, Switzerland: World Health Organization. Retrieved from: https://www.who.int/hrh/news/2019/2020year-of-nurses/en/.

The Family and Culture

Raquel Martinez-Campos

LEARNING OBJECTIVES

- Describe the main characteristics of contemporary family forms.
- Identify key factors influencing family health.
- Relate the impact of culture on childbearing families.
- Analyze cultural competence in relation to one's own nursing practice.
- Examine indicators of community health status and their relevance to perinatal health.

- Identify predisposing factors and characteristics of vulnerable populations.
- Compare the potential advantages and disadvantages of home visits.
- Explore telephonic nursing care options in perinatal nursing.
- Describe how home care fits into the maternity continuum of care.
- Describe the nurse's role in perinatal home care.

INTRODUCTION TO FAMILY, CULTURE, AND HOME CARE

The composition, structure, and function of the American family have changed dramatically in recent years, largely in response to economic, demographic, sociocultural, and technologic trends that influence family life and health. Despite current efforts to improve the overall health of the nation, there is widespread concern about family health and well-being as a reflection of individual, community, and national health status. Recent economic changes have further reduced the ability to access health care. In addition to facing significant barriers in accessing needed services, women and families are faced with the challenge of overcoming discrimination in health care practices. It is critical to consider racial and ethnic differences and sexual orientation when addressing the health status of women. American women with a minority racial or ethnic affiliation share poorer outcomes in a wide variety of conditions. Lesbian women may conceal sexual orientation for fear of discrimination. As cultural diversity increases and demographics change, nurses must become culturally competent to recognize and reduce or eliminate health disparities (Trinh, Agenor, Austin, & Jackson, 2017).

As perinatal health trends emerge, nurses are assuming greater roles in assessing family health status and providing care across the perinatal continuum. This continuum begins with family planning and continues with the following categories of care: preconception, prenatal, intrapartum, postpartum, newborn, interconception (between pregnancies), and the postpartum period and the first 6 weeks of the infant's life. In the community, health care ranges from individual care to group and community services, and from primary prevention to tertiary care experiences and home health. Depending on the needs of the individual family unit, independent self-management, outpatient care, home care, low-risk hospitalization, or specialized intensive care may be appropriate at different points along this continuum.

In community-based health care, both the population (group of people who may or may not interact with each other) and the aggregate (group of people within the larger population who possess some common characteristics) become the focus of intervention. Health professionals are required not only to determine health priorities, but also develop successful plans of care to be delivered in the health clinic, the community health center, or the client's home (see Community Activity). This home- and community-based delivery system presents unique challenges for perinatal and maternity nurses.

COMMUNITY ACTIVITY

- Visit the Health Resources & Services Administration (HRSA) website at https://www.hrsa.gov. What is the definition of a health center according to the HRSA? What populations do they serve? What are the different types of health centers?
- Locate a health center in your community at the HRSA website. What types of services do they provide? Do they provide primary and preventive maternal and women's health services? Is care provided regardless of a client's ability to pay?
- Visit your state center for health statistics (SCHS) website. Evaluate the health status of women and infants in your county. Vital statistics include live births, physician versus midwife attended births, out-of-wedlock births, cesarean births, low birth weight, maternal smoking, and fetal/infant mortality.

THE FAMILY IN CULTURAL AND COMMUNITY CONTEXT

The family and its cultural context play an important role in defining the work of maternity nurses. Despite modern stresses and strains, the family forms a social network that acts as a potent support system for its members. Family health-seeking behavior and relationships with providers are greatly influenced by culturally related health beliefs and values. Ultimately all these factors have the power to affect maternal and child health outcomes. The current emphasis in working with families is on wellness and empowerment for families to achieve control over their lives. Incorporating cultural competence enables professionals to

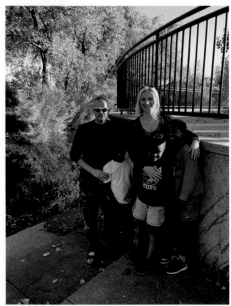

Fig. 2.1 Nuclear Family. (Courtesy Mark and Stephanie Stauder, Loveland CO.)

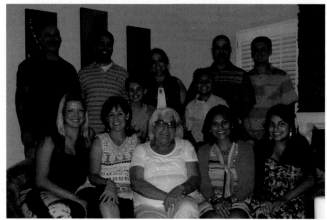

Fig. 2.2 Extended Family. (Courtesy Raquel Martinez-Campos, Lake Forest, CA.)

adapt their approaches to benefit individuals and groups from varying cultural backgrounds (Centers for Disease Control and Prevention, 2014). It is essential that nurses become culturally competent in order to provide appropriate care. To learn more, nurses can access *Culturally Competent Nursing Care: A Cornerstone of Caring*. This free, accredited, online educational program is provided by the Office of Minority Health (www.thinkculturalhealth.hhs.gov).

Defining Family

The family has traditionally been viewed as the primary unit of socialization—the basic structural unit within a community. Being the oldest and most persistent of all social institutions, the family plays a pivotal role in health care, representing the primary target of health care delivery for maternal and newborn nurses. As one of society's most important institutions, the family represents a primary social group that influences and is influenced by other people and institutions. A variety of family configurations exist. Each of these is characterized by certain structural features.

Family Organization and Structure

The nuclear family has long represented the traditional American family in which husband, wife, and their children (either biologic or adopted) live as an independent unit, sharing roles, responsibilities, and economic resources (Fig. 2.1). Today the number of families living in a nuclear family structure is steadily decreasing in response to societal changes. By race and ethnic origin, this family structure is represented as follows (U.S. Census Bureau, 2017a):

- Caucasian: 51.1% married couple (22.6% with children)
- Hispanic: 48.8% married couple (31.6% with children)
- African American: 28.4% married couple (14.1% with children)
- Asian: 59.7% married couple (36.3% with children)
- American Indian and Alaska Native: 40.1%: married couple (no data for percent children)
- Native Hawaiian and Pacific Islander: 51.3%: married couple (no data for percent children)

The majority, 69%, of America's 73.7 million children live with two parents. Of those, 47.7 million live with two married parents and 3.0 million live with two unmarried parents (U.S. Census Bureau, 2016a). Although nuclear families remain a prevalent family form, recent research

suggests that families and households in the United States are often more complex (Monte, 2017). Many nuclear families have other relatives living in the same household. These extended family members include grandparents, aunts, uncles, or other people related by blood. Members of extended families can also live in close proximity to the nuclear family (Fig. 2.2). Due to societal changes, internet access, and increased mobility, these families may also be a long-distance unit. The extended family is becoming more common as American society ages. The extended family provides social, emotional, and financial support to one another. It is therefore important for nurses to recognize the desire for people of many cultures to include their family in making important decisions even if extended family members are not physically close. This has implications for privacy and sharing individual health information under Health Insurance Portability and Accountability Act (HIPAA) rules.

Multigenerational families, consisting of three or more generations of relatives (grandparents, children, and grandchildren), are becoming increasingly common. In 2015, they made up 5.9% of all households (U.S. Census Bureau, 2015a). This type of arrangement can create stress for some as adult children must care for their parents as well as their own children. Other types of multigenerational families consist of grandparents supporting the children and grandchildren, or as sole caregivers for the grandchildren. Nonbiologic-parent families are those in which children live independently in foster or kinship care such as living with a grandparent. An estimated 7 million children in the United States live with a grandparent. Of the 4.2 million grandparents that live with a grandchild, more than 60% of those households are maintained by the grandparent (Ellis & Simmons, 2014). This category may also include adoptive children, although they are often categorized within the nuclear family.

Married-blended families, those formed as a result of divorce and remarriage, consist of unrelated family members (stepparents, stepchildren, and stepsiblings) who join to create a new household. These family groups frequently involve a biologic or adoptive parent whose spouse may or may not have adopted the child.

Cohabiting-parent families are those in which children live with two unmarried biologic parents or two adoptive parents. Hispanic children are more than twice as likely as African American children to live in cohabiting-parent families and about four times as likely as Caucasian children to live in this kind of family arrangement (U.S. Census Bureau, 2017b).

Single-parent families comprise an unmarried biologic or adoptive parent who may or may not be living with other adults. The single-parent family may result from the loss of a spouse by death, divorce, separation, or desertion; from either an unplanned or planned pregnancy; or from the adoption of a child by an unmarried woman or man. This family structure is continually on the rise. In 2016, 17.2 million (23%) children lived with their mother only,

3 million (4%) lived with only their fathers, and 2.8 million (3.7%) lived with neither of their parents (U.S. Census Bureau, 2016a). The single-parent family tends to be more vulnerable economically and socially, which can create an unstable and deprived environment for the children. This in turn affects health status, school achievement, and high-risk behaviors for these children (Laughlin, 2014). Some families become more stable with the absence of drugs, alcohol, and/or physical/emotional abuse.

Alternative families (lesbian, gay, bisexual, transgender, queer [LGBTQ]) may live together with or without children. Usually formed by same-sex couples, they can also consist of single LGBTQ parents or multiple parenting figures. Children in LGBTQ families may be the offspring of previous heterosexual unions, conceived by one member of a lesbian couple through natural or therapeutic insemination, conceived by a gay couple using a surrogate, or adopted. Approximately 858,000 same-sex couple households lived in the United States in 2015, with 17.2% of these households raising children under 18 years of age. When these children are combined with LGBTQ parents who are raising children, it is estimated that almost 2 million children are being raised by LGBTQ parents in the United States (U.S. Census, 2015b). These families could also be considered nuclear families as they often consist of two parents (either married or unmarried) with either biologic or adoptive children.

The Family in Society

The social context for the family can be viewed in relation to social and demographic trends that define the population as a whole. Racial and ethnic diversity of the population has grown dramatically, necessitating consideration of such diversity in provision of health care. According to the 2010 census, approximately 36% of the population belongs to a racial or ethnic minority group (Centers for Disease Control and Prevention [CDC], 2016).

Family Nursing

Family plays a pivotal role in health care, representing the primary target of health care delivery for maternal and newborn nurses, and primary care nurses who care for both women and men. It is crucial that nurses assist families as they incorporate new additions to their family (see Nursing Care Plan). When treating the woman and family with respect and dignity, health care providers listen to and honor perspectives and choices of the woman and family. They share information with families in ways that are positive, useful, timely, complete, and accurate. The family is supported in participating in the care and decision making at the level of their choice.

Families are viewed as part of the interprofessional health care team and as the unit of care. Because so many variables affect ways of relating, the nurse must be aware that family members may interact and communicate with each other in ways that are distinct from those of the nurse's own family of origin. Most families will hold some beliefs about health that are different from those of the nurse. Their beliefs can conflict with principles of health care management predominant in the Western health care system.

Family nursing interventions occur within nurse-family relationships through therapeutic conversation (Arnold & Boggs, 2016). This necessitates interacting with family members present during caregiving, asking about those who may be absent, and actively listening to words and noting expressions to facilitate understanding. To do this within time constraints, Wright and Leahey (1999, 2013) developed a format for a brief therapeutic interview (Table 2.1).

◎ NURSING CARE PLAN

Incorporating the Infant Into the Family

Client Problem	Expected Outcome	Nursing Interventions	Rationales
Potential decreased ability to cope due to adaptation of family to new infant.	Family members will verbalize that individual and family goals are met during a smooth transition of new family member into the home.	Assess type and amount of support available to family on daily basis during postpartum period.	To facilitate adaptation of family to situation of a new member.
		Encourage family to use past successful coping mechanisms.	To enhance ability to cope with new situation and promote self-esteem.
		Teach family about sensory needs and capabilities of infant.	To motivate family to meet infant's needs and set realistic expectations for infant's capabilities.
Need for health teaching related to addition of new family member.	Each family member will verbalize realistic expectations regarding his or her role in the family and formulate a plan to incorporate the role into overall family goals.	Assess family structure, roles, and each member's perception of his or her role in family.	To evaluate impact of new member on structure and roles of family as perceived by members.
		Evaluate individual's perception of goals and new roles during this transition.	To promote early intervention and correct any misinterpretation.
		Encourage discussion of family members' thoughts and feelings regarding this transition.	To promote open communication and trust.

When selecting a family assessment framework, an appropriate model for a perinatal nurse is one that is a health-promoting rather than an illness-care model. The low-risk family can be assisted in promoting a healthy pregnancy, childbirth, and integration of the newborn into the family. The high-risk perinatal family has illness-care needs, and the nurse can help to meet those needs while also promoting the health of the childbearing family.

A family assessment tool such as the Calgary Family Assessment Model (CFAM) (Box 2.1) can be used as a guide for assessing aspects of the family. Such an assessment is not a measurable, objective finding, but is based on the experiences of the nurse as he or she interviews and relates to the family members being interviewed.

The CFAM comprises three major categories: structural, developmental, and functional. Several subcategories are within each

TABLE 2.1 Key Ingredients of a 15-Minute (or Shorter) Family Interview

Ingredient	Exemplars
Manners	Introduce yourself to women and families, preferably by your full name (i.e., Ms., Mrs., Mr. Jones).
	Make eye contact with all members of the family.
	Inquire about relationship of persons with the women.
	Always call women by name.
Therapeutic Conversations	Interview is purposeful and time-limited.
	Provide opportunity for women and family to be acknowledged.
	Involve women in information giving and decision making.
	Routinely invite families to accompany the women to the unit/clinic.
	Invite families to ask questions during women orientation.
	Routinely consult families and women about their ideas for treatment and discharge.
Family Genograms and Ecomaps	Draw a quick genogram (and if indicated, an ecomap) for all families (see Figs. 2.4 and 2.5).
	Acknowledge that illness is a family affair.
	Include essential information such as ages, occupation, school grade, religion, ethnic background, and current health status of all family members.
Therapeutic Questions	Think of at least three questions to routinely ask all families.
	Basic themes include sharing of information; expectations of hospitalization, clinic, or home care visit; challenges; sufferings; and most pressing concerns/problems.
Commending Family and Individual Strengths	Offer at least two commendations to family on strengths, resources, or competencies that were observed or reported to the nurse. These are observations of behavior patterns rather than one-time occurrences.
	Evaluate usefulness of the interview and conclude.

From Wright, L. M., & Leahey, M. (1999). Maximizing time, minimizing suffering: The 15-minute (or less) family interview. *Journal of Family Nursing, 5*(3), 259–273.

BOX 2.1 Calgary Family Assessment Model

There are three major categories of the Calgary Family Assessment Model (CFAM): structural, developmental, and functional. Each category has several subcategories. In this box, only the major categories are listed. A few sample questions are included.

Structural Assessment

Determine the members of the family, relationship among family members, and context of family.
Genograms and ecomaps (see Figs. 2.4 and 2.5) are useful in outlining the internal and external structures of a family.

Sample Questions

- Who are the members of your family?
- Has anyone moved in or out lately?
- Are there any family members who don't live with you?

Developmental Assessment

Describe the life cycle—that is, the typical trajectory that most families experience.

Sample Questions

- Is your family the size you wanted?
- When you think back, what do you most enjoy about your life?
- What do you regret about your life?
- Have you made plans for your care as your health declines?

Functional Assessment

Evaluate the way in which individuals behave in relation to each other in instrumental and expressive aspects. (Instrumental aspects are activities of daily living; expressive aspects include communication, problem solving roles, etc.)

Sample Questions

- Which one of the family is responsible for helping with the children while the mother is caring for the newborn?
- Whose turn is it to do the shopping and fix dinner for the family?
- How can we get more family involvement in care of the household?

Data from Wright, L. M., & Leahey, M. (2013). *Nurses and families: A guide to family assessment and intervention* (6th ed.). Philadelphia: F.A. Davis.

category. The three assessment categories and the many subcategories can be conceptualized as a branching diagram (Fig. 2.3). The categories and subcategories can be used to guide the assessment that will provide data to help the nurse better understand the family and formulate a nursing care plan. The nurse asks questions of family members about themselves to gain understanding of the structure, development, and function of the family at this point in time. Not all questions within the subcategories should be asked at the first interview, and some questions may not be appropriate for all families. Although individuals are the ones interviewed, the focus of the assessment is on interaction of individuals within the family.

Graphic Representations of Families

A family genogram (family tree format depicting relationships of family members over at least three generations) (Fig. 2.4) provides valuable information about a family and can be placed in the nursing care plan for easy access by care providers. An ecomap, a graphic portrayal of social relationships of the women and family, may also help the nurse understand the social environment of the family and identify support systems available to them (Fig. 2.5). Software is available to generate genograms and ecomaps (www.interpersonaluniverse.net).

THE FAMILY IN A CULTURAL CONTEXT

Cultural Factors Related to Family Health

The culture of an individual and a group is influenced by religion, environment, and historic events and plays a powerful role in the individual's and group's behavior and patterns of human interaction. Culture is dynamic, influencing a woman throughout her entire life, from birth to death. Culture is an essential element of what defines us as people.

Cultural knowledge includes beliefs and values about each facet of life and is passed from one generation to the next. Cultural beliefs and traditions relate to food, language, religion, art, health and healing practices, kinship relationships, and all other aspects of community,

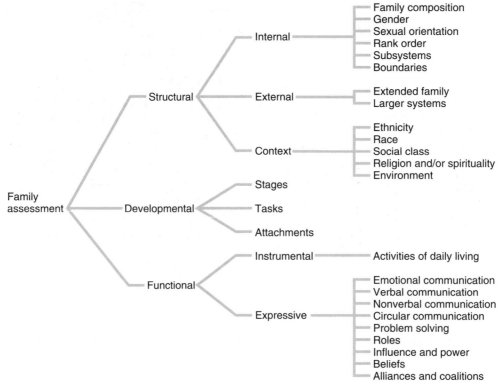

Fig. 2.3 Branching diagram of Calgary Family Assessment Model. (From Wright, L. M., & Leahey, M. [2013]. *Nurses and families: A guide to family assessment and intervention* [6th ed.]. Philadelphia: F. A. Davis.)

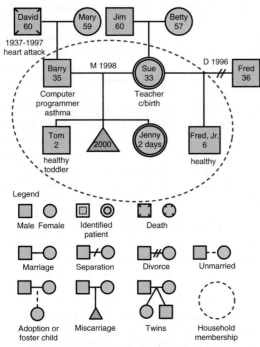

Fig. 2.4 Example of a Family Genogram.

family, and individual life. Culture has also been shown to have a direct effect on health behaviors. Values, attitudes, and beliefs that are culturally acquired may influence perceptions of illness, as well as health care–seeking behavior and response to treatment. The political, social, and economic context of people's lives is also part of the cultural experience.

Culture, the shared beliefs and values of a group, plays a powerful role in an individual's behavior, particularly when the individual is faced with health care issues. Understanding a culture can provide insight into how a person reacts to illness, pain, and invasive medical procedures, as well as patterns of human interaction and expressions of emotion. The effect of these influences must be assessed by health care professionals in providing health care and developing effective intervention strategies.

Many subcultures may be found within each culture. **Subculture** refers to a group existing within a larger cultural system that retains its own characteristics. A subculture may be an ethnic group, or a group organized in other ways. For example, in the United States and Canada, many ethnic subcultures such as African Americans, Asian Americans, Hispanic Americans, and Native Americans exist. It is important to note that subcultures also exist within these groups. In addition, the Caucasian population in America has multiple subcultures of its own. Because every identified cultural group has subcultures and because it is impossible to study every subculture in depth, greater differences may exist among and between groups than is generally acknowledged. It is important to be familiar with common cultural practices within these subgroups. However, it is also important to avoid the generalization that every person practices every cultural belief within a group because this could lead to stereotyping and misunderstanding of the nuances of various cultural groups.

Acculturation refers to the changes that occur within one group or among several groups when people from different cultures come into contact with one another. People may retain some of their own culture while adopting cultural practices of the dominant society. This familiarization among cultural groups results in overt behavioral similarity, especially in mannerisms, styles, and practices. Dress, language patterns, food choices, and health practices are often much slower to adapt to the influence of acculturation.

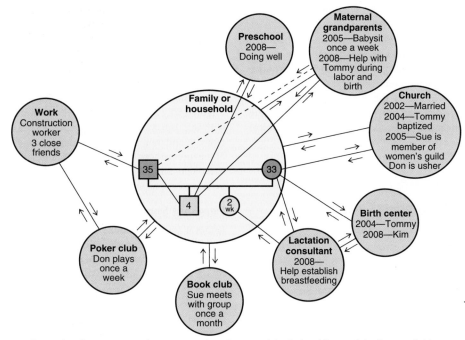

Fig. 2.5 Example of an ecomap. An ecomap describes social relationships and depicts available supports.

During times of family transitions such as childbearing, or during crisis or illness, a woman may rely on old cultural patterns even after becoming acculturated in many ways. This is consistent with the family developmental theory that states that during times of stress, people revert to practices and behaviors that are most comfortable and familiar (McGoldrick, Garcia-Prieto & Carter, 2016).

Assimilation occurs when a cultural group loses its cultural identity and becomes part of the dominant culture. Assimilation is the process by which groups "melt" into the mainstream, thus accounting for the notion of a "melting pot," a phenomenon that has been said to occur in the United States. This is illustrated by individuals who identify themselves as being of Irish or German descent, without having any remaining cultural practices or values linked specifically to that culture such as food preparation techniques, style of dress, or proficiency in the language associated with their reported cultural heritage. Spector (2017) asserts that in the United States, the melting pot, with its dream of a common culture, is a myth. Instead, a mosaic phenomenon exists in which we must accept and appreciate the differences among people.

Implications for Nursing

As our society becomes more culturally diverse, it is essential that nurses become culturally competent. Nurses must examine their own beliefs so that they have a better appreciation and understanding of their clients' beliefs. To promote culturally congruent practice, a new standard has been added to *Nursing: Scope and Standards of Practice*, 3rd Edition (American Nurses Association, 2015). Standard 8 directs nurses to practice "in a manner that is congruent with cultural diversity and inclusion principles" (Cipriano, 2016, p. 15). Understanding the concepts of ethnocentrism and cultural relativism can help nurses care for families in a multicultural society.

Ethnocentrism is the view that one's own way is best (Giger, 2016). Although the United States is a culturally diverse nation, the prevailing practice of health care is based on the beliefs and practices held by members of the dominant culture, primarily Caucasians of European descent. This practice is based on the biomedical model that focuses on curing disease states.

Pregnancy and childbirth, in this biomedical perspective, are viewed as processes with inherent risks that are most appropriately managed by using scientific knowledge and advanced technology. The medical perspective stands in direct contrast with the belief systems of many cultures. Among many women, birth is viewed as a completely normal process that can be managed with a minimum of involvement from health care practitioners. When encountering behavior in women unfamiliar with the biomedical model or those who reject it, the nurse may become frustrated and impatient and may label the women's behavior as inappropriate and believe that it conflicts with "good" health practices. If the Western health care system provides the nurse's only standard for judgment, the behavior of the nurse is ethnocentric.

Cultural relativism is the opposite of ethnocentrism. It refers to learning about and applying the standards of another's culture to activities within that culture. The nurse recognizes that people from different cultural backgrounds comprehend the same objects and situations differently. In other words, culture determines viewpoint. Cultural relativism does not require nurses to accept the beliefs and values of another culture. Instead, nurses recognize that the behavior of others can be based on a system of logic different from their own. Cultural relativism affirms the uniqueness and value of every culture.

Childbearing Beliefs and Practices

Nurses working with childbearing families care for families from many different cultures and ethnic groups. To provide culturally competent care the nurse must assess clients' beliefs and practices. When working with childbearing families, a nurse considers all aspects of culture, including communication, space, time orientation, and family roles.

Communication often creates the most challenging obstacle for nurses working with clients from diverse cultural groups. Communication is not merely the exchange of words. Instead, it involves (1) understanding the individual's language, including subtle variations in meaning and distinctive dialects; (2) appreciating individual differences in interpersonal style; and (3) accurately interpreting the volume of speech as well as the meanings of touch and gestures. For example, members of some cultural groups tend to speak loudly when they are excited, with great emotion and with vigorous and animated gestures; this is true whether their excitement is related to positive or negative events or emotions. It is important, therefore, for the nurse to avoid rushing to judgment regarding a person's intent when the client is speaking, especially in a language not understood by the nurse. Instead, the nurse should withhold an interpretation of what has been expressed until it is possible to clarify the client's intent. The nurse needs to enlist the assistance of a person who can help verify with the client the true intent and meaning of the communication (see Clinical Reasoning Case Study).

? CLINICAL REASONING CASE STUDY
Providing Culturally Appropriate Care

Isabel, a 22 year-old first-generation Mexican American, comes into your office for her initial prenatal visit. You are concerned because Isabel's fundal height is consistent with 32 weeks of gestation and this is her first prenatal visit. Isabel, who lives with her husband, four children (ages 6, 4, and 3 years, and 15 months), her mother, her aunt, and her uncle, states that she has been doing well this pregnancy and did not start prenatal care in her previous pregnancies until she was almost ready to give birth. She also comments that all the babies were full term with uneventful labors and births. In obtaining the history, you note the presence of a safety pin in Isabel's shirt and wonder what this is for. You want to provide culturally competent care to this woman and her family.

1. What is the priority concern or client need in this situation?
2. List other client needs/problems in this case.
3. Identify any additional information needed by the nurse in addressing this situation.
4. Describe the roles/responsibilities of interprofessional health team members who may be involved in this situation.

Inconsistencies between the language of clients and the language of providers present a significant barrier to effective health care. For example, there are many dialects of Spanish that vary by geographic location. Because of the diversity of cultures and languages within the U.S. and Canadian populations, health care agencies are increasingly seeking the services of *interpreters* (of oral communication from one language to another) or *translators* (of written words from one language to another) to bridge these gaps and fulfill their obligation for culturally and linguistically appropriate health care (Box 2.2). Finding the best possible interpreter in the circumstance is critically important as well. Ideally, interpreters should have the same native language and be of the same religion or have the same country of origin as the client. Interpreters should have specific health-related language skills and experience and help bridge the language and cultural barriers between the client and the health care provider. The person interpreting also should be mature enough to be trusted with private information. However, because the nature of nursing care is not always predictable and because nursing care that is provided in a home or community setting does not always allow for expert, experienced, or mature adult interpreters, ideal interpretative services sometimes are impossible to find when they are needed. In crisis or emergency situations, or when family members are extremely stressed or emotionally upset, it may be necessary to use relatives, neighbors, or children as interpreters. If this situation occurs, the nurse must ensure that the client is in agreement and comfortable with using the available interpreter to assist. Having a man or a child interpret for a woman may create embarrassment and interfere with obtaining an accurate history or detail of symptoms.

When using an interpreter, the nurse respects the family by creating an atmosphere of respect and privacy. Questions should be addressed to the woman and not to the interpreter. Even though an interpreter will of necessity be exposed to sensitive and privileged information about the family, the nurse should take care to ensure that confidentiality is maintained. A quiet location free from interruptions is ideal for interpretive services to take place. Culturally and linguistically appropriate educational materials that are easy to read, with appropriate text and graphics, should be available to assist the woman and her family in understanding health care information. To ensure understanding and avoid liability issues, it is important to make certain that the material has been translated by someone who is trained appropriately.

Personal Space

Cultural traditions define the appropriate personal space for various social interactions. Although the need for personal space varies from person to person and with the situation, the actual physical dimensions of comfort zones and taboos differ from culture to culture. Actions such as touching, placing the woman in proximity to others, taking away personal possessions, and making decisions for the woman can decrease personal security and heighten anxiety. Conversely, respecting the need for distance allows the woman to maintain control over personal space and support personal autonomy, thereby increasing her sense of security. Nurses must touch clients. However, they frequently do so without any awareness of the emotional distress they may be causing.

Time Orientation

Time orientation is a fundamental way in which culture affects health behaviors. People in cultural groups may be relatively more oriented to past, present, or future. Those who focus on the past strive to maintain tradition or the status quo and have little motivation for formulating goals. In contrast, individuals who focus primarily on the present neither plan for the future nor consider the experiences of the past. These individuals do not necessarily adhere to strict schedules and are often described as "living for the moment" or "marching to their own drummer." Individuals oriented to the future maintain a focus on achieving long-term goals.

The time orientation of the childbearing family can affect nursing care. For example, talking to a family about bringing the infant to the clinic for follow-up examinations (events in the future) may be difficult for the family that is focused on the present concerns of day-to-day survival. Because a family with a future-oriented sense of time plans far in advance, thinking about the long-term consequences of present actions, they may be more likely to return as scheduled for follow-up visits. Despite the differences in time orientation, each family can be equally concerned for the well-being of its newborn.

Family Roles

Family roles involve the expectations and behaviors associated with a member's position in the larger family system (e.g., mother, father, grandparent). Social class and cultural norms also affect these roles, with distinct expectations for men and women clearly determined by social norms. For example, culture may influence whether a man actively participates in the pregnancy and childbirth, yet maternity care practitioners working in the Western health care system expect fathers to be involved. This can create a significant conflict between the nurse and the role expectations of very traditional Mexican or Arab families, who usually view the birthing experience as a female affair (see Cultural Considerations). The way that health care practitioners manage such a family's care molds its experience and perception of the Western health care system.

BOX 2.2   Working With an Interpreter

Step 1: Before the interview
  A. Outline your statements and questions. List the key pieces of information you want/need to know.
  B. Learn something about the culture so that you can converse informally with the interpreter.

Step 2: Meeting with the interpreter
  A. Introduce yourself to the interpreter and converse informally. This is the time to find out how well he or she speaks English. Be respectful of the interpreter, regardless of proficiency or age. Some ways to show respect are to ask a cultural question to acknowledge that you can learn from the interpreter, or you could learn one word or phrase from the interpreter.
  B. Emphasize that you do want the client to ask questions, because some cultures consider this inappropriate behavior.
  C. Make sure the interpreter is comfortable with the technical terms you need to use. If not, take some time to explain them.

Step 3: During the interview
  A. Ask your questions and explain your statements (see Step 1).
  B. Make sure that the interpreter understands which parts of the interview are most important. You usually have limited time with the interpreter, and you want to have adequate time at the end for client questions.
  C. Try to get a feel for how much is "getting through." No matter what the language is, if in relating information to the client the interpreter uses far fewer or far more words than you do, something else is going on.
  D. Stop every now and then and ask the interpreter, "How is it going?" You may not get a totally accurate answer, but you will have emphasized to the interpreter your strong

desire to focus on the task at hand. If there are language problems, (1) speak slowly; (2) use gestures (e.g., fingers to count or point to body parts); and (3) use pictures.
  E. Ask the interpreter to elicit questions. This may be difficult, but it is worth the effort.
  D. Identify cultural issues that may conflict with your requests or instructions.
  F. Use the interpreter to help problem solve or at least give insight into possibilities for solutions.

Step 4: After the interview
  A. Speak to the interpreter and try to get an idea of what went well and what could be improved. This will help you to be more effective in the future with this or another interpreter.
  B. Make notes on what you learned for your future reference or to help a colleague.

Remember
Your interview is a *collaboration* between you and the interpreter. *Listen* as well as speak.

Notes:
1. The interpreter may be a child, grandchild, or sibling of the client. Be sensitive to the fact that the child is playing an adult role.
2. Be sensitive to cultural and situational differences (e.g., an interview with someone from urban Germany will likely be different from an interview with someone from a transitional refugee camp).
3. Younger females telling older males what to do may be a problem for both a female nurse and a female interpreter. This is not the time to pioneer new gender relations. Be aware that in some cultures it is difficult for a woman to talk about some topics with a husband or a father present.

Courtesy Elizabeth Whalley, PhD, San Francisco State University.

🌐 CULTURAL CONSIDERATIONS

Questions to Ask to Elicit Cultural Expectations About Childbearing

1. What do you and your family think you should do to remain healthy during pregnancy?
2. What can you do to improve your health and the health of your baby?
3. What foods will help make a healthy baby?
4. Who do you want with you during your labor?
5. What can your labor support person do to help you be most comfortable during labor?
6. What actions are important for you and your family after the baby's birth?
7. What do you and your family expect from the nurse(s) caring for you?
8. How will family members participate in your pregnancy, childbirth, and parenting?

In maternity nursing and women's health care, the nurse supports and nurtures the beliefs that promote physical or emotional adaptation to childbearing. However, if certain beliefs might be harmful, the nurse should carefully explore them with the woman and use them in the reeducation and modification process. Strategies for care delivery and providing appropriate care are presented in Box 2.3.

The nurse should take care to avoid making stereotypic assumptions about any person based on sociocultural or spiritual affiliations. Nurses should exercise sensitivity in working with every family, being careful to assess the ways in which they apply their own mixture of cultural traditions.

BOX 2.3   Strategies for Care Delivery and Providing Culturally Appropriate Care

Strategies for Care Delivery
- Break down the language barriers.
- Explain your rationale and reasons for suggestions.
- Integrate folk and Western treatments.
- Enlist the family caretaker and others.
- Get consent from the right person.
- Provide language-appropriate materials.

Providing Culturally Appropriate Care
- Ask about traditional beliefs, such as the role of hot and cold.
- Be sensitive regarding interpreters and language barriers.
- Ask about important dietary practices, particularly those related to events such as childbirth.
- Ask about group practices and beliefs.
- Ask about the woman's fears, and those of her family, regarding an unfamiliar care setting.

From Mattson, S. (2000). Providing culturally competent care: Strategies and approaches for perinatal clients. *AWHONN Lifelines, 4*(5), 37–39.

DEVELOPING CULTURAL COMPETENCE

Cultural competence has many names and definitions, all of which have subtle shades of difference, but which are essentially the same: multiculturalism, cultural sensitivity, and intercultural effectiveness.

Cultural competence involves acknowledging, respecting, and appreciating ethnic, cultural, and linguistic diversity. Culturally and linguistically appropriate services are respectful of and responsive to the health beliefs, practices, and needs of diverse clients (Office of Minority Health, 2017). Culturally competent professionals act in ways that meet the needs of the client and are respectful of ways and traditions that may be very different from their own. In today's society, it is critically important that nurses develop more than technical skill. At every level of preparation and throughout their professional lives, nurses must engage in a continual process of developing and refining attitudes and behaviors that will promote culturally competent care (Giger, 2016).

Key components of culturally competent care include:

- Recognizing that disparity exists between one's own culture and that of the client
- Educating and promoting healthy behaviors in a cultural context that has meaning for clients
- Taking abstract knowledge about other cultures and applying it in a practical way, so that the quality of service improves and policies are enacted that meet the needs of all clients
- Communicating respect for a wide range of differences, including client use of nontraditional healing practices and alternative therapies
- Recognizing the importance of culturally different communication styles, problem-solving techniques, concepts of space and time, and desires to be involved with care decisions
- Anticipating the need to address varying degrees of language ability and literacy, as well as barriers to care and compliance with treatment

In addition to issues of preserving and promoting human dignity, the development of cultural competence is of equal importance in terms of health outcomes. Nurses who relate effectively with clients are able to motivate them in the direction of health-promoting behaviors. Provider competence to address language barriers facilitates appropriate tailoring of health messages and preventive health teaching. Cross-cultural experiences also present an opportunity for the health care professional to expand cultural sensitivity, awareness, and skills.

Promoting Family Health

Functioning within the social, cultural, environmental, and economic context of the community, the family becomes an integral component of health-promotion efforts. For childbearing families, health promotion is focused primarily on early intervention through prenatal care and prevention of complications during the perinatal period. Often this early exposure to health information sets the stage for a successful birth and positive outcomes for mother, father, and baby. The nurse's role in this process is focused on collaboration with the family, identifying risk factors, and providing health information to facilitate positive health behaviors. Involving expectant mothers and fathers in identification of their learning needs is an essential first step to securing their participation in the health-promotion process.

A wide variety of strategies have been used to engage families and groups in health-promoting activities or community health programs. Some are more successful than others. Generally, participant engagement in the planning process and empowerment to create internal solutions are considered key factors in effective interventions. Many communities have organized coalitions to address specific health-promotion agendas related to sharing information, educating community members, or advocating for health policies around maternal and child health issues. The benefits of partnership with faith-based organizations for community health improvement have been demonstrated in health-promotion efforts aimed at lifestyle choices, health education, and maternal-child health outcomes.

Prepared childbirth classes are a well-established mechanism for increasing awareness of healthy behaviors during pregnancy and preparing parents for the care of themselves and their newborn during the postpartum period; these can occur through community hospitals and online courses. Mass media efforts such as those presented by the Public Education Campaign "Safe to Sleep," and AWHONN's "Go the Full 40" are advertisements with clear consumer-friendly messages designed to reach a large target audience. Other venues include public health education in newspapers and magazines, and health department programs such as the Special Supplemental Nutrition Program for Women, Infants, and Children (WIC), which offers a variety of health education and written information to mothers.

The most critical community indicators of perinatal health relate to access to care, maternal mortality, infant mortality, preterm birth, low birth weight (LBW), first-trimester prenatal care, and rates for mammography, Papanicolaou (Pap) smears, and other similar screening tests. Nurses can use these indicators as a reflection of access, quality, and continuity of health care in a community. For women and infants, access to a consistent source of care is critical. Those with a regular source of care are more likely to use preventive services and have more positive pregnancy outcomes, but many women lack access to a usual source of care or rely primarily on emergency services.

Vulnerable Populations

Assessment of population health includes indicators related to diverse groups and cultures, particularly disenfranchised or "vulnerable" community members. Vulnerability in terms of health status and health outcomes may take many forms, including sociocultural, economic, and environmental risk factors that contribute to disparities in health. Health disparities are conditions that disproportionately affect certain racial, ethnic, or other groups. African Americans, Hispanic Americans, Native Americans, Pacific Islanders, and Asian Americans are all considered vulnerable populations because of the burden of preventable disease, death, and disability compared with nonminorities (CDC, 2016).

Racial and ethnic disparities exist for a number of health conditions and services. Although some gaps are getting smaller, disparities remain. According to the 2016 National Healthcare Quality and Disparities Report (Agency for Healthcare Research and Quality [AHRQ], 2016), our system of health care distributes services inefficiently and unevenly across populations. These disparities may occur for a variety of reasons, including differences in access to care, social determinants, provider biases, poor provider-client communication, and poor health literacy. A summary of the report described health care quality and access to be suboptimal, especially for minority and low-income groups. Overall quality of health care is improving and access is improving for some; however, disparities still exist. Urgent attention needs to be directed toward diabetes care, maternal and child health care, disparities in cancer care, and quality of care.

Women

Women make up 50.8% of the U.S. population, representing a very diverse, and largely at risk, group in relation to health (U.S. Census Bureau, 2016b). Although women assume leadership for health care decision making in most families, they face significant challenges in accessing the health care system and meeting their own health needs and those of family members. There is no single contributing factor. The primary sources of health disparities for women fall into the areas of gender, socioeconomic status, and race or ethnicity. Significant gaps exist in the quality of care and outcomes for women when compared with men.

Nationally, there has been progress in improving the health care delivery system to achieve the three aims of better care, smarter spending, and healthier people, but more work needs to be done to address disparities in women's care. One of the primary factors compromising women's health is lack of access to acceptable-quality health care, which may manifest itself in many forms: lack of health insurance, living in a medically underserved area, or an inability to obtain needed services, particularly basic services such as prenatal care. From 2005 to 2012, females were significantly more likely than males to be delayed or unable to get needed medical care, dental care, or prescription medicines (AHRQ, 2015).

Many women report that they are in good to excellent health, but statistics reveal significant disparities in health status of women from all age groups and racial and ethnic backgrounds. Low levels of educational attainment (high school or lower) are also associated with lack of resources and difficulty navigating the health care system. This is particularly true of women of ethnic and racial minorities, whose limited English proficiency may compromise provider access and quality of care (AHRQ, 2015).

Racial and Ethnic Minorities

In addition to social, economic, and cultural barriers to optimal health, women who are in racial and ethnic minorities experience a disproportionate burden of disease, disability, and premature death. Significant health disparities continue to exist in the health of adult women and their infants. Although positive trends are evident, disparities persist among racial and ethnic groups in early prenatal care, an important factor in achieving healthy pregnancy outcomes.

Minority women, many of whom live in poverty, also have higher rates of chronic disease, including heart disease, cancer, hepatitis, and acquired immunodeficiency syndrome (AIDS), as well as mental health issues. Women with underlying health conditions are at especially high risk for poor obstetric outcomes for themselves and their infants. They have high rates of preterm labor and gestational hypertension, and often have intrauterine growth restriction, resulting in the birth of infants who are small for gestational age. These are the women for whom the community-based perinatal nurse will be providing care, and their needs are complex, demanding high levels of expertise and skill.

Adolescent Girls

The adolescent population in the United States is generally considered healthy. However, adolescents participate in riskier behaviors and their health is often compromised as a result.

Although adolescents are concerned about becoming pregnant, they still engage in unprotected sex. They use a variety of sources for health information such as the media, friends, and sex education, yet they are misinformed, particularly about sexually transmitted infections (STIs) and human immunodeficiency virus (HIV) transmission. These findings have significant implications for perinatal outcomes and emphasize the importance of aggressive prevention programs and community outreach related to sexuality, teen pregnancy, and substance abuse.

It is crucial that nurses engage adolescents in health education programs that will encourage them to make informed decisions about their sexual health. It is also vital that nurses be a resource to these young women.

Older Women

Although women have a greater life expectancy than men, they are more likely to have chronic illnesses, less likely to use preventive services, and ultimately spend more on health care. As nurses, it is important that we engage this population at all levels of prevention, from primary to tertiary.

Incarcerated Women

The number of incarcerated women has been growing twice as fast as that for men since 1980. Incarcerated women often have histories of intimate partner violence, including physical and/or sexual abuse; history of HIV and substance abuse, and emotional problems due to absence from family (The Sentencing Project, 2018).

Because their relationship histories are often unstable, and because they often lack the support of family, incarcerated women or those with a history of repeated incarceration frequently have difficulty providing emotional stability, secure housing, and health promotion role modeling for their children. The lifestyle choices of this group, including risky sexual relationships, illicit drug use, and smoking, place them at high risk for STIs, HIV, and AIDS; other chronic and communicable diseases; and complicated pregnancies, including incarcerated women giving birth.

Immigrant, Refugee, and Migrant Women

As of 2016, 43.7 million people in the United States, representing 13.5% of the U.S. population (PEW Research Center, 2018). This accounts for a rapidly growing diverse population for which nurses will be providing care.

An *immigrant* is an individual who moves from one country to another in an effort to take up legal residency, whereas a *refugee* is an individual who is forced to leave his or her home country, often in search of a safer and more stable living environment. Both populations are often challenged with not being able to easily access health care because they are not U.S. citizens. These women often do not seek medical care for fear of deportation. Access to care is further limited by health care policies that restrict Medicaid eligibility for these groups, although a number of states provide some prenatal, birth, and postpartum care.

Along with their profound resilience and determination, refugees and immigrants have brought rich diversity to the United States in several important dimensions, including cultural heritage and customs, economic productivity, and enhanced national vitality. In general, refugees are more likely to live in poverty than are immigrants. Over time, measures of health and well-being actually decline for the immigrant population as they become part of American society. Many of the conditions or illnesses that they acquire contribute to the persistence of disparities in maternal and neonatal health outcomes for both immigrants and refugees.

Migrant workers are those who work outside their home country or migrate within their own country seeking seasonal work. Migrant laborers and their families face many problems, including financial instability, child labor, poor housing, lack of education, language and cultural barriers, and limited access to health and social services. Poor dental health, diabetes, hypertension, malnutrition, tuberculosis, skin diseases, and parasitic infections are common health issues among migrant populations. Primary health care services are largely provided by a number of migrant health centers, of which there are more than 400 throughout the United States. In 2016 more than 957,529 seasonal and migrant farm workers and their families were served (Health Resources & Services Administration [HRSA], 2016). Routine prenatal care and screening and treatment for hypertension and diabetes are provided. Community health nurses frequently encounter the challenges of providing culturally and linguistically appropriate care while facing numerous health issues.

Numerous reproductive health issues exist for migrant women, including less consistent use of contraception and increased rates of STIs. Migrants are less likely to receive early prenatal care and have a greater incidence of inadequate weight gain during pregnancy than do other poor women.

Rural Versus Urban Community Settings

About 60 million people (19.3% of the population) live in rural areas (U.S. Census Bureau, 2016c). Generally, rural residents are older, less educated, and in poorer health than their urban counterparts. Rural communities are disproportionately affected by poverty and poor access to health care services. Fewer physicians choosing to practice in rural areas and lack of insurance present additional factors contributing to poor health in rural areas.

Rural women are especially vulnerable to financial and transportation barriers to health care. Although women in rural counties report only *fair* to *poor* health, they pay considerably more for their health care. In rural communities, women have less access to prenatal care, which contributes to higher rates of adverse pregnancy outcomes, including higher rates of preterm birth, LBW, and infant mortality. The disproportionate distribution of poverty and of variations in race/ethnicity, age, education, and availability and access to medical resources may be the link to infant mortality in rural areas.

Homeless Women

Homelessness among women is an increasing social and health issue in the United States. Although exact numbers are unknown because of the difficulty in tracking individuals without a permanent address, it is estimated that in 2017, the United States had approximately 553,742 people experiencing homelessness. For every 10,000 people in the country, 17 were experiencing homelessness. Women make up 39% of the homeless population and are often on the street to escape domestic violence (U.S. Department of Housing and Urban Development, 2017).

Families with children make up the fastest-growing group of the homeless population. Adults and children in families make up about 35% of the homeless population, and of these, 84% are headed by women (National Alliance to End Homelessness, 2017)

Health issues among the homeless are numerous and result primarily from a lack of preventive care and a lack of resources in general. Health problems include chronic illness, infectious diseases, asthma, circulatory problems, diabetes, substance abuse, and mental illness. Lifestyle factors and the vulnerability resulting from being homeless contribute to health problems. Women are at increased risk for illness and injury; many have been victims of domestic abuse, assault, and rape. Although little is known about pregnancy in this population, women do become pregnant while homeless. In addition to risk factors related to inadequate nutrition, inadequate weight gain, anemia, bleeding problems, and preterm birth, homeless women face multiple barriers to prenatal care: transportation, distance, and wait times. Most of these women underutilize available prenatal services. The unsafe environment and high-risk lifestyles often result in adverse perinatal outcomes (American College of Obstetricians and Gynecologists [ACOG], 2016). The United States has initiated programs to address these problems. For example, the U.S. Interagency Council on Homelessness and its 19 member agencies launched *Opening Doors*, the federal strategic plan to prevent and end homelessness in 2010 and updated it in 2015 (U.S. Interagency Council on Homelessness, 2015).

Implications for Nursing

Working in the community or in the home with the full spectrum of family organizational styles, vulnerable populations, and cultural groups presents challenges for nurses. Whether it involves perinatal care focused on women and their newborns, or women's health care directed toward treatment and prevention of other health conditions such as communicable diseases and sexually transmitted infections, nursing must exhibit a high degree of professionalism. Cultural sensitivity, compassion, and a critical awareness of family dynamics and social stressors that will affect health-related decision making are critical components in developing an effective nursing care plan.

Although the long-term consequences of contemporary immigration for American society are unclear, the successful incorporation of immigrant families depends on the resources, benefits, and policies that ensure their healthy development and successful social adjustment. Culturally competent health care and involvement of the immigrant community in health care programs are recommended strategies for improving the access to and effectiveness of health care for this population.

The use of camp volunteers has been effective in assisting families living in migrant worker camps to obtain prenatal, postpartum, and infant care. Working in partnership with health professionals such as nurses, lay camp aides have been used effectively for outreach and health education; however, more strategies are needed to link traditional practices with the formal health care system. Guidance and information about other health resources are available to health care providers through the National Center for Farmworker Health, Inc. (www.ncfh.org) and the Migrant Clinicians Network (www.migrantclinician.org).

Nurses working with homeless women and families are challenged to treat them with dignity and respect to establish a therapeutic relationship. Case management is recommended to coordinate the services and disciplines that may be involved in meeting the complex needs of these families. Whenever possible, general screening and preventive health services must be provided when the woman seeks treatment because this may be the only opportunity to provide health information and intervention. Building on existing coping strategies and strengths, the health care provider helps the woman and her family reconnect with a social support system. Nurses also have an important role in advocating for funding to support health services for the homeless and improve access to preventive care for all homeless populations.

CARE OF THE WOMAN AT HOME

Modern home care nursing has its foundation in public health nursing, which provided comprehensive care to sick and well clients in their own homes. Specialized maternity home care nursing services began in the 1980s when public health maternity nursing services were limited, and services had not kept pace with the changing practices of high-risk obstetrics and emerging technology. Lengthy antepartum hospitalizations for such conditions as preterm labor and gestational hypertension created nursing care challenges for staff members of inpatient units.

Many women expressed their concerns about the negative effect of antepartum hospitalizations on the family, as well as the costs and burdens of lengthy hospitalizations. Although clinical indications showed that a new nursing care approach was needed, home health care did not become a viable alternative until third-party payers (i.e., public or private organizations or employer groups that pay for health care) pushed for cost containment in maternity services.

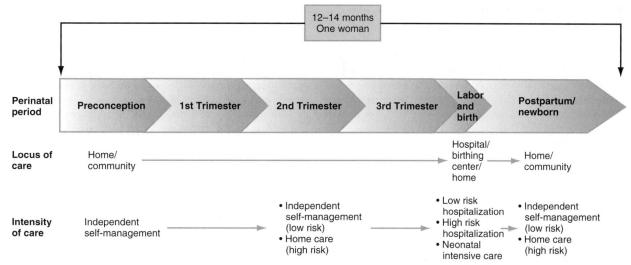

Fig. 2.6 Perinatal Continuum of Care.

In the current health care system, home care is an important component of health care delivery along the perinatal continuum of care (Fig. 2.6). The growing demand for home care is based on several factors:

- Interest in family birthing alternatives
- Shortened hospital stays
- New technologies that facilitate home-based assessments and treatments
- Reimbursement by third-party payers

As health care costs continue to rise, and because millions of American families lack health insurance, there is greater demand for innovative, cost-effective methods of health care delivery in the community. Large health care systems are developing clinically integrated health care delivery networks whose goals are (1) improved coordination of care and care outcomes; (2) better communication among health care providers; (3) increased client, payer, and provider satisfaction; and (4) reduced cost. The integration of clinical services changes the focus of care to a continuum of services that are increasingly community based.

Perinatal Continuum of Care

The perinatal continuum of care includes care before pregnancy, during pregnancy and childbirth, and the days immediately afterward (see Fig. 2.6). Continuous care across life stages and from home to hospital is crucial for health (World Health Organization, 2018). Only when attention is paid to continuity between all phases of the reproductive/perinatal health continuum, will our nation be able to ensure the health of all women across the life course (Handler & Johnson, 2016).

Communication and Technology Applications

As maternity care continues to consist of frequent and brief contacts with health care providers throughout the prenatal and postpartum periods, services that link maternity clients throughout the perinatal continuum of care have assumed increasing importance. These services include critical pathways, telephonic nursing assessments, discharge planning, specialized education programs, parent support groups, home visiting programs, nurse advice lines, and perinatal home care (Fig. 2.7). Hospitals may provide cross-training for hospital-based nurses to make postpartum home visits or to staff outpatient centers for postpartum follow-up.

Telephonic nursing through services such as warm lines, nurse advice lines, and telephonic nursing assessments is a valuable means of managing health care problems and bridging the gaps among acute,

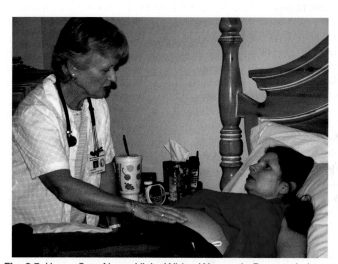

Fig. 2.7 Home Care Nurse Visits With a Woman in Preterm Labor at Home on Bed Rest. (Courtesy Shannon Perry, Phoenix, AZ.)

outpatient, and home care services. Health care professionals use the Internet and Skype to communicate with clients. Newborns in distress in rural hospitals can be assessed by neonatologists using high-definition telemedicine robots. Nursing care that occurs by telephone is interactive and responsive to immediate health care questions about particular health care needs. Warm lines are telephone lines that are offered as a community service to provide new parents with support, encouragement, and basic parenting education. Nurse advice lines, or toll-free nurse consultation services, often are supported by third-party payers or health management organization/managed care organizations (HMO/MCOs) and are designed to provide answers to medical questions. Nurse care managers are prepared to guide callers through urgent health care situations, suggest treatment options, and provide health education. Telephonic nursing assessments, or nurse consultation, assessment, and health education that take place during a telephone conversation, can be added to the nursing care plan in conjunction with skilled nursing visits, or they may comprise a separate nursing contact for the woman. Telephonic nursing assessments are commonly used after a postpartum home care visit to reassess a woman's knowledge about the signs and symptoms of adequate hydration in breastfeeding or, after initiating home phototherapy, to assess the caregiver's knowledge regarding problems with equipment.

Guidelines for Nursing Practice

The Association of Women's Health, Obstetric and Neonatal Nurses (AWHONN, 2009) defines home care as the provision of technical, psychologic, and other therapeutic support in the woman's home rather than in an institution. The scope of nursing care delivered in the home is necessarily limited to practices deemed safe and appropriate to be carried out in an environment that is physically separated from a health care institution and its resources. Nursing practice at home is consistent with federal and state regulations that direct home care practice. The nurse demonstrates practice competence through formalized orientation and ongoing clinical education and performance evaluation in the respective home care agency. Standards for practice from key specialty organizations such as AWHONN, the National Association of Neonatal Nurses (NANN), ACNM, ACOG, the American Academy of Pediatrics (AAP), and the Intravenous Nursing Society (INS) provide the basis for clinical protocols and pathways and organizational programs in home care practice. The Joint Commission (www.jointcommission.org) provides criteria for home care operations based on Centers for Medicare & Medicaid Services (CMS) regulations (www.cms.gov).

A wide range of professional health care services and products can be delivered or used in the home by means of technology and telecommunication. For example, telehealth and telemedicine make it possible for clients in the home to be interviewed and assessed by a specialist located hundreds of miles away. Home health care can be viewed as an extension of in-hospital care.

Essentially the primary difference between health care in a hospital and home care is the absence of the continuous presence of professional health care providers in a client's home. Generally, but not always, home health care entails intermittent care by a professional who visits the client's home for a particular reason and/or provides care on site for fewer than 4 hours at a time. The home health care agency maintains on-call professional staff to assist home care clients who have questions about their care and for emergencies, such as equipment failure.

Perinatal Services

Home care is best delivered by an interprofessional care team. Nurses, obstetricians, maternal-fetal medicine, pharmacy, mental health practitioners, social workers, the public health department, and case managers working together can provide comprehensive and client-centered care. Home care perinatal services may be provided by hospital-based programs, independent proprietary (for-profit) agencies, nonprofit home care agencies, and official or tax-supported agencies. Innovative programs may be supported by research grants for a period of years, but ultimately they must be sponsored by an agency with long-term funding. Home visits have advantages and disadvantages. The pregnant woman can maintain bed rest if indicated, and vulnerable neonates are not exposed to the weather or external sources of infection. The nurse can observe and interact with family members in their most natural and secure environment. Adequacy of resources and safety factors can be assessed. Teaching can be tailored to the actual home conditions, and other family members can be included. A home visit is less expensive than a day's hospitalization, but a 60- to 90-minute visit requires 2.5 to 3 hours of nursing time, including travel and documentation. Areas of challenge include limited availability of nurses with expertise in maternity care and concerns about the nurse's physical safety in the community. One alternative that is less expensive is contacting women via telephone or the internet.

Visits for outreach and health promotion are an integral part of community (or public) health nursing. In countries with national health systems, a nurse or midwife may see all women during pregnancy and after birth. In the United States, visits of this sort have been provided mainly to low-income families without health insurance and Medicaid recipients who use the clinics provided by local health departments. Until recently, private insurers did not reimburse for health promotion visits. MCOs now recognize that anticipatory guidance can be cost effective, but home visitation programs for the most part still target specific, high-risk populations such as adolescents and women at risk for preterm labor.

Home care agencies are subject to regulation by governmental and professional organizations and provide interdisciplinary services, including social work, nutrition, and occupational and physical therapy. Increasingly, their caseloads are made up of women who require high-technology care, such as infusions or home monitoring. Although the home health nurse develops the care plan, all care must be ordered by a physician. In addition, interventions must meet the insurer's criteria for reimbursement and services are limited to registered clients. Preconception care and low-risk antepartum care can usually be provided more efficiently in offices and clinics. High-risk antepartum care can be provided by home care agencies; for example, women with hyperemesis gravidarum who require parenteral nutrition may be treated at home. Conditions requiring bed rest, such as preterm labor and hypertension, are other common indications for home care. Other conditions often managed with home care may include cardiac disease, substance abuse, and diabetes in pregnancy.

Insurers may reimburse for at least one postpartum visit to families after early discharge or in the presence of high-risk factors. Many neonates who require long-term, high-technology care are also managed with home care.

Nursing Considerations

The major areas of the assessment are demographics, medical history, general health history, medication history, psychosocial assessment (Box 2.4), home and community environment, and physical assessment. There are several areas of concern when caring for a woman in the home. In home care the woman or family members are responsible for administration of medications in the absence of the nurse. A careful medication history should be obtained to see if the woman is taking her medications correctly and understands their desired action and potential side effects. It is important that women and caretakers have a clear understanding of medication regimens and are notified when medications change in any way.

Nurses have to be skilled at performing various procedures such as venipuncture and administration of intravenous medications or fluids. Nurses must be sure that women know how to respond in emergency situations. Women need to be able to have 24-hour access to resources in the community in emergency situations. Women and family members are also encouraged to learn how to perform cardiopulmonary resuscitation (CPR), especially for infants.

Verbal explanations should be supplemented with clearly written instructions. General information to promote well-being includes nutrition and common discomforts of pregnancy. The need for childbirth education and preparation can be addressed by using books or videos and supplemented by individual teaching at home. Coping with bed rest or other limitation of activity is a problem for many women with high-risk pregnancies. The nurse can share strategies that others have used such as support groups for women on bed rest using Facebook or Skype, help with time management, and provide information about support services. Teaching about infant care or the special needs of the preterm infant may be appropriate during the prenatal period.

Clear documentation of assessments, problems identified, treatments and interventions performed, and the woman's response is essential. Third-party payers base reimbursement on the nurse's written

BOX 2.4 Psychosocial Assessment

Language
- Identify the primary language spoken in the home.
- Assess whether there are any language barriers to receiving support.

Community Resources/Access to Care
- Identify primary and secondary means of transportation.
- Identify community agencies family uses for health care and support.
- Assess cultural and psychosocial barriers to receiving care.

Social Support
- Determine the people living with the pregnant woman.
- Identify who assists with household chores.
- Identify who assists with child care and parenting activities.
- Identify who the pregnant woman turns to for problems or during a crisis.

Interpersonal Relationships
- Assess the way decisions are made in the family.
- Identify the family's perception of the need for home care.
- Analyze roles of adults in caring for family members.

Caregiver
- Identify the primary caregiver for home care treatments.
- Identify other caregivers and their roles.
- Assess the caregiver's knowledge of treatments and the care process.
- Assess potential strain from the caregiver role.
- Assess the level of satisfaction with the caregiver role.

Stress and Coping
- Describe what the woman perceives as lifestyle changes and their effect on her and her family.
- Analyze the changes she and her family have made to adjust to her health condition and home health care treatments.

record of providing skilled nursing care and assessments that support the woman's continuing need for those services. The nurse must promptly inform the health care provider by telephone, fax, or electronic file of any significant changes. When new orders are transmitted by telephone, a written copy must be sent for the physician's signature.

KEY POINTS

- The family is a social network that acts as an important support system for its members.
- Family socioeconomics, response to stress, and culture are key factors influencing family health.
- The economic, religious, kinship, and political structures are embedded in the reproductive beliefs and practices of a culture.
- Nurses must develop cultural competence and integrate it into the nursing care plan.
- Of necessity, most changes aimed at improving community health involve partnerships among community residents and health workers.

- Vulnerable populations are groups who are at higher risk for developing physical, mental, or social health problems.
- Telephonic nurse advice lines, telephonic nursing assessments, and warm lines are low-cost health care services that facilitate continuous client education, support, and health care decision making, even though health care is delivered in multiple sites.
- Social and economic factors affect the scope of perinatal nursing practice. Perinatal home care is a unique nursing practice that incorporates knowledge from community health nursing, acute care nursing, family therapy, health promotion, and client education.

REFERENCES

Agency for Healthcare Research and Quality (AHRQ). (2015). 2014 *National healthcare quality and disparities report: Chartbook on women's health care* Publication No. 15-0007-10-EF. Retrieved from https://www.ahrq.gov/research/findings/nhqrdr/index.html.

American College of Obstetricians and Gynecologists (ACOG) (Reaffirmed 2016). Health care for homeless women. ACOG Committee Opinion No. 576. *Obstetrics and Gynecology, 122*(4), 936–940. https://doi.org/10.1097/01.AOG.0000435417.29567.90.

American Nurses Association. (2015). In *Nursing: Scope and standards of practice* (3rd ed.). Silver Spring, MD: Author.

Association of Women's Health, Obstetric and Neonatal Nurses (AWHONN). (2009). *Standards for professional nursing practice in the care of women and newborns* (7th ed.). Washington, DC: Author.

Centers for Disease Control and Prevention (CDC). (2014). *Practical strategies for culturally competent evaluation.* Atlanta, GA: U.S. Department of Health and Human Services.

Centers for Disease Control and Prevention (CDC). (2016). *Minority health.* Retrieved from www.cdc.gov/MinorityHealth/index.html.

Cipriano, P. F. (2016). Attaining a culturally congruent practice. *American Nurse Today, 11*(5), 15.

Ellis, R. R., & Simmons, T. (2014). *Co-resident grandparents and their grandchildren: 2012 population characteristics.* U.S. Census Bureau. Retrieved from https://www.census.gov/content/dam/Census/library/publications/2014/demo/p20-576.pdf.

Giger, J. N. (2016). *Transcultural nursing: Assessment and intervention* (7th ed.). St. Louis, MO: Mosby.

Handler, A., & Johnson, K. (2016). A call to revisit the prenatal period as a focus for action within the reproductive and perinatal care continuum. *Maternal Child Health Journal, 20,* 2217–2227. https://doi.org/10.1007/s10995-016-2187-6.

Health Resources & Services Administration (HRSA). (2016). *Health center data.* Retrieved from https://bphc.hrsa.gov/uds/datacenter.aspx?q=tall&year=2016&state=.

Laughlin, L. (2014). *A child's day: Living arrangements, nativity, and family transitions: 2011.* U.S. Census Bureau. Retrieved from https://www.2census.gov/library/publications/2014/demographics/p70-139.pdf.

McGoldrick, M., Garcia-Prieto, N. A., & Carter, B. (2016). *The expanding family life cycle: Individual, family, and social perspectives* (5th ed.). Boston: Pearson.

Monte, L. M. (2017). *Family complexity and changing household dynamics as measured in the 2014 survey of income and program participation.* SEHSD Working Paper #2017-119 U.S. Census Bureau. Retrieved from https://www.census.gov/content/dam/Census/library/working-papers/2017/demo/SEHSD-WP2017-119.pdf.

National Alliance to End Homelessness. (2017). *Children and families.* Retrieved from https://endhomelessness.org/homelesses-in-america/who-experiences-homelessness/children-and-families/.

Office of Minority Health (2017). *Cultural and linguistic competency. U.S. Department of Health and Human Services.* Retrieved from: https://minorityhealth.hhs.gov/omh/browse.aspx?lvl=1&lvlid=6.

Pew Research Center (2018). Key findings about U.S. immigrants. Washington, D.C. Retrieved from: https://www.pewresearch.org/fact-tank/2018/11/30/key-findings-about-u-s-immigrants.

Spector, R. E. (2017). *Cultural diversity in health and illness* (9th ed.). New York: Pearson.

The Sentencing Project (2018). Fact sheet: Trends in U.S. corrections. Washington, DC. Retrieved from: http://www.pewresearch.org/fact-tank/2018/11/30/key-findings-about-u-s-immigrants.

Trinh, M., Agenor, M., Austin, S. B., & Jackson, C. (2017). Health and healthcare disparities among U.S. women and men at the intersection of sexual orientation and race/ethnicity: A nationally representative cross-sectional study. *BMC Public Health, 17*(964). https://doi.10.1186/s12889-017-4937-9.

U.S. Census Bureau. (2015a). *Children characteristics: American community survey 1-year estimates.* Retrieved from https://www.census.gov/popest/data/national/asrh/2011/index.htm.

U.S. Census Bureau. (2015b). *Characteristics of same-sex couple households: 2005 to present.* Retrieved from https://www.census.gov/topics/families/same-sex-couples/data/tables.html.

U.S. Census Bureau. (2016a). *The Majority of children live with two parents.* Release Number: CB16-192. Retrieved from https://www.census.gov/newsroom/press-releases/2016/cb16-192.html.

U.S. Census Bureau. (2016b). *Population estimates.* Retrieved from www.census.gov/quickfacts/fact/table/US/PST045216.

U.S. Census Bureau. (2016c). *American community survey: 2011-2015* Release Number: CB16-210. Retrieved from www.census.gov/newsroom/press-releases/2016/cb16-210.html.

U.S. Census Bureau. (2017a). *Current population survey: Households by race and Hispanic origin of household reference person and detailed type.* Retrieved from https://www.census.gov/data/tables/2017/demo/families/cps-2017.html.

U.S. Census Bureau. (2017b). *Current population survey: Living arrangement of children under 18 and marital status of parents, by age, sex, race and Hispanic origin.* Retrieved from https://www.census.gov/data/tables/2017/demo/families/cps-2017.html.

U.S. Department of Housing and Urban Development. (2017). *The 2017 annual homeless assessment report (AHAR) to congress.* Retrieved from www.hudexchange.info/resources/documents/2017-AHAR-Part-1.pdf.

U.S. Interagency Council on Homelessness. (2015). *Opening doors: Federal strategic plan to prevent and end homelessness.* Washington, D.C. Retrieved from www.usich.gov/resources/uploads/asset_library/USICH_OpeningDoors_Amendment2015_Final.pdf.

World Health Organization [WHO], 2018. (2010). *PMNCH Knowledge summary #02 enable the continuum of care. The Partnership for Maternal, Newborn & Child Health.* Retrieved from www.who.int/pmnch/knowledge/publications/summaries/ks2/en/.

Wright, L. M., & Leahey, M. (1999). Maximizing time, minimizing suffering: The 15-minute (or less) family interview. *Journal of Family Nursing, 5*(3), 259–273.

Wright, L. M., & Leahey, M. (2013). *Nurses and families: A guide to family assessment and intervention* (6th ed.). Philadelphia: F.A. Davis Co.

3

Nursing and Genomics

Marcia Van Riper

http://evolve.elsevier.com/Lowdermilk/MWHC/

LEARNING OBJECTIVES

- Explore how advances in genetics and technology have changed health care.
- Discuss the essential competencies in genetics and genomics for all nurses.
- Describe expanded roles for nurses in genetics and genetic counseling.
- Discuss key findings of the Human Genome Project, including the ethical, legal, and social implications.
- Describe the different types of genetic testing.
- Identify genetic disorders commonly tested for in maternity and women's health nursing.

- Explore the possible benefits and risks of pharmacogenomics.
- Discuss the current status of gene therapy.
- Explain the key concepts of basic human genetics.
- Discuss the education and counseling needs of individuals and families who undergo genetic testing.
- Explore the availability of genetic testing for individuals and families from diverse backgrounds.
- Describe the role of genomics in cancer care for women.
- Identify genetics resources for nurses and other health care professionals.

This chapter presents an overview of genetics/genomics and the role of the nurse in genomic health care.

GENETICS/GENOMICS

Recent advances in genomics and technology have revolutionized health care by providing the tools needed to determine the hereditary component of many diseases as well as improve our ability to predict susceptibility to disease, onset and progression of disease, and response to medications. Moreover, these advances have led to a dramatic increase in genetic testing options, a more precise approach to health care, the development of novel therapies, and a more efficient/cost-effective use of health care resources (Doble, Schofield, Roscioli, & Mattick, 2017; Henderson & Mudd-Martin, 2018).

Since the human genome was sequenced, there has been a gradual shift from genetics to genomics. **Genetics** refers to the study of a particular gene, whereas **genomics** refers to the study of all the genes in the entire genome. **Genes** are the basic physical units of inheritance that are passed from parents to offspring and contain the information needed to specify traits. The **genome** is the entire set of genetic instructions found in a cell. Another related term is epigenetics. **Epigenetics** (which literally means over and above the genome) is "an emerging field of science that studies heritable changes caused by the activation and deactivation of genes without any change in the underlying DNA sequence of the organism." For these and other definitions of genetic terms, refer to the *Talking Glossary of Genetic Terms* (National Human Genome Research Institute [NHGRI], nd).

Genomic medicine (also known as genomic health care) has been defined as "an emerging discipline that involves using genomic information about an individual as part of their clinical care and the health outcomes and political implications of that clinical use" (NHGRI, 2018b). **Precision medicine**, also known as precision health and personalized medicine, is an emerging approach to preventing and treating illnesses that includes individual variations in genes, environment, and lifestyle (Precision Medicine Initiative, 2015). Regardless of the name used (genomic medicine, precision medicine, or personalized medicine), care is focused on the tailoring of health care to individual preferences, lifestyle, environment, and genetic variability (Alexander, 2018). With growing public interest in *personalized genomic information* (information about much or all of an individual's genome), increasing development of practice guidelines, mounting commercial pressures, and ever-increasing opportunities for individuals, families, and communities to participate in the direction and design of their genomic health care, genetic services are becoming an integral part of routine health care (Manolio, 2016).

A growing number of individuals and families have participated in *direct-to-consumer genetic testing* (testing marketed directly to consumers through television, print advertisements, and websites). Although much of the information provided by direct-to-consumer (DTC) testing companies is recreational (ancestry information, information about types of ear wax, and bitter taste perception), some of the information provided is health related and could be interpreted as diagnostic. Because of this, DTC testing provided without the involvement of competent health care professionals may be not only unhelpful, but also harmful (Burke & Trinidad, 2016; Middleton, Mendes, Benjamin, & Howard, 2017). There are ongoing efforts by the U.S. Food and Drug Administration (FDA) to regulate DTC use. A recent study conducted by Gollust, Gray, Carere, et al. (2017) found that a large percentage of the participants (over 80%) thought people should have a right to access genetic information directly, that parents should be able to get DTC testing for their children, and that genetic information should be kept private. DTC users who had a negative personal experience with DTC testing were less supportive of expanded availability of DTC without assistance from a health care professional who has expertise in genetics and genomics. In 2017, the American College of Obstetricians and Gynecologists (ACOG, 2017c) published a committee opinion paper in which their first recommendation was "Direct to consumer testing should be discouraged because of the potential harm of misinterpreted or inaccurate results."

Genetic disorders affect people of all ages, from all socioeconomic levels, and from all racial and ethnic backgrounds. Genetic disorders affect not only individuals but also families, communities, and society. Advances in genetic testing and genetically based treatments have altered the care provided to affected individuals. Improvements in diagnostic capability have resulted in earlier diagnosis and have enabled individuals who previously likely would have died in childhood to survive into adulthood. However, for most genetic conditions, therapeutic or preventive measures do not exist or are very limited. Consequently, the most useful means of reducing the incidence of these disorders is by preventing their transmission. It is standard practice to assess all pregnant women for heritable disorders to identify potential problems.

Nursing Expertise in Genetics and Genomics

Because of their front-line position in the health care system and their long-standing history of providing holistic family-centered care, nurses are likely to be one of the first health care professionals to whom individuals and families turn with questions about genetic risk and susceptibility and to seek guidance regarding the complexities of genetic testing and interpretation. Nowhere is this more apparent than in maternity and women's health care. A growing number of nurses provide information about the availability of genetic tests, answer questions about the tests, and help clients and families interpret genetic testing results. Although most of these tests are used to determine a woman's risk for having a child affected by a genetic condition with a childhood onset such as Down syndrome (DS), cystic fibrosis (CF), sickle cell disease (SCD), or spinal muscular atrophy (SMA), the number of genetic tests used to determine the presence of, or susceptibility to, adult-onset disorders (e.g., hereditary breast and ovarian cancer [HBOC], and Huntington disease [HD]) continues to rise. Additionally, nurses working in maternity and women's health are caring for an increasing number of individuals and families who are dealing with the complex ethical, legal, and social issues associated with being tested for and living with a genetic condition (Fleming, Knafl, & Van Ripe, 2017; Gee, Piercy, & Machaczek, 2017; Hodgson & McClaren, 2018; Rosell, Pena, Schoch, et al., 2016; Rowland, Plumridge, Considine, & Metcalfe, 2016; von der Lippe, Diesen, & Feragen, 2017; Whitt Hughes, Hopkins, & Maradiegue, 2016; Van Riper, Knafl, Roscigno, & Knafl, 2017).

Essential Competencies in Genetics and Genomics for All Nurses

Nearly 50 organizations, including the Association of Women's Health, Obstetric and Neonatal Nurses (AWHONN) and the National Association of Neonatal Nurses (NANN), have endorsed the *Essential Nursing Competencies and Curricula Guidelines for Genetics and Genomics* (National Human Genome Research Institute [NHGRI], 2013). According to these guidelines, which were developed by an independent panel of nurse leaders (consensus panel) from clinical, research, and academic settings and published by the American Nurses Association and the National Human Genome Research Institute (NHGRI) of the National Institutes of Health (NIH), all nurses need to have minimal competencies in genetics and genomics regardless of their academic preparation, practice setting, or specialty. Some of the competencies most relevant to nurses in the area of maternity and women's health include the following:

- Construct a pedigree from collected family history information using standardized symbols and terminology
- Develop a plan of care that incorporates genetic and genomic assessment information
- Recognize when one's own attitudes and values related to genetic and genomic science may affect care provided to clients
- Provide clients with credible, accurate, appropriate, and current genetic and genomic information, resources, services, and/or technologies that facilitate decision making
- Demonstrate in practice the importance of tailoring genetic and genomic information and services to clients based on their culture, religion, knowledge level, literacy, and preferred language
- Assess clients' knowledge, perceptions, and responses to genetic and genomic information
- Facilitate referrals for specialized genetic and genomic services for clients as needed

Expanded Roles for Maternity and Women's Health Nurses

Expanded roles for nurses with expertise in genetics and genomics are developing in many areas of maternity and women's health nursing. These areas include but are not limited to prenatal care (prenatal testing and screening, carrier testing during pregnancy, and the sharing of genetic risk information with other family members), labor and birth (the care of pregnant women who may need specialized care due to the fact they and/or the fetus they are carrying has a known genetic condition), newborn care (newborn screening, identification and care of newborns with genetic conditions and their families, and palliative care for infants with life-threatening genetic conditions and their families), and women's health care (the prevention, diagnosis, and/or treatment of genetic conditions such as HBOC, Lynch syndrome, CF, SCD, and factor V Leiden (FVL) (Kerber & Ledbetter, 2017; Metcalfe, 2018; Rogers, Lizer, Doughty, et al., 2017; Vorderstrasse, Hammer, & Dungan, 2014; Williams, Katapodi, Starkweather, et al., 2016).

Human Genome Project and Implications for Clinical Practice

The Human Genome Project (NHGRI, 2015) was a publicly funded international effort coordinated by the NHGRI (https://www.genome.gov/) at the National Institutes of Health (NIH) and the U.S. Department of Energy. When the Human Genome Project was initiated in 1990, the ultimate goal of the project was to map the human genome (the complete set of genetic instructions in the nucleus of each human cell) by 2005. Considering that the human genome consists of approximately 3 billion base pairs of DNA, many people regarded this as an impossible task. However, in 2003 an accurate and complete human genome sequence was finished and made available to scientists and researchers.

A key finding from the Human Genome Project was that all human beings are 99.9% identical at the DNA level. This finding should help discourage the use of science as a justification for drawing precise racial boundaries around groups of people. A more recent effort by the NHGRI called the **En**cyclopedia **o**f **D**NA **E**lements, or the ENCODE Project, was organized to identify the genome's functional elements (ENCODE, 2018). Researchers were able to link more than 80% of the human genome sequence to a specific biologic function, as well as map more than 4 million regulatory regions where proteins specifically interact with the DNA. This finding improved our understanding of how genes are turned on and off by proteins using sites that may be at a great distance from the genes.

Importance of Family History

Completion of the Human Genome Project and the resultant identification of the inherited causes for many diseases has resulted in renewed interest in family history. Although it is easy to be impressed by the fact that genetic testing is currently available for more than 11,000 conditions (National Center for Biotechnology Information [NCBI], 2018), family history will most likely continue to be the single most cost-effective piece of genetic information. When nurses and other clinicians conduct a family history, they can gain not only valuable information about the structure of the family and diseases that affect various individuals in the family, but also a rich understanding of family relationships, social context, occupations, lifestyle, and health habits (ACOG, 2018a). The process of collecting this information often facilitates the development of a relationship between the client/family and the clinician. In 2004, the U.S. Department of Health and Human Services launched the Family History Initiative by designating Thanksgiving Day as National Family History Day. The U.S. Surgeon General encouraged families to use their family gatherings as a time to talk about and collect important family health history. A number of family history tools are available free of charge online. One of the most widely used family history tools is the My Family Health Portrait (https://phgkb.cdc.gov/FHH/html/index.html). Another helpful tool is the family health history tool, *Does it run in the family?* that was developed by the Genetic Alliance (www.doesitruninthefamily.org). The Centers for Disease Control and Prevention (CDC) also provide valuable information about family histories, with specific focus on the importance of family health history during the preconception period and during pregnancy (https://www.cdc.gov/genomics/famhistory/index.htm).

The preconception period is an ideal time for nurses to review family history and provide personalized recommendations based on family history (Rehm, 2017). It is also one of the best times to counsel couples about carrier testing options. Finally, the preconception period is an optimal time to refer couples, when appropriate, to genetic specialists.

Gene Identification and Testing

Initial efforts to sequence and analyze the human genome have proven invaluable in the identification of genes involved in disease and in the development of genetic tests. In an effort to bridge the transition from discovery to diagnostics and treatments, the NIH launched the Genetic Testing Registry (GTR) in 2012. The GTR (www.ncbi.nlm.nih.gov/gtr) is a free online tool that can be used to obtain a list of available genetic tests. The GTR website also includes links to other resources such as *GeneReviews* and Online Mendelian Inheritance in Man (OMIM). *GeneReviews* is a collection of expert-authored, peer-reviewed disease descriptions presented in a standardized format and focused on clinically relevant and medically actionable information on the diagnosis, management, and genetic counseling of individuals and families with specific inherited conditions. OMIM is an online catalog of human genes and genetic disorders.

Genetic tests can be used to directly examine the DNA and ribonucleic acid (RNA) that make up a gene (direct or molecular testing), markers that are coinherited with a gene that causes a genetic condition (linkage analysis), the protein products of genes (biochemical testing), or chromosomes (cytogenetic testing). Cytogenetic analysis of malignant tissue has become a mainstay of oncology. Information about the most common types of genetic testing (e.g., preimplantation testing, prenatal testing, newborn screening, carrier testing, diagnostic testing, predictive testing, presymptomatic testing, and forensic testing) can be found on the Genetics

Home Reference, a website provided by the U.S. National Library of Medicine (2017) (https://ghr.nlm.nih.gov/primer).

Until 2011, the main prenatal testing options were carrier screening (used to identify people who carry one copy of a gene mutation that, when present in two copies, causes a genetic disorder), maternal serum screening (a blood test used to see if a pregnant woman is at increased risk for carrying a fetus with a neural tube defect or a chromosomal abnormality such as DS, trisomy 13, or trisomy 18), fetal ultrasound or sonogram (an imaging technique using high-frequency sound waves to produce images of the fetus inside the uterus), and invasive procedures (chorionic villus sampling and amniocentesis). Currently, prenatal testing options also include preimplantation testing (a specialized technique that can reduce the risk of having a child with a particular genetic or chromosomal disorder); expanded carrier screening panels (ethnic-specific and pan-ethnic); cell-free fetal DNA screening (uses the plasma of pregnant women to screen for DS and, in some cases, trisomy 13 and trisomy 18); prenatal microarray testing (testing performed on cells obtained through chorionic villus sampling or amniocentesis that can detect tiny bits of extra or missing genetic information known as copy number variants); whole exome sequencing (WES) (genomic technique for sequencing all of the protein-coding genes in the genome); and whole genome sequencing (WGS) (genomic technique for sequencing an organism's entire genome at a single time). The cost of sequencing a human genome dropped from $100 million in 2001 to around $1000 in 2017 (NHGRI, 2018a). The cost of sequencing has already dropped to the point that sequencing the whole genome is often cheaper and more efficient than testing a client who has a complex condition of unknown origin for a select group of genetic conditions.

Given the rapid development of prenatal testing options, many health care professionals find it challenging to keep up to date regarding best practice recommendations and guidelines. In an effort to address this issue, Post, Mottola, & Kuller (2017) published an overview of eight recently published (2016–2017) national guidelines and updates. The topics included in the guidelines and updates reviewed are carrier screening, cell-free fetal DNA screening, microarray testing, next-generation sequencing, and invasive testing. One of their key findings was that committee opinions and practice bulletins from ACOG, Society for Maternal-Fetal Medicine consult series publications, and a position statement of the American College of Medical Genetics and Genomics are largely in agreement.

Another type of genetic testing that may be seen in maternity and women's health care is predictive testing (a type of genetic testing used to clarify the genetic status of asymptomatic family members). The two types of predictive testing are presymptomatic and predispositional. Mutation analysis for HD is an example of presymptomatic testing. If the gene mutation for HD is present, symptoms of HD are certain to appear if the individual lives long enough. Testing for a *BRCA1* or *BRCA2* gene mutation to determine if a person is at increased risk for developing hereditary breast and ovarian cancer (HBOC) is an example of predispositional testing. Predispositional testing differs from presymptomatic testing in that a positive result (indicating that a *BRCA1* or *BRCA 2* mutation is present) does not indicate a 100% risk for developing HBOC.

In addition to using genetic tests to test for single-gene disorders in clients with clinical symptoms or who have a family history of a genetic disease, genetic tests are used for population-based screening. Newborn screening, a type of screening first introduced in the United States in the early 1960s, is used to identify conditions that can affect a child's long-term health or survival (Rose & Wick, 2018). Worldwide, the number of conditions screened for ranges from 5 to 60 on newborn screening panels (Taylor-Phillips, Stinton, Ferrante di Ruffano, et al., 2018). In the United States, newborn screening is a mandatory state-supported public health program; most states screen newborns for 31 core disorders and 26 secondary disorders. A complete list of conditions tested for in each state is available on the National Newborn Screening & Global Resource Center (NNSGRC) website (http://genes-r-us.uthscsa.edu).

Another type of population-based screening is carrier screening for single-gene disorders such as CF, SCD, and Tay-Sachs disease, either preconceptionally or prenatally (Rose & Wick, 2018). In the past, ACOG recommended that clinicians offer a limited number of carrier screening tests based on self-identified ethnicity or family history (Post, et al., 2017); the only carrier screening recommended as a routine offering for all women was CF screening. However, due to the growing number of carrier screening tests, increasing data about disease carrier frequency in both high- and low-risk populations and evidence of the potential benefits of expanded carrier screening, there has been an increase in the use of comprehensive carrier screening strategies. ACOG now states that ethnic-specific, pan-ethnic, and expanded carrier methods are all acceptable screening strategies with appropriate pretest counseling and selection of tests (ACOG, 2017a; ACOG, 2017b). In addition, it now recommends that all women be offered SMA carrier screening. In the future, carrier screening may include WES or WGS.

Pharmacogenomics

One of the most promising clinical applications of the Human Genome Project has been pharmacogenomic (PGx) testing (testing performed to examine an individual's genes to determine how medications are absorbed, move through the body, and are metabolized by the body). PGx testing can be used to create drug treatments that are individualized and specific to each individual. For example, prior to starting a client on Warfarin (one of the most commonly used medications in many parts of the world), PGx testing can be done to determine the most appropriate starting dose. Basing the starting dose for Warfarin on the client's genotype can help avoid toxicity and increase efficiency. Pharmacogenomic testing can also be used to target therapies. Trastuzumab (Herceptin), a monoclonal antibody that specifically targets HER2/neu overexpressing breast tumors, is an example of a drug for which an obligatory genetic test has been developed. The purpose of this obligatory genetic test is to identify the subset of women with breast cancer who overexpress HER2/neu. Women who overexpress HER2/neu are most likely the only breast cancer patients who will benefit from taking trastuzumab (www.herceptin.com/index.jsp). As of February 2018, the last update of the FDA list of pharmacogenomic biomarkers in drug labeling, over 200 drugs exist for which there are molecular biomarkers that may help assure better therapeutic outcomes for clients carrying these markers (U.S. Department of Food and Drug Administration, 2018). Nurses who have a good understanding of PGx testing can play a critical role in the optimization of drug dosage and the avoidance of drug reactions (Cheek, Bashore, & Brazeau, 2015); this is especially true during discharge planning (Haga & Mills, 2015).

Gene Therapy

Gene therapy is "an experimental technique that uses genes to treat or prevent disease" (Genetics Home Reference, 2018a). The aim of gene therapy is to correct defective genes that are responsible for disease development. Generally, gene therapy involves inserting a healthy copy of the defective gene into the somatic cells (any cell of the body except sperm and egg cells) of the affected individual. Although the early optimism about gene therapy was probably never fully justified, gene therapy has now moved from preclinical to clinical studies for many diseases

(https://www.nih.gov/news-events/news-releases/nih-researchers-tackle-thorny-side-gene-therapy). These diseases range from hemophilia and other single-gene disorders to complex disorders such as cancer, HIV, Parkinson disease, and cardiovascular disorders (Axelsen & Woldbye, 2018; Makris, 2018). Major challenges to gene therapy include determining how to target the right gene to the right location in the right cells, expressing the transferred gene at the right time, and minimizing adverse reactions.

Ethical, Legal, and Social Implications

Because of widespread concern about misuse of the information gained through genetics research, a percentage of the Human Genome Project budget was designated for the study of the ethical, legal, and social implications (ELSI) of human genome research. Two large ELSI programs were created to identify, analyze, and address the ELSIs of human genome research at the same time as basic science issues were being studied. They have focused on the possible consequences of genomic research in four main areas (Genetics Home Reference, 2018b):

- Privacy and fairness in the use of genetic information, including the potential for genetic discrimination in employment and insurance.
- The integration of new genetic technologies, such as genetic testing, into the practice of clinical medicine.
- Ethical issues surrounding the design and conduct of genetic research with people, including the process of informed consent.
- The education of health care professionals, policy makers, students, and the public about genetics and the complex issues that result from genomic research.

Both ELSI programs have excellent websites that include much educational information, as well as links to other informative sites (https://www.genome.gov/elsi/; www.ornl.gov/sci/techresources/Human_Genome/elsi/elsi.shtml). The major risk associated with genetic testing concerns what happens with the information gained through testing. It may result in increased anxiety and altered family relationships; it may be difficult to keep confidential; and it may result in discrimination and stigmatization. More important, there is a large gap between the ability to test for a genetic condition and the ability to treat that same condition. Informed consent is difficult to ensure when some of the outcomes, benefits, and risks of genetic testing remain unknown. Also, many of the tests being used continue to be imperfect—few have a 100% detection rate. Individuals and families who receive false-positive results (the test results indicate that a person or fetus is affected by a genetic condition when he or she is not) may terminate an unaffected pregnancy or undergo unwarranted extreme measures such as bilateral prophylactic mastectomy. Individuals and families who receive false-negative results (the test results indicate that a person or fetus is not affected by a genetic condition when he or she is) may fail to follow surveillance strategies designed to improve their health outcomes because they have been falsely reassured that they are not at increased risk for a specific condition.

Factors Influencing the Decision to Undergo Genetic Testing

The decision to undergo genetic testing is seldom autonomous and based solely on the needs and preferences of the individual being tested. Instead, it is often a decision based on feelings of responsibility and commitment to others. For example, a woman who is receiving treatment for breast cancer may undergo BRCA1/BRCA2 mutation testing not because she wants to find out if she carries a BRCA1 or BRCA2 mutation but, instead, because her two unaffected sisters have asked her to be tested and she feels a sense of responsibility and commitment to them. A female airline pilot with a family history of HD, who has no desire to find out if she has the gene mutation associated with HD, may undergo mutation analysis for HD because she feels she has an obligation to her family, her employer, and the people who fly with her.

Decisions about genetic testing are shaped and, in many instances, constrained by factors such as social norms where care is received, and socioeconomic status. Most pregnant women in the United States now have at least one ultrasound examination, many undergo some type of multiple-marker screening, and a growing number undergo other types of prenatal testing. The range of prenatal testing options available to a pregnant woman and her family may vary, based on where the pregnant woman receives prenatal care and her socioeconomic status. Certain types of prenatal testing may not be available in smaller communities and rural settings (e.g., chorionic villus sampling and fluorescent in situ hybridization [FISH] analysis). In addition, certain types of genetic testing may not be offered in conservative medical communities (e.g., preimplantation diagnosis). Some types of genetic testing are expensive and typically not covered by health insurance. Because of this, these tests may be available only to a relatively small number of individuals and families—those who can afford to pay for them.

Cultural and ethnic differences also have a significant impact on decisions about genetic testing. When prenatal diagnosis was first introduced, the principal constituency was a self-selected group of Caucasian, well-informed, middle- to upper-class women. Today the widespread use of genetic testing has introduced prenatal testing to women who had not previously considered genetic services. The fact that many of the women currently undergoing prenatal testing may not share mainstream U.S. views about the role of medicine and prenatal care, the meaning of *disability,* or how to respond to scientific risks and uncertainties, further amplifies the complexity of ethical issues associated with prenatal testing.

The genetic testing experience raises fundamental questions about the mutual obligations of kin. Are individuals morally obligated to alert extended family members about inherited health risks? Conversely, do extended family members have a moral obligation to participate in research designed to determine genetic risk when unwanted information about them may be generated in the process? Another important question that must be considered is "Whose gene is it?" This question is likely to stimulate a great deal of debate, especially in the area of preimplantation genetic diagnosis (when one or both parents has a known genetic abnormality and testing is performed on an embryo to determine if it also carries a genetic abnormality).

Clinical Genetics

Genetic Transmission

Human development is a complicated process that depends on the systematic unraveling of instructions found in the genetic material of the egg and the sperm. Development from conception to birth of a healthy normally developing baby occurs without incident in most cases; however, findings from a March of Dimes Global Report on Birth Defects (2006) revealed that each year 8 million children (6% of total births) are born with a serious birth defect. In the United States, birth defects occur in 1 of every 33 newborns (CDC, 2018). Factors known to increase the risk of having a baby with a birth defect include advanced maternal age, personal or family history of a birth defect, taking certain medications while pregnant, medical conditions such as diabetes mellitus and obesity, and use of recreational drugs or alcohol during pregnancy (ACOG, 2018b).

Genes and Chromosomes

The hereditary material carried in the nucleus of each of the somatic cells determines an individual's characteristics. This material, called DNA, forms threadlike strands known as *chromosomes.* Each chromosome is composed of many smaller segments of DNA referred to as *genes.* Genes or combinations of genes contain coded information that determines an individual's unique characteristics. The code is found in the specific linear order of the molecules that combine to form the strands of DNA. Genes control both the types of proteins that are made and the rate at which they are produced. Genes never act in isolation; they always interact with other genes and the environment.

All normal human somatic cells contain 46 chromosomes arranged as 23 pairs of homologous (matched) chromosomes; one chromosome of each pair is inherited from each parent. Twenty-two of the pairs of matched chormosomes, called **autosomes**, control most body traits. The twenty-third pair is called the sex chromosomes. The larger female chromosome is called the *X;* the smaller male chromosome is the *Y.* Whereas the Y chromosome is primarily concerned with sex determination, the X chromosome contains genes that are involved in much more than sex determination. Generally, the presence of a Y chromosome causes an embryo to develop as a male; in the absence of a Y chromosome, the individual develops as a female. Thus in a normal female, the homologous pair of sex chromosomes are XX, and in a normal male, the homologous pair are XY.

Homologous chromosomes (except the X and Y chromosomes in males) have the same number and arrangement of genes. In other words, if one chromosome has a gene for hair color, its partner chromosome also will have a gene for hair color and these hair-color genes will have the same loci or be located in the same place on the two chromosomes. Although both genes code for hair color, they may not code for the same hair color. Genes at corresponding loci on homologous chromosomes that code for different forms or variations of the same trait are called **alleles**. An individual having two copies of the same allele for a given trait is said to be **homozygous** for that trait. With two different alleles, the individual is **heterozygous** for the trait.

The term **genotype** typically is used to refer to the genetic makeup of an individual when discussing a specific gene pair, but at times, genotype is used to refer to an individual's entire genetic makeup or all the genes that the individual can pass on to future generations. **Phenotype** refers to the observable expression of an individual's genotype, such as physical features, a biochemical or molecular trait, and even a psychologic trait. A trait or disorder is considered *dominant* if it is expressed or phenotypically apparent when only one copy of the gene is present. It is considered *recessive* if it is expressed only when two copies of the alleles associated with the trait are present.

As more is learned about genetics and genomics, the concepts of dominance and recessivity have become more complex, especially in X-linked disorders. For example, traits considered to be recessive may be expressed even when only one copy of a gene located on the X chromosome is present. This occurs frequently in males because males have only one X chromosome, thus they have only one copy of the genes located on the X chromosome. Whichever gene is present on the one X chromosome determines which trait is expressed. Females, conversely, have two X chromosomes, so they have two copies of the genes located on the X chromosome. However, in any female somatic cell, only one X chromosome is functioning (otherwise there would be inequality in gene dosage between males and females). This process, known as *X-inactivation* or the *Lyon hypothesis,* is generally a random occurrence. That is, there is a 50-50 chance as to whether the maternal X or the paternal X is inactivated. Occasionally the percentage of cells that have the X with an abnormal or mutant gene is very high. This helps explain why hemophilia, an X-linked recessive disorder, can clinically manifest itself in a female known to be a heterozygous carrier (a female who has only one copy of the gene mutation). It also helps explain why traditional methods of carrier detection are less effective for X-linked recessive disorders; the possible range for enzyme activity values can vary greatly, depending on which X chromosome is inactivated.

Chromosomal Abnormalities

Chromosomal abnormalities are a major cause of reproductive loss, congenital problems, and gynecologic disorders. Errors resulting in chromosomal abnormalities can occur in mitosis (cell division occurring in somatic cells that results in two identical daughter cells containing a diploid number of chromosomes) or meiosis (division of a sex cell into two and four haploid cells). These errors can occur in either the autosomes or the sex chromosomes. Even without the presence of obvious structural malformations, small deviations in chromosomes can cause problems in fetal development.

The pictorial analysis of the number, form, and size of an individual's chromosomes is known as a karyotype. Cells from any nucleated, replicating body tissue (not red blood cells, nerves, or muscles) can be used. The most commonly used tissues are white blood cells and fetal cells in amniotic fluid. The cells are grown in a culture and arrested when they are in metaphase (during metaphase, the chromosomes are condensed and visible with a light microscope), and then the cells are dropped onto a slide. This breaks the cell membranes and spreads the chromosomes, making them easier to visualize. Next, the cells are stained with special stains (e.g., Giemsa stain) that create striping or "banding" patterns. These patterns aid in the analysis because they are consistent from person to person. Once the chromosome spreads are photographed or scanned by a computer, they are cut out and arranged in a specific numeric order according to their length and shape. The chromosomes are numbered from largest to smallest, 1 to 22, and the sex chromosomes are designated by the letter X or Y. Each chromosome is divided into two "arms" designated by p (short arm) and q (long arm). A female karyotype is designated as 46,XX, and a male karyotype is designated as 46,XY. Fig. 3.1 illustrates the chromosomes in a body cell and a karyotype.

Autosomal Abnormalities

Autosomal abnormalities involve differences in the number or structure of autosomal chromosomes (pairs 1 to 22). They result from unequal distribution of the genetic material during gamete (egg and sperm) formation.

Abnormalities of chromosome number. A euploid cell is a cell with the correct or normal number of chromosomes within the cell. Because most gametes are haploid (1N, 23 chromosomes) and most somatic cells are diploid (2N, 46 chromosomes), they are both considered euploid cells. Deviations from the correct number of chromosomes per cell can be one of two types: (1) polyploidy, in which the deviation is an exact multiple of the haploid number of chromosomes or one chromosome set (23 chromosomes), or (2) aneuploidy, in which the numeric deviation is not an exact multiple of the haploid set. A triploid (3N) cell is an example of a polyploidy. It has 69 chromosomes. A tetraploid (4N) cell, also an example of a polyploidy, has 92 chromosomes.

Aneuploidy is the most commonly identified chromosome abnormality in humans and the leading genetic cause of intellectual disability. A monosomy is the product of the union between a normal gamete and a gamete that is missing a chromosome. Monosomic individuals have only 45 chromosomes in each of their cells. The product of the union of a normal gamete with a gamete containing an extra chromosome is a trisomy. The most common autosomal aneuploid conditions involve trisomies. Trisomic individuals have 47 chromosomes in most or all of their cells.

The vast majority of trisomies occur during oogenesis (the process by which a premeiotic female germ cell divides into a mature egg); the incidence of these types of chromosomal errors increases exponentially with advancing maternal age. Although variation exists among trisomies with regard to the parent and stage of origin of the extra chromosome, most trisomies are maternal meiosis I (MI) errors. This means that most trisomies are caused by nondisjunction during the first meiotic division. The first meiotic division involves the segregation of homologous or similar chromosomes. One pair of chromosomes fails to separate. One resulting cell contains both chromosomes, and the other contains none. The fact that most trisomies are maternal MI errors is not that surprising, because maternal MI occurs over a long

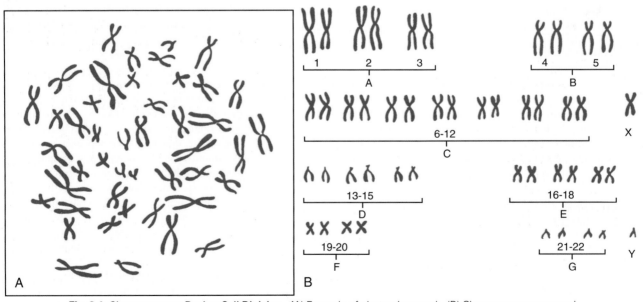

Fig. 3.1 Chromosomes During Cell Division. (A) Example of photomicrograph. (B) Chromosomes arranged in karyotype; female and male sex-determining chromosomes.

time span. It is initiated in precursor cells during fetal development, but it is not completed until the time those cells undergo ovulation after menarche.

The most common trisomy abnormality is DS. Approximately 1 in every 691 newborns has DS; there are over 400,000 individuals with DS living in the United States (CDC, 2018; http://ndsccenter.org; www.ndss.org). Approximately 95% of individuals with DS have trisomy 21 (nondisjunction) or an extra chromosome 21 (47,XX+21, female with DS; or 47, XY+21, male with DS). Another type of DS, translocation, occurs when extra chromosome 21 material is present in every cell of the individual, but it is attached to another chromosome. This type of DS affects approximately 3% to 4% of individuals with DS. In the third type of DS, mosaicism, extra chromosome 21 material is found in some but not all of the cells. Only 1% to 2% of individuals with DS have mosaicism.

Although the clinical presentation of DS is complex and variable, all individuals with DS have some level of intellectual disability; they also are at increased risk for certain health concerns (e.g., congenital heart defects, otitis media, obstructive sleep apnea, eye disease) (Bull, 2018; Martin, Smith, & Breatnach, et al., 2018). Common characteristics seen in individuals with DS are:

- Oblique palpebral fissures or an upward slant to the eyes
- Epicanthal folds or small skinfolds on the inner corners of the eyes
- Small, white, crescent-shaped spots on the irises called Brushfield spots
- A flat facial profile–often includes a depressed nasal bridge and a small nose
- Enlargement of the tongue in relationship to size of the mouth
- Small ears, which may be abnormally shaped or abnormally rotated
- Short, broad hands with a fifth finger that has one flexion crease instead of two

- A single deep crease across the center of the palm, often referred to as a simian crease
- Excessive space between the large and second toes
- Hyperflexibility, an excessive ability to extend the joints
- Muscle hypotonia or low muscle tone

Some individuals with DS have many of these characteristics, but others have only a few. Fig. 3.2 is a picture of an infant with DS who has some of the characteristics commonly associated with this genetic disorder (see "Nursing Care Plan").

Although the risk for having a child with DS increases with maternal age (incidence is approximately 1 in 1200 for a 25-year-old woman; 1 in 350 for a 35-year-old woman; and 1 in 10 for a 49-year-old woman), children with DS can be born to mothers of any age: 80% of children with DS are born to mothers younger than 35 years (National Down Syndrome Society, 2019). The risk for a mother over age 40 of having a second child with DS is about 1% (Sole-Smith, 2014).

Other autosomal trisomies that maternity nurses might see are trisomy 18 (Edwards syndrome) and trisomy 13 (Patau syndrome). Trisomy 18 is more common than trisomy 13; it occurs in about 1 of 6000 live births (Trisomy 18 Foundation, 2018) versus 1 of 16,000 live births for trisomy 13 (Genetics Home Reference, 2019d). Infants with trisomy 18 and trisomy 13 usually have severe to profound intellectual disabilities. Although both conditions have a poor prognosis, with the vast majority of affected infants dying before they reach their first birthday, a growing number of infants with these trisomies are living into their 20s and 30s (Trisomy 18 Foundation).

Infants with trisomy 18 may exhibit more than 130 different anomalies, but some of the major phenotypic features and medical complications are small for gestational age or low birth weight; craniofacial abnormalities including cleft lip and/or palate, small mouth, and small jaw; weak cry; feeding difficulties; cardiac malformations; central nervous system manifestations including hypertonia, seizures, and apnea;

⊚ NURSING CARE PLAN

The Family Living With a Neonate With Down Syndrome

Client Problem	Expected Outcome	Nursing Interventions	Rationales
Need for health teaching related to birth of a neonate with Down Syndrome	The parents will verbalize accurate information about Down Syndrome, including implications for future pregnancies.	Assess knowledge base of couple regarding the clinical signs and symptoms of Down Syndrome.	To correct any misconceptions and establish basis for teaching plan.
		Provide information throughout the genetic evaluation regarding risk status and clinical signs and symptoms of Down Syndrome.	To give parents a realistic picture of neonate's defects and assist with decision making for future pregnancies.
		Assist parents to see and describe normal aspects of infant.	To promote bonding/attachment.
Decreased ability to cope related to diagnosis of Down Syndrome as evidenced by parents' statements of guilt and shame	The parents will express an increased number of positive statements regarding their neonate with Down Syndrome.	Assist parents to list strengths and coping strategies that have been helpful in past situations.	To use appropriate strategies during this situational crisis.
		Encourage expression of feelings using therapeutic communication.	To decrease feelings of guilt and gradually increase feelings of positive self-esteem.
		Refer for further counseling as needed.	To provide more in-depth and ongoing support.
Social isolation related to full-time caretaking responsibilities for a neonate with Down Syndrome	Parents will describe a plan to use resources to prevent social isolation.	Facilitate interaction with family members and other support persons.	To facilitate effective communication and trust.
		Assist parents to identify potential caregiving resources.	To permit parents to return to a routine at home.
		Identify appropriate referrals for home care.	To provide continuity of care.

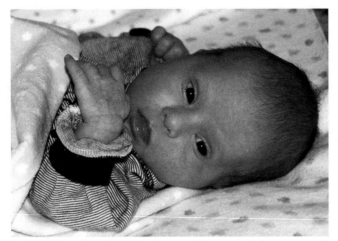

Fig. 3.2 Infant with Down Syndrome. Note upward slant to eyes, flat nasal bridge, slightly protruding tongue, and mottled skin. (Courtesy Thomas and Christie Coghill, Clayton, NC.)

and extremity malformations such as small fingernails and toenails, clenched fist with index finger overlapping the third finger, and rocker-bottom feet.

As with trisomy 18, infants with trisomy 13 have numerous abnormalities, the most common of which are central nervous system anomalies, visual abnormalities, microcephaly (small head), absent nasal bridge, cleft lip and palate, holoprosencephaly (one large eyelike structure in the center of the face due to fusion of the developing eyes), capillary hemangiomas, cardiac defects, extremity deformities including polydactyly (extra fingers or toes), renal abnormalities, and genital abnormalities.

Health care professionals can assist families who receive a prenatal diagnosis of trisomy 18 or trisomy 13 by providing up-to-date written and reliable web resources and connecting them with support groups for parents who have received a similar diagnosis (Wallace, Gilvary, Smith, & Dolan, et al., 2018). Two such groups are the Trisomy 18 Foundation (2018) and Support Organization for Trisomy 18, 13, and Related Disorders (SOFT, 2018). Families who choose to continue a pregnancy with a diagnosis of trisomy 18/13 usually want to receive expectant management with palliative care (Winn, Acharya, Peterson, & Leuthner, et al., 2018). At least half of the time, a live birth can be expected.

Nondisjunction can also occur during mitosis. If this occurs early in development, when cell lines are forming, the individual has a mixture of cells, some with a normal number of chromosomes and others either missing a chromosome or containing an extra chromosome. This condition is known as *mosaicism*. The most common form of mosaicism in autosomes is mosaic DS (http://www.mosaicdownsyndrome.com/).

Depending on when the nondisjunction occurs during development, different body tissues will have different numbers of chromosomes. The clinical characteristics of DS may be mild or with varying degrees of severity, depending on the number and location of the abnormal cells. An individual with mosaic DS may have normal intelligence. Mosaicism of both trisomy 18 and trisomy 13 has been reported. Both situations usually lead to a partial clinical expression of the phenotype. Infants who have mosaic trisomy 18 or trisomy 13 usually have a longer life span than infants with these disorders who are not mosaic.

Abnormalities of chromosome structure. Structural abnormalities can occur in any chromosome. Types of structural abnormalities include translocation, duplication, deletion, microdeletion, and inversion. Translocation results when there is an exchange of chromosomal material between two chromosomes. Exposure to certain drugs, viruses, and radiation can cause translocations, but often they arise for no apparent reason.

The two major types of translocation are reciprocal and robertsonian. Reciprocal translocations are the most common. In a reciprocal translocation, either the parts of the two chromosomes are exchanged equally (balanced translocation) or a part of a chromosome is transferred to a different chromosome, creating an unbalanced translocation because there is extra chromosomal material—extra of one chromosome but correct amount or deficient amount of the other chromosome. In a balanced translocation, the individual is phenotypically normal because there is no extra chromosome material; it is just rearranged. In an unbalanced translocation, the individual will be both genotypically and phenotypically abnormal.

In a robertsonian translocation, the short arms (p arms) of two different acrocentric chromosomes (chromosomes with very short p arms) break, leaving sticky ends that then cause the two long arms (q arms) to stick together. This forms a new, large chromosome that is made of the two long arms. The individual with a balanced robertsonian translocation has 45 chromosomes. Because the short arm of acrocentric chromosomes contains genes for ribosomal RNA and these genes are represented elsewhere, the individual usually does not show any symptoms. The individual may produce an unbalanced gamete (sperm or egg with too many or too few genes). This can lead to reproductive difficulties such as miscarriages or birth defects. Of all cases of DS, 3% to 4% occur because one parent has a balanced robertsonian translocation, a translocation between chromosomes 21 and 14. The child with this type of DS has an unbalanced translocation because there is an extra part of chromosome 21. The second most common robertsonian translocation occurs between chromosomes 13 and 14 (Homfray & Farndon, 2015).

In duplication, there is an extra chromosomal segment within the same homologous or another nonhomologous chromosome. Clinical findings are highly variable and depend on which of the chromosomal segments are involved.

Deletions result in the loss of chromosomal material and partial monosomy for the chromosome involved. Loss of chromosomal material at the end of a chromosome is referred to as a terminal deletion. In contrast, loss of chromosomal material anywhere else in the chromosome is called an interstitial deletion. The resulting clinical phenotype of either a terminal or an interstitial deletion will depend on how much of the chromosome has been lost and the number and function of the genes contained in the missing segment. Microdeletions are deletions too small to be detected by standard cytogenetic techniques. These deletions can be identified with FISH analysis. FISH technology uses a single-stranded piece of DNA with a fluorescent label that will adhere to its complementary piece of DNA in the chromosome being investigated.

Whenever a portion of a chromosome is deleted from one chromosome and added to another, the gamete produced may have either extra copies of genes or too few copies. The clinical effects produced may be mild or severe depending on the amount of genetic material involved. Two of the more common conditions are the deletion of the short arm of chromosome 5 (*cri du chat syndrome*) and the deletion of the long arm of chromosome 18. Cri du chat syndrome, so named after the typical mewing cry of the affected infant, causes severe intellectual disability with microcephaly and unusual facial appearance. Deletion of the long arm of chromosome 18 causes severe psychomotor delay with multiple organ malformations. *Velocardiofacial syndrome*, characterized by cardiac and craniofacial abnormalities, is an example of a microdeletion. In this syndrome, a very small piece of the long arm of chromosome 22 is missing.

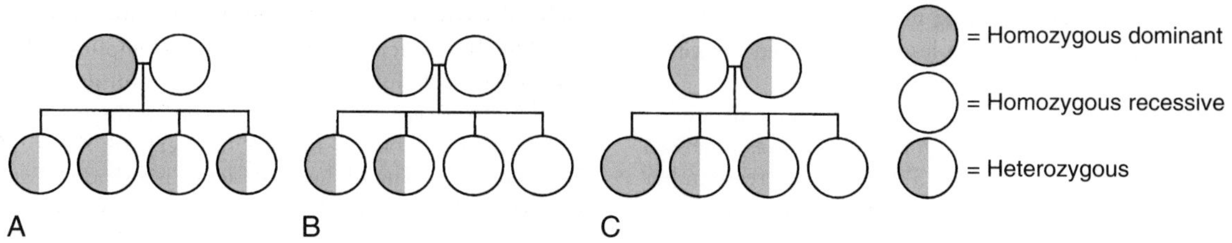

Fig. 3.3 Possible Offspring in Three Types of Matings. (A) Homozygous-dominant parent and homozygous-recessive parent. Children all heterozygous, displaying dominant trait. (B) Heterozygous parent and homozygous-recessive parent. Children 50% heterozygous, displaying dominant trait; 50% homozygous, displaying recessive trait. (C) Both parents heterozygous. Children 25% homozygous, displaying dominant trait; 25% homozygous, displaying recessive trait; 50% heterozygous, displaying dominant trait.

Microdeletions in the Y chromosome have been found in men with infertility problems.

Inversions are deviations in which a portion of the chromosome has been rearranged in reverse order. Few birth defects have been attributed to the presence of inversions, but it is suspected that inversions may be responsible for problems with infertility and miscarriages. Some inversions can be detected prenatally, and they do not occur randomly.

Sex Chromosome Abnormalities

Several sex chromosome abnormalities are caused by nondisjunction during gametogenesis in either parent. The most common deviation in females is *Turner syndrome,* or monosomy X (45,X). The affected female exhibits juvenile external genitalia with undeveloped ovaries. She is short in stature and often has webbing of the neck, a low hairline in the back, low-set ears, and lymphedema of her hands and feet. Intelligence may be impaired. There are many health concerns associated with Turner syndrome (e.g., heart defects and kidney problems). Most affected embryos miscarry spontaneously. Typically, it is the paternal X or Y that is lost. Turner syndrome is a common cause of infertility (Genetics Home Reference, 2019e).

The most common deviation in males is *Klinefelter syndrome,* or trisomy XXY (Genetics Home Reference, 2019b). The affected male typically has small testes that do not produce an adequate amount of testosterone. The shortage of testosterone usually leads to delayed or incomplete puberty, breast enlargement (gynecomastia), a reduction of facial and body hair, and infertility. Children with Klinefelter syndrome often have learning disabilities and delayed speech and language. Children and adults with Klinefelter syndrome tend to be taller than their peers. Males who have mosaic Klinefelter syndrome may be fertile.

Patterns of Genetic Transmission

Heritable characteristics are those that can be passed on to offspring. The patterns by which genetic material is transmitted to the next generation are affected by the number of genes involved in the expression of the trait. Many phenotypic characteristics result from two or more genes on different chromosomes acting together (referred to as *multifactorial inheritance*); others are controlled by a single gene (*unifactorial inheritance).* Specialists in genetics (e.g., geneticists, genetic counselors, and nurses with advanced expertise in genetics) predict the probability of the presence of an abnormal gene from the known occurrence of the trait in the individual's family and the known patterns by which the trait is inherited.

Multifactorial Inheritance

Most common congenital malformations result from multifactorial inheritance, a combination of genetic and environmental factors. Examples are cleft lip, cleft palate, congenital heart disease, neural tube

defects, and pyloric stenosis. Each malformation can range from mild to severe, depending on the number of genes for the defect present or the amount of environmental influence. A neural tube defect can range from spina bifida (a bony defect in the lumbar region of the vertebrae with little or no neurologic impairment) to anencephaly (absence of brain development, which is always fatal). Some malformations occur more often in one sex. For example, pyloric stenosis and cleft lip are more common in males, and cleft palate is more common in females.

Unifactorial Inheritance

If a single gene controls a particular trait or disorder, its pattern of inheritance is referred to as *unifactorial mendelian* or *single-gene inheritance.* The number of single-gene disorders far exceeds the number of chromosomal abnormalities. Potential patterns of inheritance for single-gene disorders include autosomal dominant, autosomal recessive, and X-linked dominant and recessive modes of inheritance (Fig. 3.3).

Autosomal dominant inheritance. Autosomal dominant inheritance disorders are those in which only one copy of a variant allele is needed for phenotypic expression. The variant allele may be a result of a mutation—a spontaneous and permanent change in the normal gene structure in which case the disorder occurs for the first time in the family. Usually an affected individual comes from multiple generations having the disorder. An affected parent who is heterozygous for the trait has a 50% chance of passing the variant allele to each offspring (see Fig. 3.3B and C). There is a vertical pattern of inheritance (i.e., there is no skipping of generations; if an individual has an autosomal dominant disorder such as HD, so must one of his or her parents). Males and females are equally affected.

Autosomal dominant disorders are not always expressed with the same severity of symptoms. For example, a woman who has an autosomal dominant disorder may show few symptoms and may not become aware of her diagnosis until after she gives birth to a severely affected child. Predicting whether an offspring will have a minor or severe abnormality is not possible. Sometimes an individual can acquire a de novo mutation (new mutation that spontaneously occurred in a gene carried by an individual germ cell) that can result in an autosomal dominant disorder. Examples of autosomal dominant disorders are FVL, HD, Marfan syndrome, neurofibromatosis, myotonic dystrophy, Stickler syndrome, Treacher Collins syndrome, and achondroplasia (dwarfism).

Factor V Leiden is the most common inherited risk factor for primary and recurrent venous thromboembolisms (Genetic Home Reference, 2019a; Kujovich, 2018; National Blood Clot Alliance, nd). It is an autosomal dominant disorder that markedly increases an individual's risk for deep vein thrombosis (blood clots in the large veins of the legs) and pulmonary emboli (blood clots that travel through the bloodstream and become embedded in the lungs), especially if the individual is a woman who (a) uses oral contraceptives, (b) is pregnant, or (c) is on hormone replacement therapy during menopause. FVL is due to a mutation in the factor V gene, which leads to activated protein C (APC) resistance.

Women who carry the FVL mutation should not take oral contraceptives. If a pregnant woman is heterozygous for FVL (has inherited one copy of the FVL mutation), she has a 5- to 8-fold increase in her chance of developing venous blood clots, but her risk increases by a factor as high as 17- to 34-fold if she is homozygous (has inherited two copies of the FVL mutation). Currently no consensus exists regarding the optimal management of FVL during pregnancy (Kujovich, 2018). Pregnant women with FVL need to undergo an individualized risk assessment so that treatment decisions about anticoagulation can be based on the number and type of thrombophilic defects, coexisting risk factors, and personal or family history of thrombosis.

FVL can be accurately detected with genetic testing, but the most cost-effective way to screen for FVL is taking a careful individual and family history. Women with a personal or close family history of venous blood clots, pulmonary emboli, early onset and recurrent preeclampsia, recurrent fetal growth restriction, recurrent pregnancy loss and stillbirth, or placental abruption should be screened for FVL.

Autosomal recessive inheritance. Autosomal recessive inheritance disorders are those in which both genes of a pair associated with the disorder must be abnormal for the disorder to be expressed. Heterozygous individuals have only one variant allele and are unaffected clinically because their normal gene (wild-type allele) overshadows the variant allele. They are known as *carriers* of the recessive trait. Because these recessive traits are inherited by generations of the same family, an increased incidence of the disorder occurs in consanguineous matings (closely related parents). For the trait to be expressed, two carriers must each contribute a variant allele to the offspring (see Fig. 3.3C). The chance of the trait occurring in each child is 25%. A clinically normal offspring may be a carrier of the gene. Autosomal recessive disorders have a horizontal pattern of inheritance rather than the vertical pattern seen with autosomal dominant disorders. That is, autosomal recessive disorders are usually observed in one or more siblings but not in earlier generations. Males and females are equally affected. Most recessive disorders tend to have severe clinical manifestations, and affected offspring may not be able to, or choose not to, reproduce. If they do, all their offspring will at least be carriers for the disorder. Most inborn errors of metabolism (IEMs), such as phenylketonuria, galactosemia, maple syrup urine disease, Tay-Sachs disease, sickle cell anemia, and CF, are autosomal recessive inherited disorders.

Inborn errors of metabolism. More than 1000 *IEMs* have been recognized. IEMs are relatively rare, but collectively, the incidence of IEMs is estimated to be as high as 1 in 800 live births (Weiner, 2017). The overall incidence and frequency for individual IEMs vary based on racial and ethnic composition of the population. IEMs occur when a gene mutation reduces the efficiency of encoded enzymes to a level at which normal metabolism cannot occur. Defective enzyme action interrupts the normal series of chemical reactions from the affected point onward. The result may be an accumulation of a damaging product, such as phenylalanine in PKU, or the absence of a necessary product, such as the lack of melanin in albinism caused by lack of tyrosinase. Diagnostic and carrier testing is available for a growing number of IEMs. In addition, many U.S. states have started screening for specific IEMs as part of their expanded newborn screening programs using tandem mass spectrometry. However, many of the deaths caused by IEMs are the result of enzyme variants not currently screened for in many of the newborn screening programs.

Phenylketonuria is a relatively uncommon autosomal recessive disorder. A deficiency in the liver enzyme phenylalanine hydroxylase results in failure to metabolize the amino acid phenylalanine, allowing its metabolites to accumulate in the blood. The incidence of this disorder ranges from 1 in every 10,000 to 250,000 births (Weiner, 2017). The highest incidence is found in Caucasians (from northern Europe and the United States). It is rarely seen in Jewish, African, or Japanese populations. Screening for PKU is routinely performed as part of state-mandated newborn screening in the United States (see Chapter 24).

Tay-Sachs disease is a lipid storage disease that occurs more commonly in Ashkenazi Jews and French Canadians from Quebec. It results from a deficiency in hexosaminidase. Until age 4 to 6 months, infants with Tay-Sachs disease appear normal; their facial features are considered very beautiful. Then the clinical symptoms appear: apathy and regression in motor and social development and decreased vision. Death occurs between ages 3 and 4 years. Only supportive treatment exists for Tay-Sachs disease.

X-linked dominant inheritance. X-linked dominant inheritance disorders occur in males and heterozygous females, but because of X inactivation, affected females are usually less severely affected than affected males and they are more likely to transmit the variant allele to their offspring. Heterozygous females (females who have one wild-type allele and one variant allele) have a 50% chance of transmitting the variant allele to each offspring. The variant allele is often lethal in affected males since, unlike affected females, they have no normal gene (wild-type allele). Mating of an affected male and an unaffected female is uncommon as a result of the tendency for the variant allele to be lethal in affected males. Relatively few X-linked dominant disorders have been identified. Two examples are vitamin D–resistant rickets and Rett syndrome.

X-linked recessive inheritance. Abnormal genes for X-linked recessive inheritance disorders are carried on the X chromosome. Females may be heterozygous or homozygous for traits carried on the X chromosome because they have two X chromosomes. Males are hemizygous because they have only one X chromosome, which carries genes with no alleles on the Y chromosome. Therefore X-linked recessive disorders are most commonly manifested in the male with the abnormal gene on his single X chromosome. Hemophilia, color blindness, and Duchenne muscular dystrophy are X-linked recessive disorders.

The male with an X-linked recessive disorder receives the disease-associated allele from his carrier mother on her affected X chromosome. Female carriers (those heterozygous for the trait) have a 50% probability of transmitting the disease-associated allele to each offspring. An affected male can pass the disease-associated allele to his daughters but not to his sons. The daughters will be carriers of the trait if they receive a normal gene on the X chromosome from their mother. They will be affected only if they receive a disease-associated allele on the X chromosome from both their mother and their father.

Fragile X syndrome (FXS), the leading inherited form of intellectual disability and autism spectrum disorder, is an X-linked disorder that has a complex pattern of inheritance (Hagerman, Berry-Kravis, Hazlett, et al., 2017). FXS is almost exclusively caused by a trinucleotide repeat expansion (CGG) at a "fragile site" on the long arm of the X chromosome. Most people have 5 to 40 CGG repeats. Individuals with FXS have more than 200 CGG repeats. The abnormally expanded CGG segment inactivates or silences the FMR1 (fragile X intellectual disability) gene, which prevents the gene from producing a protein called fragile X intellectual disability protein. Loss of this protein leads to the characteristic physical features (large ears, long face, prominent forehead, protruding ears, hypermobile joints, and macroorchidism and behavior problems (hyperactivity, impulsivity, and anxiety), as well as poor language development and seizures. Males and females can be affected by FXS, but because males have only one X chromosome, a CGG repeat expansion on one X is likely to affect males more severely than females. Also, the degree of intellectual disability tends to be milder and more variable in females than in males. Unlike DS, FXS is not generally detectable through a physical examination at birth. Delays and behavioral abnormalities gradually become apparent during the first 2 years of life, but ultimately the diagnosis of FXS can be verified only through DNA testing.

Individuals with more than 55 but fewer than 200 CGG repeats are said to be permutation carriers. These individuals were originally thought to be unaffected, but research has shown that about 20% of adult carrier females may develop premature ovarian failure (cessation of menses before 40 years of age). Elderly male permutation carriers may manifest fragile X–associated tremor/ataxia syndrome (FXTAS) (for further information on fragile X, see https://fragilex.org/).

Cancer Genomics

Gene mutations that can lead to cancer. There are three main ways that people acquire gene mutations that can lead to cancer. The first is from the environment. Known factors in the environment that cause cancer are ultraviolet (UV) light (skin cancer) and tobacco smoke (lung cancer). The second way that people acquire mutations is by chance. Normal metabolic processes can generate chemicals that damage DNA. Third, people inherit mutations from their parents; harmful hereditary mutations are thought to be a major factor in about 5% to 10% of all cancers (National Cancer Institute [NCI], 2013).

The two main types of genes that have been recognized as playing a critical role in the development of cancer are *oncogenes* and *tumor suppressor genes*. Oncogenes are mutated forms of proto-oncogenes. The main functions of proto-oncogenes are to encourage and promote normal growth and development. When proto-oncogenes mutate to become carcinogenic oncogenes, the result is excessive cell multiplication. The activation of oncogenes has been compared to a jammed accelerator in a car. Most mutations of proto-oncogenes are acquired mutations, such as mutations in the *KIT* gene which are thought to cause most cases of gastrointestinal stromal tumor (GIST). This type of cancer can be treated with drugs that target the KIT gene, such as imatinib (Gleevec). Two examples of inherited mutations of proto-oncogenes are ERBB2, located on chromosome 13, and KRAS2, located on chromosome 12. ERBB2 is involved in breast, ovarian, lung, gastric, and salivary gland cancers. KRAS2 is involved in breast, pancreatic, thyroid, colorectal, bladder, and lung cancers, as well as acute myeloid leukemia.

Tumor suppressor genes normally function to inhibit or "put the brakes on" the cell growth and division cycle. They function to prevent the development of tumors. Mutations in tumor suppressor genes cause the cell to ignore one or more of the components of the network of inhibitory signals, removing the brakes from the cell cycle. This results in a higher rate of uncontrolled growth: cancer. Acquired mutations of the tumor protein p53 gene appear in a wide range of cancers, including lung, colorectal, and breast cancer. Examples of inherited tumor suppressor genes include APC, located on chromosome 5 and involved with familial adenomatous polyposis (FAP) of the colon; BRCA1, located on chromosome 17 and associated with hereditary breast cancer and ovarian cancer; and RB1, found on chromosome 13 and involved with familial retinoblastoma.

Hereditary breast and ovarian cancer. Breast cancer is a common disease and a central concern in women's health. Hereditary mutations or variations play a key role in approximately 5% to 10% of all breast and ovarian cancers. Another 15% to 20% of female breast cancers occur in women who have a family history of breast and ovarian cancer, but do not carry a mutation in one of the genes that are known to be strongly associated with breast and ovarian cancer susceptibility.

A woman's lifetime risk of developing breast and/or ovarian cancer is greatly increased if she inherits a harmful BRCA1 or BRCA2 mutation (National Cancer Institute, 2018a). BRCA mutations are inherited in an autosomal dominant pattern, thus each offspring of an individual found to carry a BRCA mutation has a 50% chance of inheriting the same mutation. According to estimates of lifetime risk, approximately 12% of women in the general population will develop breast cancer sometime during their lifetime, compared to about 72% of women who inherit a harmful BRCA1 mutation and about 69% who inherit a harmful BRCA2 mutation. Even though only about 6% of the men who carry a harmful BRCA mutation develop breast cancer, men who carry a harmful BRCA mutation have a 50% chance of passing the mutation on to their offspring. As far as lifetime risk estimates for ovarian cancer, about 1.3% of women in the general population will be diagnosed with ovarian cancer during their lifetime, compared with 44% of women who inherit a harmful BRCA1 mutation and about 17% of women who inherit a harmful BRCA2 mutation. Carriers of BRCA1 mutations may also be at increased risk for pancreatic, prostate, peritoneal, and uterine tube cancer.

Genetic testing for HBOC has been commercially available in the United States since 1995. Some of these tests look for a specific harmful BRCA1 or BRAC2 mutation that has been inherited by another family member, while others check for harmful mutations in both genes. In addition, multigene (panel) testing that uses next-generation sequencing is available. Although some insurance policies cover these types of tests, others do not. Individuals who are considering undergoing BRCA1 and BRCA2 testing are encouraged to check their insurance coverage prior to undergoing testing. Women newly diagnosed with breast cancer are increasingly being asked to consider undergoing BRCA1 and BRCA2 testing before they make decisions about their treatment options because there is growing evidence that a woman's short-term risk of developing a second breast cancer is substantially affected by whether she carries a BRCA1 or BRCA2 mutation, and prophylactic surgery has been found to decrease the risk of breast and ovarian cancer by more than 90%. The main advantage to offering BRCA1 and BRCA2 testing before the onset of treatment is that it gives women who are found to carry a deleterious mutation the option of choosing risk-reduction surgery concurrent with therapeutic surgical treatment.

Colorectal cancer. Approximately 4.2% of men and women will be diagnosed with colorectal cancer at some point during their lifetime (National Cancer Institute, 2018). Only 10% of cases of colorectal cancer are likely to involve a mutation in one of several predisposing genes. Two examples of predisposing genes are harmful mutations in the APC tumor suppressor gene and harmful mutations in a mismatch repair gene. Mutations in the APC tumor suppressor gene have been associated with FAP, a rare autosomal dominant syndrome that accounts for about 1% of all colon cancer. It is typically diagnosed clinically. Affected individuals develop 100 to 1000 polyps in their colon by the time they are 20 to 30 years old. Genetic testing is greater than 80% sensitive. Identification of high-risk individuals guides surveillance strategies and the timing of a prophylactic colectomy. Low-risk individuals can stop the increased surveillance.

Lynch syndrome, also known as hereditary nonpolyposis colorectal cancer (HNPCC), is the most common hereditary form of colorectal and uterine cancer. About 2% to 3% of people who have colorectal cancer or uterine cancer have Lynch syndrome. Lynch syndrome is an autosomal dominant condition that results from mutations in one of many mismatch repair (MMR) genes (Genetics Home Reference, 2019c). Around 80% percent of individuals with Lynch syndrome have a mutation in either the MLH1 or MLH2 gene. Families at high risk for Lynch syndrome often have several relatives with colorectal cancer or uterine cancer. People with Lynch syndrome tend to develop cancers at an earlier age than the general populations. In addition, they have an increased risk for cancers of the stomach, small intestine, liver, gallbladder, upper urinary tract, and uncommon brain and skin cancer. Genetic testing is available for the mutations associated with Lynch syndrome. Testing should be done first on the affected family member. At-risk clients should be offered a prophylactic colectomy. Women may be offered a total abdominal hysterectomy with a salpingo-oophorectomy to decrease cancer risk. If colorectal cancer develops, a total colectomy is recommended.

GENETIC COUNSELING

It is standard practice in obstetrics to determine whether a heritable disorder exists in a couple or in anyone in either of their families. The goal of screening is to detect or define risk for disease in low-risk populations and identify those for whom diagnostic testing may be appropriate. As noted previously, the ideal time to obtain a family history is during the preconception period.

Genetic counseling is an interprofessional service that provides genetics information, education, and support to individuals and families with ongoing or potential genetic health concerns. It is typically provided by a team of genetics specialists that includes clinical geneticists (physicians), medical geneticists, genetics fellows, genetics counselors, and nurses with genetic expertise. Cytogeneticists, biochemical geneticists, and molecular geneticists support the clinical genetics team by providing laboratory expertise that helps with the diagnosis and management of individuals and families affected by genetic conditions.

Genetic counseling occurs in regional genetics centers, major medical centers, outreach or satellite genetics clinics, public health clinics, some community hospitals, and now that genetics has entered the mainstream of health care, in a wide variety of other settings. These include but are not limited to managed health care organizations, commercial facilities, and private practices. A number of specialized groups provide genetics education and counseling for individuals and families affected by specific genetic disorders, such as DS, CF, diabetes, muscular dystrophy, HD, and cancer. Genetic counseling also is offered over the Internet.

Individuals and families seek out or are referred for genetic counseling for a wide variety of reasons and at all stages of their lives. Some seek preconception or prenatal information; others are referred after the birth of a child with a birth defect or a suspected genetic condition, or after a pregnancy loss. Still others seek information because they have a family history of a genetic condition. Regardless of the setting or the individual's and family's stage of life, genetic counseling should be offered and available to all individuals and families who have questions about genetics and their health. However, there is a shortage of appropriately trained genetics professionals who can provide genetic counseling. This means that many individuals and families will not be offered genetic counseling when they undergo genetic testing. Moreover, some of the genetics education and counseling that is provided will be inadequate (see Community Focus box).

Estimation of Risk

Most families with a history of genetic disease want an answer to the following question: What is the chance that our future children will have this disease? Because the answer to this question may have profound implications for individual family members and the family as a whole, health care professionals must be able to answer this question as accurately as they can in a timely manner. In some cases, estimation of risk is rather straightforward; in other cases, it is complicated. Because of this, health care professionals should be prepared to refer families with a history of genetic disease to genetics professionals if they are at all unsure. Again, the answer to this question can have profound implications for individual family members and the family as a whole, so health care professionals must do their best to ensure that the answer is accurate.

If a couple has not yet had children but they are known to be at risk for having children with a genetic disease, they will be given an occurrence risk. Once the mating of a couple has produced one or more children with a genetic disease, the couple will be given a recurrence risk. Both occurrence and recurrence risks are determined by the mode of inheritance for the genetic disease in question. For genetic diseases caused by a factor that segregates during cell division (genes and chromosomes), risk can be estimated with a high degree of accuracy by application of mendelian principles.

In an autosomal dominant disorder, both the occurrence and recurrence risk are 50%, or one in two, that a subsequent offspring will be affected when one parent is affected and the other is not. The recurrence risk for autosomal recessive disorders is 25%, or 1 in 4, if both parents are carriers (they each have one recessive disease gene and one normal gene). Occasionally an individual homozygous for a recessive disease gene mates with an individual who is a carrier of the same recessive gene. In this case, the recurrence risk is 50%, or 1 in 2. If two individuals affected by an autosomal recessive disorder mate, all of their children will be affected. For X-linked disorders, recurrence risk is related to the sex of the child. Translocation chromosomes have a high risk for recurrence.

A number of autosomal disorders display fairly complex patterns of inheritance, making estimation of risk somewhat difficult. For example, if a child is born with a genetic disease and there has been no history of the disease in the family, the disease may have been caused by a new mutation (this is more likely if the disease in question is an autosomal dominant disorder, such as achondroplasia). If the child's genetic disease has been caused by a new mutation, the recurrence risk for the parents' subsequent children is low (1% to 2%), but it is not as low as that for the general population. Offspring of the affected child may have a substantially elevated occurrence risk.

The risk for recurrence for multifactorial conditions can be estimated empirically. An empiric risk is based not on genetics theory but, rather, on experience and observation of the disorder in other families. Recurrence risks are determined by applying the frequency of a similar disorder in other families to the case under consideration.

An important concept to be emphasized to individuals and families during a genetic counseling session is that *each pregnancy is an independent event.* For example, in monogenic disorders in which the risk factor is 1 in 4 that the child will be affected, the risk remains the same no matter how many affected children are already in the family. Families may maintain the erroneous assumption that the presence of one affected child ensures that the next three will be free of the disorder. However, "chance has no memory." The risk is 1 in 4 for each pregnancy. Conversely, in a family with a child who has a disorder with multifactorial causes, the risk increases with each subsequent child born with the disorder.

Interpretation of Risk

The guiding principle for genetics counselors has traditionally been nondirectiveness. According to the principle of nondirectiveness, the individual who is providing genetic counseling respects the right of the individual or family being counseled to make autonomous decisions. Counselors using a nondirective approach avoid making recommendations, and they try to communicate genetics information in an unbiased manner. The first step in providing nondirective counseling is becoming aware of one's own values and beliefs. Another important step is recognizing how one's values and beliefs can influence or interfere with the communication of genetics information.

If the individual who is providing genetic counseling has difficulty being nonjudgmental and objective, he or she may either intentionally or unintentionally influence the decision-making process. Individuals and families also may pressure the counselor to make decisions for them with questions such as "What would you do if you were me?" Families and individuals need education, guidance, and support throughout the counseling process. They should be given the facts and possible consequences as well as all of the assistance they need in problem solving, but the final decision regarding a course of action must be their own.

❓ CLINICAL REASONING CASE STUDY
Counseling About Genetic Risk

Camille has presented for her routine yearly physical examination and tells you she and her husband are planning to become pregnant within the next year. She confides in you that several infants have been born into her family with serious anomalies. She is interested in finding out more about her risks of having a baby with an anomaly and wants to know whom she should consult for that information.

1. What is the priority concern or client need in this situation?
2. List other client needs/problems in this case.
3. Identify any additional information needed by the nurse in addressing this situation.
4. Describe the roles/responsibilities of interprofessional health team members who may be involved in this situation.

Multiple Roles for Nurses in Genetics

Nurses play many roles in genetics. Some nurses play a key role in the identification of families in need of genetic counseling, and they collaborate with other health care professionals as part of interprofessional teams to make referrals to specialists in genetics. Other nurses take a more active role in genetic counseling.

Probably the most important of all nursing functions is to provide emotional support during all aspects of the counseling process. Feelings that are generated under the real or imagined threat posed by a genetic disorder are as varied as the individuals being counseled. Responses may include a variety of stress reactions, such as apathy, denial, anger, hostility, fear, embarrassment, grief, and loss of self-esteem. Guilt and self-blame are universal reactions. Many look on the disorder as a stigma, especially if the disorder is visible to others. Old wives' tales, superstitions, and long-held misconceptions may influence a family's reaction to a genetic disorder.

Future Promise of Genetics

Overall, the Human Genome Project and other sequencing efforts have been a huge success. Our understanding of the human genome, as well as other genomes, has grown exponentially in recent years. The increased availability of genetic testing and other genetics services gives individuals and families unprecedented opportunities to learn whether they have heightened risk for certain diseases or the potential to transmit gene mutations to their offspring. Awareness of genetic risk also can facilitate informed health care decisions and, in some cases, can promote risk reduction behaviors that have the potential to reduce morbidity and mortality. Ultimately it is hoped that advances in molecular biology and genomics will make it possible to offer diagnostic, preventive, and treatment options not only for genetic diseases, but also for common diseases such as cancer, atherosclerosis, diabetes, and Alzheimer disease.

Advances made possible through the Human Genome Project have been remarkable, but our ability to offer treatment options, even for single-gene disorders, remains very limited. Progress in the acquisition of genetics information and the development of genetics technology continue to outpace the development of therapeutic interventions. For most genetic conditions, therapeutic interventions are nonexistent or disappointingly limited. Consequently, the most useful means of reducing the incidence of genetic disorders now is preventing transmission. Only three reproductive options exist for individuals at risk for transmitting a genetic disorder: the avoidance of pregnancy; genetic diagnosis during an ongoing pregnancy; and prevention of transmission of an altered gene or genes through preimplantation genetics. For many families none of these options is viewed as acceptable.

Dialogue among pregnant women, expectant families, health care professionals, and disability advocates concerning prenatal testing for genetic disorders is urgently needed. Clinical and technical information must be complemented by social understanding of the experience of disability in contemporary society. The picture of life with a disability should be more balanced than that currently portrayed. It is critical that the voices of individuals and families living with disabilities be heard.

Nurses, as integral to the interprofessional team, are ideally positioned to help individuals and families maximize the benefits of the genetics revolution, but first, nurses need (1) a working knowledge of human genetics, (2) an awareness of recent advances in genetics and genomics, and (3) an understanding of the potential effects of genomic discoveries on individual and family well-being. More research is needed concerning the family experience of genetic testing. Nurses must understand why individuals and families decide to undergo or to forgo genetic testing. Nurses also need to be aware of how individuals and families define and manage ethical, legal, and social issues that emerge during the genetic testing experience.

KEY POINTS

- Advances in molecular biology and genomics have revolutionized health care by providing the tools needed to determine the hereditary component of many diseases.
- Increasingly, nurses, as integral to the interprofessional team, from all specialty areas, as well as all practice settings, are expected to have competencies in genetics and genomics.
- The major force behind the genetics revolution has been the Human Genome Project.
- All humans are more than 99% identical at the DNA level.
- Most of the genetic tests being offered in clinical practice are tests for single-gene disorders; however there has been a dramatic increase in genetic testing options.
- Pharmacogenomics will probably be the most immediate clinical application of the Human Genome Project.
- The decision to undergo genetic testing is often based on feelings of responsibility and commitment to others.
- Genes are the basic units of heredity responsible for all human characteristics. They comprise 23 pairs of chromosomes: 22 pairs of autosomes and 1 pair of sex chromosomes.
- Chromosomal abnormalities occur in both autosomes and sex chromosomes.
- Multifactorial inheritance includes genetic and environmental contributions.
- Advances in genetics have complex ethical, legal, and social implications.
- Cancer genetics is an important emerging field.

REFERENCES

Alexander, S. A. (2018). Primer in genetics and genomics series: Final remarks. *Biological Research for Nursing, 20*(3), 253–254.

American College of Obstetricians and Gynecologists. (2017a). Carrier screening for genetic conditions. ACOG Committee Opinion no. 690, *Obstetrics and Gynecology, 129,* e41–e55.

American College of Obstetricians and Gynecologists. (2017b). Carrier screening in the age of genomic medicine. ACOG Committee Opinion no. 690, *Obstetrics and Gynecology, 129,* e35–e40.

American College of Obstetricians and Gynecologist. (2017c). Consumer testing for disease risk. ACOG Committee Opinion no. 724, *Obstetrics and Gynecology, 130,* e270–273.

American College of Obstetricians and Gynecologists. (2018a). Originally 2011, reaffirmed 2015 and 2018. Family history as a risk assessment tool. ACOG Committee Opinion 478. Retrieved from: https://www.acog.org/-/media/Committee-Opinions/Committee-on-Genetics/co478.pdf?d-mc=1&ts=20180525T2121175010.

American College of Obstetricians and Gynecologists. (2018b). *Reducing risk of birth defects,* FAQ146. Retrieved from: https://www.acog.org/Patients/FAQs/Reducing-Risks-of-Birth-Defects.

Axelsen, T. M., & Woldbye, D. P. D. (2018). Gene therapy for Parkinson's disease, an update. *Journal of Parkinson's Disease, 8*(2), 195–215.

Bull, M. J. (2018). Improvement of outcomes for children with Down syndrome. *Journal of Pediatrics, 193,* 9–10.

Burke, W., & Trinidad, S. B. (2016). The deceptive appeal of direct-to-consumer genetics. *Annals of Internal Medicine, 164*(8), 564–565.

Centers for Disease Control and Prevention. (2018). *Birth defects: Data and statistics.* Retrieved from: https://www.cdc.gov/ncbddd/birthdefects/data.html.

Centers for Disease Control and Prevention. (2018). *Facts About Down syndrome.* Retrieved from: www.cdc.gov/ncbddd/birthdefects/DownSyndrome.html.

Cheek, D. J., Bashore, L., & Brazeau, D. A. (2015). Pharmacogenomics and implications for nursing practice. *Journal of Nursing Scholarship, 47*(6), 496–504.

Doble, B., Shofield, D. J., Roscioli, T., & Mattick, J. S. (2017). Prioritizing the application of genomic medicine. *Nature Partner Journals Genomic Medicine, 2*(35), 1–6.

ENCODE Project. (2019). *ENCyclopedia Of DNA Elements.* Bethesda, MD: National Human Genome Research Institute, *National Institutes of Health.* Retrieved from: https://www.genome.gov/10005107/encode-project/.

Fleming, L., Knafl, K., & Van Riper, M. (2017). How the child's gender matters for families having a child with congenital adrenal hyperplasia. *Journal of Family Nursing, 23*(4), 516–533.

Gee, M., Piercy, H., & Machaczek, K. (2017). Family planning decisions for parents of children with rare genetic condition: A scoping review. *Sexual & Reproductive Healthcare, 14,* 1–6.

Genetics Home Reference. (2018a). *What is gene therapy?* U.S. National Library of Science. Retrieved from: https://ghr.nlm.nih.gov/primer/therapy/genetherapy.

Genetics Home Reference. (2018b). *What were some of the ethical, legal, and social implications addressed by the Human Genome Project.* U.S. National Library of Medicine. Retrieved from: https://ghr.nlm.nih.gov/primer/hgp/elsi.

Genetics Home Reference. (2019a). *Factor V Leiden thrombophilia.* U.S. National Library of Medicine. Retrieved from: https://ghr.nlm.nih.gov/condition/factor-v-leiden-thrombophilia.

Genetics Home Reference. (2019b). *Klinefelter syndrome.* U.S. National Library of Medicine. Retrieved from: https://ghr.nlm.nih.gov/condition/klinefelter-syndrome.

Genetics Home Reference. (2019c). *Lynch syndrome.* U.S. National Library of Medicine. Retrieved from: https://ghr.nlm.nih.gov/condition/lynch-syndrome#definition.

Genetics Home Reference. (2019d). *Trisomy 13.* U.S. National Library of Medicine. Retrieved from: https://ghr.nlm.nih.gov/condition/trisomy-13#statistics.

Genetics Home Reference. (2019e). *Turner syndrome.* U.S. National Library of Medicine. Retrieved from: https://ghr.nlm.nih.gov/condition/turner-syndrome#genes.

Gollust, S. E., Gray, S. W., Carere, D. A., et al. (2017). *The Milbank Quarterly, 95*(2), 291–318.

Haga, S., & Mills, R. (2015). Nurses' communication of pharmacogenetic test results as part of discharge care. *Pharmacogenomics, 16,* 251–256.

Hagerman, R. J., Berry-Kravis, E., Hazlett, H. C., et al. (2017). Fragile X syndrome. *Nature Reviews Disease Primers, 3,* 17065.

Henderson, W. A., & Mudd-Martin, G. (2018). Genetics and genomics in nursing science. *Biological Research for Nursing, 20*(2), 117.

Hodgson, J., & McClaren, B. J. (2018). Parental experiences after prenatal diagnosis of fetal abnormality. *Seminars in Fetal & Neonatal Medicine, 23,* 150–154.

Homfray, T., Farndon, P.A. (2015). Fetal anomalies: a geneticist's approach. In A.M. Croady, S. Bower, (Eds). *Twining's textbook of fetal abnormalities* (3rd ed.). Canada: Elsevier.

Kerber, A. S., & Ledbetter, N. J. (2017). Scope and standards: Defining the advanced practice role in genetics. *Clinical Journal of Oncology Nursing, 21*(3), 309–313.

Kujovich, J.L. (1999, updated 2018). Factor V Leiden thrombophilia. In: M.P. Adam, H.H. Ardinger, R.A. Pagon, et al. (Eds.). *GeneReviews® [Internet].* Seattle (WA): University of Washington, Seattle; 1993-2019. Available from https://www.ncbi.nlm.nih.gov/books/NBK1368/.

Makris, M. (2018). Hemophilia gene therapy is effective and safe. *Blood, 131,* 952–953.

Manolio, T. A. (2016). Implementing genomics and pharmacogenomics in the clinic: The National Human Genome Research Institute's genomic medicine profile. *Atherosclerosis, 253,* 225–236.

March of Dimes. (2006). *Executive Summary: March of Dimes global report on birth defects.* Retrieved from: https://www.marchofdimes.org/materials/global-report-on-birth-defects-the-hidden-toll-of-dying-and-disabled-children-executive-summary.pdf.

Martin, T., Smith, A., Breatnach, C. R., et al. (2018). Infants born with Down syndrome: burden of disease in the early neonatal period. *The Journal of Pediatrics, 193,* 21–26.

Metcalfe, A. (2018). Sharing genetic risk information: Implications for family nurses across the life span. *Journal of Family Nursing, 21*(1), 86–105.

Middleton, A., Mendes, A., Benjamin, C. M., & Howard, H. C. (2017). Direct-to-consumer genetic testing: Where and how does genetic counseling fit. *Precision Medicine, 4*(3), 249–257.

National Blood Clot Alliance. (nd). *Factor V Leiden Resources.* Retrieved from: https://www.stoptheclot.org/learn_more/factor-v-leiden-2.htm.

National Cancer Institute. (2013). *Genetic Testing for Hereditary Cancer Syndromes.* Retrieved from: https://www.cancer.gov/about-cancer/causes-prevention/genetics/genetic-testing-fact-sheet.

National Cancer Institute. (2018). *BRCA Mutations: Cancer Risk and Genetic Testing.* Retrieved from: https://www.cancer.gov/about-cancer/causes-prevention/genetics/brca-fact-sheet.

National Center for Biotechnology Information (NCBI). (2018). *GTR: Genetic Testing Registry.* Retrieved from: https://www.ncbi.nlm.nih.gov/gtr/.

National Down Syndrome Society. (2019). *Down Syndrome Facts.* Retrieved from: https://www.ndss.org/about-down-syndrome/down-syndrome-facts/.

National Human Genome Research Institute. (2018a). *DNA Sequencing Costs: Data.* Retrieved from: https://www.genome.gov/sequencingcostsdata/.

National Human Genome Research Institute. (nd). *Talking Glossary of Genetic Terms.* Retrieved from: https://www.genome.gov/glossary/.

National Human Genome Research Institute. (2018b). *What Is Genomic Medicine?* Retrieved from: https://www.genome.gov/27552451/what-is-genomic-medicine/.

National Human Genome Research Institute (NHGRI). (2015). *All about the human genome project (HGP).* Retrieved from: https://www.genome.gov/10001772/.

National Library of Medicine. (2017). *Genetics home reference handbook: Help me understand genetics.* Retrieved from: https://ghr.nlm.nih.gov/primer.

Post, A. L., Mottola, A. T., & Kuller, J. A. (2017). What's new in prenatal genetics? A review of current recommendations and guidelines. *Obstetrical and Gynecological Survey, 72*(10), 610–617.

Precision Medicine Initiative Working Group (2015). *The precision medicine initiative cohort program: Building a research foundation for 21st century medicine.* National Institutes of Health, Washington, DC. Retrieved from: https://www.nih.gov/sites/default/files/research-training/initiatives/pmi/pmi-working-group-report-20150917-2.pdf.

Rehm, H. L. (2017). Evolving health care through personal genomics. *Nature Reviews, 18,* 259–267.

Rogers, M. A., Lizer, S., Doughty, A., Hayden, B., & Klein, C. (2017). Expanding RN scope of knowledge-genetics/genomics: The new frontier. *Journal for Nurses in Professional Development, 33*(2), 56–63.

Rose, N. C., & Wick, M. (2018). Carrier screening for single gene disorders. *Seminars in Fetal & Neonatal Medicine, 23,* 78–84.

Rosell, A. M., Pena, L. D., Schoch, K., et al. (2016). Not the end of the odyssey: Parental perceptions of whole exome sequencing (WES) in pediatric undiagnosed disorders. *Journal of Genetic Counseling, 25,* 1019–1031.

Rowland, E., Plumridge, G., Considine, A. M., & Metcalfe, A. (2016). Preparing young people for future decision-making about cancer risk in families affected or at risk from hereditary breast cancer: A qualitative interview study. *European Journal of Oncology Nursing, 25,* 9–15.

SOFT. (2018). *Trisomy 18, Trisomy 13 and related chromosome disorders.* Retrieved from: http://trisomy.org/.

Sole-Smith, V. (2014). *Doctors describe some of the known risk factors for having a child with down syndrome.* Parents. Retrieved from: http://www.parents.com/health/down-syndrome/down-syndrome-risks/.

Taylor-Phillips, S., Stinton, C., Ferrante di Ruffano, L., et al (2018). Association between use of systematic reviews and national policy recommendations on screening newborn babies for rare disease: Systematic review and meta-analysis. *British Medical Journal, 360*(k1612), 1–11. https://doi.org/10.1136/bmj.k1612.

Trisomy 18 Foundation. (2018). *What Is Trisomy 18?* Retrieved from: http://www.trisomy18.org/.

U.S. Food and Drug Administration (2018). *Table of pharacoenomic biomarkers in drug labeling. U.S.* Department of Health and Human Services. Retrieved from: https://www.fda.gov/Drugs/ScienceResearch/ucm572698.htm.

Van Riper, M., Knafl, G., Rosigno, C., & Knafl, K. (2018). Family management of childhood chronic conditions: Does it make a difference if the child has an intellectual disability. *American Journal of Medical Genetics: Part A. American Journal of Medical Genetics: Part A, 176*(1), 8291.

von der Lippe, C., Diesen, P. S., & Feragen, K. B. (2017). *Molecular Genetics and Genomic Medicine, 5*(6), 758–773.

Vorderstrasse, A. A., Hammer, M. J., & Dungan, J. (2014). *Seminars in Oncology Nursing, 30*(2), 130–136.

Wallace, S. E., Gilvary, S., Smith, M. J., & Dolan, S. M. (2018). Parent perspectives of support received from physicians and/or genetic counselors following a decision to continue a pregnancy with a prenatal diagnosis of Trisomy 13/18. *Journal of Genetic Counseling, 27*(3), 656–664.

Weiner, D. L. (2017). *Inborn Errors of Metabolism.* Medscape. Retrieved from: https://emedicine.medscape.com/article/804757-overview#showall.

Whitt, K. J., Hughes, M., Hopkins, E. S., & Maradiegue, A. (2016). The gene pool: The ethics of genetics in primary care. *Annual Review of Nursing Research, 34*(1), 119–XI.

Williams, J., Katapodi, M., Starkweather, A., et al. (2016). Advanced nursing practice and research contributions in precision medicine. *Nursing Outlook, 64*(2), 117–123.

Winn, P., Acharya, K., Peterson, E., & Leuthneer, S. (2018). Prenatal counseling and parental decision-making following a fetal diagnosis of trisomy 13 or 18. *Journal of Perinatology, 38,* 788–796.

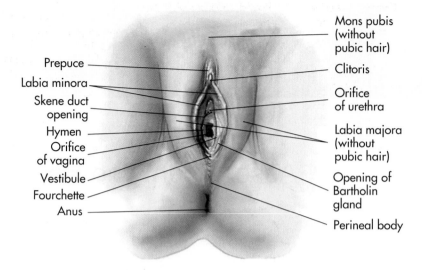

Prepuce

Labia minora

Skene duct
opening

Hymen

Orifice
of vagina

Vestibule

Fourchette

Anus

Mons pubis
(without
pubic hair)

Clitoris

Orifice
of urethra

Labia majora
(without
pubic hair)

Opening of
Bartholin
gland

Perineal body

Fig. 4.1 External Female Genitalia.

of the clitoris) and the *frenulum* (the fold of tissue under the clitoris). The labia minora join to form a thin, flat tissue called the *fourchette* underneath the vaginal opening at midline. The clitoris is located underneath the prepuce. It is a small structure composed of erectile tissue with numerous sensory nerve endings. During sexual arousal, the clitoris increases in size.

The vaginal *vestibule* is an almond-shaped area enclosed by the labia minora that contains openings to the urethra, Skene glands, vagina, and Bartholin glands. The urethra is not a reproductive organ but is discussed here because of its location. It usually is found about 2.5 cm below the clitoris. Skene glands are located on each side of the urethra and produce mucus, which aids in lubrication of the vagina. The vaginal opening is in the lower portion of the vestibule and varies in shape and size. The hymen, a connective tissue membrane that surrounds the vaginal opening, can be perforated during strenuous exercise, insertion of tampons, masturbation, or vaginal intercourse. Bartholin glands lie under the constrictor muscles of the vagina and are located posteriorly on the sides of the vaginal opening, although the ductal opening usually is not visible. During sexual arousal, the glands secrete clear mucus to lubricate the vaginal introitus.

The area between the fourchette and the anus is the **perineum**, a skin-covered muscular area that covers the pelvic structures. The perineum forms the base of the perineal body, a wedge-shaped mass that serves as an anchor for the muscles, fascia, and ligaments of the pelvis. The muscles and ligaments form a sling that supports the pelvic organs.

Internal Structures

The internal structures include the vagina, uterus, uterine tubes, and ovaries. The description of these structures follows.

The **vagina** is a fibromuscular, collapsible tubular structure that lies between the bladder and rectum and extends from the vulva to the uterus. During the reproductive years the mucosal lining is arranged in transverse folds called *rugae*. These rugae allow the vagina to expand during birth. Estrogen deprivation that occurs after birth, during lactation, and at menopause causes dryness and thinning of the vaginal walls and smoothing of the rugae. The vagina, particularly the lower segment, has few sensory nerve endings. Vaginal secretions are slightly acidic (pH 4 to 5) so that vaginal susceptibility to infections is limited. The vagina serves as a passageway for

menstrual flow, as a female organ of copulation, and as a part of the birth canal for vaginal birth. The uterine cervix projects into a blind vault at the upper end of the vagina. Anterior, posterior, and lateral pockets called fornices (singular: *fornix*) surround the cervix. The internal pelvic organs can be palpated through the thin walls of these fornices.

The *uterus* is a muscular organ shaped like an upside-down pear that is positioned midline in the pelvic cavity between the bladder and rectum and above the vagina. Four pairs of ligaments support the uterus: cardinal, uterosacral, round, and broad. Single anterior and posterior ligaments also support the uterus. The cul-de-sac of Douglas is a deep pouch, or recess, posterior to the cervix formed by the posterior ligament.

The uterus is divided into two major parts: an upper triangular portion called the *corpus* and a lower cylindric portion called the *cervix* (Fig. 4.2). The *fundus* is the dome-shaped top of the uterus and is the site at which the **uterine tubes** (fallopian tubes) enter the uterus. The **isthmus**, or lower uterine segment, is a short constricted portion that separates the corpus from the cervix.

The uterus functions as a place for reception, implantation, retention, and nourishment of the fertilized ovum, and later of the fetus during pregnancy, and for expulsion of the fetus during birth.

The uterine wall is made up of three layers: the endometrium, the myometrium, and part of the peritoneum. The endometrium is a highly vascular lining made up of three layers, the outer two of which are shed during menstruation. The myometrium is made up of layers of smooth muscles that extend in three different directions (longitudinal, transverse, and oblique) (Fig. 4.3). Longitudinal fibers of the outer myometrial layer are found mostly in the fundus, and this arrangement assists in expelling the fetus during the birth process. The middle layer contains fibers from all three directions, which form a figure-eight pattern encircling large blood vessels. These fibers assist in ligating blood vessels after birth and control blood loss. Most of the circular fibers of the inner myometrial layer are around the site where the uterine tubes enter the uterus and around the internal cervical os (opening). These fibers help keep the cervix closed during pregnancy and prevent menstrual blood from flowing back into the uterine tubes during menstruation.

The cervix is made up of mostly fibrous connective tissues and elastic tissue, making it possible for the cervix to stretch during vaginal

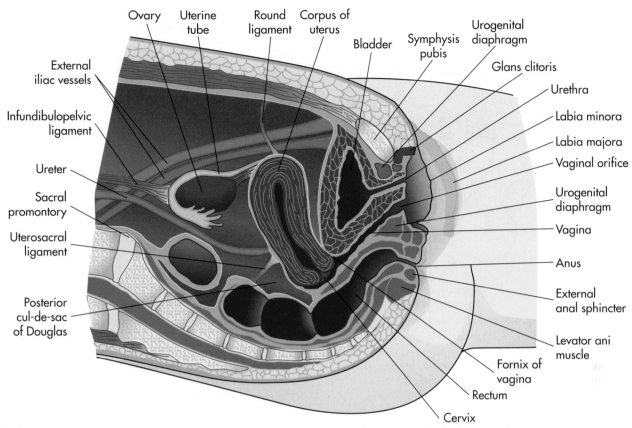

Fig. 4.2 Midsagittal View of Female Pelvic Organs With Woman Lying Supine.

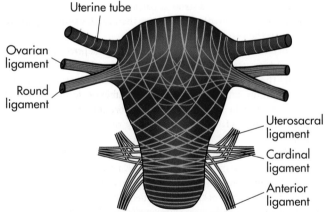

Fig. 4.3 Schematic Arrangement of Directions of Muscle Fibers. Note that uterine muscle fibers are continuous with supportive ligaments of uterus.

birth. The opening between the uterine cavity and the canal that connects the uterine cavity to the vagina (endocervical canal) is the internal os. The narrowed opening between the endocervix and the vagina is the external os, a small circular opening in women who have never been pregnant. The cervix feels firm (like the end of a nose) with a dimple in the center that marks the external os.

The outer cervix is covered with a layer of squamous epithelium. The mucosa of the cervical canal is covered with columnar epithelium and contains numerous glands that secrete mucus in response to ovarian hormones. The **squamocolumnar junction**, where the two types of cells meet, is usually located just inside the cervical os. This junction is also called the *transformation zone* and is the most common site for neoplastic changes. Cells from this site are scraped for the Papanicolaou (Pap) test (see later discussion).

The *uterine tubes* attach to the uterine fundus. The tubes are supported by the broad ligaments and range from 8 to 14 cm in length. The tubes are divided into four sections: the interstitial portion is closest to the uterus; the isthmus and the ampulla are the middle portions; and the infundibulum is closest to the ovary. The uterine tubes provide a passage between the ovaries and the uterus for the movement of the ovum. The infundibulum has fimbriated (fringed) ends, which pull the ovum into the tube. The ovum is pushed along the tubes to the uterus by rhythmic contractions of muscles of the tubes and by the current produced by the movement of the cilia that line the tubes. The ovum is usually fertilized by the sperm in the ampulla portion of one of the tubes.

The *ovaries* are almond-shaped organs located on each side of the uterus below and behind the uterine tubes. During the reproductive years they are approximately 3 cm long, 2 cm wide, and 1 cm thick; they diminish in size after menopause. Before menarche, each ovary has a smooth surface; after menarche, they are nodular because of repeated ruptures of follicles at ovulation. The two functions of the ovaries are ovulation and hormone production. **Ovulation** is the release of a mature ovum from the ovary at intervals (usually monthly). Estrogen, progesterone, and androgen are the hormones produced by the ovaries.

The Bony Pelvis

The bony pelvis serves three primary purposes: protection of the pelvic structures, accommodation of the growing fetus during pregnancy, and anchorage of the pelvic support structures. The two innominate (hip) bones (consisting of ilium, ischium, and pubis), the sacrum, and the coccyx make up the four bones of the pelvis (Fig. 4.4). Cartilage and

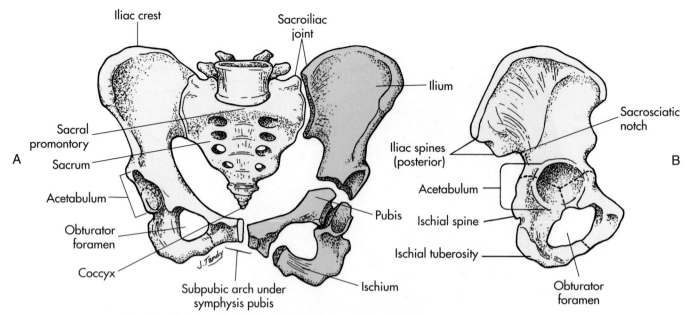

Fig. 4.4 Adult Female Pelvis. (A) Anterior view. (B) External view of innominate bone (fused).

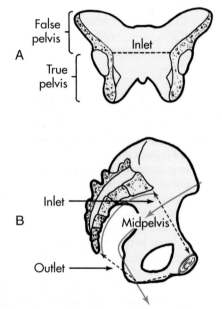

Fig. 4.5 Female Pelvis. (A) Cavity of false pelvis is shallow. (B) Cavity of true pelvis is an irregularly curved canal *(arrows)*.

ligaments form the symphysis pubis, sacrococcygeal joint, and two sacroiliac joints that separate the pelvic bones.

The pelvis is divided into two parts: the false pelvis and the true pelvis (Fig. 4.5). The false pelvis is the upper portion above the pelvic brim or inlet. The true pelvis is the lower, curved, bony canal, which includes the inlet, the cavity, and the outlet through which the fetus passes during vaginal birth. The upper portion of the outlet is at the level of the ischial spines, and the lower portion is at the level of the ischial tuberosities and the pubic arch. Variations that occur in the size and shape of the pelvis are usually related to age, race, and sex. Pelvic ossification is complete at about 20 years of age.

Breasts

The breasts are paired mammary glands located between the second and sixth ribs (Fig. 4.6). About two-thirds of the breast overlies the pectoralis muscle, between the sternum and midaxillary line, with an extension to the *tail of Spence*. The lower one-third of the breast overlies the serratus anterior muscle. The breasts are attached to the muscles by connective tissue or fascia.

The breasts of the healthy, mature woman are approximately equal in size and shape, but often are not absolutely symmetric. The size and shape vary with the woman's age, heredity, and nutrition. However, the contour should be smooth with no retractions, dimpling, or masses. Estrogen stimulates growth of the breast by inducing fat deposition in the breasts, development of stromal tissue (i.e., increase in its amount and elasticity), and growth of the extensive ductile system. Estrogen also increases the vascularity of breast tissue.

Once ovulation begins in puberty, progesterone levels increase. The increase in progesterone causes maturation of mammary gland tissue, specifically the lobules and acinar structures. During adolescence fat deposition and growth of fibrous tissue contribute to the increase in the size of the glands. Full development of the breasts is not achieved until after the end of the first pregnancy or in the early period of lactation.

Each mammary gland is made of a number of lobes that are divided into lobules. Lobules are clusters of acini. An acinus is a saclike terminal part of a compound gland emptying through a narrow lumen or duct. The acini are lined with epithelial cells that secrete colostrum and milk. Just below the epithelium is the myoepithelium (*myo*, or muscle), which contracts to expel milk from the acini.

The ducts from the clusters of acini that form the lobules merge to form larger ducts draining the lobes. Ducts from the lobes converge in a single nipple (mammary papilla) surrounded by an areola. The anatomy of the ducts is similar for each breast but varies among women. Protective fatty tissue surrounds the glandular structures and ducts. *Cooper ligaments,* or fibrous suspensory ligaments, separate and support the glandular structures and ducts. Cooper ligaments provide support to the mammary glands while permitting their mobility on the chest wall (see Fig. 4.6). The round nipple is usually slightly elevated above the breast. On each breast the nipple projects slightly upward and laterally. It contains 4 to 20 openings from the milk ducts. The nipple is surrounded by fibromuscular tissue and covered by wrinkled skin (the areola). Except during pregnancy and lactation, there is usually no discharge from the nipple.

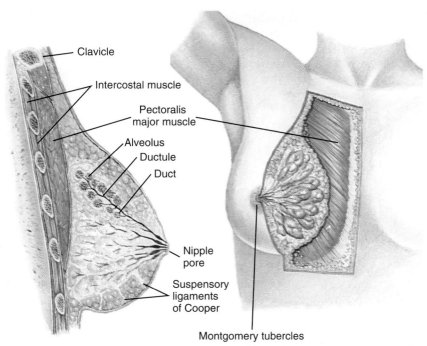

Fig. 4.6 Anatomy of the Breast, Showing Position and Major Structures. (Adapted from Seidel, H., Ball, J., Dains, J., et al. [2011]. *Mosby's guide to physical examination* [7th ed.]. St. Louis: Mosby.)

The nipple and surrounding areola are usually more deeply pigmented than the skin of the breast. The rough appearance of the areola is caused by sebaceous glands, *Montgomery tubercles,* directly beneath the skin. These glands secrete a fatty substance thought to lubricate the nipple. Smooth muscle fibers in the areola contract to stiffen the nipple to make it easier for the breastfeeding infant to grasp.

The vascular supply to the mammary gland is abundant. In the nonpregnant state there is no obvious vascular pattern in the skin. The normal skin is smooth without tightness or shininess. The skin covering the breasts contains an extensive superficial lymphatic network that serves the entire chest wall and is continuous with the superficial lymphatics of the neck and abdomen. The lymphatics form a rich network in the deeper portions of the breasts. The primary deep lymphatic pathway drains laterally toward the axillae.

Besides their function of lactation, breasts function as organs for sexual arousal in the mature adult female. The breasts change in size and nodularity in response to cyclic ovarian changes throughout reproductive life. Increasing levels of both estrogen and progesterone in the 3 to 4 days before menstruation increase the vascularity of the breasts, induce growth of the ducts and acini, and promote water retention. The epithelial cells lining the ducts proliferate in number, the ducts dilate, and the lobules distend. The acini become enlarged and secretory, and lipid (fat) is deposited within their epithelial cell lining. As a result, breast swelling, tenderness, and discomfort are common symptoms just before the onset of menstruation. After menstruation, cellular proliferation begins to regress, acini begin to decrease in size, and retained water is lost. After breasts have undergone changes numerous times in response to the ovarian cycle, the proliferation and involution (regression) are not uniform throughout the breast. In time, after repeated hormonal stimulation, small persistent areas of nodulations may develop. This normal physiologic change must be remembered when breast tissue is examined. Nodules may develop just before and during menstruation, when the breast is most active. The physiologic alterations in breast size and activity reach their minimum level about 5 to 7 days after menstruation stops. Therefore, breast self-examination (BSE) (systematic palpation of breasts to detect signs of breast cancer or other changes) is best carried out during this phase of the menstrual cycle. Although monthly BSE used to be recommended to all women, there is very little evidence that BSE or a clinical breast exam by a health care provider helps to detect breast cancer early when a woman also gets a screening mammogram (United States Preventive Task Force [USPTF], 2016). However, all women should be familiar with how their breasts normally appear and feel, and report any changes to a health care provider immediately. See the Teaching for Self-Management box: Breast Self-Examination.

MENSTRUATION AND MENOPAUSE

Menarche and Puberty

Although young girls secrete small, rather constant amounts of estrogen, a marked increase occurs between 8 and 11 years of age. The term menarche denotes first menstruation. Puberty is a broader term that denotes the entire transitional stage between childhood and sexual maturity. Increasing amounts and variations in gonadotropin and estrogen secretion develop into a cyclic pattern at least a year before menarche. In North America this occurs in most girls at about 13 years of age.

Initially, menstrual periods are irregular and unpredictable and *anovulatory* (no ovum is released from the ovary). After 1 or more years, a hypothalamic-pituitary rhythm develops and the ovary produces adequate cyclic estrogen to make a mature ovum. *Ovulatory* (ovum released from the ovary) periods tend to be regular, with estrogen dominating the first half of the cycle and progesterone dominating the second half.

Although pregnancy can occur in exceptional cases of true precocious puberty, most pregnancies in young girls occur after the normally timed menarche. All young adolescents of both sexes would benefit from knowing that pregnancy can occur at any time after the onset of menses.

TEACHING FOR SELF-MANAGEMENT

Breast Self-Examination

If you choose to perform a breast self-examination, the best time is when breasts are not tender or swollen.

How to examine your breasts:

1. Lie down and put a pillow under your right shoulder. Place your right arm behind your head (Fig. 1).

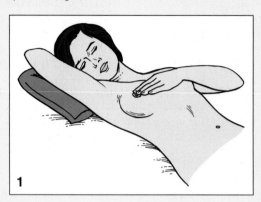

2. Use the finger pads of your three middle fingers on your left hand to feel for lumps or thickening. Your finger pads are the top third of each finger. Use circular motions of the finger pads to feel the breast tissue.

3. Press firmly enough to know how your breast feels. Use light pressure to feel the tissue just under the skin, medium pressure for a little deeper, and firm pressure to feel the breast tissue close to the chest and ribs. A firm ridge in the lower curve of the breast is normal.

4. Move around the breast in a set way, such as using an up-and-down or vertical line pattern (Fig. 2). Go up to the collar bone and down to the ribs and from your underarm on the side to the middle of your chest. Use the same technique every time. It will help you to make sure that you have gone over the entire breast area and to remember how your breast feels.

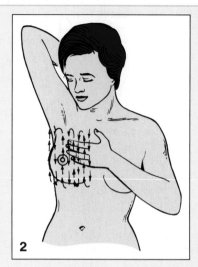

5. Now examine your left breast. Put a pillow under your left shoulder. Place your left arm behind your head and use the finger pads of your right hand, similar to the description in step 2.

6. You may want to check your breasts while standing in front of a mirror. See if there are any changes in the way your breasts look: dimpling of the skin, changes in the nipple, or redness or swelling.

7. Checking the area between the breast and the underarm, and the underarm itself is important. Examine the area above the breast to the collarbone and to the shoulder while you are standing or sitting up with your arms lightly raised.

8. If you find any changes, see your health care provider right away.

Adapted from American Cancer Society: Breast awareness and self-exam (2014). www.cancer.org.

Menstrual Cycle

Menstruation is the periodic uterine bleeding that begins approximately 14 days after ovulation. It is controlled by a feedback system of three cycles: endometrial, hypothalamic-pituitary, and ovarian. The average length of a menstrual cycle is 28 days, but variations are normal. The first day of bleeding is designated as day 1 of the menstrual cycle, or menses (Fig. 4.7). The average duration of menstrual flow is 5 days (with a range of 3 to 6 days) and the average blood loss is 50 mL (with a range of 20 to 80 mL), but this duration of flow and blood loss vary greatly. For about 50% of women, menstrual blood does not appear to clot. The menstrual blood clots within the uterus, but the clot usually liquefies before being discharged from the uterus. Uterine discharge includes mucus and epithelial cells in addition to blood.

The menstrual cycle is a complex interplay of events that occur simultaneously in the endometrium, hypothalamus, pituitary gland, and ovaries. The menstrual cycle prepares the uterus for pregnancy. When pregnancy does not occur, menstruation follows. A woman's age, physical and emotional status, and environment influence the regularity of her menstrual cycles.

Hypothalamic-Pituitary Cycle

Toward the end of the normal menstrual cycle, blood levels of estrogen and progesterone decrease. Low blood levels of these ovarian hormones stimulate the hypothalamus to secrete gonadotropin-releasing hormone (GnRH). In turn, GnRH stimulates anterior pituitary secretion of follicle-stimulating hormone (FSH). FSH stimulates development of ovarian graafian follicles and their production of estrogen. Estrogen levels begin to decrease, and hypothalamic GnRH triggers the anterior pituitary to release luteinizing hormone (LH). A marked surge of LH and a smaller peak of estrogen (day 12) (see Fig. 4.7) precede the expulsion of the ovum from the graafian follicle by about 24 to 36 hours. LH peaks at about day 13 or 14 of a 28-day cycle. If fertilization and implantation of the ovum have not occurred by this time, regression of the corpus luteum follows. Levels of progesterone and estrogen decline, menstruation occurs, and the hypothalamus is once again stimulated to secrete GnRH. This process is called the *hypothalamic-pituitary cycle.*

Ovarian Cycle

The primitive graafian follicles contain immature oocytes (primordial ova). Before ovulation, from 1 to 30 follicles begin to mature in each ovary under the influence of FSH and estrogen. The preovulatory surge of LH affects a selected follicle. The oocyte matures, ovulation occurs, and the empty follicle begins its transformation into the corpus luteum. This follicular phase (preovulatory phase) (see Fig. 4.7) of the ovarian cycle varies in length from woman to woman. Almost all variations in ovarian cycle length are the result of variations in the length of the follicular phase. On rare occasions (i.e., 1 in 100 menstrual cycles), more than one follicle is selected, and more than one oocyte matures and undergoes ovulation.

After ovulation, estrogen levels drop. For 90% of women, only a small amount of withdrawal bleeding occurs, and it goes unnoticed. In 10% of women, there is sufficient bleeding for it to be visible, resulting in what is termed *midcycle bleeding*.

The luteal phase begins immediately after ovulation and ends with the start of menstruation. This postovulatory phase of the ovarian cycle usually requires 14 days (range 13 to 15 days). The corpus luteum reaches its peak of functional activity 8 days after ovulation, secreting the steroids *estrogen* and *progesterone*. Coincident with this time of peak luteal functioning, the fertilized ovum is implanted in the endometrium. If no implantation occurs, the corpus luteum regresses and steroid levels drop. Two weeks after ovulation, if fertilization and implantation do not occur, the functional layer of the uterine endometrium is shed through menstruation.

Endometrial Cycle

The four phases of the endometrial cycle are (1) the menstrual phase, (2) the proliferative phase, (3) the secretory phase, and (4) the ischemic phase (see Fig. 4.7). During the menstrual phase shedding of the functional two-thirds of the endometrium (the compact and spongy layers) is initiated by periodic vasoconstriction in the upper layers of the endometrium. The basal layer is always retained, and regeneration begins near the end of the cycle from cells derived from the remaining glandular remnants or stromal cells in this layer.

The proliferative phase is a period of rapid growth lasting from about the fifth day to the time of ovulation. The endometrial surface is completely restored in approximately 4 days, or slightly before bleeding ceases. From this point on, an 8- to 10-fold thickening occurs, with a leveling off of growth at ovulation. The proliferative phase depends on estrogen stimulation derived from ovarian follicles.

The secretory phase extends from the day of ovulation to about 3 days before the next menstrual period. After ovulation, large amounts of progesterone are produced. An edematous, vascular, functional endometrium is now apparent. At the end of the secretory phase, the fully matured secretory endometrium reaches the thickness of heavy, soft velvet. It becomes luxuriant with blood and glandular secretions, creating a suitable protective and nutritive bed for a fertilized ovum.

Implantation of the fertilized ovum generally occurs about 7 to 10 days after ovulation. If fertilization and implantation do not occur, the corpus luteum, which secretes estrogen and progesterone, regresses. With the rapid decrease in progesterone and estrogen levels, the spiral arteries go into spasm. During the ischemic phase, the blood supply to the functional endometrium is blocked and necrosis develops. The functional layer separates from the basal layer, and menstrual bleeding begins, marking day 1 of the next cycle (see Fig. 4.7).

Other Cyclic Changes

When the hypothalamic-pituitary-ovarian axis functions properly, other tissues undergo predictable responses. Before ovulation a woman's basal body temperature is often less than 37°C (98.6°F); after ovulation, with increasing progesterone levels, her basal body temperature rises. Changes in the cervix and cervical mucus follow a generally predictable pattern. Preovulatory and postovulatory mucus is viscous (thick) so that sperm penetration is discouraged. At the time of ovulation, cervical mucus is thin and clear. It looks, feels, and stretches like egg white. This stretchable quality is termed *spinnbarkeit*. Some women have localized lower abdominal pain called *mittelschmerz* that coincides with ovulation. Some spotting may occur.

Prostaglandins

Prostaglandins (PGs) are oxygenated fatty acids classified as hormones. The different kinds of PGs are distinguished by letters (PGE and PGF), numbers (PGE$_2$), and letters of the Greek alphabet (PGF$_2\alpha$).

PGs are produced in most organs of the body, including the uterus. Menstrual blood is a potent PG source. PGs are metabolized quickly by most tissues. They are biologically active in minute amounts in the cardiovascular, gastrointestinal, respiratory, urogenital, and nervous systems. They also exert a marked effect on metabolism, particularly on glycolysis. PGs play an important role in many physiologic, pathologic, and pharmacologic reactions. PGF$_2\alpha$, PGE$_4$, and PGE$_2$ are most commonly used in reproductive medicine.

PGs affect smooth muscle contractility and modulation of hormonal activity. Indirect evidence indicates that PGs have an effect on ovulation, fertility, changes in the cervix, and cervical mucus that affect receptivity to sperm, tubal and uterine motility, sloughing of endometrium (menstruation), onset of miscarriage and induced abortion, and onset of labor (term and preterm). After exerting biologic actions, newly synthesized PGs are rapidly metabolized by tissues in such organs as the lungs, kidneys, and liver.

PGs may play a key role in ovulation. If PG levels do not rise along with the surge of LH, the ovum remains trapped within the graafian follicle. After ovulation, PGs may influence production of estrogen and progesterone by the corpus luteum.

The introduction of PGs into the vagina or the uterine cavity (from ejaculated semen) increases the motility of uterine musculature, which may assist the transport of sperm through the uterus and into the oviduct.

PGs produced by a woman cause regression of the corpus luteum and regression and sloughing of the endometrium, resulting in menstruation. PGs increase myometrial response to oxytocic stimulation, enhance uterine contractions, and cause cervical dilation. They may be a factor in the initiation of labor, the maintenance of labor, or both. They may also be involved in dysmenorrhea (see Chapter 6) and preeclampsia/eclampsia (see Chapter 27).

Climacteric and Menopause

The climacteric is a transitional phase during which ovarian function and hormone production decline. This phase spans the years from the onset of premenopausal ovarian decline to the postmenopausal time when symptoms stop. Menopause (from Latin *mensis*, month, and Greek *pauses*, to cease) refers only to the last menstrual period. However, unlike menarche, menopause can be dated with certainty only 1 year after menstruation ceases. The average age at natural menopause is 51.4 years, with an age range of 35 to 60 years. Perimenopause is a period preceding menopause that lasts about 4 years. During this time ovarian function declines. Ova slowly diminish, and menstrual cycles may be anovulatory, resulting in irregular bleeding. The ovaries stop producing estrogen, and eventually menses no longer occur.

SEXUAL RESPONSE

The hypothalamus and anterior pituitary gland in females regulate the production of FSH and LH. The target tissue for these hormones is the ovary, which produces ova and secretes estrogen and progesterone. A feedback mechanism between hormone secretion from the ovaries, the hypothalamus, and the anterior pituitary gland aids in the control of sex steroid hormone secretion.

Although the first outward appearance of maturing sexual development occurs at an earlier age in females, both females and males achieve physical maturity at approximately 17 years of age; however,

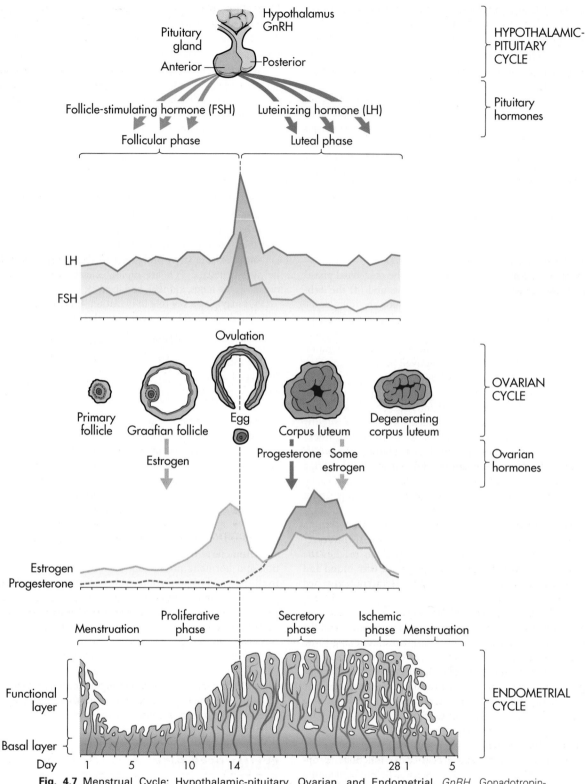

Fig. 4.7 Menstrual Cycle: Hypothalamic-pituitary, Ovarian, and Endometrial. *GnRH,* Gonadotropin-releasing hormone.

individual development varies greatly. Anatomic and reproductive differences notwithstanding, women and men are more similar than different in their physiologic response to sexual excitement and orgasm. For example, the glans clitoris and the glans penis are embryonic homologs. Little difference exists between female and male sexual response; the physical response is essentially the same whether stimulated by coitus, fantasy, or masturbation. Physiologic sexual response can be analyzed in terms of two processes: vasocongestion and myotonia (increased muscular tension).

Sexual stimulation results in increased circulation to circumvaginal blood vessels (lubrication in the female), causing engorgement and distention of the genitals. Venous congestion is localized primarily

TABLE 4.1   Four Phases of Sexual Response

Reactions Common to Both Sexes	Female Reactions	Male Reactions
Excitement Phase Heart rate and blood pressure increase. Nipples become erect. Myotonia begins.	Clitoris increases in diameter and swells. External genitalia become congested and darken. Vaginal lubrication occurs; upper two thirds of vagina lengthens and extends. Cervix and uterus pull upward. Breast size increases.	Erection of the penis begins; penis increases in length and diameter. Scrotal skin becomes congested and thickens. Testes begin to increase in size and elevate toward the body.
Plateau Phase Heart rate and blood pressure continue to increase. Respirations increase. Myotonia becomes pronounced; grimacing occurs.	Clitoral head retracts under the clitoral hood. Lower one third of vagina becomes engorged. Skin color changes occur—flush may be observed across breasts, abdomen, or other surfaces.	Head of penis may enlarge slightly. Scrotum continues to grow tense and thicken. Testes continue to elevate and enlarge. Preorgasmic emission of two or three drops of fluid appears on the head of the penis.
Orgasmic Phase Heart rate, blood pressure, and respirations increase to maximum levels. Involuntary muscle spasms occur. External rectal sphincter contracts.	Strong rhythmic contractions are felt in the clitoris, vagina, and uterus. Sensations of warmth spread through the pelvic area.	Testes elevate to maximum level. Point of "inevitability" occurs just before ejaculation and an awareness of fluid in the urethra. Rhythmic contractions occur in the penis. Ejaculation of semen occurs.
Resolution Phase Heart rate, blood pressure, and respirations return to normal. Nipple erection subsides. Myotonia subsides.	Engorgement in external genitalia and vagina resolves. Uterus descends to normal position. Cervix dips into seminal pool. Breast size decreases. Skin flush disappears. Women do not have a refractory period before they can have another orgasm.	Fifty percent of erection is lost immediately with ejaculation; penis gradually returns to normal size. Testes and scrotum return to normal size. Refractory period (time needed for erection to occur again) varies according to age and general physical condition.

in the genitalia, but it also occurs to a lesser degree in the breasts and other parts of the body. Arousal is characterized by myotonia, resulting in voluntary and involuntary rhythmic contractions. Examples of sexually stimulated myotonia are pelvic thrusting, facial grimacing, and spasms of the hands and feet (carpopedal spasms).

Although other sex researchers have noted various sexual response cycles, the sexual response cycle is classically divided into four phases: excitement, plateau, orgasm, and resolution, according to the seminal work of Masters and Johnson (1966). The four phases occur progressively, with no sharp dividing line between any two phases. The time, intensity, and duration for cyclic completion also vary for individuals and situations, and there are other models to explain sexual response, though less prevalent than the Masters and Johnson model. Sexuality and sexual response may change during pregnancy and postpartum, emphasizing the need to discuss with women possible sexual changes during this time. Specific issues related to this period (and prior procedures such as episiotomy) must be considered in counseling to promote healthy sexuality during the postpartum period. Despite these alternate models of sexual response, it is still common to describe the classic four stages in which specific body changes take place in sequence, and this description is useful in educating and talking with women who may have concerns about possible sexual dysfunction (Table 4.1).

REASONS FOR ENTERING THE HEALTH CARE SYSTEM

Women enter the health care system for varied reasons, including those specifically related to women's reproductive health, but also for general well-woman care. Nurses play a key role in working with women who enter the health system (Box 4.1). Women's health needs and concerns are common reasons for women to enter the health care system. These

BOX 4.1   Role of Nurses in Women's Health Promotion and Illness Prevention

Registered nurses work with women to promote wellness by:
- Integrating various modalities of care ("integrative nurse coaching")
- Collaborating with interprofessional health care team
- Providing care in the community; working with individuals, families, communities
- Working to influence health policy

Advanced practice nurses work with women to promote wellness by:
- Providing comprehensive primary care
- Coordinating care in communities (from hospitals to home to communities)
- Working with social service resources for clients in the community; influencing health policy

may include preconception counseling and care, pregnancy, menstrual problems, well and sick care, fertility control and infertility, and termination of unwanted pregnancy.

BARRIERS TO ENTERING THE HEALTH CARE SYSTEM

Financial Issues

Access to care varies greatly depending on type and size of the system, source of payment for services, private versus public programs, availability of and accessibility to providers, individual preferences, and insurance coverage or ability to pay. The existing system in the United States continues to be oriented to treatment of acute or episodic conditions rather than to the promotion of health and comprehensive care, despite the fact that people are discharged earlier from hospitals, requiring more care in homes and community settings. With a greater focus on preventive health care services, nurses, advanced practice nurses (including nurse practitioners [NPs]), nurse-midwives, and clinical nurse specialists, are critical to the provision of high-quality, safe, effective, and accessible health care (see Box 4.1).

Social Determinants of Health

Healthy People 2020 highlights the importance of addressing the social determinants of health by including "Create social and physical environments that promote good health for all" as one of the four overarching goals for the decade (CDC, 2014). Social determinants of health are conditions in the environments in which people are born, live, learn, work, play, worship, and age that affect a wide range of health functioning, and quality-of-life outcomes and risks (CDC Healthy People 2020). Health care is dependent not only on single interventions, but also on factors apart from any care we can provide. Poverty, education, nutrition, exercise, smoking, drinking, drug use, etc., are potent social determinants of a woman's health.

In the United States, disparity among races and socioeconomic classes affects many facets of life, including health. Inadequate finances are associated with lack of access to care, delay in seeking care, limited prevention activities, and little accurate information about health and the health care system. Many impoverished women have traditionally been underinsured or uninsured, and rules about health insurance and who and what is covered remains problematic even with the Affordable Care Act.

The field of health care continues to operate under a "risk factor" paradigm that focuses on behavior modification for high-risk groups as the core strategy for preventing disease. This approach has not proven to be effective, mostly due to individuals not being in control of the factors that make them sick and responding unconsciously to environmental cues. Health care must go beyond paying attention to risk factors and should address the social determinants that impact a woman and her family's health by beginning early and broadening the scope of interventions, thus making entire families and communities healthier. Although health care providers generally recognize that social determinants (e.g., income, education, and social status) influence the health of their clients, many are unsure of how they can intervene. There are actions that care providers can take to address social determinants in their clinical practice to improve client health and reduce inequities. Nurses can be alert to clinical flags, ask clients about social challenges in a sensitive and caring way, and help them access benefits and support services. At the practice level, nurses can offer culturally safe services, use client navigators where possible, and ensure that care is accessible. In addition, there are growing numbers of clinical decision aids, and practice guidelines and other tools are now available to assist nurses in addressing the social determinants in their day-to-day practice.

Gender influences communications between health care professionals and patients and may influence differences in access to health care in general. There are male-female disparities in receipt of major diagnostic and therapeutic interventions, especially with cardiac and kidney problems. Women tend to use primary care services more often than do men. The gender of the provider may play a role. The concept of "gender concordance," in which the patient's gender matches the health care provider's gender, was found to be important for women seeking Pap tests (Lin & Chen, 2014).

Sexual orientation may create another barrier. Nurses and other health care professionals need to understand the specific health care needs and issues related to sexual orientation, particularly since many lesbian, gay, bisexual, transgender, and queer (LGBTQ) individuals feel stigmatized and are reluctant to seek health care (Olshansky & Zender, 2015). Some lesbians may not disclose their sexual orientation to health care professionals because they feel they may be at risk for hostility, inadequate health care, or breach of confidentiality. In many health care settings heterosexuality is assumed and the setting may be one in which the woman does not feel welcome (magazines, brochures reflect heterosexual couples or the health care provider shows discomfort interacting with the woman). Lesbians may hold beliefs that are incorrect (e.g., that they have immunity to human immunodeficiency virus [HIV], sexually transmitted infections [STIs], and certain cancers [e.g., cervical]). The perceived lack of risk can result in some lesbians avoiding seeking health care, as well as in health care providers giving incorrect advice or not providing appropriate screening for these women. Not all gynecologic cancers are caused by sexual activity; woman (and that includes lesbians) who have never had children may be more at risk for breast, ovarian, or endometrial cancers. Their risk for heart disease, lung cancer, and colon cancer is not different from that of heterosexual women. To offset stereotypes, it is necessary for providers to develop an approach that does not assume that all patients are heterosexual. More content in this area needs to be included in nursing curricula.

COMMUNITY ACTIVITY

- Visit the National Women's Health Resource Center website at www.healthywomen.org. Go to the conditions and treatments link and select a condition. Review the client information sections about diagnosis, treatment, prevention, facts to know, questions to ask, and lifestyle tips.
- Visit the WomensHealth.gov and go to the various women's health topics and publications. Review the information to see what areas of women's health might be of interest to you, including how you might advocate in the community on behalf of a women's health issue.

CARING FOR THE WELL WOMAN ACROSS THE LIFE SPAN: THE NEED FOR HEALTH PROMOTION AND DISEASE PREVENTION

Maintaining optimal health is a goal for all women. Essential components of health maintenance are the identification of unrecognized problems and potential risks and the education and health promotion needed to reduce them. Current trends in the health care of women have expanded beyond a reproductive focus. A holistic approach to women's health care goes beyond only reproductive needs and includes a woman's health needs throughout her lifetime, with attention to physical, mental, emotional, social, and spiritual health. Women's health is considered to be part of the primary health care delivery system with assessment and screening focusing on a multisystem evaluation that emphasizes the maintenance and enhancement of wellness. Prevention of cardiovascular disease, promotion of mental health, and prevention of cancers beyond just reproductive-related cancers are all components of well-woman care. It is important to consider all aspects of women's health, particularly in light of the fact that the leading causes of death in women in the United States include more than just reproductive health conditions (Box 4.2).

Even when focusing on reproductive health, it is critical to take a holistic approach to the health of women. This is especially important for women in their childbearing years because conditions that increase a woman's health risks are related not only to her well-being, but also to the well-being of both mother and baby in the event of a pregnancy.

BOX 4.2 Top 10 Leading Causes of Death in Women in the United States

1. Heart disease
2. Cancer
3. Chronic lower respiratory diseases
4. Stroke
5. Alzheimer's disease
6. Unintentional injuries
7. Diabetes
8. Influenza and pneumonia
9. Kidney disease
10. Septicemia

Data from Centers for Disease Control and Prevention (2018). Leading causes of death in females, United States, 2015. Retrieved from: https://www.cdc.gov/women/lcod/2015/index.htm.

Prenatal care is an example of prevention that is practiced after conception. However, prevention and health maintenance are needed before conception because many of the mother's risks can be identified and eliminated, or at least modified.

As a female progresses through developmental ages and stages, she is faced with conditions that are age related. An overview of conditions and circumstances that increase health risks in women across the life span is presented in the next section.

Age

Adolescents

All teenagers undergo progressive development of sex characteristics. They experience the developmental tasks of adolescence such as establishing identity and sexual orientation, emancipating from family, and establishing career goals. Some of these processes can produce great stress for the adolescent, and the health care provider should treat her very carefully. Female teenagers who enter the health care system usually do so for screening or because of a problem such as episodic illness or accident. Previous guidelines recommended that young women should be screened with Pap tests at 18 years of age or when they become sexually active. Current guidelines suggest that Pap tests begin at 21 years of age (United States Preventive Services Task Force [USPSTF], 2018), but controversy exists about the evidence to support these new guidelines, with some health care providers advising earlier testing, especially if a woman is sexually active at a younger age. Gynecologic problems are often associated with menses (either bleeding irregularities or dysmenorrhea), vaginitis or leukorrhea, sexually transmitted infections (STIs), contraception, or pregnancy. The adolescent is also at risk for use of street drugs (e.g., marijuana, cocaine, etc); for eating disorders; and for stress, depression, and anxiety.

Many women first enter the health care delivery system for a Pap test or for contraception. Visits to the nurse may be their only contact with the system unless they become ill. Some women postpone examination until a specific need arises such as pregnancy, infertility, pain, abnormal bleeding, or vaginal discharge. Recently the availability of the human papillomavirus (HPV) vaccine has created another reason for young women to enter the health care system (Berg, Taylor, & Woods, 2015).

Teen pregnancy. Most young women begin having sex in the mid- to late teens. The average age at first intercourse is 17 (Guttmacher Institute, 2017), meaning that many begin sexual activity at an earlier age. In 2017, the birth rate to teens in the age range of 15 to 17 dropped by 10%, and for teens in the age range of 18 to 19, the birth rate dropped by 6% (CDC, 2019).

Effective educational programs about sex and family life are imperative to control the rate of teen pregnancy and STIs. The nurse can provide information regarding the need for child spacing, methods of family planning that are consistent with religious and personal preferences, noncontraceptive benefits of certain methods, the appropriate use of methods selected, and the protection of future fertility when so desired.

Teen pregnancy, especially for those 16 years of age and younger, often introduces additional stress into a typically challenging developmental period. The emotional level of such teens is commonly characterized by impulsiveness and self-centered behavior, and they often place primary importance on the beliefs and actions of their peers. In attempts to establish a personal and independent identity, many teens do not realize the consequences of their behavior; their thinking processes do not include planning for the future.

Teens usually lack the financial resources to support a pregnancy and may not have the maturity to avoid teratogens or seek prenatal care and instruction or follow-up care. Children of teen mothers may be at risk for abuse or neglect because of the teen's inadequate knowledge of growth, development, and parenting. Implementation of specialized adolescent programs in schools, communities, and health care systems is demonstrating continued success in reducing the birth rate in teens.

Young and Middle Adulthood

Because women 20 to 40 years of age have a need for contraception, pelvic and breast screening, and pregnancy care, they may prefer to use their gynecologic or obstetric provider as their primary care provider. During these years the woman may be "juggling" family, home, and career responsibilities, with resulting increases in stress-related conditions. Health maintenance includes not only pelvic and breast screening, but also promotion of a healthy lifestyle (i.e., good nutrition, regular exercise, no smoking, moderate or no alcohol consumption, sufficient rest, stress reduction, and referral for medical conditions and other specific problems). Common conditions requiring well-woman care include vaginitis, urinary tract infections (UTIs), menstrual variations, obesity, sexual and relationship issues, and pregnancy.

Parenthood after 35 years of age. The woman older than 35 years of age does not have a different physical response to a pregnancy per se, but rather has had health status changes as a result of time and the aging process. These changes may be responsible for age-related pregnancy conditions. For example, a woman with type 2 diabetes may not have had expression of her diabetes at 22 years of age but may have full-blown disease at 38 years of age. Other chronic or debilitating diseases or conditions increase in severity with time, and these in turn may predispose to increased risks during pregnancy. Of significance to women in this age group is the risk for certain genetic anomalies (e.g., Down syndrome). The opportunity for genetic counseling should be available to all women (see Chapter 6).

Late Reproductive Age

Women of later reproductive age are often experiencing change and reordering personal priorities. In general, the goals of education, career, marriage, and family have been achieved and now the woman has increased time and opportunity for new interests and activities. Divorce rates are high at this age, and children leaving home may produce an "empty nest syndrome," resulting in increased levels of depression. Chronic diseases also become more apparent. Most problems for the well woman are associated with perimenopause (e.g., bleeding irregularities and vasomotor symptoms). Health maintenance screening continues to be of importance because some conditions such as breast disease or ovarian cancer occur more often during this stage.

APPROACHES TO CARE AT SPECIFIC STAGES OF A WOMAN'S LIFE

There are certain specific approaches to care of women at different stages of their lives. Several of these approaches are described next.

Preconception Counseling and Care

Preconception health promotion provides women and their partners with information that is needed to make decisions about their reproductive future. Preconception care guides couples on how to avoid unintended pregnancies, identify and manage risk factors in their lives and their environment, and identify healthy behaviors that promote the well-being of the woman and her potential fetus. It has been estimated that 32% of pregnant women experience some complications of pregnancy, including mental health issues (mostly depression) and factors that lead to the need for cesarean birth (CDC, 2016a). In addition, 9.93% of births were preterm infants in 2017, which represents a 1% rise since 2016. The percentage of low birthweight (LBW) infants also rose, from 8.17% in 2016 to 8.28% in 2017 (Martin, Hamilton, Osterman, et al., 2018).

Activities that promote healthy mothers and babies are ideally initiated before the period of critical fetal organ development, which is between 17 and 56 days after fertilization. By the end of the eighth week after conception and certainly by the end of the first trimester, any major structural anomalies in the fetus are already present. Because many women do not realize that they are pregnant and do not seek prenatal care until well into the first trimester, the rapidly growing fetus may be exposed to many types of intrauterine environmental hazards during this most vulnerable developmental phase. These hazards include drugs, viruses, and chemicals. In many instances, counseling can promote behavior modification before damage is done, or the woman can make an informed decision about her willingness to accept potential hazards.

Preconception care is important for women who have had a problem with a previous pregnancy (e.g., miscarriage or preterm birth). Although causes are not always identifiable, in many cases problems can be discovered and treated and do not recur in subsequent pregnancies. Preconception care is also important to minimize fetal malformations. For example, the offspring of women who have preexisting diabetes mellitus have significantly more congenital anomalies than do children of mothers without diabetes. The rate of malformation is greatly reduced when the woman with preexisting diabetes has excellent blood glucose control at the time she becomes pregnant and maintains euglycemia (normal blood glucose level) throughout the period of organ development in the fetus. The incidence of neural tube defects (NTDs) such as spina bifida and anencephaly is decreased significantly with the daily intake of 400 mcg of supplemental folic acid.

The components of preconception care such as health promotion, risk assessment, and interventions are outlined in Box 4.3.

PREGNANCY

A woman's entry into health care is often associated with pregnancy, for either diagnosis or actual prenatal care. Early entry into prenatal care (i.e., within the first 12 weeks of pregnancy) allows for identification of the woman at risk for complications and initiation of measures to prevent problems or treat them if they arise. The US Department of Health and Human Services and the National Institute of Child Health and Human Development (2016) emphasized the importance of early and consistent prenatal care to improve outcomes for both mother and infant. Major goals of prenatal care are listed in Box 4.4 and should be addressed in the first visit. Extensive discussion of pregnancy is found in Part 3.

BOX 4.3 Components of Preconception Care

Health Promotion: General Teaching
- Nutrition
  - Healthy diet, including folic acid
  - Optimal weight
- Exercise and rest
  - Avoidance of substance abuse (tobacco, alcohol, "recreational" drugs)
  - Use of risk-reducing sex practices
  - Attending to family and social needs

Risk Factor Assessment
- Chronic diseases
  - Diabetes, heart disease, hypertension, asthma, thyroid disease, kidney disease, anemia, mental illness
- Infectious diseases
  - HIV/AIDS, other sexually transmitted infections, vaccine-preventable diseases (e.g., rubella, hepatitis B)
- Reproductive history
  - Contraception
  - Pregnancies—unplanned pregnancy, pregnancy outcomes
  - Infertility
- Genetic or inherited conditions (e.g., sickle cell anemia, Down syndrome, cystic fibrosis)
- Medications and medical treatment
  - Prescription medications (especially those contraindicated in pregnancy), over-the-counter medication use, radiation exposure
- Personal behaviors and exposures
  - Smoking, alcohol consumption, illicit drug use
  - Overweight or underweight; eating disorders
  - Folic acid supplement use
  - Spouse or partner and family situation, including intimate partner violence
  - Availability of family or other support systems
  - Readiness for pregnancy (e.g., age, life goals, stress)
  - Environmental (home, workplace) conditions
  - Safety hazards
  - Toxic chemicals
  - Radiation

Interventions
- Anticipatory guidance or teaching
  - Treatment of relevant medical conditions
  - Medications
  - Cessation or reduction in substance use and abuse
  - Immunizations (e.g., rubella, hepatitis)
- Nutrition, diet, weight management
- Exercise
- Referral for genetic counseling
- Referral to and use of:
  - Family planning services
  - Family and social needs management

AIDS, Acquired immunodeficiency syndrome; *HIV,* human immunodeficiency virus.

BOX 4.4 Major Goals of Prenatal Care

- Define health status of the mother and fetus.
- Determine the gestational age of the fetus, and monitor fetal development.
- Identify the woman at risk for complications, and minimize the risk whenever possible.
- Provide appropriate education and counseling.

Fertility Control and Infertility

Although the unintended pregnancy rate is slowly decreasing, the problem of unintended pregnancies remains significant (Guttmacher Institute, 2019). The majority of these occur in women who either do not use contraception or who experienced a contraceptive failure. Education is the key to encouraging women to make family planning choices based on preference and actual benefit-to-risk ratios. Providers can influence the user's motivation and ability to use the method correctly (see Chapter 8).

Women also enter the health care system because of their desire to become pregnant. Many couples have delayed starting their families until they are in their 30s or 40s, which allows more time to be exposed to factors that affect fertility negatively (including age-related infertility for the woman). In addition, STIs, which can predispose to decreased fertility, are becoming more common, and many women and men are in workplaces and home settings where they may be exposed to reproductive environmental hazards.

Infertility can cause emotional pain for many couples, and the inability to produce offspring sometimes results in feelings of failure and places inordinate stress on the couple's relationship. Much time, money, and emotional investment can be used for testing and treatment in efforts to build a family.

Steps toward prevention of infertility should be undertaken as part of ongoing routine health care, and information about how women may prevent some causes of infertility is especially appropriate in preconception counseling. Primary care providers can undertake initial evaluation and counseling before couples are referred to specialists. For additional information about infertility, see Chapter 9.

Menstrual Problems

Irregularities or problems with the menstrual period are among the most common concerns of women and often cause them to seek help from the health care system. Common menstrual disorders include amenorrhea, dysmenorrhea, premenstrual syndrome, endometriosis, and menorrhagia or metrorrhagia. Simple explanation and counseling may handle the concern; however, history and physical examination must be completed, as well as laboratory or diagnostic tests, if indicated. Questions from the woman should never be considered inconsequential, and age-specific reading materials are recommended, especially for teens. See Chapter 6 for an in-depth discussion of menstrual problems.

Perimenopause

The body responds to this natural transition in a number of ways, most of which are caused by the decrease in estrogen. Most women seeking health care during the perimenopausal period do so because of irregular bleeding. Others are concerned about vasomotor symptoms (hot flashes and flushes). Although fertility is greatly reduced during this period, women are urged to maintain some method of birth control because pregnancies still can occur. All women need to have factual information, the dispelling of myths, a thorough examination, and periodic health screenings thereafter.

IDENTIFICATION OF RISK FACTORS TO WOMEN'S HEALTH

In caring for women at all stages of life, it is important to understand the various and complex risk factors that can affect a woman's health. This section describes these risk factors. A thorough and systematic health history can elicit information about risk factors that exist for each woman.

Social, Cultural, and Genetic Factors

Differences exist among people from different socioeconomic levels and ethnic groups with respect to risk for illness and distribution of disease and death. Some diseases are more common among people of selected ethnicity (e.g., sickle cell anemia in African Americans, Tay-Sachs disease in Ashkenazi Jews, adult lactase deficiency in Chinese individuals, β-thalassemia in Mediterranean individuals, and cystic fibrosis in northern Europeans). Cultural and religious influences might also increase health risks because the woman and her family may have life and societal values, and a view of health and illness, that dictate practices different from those expected in the Judeo-Christian Western model. These may include food taboos or frequencies, methods of hygiene, effects of climate, care-seeking behaviors, willingness to undergo screening and diagnostic procedures, and conflicts in values.

Socioeconomic status affects birth outcomes. The rates of perinatal and maternal deaths, preterm births, and LBW infants are considerably higher in disadvantaged populations. Social consequences for poor women as single parents are great because many mothers with few skills are caught in the bind of insufficient income to afford child care. These families generate fewer and fewer resources and increase their risks for health problems. Multiple roles for women in general produce overload, conflict, and stress, resulting in higher risks for mental health problems.

Substance Use and Abuse

Use of illicit drugs and inappropriate use of prescription drugs continue to increase and are found in all ages, races, ethnic groups, and socioeconomic levels. Addiction to substances is seen as a biopsychosocial disease, with several factors leading to risk. These include biogenetic predisposition, lack of resilience to stressful life experiences, and poor social support. Women are less likely than men to abuse drugs, but the rate in women is increasing significantly. Chapter 31 includes content on pregnancy-related effects of substances. Chapter 35 includes content on neonatal-related effects of substances.

Prescription Drug Use

Psychotherapeutic medications such as stimulants, sleeping pills, tranquilizers, and pain relievers are used by an estimated 2.3% of American women (Substance Abuse and Mental Health Services Administration, 2015). Such medications can bring relief from undesirable conditions such as insomnia, anxiety, and pain. Because the medications have mind-altering capacity, misuse can produce psychologic and physical dependency in the same manner as illicit drugs. Risk-to-benefit ratios should be considered when such medications are used for more than a very short period. Depression and anxiety are the most common mental health problems in women (depression used to be considered the most common, but recently it is noted that depression occurs comorbidly with anxiety). Many kinds of medications are used to treat depression and anxiety. All of these psychotherapeutic drugs can have some effect on the fetus and must be monitored very carefully.

Illicit Drug Use

Marijuana. Marijuana is a substance derived from the cannabis plant. It is usually rolled into a cigarette and smoked, but it also may be mixed into food and eaten. Marijuana produces distorted perceptions, difficulty with problem solving as well as with thinking and memory, altered state of awareness, relaxation, mild euphoria, reduced inhibition, and mood changes (National Institute on Drug Abuse, 2016a). Marijuana is the most frequently used illicit drug, although a number of states have legalized it for recreational use.

Cocaine. Cocaine is a powerful central nervous system (CNS) stimulant that is addictive because of the tremendous sense of euphoria that it creates. It can be snorted, smoked, or injected (National Institute on Drug Abuse, 2016b). Crack or rock cocaine is a form of the drug that is exceedingly potent and even more highly addictive. (Some say that an individual is "hooked" after the first use or at least after two or three "hits.") After ingestion of cocaine, an intensely pleasurable high results that is followed by an uncomfortable low; this increases the urge to continue taking the drug.

Predisposing factors and problems associated with cocaine use are polydrug use; poor nutrition; poverty; STIs; hepatitis B infection; dysfunctional family systems; employment difficulties; stress; anger; poor self-esteem; and previous or present physical, emotional, and sexual abuse. Cocaine use is especially concentrated among poor women of color.

Cocaine affects all major body systems. Among other complications, it produces cardiovascular stress (including tachycardia and hypertension) that can lead to heart attack or stroke, liver disease, CNS simulation that can cause seizures, and even perforation of the nasal septum. Needle-borne diseases such as hepatitis B and acquired immunodeficiency syndrome (AIDS) are common among cocaine users.

Opiates. The opiates include opium, heroin, meperidine, morphine, codeine, and methadone. Heroin is one of the most commonly abused drugs of this class. It is usually taken by intravenous injection but can be smoked or "snorted." The signs and symptoms of heroin use are euphoria, relaxation, relief from pain, "nodding out" (apathy, detachment from reality, impaired judgment, and drowsiness), constricted pupils, nausea, constipation, slurred speech, and respiratory depression.

Opiate use has become a priority problem area for the U.S. Department of Health and Human Services with the recognition that prescription drugs, of which some opiates are a part, contribute to this serious abuse of opiates. Drug overdose, much of which occurs due to opiate abuse, is the leading cause of death due to injury (U.S. Department of Health & Human Services, 2019).

Methamphetamine. Methamphetamine is a relatively cheap and highly addictive stimulant. Over the past few years, use of this dangerous drug has decreased. Methamphetamine makes many users feel hypersexual and uninhibited, leading to more sex and less protection from pregnancy and STIs.

The active metabolite of methamphetamine is amphetamine, a CNS stimulant known as both "speed" and "meth." The crystalline form, which is smoked, is known as "ice." Methamphetamine causes a person to experience an elevated mood state as well as increased energy and creates addiction within a short period. It can lead to cardiac problems, including irregular heartbeat and hypertension, and over time can create cognitive and mental, as well as dental, problems (National Institute on Drug Abuse, 2014). Most of the effects of amphetamines are similar to those of cocaine.

Other illicit drugs. A number of street drugs pose risks to users. A few are derived from organic materials, but more and more are produced synthetically in laboratories. Sedatives such as "downers," "yellow jackets," or "red devils" are used to come off of "highs." Hallucinogens alter perceptions and body function. Lysergic acid diethylamide (LSD) produces vivid changes in sensation, often with agitation, euphoria, paranoia, and a tendency toward antisocial behavior. Its use may lead to flashbacks, chronic psychosis, and violent behavior.

Phencyclidine (PCP) is a synthetic drug known by various names ("peace pill," "elephant," "angel dust," "hog"). PCP causes a person to experience dissociative symptoms that include distorted perceptions and detached feelings, memory loss, depression, delusions, hallucinations, anxiety, panic, and disordered thinking. High doses can cause seizures, coma, and possibly death (National Institute on Drug Abuse, 2016c). Because some effects mimic the signs and symptoms of schizophrenia, a user may be admitted to a psychiatric unit.

Alcohol Consumption

Current data estimates that 5.3 million women drink to such an extent that it endangers their health (National Institute on Alcohol Abuse and Alcoholism, 2018). About one-third of alcoholics are women, and many relate the onset of their drinking problem to stressful events. Women who are problem drinkers are often depressed, have more motor vehicle injuries, and have a higher incidence of attempted suicide than do women in the general population. They are also at risk for alcohol-related liver damage. Early case finding and treatment are important in alcoholism for both the ill individual and family members.

Cigarette Smoking

Tobacco use is the leading cause of preventable death and illness. Smoking is linked to cardiovascular disease, various types of cancers (especially lung and cervical), chronic lung disease, and negative pregnancy outcomes. Premature death is estimated to occur in 480,000 people annually because of either smoking or being exposed to secondhand smoke, with cigarette smoking being the leading cause of preventable deaths. However, it is also estimated that 34.3 million adults in the United States smoke; 12.2% of women are smokers (CDC, 2018a). Women who smoke decrease their life span by 14.5 years compared with nonsmokers, but recent data indicate that the sooner a person quits smoking, the sooner he or she can decrease their risk for early death (ACS, 2018b). Box 4.11 includes guidelines for smoking cessation.

Tobacco contains nicotine, which is an addictive substance that creates physical and psychologic dependence. Recently, alternatives to cigarettes have been used, including electronic cigarettes (e-cigarettes), smokeless tobacco, and water pipes. These alternative methods, however, may cause serious side effects due to the chemicals used in them and may have deleterious effects on the developing fetus (England, Bunnell, Pechacek, et al., 2015).

Cigarette smoking impairs fertility in both women and men, may reduce the age for menopause, and increases the risk for osteoporosis after menopause. Passive, or secondhand, smoke (environmental tobacco smoke) contains similar hazards and presents additional problems for the smoker and harm for the nonsmoker. Smoking during pregnancy may have adverse consequences for the infant, such as LBW, preterm birth, stillbirth, sudden infant death syndrome (SIDS), ectopic pregnancy, and orofacial clefts (CDC, 2018b).

Caffeine

Caffeine is found in society's most popular drinks: coffee, tea, and soft drinks. It is a stimulant that can affect mood and interrupt body functions by producing anxiety and sleep interruptions. Heart dysrhythmias may be made worse by caffeine, and there can be interactions with certain medications such as lithium. Birth defects have not been related to caffeine consumption; however, high intake has been related to a slight decrease in birth weight and may also increase the risk for miscarriage. The March of Dimes (2015) recommends that pregnant women, or women who are trying to conceive, limit their caffeine intake to no more than 200 mg/day, which is the equivalent of one 12-ounce cup of coffee.

Nutrition Problems and Eating Disorders

Good nutrition is essential for optimal health. A well-balanced diet helps prevent illness and also is used to treat certain health problems. Conversely, poor eating habits, eating disorders, and obesity are linked to disease and debility. *Dietary Guidelines for Americans* (Office of Disease Prevention and Health Promotion [ODPHP], 2018) provides evidence-based recommendations to promote health and reduce risks for chronic diseases through diet and physical activity.

This guide contains resources for health professionals and consumers on dietary guidelines. Previously, the U.S. government advocated the Food Pyramid, followed by MyPlate. The current recommendations include five guidelines: (1) Follow a healthy eating pattern across the life span, (2) focus on variety, nutrient density, and amount, (3) limit calories from added sugars and saturated fats, and reduce sodium intake, (4) shift to healthier food and beverage choices, and (5) support healthy eating patterns for all.

In addition to specific guidelines for healthy eating, environmental factors play an important role in nutrition. Environmental factors are part of what is referred to as social determinants of health, in which the availability of resources is a critical factor in nutrition and health.

Nutritional Deficiencies

Overt disease caused by a lack of certain nutrients is rarely seen in the United States. However, insufficient amounts or imbalances of nutrients do pose problems for individuals and families. Overweight or underweight status, malabsorption, listlessness, fatigue, frequent colds and other minor infections, constipation, dull hair and nails, and dental caries are examples of problems that can be related to nutrition and indicate the need for further nutritional assessment. Poor nutrition, especially related to obesity and high fat and cholesterol intake, may lead to more serious conditions such as heart diseases, malignant neoplasms, cerebrovascular diseases, and diabetes.

Other dietary extremes also produce risk. For example, insufficient amounts of calcium can lead to osteoporosis, too much sodium can aggravate hypertension, and megadoses of vitamins can cause adverse effects in several body systems. Fad weight-loss programs and yo-yo dieting (repeated and cyclic weight gain and weight loss) result in nutritional imbalances and, in some instances, medical problems. Such diets and programs are not appropriate for weight maintenance. Adolescent pregnancy produces special nutritional requirements because the metabolic needs of pregnancy are superimposed on the teen's own needs for growth and maturation at a time when eating habits are not ideal. NTDs are more common in infants born to women with a diet poor in folate. In their childbearing years, women should ingest at least 0.4 mg (400 mcg) of folic acid daily in addition to consuming a diet rich in folate-containing foods (CDC, 2018a).

Obesity

During the past 20 years, obesity has increased dramatically in the United States. More than one-third of women in the United States are obese (body mass index [BMI] of 30 or greater), with adults 40 to 59 years of age having the highest prevalence. The BMI is defined as a measure of an adult's weight in relation to his or her height, specifically the adult's weight in kilograms divided by the square of his or her height in meters. It is estimated that over one third of adults are obese, with even higher rates of obesity for Hispanic and non-Hispanic blacks (CDC, 2018c). Overweight and obesity are known risk factors for premature death, diabetes, heart disease, stroke, hypertension, type 2 diabetes, gallbladder disease, diverticular disease, some anemias, oral disease, constipation, osteoarthritis, gout, osteoporosis, respiratory dysfunction, sleep apnea, and some types of cancer (uterine, breast, esophageal, colorectal, kidney, and pancreatic) (ACS, 2018a). In addition, obesity is associated with high cholesterol, menstrual irregularities, hirsutism (excess body/facial hair), stress incontinence, depression, complications of pregnancy, increased surgical risk, and shortened life span. Chapter 32 includes information on obesity in pregnancy.

Eating Disorders

Eating disorders are estimated to have a prevalence of 30 million people in the United States, with women having a higher rate than men.

Eating disorders are considered a mental illness, and the mortality rate is the highest of all mental illnesses (National Association of Anorexia Nervosa and Associated Disorders, 2019).

Anorexia nervosa and bulimia are two forms of eating disorders, although there are additional forms, such as binge eating disorders or other specified feeding or eating disorders. Some women, especially adolescents, do not have symptoms that lend themselves to a diagnosis of anorexia nervosa or bulimia, but they do fall under an unspecified category and require accurate diagnosis and prompt treatment (Sammarco, 2016). Eating disorders can affect not only the woman, but her family as well. Treatment must be personalized, including nutritional and behavioral/psychotherapeutic approaches. It is important to involve an interprofessional health care team in managing women with eating disorders.

It is important to assess for and treat women with eating disorders early because they are at increased risk for serious physical problems as well as diminished quality of life (Sammarco, 2016). Eating disorders during pregnancy are also associated with increased risk to the pregnant woman and her fetus.

Anorexia nervosa. Some women have a distorted view of their bodies and, no matter what their weight, perceive themselves to be much too heavy. As a result, they undertake strict and severe diets and rigorous extreme exercise. This chronic eating disorder is known as *anorexia nervosa*. Women can carry this condition to the point of starvation, with resulting endocrine and metabolic abnormalities. If not corrected, significant complications of dysrhythmias, amenorrhea, cardiomyopathy, and heart failure occur and, in the extreme, can lead to death. The condition commonly begins during adolescence in young women who have some degree of personality disorder. They gradually lose weight over several months, have amenorrhea, and are abnormally concerned with body image. A coexisting depression usually accompanies anorexia.

There are no specific tests to diagnose anorexia nervosa. A medical history, physical examination, and screening tests help identify women at risk for eating disorders. Several tools are available to use in primary care settings. The SCOFF questionnaire, developed by Morgan, Reid, and Lacey (1999) is still in use and is easy to administer and can help the nurse decide whether an eating disorder is likely, and whether the woman needs further assessment and possibly psychiatric and medical intervention (Hautala, Junnila, Alin, et al., 2009). See Box 4.5 for a description of the SCOFF.

Bulimia nervosa. Bulimia refers to secret, uncontrolled binge eating alternating with methods to prevent weight gain: self-induced vomiting, laxatives or diuretics, strict diets, fasting, and rigorous exercise. During a binge episode, a large number of calories are consumed, usually consisting of sweets and "junk foods." Binges occur at least twice per week. Bulimia usually begins in early adulthood (18 to 25 years of age) and is found primarily in females. Complications can include dehydration and electrolyte imbalance, gastrointestinal abnormalities, and cardiac dysrhythmias. Unlike those with anorexia, individuals with bulimia may feel shame or disgust about their disorder and tend to seek help earlier. The SCOFF screening assessment also can be used to assess clients with bulimia (see Box 4.5).

Lack of Exercise

Exercise contributes to good health by lowering risks for a variety of conditions that are influenced by obesity and a sedentary lifestyle. It is effective in the prevention of cardiovascular disease and in the management of chronic conditions such as hypertension, arthritis, diabetes, respiratory disorders, and osteoporosis. Exercise also contributes to stress reduction and weight maintenance. Women report that engaging in regular exercise improves their body image and self-esteem and

---

BOX 4.5   Screening for Eating Disorders

SCOFF Questions

Each question scores 1 point. A score of 2 or more indicates the person may have anorexia nervosa or bulimia.

1. Do you make yourself **S**ick (i.e., induce vomiting) because you feel too full?
2. Do you worry about loss of **C**ontrol over the amount you eat?
3. Have you recently lost more than **O**ne stone (6.4 kg [14 lb]) in a 3-month period?
4. Do you think you are too **F**at even if others think you are too thin?
5. Does **F**ood dominate your life?

From Morgan, J. F., & Lacey, J. (1999). The SCOFF questionnaire: Assessment of a new screening tool for eating disorders. *British Medical Journal, 319*(7223), 1467–1468.

---

acts as a mood enhancer. Aerobic exercise produces cardiovascular involvement because an increased amount of oxygen is delivered to working muscles. Anaerobic exercise such as weight training improves individual muscle mass without stress on the cardiovascular system. Because women are concerned about both cardiovascular and bone health, weight-bearing aerobic exercises such as walking, running, racket sports, and dancing are preferred. However, excessive or strenuous exercise can lead to hormone imbalances, resulting in amenorrhea and its consequences. Physical injury is also a potential risk.

Physical activity and exercise counseling for persons of all ages should be undertaken at schools, work sites, and primary care settings. Specific recommendations include 20 to 30 minutes of moderate activity at least three times per week. Few Americans exercise this often, and physical inactivity increases with age, especially during adolescence and early adulthood. Even small increases in activity can be beneficial. During pregnancy, an ongoing exercise regimen can be continued but intensity and duration should be decreased. Sedentary women should obtain medical clearance to initiate exercise during pregnancy and should begin with low-intensity and low-impact workouts.

Stress

The lifestyles of many American women lead to increasing levels of stress and, as a result, is prone to a variety of stress-induced complaints and illnesses. Stress often occurs because of multiple roles in which coping with job and financial responsibilities conflicts with parenting and duties at home. To add to this burden, women are socialized to be caregivers, which is emotionally draining, creating additional stress. They also may find themselves in positions of minimal power that do not allow them control over their everyday environments. Some stress is normal and contributes to positive outcomes. Many women thrive in busy surroundings. However, excessive or high levels of ongoing stress trigger physical reactions such as rapid heart rate, elevated blood pressure, slowed digestion, release of additional neurotransmitters and hormones, muscle tension and a weakened immune system. Consequently, constant stress can contribute to clinical illnesses such as flare-ups of arthritis or asthma, frequent respiratory or other infections, gastrointestinal upsets, cardiovascular problems, and infertility. Box 4.6 lists symptoms that may be related to chronic or extreme stress. Psychologic symptoms such as anxiety, irritability, eating disorders, depression, insomnia, and substance abuse have also been associated with stress.

Because it is neither possible nor desirable to avoid all stress, women must learn how to manage it. The nurse should assess each woman for signs of stress using therapeutic communication skills to determine risk factors and the woman's ability to function. Some women must be referred for counseling or other mental health therapy. Women experiencing major life changes such as separation and divorce, bereavement, serious illness, and unemployment also need special attention.

BOX 4.6   Stress Symptoms

Physical
- Perspiration/sweaty hands
- Increased heart rate
- Trembling
- Nervous tics
- Dryness of throat and mouth
- Tiring easily
- Urinating frequently
- Sleeping problems
- Diarrhea, indigestion, vomiting
- Butterflies in stomach
- Headaches
- Premenstrual tension
- Pain in the neck and lower back
- Loss of appetite or overeating
- Susceptibility to illness

Behavior
- Stuttering and other speech difficulties
- Crying for no apparent reason
- Acting impulsively
- Startling easily
- Laughing in a high-pitched and nervous tone of voice
- Grinding teeth
- Increased smoking
- Increased use of drugs and alcohol
- Being accident-prone
- Losing appetite or overeating

Psychologic
- Feeling anxious
- Feeling scared
- Feeling irritable
- Feeling moody
- Low self-esteem
- Fear of failure
- Inability to concentrate
- Embarrassed easily
- Worrying about the future
- Preoccupation with thoughts or tasks
- Forgetfulness

Adapted from State University of New York Counseling Center. (2002). *Stress management.* University of Buffalo, NY: State University of New York.

Many centers offer support groups to help women prevent or manage stress. Social support and good coping skills can improve a woman's self-esteem and give her a sense of mastery. Anticipatory guidance for developmental or expected situational crises can help her plan strategies for dealing with potentially stressful events. Role playing, relaxation techniques, biofeedback, meditation, desensitization, imagery, assertiveness training, yoga, diet, exercise, and weight control are all techniques nurses can include in their repertoire of supportive skills.

Depression, Anxiety, and Other Mental Health Conditions

Women experience depression and/or anxiety frequently. Women are twice as likely as men to suffer from anxiety panic attacks and suffer more major depression than men (Anxiety and Depression Association of America, 2018). Nurses must be alert to the symptoms of serious mental disorders such as depression and anxiety and make referrals to mental health practitioners when necessary. In addition, depression is sometimes described as a cotraveler because it exists comorbidly with other physical conditions. Depression and/or anxiety create difficulties for quality of life and, at the extreme, a risk for suicide. Recent research indicates that persons with comorbid anxiety and depression are at greater risk for developing cardiac disease. In addition to depression and anxiety, women experience other mental health disorders, such as bipolar disease (Cohen, Edmundson, & Kronish, 2015).

Sleep Disorders

Many women suffer from sleep disorders, including difficulty initiating sleep or staying asleep, and experiencing nonrestorative sleep. During pregnancy and postpartum, many factors can negatively affect sleep, and restless leg syndrome may result. Sleep disorders are correlated with physical and mental health problems, including depression, pain, and fibromyalgia. Women experience sleep and sleep problems at various stages across the life span (Shaver, 2015). It is important that the nurse talk with the woman about her sleep patterns and discuss ways to improve sleep, such as avoiding alcohol before going to sleep and sleeping in a regular pattern.

Environmental and Workplace Hazards

Environmental hazards in the home, the workplace, and the community can contribute to poor health at all ages. Categories and examples of health-damaging hazards include the following: (1) pathogenic agents, including viruses, bacteria, fungi, parasites; (2) natural and synthetic chemicals, including natural toxins from animals, insects, and plants, consumer and industrial products such as pesticides and hydrocarbon gases, medical and diagnostic devices, tobacco, fuels, and drug and alcohol abuse; (3) radiation, including radon, heat waves, sound waves; (4) food substances, including added components that are not necessary for nutrition; and (5) physical objects, including moving vehicles, machinery, weapons, water, and building materials.

Environmental hazards can affect fertility, fetal development, live birth, and the child's future mental and physical development. Children are at special risk for poisoning from lead found in paint and soil. Everyone is at risk from air pollutants such as tobacco smoke, carbon monoxide, smog, suspended particles (dust, ash, and asbestos), and cleaning solvents; noise pollution; pesticides; chemical additives; and poor preparation of food. Workers also face safety and health risks caused by ergonomically poor work stations and stress. It is important that risk assessments continue to be in effect to identify and understand environmental problems in public health. The March of Dimes (http://www.marchofdimes.org) provides information about various risks posed in the environment to pregnant women and their fetuses.

Risky Sexual Practices

Potential risks related to sexual activity include undesired pregnancy and STIs. The risks are particularly high for adolescents and young adults who engage in sexual intercourse at earlier and earlier ages. Adolescents report many reasons for wanting to be sexually active: peer pressure, desire to love and be loved, experimentation, to enhance self-esteem, and to have fun. However, many teenagers do not have the decision-making or values-clarification skills needed to take this important step. They may also lack knowledge about contraception and STIs. Many do not believe that becoming pregnant or getting an STI will happen to them.

Although some STIs can be cured with antibiotics, many cause significant problems. Possible sequelae include infertility, ectopic pregnancy, neonatal morbidity and mortality, genital cancers, AIDS, and even death. Choice of contraceptive method has an impact on the risk for contracting an STI. No method of contraception offers complete protection, unless it is abstinence that is consistently used. (See Chapter 7 for a discussion of STIs and Chapter 8 for a discussion of contraception.)

Prevention of STIs is predicated on the reduction of high-risk behaviors by educating toward a behavioral change. Behaviors of concern include multiple and casual sexual partners and unsafe sexual practices. The abuse of alcohol and drugs is a high-risk behavior, resulting in impaired judgment and thoughtless acts. Behavioral changes must come from within; therefore the nurse must provide sufficient information for the individual or group to "buy into" the need for change. Education is a powerful tool in health promotion and prevention of STIs and pregnancy. However, it works best when delivered in a way that considers the language, culture, and lifestyle of the intended listener.

> **! NURSING ALERT**
>
> A comprehensive sexual assessment should be integrated into all health histories.

Medical Conditions

Most women of reproductive age are relatively healthy. Heart disease; lung, breast, colon, and other non gynecologic cancers; chronic lung disease; and diabetes are all concerns for adult women because they are among the leading causes of death in women. Certain medical conditions during pregnancy can have deleterious effects on both the woman and the fetus.

Gynecologic Conditions

Women are at risk throughout their reproductive years for pelvic inflammatory disease, endometriosis, STIs and other vaginal infections (see Chapter 7), uterine fibroids, uterine deformities such as bicornuate uterus, ovarian cysts, interstitial cystitis, and urinary incontinence related to pelvic relaxation. See Clinical Reasoning Case Study on cardiovascular disease in women. Uterine deformities, in fact, are conditions that are congenital and are therefore present in some women at times other than the reproductive years. These gynecologic conditions may contribute negatively to pregnancy by causing infertility, miscarriage, preterm birth, and fetal and neonatal problems. Gynecologic cancers also affect women's health, although the risk for most cancers

> **? CLINICAL REASONING CASE STUDY**
>
> ***Cardiovascular Disease—The Leading Cause of Death in Women***
>
> Selena is a 56-year-old Hispanic menopausal client who presents for her annual well-woman examination. She is a nonsmoker and nondrinker who lives a sedentary lifestyle. She does not exercise. Her mother died of a heart attack at age 60.
>
> Body mass index (BMI) at today's visit is 33, blood pressure (BP) 150/100 mm Hg, high-density lipoprotein (HDL) 25 mg/dL.
>
> She says she knows that she is overweight and should probably exercise and lose weight. How would you respond to her statement?
>
> 1. What is the priority concern or client need in this situation?
> 2. List other client needs/problems in this case.
> 3. Identify any additional information needed by the nurse in addressing this situation.
> 4. Describe the roles/responsibilities of interprofessional health team members who may be involved in this situation.

4

Assessment and Health Promotion

Amy Nichols

ⓔ http://evolve.elsevier.com/Lowdermilk/MWHC/

LEARNING OBJECTIVES

- Describe the structures and functions of the female reproductive system.
- Compare phases of the menstrual cycle in terms of hormonal, ovarian, and endometrial response.
- Describe the phases of the sexual response cycle.
- Explore common reasons that women enter the health care system.
- Analyze barriers that may affect a woman's decision to seek health care.
- Evaluate risk factors for women's health in the childbearing years.
- Describe the components of the history and physical examination.

- Describe how to adapt the history and physical examination for women with special needs.
- Describe how to screen for signs of abuse and how to refer to community agencies.
- Explain the procedure for assisting with and collecting specimens for Papanicolaou (Pap) testing.
- Outline the health-screening and immunization recommendations for women across the life span.
- Discuss anticipatory guidance that prevents disease and promotes health and self-management.

Care of the well woman is focused on health promotion and illness prevention, recognizing that a woman is a biopsychosocial-spiritual being, requiring a holistic approach to nursing care. Health promotion is the motivation to increase well-being and actualize health potential. Illness prevention is the desire to avoid illness, detect it early, or maintain optimal functioning when illness is present. To encourage appropriate health-promotion activities, it is important to conduct systematic health assessments and screenings. This chapter presents an overview of the nurse's role in encouraging health promotion and illness prevention in women across the lifespan. It provides guidelines for how to conduct a complete history and physical examination, including a schedule of screening tests recommended for women at different stages of their lives. As background to understanding assessment, a review of female anatomy and physiology as well as the menstrual cycle is presented. Barriers that women encounter when they try to enter the health care system include social determinants of health as risk factors. Anticipatory guidance suggestions, including nutrition, exercise, and stress management, are included. Examples of health-promotion efforts in the community are presented in an effort to call attention to community health approaches to care, especially because much of well-woman care occurs in community settings and outpatient offices and clinics.

FEMALE REPRODUCTIVE SYSTEM

The female reproductive system consists of external structures visible from the pubis to the perineum and internal structures located in the pelvic cavity. The external and internal female reproductive structures develop and mature in response to estrogen and progesterone. This process starts in fetal life and continues through puberty and the childbearing years. Reproductive structures atrophy with age or in response to a decrease in ovarian hormone production. A complex nerve and blood supply support the functions of these structures. The appearance of the external genitalia varies greatly among women. Heredity, age, race, and the number of children a woman has borne influence the size, shape, and color of her external organs.

External Structures

The external genital organs, or *vulva*, include all structures visible externally from the pubis to the perineum. These include the mons pubis, labia majora, labia minora, clitoris, vestibular glands, vaginal vestibule, vaginal orifice, and urethral opening. The external genital organs are illustrated in Fig. 4.1.

The mons pubis is a fatty pad that lies over the anterior surface of the symphysis pubis. In the postpubertal female, the mons is covered with coarse, curly hair. The labia majora are two rounded folds of fatty tissue covered with skin that extend downward and backward from the mons pubis. These labia are highly vascular structures that develop hair on the outer surfaces after puberty. They protect the inner vulvar structures. The labia minora are two flat, reddish folds of tissue visible when the labia majora are separated. There are no hair follicles on the labia minora, although many sebaceous follicles and a few sweat glands are present. The interior of the labia minora comprises connective tissue and smooth muscle and is supplied with extremely sensitive nerve endings. Anteriorly, the labia minora fuse to form the *prepuce* (the hoodlike covering is low in pregnancy. Risk factors depend on the type of cancer. The impact of developing a gynecologic problem or cancer on women and their families is shaped by a number of factors, including the specific type of problem or cancer, the implications of the diagnosis for the woman and her family, and the timing of the occurrence in the woman's and the family's lives.

Female Genital Mutilation

Female genital mutilation (FGM), infibulation (surgical closure of the labia majora), and *circumcision* are terms used to describe procedures in which part or all of the female external genitalia is removed for cultural or nontherapeutic reasons (WHO, 2019). These procedures are attempts to control women through controlling their sexuality. FGM is supposed to remove sexual desire so that the girl will not become sexually active until married. FGM is practiced in more than 45 countries, with the majority of these countries being in Africa. As emigrants from these countries arrive in North America, nurses in the United States and Canada will see clients who have had such procedures performed. Although it is illegal in the United States to perform FGM on a person younger than 18 years of age, it is estimated that 513,000 women and girls in the United States have experienced or are at risk for FGM (Office of Women's Health, 2018).

Female circumcision occurs in women of many different ethnic, cultural, and religious backgrounds. Although circumcision is usually performed during childhood, some communities circumcise infants or older females. The procedure involves the removal of a portion of the clitoris but may extend to the removal of the entire clitoris and labia minora. In addition, the labia majora, which are often stitched together over the urethral and vaginal openings, may be affected.

The extent of the circumcision site affects the seriousness of complications. Common complications include bleeding, pain, local scarring, keloid or cyst formation, and infection. Impaired drainage of urine and menstrual blood may lead to chronic pelvic infections, pelvic and back pain, and chronic UTIs. Some women may require surgery before vaginal examination, intercourse, or childbirth if the vaginal opening is obstructed.

FGM in the United States is punishable by fines, imprisonment, and deportation. An obstetric care provider may incise the closed labia to deliver a baby or remove cysts but may not sew the labia back to its previous state, reinfibulation. If performed on a minor, FGM is considered child abuse in the United States. FGM is recognized internationally as a violation of the human rights of girls and women. It reflects deep-rooted inequality between the sexes and constitutes an extreme form of discrimination against women. FGM is nearly always carried out on minors and it is a violation of the rights of children. The practice also violates a person's rights to health, security, and physical integrity; the right to be free from torture and cruel, inhuman, or degrading treatment; and the right to life when the procedure results in death (WHO, 2018).

Nurses are providing care to a growing number of women who have emigrated from the Middle East, Asia, and Africa, where female circumcision is more common. Nurses must be sensitive to the unique needs of these clients, especially if these women have concerns about maintaining or restoring the intactness of the circumcision after childbirth.

Human Trafficking

Human trafficking is actually a form of slavery in which people are forced into the United States from other countries to become part of the unpaid labor force, usually in sweatshops or in domestic work, or to serve as sex slaves (Green, 2016). Human trafficking poses a serious risk to the health and wellbeing of women. See Chapter 5 for more detailed information on human trafficking.

Intimate Partner Violence

Intimate partner violence (IPV) is the most common form of violence experienced by women worldwide. IPV is a serious risk factor for women's health. Chapter 5 provides more detail about this serious women's health issue.

LEGAL TIP

Reporting Requirements for Domestic Violence

Domestic violence is considered a crime in all states, but it varies by state between being a misdemeanor or a felony offense; in the majority of states, domestic violence is a misdemeanor. Forty states and the District of Columbia have laws that mandate reporting by health care providers in situations in which the woman has an injury that may be caused by a deadly weapon. Some states also require reports when there is a reason to believe that the woman's injury may have resulted from an illegal act or act of violence. Because of the wide variation from state to state in mandatory reporting, nurses must be knowledgeable about the reporting requirements of the state in which they practice.

HEALTH ASSESSMENT

Trends in women's health have expanded beyond a reproductive focus to include a holistic approach to health care across the life span and place women's health within the scope of primary care. Women's health assessment and screening focus on a systems evaluation that begins with a careful history and physical examination. During assessment and evaluation, the responsibility for self-care and management, health promotion, and enhancement of wellness is emphasized. Nursing care includes assessment, planning, education, counseling, and referral as needed, as well as commendations for good self-care that the woman has practiced. This enables women to make informed decisions about their own health care.

In a market-driven system such as managed care, specific guidelines may be provided for health screening by the insurer or the managed care organization. A nurse often takes the history, orders diagnostic tests, interprets test results, makes referrals, coordinates care, and directs attention to problems requiring medical intervention. Advanced practice nurses who have specialized in women's health, such as NPs, clinical nurse specialists, and nurse-midwives, perform complete physical examinations, including gynecologic examinations.

Interview

Contact with the woman usually begins with an interview, which is an integral part of the history. This interview should be conducted in a private, comfortable, and relaxed setting (Fig. 4.8). If a person wants to accompany the woman to her interview (e.g. a partner, spouse), the woman must give her permission to have that person accompany her. The nurse is seated and makes sure that the woman is comfortable. The woman is addressed by her title and name (e.g., Mrs. Martinez), and the nurse introduces herself or himself using name and title. It is important to phrase questions in a sensitive and nonjudgmental manner. Body language should match oral communication. The nurse is aware of a woman's vulnerability and assures her of strict confidentiality. For many women, fear, anxiety, and modesty make the examination a dreaded and stressful experience. Many women are uninformed, misguided by myths, or afraid they will appear ignorant by asking questions about sexual or reproductive functioning. The woman is assured that no question is irrelevant. Cultural considerations must be addressed in the interview process (see Cultural Considerations box).

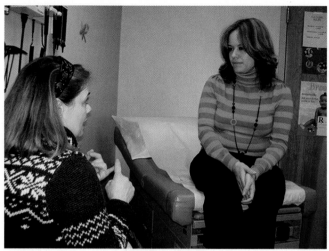

Fig. 4.8 Nurse Interviews Woman as Part of History-taking Prior to Physical Examination. (Courtesy Ed Lowdermilk, Chapel Hill, NC.)

🌐 CULTURAL CONSIDERATIONS

Communication Variations

- Conversational style and pacing: Silence may show respect or acknowledgment that the listener has heard. In cultures in which a direct "no" is considered rude, silence may mean no. Repetition or loudness may mean emphasis or anger.
- Personal space: Cultural conceptions of personal space differ. Based on one's culture, for example, someone may be perceived as distant for backing off when approached, or aggressive for standing too close.
- Eye contact: Eye contact varies among cultures from intense to fleeting. Consistent with the effort to refrain from invading personal space, avoiding direct eye contact may be a sign of respect.
- Touch: The norms about how people should touch each other vary among cultures. In some cultures, physical contact with the same sex (embracing, walking hand in hand) is more appropriate than that with an unrelated person of the opposite sex.
- Time orientation: In some cultures, involvement with people is more valued than being "on time." In other cultures, life is scheduled and paced according to clock time, which is valued over personal time.

Data from Galanti, G. (2008). *Caring for patients from different cultures* (4th ed.). Philadelphia: University of Pennsylvania Press. Striving for cultural competence: Providing care in the changing face of the U.S. *AWHONN Lifelines, 4*(3), 48–52.

The history begins with an open-ended question such as "What brings you into the office/clinic/hospital today?" and is furthered by other questions such as "Anything else?" and "Tell me about it." Additional ways to encourage women to share information include:

- **Facilitation:** Using a word or posture that communicates interest such as leaning forward, making eye contact, or saying "Mm-hmmm" or "Go on"
- **Reflection:** Repeating a word or phrase that a woman has used
- **Clarification:** Asking the woman what is meant by a stated word or phrase
- **Empathic responses:** Acknowledging the feelings of a woman by statements such as "That must have been frightening"
- **Confrontation:** Identifying something about the woman's behavior or feelings not expressed verbally or apparently inconsistent with her history

- **Interpretation:** Putting into words what you infer about the woman's feelings or about the meaning of her symptoms, events, or other matters

Direct questions may be necessary to elicit specific details. These should be worded in language that is understandable to the woman and expressed neutrally so that the woman will not be led into a specific response. The nurse asks about one item at time and proceeds from the general to the specific.

Nurses need to develop rapport and trust with their clients as they take a history; because communication within a caring context is core to nursing practice, nurses are well suited to taking a comprehensive client history. Nurses should ask questions incrementally to build a comprehensive understanding. They should also share insights with the woman by eliciting her concerns or thoughts as well as offering clarification.

Cultural Considerations

Recognizing signs and symptoms of disease and deciding when to seek treatment are influenced by cultural perceptions. It is essential that nurses have respect for the rich and unique qualities that cultural diversity brings to individuals. In recognizing the value of these differences, the nurse can modify the plan of care to meet the needs of each woman.

To understand the woman's point of view, it is important to ask the right questions. Galanti (2008) suggests the use of the four Cs of cultural competence:

1. Call—What do you call your problem?
2. Cause—What do you think caused your problem?
3. Cope—How do you cope with your condition?
4. Concerns—What are your concerns regarding your condition?

Using the four Cs of cultural competence along with cultural proficiency, biomedical values, and evidence-based practice allows the nurse to individualize care with a client-centered approach.

Modifications may be necessary for the physical examination. In some cultures, it may be considered inappropriate for the woman to disrobe completely for the physical examination. In many cultures a female examiner is preferred. Communication may be hindered by different beliefs even when the nurse and woman speak the same language (see Cultural Considerations box: Providing Culturally Appropriate Care in Chapter 2).

Women With Special Needs

Women With Disabilities

Women with emotional or physical disorders have special needs. Women who have vision, hearing, emotional, or physical disabilities should be respected and involved in the assessment and physical examination to the full extent of their abilities. The nurse should communicate openly and directly with sensitivity. It is often helpful to learn about the disability directly from the woman while maintaining eye contact (if eye contact is culturally appropriate). Family and significant others should be relied on only when absolutely necessary. The assessment and physical examination can be adapted to each woman's individual needs.

Communication with a woman who is hearing impaired can be accomplished without difficulty. Most of these women read lips, write, or both; thus an interviewer who speaks and enunciates each word slowly and in full view may be easily understood. If a woman is not comfortable with lip reading, she may use an interpreter. In this case it is important to continue to address the woman directly, avoiding the temptation to speak directly with the interpreter.

The visually impaired woman needs to be oriented to the examination room and may have her guide dog with her. As with all women, the

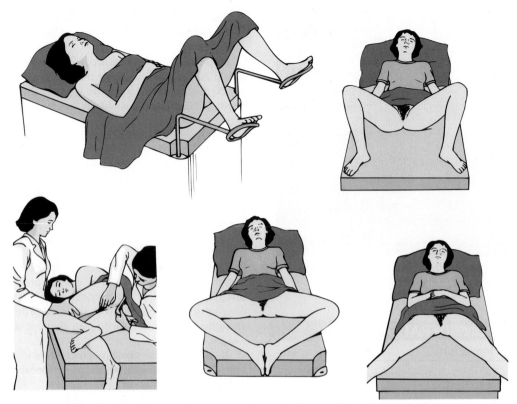

Fig. 4.9 Lithotomy and Variable Positions for Women Who Have a Disability.

visually impaired woman needs a full explanation of what the examination entails before proceeding. Before touching her, the nurse explains, "Now I am going to take your blood pressure. I am going to place the cuff on your right arm." The woman can be asked if she would like to touch each of the items that will be used in the examination.

Many women with physical disabilities cannot comfortably lie in the lithotomy position for the pelvic examination. Several alternative positions may be used, including a lateral (side-lying) position, a V-shaped position, a diamond-shaped position, and an M-shaped position (Piotrowski & Snell, 2007) (Fig. 4.9). The woman can be asked what has worked best for her previously. If she has never had a pelvic examination, or has never had a comfortable pelvic examination, the nurse proceeds by showing her a picture of various positions and asking her which one she prefers. The nurse's support and reassurance can help the woman relax, which will make the examination go more smoothly.

Women in Abusive Situations

Nurses should screen all women entering the health care system for potential abuse and human trafficking. Screening women for potential abuse can have beneficial consequences with minimal negative outcomes. Help for the woman may depend on the sensitivity with which the nurse screens for abuse, the discovery of abuse, and subsequent intervention. The nurse must be familiar with the laws governing abuse in the state in which she or he practices.

Pocket cards listing emergency numbers (abuse counseling, legal protection, and emergency shelter) may be available from the local police department, a women's shelter, or an emergency department. It is helpful to have these on hand in the setting where screening is done. An abuse-assessment screen (Fig. 4.10) can be used as part of the interview or written history. If a male partner is present, he should be asked to leave the room because the woman may not disclose experiences of abuse in his presence, or he may try to answer

questions for her to protect himself. The same procedure would apply for partners of lesbians, parents of teens, or adult children of older women.

Fear, guilt, and embarrassment may keep many women from giving information about family violence. Clues in the history and evidence of injuries on physical examination should give a high index of suspicion. The areas most commonly injured in women are the head, the neck, the chest, the abdomen, the breasts, and the upper extremities. Burns and bruises in patterns resembling hands, belts, cords, or other weapons may be seen, as well as multiple traumatic injuries. Attention should be given to women who repeatedly seek treatment for somatic complaints such as headaches, insomnia, choking sensation, hyperventilation, gastrointestinal symptoms, and pain in the chest, back, and pelvis. During pregnancy the nurse should assess for injuries to the breasts, the abdomen, and the genitals. (See Chapter 5 for further discussion of violence.)

Adolescents (Ages 13 to 19 Years)

As a young woman matures, she should be asked the same questions that are included in any history. Particular attention should be paid to hints about risky behaviors, eating disorders, and depression. Do not assume that a teenager is not sexually active. After rapport has been established, it is best to talk to a teen with the parent (partner or friend) out of the room. Questions should be asked with sensitivity and in a gentle and nonjudgmental manner.

A teen's first speculum examination is the most important because she will develop perceptions that will remain with her for future examinations. What the examination entails should be discussed with the teen while she is dressed. Models or illustrations can be used to show exactly what will happen. All of the necessary equipment should be assembled so that there are no interruptions. Pediatric speculums that are 1 to 1.5 cm wide can be inserted with minimal discomfort. If the teen is sexually active, a small adult speculum may be used.

ABUSE ASSESSMENT SCREEN

- Are you with a spouse or partner who threatens or physically hurts you?
  - Yes _____   No _____

- Are you with a spouse or partner who emotionally hurts you?
  - Yes _____   No _____

- Within the past year or in this pregnancy (if the woman is pregnant) has anyone hit, slapped, kicked, or otherwise hurt you?
  - Yes _____   No _____
  - If yes, by whom _____
  - Number of times _____
  - Mark the area of injury on the body map.

- Has anyone forced you to have sexual activities that made you uncomfortable?
  - Yes _____   No _____
  - If yes, by whom _____
  - Number of times _____

- Are you afraid of your partner or anyone you listed above?
  - Yes _____   No _____

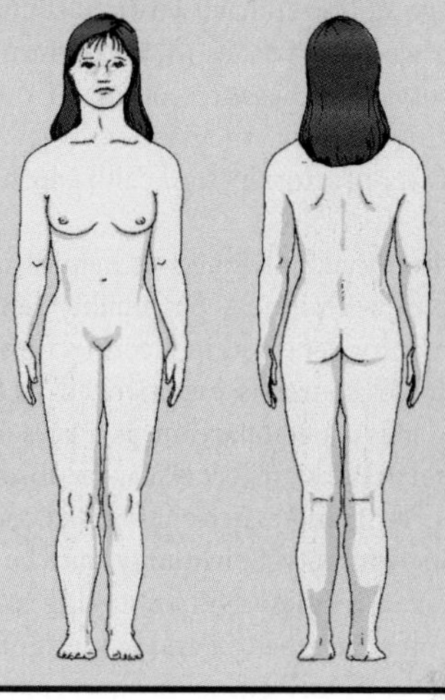

Fig. 4.10 Abuse Assessment Screen. Screening for intimate partner violence. (Adapted from American College of Obstetricians and Gynecologists [ACOG]. [2012]. *Are you being abused? Screening tools for domestic violence.* Retrieved from www.acog.org/About_ACOG/ACOG_Departments/Violence_Against_Women/Are_you_Being_Abused.)

Injury prevention should be a part of the counseling at routine health examinations, with special attention to seat belts, not texting or using cell phone while driving, helmets, firearms, recreational hazards, and sports involvement. The use of drugs and alcohol and the nonuse of seat belts contribute to motor vehicle injuries, accounting for the greatest proportion of accidental deaths in women. Contraceptive use and STI prevention information may be needed for teens who are sexually active.

To provide developmentally appropriate care, it is important to review the major tasks for women in this stage of life. Major tasks for teens include values assessment; education and work goal setting; formation of peer relationships that focus on love, commitment, and becoming comfortable with sexuality; and separation from parents. Individuality may be reflected in areas such as sexuality, politics, and career choices. Conflict exists between making and keeping commitments to keep options open. The teen is egocentric as she progresses rapidly through emotional and physical changes. Her feelings of invulnerability may lead to serious misconceptions, such as that unprotected sexual intercourse will not lead to pregnancy.

Midlife and Older Women (Ages 50 Years and Older)

The assessment of women ages 50 and older presents unique challenges. Women may be experiencing major lifestyle changes, such as children leaving home, caring for their aging parents, job change, retirement, separation, divorce or death of a partner, and aging-related changes and health problems. The nurse uses reflection and empathy to communicate in an open and caring manner. It may be necessary to schedule a longer appointment time because older women have longer histories or have a need to talk. Some women may fail to report symptoms because they fear their complaints will be attributed to old age, or they feel that they have lived with a chronic condition (e.g., incontinence, dyspareunia, interstitial cystitis, decreased libido, depression)

for so long that nothing can be done. Women may choose to ignore a problem if they have symptoms that are life threatening (e.g., chest pain or a breast lump) because they traditionally put the needs of others first. As a result, the nurse should encourage the woman to express her concerns and fears and reassure her that her problems are important and will be addressed. Exercise, hormone therapy, diet, vitamins, calcium with vitamin D supplementation, daily aspirin, BSE, Pap and mammogram recommendations, colonoscopy, immunization updates, and sun protection should be discussed.

Functional assessment is included as part of the history in women older than 70 years and those with disabilities. In the review of systems, the nurse should ask about self-management activities such as walking, getting to the bathroom, bathing, hair combing, dressing, and eating. Questions about driving, using public transportation, using the telephone or the Internet, doing laundry, buying groceries, taking medications, and meal preparation should be included.

Sexual assessment continues to be important in women 50 and older. Unless directly asked, women may omit mention of sexual concerns. Questions asked with sensitivity may invite responses regarding changes in sexual desire or response, or physical issues that challenge her sexual enjoyment. Open and reflective questions also affirm a woman's right to sexual enjoyment throughout the life span.

Women older than 50 years commonly experience menopause and have physical changes associated with decreased estrogen. Physical changes can result in increased discomfort during the pelvic examination. It is important to be both gentle and thorough during the examination. A small adult speculum may be used to view the cervix. The uterus in a menopausal woman is small and firm, and the ovaries are nonpalpable. In postmenopausal women the specimen from the vaginal pool may be useful to detect endometrial cells. A woman with palpable adnexal masses or vaginal bleeding after menopause needs immediate gynecologic referral.

A respectful and reassuring approach toward caring for women ages 50 and older will ensure their continued participation in seeking health care. Because the risk of breast, ovarian, uterine, cervical, colon, and skin cancers increases with age, the nurse has the opportunity to educate women about the importance of preventive screening. It is the nurse's responsibility to ensure a positive health care experience that encourages future visits for prevention and chronic and acute care.

Advance directives can be introduced on any entry into a health care system. It is a good idea to have a formal statement in the medical record regarding a woman's wishes in the event of accident or illness regarding life-maintaining measures or organ donation. Most states have laws formalizing such statements in writing. A woman can designate the durable power of attorney for health care authority to a trusted relative or friend.

Many women find that spirituality is helpful in maintaining wellness as well as coping with illness. Spirituality refers to the essence of our being and humanity, reflected in a connection to a Sacred Source. The concept of Sacred Source is experienced in different ways, with some experiencing it as a person, some as a presence, and some as an indescribable mystery (Burkhardt & Nagai-Jacobson, 2013). The idea of connection is important, and experiencing this connection in a sacred space is central to spirituality. Spirituality may be experienced within a context of organized religion. Nurses, taking a holistic approach to women's wellness, must be sensitive and nonjudgmental to the spiritual aspect of their clients. In an optimal healing approach to care, nurses can facilitate and encourage the client to express her spirituality in a way that is comfortable for her. Box 4.7 presents a spiritual wellness self-assessment guide.

Healthy Aging

Women in the United States can expect on average to live to be 80 years old and may spend one-third of their lives as postmenopausal women. With a healthy lifestyle, many women are living to be 100 years old or older. Proper nutrition, exercise, and mental and social stimulation are critical to keeping the body healthy and the mind active and alert into old age.

History

At a woman's first visit, she is often expected to fill out a form with biographic and historical data before meeting with the examiner. This information aids the health care provider in completing the history during the interview. Most forms include information about these categories:

- Biographic data
- Reason for seeking care
- Present health or history of present illness
- Past health
- Family history
- Screening for abuse
- Review of systems
- Functional assessment (activities of daily living)

Box 4.8 describes a complete health history.

Physical Examination

In preparation for the physical examination, the woman is instructed to undress and is given a gown to wear during the examination. She is usually given the opportunity to undress privately. Objective data are recorded by system or location. A general statement of overall health status is a good way to start. Findings are described in detail.

- General appearance: age, race, gender, state of health, posture, height, weight, development, dress, hygiene, affect, alertness, orientation, cooperativeness, and communication skills
- Vital signs: temperature, pulse, respiration, blood pressure
- Skin: color; integrity; texture; hydration; temperature; edema; excessive perspiration; unusual odor; presence and description of lesions; hair texture and distribution; nail configuration, color, texture, and condition; presence of nail clubbing
- Head: size, shape, trauma, masses, scars, rashes, or scaling; facial symmetry; presence of edema or puffiness
- Eyes: pupil size, shape, reactivity, conjunctival injection, scleral icterus, fundal papilledema, hemorrhage, lids, extraocular movements, visual fields and acuity
- Ears: shape and symmetry, tenderness, discharge, external canal, and tympanic membranes; hearing—Weber should be midline (loudness of sound equal in both ears) and Rinne negative (no conductive or sensorineural hearing loss); should be able to hear whisper at 3 feet
- Nose: symmetry, tenderness, discharge, mucosa, turbinate inflammation, frontal or maxillary sinus tenderness; discrimination of odors
- Mouth and throat: hygiene; condition of teeth; dentures; appearance of lips, tongue, buccal and oral mucosa; erythema; edema; exudate; tonsillar enlargement; palate; uvula; gag reflex; ulcers
- Neck: mobility, masses, range of motion, tracheal deviation, thyroid size, carotid bruits
- Lymphatic: cervical, intraclavicular, axillary, trochlear, or inguinal adenopathy; size, shape, tenderness, and consistency
- Breasts: skin changes, dimpling, symmetry, scars, tenderness, discharge, masses; characteristics of nipples and areolae
- Heart: rate, rhythm, murmurs, rubs, gallops, clicks, heaves, or precordial movements
- Peripheral vascular: jugular vein distention, bruits, edema, swelling, vein distention, or tenderness of extremities

---

BOX 4.7 Spiritual Wellness Self-Assessment

1. How do you describe your purpose in life?
2. What activities do you do regularly that bring you joy?
3. What goals do you have for 6 months from now?
4. What goals do you have for 2 years from now?
5. What activities make you feel nourished?
6. What kinds of things do you do for yourself every day?
7. What do you hope for in the future?
8. Are there people you can reach out to?
9. On whom can you count for encouragement and/or support?
10. Are there others to whom you give encouragement and/or support?
11. Who loves you?
12. Whom do you love or care about?
13. In what areas are you growing?
14. How do you go about forgiving yourself?
15. How do you go about forgiving others?
16. To whom do you confide your hopes, dreams, and pain?
17. Do you believe in some kind of higher power?
18. What do you hope for in the future?
19. When do you reach out to people?
20. Do you look forward to getting up in the morning?
21. Would you like to live to be 100?

The more questions you answer in the positive, the higher the level of spiritual wellness.

Adapted from Condon, M. (2004). *Women's health: Body, mind, spirit: An integrated approach to wellness and illness.* Upper Saddle River, NJ: Prentice-Hall.

BOX 4.8 Health History and Review of Systems

Identifying data: Name, age, race, sex, marital status, occupation, religion, and ethnicity

Reason for seeking care: A response to the question, "What problem or symptom brought you here today?" If the woman lists more than one reason, focus on the one she thinks is most important.

Present health: Current health status is described with attention to the following:

- *Use of safety measures:* seat belts, bicycle helmets, designated driver
- *Exercise and leisure activities:* regularity
- *Sleep patterns:* length and quality
- *Sexuality:* Is she sexually active? With men, women, or both? Risk-reducing sex practices?
- *Diet, including beverages:* 24-h dietary recall; caffeine: coffee, tea, cola, or chocolate intake
- *Nicotine, alcohol, illicit or recreational drug use:* type, amount, frequency, duration, and reactions
- *Environmental and chemical hazards:* home, school, work, and leisure setting; exposure to extreme heat or cold, noise, industrial toxins such as asbestos or lead, pesticides, diethylstilbestrol (DES), radiation, cat feces, or cigarette smoke

History of present illness: A chronologic narrative that includes the onset of the problem, the setting in which it developed, its manifestations, and any treatments received are noted. The woman's state of health before the onset of the present problem is determined. If the problem is long standing, the reason for seeking attention at this time is elicited. The principal symptoms should be described with respect to the following:

- Location
- Quality or character
- Quantity or severity
- Timing (onset, duration, frequency)
- Setting
- Factors that aggravate or relieve
- Associated factors
- Woman's perception of the meaning of the symptom

Past Health

- *Infectious diseases:* measles, mumps, rubella, whooping cough, chickenpox, rheumatic fever, scarlet fever, diphtheria, polio, tuberculosis (TB), hepatitis
- *Chronic disease and system disorders:* arthritis, cancer, diabetes, heart, lung, kidney, seizures, thyroid, stroke, ulcers, sickle cell anemia
- *Adult injuries, accidents*
- *Hospitalizations, operations, blood transfusions*
- *Obstetric history*
- *Allergies:* medications, previous transfusion reactions, environmental allergies
- *Immunizations:* diphtheria, pertussis, tetanus, polio, hepatitis B, varicella, influenza, pneumococcal vaccine, last TB skin test, measles, mumps, rubella (MMR)
- *Last date of screening tests:* Pap test, mammogram, stool for occult blood, sigmoidoscopy or colonoscopy, hematocrit, hemoglobin, rubella titer, urinalysis, cholesterol test; electrocardiogram; last vision, dental, hearing examination
- *Current medications:* name, dose, frequency, duration, reason for taking, and compliance with prescription medications; home remedies, over-the-counter drugs, vitamin and mineral or herbal supplements, or recreational drugs used over a 24-hour period

Family history: Information about the ages and health of family members may be presented in narrative form or as a family tree or genogram: age, health or death of parents, siblings, spouse, children. Check for history of diabetes; heart disease; hypertension; stroke; respiratory, renal, or thyroid problems; cancer; bleeding disorders; hepatitis; allergies; asthma; arthritis; TB; epilepsy; mental illness; human immunodeficiency virus infection; or other disorders.

Screen for abuse: Has she ever been hit, kicked, slapped, or forced to have sex against her wishes? Has she been verbally or emotionally abused? Does she have a history of childhood sexual abuse? If yes, has she received counseling or does she need referral? Does she feel safe in her current relationship? Does she feel safe in her home? Are there any signs of being trafficked?

Review of systems: It is probable that all questions in each system will not be included every time a history is taken. Some questions regarding each system should be included in every history. The essential areas to be explored are listed in the following head-to-toe sequence. If a woman gives a positive response to a question about an essential area, more detailed questions should be asked.

- *General:* weight change, fatigue, weakness, fever, chills, or night sweats
- *Skin:* skin, hair, and nail change; itching, bruising, bleeding, rashes, sores, lumps, or moles
- *Lymph nodes:* enlargement, inflammation, pain, suppuration (pus), or drainage
- *Head:* trauma, vertigo (dizziness), convulsive disorder, syncope (fainting); headache: location, frequency, pain type, nausea and vomiting, or visual symptoms present
- *Eyes:* glasses, contact lenses, blurriness, tearing, itching, photophobia, diplopia, inflammation, trauma, cataracts, glaucoma, or acute visual loss
- *Ears:* hearing loss, tinnitus (ringing), vertigo, discharge, pain, fullness, recurrent infections, or mastoiditis
- *Nose and sinuses:* trauma, rhinitis, nasal discharge, epistaxis, obstruction, sneezing, itching, allergy, or smelling impairment
- *Mouth, throat, and neck:* hoarseness, voice changes, soreness, ulcers, bleeding gums, goiter, swelling, or enlarged nodes
- *Breasts:* masses, pain, lumps, dimpling, nipple discharge, fibrocystic changes, or implants; breast self-examination practice; date of last mammogram
- *Respiratory:* shortness of breath, wheezing, cough, sputum, hemoptysis, pneumonia, pleurisy, asthma, bronchitis, emphysema, or TB; date of last chest x-ray
- *Cardiovascular:* hypertension, rheumatic fever, murmurs, angina, palpitations, dyspnea, tachycardia, orthopnea, edema, chest pain, cough, cyanosis, cold extremities, ascites, intermittent claudication (leg pain caused by poor circulation to the leg muscles), phlebitis, or skin color changes
- *Gastrointestinal:* appetite, nausea, vomiting, indigestion, dysphagia, abdominal pain, ulcers, hematochezia (bleeding with stools), melena (black, tarry stools), bowel-habit changes, diarrhea, constipation, bowel movement frequency, food intolerance, hemorrhoids, jaundice, or hepatitis; sigmoidoscopy, colonoscopy, barium enema, ultrasound
- *Genitourinary:* frequency, hesitancy, urgency, polyuria, dysuria, hematuria, nocturia, incontinence, stones, infection, or urethral discharge; menstrual history (e.g., age at menarche, length and flow of menses, last menstrual period [LMP], dysmenorrhea, intermenstrual bleeding, age at menopause or signs of menopause), dyspareunia, discharge, sores, itching
- *Sexual health and sexual activity:* with men, women, or both; contraceptive use; sexually transmitted infections
- *Peripheral vascular:* coldness, numbness and tingling, leg edema, claudication, varicose veins, thromboses, or emboli
- *Endocrine:* heat and cold intolerance, dry skin, excessive sweating, polyuria, polydipsia, polyphagia, thyroid problems, diabetes, or secondary sex characteristic changes
- *Hematologic:* anemia, easy bruising, bleeding, petechiae, purpura, or transfusions
- *Musculoskeletal:* muscle weakness, pain, joint stiffness, scoliosis, lordosis, kyphosis, range-of-motion instability, redness, swelling, arthritis, or gout
- *Neurologic:* loss of sensation, numbness, tingling, tremors, weakness, vertigo, paralysis, fainting, twitching, blackouts, seizures, convulsions, loss of consciousness or memory
- *Mental status:* moodiness, depression, anxiety, obsessions, delusions, illusions, or hallucinations
- *Functional assessment:* ability to care for self

TABLE 4.2 Female Reproductive Physical Assessment Across the Life Cycle

	Adolescent	Adult	Postmenopausal
Breasts	Tender when developing; buds appear; small, firm; one side may grow faster; areola diameter increases; nipples more erect	Grow to full shape in early adulthood; nipples and areola become pinker and darker	Become stringy, irregular, pendulous, and nodular; borders less well delineated; may shrink, become flatter, elongated, and less elastic; ligaments weaken; nipples are positioned lower
Vagina	Vagina lengthens; epithelial layers thicken; secretions become acidic	Growth complete by age 20	Introitus constricts; vagina narrows, shortens, loses rugation; mucosa is pale, thin, and dry; walls may lose structural integrity
Uterus	Musculature and vasculature increase; lining thickens	Growth complete by age 20	Size decreases; endometrial lining thins
Ovaries	Increase in size and weight; menarche occurs between 8 and 16 years of age; ovulation occurs monthly	Growth complete by age 20	Size decreases to 1-2 cm; follicles disappear; surface convolutes; ovarian function ceases between 40 and 55 years of age
Labia majora	Become more prominent; hair develops	Growth complete by age 20	Labia become smaller and flatter; pubic hair sparse and gray
Labia minora	Become more vascular	Growth complete by age 20	Become shinier and drier
Uterine tubes	Increase in size	Growth complete by age 20	Decrease in size

- Lungs: chest symmetry with respirations, wheezes, crackles, rhonchi, vocal fremitus, whispered pectoriloquy, percussion, and diaphragmatic excursion; breath sounds equal and clear bilaterally
- Abdomen: shape, scars, bowel sounds, consistency, tenderness, rebound, masses, guarding, organomegaly, liver span, percussion (tympany, shifting, dullness), or costovertebral angle tenderness
- Extremities: edema, ulceration, tenderness, varicosities, erythema, tremor, or deformity
- Genitourinary: external genitalia, perineum, vaginal mucosa, cervix; inflammation, tenderness, discharge, bleeding, ulcers, nodules, or masses; internal vaginal support, bimanual and rectovaginal palpation of cervix, uterus, and adnexa
- Rectal: sphincter tone, masses, hemorrhoids, rectal wall contour, tenderness, and stool for occult blood
- Musculoskeletal: posture, symmetry of muscle mass, muscle atrophy, weakness, appearance of joints, tenderness or crepitus, joint range of motion, instability, redness, swelling, or spinal deviation
- Neurologic: mental status, orientation, memory, mood, speech clarity and comprehension, cranial nerves II to XII, sensation, strength, deep tendon and superficial reflexes, gait, balance, and coordination with rapid alternating motions

Table 4.2 highlights physical assessment findings that differ in women across the life span.

Pelvic Examination

Many women fear the gynecologic portion of the physical examination. The nurse can be instrumental in allaying these fears by providing information and assisting the woman to express her feelings to the examiner (Box 4.9).

The woman is assisted into the lithotomy position (see Fig. 4.9) for the pelvic examination. When she is in the lithotomy position, her hips and knees are flexed, with buttocks at the edge of the table, and her feet are supported by heel or knee stirrups.

Some women prefer to keep their shoes or socks on, especially if the stirrups are not padded. Many women express feelings of vulnerability and strangeness when in the lithotomy position. During the procedure the nurse assists the woman with relaxation techniques.

Many women find it distressing to attempt to converse in the lithotomy position. Most women appreciate an explanation of the procedure as it unfolds, as well as coaching for the types of sensations they may

BOX 4.9 Procedure: Assisting With Pelvic Examination

1. Perform hand hygiene.
2. Assemble equipment (see photo below).

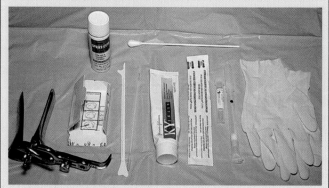

Equipment used for pelvic examination. (Courtesy Michael S. Clement, MD, Mesa, AZ.)

3. Ask the woman to empty her bladder before the examination (obtain clean-catch urine specimen as needed).
4. Assist with relaxation techniques. Have the woman place her hands on her chest at about the level of the diaphragm and breathe deeply and slowly.
5. Encourage the woman to become involved with the examination if she shows interest. For example, a mirror can be placed so that she can see the area being examined.
6. Assess for and treat signs of problems such as supine hypotension.
7. Warm the speculum in warm water if a prewarmed one is not available.
8. Instruct the woman to bear down when the speculum is being inserted.
9. Apply gloves and assist the examiner with collection of specimens for cytologic examination, such as a Pap test. After handling specimens, remove gloves and wash hands.
10. Put gloves on. Lubricate the examiner's fingers with water or water-soluble lubricant before bimanual examination.
11. Assist the woman at completion of the examination to a sitting position and then a standing position.
12. Provide tissues to wipe lubricant from perineum.
13. Provide privacy for the woman while she is dressing.

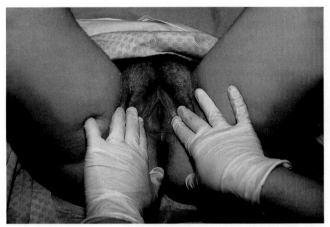

Fig. 4.11 External Examination: Separation of the Labia. (From Wilson, S., & Giddens, J. [2013]. *Health assessment for nursing practice* [5th ed.]. St. Louis: Mosby.)

expect. Generally, however, women prefer not to have to respond to questions until they are again upright and at eye level with the examiner. Being asked questions during the procedure, especially if they cannot see their questioner's eyes, may make women tense.

External inspection. The examiner wears gloves and sits at the foot of the table for the inspection of the external genitalia and the speculum examination. In good lighting, the external genitalia (clitoris, labia, and perineum) are examined and inspected for sexual maturity, and lesions indicative of STIs are noted. After childbirth or other trauma, healed scars may be present.

External palpation. Before touching the woman, the examiner explains what is going to be done and what the woman should expect to feel (e.g., pressure). The examiner may touch the woman in a less sensitive area such as the inner thigh to alert her that the genitalia examination is beginning. This gesture may put the woman more at ease. The labia are spread apart to expose the structures in the vestibule: urinary meatus, Skene glands, vaginal orifice, and Bartholin glands (Fig. 4.11). To assess Skene glands, the examiner inserts one finger into the vagina and "milks" the area of the urethra. Any exudate from the urethra or the Skene glands is cultured. Masses and erythema of either structure are assessed further. Ordinarily the openings to the Skene glands are not visible; prominent openings may be seen if the glands are infected (e.g., with gonorrhea). During the examination the examiner keeps in mind the data from the review of systems such as history of burning on urination.

The vaginal orifice is examined. Hymenal tags are normal findings. With one finger still in the vagina, the examiner repositions the index finger near the posterior part of the orifice. With the thumb outside the posterior part of the labia majora, the examiner compresses the area of Bartholin glands located at the 8-o'clock and 4-o'clock positions and looks for swelling, discharge, and pain.

The support of the anterior and posterior vaginal wall is assessed. The examiner spreads the labia with the index and middle finger and asks the woman to strain down. Any bulge from the anterior wall (urethrocele or cystocele) or posterior wall (rectocele) is noted and compared with the history, such as difficulty starting the stream of urine or constipation.

The perineum (area between the vagina and anus) is assessed for scars from old lacerations or episiotomies, thinning, fistulas, masses, lesions, and inflammation. The anus is assessed for hemorrhoids, hemorrhoidal tags, and integrity of the anal sphincter. The anal area is also assessed for lesions, masses, abscesses, and tumors. If there is a history

of STI, the examiner may want to obtain a culture specimen from the anal canal at this time. Throughout the genital examination the examiner notes any odor, which may indicate infection or poor hygiene.

Vulvar self-examination. The pelvic examination provides a good opportunity for the practitioner to emphasize the need for regular **vulvar self-examination** (**VSE**) and to teach this procedure. Because there has been a dramatic increase in cancerous and precancerous conditions of the vulva, VSE should be an integral part of preventive health care for all women who are sexually active or 18 years of age or older. VSE should be performed monthly between menses or more often if there are symptoms or a history of serious vulvar disease. Most lesions, including malignancy, condyloma acuminatum (wart like growth), and Bartholin cysts, can be seen or palpated and are easily treated if diagnosed early.

The VSE can be performed by the practitioner and woman together by using a mirror. A simple diagram of the anatomy of the vulva can be given to the woman, with instructions to perform the examination herself that evening to reinforce what she has learned. She does the examination in a sitting position with adequate lighting, holding a mirror in one hand and using the other hand to expose the tissues surrounding the vaginal introitus. She then systematically examines the mons pubis, clitoris, urethra, labia majora, perineum, and perianal area and palpates the vulva, noting any changes in appearance or abnormalities such as ulcers, lumps, warts, and changes in pigmentation.

Internal examination. A vaginal speculum consists of two blades and a handle. Specula come in a variety of types and styles. A vaginal speculum is used to view the vaginal vault and cervix. The speculum is gently placed into the vagina and inserted to the back of the vaginal vault. The blades are opened to reveal the cervix and are locked into the open position. The cervix is inspected for position and appearance of the os: color, lesions, bleeding, and discharge (Fig. 4.12). Cervical findings that are not within normal limits include ulcerations, masses, inflammation, and excessive protrusion into the vaginal vault. Anomalies such as a cockscomb (a protrusion over the cervix that looks like a rooster's comb), a hooded or collared cervix (seen in diethylstilbestrol [DES] daughters), or polyps are noted.

Collection of specimens. The collection of specimens for cytologic examination is an important part of the gynecologic examination. Infection can be diagnosed by examination of specimens collected during the pelvic examination. These infections include candidiasis, trichomoniasis, bacterial vaginosis, group B streptococcus, gonorrhea, chlamydia, and herpes simplex virus. Once the diagnoses have been made, treatment can be instituted.

Papanicolaou test. Carcinogenic conditions, whether potential or actual, can be determined by examination of cells from the cervix collected during the pelvic examination (i.e., a Pap test) (Box 4.10).

Vaginal wall examination. After the specimens are obtained, the vagina is viewed when the speculum is rotated. The speculum blades are unlocked and partially closed. As the speculum is withdrawn, it is rotated; the vaginal walls are inspected for color, lesions, rugae, fistulas, and bulging.

Bimanual palpation. The examiner stands for this part of the examination. A small amount of lubricant is placed on the first and second fingers of the gloved hand for the internal examination. To avoid tissue trauma and contamination, the thumb is abducted, and the ring and little fingers are flexed into the palm (Fig. 4.13).

The vagina is palpated for distensibility, lesions, and tenderness. The cervix is examined for position, shape, consistency, motility, and lesions. The fornix around the cervix is palpated.

The other hand is placed on the abdomen halfway between the umbilicus and symphysis pubis and exerts pressure downward toward the pelvic hand. Upward pressure from the pelvic hand traps reproductive

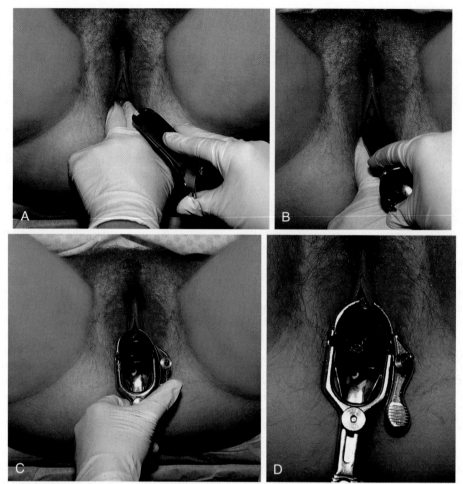

Fig. 4.12 Insertion of Speculum for Vaginal Examination. (A) Opening of the introitus. (B) Oblique insertion of the speculum. (C) Final insertion of the speculum. (D) Opening of the speculum blades. (From Wilson, S., & Giddens, J. [2013]. *Health assessment for nursing practice* [5th ed.]. St. Louis: Mosby.)

structures for assessment by palpation. The uterus is assessed for position, size, shape, consistency, regularity, motility, masses, and tenderness.

With the abdominal hand moving to the right lower quadrant and the fingers of the pelvic hand in the right lateral fornix, the adnexa is assessed for position, size, tenderness, and masses. The examination is repeated on the woman's left side.

Just before the intravaginal fingers are withdrawn, the woman is asked to tighten her vagina around the fingers as much as she can. If the muscle response is weak, the woman is assessed for her knowledge of Kegel exercises.

Rectovaginal palpation. To prevent contamination of the rectum from organisms in the vagina (e.g., *Neisseria gonorrhoeae*), it is necessary to change gloves, add fresh lubricant, and then reinsert the index finger into the vagina and the middle finger into the rectum (Fig. 4.14). Insertion is facilitated if the woman strains down. The maneuvers of the abdominovaginal examination are repeated. The rectovaginal examination permits assessment of the rectovaginal septum, the posterior surface of the uterus, and the region behind the cervix and the adnexa. The vaginal finger is removed and folded into the palm, leaving the middle finger free to rotate 360 degrees. The rectum is palpated for rectal tenderness and masses.

After the rectal examination the woman is assisted into a sitting position, given tissues or wipes to cleanse herself, and afforded privacy to dress. The examiner returns after the woman is dressed to discuss findings and the plan of care.

Pelvic Examination During Pregnancy

The pelvic examination during pregnancy is done in the same way as it is during a routine examination on a nonpregnant woman. Chapter 14 describes more details about the pelvic examination of a pregnant woman. As the pregnancy progresses, the nurse inspects the woman's abdomen, palpates fetal size and position, auscultates fetal heart tones, and measures fundal height at each visit.

Pelvic Examination After Hysterectomy

The pelvic examination after hysterectomy is done much as it is done on a woman with a uterus. Vaginal screening using the Pap test is not recommended in women who have had a total hysterectomy with removal of the cervix for benign disease. Because of the epidemic of HPV, which causes vaginal intraepithelial neoplasia, sampling of the vaginal walls after hysterectomy may still be practiced, with schedules varying from every year to every 2 to 3 years.

Laboratory and Diagnostic Procedures

The following laboratory and diagnostic procedures are ordered at the discretion of the clinician, considering the client and family history: hemoglobin, fasting blood glucose, total blood cholesterol, lipid profile, urinalysis, syphilis serology (Venereal Disease Research Laboratories [VDRL] or rapid plasma reagent [RPR]) and other screening tests for STIs, mammogram, tuberculosis skin testing, hearing, visual

BOX 4.10 Procedure: Papanicoloau Test

- In preparation, make sure the woman empties her bladder, has not douched, used vaginal medications, or had sexual intercourse for 24-48 hours before the procedure. Reschedule the test if the woman is menstruating. Midcycle is the best time for the test.
- Explain to the woman the purpose of the test and what sensations she will feel as the specimen is obtained (e.g., pressure but not pain).
- The woman is assisted into a lithotomy position. A speculum is inserted into the vagina.
- The cytologic specimen is obtained before any digital examination of the vagina is made or endocervical bacteriologic specimens are taken. A cotton swab may be used to remove excess cervical discharge before the specimen is collected.
- The specimen is obtained by using an endocervical sampling device (Cytobrush, Cervex-brush, spatula, or broom) (Figs. A and B). If the two-sample method of obtaining cells is used, the Cytobrush is inserted into the canal and rotated 90-180 degrees, followed by a gentle smear of the entire transformation zone by using a spatula. Broom devices are inserted and rotated 360 degrees five times. They obtain endocervical and ectocervical samples at the same time. If the woman has had a hysterectomy, the vaginal cuff is sampled. Areas that appear abnormal on visualization will require colposcopy and biopsy. If using a one-slide technique, the spatula sample is smeared first. This is followed by applying the Cytobrush sample (rolling the brush in the opposite direction from which it was obtained), which is less subject to drying artifact; then the slide is sprayed with preservative within 5 seconds.
- The ThinPrep or SurePath Pap test is a liquid-based method of preserving cells that reduces blood, mucus, and inflammation. The Pap specimen is obtained in the manner described above except that the cervix is not swabbed before collection of the sample. The collection device (brush, spatula, or broom) is rinsed in a vial of preserving solution that is provided by the laboratory. The sealed vial with solution is sent off to the appropriate laboratory. A special processing device filters the contents, and a thin layer of cervical cells is deposited on a slide, which is then examined microscopically. The AutoPap and Papnet tests are similar to the ThinPrep test. If cytology is abnormal, liquid-based methods allow follow-up testing for human papillomavirus (HPV) DNA with the same sample.
- Label the slides or vial with the woman's name and site. Include on the form to accompany the specimens the woman's name, age, parity, and chief complaint or reason for taking the cytologic specimens.
- Send specimens to the pathology laboratory promptly for staining, evaluation, and a written report, with special reference to abnormal elements, including cancer cells.

- Advise the woman that repeated tests may be necessary if the specimen is not adequate.
- Instruct the woman concerning routine checkups for cervical and vaginal cancer. Women vaccinated against HPV should follow the same screening guidelines as unvaccinated women. Current recommendations of the US Preventive Services Task Force (USPSTF, 2018) and the American Cancer Society (ACS, 2019) for Pap tests are that women ages 21 through 65 be screened every 3 years, or for women ages 30 through 65 every 5 years (if they had a Pap test plus HPV test that were both negative). These guidelines recommend no screening in women younger than 21, although if a girl becomes sexually active, the guidelines recommend that she get a Pap test within 3 years of initiating sexual activity or at age 21—whichever comes first. Women with high risk factors such as exposure to diethylstilbestrol (DES) in utero, those treated for cervical intraepithelial neoplasia (CIN) 2, CIN 3, cervical cancer, or human immunodeficiency virus (HIV) may need more frequent screening.
- Young women who have been treated with excisional procedures for dysplasia have an increase in premature births. A large majority of the cervical dysplasias in adolescents caused by HPV resolve on their own without treatment. It is important to avoid unnecessary instrumentation and procedures that negatively affect the cervix. Women who have had a complete hysterectomy for noncancerous reasons who have no history of high-grade CIN may have routine cervical cytology testing discontinued. Women who are older than 65 years who have not had serious cervical precancer or cancer in the past 20 years may discontinue cervical cancer screening (ACS, 2014).
- Record the examination date on the woman's record.
- Communicate findings to the woman per agency protocol.

Adapted from American Cancer Society. (2019). *Chronological history of ACS recommendations for early detection of cancer in asymptomatic people.* Available from www.cancer.org; American Cancer Society (2019). Cancer facts and figures 2019. Retrieved from: https://www.cancer.org/research/cancer-facts-statistics/all-cancer-facts-figures/cancer-facts-figures-2019.html; American College of Obstetricians and Gynecologists (2018). Practice advisory: Cervical cancer screening (update); Retrieved from: https://www.acog.org/Clinical-Guidance-and-Publications/Practice-Advisories/Practice-Advisory-Cervical-Cancer-Screening-Update; and U.S. Preventive Services Task Force. (2018). Final recommendation: Cervical cancer screening. Retrieved from: https://www.uspreventiveservicestaskforce.org/Page/Document/RecommendationStatementFinal/cervical-cancer-screening2.

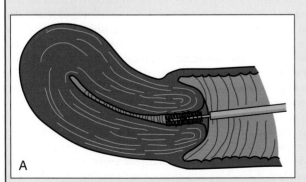

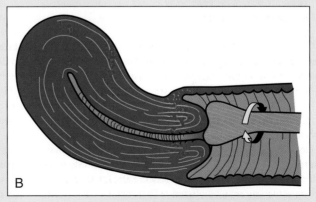

A, Cytobrush. B, Broom device. (From Lentz, G. M., Lobo, R. A., Gershenson D. M., & Katz, V. [2012]. *Comprehensive gynecology* [6th ed.]. St. Louis: Mosby.)

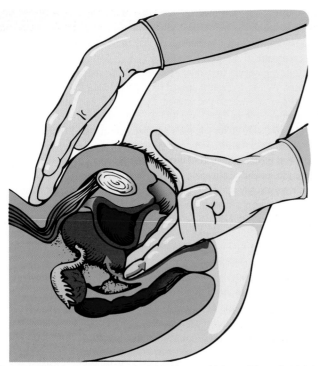

Fig. 4.13 Bimanual Palpation of the Uterus. (Adapted from Seidel, H., Ball, J., Dains, J., et al. [2011]. *Mosby's guide to physical examination* [7th ed.]. St. Louis: Mosby.)

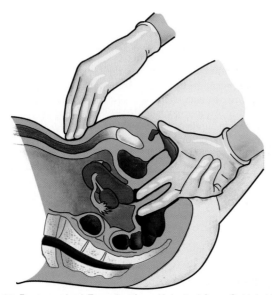

Fig. 4.14 Rectovaginal Examination. (Adapted from Seidel, H., Ball, J., Dains, J., et al. [2011]. *Mosby's guide to physical examination* [7th ed.]. St. Louis: Mosby.)

acuity, electrocardiogram, chest x-ray, pulmonary function, fecal occult blood, flexible sigmoidoscopy, and bone mineral density (dual energy x-ray absorptiometry [DEXA] scan). Results of these tests may be reported in person, by phone call, or by letter. Tests for HIV, hepatitis B, and drug screening may be offered with informed consent in high-risk populations. These test results are usually reported in person. The CDC (2015) recommends one time hepatitis C testing for persons born from 1945 through 1965.

To promote wellness and prevent illness, it is imperative that women adhere to specific screening guidelines to detect conditions that, if found early, are amenable to treatment and/or cure. Table 4.3 summarizes the screening procedures for women across the life span.

ANTICIPATORY GUIDANCE FOR HEALTH PROMOTION AND ILLNESS PREVENTION

Over the past several decades women have made tremendous strides in education, careers, policymaking, and overall participation in today's complex society. There have been costs for these advances, and although women are living longer, they may not be living better.

As a result, the health care system must pay greater attention to the health consequences for women. In addition, women must be active participants in their own health promotion and illness prevention.

Nurses have a major opportunity and responsibility to help women understand risk factors and to motivate them to adopt healthy lifestyles that prevent disease. Lifestyle factors that affect health over which the woman has some control include diet; substance use and abuse; exercise; sunlight exposure; stress management; and sexual practices. Other influences, such as genetic and environmental factors, may be beyond the woman's control, although some opportunities for prevention exist (e.g., through environmental legislation activism or genetic counseling services).

Knowledge alone is not enough to bring about healthy behaviors. The woman must be convinced that she has some control over her life and that healthy lifestyle habits, including periodic health examinations, are a sound investment. She must believe in the efficacy of prevention, early detection, and therapy and in her ability to perform self-management practices, such as BSE. Many people believe that they have little control over their health, or they become immobilized by fear and anxiety in the face of life-threatening illnesses, such as cancer, so they delay seeking treatment. The nurse must explore the reality of each woman's perceptions about health behaviors and individualize teaching if it is to be effective. In an earlier section of this chapter, risk factors to women's health were described. The following section describes actions that women can take to promote their health and prevent illness, along with the nurse's role in facilitating such actions.

Nutrition

Dietary Guidelines for Americans provides evidence-based recommendations to promote health and reduce risks for chronic diseases through diet and physical activity. This guide, published by the government, contains resources for health professionals and consumers on dietary guidelines. The Food Guide Pyramid has been replaced by MyPlate (myplate.gov), a guide to healthy eating recommended by the *Dietary Guidelines for Americans* (U.S. Department of Health and Human Services and U.S. Department of Agriculture, 2015). These guidelines recommend that half of the plate be filled with fruits and vegetables, one-quarter with grains, and one quarter with protein.

Folic acid helps reduce high levels of homocysteine, an amino acid that damages the heart and blood vessels and increases the risk of heart disease, stroke, and dementia. Folic acid is present in citrus fruits, broccoli, spinach, asparagus, peas, lettuce, beans, whole grains, and orange juice. It is in many fortified grains and pasta or can be taken as a daily vitamin supplement (USDA, 2017).

Antioxidants are thought to be effective in helping to prevent oxidative damage in the body such as cancer, heart disease, and stroke; however, more research is needed in this area. Vitamins C and E, selenium (a mineral), and a group known as β-carotenes (carotenoids) can be found in a diet containing fruits, vegetables, and whole grains.

TABLE 4.3 Health Screening Guidelines and Immunization Recommendations for Women Ages 18 Years and Older

Assessment	Recommendation[a]
Physical Examination	
Blood pressure	Every visit, but at least every 2 years
Height and weight	Every visit, but at least every 2 years
Pelvic examination	Annually until age 70; recommended for any woman who has ever been sexually active
Breast Examination	
Clinical examination	Every 3 years, ages 20-39; after age 40 with periodic examination, preferably annually
High risk	Annually after age 18 with history of premenopausal breast cancer in first-degree relative
Risk Groups	
Skin examination	Family history of skin cancer or increased exposure to sunlight every 3 years between ages 20 and 40; annually after age 40; monthly mole self-examinations also recommended
Oral cavity examination	History of mouth lesions or exposure to tobacco or excessive alcohol at least annually
Laboratory and Diagnostic Tests	
Blood cholesterol (fasting lipoprotein analysis)	Between ages 20 and 45 only if high risk; beginning at age 45 if level is within normal limits, every 5 years; more often if abnormal levels or have risk factors for coronary artery disease
Papanicolaou (Pap) test	Between ages 21 and 65—every 3 years with Pap test done Between ages 30 and 65—every 5 years if Pap test plus human papillomavirus (HPV) test done After age 65 and 3 negative tests and no risks and after total hysterectomy for benign disease—women may choose to stop screening
Mammography[b]	Every 1-2 years between ages 40 and 49 or earlier if at high risk Annually after age 40 Annually after age 50 Biennially, ages 50-74 After age 75, discuss with your health care provider
Colon cancer screening	Use one of these three methods: • Fecal occult blood test annually ages 50-74 • Flexible sigmoidoscopy every 5 years ages 50-74 • Colonoscopy every 10 years ages 50-74 Screen more often if family history of colon cancer or polyps After age 75, discuss with your health care provider
Hearing screen	Starting at age 18, then every 10 years until 49 Every 3 years after age 50 Annually with exposure to excessive noise or when loss is suspected
Vision screen	At least once between ages 20 and 29; at least twice between ages 30 and 39 Every 2-4 years between ages 40 and 64; every 1-2 years after age 65
Risk Groups	
Fasting blood sugar	Annually with family history of diabetes or gestational diabetes or if significantly obese; every 3-5 years for all women older than 45 years
Thyroid-stimulating hormone (TSH) test	As determined by the health care provider
Chlamydia test	If sexually active, yearly until age 25; after age 25, test as needed when sexually active with new or multiple partners
Sexually transmitted infection test (e.g., gonorrhea, syphilis, herpes)	As needed if sexually active with multiple partners and engaging in risky sexual behaviors
Human immunodeficiency virus (HIV) test	At least once between ages 18 and 64 to determine HIV status; test if there is a high risk for HIV infection
Tuberculin skin test	Annually with exposure to persons with tuberculosis or in risk categories for close contact with the disease
Endometrial biopsy	At menopause for women at risk for endometrial cancer; repeat as needed
Bone mineral density testing	All women ages 65 and older at least once; repeat testing as needed; younger women with risk for osteoporosis may need periodic screenings
Hepatitis C testing	All people born between 1945 and 1965, one test
Immunizations	
Tetanus-diphtheria-pertussis (Td/Tdap)	Tdap vaccine once, then booster is given every 10 years
Measles, mumps, rubella	Once if born after 1956 and no evidence of immunity

Continued

TABLE 4.3	Health Screening Guidelines and Immunization Recommendations for Women Ages 18 Years and Older—cont'd	
Hepatitis A	Primary series of two injections for all who are in risk categories
Hepatitis B	Primary series of three injections for all who are in risk categories
Influenza	Annually
Pneumococcal	1 or 2 doses between ages 19 and 64; 1 dose after age 65
Herpes zoster (shingles)	Age 50 years or older: 2-dose series RZV 2–6 months apart (minimum interval: 4 weeks; repeat dose if administered too soon)
Human papillomavirus (HPV) vaccine	Primary series of three injections for girls ages 9 to women 26 years old; intended for those not previously exposed to HPV

aThe information in this table is only a guide; health care providers will individualize the timing of tests and immunizations for each woman.
bNote: No consensus has been reached regarding mammograms for women between 40 and 49 years of age; therefore, various recommendations are listed. Women are urged to discuss circumstances with their health care providers.
Data from American Cancer Society (ACS). (2019). Cancer facts and figures 2019. Retrieved from: https://www.cancer.org/research/cancer-facts-statistics/all-cancer-facts-figures/cancer-facts-figures-2019.html; Centers for Disease Control and Prevention (CDC), Advisory Committee on Immunization Practices. (2019). *Recommended adult immunization schedule, United States.* Retrieved from https://www.cdc.gov/vaccines/schedules/hcp/imz/adult.html; CDC. (2015). *Viral hepatitis.* Retrieved from: https://www.cdc.gov/hepatitis/hcv/guidelinesc.htm; and American College of Obstetricians and Gynecologists (ACOG). (2019). *Practice advisory: Cervical cancer screening update.* Retrieved from: https://www.acog.org/Clinical-Guidance-and-Publications/Practice-Advisories/Practice-Advisory-Cervical-Cancer-Screening-Update.

Most women do not recognize the importance of calcium to health, and their diets are insufficient in calcium. Women who are unlikely to have enough calcium in the diet may need calcium supplements in the form of calcium carbonate with vitamin D, which contains more elemental calcium than do other preparations. The most recent recommendations from the Department of Health and Human Services and the Department of Agriculture (2015) are that women do need calcium supplements along with vitamin D. Postmenopausal women, in particular, need calcium to prevent osteoporosis.

The diet can be assessed by using a standard assessment form that focuses on a 24-hour recall by the woman. Following that assessment, the woman is asked to describe her food likes and dislikes, including cultural variations and typical food portions and dietary habits. This information is then discussed and can be incorporated into nutrition counseling.

Exercise

Physical activity and exercise counseling for persons of all ages should be undertaken at schools, worksites, and primary care settings. Specific recommendations include 150 minutes per week of moderate exercise or 75 minutes per week of vigorous exercise. For moderate exercise, this can be practically achieved through 30 minutes a day, five times a week. The American Heart Association (AHA) notes that dividing the 30 minutes per day into two or three segments of 10 to 15 minutes each is also beneficial (AHA, 2018). Few Americans exercise this often, and physical inactivity increases with age, especially during adolescence and early adulthood. Even small increases in activity can be beneficial. The nurse should stress the importance of daily exercise throughout life for weight management and health promotion, suggesting exercises that are enjoyable to the individual (Fig. 4.15). Physical activity builds healthy bones, muscles, and joints and reduces the risk of colon and breast cancer. It also reduces feelings of depression and anxiety and improves mood and promotes a feeling of well-being.

Activities do not need to be strenuous to bring health benefits. What is important is to include activities as part of a regular health routine. Activities that are especially beneficial when performed regularly include brisk walking, hiking, stair climbing, aerobic exercise, jogging, running, bicycling, rowing, swimming, soccer, and basketball. Before beginning any planned activity program, a woman should see

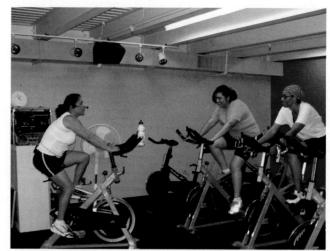

Fig. 4.15 Exercise Should Be a Part of One's Regular Health Routine. A cycle class is fun and provides moderate to vigorous exercise. (Courtesy Shari Rivera Sharpe, Chapel Hill, NC.)

her primary care NP or physician for a thorough medical evaluation to prevent potential injuries or harm.

For women who are sedentary or are not able to exercise vigorously, even moderate- and low-intensity activities, when performed daily, can have long-term health benefits such as lowering the risk of cardiovascular disease. Regular physical activity can reduce or eliminate some of these risk factors by lowering blood pressure, maintaining a reasonable weight or facilitating weight loss, and lowering cholesterol levels to below 200 mg/dL.

Home maintenance, yard work, and gardening are other activities that promote health and a sense of well-being, especially for older adults. Attention to safety factors and wearing clothing and shoes appropriate to each activity are advised. Care should be taken not to aggravate existing conditions or create muscle and joint discomfort by an overly aggressive approach to exercise.

Kegel Exercises

Kegel exercises, or pelvic muscle exercises, were developed to strengthen the supportive pelvic floor muscles to control or reduce incontinent urine loss. These exercises also are beneficial during pregnancy and postpartum. They strengthen the muscles of the pelvic floor, providing support for the pelvic organs and control of the muscles surrounding the vagina and urethra. Educational strategies for teaching women how to perform Kegel exercises are described in the Teaching for Self-Management box.

TEACHING FOR SELF-MANAGEMENT

Kegel Exercises

Description and Rationale
Kegel exercises, or pelvic muscle exercise, is a technique used to strengthen the muscles that support the pelvic floor. This exercise involves regularly tightening (contracting) and relaxing the muscles that support the bladder and urethra. By strengthening these pelvic muscles a woman can prevent or reduce accidental urine loss.

Technique
The woman needs to learn how to target the muscles for training and how to contract them correctly. One suggestion for teaching is to have the woman pretend she is trying to prevent the passage of intestinal gas. Have her use this tightening motion on the muscles around her vagina and the upper pelvis. She should feel these muscles drawing inward and upward. Other suggested techniques are to have the woman pretend she is trying to stop the flow of urine in midstream or to have her think about how her vagina is able to contract around and move up the length of the penis during intercourse.

The woman should avoid straining or bearing-down motions while performing the exercise. She should be taught how bearing down feels by having her take a breath, hold it, and push down with her abdominal muscles as though she were trying to have a bowel movement. Then the woman can be taught how to avoid straining down by exhaling gently and keeping her mouth open each time she contracts her pelvic muscles.

Specific Instructions
1. Each contraction should be as intense as possible without contracting the abdomen, thighs, or buttocks.
2. Contractions should be held for at least 10 seconds. The woman may have to start with as little as 2 seconds per contraction until her muscles get stronger.
3. The woman should rest for 10 seconds or more between contractions so that the muscles have time to recover and each contraction can be as strong as she can make it.
4. The woman should feel the pulling up over the three muscle layers so that the contraction reaches the highest level of her pelvis.

Data from Sampselle, C. (2003). Behavior interventions in young and middle-aged women: Simple interventions to combat a complex problem. *American Journal of Nursing, 103*(Suppl), 9–19; Sampselle, C. (2000). Behavioral interventions for urinary incontinence in women: Evidence for practice. *Journal of Midwifery & Women's Health, 45*(2), 94–103; Sampselle, C., Wyman, J., Thomas, K., Newman, D. K., Gray, M., Dougherty, M., et al. (2000). Continence for women: A test of AWHONN's evidence-based protocol. *Journal of Obstetric, Gynecologic, and Neonatal Nursing, 29*(1), 312–317.

Stress Management

Because it is neither possible nor desirable to avoid all stress, women must learn how to manage it. The nurse should assess each woman for signs of stress, using therapeutic communication skills to determine risk factors and the woman's ability to function. Box 4.6 lists symptoms of stress. Some women need referral for counseling or other mental health therapy. Nurses must be alert to the symptoms of serious mental disorders such as depression and anxiety and make referrals to mental health practitioners when necessary. Women experiencing major life changes such as separation and divorce, bereavement, serious illness, and unemployment also need special attention.

For many women, the nurse is able to provide comfort, reassurance, and advice concerning helping resources, such as support groups. Many centers offer support groups to help women prevent or manage stress. Social support and good coping skills can improve a woman's self-esteem and give her a sense of mastery. Anticipatory guidance for developmental or expected situational crises can help her plan strategies for dealing with potentially stressful events. Role playing, relaxation techniques, biofeedback, meditation, desensitization, imagery, assertiveness training, yoga, diet, exercise, and weight control are all techniques nurses can include in their repertoire of helping skills. Some women must be referred for counseling or other mental health therapy. Careful follow-up of all women experiencing difficulty in dealing with stress is important.

Substance Use Cessation

All women of all ages will receive substantial and immediate benefits from smoking cessation. However, this task is not easy, and most people stop several times before they accomplish their goal. Many are never able to do so. Box 4.11 describes an intervention, referred to as the five *A*s, to encourage smoking cessation. Those who wish to stop smoking can also be referred to a smoking-cessation program where individualized methods can be implemented. At the very least, individuals should be guided to self-help materials available from the March of Dimes, the American Lung Association, and the ACS.

New approaches to increase cessation among smokers and to discourage smoking among young women—especially in adolescence and during pregnancy—are needed. Health care providers can have a positive effect on smoking behavior and should attempt to motivate smokers to stop.

Counseling women who appear to be drinking alcohol excessively or using drugs may include promoting strategies to increase self-esteem and teaching new coping skills to resist and maintain resistance to alcohol abuse and drug use. Appropriate referrals should be made, with the health care provider arranging the contact and then following up to be sure that appointments are kept. General referral to sources of support also should be provided. National groups that provide information and support for those who are chemically dependent have local branches or contacts that can be found on the Internet.

Anticipatory guidance includes teaching about the health and safety risks of alcohol and mind-altering substances and discouraging drug experimentation among preteen and high school students, because the use of drugs at an early age tends to be a predictor of greater involvement later.

Sexual Practices That Reduce Risk

Prevention of STIs has been discussed earlier in this chapter. The nurse plays an important role in educating women about how to practice safer sex. Chapter 7 includes more detail related to STI prevention. In addition to the prevention of STIs, women of childbearing years need information regarding contraception and family planning (see Chapter 8). A comprehensive sexual assessment should be integrated into all health histories. Women and girls also will benefit from being encouraged to be vaccinated with the HPV series of three vaccinations to prevent cervical cancer.

Health Screening Schedule

Periodic health screening includes history, physical examination, education, counseling, immunizations, and selected diagnostic and

BOX 4.11   Interventions for Smoking Cessation: the Five *As*

Ask

What was her age when she started smoking?

How many cigarettes does she smoke a day? When was her last cigarette?

Has she tried to quit?

Does she want to quit?

Assess

What were her reasons for not being able to quit before, or what made her start again?

Does she have anyone who can help her?

Does anyone else smoke at home?

Does she have friends or family who have quit successfully?

Advise

Give her information about the effects of smoking on pregnancy and her fetus, on her own health, and on the members of her household.

Assist

Provide support; give self-help materials.

Encourage her to set a quit date.

Refer to a smoking cessation program, or provide information about nicotine replacement products (not recommended during pregnancy) if she is interested.

Teach and encourage use of stress-reduction activities.

Provide for follow-up with a phone call, letter, or clinic visit.

Arrange Follow-up

Arrange to follow the woman to find out about her smoking-cessation status.

Make a phone call around the time of her quit date. Assess her status at every prenatal visit.

Congratulate her on her success or provide support for her if she relapses.

Referral to intensive treatment may be necessary.

From Fiore, M. C., Jaen, C. R., Baker, T. B., et al (2008). *Treating tobacco use and dependence: 2008 update. Clinical practice guideline.* Rockville, MD: U.S. Department of Health and Human Services, Public Health Service. Retrieved from http://www.surgeongeneral.gov/tobacco/treating_tobacco_use08.pdf.

laboratory tests. This regimen provides the basis for overall health promotion, prevention of illness, early diagnosis of problems, and referral for appropriate management. Such screening should be customized according to a woman's age and risk factors. In most instances it is completed in health care offices, clinics, or hospitals; however, portions of the screening are now being carried out at events such as community health fairs. An overview of health screening recommendations and immunizations for women 18 years and older is provided in Table 4.3.

Health Risk Prevention

Simple safety factors often are forgotten or perceived not to be important, yet injuries continue to have a major effect on the health status of all age groups. Being aware of hazards and implementing safety guidelines will reduce risks. The nurse should frequently reinforce the following commonsense concepts that will protect the individual:

- Wear seat belts at all times in a moving vehicle.
- Avoid cell phone use (talking or texting) when driving.
- Wear safety helmets when riding a motorcycle, bicycle, or inline skates.
- Follow driving "rules of the road."
- Place smoke alarms throughout the home and workplace.
- Avoid secondhand smoke.
- Lock doors and windows to ensure personal safety.
- Reduce noise pollution or safeguard against hearing loss.
- Protect skin and eyes from ultraviolet light with the use of sunscreen, protective clothing, sunglasses, and a hat.
- Practice water safety.
- Never walk or run alone, especially at night.
- Consider storing personal health information (PHI) in a digital database that can be accessed from anywhere you travel.
- Never share computer passwords with strangers, to safeguard financial, personal, and health data.
- Take precautions and avoid dangerous situations.

Health Protection

Nurses can make a difference in stopping violence against women and preventing further injury. Educating women that abuse is a violation of their rights and facilitating their access to protective and legal services constitutes a first step. Encouraging health care institutions to implement appropriate domestic violence screening programs also is of great value (see Chapter 5). Other helpful measures for women to discourage their entry into abusive relationships include promoting assertiveness and self-defense courses; suggesting support and self-help groups that encourage positive self-regard, confidence, and empowerment; and recommending educational and skills development classes that will enhance independence and self-care.

Numerous national and local organizations provide information and assistance for women in abusive situations. All nurses who work in women's health care should become familiar with local services and legal options.

KEY POINTS

- Normal feedback regulation of the menstrual cycle depends on an intact hypothalamic-pituitary-gonadal mechanism.
- The female's reproductive tract structures and breasts respond predictably to changing levels of sex steroids across her life span.
- The myometrium of the uterus is uniquely designed to expel the fetus and promote hemostasis after birth.
- The changing status and roles of women affect their health, needs, and ability to cope with problems.
- Anticipatory guidance is enhanced in a private, safe environment in which the interaction is culturally sensitive, nonjudgmental, and confidential.

- Culture, religion, socioeconomic status, personal circumstances, the uniqueness of the individual, and the stage of development influence a person's recognition of need for care and the response to the health care system and therapy.
- Preconception counseling allows identification and possible remediation of potentially harmful personal and social conditions, medical and psychologic conditions, environmental conditions, and barriers to care before pregnancy occurs.
- Conditions that increase a woman's health risks also increase risks for her offspring.
- Effective educational programs about sex and family life are imperative to control the rate of teen pregnancy and STIs.

- Health promotion and prevention of illness assist women to actualize health potential by increasing motivation, providing information, and suggesting how to access specific resources.
- Identification of risk factors is an essential part of health assessment; (e.g., intimate partner violence, smoking, obesity).

- Periodic health screening, including history, physical examination, and diagnostic and laboratory tests, provides the basis for overall health promotion, prevention of illness, early diagnosis of problems, and referral for management.

REFERENCES

American Cancer Society. (2014). *Breast awareness and self exam.* Available at: www.cancer.org/cancer/breastcancer/moreinformation/breastcancerearlydetection/breast-cancer-early-detection-acs-recs-bse.

American Cancer Society. (2018a). *Does body weight affect cancer risk?* https://www.cancer.org/cancer/cancer-causes/diet-physical-activity/body-weight-and-cancer-risk/effects.html.

American Cancer Society. (2018b). *Health risks of smoking tobacco.* https://www.cancer.org/cancer/cancer-causes/tobacco-and-cancer/health-risks-of-smoking-tobacco.html.

American Heart Association. (2018). *American Heart Association recommendations for physical activity in adults.* http://www.heart.org/en/healthy-living/fitness/fitness-basics/aha-recs-for-physical-activity-in-adults.

Anxiety and Depression Association of America. (2018). *Facts and statistics.* https://adaa.org/about-adaa/press-room/facts-statistics.

Berg, J. A., Taylor, D., & Woods, N. F. (2015). Women at midlife. In E. F. Olshansky (Ed.), *Women's health and wellness across the lifespan.* Philadelphia, PA: Wolters Kluwer.

Burkhardt, M. A., & Nagai-Jacobson, M. G. (2012). Spirituality and health. In B. M. Dossey, & L. Keegan (Eds.), *Holistic nursing: A handbook for practice* (6th ed.). Burlington, MA: Jones and Bartlett.

Centers for Disease Control and Prevention. (2014). *Social determinants of health.* http://www.cdc.gov/socialdeterminants/Definitions.html.

Centers for Disease Control and Prevention. (2015). Viral hepatitis. Retrieved from https://www.cdc.gov/hepatitis/hcv/guidelinesc.htm.

Centers for Disease Control and Prevention. (2016). *Chronic disease prevention and health promotion: Tobacco use.* Available at: www.cdc.gov/chronicdisease/resources/publications/aag/osh.htm.

Centers for Disease Control and Prevention. (2016a). *Birthweight and gestation.* Atlanta, GA: CDC. http://www.cdc.gov/nchs/fastats/birthweight.htm.

Centers for Disease Control and Prevention. (2018a). Current Cigarette Smoking Among Adults—United States, 2017. *Morbidity and Mortality Weekly Report, 67*(44), 1225–1232.

Centers for Disease Control and Prevention. (2018b). Health effects of cigarette smoking. Retrieved from https://www.cdc.gov/tobacco/data_statistics/fact_sheets/health_effects/effects_cig_smoking/index.htm.

Centers for Disease Control and Prevention. (2018c). *Overweight and obesity.* https://www.cdc.gov/obesity/data/adult.html.

Centers for Disease Control and Prevention. (2019). About teen pregnancy. Retrieved from https://www.cdc.gov/teenpregnancy/about/index.htm.

Cohen, B. E., Edmonsdon, D., & Kronish, I. M. (2015). State of the art review: depression, stress, anxiety, and cardiovascular disease. *American Journal of Hypertension, 11,* 1295–1302.

England, L. C., Bunnell, R. E., Pechacek, T. F., et al. (2015). Nicotine and the developing human: A neglected element in the electronic cigarette debate. *American Journal of Preventive Medicine, 49*(2), 286–293.

Galanti, G. (2008). *Caring for patients from different cultures* (4th ed.). University of Pennsylvania.

Gøtzsche, Peter, C., & Jørgensen, Karsten, J. (2013). *Screening for Breast Cancer with Mammography.* Cochrane Library. http://onlinelibrary.wiley.com/doi/.

Green, C. (2016). Human trafficking: preparing for a unique patient population. *American Nurse Today, 11*(1). https://www.americannursetoday.com/human-trafficking-preparing-unique-patient-population/.

Guttmacher Institute. (2017). Adolescent sexual and reproductive health in the United States. Retrieved from https://www.guttmacher.org/fact-sheet/american-teens-sexual-and-reproductive-health?gclid=Cj0KCQjwtMvlBRDmARIsAEoQ8zRYghuxOj-lNjxii7ddNhY_zedQ8DOdV_dAjmTBhLd5Xfn4VLUxlGMaAgvsEALw_wcB.

Guttmacher Institute. (2019). Unintended pregnancy in the United States. Retrieved from https://www.guttmacher.org/fact-sheet/unintended-pregnancy-united-states.

Hautala, L., Junnila, J., Alin, J., et al. (2009). Uncovering hidden eating disorders using the SCOFF questionnaire: Cross-sectional survey of adolescents and comparison with nurse assessments. *International Journal of Nursing Studies, 46*(11), 1439–1447.

Lin, T. F., & Chen, J. (2014). Effect of physician gender on demand for Pap tests. *Economics Research International, 8.*

March of Dimes. (2015a). *Caffeine during pregnancy.* https://www.marchofdimes.org/pregnancy/caffeine-in-pregnancy.aspx.

March of Dimes. (2015b). *Caffeine in pregnancy.* https://www.marchofdimes.org/pregnancy/caffeine-in-pregnancy.aspx.

Martin, J.A., Hamilton, B.E., Osterman, M.J.K., et al. (2018). Births: Final data for 2017. *National Vital Statistics Reports, 67*(8). Retrieved from https://www.cdc.gov/nchs/data/nvsr/nvsr67/nvsr67_08-508.pdf.

Masters, W., & Johnson, V. (1966). *Human sexual response.* New York: Bantam Books.

Morgan, J., Reid, F., & Lacey, J. (1999). The SCOFF questionnaire: Assessment of a new screening tool for eating disorders. *BMJ, 319*(7223), 1467–1468.

National Association of Anorexia Nervosa and Associated Disorders. (2019). Eating disorder statistics. Retrieved from https://anad.org/education-and-awareness/about-eating-disorders/eating-disorders-statistics/.

National Institute on Alcohol Abuse and Alcoholism. (2018). Alcohol facts and statistics. Retrieved from https://www.niaaa.nih.gov/alcohol-health/overview-alcohol-consumption/alcohol-facts-and-statistics.

National Institute on Drug Abuse. (2014). *Drug facts: Methamphetamine.* Retrieved from: https://www.drugabuse.gov/publications/drugfacts/methamphetamine.

National Institute on Drug Abuse. (2016a). *Drug facts: Marijuana.* Retrieved from: https://www.drugabuse.gov/publications/drugfacts/marijuana.

National Institute on Drug Abuse. (2016b). *What is cocaine?.* Retrieved from: https://www.drugabuse.gov/publications/drugfacts/cocaine.

National Institute on Drug Abuse. (2016c). *What are hallucinogens?.* Retrieved from: https://www.drugabuse.gov/publications/drugfacts/hallucinogens.

Office of Disease Prevention and Health Promotion. (2018). https://health.gov/dietaryguidelines/.

Office of Women's Health. (2018). *Female genital mutilation.* https://www.womenshealth.gov/a-z-topics/female-genital-cutting.

Olshansky, E. F., & Zender, R. (2015). Wellness for special populations of women. In E. F. Olshansky (Ed.), *Women's health and wellness across the lifespan.* Philadelphia: Wolters Kluwer.

Piotrowski, K., & Snell, L. (2007). Health needs of women with disabilities across the lifespan. *Journal of Obstetric, Gynecologic, and Neonatal Nursing, 36*(1), 79–87.

Sammarco, A. (2016). *Women's health issues across the life cycle: A quality of life perspective.* Burlington, MA: Jones & Bartlett.

Shaver, J. L. F. (2015). Promoting healthy sleep. In E. F. Olshansky (Ed.), *Women's health and wellness across the lifespan.* Philadelphia: Wolters Kluwer.

Substance Abuse and Mental Health Services Administration (SAMHSA). (2015). *Specific populations and prescription drug misuse and abuse.* Retrieved from: https://www.samhsa.gov/prescription-drug-misuse-abuse/specific-populations.

U.S. Department of Agriculture. (2017). *Choose my.plate.com.* https://www.choosemyplate.gov/ten-tips-build-healthy-meal.

U.S. Department of Health and Human Services. (2019). What is the U.S. opioid epidemic? Retrieved from https://www.hhs.gov/opioids/about-the-epidemic/index.html.

U.S. Department of Health and Human Services and U.S. Department of Agriculture. *2015–2020 Dietary Guidelines for Americans* (8th ed.). December 2015. Available at: https://health.gov/dietaryguidelines/2015/guidelines/.

US Department of Health & Human Services/National Institute of Child Health & Human Development. (2016). *What is prenatal care and why is it important?* Retrieved from: https://www.nichd.nih.gov/health/topics/pregnancy/conditioninfo/Pages/prenatal-care.aspx.

US Department of Justice, Office on violence against women. (2015). *Domestic violence.* Washington, DC: Dept. of Justice. Retrieved from: https://www.justice.gov/ovw/domestic-violence.

U.S. Preventive Services Task Force. (2013). Final recommendation statement screening for intimate partner violence of elderly and vulnerable adults. Available at: www.uspreventiveservicestaskforce.org/uspstf12/ipvelder/ipvelderfinalrs.htm.

U.S. Preventive Services Task Force. (2016). Breast cancer screening. Retrieved from https://www.uspreventiveservicestaskforce.org/Page/Document/UpdateSummaryFinal/breast-cancer-screening.

U.S. Preventive Services Task Force. (2016). Breast cancer screening. Retrieved from https://www.uspreventiveservicestaskforce.org/Page/Document/UpdateSummaryFinal/breast-cancer-screening.

U.S. Preventive Services Task Force. (2018). Cervical cancer screening. Retrieved from https://www.uspreventiveservicestaskforce.org/Page/Document/UpdateSummaryFinal/cervical-cancer-screening2.

World Health Organization. (2019). Classification of female genital mutilation. Retrieved from https://www.who.int/reproductivehealth/topics/fgm/overview/en/.

5

Violence Against Women

Melissa Schwartz Beck, Carol Ann King, Michelle Taylor Skipper

http://evolve.elsevier.com/Lowdermilk/MWHC/

LEARNING OBJECTIVES

- Describe the beliefs and practices that historically have perpetuated violence against women.
- Examine the prevalence and effects of intimate partner violence, including during pregnancy.
- Discuss theories of violence and how they can be used in assessment and intervention for women who are abused.
- Develop a nursing care plan for a woman who is experiencing intimate partner violence.

- Review the dynamics of sexual assault.
- Describe the rape-trauma syndrome.
- Develop a nursing care plan for a woman in the acute phase of rape-trauma syndrome.
- Evaluate resources available to women experiencing abuse.
- Describe human sex trafficking and implications for health care professionals.

Beginning with the second wave of the women's movement in the mid-1960s, the protection of women and their families from all forms of partner violence has risen in priority in the United States and other Western European countries. In the 1970s the United Nations (UN) identified the eradication of all forms of violence against women (VAW) as one of the most important strategies for women to attain equality with men (Walker, 2017). The UN defines VAW as "any act of gender-based violence that results in, or is likely to result in, physical, sexual or mental harm or suffering to women, including threats of such acts, coercion or arbitrary deprivation of liberty whether occurring in public or private life" (World Health Organization [WHO], 2016). VAW takes many different forms, including but not limited to intimate partner violence (IPV), sexual violence (SV), sexual harassment at school or work, marital and nonmarital rape, dowry-related violence, human trafficking, sexual exploitation, and female genital mutilation (Centers for Disease Control and Prevention [CDC], 2014; WHO, 2016). In this chapter, we replace the older term of "victim" with "survivor," referring to someone who is not deceased. It is a newer term to empower women living with IPV (Basile, Smith, Breiding, et al., 2014). Although IPV can be experienced by men and women, this chapter will focus on IPV, SV, and trafficking of women.

INTIMATE PARTNER VIOLENCE

Intimate partner violence (IPV) refers to "behavior by an intimate partner or ex-partner that causes physical, sexual or psychological harm, including physical aggression, sexual coercion, psychological abuse and controlling behavior" (WHO, 2017). IPV can vary in severity and frequency. It occurs on a continuum, ranging from one incident that might or might not have a lasting impact to chronic and severe episodes over several years (CDC, 2014). Although IPV is the preferred term, *partner abuse*, spousal abuse, and domestic or family violence are also common terms. Older terms such as wife battering or spouse battering are generally not used. *Battery* has

been used in the past to refer to physical contact with another with the intent of harm, but the WHO (2017) has an updated definition of battery to refer to an escalation of violence with increasing threats and increasing terror. Battery consists of slapping, punching the face or head, kicking, stomping, choking, pushing, breaking of bones, burns from irons, and mutilation from knives and guns.

IPV is a complex, stigmatizing problem involving issues of emotional distress, personal safety, and social isolation. In many places in the United States and abroad, IPV has been socially tolerated or ignored. Lack of reporting and inconsistent definitions have made it difficult to get an accurate count of the number of survivors, and there are wide ranges of estimates (Smith, Chen, Basile, et al., 2017).

IPV is the most common form of VAW, with half of the countries in developing regions reporting 30% of all women having experienced IPV (UN, 2015; WHO, 2016, 2017). High-income countries estimate a 23.2% prevalence of IPV (WHO, 2017). The WHO (2017) estimates a prevalence of 24.6% in the Western Pacific Region to a high of 37.7% in the Southeast Asian Region. Prevalence is high in Africa, with one-quarter of countries in the region reporting an incidence of 50% (UN, 2015). Oceana, a collection of islands in the South Pacific, has the greatest incidence, reaching more than 60% incidence of IPV (UN, 2015).

In the United States, the National Intimate Partner and Sexual Violence Survey (NISVS), an ongoing random-digit-dial telephone survey of all 50 states and the District of Columbia, collects data on SV, stalking, and IPV. Questions on violence between same-sex partners, information not previously tracked, has been included to the NISVS survey to aid in understanding IPV. Among reportable states (seven states), the prevalence of some form of IPV (SV, physical violence, and/or stalking) during a woman's lifetime ranges between 28.0% and 42.4% (Smith et al., 2017). Abuse, which may be physical, sexual, psychologic, or financial, can continue after the relationship ends. One partner behaves in a way that injures, intimidates, humiliates, frightens, or terrorizes the other partner. These behaviors can be subtle, slowly occurring over time. Emotional abuse may include name-calling, acting in a jealous or possessive manner, trying to isolate the woman from her family or friends, putting her down in front of others, threatening her children or alienating her children from her, not wanting her to go out or go to work, or insisting that she account for every minute she is away from home (Breiding, Smith, Walters, et al., 2014; CDC, 2014). Even if physical violence is never or rarely used, threats can be as effective as actual violence, causing mental or emotional harm (CDC, 2014). If the abuser becomes physically violent, the threat of recurrence always exists.

Abusive relationships exist in couples who are dating, living together, or married (Breiding, et al., 2014; CDC, 2014). Women are at greater risk for IPV during pregnancy, and the majority of women who experience IPV during pregnancy have been battered before, but, for some, abuse begins with pregnancy (Domestic Shelters, 2015). (see later discussion in section Intimate Partner Violence in Pregnancy). Cyber dating abuse (CDA), an emerging phenomenon, is composed of behaviors used to control a partner or ex-partner through electronic means (Borrajo, Gámez-Guadix, & Calvete, 2015). Technology such as digital photos, videos, apps, and social media have all been used to engage in harassing and unsolicited or nonconsensual sexual interactions (Rape, Abuse, and Incest National Network [RAINN], 2018). Borrajo et al. (2015) conducted an online survey of 704 young adults in Spain between 18 and 30 years of age. About 20% of the sample, including males and females, were involved in some type of online aggressive behavior, and the consequences were more harmful to women.

Abused women have a higher incidence of social and family problems, substance abuse, menstrual and other reproductive disorders, STIs, musculoskeletal and gastrointestinal (GI) disorders, chest pain, abdominal pain, UTIs, and headaches (Association of Women's Health, Obstetric and Neonatal Nurses [AWHONN], 2015; Smith et al., 2017; WHO, 2017). Prolonged exposure to acute or chronic stress such as IPV is linked with structural changes in the brain that are currently associated with mental health problems, emotion regulation, and cognitive problems. Based on the review of multiple large population-based surveys, the WHO developed a global plan of action to encourage individuals to use health systems to respond to, prevent, and lead efforts to address VAW and girls (WHO, 2016).

The financial cost of IPV is high for both survivors and society as a whole (King, Murray, Crowe, et al., 2017). Cost refers to the cost of health care related to the emotional healing process, but also costs associated with legal fees, shelters, foster care, sick leave, and loss of work.

Historical Perspective

Women have been treated inhumanely throughout history. Addressing the issue of VAW continues to be of great societal concern.

The first shelter for women opened in London in 1971, and books and articles on domestic violence began to appear in the 1970s. Battered woman syndrome was described by Lenore Walker in 1979, and battered women programs emerged in the 1980s. In the 1990s the American Nurses Association issued a position statement against VAW, the American Medical Association declared that physicians were liable if they did not recognize IPV, and The Joint Commission (TJC) issued standards to identify and manage IPV clients. The National Domestic Violence Hotline was established in 1996. The CDC promotes the phrase IPV over domestic violence (CDC, 2017a). Health care providers, law enforcement, the legal system, and the general public are slowly acknowledging IPV, but power imbalances, persistent beliefs that family problems are private matters, the survivor's feelings of shame, and fear continue to keep women from disclosing abuse (U.S. Department of Health & Human Services, 2017b; WHO, 2016).

THEORIES, PERSPECTIVES, FRAMEWORKS, AND MODELS THAT SEEK TO EXPLAIN INTIMATE PARTNER VIOLENCE

Walker Cycle Theory of Violence

In the late 1970s little was known about IPV. Lenore Walker, a pioneer in the field, interviewed 120 survivors, from which she generated the phrase "battered woman syndrome" to identify by a survivor characteristics such as learned helplessness and abuser characteristics such as mental health problems. The Walker cycle theory of violence states there are three distinct phases associated with the recurrent battery of women: (1) tension building accompanied with rising sense of danger, (2) the acute battering incident, and (3) loving contrition. Phase I, tension building, consists of gradual escalation of tension displayed by discrete actions such as name-calling, other mean intentional behaviors, and/or physical abuse. The woman attempts to placate the batterer and/or use general anger reduction techniques. Phase II, the acute battering incident, is characterized by an uncontrollable discharge of verbal and or physical aggression. Most injuries occur in the second phase. The acute battering phase concludes when the batterer stops, usually commencing with a sharp reduction in tension. Phase III, loving contrition, sometimes referred to as the honeymoon phase, is characterized by a period of peace and regret. The batterer may himself believe he will never be violent again. Walker's continued research demonstrates that phase III could also be characterized by a lack of violence and tension with no observable loving-contrition behavior and still be a strengthening period for the woman (Walker, 2017). In phase I, tension building, a period of arguments and verbal abuse again leads to battery.

The cycle of violence has been widely used by health care workers and domestic violence advocates; however, limitations to the cycle of violence have been identified. For example, the cycle may not apply to sexual, emotional, financial, and mental abuse that is also experienced by women. The cycle of violence may describe violence occurring early in a relationship, because the tension and battery phases may last longer with no honeymoon phase as is seen with chronic or long-term abuse (WomanSafe, 2018).

Feminist Perspective

One contemporary view of violence is derived from feminist theory, with a recent explanation including the intersection between violence against both women and children (Namy, Carlson, O'Hara et al., 2017). The influence of gender and the power dynamics that occur within gendered relationships are emphasized as important in understanding why men engage in violent behavior, including IPV and violence against children (VAC). In numerous cases, power and control tactics were central events leading to the violence. The power and control wheel developed by the Duluth, Minnesota, Domestic Abuse Intervention Project (Domestic Abuse Intervention Programs, 2017) identifies ways that men may exercise the power and control that underlie many types of IPV and has been used to help women, men, and care providers understand violence (Fig. 5.1).

As our understanding of the complexity of VAW has evolved over time, so has the need for an evolving feminist viewpoint. Although the traditional feminist theory has been useful in explaining some cases of IPV, it does not adequately frame all examples of IPV. Cannon, Lauve-Moon, & Buttell, (2015) re-theorized IPV using poststructural feminism, queer, and sociology of gender to account for heterosexual female perpetration and same-sex IPV. Poststructural feminism suggests that the power of a woman to enact violence may stem from the woman's history merged with her own motivations for and experiences of violence (Cannon et al., 2015).

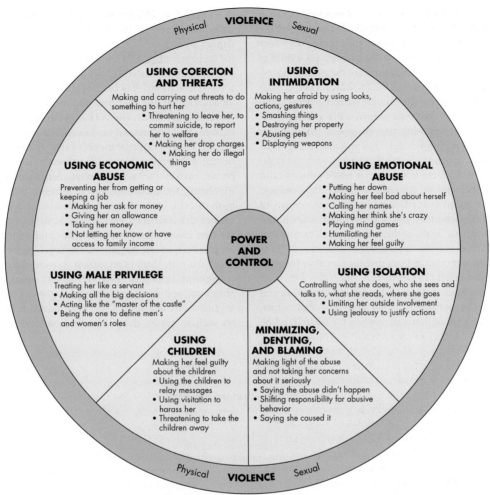

Fig. 5.1 Model of how power and control issues perpetuate battering. (Developed by the Duluth Domestic Abuse Intervention Project, Duluth, MN.)

The queer theoretical approach, like poststructural feminism, uses conceptualization of power from personal experience and drive but adds social location to explain violence within the lesbian, gay, bisexual, transgender, and queer (LGBTQ) population. The lesbian abuser does not use patriarchy to control; instead, violence in same-sex relationships is seen as a tactic available to the LGBTQ population based on their social location. The social location represents the LGBTQ placement in a society that privileges heterosexuality who may access more dominant forms of power. In this way, the lesbian batterer's violence does not represent patriarchy but a relationship tactic (Cannon et al., 2015).

Theories of gender have shifted over the past 30 years survivor's. A shift consistent with poststructural understandings reimagines power as fluid rather than static. Theoretic shifts also deconstruct the gender binary to focus on the differences between men and women that align with heterosexual expectations. Sociology of gender conceptualizes sex through masculine and feminine traits that can be embodied by both men and women. The hegemonic gender structure associates power and violence with masculinity, and it is assumed that both men and women can embody or practice masculinity. The sociology of gender provides a framework that both males and females can perpetrate IPV (Cannon et al., 2015).

Theory of Learned Helplessness

Martin Seligman's theory of learned helplessness evolved from an experiment using pavlovian conditioning, where dogs given electric shocks heralded by a tone were to learn to escape the shock by jumping over a barrier, but instead the dogs failed to escape and passively waited the shock out (Maier & Seligman, 2016). Not to be confused with being helpless, learned helplessness represents having lost the ability to predict that what one does will make a particular outcome occur (Walker, 2017). Seligman et al. continued studying learned helplessness with humans, yielding similar results. Later, he began to work on "positive psychology," the study of the causes and consequences of positive events, among them having control as opposed to being helpless (Maier & Seligman, 2016). Lenore Walker used this theory to provide insight into how an abusive situation can become paired in an identifiable pattern with positive parts of a relationship (Walker, 2017). This theory can be used to understand the development of coping strategies and explain why women find it hard to leave an abusive relationship. Walker's research suggests women exchange their escape skills to develop coping strategies and, until they are able to believe they can safely escape, breaking the learned helplessness, they will not be able to leave the relationship psychologically. It is not that women cannot use their skills to escape the batterer, stop the abuse, or even defend themselves, but they cannot predict that what they do will result in a desirable outcome. Understanding the theories of learned helplessness and positive psychology can provide direction for prevention and intervention when caring for the battered woman (Walker, 2017).

Socioecologic Model

The CDC uses the four-level socioecologic model, a framework used in public health research and practice, to understand violence and the effect of potential prevention strategies (CDC, 2015; Golden, McLeroy, Green, et al., 2015). The model provides a visual depiction of the dynamic relationships that occur between individuals, groups, and their environments (Golden et al., 2015). The first level, *individual*, identifies the biologic and personal history that may increase the risk of becoming a perpetrator or experiencing violence (CDC, 2015). Level 2, *relationship*, assesses the person's closest social circle (peers), partners, and family members that could influence their behavior. Prevention strategies at this level may include mentoring, peer programs, parenting, or family-focused prevention programs designed to promote healthy relationships. The third level, *community*, explores settings, such as neighborhoods, schools, and workplaces where social relationships occur. Prevention strategies at this level are designed to impact the social and physical environment. Examples might include the improvement of economic and housing opportunities and policies within schools and the workplace. Level 4, *societal*, looks at the broad societal factors that help to create a climate where violence is encouraged or inhibited. These factors include social and cultural standards that support violence as an acceptable way to resolve conflict (CDC, 2015).

Ecologic models include the external influences of environmental factors such as public policy and culture, along with individual factors, that influence human behavior within a framework for understanding the interacting detriments of health problems (Sabbah, Chang, & Campbell-Heider, 2017). Sabbah and colleagues (2017) explored Jordanian studies on IPV and suggest the ecologic model is well suited for understanding violence in Jordan because it includes gender-based and nongender-related factors to understand IPV within a patriarchal society. The model has been adapted to investigate determinants for violence in various countries and for specific age groups and settings (Sabbah et al., 2017). The WHO (2018) uses an ecologic framework to examine and understand various communities.

Fig. 5.2 is an ecologic model of IPV. The individual woman is at the center of the model. Her unique characteristics, such as age, life experience, race/ethnicity, social class, education, personality, emotional well-being, finances, and others, influence who she is and how she is in the world. In her immediate environment is her intimate partner, his/her characteristics, and the characteristics of their relationship. At the next level *(microsystem)* are her children, family, friends, and the people, such as her neighbors, employer, or coworkers, and activities in her daily life that are important. Surrounding the social network are community resources such as women's groups, violence prevention programs, and local resources *(mesosystem)*. The *exosystem* refers to organizations and formal agencies, health care systems, and providers such as nurses, the police, and the legal system, all of which are

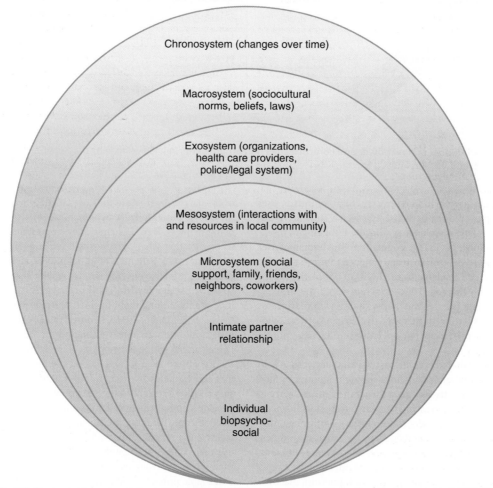

Fig. 5.2 Ecologic Framework for Intimate Partner Violence. (Adapted from Bronfenbrenner, U. [1979]. *The ecology of human development: Experiments by nature and design.* Cambridge, MA: Harvard University Press; Bronfenbrenner, U. [2005]. *Making human beings human: Bioecological perspectives on human development.* Thousand Oaks, CA: Sage; Heise, L. [1998]. Violence against women: An integrated, ecological framework. *Violence Against Women, 4*[3], 262–290; Campbell, R., Dworkin, E., & Cabral, G. [2009]. An ecological model of the impact of sexual assault on women's mental health. *Trauma Violence and Abuse, 10*[3], 225–246.)

influenced by the larger sociocultural beliefs, myths, and media (*macrosystem*). Finally, the *chronosystem* represents the influence of events over time.

For example, a woman experiencing IPV over time may develop chronic depression and hopelessness, finding it more difficult to mount the energy needed to change or leave the relationship. Her partner interactions may have pushed away her friends, and her emotional state makes it difficult to rebuild relationships. Perhaps her family or friends are influenced by social or cultural expectations not to interfere in someone else's marriage, express disbelief, or blame the woman (Sylaska & Edwards, 2014). The woman is socially isolated. She may hear about IPV issues from a local women's group, helping to destigmatize her perception of the issue. If she risks disclosing her experience to a nurse and receives validation and support, she may be more likely to seek help again in the future, perhaps with the health care system or with another social agency. The nurse who interacted with the woman is also influenced by that experience in providing support to a survivor of IPV. All facets of the model are influenced by one another, and those influences change over time.

Sociologic Perspective

The social structure and conditions in Western society provide the basis for many of the prevailing attitudes toward violent behavior. U.S. history is filled with examples of violence, such as war, as a means of social control. Social acceptance and promotion of violence in men are double standards because women are expected to be nonviolent. Psychologic theories suggest gender-based behaviors can influence social beliefs and responses to particular behaviors. Because men are socially expected to be aggressive, their violence is sometimes treated with more leniency and less stigma than violence in women, particularly in the justice system. The use of physical force in normal societal encounters can lead to the acceptance of violence in society.

Many factors contribute to violence. Family dynamics in which there are certain roles assumed within the family, the amount of time spent together, the degree of privacy, emotional involvement, and stress and conflict may all contribute to violence.

Power and violence, or even the threat of physical force, contribute to the persistent patriarchal view of a woman's place in the home and in the rest of society. Gender inequality, in both economic opportunities and physical strength, is the root of violence experienced by women and girls and equality is essential to the prevention of violence (WHO, 2016).

Some research suggests violence in the family of origin may be a predictor of IPV in the future; however, there is also research to support that exposure to violence as a child does not deterministically lead to violent behaviors in young adulthood (Kaufman-Parks, DeMaris, Giordano, et al., 2017). In families in which violence occurs, both the lack of emotional support experienced by children and the awareness that people who love each other can be violent are important factors. Children in these environments do not have role models to help them develop mental models of healthy family dynamics. However, abuse as a child does not consistently determine later violent behavior because many children who were abused grow up to avoid violent behavior.

The literature on the characteristics and dynamics of IPV are growing. Theories from biology, psychology, and sociology provide insight into the various aspects of VAW. No single theory can fully explain this complex problem. The following provides a brief overview of biologic factors and psychologic and sociologic perspectives.

Biologic Factors

A complete explanation of the biologic perspective is beyond the scope of this chapter, but evidence indicates that neurobiologic and hormonal factors, such as testosterone, influence aggression in men. Areas in the brain believed to play a role in aggressive behavior are the limbic system, frontal lobes, and hypothalamus. Changes in structural functioning of the limbic system, such as occur with brain lesions, substance use, epilepsy, and head injuries, affect the emotional experience and behavior of the individual and thus can increase or decrease the potential for aggressive behavior. Recent evidence from the experiences of professional football players has elucidated the condition referred to as chronic traumatic encephalopathy (CTE), in which brain degeneration is a result of head trauma leading to numerous symptoms, including aggression (Mayo Clinic, 2018).

Neurochemical factors also can play a role in aggressive behavior so that dysfunction or dysregulation of certain neurotransmitters can result in aggression. Increased levels of norepinephrine and L-dopa foster aggressive behavior. Reducing the levels of serotonin in animals causes aggressive behavior. The amino acid γ-aminobutyric acid (GABA) inhibits aggressive behavior.

The myth that abuse is committed by people who have some type of mental illness perpetuates the notion that violence occurs only among families suffering with mental illness. This myth is not supported by evidence and accounts for only a very small percentage of IPV cases. Hahn and colleagues (2015) conducted a secondary data analysis from the National Epidemiologic Survey on Alcohol and Related Conditions investigating the relationship between post-traumatic stress disorder (PTSD) and IPV. Findings from this study suggest heterosexual men who reported lifetime PTSD had significantly higher risk of IPV perpetration. Studies on PTSD in veterans, military, and civilian communities also showed increased incidence of IPV in men with PTSD symptoms (Hahn, Aldarondo, Silverman, et al., 2015). A diagnosis of alcohol abuse is frequently found in abusers; it should not be misconstrued as the cause of violence. Although there is no diagnostic profile of an abuser, Box 5.1 provides some characteristics of men who abuse. Awareness of these characteristics can help nurses and other health care professionals in assessing clients' relationships.

Women with severe and persistent mental illness are likely to be more vulnerable to being involved in controlling and violent relationships. However, numerous mental health problems (such as depression, psychophysiologic illnesses, substance abuse, eating disorders, PTSD,

---

BOX 5.1   Characteristics of a Potential Male Abuser

- Low self-esteem
- Problems with abandonment, loss, helplessness, dependency, insecurity, and intimacy
- Inadequate verbal skills, especially difficulty expressing feelings
- Deficits in assertiveness
- Personality disorders frequently diagnosed
- Low frustration tolerance (loses temper easily)
- Higher incidence of growing up in an abusive or violent home
- Denies, minimizes, blames, and lies about own actions
- Violence is consistent with his view of himself and the world; it is an acceptable way of dealing with everyday life
- Inability to empathize with others
- Rigidity in male and female behaviors (sex-role stereotypes)
- Perception of self as "special" and deserving special attention for being the provider/protector
- Substance abuse problems are common
- Displays of an unusual amount of jealousy (e.g., expects partner to spend all of her time with him or to keep him informed of her whereabouts)

and anxiety reactions) experienced by women with abusive partners are more likely to be consequences of long-term abuse rather than causes (WHO, 2017). Relationship violence differs by severity and frequency, the individual's characteristics, and whether it is confined to the family or occurs outside the family. Women's experiences of violence vary widely. Although there may be shared characteristics, each person's experience and response is individual. Although there may be shared characteristics, each person's experience and response is individual.

Women Experiencing Intimate Partner Violence
Characteristics of Women in Abusive Relationships

Every segment of society has people experiencing abuse. Race, religion, social background, age, and educational level do not differentiate women at risk. Poor and uneducated women tend to be disproportionately represented because they are seen in emergency departments (EDs), are financially more dependent, have fewer resources and support systems, and may have fewer problem-solving skills. Women with educational or financial resources have been hidden from public awareness but can just as easily be survivors of violence. They may be disadvantaged in other ways in that they do not fit the stereotype of an abused woman and find it difficult to come to terms with the idea that they are in an abusive relationship (United States Department of Health & Human Services, 2018).

The value women place on their social roles may have some influence in IPV. Traditional feminine characteristics such as compassion, sympathy, and yielding often result in greater tolerance of male dominance and more acceptance of partner violence. In contrast, the traits of assertiveness, independence, and willingness to take a stand have been viewed as more characteristic in women who are in nonviolent relationships. There is little research that tells us how these characteristics might change if independent, assertive women found themselves in abusive relationships. Although women who are in abusive relationships may appear passive or even helpless to an outside observer, their behaviors can represent attempts to reduce the risk of violence as they survive day to day. Therefore it is important not to attach causation to traditional feminine characteristics.

Survivors of IPV may believe they are to blame for their situations because they are "not good enough, not efficient enough, not pretty enough." The woman may blame herself for bringing on the violent behavior in her relationship because she believes she must try harder to please the abuser. In many cases a traumatic bonding with the man hinges on loyalty, fear, and terror. Some women have low self-esteem. Some may have histories of domestic violence in their families of origin. Often, abused women are socially isolated. This may be the result of stigma, fear, restrictions placed on them by their partners, or partner behaviors that discourage others from being involved.

Some survivors of IPV may be formally diagnosed as having PTSD if their symptoms meet the criteria in the *Diagnostic and Statistical Manual of Mental Disorders* (American Psychiatric Association [APA], 2013). Some characteristics of PTSD sufferers include a reexperiencing of the traumatic event through dreams, flashbacks, or recollections. They also may have a distorted sense of self-blame or blame of others, become estranged from others, have diminished interest in activities, difficulty sleeping, or being aggressive, reckless, or engage in self-destructive behavior (APA, 2013).

Every year, in the United States, more than 1800 people are killed by an intimate partner and approximately 85% are women (United States Department of Justice, 2015). Most women report IPV to at least one person in their social network, often a family member or friend. They disclose less frequently to health professionals. In a study on disclosure, the most helpful reactions were found to be emotional support, allowing the woman to talk, giving helpful advice, and providing useful or practical support. Negative responses included encouraging the woman to leave the abuser, giving unhelpful advice or minimizing the problem, avoiding the survivor, or showing annoyance when the woman did not leave or take advice, or being angry at the abuser (Sylaska & Edwards, 2014).

Health professionals can also become frustrated by women they see repeatedly who have numerous signs of abuse but seem unable to liberate themselves from the battering relationships. As with other human dynamics that are not easily explained, health professionals and others may rationalize the woman's behaviors to justify their own lack of involvement. A number of misconceptions are used to account for the woman's perceived self-destructive behavior. If nurses and other professionals believe these misconceptions, they may become judgmental (such as blaming the survivor) or respond in unhelpful ways, rather than being empathic and empowering women to take control over their lives (Kulkarni, Herman-Smith, & Caldwell Ross, 2015). Empowerment is built on respect for the woman. Providing supportive empathy, validation, and information that can be lifesaving is empowering behavior. Table 5.1 lists some myths and facts about IPV.

TABLE 5.1 Myths and Facts About Intimate Partner Violence

Myths	Facts
Intimate partner violence (IPV) occurs in a small percentage of the population.	Half of the countries in developing regions report 30% of all women have experienced IPV.
Being pregnant protects a woman from IPV.	Research suggests that pregnant women are more at risk for IPV. Sometimes abuse begins with pregnancy.
IPV occurs only in "problem" or lower-class families.	IPV can happen to anyone regardless of social class.
Abuse can occur only face to face.	Internet and mobile phones have been used by both men and women to harass, monitor, and control their partner.
Only people who come from abusive families end up in abusive relationships.	Not all "at-risk" persons become involved in violence, and some perpetrators had no history of previous violence or exposure to violence.
Women would leave the relationship if the abuse were really that bad.	Only the woman knows what is safest for her and her children
Only war veterans have posttraumatic stress disorder (PTSD)	Some survivors of IPV may be formally diagnosed as having PTSD if their symptoms meet the criteria in the *Diagnostic and Statistical Manual of Mental Disorders*
Only men with psychologic problems abuse women.	Many batterers are successful professionals. Research indicates only a small number of abusers have psychologic problems.

Data from Department of Health & Human Services (2018). Relationships and safety. Office of Women's Health. Retrieved from: https://www.womenshealth.gov/relationships-and-safety.

Intimate Partner Violence During Pregnancy

The prevalence of IPV during pregnancy may vary, but it is estimated that 300,000 pregnant women in the United States are affected by IPV annually (Domestic Shelters, 2015). Research suggests the risk factors for IPV associated with pregnancy encompass the time frame of 1 year before conception to the year following the birth of a child (Van Parys, Deschepper, Michielsen, et al., 2014). Four different patterns of violence around the time of pregnancy have been identified: (1) commencement of violence with pregnancy, (2) violence before and during pregnancy where violence is either unchanged, decreases, or increases, (3) termination of violence during pregnancy, and (4) no violence before or during pregnancy. Little is understood about how violence may change with pregnancy and why some women experience increased violence whereas, for others, pregnancy may provide protection (Van Parys et al., 2014). In the United States the Pregnancy Risk Assessment Monitoring System (PRAMS), a surveillance project of the CDC and state health departments, reported that, between 2012 and 2013, women reported a decrease in IPV 12 months before pregnancy and during the pregnancy (CDC, 2017b). Thus pregnancy may be protective for some women.

Physical assault to the abdomen or sexual trauma experienced during pregnancy may increase the risk of spontaneous abortion, preterm delivery (PTD), low birth weight (LBW), or neonatal death (Donovan, Spracklen, Schweizer, et al., 2016; WHO, 2017).

Cultural Considerations

IPV is seen in all countries, cultures, races, ethnicities, religions, and socioeconomic backgrounds (WHO, 2016). In the United States, Asian women report less contact SV, physical violence, and/or stalking by an intimate partner than do other racial groups (Smith et al., 2017). American Indian and Alaska Native women report significantly more instances of IPV than do women of any other racial background (Smith et al., 2017). Reporting rates may not reflect the magnitude of the problem because many women do not disclose violence out of fear or embarrassment or because they are not asked about IPV by their health care providers (WHO, 2016).

Since 1994 there has been a growing official acknowledgment of IPV across the globe. In 1994 the United States enacted the Violence Against Women Act (VAWA), followed by Guatemala and El Salvador in 1996, China in 1997, Colombia in 2000, and Japan in 2001. The United Nations High Commission for Refugees (2019) produced a report, noting that Mexico first passed a law prohibiting violence against women in 2017. Women from almost all cultures identify fear as a common factor in IPV.

An important cultural consideration relates to refugees and immigrants. Immigrant women face unique challenges related to their noncitizen status as well as their unfamiliarity with the health care and legal systems (U.S. Department of Health & Human Services, 2017b). The objectification of women and power inequalities in human social arrangements support the abuse of women. These are especially apparent in any social or cultural system of oppression. The cross-cultural meaning of violence is difficult to ascertain because cultures also differ in their perceptions and definitions of abuse. Finding accurate data about the incidence and prevalence of violence in ethnic groups has been challenging because the groups are infrequently represented in research studies and violence may be underreported as a result of cultural norms. For example, groups that distrust police or immigration officials may not report abuse because they fear repercussions.

Nurses must be sensitive to immigrant women and their intimate partners because acculturation is gradual and cultural expectations from their birth countries may heavily influence beliefs and behaviors. Nurses must consider all forces that shape a woman's identity—ethnicity, race, class, language, citizenship, religion, and culture—while recognizing that abuse is against the law and injurious to the health and well-being of women and children (and men). Becoming familiar with the client's cultural influences and increasing the numbers of nurses from various ethnic groups will increase the opportunity to provide culturally appropriate care.

Special Populations

Teen Pregnancy

Pregnant adolescents are at risk for being abused by their partners. Compounding the situation, inexperience may leave these young women feeling trapped. They may ignore the abuse because their partners' jealous and controlling behavior is interpreted as love and commitment.

Women With Disabilities

The 2010 NISVS reported that women with disabilities were significantly more likely to report experiencing rape, SV, physical violence, stalking, and psychologic aggression than women without disabilities (Breiding & Armour, 2015). Screening women with disabilities in private might be challenging because there is increased dependence on the partner for transportation, communication, and assistance transferring. A woman who has disabilities may be further hindered from leaving a relationship due to financial and physical dependence on the partner (Breiding & Armour, 2015).

Lesbian, Gay, Bisexual, Transgender, or Queer Persons

According to the CDC, people who identify as gay, lesbian, and bisexual experience IPV at rates equal to or greater than the general population (IPV can occur between same-sex couples and does not require sexual intimacy) (CDC, 2014). In addition to abuse experienced by heterosexual women, abusers in lesbian, gay, bisexual, transgender, or

 CLINICAL REASONING CASE STUDY

Intimate Partner Violence

Elena, a 17-year-old Hispanic client, is in the clinic for her 20th week prenatal visit. She missed her last two appointments. She is accompanied by her boyfriend, with whom she lives. The nurse suggests that he wait outside while she asks intake questions about Elena's health. Elena looks down and says quietly, "It's fine if he stays, really it is." The nurse notices that he is very attentive to Elena, is very nice to the nurse, and answers for Elena most of the time she is asked a question. The nurse explains that the clinic has a policy that the interviews are done in private. He reluctantly leaves the room. After some routine questions about her general health since her last prenatal visit, the nurse asks her about intimate partner violence and safety. "Have you been hit, slapped, kicked, or in other ways physically hurt by someone?" Elena shakes her head and says, "No" in a quiet voice. The nurse notices Elena glance at a small bruise on the inner part of her arm. The nurse asks Elena if she is being physically hurt or threatened in her relationship. She gets teary but says, "No."

1. What is the priority concern or client need in this situation?
2. List other client needs/problems in this case.
3. Identify any additional information or assessment data that is needed by the nurse in planning care for this client.
4. What nursing actions are appropriate in this situation?
   a. What is the priority nursing action?
   b. Describe other nursing interventions that are important to providing optimal client care.
5. Describe the roles/responsibilities of the interprofessional health care team members (other than nurses) who may be involved in providing care for this client.

queer (LGBTQ) relationships may use additional behaviors of control, such as pressuring of sharing their identity with friends, family, work, and other support systems and use of LGBTQ stereotypes to maintain control, withhold access to hormones, isolate the survivor from LGBTQ communities, and tell them that no one will help them because of their sexual identity (LGBTQ Domestic Violence; n.d.).

CARE MANAGEMENT

The nurse has an important role in assisting survivors of IPV, as well as perpetrators, whether male or female. Preparation for that role begins with the nurse's own self-assessment. An exploration of the nurse's attitudes toward women in abusive situations, as well as awareness of thoughts and emotions that can lead to unhelpful communication, and knowledge about the many aspects of IPV are important in preparing to care for women in abusive relationships.

Women experiencing IPV may be reluctant to seek help for various reasons. These include the need to avoid the stigma associated with the nature of the family violence; the fear that they will not be believed; the fear of reprisal from their spouses or partners; and, in some states in which battering is a reportable crime, the desire to avoid involvement with police.

Exactly what drives a woman to seek assistance is not clear. The Institute for Family Studies (Whiting, 2016) notes four specific reasons that a woman may leave an abusive relationship: (1) realizing that the abuse is really happening and choosing to seek a situation in which healthy growth can occur, (2) getting to a point at which she wants to accept support, (3) concern for the welfare and protection of her children, and (4) becoming fearful for their and their children's lives and experiencing exhaustion.

Assessment

Clients seen in any women's health care setting may be at risk for abuse. Nurses and other health care professionals are encouraged to assess for abuse in all women entering the health care system. The health care setting may provide the only contact that a socially isolated woman makes with someone outside the relationship. Failure to identify IPV and to recognize the risk of serious injury or even death further endangers the lives of women and their children.

LEGAL ASPECTS: Mandatory Reporting of Domestic Violence

Domestic violence is considered a crime in all states, but it varies between being categorized a misdemeanor and a felony, the majority calling it a misdemeanor. Mandatory reporting of domestic violence is controversial. Mandatory reporting is considered appropriate in child abuse because a minor is unable to make an informed decision about his or her own safety. In domestic violence situations involving adults, mandatory reporting takes away a woman's right to make informed decisions and may put her in danger. The Association of Women's Health, Obstetric and Neonatal Nursing (AWHONN) and the American College of Obstetricians and Gynecologists (ACOG) oppose mandatory reporting (AWHONN, 2015). Few states have mandatory reporting for domestic violence of any kind. Forty states and the District of Columbia have laws that mandate reporting by health care providers only in situations where the woman has an injury that may be caused by a deadly weapon. Some states require reports when there is a reason to believe that the woman's injury may have resulted from an act of violence or illegal act. Because of the wide variation from state to state in mandatory reporting, nurses must be knowledgeable about the reporting requirements of the state in which they practice. A useful resource for nurses, a quick chart on the state statutes and policies on domestic violence and health care can be found at http://www.acf.hhs.gov/sites/default/files/fysb/state_compendium.pdf.

A woman suspected of being emotionally abused or physically threatened or abused should be interviewed and examined in private. Some women with male partners may feel safer with a female health care provider. Nurses should *never* ask about abuse with a partner present because this may place the woman in danger and decrease the likelihood for disclosure. When one is taking a psychosocial history, the following information provides clues to violence or potential for violence: Does the woman feel safe at home with her partner, how do the woman and her partner resolve conflict, what happens when the woman's partner becomes angry, does fighting occur during disagreements, and, if fighting occurs, does it ever escalate to restraining or physical means? It may help the woman to disclose information if these events are normalized by the nurse stating, "Many people [families] have difficulty in expressing anger or dealing with conflict. What is that like for you and your partner?" The nurse listens for any evidence of power and control in the relationship. While inquiring about abuse, trauma, or injuries, the nurse should ask directly if the woman has been injured by her spouse or partner: "Have you ever been physically abused by your partner or someone important to you?" Confusion can occur when vague terms like "he disrespects me" or even labels like "domestic violence" or "abuse" are used. The following are examples of direct questions the nurse can ask:

- Has your partner hit, slapped, kicked, or otherwise hurt you?
- Do you (or did you) feel controlled or isolated by your partner?
- Do you feel safe in your relationship? Do you ever feel afraid of your partner?
- Has your partner or anyone forced you to have sexual activities that made you uncomfortable?

Women who are safe in a current relationship may still carry the physical and emotional consequences of previous trauma.

- Has any of this happened to you in previous relationships?

These questions give a woman permission to disclose sensitive information (The Center for Research on Women with Disabilities, 2018). Additional suggested questions for women with disabilities include:

- Within the past year, has anyone prevented you from using a wheelchair, cane, respirator, or other assistive devices?
- Within the past year, has anyone you depend on refused to help you with an important personal need, such as taking your medicine, getting to the bathroom, getting out of bed, bathing, getting dressed, or getting food or drink?

Assessment tools such as the one in Fig. 4.10 give the nurse useful information and are an important part of the interview. Patterns of violence in relationships can change over time, which is why the nurse should ask about potential violence since the previous client visit.

There are many cues to abuse. These cues include delay in seeking medical assistance (hours or days), missed appointments, vague explanation of injuries, nonspecific somatic complaints, social isolation, lack of eye contact, a spouse or partner who does not want to leave the woman alone with the primary health care provider, spouse or partner or nurse or other staff person, and substance abuse.

For some abused women, day-to-day survival is exhausting. They may cope by denying to the nurse the probabilities of impending abuse, severity of injury, future recurrence, and death. Women may be embarrassed about their abusive relationships and believe the abuse is caused by their inadequacies. Other abused women may cope by denying to themselves that their partner's violent behavior will happen again. By asking a woman directly about abuse, telling her that similar injuries are common in women who have been abused, and pointing out that she is not responsible for another's violent behavior, the nurse may help her to disclose the violence she is experiencing.

In the United States a pregnant woman may be accompanied by her spouse or partner to the antepartum appointment. This is especially true if the woman does not speak English and the spouse or partner does. The use of an interpreter is preferred over the partner, child, or other person accompanying the woman; it may be useful for the interpreter to be a woman and important that the interpreter communicate the nurse's sensitivity and concern accurately. All women should be seen for some part of the visit without the partner or children present.

During pregnancy, the nurse should assess for abuse at each prenatal visit and on admission to labor birth unit. Assessment for abuse continues after birth because abuse may begin or escalate then; well-baby clinics and pediatric settings may be important settings for screening women for abuse.

Assessment techniques are straightforward but do require the nurse to be comfortable asking about this socially stigmatized issue. Of utmost importance for women who disclose that they are experiencing or have experienced IPV (or sexual assault, another hidden trauma) is to validate that they have been heard. The nurse might say something like, "What you have just told me is very important. I'm glad you have shared this with me; no one has the right to hurt you this way." It can be demoralizing when, despite taking the risk to disclose, the health care professional does not consider violence a health problem and is reluctant to talk about it (WHO, 2016). The next important step is to establish the woman's safety at the moment and in the future. Psychosocial assessment findings may indicate symptoms of anxiety, insomnia, eating disorders, self-directed abuse, risky sexual behaviors, depression, smoking, and drug or alcohol abuse (CDC, 2017c; WHO, 2017). During the physical examination, the woman should be observed for injuries to the face, breasts, abdomen, and buttocks. These injuries may be old or new and may range from minor bruising to serious. Other physical signs include fractures that required significant force or that would rarely occur by accident; multiple injuries at various stages of healing; and patterns left by whatever might inflict injury, such as teeth, utensils, fists, or hot objects.

Nursing Interventions

A therapeutic relationship and skillful interviewing help women disclose and describe their abuse. Language is important when talking with women. A major factor in addressing abuse is to identify the woman as a survivor, not a victim. Victim connotes someone who is harmed, is made to suffer, and may have little or no control. Survivor is an empowering term that connotes coping and decision making in relation to taking control of one's life. The nurse might ask the woman how she sees herself. Women who have identified their abuse may appear passive, hostile, anxious, depressed, or hysterical because they may think they are at the mercy of the partner's temper. In addition, they may be embarrassed, afraid, angry, sad, or shocked. Transitioning to a different self-image takes time, persistence, and support. A tool that provides a framework for sensitive nursing interventions is the *ABCDES* of caring for the abused woman:

- *A* is reassuring the woman that she is not *alone*. The isolation and denigration by the abuser keep her from knowing that others are in the same situation and that health care providers can help.
- *B* is expressing the *belief* that violence against the woman is not acceptable in any situation and that it is not her fault; no one deserves to be hurt or mistreated. This may be the first step in empowering her to think about self-protection and acceptable boundaries.
- *C* is *confidentiality* of the information being shared, particularly because the woman may believe that if the abuse is reported, the perpetrator will retaliate (and in reality, this may happen). Explain the mandatory reporting laws, when applicable.
- *D* is for descriptive *documentation* and includes the following: (1) the woman's quoted statement, "My husband punched me," a clear statement by the woman about the abuse. It should not include her

---

BOX 5.2 Documenting Abuse

Documentation can be useful to women later in court should they choose to press charges or obtain child support, custody, or alimony. Medical records are most helpful if the examiner:

- Takes photographs of the injuries known or believed to have been caused by domestic violence.
- Writes clearly.
- Sets off the woman's words in quotation marks and uses such phrases as "client states" to indicate the information recorded reflected the woman's words. Describes the offender and the event in the words of the woman (e.g., the client said, "My husband kicked me in the stomach.").
- Avoids such legalistic phrases as "woman claims" or "woman alleges" that cast doubt about the truth of the statements. Avoids terms such as "alleged perpetrator." If the health care provider's observations differ from the woman's account of the victimization, states the reason for the difference.
- Does not summarize a client's report in conclusive terms that lack the supporting factual information (e.g., "the client is a battered woman"), because it will render the report inadmissible. In the same theme, does not place the term "domestic violence" in the diagnosis section of the medical record because it does not convey factual information and is not medical terminology.
- Describes the woman's demeanor, whether she is crying, shaking, angry, calm, laughing, or sad, even if it belies the evidence of abuse.
- Records the time of day of the examination and indicates whenever possible how much time has passed since the abuse.

---

subjective opinion, such as "I provoked the abusive behavior"; (2) accurate descriptions of injuries and a history of the first, worst, and most recent incident of violence may be included; and (3) the woman's consent, evidence, or photographs (Box 5.2).

- *E* is for *education*, especially that violence is likely to recur and escalate. Educate about options including community resources such as where a woman can be referred for help and information about local shelters; for example, National Domestic Violence/Abuse Hotline—800-799-SAFE. Ask if she knows how to obtain a restraining order.
- *S* is for *safety*, the most significant part of the intervention because one of the most dangerous times for a woman is when she decides to leave. Tell the woman to call 911 if she is in imminent danger and to consider alerting neighbors to call the police if they hear or see signs of conflict. A safety plan should be developed. The safety plan will be adapted based on whether the woman chooses to stay in the relationship or leave. The woman may be conflicted and need support as she goes through a decision-making process. The woman can be offered a telephone to call the shelter if she chooses. If she chooses to go back to the abuser, a safety plan includes necessities for a quick escape: a bag packed with personal items for an overnight stay (can be hidden or left with a neighbor), money or a checkbook, an extra set of car keys, and any legal documents to use for identification. Legal options, such as those for restraining orders or arrest of the perpetrator, also are important aspects of the safety plan. A restraining order can be obtained 24 hours a day from the county court or police department. Use of a restraining order may escalate violence but is a critical step in documenting IPV. Many communities have hotlines for battered women that offer counseling. There is some evidence in high-income countries that advocacy and counseling interventions can improve access to services for survivors of IPV and be effective in reducing violence (WHO, 2017). "Safety conferencing" is a way of building the individual and collective strength to assist women to reshape connections, make sound choices, and promote their safety (see Nursing Care Plan).

◎ NURSING CARE PLAN

The Woman Experiencing Intimate Partner Violence

Client Problem	Expected Outcome	Nursing Interventions	Rationales
Risk of harm to self and/or family members related to history of abuse by partner as evidenced by physical and/or emotional injuries	Woman will identify dynamics of violence in her unique relationship and develop a plan for safety.	Provide opportunity for woman to verbalize her feelings in a nonthreatening atmosphere. Be alert for cues indicative of abuse. Provide information on options available to women experiencing intimate partner violence (IPV) (e.g., counseling, shelters, legal assistance).	To give emotional support. To provide information related to interventions. To provide information in developing a plan for safety for herself and any children/family members. To give further information and share experiences.
Decreased self-esteem related to stigma of abuse as evidenced by behaviors of withdrawal	Woman will demonstrate an increase in social contacts and social support	Refer to social services and support groups. Provide private opportunity to express feelings of decreased self-esteem. Support opportunities for social interaction. Encourage interaction with groups for socialization and support.	To initiate and maintain a therapeutic relationship. To increase feelings of self-worth and self-confidence. To increase number of supportive social contacts.
Compromised coping by woman and her family related to situational crisis of IPV	Family will identify feelings and the need for support during this situational crisis.	Provide an appropriate time and place for therapeutic communication. Identify effective coping mechanisms. List support systems available. Refer the woman and family to counseling and social services.	To promote trust and allow expression of feelings. To provide the family with a foundation of familiar interventions. To assist the family to use outside resources when reasonable and available. To provide ongoing support.

One part of safety planning is trying to sort out the potential danger in a relationship. A validated danger assessment tool (Fig. 5.3) was designed to assess the level of violence in a relationship and to identify abused women who are at risk of being murdered (Campbell, 2018). The nurse and the abused woman can go through the tool collaboratively. Online training and permission to use the tool are available at https://www.dangerassessment.org/DATools.aspx.

If the woman is pregnant, collaboration with maternity nurses who will be involved in her care during the pregnancy may be helpful. Each nurse can plan care that will point out the woman's strengths and increase her self-esteem. The spouse or partner may attend prenatal visits and classes and is included in other ways if the woman chooses to stay with him. The first days after birth are particularly crucial because the mother is physically and emotionally vulnerable and usually tired, and the baby's crying may be intolerable to both the father and mother. The danger of abuse to mother and child is acute during this time. Facilitating the woman's establishment of a support network of maternity and pediatric staff, community health nurses, and shelter and parental crisis center personnel is important during this crucial period. Referral to resources and provision for follow-up examination by health care providers also should be part of the nursing intervention.

It is important to remember that many women have been abused for a long time, which may make it difficult for them to seek and accept help. Women in repeatedly abusive situations may have lost their ability to perceive the possibility of success and may have become very passive. In addition to understanding the many reasons women stay in abusive relationships, recognizing that the most dangerous period for a woman is when she is in the process of leaving may help nurses to be less judgmental about the woman's dilemma.

A woman may indicate her readiness to leave the relationship when she believes that she is capable of planning for herself, investing in herself, and recognizing that the abuse is part of a continuing pattern. She also needs to believe that she will have economic and other resources to "make it" on her own. Going to a shelter may be an option; however, shelter stays are typically limited to 30 to 90 days, and therefore a long-term plan must be in place. In addition, her being in a shelter may make the spouse or partner angrier. Nurses can be helpful in directing women to sources of information, continuing to be expert listeners, and offering encouragement as women struggle in their decision-making process toward freedom and control in their lives.

Prevention

Screening is a common approach to preventing the progression of health problems. Research suggests that screening increases the identification of women experiencing IPV; however, rates are low relative to best estimates of IPV in women seeking health care (O'Doherty et al., 2015). Currently, because research is limited and screening studies were not paired with interventions, there is insufficient evidence to say that universal screening prevents further incidents of IPV in asymptomatic women (O'Doherty et al., 2015). Nevertheless, major health care organizations, including the U.S. Preventive Services Task Force (2013), recommend screening of all women of childbearing age. Because IPV has been linked to many other health problems such as headaches, abdominal pain, back pain, GI disorders, limited mobility, chronic pain, arthritis, STIs, reproductive health problems, substance abuse, depression, PTSD, and suicide, women with any of these symptoms should be carefully assessed (Smith et al., 2017; WHO, 2016, 2017).

Nurses can make a difference in stopping the violence and preventing further injury. Educating women that abuse is a violation of their rights and facilitating their access to protective and legal services constitute a first step. Other measures that may help women to discourage the risk of abusive relationships are promoting assertiveness and self-defense courses; suggesting support and self-help groups that encourage positive self-regard, confidence, and empowerment; and recommending educational and skills development classes that will enhance independence or at least the ability to take care of oneself. Classes for learning English can be particularly helpful to immigrant women. Nurses can offer information on local classes. Helping children to gain problem-solving and conflict management skills may eliminate the need for violent solutions to life stresses.

DANGER ASSESSMENT

Jacquelyn C. Campbell, Ph.D., R.N.
Copyright, 2003; www.dangerassessment.com

Several risk factors have been associated with increased risk of homicides (murders) of women and men in violent relationships. We cannot predict what will happen in your case, but we would like you to be aware of the danger of homicide in situations of abuse and for you to see how many of the risk factors apply to your situation.

Using a calendar, please mark the approximate dates during the past year when you were abused by your partner or ex-partner. Write on that date how bad the incident was according to the following scale:

1. Slapping, pushing; no injuries and/or lasting pain
2. Punching, kicking; bruises, cuts, and/or continuing pain
3. "Beating up"; severe contusions, burns, broken bones
4. Threat to use weapon; head injury, internal injury, permanent injury
5. Use of weapon; wounds from weapon

(If **any** of the descriptions for the higher number apply, use the higher number.)

Mark **Yes** or **No** for each of the following. ("He" refers to your husband, partner, ex-husband, ex-partner, or whoever is currently physically hurting you.)

_____ 1. Has the physical violence increased in severity or frequency over the past year?

_____ 2. Does he own a gun?

_____ 3. Have you left him after living together during the past year?
3a. (If you have *never* lived with him, check here _____)

_____ 4. Is he unemployed?

_____ 5. Has he ever used a weapon against you or threatened you with a lethal weapon?
(If yes, was the weapon a gun?_____)

_____ 6. Does he threaten to kill you?

_____ 7. Has he avoided being arrested for domestic violence?

_____ 8. Do you have a child that is not his?

_____ 9. Has he ever forced you to have sex when you did not wish to do so?

_____ 10. Does he ever try to choke you?

_____ 11. Does he use illegal drugs? By drugs, I mean "uppers" or amphetamines, "meth", speed, angel dust, cocaine, "crack", street drugs or mixtures.

_____ 12. Is he an alcoholic or problem drinker?

_____ 13. Does he control most or all of your daily activities? For instance: does he tell you who you can be friends with, when you can see your family, how much money you can use, or when you can take the car? (If he tries, but you do not let him, check here: _____)

_____ 14. Is he violently and constantly jealous of you? (For instance, does he say "If I can't have you, no one can.")

_____ 15. Have you ever been beaten by him while you were pregnant? (If you have never been pregnant by him, check here: _____)

_____ 16. Has he ever threatened or tried to commit suicide?

_____ 17. Does he threaten to harm your children?

_____ 18. Do you believe he is capable of killing you?

_____ 19. Does he follow or spy on you, leave threatening notes or messages on answering machine, destroy your property, or call you when you don't want him to?

_____ 20. Have you ever threatened or tried to commit suicide?

_____ Total "Yes" Answers

**Thank you. Please talk to your nurse, advocate or counselor about
what the Danger Assessment means in terms of your situation.**

Fig. 5.3 Danger Assessment Tool. (From Campbell, J. [2004]. *Danger assessment.* Available at www.danger-assessment.org; Campbell, J., Webster, D., & Glass, N. [2009]. The danger assessment: Validation of a lethality risk assessment instrument for intimate partner femicide. *Journal of Interpersonal Violence, 24*(4), 653–674.)

Encouraging schoolchildren to form Students Against Violence Everywhere (SAVE) groups (http://nationalsave.org/), which is a nationwide pro-peace effort that promotes justice, respect, and love, gives them an appreciation for these qualities in all facets of life. Adolescents benefit from discussion about sex roles, their relationships, and the consequences of the "macho" concept. School nurses can be instrumental in developing and implementing informational activities for adolescents. Other means of prevention are to advocate programming and research against violence and to promote legislation and policies toward stopping violent acts (WHO, 2016).

SEXUAL VIOLENCE

Sexual violence is a broad term that includes a wide range of sexual victimization, including sexual harassment, sexual assault, and rape (CDC, 2014). Sexual harassment includes unwelcome sexual remarks, contact, or behavior such as exhibitionism that makes the work or other environment uncomfortable or difficult (CDC, 2014). Sexual assault refers to any type of sexual contact with someone who cannot consent, such as someone who is underage, has an intellectual disability, or has passed out (U.S. Department of Health & Human Services, 2017a). Sexual assault can include rape, attempted rape, sexual coercion, sexual contact with a child, fondling, or unwanted touching above or under clothes. It can also include voyeurism, peeping, sexual harassment or threats, or forcing someone to pose for sexual pictures (U.S. Department of Health & Human Services, 2017a). It also includes exhibitionism, exposing someone to pornography, or displays of images taken of the person in a private context (CDC, 2014). Rape is a legal term that is defined differently by each state. The U.S. Department of Justice Archives (2017) defines rapes as "the penetration, no matter how slight, of the vagina or anus with any body part or object, or oral penetration by a sex organ of another person, without consent of the person." It usually refers to forced sexual intercourse or penetration of the mouth, anus, or vagina by a body part or object without consent; it may or may not include the use of a weapon. It involves the use of force, threats, or a person who is incapable of giving consent. The term is a legal and not a medical one. Molestation, a crime of sexual acts with children up to the age of 18, consists of touching private parts, exposure of genitals, taking pornographic pictures, rape, and inducement of sexual acts with molester or other children. Molestation also applies to incest by a relative with a minor family member and any unwelcome sexual acts with adults that are not rape (Hill & Hill, 2018a). Statutory rape involves penetration as described previously by a person who is 18 years or older of a person younger than the age of consent, and the specifics vary from state to state (Findlaw, 2017; Hill & Hill, 2018b).

IPV is a serious, preventable public health problem that affects millions of people in the United States (CDC, 2017a). The NISVS reported almost one of five women experienced completed or attempted rape at some time in their lives, and approximately one in three women experienced some form of contact SV during their lifetime (Smith et al., 2017). For the period of 1995 to 2013, college-aged females (18 to 24) had the highest rate of rape and sexual assault compared with females in any other age group (Sinozich & Langston, 2014). Rape may occur within intimate, casual, or work relationships. Rape can also occur in institutional settings such as college campuses, long term care settings, the military, and prisons. Rapists may be intimate partners or spouses. They may be family members or acquaintances such as friends, neighbors, or dates, or they may be strangers, police, prison guards, or military members.

The CDC divides SV into five categories: rape or penetration of person, person was made to penetrate someone else, nonphysically pressured (verbally or through intimidation) unwanted penetration, unwanted sexual contact, and noncontact unwanted sexual experiences (CDC, 2017a). The WHO defines SV as "any act, attempt to obtain a sexual act, or other act directed against a person's sexuality using coercion, by any person regardless of their relationship to the survivor, in any setting" (WHO, 2016). SV includes rape, defined as "physically forced or otherwise coerced penetration of the vulva or anus with a penis, other body part or object" (WHO, 2016).

Why Do Some People Rape?

Multiple theories exist on the causes of SV from the perspective of the perpetrator. Not everyone identified as "at risk" becomes involved in violence. Individual risk factors may include low self-esteem, young age, low academic achievement, low income, heavy alcohol or drug use, depression, emotional dependence and insecurity, anger, desire for power, belief in strict gender roles, borderline or antisocial personality traits, prior history of being physically abused, being physically abused as a child, aggressive behavior as a child, or having experienced poor parenting (WHO, 2017). For some, risk factors might not be present (Perry, 2017).

Acquaintance rape involves persons who know one another such as friend, neighbor, family member, classmate, date, or acquaintance. If there is a relationship, then trust is violated. Survivors may fear retaliation from the assailant or harassment from family or friends who know the person (Rape, Abuse, and Incest National Network [RAINN]).

Stranger rape is the least common type of rape. The assailant may be a total stranger who suddenly attacks the survivor in a public place or in the home. Other stranger rapes occur when the assailant has brief contact with the survivor prior to the assault (e.g., engaging the person in conversation to earn trust at a bar or party). Women are more likely to report stranger rape than acquaintance rape.

Sexual assault and rape are considered forcible when there is threat or actual use of force on an unwilling person. An incapacitated sexual assault or rape occurs when the survivor is under the influence of alcohol or drugs, rendering the person unconscious or otherwise unable to give consent. Alcohol is the most common drug associated with sexual assault. Alcohol makes it more difficult for women to identify potentially dangerous situations and to resist unwanted sexual advances. A drug-facilitated sexual assault occurs when alcohol and/or drugs are taken unwillingly or unknowingly. The use of date rape drugs such as flunitrazepam (Rohypnol, or "roofies"), γ-hydroxybutyrate (GHB), ketamine, and carisoprodol (Soma) incapacitates the survivor and may produce amnesia. These drugs are potentiated by alcohol, and the combination can be lethal. The frequency with which these drugs are used can be underestimated because they are rapidly excreted, and lab testing has to be done within a few hours of ingestion. Signs indicating that a woman may have been drugged include having no recall after taking a drink laced with the drug, feeling as if sex has occurred but not having any memory of the incident, feeling more intoxicated than what would be a usual response to the amount of alcohol consumed, or feeling fuzzy on awakening (U.S. Department of Health and Human Services [USDHHS], Office of Women's Health, 2018).

Not all women report sexual assault to police. Many factors deter a woman from reporting the crime, so data regarding sexual assaults may underestimate the magnitude of the problem. Women do not report rape because of the associated stigma; embarrassment; guilt that in some way they provoked the assault; fear of retribution from the rapist or his friends; dread of being humiliated and figuratively "raped" again by the criminal justice system publicly; distrust of law enforcement; involvement in illegal substance use; and discouragement generated by the dismally small number of convictions. Rape survivors often fear the reactions of spouses, lovers, friends, family, and children and prefer to suffer alone (Sinozich and Langton, 2014).

Mental Health Consequences of Sexual Assault

Any type of sexual assault and especially rape can produce long-term psychologic consequences similar to those experienced by military combat veterans or others who experience acute traumatic events. Most sexual assaults result in at least minor physical injuries, including genital trauma, which may or may not be apparent (Zilkens, Smith, Phillips, 2017). However, the psychologic effect can be severe. Sexual assault and rape are associated with acute stress reaction and the possibility of depression, rape-trauma syndrome (RTS) and PTSD, substance abuse, suicidality, and a host of physical disorders, including chronic pelvic pain and sexual dysfunction (Parker, Sricharoenchai, Raparla, et al., 2015). One-third of women seek counseling as a direct result of their sexual assault (Carbone-Lopez, Slocum, & Kruttschnitt, 2015; Wilson & Miller, 2016).

Why is rape so traumatic? Survivors may have been threatened by a weapon, pushed, shoved, overpowered, or coerced. The assailant may have threatened to return and kill the survivors if the incident is reported to anyone. In the aftermath, survivors can be frightened, angry, embarrassed, feel shame, face stigma, and lack support from families and communities. They can feel betrayed if there was a preexisting relationship with the assailant. Some may withdraw, feeling socially isolated, unable to tell the people closest to them, fearful of being judged or rejected. Some survivors are afraid to return to their homes, workplace, or wherever the assault happened. The emotional suffering can take over women's lives and, although some seek support from family, friends, health care professionals, or police, others may carry this experience silently, never telling anyone (Boyle, 2017).

Rape-Trauma

When humans experience fear, horror, or helplessness after a life-threatening traumatic event such as rape or combat, there is an intense initial stress response. In the first few hours and days, an initial neurobiologic dysregulation in the brain interferes with learning new information, making memories, responding to stress, and regulating the level of arousal. In some survivors this dysregulation and other neurobiologic changes persist. For example, in most trauma, survivor's cortisol levels in the brain rise in response to stress. Emerging research suggests that in people who then develop PTSD, brain cortisol levels, rather than being elevated during stressful events, are low. Some theories suggest that the brain may become oversensitive to cortisol, and minor stress events may cause the person to overreact and major traumas may produce an underreaction. Variations in brain function and structure are important in understanding the trauma-related symptoms seen in some but not all rape survivors. Why do some survivors not recover? Suggested possibilities include genetic differences, neuroanatomic differences, sex differences, personality styles, past exposures to stress, and the characteristics and context of the specific trauma and subsequent experiences. Researchers are working on finding specific neurobiopsychologic strategies such as medications and/or therapies that can prevent and treat trauma sequelae such as PTSD (Stein, Wilmot, & Solomon, 2016).

The neurobiologic changes that occur produce an array of symptoms. In the 1970s RTS was identified as a cluster of characteristic symptoms and related behaviors seen in the weeks and months after a rape (Asagba, 2015). Understanding the pattern of responses that survivors may experience is crucial in helping the nurse provide woman-centered supportive, responsive care and to enhance their safety (WHO, 2016).

Acute Phase: Disorganization

The assault itself marks the beginning of the acute phase of RTS, which can last for several days or up to 3 weeks. Reactions such as shock, denial, and disbelief are common (Pegram & Abbey, 2016).

The rape survivor feels embarrassed, degraded, fearful, angry, and vengeful, and she can blame herself. The survivor can feel unclean and want to bathe and douche, although this can destroy evidence. Fear is the primary feeling. Observable reactions can be controlled, expressed, or disoriented. In *controlled emotions* the survivor hides her emotions; has a subdued, calm demeanor; and seems to act as if nothing happened. She may answer questions and interact in a matter-of-fact way. Her affect seems incongruent with what she has just experienced. The second type of acute phase reaction is *expressed emotions*. Here the survivor can appear agitated or hysterical. She can be restless, crying, tense, or anxiously smiling. Her affect can change rapidly from crying to being calm and controlled. She relives the scene over and over in her mind and considers things she "should have done." *Shocked disbelief* or *disorientation* marks the third type of reaction. The survivor can feel disoriented, have difficulty concentrating or making decisions, and have poor recall of the event. Memory can be fragmented, and intrusive thoughts can provide bits and pieces of information. Physiologically she can be uncomfortable, experiencing skeletal muscle pain or tension, GI irritability, sighing, hyperventilation, and flushing (Pegram & Abbey, 2016).

Outward Adjustment Phase

During the adjustment phase, the survivor may appear to have resolved her crisis. She may return to a job or to maintaining a household, or both, but she is denying and suppressing her thoughts and feelings. She needs this time to regain some control in her life. She may move, change jobs, buy a weapon to protect herself, or install an alarm system in her home. She may not be able to stop talking about the assault, letting it dominate her life, or she may minimize or suppress the event, refusing to discuss it and acting as if it did not happen. She may try to analyze the details of how it happened, trying to explain how it happened and what the rapist was thinking. She may seek safety by fleeing her job or her home or making other radical changes. She may experience fear, anxiety, phobias, mood swings, anger and rage, depression, insomnia, hypervigilance, and continued flashbacks. She may withdraw from support systems and be afraid to leave her home or go to certain places. She may develop sexual problems, such as avoidance, decreased sexual drive, or perception of painful intercourse.

Long-Term Process: Reorganization Phase

The third phase is reorganization. Denial and suppression are difficult to maintain. Disclosing personal thoughts and feelings has a profound effect on improving health and reducing stress. As a rape survivor's suppression of feelings and emotions starts to deteriorate, she becomes depressed and anxious. Her own healthy spirit pressures her to discuss the rape with someone. Because she is losing her control of denial, her fears start to surface; she may be afraid to be alone or in a crowd or may fear being attacked from behind. Nightmares and eating disorders are common in these last two phases.

The recovery process can take years and can be difficult and painful. The survivor has progressed through recovery when the physical distress and the constant memories of the rape have diminished. She no longer blames herself for what happened and can truly call herself a survivor. These phases are not necessarily linear, and survivors can move back and forth between the phases, because recovery is a process. RTS can meet the criteria for PTSD and be formally diagnosed, but this is not inevitable, because many survivors proceed through the recovery process to a well-adjusted "new normal," noting that as many as 90% of survivors do not develop long-term PTSD (Sereen, 2018).

CARE MANAGEMENT

Nurses in women's health care settings and EDs are most likely to see rape survivors in the acute phase. However, all women who manifest any of the signs of other phases should be assessed for posttraumatic experiences. It is important to remember that sexual assault acute care has a dual purpose. First and foremost is to address the health care needs of the woman. The second purpose is to facilitate the collection of evidence and documentation of findings for use by the justice system. Health care is the nurse's first priority (Destiny, 2017).

Facilities that provide initial treatment for rape survivors vary in protocols and resources. In its 1992 guidelines, The Joint Commission (TJC) required EDs and ambulatory care departments to have protocols on physical assault; rape or sexual assault; and domestic abuse of older adults, spouses, partners, and children. These protocols must address client consent, examination, and treatment guidelines and the health care facility's responsibility for collecting evidence, photographing injuries, and releasing evidence to law enforcement officials. In addition, the EDs and ambulatory care departments must provide to survivors a referral list of community-based and private service agencies dealing with family violence. The nurse interacting with the sexual assault client should be guided by the particular treatment center's protocol. The *National Protocol for Sexual Assault Medical Forensic Exams* identifies the unique roles of the many different professionals, including sexual assault nurse examiners (SANEs), physicians, police, forensic specialists, prosecutors, and counseling advocacy in the aftercare of a sexual trauma survivor (U.S. Department of Justice & Office of Violence Against Women, 2018). Agency or state recommendations for care are continually evolving as new research and forensic techniques emerge.

Many treatment centers have initiated the use of SANEs as described in the aforementioned protocols. A SANE is educated in the specialty of forensic nursing and is prepared to examine clients; recognize, collect, and preserve evidence; counsel the client; link the client with vital community resources; follow up cases; and, if necessary, testify in court. When cared for by a SANE, survivors receive better quality care, receive appropriate prophylaxis for infection and pregnancy, and are more satisfied than when cared for in settings without SANEs (Destiny, 2017). Information on becoming a certified SANE, which requires a 40-hour course, is available at http://www.forensicnurses.org/. If a SANE is not available in a particular facility, TJC member organizations must implement a plan for educating an appropriate staff member about identifying, treating, and referring abuse survivors. Additional resources can include a social worker who is called when a woman who has been raped is admitted. A local rape crisis center may have volunteers on call who can provide emotional support; provide transportation; help the woman interact with her family, friends, and various authorities; inform her of RTS; and find other resources for her as needed. Male volunteers may counsel male members of the survivor's family and her male friends (Destiny, 2017).

What to Tell a Woman Who Chooses to Stay in a Relationship

Only the woman knows what is safest for her and her children (National Center for PTSD, 2015). Safety planning is something the nurse can share with the client and might include informing her to leave the situation if she feels her or her children are in danger. Box 5.3 lists actions that the nurse can take in assisting a woman who chooses to stay in her relationship.

Psychologic First Aid

When survivors seek help from people in their social network, from the police or from health care settings, the response they get is critical to their healing process. The goal of supportive care is to help survivors to feel less threatened, feel safer, and have lower levels of PTSD. Negative experiences

---

BOX 5.3   Nursing Actions to Assist a Woman Who May Be in Danger

- Identify safe places within the home to go if conflict arises.
- Avoid rooms with weapons such as the kitchen, and avoid rooms with no exits such as a closet.
- Consider a code word to use as a distress signal to alert family members, children, and friends.
- Pack and hide a suitcase with copies of important legal documents (driver's license, social security cards, birth certificates, and medical records showing previous injuries).
- Make a list of places along with their phone numbers that would provide shelter in case of emergency.
- Provide and instruct her to memorize the National Domestic Violence Hotline 1800-799-SAFE (7233).
- Encourage her to talk to someone she can trust even if she does not want to share all the details.
- Talk to neighbors, and consider telling them to call the police if they hear fighting or loud noises.
- Consider explaining the situation to a work advisor so safety planning can occur within the workplace (National Center for PTSD, 2015).

Data from National Center for PTSD. (2015). *Intimate partner violence.* Retrieved from: https://www.ptsd.va.gov/public/types/violence/domestic-violence.asp.

---

in the law enforcement and health care systems are associated with an increase in PTSD. Research indicates that survivors who report and have negative experiences have worse mental health outcomes. The neurobiology of trauma can create for survivors a flood of intrusive thoughts. Interviewers, whether law enforcement or health care professionals, may try to clarify the survivor's fragmented story that comes out in bits and pieces. Such retelling may create additional stress for the survivor.

The health care professional may be one of the first people to talk with a survivor of sexual trauma (WHO, 2016). Initial distress is not abnormal, and most sexual assault survivors are able to recover. Even though there is limited evidence for specific treatments to prevent PTSD in sexual assault survivors, trauma experts suggest that one promising approach is psychologic or emotional first aid (Harning, 2015). Litz & Salters-Pedneault (2008) outlined eight core goals that are consistent with and can be easily adapted to nursing practice. They are to (1) respond when a survivor reaches out to you or when you initiate contact with the survivor, in a nonintrusive, compassionate, and helpful manner; (2) enhance the survivor's safety and provide physical and emotional comfort; (3) stabilize by calming and orienting the survivor if she is emotionally overwhelmed; (4) identify immediate needs and concerns and gather information; (5) offer practical help in addressing needs; (6) offer to help establish contact with personal supports; (7) provide information about stress and coping responses to sexual assault; and (8) link the survivor with community and other services. Nurses who understand postassault experiences can influence the responses of their nursing units, hospital, or institution and community.

Sexual Assault Examination

Because sexual assault is a crime, the first nurse to see the sexually assaulted client must consider the need to preserve evidence. However, the preservation of evidence should not overshadow a survivor's rights to be treated as a human being with respect, courtesy, and dignity. Client-centered care takes into consideration the psychologic needs of the survivor, and the nurse adapts the examination accordingly. There are short-term and long-term physical, emotional, and legal implications of this examination. Details are described in the National Protocol for Sexual Assault Medical Forensic Exams, Adults and Adolescents (https://www.ncjrs.gov/pdffiles1/ovw/241903.pdf). The following discussion is an overview of the protocol.

Any health care and/or evidence collection is done only with the permission of the woman. She should be informed of all the steps involved in the sexual assault examination, treatment, and follow-up care. Written informed consent for medical care and human immunodeficiency virus (HIV) testing must be obtained. In addition, consent must be obtained for collection and storage of sexual offense evidence, including forensic photography. A signed consent for release of evidence must be obtained. Unless there is a court order, medical records are confidential. The woman can choose to stop her care or the evidence examination at any time. Informed consent includes information on what will happen during the examination, what tests will be done, what treatments can be offered, what risks occur without treatment, and what evidence collection may provide. It is important for the nurse to remember that the examination cannot determine if an assault (nonconsensual sexual encounter) has happened. That is a legal determination that happens in court. The examination provides information that may or may not be consistent with sexual contact. Not all sexual assaults produce trauma, and not all sexual trauma is nonconsensual.

History. History taking is an important step in early care. History includes a statement of the traumatic event whether or not evidence will be collected. The woman needs privacy but should not be left alone. It is important to tell the woman that she is safe, that the incident is not her fault, and that she is not alone in what she has experienced. She also needs assurance of confidentiality and may need a great deal of support and patience in verbalizing the offender's acts. For example, giving the woman permission to describe the situation however she chooses and restating what the client has said (without minimizing) tells the woman she has been heard and ensures that what the nurse documents accurately reflects what she said. It also is important to obtain sexual, gynecologic, and obstetric histories (see Chapter 4).

The medical record in a sexual assault case is likely to be used in court. A key feature used in court to establish rape is the absence of consent. The survivor who is developmentally delayed, who is unconscious or otherwise physically unable to move, who has been drugged without her knowledge, or who is a minor (statutory rape) is not capable of giving consent. Bribery, threat, or coercion implies the lack of consent. The nurse's documentation is an important part of the medical record. The wording of the history should reflect the woman's report, and her exact words should be used as often as possible. When documenting, it is important for the nurse to remember that care is provided to the woman without judgment. Thus nurses should avoid using legal terms or words that suggest value judgments when documenting or referring to the woman. For example, use of the term "alleged" or "claims" suggests that the nurse questions the woman's report. It is not the role of the nurse to determine whether a sexual assault occurred but to treat the woman as any other trauma survivor. The court must prove absence of consent.

Physical examination and laboratory tests. The nurse can assist with or, if trained, perform the physical examination, which is conducted after the procedure is explained to the woman and consent is obtained. Some survivors may view the examination as a second traumatic event. Preservation of the woman's dignity is of utmost importance during the examination. The woman may choose a female attendant, rape counselor, or other person to remain with her during the examination. The room where the examination is performed should be equipped with standard examination equipment, comfort supplies for the woman, a sexual assault evidence collection kit, a method to dry evidence, a camera, lab testing supplies, a light source, and an anoscope. Some settings also have a colposcope, a microscope, and toluidine blue dye (U.S. Department of Justice & Office of Violence against Women, 2018). The health care provider (physician, nurse practitioner, physician assistant, or nurse midwife) informs her of every step of the procedure. The content of the examination is based on the history. For example, if there was oral penetration but no removal of clothing and genital contact, a speculum exam may not be appropriate. However, many survivors do not recall what happened during parts or all of the assault, and examination of all orifices is suggested. A standardized sexual assault evidence collection kit is used to obtain and package specimens. The kit gives detailed instructions on how to collect and package specimens and other evidence.

If the woman needs to urinate or defecate prior to the examination, the nurse should ask her to avoid wiping away vaginal or other secretions until after evidence is collected. It is important to collect the first voided specimen for possible drug-facilitated sexual assault testing, and document the time it was collected. If the woman has a tampon or contraceptive device in the vagina, she should not remove or discard them. The woman remains clothed while her vital signs and blood pressure are determined, and her clothing is inspected for stains, tears, and foreign material. Clothing is handled only by the woman and, if pertinent to the assault, may be collected, allowed to air dry, and sealed in a bag to be checked for evidence. She is assisted to undress and is draped for the physical examination. Her body is inspected for bruises, swelling, scratches, lacerations, or other wounds. A head-to-toe examination is performed as indicated. Survivors can have injuries to other parts of the body, including the head, face, and neck. An ultraviolet light (Wood lamp) is used to find dried secretions on the survivor's skin. External genitals, thighs, buttocks, and lower abdomen are assessed, and, if there are injuries, bruises, or marks, photographs can be taken or drawings made. Pubic and scalp hair is combed for collection. Perianal, oral, and vaginal swabs are collected. If the survivor scratched her attacker, her nails are scraped to obtain material that can aid in identification.

A speculum examination, often using magnification, is performed gently to detect tears or bruises and to collect appropriate specimens. Many survivors have some type of genital injury, even if it is asymptomatic. A bimanual pelvic examination is not usually performed for evidence collection if a SANE is doing the examination. Internal pelvic assessment may be done by the nurse practitioner, nurse midwife, physician's assistant, or physician if internal injury is suspected.

Laboratory tests can include oral swabs for the survivor's deoxyribonucleic acid (DNA) to distinguish her DNA from the suspect's DNA; a urine or blood pregnancy test; blood tests for hepatitis B virus; and oral or blood tests for HIV. A preexisting pregnancy will affect treatment decisions for possible HIV prophylaxis. Testing for HIV is a typical part of the sexual assault exam; however, HIV status should be checked within 72 hours if the assault was high risk. Cultures for gonorrhea, chlamydia, and syphilis are not recommended because women are treated prophylactically, test results will not change treatment, and testing can have negative consequences in court (U.S. Department of Justice & Office of Violence Against Women, 2018).

During the examination, the woman's emotional status is assessed, and findings are recorded: reactions she exhibits to the assault; her orientation to time and place; and her attention span, affect, and verbal description and feelings about the assault. The availability of family or peer-support systems is assessed. She is asked about her plans to report the crime to the police. After the examination, the woman should be allowed to shower and offered fresh clothes or a gown. She can be given time to rest and to talk with the nurse, rape crisis counselor, family, or friends.

It is important that the chain of custody be maintained. *Chain of custody* is a legal term that refers to the continual guarding of evidence and describes evidence from the moment that it is first collected until it appears in court. All items of evidence are individually labeled with the name of examiner, client, date, and source. The evidence is never left unattended or with the family, woman, or support person such as an advocate. During the examination, chain of custody is the responsibility of the examiner. When evidence is turned over to the next custodian, each person signs that the evidence was given and received. Signing indicates that no one touched or tampered with the evidence during that person's watch. This ensures that the evidence can be used in court.

Immediate care. Consent is needed for treatment and medical management that includes (1) treating the physical injuries, including tetanus toxoid booster if indicated; (2) providing prophylactic antibiotic therapy for STIs (e.g., chlamydia, gonorrhea); and (3) providing prophylaxis for pregnancy if the woman is not pregnant. If physical trauma is life threatening, appropriate intervention takes precedence over collecting evidence. A pregnancy test should be done on all women at risk for pregnancy (with their consent). Most pregnancy tests are sensitive by 9 days after conception. If the woman is at risk for pregnancy and the pregnancy test is negative, emergency contraception should be offered to her. Emergency contraception (see Chapter 8) is most effective if used within 120 hours after intercourse. The earlier it is taken, the more effective. The woman should be advised that emergency contraception does not guarantee pregnancy prevention and that she should repeat the pregnancy test if she has not had a menstrual period within 3 to 4 weeks. She is informed about the availability of abortion or menstrual extraction as a backup measure. If the woman is pregnant, she will be assessed for the presence any pregnacy-related complications such as vaginal bleeding or uterine contractions, depending on her gestational age.

The woman can be provided with prophylactic antibiotic therapy to prevent STIs, hepatitis B postexposure prophylaxis (PEP), and, if there is a high risk of exposure (e.g., if the assailant is known to be infected with HIV), the PEP for HIV may be offered.

Discharge. The woman is discharged with medications and printed instructions about their use, printed instructions for self-care, and names and telephone numbers of resource people if she requires assistance. Money and transportation to wherever she is staying (an alternative place may be found for her) add to the woman's comfort and perception of being in control. A medical follow-up examination is scheduled in 1 to 2 weeks for cultures for gonorrhea and other STIs; at 6 weeks for assessment of healing injuries; and at 6, 12, and 24 weeks for repeated serology tests for syphilis and HIV infection if initial test results were negative. The woman and her counselor determine whether there is a need for an additional medical or psychologic follow-up examination between the scheduled visits. The woman has a choice of site for follow-up testing. Some women choose to continue with the health care provider who first performed the examination, some prefer their primary health care provider, and others need referral to a clinic in the area (city, state) in which they live.

Nurses must be aware that responses to sexual assault are variable. Self-blame and humiliation can alternate with anger and fear. The woman needs to be reassured again before she leaves that her feelings are normal and that she is not alone. The initial care of a woman will affect her recovery and her decision to return for follow-up care. With kindness, skill, and empathy, nurses can assist women through an examination that is as nontraumatic as possible.

After discharge. Follow-up care includes contacting the woman on a regular basis until she indicates this is no longer needed. This is done by the health care provider (or other designated health care professional such as a nurse) to whom the woman was referred after the assault. Education in prevention strategies is often offered by community agencies or rape-awareness groups. The focus of the classes is usually on increasing women's awareness of situations that put them at high risk for rape or sexual assault. Other courses teach self-defense methods or how to change personal behaviors to reduce the risk of being assaulted, such as avoiding being alone in isolated places and being alert to unusual activities or persons in one's environment. Still other courses focus on changing societal attitudes about rape. Nurses can play a role in preventive education by offering courses or participating in courses offered by community or health care groups. Nurses must be knowledgeable about the epidemiology of sexual assault, reporting requirements, and services available in their community for survivors and should screen all women for a history of assault and any sequelae.

HUMAN TRAFFICKING

The International Labor Organization (ILO) estimates 20.9 million people are in forced labor globally, trafficked for work and sexual exploitation or held in slavery-like situations (ILO, 2014). Women and girls represent 11.4 million (55%) of persons in captivity. The prevalence is highest in the Asia-Pacific region (56% of global total), with the second highest number in Africa at (18%) and the lowest number in developed economies such as the United States. Globally, two-thirds (approximately $99 billion) is generated by forced sexual exploitation. Persons forced into labor exploitation, including domestic work, agriculture, and other economic activities, generate $51 billion in profits annually. Illegal profits, although difficult to estimate, are estimated to be more than $150 billion worldwide (ILO, 2014).

In 2000 the Trafficking Victim's Protection Act (TVPA) defined human trafficking as a crime involving the exploitation of someone for the purpose of compelled labor or a commercial sex act through the use of force, fraud, or coercion (U.S. Department of State, 2000). Sex trafficking is when a commercial sex act is performed under force, fraud, or coercion in exchange for the promise of something of value, such as a job or place to reside (National Human Trafficking Resource Center [NHTRC], 2016; USDHHS, 2017). Human trafficking, best known at the transnational level, does not need to involve the physical movement of a person and can originate and remain in a local area (USDHHS). Sex trafficking may be based out of brothels, hotels/motels, truck stops, hostess/strip clubs, streets, and escort services (Pourciau & Vallette, 2014; USDHHS, 2017).

Captives of sex trafficking can be male or female, but the vast majority are girls and women, many lured by false promises, such as the offer of a job or marriage (ILO, 2014; USDHHS, 2017). Sometimes they are kidnapped by traffickers, whereas others are sold into the sex trade by parents, spouses, or partners. Traffickers may subject their captives into debt-bondage, an illegal practice in which the traffickers tell the enslaved that they owe them money and must pledge their personal service as repayment. Traumatic bonding is a form of coercive control in which the perpetrator instills in the person fear, as well as gratitude for being allowed to live (USDHHS).

Captives of human trafficking may have varied experiences with health care services (Lederer & Wetzel, 2014). Some captives are able to receive regular health care services or allowed to seek medical assistance. Captives rarely self-identify for fear of retaliation by the trafficker, fear of arrest or report to social services, and lack of transportation and understanding from health care providers (NHTRC, 2016).

Health care professionals, especially providers and nurses in gynecologic and emergency department settings, are "first responders" and have unique opportunities to intervene (Lederer & Wetzel, 2014). Captives might interact with health care providers for violence-related injuries, serious illness, disease, pregnancy, birth control, abortion, substance abuse, addiction, and psychologic problems. Based on the reported symptoms of survivors, signs of being kicked, punched, or beaten and of forced sex should be "red flags." Although these signs may also appear with IPV, the additional history of multiple abortions, treatment for STIs, extreme forms of violence (stabbing, gunshot wounds, strangulation), or serious communicable diseases may help to differentiate sex trafficking from IPV (Lederer & Wetzel, 2014), in all settings, it is important that health care professionals are alert to signs and symptoms of possible trafficking, such as being accompanied to the visit by another person who appears very controlling, showing signs of being fearful, not being comfortable with answering questions, difficulty communicating, presenting with signs of abuse, and lacking documentation of citizenship (Polaris, 2018). These health care professionals include nurses, nurse practitioners, nurse midwives, physician's assistants, and physicians. Asking directly if the client is a survivor of trafficking is not advised; rather, a series of probing questions can help unveil the trafficking situation (Lederer & Wetzel, 2014). Building trust is a crucial first step for the professional and requires patience and cultural sensitivity. Some women may come alone, and, if trust is developed, contact information for rescue and services can be given. Traffickers often accompany their captive, and, if possible, separation should be done discretely (AWHONN, 2016; Lederer & Wetzel, 2014).

In 2000 the U.S. government enacted the Trafficking Victims Protection Act, which makes trafficking, including sex trafficking, a federal crime. Health care providers play a critical role in identifying perpetrators and survivors of this crime. The NHTRC (1-888-373-7888) can provide assistance.

COMMUNITY ACTIVITY

- Research the laws regarding intimate partner violence in your state. Is it considered a misdemeanor or felony crime? Is mandatory reporting of domestic violence by health care providers required? What is the definition of statutory rape in your state? Visit http://www.futureswithoutviolence.org for information on state statutes and policies on domestic violence.
- What are the resources for survivors of intimate partner violence in your community?
- Visit https://polarisproject.org/get-assistance/national-human-trafficking-hotline. Find out about the National Human Trafficking Resource Center and the resources and services that may be available in your community.

KEY POINTS

- Violence against women is a major social and health care problem in the United States, costing thousands of lives and billions of dollars in direct and indirect health care costs.
- IPV includes physical, sexual, emotional, psychologic, and economic abuse against men and women in heterosexual or homosexual relationships.
- To provide effective care, nurses must increase awareness of their own beliefs and values regarding abuse of women.
- Theoretic frameworks—psychologic, sociologic, biologic, and feminist perspectives—provide the foundation for understanding the complexity of the abuse of women.
- Cultural influences regarding violent behaviors and relationships sensitize the nurse to the special needs of women from various ethnic groups.
- IPV affects young, middle-aged, and older women of all races; all socioeconomic, educational, and religious groups; and pregnant women.

- All states have mandatory reporting of the abuse of children and older adults; some states have initiated mandatory reporting of intimate partner violence. Mandatory reporting is controversial and takes away the right for women to choose.
- Rape is a legal term defined differently by each state but usually refers to penetration of an orifice against someone's will.
- Nurses in all professional areas should respond with sensitivity and caring to women who experience abuse.
- Follow-up and interprofessional care are important in all instances of abuse.
- Nurses should be knowledgeable about reporting requirements and available community services for women who have been sexually assaulted.
- Health care professionals may have an opportunity to identify survivors of human sex trafficking, intervene to help them obtain necessary health services, and provide information about ways to escape from their situation.

REFERENCES

American Psychiatric Association. (2013). *Diagnostic and statistical manual of mental disorders* (5th ed.). Arlington, VA: American Psychiatric Association.

Asagba, R. B. (2015). Developing logotherapeutic strategies as effective interventions for victims of sexual assault. *Gender and Behavior, 13*(2), 6795–6802.

Association of Women's Health, Obstetric and Neonatal Nurses (AWHONN). (2015). *Intimate partner violence.* Retrieved from: http://www.jognn.org/article/S0884-2175(15)31805.0/pdf.

Association of Women's Health, Obstetric, and Neonatal Nurses (AWHONN). (2016). Human trafficking. *Journal of Obstetric, Gynecologic, and Neonatal Nursing, 45,* 458–460.

Basile, K. C., Smith, S. G., Breiding, M. J., Black, M. C., & Mahendra, R. (2014). *Sexual violence surveillance: Uniform definitions and recommended data elements.* National Center for Injury Prevention and Control Division of Violence Prevention. Retrieved from: https://www.cdc.gov/violenceprevention/pdf/sv_surveillance_definitionsl-2009-a.pdf.

Borrajo, E., Gámez-Guadix, M., & Calvete, E. (2015). Justification beliefs in violence, myths about love and cyber dating abuse. *Psicothema, 116*(2), 565–585.

Boyle, K. (2017). Sexual assault and identity disruption: A sociological approach to postrraumatic stress. *Society and Mental Health, 7*(2), 69–84.

Breiding, M. J., & Armour, B. S. (2015). The association between disability and intimate partner violence in the United States. *Annals of Epidemiology, 25*(6), 455–457. https://doi.org/10.1016/j.annepidem.2015.03.017.

Breiding, M. J., Smith, S. G., Walters, M. L., Chen, J., & Merrick, M. T. (2014). *Prevalence and characteristics of sexual violence, stalking, and intimate partner violence victimization-National Intimate partner and sexual violence, United States, 2011.* Retrieved from: https://www.cdc.gov/mmwr/preview/mmwrhtml/ss6308a1.htm?s_cid=ss6308a1_e.

Campbell, J. (2018). *Danger assessment.* Johns Hopkins School of Nursing. Retrieved from: https://www.dangerassessment.org/about.aspx.

Cannon, C., Lauve-Moon, K., & Buttell, F. (2015). Re-theorizing intimate partner violence through post-structural feminism, queer theory, and the sociology of gender. *Social Sciences, 4*(3), 668–687.

Carbone-Lopez, K., Slocum, L. A., & Kruttschnitt, C. (2015). "Police wouldn't give you no help": Female offenders on reporting sexual assault to police. *Violence Against Women, 22*(3), 366–396.

Centers for Disease Control and Prevention. (2014). *Sexual violence: Definitions.* Retrieved from: https://www.cdc.gov/violenceprevention/sexualviolence/definitions.html.

Centers for Disease Control and Prevention. (2015). *The social-ecological model: A framework for prevention.* Retrieved from: https://www.cdc.gov/violenceprevention/overview/social-ecologicalmodel.html.

Centers for Disease Control and Prevention. (2017a). *Intimate partner violence: Definitions.* Retrieved from: https://www.cdc.gov/violenceprevention/intimatepartnerviolence/definitions.html.

Centers for Disease Control and Prevention. (2017b). PRAMS Pregnancy Risk Assessment Monitoring System. (2017). *Prevalence of selected maternal and child health indicators-United States, all sites, pregnancy assessment monitoring system (PRAMS), 2012-2013. Retrieved from:* https://www.cdc.gov/prams/pramstat/pdfs/mch-indicators/PRAMS-All-Sites_508tagged.pdf.

Centers for Disease Control and Prevention. (2017c). *Intimate partner violence: Consequences.* Retrieved from: https://www.cdc.gov/violenceprevention/intimatepartnerviolence/consequences.html.

Center for Research on Women with Disabilities. (2018). *Investigating violence.* Retrieved from: https://www.bcm.edu/research/centers/research-on-women-with-disabilities/topics/violence/violence-against-women-with-disabilities.

Destiny, C. D. (2017). When there is no sexual assault nurse examiner: Emergency nursing care for female adult sexual assault patients. *Journal of Emergency Nursing, 43*(4), 308–315.

Domestic Abuse Intervention Programs. (2017). *The Duluth model. Duluth, MN.* Retrieved from: https://www.theduluthmodel.org/wheels/.

Domestic Shelters. (2015). *When pregnancy triggers violence: Facts to know about the danger of abuse during pregnancy.* Retrieved from: https://www.domesticshelters.org/domestic-violence-articles-information/when-pregnancy-triggers-violence.WI6x4hsrKqE.

Donovan, B. M., Spracklen, C. N., Schweizer, M. L., Ryckman, K. K., & Saftlas, A. F. (2016). Intimate partner violence during pregnancy and the risk for adverse infant outcomes: A systematic review and meta–analysis. *BJOG: An International Journal of Obstetrics & Gynecology, 123*(8) 1289–1129.

Findlaw. (2017). *Statutory rape.* Retrieved from: http://criminal.findlaw.com/criminal-charges/statutory-rape.html.

GLBTQ Domestic Violence Project (N.D.). *Domestic violence.* Retrieved from: http://www.glbtqdvp.org/our-work/domestic-violence/

Golden, S. D., McLeroy, K. R., Green, L. W., Earp, J. A. L., & Lieberman, L. D. (2015). Upending the social ecological model to guide health promotion efforts toward policy and environmental change. *Health Education & Behavior, 42*(1), 8S–14S.

Hahn, J. W., Aldarondo, E., Silverman, J. G., McCormick, M. C., & Koenen, K. C. (2015). Examining the association between posttraumatic stress disorder and intimate partner violence perpetration. *Journal of Family Violence, 30*(6), 743–752.

Harning, A. T. (2015). Provide emotional first aid when responding to sexually assaulted patients. *Journal of Emergency Services.* Retrieved Sept. 6, 2018 from: https://www.jems.com/articles/print/volume-40o-sexually-assaulted-patients.html/issue-10/features/provide-emotional-first-aid-when-responding-t.

Hill, G., & Hill, K. (2018a). *Molestation.* Retrieved from: Law.com. http://dictionary.law.com/Default.aspx?selected=1274.

Hill, G., & Hill, K. (2018b). *Statutory rape.* Retrieved from: Law.com. http://dictionary.law.com/Default.aspx?typed=statutory%20rape&type=1.

International Labour Office. (2014). *Profits and poverty: The economics of forced labour.* Retrieved from: http://www.ilo.org/wcmsp5/groups/public/---ed_norm/---declaration/documents/publication/wcms_243391.pdf.

Kaufman-Parks, A. M., DeMaris, A., Giordano, P. C., Manning, W. D., & Longmore, M. A. (2017). Familial effects on intimate partner violence perpetration across adolescence and young adulthood. *Journal of Family Issues.* Advance online publication. https://doi.org/10.1177/0192513X17734586.

King, K., Murray, C. E., Crowe, A., Hunnicutt, G., Lundgren, K., & Olson, L. (2017). The costs of recovery: Intimate partner violence survivors' experiences of financial recovery from abuse. *The Family Journal, 25*(3), 230–238.

Kulkarni, S., Herman-Smith, R., & Ross, T. C. (2015). Measuring intimate partner violence (IPV) service providers' attitudes: The development of the Survivor-Defined Advocacy Scale (SDAS). *Journal of Family Violence, 30*(7), 911–921.

Lederer, L. J., & Wetzel, C. A. (2014). The health consequences of sex trafficking and their implications for identifying victims in healthcare facilities. *Annals Health Law, 23*, 61–91.

Litz, B. T., & Salters-Pedneault, K. (2008). Training psychologists to assess, manage, and treat posttraumatic stress disorder: An examination of the National Center for PTSD Behavioral Science Division training program. *Training and Education in Professional Psychology, 2*(2), 67–74.

Maier, S. F., & Seligman, M. E. (2016). Learned helplessness at fifty: Insights from neuroscience. *Psychological Review, 123*(4), 349.

Mayo Clinic. (2018). Chronic traumatic encephalopathy. *Patient care and health information.* Mayo Foundation for Medical Education and Research. Retrieved from: https://www.mayoclinic.org/diseases-conditions/chronic-traumatic-encephalopathy/symptoms-causes/syc-20370921.

Namy, S., Carlson, C., O'Hara, K., Nakuti, J., Bukuluki, P., Lwanyaaga, J., et al. (2017). Toward a feminist understanding of intersecting violence against women and children in the family. *Social Science and Medicine, 184*, 40–48.

National Center for PTSD. (2015). *Intimate partner violence.* Retrieved from: https://www.ptsd.va.gov/public/types/violence/domestic-violence.asp.

National Human Trafficking Resource Center (NHTRC). (2016). *Recognizing and responding to human trafficking in a healthcare context.* Retrieved from: https://humantraffickinghotline.org/resources/recognizing-and-responding-human-trafficking-healthcare-context.

O'Doherty, L., Hegarty, K., Ramsay, J., Davidson, L. L., Feder, G., & Taft, A. (2015). Screening women for intimate partner violence in healthcare settings. *Cochrane Database of Systematice Reviews, 2015* (7) Art. No.: CD007007. doi:0.1002/14651858.CD007007.pub3.

Parker, A. M., Sricharoenchai, T., Raparla, S., Schneck, K. W., Bienvenu, O. J., & Needham, D. M. (2015). Posttraumatic stress disorder in critical illness survivors: A metaanalysis. *Critical Care Medicine, 43*(5), 1121–1129.

Pegram, S. E., & Abbey, A. (2016). Associations between sexual assault severity and psychological and physical health outcomes: Similarities and differences among African American and Caucasian survivors. *Journal of Interpersonal Violence.* Advance Online First. https://doi.org/10.1177/0886260516673626.

Perry, A. G. (2017). Community-based nursing practice. In P. Potter, A. Perry, P. Stockert, & A. Hall (Eds.), *Fundamentals of nursing.* St. Louis: Elsevier.

Polaris. (2018). *Recognize the signs.* Retrieved from: https://polarisproject.org/human-trafficking/recognize-signs.

Pourciau, C. A., & Vallette, E. (2014). Violence. In M. A. Nies, M. McEwen, & M. (Eds.), *Community/public health nursing: Promoting the health of populations* (6th ed.). St. Louis: Elsevier.

Rape, Abuse, and Incest National Network. (2018). *Types of sexual violence.* Retrieved from: https://www.rainn.org.

Sabbah, E. A., Chang, Y. P., & Campbell–Heider, N. (2017). Understanding intimate partner violence in Jordan: Application of the ecological model. *Perspectives in Psychiatric Care, 53*(3), 156–163.

Sereen, J. (2018). *Posttraumatic stress disorder in adults: Epidemiology, pathophysiology, clinical manifestations, course, assessment, and diagnosis. UpToDate.* Retrieved from: https://www.uptodate.com/contents/posttraumatic-stress-disorder-in-adults-epidemiology-pathophysiology-clinical-manifestations-course-assessment-and-diagnosis.

Sinozich, S., & Langston, L. (2014). *Rape and sexual assault victimization among college-age females, 1995.2013.* US Department of Justice, Office of

Justice Programs, Bureau of Justice Statistics. Retrieved from: https://assets.documentcloud.org/documents/1378364/rsavcaf9513.pdf.

Smith, S. G., Chen, J., Basile, K. C., Gilbert, L. K., Merrick, M. T., Patel, N., et al. (2017). *The national intimate partner and sexual violence survey (NISS): 2010-2012 state report*. Atlanta, GA: National Center for Injury Prevention and Control for Division of Violence Prevention. Retrieved from: https://stacks.cdc.gov/view/cdc/46305.

Stein, J. Y., Wilmot, D. V., & Solomon, Z. (2016). Does one size fit all? Nosological, clinical, and scientific implications of variations in PTSD Criterion A. *Journal of Anxiety Disorders, 43*, 106–117.

Sylaska, K. M., & Edwards, K. M. (2014). Disclosure of intimate partner violence to informal social support network members: A review of the literature. *Trauma, Violence, & Abuse, 15*(1), 3–21.

United Nations [UN]. (2015). *Violence against women. The world's women 2015*. Retrieved from: https://unstats.un.org/unsd/gender/chapter6/chapter6.html.

United Nations High Commission for Refugees. (2019). Mexico: Domestic violence, including legislation; protection and support services offered to victims by the state and civil society, including Mexico City (2015-July 2017). Retrieved from: https://www.refworld.org/docid/59c116e24.html.

U.S. Census Bureau. (2018). *About Hispanic origin*. Retrieved from: https://www.census.gov/topics/population/hispanic-origin/about.html.

U.S. Department of Health and Human Services [USDHHS]. (2017). *Fact sheet: Human trafficking*. Retrieved from: https://www.acf.hhs.gov/otip/resource/fshumantrafficking.

U.S. Department of Health & Human Services. (2018). *Relationships and safety*. Office of Women's Health. Retrieved from: https://www.womenshealth.gov/relationships-and-safety.

U.S. Department of Health and Human Services, Office on Women's Health. (2017a). *Sexual assault*. Retrieved from: https://www.womenshealth.gov/a-z-topics/sexual-assault.

U.S. Department of Health and Human Services, Office on Women's Health. (2017b). *Violence against immigrant and refugee women*. Retrieved from: https://www.womenshealth.gov/relationships-and-safety/other-types/immigrant-and-refugee-women.

U.S. Department of Health and Human Services, Office of Women's Health. (2018). *Date-rape drugs*. Retrieved from: https://www.womenshealth.gov/a-z-topics/date-rape-drugs.

U.S. Department of Justice. Federal Bureau of Investigation. (2015). *Reporting Program Data: Supplementary Homicide Reports, 2013*. Ann Arbor, MI: Inter-university Consortium for Political and Social Research. https://doi.org/10.3886/ICPSR36124.v1.

U.S. Department of Justice, & Office of Violence Against Women. (2018). *Sexual assault*. Washington, D.C. Retrieved Sept. 6, 2018 from: https://www.justice.gov/ovw/sexual-assault.

U.S. Department of Justice Archives. (2017). *An updated definition of rape*. Retrieved from: https://www.justice.gov/archives/opa/blog/updated-definition-rape.

U.S. Department of State. (2000). *Victims of trafficking and violence protection act of 2000*. Retrieved from: https://www.state.gov/j/tip/laws/61124.htm.

U.S. Preventive Services Task Force. (2013). *Final recommendation statement: Intimate partner violence and abuse of elderly and vulnerable adults: Screening*. Retrieved from: https://www.uspreventiveservicestaskforce.org/Page/Document/RecommendationStatementFinal/intimate-partner-violence-and-abuse-of-elderly-and-vulnerable-adults-screening.

Van Parys, A. S., Deschepper, E., Michielsen, K., Temmerman, M., & Verstraelen, H. (2014). Prevalence and evolution of intimate partner violence before and during pregnancy: A cross-sectional study. *BMC Pregnancy and Childbirth, 14*, 294. https://doi.org/10.1186/1471-2393-14-294.

Walker, L. E. (2017). *The battered woman syndrome* (4th ed.). New York: Springer Publishing Co.

Whiting, J. (2016). *Four factors that help women leave abusive relationships*. Institute for Family Studies. Retrieved from: https://ifstudies.org/blog/four-factors-that-help-women-leave-abusive-relationships.

Wilson, L. C., & Miller, K. E. (2016). Meta-analysis of the prevalence of Unacknowledged rape. *Trauma, Violence, & Abuse, 17*(2), 149–159.

WomanSafe. (2018). *WomanSafe: The greenhouse*. Retrieved from: http://womensafe.org/who-we-are/.

WomanSafe, Inc. (2015). The cycle of violence. Retrieved from: http://www.womensafe.org/get-help/links-and-literature-resources/the-cycle-of-violence.

Wong, J.Y.H., Fong, D.Y.T., Lai, V., & Tiwari, A. (2014). Bridging intimate partner violence and the human brain: A literature review. *Trauma, Violence, & Abuse, 15*(1), 22–33.

World Health Organization. (2016). *Global plan of action: Health systems address violence against women and girls*. Retrieved from: http://apps.who.int/iris/bitstream/10665/251664/1/WHO-RHR-16.13-eng.pdf?ua=1.

World Health Organization [WHO]. (2017). *Violence against women*. Retrieved from: http://www.who.int/mediacentre/factsheets/fs239/en/.

World Health Organization [WHO]. (2018). *The ecological framework*. Retrieved from: http://www.who.int/violenceprevention/approach/ecology/en/.

Zilkens, R. R., Smith, D. A., Phillips, M. A., Mukhtar, S. A., Semmens, J. B., & Kelly, M. C. (2017). Genital and anal injuries: A cross-sectional Australian study of 1266 women alleging recent sexual assault. *Forensic Science International, 275*, 195–202.

6

Reproductive System Concerns

Robin Webb Corbett

 http://evolve.elsevier.com/Lowdermilk/MWHC/

LEARNING OBJECTIVES

- Describe and differentiate signs and symptoms of common menstrual disorders.
- Describe premenstrual syndrome (PMS) and premenstrual dysphoric disorder (PMDD).
- Relate the symptoms of endometriosis to the associated pathophysiology.
- Develop a nursing care plan for a woman with endometriosis.
- Summarize the therapies for menstrual disorders and menopausal symptoms, including risks and benefits.

- Differentiate the various causes of abnormal uterine bleeding.
- Identify health risks of perimenopausal women.
- Describe the common signs and symptoms of perimenopause.
- Develop a teaching plan for managing symptoms in menopausal women.
- Examine the risks and benefits of menopausal hormone therapy.
- Summarize client teaching strategies for prevention of osteoporosis.

The reproductive system consists of many components, and problems may occur at any point in the menstrual cycle. Many factors—including anatomic abnormalities, physiologic imbalances, and lifestyle—can affect the menstrual cycle. The average woman is likely to have some concerns related to her menstrual and gynecologic health at some point in her life and will experience bleeding, pain, discharge, or infections associated with her reproductive organs or functions. This chapter provides information on common menstrual problems; abnormal bleeding problems; and problems associated with peri- and postmenopause.

MENSTRUAL DISORDERS

Knowledge of the normal parameters of menstruation is essential to the assessment of experiences and disorders related to the menstrual cycle, which depends on a complex interplay between the reproductive, neurologic, and endocrine systems. The hypothalamus produces gonadotropin-releasing hormone (GnRH), which stimulates the pituitary gland to produce follicle-stimulating hormone (FSH) and luteinizing hormone (LH). In turn, FSH and LH stimulate the ovaries to produce first estrogen and then progesterone. In response to the hormones, the endometrium or lining of the uterus, proliferates and then sheds. Chapter 4 provides additional information on the menstrual cycle and endocrine physiology.

Normal menstrual patterns are averages based on observations and reports from large groups of healthy women. When counseling an individual woman, remember that these values are averages only. Generally a woman's menstrual cycle stabilizes at every 28 days within 1 to 2 years after puberty, with a range from 26 to 34 days. Although no woman's cycle is exactly the same length every month, the typical month-to-month variation in an individual's cycle is usually plus or minus 2 days. However, greater but still normal variations are noted frequently.

During her reproductive years a woman may have more than one physiologic variation in her menstrual cycle. It is essential that nurses understand the physiologic variations that occur in several age groups. Menstrual cycle length is most irregular at the extremes of the reproductive years, including the 2 years after menarche and the 5

years before menopause, when anovulatory cycles are most common. Irregular bleeding, both in length of cycle and amount, is the rule rather than the exception in early adolescence. It takes approximately 15 months for completion of the first 10 cycles and an average of 20 cycles before ovulation occurs regularly. Cycle lengths of 15 to 45 days are not unusual; during the first 2 years after menarche, intervals of 3 to 6 months between menses can be normal.

Once the irregular nature of menses in the first 1 to 2 years after menarche subsides and a cyclic, predictable pattern of monthly bleeding is established, women may worry about any deviation from that pattern or from what they have been told is normal for all menstruating women. Women may be influenced by myths and misunderstandings about the menstrual cycle and what is considered "normal." A woman may be concerned about her ability to conceive and bear children without this monthly evidence. Amenorrhea or excess menstrual bleeding can be a source of severe distress and concern for a woman.

Amenorrhea

Amenorrhea, the absence of menstrual flow, is a clinical sign of a variety of disorders. Generally, the following circumstances should be evaluated: (1) the absence of both menarche and secondary sexual characteristics by 13 years of age, (2) the absence of menses by 15 years of age, regardless of normal growth and development (primary amenorrhea), (3) the absence of menstruation within 5 years of breast development, or (4) a 6-month or more absence of menses after a period of menstruation (secondary amenorrhea) (Lobo, 2017b; Marsh & Grimstad, 2014).

A moderately obese girl (20% to 30% above ideal weight) may have early-onset menstruation, whereas delay of onset is known to be related to malnutrition (starvation, such as that with anorexia). Girls who exercise strenuously before menarche can have delayed onset of menstruation until about 18 years of age (Lobo, 2017b).

Although amenorrhea is not a disease, it is often a sign of one. Still, most commonly and most benignly, amenorrhea is a result of pregnancy. It can also result from anatomic abnormalities such as outflow tract obstruction. Amenorrhea can be caused by endocrine dysfunction such as anterior pituitary disorders, polycystic ovarian syndrome, hypothyroidism, or hyperthyroidism. Amenorrhea may result from chronic diseases such as type 1 diabetes; medications such as phenytoin (Dilantin); drug abuse (e.g., alcohol, opiates, marijuana, cocaine); or oral contraceptive use.

Hypogonadotropic Amenorrhea

Hypogonadotropic amenorrhea reflects a problem in the central hypothalamic-pituitary axis. In rare instances, a pituitary lesion or genetic inability to produce FSH and LH is at fault. However, women without a lesion with low levels of gonadotropins may have primary pituitary failure, which was referred to as *hypogonadotropic hypogonadism* (Lobo, 2017b). GnRH stimulation results in increased FSH and LH levels. This suggests a hypothalamic defect with lack of adequate GnRH synthesis or a defect in a central nervous system (CNS) neurotransmitter.

Hypogonadotropic amenorrhea often results from hypothalamic suppression as a result of stress or a sudden and severe weight loss, an eating disorder, strenuous exercise, or mental illness (Gelson & Prakash, 2016; Marsh & Grimstad, 2014). Research on the interaction between nervous system or neurotransmitter functions and hormone regulation throughout the body has demonstrated a biologic basis for the relation of stress to physiologic processes. Women who are more than 20% underweight for height or who have had rapid weight loss and those with eating disorders such as anorexia nervosa may report amenorrhea. Amenorrhea is one of the classic signs of anorexia nervosa, and the interrelation of disordered eating, amenorrhea, and premature osteoporosis has been described as the female athlete triad (Marsh & Grimstad; Mielke, Parsons, & Greenberg, 2015). A loss of calcium from bone, comparable to that seen in postmenopausal women, may occur with this type of amenorrhea.

Exercise-associated amenorrhea can occur in women undergoing vigorous physical training and is thought to be associated with many factors, including body composition (height, weight, and percentage of body fat); type, intensity, and frequency of exercise; nutritional status; and the presence of emotional or physical stressors. Women who participate in sports emphasizing low body weight are at greatest risk, including the following activities (Lobo, 2017b; Marsh & Grimstad, 2014):

- Sports in which performance is subjectively scored (e.g., dance, gymnastics)
- Endurance sports favoring participants with low body weight (e.g., distance running, cycling)
- Sports in which body contour–revealing clothing is worn (e.g., swimming, diving, volleyball)
- Sports with weight categories for participation (e.g., rowing, martial arts)
- Sports in which prepubertal body shape favors success (e.g., gymnastics, figure skating)

Assessment of amenorrhea begins with a thorough history and physical examination. Specific components of the assessment process depend on the client's age—adolescent, young adult, or perimenopausal—and whether she has menstruated previously.

An important initial step, often overlooked, is to be sure that the woman is not pregnant. Once pregnancy has been ruled out by a β-human chorionic gonadotropin (β-hCG) pregnancy test, diagnostic tests may include a complete blood count (CBC), urinalysis, and serum chemistries in order to rule out any systemic conditions. Tests including FSH level, thyroid-stimulating hormone (TSH), estradiol (E2) and prolactin levels, radiographic or computed tomography (CT) scan of the sella turcica, a progestational challenge, and possibly pelvic sonography are performed (Gelson & Prakash, 2016; Lobo, 2017b; Marsh & Grimstad, 2014).

Management

When amenorrhea is caused by hypothalamic disturbances, the nurse is an ideal health professional to help women because many of the causes are potentially reversible (e.g., stress, weight loss for nonorganic reasons). Counseling and education are primary interventions and appropriate nursing roles. When an etiology is known, predisposing a woman to hypothalamic amenorrhea, initial management involves addressing the etiology. Together the woman and nurse plan how the woman can decrease or discontinue medications known to affect menstruation, correct weight loss, deal more effectively with psychologic stress, address emotional distress, and alter exercise routines (Gelson & Prakash, 2016).

The nurse works with the woman to help her identify, cope with, and eliminate sources of stress in her life. Deep-breathing exercises and relaxation techniques are simple yet effective stress-reducing measures. Referral for biofeedback or massage therapy may also be useful. In some instances, referrals for psychotherapy may be indicated.

If a woman's exercise program is thought to contribute to her amenorrhea, several options exist for management. She may decide to decrease the intensity, frequency, or duration of her training or modify her diet to include the appropriate nutrition for her age. Accepting the former alternative may be difficult for one who is committed to a strenuous exercise regimen. The woman and nurse may have several sessions before the woman elects to try exercise reduction. Many young female athletes may not understand the consequences of low bone density or osteoporosis; nurses can point out the connection between low bone density and stress fractures. The nurse and woman should also investigate other factors that may be contributing to the amenorrhea and develop plans for altering lifestyle and decreasing stress. If necessary, referral to other health care providers—for example, psychologists or psychiatric nurse practitioners—may be indicated.

Research on recommended dosages of calcium, vitamin D, and potassium is inconclusive for women experiencing amenorrhea associated with the female athlete triad. Oral contraceptives may be helpful in amenorrheic women but are usually not used in young women with amenorrhea associated with the female athlete triad unless there are specific issues that warrant such treatment, which are best discussed with the woman's health care provider.

Cyclic Perimenstrual Pain and Discomfort

Cyclic perimenstrual pain and discomfort (CPPD) is the term used to describe women's symptoms of discomfort during the menstrual cycle (Fisher, Hickman, Adams, & Sibbritt, 2018). This concept includes dysmenorrhea, premenstrual syndrome (PMS), and premenstrual dysphoric disorder (PMDD) as well as symptom clusters that occur before and after the menstrual flow starts. Symptoms occur cyclically and can include mood swings as well as pelvic pain and physical discomfort. These symptoms can range from mild to severe and can last 1 or 2 days or up to 2 weeks. CPPD is a health problem that can have a significant effect on a woman's quality of life with 80% to 97% of women having at least one symptom of CPPD during their reproductive years (Fisher et al.). The following discussion focuses on the three main conditions of CPPD: (1) dysmenorrhea, (2), PMS, and (3) PMDD.

Dysmenorrhea

Dysmenorrhea, pain during or shortly before menstruation, is one of the most common gynecologic problems in women of all ages. Many adolescents have dysmenorrhea in the first 3 years after menarche. Young adult women 17 to 24 years of age are most likely to report painful menses. Approximately 75% of women report some level of discomfort associated with menses, and approximately 15% report severe dysmenorrhea (Mendiratta, 2017). However, the degree of disruption in women's lives is difficult to determine. Researchers have estimated that as many as 10% of women with dysmenorrhea have severe enough pain to interfere with their functioning for 1 to 3 days a month. Menstrual problems, including dysmenorrhea, are relatively more common in women who smoke and are obese (Iacovides, Avidon, & Baker, 2015). Severe dysmenorrhea is also associated with early menarche, nulliparity, and lack of physical exercise (Mendiratta). Traditionally dysmenorrhea is differentiated as primary or secondary (Rabinerson,

Hiersch, & Gabbary-Gen-Ziv, 2018). Symptoms usually begin before or with menstruation, The range and severity of symptoms differ from woman to woman and from cycle to cycle in the same woman. Symptoms of dysmenorrhea may last several hours or several days.

Pain is usually located in the suprapubic area or lower abdomen. Women describe the pain as sharp, cramping, gripping, or as a steady dull ache. In some women pain radiates to the lower back or upper thighs.

Primary dysmenorrhea. Primary dysmenorrhea is a condition associated with the ovulatory cycle. Research has shown that it has a biochemical basis and arises from the release of prostaglandins with menses. During the luteal phase and subsequent menstrual flow, prostaglandin F_2-alpha ($PGF_{2\alpha}$) is secreted. Excessive release of $PGF_{2\alpha}$ increases the amplitude and frequency of uterine contractions and causes vasospasm of the uterine arterioles, resulting in ischemia and cyclic lower abdominal cramps. Systemic responses to $PGF_{2\alpha}$ include backache, weakness, diaphoresis, gastrointestinal symptoms (anorexia, nausea, vomiting, and diarrhea), and CNS symptoms (dizziness, syncope, headache, and poor concentration). Pain usually begins immediately prior to or at the onset of menstruation and lasts 12 to 72 hours, with the most severe pain on day 1 or 2 of the menses (Iacovides, et al., 2015; Mendiratta, 2017).

Primary dysmenorrhea usually appears 6 to 24 months after menarche, when ovulation is established. Anovulatory bleeding, common in the first few months or years after menarche, is painless. Because both estrogen and progesterone are necessary for primary dysmenorrhea to occur, it is experienced only with ovulatory cycles. This problem is more common among women in their late teens and early 20s than in older age groups, as the incidence declines with age. Psychogenic factors may influence symptoms, but symptoms are definitely related to ovulation and do not occur when ovulation is suppressed.

Management. Management of primary dysmenorrhea depends on the severity of the problem and the individual woman's response to various treatments. Important components of nursing care are information and support. Because menstruation is so closely linked to reproduction and sexuality, menstrual problems such as dysmenorrhea can have a negative influence on sexuality and self-worth. Nurses can correct myths and misinformation about menstruation and dysmenorrhea by providing facts about what is normal. Women need support to foster their feelings of positive sexuality and self-worth.

Often, nurses can offer more than one alternative for alleviating menstrual discomfort and dysmenorrhea, which gives women options and a chance to try various remedies and to decide which works best for them. Several of these alternatives are discussed in the following paragraphs.

The application of heat to the lower abdomen in the form of a patch, wrap, or heating pad can reduce discomfort. The heat minimizes cramping by increasing vasodilation and muscle relaxation and minimizing uterine ischemia. Aerobic exercise has also been found to help alleviate pain (Mendiratta, 2017). Relaxation training, biofeedback, transcutaneous electrical nerve stimulation (TENS), Lamaze breathing (notably a childbirth method, but also a technique that can help with pain reduction), yoga, hypnotherapy, imagery, and desensitization are also used to decrease menstrual discomfort, although evidence is insufficient to determine their effectiveness (Chien, Chang, and Liu, 2013; Mendiratta, 2017) (Fig. 6.1).

Exercise helps relieve menstrual discomfort through increased vasodilation and subsequent decreased ischemia. It also releases endogenous opiates (specifically beta-endorphins), suppresses prostaglandins, and shunts blood flow away from the viscera, resulting in reduced pelvic congestion. One specific exercise that nurses can suggest is pelvic rocking.

In addition to maintaining good nutrition at all times, specific dietary changes can help to modify some of the systemic symptoms associated with dysmenorrhea. A decreased intake of salt and refined sugar intake 7 to 10 days before the expected menses

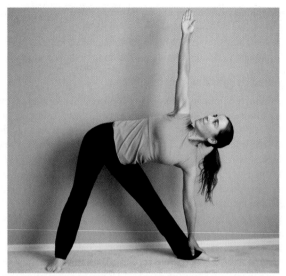

Fig. 6.1 Yoga Asana: Triangle Pose. Helpful for assisting digestion and stretching and strengthening the spine; also used for dysmenorrheal and pelvic congestion. (Courtesy Julie Perry Nelson, Loveland, CO.)

may reduce fluid retention. Natural diuretics such as asparagus, cranberry juice, peaches, parsley, or watermelon may help reduce edema and related discomforts. A low-fat vegetarian diet and vitamin E intake may also help to minimize dysmenorrheal symptoms (Mendiratta, 2017).

Medications used to treat primary dysmenorrhea include prostaglandin synthesis inhibitors, primarily nonsteroidal antiinflammatory drugs (NSAIDs) (Iacovides, et al., 2015; Mendiratta, 2017) (Table 6.1). NSAIDs are most effective if started several days before the menses or at least by the onset of bleeding. All NSAIDs have potential gastrointestinal side effects, including nausea, vomiting, and indigestion. Women taking NSAIDs should be instructed to report dark-colored stool, because this may be an indication of gastrointestinal bleeding.

Over-the-counter (OTC) preparations that are indicated for primary dysmenorrhea contain the same active ingredients (e.g., ibuprofen or naproxen sodium) as prescription preparations. However, the labeled recommended dose may be subtherapeutic. Preparations containing acetaminophen are even less effective because acetaminophen does not have the antiprostaglandin properties of NSAIDs (Yucel, Baket, Balci, et al., 2018).

> **! NURSING ALERT**
>
> If one NSAID is ineffective, often a different one may be effective. If the second drug is unsuccessful after a 6-month trial, combined oral contraceptive pills (OCPs) may be used. Women with a history of aspirin sensitivity or allergy should avoid all NSAIDs.

OCPs are associated with less severe primary dysmenorrhea and are an appropriate choice for women who want to use a contraceptive agent (DeSanctis, Soliman, Bernasconi, et al., 2015). The benefits of their use are attributed to decreased prostaglandin synthesis associated with an atrophic decidualized endometrium. Combined OCPs, which contain both estrogen and progesterone, are effective in relieving symptoms of primary dysmenorrhea for approximately 90% of women. No single OCP, including low-dose and extended-cycle OCPs, has been shown to be superior to another for the relief of primary dysmenorrhea (Mendiratta, 2017). OCPs are a

TABLE 6.1 Nonsteroidal Antiinflammatory Agents Used to Treat Dysmenorrhea

Drug	Brand Name and Status	Recommended Dosage (Oral)[a]	Common Side Effects[b]	Comments	Contraindications
Diclofenac	Cataflam Rx	100 mg initially, then 50 mg q8h	Nausea, diarrhea, constipation, abdominal distress, dyspepsia, heartburn, flatulence, dizziness, tinnitus, itching, rash	Enteric-coated; immediate release	**For all NSAIDs:** Do not give if woman has hemophilia or bleeding ulcers; do not give if woman has had an allergic or anaphylactic reaction to aspirin or another NSAID; do not give if woman is taking anticoagulant medication
Ibuprofen	Motrin Rx, Advil OTC, Nuprin OTC, Motrin IB OTC	400 mg q6-8h, 200 mg q4-6h up to 1200 mg/day	See diclofenac	If GI upset occurs, take with food, milk, or antacids; avoid alcoholic beverages; do not take with aspirin; stop taking and call care provider if rash occurs	
Ketoprofen	Orudis Rx	25-50 mg q6-8h up to 300 mg/day	See diclofenac	See ibuprofen	
	Orudis KT OTC, Actron OTC	12.5 mg q6-8h up to 75 mg/day			
Meclofenamate	Meclomen Rx	100 mg tid up to 300 mg	See diclofenac	See ibuprofen	
Mefenamic acid	Ponstel Rx	500 mg initially, then 250 mg/day	See diclofenac	Very potent and effective prostaglandin-synthesis inhibitor; antagonizes already formed prostaglandins; increased incidence of adverse GI side effects	
Naproxen	Naprosyn Rx	500 mg initially, then 250 mg q6-8h or 500 mg q h (long-acting formula) not to exceed 1250 mg/day on first day; subsequent doses not to exceed 100 mg/day	See diclofenac	See ibuprofen	
Naproxen sodium	Anaprox Rx	550 mg initially, then 275 mg q6-8h or 550 mg q12h up to 1375 mg/day	See diclofenac	See ibuprofen	
	Aleve OTC	440 mg initially, then 220 mg q6-8h up to 660 mg/day			
Celecoxib	Celebrex	400 mg initially, then 200 mg bid	See diclofenac	See ibuprofen	

[a]Dosages are current recommendations and should be verified before use. Recommended doses for over-the-counter preparations are generally less than recommendations for therapeutic doses. As-needed dosing is recommended by manufacturer; scheduled dosing may be more effective.
[b]Risk with all NSAIDs is gastrointestinal ulceration, possible bleeding, and prolonged bleeding time. Incidence of side effects is dose related. Reported incidence is 1% to 10%.
GI, Gastrointestinal; *NSAIDs,* nonsteroidal antiinflammatory drugs; *OTC,* over the counter.
Data from Calis, K. A. (2016). Dysmenorrhea medication. *Medscape.* Retrieved from http://emedicine.medscape.com/article/253812-medication#2; Mendiratta, V. (2017). Primary and secondary dysmenorrhea, premenstrual syndrome, and premenstrual dysphoric disorder. In R. A. Lobo, D. M. Gershenson, G. M. Lentz, et al. (Eds.), *Comprehensive gynecology* (7th ed.). Philadelphia: Elsevier.

particularly good choice for therapy because they combine contraception with a positive effect on dysmenorrhea, menstrual flow, and menstrual irregularities. Adolescents may benefit from use of the long-acting injectable contraceptive (depot medroxyprogesterone), but more research is needed. Since OCPs have side effects, (e.g., risk of venous thromboembolism), women may not wish to use them for dysmenorrhea, and they may be contraindicated for some women. (See Chapter 8 for a complete discussion of OCPs.) Hormonal intrauterine devices (IUDs) have been demonstrated to decrease dysmenorrhea. Specifically, levonorgestrel IUDs have been associated with fewer reports of dysmenorrhea (Yucel, Baket, Balci, et al., 2018).

Alternative and complementary therapies are increasingly popular and used in developed countries. Therapies such as acupuncture, acupressure, aromatherapy (lavender), biofeedback, desensitization, hypnosis, massage, reiki, relaxation exercises, therapeutic touch, and yoga have been used to treat pelvic pain (Fisher et al., 2018). Herbal preparations have long been used for managing menstrual problems, including dysmenorrhea (Table 6.2). However, it is essential that women understand that these therapies are not without potential toxicity and may cause drug interactions.

Vitamin D has been shown to reduce the symptoms of dysmenorrhea and PMIS (Bahrami, et al., 2018). Aerobic exercise has also been shown to improve primary dysmernorrhea (Dehnavi, Jafarnejad, & Kamali, 2017).

> ### ! NURSING ALERT
>
> Nurses must routinely ask women about their use of herbal and other alternative therapies and must document this.

Secondary dysmenorrhea. **Secondary dysmenorrhea** is menstrual pain that develops later in life than primary dysmenorrhea, typically after 25 years of age. It is associated with pelvic pathology such as adenomyosis, endometriosis, pelvic inflammatory disease, endometrial polyps, or submucous or interstitial myomas (fibroids). Women with secondary dysmenorrhea often have other symptoms that may suggest the underlying cause. For example, heavy menstrual flow with dysmenorrhea suggests a diagnosis of leiomyomata, adenomyosis, or endometrial polyps. Pain associated with endometriosis often begins a few days before menses but can be present at ovulation and continue through the first days of menses or start after menstrual flow has begun. In contrast to primary dysmenorrhea, the pain of secondary dysmenorrhea is often characterized by dull lower abdominal aching that radiates to the back or thighs. Often women experience feelings of bloating or pelvic fullness. In addition to a physical examination with a careful pelvic examination, diagnosis may be assisted by ultrasound examination, dilation and curettage (D&C), endometrial biopsy, or laparoscopy. Treatment is directed toward removal of the underlying pathology. Many of the measures described for pain relief of primary dysmenorrhea are also helpful for women with secondary dysmenorrhea.

Premenstrual Syndrome

Approximately 75% of women experience premenstrual symptoms at some time in their reproductive lives (Menditratta, 2017). Establishing a universal definition of premenstrual syndrome (PMS) is difficult, given that so many symptoms have been associated with the condition and at least two different syndromes have been recognized: PMS and premenstrual dysphoric disorder (PMDD).

PMS is a complex, poorly understood condition that includes one or more of a large number (more than 150) of physical and psychologic symptoms beginning in the luteal phase of the menstrual cycle, occurring to such a degree that lifestyle or work is affected, and followed by a symptom-free period. Symptoms include fluid retention (abdominal bloating, pelvic fullness, edema of the lower extremities, breast tenderness, and weight gain), behavioral or emotional changes (depression, crying spells, irritability, panic attacks, and impaired ability to concentrate), premenstrual cravings (sweets, salt, increased appetite, and food binges), headache, fatigue, and backache.

TABLE 6.2 Herbal Medicinals Taken Orally for Menstrual Disorders

Symptoms or Indications	Herbal Therapy[a]	Action
Menstrual cramping, dysmenorrhea	Black haw	Uterine antispasmodic
	Fennel	Uterotonic
	Catnip	Uterine antispasmodic
	Dong quai	Uterotonic; antiinflammatory
	Ginger	Antiinflammatory
	Motherwort	Uterotonic
	Wild yam	Uterine antispasmodic
	Valerian	Uterine antispasmodic
Premenstrual discomfort, tension	Black cohosh root	Estrogen-like luteinizing hormone suppressant; binds to estrogen receptors
	Chamomile	Antispasmodic
Breast pain	Chaste tree fruit	Decreases prolactin levels
	Bugleweed	Antigonadotropic; decreases prolactin levels
	Vitex agnus castus)	Decreases prolactin levels
Menorrhea, metrorrhagia	Lady's mantle	Uterotonic
	Raspberry	Uterotonic
	Shepherd's purse	Uterotonic

[a]Many herbs do not have rigorous scientific studies backing their use; most uses and properties of herbs have not been validated by the U.S. Food and Drug Administration.
Data from National Center for Complementary and Alternative Medicine. (2017). *Herbs at a glance.* Retrieved from https://nccih.nih.gov-/health/herbsataglance.htm. Zahid, H., Rizvani, G.H., & Ishaqe, S. (2017). Phytopharmacological review of vitex-agnus castus: a potential medicinal plant. *Chinese Herbal Medicines,* 8, 24–29.

All age-groups are affected, with women in their 20s and 30s most frequently reporting symptoms. Ovarian function is necessary for the condition to occur because it does not occur before puberty, after menopause, or during pregnancy. The condition is not dependent on the presence of monthly menses: women who have had a hysterectomy without bilateral salpingo-oophorectomy (BSO) still can have cyclic symptoms.

PMDD is a more severe variant of PMS in which women have marked irritability, dysphoria, mood lability, anxiety, fatigue, appetite changes, and a sense of feeling overwhelmed (Menditratta, 2017). The most common symptoms are those associated with mood disturbances, and PMDD is listed as a condition in the *Diagnostic and Statistical Manual of Mental Disorders,* Fifth Edition (DSM-5) (American Psychiatric Association [APA], 2014).

For a diagnosis of PMDD, the following criteria must be met (APA, 2014):
- Five or more affective and physical symptoms are present in the week before menses and begin to improve in the follicular phase of the menstrual cycle.
- At least one of the symptoms is marked affective lability, marked irritability or anger, depressed mood or feelings of hopelessness, self-deprecating thoughts, and/or anxiety.

- One or more of the following additional symptoms is/are present: decreased interest in usual activities, subjective difficulty concentrating; lethargy; marked change in appetite (overeating, food cravings); hypersomnia or insomnia; feeling overwhelmed; physical symptoms of breast tenderness, muscle pain, bloating, weight gain.
- Symptoms interfere markedly with work or interpersonal relationships.
- Symptoms are not caused by an exacerbation of another condition or disorder.
- Must confirm that symptoms are occurring, evidenced through daily ratings.
- Symptoms are not caused by physiologic effects of a substance or a specific medical treatment.

These criteria must be confirmed by prospective daily ratings for at least two menstrual cycles.

The causes of PMS and PMDD continue to be investigated, but there is general agreement that they are distinct psychiatric and medical syndromes rather than an exacerbation of an underlying psychiatric disorder. They do not occur if there is no ovarian function. A number of biologic and neuroendocrine etiologies have been suggested; however, none have been conclusively substantiated as the causative factor. It is likely that biologic, psychosocial, and sociocultural factors contribute to PMS and PMDD.

Management

There is little agreement on management. A careful, detailed history and daily log of symptoms and mood fluctuations spanning several cycles may give direction to a plan of management. Any changes that help a woman with PMS exert control over her life have a positive effect. For this reason, lifestyle changes are often effective in its treatment.

Education is an important component of the management of PMS. Nurses can advise women that self-help modalities often result in significant symptom improvement. Women have found a number of complementary and alternative therapies to be useful in managing the symptoms of PMS. Diet and exercise changes can provide symptom relief for some women. Nurses can suggest that women do not smoke and limit their consumption of refined sugar, salt, red meat, alcohol, and caffeinated beverages. Women can be encouraged to include whole grains, legumes, seeds, nuts, vegetables, fruits, and vegetable oils in their diets; reduce the amount of salt, sugar, and caffeine in their diets; and incorporate 60 minutes or more of physical exercise daily (a monthly program that varies in intensity and type of exercise according to PMS symptoms is best). Women who exercise regularly seem to have less premenstrual anxiety than do nonathletic women. Researchers believe that aerobic exercise increases beta-endorphin levels to offset symptoms of depression and elevate mood.

Use of natural diuretics may also help to reduce fluid retention (see the "Management" section on dysmenorrhea earlier in the chapter for more information). Nutritional supplements may assist in symptom relief. Supplementation of calcium and vitamin B_6 have been shown to be moderately effective in relieving symptoms, to have few side effects, and to be safe. High doses of vitamin D have also been associated with a decrease in symptoms (Bahrami, Avan, Sadeghnia, et al., 2018). Daily supplements of evening primrose oil are reportedly useful in relieving breast symptoms with minimal side effects, but research reports are conflicting. Chasteberry has been found to alleviate symptoms of PMS (Jafari & Orenstein, 2015). Inhalation aromatherapy (lavender oil) may be useful in helping women cope with PMS (Uzuncakman & Alkaya, 2018). Other herbal therapies have long been used to treat PMS; however, research on their effectiveness is lacking, or studies are flawed.

Nurses can explain the relation between cyclic estrogen fluctuation and changes in serotonin levels, as these can also lead to mood changes. Serotonin is one of the brain chemicals that help one to cope with normal life stresses. Different management strategies recommended for PMS help to produce a more stable mood by maintaining serotonin levels. Support groups or individual or couples counseling may be helpful. Stress-reduction techniques may also help with symptom management.

If these strategies do not provide significant symptom relief in 1 to 2 months, medication is often added. Many medications have been used in treatment of PMS, but no single medication alleviates all PMS symptoms. Medications often used in the treatment of PMS include diuretics, prostaglandin inhibitors (NSAIDs), progesterone, and OCPs. These have been used mainly for the physical symptoms. Studies of progesterone have not shown that it is an effective treatment (Mendiratta, 2017). Serotonergic-activating agents, including the selective serotonin reuptake inhibitors (SSRIs)—such as fluoxetine (Prozac or Sarafem), sertraline (Zoloft), citalopram (Celexa), escitalopram (Lexapro), and paroxetine (Paxil CR)—are approved by the U.S. Food and Drug Administration (FDA) as agents that may be used to treat PMS and are the first-line pharmacologic therapy (Mendiratta). Use of these medications during the luteal phase of the menstrual cycle is less expensive and has fewer side effects than drugs used before the development of these serotonergic activating agents (Mendiratta). Common side effects are headaches, sleep disturbances, dizziness, weight gain, dry mouth, and decreased libido.

Endometriosis

Endometriosis is characterized by the presence and growth of endometrial tissue outside of the uterus. The tissue may be implanted on the ovaries; anterior and posterior cul-de-sac; broad, uterosacral, and round ligaments; rectovaginal septum; sigmoid colon; appendix; pelvic peritoneum; cervix; and inguinal area (Fig. 6.2). Endometrial lesions have been found in the vagina and surgical scars and on the vulva, perineum, and bladder. They have also been found on sites far from the pelvic area, such as the thoracic cavity, gallbladder, and heart. A cystic lesion of endometriosis found in the ovary is sometimes described as a chocolate cyst because of the dark coloring of the contents of the cyst, which is caused by the presence of old blood.

Endometrial tissue contains uterine glands and stroma (connective tissue) and responds to cyclic hormone stimulation in the same way that the uterine endometrium does but often out of phase with it. The tissue grows during the proliferative and secretory phases of the cycle. During or immediately after menstruation the tissue bleeds, resulting in an inflammatory response with subsequent fibrosis and adhesions to adjacent organs.

The overall incidence of endometriosis is 5% to 15% in reproductive-age women, 30% to 45% in infertile women, and 33% in women with chronic pelvic pain (Advincula, Troung, & Lobo, 2017b). Although the condition usually develops in the third or fourth decade of life, endometriosis has been found in adolescents with disabling pelvic pain or abnormal vaginal bleeding. Endometriosis may worsen with repeated cycles, or it may remain asymptomatic and undiagnosed, eventually disappearing after menopause. However, it has been reported to occur in about 5% of postmenopausal women receiving menopausal hormone therapy. Endometriosis was previously considered to be a rare occurrence in adolescents, but currently it is estimated that approximately 50% of teens with pelvic pain are found to have endometriosis (Advincula et al., 2017).

Several theories concerning the cause of endometriosis have been suggested. However, the etiology and pathology of this condition

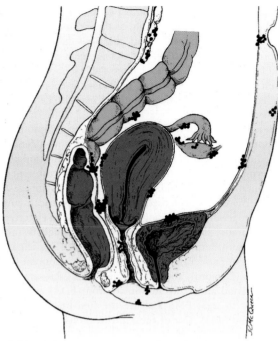

Fig. 6.2 Common Sites of Endometriosis. (From Lentz, G. M., Lobo, R. A., Gershenson, D. M., et al. [Eds.]. [2012]. *Comprehensive gynecology* [6th ed.]. Philadelphia: Elsevier.)

continue to be poorly understood. One of the most widely accepted theories is transplantation or retrograde menstruation. According to this theory, during menstruation endometrial tissue is refluxed through the uterine tubes (also referred to as the fallopian tubes) into the peritoneal cavity, where it implants on the ovaries and other organs. Retrograde menstruation has been documented in a number of menstruating women. For most women endometrial tissue outside the uterus is destroyed before it can implant or seed in the peritoneal cavity or elsewhere. A recent theory is that there is an interaction between the amount of retrograde menstruation and an individual woman's immunologic response, which may be influenced by ethnic and genetic variability (Advincula et al., 2017).

There is a wide variation of symptoms among women with endometriosis. It is interesting that often the extent of pain is not correlated with the severity of endometriosis (Advincula et al., 2017). The major symptoms are pelvic pain, dysmenorrhea, and dyspareunia (painful intercourse). Women may also have chronic noncyclic pelvic pain, pelvic heaviness, or pain radiating into the thighs. Many women report bowel symptoms such as diarrhea, pain with defecation, and constipation caused by avoiding defecation because of the pain. Other symptoms include abnormal bleeding (heavy menstrual bleeding, or premenstrual staining) and pain during exercise as a result of adhesions (Advincula et al.).

Impaired fertility may result from adhesions around the uterus that pull the uterus into a fixed, retroverted position. Adhesions around the uterine tubes may block the fimbriated ends or prevent the directional movement of the tubal cilia that carry the ovum to the uterus.

Management

Treatment is based on the severity of symptoms and the goals of the woman or couple. Women without pain who do not want to become pregnant need no treatment. In women with mild pain who may desire a future pregnancy, treatment may be limited to the use of NSAIDs during menstruation (see earlier discussion of these medications).

Suppression of endogenous estrogen production and subsequent endometrial lesion growth is the cornerstone of management of the disease. Two main classes of medications are used to suppress endogenous estrogen levels: GnRH agonists and androgen derivatives. GnRH agonist therapy (leuprolide [Lupron], nafarelin acetate [Synarel], or goserelin acetate [Zoladex]) acts by suppressing pituitary gonadotropin secretion. FSH and LH stimulation of the ovary declines markedly, and ovarian function decreases significantly. A medically induced menopause develops, resulting in anovulation and amenorrhea. Shrinkage of already established endometrial tissue, significant pain relief, and interruption in further lesion development follow. The hypoestrogenism results in hot flashes in almost all women. Trabecular bone loss is common, although most loss is reversible within 12 to 24 months after the medication is stopped (Advincula et al., 2017).

Leuprolide (3.75-mg intramuscular injection given once a month) (Dewel, 2015), nafarelin (200 mg administered twice daily by nasal spray) (MedicineNet.com), and goserelin (3.6 mg every 28 days by subcutaneous implant) (Dewel; Drugs.com, 2017) are effective and well tolerated. These medications reduce endometrial lesions and pelvic pain associated with endometriosis and have posttreatment pregnancy rates similar to those of danazol (Danocrine) therapy. Common side effects of these drugs are those of natural menopause—hot flashes and vaginal dryness. Occasionally women report headaches and muscle aches. Treatment is usually limited to 6 months to minimize bone loss. It is possible, although unlikely, for a woman to become pregnant while taking a GnRH agonist. Because the potential teratogenicity of this drug is unclear, women should use a barrier contraceptive during treatment.

Danazol, a mildly androgenic synthetic steroid, suppresses FSH and LH secretion, thus producing anovulation and hypogonadotropism. This results in decreased secretion of estrogen and progesterone and regression of endometrial tissue. Danazol can produce side effects severe enough to cause a woman to discontinue the drug. Such effects include masculinizing traits (weight gain, edema, decreased breast size, oily skin, hirsutism, and deepening of the voice), all of which often disappear when treatment is discontinued. Other side effects are amenorrhea, hot flashes, vaginal dryness, insomnia, and decreased libido. Migraine headaches, dizziness, fatigue, and depression are also reported. Danazol treatment has been reported to adversely affect lipids, with a decrease in high-density lipoprotein (HDL) levels and an increase in low-density lipoprotein (LDL) levels. Danazol should never be prescribed when pregnancy is suspected, and barrier contraception should be used with it because ovulation may not be suppressed. Danazol can produce pseudohermaphroditism in female fetuses. The medication is contraindicated in women with liver disease and should be used with caution in women with cardiac and renal disease. Danazol is less frequently used than other medical therapies to treat endometriosis (Advincula et al., 2017).

Women who have early symptomatic disease and can postpone pregnancy may be treated with continuous OCPs that have a low estrogen-to-progestin ratio and will help to shrink endometrial tissue. The OCPs are taken continuously for 6 to 12 months without any withdrawal time for the OCP. This approach is believed to lead to a more complete suppression, thus decreasing the endometriosis (Advincula et al., 2017). There can be some breakthrough bleeding, however. Any low-dose OCP can be used if taken for 15 weeks, followed by 1 week of withdrawal. This therapy is associated with minimal side effects and can be taken for extended periods.

Continuous combined hormonal therapy (HT; OCPs, estrogen/progestin patch, estrogen/progestin vaginal ring) for menstrual suppression and administration of NSAIDs comprise the usual treatment for adolescents younger than 16 years of age who have endometriosis.

GnRH agonist therapy for severe symptoms may have possible adverse effects on bone mineralization in adolescents; thus bone mineral density should be carefully monitored. For women who have problems tolerating OCPs, changing to a progestin (norethisterone acetate [NETA]) at 2.5 mg/d decreases symptomatic endometriosis (Vercellini, Ottolini, Frattarulolo, et al., 2018). It has been shown that women who cannot tolerate progestins may switch to OCPs, although better results were seen with the OCP-to-progestin change.

Surgical intervention is often needed for severe, acute, or incapacitating symptoms. Decisions regarding the extent and type of surgery are influenced by a woman's age, desire for children, and location of the disease. For women who do not want to preserve their ability to have children, the only definitive cure is total abdominal hysterectomy (TAH) with bilateral salpingectomy and oophorectomy (BSO). In women who want children and in whom the disease does not prevent childbearing, reproductive capacity should be retained through careful removal by laparoscopic surgery or laser therapy (coagulation, vaporization, or resection) of all endometrial tissue possible with retention of ovarian function (Advincula et al., 2017).

Regardless of the type of treatment (short of TAH with BSO), endometriosis recurs in approximately 40% of women. Thus, in many women, endometriosis is a chronic disease with conditions such as chronic pain or infertility. Counseling and education are critical components of nursing care for those with endometriosis. Women need an honest discussion of treatment options, with review of the potential risks and benefits of each. Because pelvic pain is a subjective, personal experience that can be frightening, support is important. Sexual dysfunction resulting from dyspareunia is common and may necessitate referral for counseling. Support groups for women with endometriosis may be found in some locations. Resolve (www.resolve.org), an organization for infertile couples, or the Endometriosis Association (http://endometriosisassn.org/) may also be helpful. The nursing care discussed in the previous section on dysmenorrhea is appropriate for managing chronic pelvic pain and dysmenorrhea experienced by women with endometriosis (see Nursing Care Plan).

Alterations in Cyclic Bleeding

Women often experience changes in amount, duration, interval, or regularity of menstrual bleeding. Common concerns include menstruation that is infrequent (oligomenorrhea), is scanty at normal intervals (hypomenorrhea), is excessive (menorrhagia), or occurs between periods (metrorrhagia).

Oligomenorrhea/Hypomenorrhea

The term oligomenorrhea is often used to describe decreased menstruation, either in amount, duration, or both. However, oligomenorrhea more correctly refers to infrequent menstrual periods characterized by intervals of 40 to 45 days or longer and hypomenorrhea to scanty bleeding at normal intervals. The causes of oligomenorrhea are often abnormalities of hypothalamic, pituitary, or ovarian function. Oligomenorrhea can also be physiologic or part of a woman's normal pattern for the first few years after menarche or for several years before menopause.

Treatment is aimed at reversing the underlying cause if possible. HT using progestins, with or without estrogens, may also be used to prevent complications of unopposed estrogen production (endometrial hyperplasia or carcinoma) or of absent estrogen (vaginal dryness, hot flashes or flushes, or osteoporosis).

Women with menstruation characterized by prolonged intervals between cycles need education and counseling. The cause of the condition and the rationale for a specific treatment should be discussed, as should advantages and disadvantages of HT. If a woman chooses medical intervention, she should be provided with written instructions, taught how to take the medications, and made aware of their side effects. Teaching and counseling should emphasize the importance of the woman keeping careful records of her vaginal bleeding.

One of the most common causes of scanty menstrual flow is OCPs. If a woman is considering OCPs for contraception, it is important to explain in advance that the use of OCPs can decrease menstrual flow by as much as two-thirds. This effect is caused by the continuous action of the progestin component, which produces a decidualized endometrium with atrophic glands.

Hypomenorrhea also may be caused by structural abnormalities of the endometrium or the uterus that result in partial disintegration of the endometrium. These conditions include Asherman syndrome, in which adhesions resulting from curettage or infection obliterate the endometrial cavity, and congenital partial obstruction of the vagina.

Metrorrhagia

Metrorrhagia, or intermenstrual bleeding, refers to any episode of bleeding—whether spotting, menses, or hemorrhage—that occurs at a time other than the normal menses. In *mittelstaining,* also referred to as *mittelschmerz,* a small amount of bleeding or spotting occurs at the time of ovulation (14 days before onset of the next menses); this

---

◎ NURSING CARE PLAN

The Woman With Endometriosis

Client Problem	Expected Outcome	Nursing Interventions	Rationales
Discomfort related to menstruation secondary to endometriosis	Stacey will verbalize a decrease in intensity and frequency of pain during each menstrual cycle.	Assess location, type, and duration of pain and history of discomfort.	To determine severity of dysmenorrhea
		Administer nonsteroidal anti-inflammatory drugs as indicated.	To assist with pain relief
		Administer hormone-altering medications as ordered.	To suppress ovulation and subsequently suppress endometrial tissue lesion growth
		Provide information about use of non-pharmacologic methods such as heat.	To increase blood flow to the pelvic region
Need for health teaching related to insufficient understanding about disease process and prescribed therapy and the effects on self-care	Stacey will verbalize correct understanding of endometriosis and the use of self-care methods and prescribed therapies.	Assess woman's current understanding of the disorder and related therapies.	To validate the accuracy of knowledge base
		Give information to woman regarding the disorder and treatment regimen.	To empower the woman to become a partner in her own care
Decreased self-esteem related to inability to get pregnant	Stacey will verbalize positive feelings of self-worth.	Provide therapeutic communication. Include husband as appropriate. Refer to support group.	To validate feelings and provide support To enhance feelings of self-worth through group communication

is considered normal. The cause of mittelstaining is not known; however, its common occurrence can be documented by its repetition in the menstrual cycle.

Women taking OCPs may have midcycle bleeding or spotting. (See Chapter 8 for a discussion of the side effects of OCPs.) If the OCP does not maintain a sufficiently hypoplastic endometrium, the endometrium will begin to shed, usually in small amounts at a time, a process termed *breakthrough bleeding*, which is most common in the first three cycles of OCPs. The reduced-potency OCPs (which are safer) lower the amounts of available hormones, making it more important that blood levels be kept constant. Taking the pill at exactly the same time each day may alleviate the woman's problem. If the spotting continues, a different formulation of the OCP that increases either the estrogen or progestin component of the pill can be tried.

Progestin-only contraceptive methods (oral and injectable) may also cause midcycle bleeding, especially in the first several cycles. Women should be advised of this and counseled to report continuation of breakthrough bleeding after the first three to six cycles to their health care provider.

The causes of intermenstrual bleeding are varied (Table 6.3). It is important for the nurse to consider the possibility that any woman who has not undergone menopause and seeks care for intermenstrual bleeding is or may recently have been pregnant.

Treatment of intermenstrual bleeding depends on the cause and may include reassurance and education concerning mittelstaining, observation of three menstrual cycles for a suspected functional ovarian cyst, adjustment of an OCP, removal of foreign bodies, and treatment for vaginal infection. More complex treatment may consist of removal of polyps; evaluation and treatment of an abnormal Papanicolaou (Pap) test, including colposcopy, biopsy, cautery, cryosurgery, or conization; and surgery, chemotherapy, or radiation treatment for malignancy. Important nursing roles include reassurance, counseling, education, and support.

Menorrhagia

Menorrhagia (hypermenorrhea) is defined as excessive menstrual bleeding, in either duration or amount. The causes of heavy menstrual bleeding are many, including hormonal disturbances, systemic disease, benign and malignant neoplasms, infection, and contraception (IUDs). A single episode of heavy bleeding may occur, or a woman may have regular flooding as a pattern in which she changes tampons or pads every few hours for several days. Hemoglobin and hematocrit are objective indicators of actual blood loss and should always be assessed.

A single episode of heavy bleeding may signal an early pregnancy loss. This type of bleeding is often thought to be a period that is heavier than usual, perhaps delayed, and is associated with abdominal pain or pelvic discomfort. When early pregnancy loss is suspected, a hematocrit and serum β-hCG pregnancy test should be done.

Infectious and inflammatory processes such as acute or chronic endometritis and salpingitis may cause heavy menstrual bleeding. Although rare, systemic diseases of nonreproductive origin such as blood dyscrasias, hypothyroidism, and lupus erythematosus can also cause hypermenorrhea. In obese women, anovulation caused by increased peripheral conversion of androstenedione to estrogen may develop and manifest as menorrhagia. Medications may also cause abnormal bleeding. Chemotherapy, anticoagulants, neuroleptics, and steroid hormone therapy have all been associated with excessive flow.

Uterine leiomyomas (fibroids or myomas) are a common cause of heavy menstrual bleeding. Fibroids are benign tumors of the smooth muscle of the uterus; their cause is unknown. Fibroids occur

TABLE 6.3　Causes of Intermenstrual Bleeding

Reproductive Disorder	Pregnancy Problems	Infections
Functional ovarian cyst	Pregnancy implantation	Endometritis
Cervical erosion	Miscarriage	Sexually transmitted infections
Leiomyoma	Ectopic pregnancy	ted infections
Uterine or endocervical polyps	Molar pregnancy	
Trauma	Retained placenta after miscarriage, or induced abortion	
Foreign body		
Malignancy of reproductive tract	Retained placenta after birth	

in approximately 70% of women, with about 50% having symptoms (Ryntz & Lobo, 2017b). Other uterine growths ranging from endometrial polyps to adenocarcinoma and endometrial cancer are common causes of heavy menstrual and intermenstrual bleeding.

Treatment for heavy menstrual bleeding depends on the cause of the bleeding. If the bleeding is related to the contraceptive method (e.g., an IUD), the health care professional can provide factual

⚠ NURSING ALERT

If the woman herself considers the amount or duration of bleeding to be excessive, the problem should be investigated.

information and reassurance and also discuss other contraceptive options.

If there is no known cause for the bleeding and anatomic causes have been ruled out, therapy is aimed at reducing the amount of heavy bleeding using medical rather than surgical approaches. Current options for treatment include estrogens, progestogen, NSAIDS, antifibrinolytic agents, and GnRH (Hartmann, Fonnesbeck, Surawicz, et al., 2017; Ryntz & Lobo, 2017b). Nurses should focus on the correct administration of these treatments and on reducing potential adverse side effects, such as gastrointestinal distress with NSAIDs.

If bleeding is related to the presence of fibroids, the degree of disability and discomfort associated with the fibroids and the woman's plans for childbearing influence treatment decisions (Fortin, Flyckt, & Falcone, 2018). Treatment options include pharmacologic and surgical management. Most fibroids can be managed by frequent examinations to judge growth, if any, and correction of anemia if present. It is important to warn women with bleeding between menses to avoid using aspirin because of its tendency to increase bleeding. Pharmacologic treatment is directed toward temporarily reducing symptoms, shrinking the myoma, and reducing its blood supply. This reduction is often accomplished with the use of a GnRH agonist or ulipristal acetate (UPA) (Piecak, Milart, Wozniakowska, & Pazkowski, 2017). There is evidence that following cessation of treatment, blood loss may return to levels that existed prior to treatment (Ryntz & Lobo, 2017). If the woman wishes to retain her childbearing potential, a myomectomy may be performed. Myomectomy, or removal of the tumors by laparoscopic or hysteroscopic resection or laser surgery, is particularly difficult if multiple myomas must be removed. One in four women will have a hysterectomy performed within 20 years of having a myomectomy. If the woman does not want to preserve her childbearing potential or if she has severe symptoms (severe anemia, severe pain, considerable disruption of lifestyle), uterine artery embolization (UAE) (a procedure that blocks blood supply to fibroid), or hysterectomy (removal of uterus) may be performed. Neither procedure is considered to be very effective unless the cause of the excessive bleeding is fibroids (Ryntz & Lobo). Important nursing roles include reassurance, counseling, education, and support.

Abnormal Uterine Bleeding

Abnormal uterine bleeding (AUB) is any form of uterine bleeding that is irregular in amount, duration, or timing and is not related to regular menstrual bleeding; it affects nearly one-third of women of reproductive age (Lam, Anderson, Lopes, et al, 2017). Box 6.1 lists possible causes of AUB (Cheong, Cameron, & Critchely, 2017; Munro, Critchley, Broder, et al., 2011).

AUB can be anovulatory or ovulatory, but it is most commonly caused by anovulation. When no surge of LH occurs or if insufficient progesterone is produced by the corpus luteum to support the endometrium, it will begin to involute and shed. This process most often occurs at the extremes of a woman's reproductive years, when the menstrual cycle is just becoming established at menarche or when it draws to a close at menopause. AUB also occurs with any condition that gives rise to chronic anovulation associated with continuous estrogen production. Such conditions include obesity, hyperthyroidism and hypothyroidism, polycystic ovarian syndrome, and any of the endocrine conditions discussed in the sections on amenorrhea and infrequent menstruation.

Management

The most effective medical treatment of acute bleeding episodes of AUB is oral or intravenous estrogen. D&C may be done if the bleeding has not stopped within 12 to 24 hours. An oral conjugated estrogen and progestin regimen is usually given for at least 3 months after the acute phase has passed. Such long-term treatment will help prevent recurrence of the pattern of AUB and hemorrhage. If the woman desires contraception, she should continue to take OCPs. If she has no need for contraception, the treatment may be stopped to assess the woman's bleeding pattern. If her menses do not resume, a progestin regimen (e.g., medroxyprogesterone, 10 mg each day for 10 days before the expected date of her menstrual period) may be prescribed after ruling out pregnancy. This is done to prevent persistent anovulation with chronic unopposed endogenous estrogen hyperstimulation of the endometrium, which can result in eventual atypical tissue changes. This approach usually successfully leads to regular withdrawal bleeding (Ryntz & Lobo, 2017).

Nursing roles include informing clients of their options, counseling and education as indicated, and referring to the appropriate specialists and health care services. If the recurrent, heavy bleeding is not controlled by hormone therapy or D&C, ablation of the endometrium through laser treatment may be performed.

Nursing assessments for women who have a menstrual disorder include the following:

- Taking a thorough menstrual, obstetric, sexual, and contraceptive history

---

BOX 6.1 Possible Causes of Abnormal Uterine Bleeding

Pregnancy-Related Conditions
- Threatened or spontaneous miscarriage
- Retained products of conception after elective abortion
- Ectopic pregnancy
- Placenta previa/placental abruption
- Trophoblastic disease

Lower Reproductive Tract Infections
- Cervicitis
- Endometritis
- Myometritis
- Salpingitis

Benign Anatomic Abnormalities
- Adenomyosis
- Leiomyomata
- Polyps of the cervix or endometrium

Neoplasms
- Endometrial hyperplasia
- Cancer of cervix and endometrium
- Hormonally active tumors (rare)
- Vaginal tumors (rare)

Malignant Lesions
- Cervical squamous cell carcinoma
- Endometrial adenocarcinoma

- Estrogen-producing ovarian tumors
- Testosterone-producing ovarian tumors
- Leiomyosarcoma

Trauma
- Genital injury (accidental, coital trauma, sexual abuse)
- Foreign body
- Lacerations

Systemic Conditions
- Adrenal hyperplasia and Cushing disease
- Blood dyscrasias
- Coagulopathies
- Hypothalamic suppression (from stress, weight loss, excessive exercise)
- Polycystic ovarian syndrome
- Thyroid disease
- Pituitary adenoma or hyperprolactinemia
- Severe organ disease (renal or liver failure)

Iatrogenic Causes
- Medications with estrogenic activity
- Anticoagulants
- Exogenous hormone use (oral contraceptives, menopausal hormone therapy)
- Selective serotonin reuptake inhibitors
- Tamoxifen
- Intrauterine devices
- Herbal preparation (ginseng)

Modified from Ryntz, T., & Lobo, R. A. (2017). Abnormal uterine bleeding: Etiology and management of acute and chronic excessive bleeding. In R. A. Lobo, D. M. Gershenson, G. M. Lentz, et al. (Eds.), *Comprehensive gynecology* (7th ed.). Philadelphia: Elsevier.

- Exploring the woman's perceptions of her condition, cultural or ethnic influences, lifestyle, and patterns of coping
- Evaluating the amount of pain or bleeding experienced and its effect on daily activities
- Noting any home remedies and prescriptions to relieve discomfort. A symptom diary, in which the woman records emotions, behaviors, physical symptoms, diet, and exercise and rest patterns, is a useful diagnostic tool.

In addition to the medical, surgical, and nursing interventions discussed with each problem, additional nursing interventions may include the following:

- Accepting the woman's symptoms as valid
- Correlating data from the daily diary of emotional status, subjective feelings, and physical state with physiologic changes
- Encouraging the woman to express her feelings about her symptoms
- Providing information about therapeutic options (pharmacologic and nonpharmacologic) so the woman or the couple can make the choices considered best
- Providing information about local support groups

MENOPAUSE

With the increasing life span of American women, most can expect to live one-third of their lives after their reproductive years. As they age, many women experience transitions that present challenges—such as changing health, work, or marital status—that require adaptation. At no time is this more true than during menopause and the changes associated with it. In the United States, menopause usually occurs during the late 40s and early 50s, with a mean age of 51.4 years (Pace & Secor, 2019). The average age for the onset of the perimenopausal transition is 46 years; 95% of women experience the onset between ages 42 and 58 years (O'Neill & Eden, 2017). The average duration of the perimenopause period is 4 to 8 years, with 95% of women reaching postmenopause by age 58 (Lobo, 2017a; Pace & Secor). Cigarette smoking and a history of short intermenstrual intervals seem to decrease the age at onset of menopause. African American and Hispanic women in the United States experience menopause earlier than Caucasian women. However, heredity is the major determinant of age at menopause; genetics may explain most of the variation in age at the onset of menopause (Lobo, 2017a).

Perimenopause is the period that encompasses the transition from normal ovulatory cycles to the cessation of menses; it is marked by irregular menstrual cycles. Another term used to signal the period when a woman moves from the reproductive stage of life through the perimenopausal transition and menopause to the postmenopausal years is the **climacteric**. *Menopause* refers to the complete cessation of menses and is a single physiologic event said to occur when women have not had menstrual flow or spotting for a year; it can be identified only in retrospect. **Surgical menopause** occurs with hysterectomy and bilateral oophorectomy. **Postmenopause** is the time after menopause.

Although all women have similar hormonal changes with menopause, the experience of each woman is influenced by her age, cultural background, health, type of menopause (spontaneous or surgical), childbearing desires, and relationships. Women may view menopause as a major change in their lives—either positive, such as freedom from troublesome dysmenorrhea and the need for contraception, or negative, such as feeling "old" or losing one's childbearing potential.

Physiologic Characteristics

Knowledge of the normal changes that occur during perimenopause is essential in assessing menopausal experiences and problems. Natural menopause is a gradual process with progressive increases in anovulatory cycles and eventual cessation of menses. In the 2 to 8 years preceding menopause, subtle hormonal changes eventually lead to altered menstrual function and later to amenorrhea. When women are in their 40s, anovulation occurs more often, menstrual cycles increase in length, and ovarian follicles become less sensitive to hormonal stimulation from FSH and LH. Because of these changes, a follicle is stimulated to the point that an ovum grows to maturity and is released in some months, whereas in other months no ovulation takes place. Without ovulation and release of an ovum, progesterone is not produced by the corpus luteum. The lining continues to grow until it lacks a sufficient blood supply, at which point it bleeds. During this time a woman's cycle becomes more irregular. She may miss periods; have shorter or lighter periods or longer, heavier periods; and have clotting. FSH levels become elevated, reflecting an attempt to stimulate a follicle to produce estrogen.

Physical Changes During the Perimenopausal Period

Bleeding

During the perimenopausal years, women may have longer menstrual periods that differ in the type of bleeding. They may have 2 to 3 days of spotting followed by 1 to 2 days of heavy bleeding, or they may have regular menses followed by 2 to 3 days of spotting. Such symptoms are characteristic of degenerating corpus luteum function. After menopause, women continue to have small amounts of circulating estrogen. Although the ovaries do not produce estrogen, androgens (androstenedione and testosterone) are produced for some time after menopause. Androgens produced by the adrenal glands are converted to estrone, a form of estrogen, in the liver and fat cells. With advanced age the ovaries stop producing androstenedione, which further limits the amount of estrone in the body. Obese women are more likely to have dysfunctional uterine bleeding and endometrial hyperplasia because those with more body fat have higher circulating levels of estrone. This occurs because the estrogen that is stored in the body's fat cells is converted into a form of estrogen (estrone) that is available to the estrogen receptors within the endometrium.

Genital Changes

The vagina and urethra are estrogen-sensitive tissues, and low levels of estrogen can cause atrophy of both. Age-related vaginal changes not affected by estrogen also occur. Through both processes the vaginal membranes thin, hold less moisture, and lubricate more slowly. However, not all women have symptoms of genital atrophy. Women who are sexually active have less vaginal atrophy and fewer problems related to intercourse. Thin women tend to have more symptoms related to reduced estrogen levels, such as vaginal dryness, because of lack of adipose tissue and thus stored estrogen. Additionally, vaginal pH increases, the growth of *Lactobacillus* can be depressed, and other bacteria tend to multiply. This combination of factors can lead to vaginitis.

Dyspareunia (painful intercourse) can occur because the vagina becomes smaller, the vaginal walls become thinner and drier, and lubrication during sexual stimulation takes longer. Intercourse becomes painful and may result in postcoital bleeding. Some women decide to forgo intercourse altogether.

In some women these changes—the shrinking of the uterus, the vulva, and the distal portion of the urethra—associated with aging lead to disturbing symptoms, including urinary frequency, dysuria, uterine prolapse, and stress incontinence. Vaginal relaxation with cystocele, rectocele, and uterine prolapse is not caused by reduced estrogen levels but may be a delayed result of childbearing or another cause of weakness of the pelvic support structures. Urinary frequency sometimes occurs after menopause because the distal portion of the urethra, which has the same embryologic origin as the reproductive organs, shortens and shrinks. Irritants have easier access to the urinary tract with its short urethra and may cause frequency and urinary tract infections.

Urinary incontinence and uterine displacement are two other common age-related rather than menopause-related findings in the postmenopausal period. These conditions are discussed in Chapter 11.

Vasomotor Instability

Investigators have devoted significant attention to identifying ovarian, hypothalamic, and pituitary hormonal mechanisms that produce symptoms related to menopause. Two symptoms appear to increase in incidence as women progress through menopause: hot flashes and night sweats. Many of the other changes commonly associated with menopause—such as decrease in size of genital structures, skin changes, and changes in breast size—are more correctly attributed to aging.

Vasomotor instability in the form of hot flashes or flushes is a result of fluctuating estrogen levels and is the most common disturbance of the perimenopausal years, occurring in up to 75% of women having natural menopause (Lobo, 2017a; Noble, 2018; Pace & Secor, 2019) and 90% of women who have a surgical menopause. In the United States, Hispanic and African American women report a higher incidence of these symptoms than do Caucasian women; Asian women have the lowest incidence (Lobo, 2017a; Pace & Secor, 2019). Vasomotor instability occurs most frequently in the first two postmenopausal years; the number of episodes decreases over time. However, some women have hot flashes before menopause and continue to have them for 10 or more years afterward. During this time women experience changeable vasodilation and vasoconstriction as a hot flush (visible red flush of skin and perspiration) or hot flash (sudden warm sensation in neck, head, and chest) and night sweats. For some women, hot flashes may be an infrequent, possibly pleasant, sensation of warmth; for others, they may be an intensely unpleasant sensation of heat or warmth that can occur 20 to 50 times a day, create intense anxiety, and significantly compromise quality of life. Several factors can precipitate or aggravate an episode, including being in a crowded or warm room, ingesting alcohol or a hot drink, spicy foods, proximity to a heat source, and stress.

Night sweats, characterized by profuse perspiration and heat radiating from the body during the night, are another form of vasomotor instability experienced by many women. Their sleep may be interrupted nightly because their nightclothes and bed linens are soaked. Thereafter such women may find that they are not able to go back to sleep. Sleep deprivation is a primary complaint of women experiencing hot flashes (Lobo, 2017a; O'Neill & Eden, 2017; Pace & Secor, 2019). Other problems associated with perimenopausal fluctuations of vasoconstriction or vascular spasms include dizziness, numbness and tingling in fingers and toes, and headaches.

Mood and Behavioral Responses

The tendency to associate hormonal changes with psychologic symptoms in midlife—which has been prevalent in the medical literature for decades and continues today—was fueled by a belief that postmenopausal women have "estrogen deficiency." However, there is no concrete evidence that menopause has a deleterious effect on the mental health of midlife women. Reviews of epidemiologic studies on menopause and depression found no causal association between the two, but there

is an increased incidence of depression in menopausal women (Lobo, 2017a). Women with hot flashes and night sweats do report insomnia, fatigue from loss of sleep, and depressed mood. They complain of feeling more emotionally labile, nervous, or agitated, with less control of their emotions. However, the interaction of psychologic, biologic, and sociocultural factors is so complex that it is difficult to determine whether a woman's reported mood shifts are the result of hormonal changes, normal aging, or cultural conditioning. Most likely a woman's psychologic makeup, cultural background, intercurrent stresses, and changing life roles and circumstances are more important than estrogen levels. Dealing with teenage children; having teenagers leave home; helping aging parents; becoming widowed or divorced; the onset of a major illness or disability in the woman herself or illness, disability, or death in a spouse, relative, or friend; grieving for friends and family who are ill or dying; retirement; and financial insecurity are among the many stresses of women in their 40s and 50s.

Cultural messages also influence a woman's perception of menopause. Experiences with menopause are not universal and vary among cultural groups. Many women have accepted childbearing and child rearing as their major role in life; for them, the inability to bear children represents a significant loss. Others see menopause as the first step to old age and associate it with a loss of attractiveness, physical mobility, and energy. Western culture values youth and physical attractiveness; the wisdom gained from life experience is not valued, and older adults lose status, function, and role. No rituals give older women a special place and function. In cultures in which postmenopausal women gain status—such as India, the Far East, and the South Pacific islands—depression among menopausal women is not observed. Western women, however, may have little to compensate for their losses.

For other women, menopause is not a loss or a symbol of loss but a relief. Menopause means relief from the fear of pregnancy, the discomfort and bother of menstruation, and the inconveniences of contraception.

The ability to cope with any stress involves three factors: the person's perception or understanding of the event, the support system, and coping mechanisms. Nurses counseling a woman in the perimenopausal years must therefore assess her understanding of perimenopausal changes, her perceptions of stressful experiences, her support systems, and her coping skills.

Health Risks of Perimenopausal Women

Osteoporosis and coronary heart disease are the major health risks of perimenopausal women. These conditions are the focus of the following discussion.

Osteoporosis

Aging is associated with a progressive decrease in bone density in both men and women. Osteoporosis is a generalized metabolic disease characterized by decreased bone mass and an increased incidence of bone fractures. Normally there is a dynamic balance between bone formation (osteoblastic activity) and bone resorption (osteoclastic activity). Because one of the functions of estrogen is to stimulate the osteoblasts, the postmenopausal decrease in estrogen levels causes an imbalance between bone formation and resorption. Old bone deteriorates faster than new bone is formed, resulting in a slow thinning of the bones. Estrogen is also required for the conversion of vitamin D to calcitonin, which is essential in the absorption of calcium by the intestine. Reduced calcium absorption from the gut, in addition to the thinning of the bones, places postmenopausal women at risk for problems associated with osteoporosis.

Osteoporosis is a major health problem in the United States, affecting more than 25 million women (Berman, Pope, & Kessenich, 2019). It is one of the key diseases that predominantly affect women. In fact, half of all women aged 50 and older will break a bone due to osteoporosis in their lifetimes and 2 million bone breaks are caused by osteoporosis every year. Approximately 50% of U.S. women have some degree of osteoporosis, placing women who are older than 50 at particular risk in their lifetimes for breaking a bone as a result of osteoporosis. One in two Caucasian women will have changes severe enough to predispose them to fractures. In the United States, the incidence of osteoporosis-related fractures has increased (Berman et al.).

Less than 50% of women with a hip fracture return to their previous level of function, with 1-year mortality rates ranging from 12% to 20% (Berman et al., 2019). During the first 5 to 6 years after menopause, women lose bone six times more rapidly than men. By age 65, one-third of women have had a vertebral fracture; by age 81, one-third have had a hip fracture. By the time women reach age 80, they have lost 47% of their trabecular bone, concentrated in the vertebrae, the pelvis and other flat bones, and the epiphyses (Berman et al.). The most well-defined risk factor for osteoporosis is the loss of the protective effect of estrogen associated with the cessation of ovarian function, particularly at menopause. Women at risk are likely to be Caucasian or Asian, small-boned, and thin. Obese women have higher estrogen levels resulting from the conversion of androgens in adipose tissue; mechanical stress from extra weight also helps preserve bone mass. A family history of the disease is common. Much more research must be done to determine genetic testing for those at higher risk for osteoporosis.

Inadequate calcium intake is a risk factor, particularly during adolescence and into the third and fourth decades, when peak bone mass is attained. An excessive caffeine intake increases calcium excretion, causing a systemic acidosis that stimulates bone resorption. Vitamin D deficiency can affect the physiologic regulation and stimulation of intestinal absorption of calcium (National Osteoporosis Foundation [NOF], 2019). Smoking is associated with earlier and greater bone loss and decreases estrogen production. Excessive alcohol intake interferes with calcium absorption and depresses bone formation. A greater intake of phosphorus than of calcium, which occurs with soft drink consumption, may be a risk factor. Other risk factors include steroid

therapy and disorders such as hypogonadism, hyperthyroidism, and diabetes mellitus.

The first sign of osteoporosis is often a loss of height, resulting from vertebral fracture and collapse (Fig. 6.3). Back pain, especially in the lower back, may or may not be present. Later signs include "dowager's hump," where the vertebrae can no longer support the upper body in an upright position, and fractured hip, where the fracture often precedes a fall. Damage to the vertebrae usually precedes bone loss in the hip by an average of 10 years. Osteoporosis cannot be detected by radiographic examination until 30% to 50% of the bone mass has been lost; thus routine screening is not warranted in women younger than age 65. However, bone density testing is recommended for women who are 65 and postmenopausal women 50 to 69 years of age based on risk factors (Berman, et al., 2019; U.S. Preventive Health Services Task Force, 2011).

🏠 COMMUNITY ACTIVITY

- Visit the Office of Women's Health website at www.WomensHealth.gov. Select menopause from the list of topics on women's health issues to understand better the resources available to women who have questions about menopause.
- Visit the National Osteoporosis Foundation website at https://www.nof. org/. Review the client information regarding osteoporosis, prevention, management, and finding a doctor. What are the resources for women with osteoporosis in your community?
- Visit the North American Menopause Society (NAMS) website at www.menopause.org. Review Memo Note and the Menopause Guidebook. How can this information help you in teaching your clients about how to manage menopausal symptoms?

Coronary Heart Disease

A woman's risk of developing and dying of cardiovascular disease increases after menopause. Diseases of the heart are the leading cause of death for U.S. women. The lifetime risk of death from coronary heart disease is 31% in postmenopausal women, in contrast to a 3% risk of death from breast cancer (Lobo, 2017a). Known risk factors for coronary heart disease include obesity, cigarette smoking, elevated cholesterol levels, hypertension, diabetes mellitus, family history of cardiac disease, alcohol abuse, and the effects of aging on the cardiovascular system (Lobo). Estrogen has a favorable effect on circulating lipids, decreasing LDL and total cholesterol and increasing HDL. It has a direct anti-atherosclerotic effect on arteries. Postmenopausal women are at risk for coronary artery disease because of changes in their lipid metabolism: a decline in serum levels of HDL cholesterol, and an increase in LDL levels (Lobo). These changes can be reduced by diet and exercise.

Menopausal Hormonal Therapy

Until 2002 **menopausal hormonal therapy** (MHT)—either as *estrogen therapy (ET)*, in which a woman takes only estrogen, or *HT*, in which she takes both estrogen and progestins—was widely prescribed for discomforts associated with the perimenopausal years, including hot flashes and vaginal and urinary tract atrophy. Findings from the Women's Health Initiative (WHI), a study by the National Institutes of Health (NIH), documented an increase in heart disease with the continuous use of combined estrogen plus progestin (NIH, 2010). There is also an increased risk for breast cancer in women taking HT, although that risk returns to normal 5 years after its discontinuation (American Cancer Society [ACS], 2017). These findings changed the way HT is

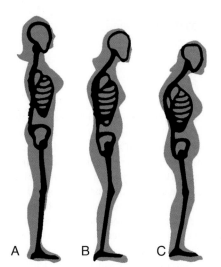

Fig. 6.3 Skeletal changes secondary to osteoporosis assessed by height and body shape at (A) age 55 years; (B) age 65 years; and (C) age 75 years.

used. Many women stopped taking HT and sought alternative therapies to treat their menopausal symptoms. Others chose to continue with the HT but had questions about the available regimens and associated risks.

The North American Menopause Society (NAMS) (2017) supports the use of ET before the age of 60 years and within 10 years after menopause at the lowest effective dose to individually treat menopausal symptoms. Risks associated with the long-term use of estrogen-progesterone therapy include stroke, venous thromboembolism, coronary heart disease, and dementia (NAMS).

Recommendations from the American College of Obstetricians and Gynecologists (ACOG) (2012, updated 2018) continue to support the use of MHT but encourage greater use of nonhormonal alternatives, such as SSRIs as well as selective serotonin-norepinephrine reuptake inhibitors (SNRIs). The recommendations also mention the use of drugs such as SSRIs, SNRIs, gabapentin, clonidine or oxybutynin to decrease vasomotor symptoms. Vaginal creams and lubricants are effective in treating vaginal dryness and atrophy (Noble, 2018). More research is needed regarding safety and effectiveness of bioidentical hormones (Noble; Thompson, Ritenbaugh, & Nichter, 2017). (See later discussion on bioidentical hormones.)

Decision to Use Hormone Therapy

All women considering ET or HT must understand that studies on HT are ongoing and there is still much to be learned. Nurses can provide information and counseling to assist women in making decisions regarding HT use. Important teaching points include the following:

- For women taking HT for short-term (1 to 3 years) relief of menopausal discomforts who do not have increased risks for cardiovascular disease, the benefits may outweigh the risks. The decision to use HT should be made between a woman and her health care provider.
- If used, MHT should be taken at the lowest effective dose for the shortest possible duration.
- When a woman decides to stop HT, symptoms will recur whether the medication is tapered or discontinued abruptly. NAMS makes

no recommendation on how to discontinue the medication, although some clinicians recommend a gradual withdrawal.

- Older women who are taking or considering HT only for the prevention of cardiovascular disease should be counseled on other methods to reduce their risks of cardiovascular disease.
- Alternatively beneficial cardiovascular effects may be associated with HT for younger, more recently menopausal women, but more research is needed in this area.
- Women who are taking HT only for the prevention of osteoporosis or other chronic conditions should be counseled regarding their personal risks and benefits in continuing the therapy. These women should be reassured that there are effective alternatives for long-term prevention. Bone density studies may also be indicated to determine the degree of risk in an individual woman (U.S. Preventive Health Services Task Force, 2011).
- Oral estrogens are associated with an increased incidence of gallbladder disease, and women with a known history of gallbladder disease should consider the use of transdermal routes (NAMS, 2017)

Side Effects

Side effects associated with estrogen use include headaches, nausea and vomiting, bloating, ankle and foot swelling, weight gain, breast soreness, brown spots on the skin, eye irritation with contact lenses, and depression. The type of estrogen used for postmenopausal HT is much less potent than the ethinyl estradiol used in OCPs and has fewer serious side effects. Side effects that occur with MHT may disappear with a change in estrogen preparation or a decrease in the dose prescribed.

Treatment Guidelines

Research in HT continues; however, nurses who counsel women about HT must understand what is available and teach women who choose to continue HT how to take the medications correctly. Thus the following discussion about the different regimens of HT is included.

There are many different estrogen preparations available as well as ways to administer them. There are oral tablets, topical creams, transdermal preparations, suppositories, and vaginal rings (Table 6.4).

TABLE 6.4   Hormone Medications for Menopausal Symptoms

Medication Name	Composition	Available Doses
Estrogens		
Oral		
Premarin	Conjugated estrogens	0.3 mg; 0.45 mg; 0.625 mg; 0.9 mg; 1.25 mg
Cenestin, Congest	Synthetic conjugated estrogens, A	0.3 mg; 045 mg; 0.625 mg; 0.9 mg; 1.25 mg; 0.3 mg; 0.625 mg; 0.9 mg, 1.25 mg, 2.5 mg; 0.3 mg, 0.625 mg, 0.9 mg, 1.25 mg; 0.3 mg, 0.625 mg, 0.9 mg, 1.25 mg
Enjuvia	Synthetic conjugated estrogens, B	0.3 mg; 0.45 mg; 0.625 mg; 0.9 mg; 1.25 mg
Estrace, various generics	Micronized estradiol	0.5 mg; 1 mg; 2 mg
Menest	Esterified estrogens	0.3 mg; 0.625 mg; 1.25 mg; 2.5 mg
Femtrace	Estradiol acetate	0.45 mg; 0.9 mg; 1.8 mg
Ortho-Est	Estropipate	0.625 mg; 1.25 mg; 2.5 mg
Transdermal		
Estraderm	Estradiol reservoir patch	0.05 mg; 0.1 mg twice weekly
Climera, Esclim, Estradot	Estradiol matrix patch	0.025 mg; 0.0375 mg; 0.05 mg; 0.075 mg; 0.1 mg once weekly
Vivelle	Estradiol matrix patch	0.05 mg; 0.1 mg twice weekly
Vivelle-Dot	Estradiol matrix patch	0.025 mg; 0.0375 mg; 0.05 mg; 0.1 mg twice weekly
Menostar	Estradiol matrix patch	0.014 mg once weekly

TABLE 6.4   Hormone Medications for Menopausal Symptoms—cont'd

Medication Name	Composition	Available Doses
Alora	Estradiol matrix patch	0.0025 mg; 0.05 mg; 0.075 mg; 0.1 mg twice weekly
Divigel	Estradiol gel 0.1%	0.003 mg; 0.009 mg; 0.027 mg daily
EstroGel	Estradiol gel 0.06%	0.035 mg daily
Elestrin	Estradiol gel 0.06%	0.0125 mg daily
Evamist	Estradiol spray	0.021 mg per spray daily; may increase to 2 or 3 sprays daily
Estrasorb	Estradiol emulsion	0.05 mg/2 packets daily
Vaginal		
Premarin cream	Conjugated estrogens	0.5-2 g/day (0.0625 mg/g)
Estrace cream	Estradiol	1 g/day (0.1 mg/g)
Femring vaginal ring	Estradiol acetate	12.4 mg or 24.8 mg; releases 0.05 mg/day or 0.10 mg/day for 90 days
Estring vaginal ring	Estradiol	2 mg; releases 7.5 mcg daily for 90 days
Vagifem vaginal tablet	Estradiol hemihydrate	25-mcg tablet twice a week
Progestogens		
Oral		
Provera	Medroxyprogesterone acetate	2.5 mg; 5 mg; 10 mg
Aygestin	Norethindrone acetate	5 mg
Micronor	Norethindrone	0.35 mg
Norgestrel	Ovrette	0.075 mg
Progesterone capsule (in peanut oil)	Prometrium	100 mg; 200 mg
Intrauterine		
Levonorgestrel	Mirena	Approximately 20 mcg/day
Vaginal		
Progesterone gel	Prochieve 4%	45 mg/applicator
Combination Estrogen-Progestin		
Oral		
Premphase	Conjugated estrogens (E)	0.625 mg E daily for 28 days
	Medroxyprogesterone acetate (P)	5 mg P on day 14 through day 28
Prempro	Conjugated estrogens (E)	0.0625 mg E plus 2.5 or 5 P daily
	Medroxyprogesterone acetate (P)	0.3 mg or 0.45 mg E plus 1.5 P daily
Activella	Estradiol (E) and norethindrone acetate (NETA)	1 mg E plus 0.5 mg NETA daily
Femhrt	Ethinyl estradiol and norethindrone acetate (NETA)	2.5 mcg E plus 0.5 mg NETA daily
Transdermal		
CombiPatch	Estradiol/norethindrone acetate (NETA)	0.05 mg estradiol/0.14 mg NETA or 0.05 mg estradiol/0.25 mg NETA twice weekly
Climera Pro	Estradiol and levonorgestrel	0.045 mg/0.015 mg weekly

PMS, premenstrual syndrome
Modified from North American Menopause Society. (2012). *Hormone products for postmenopausal use in the United States and Canada*. Retrieved from www.menopause.org/docs/professional/htcharts.pdf?sfvrsn=6. Copyright © The North American Menopause Society, November 19, 2012.

There are multiple dosing regimen options for combining progesterone with estrogen for women who have a uterus. According to NAMS, ET is the treatment of choice for vulvar and vaginal atrophy, and low-dose local vaginal ET is best if the woman is only experiencing vaginal symptoms. In addition, NAMS (2017) recommends transdermal or low-dose estrogen for women at risk for venous thromboembolism or stroke, although this recommendation is given with caution because there is still not enough research. There is evidence to recommend keeping exposure to progesterone at a minimum. An oral continual-cyclic regimen that is most commonly prescribed includes estrogen on days 1 to 28 and a progestogen (e.g., medroxyprogesterone) on days 14 to 28. Women usually do not have cyclic bleeding with this regimen and are less likely to have progestin side effects.

There are also multiple regimen options for ET for women who have had a hysterectomy. The transdermal estrogen patch is applied once or twice a week to a hairless area of skin. Transdermal gels and sprays are applied daily. Any site on the trunk or upper arms provides adequate absorption. Sites should be rotated. The patches should not be placed on the breasts because of their sensitivity. Some women report minor skin irritation and reddening at the patch site. Generally transdermal estrogen offers the same relief of menopausal symptoms as the oral preparation. The transdermal method of delivery of estrogen does not have the same side effects such as breast tenderness and fluid retention. Oral progestin therapy can be used with transdermal ET. Combined estrogen-progestin transdermal patches also are available.

Vaginal creams and tablets are inserted daily or twice a week. Usually these local administrations of low-dose estrogen are used for vaginal symptoms of dryness and atrophy. Vaginal rings are inserted and left in place for 90 days. Although minimal systemic absorption is possible, there are no reports of adverse effects when a low dose is used (NAMS, 2017).

Bioidentical and Custom-Compounded Hormones

Bioidentical hormones, sometimes referred to as natural hormones, are structurally identical to those produced by the ovary. Bioidentical hormone preparations are available as government-approved, well-tested brand-name prescription medications. Others are made at compounding pharmacies. Custom-compounded hormones are custom mixes of one or more hormones in varying amounts. These mixes can provide individualized doses and mixtures of hormones that are not available commercially. They also include ingredients that are nonhormonal (e.g., dyes, preservatives). The risks are that these mixtures have not been studied to confirm whether appropriate absorption occurs or if predictable levels can be detected in blood and tissue (NAMS, 2017). Preparations may vary from one pharmacy to another, meaning that a woman may not get consistent amounts of medication. These preparations are not approved by any regulatory agency (NAMS). Although these hormones may relieve menopausal symptoms, more research is needed to determine their effects on the body. Women who choose to take these hormones must understand and accept the potential risks. Expense is also an issue, because these drugs are often more expensive and are not covered by third-party payers.

Controversy continues in regard to the use of herbal preparations and bioidentical hormone therapy for menopause. ACOG (2012, updated 2018) concluded that there is not enough evidence to support the efficacy and safety of compounded bioidentical hormones as better than conventional HT, and customized preparations are too variable (i.e., lacking standardization), creating greater risks and difficulty in determining correct dosages.

Alternative Therapies

Many complementary and alternative therapies are useful for relieving some of the changes associated with altered estrogen levels. Homeopathy, acupuncture, and herbs have been used with varying degrees of success for menopausal problems such as heavy bleeding, hot flashes, irritability, and headaches.

Homeopathy views menopausal symptoms as the body's efforts to heal itself from the hormonal changes it is experiencing. Examples of remedies commonly prescribed during menopause by homeopaths are sepia, made from the inky juice of the cuttlefish, to relieve symptoms such as dry mouth, eyes, and vagina; nux vomica, derived from the poison nut, to relieve backaches, constipation, and frequent awakenings; and pulsatilla, made from the windflower, to relieve severe menstrual symptoms and hot flashes. Homeopathic remedies are subject to regulation by the FDA, although the FDA does not require proof of effectiveness. More study is needed to determine the effectiveness of homeopathic remedies.

Acupuncture may provide some relief of hot flashes and other symptoms. Women should make informed decisions in selecting their acupuncture therapists. Persons who administer acupuncture should be certified by the National Commission for the Certification of Acupuncture in the state where they practice, and should carry malpractice insurance. The American Association of Acupuncturists and Oriental Medicine will supply a list of acupuncturists in a given state.

Herbal therapy has also been used to treat menopausal discomforts. Herbs can be ingested as teas or tinctures. Many herbal preparations also are available in capsule form. It is important that women understand the mechanisms of action, contraindications, and potential side effects of each herb.

> ### ⚡ SAFETY ALERT
>
> Most herbal preparations have not undergone long-term testing for safety and efficacy. Benefits and risks are not completely known. Women should always consult with their health care provider before beginning herbal therapy. Questions regarding the use of herbal therapy and other supplements must be a component of a client history and discussions with her provider.

In addition to resolving physical symptoms, herbs also are used to combat mood swings and depression. Ginseng has been claimed to be helpful in alleviating hot flashes, although research studies have not supported this assertion. Women should be advised against prolonged use of ginseng in high doses because it can increase blood pressure. Oriental herbal teas composed of licorice, ginseng, coptis, red raspberry leaf, and Chinese rhubarb may be of some help in relieving hot flashes.

Dong quai, black cohosh, sage and other herbs have been recognized as possibly helping to alleviate menopausal symptoms, although evidence is lacking to support their use. Systematic clinical trials are needed to support the use of these alternative therapies.

Some plant foods contain **phytoestrogens** (isoflavones) and are capable of interacting with estrogen receptors in the body. These foods include red clover, wild yams, dandelion greens, cherries, alfalfa sprouts, black beans, and soybeans. Use of soy-rich foods as an alternative to traditional HT for menopause has been studied. NAMS (2017), in a report on the role of isoflavones in menopause, concluded that more study is needed to demonstrate evidence for beneficial effects on menopausal symptoms.

For women who want to add soy to their diets, tofu, roasted soy nuts, and soy milk are good sources. Foods should be added gradually because some women have gastrointestinal (GI) discomfort from the high fiber content of these foods. Spreading out the daily intake over several meals may be the best way to include soy products in the diet.

Vitamin E is a popular alternative among women who do not take HT. Nihira (2012) reviewed a variety of treatments for hot flashes, and included vitamin E as a possible treatment. Vitamin E is found in a variety of foods, including spinach, peanuts, wheat germ, vegetable oils, and soybeans, or it may be taken as a supplement. Dosage varies widely, from 400 to 800 international units (IU) per day.

Layered clothing, ice packs, ice water, and fans may offer symptomatic relief from hot flashes (see box Teaching for Self-Management: Comfort Measures for Menopausal Symptoms). Women can be counseled to avoid hot curries and other spicy foods. Reassurance that hot flashes will not last forever may be of comfort even if the duration of the problem cannot be predicted accurately. Many women find that hot flashes lessen in frequency and intensity or disappear within 4 to 6 years after menopause.

TEACHING FOR SELF-MANAGEMENT
Comfort Measures for Menopausal Symptoms

Hot Flashes/Flushes
During the Day
- Wear layered clothing so you can take things off if you get warm.
- Avoid "triggers" that bring on a flash/flush; these include vigorous exercise on hot days, spicy foods, caffeine, hot beverages, and alcohol.
- Splash your face with cool water, drink ice water, or take a cool shower.
- Try slow, deep breathing.

At Night
- Sleep in cotton clothes, use cotton sheets, and keep the room cool.
- Avoid heavy blankets that will make you too warm at night.
- Keep a thermos of water by the bed.

Insomnia
- Avoid caffeine, alcohol, or tobacco in the evening.
- Avoid liquids after dinner.
- Exercise regularly but limit exercise to the daytime and early evening.
- Develop a bedtime routine.
- Try drinking warm milk or taking a hot bath.
- Use your bed only for sleeping or sexual activity and not for watching TV or reading, etc.
- Encourage your body's circadian rhythm.

- If you cannot sleep, get up and do something else until you feel tired.
- Avoid naps during the day.
- Sprinkle lavender oil on your pillow.
- Drink chamomile tea (do not use if allergic to ragweed or chrysanthemums).

Headaches
- Try to avoid stress and get plenty of rest.
- Eat or drink foods that contain natural diuretics (parsley).

Urogenital Symptoms
- Drink lots of water (i.e., at least 8 glasses a day), and empty your bladder frequently.
- Practice Kegel exercises daily.
- Wear cotton underwear and avoid wearing a wet bathing suit for a prolonged time.
- Use a water-soluble lubricant for vaginal dryness.

Nervousness, Irritability
- Practice yoga or other meditation exercises.
- Do relaxation or deep-breathing exercises.
- Practice guided imagery.

Data from Wilson, C., McClure, R.A., Kostas-Polston, E.A. (2017). Perimenstrual and Pelvic Symptoms and Syndromes. In I. M. Alexander, V. Mallard-Johnson, E. Kostas-Polson, C. I. Fogel, N. F. Woods (Eds.), *Womens' health care in advanced practice nursing*. (2nd ed.). New York: Springer.

CARE MANAGEMENT

Most women know little about menopause, and misinformation can cause anxiety. They must know what to expect, why it happens, and measures to make them more comfortable. Women appreciate the opportunity to discuss what they are experiencing. They need to know that their discomforts have a normal physiologic basis and that other women experience similar discomforts.

Planning for nursing care requires knowledge of the perimenopausal period as well as great sensitivity on the part of the nurse. Treatment must be individualized for each woman. A thorough health history, physical examination, and laboratory tests are essential to distinguish pathologic conditions from the normal perimenopausal experiences. Menopause clinics are needed where research on the effects of various treatments can be developed and evaluated and where care by interprofessional health care teams—such as endocrinology, radiology, psychosocial resources, exercise physiology, and nutrition—can be effectively coordinated. Women's support groups also are needed. Sexual counseling, nutrition, exercise, and support are topics that are included for further discussion.

Sexual Counseling

Sexuality is a lifelong behavior and, contrary to common stereotypes, it does not end with menopause. Many women remain sexually active throughout their lives. However, women and their partners may change their expressions of sexuality during and after menopause depending on physical changes, changes in the partner, and cultural beliefs and practices. Some women report declines in interest and desire. Such instances of decreasing interest in sexuality with aging may be influenced more by culture and prevailing attitudes than by nature and physiology (hormones). Although some women report that it takes longer to reach orgasm and that the orgasm is not as intense as it once was, the capacity for orgasm remains unchanged. There is no way to prevent the inevitable aging of the body. For people who see aging as loss, sexuality may become difficult to incorporate into what they perceive to be a less attractive identity. A fear of rejection may also arise.

Changes in a male partner may influence whether he continues to want to engage in sexual activity. As men age, they too take longer to reach orgasm; erections take longer to occur and are less firm. Men may believe that they are becoming impotent or ill and thus give up sexual activity, viewing it as too frustrating. Women may believe that their partners are losing interest in them. Couples may need counseling to understand these changes. Although women tend to outlive men, that is not always the case, and some men may lack available female partners.

The two most important influences on older women's sexual activity are the strength of a relationship and the physical condition of each partner. The lack of available male partners can have a negative effect on sexual expression for many midlife and older women. Women generally outlive men, and older widowed and divorced women frequently have fewer opportunities to develop relationships because they are less sought after. In counseling older women who do engage in intercourse, the nurse cannot assume that new or nonmonogamous partners are free of STIs; therefore they should inform women of their risk for human immunodeficiency virus (HIV) infection and other STIs and the need to use condoms.

As long as they remain able to bear children, some women view intercourse as part of their spousal responsibility. When menopause frees them from this duty, they may choose to forego intercourse. For other women—who no longer have to be concerned with contraception, fear of pregnancy, or being interrupted by menses—libido may increase.

Older lesbian women have largely been silent about their sexual needs, and their unusual social circumstances have not been acknowledged or recognized. Although lesbian women in midlife and in later years do not face the problem of a lack of available male partners, they are faced with the negative attitudes that go with being old, female, and lesbian—all of which can adversely affect sexuality and sexual expression.

Nurses must offer all women accurate information on matters such as appropriate contraception, sexuality, and the physiology of menopause as well as support and nonjudgmental guidance. Women need advice about contraception because ovulation may not cease for a year after the last menstrual cycle, and menopausal women can still become pregnant. The nurse's attitude toward sex and the older woman is important. Negative attitudes can reinforce the woman's misgivings about maintaining an active and satisfying sex life. The nurse can reassure the woman grieving over her lost youth and attractiveness, explaining that the desire for sex into old age is natural and that her body still has the capacity for sexual satisfaction. Only minor adjustments may be required.

Muscle tone around the reproductive organs decreases after menopause. Kegel exercises (see Chapter 4 for more detailed information) strengthen these muscles, improve tone, and, if practiced regularly, help prevent prolapsed uterus and stress incontinence. This is a low-cost, effective, noninvasive intervention to control symptoms. However, symptoms return if exercises are discontinued.

Water-soluble lubricating jelly (e.g., K-Y, Femglide, Aqualube) can aid in providing relief from painful intercourse. It may be applied directly to the vulva and the penis. Vaginal moisturizers may be water based but also contain other products such as vitamin E and aloe (e.g., K-Y Longlasting, Replens, Astroglide). They are inserted into the vagina using a prefilled applicator. Oil-based lubricants such as petroleum jelly (Vaseline) should not be used because they clog vaginal glands, which can then become sites for bacterial infection.

Prolonged hospitalization of an older adult partner may have a significant effect on the couple's sexual relationship. They may have difficulty renewing sexual activity when the separation is over and may need counseling or referral. In the event that a couple is admitted to a nursing home, the nurse should encourage placement of the couple together. With the aging of the American population and changing attitudes about the appropriateness of lifelong sexual expression, long-term care, extended care, and full-time care facilities are more receptive to providing opportunities for sexual activity between marital partners.

Sometimes more in-depth counseling is needed. The nurse can refer couples to a sex counselor or other appropriate health care provider as needed.

Nutrition

Obesity and osteoporosis are common health problems of midlife and older women. As women move out of their childbearing years, they may need to change their diets. Because metabolic rates decrease with age and many women exercise less, fewer calories are needed for weight maintenance as women age. In general, foods chosen should be high in nutrients, fiber, and calcium but moderate in calories and low in fat to allow adequate nutritional intake while maintaining body weight. Nurses can suggest that women substitute skim for whole milk or chicken without skin for steak. Excessive protein should be avoided. Fat-free milk and yogurt are good sources of calcium and vitamin D.

Women should avoid excessive intake of alcohol, soft drinks, and caffeinated coffee.

Calcium is an essential part of any therapeutic regimen for women with osteoporosis and those who want to prevent osteoporosis. The best source of calcium is milk and other dairy products. Other foods that contain calcium (sesame seeds, spinach, greens, broccoli, and seaweed) are often difficult to eat in quantities sufficient to meet daily requirements. Calcium supplements are recommended when a woman's diet does not supply recommended amounts of calcium. Although calcium cannot reverse loss of bone mass or prevent fractures, calcium supplementation may retard the development of osteoporosis after menopause. Menopausal women without contraindications to calcium supplementation (history of kidney stones, kidney failure, hypercalcemia) should be encouraged to consume a diet that has 1200 to 1500 mg of calcium a day or to add an amount of calcium supplementation that will increase their daily intake to this level. Calcium supplements are best taken in divided doses and with meals because of the increase in acid secretions and extended time in the stomach. At least 8 ounces of water to increase solubility is recommended. Calcium supplements should not be taken with caffeinated beverages. Calcium is most commonly available as calcium carbonate, calcium lactate, and calcium phosphate.

The Institute of Medicine (IOM) (2010) recommends 600 IU of vitamin D for healthy adults up to age 70 and 800 IU for those who are 71 years of age and older. The International Osteoporosis Foundation (IOF) (2017), however, recommends that women below age 50 take 400 to 800 IU daily and those older than age 50 take vitamin D 800 to 1000 IU daily. Sources of vitamin D include sunlight, food (e.g., fortified dairy products, fatty fish, liver, egg yolks), and supplements. Usually a supplement is needed to get the required daily dose. A combination of vitamin D and calcium is available, and most multivitamins contain some vitamin D.

Exercise

All too often midlife women are sedentary—the demands of family and work constraints increase, and energy levels decrease. Unfortunately when they get little or no exercise, women become predisposed to weight gain, and this does not help to prevent cardiac disease or osteoporosis. Exercise alone cannot prevent or reverse osteoporosis, but data indicate that weight-bearing exercise, such as walking and stair climbing, may delay bone loss and increase bone mass at any age. Aerobics and strength training have positive effects on midlife women's health, including cardiorespiratory function, weight, bone density, and quality of life.

Water aerobics is excellent for cardiovascular fitness and is a good choice for older women who may be unable to engage in weight-bearing exercises. The nurse can help women plan an exercise program. Examples of exercises are available from the NOF (Fig. 6.4).

Medications for Osteoporosis

In addition to calcium and exercise, there are a number of FDA-approved medications for preventing and treating osteoporosis. The medications assist in delaying bone loss, increasing bone mass, and preventing fractures. These include salmon calcitonin (Miacalcin); bisphosphonates (alendronate sodium [Fosamax], risedronate sodium [Actonel]), ibandronate [Boniva], zoledronic acid [Reclast]); estrogen agonist/antagonists such as raloxifene (Evista), parathyroid hormone (teriparatide [Forté o]), and ET or HT (Cosman, F., de Beur, S.J., et al., 2014).

Calcitonin reduces the rate of bone turnover and stabilizes bone mass in women with osteoporosis and may have some analgesic

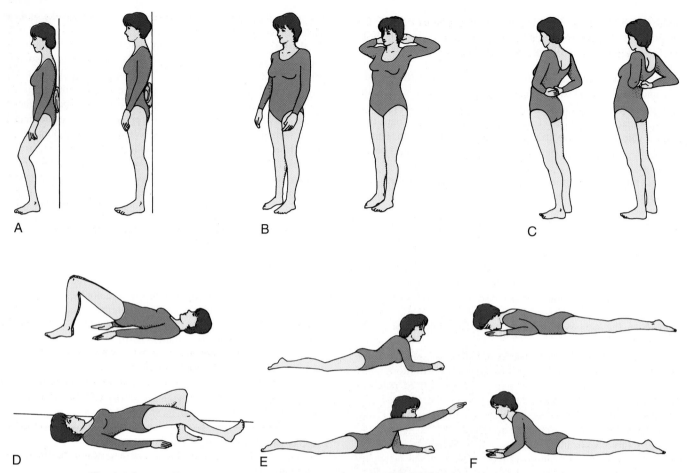

Fig. 6.4 Posture Exercises. (A) Wall standing and pelvic tilt. (B) Isometric posture correction. (C) Standing back bend. (D) The bridge. (E) The elbow prop. (F) Prone press-ups with deep breathing. (From *Boning Up on Osteoporosis* [2013]. Courtesy the National Osteoporosis Foundation.)

effects. Although calcitonin can reduce the incidence of spinal fractures, no data are available about its use to protect against hip fractures. Calcitonin may be used with women who are at least 5 years postmenopausal and in whom estrogen is contraindicated or not tolerated. The drug usually is administered intranasally on a daily basis; subcutaneous administration is also available. The medication is considered safe; however, side effects of nausea, vomiting, anorexia, and rhinitis (if used intranasally) have been reported (Cosman, F., de Beur, S.J., et al., 2014).

Bisphosphonates are approved for prevention and treatment of osteoporosis, especially in reducing the incidence of spinal fractures. Side effects include GI problems such as difficulty swallowing, inflammation of the esophagus, and gastric ulcer. Depending on the medication used, the oral drugs may be taken daily or monthly. Some formulations contain vitamin D (Cosman, F., de Beur, S.J., et al., 2014). Alendronate is available in the United States in a generic preparation. Ibandronate is available as an intravenous injection every 3 months; zoledronic acid is given intravenously yearly for treatment of osteoporosis and every 2 years for prevention (Cosman, F., de Beur, S.J., et al., 2014).

Raloxifene is approved by the FDA for osteoporosis prevention and treatment in postmenopausal women only. This medication seemingly preserves the beneficial effects of estrogen, including

> **⬤ MEDICATION ALERT**
>
> Because food and certain minerals reduce the absorption of bisphosphonates, women must take alendronate sodium and risedronate sodium on an empty stomach with 6-8 ounces of plain water only at least 30 min before eating or drinking to improve absorption; remaining upright for these 30 min also is recommended (Cosman, F., deBeur, S.J., et al., 2014).

protection against cardiovascular diseases and osteoporosis, without stimulating breast and uterine tissues. Studies have shown that raloxifene may lower the risk of breast cancer in a high-risk population with lesser side effects than tamoxifen (Sandadi, Rock, Orr, & Valea, 2017). The medication modestly increases bone density. Calcium supplements up to 1500 mg daily should be taken if dietary intake is inadequate.

Parathyroid hormone is approved for the treatment of osteoporosis in postmenopausal women at high risk for fractures. It is administered by daily subcutaneous injection. It can be used for a maximum of 2 years. The drug is well tolerated although some women report dizziness and leg cramps (Cosman, F., de Beur, S.J., et al., 2014).

Estrogen/hormone therapy is approved for the prevention of osteoporosis. It should be used in the lowest effective doses for the shortest treatment time. The FDA recommends that it not be used solely for the prevention of osteoporosis until after approved nonestrogen treatments have been tried (Cosman, F., de Beur, S.J., et al., 2014).

Midlife Support Groups

Nurses should be familiar with local resources and direct women to classes that supply appropriate information and support. They can encourage women to develop a supportive network with other women with whom they can share their concerns (Fig. 6.5).

Women's centers and clinics may have support groups and classes for women who want to discuss menopause and other midlife events. If no group or class is available in the community, nurses should consider starting one.

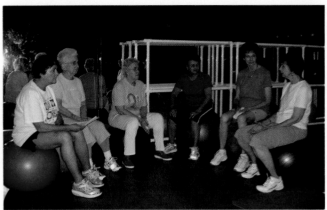

Fig. 6.5 Midlife Women Can Develop a Supportive Network. (Courtesy Dee Lowdermilk, Chapel Hill, NC.)

▊ KEY POINTS

- Menstrual disorders diminish the quality of life for affected women and their families.
- Pregnancy is the most common cause of amenorrhea.
- Dysmenorrhea is one of the most common gynecologic problems in women.
- PMS is a disorder with symptoms that begin in the luteal phase of the menstrual cycle and end with the onset of menses.
- Endometriosis is characterized by secondary amenorrhea, dyspareunia, abnormal uterine bleeding, and infertility.
- Perimenopause is a normal developmental phase during which a woman passes from the reproductive to the nonreproductive stage of life.
- During perimenopause women seek care for symptoms that arise from bleeding irregularities, vasomotor instability, fatigue, genital changes, and changes related to sexuality.

- MHT, if used, should be taken at the lowest effective dose for the shortest possible time.
- Alternative therapies are beneficial in relieving discomforts associated with menstrual disorders and menopause.
- Osteoporosis, a progressive loss of bone mass that results from decreasing levels of estrogen after menopause, can be prevented or minimized with lifestyle changes and medication.
- Postmenopausal women are at increased risk for coronary artery disease because of changes in lipid metabolism.
- Sexuality and the capacity for sexual expression continue after menopause.
- Postmenopausal women may have to adjust their diet due to slowing metabolism and should continue to exercise regularly.

REFERENCES

Advincula, A., Troung, M., & Lobo, R. A. (2017). Endometriosis: Etiology, pathology, diagnosis, management. In R. A. Lobo, D. M. Gershenson, G. M. Lentz, et al. (Eds.), *Comprehensive gynecology* (7th ed.). Philadelphia: Mosby.

American College of Obstetricians and Gynecologists. (2012, reaffirmed 2018). Committee opinion no. 532: Compounded bioidentical menopausal hormone therapy. *Obstetrics & Gynecology, 120*(2 Pt 1), 411–415.

American Psychiatric Association. (2014). *Diagnostic and statistical manual of mental disorders* (5th ed.). Washington, DC: Arlington.

Bahrami, A., Avan, A., Sadeghnia, H. R., Esmaeili, H., Tayefi, M., Ghasemi, F., Ghayour-Mobarhan, M., et al. (2018). High dose vitamin D supplementation can improve menstrual problems, dysmenorrhea, and premenstrual syndrome in adolescents. *Gynecological Endocrinology*, 1–5.

Berman, N. R., Pope, R. S., & Kessenich, C. R. (2019). Osteoporosis and evaluation of fracture risk. In Carcio HA, & M. Secor (Eds.), *Advanced health assessment of women : Clinical skills and procedures* (4th ed.). New York: NY Springer Publishing.

Cheong, Y., Cameron, I. T., & Critchley, H. (2017). Abnormal Uterine Bleeding. *British Medical Bulletin, 123*, 103–114.

Chien, L. W., Chang, H. C., & Liu, C. F. (2013). Effect of yoga on serum homocysteine and nitric oxide levels in adolescent women with and without dysmenorrhea. *The Journal of Alternative and Complementary Medicine, 19*(1), 20–23.

Cosman, F., de Beur, S. J., LeBoff, M. S., Lewiecki, E. M., Tanner, B., Randall, S., et al. (2014). Clinician's guide to prevention and treatment of osteoporosis. *Osteoporosis International, 25*(10), 2359–2381.

Dehnavi, Z. M., Jafarnejad, F., & Kamali, Z. (2018). The effect of aerobic exercise on primary dysmenorrhea: a clinical trial study. *Journal of Education and Health Promotion*, 7.

DeSanctis, V., Soliman, A., Bernasconi, S., Bianchin, L., Bona, G., Bozzola, M., et al. (2015). Primary dysmenorrhea in adolescents: Prevalence, impact, and recent knowledge. *Pediatric Endocrinology Reviews, 13*(2), 512–520. https://www.ncbi.nlm.nih.gov/pubmed/26841639.

Dewel, D. (2015). Drugs affecting the reproductive system. In T. M. Woo, & M. V. Robinson (Eds.), *Pharmacotherapeutics for advanced practice prescribers* (4th ed.). Philadelphia: F.A. Davis.

Drugs.com. (2017). *Goserelin dosage.* https://www.drugs.com/dosage/goserelin.html.

Fisher, C., Hickman, L., Adams, J., & Sibbritt, D. (2018). Cyclic perimenstrual pain and discomfort and australian women's associated use of complementary and alternative medicine: a longitudinal study. *Journal of Women's Health, 27*(1), 4–50.

Fortin, C., Flyckt, R., & Falcone, T. (2018). Alternatives to hysterectomy: The burden of fibroids and the quality of life. *Best Practice & Research Clinical Obstetrics and Gynaecology, 46*, 31–42.

Gershenson, G. M. Lentz, et al. (Eds.), Comprehensive gynecology (7th ed.). Philadelphia: Mosby.

Hartmann, K. E., Fonnesbeck, C., Surawicz, T., Krishnaswami, S., Andrews, J. C., Wilson, J. E., et al. (2017). *Management of Uterine Fibroids. Comparative Effectiveness Review No. 195*. Rockville, MD: agency for healthcare research and quality (Prepared by the Vanderbilt Evidence-based Practice Center under Contract No. 290-2015-00003-I.) AHRQ Publication No. 17(18)-EHC028-EF.

Healthwise (2015). *Pelvic rocking*. WebMD. http://www.webmd.com/fitness-exercise/pelvic-rocking.

Iacovides, S., Avidon, I., & Baker, F. C. (2015). What we know about primary dysmenorrhea today: a critical review. *Human Reproduction Update*, *21*(6), 762–778.

Institute of Medicine. (2010). *Dietary reference intakes for calcium and vitamin D*. Retrieved from http://www.nationalacademies.org/hmd/~/media/Files/Report%20Files/2010/Dietary-Reference-Intakes-for-Calcium-and-Vitamin-D/Vitamin%20D%20and%20Calcium%202010%20Report%20Brief.pdf.

International Osteoporosis Foundation. (2017). *IOM statement on new IOM dietary reference intakes from calcium and vitamin D*. Retrieved from https://www.iofbonehealth.org/iof-statement-new-iom-dietary-reference-intakes-calcium-and-vitamin-d.

Jafari, M., & Orenstein, G. (2015). Women and herbal medicine. In E. F. Olshansky (Ed.), *Women's health and wellness across the lifespan*. Philadelphia: Wolters Kluwer.

Lam, C., Anderson, B., Lopes, V., Schulkin, J., & Matteson, K. (2017). Assessing abnormal uterine bleeding: are physicians taking a meaningful clinical history? *Journal of Women's Health, 26*(7), 762–767.

Lobo, R. A. (2017a). Menopause and care of the mature woman Endocrinology, consequences of estrogen deficiency, effects of hormonal therapy and other treatment options. In R. A. Lobo, D. M. Gershenson, G. M. Lentz, et al. (Eds.), *Comprehensive gynecology* (7th ed.). Philadelphia: Mosby.

Lobo, R. A. (2017b). Primary and secondary amenorrhea and precocious puberty. In R. A. Lobo, D. M. Gershenson, G. M. Lentz, et al. (Eds.), *Comprehensive gynecology* (7th ed.). Philadelphia: Mosby.

Marsh, C. A., & Grimstad, F. W. (2014). Primary amenorrhea: Diagnosis and management. *Obstetrical & Gynecological Survey, 69*(10), 603–612.

MedicineNet.com. (2017). *Nafarelin, Synarel*. http://www.medicinenet.com/nafarelin/page3.htm.

Medscape. (2017). Leuprolide. http://reference.medscape.com/drug/lupron-leuprolide-342221.

Mendiratta, V. (2017). Primary and secondary dysmenorrhea, premenstrual syndrome, and premenstrual dysphoric disorder. In R. A. Lobo, D. M.

Gershenson, G. M. Lentz, et al. (Eds.), *Comprehensive gynecology* (7th ed.). Philadelphia: Mosby.

Mielke, R., Parsons, K., & Greenberg, C. S. (2015). Puberty through early adulthood. In E. F. Olshansky (Ed.), *Women's health and wellness across the lifespan*. Philadelphia: Wolters Kluwer.

Munro, M. G., Critchley, H. O. D., Broder, M. S., & Fraser, I. S. (2011). FIGO classification system (PALM-COEIN) for causes of abnormal uterine bleeding in nongravid women of reproductive age. *International Journal of Gynecology & Obstetrics, 113*(1), 3–13.

National Osteoporosis Foundation. (2019). *Calcium and vitamin D*. Retrieved from https://www.nof.org/patients/treatment/calciumvitamin-d/.

Noble, N. (2018). Symptom management in women undergoing the menopause. *Nursing Standard, 332*(22), 55–62.

O'Neill, S., & Eden, J. (2017). The pathophysiology of menopausal symptoms. *Obstetrics, gynaecology and reproductive medicine, 27*(10), 303–310.

Pace, D., & Secor, M. (2019). Assessment of Menopausal Status. In Carcio HA, & M. Secor (Eds.), *Advanced health assessment of women : Clinical skills and procedures* (4th ed.). New York: Springer Publishing.

Piecak, K., Milart, P., Woźniakowska, E., & Paszkowski, T. (2017). Ulipristal acetate as a treatment option for uterine fibroids. *Menopause Review/Przegląd Menopauzalny, 16*(4), 133–136.

Rabinerson, D., Hiersch, L., & Gabbay-Ben-Ziv, R. (2018). Dysmenorrhea – Its prevalence, causes, influence on the affected women and possible treatments. *Harefua, 157*(2), 91–94. https://www.ncbi.nlm.nih.gov/pubmed/29484863.

Ryntz, T., & Lobo, R. A. (2017). Abnormal uterine bleeding: etiology and management of acute and chronic excessive bleeding. In R. A. Lobo, D. M. Gershenson, G. M. Lentz, et al. (Eds.), *Comprehensive gynecology* (7th ed.). Philadelphia: Mosby.

Sandadi, S., Rock, D., Orr, J., & Valea, F. (2017). Breast diseases, detection, management and surveillance of breast disease. In R. A. Lobo, D. M. Gershenson, G. M. Lentz, et al. (Eds.), *Comprehensive gynecology* (7th ed.). Philadelphia: Mosby.

Vercellini, P., Ottolini, F., Frattaruolo, M. P., Buggio, L., Roberto, A., & Somigliana, E. (2018). Shifting from oral contraceptives to Norethisterone Acetate, or vice versa, because of drug intolerance: does the change benefit women with endometriosis? *Gynecologic and Obstetric Investigation*.

Yucel, N., Baskent, E., Balci, B. K., & Goynumer, G. (2018). The levonorgestrel-releasing intrauterine system is associated with a reduction in dysmenorrhea and dyspareunia, a decrease in CA 125 levels, and an increase in the quality of life in women with suspected endometriosis. *Australian and New Zealand Journal of Obstetrics and Gynaecology*.

7

Sexually Transmitted and Other Infections

Cheryl L. Kovar

http://evolve.elsevier.com/Lowdermilk/MWHC/

LEARNING OBJECTIVES

- Describe the prevention of sexually transmitted infections in women, including risk-reduction measures.
- Differentiate the signs, symptoms, diagnosis, and management of nonpregnant and pregnant women with selected sexually transmitted bacterial infections (chlamydia, gonorrhea, syphilis).
- Examine the care of nonpregnant and pregnant women with selected sexually transmitted viral infections (human immunodeficiency virus [HIV]; hepatitis A, B, and C; human papillomavirus; genital herpes).
- Compare and contrast the signs, symptoms, and management of selected vaginal infections in nonpregnant and pregnant women.

- Discuss the effect of group B streptococcus (GBS) on pregnancy and the management of pregnant women with GBS.
- Identify the effects of TORCH (toxoplasmosis, other, rubella, cytomegalovirus, and herpes) infections on pregnancy and the fetus.
- Describe the health consequences (e.g., ectopic pregnancy, infertility) for women who are diagnosed with reproductive tract infections.
- Develop a nursing care plan for a woman who is 12 weeks pregnant and has been diagnosed with HIV.
- Review the principles of infection control for HIV and blood-borne pathogens.

Reproductive tract infection is a term that encompasses both sexually transmitted infections (STIs) and other common genital tract infections (Marrazzo & Park, 2018). STIs include those due to more than 30 organisms that cause infections or infectious disease syndromes primarily through intimate contact (World Health Organization [WHO], 2019) (Box 7.1). These causative organisms include a wide spectrum of bacteria, viruses, protozoa, and ectoparasites (organisms that live on the outside of the body, such as a louse). Overall, STIs are a direct cause of tremendous human suffering; they place heavy demands on health care services and their treatment costs society almost $16 billion annually (Centers for Disease Control and Prevention [CDC], 2017a). Although the U.S. Surgeon General has targeted STIs as a priority for prevention and control efforts, STIs are among the most common health problems in the United States, especially for young people. The CDC estimate that almost 20 million Americans are infected with new STIs every year, and almost half of those infected are between the ages of 15 and 24. About 46% of chlamydial infections for this age group occur in young women who, if untreated, could face serious long-term consequences, specifically infertility. This is a major public health concern, as it is estimated that untreated STIs cause infertility in more than 20,000 women each year (CDC).

The most common STIs in women are chlamydia, gonorrhea, human papillomavirus (HPV), herpes simplex virus type 2, syphilis, and human immunodeficiency virus (HIV) infection; these are discussed in this chapter. Common vaginal infections are also discussed. Neonatal effects of STIs are discussed in Chapter 35.

PREVENTION

Preventing infection (primary prevention) is the most effective way of reducing the adverse consequences of STIs for women and for society. Because some STIs have serious and potentially lethal effects and some are incurable, primary prevention is critical. Prompt diagnosis and treatment of current STIs (secondary prevention) can also prevent personal complications and transmission to others.

Preventing the spread of STIs requires that women at risk for transmitting or acquiring infections change their behavior. A critical first step is for the nurse to include questions about a woman's sexual history, including risky sexual and drug-related behaviors as a part of the client's assessment. The six Ps regarding STIs—Partners, Prevention of pregnancy, Protection, Practices, and Past history—approach to obtaining a sexual history is an example of an effective strategy for eliciting information concerning six key areas of interest (CDC, 2015b) (Box 7.2). Techniques that are effective in providing prevention counseling include using open-ended questions, using understandable language, and reassuring the woman that treatment will be provided regardless of factors such as ability to pay, language spoken, or lifestyle (Marrazzo & Park, 2018). Prevention messages should include descriptions of specific actions to be taken to avoid acquiring or transmitting STIs (e.g., correct and consistent use of a latex or polyurethane condom with each sexual act) and should be individualized for each woman, based on her specific risk factors.

To be motivated to take preventive actions, a woman must believe that acquiring an STI will have serious consequences for her and that she is currently at risk for infection. However, most individuals tend to underestimate their personal risk of infection in a given situation; thus many women, and especially adolescents, may not perceive themselves as being at risk for contracting an STI. Advice that they should carry condoms may not be well received. Although levels of awareness of STIs are generally high, widespread misconceptions or specific gaps in knowledge also exist. Therefore nurses have a responsibility to ensure that their clients have accurate, complete knowledge about the transmission and symptoms of STIs and behaviors that place them at risk for contracting an infection.

Primary preventive measures are individual activities aimed at deterring infection. Risk-free options include complete abstinence

BOX 7.1 Selected Sexually Transmitted Infections

Bacteria
- Chlamydia
- Gonorrhea
- Syphilis

Viruses
- Human immunodeficiency virus
- Herpes simplex virus types 1 and 2
- Cytomegalovirus
- Viral hepatitis types A and B
- Human papillomavirus

Protozoa
- Trichomoniasis

Parasites
- Pediculosis
- Scabies

Data from Planned Parenthood. (2018). *Sexually transmitted diseases (STDs).* Retrieved from https://www.plannedparenthood.org/learn/stds-hiv-safer-sex; World Health Organization. (2019). *Sexually transmitted infections (STIs).* Retrieved from http://who.int/mediacentre/factsheets/fs110/en/

from sexual activities that transmit semen, blood, or other body fluids or that allow skin-to-skin contact (Marrazzo & Park, 2018).

Risk Reduction Measures

An essential component of primary prevention is counseling women regarding risk-reduction practices, including reduction of the number of partners, low-risk sex, avoiding the exchange of body fluids, and vaccination (CDC, 2015b). Sexually active people may also benefit from carefully examining a partner for lesions, sores, ulcerations, rashes, redness, discharge, swelling, and odor before initiating sexual activity. Other preventive measures include education on the influence of drugs or alcohol abuse on sexual behavior and partner selection. Douching has also been associated with an increased risk of pelvic inflammatory disease (PID) and ectopic pregnancy (Marrazzo & Cates) (Table 7.1). See the Critical Reasoning Case Study for an analysis of the nurses' role in counseling a pregnant woman about STIs.

 CLINICAL REASONING CASE STUDY

Counseling for Sexually Transmitted Infection in Pregnancy

Shawanda is an 18-year-old African American, gravida 1 para 0, who has come to the prenatal clinic for her first visit. She has a history of marijuana use. She says that her current boyfriend is her support person but that he is not the father of the baby. Shawanda is unemployed and living with her mother. She has been given an explanation of the prenatal laboratory tests that will be done during her examination. She says that she does not see why she has to have the tests for sexually transmitted infections (STIs) because she has not had these infections.

1. What is the priority concern or client need in this situation?
2. List other client needs/problems in this case.
3. Identify any additional information needed by the nurse in addressing this situation.
4. Describe the roles/responsibilities of interprofessional health team members who may be involved in this situation.

BOX 7.2 The Six Ps Regarding Sexually Transmitted Infections: Partners, Practices, Prevention of Pregnancy, Protection, and Past History

1. Partners
   - Do you have sex with men, women, or both?
   - In the past 2 months, how many partners have you had sex with?
   - In the past 12 months, how many partners have you had sex with?
   - Is it possible that any of your sex partners in the past 12 months had sex with someone else while they were still in a sexual relationship with you?
2. Practices
   - To understand your risks for STIs, I need to understand the kind of sex you have had recently.
   - Have you had vaginal sex, meaning penis-in-vagina sex? If yes, Do you use condoms: never, sometimes, or always?
   - Have you had anal sex, meaning penis-in-rectum/anus sex? If yes, Do you use condoms: never, sometimes, or always?
   - Have you had oral sex, meaning mouth-on-penis/vagina?

   For condom answers:
   - If never: Why don't you use condoms?
   - If sometimes: In what situations (or with whom) do you use condoms?
3. Prevention of pregnancy
   What are you doing to prevent pregnancy?
4. Protection from STIs
   What do you do to protect yourself from STIs and HIV?
5. Past history of STIs
   Have you ever had an STI?
   Have any of your partners had an STI?
   Additional questions to identify HIV and viral hepatitis risk include
   Have you or any of your partners ever injected drugs?
   Have you or any of your partners exchanged money or drugs for sex?
   Is there anything else about your sexual practices that I need to know?

HIV, Human immunodeficiency virus; *STI,* sexually transmitted infection. From Centers for Disease Control and Prevention (CDC). (2015). *Sexually transmitted diseases treatment guidelines 2015.* Retrieved from https://www.cdc.gov/std/tg2015/clinical.htm#box1.

Reproductive Coercion

It is essential that nurses are nonjudgmental in their approach to all women when counseling them about the prevention of STIs. Not all women are in safe and healthy relationships and some may be experiencing reproductive coercion, defined as any behavior that interferes with a woman's right to make any and all decisions regarding her health, sexual or otherwise (Grace & Anderson, 2016). That is, she is entitled to control her behavior and maintain power over any relationship related to her sexual and reproductive health (ACOG, 2016). The most common forms of reproductive coercion include "contraceptive sabotage, pressure or coercion to become pregnant, or controlling the outcome of a pregnancy" (Grace & Anderson, p. 1). Reproductive coercion has been found to be related to STIs (Decker, Miller, McCauley, et al., 2014). This can occur when the male partner refuses to use a condom or to allow the woman to use a female condom as a barrier to potential transmission of an STI. There are evidence-based interventions that can be helpful in such situations, such as clinician-delivered education and counseling and the use of safety cards when one is working with a client who may find herself in such a situation (Clark, Allen, Goyal, et al., 2014; Tancredi, Silverman, Decker, et al., 2015).

TABLE 7.1 Risk-Reduction Practices

Safest	Low but Potential Risk	High Risk (Unsafe)
Abstinence	Wet kissing[a]	Unprotected anal intercourse; unprotected vaginal intercourse
Self-masturbation	Vaginal intercourse with condom; anal intercourse with condom	Oral-anal contact
Monogamous (both partners and no high-risk activities) and tested negative for HIV and other STIs	Monogamous (both partners and no high-risk activities) but not tested for HIV or other STIs	Multiple sexual partners, no HIV or STI testing
Hugging, massage, touching (assuming no break in skin)	Oral sex with woman wearing female condom, dental dam or plastic wrap	Any sex (fisting, rough vaginal or anal intercourse, rape) that causes tissue damage or bleeding
Dry kissing	Oral sex with man wearing condom	Oral sex on man or woman without a latex or plastic barrier
Mutual masturbation without contact with semen or vaginal secretions, blood, and no broken skin	Mutual masturbation on healthy intact skin or use of latex or plastic barrier	Sharing sex toys, douche equipment
Sexual fantasy		Sharing needles, using illicit drugs, alcohol abuse
Erotic conversation, books, movies		Blood contact, including menstrual blood
Erotic bathing, showering		
Eroticizing feet, fingers, buttocks, abdomen, ears		

[a]Assumes no breaks in skin.

HIV, Human immunodeficiency virus; *STI,* sexually transmitted infection.

From Marrazzo, J.M., & Park, I.U. (2018). Reproductive tract infections, including HIV and other sexually transmitted infections. In R.A. Hatcher, A.L. Nelson, J. Trussell, C. Cwiak, P. Cason, M.S. Policar, A.B. Edelman, A.R.A. Aiken, J.M. Marrazzo, D. Kowal (Eds.), *Contraceptive technology* (21st ed.). New York: Ayer Company Publishers, Inc.

The physical barrier promoted for the prevention of sexual transmission of HIV and other STIs is the condom (male and female). Nurses can help motivate clients to use condoms by initiating a discussion about them. This gives women permission to discuss any concerns, misconceptions, or hesitations they may have about using condoms. Information to be discussed includes the importance of using latex or plastic male condoms rather than natural skin condoms for STI protection. The nurse should remind women to use a condom with every sexual encounter, to use each only once, to use a condom that has not reached its expiration date, and to handle it carefully to avoid damaging it with fingernails, teeth, or other sharp objects. Condoms should be stored away from high heat. Women should also be taught the differences among condoms: price ranges, sizes, and where they can be purchased. Explicit instructions for how to apply a male condom are included in Box 8.3.

The female condom—a lubricated polyurethane sheath with a ring on each end, one inserted into the vagina and the other covering the labia (see Fig. 8.7)—has been shown in laboratory studies to be an effective mechanical barrier to viruses, including HIV. The Food and Drug Administration has approved labeling on the female condom that it may prevent HIV/AIDS and other STIs, although this is only for vaginal, not anal, sex (Nelson & Harwood, 2018). According to the CDC (2015b), when used correctly and consistently, the female condom may reduce STI risk, and its use is recommended when a male condom cannot be used properly. What is important and should be stressed by nurses is that a condom must be used consistently for every act of sexual intimacy when there is a possibility of transmitting disease.

Despite concern about the potential for cervicovaginal epithelial disruption with nonoxynol-9 (N-9)–based spermicides, interest in vaginally applied chemical barriers that provide dual contraceptive and protection against bacterial STIs remains. Evidence has shown, however, that vaginal spermicides do not protect against certain STIs, such as cervical gonorrhea and chlamydia, and are not effective in preventing HIV infection. Condoms lubricated with N-9 are not recommended for the prevention of HIV and other STIs (CDC, 2015b).

A key issue in condom use as a preventive strategy is to stress to women that in any sexual encounter, the male partner must comply with the woman's suggestion or request that a condom be used. Moreover, condom use must be renegotiated with every sexual contact, and a woman must address the issue of control of sexual decision making every time she asks a male partner to use a condom. The concept of reproductive coercion may play into this situation, as some women may fear that their partner would be offended if the issue of condom use were brought up. The woman may fear rejection and abandonment, conflict, potential violence, or loss of economic support if she suggested the use of a condom. Nurses should offer strategies to enhance a woman's negotiation and communication skills in this regard. It can be suggested that she speak with her partner about condom use at a time removed from sexual activity, which may make it easier to bring up the subject. Role-playing possible partner reactions with a woman and discussing alternative responses can be helpful. Asking a woman who appears particularly uncomfortable to rehearse how she might approach the topic can be useful, particularly when she fears that her partner may be resistant.

Finally, women should be counseled to watch out for situations in which it is difficult to talk about and to practice safer sex. These include romantic times when condoms are not available and when alcohol or drugs make wise decisions about safer sex impossible.

Preexposure vaccination is an effective method for the prevention of some STIs, such as hepatitis B and human papillomavirus (HPV). Hepatitis B vaccine is recommended for unvaccinated, uninfected women being evaluated or treated for STIs (CDC, 2015b).

SEXUALLY TRANSMITTED BACTERIAL INFECTIONS

Chlamydia

Chlamydia trachomatis is the most commonly reported STI in American women. In 2016 almost 1.6 million cases were reported; the rate of infection among women was twice that among men (CDC, 2015b). These infections are often silent and highly destructive; their sequelae and complications can be very serious. In women, chlamydial infections are difficult to diagnose; the symptoms, if present, are nonspecific; and the organism is expensive to culture.

Early identification of *C. trachomatis* is important because untreated infection often leads to acute salpingitis or pelvic inflammatory disease (PID). PID is the most serious complication of chlamydial infections, and past chlamydial infections are associated with an increased risk of ectopic pregnancy and tubal factor infertility. Furthermore, chlamydial infection of the cervix causes inflammation, which results in microscopic cervical ulcerations and thus may increase the risk of acquiring HIV infection. More than half of infants born to mothers with chlamydia will develop conjunctivitis or pneumonia after perinatal exposure to the mother's infected cervix. *C. trachomatis* is the most common infectious cause of ophthalmia neonatorum. Neonatal ocular prophylaxis with silver nitrate solution or antibiotic ointment does not prevent perinatal transmission from mother to infant, nor does it adequately treat chlamydial infection (see Chapter 35).

Sexually active women ages 20 to 24 years have the highest rates of infection. In 2016, the rates were highest among black women, at more than five times the rate among white women. American Indian, Alaska Native, and Hispanic women also had higher rates than white women (CDC, 2015b). Women older than 30 years have the lowest rates of infection. Risky behaviors, including multiple partners and nonuse of barrier methods of birth control, increase a woman's risk of chlamydial infection.

Screening and Diagnosis

In addition to obtaining information regarding the presence of risk factors, the nurse should inquire about the presence of any symptoms. The CDC guidelines (CDC, 2014) recommend yearly screening of all sexually active women under age 25 years and of women older than 25 years who are at high risk (e.g., those with new or multiple partners). In addition, whenever possible, all women with two or more of the risk factors for chlamydia should be screened. All pregnant women should be screened for chlamydia at the first prenatal visit. Screening late in the third trimester (36 weeks) may be repeated if the woman was positive previously or if she is younger than 25 years, has a new sex partner, or has multiple sex partners.

Although chlamydial infections are usually asymptomatic, some women may experience spotting or postcoital bleeding, mucoid or purulent cervical discharge, or dysuria. Bleeding results from inflammation and erosion of the cervical columnar epithelium.

Laboratory diagnosis of chlamydia is by culture (expensive and labor-intensive), deoxyribonucleic acid (DNA) probe (relatively less expensive but less sensitive), or enzyme immunoassay (also relatively less expensive but less sensitive). The CDC recommends the nucleic acid amplification test (NAAT—expensive but with relatively higher sensitivity) of urinary, vaginal, or endocervical specimens (CDC, 2015b).

Management

The CDC recommendations for treatment of urethral, cervical, and rectal chlamydial infections are azithromycin or doxycycline (CDC, 2015b) (Table 7.2). Azithromycin is often prescribed when compliance may be a problem because only one dose is needed. If the woman is pregnant, azithromycin or amoxicillin is used. Pregnant women should be retested in 3 to 4 weeks to determine if treatment was effective (test of cure). In addition, all pregnant women who have a chlamydial infection should be retested 3 months after treatment (CDC). Women who have a chlamydial infection and are also infected with HIV should be treated with the same regimen as those who are not infected with HIV.

Because chlamydia is often asymptomatic, the woman should be cautioned to take all medication prescribed. All exposed sexual partners should also be treated. Nonpregnant women treated with doxycycline or azithromycin do not have to be retested unless symptoms continue, adherence was in question, or reinfection is suspected (CDC, 2015b).

Gonorrhea

Gonorrhea is second to only chlamydia in reported cases. In 2016, 468,514 cases of gonorrhea were reported in the United States (CDC, 2017a). The incidence of drug-resistant cases of gonorrhea (i.e., that do not respond to the antimicrobials used in treatment) is increasing dramatically in the United States. Declining susceptibility to cefixime (an oral cephalosporin antibiotic) has resulted in a change to the 2015 CDC treatment guidelines.

Gonorrhea is caused by the aerobic gram-negative diplococcus *Neisseria gonorrhoeae*. It is almost exclusively transmitted by sexual contact. The principal means of transmission is genital-genital contact; however, it is also spread by oral-genital and anal-genital contact. In females, there is also evidence that infection can spread from vagina to rectum.

Age is an important risk factor associated with gonorrhea. In the United States the highest reported rates of infection differ slightly according to gender, with the highest rates of infection in the 20- to 24-year age group among both men and women. The difference is demonstrated in the second-highest age group for women (15 to 19 years) compared with men, in whom the second-highest rate of infection was found in the 25- to 29-year age group. In 2016, the rate among blacks was almost nine times higher than that among whites. American Indian, Alaska Native, and Hispanic rates were also higher than the rate for whites (CDC, 2017a).

Women with gonorrheal infection are often asymptomatic. When symptoms are present, they are often less specific than symptoms in men. Women may have a purulent endocervical discharge, but this is more often minimal or absent. Menstrual irregularities may be the presenting symptom, or women may complain of pain—chronic or acute severe pelvic or lower abdominal pain or longer, more painful menses. Infrequently, dysuria, vague abdominal pain, or low backache prompts a woman to seek care. Gonococcal rectal infection may occur in women after anal intercourse. Individuals with rectal gonorrhea may be completely asymptomatic or, conversely, have severe symptoms with profuse purulent anal discharge, rectal pain, and blood in the stool. Rectal itching, fullness, pressure, and pain are also common symptoms, as is diarrhea. A diffuse vaginitis with vulvitis is the most common form of gonococcal infection in prepubertal girls. There may be few signs of infection; on the other hand, vaginal discharge, dysuria, and swollen, reddened labia may be present.

Gonococcal infections in pregnancy can affect mother and fetus. In women with cervical gonorrhea, salpingitis may develop in the first trimester. Perinatal complications of gonococcal infection include prelabor rupture of membranes, preterm birth, chorioamnionitis, neonatal sepsis, intrauterine growth restriction, and maternal postpartum sepsis. Ophthalmia neonatorum, the most common manifestation of neonatal gonococcal infection, is highly contagious; if untreated, it may lead to blindness of the newborn (see Chapter 35). In an effort to prevent ophthalmia neonatorum, antibiotic ointment (e.g., erythromycin) is routinely applied to the eyes of all newborns soon after birth (see Chapter 24).

Screening and Diagnosis

Because gonococcal infections in women are often asymptomatic, the CDC recommends the screening of all sexually active women younger than 25 years of age who are at risk for gonorrhea due to multiple sex partners or a new sex partner (CDC, 2015b). All pregnant women should be screened at the first prenatal visit, and infected women and those not infected but identified with risky behaviors should be rescreened at 36 weeks of gestation. Gonococcal infection cannot be diagnosed reliably by clinical signs and symptoms alone. Individuals may have "classic" symptoms, vague symptoms that can be attributed to a number of conditions, or no symptoms at all.

Specific diagnosis of infection with *N. gonorrhoeae* can be performed by testing endocervical, vaginal, or urinary specimens. Culture and nonculture tests (nucleic acid hybridization tests and NAATs) are

TABLE 7.2	Sexually Transmitted Infections and Recommended Drug Therapies for Women[a]			
Disease	**Nonpregnant Women (13-17 Years)**	**Nonpregnant Women (>18 Years)**	**Pregnant Women**	**Lactating Women[b]**
Chlamydia	*Recommended:* azithromycin, 1 g PO once *or* doxycycline, 100 mg PO bid for 7 days	*Recommended:* azithromycin, 1 g PO once *or* doxycycline, 100 mg PO bid for 7 days	*Recommended:* azithromycin, 1 g PO once *or* amoxicillin, 500 mg PO tid for 7 days.	*Recommended:* azithromycin, 1 g PO once *or* amoxicillin, 500 mg PO tid for 7 days.
Gonorrhea	*Recommended:* ceftriaxone, 125 mg IM once (adolescents who weigh >45 kg can be treated with any regimen recommended for adults), plus treatment for chlamydia as above	*Recommended:* ceftriaxone, 250 mg IM once, plus treatment for chlamydia as above	*Recommended:* ceftriaxone, 250 mg IM once, plus treatment for chlamydia as above.	*Recommended:* ceftriaxone, 250 mg IM once, plus treatment for chlamydia as above.
Syphilis	Primary, secondary, early latent disease: *Recommended:* benzathine penicillin G, 2.4 million units IM once Late-latent or unknown-duration disease: *Recommended:* benzathine penicillin G, 7.2 million units total, administered as three doses, 2.4 million units each, at 1-wk intervals Penicillin allergy: doxycycline, 100 mg PO qid for 14 days *or* tetracycline, 500 mg PO qid for 14 days	Primary, secondary, early latent disease: *Recommended:* benzathine penicillin G, 2.4 million units IM once Late-latent or unknown-duration disease: *Recommended:* benzathine penicillin G, 7.2 million units total, administered as three doses, 2.4 million units each, at 1-wk intervals Penicillin allergy: doxycycline, 100 mg PO qid for 14 days *or* tetracycline, 500 mg PO qid for 14 days	Primary, secondary, early latent disease: *Recommended:* benzathine penicillin G, 2.4 million units IM once (some experts recommend a second dose of benzathine penicillin, 2.4 million units, 1 wk later) Late-latent or unknown-duration disease: *Recommended:* benzathine penicillin G, 7.2 million units total, administered as three doses, 2.4 million units each, at 1-wk intervals No proven alternatives to penicillin in pregnancy. Pregnant women who have a history of allergy to penicillin should be desensitized and treated with penicillin.	Primary, secondary, early latent disease: *Recommended:* benzathine penicillin G, 2.4 million units IM once
Human papillomavirus	*Recommended for external genital warts:* Client-applied: podofilox, 0.5% solution, or gel to wart bid for 3 days followed by 4-day rest for ≤4 cycles *or* imiquimod, 5% cream, at bedtime 3 times a week for ≤16 weeks *or* sinecatechins 15% ointment tid for ≤16 wk Provider-applied: cryotherapy with liquid nitrogen or cryoprobe *or* podophyllin resin, 10%-25% in tincture of benzoin compound weekly (wash off in 1-4 h). Repeat weekly as necessary *or* TCA or BCA 80%-90% weekly	*Recommended for external genital warts:* Client-applied: podofilox, 0.5% solution, or gel to wart bid for 3 days followed by 4-day rest for ≤4 cycles *or* imiquimod, 5% cream, at bedtime 3 times a week for ≤16 weeks *or* sinecatechins 15% ointment tid for ≤16 wk Provider- applied: cryotherapy with liquid nitrogen or cryoprobe *or* podophyllin resin, 10%-25% in tincture of benzoin compound weekly (wash off in 1-4 h). Repeat weekly as necessary *or* TCA or BCA 80%-90% weekly	*Recommended for external genital warts:* Provider-applied: cryotherapy with liquid nitrogen or cryoprobe *or* TCA or BCA 80%-90% weekly imiquimod, podophyllin (Podocon-25), sinecatechins, and podofilox should not be used in pregnancy.	*Recommended for external genital warts:* Provider-applied: cryotherapy with liquid nitrogen or cryoprobe *or* TCA or BCA 80%-90% weekly imiquimod, podophyllin, sinecatechins, and podofilox should not be used during lactation.

Continued

TABLE 7.2 Sexually Transmitted Infections and Recommended Drug Therapies for Women[a]—cont'd

Disease	Nonpregnant Women (13-17 Years)	Nonpregnant Women (>18 Years)	Pregnant Women	Lactating Women[b]
Genital herpes simplex virus (HSV-1 or HSV-2)	Primary infection: acyclovir, 400 mg PO tid for 7-10 days or acyclovir, 200 mg PO 5 times a day for 7-10 days or famciclovir, 250 mg PO tid for 7-10 days or valacyclovir, 1 g PO bid for 7-10 days Recurrent infection: acyclovir, 400 mg PO tid for 5 days or acyclovir, 800 mg PO bid for 5 days or acyclovir, 800 mg PO tid for 2 days or famciclovir, 125 mg PO bid for 5 days or famciclovir 1000 mg PO bid for 1 day or famciclovir, 500 mg once, then 250 mg bid for 2 days or valacyclovir, 500 mg PO bid for 3 days or valacyclovir, 1 g PO qd for 5 days Suppression therapy: Take daily for 1 year or more: acyclovir, 400 mg PO bid or famciclovir, 250 mg PO bid or valacyclovir, 500 mg PO once a day or valacyclovir, 1 g PO qd	Primary infection: acyclovir, 400 mg PO tid for 7-10 days or acyclovir, 200 mg PO 5 times a day for 7-10 days or famciclovir, 250 mg PO tid for 7-10 days or valacyclovir, 1 g PO bid for 7-10 days Recurrent infection: acyclovir, 400 mg PO tid for 5 days or acyclovir, 800 mg PO bid for 5 days or acyclovir, 800 mg PO tid for 2 days or famciclovir, 125 mg PO bid for 5 days or famciclovir, 1000 mg PO bid for 1 day or famciclovir 500 mg once, then 250 mg bid for 2 days or valacyclovir, 500 mg PO bid for 3 days or valacyclovir, 1 g PO qd for 5 days Suppression therapy: Take daily for 1 year or more: acyclovir, 400 mg PO bid or famciclovir, 250 mg PO bid or valacyclovir, 500 mg PO qd or valacyclovir, 1 g PO qd	No increase in birth defects beyond the general population has been found with acyclovir use in pregnancy. Acyclovir, 400 mg PO tid for 7 days for first episode or severe recurrent infection; may be given intravenously if infection is severe. Begin suppression therapy 4 wk before the birth for women with recurrent infections can reduce the need for a cesarean birth.	Acyclovir usually considered compatible with breastfeeding Acyclovir, 400 mg PO tid for 7 days

[a]List is not inclusive of all drugs that may be used as alternatives.
[b]These medications are usually compatible with breastfeeding.
BCA, Bichloroacetic acid; *bid,* twice daily; *HSV,* herpes simplex virus; *IM,* intramuscular; *IV,* intravenous; *qid,* four times daily; *TCA,* trichloroacetic acid; *tid,* three times daily.
Centers for Disease Control and Prevention (CDC). (2015b). 2015 Sexually transmitted disease treatment guidelines. *MMWR Morbidity and Mortality Weekly Report, 64*(3), 1–140.

available for the detection of genitourinary infection with *N. gonorrhoeae.* Cultures should be obtained from the endocervix, rectum, and, when indicated, the pharynx, as NAAT testing has not received approval from the U.S. Food and Drug Administration (FDA) in these sites. Thayer-Martin cultures are recommended to diagnose gonorrhea in women. NAATs allow testing of the widest variety of specimen types including endocervical swabs, vaginal swabs, and urine (CDC, 2015b). Because coinfection is common, any woman suspected of having gonorrhea should have a chlamydial culture and a serologic test for syphilis if one has not been done in the previous 2 months.

Management

Management of gonorrhea is straightforward; with appropriate antibiotic therapy, the cure is usually rapid (see Table 7.2). Single-dose efficacy is a major consideration in selecting an antibiotic regimen for women with gonorrhea. Another important consideration is the high percentage of women with coexisting chlamydial infections. The treatment of choice for uncomplicated urethral, endocervical, and rectal infections in pregnant and nonpregnant women is dual therapy with ceftriaxone (an injectable cephalosporin) and azithromycin; this is now the only CDC-recommended treatment regimen for gonorrhea (CDC, 2017a). Pregnant women should be retested after 3 to 4 weeks to determine if treatment was effective (test of cure). In addition, all pregnant women who have chlamydial infection diagnosed should be retested 3 months after treatment (CDC, 2015b). All women with both gonorrhea and syphilis should be treated for syphilis according to CDC guidelines (see discussion of syphilis in this chapter).

Gonorrhea is a highly communicable disease. It is important to notify partners if a woman is diagnosed with a gonorrheal infection. Recent (past 30 days) sexual partners should be examined, cultured, and treated with appropriate regimens. Most treatment failures result from reinfection. The woman must be informed of this, as well as of the consequences of reinfection in terms of chronicity, complications, and potential infertility. Women are counseled to use condoms. All clients with gonorrhea should be offered confidential counseling and testing for HIV infection.

LEGAL TIP

Reporting Communicable Diseases

Syphilis (including congenital syphilis), gonorrhea, chlamydia, chancroid, HIV infection, and AIDS are reportable diseases in every state. Because the requirements for reporting other STIs differ by state, health care providers should be familiar with the reporting requirements applicable within their states because these providers are legally responsible for reporting all cases to the health authorities, usually the local health department in the client's county of residence. Infected women should be informed that their cases will be reported, told why, and informed of the possibility of being contacted by a health department epidemiologist.

Syphilis

Syphilis is caused by *Treponema pallidum,* a motile spirochete. Transmission is thought to be by entry into the subcutaneous tissue through microscopic abrasions that can occur during sexual intercourse. The disease can also be transmitted through kissing, biting, and oral-genital sex. Transplacental transmission can occur at any time during pregnancy; the degree of risk is related to the number of spirochetes in the maternal bloodstream. See Chapter 35 for a description of congenital syphilis.

In 2015 to 2016, a total of 88,042 cases of syphilis were reported in the United States; these included 27,814 cases of primary and secondary syphilis. In women, the rates of primary and secondary syphilis were highest in those aged 20 to 24 years. The rates were highest among black women (CDC, 2017a).

Syphilis is a complex disease that can lead to serious systemic disease and even death when untreated. Infection manifests itself in distinct stages with different symptoms and clinical signs and symptoms. *Primary* syphilis is characterized by a primary lesion, the chancre that appears 5 to 90 days after infection. This lesion often begins as a painless papule at the site of inoculation and then erodes to form a nontender, shallow, indurated, clean ulcer several millimeters to centimeters in size (Fig. 7.1A). *Secondary* syphilis occurs 6 weeks to 6 months after the appearance of the chancre and is characterized by a widespread symmetric maculopapular rash on the palms and soles and generalized lymphadenopathy. The infected individual may also experience fever, headache, and malaise. Condylomata lata (broad, painless, pink-gray wart like infectious lesions) may develop on the vulva, perineum, or anus (see Fig. 7.1B). If the woman is untreated, she enters a latent phase that is usually asymptomatic. Latent infections are those that lack clinical manifestations but are detected by serologic testing. If the infection was acquired in the preceding year, the infection is termed an *early latent* infection. If it is left untreated, *tertiary* syphilis will develop in about one-third of such women. Neurologic, cardiovascular, musculoskeletal, or multiorgan-system complications can develop in the tertiary stage.

Screening and Diagnosis

All women who are diagnosed with another STI or with HIV should be screened for syphilis. All pregnant women should be screened

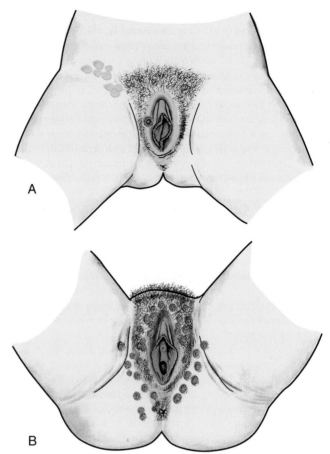

Fig. 7.1 Syphilis. (A) Primary stage: chancre with inguinal adenopathy. (B) Secondary stage: condylomata lata.

for syphilis at the first prenatal visit and again early in the third trimester and at the time of giving birth if they are at high risk. Diagnosis is dependent on microscopic examination of primary and secondary lesion tissue and serology during latency and late infection. Dark-field examinations and tests to detect *T. pallidum* directly from lesion exudate or tissue are the definitive methods for diagnosing early syphilis. A test for antibodies may not be reactive in the presence of active infection because it takes time for the body's immune system to develop antibodies to any antigen. Up to one-third of people with early primary syphilis may have nonreactive serologic tests. Two types of serologic tests are used: nontreponemal and treponemal. Nontreponemal antibody tests, such as the Venereal Disease Research Laboratories (VDRL) or the rapid plasma reagin (RPR) test, are used as screening tests. False-positive results are not unusual, particularly when acute infection, autoimmune disorders, malignancy, pregnancy, and drug addiction exist and after immunization or vaccination. The treponemal tests—fluorescent treponemal antibody-absorbed (FTA-ABS), and the *T. pallidum* passive particle agglutination (TP-PA) assay—are used to confirm positive results. Test results in clients with early primary or incubating syphilis can be negative. Seroconversion usually takes place 6 to 8 weeks after exposure, so testing should be repeated in 1 to 2 months when a suggestive genital lesion exists. Tests for coexisting STIs (e.g., chlamydia and gonorrhea) should be done (e.g., NAATs and cultures) and HIV testing offered if indicated (CDC, 2015b).

Management

Penicillin G is the preferred drug for treating syphilis (see Table 7.2). It is the only proven therapy that has been widely used to treat neurosyphilis, congenital syphilis, or syphilis during pregnancy. Intramuscular benzathine penicillin G is used to treat primary, secondary, and early latent syphilis. Although doxycycline, tetracycline, and erythromycin are alternative treatments for penicillin-allergic clients, both tetracycline and doxycycline are contraindicated in pregnancy, and erythromycin is unlikely to cure a fetal infection. Therefore pregnant women should, if necessary, receive skin testing and be treated with penicillin or be desensitized (CDC, 2015b). Specific protocols are recommended in the treatment guidelines (https://www.cdc.gov/std/tg2015/clinical.htm).

🖉 MEDICATION ALERT

Clients treated for syphilis with penicillin may experience a Jarisch-Herxheimer reaction. This acute febrile reaction is often accompanied by headache, myalgias, and arthralgias that develop within the first 24 hrs of treatment. The reaction can be treated symptomatically with analgesics and antipyretics. If the treatment precipitates this reaction in the second half of pregnancy, women are at risk for preterm labor and birth. They should be advised to contact their health care provider if they notice any change in fetal movement or have any contractions.

Monthly follow-up is mandatory so that repeated treatment may be given if needed. The nurse should emphasize the necessity of long-term serologic testing even in the absence of symptoms. The woman should be advised to practice sexual abstinence until treatment is completed, all evidence of primary and secondary syphilis is gone, and serologic evidence of a cure is demonstrated. Women should be told to notify all partners who may have been exposed. They should be informed that the disease is reportable. Preventive measures should be discussed.

Pelvic Inflammatory Disease

Pelvic inflammatory disease (PID) is an infectious process that most commonly involves the uterine (fallopian) tubes (salpingitis), uterus (endometritis), and, more rarely, the ovaries and peritoneal surfaces. Multiple organisms have been found to cause PID, and most cases are associated with more than one organism. In the past, the most common causative agent was thought to be *N. gonorrhoeae;* however, *C. trachomatis* is now estimated to cause half of all cases of PID. In addition to gonorrhea and chlamydia, a wide variety of anaerobic and aerobic bacteria are recognized to cause PID. PID encompasses a wide variety of pathologic processes; the infection can either be acute, subacute, or chronic and can have a wide range of symptoms.

Most PID results from ascending spread of microorganisms from the vagina and endocervix to the upper genital tract. This spread most frequently happens at the end of or just after menses following reception of an infectious agent. During the menstrual period several factors facilitate the development of an infection: the cervical os is slightly open, the cervical mucous barrier is absent, and menstrual blood is an excellent medium for growth. PID also can develop after a miscarriage or an induced abortion, pelvic surgery, or birth.

Risk factors for acquiring PID are those associated with the risk of contracting an STI, including young age (most cases of acute PID are in women younger than age 25), nulliparity, multiple partners, high rate of new partners, and a history of STIs and PID. Women who use intrauterine devices (IUDs) may be at increased risk for PID up to 3 weeks after insertion (Gardella, Eckert, & Lentz, 2017). PID tends to recur.

Women who have had PID are at increased risk for ectopic pregnancy, infertility, and chronic pelvic pain. After a single episode of PID, a woman's risk for ectopic pregnancy increases sevenfold compared with the risk for women who have never had PID. Other problems associated with PID include dyspareunia (painful intercourse), pyosalpinx (pus in the uterine tubes), tubo-ovarian abscess, and pelvic adhesions.

The symptoms of PID vary depending on whether the infection is acute, subacute, or chronic; however, pain is common to all types of infections. It may be dull, cramping, and intermittent (subacute) or severe, persistent, and incapacitating (acute). Women may also report one or more of the following: fever, chills, nausea and vomiting, increased vaginal discharge, symptoms of a urinary tract infection, and irregular bleeding. Abdominal pain is usually present (Gardella, et al., 2017).

Screening and Diagnosis

PID is difficult to diagnose because of the accompanying wide variety of symptoms. The CDC recommends treatment for PID in all sexually active young women and others at risk for STIs if the following criteria are present and no other cause or causes of the illness are found: lower abdominal tenderness, bilateral adnexal tenderness, and cervical motion tenderness. Other criteria for diagnosing PID include an oral temperature of 38.3°C (100.9°F) or above, abnormal cervical or vaginal discharge, elevated erythrocyte sedimentation rate, elevated C-reactive protein, and laboratory documentation of cervical infection with *N. gonorrhoeae* or *C. trachomatis* (CDC, 2015b).

Management

Perhaps the most important nursing intervention is prevention. Primary prevention includes education about preventing the acquisition of STIs, and secondary prevention involves preventing a lower genital tract infection from ascending to the upper genital tract. Instructing women in self-protective behaviors such as practicing risk-reduction measures and using barrier methods is critical. Also important is the detection of asymptomatic gonorrheal and chlamydial infections through routine screening of women with risky behaviors or specific risk factors such as age.

Although treatment regimens vary with the infecting organism, a broad-spectrum antibiotic is generally used (Box 7.3). Treatment for mild to moderately severe PID may be oral medication or may involve a combination of oral and parenteral agents, and such regimens can be administered in inpatient or outpatient settings (CDC, 2015b). Comfort measures include analgesics for pain and all other nursing measures applicable to a woman confined to bed. The woman should have as few pelvic examinations as possible during the acute phase of the disease. During the recovery phase the woman should restrict her activity and make every effort to get adequate rest and eat a nutritionally sound diet. Follow-up laboratory work after treatment should include endocervical cultures for a test of cure.

Health education is central to the effective management of PID. The nurse should explain to women the nature of their disease and encourage them to comply with all therapy and prevention recommendations, emphasizing the necessity of taking all medication even if symptoms disappear. The nurse should counsel women to refrain from sexual intercourse until their treatment is complete and provide contraceptive counseling. A woman with a history of PID may choose an IUD as her contraceptive method.

The potential or actual loss of reproductive ability can be devastating and can adversely affect a woman's self-concept. The woman may need help in adjusting her self-concept to fit reality and accept alterations in a way that promotes health. Because PID is so closely tied to sexuality, body image, and self-concept, the woman diagnosed with it will need supportive care and should be encouraged to discuss her feelings. Referral to a support group or for counseling may be appropriate.

SEXUALLY TRANSMITTED VIRAL INFECTIONS

Human Papillomavirus

HPV infections, also known as *condylomata acuminata,* or *genital warts,* is the most common viral STI seen in ambulatory health care

BOX 7.3 Treatment of Pelvic Inflammatory Disease

Parenteral Treatment

Cefotetan, 2 q IV q 12 hours
PLUS
doxycycline, 100 mg PO or IV q 12 hours for 14 days
OR Cefoxitin, 2 g IV q 6 hours
PLUS
doxycycline, 100 mg PO or IV q 12 hours for 14 days
OR
Clindamycin, 900 mg IV q 8 hours
PLUS
Gentamicin, loading dose IV or IM (2 mg/kg) followed by maintenance dose (1.5 mg/kg) q 8 hours
Parenteral therapy can be discontinued 24 hours after clinical improvement. Ongoing oral therapy consisting of doxycycline 100 mg PO or clindamycine 450 mg PO qid for 14 days

Intramuscular/Oral Treatment

Ceftriaxone 250 mg IM single dose
PLUS
Doxycycline 100 mg PO bid for 14 days
WITH OR WITHOUT
Metronidazole 500 mg PO bid for 14 days
OR
Cefoxitin 2 g IM single dose and probenecid 1 g PO concurrently in single dose
PLUS
Doxycycline 100 mg PO bid for 14 days
WITH OR WITHOUT
Metronidazole 500 mg bid for 14 days
OR
Other parenteral third-generation cephalosporin (ceftizoxime or cefotaxime)
PLUS
Doxycycline 100 mg PO bid for 14 days
WITH OR WITHOUT
Metronidazole 500 mg PO bid for 14 days

IM, Intramuscular; *IV,* intravenous; *PO,* per os. Centers for Disease Control and Prevention (CDC). (2015b). 2015 Sexually transmitted disease treatment guidelines. *Morbidity and Mortality Weekly Report, 64*(3), 1–140.

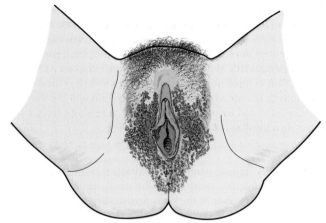

Fig. 7.2 Human Papillomavirus Infection. Genital warts or condylomata acuminata.

as the vaginal introitus, the lesions may appear to have multiple, fine fingerlike projections. Vaginal lesions are often multiple. Flat-topped papules, 1 to 4 mm in diameter, are seen most often on the cervix and are often visualized only under magnification. Warts are usually flesh-colored or slightly darker on Caucasian women, black on African American women, and brownish on Asian women. The lesions are often painless but may be uncomfortable, particularly when they are very large, inflamed, or ulcerated. Chronic vaginal discharge, pruritus, or dyspareunia can occur.

HPV infections are thought to be more frequent in pregnant than in nonpregnant women, with an increase in incidence from the first to the third trimester. Furthermore, a significant proportion of preexisting HPV lesions enlarge greatly during pregnancy, a proliferation presumably resulting from the relative state of immunosuppression present during pregnancy. Lesions can become so large during pregnancy that they affect urination, defecation, mobility, and fetal descent; they can obstruct the birth canal, although birth by cesarean is rarely necessary (CDC, 2015b). Cesarean birth may be performed when extensive growths are present. Initial observation of large growths can be misleading, suggesting that the entire vagina is involved. However, all of the growth may derive from one stalk; in such cases it may be possible to push the large mass to the side, allowing the baby to pass through.

Screening and Diagnosis

A woman with HPV lesions may complain of symptoms such as a profuse irritating vaginal discharge, itching, dyspareunia, or postcoital bleeding. She also may report "bumps" on her vulva or labia. History of a known exposure is important; however, because of the potentially long latency period and the possibility of subclinical infections in men, the lack of a history of known exposure cannot be used to exclude a diagnosis of HPV infection.

Physical inspection of the vulva, perineum, anus, vagina, and cervix is essential whenever HPV lesions are suspected or seen in one area. Because speculum examination of the vagina may block some lesions, it is important to rotate the speculum blades until all areas have been visualized. When lesions are visible, the characteristic appearance previously described is considered diagnostic. In many instances, however, cervical lesions are not visible, and some vaginal or vulvar lesions may also be unobservable to the naked eye. Because of the potential spread of vulvar or vaginal lesions to the anus, gloves should be changed between vaginal and rectal examinations.

Viral screening and typing for HPV is available but not standard practice. History, evaluation of signs and symptoms, the Papanicolaou (Pap) test, and physical examination are used in making a diagnosis. The HPV-DNA test can be used in combination with the Pap test to screen for types of HPV that are likely to cause cancer in women older

settings. There are approximately 100 types of HPV, which is a double-stranded DNA virus; about 40 of these types have been found to be causes of anogenital infections. There are several that can cause genital cancers, with two specific types (16 and 18) being highly oncogenic, meaning that they pose highest risk for causing cancers of the cervix, vagina, vulva, penis, and oropharyngeal area (CDC, 2015b). HPV is the primary cause of cervical neoplasia.

An estimated 79 million Americans are infected with HPV, and about 14.1 million new infections occur every year. HPV is not a nationally reportable condition, and the CDC estimates that almost 50% of all sexually active women will become infected in their lifetimes. Most HPV infections are asymptomatic, and it has now been found that most appear to resolve spontaneously within a few years. The highest rate of HPV infection occurs in women aged 20 to 24 years. HPV types 6 and 11 are responsible for approximately 90% of genital warts (CDC, 2017a).

HPV lesions in women are most commonly seen in the posterior part of the introitus; however, lesions are also found on the buttocks, vulva, vagina, anus, and cervix (Fig. 7.2). Typically the lesions are small—2 to 3 mm in diameter and 10 to 15 mm in height. They appear as soft, papillary swellings occurring singly or in clusters in the genital and anorectal regions. Lesions resulting from infections of long duration may appear as a cauliflower-like mass. In moist areas such than age 30 or in those with abnormal Pap test results (American Cancer Society [ACS], 2016). The only definitive diagnostic test for the presence of HPV is histologic evaluation of a biopsy specimen.

HPV lesions must be differentiated from molluscum contagiosum and condylomata lata. Molluscum contagiosum lesions are half-domed, smooth, flesh-colored to pearly white papules with depressed centers. Condylomata lata are a form of secondary syphilis and the lesions are generally flatter and wider than genital warts. A serologic test for syphilis confirms the diagnosis of secondary syphilis.

Management

Untreated HPV infection resolves spontaneously in young women because their immune systems may be strong enough to fight the HPV infection. However, if the virus persists, depending on the type of virus, genital warts or cancer can develop months or years after the woman has been infected with HPV (CDC, 2017a). No therapy has been shown to eradicate HPV. The goal of treatment for genital warts is removal of the warts and relief of signs and symptoms. Treatment for cervical cancer is discussed in Chapter 11.

Treatment of genital warts should be guided by the preference of the woman, available resources, and the experience of the health care provider. The woman must often make multiple office visits, and many different treatment modalities will be used. None of the treatments is superior to all other treatments, and no one treatment is ideal for all warts (CDC, 2017a).

Available treatments are outlined in Table 7.2. Imiquimod, podophyllin, podofilox, and sinecatechins should not be used during pregnancy. Because the lesions can proliferate and become friable during pregnancy, many experts recommend their removal by using cryotherapy or various surgical techniques during pregnancy (CDC, 2017a).

Women with discomfort associated with genital warts may find that bathing with an oatmeal solution and drying the area with a hair

---

EVIDENCE-BASED PRACTICE

Age-Based Cervical Screening Recommendations Using Cytology and/or Human Papillomavirus Typing

Ask the Question
How does cytology screening (conventional or liquid-based) compare to HPV testing in sensitivity and specificity for detection and treatment of cervical cancer? Does age make a difference in recommendations?

Search for the Evidence
Search Strategies English language reviews, systematic reviews, meta-analyses, and practice guidelines on cervical cytology and HPV typing were included.

Databases Used Cochrane Database of Systematic Reviews, National Guideline Clearinghouse (AHRQ), PubMed, UpToDate, Cumulative Index to Nursing and Allied Health Literature (CINAHL) and the professional websites for American College of Obstetricians and Gynecologists (ACOG) and Association of Women's Health, Obstetric, and Neonatal Nursing (AWHONN)

Critical Appraisal of the Evidence
El Zein, Richardson, & Franco (2016); Goodman (2015); Kessler (2017); Wuerthner & Avila-Wallace (2016):
- Cervical abnormalities that may progress to cervical cancer are caused by certain high-risk oncogenic HPV types.
- Cervical screening includes conventional Papanicolaou (Pap) slide preparation, liquid-based cytology (LBC), and HPV testing.
- High-risk HPV testing (primary screening) had the highest sensitivity for detecting cervical neoplasia but has the lowest specificity.
- Using HPV testing first with follow-up cytology for high-risk HPV results enhances the detection of severe precancerous cervical changes (cervical intraepithelial neoplasia, severe [CIN 3]). The incidence of cervical cancer was lower in women first screened with HPV testing compared with cytology alone.
- The major benefit from using HPV testing as the primary screen may be a longer screening interval for a low-risk population.
- Ongoing research in HPV subtypes, markers, and clinical history can further focus screening targets.
- In women below 30 years of age, most HPV infections resolve within 8 months.

ACOG (2016):
- Cervical cancer screening should begin at 21 years of age. Unless HIV-positive or otherwise immunocompromised, women below 21 years of age should not be screened regardless of the age of sexual initiation or whether other behavior-related risk factors are present.

- Cytology screening alone is recommended every 3 years for women 21-29 years old. Annual screening should not be performed.
- For women ages 30-65, cytology and HPV testing are recommended every 5 years. Alternately, cytology alone every 3 years is acceptable. Annual screening should not be performed.
- In the presence of hysterectomy and no history of cervical intraepithelial neoplasia, moderate (CIN 2) or higher, screening may be discontinued and not restarted for any reason.
- Screening may be discontinued for women after age 65 if adequate testing has been negative for 10 years, with the most recent test being performed within the past 5 years.

Apply the Evidence: Nursing Implications
Kessler (2017):
- Nurses must stay informed about current cervical screening guidelines so that clients can be educated as well. Clients should know that the HPV vaccine is safe and that it prevents cancer.
- Nurses should be aware of effective behavior-change models to promote cervical cancer prevention strategies. For college-aged young adults, there is a gap in the number who have received the HPV vaccination. Nurses working in college settings are in a position to implement behavior-change models to affect the health of this particular population.
- Nurses have an opportunity to educate clients about risk factors of cervical cancer, including HPV positivity, past or current chlamydial infection, a diet low in fruits and vegetables, smoking, positive family history of cervical cancer, and three or more full-term pregnancies.

References
American College of Obstetricians and Gynecologists. (2016). Practice bulletin number 168: Cervical cancer screening and prevention. *Obstetrics and Gynecology, 128*(4), 923–925.
El Zein, M., Richardson, L., & Franco, E. L. (2016). Cervical cancer screening of HPV vaccinated populations: Cytology, molecular testing, both or none. *Journal of Clinical Virology, 76*(1), S62–S68.
Goodman, A. (2015). HPV testing as a screen for cervical cancer. *The British Medical Journal, 350*, 1–14. h2372.
Kessler, T. (2017). Cervical cancer: Prevention and early detection. *Seminars in Oncology Nursing, 33*(2), 172–183.
Wuerthner, B. A., & Avila-Wallace, M. (2016). Cervical cancer: Screening, management, and prevention. *The Nurse Practitioner, 41*(9), 18–23.

Jennifer Taylor Alderman

dryer on a cool or low setting provides some relief. Keeping the area clean and dry also decreases growth of the warts. Cotton underwear and loose-fitting clothes that decrease friction and irritation may also decrease discomfort. Women should be advised to maintain a healthy lifestyle to aid the immune system; women can be counseled regarding diet, rest, stress reduction, and exercise.

Client counseling is essential to reduce the prevalence of HPV and to improve the management of HPV in women who are infected. Women need to know that HPV infection is very common and, in most cases, will clear up spontaneously. Some infections will progress to genital warts, precancerous lesions, or cancers. Women must understand how the virus is transmitted, that no immunity is conferred with infection, and that reacquisition of the infection is likely with repeated contact. Because HPV is highly contagious, the majority of partners of women with HPV will be infected even if they are asymptomatic. All sexually active women with multiple partners or a history of HPV should be encouraged to use latex condoms consistently and correctly for intercourse in order to decrease the risk of acquisition or transmission of genital HPV (CDC, 2017a).

Instructions for all medications and treatments must be detailed. Women should be told that treatments are for the conditions caused by the virus but not HPV itself. Women should be informed before treatment of the possibility of posttreatment pain associated with specific therapies. The importance of the thorough treatment of concurrent vaginitis or a coexisting STI should be emphasized. The link between cervical cancer and some HPV infections and the need for close follow-up should be discussed. Annual health examinations are recommended to assess disease recurrence and screen for cervical cancer. Women 21 years of age and older should be counseled to have regular Pap screening, as recommended for women without genital warts (CDC, 2017a). Preventive strategies such as those presented in the following section should also be discussed.

Prevention

Preventive strategies include abstinence from all sexual activity, staying in a long-term monogamous relationship, limiting the number of sexual partners, and prophylactic vaccination (CDC, 2017a).

Gardasil 9, a 9 valent vaccine, is available in the U.S. This vaccine was previously recommended for 9- to 26-year-old females and then became available to males. Recently it has been approved for females and males ages 9 through 45 (U.S. Food & Drug Administration, 2018) and are safe and effective in protecting against some of the most common types of HPV that can lead to genital warts and cancers. Gardasil 9 protects against types 6, 11, 16, 18, 31, 33, 35, 45, 52, and 58. The vaccine is most effective if given before the woman has her first sexual contact (Meites, Kempe & Markowitz, 2016). The vaccine can be given to girls and boys as early as 9 years of age and can also be given to young women and men ages 15 to 26 years if they did not receive the vaccine previously. The vaccine is given in a 2-dose schedule for girls and boys who initiate the vaccine series at age 9 to 14 years. The 3 dose schedule remains for those who are immunocompromised or initiate the vaccine series at age 15 to 45 years.

Genital Herpes Simplex Virus

Genital herpes simplex virus (HSV) infection results in painful recurrent genital ulcers and is caused by two antigen subtypes of herpes simplex virus: herpes simplex virus 1 (HSV-1) and herpes simplex virus 2 (HSV-2). HSV-2 is usually transmitted sexually and HSV-1 nonsexually. Although HSV-1 is more commonly associated with gingivostomatitis and oral labial ulcers (fever blisters/cold sores) and HSV-2 with genital lesions, neither type is exclusively associated with the respective sites.

Although HSV infection is not a reportable disease, so its true prevalence is unknown and many people with genital HSV may not have received a clinical diagnosis; however, it remains one of the most prevalent STIs. Non-Hispanic black women have the highest rates of any racial group (CDC, 2017a). Women between the ages of 15 and 34 are most likely to become infected, especially if they have multiple sex partners.

Many persons infected with HSV-2 are asymptomatic and therefore undiagnosed. They can transmit the infection while unaware that they are infected.

An initial HSV genital infection is characterized by multiple painful lesions, fever, chills, malaise, and severe dysuria and may last 2 to 3 weeks. Women generally have a more severe clinical course than men. Women with primary genital herpes have many lesions that progress from macules to papules and then form vesicles, pustules, and ulcers that crust and heal without scarring (Fig. 7.3). These ulcers are extremely tender, and primary infections may be bilateral. Women can also have itching, inguinal tenderness, and lymphadenopathy. Severe vulvar edema may develop, and women may have difficulty sitting. HSV cervicitis is also common with initial HSV-2 infections. The cervix may appear normal or be friable, reddened, ulcerated, or necrotic. A heavy watery-to-purulent vaginal discharge is common. Extragenital lesions may be present because of autoinoculation. Urinary retention and dysuria may occur secondary to autonomic involvement of the sacral nerve root.

Women with recurrent episodes of HSV infections commonly have only local symptoms that are usually less severe than those associated with the initial infection. Systemic symptoms are usually absent, although the characteristic prodromal genital tingling is common. Recurrent lesions are unilateral, less severe, and usually last 5 to 7 days. Lesions begin as vesicles and progress rapidly to ulcers. Few women with recurrent disease have cervicitis.

During pregnancy, maternal infection with HSV-2 can have adverse effects on both the mother and fetus. Viremia occurs during the primary infection, and congenital infection is possible though rare. Primary infections during the first trimester have been associated with increased rates of miscarriage (CDC, 2017a). The most severe complication of HSV infection is neonatal herpes, a potentially fatal or severely disabling disease occurring in 1 in 2000 to 10,000 live births. Most mothers of infants who contract neonatal herpes lack histories of clinically evident genital herpes. The risk of neonatal infection is highest among women with primary herpes infection who are near term and is low among women with recurrent herpes (CDC, 2015a).

Screening and Diagnosis

A detailed client history is important when attempting to diagnose herpes. A history of exposure to an infected person is important, although infection from an asymptomatic individual is possible. A history of having viral symptoms such as malaise, headache, fever, or myalgia is

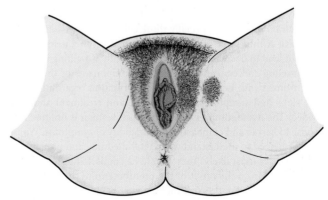

Fig. 7.3 Herpes Genitalis.

suggestive. Local symptoms such as vulvar pain, dysuria, itching, or burning at the site of infection and painful genital lesions that heal spontaneously are also highly suggestive of HSV infection. The nurse should ask about a history of a primary infection, prodromal symptoms, vaginal discharge, and dyspareunia. Women should be asked whether they or their partners have had genital lesions.

During the physical examination the health care provider assesses for inguinal and generalized lymphadenopathy and elevated temperature. The entire vulvar, perineal, vaginal, and cervical areas should be carefully inspected for vesicles or ulcerated or crusted areas. A speculum examination may be very difficult for the woman because of the extreme tenderness often associated with herpes infections. Any suggestive or recurrent lesions found during pregnancy should be cultured to verify HSV. Although a diagnosis of herpes infection may be suspected from the history and physical, it is confirmed by laboratory studies. A viral culture is obtained by swabbing exudate during the vesicular stage of the disease. Type-specific serologic tests for HSV-2 antibodies are also available (CDC, 2015b).

Management

Genital herpes is a chronic and recurring disease for which there is no known cure. Management is directed toward specific treatment during primary and recurrent infections, prevention of recurrences, self-help measures, and psychologic support.

Systemic antiviral medications partially control the symptoms and signs of HSV infections when used for the primary or recurrent episodes or as daily suppressive therapy. However, these medications do not eradicate the infection, nor do they alter subsequent risk or frequency of recurrences after the medication is stopped. Three antiviral medications provide clinical benefit: acyclovir, valacyclovir, and famciclovir. Treatment recommendations are given in Table 7.2. The safety of acyclovir, valacyclovir, and famciclovir therapy during pregnancy has not been established; however, acyclovir may be used to reduce the symptoms of HSV if the benefits to the woman outweigh the potential harm to the fetus (CDC, 2015b). Continued investigation of HSV therapy with these medications in pregnancy is needed.

Cleaning lesions twice a day with saline helps prevent secondary infection. Bacterial infection must be treated with appropriate antibiotics. Measures that may increase comfort for women when lesions are active include warm sitz baths with baking soda; keeping lesions dry by blowing the area dry with a hair dryer set on cool or patting dry with a soft towel; wearing cotton underwear and loose clothing; using drying aids such as hydrogen peroxide, Burow solution, or oatmeal baths; applying cool, wet black teabags to lesions; and applying compresses with an infusion of cloves or peppermint oil and clove oil to lesions.

Oral analgesics such as aspirin, acetaminophen, or ibuprofen may be used to relieve pain and systemic symptoms associated with initial infections. Because the mucous membranes affected by herpes are extremely sensitive, any topical agents should be used with caution. Nonantiviral ointments, especially those containing cortisone, should be avoided. A thin layer of lidocaine ointment or an antiseptic spray may be applied to decrease discomfort, especially if walking is painful.

Counseling and education are critical components of the nursing care of women with herpes infections. Information regarding the etiology, signs and symptoms, transmission, and treatment should be provided. The nurse should explain that each woman is unique in her response to herpes and emphasize the variability of symptoms. Women should be helped to understand when viral shedding and transmission to a partner are most likely. They should be counseled to refrain from sexual contact from the onset of the prodrome until the lesions have completely healed. Suppressive therapy may be an option because it can decrease the risk of transmission to partners (CDC, 2015b).

Some authorities recommend consistent use of condoms for all persons with genital herpes. Condoms may not prevent transmission, particularly male-to-female transmission; however, this does not mean that the partners should avoid all intimacy. Women can maintain close contact with their partners who should be aware of the need to avoid contact with the woman's herpetic lesions. They should be taught how to look for herpetic lesions using a mirror and a good light source and a wet cloth or finger covered with a finger cot to rub lightly over the labia. The nurse should make sure to explain that when lesions are active, it is important to avoid sharing intimate articles such as washcloths that come into contact with the lesions. Only plain soap and water or hand sanitizer are needed to clean hands that have come into contact with herpetic lesions; isolation is neither necessary nor appropriate.

Stress, menstruation, trauma, febrile illnesses, chronic illnesses, and ultraviolet light have all been found to trigger genital herpes. Women may wish to keep a diary to identify stressors that seem to be associated with recurrent herpes attacks so that they can then avoid these stressors when possible. The role of exercise in reducing stress can be discussed. Referral for stress-reduction therapy, yoga, or meditation classes may be indicated. It may be helpful to avoid exposure to sun and excessive heat, including hot baths; and to use a lubricant to reduce friction during sexual intercourse. Women in their childbearing years should be counseled regarding the risk of herpes infection during pregnancy. They should be instructed to use condoms if there is any risk of contracting an STI from a sexual partner. If they become pregnant while taking acyclovir, the risk of birth defects does not appear to be higher than for the general population; however, continued use should be based on whether the benefits for the woman outweigh the possible risks to the fetus. Acyclovir does enter breast milk, but the amount of medication ingested during breastfeeding is very low and is usually not a health concern (CDC, 2015b).

Because neonatal HSV infection is such a devastating disease, prevention is critical. Recommendations include carefully examining and questioning all women about symptoms of HSV infection at the onset of labor. If visible lesions are not present at onset of labor, vaginal birth is acceptable. Cesarean birth is recommended if visible lesions are present (CDC, 2015b). Some authorities recommend cesarean birth also if prodromal symptoms (like genital tingling) are present, even if there are no visible lesions. Infants who are born through an infected vagina should be carefully observed and their body fluids cultured (see Chapter 35).

The emotional effect of contracting an incurable STI such as herpes is considerable. At diagnosis, many emotions may surface—helplessness, anger, denial, guilt, anxiety, shame, or inadequacy. Women need the opportunity to discuss their feelings and also need help in learning to live with the disease. Herpes can affect a woman's sexuality, her sexual practices, and her current and future relationships. Women may need help in raising the issue with their partners or future partners. The partners may also benefit from counseling.

Viral Hepatitis

Five different viruses (hepatitis viruses A, B, C, D, and E) account for almost all cases of viral hepatitis in humans. Hepatitis viruses A, B, and C are discussed. Hepatitis D and E viruses, common among intravenous drug users (IDUs) and recipients of multiple blood transfusions, are not included in this discussion.

Hepatitis A

Hepatitis A virus (HAV) infection is acquired primarily through a fecal-oral route by ingestion of contaminated food, particularly milk, shellfish, or polluted water, or person-to-person contact (CDC, 2015b). Risk factors for hepatitis A include sexual and household contacts with others who have hepatitis A; children as well as caregivers exposed to hepatitis A in nursery, daycare, or preschool; men who have sex with men (MSM); IDUs; international travelers; and persons exposed to a common-source food or water outbreak. Transmission of HAV during sexual activity probably results from fecal-oral contact (CDC, 2015b). HAV infection is characterized by flulike symptoms, with malaise, fatigue, anorexia, nausea, pruritus, fever, and right upper quadrant pain. Serologic testing to detect the immunoglobulin M (IgM) antibody is done to confirm acute infections. The IgM antibody is detectable 5 to 10 days after exposure and can remain positive for up to 6 months. Because HAV infection is self-limited and does not result in chronic infection or chronic liver disease, treatment is usually supportive. Women who become dehydrated from nausea and vomiting or who have fulminating hepatitis A may need to be hospitalized. Medications and other ingested substances that might cause liver damage or are metabolized in the liver (e.g., acetaminophen, ethyl alcohol) should be avoided. No specific diet or activity restrictions are necessary. Hepatitis A vaccine and immunoglobulin (Ig) for intramuscular administration are effective in preventing most hepatitis A infections (CDC, 2015b). Food-related HAV outbreaks are reportable and local health departments and the CDC are involved in locating the source of infection and as many infected individuals as possible.

Hepatitis B

Hepatitis B virus (HBV) is the virus most threatening to the fetus and neonate. It is caused by a large DNA virus and is associated with three antigens and their antibodies: hepatitis B surface antigen (HBsAg), HBV antigen (HBeAg), HBV core antigen (HBcAg), antibody to HBsAg (anti-HBs), antibody to HBeAg (anti-HBe), and antibody to HBcAg (anti-HBc). Screening for active or chronic disease or disease immunity is based on testing for these antigens and their antibodies.

Populations at risk include women of Asian, Pacific Island (Polynesian, Micronesian, Melanesian), or Alaska Native–Inuit descent, and women born in Haiti or sub-Saharan Africa. Women who have a history of acute or chronic liver disease, who work or receive treatment in a dialysis unit, or who have household or sexual contact with a hemodialysis client are at greater risk. Women who work or live in institutions for the mentally challenged are considered to be at risk, as are women with a history of multiple blood transfusions. Health care workers and public safety workers exposed to blood in the workplace are at risk. Behaviors such as having multiple sexual partners and a history of intravenous drug use increase the risk of contracting HBV infections. Drug abusers who share needles are at risk, as are health care workers who are exposed to blood and needlesticks.

HBsAg has been found in blood, saliva, sweat, tears, vaginal secretions, and semen. Perinatal transmission most often occurs in infants of mothers who have acute hepatitis infection late in the third trimester or during the intrapartum or postpartum period from exposure to HBsAg-positive vaginal secretions, blood, amniotic fluid, saliva, and breast milk. HBV has also been transmitted by artificial insemination.

Although HBV can be transmitted via blood transfusion, the incidence of such infections has decreased significantly since testing of blood for HBsAg became routine.

HBV infection is a disease of the liver and is often a silent infection. In an adult the course can be sudden and severe and the outcome fatal. Symptoms of HBV infection are similar to those of hepatitis A: arthralgias, arthritis, lassitude, anorexia, nausea, vomiting, headache, fever, and mild abdominal pain. Later the woman may have clay-colored stools, dark urine, increased abdominal pain, and jaundice. Some individuals with HBV have persistence of HBsAg and become chronic hepatitis B carriers.

Screening and Diagnosis

All women at high risk for contracting HBV should be screened regularly at routine appointments. However, screening only individuals at high risk may not identify up to 50% of HBsAg-positive women. Screening for the presence of HBsAg is recommended for all pregnant women at the first prenatal visit regardless of whether they have been tested previously. Screening is recommended for women at high risk or in areas of the country with large numbers of Hepatitis B+ women (just like HIV testing), and women are automatically tested during the third trimester (or on admission for birth) if they had no prenatal care or if lab results are not available (CDC, 2015b).

If HBsAg persists in the blood, the woman is identified as a carrier. If the HBsAg test result is positive, further laboratory studies may be ordered: anti-HBe, anti-HBc, serum glutamic-oxaloacetic transaminase (SGOT), alkaline phosphatase, and a liver panel.

Management

There is no specific treatment for hepatitis B. Recovery is usually spontaneous in 3 to 16 weeks. Pregnancies complicated by acute viral hepatitis are managed on an outpatient basis. Women should be advised to increase rest periods; eat a high-protein, low-fat diet; and increase their fluid intake. They should avoid alcohol and medications metabolized in the liver. Pregnant women with a definite exposure to HBV should be given hepatitis B immune globulin and should begin the hepatitis B vaccine series within 14 days of the most recent contact to prevent infection (CDC, 2015b). Vaccination during pregnancy is not thought to pose risks to the fetus.

All unvaccinated women at high or moderate risk of hepatitis should be informed of the availability of hepatitis B vaccine. Vaccination is recommended for all individuals who have had multiple sex partners within the past 6 months, IDUs, residents of correctional or long-term care facilities, people seeking care for an STI, prostitutes, women whose partners are IDUs or bisexual, and women whose occupation exposes them to high risk should be vaccinated. The vaccine is given in a series of three (four if rapid protection is needed) doses over a 6-month period, with the first two doses given at least 1 month apart. The vaccine is given in the deltoid muscle (CDC, 2015b).

Client education includes explaining the meaning of hepatitis B infection, including transmission, state of infectivity, and sequelae. The nurse also should explain the need for immunoprophylaxis for household members and sexual contacts. To decrease transmission of the virus, women with hepatitis B or those who test positive for HBV should be advised to maintain a high level of personal hygiene (e.g., wash hands after using the toilet; carefully dispose of tampons, pads, and bandages in plastic bags; do not share razor blades, toothbrushes, needles, or manicure implements; have male partner use a condom if unvaccinated and without hepatitis; avoid sharing saliva through kissing or sharing of silverware or dishes; and wipe up blood spills immediately with soap and water). They should inform all health care providers of their carrier state. Postpartum women should be reassured that breastfeeding is not contraindicated if their infants received prophylaxis at birth and are currently on the immunization schedule (see Chapter 24).

Hepatitis C

Hepatitis C virus (HCV) infection has become an important health problem as increasing numbers of persons acquire the disease. The CDC estimates that individuals born between 1945 and 1965 make up about 75% of all HCV infections. Hepatitis C is responsible for nearly 50% of the cases of chronic viral hepatitis. Risk factors include having STIs such as HBV and HIV, multiple sexual partners, history of blood transfusions, and history of intravenous drug use. HCV is readily transmitted through exposure to blood and much less efficiently via semen, saliva, or urine (CDC, 2015a).

Most clients with HCV are asymptomatic or have general influenza-like symptoms similar to those of HAV. Previously HCV testing was done on people based on known risk factors and clinical manifestations. The CDC recommends one-time testing of adults born between 1945 and 1965 be instituted without prior determination of HCV risk factors (CDC, 2015a). HCV infection is confirmed by the presence of anti-C antibody during laboratory testing.

Currently there is no vaccine to prevent HCV. Its transmission through breastfeeding has not been reported. The CDC (2017d) does not recommend routine testing for HCV in pregnant women unless they are considered to be at high risk.

The U.S. FDA (USFDA, 2017) has approved several drugs for the treatment of hepatitis C, although more study is needed to determine the safety of these drugs during pregnancy.

Human Immunodeficiency Virus

Approximately 25% of people currently living with HIV infection are women; however, over the past 10 years there has been an estimated decrease of 40% of newly diagnosed cases of HIV infection among women. The largest proportion of HIV infection is found among African American women, followed by Caucasian and Hispanic/Latinas. There is also a high prevalence of HIV infection among transgender women (CDC, 2019).

Severe depression of the cellular immune system associated with HIV infection characterizes acquired immunodeficiency syndrome (AIDS). Although behaviors that place women at risk have been well documented, all women should be assessed for the possibility of HIV exposure. The most commonly reported opportunistic diseases are *Pneumocystis (jirovecii)* pneumonia (PCP), candidal esophagitis, and wasting syndrome. Other viral infections such as HSV and cytomegalovirus infections seem to be more prevalent among women than men. There is a higher incidence of adnexal masses in women with PID who are also HIV-positive, but antibiotics are often as effective in HIV-positive women with PID as they are in HIV-negative women with PID (Gardella, Eckert, & Lentz, 2017). The clinical course of HPV infection in women with HIV infection is accelerated, and recurrence is more frequent in non–HIV-infected women.

Once HIV enters the body, seroconversion to HIV positivity usually occurs within 6 to 12 weeks. Although HIV seroconversion may be totally asymptomatic, it is usually accompanied by a viremic influenza-like response. Symptoms include fever, headache, night sweats, malaise, generalized lymphadenopathy, myalgias, nausea, diarrhea, weight loss, sore throat, and rash.

Laboratory studies may reveal leukopenia, thrombocytopenia, anemia, and an elevated erythrocyte sedimentation rate. HIV has a strong affinity for surface-marker proteins on T lymphocytes. This affinity leads to significant T-cell destruction. Both clinical and epidemiologic studies have shown that declining CD4 levels are strongly associated with increased incidence of AIDS-related diseases and death in many different groups of HIV-infected people.

Transmission of the virus from mother to child can occur throughout the perinatal period. Exposure may occur to the fetus through the maternal circulation as early as the first trimester of pregnancy, to the infant during labor and birth by inoculation or ingestion of maternal blood and other infected fluids, or to the infant through breast milk (CDC, 2019).

Screening and Diagnosis

Screening, teaching, and counseling regarding HIV risk factors, indications for being tested, and testing are major roles for nurses caring for women today. A number of behaviors place women at risk for HIV infection, including intravenous drug use, high-risk sexual behavior, multiple sex partners, and a history of multiple STIs. HIV infection is usually diagnosed by using HIV-1 and HIV-2 antibody tests. Antibody testing is first done with a sensitive screening test such as the enzyme immunoassay (EIA). Reactive screening tests must be confirmed by an additional test, such as the Western blot or an immunofluorescence assay. If a positive antibody test is confirmed by a supplemental test, it means that a woman is infected with HIV and is capable of infecting others. HIV antibodies are detectable in at least 95% of individuals within 3 months after infection. Although a negative antibody test usually indicates that a person is not infected, antibody tests cannot exclude recent infection. The FDA has approved six rapid HIV antibody screening tests for clinical use. These use a blood sample obtained by fingerstick or venipuncture, an oral fluid sample, or a urine sample to provide test results within 20 minutes; they have sensitivity and specificity rates of more than 99%. If the results are reactive, further testing is necessary (CDC, 2019). Quicker results mean that clients do not have to make extra visits for follow-up standard tests, and the oral test provides an option for clients who do not want to have a blood test.

The CDC (2017a) recommends offering HIV testing to all women whose behavior places them at risk for HIV infection. It may be useful to allow women to self-select for HIV testing. On entry to the health care system, a woman can be handed written information about the risk factors for HIV and asked to inform the nurse if she believes she is at risk. She should be told that she does not have to say why she may be at risk, only that she thinks she might be.

Counseling for HIV Testing

HIV testing presents nurses with an opportunity to conduct HIV/STI prevention counseling and to communicate risk-reduction messages (CDC, 2017a). It is a nursing responsibility to assess a woman's understanding of the information such a test would provide; and to make sure that the woman thoroughly understands the emotional, legal, and medical implications of a positive or negative result before she is ready to take an HIV test.

Unless rapid testing is done, there is generally a 1- to 3-week waiting period after HIV testing, which can be a very anxious time for the woman. The nurse can help by informing her that this time period between blood drawing and test results is routine. Whatever the results may be, they must always be communicated in person, and women must be informed in advance that such is the procedure. Whenever possible, the person who provided the pretest counseling should also give the woman her test results.

When some women are informed of negative results, they may escalate their risk behaviors because they equate negativity with immunity. Others may believe that negative means "bad" and positive means "good." Women's reactions to a negative test should be explored, as by asking, "How do you feel?" Counseling regarding HIV-negative results provides another opportunity to offer education. Emphasis can be placed on ways in which a woman can remain free of HIV. She should be reminded that if she has been exposed to HIV in the past 6 months, she should be retested, and that if she continues to engage in high-risk behaviors, she should have ongoing testing.

When test results are being provided to an HIV-positive woman, privacy with no interruptions is essential. Adequate time for the counseling session should be provided. The nurse must make sure that the woman understands what a positive test means and review its reliability. Risk-reduction practices should be reemphasized. Referral for appropriate medical evaluation and follow-up should be made, and the need or desire for psychosocial or psychiatric referrals should be assessed.

It is important to stress early medical evaluation so that a baseline assessment can be made and prophylactic medication begun. If possible, the nurse should make a referral or appointment for the woman at this session.

Management

During the initial contact with an HIV-infected woman, the nurse should assess the woman's knowledge about HIV infection and assure her health care provider that she is being cared for by a medical practitioner or facility with expertise in caring for people with HIV infections, including AIDS. A mental health referral may be needed. Resources such as counseling for financial assistance, legal advocacy, suicide prevention, and death and dying may be appropriate. All women who are drug users should be referred to a substance-abuse program. A major focus of counseling is the prevention of HIV transmission to partners.

For the HIV-positive woman, pregnancy can be associated with an adverse health risk; thus it is important to consider the effectiveness of the woman's contraceptive method (Curtis, Tepper, Jatlaoui, et al., 2016). According to the CDC, nurses counseling seropositive women who are well and on antiretroviral (ARV) medication wishing contraceptive information can recommend the copper intrauterine device (IUD) and levonorgestrel-releasing intrauterine system (LNG) IUD. For those who are not clinically well or on ARV medication, the LNG IUD is preferred over the copper IUD. For women who are not clinically well and are not on ARV medication, the nurse can recommend the contraceptive implant, injectable progestin, or combined hormonal contraceptives (i.e., oral contraceptive, patch, or vaginal ring). These are not recommended for women who are on ARV medication owing to possible drug interactions between the method and the ARV drugs. Female condoms or abstinence can be used by women whose male partners refuse to use condoms. Women should be reminded that of the methods suggested, only condoms offer protection from HIV infection and other STIs.

There is no cure for HIV infection. Opportunistic infections, and concurrent diseases are managed vigorously with treatment specific to the infection or disease. Routine gynecologic care for HIV-positive women should include a pelvic examination every 6 months. Thorough Pap screening is essential because of the greatly increased incidence of abnormal findings on examination. In addition, HIV-positive women should be screened for syphilis, gonorrhea, chlamydia, and other vaginal infections and treated if such infections are present. General health promotion strategies are an important part of care (e.g., smoking cessation, sound nutrition) as is antiretroviral therapy. Discussion of the medical care of HIV-positive women or those with AIDS is beyond the scope of this chapter because of the rapidly changing recommendations. The reader is referred to the CDC (www.cdc.gov), CDC National AIDS hotline (800-342-2437), and internet websites such as the HIV/AIDS Treatment Information Service (www.hivatis.org) for current information and recommendations.

HIV and Pregnancy

HIV counseling and testing should be offered to all women at their initial prenatal care visit as part of routine prenatal testing unless the woman opts out of the screening. Universal testing versus selective testing for maternal HIV is recommended because it results in a greater number of women being screened and treated and can reduce the likelihood of perinatal transmission while also maintaining women's health. The CDC also recommends retesting in the third trimester for women known to be at high risk for HIV and rapid HIV testing in labor for women with unknown HIV status (CDC, 2017a).

Perinatal transmission of HIV has decreased significantly since 2004 because of the administration of antiretroviral prophylaxis (e.g., zidovudine) to pregnant women in the prenatal and the perinatal periods. Treatment of HIV-infected women with triple-drug antiretroviral therapy (ART) or highly active antiretroviral therapy (HAART) during pregnancy has been reported to decrease mother-child transmission to 1% to 2% (CDC, 2019). All HIV-infected women should be treated with a combination of ART during pregnancy regardless of their CD4 cell counts (Hughes & Cu-Uvin, 2018). Women who are infected with HIV and need treatment for their own health should start therapy as soon as possible, even in the first trimester; women who are taking the therapy as prophylaxis usually start therapy after the first trimester.

Antiretroviral therapy is administered orally and continued throughout pregnancy. The major side effect is bone marrow suppression. Periodic hematocrits, white blood cell counts, and platelet counts should be performed. Women who are HIV-positive should also be vaccinated against hepatitis B, pneumococcal infection, *Haemophilus influenzae* type B, and viral influenza. To support any pregnant woman's immune system, appropriate counseling regarding optimal nutrition, sleep, rest, exercise, and stress reduction is provided. Condom use is encouraged to minimize further exposure to HIV from a sexual partner who may be a source.

In the intrapartum period, ART is recommended and the decision to have a cesarean birth versus a vaginal birth is dependent on the degree of viral load. The U.S. Department of Health and Human Services Clinical Guidelines Portal (USHHS, 2019) recommends a scheduled cesarean birth at 38 weeks of gestation for women with a viral load of more than 1000 copies per milliliter. A vaginal birth may be an option for HIV-infected women who have viral loads of fewer than 1000 copies per milliliter at 36 weeks, if a woman has ruptured membranes and labor is progressing rapidly, or if she declines a cesarean birth. Intravenous zidovudine is recommended during the intrapartum period for HIV-infected pregnant women except for those with a low viral load (<1000 copies) who have been on HAART during pregnancy. The drug is administered at least 3 hours before a scheduled cesarean birth and continued until the cord is clamped. It should be given during labor if the woman is having a vaginal birth and to the infant for 6 weeks after birth. Fetal scalp electrode and scalp pH sampling should be avoided because these procedures may serve to inoculate the virus into the fetus. Similarly, the use of forceps or a vacuum extractor should be avoided when possible. For women infected with HIV, the avoidance of breastfeeding is recommended in the United States and most other developed countries (Department of Health and Human Services).

Women who are infected with HIV but are without symptoms may have an unremarkable postpartum course. Immunosuppressed women with symptoms may be at increased risk for postpartum UTIs, vaginitis, postpartum endometritis, and poor wound healing. Good perineal hygiene should be stressed. Women who are HIV-positive but were not on antiretroviral drugs before pregnancy should be tested in the postpartum period to determine whether therapy that was initiated in pregnancy should be continued. After the initial bath, the newborn may be with the mother. In planning for discharge, comprehensive care and support services must be arranged. After discharge the woman and her infant are referred to health care providers who are experienced in treating HIV, AIDS, and associated conditions and follow-up.

Zika Virus

The Zika virus is spread by bites from the *Aedes* mosquito. It is also spread via sexual contact by semen. Women who become pregnant and are infected by the Zika virus have an increased risk of giving birth to an infant with microcephaly. Zika virus has also been associated with risk for Guillain-Barré syndrome, a neurologic condition that can lead to muscle weakness and possibly paralysis. The *Aedes* mosquito has been found predominantly in Africa, Southeast Asia, the Caribbean, Central America, South America, and the Pacific Islands, with a few recent cases found in the southeastern United States (CDC, 2018a). Pregnant women and women considering becoming pregnant should avoid traveling to areas that are known to harbor the *Aedes* mosquito. Women should use condoms or abstain from sex with male partners who have traveled to areas identified with transmission of the Zika virus (CDC, 2018d; Moreira, Peixoto, Siqueira, et al, 2017).

Testing for Zika virus varies depending on whether pregnant women have symptoms or have been exposed. Asymptomatic pregnant women with ongoing possible Zika virus exposure should be offered Zika virus nucleic acid amplification test (NAAT) testing three times during pregnancy. Asymptomatic pregnant women who have had recent possible Zika exposure (through travel or sexual exposure) but who do not have ongoing exposure are not routinely recommended to have Zika virus testing. Pregnant women who have had recent possible Zika virus exposure and have a fetus with prenatal ultrasound findings consistent with congenital Zika virus syndrome should receive Zika virus testing to assist in establishing the etiology of the birth defects. Testing for this group of women should include both NAAT and immunoglobulin (Igm) tests (Oduyebo T, Polen KD, Walke HT, et al., 2017).

Vaginal Infections

Vaginal discharge and itching of the vulva and vagina are among the most frequent reasons a woman seeks help from a health care provider. Women complain more often of vaginal discharge than of any other gynecologic symptom. Vaginal discharge resulting from infection must be distinguished from normal secretions. Women who have adequate endogenous or exogenous estrogen will have vaginal secretions. Normal vaginal secretions, or leukorrhea, are clear to cloudy and may turn yellow after drying; the discharge is slightly slimy, is nonirritating, and has a mild, inoffensive odor. Normal vaginal secretions are acidic, with a pH of 3.8 to 4.5. Normal vaginal secretions contain lactobacilli and epithelial cells. The amount of leukorrhea differs with phases of the menstrual cycle, with greater amounts occurring at ovulation and just before menses. Leukorrhea is also increased during pregnancy.

Vaginitis or abnormal vaginal discharge is an infection caused by a microorganism. The most common vaginal infections are bacterial vaginosis, candidiasis, and trichomoniasis. Although streptococcus B is considered normal vaginal flora, it may also cause infection. Vulvovaginitis, or inflammation of the vulva and vagina, may be caused by vaginal infection or copious amounts of leukorrhea, which can cause tissue maceration. Chemical irritants, allergens, and foreign bodies that produce inflammatory reactions can also cause vulvovaginitis.

Bacterial Vaginosis

Bacterial vaginosis (BV)—formerly called nonspecific vaginitis, *Haemophilus vaginitis*, or *Gardnerella*—is the most common cause of vaginal symptoms today (Gardella, Eckert, & Lentz, 2017). The prevalence is most common in women of childbearing age, or ages 14 to 49 in the United States. Women with new or multiple sexual partners, those who douche or do not use condoms, and those who lack vaginal lactobacilli (women who have never been sexually active are rarely affected) are at higher risk for infection. BV can increase susceptibility to STIs such as chlamydia, gonorrhea, genital herpes, and HIV (CDC, 2017a). BV is associated with preterm labor and birth. The exact etiology of BV is unknown. It is a syndrome in which normal H_2O_2-producing lactobacilli are replaced with high concentrations of anaerobic bacteria (*Gardnerella* and *Mobiluncus*). With the increased amount of anaerobes, the level of vaginal amines is increased, and the normal acidic pH of the vagina is altered. Epithelial cells slough, and numerous bacteria attach to their surfaces (clue cells). When the amines are volatilized, the characteristic odor of BV occurs.

Many women with BV complain of the characteristic "fishy odor." The odor may be noticed by the woman or her partner after heterosexual intercourse because semen releases the vaginal amines. When present, the BV discharge usually appears profuse, thin, and white, gray, or milky. Some women may also experience mild irritation or pruritus.

Screening and Diagnosis

A focused history may help distinguish BV from other vaginal infections if the woman is symptomatic. Reports of fishy odor and increased thin vaginal discharge are most significant, and a report of increased odor after intercourse is also suggestive of BV.

Microscopic examination of vaginal secretions is always performed (Table 7.3). Both normal saline and 10% potassium hydroxide (KOH) smears are made. The presence of more than 20% clue cells (vaginal epithelial cells coated with bacteria) on wet saline smear is highly diagnostic because the phenomenon is specific to BV. Vaginal secretions are tested for pH and amine odor. Nitrazine paper is sensitive enough to detect a pH of 4.5 or greater. The fishy odor of BV will be released when KOH is added to vaginal secretions on the lip of the withdrawn speculum (CDC, 2015b).

Management

Treatment of bacterial vaginosis with oral metronidazole (Flagyl) is most effective (CDC, 2015b). Table 7.4 outlines treatment guidelines. The side effects of metronidazole are numerous, including a sharp, unpleasant metallic taste in the mouth; a furry tongue; central nervous system reactions; and urinary tract disturbances. When oral metronidazole is taken, the woman is advised not to drink alcoholic beverages or she will experience the severe side effects of abdominal distress, nausea, vomiting, and headache. Gastrointestinal symptoms are common but less severe if alcohol is not consumed. The treatment of sexual partners is not routinely recommended (CDC, 2015b).

Metronidazole is not recommended if the woman is breastfeeding. However, if it is necessary to prescribe it, the woman can suspend breastfeeding (pump and discard to maintain milk supply) during treatment and for 12 to 24 hours after the last dose to reduce the infant's exposure to metronidazole (CDC, 2015b).

TABLE 7.3 Wet Mount Tests for Vaginal Infections

Infection	Test	Positive Findings
Trichomoniasis	Use NAAT testing as preferred method Saline wet mount (vaginal secretions mixed with normal saline on a glass slide and if used, must be read within 1 hour of collection)	Presence of many white blood cell protozoa
Candidiasis	KOH prep (vaginal secretions mixed with KOH on a glass slide)	Presence of hyphae and pseudohyphae (buds and branches of yeast cells)
Bacterial vaginosis	Normal saline wet mount	Presence of clue cells (vaginal epithelial cells coated with bacteria)
	Whiff test (vaginal secretions mixed with KOH)	Release of fishy odor

KOH, Potassium hydroxide.
Data from Centers for Disease Control and Prevention (CDC). (2017b). 2015 Sexually transmitted disease treatment guidelines. *Morbidity and Mortality Weekly Report, 64*(3), 1–140.

Candidiasis

Vulvovaginal candidiasis (VVC), or yeast infection, is the second most common type of vaginal infection in the United States. Although vaginal candidiasis infections are common in healthy women, those seen in women with HIV infection are often more severe and persistent. Genital candidiasis lesions may be painful, coalescing ulcerations necessitating continuous prophylactic therapy.

The most common organism is *Candida albicans*; estimates indicate that more than 90% of the yeast infections in women are caused by this organism. However, since 2004, the incidence of non–*C. albicans* infections has risen steadily. Women with chronic or recurrent infections are often infected with these organisms (Gardella, Eckert, & Lentz, 2017).

Numerous factors have been identified as predisposing a woman to yeast infections, including antibiotic therapy, particularly broad-spectrum antibiotics such as ampicillin, tetracycline, cephalosporins, and metronidazole; diabetes, especially when uncontrolled; pregnancy; obesity; diets high in refined sugars or artificial sweeteners; use of corticosteroids and exogenous hormones; and immunosuppressed states. Clinical observations and research have suggested that tight-fitting clothing and underwear or pantyhose made of nonabsorbent materials create an environment in which a vaginal fungus can grow.

TABLE 7.4 Vaginal Infections and Drug Therapies for Women

Disease	Nonpregnant Women (13-17 Years)	Nonpregnant Women (>18 Years)	Pregnant Women	Lactating Women
Bacterial vaginosis	*Recommended:* metronidazole, 500 mg bid for 7 days (no alcohol) *or* metronidazole gel 0.75%, 5 g intravaginally bid for 7 days *or* clindamycin cream 2%, 5 g intravaginally at bedtime for 7 days (less effective)	*Recommended:* metronidazole, 500 mg bid for 7 days (no alcohol) *or* metronidazole gel 0.75%, 5 g intravaginally bid for 7 days *or* clindamycin cream 2%, 5 g intravaginally at bedtime for 7 days (less effective)	High-risk asymptomatic or symptomatic women *Recommended:* metronidazole, 500 mg PO bid for 7 days (no alcohol) *or* metronidazole, 250 mg PO tid for 7 days *or* clindamycin, 300 mg PO bid for 7 days	*Recommended:* clindamycin cream or ovules
Trichomoniasis	*Recommended:* metronidazole, 2 g PO once *or* tinidazole, 2 g PO once	*Recommended:* metronidazole, 2 g PO once	*Recommended:* metronidazole, 2 g PO once	Metronidazole not recommended during lactation; stop breastfeeding treat, resume breastfeeding in 12-24 h after drug completed Tinidazoles: Stop breastfeeding and resume 3 days after treatment Pump and discard milk to maintain supply
Candidiasis	Numerous OTC intravaginal agents: butoconazole, clotrimazole, miconazole, tioconazole, terconazole; treatment with "azole" drugs more effective than nystatin Dose varies by agent from one dose only to one dose taken for 3-7 days *Oral agent:* fluconazole 150-mg oral tablet once	Numerous OTC intravaginal agents: butoconazole, clotrimazole, miconazole, tioconazole, terconazole; treatment with "azole" drugs more effective than nystatin Dose varies by agent from one dose only to one dose taken for 3-7 days *Oral agent:* fluconazole 150-mg oral tablet once	OTC "azole" intravaginal agents: butoconazole, clotrimazole, miconazole, terconazole Use for 3-7 days Oral agents not recommended	OTC "azole" intravaginal agents: butoconazole, clotrimazole, miconazole, terconazole Use for 3-7 days

OTC, Over the counter.
Data from Centers for Disease Control and Prevention (CDC). (2015b). 2015 Sexually transmitted disease treatment guidelines. *Morbidity and Mortality Weekly Report, 64*(3), 1–140.

The most common symptom of yeast infections is vulvar and possibly vaginal pruritus. The itching can be mild or intense, interfere with rest and activities, and may occur during or after intercourse. Some women report a feeling of dryness. Others may experience painful urination as the urine flows over the vulva, which usually occurs in those who have excoriations resulting from scratching. Most often the discharge has a thick, white, lumpy, and cottage cheese–like consistency. The discharge may be found in patches on the vaginal walls, cervix, and labia. Commonly the vulva is red and swollen, as are the labial folds, vagina, and cervix. Although there is no characteristic odor with yeast infections, sometimes a yeasty or musty smell is noted.

Screening and Diagnosis

In addition to a complete record of the woman's symptoms, their onset, and course, the history is a valuable screening tool for identifying predisposing risk factors. Physical examination should include a thorough inspection of the vulva and vagina. A speculum examination is always done. Commonly health care practitioners will obtain saline and KOH wet smears and check vaginal pH (see Table 7.3). Vaginal pH is normal with a yeast infection; if the pH is greater than 4.5, trichomoniasis or BV should be suspected. The characteristic pseudohyphae (bud or branching of a fungus) may be seen on a wet smear done with normal saline; however, they may be confused with other cells and artifacts.

Management

A number of antifungal preparations are available for the treatment of *C. albicans*. Many of these medications (e.g., miconazole [Monistat] and clotrimazole [Gyne-Lotrimin]) are available as over-the-counter (OTC) agents. Exogenous lactobacillus (in the form of dairy products [yogurt] or powder, tablet, capsule, or suppository supplements) and garlic have been suggested for the prevention and treatment of vulvovaginal candidiasis, but research is inconclusive and no recommendations have been developed for use in practice (Gardella, Eckert, & Lentz, 2017). The first time a woman suspects that she may have a yeast infection she should see a health care provider for confirmation of the diagnosis and treatment recommendations. If she has another infection, she may wish to purchase an OTC preparation and self-treat. If she elects to do this, she should always be counseled to seek care for numerous recurrent or chronic yeast infections. If vaginal discharge is extremely thick and copious, vaginal debridement with a cotton swab followed by application of vaginal medication may be effective.

Women who have extensive irritation, swelling, and discomfort of the labia and vulva may find sitz baths helpful in decreasing inflammation and increasing comfort. Adding colloidal oatmeal powder to the bath may also increase the woman's comfort. Not wearing underpants to bed may help decrease symptoms and prevent recurrences. Completing the full course of treatment prescribed is essential to removing the pathogen. Women should be instructed to continue the medication even during menstruation and to avoid using tampons during menses because the tampon will readily absorb the medication. If possible, women should avoid intercourse during treatment; if abstinence is not feasible, the woman's partner should use a condom to prevent the introduction of more organisms (see the Teaching for Self-Management box).

Trichomoniasis

Trichomonas vaginalis is almost always an STI and is also a common cause of vaginal infection (5%-50% of all vaginitis) and discharge (Gardella, Eckert, & Lentz, 2017).

Trichomoniasis is caused by *T. vaginalis,* an anaerobic one-celled protozoan with characteristic flagellae. Although trichomoniasis

TEACHING FOR SELF-MANAGEMENT
Prevention of Genital Tract Infections

- Practice genital hygiene.
- Choose underwear or hosiery with a cotton crotch.
- Avoid tight-fitting clothing (especially tight jeans).
- Select cloth car seat covers instead of vinyl or cover the vinyl with a towel or other cotton cloth
- Limit time spent in damp exercise clothes (especially swimsuits, leotards, and tights).
- Limit exposure to bath salts or bubble bath.
- Avoid colored or scented toilet tissue.
- If sensitive, discontinue use of feminine deodorant sprays.
- Use condoms.
- Void before and after intercourse.
- Decrease dietary sugar.
- Drink yeast-active milk and eat yogurt (with lactobacilli).
- Do not douche.

TABLE 7.5 Maternal and Fetal Effects of Common Sexually Transmitted Infections

Infection	Maternal Effects	Fetal Effects
Chlamydia	Prelabor rupture of membranes Preterm labor Postpartum endometritis	Low birth weight
Gonorrhea	Miscarriage Preterm labor Prelabor rupture of membranes Chorioamnionitis Postpartum endometritis Postpartum sepsis	Preterm birth IUGR
Group B streptococcus	Urinary tract infection Chorioamnionitis Postpartum endometritis Sepsis Meningitis (rare)	Preterm birth
Herpes simplex virus	Intrauterine infection (rare)	Congenital infection (rare)
Human papillomavirus	Dystocia from large lesions Excessive bleeding from lesions after birth trauma	None known
Syphilis	Miscarriage Preterm labor	IUGR Preterm birth Stillbirth Congenital infection

IUGR, Intrauterine growth restriction.
Data from Gilbert, E. (2011). *Manual of high risk pregnancy & delivery* (5th ed.). St. Louis: Mosby; Duff, P., Sweet, R., & Edwards, R. (2013). Maternal and fetal infections. In R. K. Creasy, R. Resnik, J. D. Iams, C. J. Lockwood, T. R. Moore, & M. F. Greene (Eds.), *Creasy and Resnik's maternal-fetal medicine: Principles and practice* (7th ed.). Philadelphia: Saunders.

may be asymptomatic, commonly women have a characteristic yellowish to greenish discharge that is frothy, mucopurulent, copious, and malodorous. Inflammation of the vulva, vagina, or both may be present, and the woman may complain of irritation and pruritus. Dysuria and dyspareunia are often present. Typically the discharge worsens during and after menstruation. Often the cervix and vaginal walls will demonstrate the characteristic "strawberry spots" or tiny petechiae, and the cervix may bleed on contact. In severe infections, the vaginal walls, cervix, and occasionally also the vulva may be acutely inflamed.

Screening and Diagnosis

In addition to obtaining a history of current symptoms, a careful sexual history should be obtained. Any history of similar symptoms in the past and the treatment that was used should be noted. The nurse should determine whether the woman's partner or partners were treated and whether she had subsequent relations with new partners.

The use of highly sensitive and specific tests is recommended for detecting *T. vaginalis*. Among women, NAAT is highly sensitive, often detecting three to five times more *T. vaginalis* infections than wet-mount microscopy, a method with poor sensitivity (51%-65%). Among women, vaginal swab and urine have up to 100% concordance. Clinicians using wet mounts should attempt to evaluate slides immediately because sensitivity declines as evaluation is delayed, decreasing by up to 20% within 1 hour after collection (CDC, 2015b). Because trichomoniasis is an STI, once diagnosis has been confirmed, appropriate laboratory studies for other STIs should be carried out.

Management

The recommended treatment is metronidazole or tinidazole orally in a single dose (CDC, 2015b) (see Table 7.4). When oral metronidazole is taken, the woman is advised not to drink alcoholic beverages. Although the male partner is usually asymptomatic, it is recommended that he receive treatment also because he often harbors the trichomonads in the urethra or prostate. It is important that nurses discuss the significance of partner treatment with their clients, because if they are not treated it is likely that the infection will recur. Nurses must also counsel the women to abstain from sex until they and their partners have been treated (i.e., when therapy has been completed and any symptoms have resolved).

Women with trichomoniasis must understand the sexual transmission of this disease. They must know that the organism may be present without any associated symptoms, perhaps for several months, and that it is not possible to determine when they became infected. Women should be informed of the necessity for treating all sexual partners and helped with ways of raising this issue with them.

Group B Streptococcus

Group B streptococcus (GBS) may be considered a part of the normal vaginal flora in a woman who is not pregnant; it is present in about 25% of healthy pregnant women (CDC, 2018b). GBS infection has been associated with poor pregnancy outcomes. These infections are important factors in neonatal morbidity and mortality, usually resulting from vertical transmission from the birth canal of the infected mother to the infant during birth (CDC, 2018b).

Risk factors for neonatal GBS infection include positive prenatal culture for GBS in the current pregnancy; preterm birth of less than 37 weeks of gestation; prelabor rupture of membranes for a duration of 18 hours or more; intrapartum maternal fever higher than 38°C (100.4°F); and a positive history of early-onset neonatal GBS (CDC, 2018b).

To decrease the risk of neonatal GBS infection, it is recommended that all women be screened at 35 to 37 weeks of gestation for GBS using a rectovaginal culture, and that intravenous antibiotic

prophylaxis (IAP) be offered during labor to all who test positive. If a culture is not available at the onset of labor or if a risk factor is present, IAP is also offered. IAP is not recommended before a cesarean birth if labor or rupture of membranes has not occurred. The recommended treatment is penicillin G, 5 million units IV loading dose, and then 2.5 million units IV q 4 h during labor. Ampicillin, 2 g IV loading dose, followed by 1 g IV q 4 h, is an alternative therapy (CDC, 2016).

CONCERNS OF THE LESBIAN, GAY, BISEXUAL, AND TRANSSEXUAL COMMUNITY

It is important to note that persons in the lesbian, gay, bisexual, and transsexual (LGBT) community are at risk for STIs. In women's health, it is particularly important to understand the specific issues related to women who have sex with women (WSW). The CDC (2017g) has issued guidelines that are specific to WSW as well as other populations. WSW are at risk for acquiring bacterial, viral, and protozoal infections from current and prior partners, both male and female. They should not be presumed to be at low or no risk for STIs because of their sexual orientation. It is critical for effective screening that health care providers discuss sexual orientation with their clients in an open, accepting manner.

MATERNAL AND FETAL EFFECTS OF SEXUALLY TRANSMITTED INFECTIONS

Sexually transmitted infections in pregnancy are responsible for significant morbidity and mortality. Some consequences of maternal infection, such as infertility and sterility, last a lifetime. Congenitally acquired infection may affect a child's length and quality of life. Table 7.5 describes the effects of several common STIs on the pregnant woman and the fetus. It is difficult to predict these effects with certainty. Factors such as coinfection with other STIs and when in pregnancy the infection was acquired and treated can affect outcomes.

TORCH INFECTIONS

*T*oxoplasmosis, *o*ther infections (e.g., hepatitis), *r*ubella, *c*ytomegalovirus (CMV), and *h*erpes simplex, known collectively as **TORCH infections,** form a group of organisms capable of crossing the placenta. TORCH infections can affect a pregnant woman and her fetus. Generally, all TORCH infections produce influenza-like symptoms in the mother, but fetal and neonatal effects are more serious. TORCH infections and their maternal and fetal effects are shown in Table 7.6. Neonatal effects are discussed in Chapter 35.

 CARE MANAGEMENT

Women may delay seeking care for STIs and other infections because they fear social stigma, have little accessibility to health care services, are asymptomatic, or are unaware that they have an infection. A comprehensive assessment focuses on lifestyle issues that are often personal or sensitive. A culturally sensitive, nonjudgmental approach is essential to facilitate accurate data collection. Throughout this chapter the discussion for each STI has included essential areas of assessment, including signs and symptoms of the current problem, history (medical, personal, and social, and lifestyle behaviors), diagnostic tests, and physical examination.

TABLE 7.6   TORCH Infections: Maternal and Fetal

Infection	Maternal Effects	Fetal Effects	Counseling: Prevention, Identification, and Management
Toxoplasmosis (protozoa)	Most infections asymptomatic Acute infection similar to mononucleosis Woman immune after first episode (except in immunocompromised clients)	Congenital infection is most likely to occur when maternal infection develops during the third trimester. The risk of fetal injury, however, is greatest when maternal infection occurs during the first trimester.	Good handwashing technique should be used. Eating raw or rare meat and exposure to litter used by infected cats should be avoided; *Toxoplasma* titer should be checked if there are cats in the house. If titer is rising during early pregnancy, therapeutic abortion may be considered an option.
Other infections			
Hepatitis A (infectious hepatitis) (virus)	Liver failure (extremely rare) Low-grade fever, malaise, poor appetite, right upper quadrant pain and tenderness, jaundice, and light-colored stools	Perinatal transmission virtually never occurs.	Spread by fecal-oral contact especially by culinary workers; gamma globulin can be given as prophylaxis for hepatitis A. Hepatitis A vaccine is available.
Hepatitis B (serum hepatitis) (virus)	May be transmitted sexually Approximately 10% of clients become chronic carriers. Some people with chronic hepatitis B eventually develop severe chronic liver disease, such as cirrhosis or hepatocellular carcinoma.	Infection occurs during birth. Maternal vaccination during pregnancy should present no risk for fetus; however, data are not available.	Generally passed by contaminated needles, syringes, or blood transfusions; also can be transmitted PO or by coitus (but incubation period is longer); hepatitis B immune globulin can be given prophylactically after exposure. Hepatitis B vaccine recommended for populations at risk
Rubella (3-day or German measles) (virus)	Rash, fever, mild symptoms such as headache, malaise, myalgias, and arthralgias; postauricular lymph nodes may be swollen; mild conjunctivitis.	Approximately 50%-80% of fetuses exposed to the virus within 12 weeks after conception will show signs of congenital infection. Very few fetuses are affected if infection occurs after 18 weeks of gestation. The most common fetal anomalies associated with congenital rubella syndrome are deafness, eye defects (e.g., cataracts or retinopathy), central nervous system defects, and cardiac defects.	Vaccination of pregnant women is contraindicated; non-immune women should be vaccinated in the early postpartum period; pregnancy should be prevented for 1 month after vaccination. Women may breastfeed after vaccination and the vaccine can be administered along with immunoglobulin preparations such as Rh immune globulin.
Cytomegalovirus (CMV) (a herpesvirus)	Most adults are asymptomatic or have only mild influenza-like symptoms. The presence of CMV antibodies does not totally prevent reinfection.	The fetus can be infected transplacentally. Infection is much more likely with a primary maternal infection. The most common indications of congenital infection include hepatosplenomegaly, intracranial calcifications, jaundice, growth restriction, microcephaly, chorioretinitis, hearing loss, thrombocytopenia, hyperbilirubinemia, and hepatitis.	The virus is transmitted by transplantation of an infected organ, transfusion of infected blood, sexual contact, or contact with contaminated saliva or urine. Virus may be reactivated and cause disease in utero or during birth in subsequent pregnancies; fetal infection may occur during passage through infected birth canal. Prevention includes use of CMV-negative blood products if transfusion of pregnant women is necessary and teaching all women to wash hands carefully after handling infant diapers and toys.
Herpes Genitalis (herpes simplex virus, type 1 or type 2 [HSV-1 or HSV-2])	Primary infection with painful blisters, tender inguinal lymph nodes, fever, viral meningitis (rare). Recurrent infections are much milder and shorter.	Transplacental infection resulting in congenital infection is rare and usually occurs with primary maternal infection. The risk mainly exists with infection late in pregnancy.	As many as two-thirds of women with HSV-2 antibodies acquired the infection asymptomatically; however, asymptomatic women can give birth to seriously infected neonates. Risk of transmission is greatest during vaginal birth if woman has active lesions; thus cesarean birth is recommended. Acyclovir can be used to treat recurrent outbreaks during pregnancy or as suppressive therapy late in pregnancy to prevent an outbreak during labor and birth.

TORCH, Toxoplasmosis, Other infections, Rubella, Cytomegalovirus, Herpes genitalis.
Data from Duff, P., Sweet, R., & Edwards, R. (2013). Maternal and fetal infections. In R. K. Creasy, R. Resnik, J. D. Iams, C. J. Lockwood, T. R. Moore, & M. F. Greene (Eds.), *Creasy and Resnik's maternal-fetal medicine: Principles and practice* (7th ed.). Philadelphia: Saunders.

Concerns of the Lesbian, Gay, Bisexual, Transgender, and Queer Community

It is important to note that persons in the LGBTQ community are at risk for STIs. In women's health, it is particularly important to understand the specific issues related to WSW. The CDC (2017c) has issued guidelines that are specific to WSW as well as other populations. WSW are at risk for acquiring bacterial, viral, and protozoal infections from current and prior partners, both male and female. They should not be presumed to be at low or no risk for STIs because of their sexual orientation. It is critical for effective screening that health care providers discuss sexual orientation with their clients in an open, accepting manner. Becoming knowledgeable regarding the health needs of the LGBTQ population is facilitated by a review of some of the available resources, which identify the top ten health issues of each group of the LGBTQ community.

Infection Control

Interrupting the transmission of infection is crucial to STI control. Many STIs are reportable; all states require syphilis (including congenital syphilis), gonorrhea, chlamydia, HIV infection, and AIDS be reported to public health officials. Many other states require that other STIs such as genital herpes and genital warts be reported. In addition, all states require that AIDS cases be reported. In 2018, a total of 46 state laboratories and Washington, D.C. were required to report viral load and CD4 data for people who have HIV infections (CDC, 2018c).

Infection-control measures are essential to protect care providers and to prevent health personnel–related infection of clients regardless of the infectious agent. The risk for occupational transmission varies with the disease. Even when the risk is low, as with HIV, the existence of any risk warrants reasonable precautions. Precautions against

---

◎ NURSING CARE PLAN

Sexually Transmitted Infections

Client Problem	Expected Outcome	Nursing Interventions	Rationales
Need for health teaching related to practicing prevention of sexually transmitted infections (STIs) as evidenced by client's positive diagnosis of STI	Woman will verbalize which health practices directly led to a positive diagnosis of an STI.	Assess woman's sexual history and sexual health practices. Provide information about transmission of disease, including cause, symptoms, and treatment for both partners. Discuss the use and importance of safe sexual practices.	To provide database for current problem To enhance woman's knowledge base and correct any misinformation To raise woman's awareness and motivation to avoid future risk-taking behaviors
Anxiety related to diagnosis of STI	Woman will report decreased level of anxiety.	Provide opportunity for therapeutic communication. Assist woman to identify effective coping mechanisms. Refer to support groups.	To promote trust and expression of feelings To decrease anxiety To share feelings and common effective strategies
Problems with sexuality related to fear of STI	Woman will understand and verbalize how to have sexual relations while protecting herself against STIs	Allow woman to discuss her fears and to discuss plan to make sure she uses safe sexual practices	To clarify her fears and ensure she has correct knowledge To provide her with a plan to make sure she practices safe sex.

TEACHING FOR SELF-MANAGEMENT

Sexually Transmitted Infections

- Take your medication as directed.
- Use comfort measures for symptom relief as suggested by your health care provider.
- Keep your appointment for repeat testing or checkups after your treatment to make sure your infection is cured.
- Inform your sexual partner(s) of the need to be tested and treated, if necessary.
- Abstain from sexual intercourse until your treatment is completed or for as long as you are advised by your health care provider.
- Use sex practices that decrease risk when sexual intercourse is resumed.
- Call your health care provider immediately if you notice bumps, sores, rashes, or discharges.
- Keep all future appointments with your health care provider, even if things appear normal.

LEGAL TIP

Sexually Transmitted Infection Reporting

The primary health care provider is legally responsible for reporting all cases of those diseases identified as reportable and should know what the requirements are in the state in which she or he practices. The woman must be informed when a case will be reported and be told why. Failure to inform the woman that the case will be reported is a serious breach of professional ethics.

---

airborne disease transmission are available in all health care agencies. Standard precautions (to use for infection control when caring for everyone) and additional precautions for labor and birth settings are listed in Box 7.4.

BOX 7.4   Standard Precautions

Medical history and examination cannot reliably identify everyone infected with human immunodeficiency virus (HIV) or other blood-borne pathogens. Standard precautions should therefore be used consistently in the care of all clients. These precautions apply to blood, body fluids, and all secretions and excretions except sweat, nonintact skin, and mucous membranes. The following infection-control practices should be applied during the delivery of health care to reduce the risk of transmission of microorganisms from known and unknown sources of infection:

1. *Hand hygiene.* During the delivery of health care, avoid unnecessary touching of surfaces in close proximity to the client to prevent both contamination of clean hands from environmental surfaces and transmission of pathogens from contaminated hands to surfaces. Wash dirty or contaminated hands with either a nonantimicrobial or an antimicrobial soap and water. If hands are not visibly soiled, decontaminate hands with an alcohol-based hand rub, or hands may be washed with an antimicrobial soap and water. Perform hand hygiene (1) before having direct contact with clients; (2) after contact with blood, body fluids, or excretions, mucous membranes, nonintact skin, or wound dressings; (3) after contact with a client's intact skin (e.g., when taking a pulse or blood pressure or lifting a client); (4) if hands will be moving from a contaminated body site to a clean body site during client care; (5) after contact with inanimate objects (including medical equipment) in the immediate vicinity of the client; and (6) after removing gloves. Wash hands with nonantimicrobial or antimicrobial soap and water if contact with spores (e.g., *Clostridium difficile* or *Bacillus anthracis*) is likely to have occurred. The physical action of washing and rinsing hands under such circumstances is recommended because alcohols, chlorhexidine, iodophors, and other antiseptic agents have poor activity against spores. Do not wear artificial fingernails or extenders if duties include direct contact with clients at high risk for infection and associated adverse outcomes.

2. *Personal protective equipment (PPE).* Observe the following principles of use:

3. *Gloves.* Wear gloves when a reasonable possibility exists for contact with blood or other potentially infectious materials, mucous membranes, nonintact skin, or potentially contaminated intact skin (e.g., of a client incontinent of stool or urine). Gloves should be worn during infant eye prophylaxis, care of the umbilical cord, circumcision site, parenteral procedures, diaper changes, contact with colostrum, and postpartum assessments. Wear gloves with fit and durability appropriate to the task. Remove gloves after contact with a client or the surrounding environment (including medical equipment) using proper technique to prevent hand contamination. Do not wear the same pair of gloves for the care of more than one client. Change gloves during client care if the hands will move from a contaminated body site (e.g., perineal area) to a clean body site (e.g., face).

4. *Gowns.* Wear a gown that is appropriate to the task to protect the skin and prevent soiling or contamination of clothing during procedures and client-care activities when contact with blood, body fluids, secretions, or excretions is anticipated. Remove the gown and perform hand hygiene before leaving the client's environment. Do not reuse gowns, even for repeated contacts with the same client. Routine donning of gowns on entrance into a high-risk unit (e.g., intensive care unit [ICU] or neonatal intensive care unit [NICU]) is not indicated.

5. *Mouth, nose, eye protection.* Use PPE to protect the mucous membranes of the eyes, nose, and mouth during procedures and client-care activities that are likely to generate splashes or sprays of blood, body fluids, secretions, and excretions. Select masks, goggles, face shields, and combinations of each according to the need anticipated by the task performed.

6. *Respiratory hygiene and cough etiquette.* Post signs at entrances and in strategic places (e.g., elevators, cafeterias) within ambulatory and inpatient settings with instructions to clients and others with symptoms of a respiratory infection to cover mouth and nose when coughing or sneezing, use and dispose of tissues, and perform hand hygiene after hands have been in contact with respiratory secretions. Provide tissues and no-touch receptacles (e.g., foot pedal–operated lid or open, plastic-lined wastebasket) for disposal of tissues. Provide resources and instructions for performing hand hygiene in or near waiting areas in ambulatory and inpatient settings; provide conveniently located dispensers of alcohol-based hand rubs and, where sinks are available, supplies for handwashing. During periods of increased respiratory infections in the community, offer masks to coughing clients and other symptomatic individuals (e.g., people who accompany ill clients) on entry into the facility, and encourage them to maintain special separation, ideally a distance of at least 3 feet, from others in common waiting areas.

7. *Safe injection practices.* The following recommendations apply to the use of needles, cannulas that replace needles, and, where applicable, intravenous delivery systems:

8. Use aseptic technique to prevent contamination of sterile injection equipment. Needles, cannulas, and syringes are sterile, single-use items; they should not be reused for another client. Use fluid infusion and administration sets (i.e., intravenous bags, tubing, and connectors) for one client only, and dispose appropriately after use. Use single-dose vials for parenteral medications whenever possible. If multidose vials must be used, both the needle (or cannula) and the syringe used to access the multidose vial must be sterile. Do not keep multidose vials in the immediate client treatment area and store in accordance with the manufacturer's recommendations; discard if sterility is compromised or questionable.

Modified from Siegel, J. D., Rhinehart, E., Jackson, M., et al. (2007). Guideline for isolation precautions: Preventing transmission of infectious agents in healthcare settings. Retrieved from www.cdc.gov/ncidod/dhqp/pdf/isolation2007.pdf.

■ KEY POINTS

- Reproductive tract infections include STIs and common genital tract infections.
- Young sexually active women who do not practice risk-reducing sexual behaviors and have multiple partners are at greatest risk for STIs and HIV.
- Risk-reduction sexual practices are key strategies for the prevention of STIs.
- STIs are responsible for substantial morbidity and mortality and a heavy economic burden in the United States.
- HIV is transmitted through body fluids, primarily blood, semen, vaginal secretions, and breast milk.
- Prevention of mother-to-newborn HIV transmission is most effective when the woman receives antiretroviral drugs during pregnancy, labor, and birth and the infant receives the drugs after birth.

- STIs and vaginitis are biologic events for which all individuals have a right to expect objective, compassionate, and effective health care.
- Pregnancy confers no immunity against infection, and both mother and fetus must be considered when the pregnant woman contracts an infection.
- HPV is the most common viral STI.
- Syphilis has reemerged as a common STI, affecting black women more than any other ethnic or racial group.
- Because history and examination cannot reliably identify everyone with HIV or other blood-borne pathogens, blood and body-fluid precautions should be used consistently for everyone all the time.
- Chlamydia is the most common STI in women in the United States and one of the most common causes of PID.
- Viral hepatitis has several forms of transmission; HBV infections carry the greatest risk.

REFERENCES

American Cancer Society. (2016). *The American Cancer Society guidelines for the prevention and early detection of cervical cancer.* Retrieved from: https://www.cancer.org/cancer/cervical-cancer/prevention-and-early-detection/cervical-cancer-screening-guidelines.html.

American College of Obstetricians and Gynecologists. (2016). ACOG committee opinion no.168: Cervical cancer screening and prevention. *Obstetrics and Gynecology, 128*(4), e111–e130.

Centers for Disease Control and Prevention. (2018). *State laboratory reporting laws: Viral load and CD4 requirements.* Available at: https://www.cdc.gov/hiv/policies/law/states/reporting.html.

Centers for Disease Control and Prevention. (2018a). *Areas with Zika.* Retrieved from: http://www.cdc.gov/zika/about/index.html.

Centers for Disease Control and Prevention. (2018b). *Group B strep (GBS): Prevention in newborns.* Retrieved from: http://www.cdc.gov/groupbstrep/about/prevention.html.

Centers for Disease Control and Prevention. (2017b). *Sexually transmitted disease surveillance 2016.* Atlanta: U.S. Department of Health and Human Services. Retrieved from: https://www.cdc.gov/std/stats16/CDC_2016_STDS_Report-for508WebSep21_2017_1644.pdf.

Centers for Disease Control and Prevention. (2015b). 2015 Sexually transmitted diseases treatment guidelines. Retrieved from: https://www.cdc.gov/std/tg2015/clinical.htm.

Centers for Disease Control and Prevention. (2014) Chlamydia - CDC fact sheet. Retrieved from https://www.cdc.gov/std/chlamydia/stdfact-chlamydia.htm.

Centers for Disease Control and Prevention. (2015a). Guidelines For Viral Hepatitis Surveillance and Case Management. Available at: https://www.cdc.gov/hepatitis/statistics/surveillanceguidelines.htm.

Centers for Disease Control and Prevention. (2019). *HIV Surveillance Report, 2016.* Retrieved from: http://www.cdc.gov/hiv/library/reports/hiv-surveillance.html. https://www.cdc.gov/hiv/library/reports/hiv-surveillance.html.

Centers for Disease Control and Prevention (CDC). (2017a). *Bacterial vaginosis - CDC fact sheet.* Retrieved from: https://www.cdc.gov/std/bv/stdfact-bacterial-vaginosis.htm.

Centers for Disease Control and Prevention. (2018d). *Zika travel information.* Retrieved from: https://wwwnc.cdc.gov/travel/page/zika-travel-information.

Clark, L. E., Allen, R. H., Goyal, V., et al. (2014). Reproductive coercion and co-occurring intimate partner violence in obstetrics and gynecology patients. *American Journal of Obstetrics and Gynecology, 210*(1), 42.e1–42.e8.

Curtis, K. M., Tepper, J. k, Jatlaoui, T. C., et al. (2016). U.S. Medical Eligibility Criteria for Contraceptive Use, 2016. *Morbidity and mortality weekly report, 65*(3), 1–108.

Decker, M. R., Miller, E., McCauley, H. L., et al. (2014). Recent partner violence and sexual and drug-related STI/HIV risk among adolescent and young adult women attending family planning clinics. *Sexually Transmitted Infections, 90*(2), 145–149.

Gardella, C., Eckert, L. O., & Lentz, G. M. (2017). Genital tract infections: Vulva, vagina, cervix, toxic shock syndrome, endometritis, and salpingitis. In R. A. Lobo, D. M. Gershenson, G. M. Lentz, et al. (Eds.), *Comprehensive gynecology* (7th ed.). Philadelphia: Mosby.

Grace, K. T., & Anderson, J. C. (2016). Reproductive coercion: A systematic review. *Trauma, Violence & Abuse, 19*(4), 371–390.

Hughes, B., & Cu-Uvin, S. (2018). *Antiretroviral and intrapartum management of pregnant HIV-infected women and their infants in resource-rich setting.* Retrieved from: www.uptodate.com/contents/antiretroviral-treatment-of-pregnant-hiv-infected-women-and-antiretroviral-prophylaxis-of-their-infants-in-resource-rich-settings.

Marrazzo, J.M., & Park, I.U. (2018). Reproductive tract infections, including HIV and other sexually transmitted infections. In R.A. Hatcher, A.L. Nelson, J. Trussell, C. Cwiak, P. Cason, M.S. Policar, A.B. Edelman, A.R.A. Aiken, J.M. Marrazzo, D. Kowal (Eds.). *Contraceptive technology* (21st ed.). New York: Ayer Company Publishers, Inc.

Meites, E., Kempe, A., & Markowitz, L. E. (2016). Use of a 2-dose schedule for human papillomavirus vaccination — updated recommendations of the advisory committee on immunization practices. *Morbidity and mortality weekly report, 65*(49), 1405–1408.

Moreira, J., Peixoto, T. M., Siqueira, A. M., et al., C. C. (2017). Sexually acquired Zika virus: A systematic review. *Clinical Microbiology and Infection, 23*(5), 296–305.

Nelson, A. & Harwood, B. (2018). Vaginal barriers and spermicides. In R.A. Hatcher, A.L. Nelson, J. Trussell, C. Cwiak, P. Cason, M.S. Policar, A.B. Edelman, A.R.A. Aiken, J.M. Marrazzo, D. Kowal (Eds.). *Contraceptive technology* (21st ed.). New York: Ayer Company Publishers, Inc.

Oduyebo, T., Polen, K.D., Walke, H.T., et al (2017). Update: Interim Guidance for Health Care Providers Caring for Pregnant Women with Possible Zika Virus Exposure—United States (Including U.S. Territories), July 2017. *Morbidity and mortality weekly report* 2017;66:781–793.

Tancredi, D. J., Silverman, J. G., Decker, M. R., et al. (2015). Cluster randomized controlled trial protocol: Addressing reproductive coercion in health settings (ARCHES). *BMC Women's Health, 15*(57), 1–16.

U.S. Food and Drug Administration (FDA). (2018). FDA approves expanded use of Gardasil 9 to include individuals 27 through 45 years old. Retrieved from: https://www.fda.gov/newsevents/newsroom/pressannouncements/ucm622715.htm.

U.S. Department of Health and Human Services. (2019). *Recommendations for the use of antiretroviral drugs in pregnant women with HIV infection and interventions to reduce perinatal HIV transmission in the United States.* Retrieved from: https://aidsinfo.nih.gov/guidelines/html/3/perinatal- guidelines/182/transmission-and-mode-of-delivery.

U.S. Food and Drug Administration (FDA). (2017). *FDA approves two hepatitis C drugs for pediatric patients.* Retrieved from: https://www.fda.gov/NewsEvents/Newsroom/PressAnnouncements/ucm551407.htm.

World Health Organization. (2019). *Sexually transmitted infection (STIs).* Retrieved from: http://who.int/mediacentre/factsheets/fs110/en/.

8

Contraception and Abortion

Lisa L. Ferguson

 http://evolve.elsevier.com/Lowdermilk/MWHC/

LEARNING OBJECTIVES

- Compare various methods of contraception.
- Identify the advantages and disadvantages of commonly used methods of contraception.
- Describe the common nursing interventions that facilitate contraceptive use.
- Examine the various ethical, legal, cultural, and religious considerations of contraception.

- Describe the techniques used for medical and surgical interruption of pregnancy.
- Discuss the various techniques and ethical and legal considerations of elective abortion.
- Develop a plan of care for a woman who needs emergency contraception.

CONTRACEPTION

The capability of Americans to engage in effective family planning as a result of the modern era of contraception is considered one of the 10 greatest public health achievements of the 20th century. Nevertheless, nearly half of all U.S. pregnancies are not planned (Guttmacher Institute, 2016; Mosher, Jones, & Abma, 2015). Among adolescent women, approximately 75% of those who became pregnant did not intend to do so, giving the United States the dubious distinction of having the highest unintended teen pregnancy rate when compared with equally high-income countries (Finer & Zolna, 2016; Wilkinson, Clark, Rafie, et al., 2017). The nurse can play a vital role in prevention of unwanted pregnancy through counseling and education regarding family planning, contraception, and effective birth control.

Family planning is the conscious decision on when to conceive or to avoid pregnancy throughout the reproductive years. **Contraception** is defined as the intentional prevention of pregnancy during sexual intercourse. **Birth control** is the device and/or practice used to decrease the risk of conceiving or bearing offspring.

With the wide assortment of birth control options available, it is possible for a woman to use several different contraceptive methods at various stages throughout her fertile years. Nurses interact with the individual, as well as the couple, to compare and contrast available contraceptive options. Factors to consider include reliability, relative cost of the method, any protection from sexually transmitted infections (STIs), the individual's comfort level with the method, and the partner's willingness to use a particular birth control method. Those who use contraception can still be at risk for pregnancy if their chosen contraceptive method is not used correctly or if it is less reliable than other methods. Expanding access to contraception, especially long-acting reversible methods, and improving accurate and reliable use of birth control methods can decrease the chance of unintended pregnancy (CDC, 2015b).

🏠 COMMUNITY ACTIVITY

Nurses provide discharge planning after birth; they commonly staff family planning clinics and provide contraceptive information to those clients and others in the community. Education concerning contraceptive use in the postpartum period is a common component of discharge planning in many countries, with wide variation among health care delivery systems. Education at this time assumes women's receptiveness to information about contraception and that education or receptiveness to such information could be less at a later period. However, clinical trials have not demonstrated that education in the immediate postpartum period is effective. Contact a clinic in your community to see if you can talk with one of the nurses about their procedures in caring for postpartum women, focusing on what the nurses do related to education about family planning.

📋 CARE MANAGEMENT

An interprofessional approach may assist a woman in choosing and correctly using an appropriate contraceptive method. Nurses, nurse-midwives, nurse practitioners, and other advanced practice nurses, as well as physicians and pharmacists, have the knowledge and expertise to assist a woman in making decisions about contraception that will satisfy her personal, social, cultural, religious, and interpersonal needs.

Family, friends, media, partner or partners, religious affiliation, and health care professionals influence a woman's perception of contraceptive choices. These external influences help to form a woman's unique view. The nurse assists in supporting the woman's decision based on her individual situation and ensures that she has accurate information.

Evaluation of the couple desiring contraception involves assessing the woman's reproductive history (menstrual, obstetric, gynecologic, contraceptive), physical examination, and, sometimes, current laboratory tests. The nurse must determine the woman's knowledge about reproduction, contraception, and STIs, as well as her sexual partner's commitment to any particular method.

Assessment of the client begins with the following appraisals:

- Determining the woman's knowledge about contraception and her sexual partner's commitment to any particular method
- Collecting data about the frequency of coitus, the number of sexual partners, the level of contraceptive involvement, and her or her partner's objections to any methods
- Assessing the woman's level of comfort and willingness to touch her genitals and cervical mucus
- Identifying any misconceptions, as well as religious and cultural factors, and paying close attention to the woman's verbal and nonverbal responses to hearing about the various available methods
- Considering the woman's reproductive life plan
- Completing a history (including menstrual, contraceptive, and obstetric), physical examination (including pelvic examination), and laboratory tests (as needed for identifying presence of STIs).

Informed consent is a vital component in educating a client about contraception or sterilization. The nurse often has the responsibility to document information provided and the understanding of that information by the client. The mnemonic BRAIDED may be useful (see Legal Tip).

Once the assessment is complete, client problems can be identified to help develop the nursing care plan and interventions.

LEGAL TIP

Informed Consent
- B—Benefits: information about advantages and success rates
- R—Risks: information about disadvantages and failure rates
- A—Alternatives: information about other available methods
- I—Inquiries: opportunity to ask questions
- D—Decisions: opportunity to decide or to change her mind
- E—Explanations: information about method and how it is used
- D—Documentation: information given and client's understanding

---

Education is the cornerstone of the nursing care plan and planned interventions that accomplish the goal of increasing client understanding that leads to improved adherence to the contraceptive plan and increased client satisfaction. The nurse should teach about the specific contraceptive used. After providing instruction about the contraceptive method, the nurse should ask the woman to perform a return demonstration of how a device is used, if appropriate, and assess her understanding of the method. The nurse should also provide the woman and her partner with written instructions about the contraceptive method and with contact information in case she has questions later. If a woman has difficulty understanding written instructions, offer her (and her partner, if available) graphic material as well as reliable websites and contact information (telephone number, email) for questions of the clinic if necessary, and let her know that she may return to the clinic for further instruction if needed. It is very important to provide the woman and her partner with information about backup methods of birth control and emergency contraception (EC).

Contraceptive counseling should be conducted in a private setting. The woman should feel safe and free to communicate with the nurse. Distractions should be minimized, and samples of birth control devices for interactive teaching should be available. The nurse counters myths with facts, clarifies misinformation, and fills in gaps of knowledge. The ideal contraceptive should be safe, easily available, economical, acceptable, simple to use, and promptly reversible. Although no method may ever have all these characteristics, new contraceptive technologies are being developed, and couples have more choices currently available to them than ever before.

BOX 8.1 Factors Affecting Contraceptive Method Effectiveness

- Frequency of intercourse
- Motivation to prevent pregnancy
- Understanding of how to use method
- Adherence to method
- Provision of short- or long-term protection
- Likelihood of pregnancy for the individual woman
- Consistent use of method

"Contraceptive failure rate" refers to the percentage of contraceptive users expected to have an unplanned pregnancy during the first year of use, even when they use a method consistently and correctly. Contraceptive effectiveness varies from couple to couple and depends on the properties of the method and the characteristics of the user (Box 8.1). Effectiveness of a method can be expressed as theoretic effectiveness, or how effective the method is with perfect use, and as typical effectiveness, or how effective the method is with typical use. Failure rates decrease over time, either because a user gains experience and uses a method more appropriately or because the less effective users stop using the method. Safety of a method may be affected by a woman's medical history (e.g., thromboembolic problems and contraceptive methods containing estrogen). In most instances, pregnancy would be more dangerous to the woman with medical problems than a particular contraceptive method, but thromboembolic problems are an example of why a certain type of contraception should be avoided. On the other hand, the use of many contraceptive methods is associated with health promotion effects. For example, barrier methods, such as the male condom, offer some protection from acquiring STIs, and oral contraceptives lower the incidence of ovarian and endometrial cancer.

⚡ SAFETY ALERT

Make sure the woman has a backup method of birth control and contraceptive pills (CPs) readily available during the initial learning phase when she uses a new method of contraception to help prevent an unintentional conception.

❓ CLINICAL REASONING CASE STUDY

Contraception for Adolescents

Maria is a 16-year-old Hispanic client who comes to the family planning clinic seeking contraception. She has recently become sexually active and tells the nurse that she is concerned that her mother will find out. She also has many questions about the type of contraception to use. She seeks the nurse's advice to help in her decision making.

1. What is the priority concern or client need in this situation?
2. List other client needs/problems in this case.
3. Identify any additional information needed by the nurse in addressing this situation.
4. Describe the roles/responsibilities of interprofessional health team members who may be involved in this situation.

METHODS OF CONTRACEPTION

The following discussion of contraceptive methods provides the nurse with information needed for client teaching (Fig. 8.1).

The most effective contraceptive methods are the long-acting, reversible contraceptive (LARC) methods (e.g., contraceptive

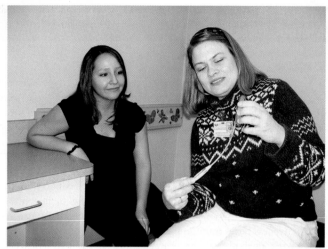

Fig. 8.1 Nurse Counseling Woman About Contraceptive Methods. (Courtesy Dee Lowdermilk, Chapel Hill, NC.)

implants, intrauterine devices [IUDs]). With these methods, theoretic and typical pregnancy rates are the same because the method requires no user intervention after correct insertion. Other effective methods include those that prevent pregnancy through exogenous hormones (estrogen and/or progestins), such as contraceptive injections, oral contraceptive pills, contraceptive patches, and vaginal rings. Each of these methods involves user interventions, so typical use pregnancy rates are higher than pregnancy rates with perfect use. The least effective contraceptive methods include the barrier methods and natural family planning (NFP).

Coitus Interruptus

Coitus interruptus (withdrawal) involves the male partner withdrawing the penis from the woman's vagina before he ejaculates. Although coitus interruptus is one of the least effective methods of contraception, it is a good choice for couples who do not have another contraceptive available (CDC, 2017a). Effectiveness is similar to barrier methods and depends on the man's ability to withdraw his penis before ejaculation. The percentage of women who will experience an unintended pregnancy (failure rate) within the first year of typical use of withdrawal is approximately 22% (Rivlin & Westhoff, 2017). Coitus interruptus does not protect against STIs or human immunodeficiency virus (HIV) infection.

Fertility Awareness–Based Methods (Natural Family Planning)

Fertility awareness–based (FAB) methods of contraception, also known as periodic abstinence or NFP, depend on identifying the beginning and end of the fertile period of the menstrual cycle. These methods provide contraception by relying on avoidance of intercourse during fertile periods. NFP methods are the only contraceptive practices acceptable to the Roman Catholic Church. When women who want to use FABs are educated about the menstrual cycle, three phases are identified:
1. Infertile phase: before ovulation
2. Fertile phase: approximately 5 to 7 days around the middle of the cycle, including several days before and during ovulation and the day afterward
3. Infertile phase: after ovulation

The human ovum can be fertilized no later than 12 to 24 hours after ovulation (Cunningham, Leveno, Bloom, et al., 2018). Motile sperm have been recovered from the uterus and the oviducts as long as 60 hours after coitus, but their ability to fertilize the ovum probably lasts no longer than 24 to 48 hours. One problem with FAB methods is that the exact time of ovulation cannot be predicted accurately, and couples may find it difficult to exercise restraint for several days before and after ovulation. In addition, women with irregular menstrual periods have the greatest risk of failure with FAB methods.

Although ovulation can be unpredictable in many women, teaching the woman how she can directly identify her fertility patterns is an empowering tool. There are nearly a dozen categories of FAB methods. To prevent pregnancy, each one uses a combination of charts, records, calculations, tools, observations, and either abstinence or barrier methods of birth control during the fertile period in the menstrual cycle. The charts and calculations associated with these methods can also be used to increase the likelihood of detecting the optimal timing of intercourse to achieve conception. Signs used to determine the time of fertility include menstrual bleeding, cervical mucus, and basal body temperature (BBT), as described later in the chapter.

Advantages of these methods include low to no cost, heightened awareness and understanding of personal fertility, increased self-reliance, absence of chemicals, instant availability, increased involvement and intimacy with partner, and the ability of the couple to follow religious/cultural traditions. In addition, these methods can be used to establish fertile days for conception in the couple who wants to achieve pregnancy. Disadvantages of FABs include difficulty with adherence to strict record-keeping, requirement of male partner support, lower typical effectiveness than other methods, decreased effectiveness in women with irregular cycles (particularly adolescents who have not established regular ovulatory patterns), decreased spontaneity of coitus, and no protection from STIs, including HIV infection. The typical failure rate for most FAB methods is 24% during the first year of use (Rivlin & Westhoff, 2017).

FAB methods involve several techniques to identify fertile days. The following discussion includes the most common techniques and some promising techniques for the future. Recently various smartphone apps have been developed to assist with following FAB methods, and these apps are currently being studied to understand their effectiveness (Jennings & Polis, 2018).

Calendar-Based Methods

Calendar rhythm method. Practice of the calendar rhythm method is based on the number of days in each cycle, counting from the first day of menses. With this method the fertile period is determined after accurately recording the lengths of menstrual cycles for at least 6 months. The beginning of the fertile period is estimated by subtracting 18 days from the length of the shortest cycle. The end of the fertile period is determined by subtracting 11 days from the length of the longest cycle (Jennings & Polis, 2018). If the shortest cycle is 24 days and the longest is 30 days, application of the formula to calculate the fertile period is as follows:

Shortest cycle: 24 − 18 = sixth day
Longest cycle: 30 − 11 = ninteenth day

To avoid conception the couple would abstain from sexual intercourse during the fertile period—days 6 through 19. If the woman has very regular cycles of 28 days each, the formula indicates the fertile days to be as follows:

Shortest cycle: 28 − 18 = tenth day
Longest cycle: 28 − 11 = seventeenth day

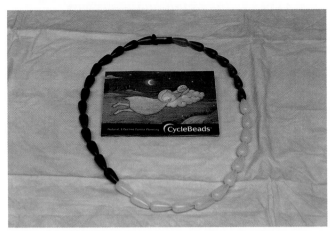

Fig. 8.2 CycleBeads. Red bead marks the first day of the menstrual cycle. White beads mark days that are likely to be fertile days; therefore unprotected intercourse should be avoided. Brown beads are days when pregnancy is unlikely and unprotected intercourse is permitted. (Courtesy Dee Lowdermilk, Chapel Hill, NC.)

To avoid pregnancy the couple avoids sexual intercourse from days 10 through 17 because ovulation occurs on day 14 plus or minus 2 days. A major drawback of the calendar method is that one is trying to predict future events with past data. The unpredictability of the menstrual cycle also is not taken into consideration. The calendar rhythm method is most useful as an adjunct to the BBT or the cervical mucus method.

Standard days method. The Standard Days Method (SDM) is essentially a modified form of the calendar rhythm method that has a "fixed" number of days of fertility for each cycle (i.e., days 8 to 19) (Jennings & Polis, 2018). A CycleBeads necklace—a color-coded string of beads—can be purchased as a concrete tool to track fertility (Fig. 8.2). Day 1 of the menstrual flow is the first day to begin counting. Women who use this device are taught to avoid unprotected intercourse on days 8 to 19 (white beads on CycleBeads necklace). Although this method is useful to women whose cycles are regular and occur at 26- to 32-day intervals, the SDM is unreliable for those who have longer or shorter cycles (Contracept.org, 2016a). The typical failure rate for the SDM is reported as 12%, but it is difficult to

measure effectiveness rates of this method, which is so dependent upon the persons using it, and the failure rate may be even higher than initially stated (Marston & Church, 2016).

Symptoms-Based Methods

TwoDay Method. The TwoDay Method is based on the monitoring and recording of cervical secretions (Jennings & Polis, 2018). Unlike other methods that rely on this indicator, such as the ovulation mucus method or the symptothermal method, it does not involve analyzing the characteristics of the secretions (e.g., amount, color, consistency, slipperiness, stretchability, or viscosity) (Contracept.org, 2016b). Each day the woman asks herself, (1) "Did I note secretions today?" and (2) "Did I note secretions yesterday?" If the answer to either question is yes, she should avoid coitus or use a backup method of birth control. If the answer to both questions is no, her probability of getting pregnant is very low. After 2 days without secretions, the woman may resume unprotected intercourse. The TwoDay Method appears to be simpler to teach, learn, and use than other natural methods. The method can be an effective alternative for low-literacy populations or for programs that find current NFP methods too time consuming or otherwise not feasible to incorporate into their services. Studies have found the typical failure rate of the TwoDay Method to be 14% (Jennings & Polis, 2018).

Cervical mucus ovulation detection method. The cervical mucus ovulation detection method (i.e., Billings method or ovulation method) requires that the woman recognize and interpret the cyclic changes in the amount and consistency of cervical mucus that characterize her own unique pattern of changes at the time of ovulation. Cervical mucus transforms prior to and during ovulation to facilitate and promote the viability and motility of sperm. Without adequate cervical mucus, coitus does not result in conception. This method requires that a woman check the quantity and character of mucus on the vulva or introitus with her fingers or tissue paper each day for several months and evaluate the mucus for cloudiness, tackiness, and slipperiness. This way she can learn how her cervical mucus responds to ovulation during her menstrual cycles. To ensure an accurate assessment of changes, the cervical mucus should be free from semen, contraceptive gels or foams, and blood or discharge from vaginal infections for at least one full cycle. Other factors that create difficulty in identifying mucus changes include douches and vaginal deodorants, being in a sexually aroused state (which thins the

---

◎ NURSING CARE PLAN

Sexual Activity and Contraception

Client Problem	Expected Outcome	Nursing Interventions	Rationales
Need for Health Teaching related to contraceptive alternatives	Woman and partner will verbalize understanding of different methods of contraception and will choose the method best suited for their needs.	Provide information regarding reliability, use, indications, contraindications, and side effects of different methods of contraception. Use privacy and therapeutic communication during discussion of sexual activity and methods of contraception.	To facilitate the decision-making process To provide clarification of information and client trust of caregiver
Potential for sexually transmitted infection	Woman and her partner will remain free of STIs.	Provide information regarding sex practices to reduce risk of STIs and use of barrier methods.	To raise client awareness of methods to prevent infection
Risk for unplanned and/or unwanted pregnancy related to contraceptive failure as a result of incorrect use of chosen method	Woman and partner will verbalize intent and understanding to use chosen contraception correctly.	Review information given regarding use, reliability, and side effects of chosen contraceptive method.	To ensure woman's and partner's understanding
		Provide list of informational resources.	To promote consistency of use of chosen method
		Encourage ongoing effective communication with health care provider.	To promote trust

STIs, Sexually transmitted infections.

mucus), and taking medications such as antihistamines (which dry the mucus). Intercourse is considered safe without restriction beginning the fourth day after the last day of wet, clear, slippery mucus, which would indicate that ovulation occurred 2 to 3 days previously.

Some women find this method unacceptable if they are uncomfortable touching their genitals. Whether or not a woman wants to use this method for contraception, it is to her advantage to learn to recognize mucus characteristics at ovulation. Self-evaluation of cervical mucus can be highly accurate and useful diagnostically for any of the following purposes:

- To alert the couple to the reestablishment of ovulation while breast-feeding and after discontinuation of oral contraception
- To note anovulatory cycles at any time and at the beginning of menopause
- To assist couples in planning a pregnancy

Basal body temperature method. The BBT is the lowest body temperature of a healthy person, taken immediately after waking and before getting out of bed. The BBT usually varies from 36.2°C to 36.3°C (97.16°F to 97.34°F) during menses and for approximately 5 to 7 days afterward (Fig. 8.3).

About the time of ovulation, a slight drop in temperature (approximately 0.5°C [0.9°F]) may occur in some women just prior to

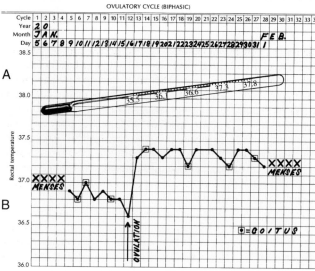

Fig. 8.3 (A) Special thermometer for recording basal body temperature, marked in tenths to enable person to read more easily. (B) Basal temperature record shows drop and sharp rise at time of ovulation. Biphasic curve indicates ovulatory cycle.

TEACHING FOR SELF-MANAGEMENT

Cervical Mucus Characteristics

Setting the Stage
- Show charts of menstrual cycle along with changes in the cervical mucus.
- Have the woman practice with raw egg white.
- Supply her with a BBT log and graph if she does not already have one.
- Explain that assessment of cervical mucus characteristics is best when mucus is not mixed with semen, contraceptive jellies or foams, or discharge from infections. Tell her to refrain from douching before the assessment.

Content Related to Cervical Mucus
- Explain to the woman (couple) how cervical mucus changes throughout the menstrual cycle.
  - Postmenstrual mucus: scant
  - Preovulation mucus: cloudy, yellow or white, sticky
  - Ovulation mucus: clear, wet, sticky, slippery
  - Postovulation fertile mucus: thick, cloudy, sticky
  - Postovulation, postfertile mucus: scant

- Right before ovulation, the watery, thin, clear mucus becomes more abundant and thick (Fig. A). It feels similar to a lubricant and can be stretched 5+ cm between the thumb and forefinger; this quality of mucus is called spinnbarkeit (Fig. B), and its presence indicates the period of maximal fertility. Sperm deposited in this type of mucus can survive until ovulation occurs.

Assessment Technique
- Stress that good handwashing is imperative to begin and end all self-assessments.
- Start observation from last day of menstrual flow.
- Assess cervical mucus several times a day for several cycles. Mucus can be obtained from vaginal opening; reaching into the vagina to the cervix is unnecessary.
- Record the findings on the same record on which the basal body temperature is entered.

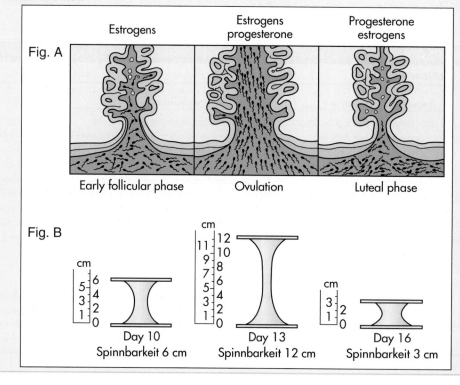

ovulation, but other women may have no decrease at all. After ovulation, in concert with the increasing progesterone levels of the early luteal phase of the cycle, the BBT increases slightly (approximately 0.4°C to 0.8°C [0.72°F to 1.4°F]). Before ovulation, 35.5°C to 36.6°C (96°F to 98°F) is normal in many women. After ovulation, temperature increases to 36.1°C to 37.2°C (97°F to 99°F). The temperature remains on an elevated plateau until 2 to 4 days before menstruation. Then BBT decreases to the low levels recorded during the previous cycle unless pregnancy has occurred. In pregnant women the temperature remains elevated. If ovulation fails to occur, the pattern of lower body temperature continues throughout the cycle.

To use this method, the fertile period is defined as the day of first temperature drop, or first elevation, through 3 consecutive days of elevated temperature. Abstinence begins the first day of menstrual bleeding and lasts through 3 consecutive days of sustained temperature rise (at least 0.2°C [0.18°F]). The decrease and subsequent increase in temperature are referred to as the *thermal shift*. When the entire month's temperatures are recorded on a graph, the pattern described is more apparent. It is more difficult to perceive day-to-day variations without the entire picture (see Fig. 8.3). Either a glass mercury thermometer or a digital thermometer may be used for BBT, but the thermometer must measure the temperature within 0.1 degree. The glass mercury thermometer needs no batteries but is fragile and can break. A digital thermometer will require batteries but may have a history recall function and an audible beep when the temperature assessment is finished.

Infection, fatigue, less than 3 hours of sleep per night, awakening late, and anxiety may cause temperature fluctuations and alter the expected pattern. If a new BBT thermometer is purchased, this fact is noted on the chart because the readings may vary slightly. Jet lag, alcohol consumed the evening before, or sleeping in a heated waterbed must also be noted on the chart because each affects the BBT. Therefore the BBT alone is not a reliable method of predicting ovulation.

Digital thermometers that monitor temperature throughout the day combined with an accelerometer to monitor movement have been cleared for use by the U.S. Food and Drug Administration (FDA). One such device, DuoFertility, can be worn by the woman with data uploaded wirelessly to a computer through a companion device (DuoFertility, n.d.). Other "wearable" devices available are Ava bracelet, worn only at night and boasting 89% accuracy rate; Wink, an oral thermometer that vibrates to remind you to take your temperature and wirelessly sync to the Kindara app; Yono, an in-ear device that uploads temperature data once in its cradle; Tempdrop, worn on the arm and uploadable to multiple different apps; and Daysy, an oral thermometer which connects directly to a smartphone and claims to be 99.3% effective (Peck, 2017). These devices' use in FAB methods needs further research.

Symptothermal method. The symptothermal method combines the BBT and cervical mucus methods with awareness of secondary phase–related signs and symptoms of the menstrual cycle. The woman gains fertility awareness as she learns the signs and symptoms that mark the phases of her cycle. Secondary signs and symptoms include increased libido, midcycle spotting, mittelschmerz (cramplike pain prior to ovulation), pelvic fullness or tenderness, and vulvar fullness.

The woman is taught to palpate her cervix to assess for changes indicating ovulation: the cervical os dilates slightly, the cervix softens and rises in the vagina, and cervical mucus is copious and slippery. The woman notes days on which coitus, changes in routine, illness, and other changes that might affect BBT have occurred (see Fig. 8.4). Calendar calculations and cervical mucus changes are used to estimate the onset of the fertile period; changes in cervical mucus or the BBT are used to estimate the end of the fertile period.

BIOLOGIC MARKER METHODS

Home Predictor Test Kits for Ovulation

Although the methods previously discussed are based on characteristics of ovulation, they do not prove that ovulation actually occurred or indicate the exact timing. The urine predictor test for ovulation is a major addition to the NFP and fertility-awareness methods to help women who desire to become pregnant (Fig. 8.5). The urine predictor test for ovulation detects the sudden surge of luteinizing hormone (LH) that occurs approximately 12 to 24 hours before ovulation. Unlike BBT, this test is not affected by illness, emotions, or physical activity. For home use, a test kit contains sufficient material for several days' testing during each cycle. A positive response indicating an LH surge is noted by a color change that is easy to interpret. Directions for use of urine predictor test kits vary with the manufacturer. Research continues on the efficacy of available home test kits and devices for the prevention of pregnancy (Leiva, Burhan, Kyrillos, et al., 2014).

Marquette Model

The Marquette Model (MM) is an NFP method that was developed through the Marquette University College of Nursing Institute for NFP (Marquette University, 2018). The MM uses cervical monitoring along with the ClearBlue Fertility Monitor. The ClearBlue monitor is a handheld device that uses test strips to measure urinary metabolites of estrogen and LH. The monitor provides the user with "low," "high," and "peak" fertility readings. The MM incorporates the use of the monitor as an aid to learning NFP and fertility awareness. Three studies on the efficacy of the MM have shown typical use failure rates of 10% to 12% (Marquette University, 2018).

Applications for Fertility Awareness–Based Methods

Dynamic Optimal Timing

For women with menstrual cycles between 20 and 40 days, a mobile application is currently in the testing phase. Dynamic Optimal Timing (DOT) uses a complex algorithm to predict the best days of fertility, whether one intends to become or avoid becoming pregnant. The only data point required is the menstrual start date (Cycle Technologies, 2017).

NaturalCycles

This app is used in conjunction with the basal body thermometer to predict ovulation and a woman's fertile window. Data required for this app are daily BBTs and date of menstruation. The typical-use failure rate for this method is 7.5%, significantly lower than the 24% attributed to FAB methods overall (Scherwitzl, Danielsson, Sellberg, & Scherwitzl, 2016; Scherwitzl, Hirschberg, & Scherwitzl, 2015).

Spermicides and Barrier Methods

Barrier contraceptives have gained in popularity not only as a contraceptive method but also as protection against the spread of STIs such as HIV and herpes simplex virus (HSV). Spermicides serve as chemical barriers against semen and inhibit the ability of sperm to fertilize the ovum.

The nurse should remember that any user of a barrier method of contraception must also be aware of EC options in case there is a failure of the method. An example of a barrier method failure would be if a condom broke during intercourse. In this instance, EC would be indicated to prevent unplanned pregnancy.

Spermicides

Spermicides such as nonoxynol-9 (N-9) work by reducing the sperm's mobility. The chemicals attack the sperm flagella and body, thereby preventing the sperm from reaching the cervical os. N-9, the most commonly used spermicidal chemical in the United States, is a surfactant that

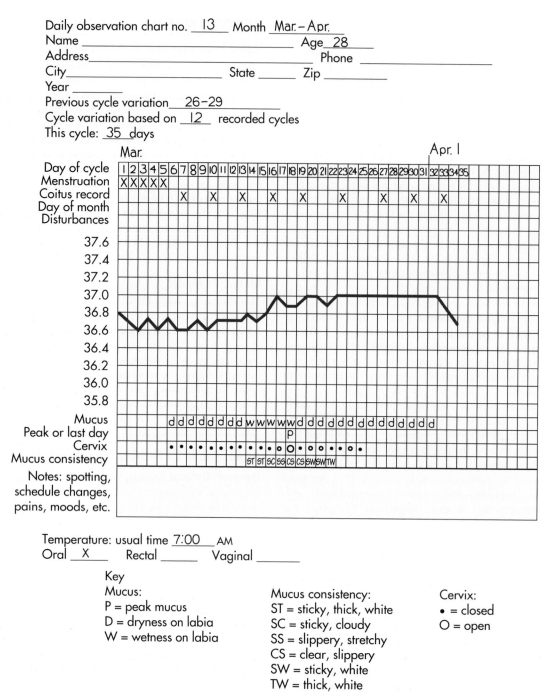

Fig. 8.4 Example of a Completed Symptothermal Chart.

destroys the sperm cell membrane. Results from data analyses suggest that frequent use (more than two times a day) of N-9 or the use of N-9 as a lubricant during anal intercourse may increase the transmission of HIV and can cause lesions (World Health Organization [WHO], 2018). There is no evidence that the addition of spermicides to male condoms decreases the risk of subsequent pregnancy. Women with high-risk behaviors that increase their likelihood of contracting HIV and other STIs are advised to avoid the use of spermicidal products containing N-9, including lubricated condoms, diaphragms, and cervical caps to which N-9 is added (WHO). Intravaginal spermicides are marketed and sold without prescriptions as aerosol foams, tablets, suppositories, creams, films, and gels (Fig. 8.6). Preloaded, single-dose applicators small enough to be carried in a small purse are available. Effectiveness of spermicides

depends on consistent and accurate use. Clients should be cautioned against misunderstanding terms: contraceptive gel differs from fruit jelly, and cosmetics or hair products containing the nonspermicidal forms of nonoxynol are not adequate substitutes for contraception. The spermicide should be inserted high into the vagina so that it makes contact with the cervix. Some spermicide should be inserted at least 15 minutes before, and no longer than 1 hour before, sexual intercourse. Spermicide must be reapplied for each additional act of intercourse, even if a barrier method is used. Studies have shown varying effectiveness rates for spermicidal use alone. Typical failure rate in the first year of spermicidal use alone is 29% (Rivlin & Westhoff, 2017). Some female barrier methods (e.g., diaphragm, cervical caps) offer more effective protection against pregnancy with the addition of spermicides (Mayo Clinic, 2018a).

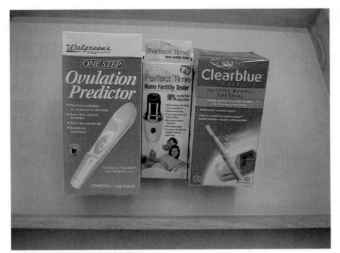

Fig. 8.5 Examples of Ovulation Prediction Tests. (Courtesy Shannon Perry, Phoenix, AZ.)

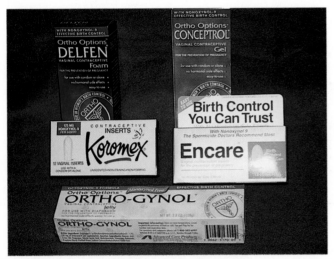

Fig. 8.6 Spermicides. (Courtesy Marjorie Pyle, RNC, Lifecircle, Costa Mesa, CA.)

Condoms

The male condom is a thin, stretchable sheath that covers the penis. A condom is applied before genital, oral, or anal contact and is removed when the penis is withdrawn from the partner's orifice after ejaculation. Condoms are made of latex rubber, which provides a barrier to sperm and some STIs; polyurethane (strong, thin plastic); or natural membranes (animal tissue). In addition to providing a physical barrier for sperm, nonspermicidal latex condoms provide a barrier for STIs as follows: *Neisseria gonorrhoeae,* 90%; *Chlamydia trachomatis* and *Treponema pallidum,* 50% to 90%; *Haemophilus ducreyi,* 10% to 50%; HIV and hepatitis B, 90%; cytomegalovirus (CMV), 50% to 90%; HSV-2, 10% to 50%; human papillomavirus (HPV), 0%; and trichomonas, 30% (Marfatia, Pandya, & Mehta, 2015). Condoms lubricated with N-9 are not recommended for preventing STIs or HIV and do not increase protection against pregnancy. Latex condoms break down with oil-based lubricants (e.g., petroleum jelly and suntan oil) and should be used only with water-based or silicone lubricants (Cornell University, 2017). Because of the growing number of people with latex allergies, condom manufacturers have begun using polyurethane, which is thinner and stronger than latex.

Although polyurethane condoms are as effective for STI prevention as latex condoms, they are more likely to slip or lose contour when compared with latex condoms. With perfect use, therefore latex condoms offer better protection against pregnancy. Polyurethane condoms do offer equivalent pregnancy protection as most barrier products. A small percentage of condoms are made from lamb cecum (natural skin). Natural skin condoms do not provide the same protection against STIs and HIV infection as latex condoms. Natural skin condoms contain small pores that could allow passage of viruses such as hepatitis B, HSV, and HIV and are not recommended generally.

A functional difference in condom shape is the presence or absence of a sperm reservoir tip. To enhance vaginal stimulation, some condoms are contoured and rippled or have ribbed or roughened surfaces. Thinner construction increases heat transmission and sensitivity. A wet jelly or dry powder lubricates some condoms. Condoms must be discarded after each single use. They are available without a prescription and from a variety of sources, including vending machines. Typical failure rate for the first year of use of the male condom is 15% (Rivlin & Westhoff, 2017). To prevent unintended pregnancy and the spread of STIs, it is essential that condoms be used consistently and correctly. Instructions, such as those listed in Box 8.2, can be used for client teaching. Effective condom use is a skill that must be taught.

The female condom is a vaginal sheath made of nitrile, a nonlatex synthetic rubber, with flexible rings at both ends (Fig. 8.7A). Female condoms offer the following protection percentages: HIV and CMV, 100%, and other STIs, 95% (Marfatia et al., 2015). The closed end of the pouch is inserted into the vagina and anchored around the cervix; the open ring covers the labia. Women whose partner will not wear a male condom can use this device as a protective mechanical barrier. Rewetting drops or oil- or water-based lubricants can be used to help decrease the distracting noise that is produced during penile thrusting. The female condom is available in one size, is intended for single use only, and is sold over the counter. Male condoms should not be used concurrently because the friction from both sheaths can increase the likelihood of either or both tearing (Cornell University, 2017). Typical failure rate in the first year of female condom use is 21% (Rivlin & Westhoff, 2017).

Diaphragms

The traditional contraceptive diaphragm is a shallow dome-shaped latex or silicone device with a flexible rim that covers the cervix. There are four types of traditional diaphragms: coil spring, arcing spring, flat spring, and wide seal rim. Available in many sizes, this diaphragm should be the largest size the woman can wear without her being aware of its presence. The typical failure rate of the diaphragm combined with spermicide ranges from 13% to 17%, but the failure rate

BOX 8.2   Male Condoms

Mechanism of Action

- Sheath is applied over the erect penis before insertion or loss of preejaculatory drops of semen. Used correctly, condoms prevent sperm from entering the cervix. Spermicide-coated condoms cause ejaculated sperm to be immobilized rapidly, thus increasing contraceptive effectiveness.

Failure Rate

- Typical users: 18%
- Correct and consistent users: 2%

Advantages

- Safe
- No side effects
- Readily available
- Premalignant changes in cervix can be prevented or reduced in women whose partners use condoms
- Method of male nonsurgical contraception

Disadvantages

- Must interrupt lovemaking to apply sheath
- Sensation may be altered
- If used improperly, spillage of sperm can result in pregnancy
- Condoms occasionally may tear during intercourse

STI Protection

- If a condom is used throughout the act of intercourse and there is no unprotected contact with female genitals, a latex rubber condom, which is impermeable to viruses, can act as a protective barrier against STIs.

Nursing Considerations

Teaching should include the following instructions:

- Use a new condom (check expiration date) for each act of sexual intercourse or other acts between partners that involve contact with the penis.
- Place condom after penis is erect and before intimate contact.
- Place condom on head of penis (Fig. A), and unroll it all the way to the base (Fig. B).

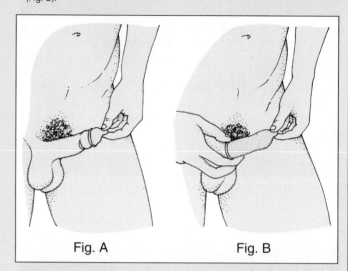

Fig. A   Fig. B

- Leave an empty space at the tip (see Fig. A); remove any air remaining in the tip by gently pressing air out toward the base of the penis.
- If a lubricant is desired, use water-based products such as K-Y lubricating jelly. Do *not* use petroleum-based products because they can cause the condom to break.
- After ejaculation, carefully withdraw the still-erect penis from the vagina, holding on to condom rim; remove and discard the condom.
- Store unused condoms in cool, dry place.
- Do not use condoms that are sticky, brittle, or obviously damaged.

STI, Sexually transmitted infection.

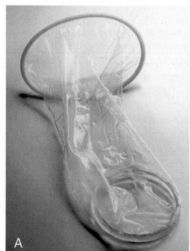
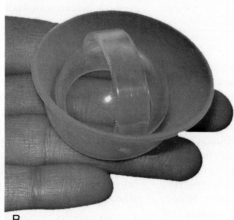
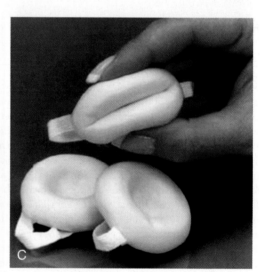

Fig. 8.7 Barrier Methods. (A) Female condom (FC2). (B) FemCap. (C) Contraceptive sponge. (A, Courtesy The Female Health Company, Chicago; B, courtesy FemCap, Del Mar, CA; C, Today vaginal contraceptive sponge. Courtesy Mayer Laboratories, Inc., 2014.)

can be decreased to 4% to 8% with correct and consistent use (Rivlin & Westhoff, 2017). Effectiveness of the diaphragm is less when used without spermicide. Women at high risk for HIV should avoid use of N-9 spermicides with the diaphragm (WHO, 2018). A newer diaphragm, Caya, is a one-size-fits-many silicon device with a nylon rather than metal rim. This device will fit women who formerly used a traditional diaphragm in sizes 65 to 80 mm (HPSRx Enterprises, Inc., 2017a). Spermicide used with Caya must be water based, and the diaphragm is recommended to stay in place for 6 hours after intercourse (HPSRx Enterprises, Inc., 2017b).

The woman is advised that she needs an annual gynecologic examination to assess the fit of the diaphragm. The device should be inspected before every use, should be replaced every 2 years, and in the case of the traditional diaphragm, may have to be refitted for a 20% weight fluctuation, after any abdominal or pelvic surgery, and after every pregnancy. Because various types of diaphragms are on the market, the nurse should use the package insert for teaching a woman how to use and care for the diaphragm (see the Teaching for Self-Management box).

Disadvantages of diaphragm use include the reluctance of some women to insert and remove it. Although it can be inserted up to 6 hours before intercourse, a cold diaphragm and a cold gel temporarily reduce vaginal response to sexual stimulation if insertion of the diaphragm occurs immediately before intercourse. Some women or couples object to the messiness of the spermicide. These annoyances of diaphragm use, along with failure to insert the device once foreplay has begun, are the most common reasons for failures of this method. Side effects may include irritation of tissues related to contact with spermicides. The male could also have a reaction to the spermicide. The diaphragm is not a good option for women with poor vaginal muscle tone or recurrent urinary tract infections. For proper placement, the diaphragm must rest behind the pubic symphysis and completely cover the cervix. To decrease the chance of exerting urethral pressure, the woman should be reminded to empty her bladder before diaphragm insertion and immediately after intercourse. Diaphragms are contraindicated for women with pelvic relaxation (uterine prolapse) or a large cystocele. Women with a latex allergy should not use latex diaphragms.

Toxic shock syndrome (TSS), although reported in very small numbers, can occur in association with the use of the contraceptive diaphragm and cervical caps (U.S. Department of Health and Human Services, 2017). The nurse should instruct the woman about ways to reduce her risk for TSS. These measures include prompt removal 6 to 8 hours after intercourse, not using the diaphragm or cervical caps during menses, and learning and watching for danger signs of TSS (Mayo Clinic, 2018d).

⚡ SAFETY ALERT

The nurse should inform the woman who uses a diaphragm or cervical cap as a contraceptive method to be alert for signs of TSS. The most common signs include a sunburn type of rash, diarrhea, dizziness, faintness, weakness, sore throat, aching muscles and joints, sudden high fever, and vomiting (Mayo Clinic, 2018a).

Cervical Caps

The FemCap (see Fig. 8.7B) is the only type of cervical cap available in the United States (Mayo Clinic, 2018a). It comes in three sizes and is made of silicone rubber. The cap fits snugly around the base of the cervix, close to the junction of the cervix and vaginal fornices. It is recommended that the cap remain in place no less than 6 hours and not more than 48 hours at a time. It is left in place at least 6 hours after the last act of intercourse. The seal provides a physical barrier to sperm; spermicide inside the cap adds a chemical barrier. The extended period of wear may be an added convenience for women.

TABLE 8.1 Hormonal Contraception

Composition	Route of Administration	Duration of Effect
Combination estrogen and progestin (synthetic estrogens and progestins in varying doses and formulations)	Oral Transdermal Vaginal ring insertion	24 hours; extended cycle 12 weeks 7 days 3 weeks
Progestin only		
Norethindrone, norgestrel	Oral	24 hours
Medroxyprogesterone acetate	Intramuscular injection; subcutaneous injection	3 months
Progestin, etonogestrel	Subdermal implant	Up to 3 years
Levonorgestrel	Intrauterine device	Up to 5 years

Instructions for the actual insertion and use of the cervical cap closely resemble those for a contraceptive diaphragm. Some of the differences are that the cervical cap can be inserted hours before sexual intercourse without a later need for additional spermicide, the cervical cap requires less spermicide than the diaphragm when initially inserted, and no additional spermicide is required for repeated acts of intercourse. Effectiveness of the first-generation FemCap has been found to be similar to the diaphragm (Rivlin & Westhoff, 2017).

The angle of the uterus, the vaginal muscle tone, and the shape of the cervix may interfere with the cervical cap's ease of fitting and use. Correct fitting requires time, effort, and skill from both the woman and the clinician. The woman must check the cap's position before and after each act of intercourse.

Because of the potential risk of TSS associated with the use of the cervical cap, another form of birth control is recommended for use during menstrual bleeding and up to at least 6 weeks postpartum. The cap should be refitted after any gynecologic surgery or birth and after major weight losses or gains. Otherwise, the size should be checked at least once a year.

Women who are not good candidates for wearing the cervical cap include those with abnormal Papanicolaou (Pap) test results, those who cannot be fitted properly with the existing cap sizes, those who find the insertion and removal of the device too difficult, those with a history of TSS, those with vaginal or cervical infections, and those who experience allergic responses to the latex cap or spermicide. Failure rates the first year of use are 20% in nulliparous and 40% in multiparous women (University of Michigan, 2018).

Contraceptive Sponge

The vaginal sponge is a small, round polyurethane sponge that contains N-9 spermicide (see previous discussion of N-9) (see Fig. 8.7C). It is designed to fit over the cervix (one size fits all). The side that is placed next to the cervix is concave for better fit. The opposite side has a woven polyester loop to be used for removal of the sponge.

The sponge must be moistened with water before it is inserted. It provides protection for up to 24 hours and for repeated instances of sexual intercourse. The sponge should be left in place for at least 6 hours after the last act of intercourse. Wearing it longer than 24 to 30 hours may put the woman at risk for TSS (Mayo Clinic, 2019a). The failure rate for typical use is more than that of the diaphragm (Center for Young Women's Health, 2016).

Hormonal Methods

More than 100 different hormonal contraceptive formulations are available in the United States (Golobof & Kiley, 2016). General classes are described in Table 8.1. Because of the wide variety of preparations available, the woman and the nurse must read the package insert for information about specific products prescribed. Formulations include combined estrogen-progestin medications and progestational agents. The formulations are administered orally, transdermally, vaginally, by implantation, by injection, or by intrauterine insertion.

Combined Estrogen-Progestin Contraceptives

Oral contraceptives. The normal menstrual cycle is maintained by a feedback mechanism. Follicle-stimulating hormone (FSH) and LH are secreted in response to fluctuating levels of ovarian estrogen and progesterone. Regular ingestion of combined oral contraceptive pills (COCs) suppresses the action of the hypothalamus and anterior pituitary, leading to insufficient secretion of FSH and LH; therefore follicles do not mature, and ovulation is inhibited.

Other contraceptive effects are induced by the combined steroids. Maturation of the endometrium is altered, making it a less favorable site for implantation. COCs also have a direct effect on the endometrium, so that from 1 to 4 days after the last COC is taken, the endometrial tissue sloughs and bleeding occurs as a result of hormone withdrawal. The withdrawal bleeding is usually less profuse than that of normal menstruation and may last only 2 to 3 days. Some women have no bleeding at all. The cervical mucus remains thick from the effect of the progestin (Golobof & Kiley, 2016).

Cervical mucus under the effect of progesterone does not provide as suitable an environment for sperm penetration as does the thin, watery mucus at ovulation. The possible effect, if any, of altered tubal and uterine motility induced by COCs is not clear.

Monophasic pills provide fixed dosages of estrogen and progestin. Multiphasic pills (e.g., biphasic and triphasic oral contraceptives) alter the amount of progestin and sometimes the amount of estrogen within each cycle. These preparations reduce the total dosage of hormones in a single cycle without losing contraceptive efficacy (Golobof & Kiley, 2016). To maintain adequate hormonal levels for contraception and enhance compliance, COCs should be taken at the same time each day. The overall user effectiveness rate of COCs is 91% (Golobof & Kiley, 2016).

Advantages. Because taking the pill does not relate directly to the sexual act, the acceptability of the pill may be increased. Improvement in sexual response may occur once the possibility of pregnancy is not an issue. For some women it is convenient to know when to expect the next menstrual flow.

The noncontraceptive health benefits of COCs include regulation of menorrhagia and irregular cycles, treatment of endometriosis, and reduced incidence of dysmenorrhea and premenstrual syndrome (PMS). Oral contraceptives also offer protection against endometrial cancer and ovarian cancer, improve hirsutism and acne, protect against the development of functional ovarian cysts, and increase bone mass (Golobof & Kiley, 2016). Oral contraceptives are considered a safe option for nonsmoking women until menopause. Perimenopausal women can benefit from regular bleeding cycles, a regular hormonal pattern, and the noncontraceptive health benefits of oral contraceptives.

A pelvic examination and Pap test are not necessary before initiating COCs (CDC, 2016). If STI screening is indicated, a urine-based test can be used for some infections (e.g., chlamydia, gonorrhea); others require a pelvic examination and cultures of vaginal or cervical secretions or blood tests (CDC, 2015a). Most health care providers assess the woman 3 months after beginning COCs to detect any complications.

Use of oral hormonal contraception can be initiated at any time during the menstrual cycle without any restrictions, as long as the woman is not pregnant (CDC, 2016). This is known as the Quick Start method and offers faster, more reliable pregnancy protection, increased continuation rates, and virtually no difference in breakthrough bleeding patterns than conventional start methods (wherein the pill must be started at the first day of the menstrual period). Taken exactly as directed, oral contraceptives prevent ovulation, and pregnancy cannot occur; the overall effectiveness rate is almost 100%. Almost all failures (i.e., pregnancy occurs) are caused by omission of one or more pills during the cycle. The typical failure rate of COCs due to omission is 9% (Cwiak & Edelman, 2018).

Disadvantages and side effects. Since hormonal contraceptives have come into use, the amount of estrogen and progestational agent contained in each tablet has been reduced considerably. This is important because adverse effects are, to a degree, dose related (Golobof & Kiley, 2016).

Women must be screened for conditions that present absolute or relative contraindications to oral contraceptive use. Contraindications for COC (see Contraindications for Combined Oral Contraceptives box).

Contraindications to Combined Oral Contraceptive Use

History of thromboembolic disorders
Cerebrovascular or coronary disease
Breast cancer
Positive antiphospholipid antibodies
Migraine with aura
Multiple sclerosis with prolonged immobility
Gallbladder disease
Acute or flare-up of viral hepatitis
Liver cancer
Pregnancy
Severe cirrhosis
Hepatocellular tumor
Complicated solid organ transplantation
Use of fosamprenavier, rifampin, or rifabutin
Use of certain anticonvulsants
Lactation and nonlactation less than 6 weeks postparum
Smoking if older than 35 years
Surgery with prolonged immobilization or any surgery on the legs
Hypertension (140/90 HG)
Diabetes mellitus (more than 20 years' duration) with vascular disease or nephropathy, neuropathy, or retinopathy

From Centers for Disease Control and Prevention (CDC). (2016). *U.S. selected practice recommendations for contraceptive use, 2016.* Available at: https://www.cdc.gov/mmwr/volumes/65/rr/pdfs/rr6503.pdf.

Certain side effects of COCs are attributable to estrogen, progestin, or both. Serious adverse effects documented with high doses of estrogen and progesterone include stroke, myocardial infarction, thromboembolism, hypertension, gallbladder disease, and liver tumors. Common side effects of estrogen excess include nausea, breast tenderness, fluid retention, and chloasma. Side effects of estrogen deficiency include early spotting (days 1 to 14), hypomenorrhea, nervousness, and atrophic vaginitis leading to painful intercourse (dyspareunia). Side effects of progestin excess include increased appetite, tiredness, depression, breast tenderness, vaginal yeast infection, oily skin and scalp, hirsutism, and postpill amenorrhea. Side effects of progestin deficiency include late spotting and breakthrough bleeding (days 15 to 21), heavy flow with clots, and decreased breast size. One of the most common side effects of combined COCs is bleeding irregularities (Golobof & Kiley, 2016).

If a woman experiences unpleasant or unsafe side effects when taking a particular COC, the health care provider may prescribe an alternative COC that has a different mix of estrogen and progestin. The ideal COC for a woman contains the lowest dose of hormones that prevents ovulation and that has the fewest and least harmful side effects. There is no way to predict the right dosage for any particular woman. Issues to consider in prescribing oral contraceptives include history of oral contraceptive use, side effects during past use, menstrual history, and drug interactions.

There is no evidence of a relationship between use of oral contraceptives and the development of diabetes or glucose intolerance. The risks and benefits should be assessed before prescribing oral contraceptives for women who have diabetes with vascular problems.

 MEDICATION ALERT

Over-the-counter medications, as well as some herbal supplements (such as St. John's wort), can alter the effectiveness of combined oral contraceptive pills (COCs). Women should be asked about their use when COCs are being considered for contraception.

No strong pharmacokinetic evidence exists that shows a relation between broad-spectrum antibiotic use and altered hormonal levels among oral contraceptive users, although potential antibiotic interaction can occur. (Mørch, Skovlund, Hannaford, Iversen, Fielding, & Lidegaard, 2017).

After discontinuing oral contraception, return to fertility usually happens quickly (Golobof & Kiley, 2016). Many women ovulate the next month after stopping oral contraceptives, although it may take longer for ovulation to occur in some women. Women who discontinue oral contraception for a planned pregnancy commonly ask whether they should wait before attempting to conceive. There is a lack of evidence to support delaying attempts to achieve pregnancy after discontinuing oral contraceptive use. Little evidence suggests that oral contraceptives cause postpill amenorrhea.

Nursing interventions. Many different preparations of oral hormonal contraceptives are available. The nurse reviews prescribing information with the woman, individualizing this education and prescribing instructions based on the specific oral contraceptive that is prescribed for her. Because of the wide variations, each woman must be clear about the unique dosage regimen for the preparation prescribed

TEACHING FOR SELF-MANAGEMENT
Use and Care of the Diaphragm

Inspection of the Diaphragm
You must inspect your diaphragm carefully before each use. The best way to perform this inspection is as follows:
- Hold the diaphragm up to a light source. Carefully stretch the diaphragm at the area of the rim, on all sides, making sure there are no holes. Remember, sharp fingernails can puncture the diaphragm.
- Another way to check for pinholes is to carefully fill the diaphragm with water. If any problem develops, you will see it immediately.
- A diaphragm that is puckered, especially near the rim, could mean thin spots.
- If you see any of these problems, do not use the diaphragm; avoid sexual intercourse or use another method of birth control; consult your health care provider about replacing the diaphragm.

Preparation of the Diaphragm
Rinse off the cornstarch, which is used to protect the diaphragm when it is stored. Your diaphragm must always be used with a spermicidal lubricant (in the form of contraceptive jelly or cream that is made especially for use with the diaphragm) to be effective. Pregnancy cannot be prevented effectively by the diaphragm alone.

Always empty your bladder before inserting the diaphragm. Place approximately 2 teaspoons of contraceptive jelly or contraceptive cream on the side of the diaphragm that will rest against the cervix (or whichever way you have been instructed). Spread it around to coat the surface and the rim. This measure aids in insertion and offers a more complete seal. Many women also spread some jelly or cream on the other side of the diaphragm (Fig. A).

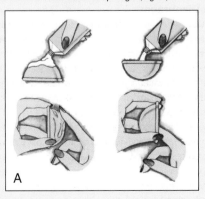

A

Positions for Insertion of the Diaphragm
Squatting: Squatting is the most commonly used position, and most women find it satisfactory.

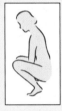

Leg-up method: Another position is to raise the left foot (if right hand is used for insertion) on a low stool, and, while in a bending position, insert the diaphragm.

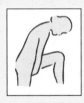

Chair method: Another practical method for diaphragm insertion is to sit far forward on the edge of a chair.

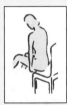

Reclining: You may prefer to insert the diaphragm while in a semireclining position in bed.

TEACHING FOR SELF-MANAGEMENT—cont'd

Use and Care of the Diaphragm

Insertion of the Diaphragm

1. The diaphragm can be inserted up to 6 h before intercourse. Hold the diaphragm between your thumb and fingers. The dome can be either up or down, as directed by your health care provider. Place your index finger on the outer rim of the compressed diaphragm (Fig. B).

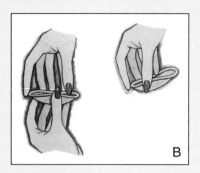

B

2. Use the fingers of the other hand to spread the labia (lips of the vagina). This action will assist in guiding the diaphragm into place.
3. Insert the diaphragm into the vagina. Direct it inward and downward as far as it will go to the space behind and below the cervix (Fig. C).

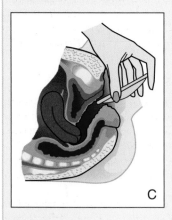

C

4. Tuck the front of the rim of the diaphragm behind the pubic bone so that the rubber hugs the front wall of the vagina (Fig. D).

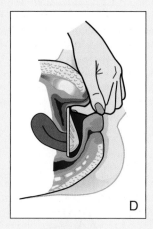

D

5. Feel for your cervix through the diaphragm to be certain it is properly placed and securely covered by the rubber dome (Fig. E).

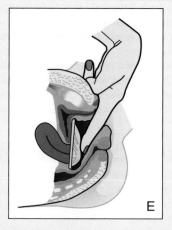

E

General Information

Regardless of the time of the month, you must use your diaphragm every time intercourse takes place. The cervix moves its position throughout the month, requiring that the angle of insertion of the diaphragm will change slightly. Your diaphragm must be left in place for at least 6 hours after the last intercourse. If you remove your diaphragm before the 6-h period, you will greatly increase your chance of becoming pregnant. If you have repeated intercourse, you must add more spermicide for each act of intercourse.

Removal of the Diaphragm

The only proper way to remove the diaphragm is to insert your forefinger up and over the top side of the diaphragm and slightly to the side.

Next, turn the palm of your hand downward and backward, hooking the forefinger firmly on top of the inside of the upper rim of the diaphragm, breaking the suction.

Pull the diaphragm down and out. This technique prevents tearing the diaphragm with the fingernails. You should not remove the diaphragm by trying to catch the rim from below the dome (Fig. F).

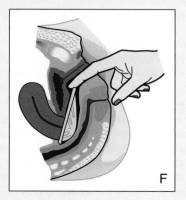

F

Care of the Diaphragm

When using a vaginal diaphragm, avoid using oil-based products, such as certain body lubricants, mineral oil, baby oil, vaginal lubricants, or vaginitis preparations. These products can weaken the rubber.

A little care means longer wear for your diaphragm. After each use, wash the diaphragm in warm water and mild soap. Do not use detergent soaps, cold-cream soaps, deodorant soaps, and soaps containing oil products because they can weaken the rubber.

After washing, dry the diaphragm thoroughly. Remove all water and moisture with a towel. Then dust the diaphragm with cornstarch. Do not use scented talc, body powder, baby powder, or similar products because they can weaken the rubber.

To clean the introducer (if one is used), wash with mild soap and warm water, rinse, and dry thoroughly.

Place the diaphragm back in the plastic case for storage. Do not store it near a radiator or heat source or in a location that is exposed to light for an extended period.

for her. Directions for care after missing one or two pills also vary. It is important that the woman speak with her health care provider about the best way to manage missing any pills.

Withdrawal bleeding tends to be short and scanty when some combination pills are taken. A woman may see no fresh blood at all. A drop of blood or a brown smudge on a tampon or the underwear counts as a menstrual period.

All women choosing to use oral contraceptives should be provided with a second method of birth control and be instructed in and comfortable with this backup method. Most women stop taking oral contraceptives for nonmedical reasons.

The nurse also reviews the signs of potential complications associated with the use of oral contraceptives (see Signs of Potential Complications). Oral contraceptives do not protect a woman against STIs or HIV. A barrier method such as condoms and spermicide should be used to provide this protection.

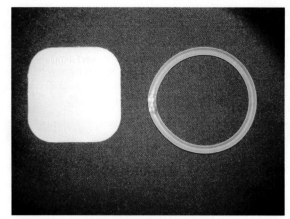

Fig. 8.8 Hormonal Contraceptive Transdermal Patch and Vaginal Ring. (Courtesy Dee Lowdermilk, Chapel Hill, NC.)

SIGNS OF POTENTIAL COMPLICATIONS

Oral Contraceptives

When oral contraceptives are initially prescribed and at follow-up visits throughout hormone therapy, alert the woman to stop taking the pill and to report any of the following symptoms to the health care provider immediately. The pneumonic, ACHES, is useful to help clients remember this information:

A—Abdominal pain may indicate a problem with the liver or gallbladder.

C—Chest pain or shortness of breath may indicate possible clot problem within the lungs or heart.

H—Headaches (sudden or persistent) may be caused by cardiovascular accident or hypertension.

E—Eye problems may indicate vascular accident or hypertension.

S—Severe leg pain may indicate a thromboembolic process.

Oral Contraceptive 91-Day Regimen

Some women prefer to take COCs in 3-month cycles and have fewer menstrual periods. Levonorgestrel (LNG)/ethinyl estradiol (Seasonale, Seasonique), FDA approved for extended cycle use, contains both estrogen and progestin and is taken in 3-month cycles of 12 weeks of active pills (pills that contain hormones) followed by 1 week of inactive pills (pills that don't contain hormones). Menstrual periods occur during the 13th week of the cycle. There is no protection from STIs, and risks are similar to COCs. Other monophasic COCs may be prescribed for extended cycle use and must be taken on a daily schedule, regardless of the frequency of intercourse (Golobof & Kiley, 2016).

Transdermal Contraceptive System

Available by prescription only, the contraceptive transdermal patch delivers continuous levels of norelgestromin (progestin) and ethinyl estradiol. The patch can be applied to intact skin of the upper outer arm, upper torso (front and back, excluding the breasts), lower abdomen, or buttocks (Fig. 8.8). Application is on the same day once a week for 3 weeks, followed by a week without the patch. Withdrawal bleeding occurs during the "no-patch" week. Mechanism of action, efficacy, contraindications, skin reactions, and side effects are similar to those of COCs. The typical failure rate during the first year of use is less than 9% in women weighing less than 198 pounds (90 kg) (CDC, 2016).

Vaginal Contraceptive Ring

Available only with a prescription, the vaginal contraceptive ring is a flexible ring (made of ethylene vinyl acetate copolymer) worn in the vagina to deliver continuous levels of etonogestrel (progestin) and ethinyl estradiol (see Fig. 8.8). One vaginal ring remains in the vagina for 3 weeks, followed by a week without the ring. The ring is inserted by the woman and does not have to be fitted. Some wearers may experience vaginitis, leukorrhea, and vaginal discomfort. Withdrawal bleeding occurs during the "no-ring" week. If the woman or partner notices discomfort during coitus, the ring can be removed from the vagina, but only up to 3 hours to still be effective when reinserted. Mechanism of action, efficacy, contraindications, and side effects are similar to those of COCs. The typical failure rate of the vaginal contraceptive ring is reportedly less than 9% during the first year of use (Nanda & Burke, 2018).

Progestin-Only Contraceptives

Progestin-only methods impair fertility by inhibiting ovulation, thickening and decreasing the amount of cervical mucus, thinning the endometrium, and altering cilia in the uterine tubes (American College of Obstetricians and Gynecologists [ACOG], 2019). The mechanism of action in progestin-only pills can vary among women and can also vary in one woman from cycle to cycle (Raymond & Grossman, 2018).

Oral progestins (minipill). Oral progesterones, also referred to as "minipills," contain only progesterone hormones. Effectiveness is increased if minipills are taken correctly. Because the dose of progesterone is low, the minipill must be taken at the same time every day (ACOG, 2019). Users often complain of irregular vaginal bleeding.

Injectable progestins. There are two formulations of injectable progestins, referred to as medroxyprogesterone acetate (DMPA or Depo-Provera). There is a 150 mg intramuscular injections given in the deltoid or gluteus maximus muscle, and a 104 mg subcutaneous injection. These are both considered to be long-acting reversible contraceptives, (LARCs), as are intrauterine devices (IUDs), discussed later in the chapter. DMPA should be initiated during the first 5 days of the menstrual cycle and administered every 11 to 13 weeks (Wu & Bartz, 2018).

⊘ MEDICATION ALERT

When administering an intramuscular injection of progestin (e.g., Depo-Provera), do not massage the site after the injection, because this action can hasten the absorption and shorten the period of effectiveness.

Advantages of DMPA include a contraceptive effectiveness comparable to that of perfect use of COCs, long-lasting effects, requirement of injections only four times a year, and the improbability of lactation being impaired. Side effects at the end of a year include possible decreased bone mineral density, weight gain, and irregular vaginal spotting (Wu & Bartz, 2018). Other disadvantages include no protection against STIs (including HIV). Return to fertility may be delayed as long as up to 10 months after discontinuing DMPA. The typical failure rate is 6% in the first year of use (Wu & Bartz, 2018).

> ### 💊 MEDICATION ALERT
>
> Women who use DMPA may lose bone mineral density no different than that seen in pregnancy and breastfeeding mothers. The World Health Organization (WHO) and American College of Obstetricians and Gynecologists (ACOG) currently support long-term use of Depo-Provera in women aged 18-45. Data on adolescents using DMPA and its effect on bone density are not clear. Women who receive depot medroxyprogesterone acetate (DMPA) should be counseled about calcium intake and exercise (Wu & Bartz, 2018).

Implantable progestins. Contraceptive implants consist of one or more nonbiodegradable flexible tubes or rods that are inserted under the skin of a woman's arm. These implants contain a progestin hormone and are effective for contraception for at least 3 years. They must be removed at the end of the recommended time. The only FDA-approved implant in the United States is a single-rod etonogestrel implant (Nexplanon). Its predecessor, Implanon, was discontinued at the advent of Nexplanon use. Nexplanon is radiopaque, a feature that Implanon lacked. Three other devices used worldwide are unavailable in the United States. One of these is Norplant, which was frequently used in the United States, but due to difficulties in insertion and removal (because it contains six rods), it is no longer used (Rivlin & Westhoff, 2017).

Insertion and removal of the single-rod etonogestrel capsule are minor, in-office surgical procedures including a local anesthetic, a small incision, and no sutures. The capsule is injected subdermally in the inner aspect of the nondominant upper arm. Implants will prevent some, but not all, ovulatory cycles and will thicken cervical mucus. Other advantages include reversibility and long-term continuous contraception that is not related to frequency of coitus. The Nexplanon can be inserted immediately following birth in breastfeeding women without affecting lactation. Irregular menstrual bleeding is the most common side effect. Less common side effects include headaches, nervousness, nausea, skin changes, and vertigo. No STI protection is provided with the implant method, so condoms should be used for protection. Implants are understood to be as effective, perhaps even more so, than sterilization and intrauterine devices (IUDs), so they are considered to be the most effective contraceptive methods available (Rivlin & Westhoff, 2017).

Emergency Contraception

EC is available in more than 100 countries, and in approximately one-third of these countries it is available without a prescription. In the United States, levonorgestrel-releasing intrauterine system (LNG-IUS) tablets are the only EC method available without a prescription, found on store shelves, and sold without age restriction. This method carries names such as Plan B One-Step, Take Action, Aftera, Next Choice One-Dose, and My Way and are located in the family planning aisle.

Ulipristal acetate, marketed as Ella, is available by prescription from a health care provider and, in only eight states, it is available from a pharmacist without a prescription (Guttmacher Institute, 2018a). Other options that the FDA has determined to be safe for EC include high doses of oral estrogen or COCs and insertion of a copper IUD

(Cu IUD) (Reproductive Health Technologies Project, 2016). These options continue to be available by prescription only. States differ in allowing pharmacists to dispense EC, and some states have effected refusal legislation (Guttmacher Institute).

Oral EC should be taken by a woman as soon as possible but within 5 days of unprotected intercourse or birth control mishap (broken condom, dislodged ring or cervical cap, missed oral CPs, late for injection, and so on) to prevent unintended pregnancy (WHO, 2017). If taken before ovulation, EC prevents ovulation by inhibiting follicular development. If taken after ovulation occurs, there is little effect on ovarian hormone production or the endometrium. Oral medication regimens with ECPs consists of combined estrogen (0.1 to 0.12 mg ethinyl estradiol) and progestin (levonorgesterl 0.5-0.6mg) pills (Trussell, Cleland, & Schwarz, 2018). To minimize the side effect of nausea that occurs with high doses of estrogen and progestin, the woman can be advised to take an over-the-counter antiemetic 1 hour before each dose. Women with contraindications for estrogen use should use progestin-only EC. No medical contraindications for EC exist except current pregnancy (CDC, 2016). If the woman does not begin menstruation within 21 days after taking the pills, she should be evaluated for pregnancy. EC is ineffective if the woman is pregnant, because the pills do not disturb an implanted pregnancy. Risk of pregnancy is reduced by as much as 95% if the woman takes ECPs within 5 days of intercourse (WHO, 2017). There are no data available for effectiveness of ECPs after 120 hours (Rivlin & Westhoff, 2017).

> ### 💊 MEDICATION ALERT
>
> Emergency contraception will not protect a woman against pregnancy if she engages in unprotected intercourse in the days or weeks that follow treatment. Because ingestion of emergency contraceptive pills may delay ovulation, the woman should be cautioned that she needs to establish a reliable form of birth control to prevent unintended pregnancy. Information about emergency contraception method options and access to providers is available at www.NOT-2-LATE.com or by calling 1-888-NOT-2-LATE.

IUDs containing copper (see later discussion) provide another emergency contraception option. The IUD should be inserted within 5 days of unprotected intercourse (WHO, 2017). This method is suggested only for women who wish to have the benefit of long-term contraception. The risk of pregnancy is reduced by as much as 99% with emergency insertion of the copper-releasing IUD (Rivlin & Westhoff, 2017).

Contraceptive counseling should be provided to all women requesting emergency contraception, including a discussion of modification of risky sexual behaviors to prevent STIs and unwanted pregnancy.

Intrauterine Devices

An IUD is a small T-shaped device with bendable arms for insertion through the cervix (Fig. 8.9). Once the trained health care provider inserts the IUD against the uterine fundus, the arms open near the fallopian tubes to maintain position of the device and to adversely affect the sperm motility and irritate the lining of the uterus. Two strings hang from the base of the stem through the cervix and protrude into the vagina for the woman to feel for assurance that the device has not been dislodged. The woman should have had a negative pregnancy test, treatment for dysplasia if present, cervical cultures to rule out STIs, and a consent form signed before IUD insertion. Advantages to choosing this method of contraception include long-term protection from pregnancy, although in rare cases an ectopic pregnancy can occur (Mayo Clinic, 2018), possible decrease in menstrual symptoms in those with fibroids or adenomyosis

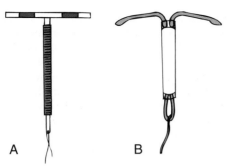

Fig. 8.9 Intrauterine Devices (IUDs). (A) Copper T 380A. (B) Levonorgestrel-releasing IUD.

and decreased blood loss in those at risk for anemia (LNG only), very effective, cost effective, insertion without time restrictions (although some providers prefer to insert the IUD during menstruation when the cervix is dilated and there is no chance of pregnancy), suitable for those with estrogen contraindications, and immediate return to fertility when removed. Disadvantages include unintentional expulsion of the device, increased risk of infection in the first month, increased bleeding (Copper T only), and unpredictable bleeding patterns (LNG only). IUDs offer no protection against HIV or other STIs (Dean & Schwarz, 2018).

There are five FDA-approved IUDs: the ParaGard Copper T 380A and the levonorgestrel hormonal intrauterine systems Mirena, Liletta, Kyleena, and Skyla. The ParaGard Copper T 380A is made of radiopaque polyethylene and fine solid copper and is approved and effective for 10 years of use, but may be effective for longer than 10 years. The copper primarily serves to cause an immune response creating an unreceptive setting for sperm and interferes with oocyte division and development of fertilizable ova (Dean & Schwarz, 2018).

Mirena, Liletta, and Skyla release LNG from their vertical reservoirs. Effective for up to 5 years for Mirena and 3 years for Skyla and Liletta, they impair sperm motility, thicken cervical mucus, decrease the lining of the uterus, and have some anovulatory effects. Uterine cramping and bleeding are usually decreased with these devices, although irregular spotting is common in the first few months following insertion. The typical failure rate in the first year of use is 0.2% (Bayer, 2018).

Nursing Interventions

The woman should be taught to check for the presence of the IUD strings after menstruation to rule out expulsion of the device. If pregnancy occurs with the IUD in place, an ultrasound is needed to rule out ectopic pregnancy. Early removal of the IUD helps to decrease the risk of spontaneous miscarriage or preterm labor (ACOG, 2016). In some women who are allergic to copper, a rash develops, necessitating the removal of the copper-bearing IUD. Signs of potential complications to be taught to the woman are listed in the Signs of Potential Complications box.

EVIDENCE-BASED PRACTICE BOX

Emergency Contraception and Obesity

Ask the Question
What is the best EC for overweight and obese women?

Search for the Evidence
Search Strategies English language research–based publications since 2014 on emergency contraception, overweight, and obesity were included.
Databases Used Cochrane Collaborative Database, National Guideline Clearinghouse, Agency for Healthcare Quality and Research (AHRQ), Cumulative Index of Nursing and Allied Health Literature (CINAHL), PubMed, UpToDate, and the professional websites for American College of Obstetricians and Gynecologists (ACOG) and Association of Women's Health, Obstetric, and Neonatal Nurses (AWHONN)

Critical Appraisal of the Evidence
In the United States, 27% of reproductive-aged women are overweight; 35% are obese. Approximately half of all pregnancies are unintended and occur mostly due to the failure of the contraceptive method (Morse & Pathak, 2018). Three options for emergency contraception are:
- Levonorgetrel (LNG) EC, a progestin commonly used in oral contraceptives, causes a delay in ovulation when taken at a higher dose (e.g., Plan B). It cannot interfere with an established pregnancy or harm an embryo (Morse & Pathak, 2018).
- Ulipristal acetate (UPA) is a progesterone receptor modulator, which interrupts the action of endogenous progesterone that is necessary to ovulate and maintain pregnancy (e.g., Ella). It can delay ovulation when taken up to 120 hours after intercourse. UPA is more effective than LNG EC, particularly in obese women (Morse & Pathak, 2018).
- Cu (copper) IUD (Paragard) prevents pregnancy for up to 7 days after intercourse and can be very effective for up to 10 years. It is the only method of the three that provides ongoing contraception. It is the most effective method of EC. Its effectiveness does not change based on weight or body mass index

(BMI). It requires a skilled health care provider for insertion (ACOG, 2017; Morse & Pathak, 2018).
Being overweight and obese negatively affects the ability of oral EC to prevent pregnancy.
- Obese women have an increased risk of pregnancy of approximately fourfold after using levonorgestrel emergency contraceptive pill (LNG ECP), compared with normal weight women (Jatlaoui & Curtis, 2016).
- Obese women have an increased risk of pregnancy of approximately twofold after taking UPA, when compared with women of normal weight (Jatlaoui & Curtis, 2016).

Apply the Evidence: Nursing Implications
- A client's preferences and priorities should be assessed when providing contraceptive counseling.
- Oral EC is one of the few types of contraception that decreases in efficacy as weight/BMI increases.
- The first-choice EC for obese women would be a Cu IUD insertion, when available and acceptable to the women. Women should be informed that it acts to prevent implantation. If oral EC is preferred, UPA is a better choice than LNG EC.
- All women should be counseled about EC and given educational materials (ACOG, 2017). Women should understand the risks of pregnancy versus any risks posed by contraceptive methods. Pregnancy is riskier (Morse & Pathak, 2018).

References
American College of Obstetricians and Gynecologists (ACOG). (2017). Access to emergency contraception. Committee Opinion No. 707. *Obstetrics and Gynecology, 130*(1), 251–252.
Jatlaoui, T. C., & Curtis, K. M. (2016). Safety and effectiveness for emergency contraceptive pills among women with obesity: A systematic review. *Contraception, 94*(6), 605–611.
Morse, J. E., & Pathak, P. R. (2018). Contraceptive care of obese women. *Obstetrical and Gynecological Survey, 73*(1), 56–66.

Jennifer Taylor Alderman

Sterilization

Sterilization refers to surgical procedures intended to render a person infertile. Most procedures involve the occlusion of the passageways for the ova and sperm (Fig. 8.10). For the woman, the oviducts (uterine tubes) are occluded; for the man, the sperm ducts (vas deferens) are occluded. Only surgical removal of the ovaries (oophorectomy) or uterus (hysterectomy) or both will result in absolute sterility for the woman. All other sterilization procedures have a small but definite failure rate (i.e., pregnancy may result).

Female Sterilization

Female sterilization (bilateral tubal ligation [BTL]) may be done immediately after birth (within 24 to 48 hours), concomitant with induced abortion, or as an interval procedure (during any phase of the menstrual cycle). If sterilization is performed as an interval procedure, the health care provider must be certain that the woman is not pregnant. Half of all female sterilization procedures are performed immediately after a pregnancy. Sterilization procedures can be safely done on an outpatient basis.

Tubal occlusion. A laparoscopic approach or a minilaparotomy can be used for tubal ligation (Fig. 8.11), tubal electrocoagulation, or the application of bands or clips. Electrocoagulation and ligation are considered to be permanent methods. Use of the bands or clips has the theoretic advantage of possible reversal and return to fertility if the woman desires to become pregnant in the future.

For the minilaparotomy, the woman is admitted the morning of surgery, having received nothing by mouth since midnight. Preoperative sedation is given. The procedure can be carried out with a local anesthetic, but a regional or general anesthetic can also be used. A small incision is made in the abdominal wall below the umbilicus. The woman may experience sensations of tugging, but no pain, and the operation is completed within 20 minutes. She may be discharged several hours later if she has recovered from anesthesia or next day if done postpartum. Any abdominal discomfort usually can be controlled with a mild analgesic (e.g., acetaminophen). Within days the scar is almost invisible (see the Teaching for Self-Management box: What to Expect After Tubal Ligation). As with any surgery, there is always a possibility of complications of anesthesia, infection, hemorrhage, and trauma to other organs.

Transcervical sterilization. Hysteroscopic techniques can be used to inject occlusion agents into the uterine tubes. One FDA-approved device is the Essure system, an interval sterilization method (not intended for the postpartum period). The Essure device contains polyester fibers within a metal coil. A trained health care professional inserts a small catheter holding the device through the vagina and cervix and into the fallopian tubes. The device works by stimulating the woman's own scar tissue formation to occlude the uterine tubes and prevent conception (Mayo Clinic, 2018c). An advantage is that the nonhormonal form of contraception can be inserted during an outpatient procedure in a provider's office or a clinic without anesthesia. Analgesia is recommended to decrease mild to moderate discomfort associated with tubal spasm. The transcervical approach is advantageous for obese women and those with abdominal adhesions as it eliminates the need for abdominal surgery. Because the procedure is not immediately effective, it is essential that the woman and her partner use another form of contraception until tubal blockage is proven. It may take up to 3 months for tubal occlusion to fully occur, and success must be confirmed by hysterosalpingogram. Other disadvantages include possible expulsion and perforation. The 1-year pregnancy rate is 0.1% (Mayo Clinic, 2018c). The U.S. Food and Drug Administration (2018a) reported that Bayer announced it is discontinuing Essure, although providers can continue to implant Essure for up to one year past the sale date.

Tubal reconstruction. Restoration of tubal continuity (reanastomosis) and function is technically feasible except after laparoscopic tubal electrocoagulation. However, sterilization reversal is costly, difficult (requiring microsurgery), and uncertain. The success rate varies with the extent of tubal destruction and removal. There may be an increased risk of ectopic pregnancy after tubal reanastomosis.

Male Sterilization

Vasectomy is the surgical interruption of a man's vas deferens, which is responsible for transporting mature sperm to the urethra (Amory, 2016). It is considered the easiest and most commonly used operation for male sterilization. Vasectomy can be carried out with local anesthesia on an outpatient basis. It is considered a permanent method of sterilization because reversal is successful.

Two methods are used for scrotal entry: conventional (scalpel incision) and no-scalpel (small puncture) vasectomy. The surgeon identifies and immobilizes the vas deferens through the scrotum. Then the vas is ligated or cauterized (see Fig. 8.10B). Surgeons vary in their techniques to occlude the vas deferens: ligation with sutures, division, cautery, application of clips, excision of a segment of the vas, fascial interposition, or some combination of these methods.

The man is instructed in self-care to promote a safe return to routine activities. To reduce swelling and relieve discomfort, ice packs are applied to the scrotum intermittently for a few hours after surgery. A scrotal support may be applied to decrease discomfort. Moderate inactivity for approximately 2 days is advisable because of local scrotal tenderness. The skin suture can be removed 5 to 7 days after surgery. Sexual intercourse may be resumed as desired; however, sterility is not immediate. Some sperm will remain in the proximal portions of the sperm ducts after vasectomy. One week to several months are required to clear the ducts of sperm; therefore some form of contraception is needed until the sperm count in the ejaculate on two consecutive tests is down to zero.

Vasectomy has no effect on potency (ability to achieve and maintain erection) or volume of ejaculate. Endocrine production of testosterone continues, so secondary sex characteristics are not affected. Sperm production continues, but sperm are unable to leave the epididymis and are lysed by the immune system. Less common are painful granulomas from accumulation of sperm.

Complications after bilateral vasectomy are uncommon and usually not serious. It is considered a safe and highly effective procedure (Hou & Roncari, 2018).

Tubal reconstruction. Microsurgery to reanastomose can be accomplished, but the pregnancy rates are 30 to 90%, depending on the procedure (Mayo Clinic, 2019a). The rate of success decreases as the time since the procedure increases. The vasectomy may result in permanent changes in the testes that leave men unable to father children. The changes are those ordinarily seen only in older adults (e.g., interstitial

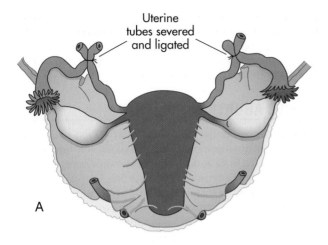

A

Fig. 8.10 Sterilization. (A) Uterine tubes severed and ligated (tubal ligation). (B) Sperm duct severed and ligated (vasectomy).

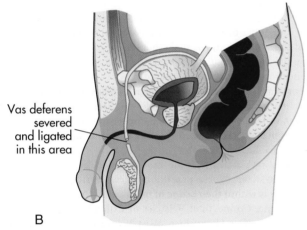

B

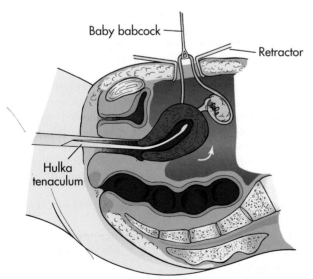

Fig. 8.11 Use of Minilaparotomy to Gain Access to Uterine Tubes for Occlusion Procedures. Tenaculum is used to lift uterus *(arrow)* toward incision.

TEACHING FOR SELF-MANAGEMENT
What to Expect After Tubal Ligation

- You should expect no change in hormones and their influence.
- Your menstrual period will be about the same as before the sterilization.
- You may feel pain at ovulation.
- The ovum disintegrates within the abdominal cavity.
- It is highly unlikely that you will become pregnant.
- You should not have a change in sexual functioning; you may enjoy sexual relations more because you will not be concerned about becoming pregnant.
- Sterilization offers no protection against STIs; therefore you may need to use condoms.

fibrosis [scar tissue between the seminiferous tubules]). In some men, antibodies develop against their own sperm (autoimmunization). The role of antisperm antibodies in fertility after vasectomy reversal has not been completely determined.

Informed Consent

All states have strict regulations for informed consent. Many states permit voluntary sterilization of any mature, rational woman without reference to her marital or pregnancy status. Although the partner's consent is not required by law, the man or woman is encouraged to discuss the situation with the partner, and health care providers may request the partner's consent. Sterilization of minors or mentally incompetent individuals is restricted by most states and often requires the approval of a board of eugenicists or other court-appointed individuals (see Legal Tip).

LEGAL TIP

Sterilization

If federal funds are used for female or male sterilization:

- The person must be age 21 years or older.
- Informed consent must include an explanation of the risks, benefits, and alternatives; a statement that describes sterilization as a permanent, irreversible method of birth control; and a statement that mandates a 30-day waiting period between giving consent and the sterilization.
- Informed consent must be in the man's or woman's native language, or an interpreter must be provided to read the consent form to the man or woman.

Nursing Interventions

The nurse plays an important role in assisting people with decision making so all requirements for informed consent are met. The nurse also provides information about alternatives to sterilization, such as contraception. The nurse acts as a "sounding board" for people who are exploring the possibility of choosing sterilization and their feelings about and motivation for this choice. The nurse records this information, which may be the basis for referral to a family planning clinic, a psychiatric social worker, or another professional health care provider.

Information must be given about what is entailed in various procedures, how much discomfort or pain can be expected, and what type of care is needed. Many individuals fear sterilization procedures because of the imagined effect on their sex life. They need reassurance concerning the hormonal and psychologic basis for sexual function and that uterine tube occlusion or vasectomy has no biologic sequelae in terms of sexual adequacy. Preoperative care consists of health assessment, which includes a psychologic assessment, physical examination, and laboratory tests. The nurse assists with the health assessment, answers questions, and confirms the client's understanding of printed instructions (e.g., nothing by mouth after midnight). Ambivalence and extreme fear of the procedure are reported to the health care provider.

Postoperative care depends on the procedure performed (e.g., laparoscopy, laparotomy for tubal occlusion, or vasectomy). General care includes recovery after anesthesia, monitoring of vital signs and fluid and electrolyte balance (intake and output, laboratory values), prevention of or early identification and treatment for infection or hemorrhage, control of discomfort, and assessment of emotional response to the procedure and recovery.

Discharge planning depends on the type of procedure performed. In general, the client is given written instructions about observing for and reporting symptoms and signs of complications, the type of recovery to be expected, and the date and time for a follow-up appointment.

Breastfeeding: Lactational Amenorrhea Method

The *lactational amenorrhea method (LAM)* can be a highly effective, *temporary* method of birth control. It is more popular in underdeveloped countries and traditional societies, where breastfeeding is used to prolong birth intervals. The method has seen limited use in the United States because most American women do not establish breastfeeding patterns that provide maximum protection against pregnancy.

When the infant suckles at the mother's breast, a surge of prolactin hormone is released, which inhibits estrogen production and suppresses ovulation and the return of menses. LAM works best if the mother is exclusively or almost exclusively breastfeeding, if the woman has not had a menstrual flow since giving birth, and if the infant is younger than 6 months of age. Effectiveness is enhanced by frequent feedings at intervals of less than 4 hours during the day and no more than 6 hours during the night, long duration of each feeding, and no bottle supplementation or limited supplementation by spoon or cup. The woman should be counseled that disruption of the breastfeeding pattern or supplementation can increase the risk of pregnancy. The typical failure rate is 1% to 2% (CDC, 2017b).

Future Trends

Contraceptive options are more limited in the United States and Canada than in some other industrialized countries. Lack of funding for research, governmental regulations, conflicting values about contraception, and high costs of liability coverage for contraception have been cited as blocks to new and improved methods. Existing methods of contraception are being improved; however, and a variety of new methods are being developed.

In development are techniques to make current contraceptive use easier: a vaginal ring which can be used for 1 year, self-administered injectables (available in Europe and Uganda), and a pill taken only at the time of intercourse. Over-the-counter CPs are a topic that is being investigated, although it is likely to be fraught with much controversy (Upadhya, Santelli, Raine-Bennett, et al., 2017). In states such as Oregon and California, pharmacists can now prescribe hormonal contraception without a woman visiting a health professional for a prescription. This newer legislation may open the door for similar laws in the rest of the United States but may also discourage manufacturers from applying for over-the-counter status of hormonal contraception (Yang, Kozhimannill, & Snowden, 2016). Spermicidal microbicides are being evaluated. Male hormonal methods are also being investigated, including hormonal injections (testosterone and progestin), targeted gene therapy, gonadotropin-releasing hormone antagonists, antisperm compounds, temporary vas occlusion, vas muscle inhibitor, immunologic methods, ultrasonic massage, internal/external heat, and contraceptive vaccines (Wang, Sitruk-Ware, & Serfaty, 2016).

INDUCED ABORTION

Induced abortion is the purposeful interruption of a pregnancy before 20 weeks of gestation. (Spontaneous abortion or miscarriage is discussed in Chapter 28.) If the abortion is performed at the woman's request, the term elective abortion is usually used; if performed for reasons of maternal or fetal health or disease, the term therapeutic abortion applies. Many factors contribute to a woman's decision to have an abortion. Indications include (1) preservation of the life or health of the mother, (2) genetic disorders of the fetus, (3) rape or incest, and (4) the pregnant woman's request. The control of birth, dealing as it does with human sexuality and the question of life and death, is one of the most emotional components of health care. It has been the most controversial social issue in the last half of the 20th century and the beginning of the 21st century in the United States. Regulations exist to protect the mother from the complications of abortion.

Abortion is regulated in most countries, including the United States. Before 1970 legal abortion was not widely available in the United States. However, in January 1973, the U.S. Supreme Court set aside previous antiabortion laws and legalized abortion as a result of the *Roe vs Wade* decision (U.S. Reports, 1973).

Currently 41 states legislate that abortion be performed by a licensed physician. Nurse practitioners can perform abortions (if the practice is within their scope of practice) in the states of California, Colorado, Connecticut, District of Columbia, Montana, Oregon, Vermont, New Hampshire, West Virginia, and Rhode Island. Congress has legislated that Medicaid funds can be used only to pay for abortion when a woman's life is endangered. States vary on the financing of abortion, with 17 states using their own funds to pay for abortions, depending on the circumstances surrounding the procedure. States also vary regarding parental notification if a minor is requesting an abortion and/or consent regarding abortion, with 37 states providing legislation for some type parental involvement in the abortion of a fetus. Individual health care providers may refuse to participate in abortion in 45 states (Guttmacher Institute, 2018b).

In 1992 the U.S. Supreme Court made another landmark ruling, this time allowing states to restrict early abortion services as long as the restrictions did not place an "undue burden" on the woman's ability to choose abortion. Since then many bills have been introduced to limit access and funds for women seeking abortion. The Supreme Court will again play a major role in deciding the future of abortions as states introduce bills to limit or ban access to abortions.

> **LEGAL TIP**
>
> **Induced Abortion**
>
> It is important for nurses to know the laws regarding abortion in their country or state of practice before they offer abortion counseling or nursing care to a woman choosing an abortion. Many states enforce a mandatory delay or state-directed counseling before a woman may legally obtain an abortion.

Incidence

In 2014 in the United States there were nearly 4.9 million pregnancies, and approximately 19% of these pregnancies were terminated. The numbers of abortions in the United States have decreased from 1.06 million abortions in 2011 to 926,200 abortions in 2014. Most terminations were performed in women who were unmarried (46%). Non-Hispanic white women comprised 39% of those who experienced elective abortion; non-Hispanic African-American women comprised 28% of those who experienced elective abortions, Hispanic women comprised 25%, and women of other races accounted for 9% of abortions (Guttmacher Institute). Most abortions occur in women who already have children, and abortion rates tend to be higher in women whose income is below the poverty level (Guttmacher Institute, 2018c).

Decision to Have an Abortion

Rates of biologic complications after abortions such as ectopic pregnancy, infection, or hemorrhage tend to be low if the woman aborts during the first trimester. Psychologic sequelae of induced abortion are rare with no evidence of a correlation between abortion and mental health issues. The decision to have an abortion should be the woman's, based on her own values and situation.

Nurses and other health care providers often struggle with the same values and moral convictions as those of the pregnant woman. The conflicts and doubts of the nurse can be readily communicated to women who are already anxious. Regardless of personal views on abortion, nurses who provide care to women seeking abortion have an ethical responsibility to counsel women about their options and to make appropriate referrals.

The Association of Women's Health, Obstetric and Neonatal Nurses (AWHONN) (2016) continues to support a nurse's right to choose whether to participate in abortion procedures in keeping with his or her "personal, moral, ethical, or religious beliefs." AWHONN also advocates that "nurses have a professional obligation to inform their employers, at the time of employment, of any attitudes and beliefs that may interfere with essential job functions."

LEGAL TIP

Institutional Policies for Nurses' Rights and Responsibilities Related to Abortion

Nurses' rights and responsibilities related to caring for abortion clients should be protected through policies that describe how the institution will accommodate the nurse's ethical or moral beliefs and what the nurse should do to avoid client abandonment in such situations. Nurses should know what policies are in place in their institutions and encourage such policies to be written.

? CLINICAL REASONING CASE STUDY

Termination of Pregnancy

Angelica is a 19-year-old single client whose contraceptive method failed. An examination determines that she is 6 weeks pregnant and is seeking termination of the pregnancy. She has many questions for the nurse in the family planning clinic: Which procedure is most likely to be chosen at this gestation? What are the risks associated with the procedure? Should her boyfriend be involved in the decision to terminate the pregnancy?

1. What is the priority concern or client need in this situation?
2. List other client needs/problems in this case.
3. Identify any additional information needed by the nurse in addressing this situation.
4. Describe the roles/responsibilities of interprofessional health team members who may be involved in this situation.

First-Trimester Abortion

Methods for performing early abortion (less than 9 weeks of gestation) include surgical (aspiration) and medical methods (mifepristone with misoprostol and methotrexate with misoprostol).

Aspiration

Aspiration (vacuum or suction curettage) is the most common procedure in the first trimester, with slightly more than 67.9% of all procedures being performed by this method (Jatlaoui, Ewing, Mandel, et al., 2016). Aspiration abortion is usually performed under local anesthesia in the health care provider's office, the clinic, or the hospital. The suction procedure for performing an early elective abortion (ideal time is 8 to 12 weeks since the last menstrual period) usually requires less than 5 minutes.

A bimanual examination is done before the procedure to assess uterine size and position. A speculum is inserted, and the cervix is anesthetized with a local anesthetic agent. The cervix is dilated if necessary, and a cannula connected to suction is inserted into the uterine cavity. The products of conception are evacuated from the uterus.

During the procedure the nurse or health care provider keeps the woman informed about what to expect next (e.g., menstrual-like cramping, sounds of the suction machine). The nurse assesses the woman's vital signs. The aspirated uterine contents must be carefully inspected by the health care provider to ascertain whether all fetal parts and adequate placental tissue have been evacuated. After the abortion the woman rests until she is ready to stand. She remains in the recovery area or waiting room for 1 to 3 hours for detection of excessive cramping or bleeding; then she is discharged.

Bleeding after the operation is normally about the equivalent of a heavy menstrual period, and cramps are rarely severe. Excessive vaginal bleeding and infection, such as endometritis or salpingitis, are the most common complications of elective abortion. Retained products of conception are the primary cause of excessive or prolonged vaginal bleeding. Evacuation of the uterus, uterine massage, and administration of oxytocin or methylergonovine (Methergine) or both may be necessary. Prophylactic antibiotics to decrease the risk of infection are commonly prescribed. Postabortion pain may be relieved with NSAIDs such as ibuprofen.

Postabortion instructions differ among health care providers (e.g., tampons should not be used for at least 3 days or should be avoided for up to 3 weeks, and resumption of sexual intercourse may be permitted within 1 week or discouraged for 2 weeks). When the woman does resume sexual intercourse, she should be sure to use contraception until she wants to become pregnant again. The woman may shower daily. Instruction is given to watch for excessive bleeding and other signs of complications and to avoid douches of any type.

⚡ SAFETY ALERT

The woman who has an induced abortion should be given clear instructions to return immediately to the health care facility or emergency department for any of the following signs and symptoms:

- Fever greater than 38°C (100.4°F)
- Chills
- Bleeding greater than two saturated pads in 2 hours or heavy bleeding lasting a few days
- Foul-smelling vaginal discharge
- Severe abdominal pain, cramping, or backache
- Abdominal tenderness (when pressure applied)

The woman may expect her menstrual period to resume 4 to 6 weeks from the day of the procedure. Information about the birth control method the woman prefers is offered, if this has not been done previously during the counseling interview that usually precedes the decision to have an abortion. Some methods can be initiated immediately, such as an IUD insertion. Hormonal methods may be started immediately or within a week. The woman must be strongly encouraged to return for her follow-up visit so complications can be detected. A pregnancy test may also be performed at that time to determine whether the pregnancy was successfully terminated.

Medical Abortion

Medical abortions are available for use in the United States for up to 9 weeks after the last menstrual period. Methotrexate, misoprostol, and mifepristone are the drugs used in the current regimens to induce early abortion. Approximately 22.2% of all reported abortion procedures in the United States in 2013 were medical procedures (Jatlaoui, et al., 2016).

Methotrexate is a cytotoxic drug that causes early abortion by blocking folic acid in fetal cells so that they cannot divide. Misoprostol (Cytotec) is a prostaglandin analog that acts directly on the cervix to soften and dilate and on the uterine muscle to stimulate contractions. Mifepristone, formerly known as RU 486, works by binding to progesterone receptors and blocking the action of progesterone, which is necessary for maintaining pregnancy (Rivlin & Westhoff, 2017).

Methotrexate and misoprostol. There is no standard protocol, but methotrexate is given intramuscularly or orally (usually mixed with orange juice). The woman returns in 3 to 7 days for vaginal placement of misoprostol. A follow-up visit is scheduled 1 week later to confirm the abortion is complete. If not, the woman is offered an additional dose of misoprostol or vacuum aspiration is performed (European Society of Human Reproduction and Embryology [ESHRE] Capri Workshop Group, 2017).

Mifepristone and misoprostol. Mifepristone can be given up to 70 days or less since the woman's last menstrual period. The FDA-approved regimen is that the woman takes 200 mg of Mifepristone by mouth; 24 to 48 later, at a location appropriate for her, she takes 800 mcg of misoprostol buccally (in the cheek pouch) (U.S. Food & Drug Administration, 2018b). Two weeks after the administration of mifepristone, the woman must return to the office for a clinical examination or ultrasound to confirm that the pregnancy has been terminated. In 2% to 5% of cases, the drugs do not work, and surgical abortion (aspiration) is needed (ESHRE Capri Workshop Group, 2017).

With any medical abortion regimen, the woman usually will experience bleeding and cramping. Side effects of the medications include nausea, vomiting, diarrhea, headache, dizziness, fever, and chills. These are attributed to misoprostol and usually subside in a few hours after administration.

Second-Trimester Abortion

Second-trimester abortion is associated with more complications and costs than first-trimester abortions. Dilation and evacuation (D&E) accounts for almost all procedures performed in the second trimester in the United States.

Dilation and Evacuation

D&E can be performed at any point up to 20 weeks of gestation, although this procedure is more commonly performed between 13 and 16 weeks of gestation. The cervix requires more dilation because the products of conception are larger. Often, osmotic dilators (e.g., laminaria) are inserted several hours or several days before the procedure, or misoprostol can be applied to the cervix. The procedure is similar to vaginal aspiration except a larger cannula is used and other instruments may be needed to remove the fetus and placenta. Nursing care includes monitoring vital signs, providing emotional support, administering analgesics, and postoperative monitoring. Disadvantages of D&E may include possible long-term harmful effects to the cervix.

CARE MANAGEMENT

The woman will need help exploring the meaning of the various alternatives and consequences to herself and her significant others. Choosing to terminate a pregnancy, regardless of the circumstances, can be stressful and cause anxiety. A calm, matter-of-fact approach on the part of the nurse can be helpful (e.g., "Yes, I know you are pregnant. I am here to help. Let's talk about all your options"). Listening to what the woman has to say and encouraging her to speak are essential. Neutral responses such as "Oh," "Uh-huh," and "Umm" and nonverbal encouragement such as nodding, maintaining eye contact, and use of touch are helpful in setting an open, accepting environment. Clarifying, restating, and reflecting statements, open-ended questions, and feedback are communication techniques that can be used to maintain a realistic focus on the situation and bring the woman's concerns into the open.

Information about all options, including abortion, referral to adoption agencies, or to support services if a woman chooses to keep her baby, should be provided. If a decision is made to have an abortion, the woman must be assured of continued support. Information about what is entailed in various procedures, how much discomfort or pain can be expected, and what type of care is needed must be given. A discussion of the various feelings, including depression, guilt, regret, and relief that the woman might experience after whatever she chooses, is needed. Information about community resources for postabortion counseling may be needed. If family or friends cannot be involved, scheduling time for nursing personnel to give the necessary support is an essential component of the plan for care.

After an abortion, studies have indicated that most women report relief, but some have temporary distress or mixed emotions, although serious psychologic sequelae are rare. Because symptoms can vary among women who have had abortions, nurses must assess women for grief reactions and facilitate the grieving process through active listening and nonjudgmental support and care.

A thorough assessment is conducted through history, physical examination, and laboratory tests and may also be performed to assess weeks of gestation for a first-timester pregnancy. The length of pregnancy and the condition of the woman must be determined to select the appropriate type of abortion procedure. An ultrasound examination should be performed before a second-trimester abortion is done. If the woman is Rh negative, she is a candidate for prophylaxis against Rh isoimmunization. She should receive $Rh_o(D)$ immune globulin within 72 hours after the abortion if she is D negative and if Coombs test results are negative (if the woman is unsensitized or isoimmunization has not developed).

The woman's understanding of alternatives, the types of abortions, and expected recovery are assessed. Misinformation and gaps in knowledge are identified and corrected. The record is reviewed by the healthcare provider for the signed informed consent, and the woman's understanding is verified. General preoperative, operative, and postoperative assessments are performed.

Counseling about abortion includes help for the woman in identifying how she perceives the pregnancy, information about the choices available (i.e., having an abortion or carrying the pregnancy to term and then either keeping the infant or placing the baby for adoption), and information about the types of abortion procedures.

■ KEY POINTS

- A variety of contraceptive methods are available with various effectiveness rates, advantages, and disadvantages.
- Women and their partners should choose the contraceptive method or methods best suited to them.
- Effective contraceptives are available through prescription and nonprescription sources.
- A variety of techniques are available to enhance the effectiveness of periodic abstinence in motivated couples who prefer this natural method.
- Hormonal contraception includes both precoital and postcoital prevention through various modalities and requires thorough client education.
- The barrier methods of diaphragm and cervical cap provide safe and effective contraception for women or couples motivated to use them consistently and correctly.

- IUDs can provide long-term (3 to 10 years) protection against pregnancy.
- Emergency contraception should be taken as soon as possible after unprotected intercourse but no later than 120 hours.
- Proper, concurrent use of spermicides and latex condoms provides protection against STIs.
- Tubal ligations and vasectomies are permanent sterilization methods used by increasing numbers of women and men.
- Induced abortion performed in the first trimester is safer than an abortion performed in the second trimester.
- The most common complications of induced abortion include infection and excessive vaginal bleeding.
- There is no evidence to support a correlation between abortion and mental health problems.

REFERENCES

American College of Obstetricians and Gynecologists. (2016/reaffirmed 2019). *Committee opinion number 672: Clinical challenges of long-acting reversible contraceptive methods*. Retrieved from: www.acog.org/-/media/Committee-Opinions/Committee-on-Gynecologic-Practice/co672.pdf?dmc=1&ts=20170215T1853475465.

American College of Obstetricians and Gynecologists. (2019). *Progestin-only hormonal birth control: Pill and injection*. Retrieved from: https://www.acog.org/Patients/FAQs/Progestin-Only-Hormonal-Birth-Control-Pill-and-Injection#take.

Association of Women's Health, Obstetric and Neonatal Nurses. (2016). *AWHONN position statement. Rights and responsibilities of nurses related to reproductive health care*. Retrieved from: http://www.jognn.org/article/S0884-2175(16)30437-3/pdf.

Bayer. (2018). *What is Skyla?*. Retrieved from: http://www.skyla-us.com/what-is-skyla.php?pse=google&matchtype=e&Keyword=skyla%20us&campaignid=626004667&adgroupid=37784901424&device=c&adposition=1t1&loc=9057284&gclid=Cj0KCQiA2NXTBRDoARIsA-JRIvLyt7mpA5ML9LELOq2JUuWs0lRAixoddOTBpIHIGDvQLYVqlX-vHmbt8aAu64EALw_wcB.

Center for Young Women's Health. (2016). *Contraceptive sponge. Division of Adolescent and Young Adult Medicine*. Division of Gynecology-Boston Children's Hospital. Retrieved from: http://youngwomenshealth.org/2013/08/22/contraceptive-sponge/.

Centers for Disease Control and Prevention (CDC). (2015a). *Sexually transmitted disease treatment guidelines, 2015*. Retrieved from: www.cdc.gov/std/tg2015/default.htm.

Centers for Disease Control and Prevention (CDC). (2015b). *Reproductive health: Unintended pregnancy prevention*. Retrieved from: https://www.cdc.gov/reproductivehealth/unintendedpregnancy/.

Centers for Disease Control and Prevention (CDC). (2016). *U.S. selected practice recommendations for contraceptive use, 2016*. Retrieved from: https://www.cdc.gov/mmwr/volumes/65/rr/pdfs/rr6503.pdf.

Centers for Disease Control and Prevention (CDC). (2017a). *Coitus interruptus (withdrawal)*. Retrieved from: https://www.cdc.gov/reproductivehealth/contraception/mmwr/mec/appendixh.html.

Centers for Disease Control and Prevention (CDC). (2017b). *Lactational amenorrhea method*. Retrieved from https://www.cdc.gov/reproductivehealth/contraception/mmwr/mec/appendixg.html.

Contracept.org. (2016a). *Fertility awareness methods: The TwoDay method*. Retrieved from: www.contracept.org/twoday-method.php.

Contracept.org. (2016b). *Fertility awareness methods: Standard days method*. Retrieved from: http://www.contracept.org/calendar.php.

Cornell University. (2017). *Cornell health: Condoms & lubricants*. Retrieved from: https://health.cornell.edu/sites/health/files/pdf-library/Condoms_Lube.pdf.

Cunningham, F., Leveno, K., Bloom, S., et al. (2018). *Williams obstetrics* (25th ed.). New York: McGraw-Hill.

Cwiak, C. & Edelman, A. (2018). Combined oral contraceptives (COCs). In R. A. Hatcher, A. L. Nelson, J. Trussell, C. Cwiak, P. Cason, M. S. Policar, A.B. Edelman, A.R.A. Aiken, J.M. Marrazzo D. Kowal (Eds.), *Contraceptive technology* (21st ed.). New York, NY: Ayer Company Publishers, Inc.

Cycle Technologies. (2017). *What we do: Our suite of family planning innovations*. Available at: www.cycletechnologies.com.

Dean, G., & Schwarz, E. B. (2018). Intrauterine devices (IUDs). In R. A. Hatcher, A. L. Nelson, J. Trussell, C. Cwiak, P. Cason, M. S. Policar, et al. (Eds.), *Contraceptive Technology* (21st ed.). New York: Ayer Company Publishers, Inc.

DuoFertility. (n.d.). *DuoFertility: Service: Quickstart guide*. Available at: www.duofertility.com/service/quick-start/guide/http://www.duofertility-com/service/quick-start-guide/

European Society of Human Reproduction and Embryology (ESHRE) Capri Workshop Group. (2017). Induced abortion. *Human Reproduction, 32*(6), 1160–1169.

Finer, L., & Zolna, M. (2016). Declines in unintended pregnancy in the United States, 2008.2011. *The New England Journal of Medicine, 374*(9), 843–852.

Golobof, A., & Kiley, J. (2016). The current status of oral contraceptives: progress and recent innovations. *Seminars in Reproductive Medicine, 34*(3), 145–151.

Guttmacher Institute. (January 2018). *Fact sheet: Induced abortion in the United States*. Retrieved from: https://www.guttmacher.org/fact-sheet/induced-abortion-united-states.

Guttmacher Institute. (January 2019). *Fact sheet. Unintended pregnancy in the United States*. Retrieved from: https://www.guttmacher.org/fact-sheet/unintended-pregnancy-united-states.

Guttmacher Institute. (March 2019a). *State laws and policies: An overview of abortion laws*. Retrieved from: https://www.guttmacher.org/state-policy/explore/overview-abortion-laws.

Guttmacher Institute. (March, 2019b). *State laws and policies: Emergency contraception*. Retrieved from: https://www.guttmacher.org/state-policy/explore/emergency-contraception.

Hou, M. Y., & Roncari, D. (2018). Permanent contraception. In R. A. Hatcher, A. L. Nelson, J. Trussell, et al. (Eds.), *Contraceptive Technology* (21st ed.). New York: Ayer Company Publishers, Inc.

HPSRx Enterprises, Inc. (2017a). *Caya: For providers*. Retrieved from: http://caya.us.com/services/for-providers/#6-hours.

HPSRx Enterprises, Inc. (2017b). *Caya: For providers: Instruction manual*. Retrieved from: http://caya.us.com/wp-content/uploads/pdf/cayaifu.pdf.

Jatlaoui, T., Ewing, A., Mandel, M., et al. (2016). Abortion surveillance—United States, 2013. *Mortality and Morbidity Weekly Report, 65*(12).

Jennnings, V. H., & Polis, C. B. (2018). Fertility awareness-based methods. In R. A. Hatcher, A. L. Nelson, J. Trussell, et al. (Eds.), *Contraceptive Technology* (21st ed.). New York: Ayer Company Publishers, Inc.

Leiva, R., Burhan, U., Kyrillos, E., et al. (2014). Use of ovulation predictor kits as adjuncts when using fertility awareness methods (FAMs): a pilot study. *Journal of the American Board of Family Medicine, 27*(3), 427–429.

Male Contraceptive Initiative. (March 2018). *Prospective.* Retrieved from: https://www.malecontraceptive.org/male-contraception-research/prospective-male-contraceptive-options/.

Marfatia, Y., Pandya, I., & Mehta, K. (2015). Condoms: Past, present and future. *Indian Journal of Sexually Transmitted Diseases and AIDS, 36*(2), 133–139.

Marquette University. (2018). *Natural family planning: Natural family planning information: efficacy of the Marquette Method of natural family planning.* Available at https://nfp.marquette.edu/efficacy.php.

Marston, C., & Church, K. (2016). Does the evidence support global promotion of the calendar-based Standard Days Method® of contraception? *Contraception, 93,* 492–497.

Mayo Clinic. (2018a). *Cervical cap.* Retrieved from: https://www.mayoclinic.org/tests-procedures/cervical-cap/about/pac-20393416.

Mayo Clinic. (2018b). *Ectopic pregnancy.* Retrieved from: https://www.mayoclinic.org/diseases-conditions/ectopic-pregnancy/symptoms-causes/syc-20372088.

Mayo Clinic. (2018c). *Essure.* Retrieved from: www.mayoclinic.org/tests-procedures/essure/about/pac-20394017.

Mayo Clinic. (2018d). *Toxic shock syndrome.* Retrieved from: https://www.mayoclinic.org/diseases-conditions/toxic-shock-syndrome/symptoms-causes/syc-20355384.

Mayo Clinic. (2019a). *Contraceptive sponge.* Retrieved from: https://www.mayoclinic.org/tests-procedures/contraceptive-sponge/about/pac-20384547.

Mayo Clinic. (2019b). *Vasectomy reversal.* Retrieved from: https://www.mayoclinic.org/tests-procedures/vasectomy-reversal/about/pac-20384537.

Mørch, L., Skovlund, C., Hannaford, P., et al. (2017). *Contemporary hormonal contraception and the risk of breast cancer.* Retrieved from: https://www.nejm.org/doi/10.1056/NEJMoa1700732.

Mosher, W., Jones, J., & Abma, J. (2015). Nonuse of contraception among women at risk of unintended pregnancy in the United States. *Contraception, 92*(2), 170–176.

Nanda, K., & Burke, A. (2018). Contraceptive patch and vaginal contraceptive ring. In R. A. Hatcher, A. L. Nelson, J. Trussell, et al. (Eds.), *Contraceptive Technology* (21st ed.). New York: Ayer Company Publishers, Inc.

Nelson, A., & Cwiak, C. (2011). Combined oral contraceptives (COCs). In R. Hatcher, J. Trussell, A. Nelson, et al. (Eds.), *Contraceptive technology (20th rev. ed.).* New York: Ardent Media.

Peck, E. (2017). *Fertility tracking tech: Wearables and apps to help couples conceive.* Retrieved from: https://www.wareable.com/health-and-wellbeing/fertility-tracking-tech-wearables-and-apps-to-help-couples-conceive.

Raymond, E. G., & Grossman, D. (2018). Progestin-only pills. In R. A. Hatcher, A. L. Nelson, J. Trussell, et al. (Eds.), *Contraceptive Technology* (21st ed.). New York: Ayer Company Publishers, Inc.

Reproductive Health Technologies Project. (2016). *Types of emergency contraception.* Retrieved from: http://rhtp.org/wp-content/uploads/2016/08/RHTP-factsheet-Types-of-Emergency-Contraception.pdf.

Rivlin, K., & Westhoff, C. (2017). Family planning. In R. A. Lobo, D. M. Gershenson, g. M. Lentz, & F. A. Valea (Eds.), *Comprehensive Gynecology* (7th ed.). Philadelphia: Mosby.

Scherwitzl, E., Hirschberg, A., & Scherwitzl, R. (2015). Identification and prediction of the fertile window using NaturalCycles. *The European Journal of Contraception and Reproductive Health Care, 20*(5), 403–408.

Scherwitzl, E., Danielsson, K., Sellberg, J., & Scherwitzl, R. (2016). Fertility awareness-based mobile application for contraception. *The European Journal of Contraception and Reproductive Health Care, 21*(3), 234–241.

Trussell, J., Cleland, K., & Schwarz, E. B. (2018). Emergency contraception. In R. A. Hatcher, A. L. Nelson, J. Trussell, et al. (Eds.), *Contraceptive Technology* (21st ed.). New York: Ayer Company Publishers, Inc.

Upadhya, K., Santelli, J., Raine-Bennett, T., et al. (2017). Over-the-counter access to oral contraceptives for adolescents. *Journal of Adolescent Health, 60*(6), 634–640.

U.S. Department of Health and Human Services. (2017a). *Lactational amenorrhea method.* Retrieved from: https://www.hhs.gov/opa/pregnancy-prevention/birth-control-methods/lam/index.html

U.S. Department of Health and Human Services. (2017b). *Diaphragm and cervical cap.* Retrieved Sept. 8, 2018 from: https://www.hhs.gov/opa/pregnancy-prevention/birth-control-methods/diaphragm-cervical-cap/index.html.

U.S. Food and Drug Administration. (2018a). *Medical devices: Products and medical procedures: Implants and prosthetics: Essure permanent birth control.* Retrieved from: www.fda.gov/MedicalDevices/ProductsandMedicalProcedures/ImplantsandProsthetics/EssurePermanentBirthControl/ucm452254.htm.

U.S. Food and Drug Administration. (2018b). *Mifeprex (mifepristone) information.* Retrieved from: https://www.fda.gov/Drugs/DrugSafety/ucm111323.htm.

U.S. Reports. (1973). *Roe v Wade, 401 U.S. 113.*

Wang, C., Sitruk-Ware, R., & Serfaty, D. (2016). It is time for new male contraceptives!. *Andrology, 4*(5), 773–775.

Wilkinson, T., Clark, P., Rafie, S., Carroll, A., & Miller, E. (2017). *Access to emergency contraception after removal of age restrictions.* Retrieved from: http://pediatrics.aappublications.org.ezproxy.uta.edu/content/140/1/e20164262.full.

World Health Organization. (2017). *Media centre: Emergency contraception.* Retrieved from: http://www.who.int/mediacentre/factsheets/fs244/en/.

World Health Organization. (2018). *Nonoxynol-9 ineffective in preventing HIV infection.* Retrieved from: http://www.who.int/mediacentre/news/notes/release55/en/.

Wu, W.J., & Bartz, D. (2018). Injectable contraceptives. In R. A. Hatcher, A. L. Nelson, J. Trussell, et al. (Eds.), *Contraceptive Technology* (21st ed.). New York: Ayer Company Publishers, Inc.

Yang, Y.T. , Kozhimannil, K. B., & Snowden, J. M. (2016). Pharmacist-prescribed birth control in Oregon and other states. *Journal of the American Medical Association, 315*(15), 1567–1568.

9

Infertility

Pat Mahaffee Gingrich

 http://evolve.elsevier.com/Lowdermilk/MWHC/

This chapter addresses infertility, associated tests, and common therapies. The available alternatives and the psychosocial implications of infertility are discussed.

INCIDENCE

Infertility is a serious medical concern that affects quality of life for approximately 18% of reproductive-age couples (Center for Disease Control [CDC], 2016). The term *infertility* implies a prolonged time to conceive, as opposed to *sterility,* which means inability to conceive. Before age 35, a fertile couple has approximately a 25% to 30% chance of conception in each ovulatory cycle; 80% can conceive within 6 months (American Society for Reproductive Medicine [ASRM] & Society for Reproductive Endocrinology and Infertility [SREI], 2017). If a couple does not achieve pregnancy after a year of unprotected intercourse, they are normally advised to seek specialized fertility evaluation. This evaluation is recommended sooner, after 6 months of attempting pregnancy, for women older than 35, or who have a known risk factor for infertility (ASRM, 2015a). *Primary infertility* refers to difficulty conceiving when there has never been a pregnancy; *secondary infertility* refers to difficulty conceiving after having had a pregnancy, regardless of the outcome. *Fecundity* refers to the ability to carry a pregnancy to a live birth (ASRM & SREI, 2017)

FACTORS ASSOCIATED WITH INFERTILITY

A normally developed reproductive tract in both the male and female partner is essential for fertility. Normal functioning of an intact hypothalamic-pituitary-gonadal axis supports gametogenesis—the formation of sperm and ova. The life spans of the sperm and the ovum are short. Although sperm remain viable in the female's reproductive tract for 48 hours or more, only a few retain fertilization potential for more than 24 hours. Ova remain viable for about 24 hours. Infertility may also be caused by something as simple as poor timing or inadequate frequency of intercourse or lack of penile penetration. The couple should be taught about the menstrual cycle, coital positions to optimize achieving conception, and the ways to detect ovulation (see Chapters 4 and 8). Basal body temperature or ovulation test kits can be useful to determine ovulation.

Probable causes of infertility include the trend toward delaying pregnancy until later in life, the cumulative reproductive organ damage from toxins and diseases such as endometriosis, obesity, smoking, and tubal infection (ASRM & SREI, 2017), and depression (Crawford, Smith, Kuwabara, & Grigorescu, 2017). Male infertility can result from unfavorable sperm production due to age over 50, physical or endocrine dysfunction, cumulative metabolic disease, or toxins (ASRM & SREI). Boxes 9.1 and 9.2 list factors affecting female and male infertility. In general, about 10% to 20% of couples will have idiopathic (unexplained) infertility (ASRM, 2015b).

Female Infertility Causes
Hormonal and Ovulatory Factors
Anovulation may be primary or secondary (see Chapter 6). Primary anovulation may be caused by a pituitary or hypothalamic hormone disorder. It is usually seen in adolescents. Secondary anovulation, usually seen in young to midlife women, is relatively common and is caused by the disruption of the hypothalamic-pituitary-ovarian axis. Besides aging, common risk factors for ovulatory dysfunction include obesity, polycystic ovarian syndrome, strenuous exercise, or endocrine dysfunction, (ASRM, 2015a).

Early menopause (before age 40) may run in families. In menopause, the ovaries do not respond to ovulation-inducing drugs. Nutritional conditions, such as eating disorders, very low weight, or poor diet can disrupt ovarian function. Cancer treatments involving ovarian surgery, radiation, and chemotherapy can decrease or halt ovarian function (ASRM, 2015a). Other risk factors for ovarian disruption include smoking; depression (Crawford et al., 2017); environmental exposure to air pollution, heavy metals, and insecticides (ASRM & SREI, 2017); and inflammation and oxidative stress (Maxia, Uccella, Ersettigh, et al., 2017). Heavy consumption of caffeine (equivalent to five cups of coffee a day) and alcohol (two drinks a day) are associated with decreased fertility (ASRM & SREI).

An increased prolactin level may cause anovulation and amenorrhea in the same way it does during lactation. Hyperprolactinemia can be a side effect of drugs; or a result of physical stressors such as cranial lesions, surgery, or injury; or severe emotional stress. Benign pituitary adenoma may also cause hyperprolactinemia.

BOX 9.1   Factors Affecting Female Fertility

Ovarian Factors
Developmental anomalies
Anovulation, primary or secondary
Pituitary or hypothalamic hormone disorder
Adrenal gland disorder
Congenital adrenal hyperplasia
Disruption of hypothalamic-pituitary-ovarian axis
Amenorrhea after discontinuing oral contraceptive pills
Premature ovarian failure
Increased prolactin levels

Uterine, Tubal, and Peritoneal Factors
Developmental anomalies
Tubal motility reduced
Inflammation within the tube
Tubal adhesions
Endometrial and myometrial tumors
Asherman syndrome (uterine adhesions or scar tissue)
Endometriosis
Chronic cervicitis
Unfavorable cervical mucus

Other Factors
Nutritional deficiencies (e.g., anemia)
Obesity
Substance abuse
Thyroid dysfunction
Genetic disorders (e.g., Turner syndrome)
Anxiety/Depression

BOX 9.2   Factors Affecting Male Fertility

Poor Sperm Quality
Substance abuse, especially tobacco
Age
Sexually transmitted infections
Exposure to workplace hazards such as radiation or toxic substances
Exposure of scrotum to high temperatures
Nutritional deficiencies
Obesity
Antisperm antibodies

Structural or Hormonal Disorders
Undescended testes
Hypospadias
Varicocele
Obstructive lesions of the vas deferens or epididymis
Low testosterone levels
Hypopituitarism
Endocrine disorders
Testicular damage caused by mumps
Retrograde ejaculation

Other Factors
Genetic disorders (e.g., Klinefelter syndrome)
Decrease in libido—heroin, methadone, selective serotonin reuptake inhibitors, barbiturates, depression
Impotence—alcohol, antihypertensives, antiseizure medications

The decline in fertility rate in women accelerates after age 35. Decreased *ovarian reserve,* or total number and quality of follicles, is thought to be the primary reason for age-associated infertility (ASRM, 2015a).

Progesterone, produced by the ovarian corpus luteum, is necessary to mature and maintain the uterine lining. Inadequate progesterone results in a thin endometrial lining, unable to nourish the implanted blastocyst.

Tubal and Peritoneal Factors

Impaired tubal patency and motility result from infections, adhesions, scarring, tumors, or intentional sterilization. One tube may be relatively shorter than the other or absent, which is often associated with an abnormally developed uterus.

Inflammation of the tube or the fimbriated ends resulting from pelvic infections may impair fertility. When infection with purulent discharge heals, scar tissue adhesions form, blocking or kinking the tube. Adhesions may not prevent the tiny sperm from passing through the tube, but may prevent a larger fertilized egg from completing the journey into the intrauterine cavity. This results in an ectopic pregnancy, which can completely destroy the tube and be life threatening if untreated. Women who have used barrier contraceptive methods, such as condoms, are more likely to conceive than those who did not, presumably because of the protective effects against tubal damage from sexually transmitted infections (STIs), especially chlamydia.

Endometriosis is the inflammatory peritoneal damage caused by endometrial tissue that has migrated out of the uterus and implanted on pelvic organs or connective tissue (see Chapter 6). Resulting adhesions can result in pelvic distortion. Inflammatory changes are a high-risk factor for ovarian dysfunction and blocked tubal transport (ASRM, 2015a).

Uterine Factors

Minor developmental anomalies of the uterus are fairly common; major anomalies occur rarely. Müllerian malformations of the uterine cavity, such as bicornuate or septate uterus (Fig. 9.1) or tumors of the endometrium and myometrium (e.g., polyps or myomas), can impair implantation and normal fetal growth. If a functional uterus can be reconstructed, pregnancy may be possible. Experimental uterine transplants are showing increasing promise for outcomes of live births, and can be removed when childbearing is complete (Flyckt, Davis, Farrrell, et al., 2017).

Asherman syndrome (uterine adhesions or scar tissue) is characterized by hypomenorrhea. The adhesions prevent normal cyclic endometrial proliferation necessary for implantation. This can result from endometriosis or surgical interventions such as too-vigorous curettage (scraping) after an elective abortion or miscarriage.

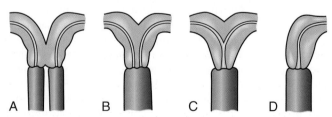

Fig. 9.1 Abnormal Uterus. (A) Complete bicornuate uterus with vagina divided by a septum. (B) Complete bicornuate uterus with normal vagina. (C) Partial bicornuate uterus with normal vagina. (D) Unicornuate uterus.

Vaginal-Cervical Factors

Endocervical mucus normally obstructs or plugs the cervix, acting as a barrier against infection, until increasing midcycle estrogen levels cause the mucus to become clear, thin, and nutritionally supportive of sperm. This change occurs around the time of ovulation and lasts approximately 48 to 72 hours (see Teaching for Self-Management box: Cervical Mucus Characteristics, Chapter 8). In the presence of vaginal or cervical infections, inflammation and white blood cells dramatically reduce the number of viable motile sperm before they enter the cervical canal. The amount of mucus and its physical changes are influenced by the presence of blood, pathogenic bacteria, and irritants such as an intrauterine device (IUD) or a polyp. Severe emotional stress, antibiotic therapy, and diseases such as diabetes mellitus diminish the supportive alkalinity of the cervical mucus.

Some women develop antisperm antibodies, causing the sperm to be clumped within the cervical mucus. This immobilizes the sperm, preventing its migration into the uterus, and thus prevents fertilization.

MALE INFERTILITY CAUSES

Structural or hormonal disorders such as undescended testes, hypospadias, varicocele (varicose veins on the spermatic vein in the scrotal sac), low testosterone levels, or previous vasectomy, can cause *azoospermia* (no sperm cells produced) or *oligospermia* (few sperm cells produced). A low sperm count may occur when spermatic fluid is ejaculated *retrograde,* or backward, into the bladder. Damage from mumps, testicular cancer, or pituitary tumors may present as infertility (ASRM, 2015b).

Similar health issues that affect women, such as nutritional problems, endocrine disorders, genetic disorders, psychologic disorders, and STIs, can also affect fertility in men. Male obesity can lead to decreased semen quality. Exposure to hazards in the environment such as radiation, heavy metals, air pollution, or insecticides also can affect sperm production (ASRM, 2015b). Exposure of the scrotum to high temperatures can cause a decrease in sperm production, as well as abnormal sperm production. Cancer treatments can decrease production or quality of sperm.

Substance use, medications, and steroids can be factors in androgen deficient infertility (Sandher & Aning, 2017). Cigarette smoking has been associated with a decrease in number and quality of sperm as well as chromosomal damage. Heroin, methadone, selective serotonin reuptake inhibitors (SSRIs), and barbiturates decrease libido. Monoamine oxidase inhibitors (MAOIs), a class of antidepressants, adversely affect spermatogenesis. In addition, some antihypertensive and antiseizure medications may cause erectile dysfunction (impotence).

Male fertility declines slowly after age 40; however, no cessation of sperm production occurs analogous to menopause in women. Advanced paternal age (>40 years old) is associated with a slightly increased risk for some autosomal dominant conditions, autism spectrum disorder, and schizophrenia in the offspring, as well as practical and ethical issues of older fatherhood (Braverman, 2017).

TRANSGENDER FERTILITY ISSUES

Transgender clients have several options for reproduction. As with cancer patients, sexually mature individuals may choose cryopreservation of their oocytes or sperm prior to gender reassignment (Martinez, 2017). Individuals with intact reproductive organs may choose to discontinue their gender-reassignment hormone therapy and proceed with fertility care according to their biological gender (Finlayson, Johnson, Chen, et al., 2016). Reversion to their previous gender appearance and the intrusive nature of fertility treatments, such as vaginal ultrasounds, can be unsettling and traumatic to the client with gender dysphoria. An interprofessional team, including medical, nursing, pharmacologic, and mental health specialists, and careful education of all staff are ideal to provide sensitive care

---

BOX 9.3 Religious and Cultural Considerations of Fertility

Religious Considerations

- Civil laws and religious proscriptions about sex must always be kept in mind by the health care professional.
- Conservative and reform Jewish couples are accepting of most infertility treatment; however, the Orthodox Jewish husband and wife may face problems with infertility investigation and management because of religious laws that govern marital relations. For example, according to Jewish law, the Orthodox couple may not engage in marital relations during menstruation and through the following 7 "preparatory days." The wife then is immersed in a ritual bath *(mikvah)* before relations can resume. Fertility problems can arise when the woman has a short cycle (i.e., a cycle of 24 days or fewer; when ovulation would occur on day 10 or earlier).
- The Roman Catholic Church regards the embryo as a human being from the first moment of existence and regards as unacceptable technical procedures such as in vitro fertilization (IVF), masturbation to collect semen for husband/partner or therapeutic donor insemination (TDI), and freezing of embryos.
- Other religious groups may have ethical concerns about infertility tests and treatments. For example, most Protestant denominations and Muslims usually support infertility management as long as IVF is done with the husband's sperm, there is no reduction of fetuses, and insemination is done with the husband's sperm. These groups are less supportive of surrogacy and use of donor sperm and eggs. Christian Scientists do not permit surgical procedures or IVF but do permit insemination with husband and donor sperm.
- Care providers should seek to understand the woman's spiritual and religious beliefs and how they affect her perception of health care, especially in relation to infertility. Women may wish to seek infertility treatment but have questions about proposed diagnostic and therapeutic procedures because of religious proscriptions. These women are encouraged to consult their minister, rabbi, priest, or other spiritual leader for advice.

Cultural Considerations

- In many cultures the responsibility for infertility is usually attributed to the woman. A woman's inability to conceive may be a result of her sins, of evil spirits, or of the fact that she is an inadequate person. The virility of a man in some cultures remains in question until he demonstrates his ability to reproduce by having at least one child.
- Families and faith-based organizations may be disapproving and unsupportive of LGBTQ families.

Modified from D'Avanzo, C. (2008). Mosby's pocket guide to cultural health assessment (4th ed.). St Louis: Mosby.

---

and support, including careful attention to inclusive language and the client's preference for pronouns.

CARE MANAGEMENT

The nurse begins assessment by obtaining data relevant to fertility through interviewing and assisting in physical examination. The database must include information to identify whether infertility is primary or secondary. Religious, cultural, and ethnic data are noted (Box 9.3). Many couples have already visited various health care providers and have read extensively on the subject. Their previous infertility experiences and knowledge should be explored and recorded.

Much of the data needed to investigate impaired fertility is of a sensitive, personal nature. Obtaining these data may be perceived as an invasion of privacy.

TABLE 9.1   Tests for Impaired Fertility

Test or Examination	Timing (Menstrual Cycle Days)	Rationale
Hysterosalpingogram	7-10	Late follicular, early proliferative phase; will not disrupt a fertilized ovum; may open uterine tubes before time of ovulation
Sonohysterogram	7-10	Same as hysterosalpingogram
Basal body temperature	Chart entire cycle	Elevation occurs in response to progesterone, documents ovulation
Ovulation detection kit	Begin on day 11 of 28-day cycle	Detects luteinizing hormone surge, 12-36 h prior to ovulation
Assessment of cervical mucus	Variable, ovulation	Cervical mucus should have low viscosity, high spinnbarkeit
Ultrasound diagnosis of follicular collapse	Ovulation	Collapsed follicle is seen after ovulation
Serum assay of plasma progesterone	20-25	Midluteal midsecretory phase; check adequacy of corpus luteal production of progesterone
Serum antimüllerian hormone (AMH)	Any day during the cycle	AMH confirms developing follicles
Hysteroscopy	Variable	Direct visualization of inside of uterus, via cervix
Laparoscopy	Variable	Direct visualization of outside of uterus, ovaries, and tubes, via abdomen

Investigation of impaired fertility begins for the woman and the man with a complete history and physical examination. A complete general physical examination is followed by a specific assessment of the reproductive tract and laboratory data. The nurse can alleviate some of the anxiety associated with diagnostic testing by explaining to clients the timing and rationale for each test (Table 9.1). Test findings that are favorable to fertility are summarized in Box 9.4.

Couples should be cautioned that all tests can be normal and conception still may not occur. Conversely, pregnancy can occur despite poor test results.

Assessment of Female Infertility

Fertility data for the woman include evaluation of the cervix, uterus, tubes, and peritoneum; detection of ovulation; assessment of immunologic compatibility; and evaluation of psychogenic factors. See Clinical Reasoning Case Study to explore how to assist women using evidence and best practices.

❓ CLINICAL REASONING CASE STUDY

Infertility

Amber is a 39-year-old accountant who has recently married for the first time. Charles is 41 and has two children from a previous marriage. Amber has a history of amenorrhea when she was in college and a member of the track team. Currently her menstrual periods are irregular. She wants to have a baby "before it's too late," and she and Charles have been having unprotected sex for almost a year. They have come to the fertility clinic today for an evaluation. Diane tells the nurse that she has heard a lot about the success of in vitro fertilization and wants to know if she will be able to have it performed.

1. What is the priority concern or client need in this situation? Support your answer with data as stated in the case.
2. List other client needs/problems in this case.
3. Identify any additional information or assessment data that is needed by the nurse in planning for this client.
4. What nursing actions are appropriate in this situation?
   a. What is the priority nursing action? (What should the nurse do first?)
   b. Describe other nursing interventions that are important for providing optimal client care.
5. Describe the roles/responsibilities of the interprofessional health care team members (other than the nurses) who may be involved in providing care for this client.

BOX 9.4   Summary of Findings Favorable to Fertility

1. Follicular development, ovulation, and luteal development are supportive of pregnancy:
   a. Basal body temperature (presumptive evidence of ovulatory cycles) is biphasic, with temperature elevation that persists for 12-14 days before menstruation.
   b. Cervical mucus characteristics change appropriately during phases of the menstrual cycle.
   c. Days 3-10 follicle-stimulating hormone (FSH) levels are low enough to verify presence of adequate ovarian follicles.
   d. Day 3 estradiol levels are low enough to verify presence of adequate ovarian follicles.
   e. Woman reports a history of regular, predictable menses with consistent premenstrual and menstrual symptoms.
   f. Any day antimüllerian hormone (AMH) is high enough to verify follicle development.
2. The luteal phase is supportive of pregnancy:
   a. Levels of plasma progesterone are adequate to indicate ovulation.
   b. Luteal phase of menstrual cycle is of sufficient duration to support pregnancy.
3. Cervical factors are receptive to sperm during expected time of ovulation:
   a. Cervical os is open.
   b. Cervical mucus is clear, watery, abundant, and slippery and demonstrates good spinnbarkeit and arborization (fern pattern) at time of ovulation.
   c. Cervical examination reveals no lesions or infections.
4. The uterus and uterine tubes support pregnancy:
   a. Uterine and tubal patency are documented by (1) spillage of dye into the peritoneal cavity, and (2) outlines of uterine and tubal cavities of adequate size and shape with no abnormalities.
   b. Laparoscopic examination verifies normal development of internal genitals and absence of adhesions, infections, endometriosis, and other lesions.
5. The male partner's reproductive structures are normal:
   a. There is no evidence of developmental anomalies of penis, testicular atrophy, or varicocele (varicose veins on the spermatic vein in the groin).
   b. There is no evidence of infection in the prostate, seminal vesicles, or urethra.
   c. Testes are more than 4 cm in largest diameter.
6. Semen is supportive of pregnancy:
   a. Sperm (number per milliliter) are adequate in the ejaculate (at least 15 mil/mL).
   b. Most sperm show normal morphology.
   c. Most sperm are motile and forward moving.
   d. No autoimmunity exists.
   e. Seminal fluid is normal (volume is at least 1.5 mL).

Detection of Ovulation

Direct proof of ovulation is pregnancy or the retrieval of an ovum from the uterine tube. Indirect or presumptive proof can be provided by over-the-counter ovulation detection kits, which test the urine for the luteinizing hormone (LH) surge at 24 to 36 hours prior to ovulation. When drawn at 1 week prior to the expected onset of the next menses, an elevated serum progesterone level gives reliable presumptive evidence of ovulation (ASRM, 2015a). Other indirect detections of ovulation include assessment of basal body temperature (BBT) and cervical mucus characteristics, as well as ultrasound imaging, described later. Occurrence of mittelschmerz (lower quadrant pain) and midcycle spotting provides unreliable presumptive evidence of ovulation.

Hormone Analysis

Serum prolactin and thyroid levels may be necessary to diagnose the cause of irregular or absent menstrual cycles. Serum progesterone levels during the second half of the menstrual cycle may help in diagnosing luteal phase deficiency, which may interfere with maintaining a future pregnancy. However, the significance of progesterone levels is controversial (Mesen & Young, 2015).

Ovarian reserve is established by testing serum follicle-stimulating hormone (FSH) and estradiol (E2) on day 3 of the cycle. High FSH and low E2 may indicate ovarian failure. Ovarian stimulation is attempted using a clomiphene citrate challenge test (CCCT). Ovarian follicle development is subsequently assessed visually using transvaginal ultrasound or via a blood test for antimüllerian hormone (AMH), produced by developing follicles (ASRM, 2015a). Poor ovarian reserve may indicate the need for donor eggs.

Imaging

Transvaginal ultrasound and *magnetic resonance imaging* (MRI) are used to assess pelvic structures (Fig. 9.2) for abnormalities such as fibroid tumors and ovarian cysts; to verify follicular development and maturity; and to assess thickness of the endometrium around the time of ovulation. *Sonohysterography* uses fluid infused into the uterus through the cervix to help define the uterine cavity and the depth of the uterine lining, using vaginal ultrasound (ASRM, 2015a).

Hysterosalpingography, a radiographic (x-ray) film examination allows visualization of the uterine cavity and tubes after the instillation of radiopaque contrast material via the cervix (Fig. 9.3). The contrast medium is gently pushed through the uterus and out into the uterine tubes, where it can sometimes have the therapeutic effect of opening a blocked tube (Mohiyiddeen, Hardiman, Fitzgerald, et al., 2015).

Hysterosalpingography is scheduled 2 to 5 days after menstruation to avoid flushing a potential fertilized ovum out through a uterine tube into the peritoneal cavity. Endometrial blood vessels are closed at this time, and all menstrual debris has been discharged. This decreases the risk of embolism or of forcing menstrual debris into the peritoneal cavity. (See Nursing Tip.)

> ### ! NURSING TIP
>
> - Referred shoulder pain may occur during a hysterosalpingogram. The referred pain is indicative of subphrenic irritation from the contrast media if it is spilled out of the patent uterine tubes. The discomfort can be managed with position change and mild analgesics. Pain usually subsides within 12-14 hours. Women with blocked tubes may have cramping for up to 48 hours.

Hysteroscopy uses a flexible scope threaded through the cervix to directly view the uterine cavity. This is the gold standard method for evaluation of leiomyomas (fibroids) and adhesions that might impair

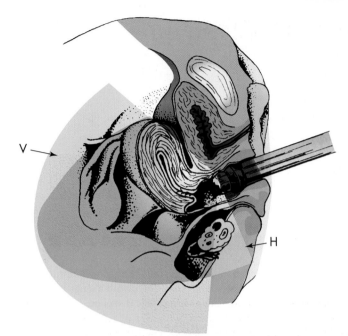

Fig. 9.2 Vaginal Ultrasonography. Major scanning planes of transducer. *H,* Horizontal; *V,* vertical.

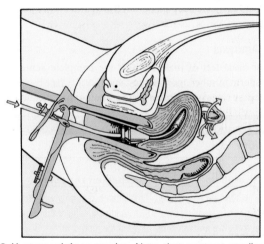

Fig. 9.3 Hysterosalpingography. Note that contrast medium flows through an intrauterine cannula and out through the uterine tubes.

implantation. It is also the most expensive and invasive, so it is not a first-line assessment method (ASRM, 2015a).

Laparoscopy is useful to view the pelvic structures intraperitoneally, outside the uterus, which may reveal endometriosis, pelvic adhesions, tubal occlusion, leiomyomas, or polycystic ovaries. It is indicated for women with symptoms, and to rule out endometriosis in long-term infertility of unknown reason (ASRM, 2015a). Performed early in the menstrual cycle, under either general or local anesthesia, a small endoscope is inserted through a small incision in the anterior abdominal wall. Cold fiberoptic light sources allow superior visualization of the internal pelvic structures (Fig. 9.4). A needle is inserted, and carbon dioxide gas is pumped into the peritoneum to elevate the abdominal wall from the organs, thereby creating an empty space that permits visualization and exploration with the laparoscope. If tubal patency is being assessed, a cannula is used to instill a dye contrast medium through the cervix.

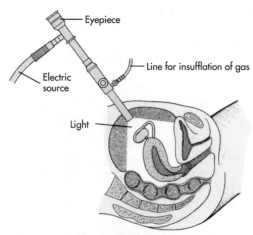

Fig. 9.4 Laparoscopy.

After surgery, deflation of most gas is done by gentle pressure on the abdomen. Trocar and needle sites are closed with a single absorbable suture or skin clip, and an adhesive bandage is applied.

Assessment of Male Infertility

Fertility assessment in the man includes evaluation of general health, penis, meatus, testes, scrotum, prostate, hair distribution, and breast development. In addition, assessment includes semen analysis, assessment of immunologic compatibility, endocrine evaluations, imaging and lab tests as indicated, genetic screening, and evaluation of psychological factors (ASRM, 2015b).

Semen Analysis

The most basic test of male fertility, the complete semen analysis, assesses sperm number, morphology, and motility (see Box 9.4). Semen is collected by ejaculation into a clean container or a plastic sheath that does not contain a spermicidal agent. The specimen is usually collected by masturbation after 2 to 5 days of abstinence from ejaculation. The semen is kept at room or body temperature and taken to the laboratory in a sealed container within 1 hour of ejaculation (ASRM, 2015b).

If results are in the fertile range, no further sperm evaluation is necessary. Poor sperm morphology may indicate a need for donor sperm. Semen analysis may reveal leukocytes from genital tract infection or clumping from antisperm antibodies of the male (ASRM, 2015b).

Ultrasonography

Scrotal ultrasound is used to examine the testes for the presence of varicocele and to identify abnormalities in the scrotum and spermatic cord. Transrectal ultrasound can be used to evaluate the ejaculatory ducts, seminal vesicles, and vas deferens for obstruction.

Other Tests

The male is assessed for other causes of infertility: hypopituitarism; nutritional deficiency; debilitating or chronic disease, including obesity and metabolic disease; trauma; exposure to environmental hazards such as radiation and toxic substances; use of tobacco, alcohol, medication, recreational drugs, or anabolic steroids; and gonadotropic inadequacy. Genetic testing may reveal other reproductive problems. Hormone analyses are done for testosterone, gonadotropin, FSH, and LH. In the presence of a mass, testicular biopsy may be warranted.

INTERVENTIONS

Assisted reproductive therapies may be indicated. The management of clients seeking medically-assisted reproduction includes psychosocial, nonmedical, medical, and surgical interventions (Zegers-Hochschild et al., 2017). Nursing interventions are an important aspect of care (see Nursing Care Plan).

◎ NURSING CARE PLAN

Infertility

Client Problems	Expected Outcome	Nursing Interventions	Rationales
Need for Health Teaching related to lack of understanding of the reproductive process with regard to conception	Woman and partner will verbalize understanding of the components of the reproductive process, common problems leading to infertility, usual infertility testing, and the importance of completing testing in a timely manner.	Assess woman's/partner's current level of understanding of the factors promoting conception. Provide information regarding factors promoting conception, including common factors leading to infertility of either partner in a supportive manner. Identify and describe the basic infertility tests and the rationale for precise scheduling.	To identify gaps or misconceptions in knowledge base. To raise woman's/partner's awareness and promote trust in caregiver. To enhance completion of the diagnostic phase of the infertility workup
Decreased Ability to Cope related to inability to conceive and infertility process	Woman and partner will identify situational stressors and positive coping methods to deal with testing and unknown outcomes.	Provide opportunities through therapeutic communication to discuss feelings and concerns. Evaluate couple's support system, including support of each other during this process. Identify support groups and refer as needed.	To identify common feelings and perceived stressors. To identify any barriers to effective coping. To enhance coping by sharing experiences with other couples experiencing similar problems
Decreased Self-Esteem and/or Grieving related to inability to conceive and feelings of hopelessness	Woman and partner will verbalize a realistic plan to decrease feelings of hopelessness.	Provide support for couple while grieving for loss of fertility. Assess for behaviors indicating possible depression, anger, and frustration. Refer to support groups.	To allow couple to work through feelings. To prevent impending crisis. To promote a common bond with other couples during expression of feelings and concerns

Psychosocial

Besides the need for safety with relatively minor office procedures, the care priority for couples seeking fertility treatment is psychologic support. Infertility is recognized as a major life stressor that can affect self-esteem, relationships, life goals, and careers. Infertility tests and interventions are occasionally painful and intrusive. Timed abstinence and intercourse can create stress and decrease pleasure with sexual activity. The medical investigation requires time (at least 3 to 4 months) and considerable financial expense. It can cause emotional distress, anger, isolation, sexual dysfunction, and strain on the couple's relationship. A high level of motivation from both partners is needed to complete the investigation. Preparatory and concurrent counseling support is recommended.

Couples frequently refer to their experience with infertility as a "roller coaster" of emotions. The stress of infertility and its treatment can exacerbate preexisting anxiety or depression. Conversely, stress can be a cause of infertility for men and women, making it difficult to identify cause and effect. Table 9.2 discusses some therapeutic nursing actions in response to emotional behaviors associated with impaired fertility.

Same-sex and transgender couples desire pregnancy and parenthood for the same reasons as do cisgender (when one's gender identity matches the sex the person was assigned at birth) couples, but may feel unaccepted and marginalized in health care settings. This adds to the stress of fertility treatments.

The nurse who is comfortable discussing intercourse and sexuality can better help couples understand why the private information about sexual activity must be shared with health care professionals. Nurses must be knowledgeable and nonjudgmental of the preferences and activities of others (including LGBTQ couples). Gender-neutral and inclusive language, as well as pictures and brochures depicting all types of families, including same-sex couples, establishes a tone of respect and safety in the health care setting.

The support systems of the couple with impaired fertility must be explored. It is important to identify support available from family and friends, support groups, and their greater spiritual community. Individuals undergoing infertility evaluation and treatment should be encouraged to share their infertility experiences with all other providers of health care, including mental health practitioners.

If the couple conceives, the nurse must be aware that previously infertile couples may continue to experience distress and anxiety. Some couples are shocked to find that they feel resentment of impending parenthood. Pregnancy, once a cherished dream, now necessitates more changes in goals, plans, and identities. Reactions of couples range from joy to feeling overwhelmed with worry and fear, to the point of considering aborting the pregnancy. The couple with long-term infertility may have idealized childbearing when they thought it was beyond their reach. A history of impaired fertility is a risk factor for pregnancy complications and postpartum depression; therefore, ongoing supportive psychological therapy should be encouraged.

Health team members must respect affected individuals' and couples' desires in choosing to stop treatment. If the couple does not conceive, they are assessed regarding their desire to be referred for help with adoption, assisted reproductive alternatives, or choosing a child-free state. The couple may find a list of agencies, support groups, and other resources in their community helpful such as ASRM (www.asrm.org) and RESOLVE (www.resolve.org).

Nonmedical Therapy

Lifestyle Changes

Simple changes in lifestyle may be effective in increasing fertility for men. Daily hot baths or tight athletic clothing can cause scrotal temperatures that are too high for efficient spermatogenesis. Loose clothing may improve sperm count. Many commonly used lubricants can diminish sperm motility and quality. Cell phones worn at the belt or hip have been linked to decreased sperm quality (Kamali, Atarod, Sarhadi, et al., 2017).

Changes in nutrition and habits may increase fertility for men and women. A well-balanced plant-based diet, exercise, and avoidance of toxins and toxic substances can increase fertility for both partners. Weight normalization, optimal nutrition, and maintaining normoglycemia maximize the chance of conception for males and females. Women who are overweight or obese have a reduced chance of

TABLE 9.2	Nursing Actions in Response to Behavior Associated With Impaired Fertility	
Behavioral Characteristic	**Nursing Action**
Surprise: Each person assumes she or he is fertile and that pregnancy is an option.	Point out resemblance to grieving process—a normal, expected reaction to loss. Refer to support group. Prepare clients for length of time it may take to grieve and for types of feelings (psychologic, somatic) to expect. Encourage and allow time to talk of past and present feelings of sexuality, self-image, and self-esteem.
Denial: "It can't happen to me!"	Allow time for denial, because it gives the body and mind time to adjust a little at a time. Do not feed into the client's denial; instead say, "It must be hard to believe such a devastating report."
Anger: Toward others (perhaps even the nurse) or themselves	Explain that the reaction to loss of control and to a feeling of helplessness is often anger, which can easily be projected onto another person. Anger is a natural feeling. Allow time to express anger at losing sense of control over bodies and destinies. A helpful approach may be, "It's OK to be angry . . . at those who are pregnant, at people who want abortions, at self, at mate, at caregivers," and so forth.
Bargaining: "If I get pregnant, I'll dedicate the child to God."	Accept bargaining statements without comment.
Depression: Isolation	Allow time for both woman and man to talk about how it feels whenever a sight, event, or word serves as a reminder of his or her own state of impaired fertility. Develop role-playing situations to practice interactions with others under various circumstances to increase the couple's ability to cope and to solve problems (increases their self-confidence). The nurse may say, "You must feel so terribly alone sometimes."
Guilt or unworthiness	Allow time to identify feelings that may be related to earlier behaviors (such as abortion, premarital sex, contact with sexually transmitted infections [STIs]).
Acceptance (resolution)	Couple or person comes to the realization that "unworthiness" and impaired fertility are unrelated. Clients need to know that grief feelings are never laid away forever; they may be activated by special reminders (such as anniversaries).

Adapted from Resolve. (n.d.). *Managing infertility stress.* Retrieved from https://resolve.org/support/managing-infertility-stress.

pregnancy following IVF and a significantly greater risk of miscarriage following infertility treatment as compared with women of normal weight (ASRM, 2015c). Even modest weight loss (5% to 10%) can be sufficient to increase their chances of achieving a successful pregnancy.

Counseling couples on optimal timing of intercourse can also help. Encouraging intercourse every 1 to 2 days, especially on the day prior to ovulation, will maximize chances of pregnancy (ASRM & SREI, 2017). Sexual counseling may help couples if there is a question of sexual dysfunction that is affecting penile penetration (e.g., vaginismus, obesity).

Complementary and Alternative Measures

Most herbal remedies have not been proven clinically to promote fertility or to be safe in early pregnancy. Women should take these only when prescribed by a physician, nurse-midwife, or nurse practitioner who has expertise in herbology. Stress management (e.g., aromatherapy, yoga, mindfulness meditation), relaxation, and nutritional and exercise counseling have increased pregnancy rates in some women (Toosi, Azbarzadeh, & Ghaemi, 2017). Integrative mind-body-spirit programs for counseling on attitudes of kindness, flexibility, curiosity, acceptance, and openness effectively decrease stress and anxiety related to infertility in couples (Pasch & Sullivan, 2017). Antioxidant vitamins E and C, selenium, zinc, coenzyme Q10, and ginseng have shown possible beneficial effects for infertility (Showell, Mackenzie-Proctor, Jordan, et al., 2017). Acupuncture can decrease anxiety and improve pregnancy rates for women undergoing IVF (Qian, Xia, Orchi, et al., 2017).

Medical Therapy
Correcting Preexisting Factors

For women, pretreatment or surgery may be indicated to optimize conditions for conception. Infections are treated with appropriate antimicrobial formulations. Surgery or hysterosalpingogram may be necessary to correct tubal blockage or pelvic distortion. Uterine fibroids may need removal via laparotomy, laparoscopy, or hysteroscopy (accessed via the cervix) (ASRM, 2017). Laparoscopic removal of endometrial adhesions and implants, and draining of hydrosalpinges (endometrial fluid pockets) can normalize reproductive function.

Drug therapy may be indicated for male infertility. Problems with the thyroid or adrenal glands are corrected with appropriate medications. Infections are identified and treated promptly with antimicrobials. Surgery may be needed to correct varicoceles, blockages, or tumors. FSH, gonadotropins, and clomiphene may be used to stimulate spermatogenesis in men with hypogonadism. Commonly used medications are summarized in the Medication Guide.

MEDICATION GUIDE

Infertility Medications

Drug	Indication	Mechanism of Action	Dosage	Common Side Effects
Clomiphene citrate	Ovulation induction, treatment of luteal phase inadequacy	Thought to bind to estrogen receptors in the pituitary, blocking them from detecting estrogen	Tablets, starting with 50 mg/day by mouth for 5 days beginning on 5th day of menses; if ovulation does not occur, may increase dose next cycle-variable dosage	Vasomotor flushes, abdominal discomfort, nausea and vomiting, breast tenderness, ovarian enlargement
Menotropins (human menopausal gonadotropins [hMG])	Ovarian follicular growth and maturation	LH and FSH in 1:1 ratio, direct stimulation of ovarian follicle; given sequentially with human chorionic gonadotropin (hCG) to induce ovulation	IM or subcutaneous injections, dosage regimen variable based on ovarian response. Initial dose is 75 International Units of FSH and 75 International Units of LH (1 ampule) daily for 7-12 days followed by 10,000 International Units hCG	Ovarian enlargement, ovarian hyperstimulation, local irritation at injection site, multifetal gestations
Follitropins (purified FSH)	Treatment of polycystic ovarian syndrome (PCOS); follicle stimulation for assisted reproductive techniques	Direct action on ovarian follicle	Subcutaneous or IM injections, dosage regimen variable	Ovarian enlargement, ovarian hyperstimulation, local irritation at injection site, multifetal gestations
Human chorionic gonadotropin (hCG)	Ovulation induction	Direct action on ovarian follicle to stimulate meiosis and rupture of the follicle	5000-10,000 International Units IM 1 day after last dose of menotropins; dosage regimen variable	Local irritation at injection site; headaches, irritability, edema, depression, fatigue
Exogenous progesterone	Treatment of luteal phase inadequacy	Direct stimulation of endometrium	Vaginal gel 8%, 1 prefilled applicator per day; after ovulation induction, continue through 10-12 weeks of pregnancy	Breast tenderness, local irritation, headaches
GnRH antagonists (ganirelix acetate, cetrorelix acetate)	Controlled ovarian stimulation for infertility treatment	Suppress gonadotropin secretion; inhibit premature LH surges in women undergoing ovarian hyperstimulation	250 mcg daily subcutaneously usually in the early to midfollicular phase of the menstrual cycle; usually followed by hCG administration	Abdominal pain, headache, vaginal bleeding, irritation at the injection site
Metformin (off-label use)	Restores cyclic ovulation and menses in many women with PCOS	Induces ovulation through reducing insulin resistance and thus affecting gonadotropins and androgens; stimulates the ovary	Initial dose is 500 mg/day and titrated up over several weeks to 1500 mg/day. Administered orally	Nausea, vomiting, diarrhea, lactic acidosis, liver dysfunction
Letrozole (off-label use)	Ovulation induction	Aromatase inhibitor that inhibits E2 production, which causes an increase in LH:FSH ratio	2.5-5 mg tablets Administered orally for 5 days beginning on day 3-5 of menses	Hot flashes, headaches, breast tenderness, may increase risk of congenital anomalies

FSH, Follicle-stimulating hormone; *IM*, intramuscular; *LH*, luteinizing hormone.
Data from Society for Assisted Reproductive Technology (SART) (2019). *Assisted reproductive technology: A patient guide.* Retrieved from: https://www.sart.org/patients-a-patients-guide-to-assisted-reproductive-technology/.

Ovarian Stimulation

If the ovarian reserve is determined to be sufficient, pharmacologic therapy is often directed at stimulating the ovary to produce follicles. The most common ovarian stimulants include the selective estrogen receptor modulator (clomiphene citrate) or gonadotropin (FSH, LH).

Assisted Reproductive Technology

Assisted reproductive technology (ART) is the manipulation of eggs, sperm, and/or embryo (Zegers-Hochschild , Adamson, Dyer, et al., 2017). In general, these treatments involve introducing sperm into the uterus or tubes, or removing the eggs from the woman, fertilizing the eggs in the laboratory, and returning the embryo or embryos to the woman or surrogate carrier. The following discussion describes the commonly used ARTs.

Intrauterine Insemination

Ovarian stimulation therapy is followed by timed intercourse. If sperm quality is low or female factors such as unfavorable cervical mucus, semen allergy, or endometriosis are suspected, the sperm can be introduced directly into the uterus using *intrauterine insemination* (IUI). This is also the preferred technique for introducing donor sperm, or sperm that has been washed.

In Vitro Fertilization

In vitro fertilization–embryo transfer (IVF-ET) is used when blockage or inflammatory changes of endometriosis are suspected to impair tubal patency or when tubes have been surgically removed. Ovarian follicles are monitored via ultrasound and removed at maturity through intravaginal needle aspiration or laparoscopic procedure. Fertilization with sperm occurs in a dish. If sperm are not available via ejaculation, they can be retrieved via needle from the testicle, epididymis, or vas deferens.

A micromanipulation technique of the follicle called *intracytoplasmic sperm injection* (ICSI) makes it possible to achieve fertilization even with few or poor-quality sperm by introducing sperm beneath the zona pellucida directly into the egg. The photo in Fig. 9.5 depicts an ultrasound photo of a 6-day-old embryo. ICSI offers the opportunity to enhance the chances of fertilization in cases of a severe male factor (i.e., poor sperm quality). Another micromanipulation option is *assisted*

hatching. In some instances, the zona pellucida is thick or tough and the embryo cannot break through, or "hatch" through this coating in the blastocystic phase of development. An infrared laser is used to create a hole in the zona pellucida so that the embryo can break through and implant.

Preimplantation genetic diagnosis (PGD) can be done on a single cell removed from each embryo after 3 to 4 days. PGD is a form of early genetic testing designed to screen for inherited diseases. Developing embryos free of the disease gene are transferred to the uterus. Couples must be counseled about their options when genetic analysis is considered.

With the availability of extended culture medium, embryos transferred at the blastocyst stage (day 5) have a significantly better chance of live birth than the older practice of transferring the embryo at the cleavage stage (day 3) (Glujovky, Fraquhar, Quintero Retamar, et al., 2016). Because of this improvement, the ASRM recommends no more than a single embryo transfer at a time for women, except in women over 37 or with other poor fertility prognoses (ASRM & SART, 2017). See the Community Activity box.

🏠 COMMUNITY ACTIVITY

Visit the Resolve website (https:\\resolve.org/). Research what Resolve is and what it offers. Review the information that is provided to clients and their families. Use this website to learn about insurance coverage for clients and the various options for treatment as well as various ways that clients come to terms with infertility. Is the information written so that it can be easily understood by a client with no medical background? Do you have suggestions for other information that could be included? How helpful do you think this website is for clients?

Gamete Intrafallopian Transfer and Zygote Intrafallopian Transfer

Gamete intrafallopian transfer (GIFT) is similar to IVF-ET. GIFT requires women to have at least one normal uterine tube. Ovulation is induced as in IVF-ET, and the oocytes are aspirated from follicles via laparoscopy (Fig. 9.6A). Semen is collected before laparoscopy. The ova and sperm are then transferred to one uterine tube (see Fig. 9.6B), permitting natural fertilization and cleavage. *Zygote intrafallopian transfer* (ZIFT) is similar to GIFT except fertilization occurs in vitro, and then the zygote is placed in the uterine tube.

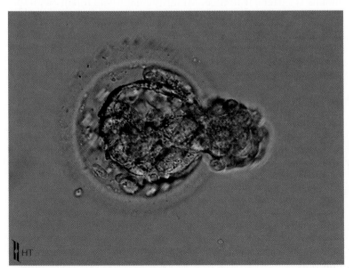

Fig. 9.5 Ultrasound photo of a 6-day-old embryo. (Courtesy Amber and Zack Gaynor, Apex, NC.)

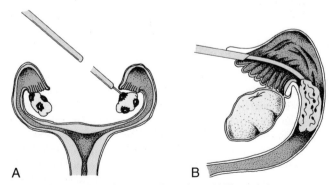

Fig. 9.6 Gamete Intrafallopian Transfer. (A) Through laparoscopy, a ripe follicle is located and fluid containing the egg is removed. (B) The sperm and egg are placed separately in the uterine tube, where fertilization occurs.

Oocyte Donation

Women who have ovarian failure or oophorectomy, who have a genetic defect, or who fail to achieve pregnancy with their own oocytes may be eligible for the use of *donor oocytes* (eggs). Oocyte donation is usually done by women who are younger than 35 years and healthy, and who are recruited and paid to undergo ovarian stimulation and oocyte retrieval. The donor eggs are fertilized in the laboratory with the sperm of the male partner or a donor. The recipient woman undergoes hormonal stimulation to allow development of the uterine lining. The embryos are then transferred to the uterus. The psychosocial issues are similar to those in therapeutic donor insemination (TDI). Historically, the courts have upheld the gestational mother as the legal mother. Sometimes the gestational mother is also a surrogate mother (see later discussion), however, which could complicate the legal aspects. It is expected that the egg donor will have no rights or responsibilities in relation to the offspring.

LEGAL TIP

Cryopreservation

Sperm, ovarian tissue, oocytes, or embryos can be cryopreserved for later use. Couples who have excess embryos frozen for later transfer must be fully informed before consenting to the procedure to make decisions regarding the disposal of embryos in the event of (1) death, (2) divorce, or (3) the decision that the couple no longer wants the embryos. Embryos can be frozen for prolonged periods, and live births have occurred from embryos frozen for 20 years (ASRM, 2016).

Sperm Donation

TDI, previously referred to as artificial insemination by donor, but now called "therapeutic donor insemination," is used when the male partner has absent or unfavorable sperm, the couple has a genetic defect, the male partner has antisperm antibodies, or it is a woman without a male partner. Men in a gay relationship may use TDI with a woman who is a surrogate in order to become parents. Donors are screened thoroughly, and their sperm stored until they have completed 6 months of testing, to account for the latency period for HIV seroconversion.

Embryo Donation

On occasion a couple decides that they do not want their frozen embryos, and they release these for other infertile couples. Infertility centers are struggling to develop guidelines and protocols to address the various legal and ethical issues associated with these procedures. Extensive medical testing of both partners who wish to release the embryos is required as well.

Surrogate Mothers and Embryo Hosts

Surrogate motherhood can be achieved by two methods. The first is for the surrogate mother to be inseminated with semen from the infertile woman's partner and to carry the baby until the birth. The baby is then formally adopted by the infertile couple. A less common method is to retrieve an ovum from the infertile woman, fertilize it with her partner's sperm, and place it into the uterus of an embryo host or gestational carrier. Same sex male couples may use a surrogate, inseminated with sperm from one or a mixture of sperm from both males. These interventions raise considerable legal and ethical issues that require extensive counseling of couples and the women who choose to become surrogates.

Success Rates and Costs of Assisted Reproductive Technology

Nurses can provide information so that couples have an accurate understanding of their realistic chances for a successful birth. Success rates for pregnancy and birth vary widely among fertility centers and practitioners. Each couple's physical status, age, whether the embryos are fresh or frozen, and whether from eggs of the woman or a donor all factor into their individual chances for pregnancy. Updated and detailed success rates of ART by clinic and procedure can be found at cdc.gov/art and sart.org, which include a patient predictor calculator for individual odds of success. In 2015, the success rate for live birth with ART transfer procedures ranged from 57% for women younger than 35 years, to 4.5% for women older than 42 years (American Society for Reproductive Medicine [ASRM] & Society for Assisted Reproductive Technology [SART], 2017). Costs vary by treatment and by region of the country: one cycle of IVF-ET averages $15,000. Table 9.3 summarizes ART procedures and their possible indications.

Risks of Assisted Reproductive Technology

ART carries the established risks associated with ovarian stimulation, such as nausea, fluid retention, or ovarian hyperstimulation; invasive procedures; psychologic stress; and general anesthesia. The more common transvaginal needle aspiration requires only local or intravenous analgesia.

ART's rapid advances are associated with many ethical and legal issues (Box 9.5). Nurses and their interprofessional healthcare team can provide anticipatory guidance about the moral distress and ethical dilemmas regarding the use of ARTs.

Couples using donated eggs or sperm need to be counseled extensively regarding the mutuality of their decision, and their grief at the loss of a biologic link to their child. Long-term issues relating to parenting the child conceived through donation include disclosure to the child and family, and unknown family health history. Couples also must be aware of the legal status of donors and surrogates in their state.

Adoption

Couples may choose to build their family through adoption of children who are not their own biologically. With increased availability of birth control and abortion and increasing numbers of single mothers keeping their babies, however, the adoption of Caucasian infants is extremely limited. Minority infants and infants with special needs, older children, and foreign adoptions are other options (Fig. 9.7). Of course, not all infertile individuals and couples are Caucasian, as infertility affects persons of all racial and ethnic backgrounds.

Prospective parents can become so focused on attempting to become pregnant with their own genetic child that they don't see alternate ways of creating a family and parenting a child. The question for potential adoptive couples to ponder is, "What is important to you—that you become parents or that you go through the experience of pregnancy and birth?" Nurses should have information on options for adoption available for couples or refer them to community resources for further assistance.

Choosing to Live Without Children

Some couples, after undergoing infertility treatments to no avail, will decide to live without children. Although this was not a choice initially, it does become a choice for some couples as they accept their infertility.

TABLE 9.3 Assisted Reproductive Technologies

Procedure	Definition	Indications
Intrauterine insemination (IUI)	Prepared sperm is placed in uterus at ovulation.	Male subfertility; cervical factor; vaginal factors
In vitro fertilization–embryo transfer (IVF-ET)	A woman's eggs are collected from her ovaries, fertilized in the laboratory with sperm, and transferred to her uterus after normal embryo development has occurred.	Tubal absence, disease, or blockage; severe male infertility; endometriosis; unexplained infertility; cervical factor; immunologic infertility
Intracytoplasmic sperm injection	Selection of one sperm cell that is injected directly into the egg to achieve fertilization. Used with IVF-ET.	Male partner is azoospermic or has a very low sperm count; couple has a genetic defect; male partner has antisperm antibodies.
Assisted hatching	The zona pellucida is penetrated chemically or manually to create an opening for the dividing embryo to hatch and implant into uterine wall. Used with IVF-ET.	Recurrent miscarriages; to improve implantation rate in women with previously unsuccessful IVF attempts; advanced age
Gamete intrafallopian transfer (GIFT)	Oocytes are retrieved from the ovary, placed in a catheter with washed motile sperm, and immediately transferred into the fimbriated end of the uterine tube. Fertilization occurs in the uterine tube.	Same as for IVF-ET, except there must be normal tubal anatomy, patency, and absence of previous tubal disease in at least one uterine tube
Zygote intrafallopian transfer (ZIFT)	This process is similar to IVF-ET; after in vitro fertilization the ova are placed in one uterine tube during the zygote stage.	Same as for GIFT
Donor oocyte	Eggs are donated by an IVF procedure, and the donated eggs are inseminated. The embryos are transferred into the recipient's uterus, which is hormonally prepared with estrogen/progesterone therapy.	Early menopause; surgical removal of ovaries; congenitally absent ovaries; autosomal or sex-linked disorders; lack of fertilization in repeated IVF attempts because of subtle oocyte abnormalities or defects in oocyte-spermatozoa interaction
Donor embryo	A donated embryo is transferred to the uterus of an infertile woman at the appropriate time (normal or induced) of the menstrual cycle.	Infertility not resolved by less aggressive forms of therapy; absence of ovaries; male partner is azoospermic or is severely compromised
Surrogate mother; embryo host	Surrogate motherhood is a process by which a woman is inseminated with semen and then carries the fetus until birth. Embryo host: a couple undertakes an IVF cycle, and the embryo(s) is transferred to the uterus of another woman (the carrier) who has contracted with the couple to carry the baby to term. The carrier has no genetic investment in the child.	Congenital absence or surgical removal of uterus; a reproductively impaired uterus, myomas, uterine adhesions, or other congenital abnormalities; a medical condition that might be life threatening during pregnancy, such as diabetes, immunologic problems, or severe heart, kidney, or liver disease; or gay male couple seeking genetic offspring
Therapeutic donor insemination (TDI)	Donor sperm are used to inseminate the female partner. Can be used with IUI, IVF-ET, GIFT or ZIFT	Male partner is azoospermic or has a very low sperm count; couple has a genetic defect; male partner has antisperm antibodies; lesbian or transgender couple

Data from American Society for Reproductive Medicine. (2017). *The international glossary on infertility and fertility care,* Retrieved from http://www.reproductivefacts.org/topics/topics-index/assisted-reproductive-technologies/.

BOX 9.5 Issues to Be Addressed by Infertile Couples Before Treatment

- Risks of multiple gestation
- Possible need for multifetal reduction
- Possible need for donor oocytes, sperm, or embryos, or for gestational carrier (surrogate mother)
- Whether to or how to disclose facts of conception to offspring
- Freezing embryos for later use
- Possible risks of long-term effects of medications and treatment on women, children, and families
- Stress management techniques and recommendation for ongoing psychologic and couples counseling

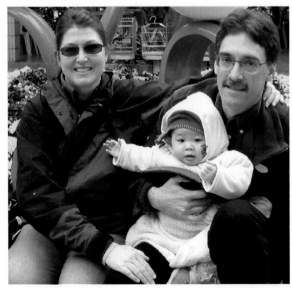

Fig. 9.7 Adoption as a Solution to Infertility. After two miscarriages, this couple chose foreign adoption. (Courtesy Shannon Perry, Phoenix, AZ.)

KEY POINTS

- Infertility is the inability to conceive and carry a child to term gestation when the couple has chosen to do so.
- Infertility affects approximately 18% of otherwise healthy adults. Infertility increases as the woman ages, especially after age 40.
- Common etiologic factors of infertility in the male include decreased sperm production; common factors in the female include ovulation disorders, tubal occlusion, and endometriosis. Obesity, smoking, or underlying disease in either partner is receiving increasing attention as causes of infertility.
- The investigation of infertility is conducted systematically and simultaneously for male and female partners.

- The individual's and couple's relationship dynamics, sexuality, and ability to cope with the psychologic and emotional effects caused by diagnostic procedures and treatment of infertility must be considered in the plan of care. Ongoing support is recommended.
- Infertility may affect LGBTQ individuals and couples as well as heterosexual individuals and couples.
- Interprofessional care is essential to optimum care for individuals and couples experiencing infertility.
- Reproductive alternatives for family building include ovarian stimulation, followed by IUI, IVF-ET, GIFT, or ZIFT, egg or sperm donation, embryo donation, gestational or surrogate motherhood, and adoption.

REFERENCES

American Society for Reproductive Medicine (ASRM). (2015a). Diagnostic evaluation of the infertile female: A committee opinion. *Fertility & Sterility, 103*(6), e18–e25.

American Society for Reproductive Medicine (ASRM). (2015b). Diagnostic evaluation of the infertile male: A committee opinion. *Fertility & Sterility, 103*(3), e44–e50.

American Society for Reproductive Medicine (ASRM). (2015c). Obesity and reproduction: A committee opinion. *Fertility & Sterility, 104*(5), 1116–1126.

American Society for Reproductive Medicine (ASRM). (2016). Defining embryo donation: An ethic committee opinion. *Fertility & Sterility, 106*(1), 56–58.

American Society for Reproductive Medicine (ASRM). (2017). Removal of myomas in asymptomatic patients to improve fertility and/or reduce miscarriage: A committee opinion. *Fertility & Sterility, 108*(3), 416–425.

American Society for Reproductive Medicine (ASRM) & Society for Assisted Reproductive Technology (SART). (2017). Guidance on the limit to the number of embryos to transfer: A committee opinion. *Fertility & Sterility, 107*(4), 901–903.

American Society for Reproductive Medicine (ASRM) & Society for Reproductive Endocrinology and Infertility (SREI). (2017). Optimizing natural fertility: A committee opinion. *Fertility & Sterility, 107*(1), 52–58.

Braverman, A. M. (2017). Old, older and too old: Age limits for medically assisted fatherhood. *Fertility and Sterility, 107*(2), 329–333.

Centers for Disease Control and Prevention. (2016). National Center for Health Statistics, Division of Vital Statistics. Infertility. From Key Statistics from the National Survey of Family Growth. Available at: https://www.cdc.gov/nchs/fastats/infertility.htm.

Center for Disease Control and Prevention (CDC), ASRM, and SART. (2017). Assisted reproductive technology national summary report. Retrieved from: https://www.cdc.gov/art/reports/2015/national-summary.html.

Crawford, S., Smith, R. A., Kuwabara, et al. (2017). Risk factors and treatment use related to infertility and impaired fecundity among reproductive-aged women. *Journal of Women's Health, 26*(5), 500–510.

Finlayson, C., Johnson, E. K., Chen, D., et al. (2016). Proceedings of the working group session on fertility preservation for individuals with gender and sex diversity. *Transgender Health, 1*(1), 99–107.

Flyckt, R., Davis, A., Farrell, R., et al. (2017). Uterine transplant: surgical innovation in the treatment of uterine factor infertility. *Journal of Obstetrics and Gynaecology of Canada, 40*(1), 86–93.

Glujovsky, D., Farquhar, C., Quinteiro Retamar, A., et al. (2016). Cleavage stage versus blastocyst stage embryo transfer in assisted reproductive technology. *In The Cochrane Database of Systemic Reviews, 2016*(6).

Kamali, K., Atarod, M., Sarhadi, S., et al. (2017). Effect of electromagnetic waves emitted from 3G+ wi-fi modems on human semen analysis. *Urologia, 84*(4), 209–214.

Martinez, F. (2017). Update on fertility preservation from the Barcelona International Society for Fertility Preservation-ESHRE=ASRM 2105 expert meeting: Indications, results and future perspectives. *Human Reproduction, 32*(9), 1802–1811.

Maxia, N., Uccella, S., Ersettigh, G., et al. (2017). Can unexplained infertility be evaluated by a new immunological four biomarkers panel? A pilot study. *Minerva Ginecologica, 70*(2), 129–137 [epub ahead of print].

Mohiyiddeen, L., Hardiman, A., Fitzgerald, C., et al. (2015). Tubal flushing for subfertility. *Cochrane Database of Systemic Reviews, 5, CD003718, 2016*(6).

Pasch, L. A., & Sullivan, K. T. (2017). Stress and coping in couples facing infertility. *Current Opinion in Psychology, 13*, 131–135.

Qian, Y., Xia, X. R., Ochin, H., et al. (2017). Therapeutic effect of acupuncture on the outcomes of in vitro fertilization: A systematic review and meta-analysis. *Archives of Gynecology and Obstetrics, 295*(3), 543–558.

Sandher, R. K., & Aning, J. (2017). Diagnosing and treating androgen deficiency in men. *Practitioner, 261*(1803), 19–22.

Showell, M. G., Mackenzie-Proctor, R., Jordan, V., et al. (2017). Antioxidants for female subfertility. *Cochrane Database of Systemic Reviews, 7, CD007807, 2017*(7).

Toosi, M., Azbarzadeh, M., & Ghaemi, Z. (2017). The effect of relaxation on mother's anxiety and maternal-fetal attachment in primiparous IVF mothers. *Journal of the National Medical Association, 109*(3), 164–171.

Zegers-Hochschild, F., Adamson, G. D., Dyer, S., et al. (2017). The international glossary on infertility and fertility care, 2017. *Human Reproduction, 32*(9): 1786–1801.

10

Problems of the Breast

Ann Schreier

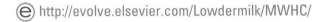

http://evolve.elsevier.com/Lowdermilk/MWHC/

LEARNING OBJECTIVES

- Discuss the pathophysiology of both benign and malignant breast disease affecting women throughout the life cycle.
- Design a nursing plan of care for the woman with a benign breast disorder.
- Understand the relevance and application of assessing risk for the development of breast cancer.

- Evaluate treatment alternatives for women with breast cancer.
- Integrate critical elements for teaching clients who have undergone medical-surgical management of malignant neoplasms of the breast.
- Examine survivorship issues for the woman and her family after treatment for breast cancer.

Problems of the breast affect women throughout most of their lives; starting at early ages with variances in breast development, through the naturally occurring changes related to aging, gaining weight, or becoming pregnant. These changes continue through menopause. Variables that can affect these changes include certain foods or hormones, both endogenous and exogenous. There are variations in the presentation and management of benign breast diseases. Understanding breast disease, along with understanding how to recognize and address risk factors, is not only critical for a woman's care, but also vital in ensuring that adequate breast cancer prevention strategies are used.

This chapter explores breast conditions, including benign and malignant breast diseases, and how breast cancer diagnosis and treatment affect women of all age groups. The unique complexities of the very young and the recent changes to care of older women are addressed. Relevant survivorship issues are discussed with implications for primary women's health care.

Nurses, as important advocates in the interprofessional health care team, provide expertise through direct care, education, support, and advocacy. They teach women about breast disease and cancer. They provide support and advocacy through the actual nursing care delivered, which includes holistic attention to all biopsychosocial and spiritual issues in helping women and their families achieve quality outcomes.

BENIGN CONDITIONS OF THE BREAST

Anatomy and physiology of the normal breast is discussed in Chapter 4. The following text focuses on the normal variations of the breasts and the most common benign breast conditions.

Anatomic Variances
Micromastia and Macromastia
Micromastia, or underdevelopment of breast tissue, is a congenital condition that can affect a woman's self-esteem. Augmentation may be done to correct the variant in development, but usually it is not done until breast development is complete. Because this procedure usually is considered to be cosmetic, it may not be covered by all insurance companies. However, if there is documentation of a congenital abnormality, it might be covered.

Macromastia, or breast hyperplasia, is a condition in which women have very large, heavy, and pendulous breasts. Like the former condition, it is not usually corrected by a plastic surgeon until after complete breast development and then only if the woman chooses to have this procedure. If done too early, the breast can continue to grow after reduction. Breast reduction mammoplasty can improve symptoms including pain in the neck, shoulders and back (Perez-Panzano, Guemes-Sanchez, & Gascon-Catalan, 2016). It should be noted that if reduction is done, breastfeeding later in life might be difficult due to removal of glandular tissue, interference with the ductal system, and nerve damage. In addition, there can be decreased nipple sensation or pain secondary to scar tissue.

Developmental Anomalies

Asymmetric breast development is often seen in adolescent women and is a normal variation unless a palpable abnormality is detected. The nurse can offer reassurance that most often breast symmetry occurs at maturity (Kriebs, 2017). A teenager may choose a prosthetic to achieve symmetry until she is fully matured. Breast asymmetry, especially if the breasts are tubular in appearance, can indicate a lack of glandular tissue. This is often associated with insufficient milk production in lactating women.

Supernumerary nipples or breasts are fairly common anomalies that are found along the breast or milk lines that go from the axilla to the groin area. Usually there is no treatment recommended, but if the extra nipples or breast tissue is bothersome, it can be removed surgically (De Silva, 2017).

Pathophysiology of Benign Breast Disease

In defining breast disorders from a pathologic standpoint, they are best understood as a heterogeneous group of lesions that may represent a palpable mass, a nonpalpable abnormality on imaging, or an incidental microscopic finding discovered during surgery. The two goals in the pathologic evaluation of a breast biopsy are to distinguish benign from malignant in situ or invasive tumors of the breast and to assess the risk of subsequent breast cancer associated with the lesion.

Nonproliferative lesions, including cysts, papillary apocrine change, epithelial calcifications (on mammography), or hyperplasia of the usual type, are not associated with an increased risk for breast cancer

(Kriebs, 2017). Proliferative lesions without atypia include intraductal papilloma, moderate hyperplasia, sclerosing adenosis, radial scar, and fibroadenomas. The estimated elevated risk for breast cancer is 1.2 to 2 times that of women who do not have these lesions (Orr & Kelley, 2016). Atypical hyperplasias are defined as proliferative lesions that possess some, but not all the features of carcinoma in situ. Atypical ductal hyperplasia (ADH) and atypical lobular hyperplasia (ALH) are the two most common, with a risk factor 4 to 5 times greater for developing breast cancer (Sasaki, Geletzke, Krass, et al., 2018).

Fibrocystic Changes

The most common benign breast problem is fibrocystic change, found in varying degrees in healthy women's breasts (De Silva, 2017). Fibrocystic changes are characterized by lumpiness, with or without tenderness, in both breasts (Orr & Kelley, 2016). A fibrocystic breast condition involves the glandular breast tissue. The sole known biologic function of these glands is the production and secretion of milk. The histologic findings associated with fibrocystic changes are part of the spectrum of normal involutional patterns of the breast (Sasaki et al., 2018).

Etiology. Fibrocystic changes tend to appear most commonly in women between the ages of 20 and 50 (Kriebs, 2017). The most significant contributing factor to a fibrocystic breast condition is a woman's normal hormonal variation during her monthly cycle. Many hormonal changes occur as a woman's body prepares each month for a possible pregnancy. The most important of these hormones are estrogen and progesterone, which directly affect the breast tissues by causing cells to proliferate. Other hormones, however, also play an important role in fibrocystic changes. Prolactin, growth factor, insulin, and thyroid hormones can affect cell growth within the breast tissue.

Clinical manifestations and diagnosis. The usual clinical presentation of fibrocystic change is lumpiness in both breasts; however, single simple cysts also can occur. Symptoms usually develop about a week before menstruation begins and subside about a week after menstruation ends. They include dull heavy pain and a sense of fullness and tenderness, often in the upper outer quadrants of the breasts, that increases in the premenstrual period. Physical examination may reveal excessive nodularity. Women in their 20s report the most severe pain. Women in their 30s have premenstrual pain and tenderness; small multiple nodules are usually present. Women in their 40s usually do not report severe pain, but cysts will be tender and often regress in size. The woman with fibrocystic change can form cysts that manifest as painful enlarging lumps in her breasts. Cysts are common in premenopausal women who are not receiving estrogen therapy and approximately one in three women experience a cyst between the ages of 35 and 50 (Kriebs, 2017). The cysts are soft on palpation, well differentiated, and movable. Deeper cysts, especially aggregations of cysts, are indistinguishable by palpation from carcinomas, which are malignant growths that infiltrate surrounding tissue.

A first diagnostic step of a breast lump is ultrasonography to determine if it is fluid filled or solid (Orr & Kelley, 2016). Fluid-filled cysts are aspirated, and the woman is monitored on a routine basis for development of other cysts. If the lump is solid and the woman is older than 35 years, mammography is obtained. A fine-needle aspiration (FNA) is a cost-effective procedure but currently core needle biopsies are preferred for suspicious lumps (Obeng-Gyasi et al., 2018).

Therapeutic management. Treatment for fibrocystic changes is usually conservative. Management can depend on the severity of the symptoms. Dietary changes and vitamin supplementation are one management approach. Although research findings are contradictory, some practitioners advocate reducing consumption of or eliminating fat methylxanthines (i.e., colas, coffee, tea, chocolate) (Kriebs, 2017). Some symptom relief may be achieved by refraining from both smoking and consuming alcohol. Recommended pain relief measures include analgesics or nonsteroidal antiinflammatory drugs (NSAIDs) such as ibuprofen, wearing a supportive bra, and applying heat to the breasts.

Most women report relief while taking oral contraceptives (De Silva, 2017). Danazol and tamoxifen have also been used with varying degrees of success for severe cases (Sasaki et al., 2018). Evening primrose oil can be effective for some women, although adequate evidence is lacking. It is important to stress that women may need to try several approaches for a number of months before noting improvement. Surgical removal of nodules is attempted only in rare cases. In the presence of multiple nodules, the surgical approach involves multiple incisions and tissue manipulation and may not prevent the development of more nodules.

Breast Pain (Mastalgia)

Breast pain occurs in many women at some time in their reproductive years, especially the perimenopausal years. The symptom of breast pain commonly is associated with fibrocystic changes that were previously discussed. Breast pain is unusual in breast cancer and, if it is present, is more likely (though uncommon) only in a locally advanced breast cancer. This is important information because many women fear that their breast pain is a symptom of cancer. However, if a woman is over 35, has a first degree relative with a history of breast cancer, and other risk factors, breast imaging is recommended (Kriebs, 2017). The character and pattern of breast pain are important in understanding how to manage this symptom. It is important to distinguish between cyclic versus noncyclic, and diffuse versus focal. Patterns can clue one into whether or not the pain is hormonal or related to a specific etiology—a cyst or trauma from external injury or surgery (Orr & Kelley, 2016).

Diagnostic procedures may include serologic tests for prolactin and human chorionic gonadotropin (hCG) levels in premenopausal women, ultrasound, mammography, and aspiration and biopsy for cysts. Treatment depends on the cause of the pain, the severity of pain and may include the measures described for pain relief related to fibrocystic changes such as dietary changes (reduced fat and methylxanthine intake), NSAIDs, hormone treatment (danazol), and evening primrose (Kriebs, 2017; Sasaki et al., 2018).

Solid Masses

A benign solid mass in contrast to a cystic mass has no fluid component. It is generally described as a smooth, round, mobile, painless lesion that is discrete on palpation. It is a pseudoencapsulated or multilobulated lesion that originates in the stroma of the breast. Solid benign masses in this category with no associated increased risk for breast cancer include fibroadenomas, radial scar, granular cell tumor, fibromatosis, pseudoangiomatous stromal hyperplasia (PASH), and hamartoma. Lipoma, a fatty tumor, is also common, whereas hemangiomas or vascular lesions are less common.

Fibroadenoma. The most common solid mass of the breast is a fibroadenoma. It is the single most common type of tumor seen in the adolescent population, although it can also occur in women in their 20s and 30s (Orr & Kelley, 2016). Fibroadenomas are discrete, usually solitary lumps less than 3 cm in diameter (Kriebs, 2017). Occasionally the woman with a fibroadenoma experiences tenderness in the tumor during the menstrual cycle. Fibroadenomas do not increase in size in response to the menstrual cycle (in contrast to fibrocystic lesions). The mass tends to remain the same size or increase in size slowly over time. Fibroadenomas increase in size during pregnancy and decrease in size as a woman ages. Diagnosis is made by a review of the client history and physical examination. Mammography, ultrasonography, or magnetic resonance imaging (MRI); and core needle biopsies may be used to determine the type of lesion. Surgical excision may be necessary if the lump is suspicious or if the symptoms are severe. Fibroadenomas do not respond to either dietary changes or hormonal therapy. Periodic observation of masses through physical examination or mammography may be all that is necessary for those masses not requiring surgical intervention (Sasaki et al., 2018).

Reactive Inflammatory Lesions

Mammary duct ectasia is the most common benign lesion in this category. Granulomatous mastitis is a rare cause for inflammation. It is characterized by granuloma and abscess formation and occurs most frequently in women over 60 (Sasaki et al., 2018). Other reactive inflammatory lesions include fat necrosis, which results from trauma to the fatty tissue of the breast; Mondor disease, which is phlebitis secondary to trauma; and diabetic mastopathy, which is an autoimmune, painful fibrotic mass commonly seen in women who are insulin dependent.

Mammary Duct Ectasia

Mammary duct ectasia characterized by dilated ducts and nipple inversion (acquired, not congenital) most commonly presents during the perimenopausal period. It is not common in postmenopausal years. The incidence is higher in women who smoke or who have diabetes. Pathologically, the ducts are dilated with thick walls. Ducts fill with epithelial secretions and common skin bacteria may enter the duct, causing mastitis. There is fibrotic stroma, rupture, and leakage of secretion into surrounding tissue that results in inflammation and fat necrosis. Characteristic signs include pain, redness of the skin, nipple inversion, and greenish nipple discharge. Fever can be present or absent. The breast tissue is thickened and inflamed, suggestive of mastitis, but abscess formation is also possible. Management includes pain medication and antibiotics. Applying heat to the breast, wearing a supportive bra, and sleeping on the unaffected side may provide comfort. It may be necessary to wear a breast pad if leaking occurs. A surgical incision and drainage are usually performed for an abscess. Recurrence rates are higher in women who smoke (Kriebs, 2017).

Nipple Discharge

Nipple discharge is a common occurrence that concerns many women. Though most nipple discharge is physiologic, each woman who presents with this problem must be evaluated carefully because in a small percentage of women, nipple discharge can be related to a serious endocrine disorder or malignancy. Bilateral serous discharge from multiple ducts, expressed during nipple stimulation, can be considered a normal finding. Spontaneous discharge, bloody discharge, or discharge from only one or two ducts must be evaluated (Kriebs, 2017).

One form of nipple discharge not related to malignancy is galactorrhea, a bilaterally spontaneous, milky, sticky discharge. It is a normal finding in pregnancy. Galactorrhea can also occur as the result of elevated prolactin levels. Increased prolactin levels can be a result of a thyroid disorder, pituitary tumor, coitus, eating, stress, trauma, or chest wall surgery. Obtaining a complete medical history on each woman is essential. Certain medications may precipitate galactorrhea. Some tranquilizers (i.e., tricyclic antidepressants), opiates, antihypertensive medications, and oral contraceptives can precipitate galactorrhea (Kriebs, 2017). Diagnostic tests include a prolactin level, a microscopic analysis of the discharge from each breast, a thyroid profile, a pregnancy test, and a mammogram. Ideally, prolactin levels should not be drawn directly after a breast examination, sexual activity, or exercise because these activities may increase the levels above the normal range.

Nipple discharge ranges from milky white to bloody and can be green or brown. Nipple discharge after menopause and in a single breast elevates the concern for a cancer diagnosis (Kriebs, 2017). Further diagnostic testing is recommended and biopsy may be warranted.

Intraductal Papilloma

Intraductal papilloma is a relatively rare, benign condition that develops in the terminal nipple ducts. The cause is unknown. It usually occurs in women between ages 30 and 50. Papillomas are usually too small to be palpated (<0.5 cm), and present with the characteristic sign of serous, serosanguineous, or bloody nipple discharge. The discharge is unilateral and spontaneous. A ductogram (imaging technique to evaluate lesions causing nipple discharge) is a common way of making the diagnosis, along with mammography and core biopsy. Because of the risk of a malignancy, surgical excision of the papilloma is recommended (Orr & Kelley, 2016).

Table 10.1 compares common manifestations of benign breast masses.

Infections of the Breast

Cellulitis with and without abscess formation is very common in women in most age groups but uncommon in younger adolescent girls. The at-risk population has some shared characteristics such as obesity, large breasts, previous surgeries, radiation, sebaceous cysts of the chest and axillae, smoking, and diabetes (Orr & Kelley, 2016). Nipple piercing has been associated with infection and abscess formation (Kriebs, 2017). The most common pathogen is *Staphylococcus aureus;* however,

TABLE 10.1 Comparison of Common Manifestations of Benign Breast Masses

Fibrocystic Changes	Fibroadenoma	Lipoma	Intraductal Papilloma	Mammary Duct Ectasia
Multiple lumps	Single lump	Single lump	Nonpalpable	Mass behind nipple
Nodular	Well delineated	Well defined	Not well delineated	Not well delineated
Palpable	Palpable	Palpable	Nonpalpable	Palpable
Movable	Movable	Movable	Nonmobile	Nonmobile
Round, smooth	Round, lobular	Round, lobular	Small, sometimes multiple	Irregular
Firm or soft	Firm	Soft	Firm or soft	Firm
Tenderness influenced by menstrual cycle	Usually asymptomatic	Nontender	Usually nontender	Painful, burning, itching
Bilateral	Unilateral	Unilateral	Unilateral	Unilateral
May or may not have nipple discharge	No nipple discharge	No nipple discharge	Serous or bloody nipple discharge	Thick, sticky nipple discharge

methicillin-resistant *Staphylococcus aureus* (MRSA) is becoming prevalent. Cellulitis of the breast presents as painful, red inflamed skin that is usually thickened. It feels warm or hot to touch. Abscess is present when there is a ballotable mass associated with these symptoms. Ultrasound images show a mixed fluid collection. If abscess is present, it can be managed by percutaneous ultrasound aspiration or, if large enough, incision and drainage. Treatment for cellulitis usually includes antibiotics.

Lactational infections are similar to cellulitis, except they occur during pregnancy and postpartum. Mastitis is discussed in Chapters 25 and 33.

 CLINICAL REASONING CASE STUDY

Breast Cancer Treatment Options

Susan is a 36-year-old with stage I breast cancer. Her family history includes her mother being diagnosed with breast cancer at age 55 and her maternal aunt diagnosed with ovarian cancer at age 48. Both succumbed to their diseases. Her menstrual periods started at age 11. She has one sibling, a sister, age 40, who has had no breast health issues. Susan is divorced, has two young children, both in elementary school, and is employed full-time as a dental assistant. She states that she is scared and doesn't want to have a mastectomy but thinks she should because she has heard that is the best treatment for long-term survival. How would you respond to this statement?

1. What is the priority concern or client need in this situation?
2. List other client needs/problems in this care.
3. What nursing actions are appropriate in this situation?
   a. What is priority nursing action?
   b. Describe other nursing interventions that are important to providing optimum care.
4. Describe the roles/responsibilities of the interprofessional health care team members who may be involved in providing care for this client.

 ## CARE MANAGEMENT FOR WOMEN WITH BENIGN BREAST CONDITIONS

Assessment of the woman with a benign breast condition should include a careful history and physical examination. The history should focus on the woman's risk factors for breast diseases, events related to the breast mass, and health maintenance practices. (Risk factors for breast cancer are discussed later in this chapter.) Information related to the breast symptoms should include how, when, and by whom the symptoms were discovered. The interval between discovery and seeking care is crucial. The following client information is documented: presence of pain, whether symptoms increase with menses, dietary habits, smoking habits, use of oral contraceptives or hormone replacement therapy, personal history of breast cancer, and family history of breast cancer. Both the American Cancer Society (ACS, 2019d) and Susan G. Komen Foundation (2017a) no longer recommend breast self-exams (BSE). It is important for the nurse to be aware, however, that many women discover breast cancer symptoms (e.g., lump) through regular daily activities. Therefore, women should be encouraged to be familiar with their breasts. Some women desire to learn BSE and nurses can provide this teaching (Kriebs, 2017). The woman's emotional status, including her stress level, fears, and concerns, and her ability to cope also should be assessed.

Physical examination may include assessment of the breasts for symmetry, masses (size, number, consistency, mobility), and nipple discharge.

Nursing actions might include the following:

- Discuss the intervals for and facets of breast screening, including professional examination and mammography (Table 10.2). Women with breast implants may need special views (called push backs) of the breast, and precautions taken not to rupture the implant during mammography.
- Provide written educational materials and refer to reliable web sites.
- Encourage the verbalization of fears and concerns about treatment and prognosis.
- Provide specific information regarding the woman's condition and treatment, including dietary changes, drug therapy, comfort measures, complementary and alternative therapies, stress management, and surgery.
- Demonstrate correct BSE technique if a woman desires to practice it (see Teaching for Self-Management box: Breast Self-Examination in Chapter 4).
- Describe pain-relieving strategies in detail, and collaborate with the primary health care provider to ensure effective pain control.
- Encourage discussion of feelings about body image.
- Refer to a stress management resource if needed to cope with long-term consequences of benign breast conditions.

TABLE 10.2	Screening Guidelines for Early Breast Cancer Detection	
Age (Years)	**Examination**	**Frequency**
Average Risk for Asymptomatic Women		
20-39	No specific examinations recommended	
40-44	Mammography	Optional to begin yearly
45-54	Mammography	Yearly
55 and older	Mammography	Every other year
High-Risk Women (>20% Lifetime Risk, Known BRCA1 or BRCA2 Mutation)		
30 and older[a]	MRI and mammogram	Yearly

[a]The best age to start should be decided between health care provider and woman after looking at her individual status.
MRI, Magnetic resonance imaging.
Modified from American Cancer Society. (2017a). *American Cancer Society recommendations for early detection of brest cancer.* Retrieved from: https://www.cancer.org/cancer/breast-cancer/screening-tests-and-early-detection/american-cancer-society-recommendations-for-the-early-detection-of-breast-cancer.html.

MALIGNANT CONDITIONS OF THE BREAST

Breast cancer is the most common cancer, other than skin cancers, with an estimated 268,600 women anticipated to be diagnosed with breast cancer in 2019 (ACS, 2019c). Non-Hispanic white women have a higher incidence than other racial/ethnic groups, but mortality rates are higher among black women. The incidence has decreased since the year 2000 and is now stable at 1:8 women at risk for breast cancer (ACS, 2019c). Statistics suggest that about 79% of breast cancers are found in women over the age of 50. There are 3.1 million survivors of breast cancer, with statistics indicating a survival rate of 83% at 10 years after diagnosis (ACS, 2019c), which has implications for women's primary health care and prevention of second malignancies. Although the exact cause for breast cancer remains unknown, at least 15% are related to a genetic mutation.

Etiology of Breast Cancer and Risk Factors

The risk factors are considered a mosaic of statistical data points that, when put together and used correctly, can help one understand which groups of women need more heightened surveillance in high-risk clinics or referral to a genetic counselor for genetic testing. Some risk factors cannot change, such as gender, age, the time of menarche, menopause, and time of first live birth. The length of time on unopposed estrogen is a significant risk factor. Having a personal history of breast cancer is a constant risk factor, leading to a risk for developing a second malignancy. Breast cancer affects predominantly women, but 1% of all breast cancers occur in men. Geographic differences are related to breast cancer risk. For instance, when women from Japan, where there is one of the lowest rates of breast cancer, move to Western countries, their risk equalizes to that of the native population. Whether this is due to diet or other environmental exposure is not yet clear but may be a combination of the two. Experiencing a first pregnancy after age 40 is another risk factor. Having fibrocystic disease with any of the previously discussed proliferative diseases with atypia increases one's risk fourfold. Higher breast density may make interpretation of mammography more difficult. Legislation has mandated that radiologists need to communicate this information to women, probably more as a liability protection.

Relative factors such as maintaining one's ideal body weight is important in that heavier women have higher circulating estrogens and that regular exercise reduces risk by about 20%. Dietary risk factors include high saturated fats and moderate to high alcohol consumption. The use of exogenous hormones such as oral contraception or hormone replacement for postmenopausal support becomes a risk factor when used for more than 10 years. Diethylstilbestrol (DES), a drug used years ago to maintain pregnancy, is slightly correlated with elevated risk.

Genetic Considerations

Having a genetic mutation, either BRCA1 or BRCA2, may create an 85% chance of developing breast cancer in a woman's lifetime. There are other mutations such as the Li-Fraumeni syndrome and Cowden syndrome, which have different family pedigrees. Genetic testing is complex and it is very important that this be done in conjunction with genetic counseling. Not all women with family history of cancer are at risk, and there are statistical models that help determine the risk-benefit ratio of testing for a genetic mutation. Also, if the estimated risk determines that there is probability for a mutation, it is suggested that the living family member with breast cancer be tested first. This helps validate whether additional testing is needed in the family. After testing, if the result is negative, the genetics team can determine the tested family members' estimated risk for subsequent development of breast cancer. This information uniquely tailors surveillance for women who remain at greater than a 20% risk. Women and men who carry a mutation have

---

> **BOX 10.1 Risk Factors Included in the Breast Cancer Risk Assessment Tool**
>
> - Woman's age
> - Number of first-degree relatives affected
> - Age of woman at menarche
> - Age of woman at first live birth
> - Number of breast biopsies
> - History of atypical hyperplasia in biopsy specimens

choices to make in how they manage their lives. They can be followed in a dedicated high-risk clinic with biannual clinical breast examinations by an expert, along with imaging that may include diagnostic mammography and breast MRI (National Cancer Institute [NCI], 2018a).

The Breast Cancer Risk Assessment Tool (Gail Model), a risk calculator used in the first- and second-generation national prevention trials, can quantify risk for development of breast cancer at 5 years and then a lifetime risk (up to age 90). (Risk factors are listed in Box 10.1; the tool is available at www.cancer.gov/bcrisktool.)

Chemoprevention

Some drugs are used for prevention of breast cancer, although research is ongoing to test their efficacy. Current evidence and clinical guidelines suggest that women at increased risk for estrogen receptor positive breast cancer or carriers of BRCA1 or BRCA2 mutations can be offered chemoprevention with either tamoxifen or raloxifene (Vogel, 2018). Both these drugs are taken once daily, but have very different side effect profiles. Tamoxifen can cause hot flashes, weight gain, cataracts, chemical hepatitis, and blood clots and carries a small risk for uterine cancer. Because there is an increased risk of uterine cancers with tamoxifen, regular clinical follow-up is needed (Vogel, 2018). Raloxifene can contribute to heart disease or stroke. Raloxifene is a good choice for healthier women who might be at risk for osteopenia. Tamoxifen is available for pre- and postmenopausal women, whereas raloxifene is available only for postmenopausal women. (See Medication Guides later in this chapter.) Providing comprehensive information on these drugs helps women to make informed decisions, empowering them to take charge of their lives.

Pathophysiology of Malignant Breast Disease

Although breast cancer presents within the breast, it is, in fact, considered to be a systemic disease because as it is growing in the breast, invasive tumors have the capability of traveling elsewhere in the body. Tumors are classified by location in the breast and histological type (NCI, 2018b). Generally breast cancer is either ductal or lobular. Genetic alterations, either inherited or spontaneous, are found in the epithelial cells, compromising ductal or lobular tissue.

By far the most frequently occurring cancer of the breast is invasive ductal carcinoma. Ductal carcinoma originates in the lactiferous ducts and invades surrounding breast structures. The tumor is usually unilateral, not well delineated, solid, nonmobile, and nontender.

Lobular carcinoma originates in the lobules of the breasts. This type of breast cancer can be nonpalpable and appear smaller on imaging studies than its actual size.

Nipple carcinoma (Paget disease) originates in the nipple. It usually occurs with invasive ductal carcinoma and can cause bleeding, oozing, and crusting of the nipple.

A rarer form of breast cancer is known as inflammatory breast cancer, which is diagnosed by the appearance of a rash or reddish skin of the breast. It can be misdiagnosed as mastitis. A skin punch biopsy

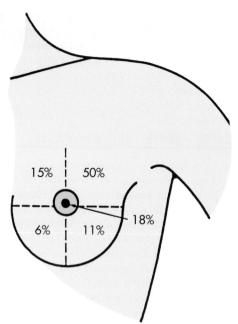

Fig. 10.1 Relative Location of Malignant Lesions of the Breast. (Modified from DiSaia, P., & Creasman, W. [2007]. *Clinical gynecologic oncology* [7th ed.]. St. Louis: Mosby.)

TABLE 10.3 **Staging of Breast Cancer**
After a diagnosis of breast cancer is established, the stage of the cancer is then determined.
Staging is based on the following 3 factors:
The TNM System, which consists of:
Size and location of the Tumor (T)
Size and location of Lymph Nodes (N), indicating that cancer has spread to nodes
Presence of Metastasis (M), indicating spread of cancer to other parts of the body
The Grading System, which consists of:
Likelihood of the cancer growing and spreading to other parts of the body
The Biomarker Testing, which consists of:
Determination of whether cancer cells have certain receptors within the body

From National Cancer Institute (2018). Breast cancer treatment (PDQ)—patient version. Retrieved from: https://www.cancer.gov/types/breast/patient/breast-treatment-pdq.

is performed, and the pathology report will state that there are breast cancer cells in the dermal lymphatic channels. It is usually aggressive and is classified as stage II breast cancer from its onset. There are also other types of less common forms of breast cancers such as mucinous and malignant phyllodes tumors.

Breast cancer can invade surrounding tissues in such a way that the primary tumor can have tentacle-like projections (referred to as being a spiculated mass). This invasive growth pattern can result in the irregular tumor border felt on palpation. As the tumor grows, fibrosis develops around it and can shorten Cooper ligaments, which results in the characteristic peau d'orange (orange peel–like skin) changes and edema associated with some breast cancers. If the breast cancer invades the lymphatic channels, tumors can develop in the regional lymph nodes, often occupying the axillary lymph nodes. The tumor may invade the outer layers of skin, creating ulcerations. Fig. 10.1 indicates the portions of the breast where most breast cancers originate.

The rate of breast cancer growth depends on the effects of estrogen and progesterone and other prognostic factors such as its grade, Ki67 score (a proliferative marker), human epidermal growth factor receptor 2 (HER2)/neu receptor status, and other variables. For purpose of prognosis, three subtypes are identified: Hormone receptor positive, HER2 positive, and triple negative (ER, PR, HER2/neu negative). To determine the likelihood of recurrence and metastasis, two genetic profile tests may be performed (Oncotype DX and MammaPrint). With results from these tests, clinicians can identify those who will benefit from adjuvant chemotherapy (NCI, 2018b).

Metastasis results from seeding of the breast cancer cells into the blood and lymph systems, leading to tumor development in the bones, the lungs, the brain, and the liver. Breast cancer can be small or large—the size does not always equate with aggressiveness. Some aggressive small tumors spread quickly, and some large tumors spread very slowly.

Clinical Manifestations and Diagnosis

When breast cancer is detected either as a palpable lump or ill-defined thickening in the breast, it is usually painless. One might see nipple retraction, skin dimpling or skin changes to the nipple, or redness with edema and pitting of the skin, which is suggestive of a locally advanced and aggressive form of breast cancer. Lymph nodes are always clinically examined to determine extent of the clinical stage. Clinical staging helps to understand the parameters of the breast problem and whether lymph node involvement is suspected. The clinical stage is what helps providers decide on how to proceed with treatment. This stage is determined by a combination of the TNM system, the grading system, and a biomarker determination (NCI, 2018a) (Table 10.3). It sorts stage by size of *t*umor, lymph *n*ode, and whether *m*etastasis is involved. It is the pathologic stage, which is determined after surgery, that really correlates with overall prognosis and one's risk for recurrence at 2, 5, or 10 years.

Screening

Guidelines for breast cancer screening continue to evolve as new evidence is generated. BSE, once standard, has been scrutinized for its benefit in early detection and overall survival and is no longer recommended as a monthly examination (ACS, 2019d). Clinical breast examinations are omitted by many clinicians, evidenced by lack of documentation in medical records and by client reports that this is not part of an annual examination. These two factors are significant in that women are often referred to breast clinics prematurely by their health care providers because there is a lack of understanding of normal variation versus real disease. Guidelines for screening mammography have changed. While the U.S. Preventive Services Task Force (2016) recommends baseline mammography in average risk women at age 50, and then every 2 years, there is lack of consensus on these guidelines. For example, the ACS (2019d) continues to recommend that women may opt for mammography beginning at age 40 and annually. Nelson, Cantor, Humphrey, et al. (2016) concluded from a review of mammography screening trials and observational studies that mammography between ages of 40 and 69 results in a reduced mortality and detection of early stage breast cancer. However, there are a greater number of false positives particularly for women between ages of 40 and 49 and some overtreatment occurs. Screening studies include primarily white women and results are not applicable to minorities. The nurse should keep in mind that those women at increased risk need to consult with a health care provider for recommendations.

Screening guidelines based on risk are outlined in Table 10.2. Nurses are key to educating women about screening. There is growing evidence among geriatric oncologists of the need to comprehensively assess older women. Screening decisions are individually based on decisions between the woman and her health care provider.

When caring for a woman with breast cancer, as in all situations, her cultural and ethnic background must be taken into account (see the Cultural Considerations box).

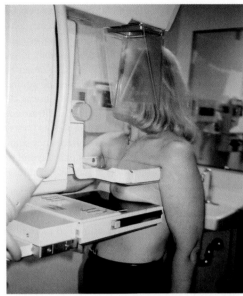

Fig. 10.2 Mammography. (Courtesy Shannon Perry, Phoenix, AZ.)

⊕ CULTURAL CONSIDERATIONS

Breast Screening Practices

Reasons for rates of screening for breast cancer vary across minority groups. For example, African-American women have reported feeling discomfort with impersonal care from providers and lack of support from the health care system.

Hispanic/Latina women may lack a regular health care provider and/or insurance coverage; they may lack accessibility to screening facilities and have difficulty taking time off work. Asian women may be unaware of mammography tests. Gender and modesty concerns that are common to their culture may prevent them from seeking screening. All women from various ethnic groups may experience "implicit bias" from health care providers.

Interventions that will encourage minority women to participate in early breast cancer screening practices begin with the development of culturally sensitive community education programs designed to help women overcome barriers to reaching optimal levels of health. Programs should be designed to educate small groups of women about risk factors for breast cancer, prevention strategies, and early detection methods. Recruitment of women may be communicated through fliers in neighborhoods, women's groups, churches, clubs, and organizations. Use of incentives to reward participation may be helpful. Nurses and guest speakers of similar ethnicity as the attending group who are breast cancer survivors are valuable in providing meaningful information and support, and providing past, present, and future perspective to the educational content. Nurses and all health care providers should learn about implicit bias that can occur in health care settings.

Data from Lee-lin, F., Pedhiwala, N., Nguyen, T., & Menon, U. (2015). Breast health intervention effects on knowledge and beliefs over time among Chinese American immigrants—a randomized controlled study. *Journal of Cancer Education, 30*(3), 482–489 and Torres, E., Richman, A. R., Schreier, A. M., et al. (2017). An evaluation of a rural community-based breast education and navigation program: Highlights and lessons learned. *Journal of Cancer Education.*

Mammography

Mammography remains the gold standard for breast cancer screening and early detection. New technologies that are considered for breast cancer screening must equal or exceed the performance of screen-film mammography to be accepted as screening tools. In other words, these technologies must demonstrate identification of more breast cancers that are missed by mammography, such as a higher fraction of early-stage cancers (stages 0 and I), and be cost-effective, noninvasive, and available and acceptable to clients. Full-field digital mammography (FFDM) is much like standard film mammography in that x-rays are used to produce an image of the breast. Digital mammogram is standard screening (Bassett & Lee-Felker, 2018).

Breast tomosynthesis or three-dimensional (3D) mammography is often recommended for women less than 50 years old, for women with high-density breasts, or for women who are not yet menopausal or have been in menopause for less than a year. For women in these groups, 3D mammography detects more abnormalities that would otherwise go undetected, and results in fewer false positives. These images enable the radiologist to enlarge the image as well as lighten and darken the background contrast and to find abnormalities that may go undetected with film mammography. An additional method to assist radiologists with reading mammograms, which can be important for facilities that do not have dedicated breast imaging radiologists, is computer-aided detection (CAD). For nearly two decades this device has been in use to help radiologists find suspicious changes on mammography studies. This can be especially important for film mammography evaluation. CAD electronically scans the mammogram first. It can detect tumors or other breast abnormalities and flag them for the radiologist to further investigate (Bassett & Lee-Felker, 2018).

A screening mammogram (Fig. 10.2) is performed on women who do not have any signs or symptoms of a breast abnormality. Diagnostic mammograms are performed when a screening mammogram identifies something warranting further inspection or if the woman, her health care provider or nurse finds a sign such as a lump, nipple discharge, or other breast symptom that is new.

One of the most valuable uses of mammography is the identification of calcifications within the breast. Though most are benign, some can be an early sign of breast cancer. There are two types of calcifications:

- Macrocalcifications—mineral deposits that are most likely changes in the breast caused by aging of the breast arteries, old injuries, or inflammation. They appear as large white dots or dashes. These deposits are related to noncancerous conditions and do not require a biopsy. These types of calcifications are found in about half of women older than age 50 and in 1 in 10 women younger than 50.
- Microcalcifications—fine white specks of calcium in the breast. They may be alone or in clusters and resemble grains of sand or salt. These can be more concerning depending on their pattern and shape. Those that are tightly clustered together and have irregular edges can be a sign of ductal carcinoma in situ (DCIS) or early stage I breast cancer, and warrant biopsy.

Mammography does have its limitations. It has not proven helpful in screening younger women due to the high breast density associated with youth. Approximately 78% of breast cancer can be identified through mammography, although this number is increased to 83% among women older than age 50 (Susan G. Komen Foundation, 2017a). Ultrasound has become a valuable screening adjunct to mammography, especially for women with significant breast density. It is cost-effective, noninvasive, and widely available. Ultrasound has been helpful in distinguishing between fluid-filled masses (cysts) and solid masses (benign and malignant). It uses high-frequency sound waves to assess the breast tissue and axillae. The test is painless and noninvasive and requires no exposure to radiation. It has also been useful in performing image-guided biopsies (ACS, 2019d).

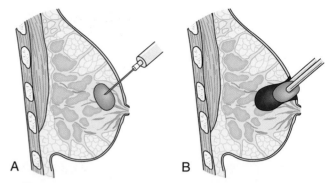

Fig. 10.3 Diagnosis. (A) Needle aspiration. (B) Open biopsy.

Magnetic Resonance Imaging

MRI has become a valuable screening adjunct to mammography and ultrasound. It may be useful in women with difficult-to-find masses, sometimes referred to as occult breast cancers. MRI is indicated for women who have silicone injects, at high risk for breast cancer, and those with a history of breast cancer (Bassett & Lee-Felker, 2018). There is growing popularity to use it for women diagnosed with breast cancer to rule out the presence of multicentric disease and determine the size of tumors (such as invasive lobular carcinomas), and it has been used increasingly for high-risk women (such as those who carry a BRCA gene mutation). It is not, however, without drawbacks. One concern with MRI is that although it helps find small, difficult-to-detect abnormalities, it has been found to lead to more unnecessary mastectomies instead of lumpectomies with radiation (Susan G. Komen, 2017b).

Positron emission tomography (PET) scans, which are based on glucose uptake metabolism, can help determine if breast cancer has spread to other parts of the body, identifying metastatic disease. Newer technologies for breast cancer screening are under development.

Biopsy

When a suspicious finding on a mammogram is noted or a lump is detected, diagnosis is confirmed by core needle biopsy (stereotactically or ultrasound-guided core) or by needle localization biopsy (Fig. 10.3). The latter procedure requires the collaborative efforts of both the radiologist and the surgeon. This often requires that the procedure take place in two different environments (radiology and surgery), so women need specific information regarding procedures, duration, and outcomes. In most facilities, core biopsies can be performed and the pathology results known the following day, providing the woman with rapid results. This is especially important because women are often highly anxious while waiting for biopsy results.

Prognosis

Nodal involvement and tumor size remain the most significant prognostic criteria for long-term survival (Fig. 10.4). Certain biologic factors include estrogen receptor assay, progesterone receptor assay, tumor *ploidy* (the amount of deoxyribonucleic acid [DNA] in a tumor cell compared with that in a normal cell), S-phase index or growth rate (the percentage of cells in the S phase of cellular division done by flow cytometric determinations of the S-phase fraction), Ki67 (another proliferation marker), and histologic or nuclear grade (Arciero & Styblo, 2018). Estrogen and progesterone receptors (ERs, PRs) are proteins in the cell cytoplasm and surface of some breast cancer cells. When these receptors are present, they bind to estrogen or progesterone, which promotes cancer cell

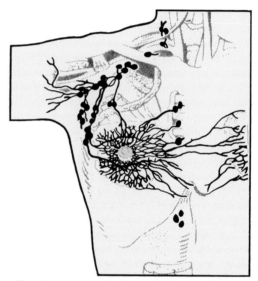

Fig. 10.4 Lymphatic Spread of Breast Cancer.

growth. A breast cancer can have ERs or PRs, or both. It is valuable to know the ER status of the cancer to predict which women will respond to hormone therapy (Arciero & Styblo). Molecular and biologic factors are valuable indicators for prognosis and treatment of breast cancer. HER2, which is associated with cell growth, is overexpressed in 30% of all breast cancers and is associated with loss of cell regulation and uncontrolled cell proliferation. Thus a positive HER2 status is associated with aggressive tumors, poor prognosis, and resistance to certain chemotherapeutic drugs (ACS, 2019a). Luminal A or B tumors are receptor-positive tumors and are for the most part less aggressive. Tumors expressing H2NU can be more aggressive. Tumors referred to as basal types or triple negative are tumors that have no receptors. The basal tumors are more aggressive and there are limited therapies, usually chemotherapy based.

CARE MANAGEMENT FOR WOMEN WITH BREAST CANCER

Breast cancer is treated in a variety of ways, using one or a combination of the following approaches: surgery, radiation, systemic therapies, and plastic surgical reconstruction. The specific treatment approach depends on the size of the abnormality and whether there is palpable lymph node involved. A woman with breast cancer is cared for by an interprofessional health care team consisting of surgeons, oncologists,

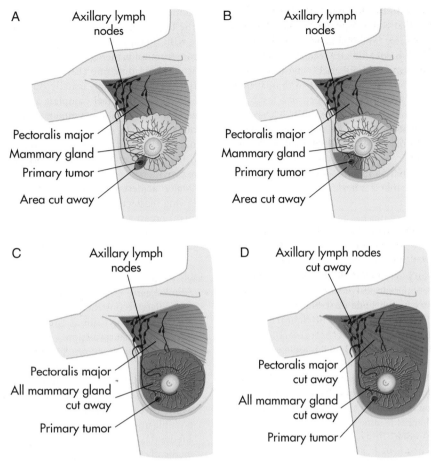

Fig. 10.5 Surgical Alternatives for Breast Cancer. (A) Lumpectomy. (B) Segmental mastectomy. (C) Total (simple) mastectomy. (D) Radical mastectomy.

radiologists, nurses, pharmacists, mental health providers, social workers, and others as needed.

Breast reconstruction, immediately with surgery or delayed, is usually an option for women with mastectomy. Delayed reconstruction is the preferred course for women with locally advanced disease that will most likely need radiation after mastectomy and those with a high chance of local recurrence. Immediate reconstruction is best suited to those women with noninvasive tumors or lymph node–negative disease.

Surgery

Surgical approaches for the treatment of breast cancer include breast-conserving surgery (BCS) and mastectomy. One option for BCS is **lumpectomy** (Fig 10.5A), which involves the removal of the small tumor and a rim of healthy tissue around it, to ensure clear margins. **Segmental mastectomy** (also called partial mastectomy) (see Fig. 10.5B), is another option, and includes *wide excision* and/or *quadrantectomy* and involves removal of the tumor, which may be larger, along with a rim of healthy tissue around it, to ensure clear margins.

BCS is used for the primary treatment of women with early-stage (I or II) breast cancer. The criteria for recommending BCS are as follows: a tumor that is relatively small compared to breast volume and will result in acceptable cosmetic outcome; no previous breast radiation; no previous mantle field radiation (area includes neck, chest, and underarm lymph nodes) as a youth; and no evidence of multicentric disease (Rivera, Klimberg, & Bland, 2018).

Mastectomy is the removal of the breast, including the nipple and areola. Women who are advised to have mastectomy instead of BCS are women who have:

- Had radiation to the breast
- Multiple tumors in the breast occupying several quadrants of the breast
- Invasive or extensive DCIS that occupies a large area of the breast tissue
- A large tumor compared to breast volume

There are several different types of mastectomies. These include:

- *Total simple mastectomy* (see Fig. 10.5C): This is removal of the breast, nipple, and areola. No lymph nodes from the axillae are taken. Recovery from this procedure, if no reconstruction is done at the same time, is usually 1 to 2 weeks. Hospitalization varies; for some it may be an outpatient procedure, whereas other women may require an overnight stay.
- *Modified radical mastectomy*: This procedure is removal of the breast, nipple, and areola as well as axillary node dissection. Recovery, when surgery is done without reconstruction, is usually 2 to 3 weeks.
- *Skin-sparing mastectomy*: This is the removal of the breast, nipple, and areola, keeping the outer skin of the breast intact. It is a special method of performing a mastectomy that allows for a good cosmetic outcome when combined with a reconstruction done at the same time. A tissue expander may also be placed as a space holder for later reconstruction.
- *Nipple-sparing mastectomy*: This kind of mastectomy is reserved for women with tumors that are not near the nipple areola area. The surgeon makes an incision on the outer side of the breast or around

the edge of the areola and hollows out the breast, removing the areola and keeping the nipple intact. Sometimes the completed reconstruction is performed at the same time, and in other cases a tissue expander is inserted as a space holder for later reconstruction.

- *Preventive/prophylactic mastectomy*: Prophylactic mastectomy is designed to remove one or both breasts in order to dramatically reduce the risk of developing breast cancer. Women who test positive for certain genetic mutations like BRCA1 and BRCA2, or who have a strong family history of breast cancer, may elect this kind of surgery. When this type of mastectomy is performed, no lymph nodes need to be removed because there is no evidence of cancer present. It is necessary to have a mammogram within 90 days before the procedure to ensure that it is healthy breast tissue being removed for preventive purposes.

If there is only one area of concern that has been biopsy-proven, and it is not so large that it occupies more than 50% of a woman's breast, then a BCS is an option. For tumors greater than 50% or multiple tumors that occupy other quadrants, total mastectomy is recommended.

Since breast cancer cells can migrate through the lymphatic tissue, axillary node biopsies are part of the surgical procedures. There are two types of node biopsies: axillary lymph node dissection (ALND) and sentinel lymph node biopsy (SLNB). When there is no clinical evidence of lymph node involvement in early stage breast cancer (I & II), SLNB is recommended (Yen, Laud, Pezzin, et al., 2018). SLNB reduces the risk of lymphedema subsequent to surgery. The sentinel node is the first node that receives lymphatic drainage from the tumor and is identified by injecting vital blue dye and radioactive dye in the area surrounding the tumor. A small incision in the axilla allows for identification of the blue-stained lymphatic channel leading to the blue sentinel node, both visually and by gamma probe. This node can then be removed and examined for the presence of tumor cells, as opposed to an entire axillary dissection. It is helpful to indicate whether nodes are positive for metastatic cells in determining the need for adjuvant systemic treatment. If the SLNB is positive, then an ALND will be performed.

For women who have a palpable lymph node that is suspected of malignancy, core biopsy of the lymph node confirms the histology. If the node has cancer, a traditional ALND at the time of her breast surgery is recommended. If the sentinel lymph node is positive, the next step will depend on how much tumor is present. The pathologic stage of the tumor combined with the lymph node biopsy determines the surgical options (e.g., lumpectomy versus mastectomy).

If a woman presents with a very large palpable locally advanced tumor, positive lymph node, or medium-sized tumor (3 cm or more) and BCS would deform her, then systemic therapy before surgery or neoadjuvant therapy is an option. This approach can downstage the tumor before surgery and, through this early systemic therapy, can prevent recurrence elsewhere. Women who choose BCS must have cancer-free margins following surgery, before proceeding to radiation treatment. Radiation treatments are 5 days a week, and the length of courses are variable (discussed in more detail later).

DCIS is an early form of noninvasive breast cancer. Although DCIS does not spread, it does require management. The surgical approach is usually a BCS (e.g., lumpectomy) followed by radiation. In invasive or extensive DCIS, segmental mastectomy with radiation or mastectomy may be recommended. If the actual tumor is small on mammogram, there is no need for lymph node assessment; if it is large, the woman may be advised to have SLNB because this procedure must be done before mastectomy. If an invasive tumor is found and no sentinel node biopsy was done, then she would be committed to an ALND.

Breast Reconstruction

The goals of surgical breast reconstruction are achievement of symmetry and preservation of body image. Surgical reconstruction can be done immediately or at a later date. Immediate reconstruction at the time of mastectomy does not change survival rates or interfere with therapy or the treatment of recurrent disease. Immediate reconstruction is increasingly the preferred option as it provides the best cosmetic outcome (Rivera et al., 2018). Women who opt for surgical reconstruction usually do so for one or more of the following reasons: to feel complete again, to avoid using an external prosthesis, to achieve symmetry, to decrease self-consciousness about appearance, and to enhance femininity. It is important to recognize that some women may choose not to have reconstruction and that choice must be supported by the nurse and other health care providers.

Major achievements have been made in breast reconstruction following mastectomy surgery. Plastic surgeons are able to rebuild a woman's breast with minimal scarring.

Women with breast cancer have two main considerations regarding reconstructive surgery—when to have surgery and what type of surgery to have. The options for when to have reconstruction are (Table 10.4):

- *Simultaneous reconstruction*: Women have the option to have immediate reconstruction of their breast(s) at the same time as their mastectomy. This is a reasonable option for women who do not need breast irradiation.
- *Delayed reconstruction*: A woman may opt for delayed reconstruction if, during her mastectomy, a plastic surgeon was not involved. Many women who did not know their options at the time of mastectomy fall into this category. More and more these women are discovering that surgically re-creating their breasts is possible and is required to be covered by insurance as a result of a federal law passed in 1998. Delayed reconstruction is preferred medically if the pathologic stage requires post-mastectomy radiation.

The types of surgical options for breast reconstruction include implants and flap procedures. Implants are made out of silicone or saline or a combination of both and can be inserted at the same time as a mastectomy, or later. They are placed underneath the chest muscle. Silicone implants have been deemed safe and are an option for women having breast reconstruction following mastectomy.

Flap procedures are done by plastic and reconstructive surgeons who specialize in microsurgery. During flap reconstruction a breast is created using tissue taken from other parts of the body, such as the abdomen, back, buttocks, or thighs, which is then transplanted to the chest by reconnecting the blood vessels to new ones in the chest region. Due to the high level of skill required for microsurgery, as well as the equipment and staff needed, these techniques are available only at specialized centers. Many health care settings are still using techniques that include transverse rectus abdominis myocutaneous (TRAM) flaps and latissimus dorsi flaps, which result in the woman sacrificing either her abdominal muscles or her upper back muscles. Although these procedures were the best options decades ago, they result in a higher risk of hernia, weakness, abdominal bulging, and limits on physical activity.

After a woman has recovered from initial reconstructive surgery, she may choose to have nipple and areolar reconstruction. Nipple reconstruction is achieved by using an autologous skin graft to construct a nipple, either from tissue from the remaining nipple or from a donor site. Tiny flaps from the new breast itself also may be used. This outpatient procedure requires local anesthesia, intravenous (IV) sedation, or a combination of both, depending on how much sensation has returned to the breast. The procedure lasts about an hour. Following this procedure, a woman may choose to have a tattoo to create an areola and match the color of the natural nipple.

TABLE 10.4   Reconstructive Breast Surgery Options

Name of Option	Brief Description	Advantages	Disadvantages
Simultaneous reconstruction	Reconstruction of the breast done at the same time as surgery to remove the cancer	• The woman wakes up with a breast mound already in place, having been spared the experience of seeing herself with no breast at all. • The process is done in the shortest time possible and is not a series of complex surgeries over a length of time.	• If there is a recurrence of the cancer, the reconstruction may need to be modified. • If there are postsurgery complications, the woman may need to have more surgeries. • Small revision surgeries or matching procedures on the opposing breast may be required. • Rarely it is determined that a woman will need radiation, which can compromise reconstructed breast tissue.
Staged reconstruction	This reconstruction involves placement of a temporary tissue expander at time of mastectomy. The expander gradually stretches the muscle and skin in preparation for either an implant or flap reconstruction.	• The surgeon creates a natural "pocket" in which a permanent implant or a tissue flap may be placed. • The overall result is more symmetric, natural, and aesthetically pleasing. • It allows a woman to complete radiation treatment while having a "placeholder" implanted. • It allows enough time to make sure all of the cancer has been treated.	• It takes longer to "complete" the breast cancer process. • During the time of temporary tissue expansion, the breasts do not look natural. • Small revision surgeries or matching procedures on the opposing breast may be required.
Delayed reconstruction	This reconstruction happens after all of the recommended treatment is completed.	• Some women are not comfortable weighing all the options at once when they are struggling with a diagnosis of cancer. • Some women need time to come to terms with losing their breast(s). • Some women who are overweight, smokers, or who have high blood pressure may be advised to wait. • It allows enough time to make sure all of the cancer has been treated.	• It takes longer to "complete" the breast cancer treatment. • Women may not feel whole without their breast(s).
Implant	A breast implant is a silicone shell filled with either silicone gel or saline.	• The recovery from the initial expander placement surgery and from the permanent implant placement surgery is usually quicker than flap surgery. • It may be easier to control the final size of the reconstructed breast with implant reconstruction. • There are no additional scars on the woman's body other than those on the breasts. • For women without excess fatty tissue and who do not require radiation treatment, implants are a good choice, one with good final results.	• Because most women require placement of an expander first followed by secondary replacement of the expander with an implant, this type of reconstruction almost always requires at least two surgical stages and multiple visits to the plastic surgeon's office between these stages for tissue expansion. • It is important to realize that for women who are having a unilateral (one-sided) mastectomy, matching the other natural breast with an implant can be difficult. The shape and feel of an implant are not exactly like that of a natural breast. • In the short term, implants can become infected or malpositioned and require surgery to correct these problems. • Implant-based reconstruction is not generally recommended if women require radiation, due to the risk of complications. In the longer term, implants can develop capsular contracture (tightening of the soft tissues around the implant), implant malposition, and implant rupture. • In the case of complications, secondary procedures may be required.

Continued

TABLE 10.4   Reconstructive Breast Surgery Options—cont'd

Name of Option	Brief Description	Advantages	Disadvantages
Deep inferior epigastric perforator (DIEP) flap, superficial inferior epigastric artery (SIEA) flap, bilateral simultaneous superior gluteal artery perforator (SGAP) flap	The DIEP flap is the technique in which skin and tissue (no muscle) are taken from the abdomen in order to re-create the breast. Other flap techniques, called the SIEA flap and the SGAP flap, take tissue from the lower abdomen or lateral buttock regions.	• Because the reconstruction involves using the woman's own tissues, the risks of implant reconstruction are avoided, particularly in the case of radiation. • Most women have less postoperative pain than after a TRAM flap and are therefore able to leave the hospital sooner and return to normal activities more quickly than after a TRAM flap. • Because the abdominal muscle is not removed as in the TRAM flap, women have much less risk of developing hernias, bulges, and core weakness at the site where the flap is removed. This advantage is much greater in bilateral (both sides) reconstruction. • It is typically easier to match the contralateral natural breast with the woman's own tissue when compared with implant reconstruction. • Women essentially end up with a "tummy tuck," "bottom lift," or other cosmetic benefits at the same time as the breast reconstruction.	• DIEP/SIEA/SGAP flap reconstruction generally requires a longer and more challenging surgery at the first stage when compared with implants or TRAM flaps. • Women will have a scar across the lower abdomen or the upper part of the buttock where the flap is obtained. However, this does not differ from the TRAM flap as the abdominal scars are equivalent. • Small revision surgeries or matching procedures on the opposing breast or donor site may be required. • Women who smoke, are obese, or who have diabetes are not ideal candidates for this type of surgery.
Transverse rectus abdominis myocutaneous (TRAM) flap	In a pedicle TRAM flap, the tissue remains attached to its original site, retaining its blood supply. The flap, consisting of the skin, fat, and muscle with its blood supply, is tunneled beneath the skin to the chest, creating a pocket for an implant or, in some cases, creating the breast mound itself, without need for an implant. The free TRAM flap involves less muscle.	• Shorter and less complex surgery than the other flaps	• This was state of the art decades ago and has since been replaced by other, more advanced procedures. • The woman may have more postoperative pain and longer hospital stays. • There is a risk of abdominal bulge or hernias, and as a result there might be a limit to how much weight the woman can lift. • Other newer procedures may offer more natural results.

Data from Rivera, A. E., Klimberg, V. S., & Bland, K. I. (2018). Breast conservation therapy for invasive breast cancer. In K. I. Bland, E. M. Copeland, V. S. Klimberg, & W. J. Gradishar (Eds.). *The breast: Comprehensive management of benign and malignant diseases* (5th ed.). Philadelphia: Elsevier.

Radiation

Radiation is recommended for women who have BCS and for some following a mastectomy with the goal of decreasing incidence of local recurrence (NCI, 2018b). Radiation to the breast destroys tumor cells remaining after manipulation and handling of the tumor during surgery. There are different options for doses and scheduling of radiation. The usual recommended radiation dose is 45 to 50 Gy in 1.8- to 2-Gy fractions over 5 to 6 weeks, but for some women a shorter course (3 to 4 weeks) for a total of 42.5 Gy is effective (NCI). The risk of local recurrence depends on extent of breast resection, tumor margins, technical details of radiation therapy, and use of adjuvant systemic therapy. Although radiation after BCS is standard protocol, some large breast tumors (due to the disease being locally advanced) may be irradiated before surgery to facilitate easier surgical removal. Side effects of radiation therapy include swelling and heaviness in the breast, sunburn-like skin changes in the treated area, and fatigue. Changes to the breast tissue and skin usually, but not always, resolve in 6 to 12 months.

The breast may become smaller and firmer after radiation therapy. Radiation therapy in the area of the axilla can cause lymphedema of the arm on the affected side. Close medical follow-up is important after conservative surgery and radiation. Recommended guidelines include a breast physical examination every 4 to 6 months for 5 years and then yearly. A mammogram is recommended 6 months after radiation and then annually (National Comprehensive Cancer Network [NCCN], 2018a).

A variety of radiation methods are widely used. These include accelerated therapy and brachytherapy.

• *Accelerated breast radiation.* External beam radiation for 6 weeks, 5 days a week, can be inconvenient for a woman. Research has been conducted to develop ways to shorten this time frame and still deliver the therapy needed to prevent recurrence of this disease. Accelerated radiation was created with this goal in mind and delivers a slightly larger dose of radiation over a 3-week period. Skin changes (resembling sunburn) can be slightly more prevalent because of the more intense period of time and corresponding dosage.

- *Brachytherapy.* Initially created for other types of cancer, like prostate, this form of radiation enables the client to complete her radiation in an even shorter time and is not delivered via external beam. Instead a deflated balloon is inserted into the space left by the lumpectomy and is filled with saline. The balloon is left in place until the margins are confirmed as clear. The balloon is removed and replaced with another balloon specifically created to allow radiation to be inserted within it. Radiation rods or seeds are inserted into the balloon each day for 5 days, and the radiation is completed, at which time the balloon is removed. This enables partial breast radiation to be delivered, recognizing that most local recurrences happen at or near the location of the original cancer.
- *Partial breast radiation.* Intraoperative radiation done at the time of surgery in the operating room. Indications are for small less aggressive tumors. This technique is still not yet standard of care.

Adjuvant Systemic Therapy

Chemotherapy administered soon after surgical removal of the tumor is referred to as adjuvant chemotherapy. The role of adjuvant chemotherapy (chemotherapy and endocrine therapy) in treating breast cancer is either to eradicate or impede the growth of micrometastatic (microscopic cell metastasis) disease. Often it is not possible to detect the presence of micrometastasis at the time of initial treatment, and when it is present, mutations can occur in the tumor cells. These mutations make tumor cells resistant to the effects of chemotherapeutic agents despite tumor sensitivity to drug therapy being greatest when the tumor burden is small. Consequently, the prediction cannot be made with confidence that all tumors of 1 cm or less can be cured with initial local and regional treatment. The early introduction of systemic adjuvant therapy, as determined by the estimated risk of tumor recurrence in certain subsets of women with node-negative disease, is a prudent course of treatment. Adjuvant therapy may help to destroy undetected cancers that were not surgically removed (Kriebs, 2017). For women diagnosed with early-stage breast cancer and favorable prognostic factors (hormone receptor positive and HER2/neu negative), a special pathology test may help determine the woman's risk of recurrence. This test, called Oncotype DX, provides a score that represents the likelihood of her specific cancer recurring. Such information can be useful for a woman whose known benefit for receiving chemotherapy may be minimal based on her prognostic factors from the tumor itself. For women with a low score, commonly only hormonal therapy is recommended, and for those with a high score, chemotherapy is strongly considered.

Neoadjuvant therapy is systemic treatment given before surgery; the goal is to reduce tumor burden, making breast-conserving treatment an option.

Hormonal Therapy

To determine whether a woman is a candidate for hormonal therapy, a receptor assay is done. After the entire tumor or a portion is removed by biopsy or excision, a pathologist examines the cancer cells for ERs and PRs.

The presence of a receptor on the cell wall indicates that the woman is positive for that type of hormone receptor. If these receptors are present, the growth of the woman's breast cancer can be influenced by estrogen, progesterone, or both. It is unknown exactly how these hormones affect breast cancer growth. Bilateral oophorectomy may benefit women diagnosed with their first breast cancer before age 50 by reducing exposure to endogenous estrogen. For women with BRCA1/BRCA2 mutations, a prophylactic salpingo-oophorectomy greatly reduces the risk of ovarian cancer and can reduce the risk of breast cancer by 50% (O'Donnell, Axilbund, & Euhus, 2018).

There are two hormonal or endocrine therapy drug classes including selective estrogen receptor modulators (SERMs) and aromatase inhibitors (AIs). Tamoxifen, the oldest and longest used, is an oral antiestrogen medication that mimics progesterone and estrogen. Tamoxifen attaches to the hormone receptors on cancer cells and prevents natural hormones from attaching to the receptors. When tamoxifen fits into the receptors, the cell is unable to grow. Tamoxifen has been shown to decrease the risk of local and distant recurrences of breast cancer about 50% and mortality by about 30% (Smith & Stearns, 2018). Adjuvant hormonal therapy with tamoxifen for 5 years is recommended for most premenopausal women with breast cancer whose tumors are hormone receptor positive. Recently, the ideal length of adjuvant endocrine therapy has been studied. For premenopausal women, some clinicians are recommending 10 years of therapy. For those who develop menopause after 5 years, AIs for 5 additional years may be considered (see Medication Guide: Tamoxifen).

MEDICATION GUIDE

Tamoxifen (Nolvadex)

Action

A selective estrogen receptor modulator that exerts antiestrogenic effects; attaches to hormone receptors on cancer cells and prevents natural hormones from attaching to the receptors

Indications

For treatment of advanced-stage or metastatic breast cancer; treatment of early-stage breast cancer after breast cancer surgery and radiation therapy; to reduce the incidence of breast cancer in women at high risk

Dosage and Route

20 mg orally, daily, but can vary depending on the reason for taking tamoxifen

Adverse Reactions

Common side effects include hot flashes, night sweats, nausea, vaginal discharge, mood swings, weight gain, and cataracts. Hair loss is an uncommon effect. Serious side effects include deep vein thrombosis, increased risk of endometrial cancer, and stroke. Symptoms of these serious side effects include abnormal vaginal bleeding, leg swelling or tenderness, chest pain, shortness of breath, weakness or numbness of extremities, sudden severe headache, and chemical hepatitis.

Nursing Considerations

The medication may be taken on an empty stomach or with food. Missed doses should be taken as soon as possible, but taking two doses at once is not recommended. A barrier or nonhormonal form of contraception is recommended in premenopausal women because tamoxifen may be harmful to the fetus if pregnancy should occur. Client counseling should concentrate on annual Pap smear (if no hysterectomy), annual eye exam, bone density testing every 3 years, and liver function tests (LFTs) every 6 months.

The National Cancer Comprehensive Network (NCCN) guidelines (2018a) recommend adjuvant hormonal therapy for women with hormone receptor–positive breast cancer regardless of menopause status, age, or HER2/neu status. The exception to this is women with lymph node–negative cancers less than or equal to 0.5 cm, or 0.6 to 1 cm in diameter with favorable prognostic features. However, adjuvant hormonal therapy can be considered for this group of patients. Women treated with hormonal therapy should receive therapy for at least 5 years for chemoprevention. Continuing hormonal therapy for 10 years can reduce risk of recurrence, but it is unclear which women would benefit most from extending therapy (Pan, Gray, Braybrooke, et al., 2017).

Raloxifene is an oral selective ER modulator. It is used to prevent osteoporosis in menopausal women. It was also used in a second-generation National Cancer Institute (NCI) prevention trial. It demonstrated the same 50% risk reduction in invasive breast cancer in postmenopausal women with a high risk for breast cancer with fewer thromboembolic events and lower risk of uterine cancer when compared with the use of tamoxifen (see Medication Guide: Raloxifene Hydrochloride).

MEDICATION GUIDE
Raloxifene Hydrochloride (Evista)

Action
A selective estrogen receptor modulator, serving as an agonist and antagonist to estrogen receptor sites

Indications
Treatment and prevention of osteoporosis; reduction in the risk of invasive breast cancer in postmenopausal women with osteoporosis; and reduction of risk of invasive breast cancer in postmenopausal women at high risk for invasive breast cancer

Dosage and Route
60 mg orally, daily

Adverse Reactions
Common side effects include hot flashes, nausea, peripheral edema, joint pain, leg cramps, flu like symptoms, sweating. Serious and life-threatening side effects can occur from existing conditions. Women who have had a heart attack or are at risk for a heart attack have increased risk of dying from a stroke. There is an increased risk of venous thromboembolism (VTE) and pulmonary embolism. Raloxifene is contraindicated in women with an active or past history of VTE.

Nursing Considerations
The medication may be taken on an empty stomach or with food. Missed doses should be taken as soon as possible, but taking two doses at once is not recommended. Counsel the woman to contact her health care provider if leg pain or feeling of warmth in lower legs, swelling of hands and feet, sudden chest pain or shortness of breath, or sudden changes in vision occur. Calcium 1500 mg plus vitamin D 400 to 800 International Units daily is recommended.

AIs are a classification of hormonal therapy in use. They suppress plasma estrogen levels in postmenopausal women by inhibiting or inactivating aromatase, the enzyme responsible for synthesizing estrogens from androgens (Smith & Sterns, 2018). AIs such as anastrozole, letrozole, and exemestane are effective agents in hormonal therapy for breast cancer. Clinical trials indicate that letrozole is better than tamoxifen in treating advanced disease in postmenopausal women, and anastrozole is at least as good. In early-stage breast cancer, adjuvant therapy with anastrozole appears to be superior to adjuvant therapy with tamoxifen in reducing recurrence in postmenopausal women. AIs appear to be well tolerated with lower incidence of adverse effects as compared with tamoxifen and thus are often recommended for postmenopausal women with hormone receptor positive breast cancer. For some women, endocrine therapy is recommended for 10 years (Smith & Stearns) (see Medication Guide: Letrozole).

MEDICATION GUIDE
Letrozole (Femara)

Action
An aromatase inhibitor; inhibits the conversion of androgens to estrogen

Indications
For adjuvant treatment of early breast cancer in postmenopausal women who have received 5 years of tamoxifen therapy; first-line treatment of postmenopausal women with hormone receptor–positive or hormone receptor–unknown locally advanced or metastatic cancer; adjuvant treatment of postmenopausal women with hormone receptor–positive early breast cancer

Dosage and Route
2.5 mg orally, daily

Adverse Reactions
Common side effects include hot flashes, nausea, increased sweating, joint or muscle pain, fluid retention, vaginal dryness, constipation, dizziness, fatigue, headache. Severe side effects include serious allergic reactions (e.g., rash, hives, difficulty breathing), vomiting, chest pain, intense bone pain, and calf pain or tenderness.

Nursing Considerations
The medication may be taken on an empty stomach or with food. Missed doses should be taken as soon as possible, but taking two doses at once is not recommended. The woman should use caution if driving or using machinery because this medication may cause drowsiness or dizziness. Women who are not postmenopausal should not take letrozole.

Chemotherapy

Chemotherapy drugs are most often given in combination regimens, which have been shown to improve or increase the disease-free survival time after therapy. The most common chemotherapy regimens used for adjuvant treatment of node-positive and node-negative tumors are listed in Box 10.2. These regimens are constantly changing in response to new evidence.

BOX 10.2 Common Chemotherapy Regimens for Adjuvant Treatment of Breast Cancer

- CAF: cyclophosphamide (**C**ytoxan), doxorubicin (**A**driamycin), **F**luorouracil
- TAC: docetaxel (**T**axotere), doxorubicin (**A**driamycin), and cyclophosphamide (**C**ytoxan)
- AC → T: doxorubicin (**A**driamycin) and cyclophosphamide (**C**ytoxan) followed by paclitaxel (**T**axol) or docetaxel (**T**axotere) (Trastuzumab may be given with the paclitaxel or docetaxel for HER2/neu-positive tumors.)
- FEC: fluorouracil, epirubicin, and cyclophosphamide (this may be followed by docetaxel)
- TC: docetaxel and cyclophosphamide
- TCH: docetaxel, carboplatin, and Herceptin for HER2/neu-positive tumors
- Less common regimens include:
  - CMF: cyclophosphamide, methotrexate, fluorouracil
  - AC: doxorubicin, cyclophosphamide
  - EC: epirubicin, cyclophosphamide
  - A → CMF: doxorubicin followed by CMF

American Cancer Society. (2017). Chemotherapy for breast cancer. Retrieved from: https://www.cancer.org/cancer/breast-cancer/treatment/chemotherapy-for-breast-cancer.html.

The decision to recommend adjuvant chemotherapy is based upon ER and HER2 receptor status, stage of disease, and genetic tumor phenotyping with either MammaPrint or Oncotype DX (Santa-Maria & Gradishar, 2018). With the advent of HER2 therapies, breast cancer survival rates have improved. The specific genotypes provide guidance to oncologists on which ER positive women will benefit from adjuvant chemotherapy. Adjuvant chemotherapy is recommended for triple negative breast cancer as this subtype is particularly aggressive with metastases occurring early (Santa-Maria & Gradishar). Premenopausal women with early stage ER positive breast cancer usually receive adjuvant chemotherapy.

Chemotherapy with multiple drug combinations is used in the treatment of recurrent and advanced breast cancer with positive results. First-line single agents for women with locally advanced or metastatic breast cancer include paclitaxel, docetaxel, epirubicin, doxorubicin, pegylated liposomal doxorubicin, capecitabine, vinorelbine, and gemcitabine. Combination regimens and sequential single agents can be used as well (NCCN, 2018a). The use of trastuzumab and pertuzumab has advanced response rates and lowered recurrences. Because chemotherapy drugs kill rapidly reproducing cells, treatment also affects normal body cells that rapidly reproduce (red and white blood cells, gastric mucosa, and hair). Thus chemotherapy can cause leukopenia, neutropenia, thrombocytopenia, anemia, gastrointestinal side effects (nausea, vomiting, anorexia, mucositis), and partial or full hair loss.

Chemotherapy treatments are usually administered in ambulatory care settings once or twice per month. During the informed consent process, before the treatment is selected, the woman and her family members should be educated about the names of the medications, routes of administration, treatment schedule, timing and ordering of medications, length of time of administration, reimbursed and unreimbursed costs of therapy, potential side effects, management of side effects, possible changes in body image (e.g., full or partial hair loss), recovery time after treatment (necessitating lost work time), and need for a caregiver to transport the woman to treatment and to care for her afterward. Depending on the medications used, the treatments can include IV, subcutaneous, and oral administration. Often a long-term central venous catheter is inserted when the women will be receiving chemotherapy for an extended period or when she will receive medications that may damage the vein. Presence of a central venous catheter, hair loss, loss of part or all of her breast, menopause, and possible infertility all have the potential to cause a change in body image and increase emotional distress.

Treatment with chemotherapy or hormonal therapy, or a combination of the two, often causes changes in reproductive function. The premenopausal woman may experience these changes along with symptoms of menopause and possible infertility. It is not known whether hormonal therapy to ease the effects of menopause is safe for women with breast cancer; therefore, it is not recommended. For this reason, the nurse must use other measures to help the woman cope with menopause (see Chapter 6).

Women receiving chemotherapy and their partners must understand that chemotherapy can be teratogenic, that is, chemotherapy agents can cause congenital birth defects. Any woman who is of childbearing age and receiving chemotherapy, even though no longer menstruating, must use birth control. Although a woman may not be menstruating, she may still be able to become pregnant.

Oral contraceptives are not recommended because they contain hormones that may assist in the growth of cancer. A birth control method must be chosen with the assistance of a gynecologist and a medical oncologist, and it must be used before chemotherapy begins and continue to be used until the medical oncologist and gynecologist believe it is safe to discontinue.

Special Groups
Young Women

Of the newly diagnosed breast cancers, approximately 12,150 will be in women under age 40 (Young Survival Coalition, 2019). The diagnosis of concomitant pregnancy and breast cancer is estimated at about 1 in 3000 (Durrani, Akbar, Heena, 2018). Although the basic treatment modalities for breast cancer are used, the unique importance in this age population requires careful consideration of their developmental tasks. Nurses can identify developmental tasks and help young women cope with their disease.

In identifying special surgical concerns for young women diagnosed with breast cancer, it is important to consider the timing and extent of the surgery offered. A younger woman is more likely than not to harbor a mutation, and therefore genetic testing may be an important aspect in deciding on a surgical plan. She may want to use the genetic results to decide whether to consider bilateral mastectomies. If chemotherapy is planned, a neoadjuvant approach would allow enough time for surgical decision making while still actively receiving treatment. Choosing a breast-conserving approach requires a careful discussion because it leaves the woman with a higher chance for recurrence.

Systemic therapy, whether adjuvant or neoadjuvant, will affect fertility. Since most chemotherapy and endocrine therapy result in ovarian suppression, clinicians should discuss with women their fertility concerns prior to treatment (Rosenberg & Partridge, 2015). It is important to include a consult to a reproductive gynecologist early after diagnosis to discuss preserving fertility.

Chapter 11 presents information about young women who are diagnosed with breast cancer during pregnancy. This is an important area for nurses to understand.

Young women with breast cancer face different challenges than do the majority of older diagnosed women. The biology of their tumors together with the genetic implications suggest a more threatening outcome. The defining difference, however, is the time of life at which the disease strikes. Independence, autonomy, integration into society, and fusion in the family are the foundations on which nursing interventions should focus in achieving the best outcomes for quality of life and survivorship.

The future might also appear different for these women. Although the risk of recurrence plagues all women with breast cancer, younger women with this disease face the possibility of second or third malignancies if they survive long term. The consideration of undergoing prophylactic surgery can be an overwhelming decision for these young women. Successful survivorship will be defined by their ability to move beyond treatments, continue to work productively, have their families, and find meaning in their lives. Young survivors may benefit from connecting with others through Young Survival Coalition (https://www.youngsurvival.org/learn/about-breast-cancer/statistics).

Women Ages 65 and Older

Although the risk of death from breast cancer is declining, the likelihood of being diagnosed with breast cancer increases with age (ACS, 2019b). Women who are 65 years of age are expected to live another 20 years. Since few women older than 65 have participated in clinical trials, the decision on treatment should be based on biologic age rather than chronologic age (NCCN, 2017). However, there are variations in treatment based on comorbidities and frailty index. The variations in treatment are largely based on comorbidities and frailty index (Mandelblatt, Cai, Luta, et al., 2017). The majority of older woman diagnosed with breast cancer will likely be estrogen receptor positive and demonstrate less aggressive forms of disease. Older women who are healthy can benefit from chemotherapy, if indicated, and from endocrine therapy (Mandelblatt et al.) For women over 70 with comorbidities, use of an AI alone without surgery is an option and does not compromise survival (Johnston & Cheung, 2015).

The overall success in treating older women is based largely on integrating geriatrics with oncology. There are available tools through NCCN that can help with providing geriatric assessments. Older women face treatment decisions based on many factors, with quality of life being a major one.

Survivorship Issues

Because women are living longer after treatment for breast cancer, survivorship issues have become very important in relation to quality of life. Evidence-based guidelines standardize surveillance and include history and physical examination every 3 to 6 months during the first 3 years, every 6 to 12 months during years 4 and 5, and annually thereafter. At that point women can be transitioned into primary care. In addition, mammography is annual, with the first at 6 months postradiation to establish a new baseline. It is recommended that women who carry a genetic mutation have MRI added to their surveillance. Routine gynecologic care is suggested. Many women suffer from sequelae of cancer treatment, including vasomotor symptoms, sexual dysfunction, infertility, osteoporosis, musculoskeletal pain, weight gain, cognitive changes, fatigue, neuropathy, and congestive heart failure. Whether a woman is in a specialty clinic or primary care, the ability of health care providers to recognize and treat these problems is critical for optimum health.

Vasomotor symptoms occur in many women treated for breast cancer, partly due to hormonal treatments. Lifestyle changes such as keeping room temperatures down, avoiding spicy food and caffeine, and dressing in layers can be useful. Hormone replacement therapy is contraindicated. Some pharmacologic agents, including antidepressants such as paroxetine, fluoxetine, citalopram, and venlafaxine, as well as anticonvulsants such as gabapentin and the antihypertensive clonidine have been used with varying success (Runowicz, Leach, Henry, et al., 2016).

Sexual dysfunction may be related to the endocrine changes that result from systemic therapy. The most commonly reported issue for women is decreased libido, followed by decreased arousal or lubrication, dyspareunia, and body image. Helping women overcome these problems requires the nurse to discuss such symptoms openly with their clients.

Osteoporosis caused by systemic chemotherapy or antiestrogen therapies is a potential major comorbidity of breast cancer treatment. The incidence of bone fractures in this population is greater than in the general population and most frequently occurs within 4 years of beginning treatment (Edwards, Gradishar, Smith, et al., 2016). With this in mind, screening for osteoporosis with dual-energy x-ray absorptiometry (DEXA) scans every 1 to 2 years is recommended in survivors 65 years or older (60 to 64 for those women deemed at risk or on AI therapy). They should be given additional counseling for weight-bearing exercises, supplemental vitamin D and calcium, smoking cessation, and avoidance of excessive alcohol intake. Bisphosphonates can treat or prevent osteoporosis in breast cancer survivors.

Weight gain is common in women treated for breast cancer. Chemotherapy causes sarcopenic obesity, characterized by lean mass loss and fat gain. Obesity is associated with an increased incidence of recurrence and mortality (Jiralerspong & Goodwin, 2016). Women are encouraged to exercise and monitor their diet to maintain a healthy weight. The ACS recommends strength training at least twice per week and 150 minutes of aerobic exercise per week.

Women treated for breast cancer report decreased cognitive function with changes in the ability to concentrate, difficulty in paying attention, and short-term memory loss. However, it is unclear as to the etiology of these changes. Current research supports an association with hormonal therapy, mood disorders (depression), and race

(Seliktar, Polek, Brooks, & Hardie, 2015). Older women and those with lower cognitive reserve are more vulnerable to the treatment effects.

Cancer-related fatigue (CRF) is a persistent feeling of emotional, physical, and cognitive exhaustion associated with cancer diagnosis and treatment that is out of proportion to the average population. It is reported as one of the most common side effects associated with treatment and has a great effect on quality of life. For breast cancer patients, fatigue is more common with later stage disease and chemotherapy (NCCN, 2018b). NCCN recommends routine screening for this symptom. It has long been known that radiation causes fatigue, but the combination of chemotherapy and other systemic therapies is considered synergistic.

Cardiotoxicity is well recognized as a side effect of breast cancer treatment. The most common cause is anthracycline-based regimens and trastuzumab; however, with the addition of taxanes, this incidence has increased. Women who are on either anthracyclines or taxanes need regular heart function monitoring and dose modifications, along with cardiac management. Exercise during and following treatment may ameliorate cardiotoxicity, but further research is needed (Sturgeon, Ky, Libonati, & Schmitz, 2014). Neuropathies, another side effect of taxanes, are chronic and may require dose modifications.

Nursing Interventions

Nursing care of a woman with breast cancer depends on the treatment chosen. Data that guide the care include a client history, physical examination, laboratory and diagnostic test results, psychosocial, and spiritual assessment. Interprofessional care, with nursing as part of that team, is essential to helping to identify need for referrals, and follow up when indicated.

Emotional Support After Diagnosis

When a woman is diagnosed with cancer, she confronts mortality and potential bodily changes. The emotional reaction to the diagnosis varies with each woman, but is often intense, and the many disruptions caused by the disease challenge the woman's and family's ability to cope. Disruptions may be caused by costs of treatment, loss of role function, lack of stress-relieving activities, spouse's or child's reaction to the diagnosis, change in body image and sexual function, disability, and pain. The woman may feel despair, fear, and shame. Health care providers are responsible for discussing the influence of breast cancer on the woman's life and in assisting her and her family in coping effectively.

Women and their families often undergo a period of psychosocial and spiritual distress after the diagnosis of cancer. It is difficult to accept the diagnosis when the woman may feel and look well. This period may be characterized by anguish and shock followed by disbelief and denial. During this time, absorbing information and education can be difficult, and the nurse should be sensitive as to how this may affect decision-making abilities. Flexibility is the key to sensitive nursing care. As the woman and family begin to accept her diagnosis, more and more information can be shared, and care planning with full client participation can take place, including the following:
- Validate and reinforce accurate information processing by the woman and her family.
- Assist in client decision making and arrange for the woman to speak with breast cancer survivors who have chosen a variety of treatment options (Box 10.3).
- Suggest approaches the woman might take to deal with the sexual concerns of her partner.
- Discuss the application of alternative therapies to alleviate stress and promote healing, such as exercise, guided imagery, meditation, and progressive muscle relaxation.

BOX 10.3 Decision-Making Questions to Ask

1. What kind of breast cancer is it (invasive or noninvasive)?
2. What is the stage of the cancer (i.e., how extensive is the spread)?
3. What further tests are recommended (e.g., estrogen receptor assay, HER2 status)?
4. What are the treatment options (pros and cons of each, including side effects)?
5. If surgery is recommended, what will the scar look like?
6. If a mastectomy is done, can breast reconstruction be done (at the time of surgery or later)?
7. How long will the woman be in the hospital? What kind of postoperative care will she need?
8. How long will treatment last if radiation or chemotherapy is recommended? What effects can the woman expect from these treatments?
9. What community resources are available for support?

Data from American Cancer Society. (2017). *Questions to ask my doctor about breast cancer.* Retrieved from: https://www.cancer.org/cancer/breast-cancer/understanding-a-breast-cancer-diagnosis/questions-to-ask-your-doctor-about-breast-cancer.html.

- Refer the woman to the ACS's Reach to Recovery program or other resources that provide trained survivor volunteers for one-on-one support (Box 10.4).
- Refer the woman to a cancer rehabilitation program, such as Encore—an exercise program run by the YWCA.

The NCCN (www.nccn.org) and the ACS (www.cancer.org) provide specific, up-to-date recommendations on breast cancer treatments on the Internet. These are invaluable resources for women to learn about scientifically tested treatment protocols for each stage of breast cancer.

COMMUNITY ACTIVITY

Research the availability of rehabilitation programs for breast cancer survivors in your community such as the American Cancer Society's (ACS's) Reach to Recovery program. Contact the agency (e.g., local ACS agency) to identify the services provided by the program and the requirements for becoming a volunteer. How are the resources and programs promoted in the community (e.g., brochures in waiting areas of clinics, newspaper ads)? Are nurses in the community involved, and if so, how? Do women who use the services provide evaluation about their experiences, and if so, how is it collected and used?

Nursing Care of the Woman Receiving Surgery for Breast Cancer

Nurses are instrumental in caring for women with breast cancer. When surgery is needed, nurses are part of the interprofessional team providing care and support during the preoperative, intraoperative, postoperative, and convalescent periods. The discussion that follows describes nursing care at each of these periods for a woman having breast-conserving surgery and axillary node dissection (see Nursing Care Plan).

NURSING CARE PLAN

The Woman Having Breast-Conserving Surgery and Axillary Node Dissection

Client Problem	Expected Outcome	Nursing Interventions	Rationales
Potential inflammation (lymphedema)	Woman will experience no swelling in her arm.	Explain the need to avoid trauma or irritation to the affected arm.	To reinforce to the woman that alterations in sensation and removal of some lymph nodes may affect ability to sense irritation or prevent infection
		Teach the woman to avoid having blood drawn from or blood pressure taken on the affected arm.	Decreased sensation and decreased lymphatic return could lead to trauma in the affected arm.
		Monitor for signs and symptoms	To provide identification and treatment of problem
Anxiety	Woman will report decreased anxiety.	Provide timely and accurate information about diagnosis and treatment.	To decrease fear of unknown
		Encourage connection with Reach to Recovery volunteer.	To facilitate verbalization of feelings with women who have similar concerns
		Teach simple breathing exercises for relaxation and access to other nonpharmacologic interventions.	To provide simple techniques to reduce anxiety
Decreased functional ability	Woman will return to her preoperative level of function.	Encourage woman to do hand, arm, and wrist exercises that can be performed in the immediate postoperative period.	To enhance fluid return and prevent muscle atrophy
		Encourage woman to perform activities of daily living as much as possible.	To encourage woman to focus on her strengths rather than her limitations
		Teach woman exercises to be performed after the axillary drains are removed.	To promote range of motion in the arm that had the axillary nodes dissected
		Teach woman to do exercises slowly and gently.	To prevent injury and pain
		Caution woman not to lift anything heavier than 10 pounds for 4 to 6 weeks.	To avoid exerting strain on affected arm

Preoperative Care

General preoperative teaching and care are given, including expectations regarding physical appearance, pain management, equipment to be used (e.g., IV therapy, drains), and emotional support. Some emotional support may be obtained by arranging for a visit from a member of an organization such as Reach to Recovery. The woman is reminded that when she awakens after surgery, her arm on the affected side will feel tight.

> **⚠ NURSING ALERT**
>
> When vital signs are taken, never apply the blood pressure cuff to the arm affected by the axillary lymph node dissection.

Immediate Postoperative Care

After recovery from anesthesia, the woman is returned to her room. Special precautions must be observed to prevent or to minimize lymphedema of the affected arm. The affected arm is elevated with pillows above the level of the right atrium. Blood is not drawn from this arm, and this arm is not used for IV therapy or any injections. Early arm movement is encouraged. Any increase in the circumference of that arm is reported immediately.

Nursing care of the wound involves observing for signs of hemorrhage: (dressing, drainage tubes, drainage reservoirs), shock, and infection. Dressings are reinforced as necessary and drainage reservoirs (e.g., Hemovac, Jackson-Pratt) are emptied at least every 8 hours. The woman is asked to turn (alternating between unaffected side and back), cough (while the nurse or the woman applies support to the chest), and deep breathe every 2 hours. Breath sounds are auscultated every 4 hours. Active range-of-motion (ROM) exercise of legs is encouraged. Parenteral fluids are given until adequate oral intake is possible. Emotional support is continued.

Care given during the immediate postoperative period is continued as necessary. Most women who undergo lumpectomy have surgery in outpatient facilities and return home a few hours after surgery. Women are discharged 24 hours or less after mastectomy without reconstruction. Women having a mastectomy with tissue expander placement will be in the hospital for 24 hours. Those having flap reconstruction at the same time will be hospitalized for 3 to 5 days. Because of the generally short time spent in the hospital, thorough teaching is important. It is best to do as much teaching as possible before surgery if the outcome is known. If this is not possible, discharge teaching should be done with the woman's caregiver present. This is to acknowledge the possibility that emotional stress or recovery from anesthesia may cause the woman to forget some of the discharge instructions. Printed information and a list of appropriate websites also should be provided for the woman and family to refer to at home.

Women who have had breast cancer surgery are usually seen by their surgeon within 5 to 7 days of surgery. This follow-up visit is important because it allows the physician to assess the outcome of surgical treatment as well as provide reinforcement of education and emotional support. A woman having simultaneous reconstruction will also be seen by her plastic surgeon within a week postoperatively.

Early ambulation is encouraged to improve circulation and ventilation and to prevent loss of bone calcium. The psychologic benefits of early mobility include resumption of self-care and activities of daily living that serve to reinforce the woman's control over her life and help her move from a sick role to the role of breast cancer survivor.

Arm exercises are encouraged at least four times daily (Box 10.5). Exercise is increased as tolerated and is stopped at the point of pain. Initially the woman alternately clenches and extends her fingers and then progresses to wrist and elbow exercises, gradually abducting her arm and raising it to and over her head. She is encouraged to exercise by assisting with her care—washing her face, brushing her teeth, and eating with her hand and arm on the affected side. Physical therapy may be prescribed to improve strength and mobility of the affected arm. Women having a sentinel node biopsy only should have full ROM back within a few days. A woman having axillary dissections will need to work more vigorously at restoring ROM. She should have returned to her baseline ROM by the end of the third week postoperatively.

It is important to discuss the appearance of the woman's breast if dressings have not been removed before discharge. Some women may not want to view their surgical site, but it is important to give them the opportunity to do so and to provide emotional support at that time. The woman should be encouraged to express her emotions and verbalize her feelings. She needs to know that it will take time to become accustomed to her change of appearance. A woman who has undergone reconstruction at the same time should be encouraged to look at herself as a work in progress—swelling, positioning of tissue expanders, appearance of flaps, and presence of multiple drains initially can be difficult to accept. Over time, when drains are out and swelling subsides, she will begin to see her new silhouette take shape.

An option for restoring body image is choosing an external prosthesis to replace the lost breast or portion of breast tissue for a client who has a mastectomy without reconstruction. The external prosthesis is inserted into a mastectomy bra. Women who choose to use a partial external prosthesis after BCS or full external prosthesis after mastectomy need information about where to obtain prostheses and an appropriate bra. Usually a temporary prosthesis is worn for the first 3 months before the woman is fitted for a permanent one. Women should be advised on how to submit the cost of the prosthesis to their insurance company. Volunteers of the Reach to Recovery program are able to provide this information, as well as a list of sources for prostheses, bathing suits, and lingerie. They can offer helpful hints and suggestions for coping with prostheses and wearing apparel. Some women find that an external prosthesis does not restore body image and seek surgical reconstruction of the missing or disfigured breast (see earlier discussion). It is also important to note that some women may choose to forgo a prosthesis as well as surgical reconstruction.

Discharge Planning and Follow-up Care

Before discharge, considerable time should be spent counseling the woman and her family about self-management. These instructions are summarized in the Teaching for Self-Management box: After a Mastectomy Without Reconstruction. Printed instructions should be given

---

BOX 10.5 Arm Exercises After Lymph Node Dissection

Exercises After Breast Surgery

It is important that the woman talk to her physician before starting any exercises. A physical therapist or occupational therapist can help design an exercise program for the woman.

Exercises in Lying Position

These exercises should be performed on a bed or the floor while lying on your back with your knees and hips bent, feet flat.

Wand Exercise

This exercise helps increase the forward motion of the shoulders. You will need a broom handle, yardstick, or other similar object to perform this exercise.

- Hold the wand in both hands with palms facing up.
- Lift the wand up over your head (as far as you can) using your unaffected arm to help lift the wand, until you feel a stretch in your affected arm.
- Hold for 5 seconds.
- Lower arms and repeat 5 to 7 times.

Elbow Winging

This exercise helps increase the mobility of the front of your chest and shoulder. It may take several weeks of regular exercise before your elbows will get close to the bed (or floor).

- Clasp your hands behind your neck with your elbows pointing toward the ceiling.
- Move your elbows apart and down toward the bed (or floor).
- Repeat 5 to 7 times

Exercises in Sitting Position

Shoulder Blade Stretch

This exercise helps increase the mobility of the shoulder blades.

- Sit in a chair very close to a table with your back against the chair back.
- Place the unaffected arm on the table with your elbow bent and palm down. Do not move this arm during the exercise.
- Place the affected arm on the table, palm down with your elbow straight.
- Without moving your trunk, slide the affected arm toward the opposite side of the table. You should feel your shoulder blade move as you do this.
- Relax your arm and repeat 5 to 7 times.

Shoulder Blade Squeeze

This exercise also helps increase the mobility of the shoulder blade.

- Facing straight ahead, sit in a chair in front of a mirror without resting on the back of the chair.
- Arms should be at your sides with elbows bent.
- Squeeze shoulder blades together, bringing your elbows behind you. Keep your shoulders level as you do this exercise. Do not lift your shoulders up toward your ears.
- Return to the starting position and repeat 5 to 7 times.

Side Bending

This exercise helps increase the mobility of the trunk/body.

- Clasp your hands together in front of you and lift your arms slowly over your head, straightening your arms.
- When your arms are over your head, bend your trunk to the right while bending at the waist and keeping your arms overhead.
- Return to the starting position and bend to the left.
- Repeat 5 to 7 times.

Exercises in Standing Position

Chest Wall Stretch

This exercise helps stretch the chest wall.

- Stand facing a corner with toes approximately 8 to 10 inches from the corner.
- Bend your elbows and place forearms on the wall, one on each side of the corner. Your elbows should be as close to shoulder height as possible.
- Keep your arms and feet in position and move your chest toward the corner. You will feel a stretch across your chest and shoulders.
- Return to starting position and repeat 5 to 7 times.

Shoulder Stretch

This exercise helps increase the mobility in the shoulder.

- Stand facing the wall with your toes approximately 8 to 10 inches from the wall.
- Place your hands on the wall. Use your fingers to "climb the wall," reaching as high as you can until you feel a stretch.
- Return to starting position and repeat 5 to 7 times.

Modified from American Cancer Society. (2017). *Exercises after breast surgery*. Retrieved from: www.cancer.org/cancer/breastcancer/moreinformation/exercises-after-breast-surgery.

---

to the woman and her family. A referral for home nursing care may be made if the woman needs assistance caring for her incision.

Education Needs for the Client and Family Undergoing Adjuvant Therapies

It is important that the woman and her family be given thorough instructions regarding side effects and avoidance of possible complications of adjuvant treatment. A common side effect of radiation therapy is skin irritation and breakdown. The woman should avoid using lotions, powders, or ointments on the skin at the radiation site unless instructed by the radiologist. The skin should be cleansed gently with mild soap and water, rinsed thoroughly, and patted dry. Skin markings that direct the placement of the radiation beam should not be removed. Soft, nonirritating clothing should be worn over the site, and the skin protected from exposure to sun and heat.

Common side effects of chemotherapy include alopecia, fatigue, nausea, vomiting, mouth sores, and immunosuppression. The woman receiving chemotherapy that produces hair loss should be encouraged to obtain a wig matching her own hair color and style before beginning treatments so that she is prepared when hair loss begins. Some women may choose not to wear a wig or a scarf. The local ACS can assist in obtaining a wig and head coverings designed for women experiencing hair loss from chemotherapy. The woman should be taught the importance of rest periods when fatigue occurs. She and her family will need to know that work and family schedules may need adjustment to accommodate needed rest. Exercise may help in increasing energy and decreasing fatigue. Nausea and vomiting should be reported to the health care provider and are treated with antiemetics. Mouth sores may be very painful, and the woman should be instructed to maintain good oral hygiene and avoid trauma to the oral mucosa by using a soft toothbrush. The mouth should be rinsed frequently with water or saline, and mouthwashes containing alcohol or glycerin should be avoided as well as spicy or irritating foods (see Box 10.4 for other suggestions). Topical anesthetic medications may be prescribed by the health care provider. The woman with immunosuppression should be instructed to use frequent handwashing and avoid crowds and other large gatherings of people, especially during cold and flu season. She should be taught to avoid eating raw fruits and vegetables (low-bacteria diet), maintain strict personal hygiene, and recognize the signs and symptoms of infection and report them to the health care provider immediately.

TEACHING FOR SELF-MANAGEMENT

After a Mastectomy Without Reconstruction

- Wash hands well before and after touching incision area or drains.
- Empty surgical drains twice a day and as needed, recording the date, time, drain sites (if more than one drain is present), and amount of drainage in milliliters in the diary you will take to each surgical checkup until your drains are removed (before discharge, you may receive a graduated container for emptying drains and measuring drainage).
- Avoid driving, lifting more than 10 pounds, or reaching above your head until given permission by the surgeon.
- Take medications for pain as soon as pain begins.
- Perform arm exercises as directed.
- Call your physician if inflammation of incision or swelling of the incision or the arm occurs.
- Avoid tight clothing, tight jewelry, and other causes of decreased circulation in the affected arm.
- Until drains are removed, wear loose-fitting underwear (e.g., camisole) and clothes, pinning surgical drains inside of clothing (you will be taught how to do this safely).
- After drains are removed and surgical sites are healing and still tender, wear a mastectomy bra or camisole with a cotton-filled, muslin temporary prosthesis. Temporary prostheses of this type are often available from Reach to Recovery.
- Avoid depilatory creams, strong deodorants, and shaving of affected chest area, axilla, and arm.
- Sponge bathe for the first 48 hours; then you may shower. Thoroughly dry yourself afterward and reapply fresh dressings.
- Return to the surgeon's office for incision check, drain inspection, and possible drain removal as directed.
- Contact Reach to Recovery or a breast center nursing staff member for assistance in obtaining external prosthesis and lingerie when dressings, drains, and staples are removed, and wound is healing and nontender.
- Contact insurance company for information about coverage of prosthesis and wig, if needed. Obtain prescriptions for prosthesis and wig to submit with receipts of purchase for these items to the insurance company. If insurance does not pay for these items, contact the hospital or agency social worker or local American Cancer Society for assistance.
- Keep follow-up visits for physical examination, mammography, and testing to detect recurrent breast cancer.
- Expect decreased sensation and tingling at incision sites and in the affected arm for weeks to months after surgery.
- Resume sexual activities as desired.
- Participate in breast cancer survivor support group if desired.
- Encourage mother, sisters, and daughters (if applicable) to have annual professional breast examinations and mammography (if appropriate).

▌KEY POINTS

- The most common benign breast problems are fibrocystic changes and fibroadenomas.
- The development of breast neoplasms, whether benign or malignant, can have a significant physical and emotional effect on a woman and her family.
- The risk of American women developing cancer of the breast is one in eight.
- An estimated 90% of all breast lumps are detected by the woman.
- Clinical breast examinations by a health care provider (starting in one's 20s), and routine screening mammograms (after age 40) are recommended by the ACS for early detection of breast cancer.
- Digital mammography is superior to traditional analog mammography.

- The primary therapy for most women with stage I or stage II breast cancer is breast-conserving surgery followed by radiation therapy.
- Adjuvant chemotherapy is most helpful to premenopausal women with breast cancer that has spread to the lymph nodes.
- Tamoxifen, along with raloxifene and anastrozole, provides the first real hope in preventing breast cancer.
- The diagnosis and treatment of breast cancer cause psychological and emotional stress for the woman and her family.
- There are more reconstruction options today than ever before.
- Of women diagnosed today with breast cancer, 85% will be long-term survivors.

REFERENCES

American Cancer Society. (2019a). *Breast cancer HER2 status*. Retrieved from: https://www.cancer.org/cancer/breast-cancer/understanding-a-breast-cancer-diagnosis/breast-cancer-her2-status.html.

American Cancer Society. (2019b). *Facts and figures 2019: U.S. cancer death rate has dropped 27% in 25 years*. Retrieved from: https://www.cancer.org/latest-news/facts-and-figures-2019.html.

American Cancer Society. (2019c). *How common is breast cancer?* Retrieved from: https://www.cancer.org/cancer/breast-cancer/about/how-common-is-breast-cancer.html.

American Cancer Society. (2019d). *Recommendations for the early detection of breast cancer*. Retrieved from: https://www.cancer.org/cancer/breast-cancer/screening-tests-and-early-detection/american-cancer-society-recommendations-for-the-early-detection-of-breast-cancer.html.

Arciero, C. A., & Styblo, T. M. (2018). Clinically established prognostic factors in breast cancer. In K. I. Bland, E. M. Copeland, V. S. Klimberg, & W. J. Gradishar (Eds.), *The breast: Comprehensive management of benign and malignant diseases* (5th ed.). Philadelphia: Elsevier.

Bassett, L., & Lee-Felker, S. (2018). Breast imaging screening and diagnosis. In K. I. Bland, E. M. Copeland, V. S. Klimberg, & W. J. Gradishar (Eds.), *The breast: Comprehensive management of benign and malignant diseases* (5th ed.). Philadelphia: Elsevier.

De Silva, N. K. (2017). Breast development and disorders in the adolescent female. *Best Practice & Research Clinical Obstetrics and Gynaecology, 48*, 40–50.

Durrani, S., Akbar, S., & Heena, H. (2018). Breast cancer during pregnancy. *Cureus, 10*(7).

Edwards, B. J., Gradishar, W. J., Smith, M. E., et al. (2016). Elevated incidence of fractures in women with invasive breast cancer. *Osteoporosis International, 27*(2), 499–507.

Jiralerspong, D., & Goodwin, P. J. (2016). Obesity and breast cancer prognosis: evidence, challenges and opportunities. *Journal of Clinical Oncology, 34*(35), 4203–4206.

Johnston, S. J., & Cheung, K. L. (2015). The role of primary endocrine therapy in older women with operable breast cancer. *Future Oncology, 11*(10), 1555–1565.

Kriebs, J. M. (2017). Breast health and disease. In B. J. Hackley, & J. M. Kriebs (Eds.), *Primary care of women*, 2nd ed. Burlington, MA: Jones and Bartlett Learning.

Mandelblatt, J. S., Cai, L., Luta, G., et al. (2017). Frailty and long-term mortality of older breast cancer patients: *CALGB 369901 (Alliance). Breast Cancer Research and Treatment, 164*(1), 107–117.

National Cancer Institute. (2018a). *BRCA mutations: cancer risk and genetic testing.* Retrieved from: https://www.cancer.gov/about-cancer/causes-prevention/genetics/brca-fact-sheet.

National Cancer Institute. (2018b). *Breast cancer treatment (PDQ®)-patient.* Version retrieved from: https://www.cancer.gov/types/breast/patient/breast-treatment-pdq.

National Comprehensive Cancer Network. (2017). *Guidelines version 2.2017 older adult oncology.* Retrieved from: https://www.nccn.org/professionals/physician_gls/pdf/senior.pdf.

National Comprehensive Cancer Network. (2018a). *Guidelines version 1.2018 invasive breast cancer.* Retrieved from: https://www.nccn.org/professionals/physician_gls/pdf/breast.pdf.

National Comprehensive Cancer Network. (2018b). *Guidelines version 2.2018 cancer related fatigue.* Retrieved from: https://www.nccn.org/professionals/physician_gls/pdf/fatigue.pdf.

Nelson, H. D., Cantor, A., Humphrey, L., et al. (2016). *Screening for breast cancer: a systematic review to update the 2009 U.S. Preventive Services Task force recommendation. Evidence synthesis no. 124.* AHRQ Publication No. 14-05201-EF-1. Rockville, MD: Agency for Healthcare Research and Quality.

Obeng-Gyasi, S., Grimm, L. J., Hwand, E. S., et al. (2018). Indications and techniques for biopsy. In K. I. Bland, E. M. Copeland, V. S. Klimberg, & W. J. Gradishar (Eds.), *The breast: Comprehensive management of benign and malignant diseases* (5th ed.). Philadelphia: Elsevier.

O'Donnell, M., Axilbund, J., & Euhus, D. M. (2018). Breast cancer genetics, syndromes, genes, pathology, counseling, testing and treatment. In K. I. Bland, E. M. Copeland, V. S. Klimberg, & W. J. Gradishar (Eds.), *The breast: Comprehensive management of benign and malignant diseases* (5th ed.). Philadelphia: Elsevier.

Orr, B., & Kelley, J. L. (2016). Benign breast diseases: Evaluation and management. *Clinical Obstetrics and Gynecology, 54*(4), 710–726.

Pan, H., Gray, R., Braybrooke, J. B., et al. (2017). 20-year risks of breast-cancer recurrence after stopping endocrine therapy at 5 years. *The New England Journal of Medicine, 377*(19), 1836–1846.

Perez-Panzano, E., Guemes-Sanchez, A., & Gascon-Catalan, A. (2016). Quality of life following symptomatic macromastia surgery: Short and long-term evaluation. *The Breast Journal, 22*(4), 397–406.

Rivera, A. E., Klimberg, V. S., & Bland, K. I. (2018). Breast conservation therapy for invasive breast cancer. In K. I. Bland, E. M. Copeland, V. S. Klimberg, & W. J. Gradishar (Eds.), *The breast: Comprehensive management of benign and malignant diseases* (5th ed.). Philadelphia: Elsevier.

Rosenberg, S. M., & Partridge, A. H. (2015). Management of breast cancer in very young women. *Breast, 24*(Suppl. 2), S154–158.

Runowicz, C. D., Leach, C. R., Henry, N. L., et al. (2016). American cancer society/american society of clinical oncology breast cancer survivorship care guideline. *Journal of Clinical Oncology, 34*(6), 611–635.

Santa-Maria, C. A., & Gradishar, W. J. (2018). Adjuvant & neoadjuvant systemic therapies for early-stage breast cancer. In K. I. Bland, E. M. Copeland, V. S. Klimberg, & W. J. Gradishar (Eds.), *The breast: Comprehensive management of benign and malignant diseases* (5th ed.). Philadelphia: Elsevier.

Sasaki, J., Geletzke, A., Krass, R., et al. (2018). Etiology and management of benign breast disease. In K. I. Bland, E. M. Copeland, V. S. Klimberg, & W. J. Gradishar (Eds.), *The breast: Comprehensive management of benign and malignant diseases* (5th ed.). Philadelphia: Elsevier.

Seliktar, N., Polek, C., Brooks, A., & Hardie, T. (2015). Cognition in breast cancer survivors: Hormones versus depression. *Journal of Psychosocial Oncology, 24*(4), 402–407.

Smith, K. J., & Stearns, V. (2018). Adjuvant endocrine therapy (Ch. 54, p. 736-751). In K. I. Bland, E. M. Copeland, V. S. Klimberg, & W. J. Gradishar (Eds.), *The breast: Comprehensive management of benign and malignant diseases* (5th ed.). Philadelphia: Elsevier.

Sturgeon, K. M., Ky, B., Libonati, H. P., & Schmitz, K. H. (2014). The effects of exercise on cardiovascular outcomes before, during and after treatment for breast cancer. *Breast Cancer Research and Treatment, 143*(2), 219–226.

Susan G. Komen Foundation. (2017a). *Screening and early detection.* Retrieved from: https://ww5.komen.org/breastcancer/earlydetectionampscreening.html.

Susan G. Komen Foundation. (2017b). *Accuracy of mammograms.* Retrieved from: https://ww5.komen.org/BreastCancer/AccuracyofMammograms.html.

U.S. Preventive Services Task Force (2016). Breast cancer screening. Retrieved from: https://www.uspreventiveservicestaskforce.org/Page/Document/UpdateSummaryFinal/breast-cancer-screening.

Vogel, V. G. (2018). Primary prevention of breast cancer. In K. I. Bland, E. M. Copeland, V. S. Klimberg, & W. J. Gradishar (Eds.), *The breast: Comprehensive management of benign and malignant diseases* (5th ed.). Philadelphia: Elsevier.

Yen, T. W. F., Laud, P. W., Pezzin, L. E., McGinley, E. L., Wozniak, E., Sparapani, R., et al. (2018). Prevalence and consequences of axillary lymph node dissection in the era of sentinel lymph node biopsy for breast cancer. *Medical Care, 56*(1), 78–84.

Structural Disorders and Neoplasms of the Reproductive System

Lecia Reardon

http://evolve.elsevier.com/Lowdermilk/MWHC/

LEARNING OBJECTIVES

- Describe the various structural disorders of the uterus and vagina.
- Discuss the pathophysiology of selected benign and malignant neoplasms of the female reproductive tract.
- Compare the common medical and surgical therapies for selected benign gynecologic conditions.
- Explain diagnostic procedures in terms the client can easily understand.
- Examine the emotional effects of benign and malignant neoplasms.
- Develop a nursing care plan for a woman who has had a hysterectomy due to endometrial cancer.

- Differentiate treatments for preinvasive and invasive conditions.
- Identify critical education needed for clients with selected benign or malignant neoplasms.
- Investigate health-promoting behaviors that reduce cancer risk.
- Assess the effects of and treatments for malignant neoplasms during pregnancy.
- Discuss the development and sequelae of gestational trophoblastic neoplasia (GTN).

Structural disorders and neoplastic disease of the female reproductive system can occur in women from the age of menarche throughout the lifespan. Both benign and malignant problems can profoundly impact the physical, reproductive, and psychologic health of the woman.

Structural problems include disorders of the uterus and vagina, effects of pelvic relaxation, urinary incontinence, and vulvodynia. Neoplasms can be benign (fibroids and cysts) or malignant (cancerous). Benign tumors usually do not endanger life, tend to grow slowly, and are not invasive. Malignant tumors (cancers) grow rapidly in a disorganized manner, invade surrounding tissues, and can cause death if untreated or detected at a late stage.

Nurses educate women and communities on preventive health care, the early detection of abnormalities, and the importance of seeking early treatment of suspected problems. Nurses are also advocates in providing supportive care to women and their families. This chapter includes an overview of female reproductive system structural disorders and neoplasms to provide the nurse a foundation to apply nursing care concepts. Nursing care concepts related to early detection, treatment methods, and education are included. An interprofessional approach provides optimum care for women with these reproductive conditions.

STRUCTURAL DISORDERS OF THE UTERUS AND VAGINA

Alterations in Pelvic Support

Alterations in pelvic support include uterine displacement and prolapse, cystoceles and rectoceles, urinary incontinence, and genital fistulas. As women age, these problems become more prevalent.

Uterine Displacement and Prolapse

The round ligaments normally hold the uterus in anteversion, and the uterosacral ligaments pull the cervix backward and upward (see Fig. 4.3). **Uterine displacement** is a variation of normal placement. The most common type is posterior displacement, or retroversion, in which the uterus is tilted posteriorly, and the cervix rotates anteriorly. Other variations include retroflexion and anteflexion (Fig. 11.1).

About 2 months postpartum the ligaments should return to normal length, but in about one-third of women, the uterus remains retroverted. This condition is rarely symptomatic, but subsequent conception may be difficult because the cervix points toward the anterior vaginal wall and away from the posterior fornix, where seminal fluid pools after coitus. If symptoms occur, they may include pelvic and low back pain, dyspareunia, and exaggeration of premenstrual symptoms.

Uterine prolapse is a more serious type of displacement. The degree of prolapse can vary from mild to complete. In complete prolapse, the cervix and body of the uterus protrude through the vagina, and the vagina is inverted (Fig. 11.2).

Uterine displacement and prolapse can be caused by congenital or acquired weakness of the pelvic support structures (often called **pelvic relaxation**). In many cases, problems can be a result of vaginal birth–related injury. Extensive damage may be noted and repaired shortly after birth. Symptoms related to pelvic relaxation most often appear during the perimenopausal period, when the effects of ovarian hormones on pelvic tissues are lost and atrophic changes begin. Pelvic trauma, stress and strain, and the aging process also are contributing factors. Other causes of pelvic relaxation include obesity, reproductive surgery, and pelvic radiation (Kirby & Lentz, 2017a).

Clinical manifestations. Symptoms of pelvic relaxation generally relate to the structure involved: urethra, bladder, uterus, vagina, cul-de-sac, or rectum. The most common complaints are pulling and

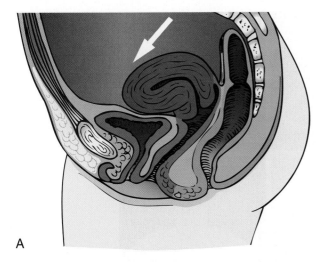

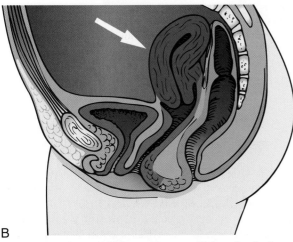

A

B

Fig. 11.1 Types of Uterine Displacements. (A) Anterior displacement. (B) Retroversion (backward displacement of the uterus).

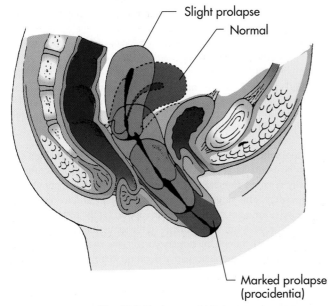

Slight prolapse

Normal

Marked prolapse (procidentia)

Fig. 11.2 Prolapse of Uterus.

dragging sensations, pressure, protrusions, fatigue, and low backache. Symptoms may be worse after prolonged standing or deep penile penetration during intercourse. Urinary incontinence can be present.

Medical and surgical management. If discomfort related to uterine displacement is a problem, several interventions can be implemented to treat this condition. Kegel exercises (see Teaching for Self-Management box: Kegel Exercises in Chapter 4) can be performed several times a day to increase muscular strength. A knee-chest position performed for a few minutes several times a day can correct a mildly retroverted uterus. A fitted pessary to support the uterus and hold it in the correct position may be inserted into the vagina (Fig. 11.3). Usually a pessary is used for only a short time because it can lead to pressure necrosis and vaginitis. After a period of treatment, most women are free of symptoms and do not require the pessary. Surgical correction is rarely indicated.

Treatment for uterine prolapse depends on the degree of prolapse. Pessaries can be useful in mild prolapse and are recommended by many health care providers as the first-line management of uterine prolapse (Bugge, Adams, Gopinath, & Reid, 2013). Estrogen therapy may be used in the older woman to improve tissue tone. If these conservative treatments do not correct the problem or the degree of prolapse is significant, vaginal hysterectomy with a vaginal vault suspension (see later discussion) is usually recommended (Kirby & Lentz, 2017a).

Nursing interventions. Nurses can teach Kegel exercises and the correct use of a pessary. Good hygiene is important when using a pessary. Some women are taught to remove the pessary at night, cleanse it, and replace it in the morning. If the pessary is always left in place, regular douching with commercially prepared solutions or weak vinegar solutions (e.g., 1 tbsp to 1 qt of water) to remove increased secretions and keep the vaginal pH at 4.0 to 4.5 can be suggested.

Cystocele and Rectocele

Cystocele and rectocele almost always accompany uterine prolapse, causing the uterus to sag even farther backward and downward into the vagina. Cystocele (Fig. 11.4A) is the protrusion of the bladder downward into the vagina that develops when supporting structures in the vesicovaginal septum are injured. Anterior wall relaxation gradually develops over time as a result of congenital defects of support structures, childbearing, obesity, or advanced age. When the woman stands, the weakened anterior vaginal wall cannot support the weight of the urine in the bladder; the vesicovaginal septum is forced downward and the bladder is stretched, resulting in an increase in capacity. With time, the cystocele enlarges until it protrudes into the vagina. Complete emptying of the bladder is difficult because the cystocele sags below the bladder neck.

Rectocele is the herniation of the anterior rectal wall through the relaxed or ruptured vaginal fascia and rectovaginal septum; it appears as a large bulge that may be seen through the relaxed introitus (see Fig. 11.4B).

Clinical manifestations. Cystoceles and rectoceles often are asymptomatic. If symptoms of cystocele are present, they include complaints of a bearing-down sensation or that "something is in my vagina." Other symptoms include urinary frequency, retention, and incontinence, as well as possible recurrent cystitis and urinary tract infections (UTIs). Pelvic examination reveals a bulging of the anterior wall of the vagina when the woman is asked to bear down. Unless the bladder neck and urethra are damaged, urinary continence is unaffected. Women with large cystoceles complain of having to push upward on the sagging anterior vaginal wall to be able to void.

Rectoceles may be small and produce few symptoms, but some are so large that they protrude outside of the vagina when the woman stands. Symptoms are absent when the woman is lying down. A rectocele causes a disturbance in bowel function, the sensation of bearing down, or the sensation that the pelvic organs are falling out. With a very large rectocele, it

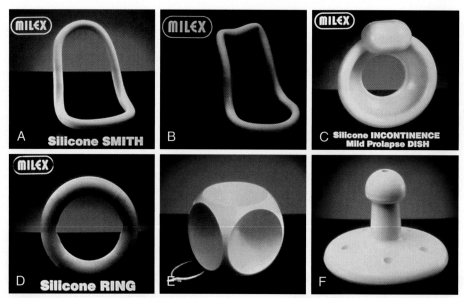

Fig. 11.3 Examples of Pessaries. (A) Smith. (B) Hodge without support. (C) Incontinence dish without support. (D) Ring without support. (E) Cube. (F) Gellhorn. (Courtesy Milex Products, Inc., a division of CooperSurgical, Trumbull, CT.)

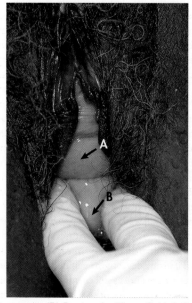

Fig. 11.4 (A) Cystocele. (B) Rectocele. (From Seidel, H., Ball, J., Dains, J., et al. [2015]. *Mosby's guide to physical examination* [8th ed.]. St. Louis: Mosby.)

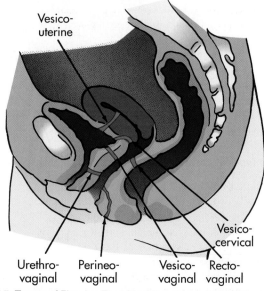

Fig. 11.5 Types of Fistulas That May Develop in the Vagina, Uterus, or Rectum. (From Monahan, F., Sands, J. K., Neighbors, M., et al. [2007]. *Phipps' medical-surgical nursing: Health and illness perspectives* [8th ed.]. St. Louis: Mosby.)

may be difficult to have a bowel movement. Each time the woman strains during bowel evacuation, the feces are forced against the thinned rectovaginal wall, stretching it more. Some women facilitate evacuation by applying digital pressure vaginally to hold up the rectal pouch.

Medical and surgical management. Treatment for a cystocele includes use of a vaginal pessary or surgical repair. An anterior repair (colporrhaphy) is the surgical procedure usually done for large symptomatic cystoceles. This involves a surgical shortening of pelvic muscles to provide better support for the bladder. An anterior repair is often combined with a vaginal hysterectomy. Physical therapy may be recommended. Use of Kegel exercises helps strengthen pelvic floor muscles and may relieve some of the symptoms of pressure caused by the cystocele (Kirby & Lentz, 2017a).

Small rectoceles may not need treatment. The woman with mild symptoms may get relief from a high-fiber (e.g., 25 g) diet and adequate fluid intake, stool softeners, or mild laxatives. Vaginal pessaries and Kegel exercises may be useful. Large rectoceles that are causing significant symptoms are usually repaired surgically. A posterior repair (colporrhaphy) is the usual procedure. This surgery is performed vaginally and involves shortening the pelvic muscles to provide better support for the rectum. Anterior and posterior repairs can be performed at the same time and with vaginal hysterectomy. Even though the surgery corrects the anatomic position, the woman may still have problems with defecation (Kirby & Lentz, 2017a).

Genital Fistulas

Genital **fistulas** are perforations between genital tract organs. Most occur between the bladder and the genital tract (e.g., vesicovaginal), between the urethra and the vagina (urethrovaginal), and between the rectum or sigmoid colon and the vagina (rectovaginal) (Fig. 11.5).

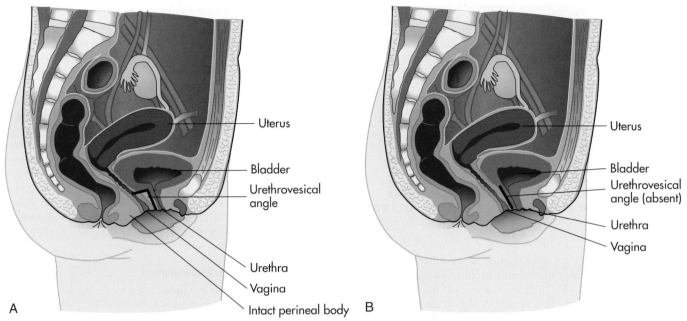

Fig. 11.6 Urethrovesical Angle. (A) Normal angle. (B) Widening (absence) of angle.

Genital fistulas may be a result of a congenital anomaly, gynecologic surgery, obstetric trauma, cancer, radiation therapy, gynecologic trauma, or infection (e.g., in the episiotomy).

Clinical manifestations. Signs and symptoms of vaginal fistulas depend on the site but can include presence of urine, flatus, or feces in the vagina. In addition, there can be odors of urine or feces in the vagina as well as irritation of vaginal tissue.

Medical and surgical management. Management of genital fistulas depends on the location. Surgical repair is the usual treatment; however, it may not be successful.

Nursing interventions. Nursing interventions for women with a mild cystocele or rectocele are similar to those suggested for women with uterine prolapse. However, nursing care of the woman with a more severe rectocele or genital fistula requires great sensitivity because the woman's reactions are often intense. She can become withdrawn or hostile because of embarrassment about odors and soiling of her clothing that are beyond her control. Her sexuality is threatened; her partner may refuse sexual intimacy.

The nurse can suggest hygiene practices that reduce odor. Commercial deodorizing douches are available, or noncommercial solutions such as diluted chlorine (e.g., 1 tsp chlorine household bleach to 1 qt water) may be used. The chlorine solution is also useful for external perineal irrigation. Sitz baths and thorough washing of the genitalia with unscented, mild soap and warm water are helpful. Sparse dusting with deodorizing powders can be useful.

If a rectovaginal fistula is present, enemas given before leaving the house may provide temporary relief from oozing of fecal material until corrective surgery is performed. Irritated skin and tissues may benefit from use of a heat lamp or application of an emollient. Hygienic care is time consuming and may need to be repeated frequently throughout the day; protective pads or pants may need to be worn. All of these activities can be demoralizing to the woman and frustrating to her and her family.

Urinary Incontinence

Urinary incontinence (UI) is defined as the involuntary leakage of urine. This condition can affect up to 75% of women across the lifespan but is more prevalent as women age (perimenopausal and postmenopausal women). Also, vaginal birth can result in this increased occurrence of urinary incontinence that rises with increased parity. Obesity and smoking also increase the risk of UI (Kirby & Lentz, 2017b).

There are three primary types of urinary incontinence that affect women: (1) stress urinary incontinence, (2) urge urinary incontinence, and (3) mixed urinary incontinence (American College of Obstetricians & Gynecologists [ACOG], 2015). Stress urinary incontinence affects urinary control due to sudden increases in intra-abdominal pressure (such as sneezing or coughing), causing involuntary urine loss. Urge incontinence is caused by disorders of the bladder and urethra, such as urethritis, urethral stricture, trigonitis, or cystitis; neuropathies, such as multiple sclerosis, diabetic neuritis, and pathologic conditions of the spinal cord; and congenital and acquired urinary tract abnormalities. Urge incontinence results from urgency to void without adequate location or time to avoid incontinence. Mixed urinary incontinence can involve both types of stress and urge incontinence and can be multifactorial in causation (ACOG).

Sometimes, stress incontinence can result from injury to bladder neck structures. A sphincter mechanism at the bladder neck compresses the upper urethra, pulls it upward behind the symphysis, and forms an acute angle at the junction of the posterior urethral wall and the base of the bladder (urethrovesical angle) (Fig. 11.6). To empty the bladder, the sphincter complex relaxes, and the trigone contracts to open the internal urethral orifice and pull the contracting bladder wall upward, forcing urine out. The angle between the urethra and the base of the bladder is lost or increased if the supporting pubococcygeus muscle is injured; this change, coupled with urethrocele, causes incontinence. Urine spurts out when the woman is asked to bear down or cough when she is in the lithotomy position.

Clinical manifestations. Involuntary leakage of urine is the main sign, with episodes commonly occurring during coughing, laughing, and exercise. Nurses may have to encourage a woman to discuss UI symptoms because she may be reluctant to discuss this problem with her health care provider (ACOG, 2015). Depression may be a comorbid factor, due to quality of life issues, including social isolation and embarrassment experienced by the woman because of UI.

Medical management. Mild to moderate UI can be significantly decreased or relieved in many women by bladder training and pelvic muscle (Kegel) exercises (ACOG, 2015). Modest weight loss can also

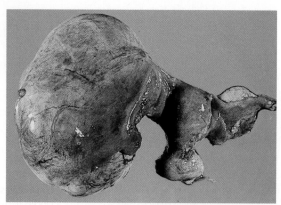

Fig. 11.7 Ovarian Cyst. (From Seidel, H., Ball, J., Dains, J., et al. [2015]. *Mosby's guide to physical examination* [8th ed.]. St. Louis: Mosby.)

improve UI symptoms in many women. Behavioral modification therapies such as reducing caffeine and scheduled voiding may reduce occurrence of UI (Muth, 2017). Other management strategies include pelvic flow support devices (i.e., pessaries), vaginal estrogen therapy, serotonin-norepinephrine reuptake inhibitors, electrical stimulation, insertion of an artificial urethral sphincter, and surgery (e.g., anterior repair) (ACOG).

Nursing interventions. Nursing care for a woman with UI includes education on UI prevention and treatment, including bladder training, pelvic muscle exercises, and guidance in lifestyle changes (e.g., losing weight, caffeine reduction, and smoking cessation). Assessment for depressive symptoms may also be warranted to ensure that quality of life and functional status concerns are addressed.

In summary, nurses should provide information and self-care education regarding UI to prevent symptoms, to manage or reduce severity of symptoms, to promote hygienic measures, and to recognize when further intervention or referral is indicated. This information can be included in women's health encounters, as well as in postpartum discharge and outpatient follow-up visits.

BENIGN NEOPLASMS

Benign neoplasms include a variety of nonmalignant cysts and tumors of the ovaries, the uterus, the vulva, and other organs of the reproductive system.

Ovarian Cysts

Functional ovarian cysts (Fig. 11.7) are dependent on hormonal influences associated with the menstrual cycle. These cysts may be classified as follicular cysts, corpus luteum cysts, theca-lutein cysts, endometrial cysts, and polycystic ovarian syndrome (PCOS). Other benign ovarian neoplasms include dermoid cysts and ovarian fibromas.

Follicular Cysts

Follicular cysts develop most commonly in normal ovaries of young women as a result of the mature graafian follicle failing to rupture, or when an immature follicle does not resorb fluid after ovulation. A cyst is usually asymptomatic unless it ruptures, in which case it causes severe pelvic pain. If the cyst does not rupture, it usually shrinks after two or three menstrual cycles.

Corpus Luteum Cysts

Corpus luteum cysts occur after ovulation and are possibly caused by an increased secretion of progesterone that results in an increase of fluid in the corpus luteum. Clinical manifestations associated with a corpus luteum cyst include pain, tenderness over the ovary, delayed menses, and irregular or prolonged menstrual flow. A rupture can cause intraperitoneal hemorrhage. Corpus luteum cysts usually disappear without treatment within one or two menstrual cycles.

Theca-Lutein Cysts

Theca-lutein cysts are uncommon—up to 50% of cases are associated with hydatidiform mole (a rare, abnormal growth of tissue from a fertilized egg or overgrowth of placental tissue. See Chapter 28 for more information on hydatidiform mole). Theca-lutein cysts develop as a result of prolonged stimulation of the ovaries by human chorionic gonadotropin (hCG). They also can occur if the woman has taken ovulation induction drugs; if she is pregnant and a large placenta is present, such as in the presence of a multiple gestation; or if she has diabetes (Dolan, Hill, & Valea, 2017). The cysts are almost always bilateral. The woman may note a feeling of pelvic fullness if the ovary is enlarged, but most women are asymptomatic.

Medical and Surgical Management

Medical interventions can be implemented for the woman with a functional cyst. In expectant management, the woman is advised to keep appointments for pelvic examinations to assess for changes in size of the cyst (enlarging or shrinking). Pharmacologic interventions such as analgesics may be prescribed for pain management. Oral contraceptives (OCs) may be ordered for several months to suppress ovulation for functional cysts. Large cysts (greater than 8 cm) or cysts that do not shrink may be removed surgically (cystectomy). Corpus luteum cysts are treated similarly. Theca-lutein cysts are usually managed conservatively (they often regress without treatment) or by removal of the hydatidiform mole (Dolan et al., 2017).

Nursing Interventions

Nursing care focuses on educating the woman about treatment options as well as pain management with analgesics or comfort measures such as heat to the abdomen or relaxation techniques. If surgery is performed, the nurse provides preoperative and postoperative care. Discharge teaching includes signs of infection, postoperative incision care, the possibility of recurrence, and advice regarding follow-up appointments.

Polycystic Ovarian Syndrome

Polycystic ovarian syndrome (PCOS) occurs when an endocrine imbalance results in high levels of estrogen, testosterone, and luteinizing hormone (LH) and decreased secretion of follicle-stimulating hormone (FSH). This syndrome is associated with a variety of problems in the hypothalamic-pituitary-ovarian axis and with androgen-producing tumors. The condition can be transmitted as an X-linked dominant or autosomal dominant trait (Stein-Leventhal syndrome). Multiple follicular cysts develop on one or both ovaries and produce excess estrogen. The ovaries often double in size (Lobo, 2017).

Clinical Manifestations

Clinical manifestations include obesity, hirsutism (excessive hair growth), irregular menses or amenorrhea, and infertility. Impaired glucose tolerance and hyperinsulinemia occur in about 40% of women with PCOS (Dolan et al., 2017). Affected women are at increased risk for metabolic syndrome, including development of type 2 diabetes mellitus, nonalcoholic fatty liver disease, and possibly cardiovascular disease (Goodman, Corbin, Futterweit, et al., 2015). PCOS is often diagnosed in adolescence when menstrual irregularities and other symptoms appear (Dolan et al).

Medical Management

The treatment for PCOS depends on symptoms that are of greatest concern to the woman. Lifestyle modifications (e.g., losing weight) and management of presenting symptoms such as infertility, irregular menses, and hirsutism are the focus. Lifestyle modifications can be very effective in regulating menses, preventing progression to type 2 diabetes mellitus, and lowering cardiovascular risk (Jayasena & Franks, 2014). OCs are the usual treatment for irregular menses, if pregnancy is not desired, because they inhibit LH and decrease testosterone levels. OCs can also lessen acne to some degree. Spironolactone, an antiandrogen, is frequently used with an OC. In severe cases, gonadotropin-releasing hormone (GnRH) analogs may be used to treat hirsutism if OCs are not effective. If pregnancy is desired, ovulation-inducing medications are given (Dolan et al., 2017). Metformin and other insulin medications for type 2 diabetes also are used to lower insulin, testosterone, and glucose levels, which in turn can reduce acne, hirsutism, abdominal obesity, amenorrhea, and other PCOS symptoms (Dolan et. al). Women with PCOS should be monitored for development of type 2 diabetes, metabolic syndrome, and risk for cardiovascular disease.

Nursing Interventions

Nurses have important roles in educating and counseling women with PCOS, including information on managing symptoms, current and possible long-term health effects, as well as psychosocial concerns. Education and counseling on lifestyle modifications such as exercise, dietary modifications, weight loss, and prescribed medications should be provided. Information about finding a support group or information on the internet may also be helpful. The nursing care plan should include assessment for potential signs of psychological distress such as depression, anxiety, or social fears. The woman may need to discuss feelings regarding PCOS symptoms, and will need emotional support if PCOS-related self-image problems exist.

Other Benign Ovarian Cysts and Neoplasms

Two other ovarian neoplasms are dermoid cysts and ovarian fibromas. Dermoid cysts are germ cell tumors, usually occurring in childhood. These cysts contain substances such as hair, teeth, sebaceous secretions, and bones. Unless the cyst is large enough to put pressure on other organs, it is usually asymptomatic. Dermoid cysts may develop bilaterally and are often attached to the ovary. Treatment is usually surgical removal.

Ovarian fibromas are solid ovarian neoplasms developing from connective tissue, and most often occurring after menopause. Fibromas range in size from small nodules to large masses weighing more than 23 kg. Most fibromas are unilateral. They are usually asymptomatic, but if large enough, they may cause ascites, feelings of pelvic pressure, or abdominal enlargement. Treatment is usually surgical removal.

Nursing care of women who have surgery for the removal of dermoid cysts and ovarian fibromas is similar to that described for functional ovarian cysts.

Uterine Polyps

Uterine polyps may be endometrial or cervical in origin. They are tumors that are on pedicles (stalks) arising from the mucosa (Fig. 11.8). The etiology is unknown, although they may develop in response to hormonal stimulus or be the result of inflammation. Polyps are the most common benign lesions of the cervix and endometrium that occur during the reproductive years. These polyps may be single or multiple. Endocervical polyps are most common in multiparous

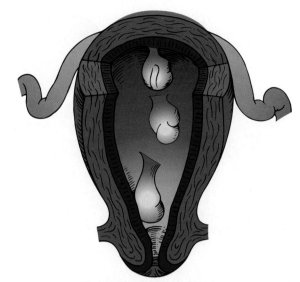

Fig. 11.8 Endometrial Polyps.

women older than 40 years. The woman may be asymptomatic or she may have premenstrual or postmenstrual staining, menorrhagia, postmenstrual spotting, or postcoital bleeding (Dolan et al., 2017).

Surgical Management

Clinical management of endometrial polyps is surgical removal. Cervical polyps are usually removed in an office or clinic procedure without anesthesia. The polyp is grasped with a clamp and twisted or cut off. All polyps should be sent for pathologic examination. Endometrial sampling (which may require local anesthesia) should be done to determine if other pathologic conditions are present (Dolan et al., 2017).

Nursing Interventions

Nursing care includes preparing the woman for what to expect during the removal procedure, encouraging relaxation and breathing exercises, and providing support during the procedure. After the procedure, the woman is advised to avoid using tampons, having sexual intercourse, and douching for up to 1 week or until the site is healed. She is taught how to identify signs of infection and to notify her health care provider if she experiences heavy bleeding (more than one pad in 1 hour).

Leiomyomas

Leiomyomas, also known as fibroid tumors, fibromas, myomas, or fibromyomas, are slow-growing benign tumors arising from the muscle tissue of the uterus (Dolan et al., 2017). They are the most common benign tumors of the reproductive system, occurring most often after age 50. They tend to occur more often in African American women and women who have never been pregnant. Fibroids also occur more often in women who are overweight (Dolan et al.). They rarely become malignant. Because their growth is influenced by ovarian hormones, these benign tumors can become quite large when the woman is pregnant or taking hormone therapy. They often spontaneously shrink after menopause when circulating ovarian hormones diminish (Dolan et al).

Clinical Manifestations

The cause of leiomyomas remains unknown, although genetic factors may be involved. Most of the tumors are found in the body of the uterus. Leiomyomas are classified according to the location in the uterine wall. Subserous leiomyomas (Fig. 11.9A) develop beneath the peritoneal surface of the uterus and appear as small or large masses that protrude from the outer uterine surface. Intramural leiomyomas

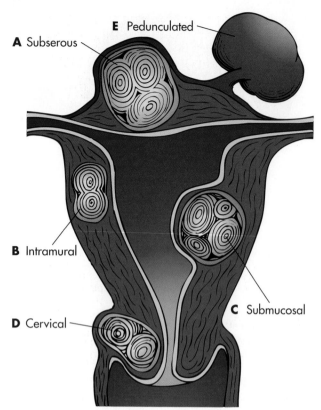

Fig. 11.9 Types of Leiomyomas. (A) Subserous. (B) Intramural. (C) Submucosal. (D) Cervical. (E) Pedunculated.

(see Fig. 11.9B) are tumors that develop within the wall of the uterus. *Submucosal* leiomyomas (see Fig. 11.9C) are the least common tumors, but often cause the most symptoms; they develop in the endometrium and protrude into the uterine cavity. Leiomyomas can develop in the cervix and on the broad ligaments (see Fig. 11.9D). They can grow on pedicles or stalks (see Fig. 11.9E). Occasionally these break off the pedicle and attach to other tissues (become parasitic).

Most women are asymptomatic; abnormal uterine bleeding is the most common symptom of fibroids. If the tumor is very large, pelvic circulation may be compromised, and surrounding viscera may be displaced. A woman may complain of backache, low abdominal pressure, constipation, urinary incontinence, or dysmenorrhea (painful menstruation). Nausea and vomiting may occur if the tumor obstructs the intestines. The woman also may notice an abdominal mass if the tumor is large. Anemia can occur if the woman has excessive bleeding. Pedunculated tumors can twist and become necrotic, causing pain (Dolan et al., 2017).

The tumors appear to be influenced by the presence of estrogen. Fibroids can affect implantation and maintenance of pregnancy. During pregnancy the tumors can produce complications such as miscarriage, preterm labor, or dystocia (difficult labor). The severity of the symptoms seems to be directly related to the size and location of the tumors.

CARE MANAGEMENT

Assessment should include a history of symptoms (which might include abnormal bleeding, abdominal pain, dysmenorrhea, pelvic fullness or heaviness, or problems with elimination) and a pelvic examination. Diagnosis is usually accomplished by a process of elimination. A pelvic examination usually identifies the presence of uterine enlargement. Negative pregnancy tests rule out pregnancy as the cause

of the symptoms. Laparoscopy may be used to differentiate ovarian masses from uterine masses. Ultrasound examination can differentiate between inflammatory masses or endometriosis and subserous fibroids.

Based on the assessment, the nurse may identify client concerns about pain, fear of malignancy, and the different surgical treatments that can be used, and their potential effects on her physical and sexual well-being. The nurse uses this information to determine nursing diagnoses as a plan of care is formulated.

Knowledge of the medical-surgical management of leiomyomas is essential in planning nursing care. This knowledge enables the nurse to work collaboratively with other members of the interprofessional team and to meet the woman's informational and emotional needs. Clinical management of benign tumors of the uterus depends on the severity of the symptoms, the age of the woman, and her desire to preserve childbearing potential.

Medical Management

Medications. If symptoms are mild, follow-up care may suffice to observe for growth or changes in size. Nonsteroidal antiinflammatory drugs (NSAIDs) may be prescribed for pain; OCs inhibit ovulation and may relieve symptoms. Medical management is based on using medications to reduce circulating levels of estrogen and progesterone. GnRH agonists may be prescribed to reduce the size of the leiomyoma. Other medications include medroxyprogesterone acetate (Depo-Provera), danazol (Danocrine), antiprogesterone (mifepristone), selective estrogen receptor modulators (SERMs), and aromatase inhibitors (Dolan et al., 2017).

Nursing interventions. The woman who prefers medication for treatment will need information about prescribed medications, their actions and side effects, and routes of administration. Women who are receiving GnRH agonists (to decrease the size of the fibroid) need instruction on the fact that regrowth will occur after the treatment is stopped. A small loss in bone mass and changes in lipid levels also can occur; therefore, long-term use is not recommended. Amenorrhea may occur; however, women who want to avoid pregnancy should use a nonhormonal or barrier method of contraception. A discussion of administration methods for GnRH agonists, including subcutaneous and intramuscular injections, intranasal administration, and subcutaneous implantation, will assist the woman in making a decision about her preferred method of administration (see Medication Guide: Infertility Medications in Chapter 9).

Uterine Artery Embolization

Uterine artery embolization (UAE) is a treatment during which polyvinyl alcohol (PVA) pellets or other embolic materials are injected into selected blood vessels to block the blood supply to the fibroid and cause shrinkage and resolution of symptoms (Dolan et al., 2017). The procedure is done under local anesthesia with conscious sedation and can be done as an outpatient procedure, although some women will have the procedure in the hospital setting and remain overnight or be discharged within 4 to 6 hours (Dolan et al.). An incision is made into the groin, and a catheter is threaded into the femoral artery to the uterine artery. An arteriogram identifies the vessels supplying the fibroid. Most fibroids are reduced in size by 50% within 3 months. Temporary amenorrhea or early menopause can occur in some women. Although symptom improvement occurs for most women, data are lacking about the effects on future fertility and pregnancy outcomes. Miscarriage, intrauterine growth restriction, and preterm birth have been reported. Complications are usually minor and of short duration. Major complications are less likely to occur with UAE compared with myomectomy (Agnihotri, 2016). There is an increase in the likelihood that further surgical intervention will be needed in a few years after the initial UAE (Agnihotri, 2016; Fonseca, Castro, Machado, et al., 2017).

Nursing interventions. Preoperative teaching includes advising the woman not to drink alcohol or smoke and not to take aspirin or anticoagulant medications before the procedure. She can expect cramping during injection of the PVA pellets. Post procedure, the nurse assesses for and teaches the woman about what to expect, including some pain, fever, malaise, and nausea and vomiting that may be caused by acute fibroid degeneration. Pain can be controlled with NSAIDs or opioid analgesics if needed. Postoperative nursing assessments include vital signs, monitoring the groin for bleeding, pain assessment, and neurovascular assessment of the affected leg. Discharge instructions should include self-care and notifying the health care provider for any suspected postprocedure complications.

Surgical Management

Surgical options to treat leiomyomas include hysterectomy and myomectomy, as well as other surgical techniques that have been developed These include laparoscopic and hysteroscopic techniques; myolysis by heat, cold, and laser; and magnetic resonance–guided focused ultrasound surgery. Not all of these techniques are suitable for every woman, nor are all of them universally available.

Laser surgery. Laser surgery or electrocauterization can be used to destroy small fibroids through a laparoscopic (abdominal) or hysteroscopic (vaginal) approach. Hysteroscopic uterine *ablation* (vaporization of tissues) can be performed under local or general anesthesia, usually as an outpatient procedure. Medical therapy using GnRH agonists to control bleeding temporarily and to suppress endometrial tissue may be given for 8 to 12 weeks before surgery. Although the uterus remains in place, the vaporization process can cause scarring and adhesions in the uterine cavity, affecting future fertility. Therefore, this procedure is for women who wish to retain their uterus but no longer desire childbearing potential (Parker & Gambone, 2016).

Risks of the procedure include uterine perforation, cervical injury, and fluid overload (caused by the leaking into blood vessels of fluid used to expand the uterus during surgery). The woman may experience postoperative cramping and a slight vaginal discharge for a few days. Before discharge, the following information is given:

- Analgesics or NSAIDs can be used for pain relief as needed.
- Normal activities can be resumed within several days.
- Vaginal discharge is to be expected for 4 to 6 weeks.
- Use of tampons and vaginal intercourse should be avoided for 2 weeks.
- The next menstrual period may be irregular.
- The woman should be reminded about the effects of ablation on her fertility, if appropriate.
- The health care provider should be called if the woman has heavy bleeding or signs of infection.

Myomectomy. If the tumor is near the outer wall of the uterus, the uterine size is no larger than the equivalent of 12 to 14 weeks of gestation, and symptoms are significant, myomectomy (removal of the tumor) may be performed (Dolan et al., 2017). Myomectomy can be performed through a laparoscopic or abdominal incision approach or a vaginal (hysteroscopic) approach. Myomectomy leaves the uterine muscle walls relatively intact, thereby preserving

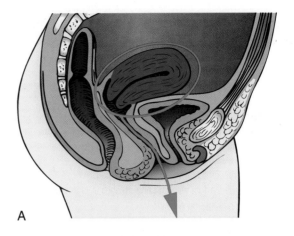

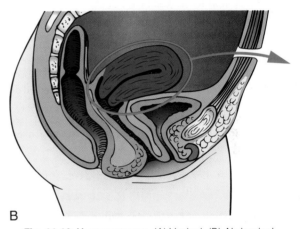

Fig. 11.10 Hysterectomy. (A) Vaginal. (B) Abdominal.

the uterus and allowing the possibility of future pregnancies. It is usually performed in the proliferative phase of the menstrual cycle to avoid interrupting a possible pregnancy. GnRH therapy may be given before surgery to reduce the size of the fibroid. Fibroids can recur after myomectomy; further treatment may be needed (Parker & Gambone, 2016).

Hysterectomy. A total hysterectomy (removal of the entire uterus) is the treatment of choice if bleeding is severe or if the fibroid is obstructing normal function of other organs. An abdominal or vaginal surgical approach depends on the size and location of the tumors. For example, abdominal hysterectomy is usually performed for leiomyomas larger than a uterus would be at 12 to 14 weeks of gestation or for multiple leiomyomas. The uterus is removed through either a vertical or transverse incision. Vaginal approaches can be used for smaller tumors. In both abdominal and vaginal approaches, the uterus is removed from the supporting ligaments (broad, round, and uterosacral). These ligaments are then attached to the vaginal cuff, allowing maintenance of normal depth of the vagina (Fig. 11.10). Alternatives to these procedures are the *laparoscopic-assisted vaginal hysterectomy (LAVH)* and the *laparoscopic-assisted supracervical hysterectomy (LASH)*. LAVH converts an abdominal procedure to a vaginal one by using a laparoscope in the abdomen to assist with removal of the uterus. LASH allows the cervix to remain.

Preoperative nursing interventions. Assessments needed before surgery include the woman's knowledge of treatment options, her desire for future fertility if she is premenopausal, the benefits and risks

BOX 11.1 Questions to Inform Consent When Surgery is Recommended

- Why is this procedure proposed for my condition/problem?
- What are the risks/benefits of the proposed surgery?
- Are there alternatives to this surgery? If so, what are the risks and benefits of these alternatives?
- How many times have you performed this surgery?
- How long will I be hospitalized? Can the procedure be done in an outpatient setting? How long will it take to recover?
- What types of anesthesia can be used?
- What hospital and surgical procedures can I expect?
- How will the surgery affect me (e.g., any changes in physical function, sexual function, or childbearing ability)?

From Wade, J., Pletsch, P., Morgan, S., & Menting, S. (2000). Hysterectomy: What do women need and want to know? *Journal of Obstetric, Gynecologic and Neonatal Nursing, 29*(1), 33–42.

of each procedure, preoperative and postoperative procedures (Boxes 11.1 and 11.2), and the recovery process. If the woman demonstrates understanding of this information, she can make an informed decision about treatment and feel a sense of control over the surgical experience. Resources on helping women to make decisions about treatment can be found at the website for the Fibroid Treatment Collective at www.fibroids.org.

⍰ CLINICAL REASONING CASE STUDY

Informed Decision Making for Treatment of Leiomyoma

Janay, a 35-year-old divorced African American woman, has a large uterine leiomyoma. She has experienced very heavy, prolonged, and painful menses for the past 2 years, and has failed conservative management, including systemic oral contraceptives to lighten menstrual symptoms. She does not want to have a hysterectomy and also wants to retain childbearing potential. She is considering a UAE that has been offered by the gynecologist to ease her symptoms. She is seeking more information and asked the nurse to provide information prior to making her decision on whether or not to proceed with UAE. What responses by the nurse would be appropriate?

1. What is the priority concern or client need in this situation?
2. List other client needs/problems in this case.
3. Identify any additional information needed by the nurse in addressing this situation.
4. Describe the roles/responsibilities of interprofessional health team members who may be involved in this situation.

Psychologic assessment is essential, particularly for a woman who is scheduled for a hysterectomy. Areas to be explored include the significance of the loss of the uterus for the woman, misconceptions about effects of surgery, and adequacy of her support system. Women who have not completed their childbearing, who believe that their self-concept is related to having a uterus (to be a complete woman), who feel that sexual functioning is related to having a uterus, or who have too little or too much anxiety about the surgery may be at risk for postoperative emotional reactions.

BOX 11.2 Preoperative Procedures for Hysterectomy

- Vaginal examination or physical examination
- Laboratory tests
  - Complete blood count, type, and crossmatch
  - Urinalysis
- Chest radiograph
- Electrocardiogram
- Teaching for postoperative routines
  - Turning, coughing, deep breathing
  - Passive and active leg exercises
  - Need for early ambulation
  - Pain relief options
- Nothing by mouth after midnight the night before surgery or as ordered
- Enema if ordered
- Douche if ordered
- Abdominal: mons or perineal hair clipping if ordered
- Removal of makeup, nail polish
- Removal of glasses, contact lenses, dentures, etc.
- Identification band in place
- Signed consent form in chart
- Have woman empty bladder immediately before surgery

Postoperative nursing interventions. Postoperative assessments and care after myomectomy and abdominal hysterectomy are similar to those for other abdominal surgery (Box 11.3). Specific to abdominal and vaginal hysterectomy are assessments for vaginal bleeding (one perineal pad saturated in less than 1 hour is excessive), urinary retention (especially after vaginal hysterectomy), perineal pain after vaginal hysterectomy, and psychologic assessments (e.g., depression).

Discharge planning and teaching. Discharge planning and teaching are similar for myomectomy and hysterectomy (see Teaching for Self-Management box: Care After Myomectomy or Hysterectomy). Myomectomy and vaginal hysterectomy may be performed in an ambulatory setting, and women may be discharged the evening of the surgery. Women who have an abdominal hysterectomy may have a 1- to 2-day stay in the hospital before being discharged.

TEACHING FOR SELF-MANAGEMENT

Care After Myomectomy or Hysterectomy

- Eat foods high in protein, iron, and vitamin C to aid in tissue healing; include foods with high fiber content; and drink six to eight 8-ounce glasses of water daily.
- Rest when tired; resume activities as comfort level permits. Avoid vigorous exercise and heavy lifting for 6 weeks. Avoid sitting for long periods. Resume driving when comfort allows or on advice from health care provider.
- Avoid tub baths, intercourse (vaginal rest), and douching until after the follow-up examination.
- When vaginal intercourse is resumed, water-soluble lubricants may decrease discomfort.
- Report the following symptoms to your health care provider: vaginal bleeding, gastrointestinal changes, persistent postoperative symptoms (cramping, distention, change in bowel habits), and signs of wound infection (redness, swelling, heat, or pain at incision site).
- Keep your follow-up appointment with your health care provider.

BOX 11.3 Postoperative Care After Hysterectomy

- Monitor vital signs every 15 minutes until stable, then every 4 hours for 48 hours
- Remind client to turn, cough, deep breathe every 2 hours for 24 hours
  - Assist her to splint incision with hands or pillow
- Incentive spirometry if ordered
- Leg exercises every 2-4 hours until ambulatory
- Assess bleeding
  - Abdominal: assess dressing or incision
  - Vaginal: perineal pad count (one saturated pad in less than 1 hour is excessive; vaginal bleeding is usually minimal)
- Check laboratory values, especially hematocrit
- Assess lung sounds
- Assess bowel sounds and monitor bowel function
- Monitor intake and output
  - Foley catheter may be in place for 24 hours after abdominal surgery
  - After vaginal hysterectomy, urinary retention may occur because of manipulation of the urethra during surgery
- Assess abdominal incision or vagina for signs of infection
- Observe for signs of complications
  - Abdominal hysterectomy: assess for signs of wound evisceration, pulmonary embolism, thrombophlebitis, pneumonia, bowel obstruction, bleeding (incisional or vaginal)
  - Vaginal hysterectomy: assess for signs of urinary tract infection, urinary retention, wound infection, vaginal bleeding
- Pain relief
  - Pharmacologic measures: patient-controlled analgesia or epidural opioids may be ordered for the first 24 hours, followed by oral analgesics and nonsteroidal antiinflammatory drugs
  - Nonpharmacologic measures: breathing and relaxation exercises, position changes, guided imagery, application of heat to the abdomen (abdominal hysterectomy), and sitz baths or ice packs for the perineum (vaginal hysterectomy); ambulation may relieve gas pains
- Psychologic assessments
  - Assess for depression or other emotional reactions
  - Assess support systems
  - Assess sexual concerns

If a hysterectomy was performed, the woman is reminded that she will experience cessation of menses. If the woman is premenopausal, she will not experience menopause at this time unless her ovaries also were removed. If the ovaries were not removed, there will be no reason for her to consider hormone replacement therapy. If the ovaries are removed, the woman will need the most current information on the risks and benefits of hormone replacement therapy (see Chapter 6). Other symptoms include pain, sleep disturbance, fatigue, anxiety, and depression.

Vaginal intercourse may be uncomfortable at first, especially after vaginal procedures. Water-soluble lubricants, relaxation exercises, and positions that control penile penetration may be beneficial. Women can be assured that this discomfort will decrease over time.

The schedule for follow-up care depends on the procedure performed, but usually a postoperative visit is scheduled within a week. Vaginal screening with cytology or Papanicolaou (Pap) test after total hysterectomy for a nonmalignant reason is not recommended (American Cancer Society [ACS], 2019a). (See Table 4.3 for Pap test recommendations.)

Vulvar Problems

Bartholin Cysts

Bartholin cysts are the most common benign lesions of the vulva. They arise from obstruction of the Bartholin duct, which causes it to enlarge. Small cysts often are asymptomatic; however, large cysts or infected cysts cause symptoms such as vulvar pain, dyspareunia (painful intercourse), and a feeling of a mass in the vulva (Gardella, Eckert, & Lentz, 2017).

Medical and surgical management. If the woman is asymptomatic, no treatment is necessary. If the cyst is symptomatic or infected, surgical incision and drainage may provide temporary relief. Cysts tend to recur; therefore, a permanent opening for drainage may be recommended. This procedure is called *marsupialization* and is the formation of a new duct opening for drainage (Gardella et al., 2017).

Nursing interventions. Nursing care after surgery includes teaching the woman about pain-relief measures such as sitz baths, heat lamps to the perineum, and the use of analgesics. The woman is taught to assess the incision site for signs of healing and infection and to take antibiotics, if prescribed, to prevent infection.

Vulvodynia

Vulvar pain is a common gynecologic problem. Vulvodynia, also called *vulvar pain syndrome* or *vulvovestibulitis*, is reportedly experienced by about 15% of women. The incidence is thought to be the same for women of all races and ethnicities (Dolan et al., 2017).

Vulvodynia is a complex condition thought to be a chronic pain disorder of the vulvar area. The term *vulvodynia* is used if pain is present with no visible abnormality or no identified neurologic diagnosis. Pain can be described as provoked (e.g., by inserting a tampon or having vaginal intercourse) or unprovoked and localized to the vestibule or generalized over the vulvar area (Dolan et al., 2017).

Etiology has not been established although psychologic and biologic theories have been proposed. The most common theory is that vulvodynia is caused by a chronic neuropathic pain syndrome. Inflammation may also be a causative factor and continues to be investigated (Dolan et al., 2017).

A feature of neuropathic pain is *allodynia*, which is a painful sensation that is from something not supposed to be painful. It commonly occurs in women with vulvodynia. Several triggers that reportedly cause allodynia in the vulvar area include use of OCs; presence of candidiasis or human papillomavirus (HPV); wearing tight-fitting underwear and pants, especially synthetic materials; sexual activity; and tampon use (Dolan et al., 2017). However, with all these triggers, research evidence is conflicting and the search for scientific evidence is ongoing.

Assessment of a woman with possible vulvodynia includes a health history that also addresses mental health issues, specifically anxiety or depression. A thorough pain assessment is essential. Questions about provoking and palliative factors, quality of the pain, radiation of the pain, strength of the pain, and the timing of pain occurrence are included. A history may elicit complaints about burning, stinging, or irritation in the vulvar area, and reports of how the woman thinks her symptoms affect her physical activities and ability for sexual intimacy.

A thorough pelvic examination is recommended to rule out other causes of pain such as infection or trauma. The vulva should be inspected for erythema, ulcerations, and hyperpigmentation (Dolan et al., 2017).

A cotton swab is used to identify areas of pain on pressure to confirm presence of allodynia. A systematic assessment (e.g., using positions of the face of a clock) is suggested, and pain should be rated as mild, moderate, or severe. A speculum (a pediatric size is recommended) is used to examine the vagina for redness, erosions, and dryness. A swab of vaginal secretions is obtained and can be tested for increased white blood cells, and pH. Cultures for *Candida* (yeast) and bacteria can be obtained. A bimanual examination may be performed (Dolan et al., 2017).

Management strategies are individualized to the woman. Often a series of therapies or a combination of therapies is implemented to find the best treatment. There is little evidence to support one therapy over another. Oral medications include gabapentin and tricyclic antidepressants. Topical therapies include the use of lidocaine 5% ointment that can be applied nightly or prophylactically (i.e., before sexual intercourse). Other therapeutic measures that are reportedly helpful for symptoms include pelvic floor exercises, biofeedback, vaginal dilator training, hypnosis, and cognitive-behavioral therapy (Dolan et al., 2017). Hygienic measures include wearing white cotton underwear, using 100% cotton menstrual pads, using soaps and detergents for sensitive skin, avoiding wearing tight clothing over the vulvar area, avoiding lubricants that contain propylene glycol, and using natural oils such as olive oil for lubricants (Mayo Clinic, 2019).

Surgery is usually not recommended until other measures have proven to be ineffective. The surgical procedure is a vestibulectomy, a difficult procedure that removes the vestibule and hymen and has a high rate of complications (Dolan et al., 2017).

Client information about vulvodynia, including how to locate support groups, is available on various websites:
- International Society for the Study of Vulvovaginal Disease: www.issvd.org
- National Vulvodynia Association: www.nva.org
- Vulval Pain Society: www.vulvalpainsociety.org

MALIGNANT NEOPLASMS

Malignant neoplasms of the reproductive system include cancers of the endometrium, the cervix, the ovary, the vulva, the vagina, and the uterine tubes. In 2019, it is estimated that 13,170 women will be diagnosed with invasive cervical cancer, and 22,530 women will be diagnosed with ovarian cancer (ACS, 2019a). Obesity is associated with increased risk for developing many cancers, including cancers of the endometrium, ovary, and cervix. Evidence suggests that being overweight increases the risk for cancer recurrence and decreases the likelihood of survival for these cancers (ACS).

Cancer of the Endometrium
Incidence and Etiology

Endometrial cancer is estimated to occur in 61,880 women in 2019 (ACS, 2019a). It is most commonly seen in perimenopausal and postmenopausal women between ages 50 and 65. Certain risk factors have been associated with the development of endometrial cancer, including obesity (especially upper body fat localization), nulliparity, infertility, late onset of menopause, diabetes mellitus, hypertension, PCOS, and family history of ovarian or breast disease (ACS; Creasman & Miller, 2018). There appears to be an increased risk for endometrial cancer in families with hereditary nonpolyposis colorectal cancer (HNPCC). Hormone imbalance, however, seems to be the most significant risk factor. Numerous studies have correlated the use of exogenous estrogens (unopposed stimulation; i.e., absence of progesterone) in postmenopausal women with an increased incidence of uterine cancer. Tamoxifen taken by women for breast cancer also has been related to

a slight increase in endometrial cancer (Creasman & Miller, 2018). Pregnancy and use of low-dose oral contraceptive pills appear to offer some protection. While the incidence of endometrial cancer in Caucasian women has been higher than that in African American and Hispanic women, in the years 2006 to 2015, the incidence rate increased by about 1% per year among white women and by about 2% per year among black women. Mortality rate is higher in African American women (ACS, 2019a).

Endometrial cancer is slow-growing and for that reason has a good prognosis if diagnosed at a localized stage. Most endometrial cancers are adenocarcinomas that develop from endometrial hyperplasia. The tumor usually develops in the fundus of the uterus and can spread directly to the myometrium and cervix, as well as to other reproductive organs. Metastasis (spread of cancer from its original site) is through the lymphatic system in the pelvis and through the blood to the liver, the lungs, and the brain.

CARE MANAGEMENT

Clinical Manifestations and Diagnoses

Assessment includes a history of physical symptoms. The cardinal sign of endometrial cancer is abnormal uterine bleeding (e.g., postmenopausal bleeding and premenopausal recurrent menorrhagia). Late signs include a mucosanguineous vaginal discharge, low back pain, or low pelvic pain. A pelvic examination may reveal the presence of a uterine enlargement or mass.

! NURSING ALERT

Women can be informed that they can identify their own risk for developing endometrial as well as ovarian, cervical, and breast cancers by filling out a confidential cancer risk assessment survey that is available at the American Cancer Society (ACS) website: www.cancer.org.

Histologic examination is used for diagnosis. A Pap test of cellular material obtained by aspiration of the endocervix identifies only one-third to one half of cases. Endometrial biopsy or fractional curettage yields the most accurate results. Fractional curettage involves scraping the endocervix and endometrium for histologic evaluation to determine the grade of neoplasm and its stage (extent). Perforation of the uterus is a possible complication of this procedure. Endometrial biopsy is more commonly performed and identifies about 90% of cases (Creasman & Miller, 2018). It is usually done on an outpatient basis under local anesthesia. A suction-type curette is used to remove tissue for sampling. It is recommended that women at risk for HNPCC have an annual biopsy or transvaginal ultrasound beginning at age 35 (ACS, 2019a). Tests to determine the spread of cancer include liver function tests, renal function tests, chest x-ray, intravenous pyelography (IVP), barium enema, computed tomography (CT), magnetic resonance imaging (MRI), bone scans, and biopsy of suspicious tissues. The International Federation of Gynecology and Obstetrics (FIGO) classification system is used to describe the stages of endometrial carcinoma (Table 11.1).

Medical and Surgical Management

Collaborative efforts are needed to work with the woman with endometrial cancer. Care management by an interprofessional team includes understanding appropriate treatment modalities.

TABLE 11.1 2009 FIGO Classification of Endometrial Carcinoma

Stage	Description
I (Includes grades 1, 2, or 3)	Tumor limited to corpus uteri
IA	No or less than half myometrial invasion
IB	Invasion equal to or more than half of the myometrium
II	Cervical stromal invasion, not extending beyond the uterus
III (Includes grades 1, 2, or 3)	Local and regional spread of tumor
IIIA	Tumor invades the serosa of the corpus uteri and/or adnexae
IIIB	Vaginal and/or parametrial involvement
IIIC	Metastases to pelvic and/or paraaortic lymph nodes
	IIIC1 Positive pelvic nodes
	IIIC2 Positive paraaortic lymph nodes with or without positive pelvic lymph nodes
IV (Includes grades 1, 2, or 3)	Tumor invasion of bladder and/or bowel mucosa and/or distant metastasis
IVA	Tumor invasion of bladder and/or bowel mucosa
IVB	Distant metastases, including intraabdominal metastasis and/or inguinal lymph nodes

From Creasman, W. T., & Miller, D. S. (2018). Adenocarcinoma of the uterine corpus. In P. J. DiSaia, W. T. Creasman, R. S. Mannel, & D. S. Mutch (Eds.), *Clinical gynecologic oncology* (9th ed.). Philadelphia: Saunders.

For stage I adenocarcinoma of the endometrium limited to the uterus, total abdominal hysterectomy (TAH) and bilateral salpingo-oophorectomy (BSO) is the usual treatment (Creasman & Miller, 2018). Radiation use in stage I continues to be studied; it can reduce the risk of recurrence, but evidence does not demonstrate improved survival rates or reduced metastasis to distant sites. It can be used when the woman is a poor surgical risk (Soliman & Lu, 2017). A **radical hysterectomy** (abdominal hysterectomy with wide excision of parametrial tissue laterally and uterosacral ligaments posteriorly), BSO, and pelvic node dissection usually are performed for stage II endometrial cancer. If nodes are positive or if there is extensive uterine disease or metastasis outside the uterus, external pelvic radiation (see External Therapy later in this chapter) is usually done postoperatively. Internal radiation therapy or brachytherapy (placement of an applicator loaded with a radiation source into the uterine cavity; see Internal Therapy later in this chapter) also may be used before surgery or combined with external radiation. Treatment of advanced stages is individualized but usually includes a TAH-BSO plus chemotherapy or radiation, or both (Soliman & Lu).

Chemotherapy is used to treat advanced and recurrent. No definitely effective treatment regimen, however, has been established (Soliman & Lu, 2017).

Progestational therapy—use of medroxyprogesterone (Depo-Provera) and megestrol (Megace)—may be effective for recurrent cancers, especially those that are estrogen receptor (ER) positive. These drugs usually do not cause acute side effects. Tamoxifen and raloxifene (see Medication Guide Guides: Tamoxifen and Raloxifene Hydrochloride in Chapter 10) are antiestrogens that have shown some effectiveness against recurrent endometrial cancer (Creasman & Miller, 2018; Soliman & Lu, 2017).

Nursing Interventions

Nursing care of the woman having surgery includes assessing her perception of the anticipated surgery, her knowledge of what to expect after surgery, and any preoperative special procedures, such as cleansing enemas or douches. In today's practice of short hospital stays, even for radical surgery, many of these preoperative procedures are performed at home before admission, so assessment of understanding becomes a critical nursing action (see Cultural Considerations box). Nursing care for the woman having a TAH-BSO is similar to the care for a woman having a hysterectomy for leiomyoma described earlier. The following section focuses on care of the woman having a radical hysterectomy (see Nursing Care Plan).

🌐 CULTURAL CONSIDERATIONS
Meaning of Cancer

A woman's culture influences the meaning she attaches to cancer screening and diagnosis of cancer. Some women may be reluctant to be screened because of language barriers, lack of knowledge about the risks of gynecologic cancers, or the belief that they are not at risk. Some women do not believe that health care providers are sensitive to their values of modesty. A woman's response to a cancer diagnosis also must be appropriate to her cultural context for it to be acceptable to her. For example, body image issues (e.g., loss of uterus), the meaning of death, and pain responses (e.g., stoic or expressive) are influenced by cultural beliefs and values. In making assessments about these issues, the nurse takes into account the influence of culture before developing a plan of care.

Modified from Guimond, M. E., & Salman, K. (2013). Modesty matters: Cultural sensitivity and cervical cancer prevention in Muslim women in the United States. *Nursing for Women's Health, 17*(3), 210–217.

Preoperative care. The nurse explains preoperative procedures for a radical hysterectomy and pelvic node dissection (see Box 11.2). Additional teaching includes information about postsurgical events such as a suprapubic drain that may remain in place for several days to a week.

Postoperative care. Assessment of vital signs usually follows a postanesthesia protocol, gradually decreasing in frequency to two to four times a day. Intravenous (IV) fluids are infused to maintain hydration and electrolyte balance and are usually discontinued when the woman is taking oral fluids well and has no elevated temperature. A regular diet is resumed as tolerated. Intake and output are monitored. The urinary catheter is usually removed the morning after surgery and the first few urinary voidings are measured.

The woman should turn and take deep breaths with assistance as needed. Incentive spirometry may be used. Breath sounds are assessed, and any deviations from normal are reported immediately. The most significant single cause of morbidity and prolonged hospitalization after major procedures is respiratory complications. Anesthesia and surgery alter breathing patterns and ability to cough. Atelectasis, pneumonia, and pulmonary embolus may occur.

To promote venous return and prevent deep vein thrombosis, the woman may wear antiembolic stockings or pneumonic pressure devices (i.e., boots) while in bed. Leg exercises and early ambulation are beneficial. Most women are encouraged to get out of bed the evening of or the day after surgery. Assistance in getting up and walking may be needed.

Hemorrhage is always a possible complication after surgery. The wound drainage tube is emptied as needed or every 4 hours, and the amount and character of drainage are recorded. Drainage from

◎ NURSING CARE PLAN

Hysterectomy for Endometrial Cancer

Client Problem	Expected Outcome	Nursing Interventions	Rationales
Anxiety about diagnosis, treatment, and prognosis of endometrial cancer as evidenced by woman's questions and concerns	Woman will identify source of anxiety and verbalize understanding of diagnosis, effects of hysterectomy, and prognosis.	Assess woman's level of understanding of procedure and its effects.	To correct any misunderstanding, provide clarification, and identify starting point for further information
		Provide information about cancer of the endometrium, individualizing information to the woman's situation.	To provide clarification concerning treatment regimen
		Provide preoperative and postoperative teaching.	To give anticipatory guidance and rationales for upcoming events
Acute pain postoperatively as evidenced by woman's verbal and nonverbal behaviors	Woman will verbalize decrease in intensity and number of painful episodes after interventions.	Assess the location and intensity of pain by using a pain scale.	To use appropriate treatment
		Administer prescribed analgesics.	To decrease perception of pain
		Use nonpharmacologic techniques such as distraction, relaxation, position changes, and heat.	To decrease perception of pain
		Monitor effectiveness of interventions.	To modify interventions if needed
Disturbed self-concept related to altered body image, as evidenced by woman's statements of fears and concerns about loss of uterus and sexual functioning	Woman will maintain a positive body image and resume sexual relationship with partner.	Encourage expression of feelings through therapeutic communication.	To provide clarification of and validity of feelings
		Encourage woman to share feelings with significant other.	To obtain emotional support and to address concerns about resumption of sexual relations
		Offer referral to sexual counselor if indicated.	To provide in-depth intervention as needed

any tube is assessed for bleeding. Vaginal drainage, if any, should be serosanguineous. Hematuria is noted and recorded. The primary health care provider is informed of any deviations from normal expectations.

Paralytic ileus may occur after surgery in which the intestines have been manipulated. Use of a nasogastric tube, limiting oral fluids, and early ambulation all support the return of gastrointestinal function. An enema or suppository may bring relief of flatus and stimulate the return of bowel function. Oral laxatives should not be given until lower bowel function has returned.

Opioid analgesics and NSAIDs are used for postoperative pain. Nursing measures such as massages, repositioning, and emotional support are all helpful adjuncts to pharmacologic control of discomfort.

Because the in-hospital convalescent period is generally short, close observation by the nurse and attention to detail are critical. Nursing actions appropriate to this period include monitoring for urinary retention after the catheter is removed, monitoring the woman's appetite and diet, monitoring bowel function, and encouraging progressive ambulation and self-care.

Discharge planning and teaching. Discharge planning begins preoperatively and continues through convalescence. Discharge instructions are similar to those that can be found in the Teaching for Self-Management box: Care After Myomectomy or Hysterectomy.

Care for the woman who has had external or internal radiation therapy is the same as that described for the woman with cervical cancer. This is discussed later in the chapter.

Nursing care for the woman undergoing chemotherapy depends on the type of drug given. If alopecia is likely, the nurse can suggest wigs, scarves, or other kinds of head coverings. If the therapy affects the appetite or causes gastrointestinal side effects, suggestions such as those in Box 11.4 may be useful.

After discharge, the woman may require continued nursing care or monitoring of her physical status or advice for managing the treatment effects of the cancer. The family is likely to provide much of the woman's care, and should therefore, be included in discussions about care management.

Psychologic care for the woman with endometrial cancer is essential. A woman needs to be able to discuss her concerns about having cancer and the potential for recurrence. She may have fears of death, permanent disfigurement, and change in functioning; altered feelings of self as a woman; and concerns regarding her femininity, sexuality, and loss of reproductive capacity. She may have questions arising from things she has heard about posthysterectomy changes, radiation therapy, or chemotherapy. Significant others should be encouraged to express their questions and concerns as well. The woman and her significant others may benefit from a referral to a community cancer support group (see the ACS website, www.cancer.org).

Cancer of the Ovary

Incidence and Etiology

Ovarian cancer is estimated to cause 13,980 deaths in 2019 (ACS, 2019a). Because the symptoms of this type of cancer are vague and definitive screening tests do not exist, ovarian cancer is often diagnosed in an advanced stage. The 5-year relative survival rate for ovarian cancer diagnosed at a localized state is about 92%; however, only about 15% of ovarian cancers are found at this stage. For advanced stages, the survival rate is about 29% (ACS). Malignant neoplasia of the ovaries occurs at all ages, including in infants and children. However, cancer of the ovary is seen primarily in women older than age 50, with the greatest number of cases found in women ages 60 to 64 years (Eisenhauer, Salani, & Copeland, 2018). Major histologic cell types occur in different age groups, with malignant germ cell tumors most common in women between 20 and 40 years of age and epithelial cancers occurring in the

BOX 11.4 Nutritional Management for Common Problems Related to Gynecologic Cancer or Treatment

Altered Taste
- Rinse mouth with baking soda solution with 1 teaspoon salt, 1 teaspoon baking soda to 1 quart (liter) water
- Use extra seasoning, spices
- Use sauces and marinades for meats
- Eat fish or chicken instead of red meat
- Eat tart foods to stimulate taste buds
- Try sugar-free mints, gum, hard sour candy

Anorexia
- Eat with family, friends
- Eat favorite foods any time
- Try new foods, recipes
- Use smaller servings
- Eat high-calorie, high-protein snacks
- Drink nutritional supplements
- Exercise before meals to stimulate appetite

Nausea and Vomiting
- Drink clear liquids
- Avoid carbonated fluids
- Avoid sweet, rich, fatty foods
- Eat cool foods rather than hot or warm foods
- Eat six to eight small meals a day
- Consume a high-calorie, high-protein diet
- Eat toast, bland foods
- Avoid lying down at least 1 h after eating
- Take antiemetics before meals

Stomatitis
- Eat small meals
- Eat soft, bland foods
- Avoid rough-textured foods (e.g., chips, crackers)
- Drink 8-10 cups of fluids a day
- Avoid citrus fruits, spicy foods
- Avoid alcohol
- Avoid very hot or very cold foods
- Drink nutritional supplements, milkshakes
- Drink through a straw if mouth is sore
- Rinse mouth frequently with baking soda solution or prescribed mouthwash
- Eat liquid or pureed foods as needed

Constipation
- Increase fiber (bran, fresh fruits, and vegetables)
- Drink 8-10 cups of fluids a day
- Eat natural laxative foods (prunes, apples)
- Avoid cheese products
- Drink warm drinks with breakfast

Diarrhea
- Limit milk to 2 cups a day
- Avoid high-fiber, spicy, fatty foods
- Eat foods high in potassium
- Increase fluid intake 12.5 cups; avoid caffeine and carbonated fluids
- Add nutmeg to food to decrease gastric motility
- Eat a high-protein, high-carbohydrate diet
- Eat small meals and snacks

Postoperative Recovery
- Eat foods high in iron
- Eat high-protein foods
- Eat foods high in vitamins C, B complex, and K
- Drink 6-8 glasses of fluids a day

Data from American Cancer Society. (2015). *Managing eating problems caused by surgery, radiation, and chemotherapy.* Retrieved from www.cancer.org.

---

perimenopausal age groups. The spread of ovarian cancer is by direct extension to adjacent organs, but distal spread can occur through the lymph system to the liver and the lungs.

The cause of ovarian cancer is unknown; however, a number of risk factors have been identified. Woman at greatest risk are those with family history of ovarian or breast cancer. Other risk factors include nulliparity, infertility, and previous breast cancer. Inherited BRCA1 and BRCA2 mutations increase the risk, but 90% of women do not have inherited ovarian cancer. Genital exposure to talc, a diet high in fat, lactose intolerance, excess body weight, smoking, physical inactivity, and use of fertility drugs have been suggested as risk factors, but research findings are inconclusive (Coleman, Ramirez, & Gershenson, 2017; Eisenhauer et al., 2018).

Non-Hispanic white women of North American or northern European descent and older women have the highest incidence of ovarian cancers. Pregnancy and use of OCs seem to have some protective benefits against ovarian cancer, whereas use of postmenopausal estrogen may increase the risk. Research has shown that preventive removal of the ovaries and uterine tubes can decrease the risk (ACS, 2019a; Coleman et al., 2017; Eisenhauer et al., 2018).

Clinical Manifestations and Diagnosis

Ovarian cancer was once called a silent disease because early warning symptoms that would send a woman to her health care provider are absent (e.g., no bleeding or other discharge and no pain). However, research has shown that some women experience symptoms that are associated with early ovarian cancer. These include abdominal bloating, noticeable increase in abdominal girth, pelvic or abdominal pain, difficulty eating or feeling full quickly, and urinary urgency or frequency (ACS, 2019a; Eisenhauer et al., 2018). The increase in abdominal girth (caused by ovarian enlargement or ascites) is usually attributed to an increase in weight or a shift in weight that is seen commonly in women entering their middle years. An ovary enlarged 5 cm or more than normal that is found during routine examination requires careful diagnostic workup. Pelvic pain, anemia, and general weakness and malnutrition are signs of late-stage disease.

Early diagnosis of ovarian cancer is uncommon. Attempts at early detection have not proven to be reliable. Taking a family history is important because it may reveal cancer of the uterus or breast. Transvaginal ultrasound, CA-125 antigen (a tumor-associated antigen) testing, and frequent pelvic examinations have all been used without a great deal of success. Research continues on the use of proteomics (study of proteins in blood) to identify ovarian cancer in its earlier stages (Eisenhauer et al., 2018). Transvaginal ultrasound and CA-125 screening currently are not recommended for routine screening in the general population but are recommended for women who are at high risk (e.g., BRCA1 mutation carriers) (ACS, 2019a). Routine pelvic examination continues to be the only practical screening method for detecting early disease, even though few cancers are detected in women without symptoms. Any ovarian enlargement should be considered highly suggestive and needs further evaluation by laparoscopy or laparotomy. Responsibility for diagnosis rests with the pathologist. The size of the tumor is not indicative of the severity of disease. Clinical staging is done surgically and gives direction to treatment and prognosis (Eisenhauer, Salani, & Copeland, 2018).

Medical and Surgical Management

Treatment depends on the stage of the disease at initial diagnosis. Surgical removal of as much of the tumor as possible is the first step in therapy for all stages. This may involve just the removal of one ovary and tube (if the cancer is limited to one ovary and childbearing is desired) or the radical excision of the uterus, ovaries, tubes, and omentum. Cytoreductive surgery (the debulking of the poorly vascularized larger tumors) also is done. The smaller the volume of tumor remaining, the better the response to adjuvant therapy. For women who are in stage II, III, or IV of this disease at the time of diagnosis, surgical cure alone is less likely. Therefore after tumor reduction surgery is performed, women with epithelial cell carcinoma will receive chemotherapy.

A platinum-based combination of antineoplastic drugs such as carboplatin and paclitaxel is recommended for most women with advanced disease. Second-look surgery is used to determine the response of the disease to chemotherapy and whether treatment should be continued; however, this procedure usually is not done unless it is part of a research protocol. Radiation has been used to treat early-stage disease, and some women have had long-term survival after debulking surgery followed by radiation therapy. It has also been used as a palliative measure in advanced disease (Eisenhauer, Salani, & Copeland, 2018).

Nursing Interventions

Generally, there is a lack of awareness of ovarian cancer symptoms and risk factors. Nurses should provide education to women and communities to help raise awareness and to identify those at risk to improve prevention and early detection.

The woman diagnosed with ovarian cancer has concerns similar to those described for the woman with endometrial or cervical cancer. Nursing interventions for the woman having surgery, chemotherapy, or external radiation therapy for ovarian cancer are described in other sections of this chapter.

Women with advanced ovarian cancer have a higher rate of recurrence; thus close follow-up for 5 years is necessary. Palliative care is offered when a cure or remission cannot be achieved. These measures alleviate symptoms of the progressing disease to provide comfort and maximal function. Nutritional support such as enteral feedings and total parenteral nutrition (TPN) are sometimes necessary due to effects on the gastrointestinal tract from the disease and treatments. Palliative care focuses on quality of life for the woman in health care settings and her home.

Transition of ovarian cancer between a goal of cure and a palliative focus can be prolonged. Thus, women with ovarian cancer can experience most or all of the grief stages described by Kübler-Ross. After diagnosis the woman can experience denial and then anger. As treatment begins, she may "bargain" for a cure. If treatment is successful and death is forestalled by remission or cure, the process of adjustment to dying ceases, and the woman again focuses on life and its challenges. When treatment fails to secure a cure or remission ends, the woman must turn again to the task of adjustment (see Legal Tip).

> **LEGAL TIP**
> **Advance Directives**
> Nurses who work with clients in hospitals with federal funding must know that because of the Patient Self-Determination Act, all clients must be asked if they have knowledge of advance directives and be provided with the information if desired. This is important to nurses working in gynecology-oncology settings, where decisions about living wills and "no codes" may be issues.

Family and friends can experience diverse feelings when grieving is prolonged. The stress may interfere with interpersonal relationships. Hospital environments can further intrude on relationships, limiting privacy and opportunities for family and friends to provide caring gestures. The nurse can encourage the woman and her family to share their feelings with each other and help them develop a support network. Referral to a cancer support group may be useful (e.g., National Ovarian Cancer Coalition, www.ovarian.org; Ovarian Cancer Research Fund Alliance https://ocrfa.org/).

Cancer of the Cervix
Incidence and Etiology

Cervical cancer is the third most common reproductive cancer. The accessible location of the cervix to both cell and tissue study and direct examination have led to a refinement of diagnostic techniques, contributing to improved diagnosis and treatment of these disorders. The incidence of invasive cancer has decreased since the 1980s, reducing mortality rates (ACS, 2019a; Salcedo, Baker, & Schmeler, 2017).

Cancer of the cervix begins as neoplastic changes in the cervical epithelium. Terms that have been used to describe these epithelial changes or preinvasive lesions include dysplasia and cervical intraepithelial neoplasia (CIN), the term currently used. CIN 1 refers to abnormal cellular proliferation in the lower one-third of the epithelium; this change tends to be self-limiting and generally regresses to normal. CIN 2 involves the lower two-thirds of the epithelium and may progress to carcinoma in situ (CIS). CIN 3 involves the full thickness of the epithelium and often progresses to CIS. Carcinoma in situ (CIS) is diagnosed when the full thickness of epithelium is replaced with abnormal cells (Massad, 2018) (Fig. 11.11). Terms used to describe neoplastic changes in abnormal cervical cytology reports are low-grade and high-grade squamous intraepithelial lesions (SILs); however, CIN continues to be a common term used in clinical practice.

Preinvasive lesions are limited to the cervix and usually originate in the squamocolumnar junction or transformation zone (Fig. 11.12). Intensive study of the cervix and the cellular changes that take place has shown that most cervical tumors have a gradual onset rather than an explosive one. Preinvasive conditions may exist for years before the development of invasive disease. These preinvasive conditions are highly treatable in many cases.

Invasive carcinoma is the diagnosis when abnormal cells penetrate the basement membrane and invade the stroma. There are two types of invasive carcinomas of the cervix: microinvasive and invasive. Microinvasive carcinoma is defined as one or more lesions that penetrate no more than 3 mm into the stroma below the basement membrane with no areas of lymphatic or vascular invasion (Massad, 2018). Invasive carcinoma describes invasion that goes beyond these parameters. The staging of invasive carcinoma extends from CIS to distant metastasis or disease outside the true pelvis.

Approximately 90% of cervical malignancies are squamous cell carcinomas; 10% are adenocarcinomas (National Cervical Cancer Coalition, 2019). Squamous cell carcinomas can spread by direct extension to the vaginal mucosa, the pelvic wall, the bowels, and the bladder.

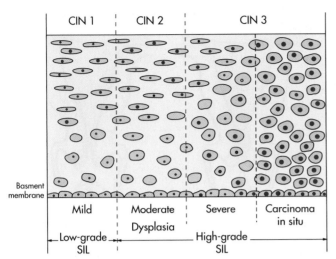

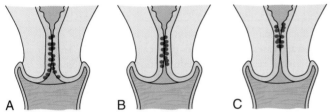

Fig. 11.11 Diagram of Cervical Epithelium Showing Progressive Changes and Various Terminology. *CIN*, Cervical intraepithelial neoplasia; *SIL*, squamous intraepithelial lesion.

Fig. 11.12 Location of Squamocolumnar Junction According to Age. The location where the endocervical glands meet the squamous epithelium becomes progressively higher with age. (A) Puberty. (B) Reproductive years. (C) Postmenopausal.

Metastasis usually occurs in the pelvis, but it can occur in the lungs and the brain through the lymphatic system.

The average age range for the occurrence of cervical cancer is 40 to 50 years; however, preinvasive conditions may exist for 10 to 15 years before the development of an invasive carcinoma. About 90% of cervical cancers are caused by HPV (Massad, 2018). A strong link has been established between HPV types 16 and 18 and cervical neoplasia (see Chapter 7 for a discussion of HPV, including preventive vaccines). Risk factors for persistent HPV infections include early age at first coitus (younger than 20 years), multiple sexual partners (more than two), a sexual partner with a history of multiple sexual partners, high parity, and belonging to a lower socioeconomic group. Potential risk factors include long-term use of OCs, cigarette smoking, and intrauterine exposure to diethylstilbestrol (DES) (ACS, 2019a; Massad, 2018; Tewari & Monk, 2018). Low levels of beta-carotene, vitamin C, and folate are being investigated as potential risk factors (Tewari & Monk, 2018).

The incidence of cervical cancer in the United States is highest in Hispanic women and lowest in Asian women, whereas the highest mortality occurs in African American women (ACS, 2019a). Factors that may influence cervical screening behaviors for these groups include lack of a health promotion or disease prevention perspective, lack of knowledge about Pap tests and availability of services, financial barriers, and failure of health care providers to recommend screening (ACS). There also is a high rate of CIN in human immunodeficiency virus–positive women, suggesting that altered immune status is a risk factor (Massad, 2018) (see Community Activity).

Clinical Manifestations and Diagnosis

Preinvasive cancer of the cervix is often asymptomatic. Abnormal bleeding, especially postcoital bleeding, is the classic symptom of invasive cancer. Other late symptoms include rectal bleeding, hematuria, back pain, leg pain, and anemia. Diagnosis includes taking a history that includes menstrual and sexual activity information, particularly sexually transmitted infections and abnormal bleeding episodes (Massad, 2018). A pelvic examination usually is normal except in late-stage cancer.

The most widely used method to detect preinvasive cancer is the Pap test, which can detect 90% of early cervical changes. According to the ACS, the American Society for Colposcopy and Cervical Pathology, and the American Society for Clinical Pathology, cervical cancer screening should begin at age 21. For women ages 21 to 29, screening should be done every 3 years with conventional or liquid-based Pap tests. For women ages 30 to 65, screening should be done every 5 years with both the HPV test and the Pap test (preferred method), or every 3 years with the Pap test alone (acceptable). Women who are 65 years or older who have had three or more consecutive negative Pap tests or more than two consecutive negative HPV and Pap tests within the past 10 years, with the most recent test occurring within 5 years; and women who have had a total hysterectomy can stop cervical cancer screening (ACS, 2019a; Moyer and U.S. Preventive Services Task Force, 2012). Women in high-risk categories should have more frequent Pap tests.

Pap test results have been recorded by using several different classification systems. The reporting system most often used today is the Bethesda system, which reports on gynecologic cytology as well as histology of cervical lesions (Box 11.5). Changes secondary to inflammation, treatment (e.g., radiation), and contraceptive devices can be reported, as well as changes caused by infections. Epithelial cell abnormalities are described in three categories: atypias, or atypical squamous cells (ASC); low-grade squamous intraepithelial lesions (LSILs); and high-grade squamous intraepithelial lesions (HSILs).

Several options for follow-up of a finding of ASC of undetermined significance (ASC-US) are suggested. These include immediate colposcopy, repeating cytology at 6 months and 12 months, or HPV testing and referral for colposcopy if the test is positive. Colposcopy is recommended for evaluation of LSIL except in adolescents; teens can be followed with cytology tests at 6 and 12 months. Follow-up for a report of HSIL includes colposcopy or loop electrosurgical excision (Massad, 2018). Colposcopy is the examination of the cervix with a stereoscopic binocular microscope that magnifies the view of the cervix. Usually a solution of 3% acetic acid is applied to the cervix for better visualization of the epithelium and

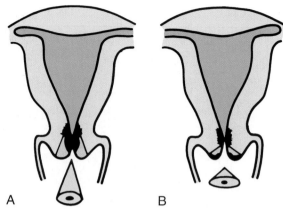

Fig. 11.13 Cone Biopsy. (A) For endocervical disease. Limits of lesion were not seen colposcopically. (B) For cervical intraepithelial neoplasia of the exocervix. Limits of lesion were identified colposcopically. (From Creasman, W. [2019]. Preinvasive disease of the cervix. In P. J. DiSaia, W. T. Creasman, R. S. Mannel, & D. S. Mutch [Eds.]. *Clinical gynecologic oncology* [9th ed.]. Philadelphia: Saunders.)

CARE MANAGEMENT

For the woman diagnosed with invasive carcinoma of the cervix, pretherapy assessment includes physical, psychologic, and educational components, regardless of whether surgery or radiation is the method of treatment. The health history includes a review of current medications because medications for other medical problems may have to be continued. Skin is assessed to identify potential pressure points; respiratory and gastrointestinal status and state of nutrition are important factors to assess. Urinalysis and complete blood count also are commonly performed. An electrocardiogram and a chest x-ray examination may be done if use of general anesthesia is anticipated for surgery or placement of internal applicators.

Psychologic assessment is important because frequently these women are emotionally distressed about the diagnosis and anticipated treatment (e.g., fear of being radioactive and fear of surgery and pain) and fear that family or significant others will become distant.

The nurse must assess the woman's knowledge and understanding of her diagnosis and the treatment regimen. This assessment will help the nurse in effectively focusing on areas where education is needed.

Medical and Surgical Management

Once the stage of disease is identified, appropriate treatment goals are established. For preinvasive lesions, several techniques are used. Because many preinvasive conditions are detected in younger women who may wish to continue childbearing, treatment is geared toward eradicating abnormal cells while attempting to preserve the structure of the cervix. Techniques available for preinvasive lesions are cryotherapy, laser therapy, and LEEP, all of which have comparable success rates in treating CIN (Massad, 2018) (Box 11.6). Five-year survival rates are more than 92% when the cancer is localized (ACS, 2019a).

Treatment for invasive cancer includes surgery, radiation therapy, and chemotherapy. Microinvasive cancer is usually treated with conization, but a hysterectomy is often done if childbearing is not desired. The choice of treatment for early-stage invasive cancer is hysterectomy or chemoradiation therapy (Tewari & Monk, 2018). A radical hysterectomy (see previous discussion) is performed if the cancer has extended beyond the cervix but not to the pelvic wall. Locally advanced stages of

to identify areas for biopsy. Colposcopy is not an invasive procedure and usually is well tolerated. However, a woman who is scheduled for colposcopy because of an abnormal Pap test may be anxious and may need explanations or written information about what to expect during the procedure.

Biopsy is the removal of cervical tissue for study; several techniques can be used. An endocervical curettage is an effective diagnostic tool in about 90% of cases. It can be performed as an outpatient procedure with little or no anesthesia. It may be uncomfortable, and interventions to help the woman relax and cope with the pain may be needed.

Conization and loop electrosurgical excision procedure (LEEP) (see later discussion) can be done as outpatient procedures, although neither is usually performed unless the biopsy is positive or the results of the colposcopy are unsatisfactory. Conization involves removal of a cone of tissue from the exocervix and endocervix (Fig. 11.13). It can be a cold knife procedure, a laser excision, or an electrosurgical excision (Fig. 11.14) (see later discussion). There are two advantages to a cone biopsy. It can be used (1) to establish the diagnosis and (2) to effect a cure. If CIS is diagnosed, and if the woman wishes to retain her childbearing capacity, conization removes the abnormal tissue; further treatment (e.g., hysterectomy) is unnecessary. The woman is monitored with Pap tests and colposcopy when indicated.

If invasive cancer is diagnosed, other diagnostic tests can assess the extent of spread (see earlier discussion under endometrial cancer). Once the extent of the cancer is known, treatment begins.

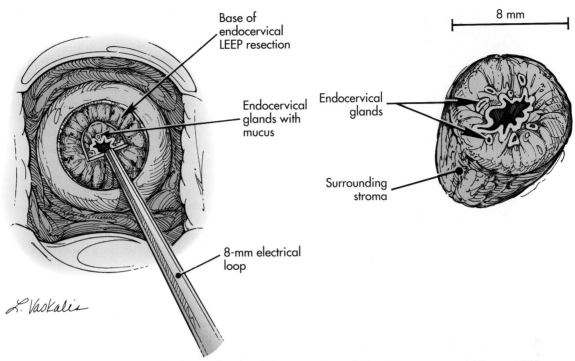

Fig. 11.14 Electrosurgical Excision. The electric loop vaporizes quickly and removes cone of tissue. *LEEP,* Loop electrosurgical excision procedure. (From Nichols, D., & Clark-Pearson, D. [2000]. *Gynecologic, obstetric, and related surgery* [2nd ed.]. St. Louis: Mosby.)

BOX 11.6 Surgical Alternatives for Preinvasive Cancer of the Cervix

Cryosurgery
- A technique to freeze abnormal cells is used, and when sloughing occurs, normal tissue is regenerated.
- Side effects occurring after treatment are usually few and not serious. A profuse watery discharge can persist for 2-4 weeks.
- Endocervical cells are thought to regenerate, leaving a normal cervical canal in most instances.
- Surveillance with frequent Pap tests and colposcopic examination must continue indefinitely after this type of conservative therapy.

Laser Ablation
- A laser mounted on a colposcope that allows precise direction of a beam of light (heat) is used to remove diseased tissue.
- For treatment of the cervix (relatively insensitive tissue), little or no anesthesia may be needed, although a burning or cramping sensation may be noticed.
- The cervix treated with CO_2 laser will show epithelial regrowth beginning by 2 days afterward. The site is usually healed in 4-6 weeks. The original architecture of the cervix is preserved, and the squamocolumnar junction remains visible; however, there can be more damage to normal tissues than with other treatments.
- Women usually have less vaginal discharge than with cryosurgery, but can have more discomfort after the procedure.

LEEP (Loop Electrosurgical Excision Procedure)
- A standard treatment for cervical intraepithelial neoplasia in the United States that uses a wire loop electrode that can excise and cauterize with minimal tissue damage (see Fig. 11.14).
- Healing is rapid, and there is only a mild discharge afterward.
- Possible complications include bleeding, cervical stenosis, infertility, and loss of cervical mucus.

---

cervical cancer usually are treated with radiation therapy, both external and internal, and chemotherapy. Late stages are usually treated with radiation and chemotherapy.

Radiation therapy. Radiation may be delivered by internal radium applications to the cervix or external radiation therapy that includes lymphatics of the pelvic side wall. In preparation for radiation therapy, the woman must maintain good nutritional status and a high-protein, high-vitamin, and high-calorie diet. Anemia, if present, should be corrected before initiating radiotherapy.

External radiation therapy and internal radiation therapy are given in various combinations for the best results and are tailored to each woman and her particular lesion. For example, external radiation may be given first to treat regional pelvic nodes and to shrink the tumor. External radiation is usually an outpatient procedure given 5 days a week for 4 to 6 weeks. Internal radiation therapy consists of one or two intracavitary treatments at least 2 weeks apart (Tewari & Monk, 2018). External radiation is provided by megavoltage machines such as cobalt, and supervoltage machines such as linear accelerators and betatron, with each having a distinct advantage of providing a more homogeneous dose to the pelvis. Before treatment begins, a localization procedure is done to determine the best way to deliver the treatments. Markings or small tattoos may be placed on the body to make sure the woman is positioned correctly to receive treatment (Viscosky & Ponto, 2018).

For internal radiation therapy, the woman may be treated in the hospital or in a special outpatient unit. If treatment is done in the hospital, she is taken to the operating room, and while she is under general or spinal anesthesia, a specially designed applicator is placed into her vagina and cervix. X-rays are taken to make sure the applicator is correctly placed. The woman is returned to her room, where the radioactive source is placed into the applicator (Fig. 11.15). The source remains in place from 12 hours to 3 days. If treatment is in the outpatient setting, the applicator is inserted into the uterus in a treatment room; use of high-dose implants shortens the treatment time and is

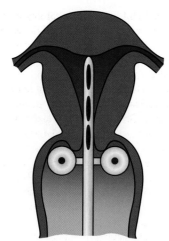

Fig. 11.15 Intracavitary Implant. Applicator in place in uterus is loaded with radium source.

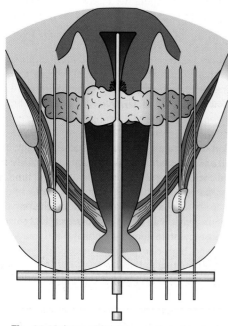

Fig. 11.16 Interstitial-Intracavitary Implant.

being used more frequently than low-dose implants because no hospital stay is required (Tewari & Monk, 2018; Viscosky & Ponto, 2018).

In advanced carcinoma of the cervix, conventional intracavitary applicators are not applicable. Interstitial therapy uses a template to guide the transperineal insertion of a group of 18-gauge hollow steel needles into the lesion (Fig. 11.16). After the needles are placed, the iridium wires are inserted when the woman is returned to her room.

Nursing interventions. Nursing care is based on assessment of the woman's concerns about the type of radiation therapy to be used. Nursing actions for external and internal radiation differ, so they are discussed separately.

External therapy. To help reduce the woman's anxiety about external radiation therapy, the nurse explains what to expect. This includes describing the equipment, which is similar to that used for x-ray examination except larger; the hyperbaric oxygen chamber, which may be used to increase cellular oxygen and thus make tumor cells more radiosensitive; the radiotherapist, who will be behind a shield, but still close by and in communication with her; the position she will be put in and asked to maintain for some minutes; and the therapy, which is painless.

During the course of therapy, the woman is counseled regarding maintaining general good health. To maintain good skin care, the woman is taught to assess her skin often; avoid soaps, ointments, cosmetics, and deodorants if the axilla is being irradiated because these may contain metals that alter the dose she receives and could lead to skin breakdown; wear loose clothing over the area and cotton underwear (or no underwear); use an air mattress or cover the mattress with foam pads or sheepskin; avoid exposing the irradiated areas to temperature extremes (e.g., hot tubs); and especially avoid removing the markings made by the radiologist. If skin becomes red or itchy, she can treat it with remedies recommended by the radiologist (e.g., aloe vera lotion, Aquaphor, or warm sitz baths). To treat skin that is broken or desquamating, the woman is shown how to use remedies prescribed by the radiologist (e.g., irrigation with warm water, application of antibiotic or lanolin ointment, exposure to air, and application of a loose dressing). The use of adhesive (or any) tape directly on the target area of skin should be avoided (Viscosky & Ponto, 2018).

To maintain good nutrition, the woman is reminded to keep a daily record of weight; use high-protein supplements; eat small, attractive, appetizing meals that are more bland than spicy; and keep the environment light, airy, clean, and quiet (especially before and after meals). A dietitian consult may be needed to help the woman and her family plan to meet her nutritional needs. If she is ill enough to be hospitalized, she may need total parenteral nutrition or tube feedings. Nausea interferes with adequate intake; therefore, the woman may take antiemetics, as necessary. High daily fluid intake (2 to 3 L) should be suggested if not contraindicated. To increase her comfort, minimize infection, and promote adequate food intake, she is encouraged to perform frequent oral hygiene. Box 11.4 provides other suggestions for nutritional problems associated with radiation treatment.

The nurse explains, as necessary, the need for routine blood studies to monitor the white blood cell count (to determine degree of immunosuppression). The woman and her family will need information about neutropenia, thrombocytopenia, and anemia and precautions to be taken. Because she is more vulnerable to infection, the woman is reminded of general measures to avoid infection (e.g., practice good hygiene, avoid people with infection, avoid large crowds, keep environment clean).

After the radiation treatment is completed, the woman needs information for self-care (see the Teaching for Self-Management box: Care After External Radiation Therapy). She should also be informed that side effects of the treatment, especially fatigue and altered taste sensations, can continue for weeks after the therapy is completed.

TEACHING FOR SELF-MANAGEMENT
Care After External Radiation Therapy

- Avoid infection and report symptoms of infection to the health care provider immediately.
- Maintain good nutrition and fluid intake.
- Anticipate possible effects of radiation for 10-14 days after the last treatment.
- Expect signs of healing to occur in about 3 weeks.
- Maintain good skin and mouth care to support a sense of well-being and prevent infection.
- Report the following symptoms to your health care provider:
  - Continued gastrointestinal symptoms (nausea, vomiting, anorexia, diarrhea)
  - Increasing skin irritation at the site of therapy (redness, swelling, pain, pruritus)
- Take medications as prescribed, and avoid any medications not prescribed or approved by the health care provider.

Internal therapy. Internal radiation therapy may require hospitalization or may be done in a special outpatient unit. Radiation safety officers determine the precautions to be observed in each situation. This discussion focuses on treatment in the hospital setting, but similar precautions are used in the outpatient setting. Printed instruction sheets are usually available, stating precautions to be followed for each type of radiation substance used. A precaution sign is placed on the door of the woman's room.

> ### ⚡ SAFETY ALERT
>
> Personnel who come into direct contact with anyone receiving radiation therapy should wear a film badge or other device to monitor the amount of exposure received.

Nurses must protect themselves from overexposure to radiation. Precautions include the following (Viscosky & Ponto, 2018):

- Careful isolation techniques: wearing gloves while handling bodily fluids and observing good handwashing technique. These behaviors reflect knowledge that alpha and beta rays cannot pass through skin but may be in body fluids and excrement.
- Careful planning of nursing activity to limit time (to 30 minutes or less per 8 hours) spent in proximity to the woman to avoid exposure to gamma rays, which can penetrate several inches of lead.

Exposure to radiation is controlled in three ways: distance, time, and shielding (with lead). For the woman with sealed radiotherapy, a movable lead screen can be placed between the area in which the therapeutic applicator is located and the personnel. The lead screen also is used to protect visitors from radiation. Increasing the distance from the source also decreases exposure (Viscosky & Ponto, 2018).

Familiarity with applicators is a must for all nurses working with people receiving radiotherapy so that if a "strange object" is found in the linen or on the floor, it is not touched. Today most hospital protocols include having a lead container and forceps in the room for use if a radioactive implant is dislodged.

The woman is prepared for insertion with the following care, which is accompanied by an explanation for each activity. To reduce the need for attention to bowel elimination for a few days, the gastrointestinal tract is usually prepared by using low-residue diet, enemas, and sometimes bowel sedation. The vaginal vault is usually prepared with an antiseptic douche, such as povidone-iodine. An indwelling urinary catheter is inserted, as ordered, to prevent bladder distention that could dislodge the applicator. Food and fluids are withheld for a specified time before the procedure in anticipation of using general anesthesia. Preoperative medications may be ordered for the morning of the procedure. Deep-breathing exercises, range-of-motion (ROM) exercises, and positioning are all demonstrated before the procedure to minimize the effects of immobilization afterward. An IV infusion will probably be started before the procedure, and IV therapy may be continued if nausea prevents adequate intake of oral fluids. The woman is assured that pain will be managed.

Explanations about restricted visitation of personnel and visitors are given in the preinsertion phase. Women are often encouraged to bring books, magazines, electronic readers, laptop computers or tablets, iPods, cell phones, or other devices or materials to the hospital to combat the boredom that isolation imposes on them. In addition, many units are equipped with televisions and CD and DVD players.

The applicator is inserted into the woman's vaginal vault during surgery. After the usual postanesthesia recovery care, the woman is returned to her room, where the applicators are loaded with the radioactive substance.

A lead shield is placed next to the bed in line with the woman's pelvic area to protect the caregivers and visitors. Vital signs are monitored every 4 hours. Active ROM and deep-breathing exercises are encouraged every 2 hours; the woman is positioned on her back and may not be permitted to turn from side to side, although log-rolling may be done occasionally to relieve back pressure. The head of the bed may or may not be elevated slightly.

The woman's diet is changed from clear liquid to low residue, as tolerated. Many individuals have difficulty eating while lying flat or even if the bed is elevated slightly. The nurse arranges the food so that it is easy to reach. Finger foods or liquids are generally more manageable. Parenteral or oral fluids are given, up to 3 L daily.

The urinary catheter remains in the bladder while the implant is in place. However, no perineal or catheter care is given. Intake and output are measured. Bathing is restricted to above the waist. Linen is changed only as absolutely necessary. Any linen or equipment used is retained in the room until therapy is complete to prevent loss of an applicator or seed. If vaginal or rectal bleeding or hematuria occurs, the health care provider is notified immediately.

Emotional support is provided by planning to be with the woman for short periods, encouraging her to verbalize concerns and needs, and encouraging family members, clergy, or others to visit for short periods daily or to communicate by telephone, texting, or video-chat. Pregnant women and children are not permitted to visit.

Many women undergoing internal radiation treatment are given medication to prevent complications and to promote comfort during the procedure. Such medications might include antibiotics to prevent urinary tract infections, heparin injections to prevent thrombophlebitis, sedatives for relaxation, antiemetics for nausea, and narcotics for pain. The woman is considered radioactive during the time the internal sources are in place (Viscosky & Ponto, 2018).

After the radium is removed the urinary catheter is removed, and the woman is assisted in getting out of bed the first time. She is usually discharged the same day. Discharge teaching can be found in the Teaching for Self-Management box: Care After Internal Radiation Therapy. The woman and her family are reassured that she is not radioactive after the treatment.

TEACHING FOR SELF-MANAGEMENT
Care After Internal Radiation Therapy

- Eat three balanced meals a day, and increase fluid to 3 L daily.
- Rest when tired, and resume normal activities as comfort permits.
- Maintain good hygiene (e.g., daily showers and daily douches until discharge stops).
- Use a vaginal dilator if needed for vaginal stenosis. Sexual intercourse may be resumed in 7-10 days or as recommended by your health care provider.
- Understand that sterility and cessation of menstruation usually occur with this procedure if you are premenopausal.
- Report any of the following to your health care provider: bleeding (vaginal, rectal, or in the urine), foul-smelling vaginal discharge, fever, abdominal distention, or pain.
- Take any prescribed medications as directed.
- Call your health care provider or clinic if there are concerns or problems.
- Keep scheduled follow-up visits to determine emotional as well as physical recovery.

Posttreatment complications range from those arising from immobilization, such as thrombophlebitis, pulmonary embolism, and pneumonia, to those arising from the treatment itself, such as hemorrhage, skin reactions (rashes or inflammation), diarrhea, cramping, dysuria, and vaginal stenosis. The woman is assessed for any of these complications before discharge.

The woman may experience sexual problems related to treatment side effects. A decrease in vaginal secretions and sensation may occur, as well as vaginal stenosis. These can contribute to decreased sexual desire, because pain and discomfort during intercourse can affect the desire to resume sexual activities. The nurse can initiate a discussion with the woman and her partner, offer information about the effects of radiation on the ability to have sexual intercourse, and offer suggestions for specific problems, such as using a water-based lubricant for vaginal dryness and using a vaginal dilator as directed by her health care provider. If necessary, the couple can be referred to other resources.

Complications of radiation therapy. Morbidity as a result of properly conducted therapy is usually minimal and most often caused by the uncontrolled tumor more than the therapy. Acute treatment complications during or shortly after therapy include irritation of the rectum, the small bowel, and the bladder; reactions in the skinfolds; and mild bone marrow suppression. Dysuria and frequency may occur. Late complications, although not common, include genital fistulas and necrosis (Yashar, 2018).

Recurrent and Advanced Cancer of the Cervix

Approximately one-third of women with invasive cervical cancer have recurrent or persistent disease after therapy. The 1-year survival rate is between 10% and 15% (Tewari & Monk, 2018). Irradiation of metastatic areas is commonly successful in providing local control and symptomatic relief.

Pelvic exenteration. Pelvic exenteration may be an option for women with recurrent advanced cancer that is confined to the pelvis. A total exenteration involves removal of the perineum, the pelvic floor, the levator muscles, and all reproductive organs. Pelvic lymph nodes, rectum, sigmoid colon, urinary bladder, and distal ureters are removed, with colostomy and ileal conduit constructed (Tewari & Monk, 2018) (Fig. 11.17A). In select cases, the procedure can be modified to either an anterior or a posterior exenteration. Anterior pelvic exenteration includes removal of all the previously mentioned pelvic viscera with sparing of the sigmoid colon and rectum. Urine is rerouted through an ileal conduit (see Fig. 11.17B). Posterior pelvic exenteration involves removal of all pelvic viscera with the exception of the bladder. The feces are rerouted through a colostomy (see Fig. 11.17C). A neovagina (new vagina) may be constructed.

Women are carefully selected for this procedure; 5-year survival rates range from 20% to 62% (Tewari & Monk, 2018). Complications resulting from this surgery are those that follow any form of major surgery—for example, pulmonary embolism, pulmonary edema, myocardial infarction, and cerebrovascular accident. Typically these complications are seen immediately after surgery. Infection originating in the pelvic cavity can occur later.

Nursing interventions. Nursing care of the woman having a pelvic exenteration depends on the structures removed. Preoperative care includes assessments similar to preparation for a radical hysterectomy. A thorough sexual assessment is needed because of the dramatic changes involved. The woman needs information about the construction of a neovagina if that is an option. She will need to be assessed for stoma site selection and information should be given about management of the colostomy and/or an ileal conduit if appropriate. Extensive preoperative bowel preparation is performed before surgery. Pain management is discussed, as is what to expect postoperatively (e.g., nasogastric tubes, arterial catheters). Significant others are included in preoperative teaching when possible so they can be informed and provide needed postoperative support.

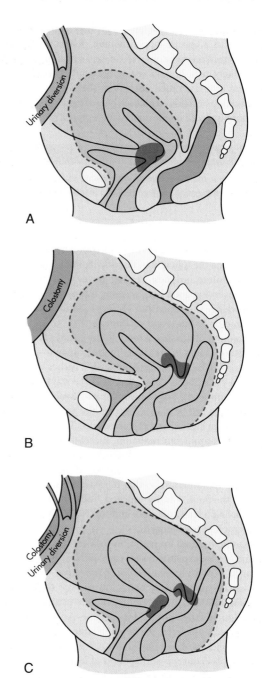

Fig. 11.17 Pelvic Exenteration Procedures. (A) Anterior exenteration. (B) Posterior exenteration. (C) Total exenteration.

Postoperative care usually begins in an intensive care unit until the woman's condition is stable. She is monitored for shock, hemorrhage, pulmonary embolus and other pulmonary complications, fluid and electrolyte imbalance, and urinary complications (Tewari & Monk, 2018). Once the woman's condition is stable, she is moved to a room on the surgical unit. Wound care consists of irrigation with half-strength normal saline, followed by drying of the area with either a hair dryer on cool setting or a heat lamp placed at least 12 inches from the perineal area. The woman is taught how to care for her colostomy or ileal conduit when she is able to begin self-care. Assessment for psychologic reactions is important. The woman will probably experience a grief reaction over the changes in her body due to surgery. She may become depressed during the long convalescence.

The woman may be discharged to a long-term care facility or to her home. She will need assistance until she regains her strength and is comfortable with performing self-care. Teaching needed for home care includes colostomy or ileal/conduit care; dietary needs for healing; perineal care, including use of perineal pads to protect clothing from discharge; ROM exercises and physical activities permitted by her health care provider; and signs of complications, especially infection and bowel obstruction.

Sexual counseling is an important aspect of care management. The changes in her body due to the surgery affect the woman's ability to function sexually. Unless she had vaginal reconstruction, she will be unable to have vaginal intercourse. Usually even with a vaginal reconstruction, vaginal intercourse is not advised until healing has taken place, usually in 12 to 18 months. Women with neovaginas may complain of decreased vaginal sensations or chronic discharge or that the vagina is too short or too long. Women with colostomies or ileal conduits may worry about leakage or odors during sexual activities or may be concerned about the changes in their appearance. They may need counseling about alternative activities for sexual expression for themselves and their partners. The woman and her partner may need referral for further sexual counseling.

Chemotherapy. Chemotherapy may be used in advanced cancer of the cervix to reduce tumor size before surgery or as adjuvant therapy for poor-prognosis tumors. In general, no long-term benefits are derived with chemotherapy, although chemotherapy concurrent with radiation therapy can improve survival (Tewari & Monk, 2018). Cisplatin is the most effective; other chemotherapeutic agents used in combination with cisplatin include carboplatin, cyclophosphamide, ifosfamide, methotrexate, mitomycin C, bleomycin, paclitaxel, topotecan, and hydroxyurea (Chu & Rubin, 2018).

Cancer of the Vulva

Incidence and Etiology

Vulvar carcinoma accounts for about 6% of all female genital malignancies and is the fourth most commonly occurring gynecologic cancer. It appears most frequently in women in their mid-60s to 70s (Herzog, 2018).

Vulvar cancers in older women do not appear to be caused by HPV infection. The incidence of vulvar cancer, specifically vulvar intraepithelial neoplasia (VIN), is increasing in younger women. Almost 20% of vulvar cancers occur in women younger than 50 years of age, and most women are in their 20s. HPV infection is thought to be responsible for most of these cancers (ACS, 2019b). Women who have a history of genital warts (condylomata acuminata), and those who smoke have an increased risk of developing VIN (ACS).

By far the majority (90%) of vulvar carcinoma is squamous cell; other vulvar neoplasms are attributed to Paget disease, adenocarcinoma of Bartholin glands, fibrosarcoma, melanoma, and basal cell carcinoma. VIN is the first neoplastic change, progressing over time to CIS and then to invasive cancer. Metastasis is by direct extension and lymphatic spread (Herzog, 2018).

Prognosis depends on the size of the lesion and the tumor grade at the time of diagnosis; 50% of women have symptoms for 2 to 16 months before seeking treatment. Fortunately, vulvar cancer grows slowly, extends slowly, and metastasizes fairly late. Even with a pattern of delayed diagnosis, survival rates are approximately 90% if nodes are negative. Survival rates drop to 40% to 50%, however, if lymph node metastasis has occurred (Herzog, 2018).

Clinical Manifestations and Diagnosis

Itching is the most common symptom of VIN. A lump or lesion is more common with invasive cancer (Herzog, 2018).

The most common site for vulvar lesions is on the labia majora. The vulvar lesion is usually asymptomatic until it is 1 to 2 cm in diameter.

When it is symptomatic, women may complain of vulvar pruritus, burning, or pain. Necrosis and infection of the lesion result in ulceration with bleeding or watery discharge.

VINs are usually multifocal in young women. Unifocal lesions are associated with invasive cancer and are more common in older women. Initially, growth is superficial but later extends into the urethra, the vagina, and the anus. In approximately 50% of late cases, superficial inguinal and femoral lymph nodes become involved (Herzog, 2018).

Simple biopsy with histologic evaluation confirms the diagnosis. The areas of pathologic involvement are identified by staining the vulva with toluidine blue (1%), allowing an absorption time of 3 to 5 minutes, and then washing with acetic acid (2% to 3%); abnormal tissue retains the dye. Biopsy is necessary to rule out such conditions as sexually transmitted infections (e.g., chancroid, granuloma inguinale, syphilis), basal cell carcinoma, and CIS. In situ malignancies are initially small, red, white, or pigmented friable papules. In Paget disease, the lesions are red, moist, and elevated. Melanomas appear as bluish black, pigmented, or papillary lesions. Melanomas metastasize through the bloodstream and lymphatics (Herzog, 2018).

Medical and Surgical Management

Treatment varies, depending on the extent of the disease. Laser surgery, cryosurgery, or electrosurgical excision may be used to treat VIN. A disadvantage to these treatments is that healing is slow and the treated area is painful. A local wide excision may be performed for localized lesions. Recurrence can occur after these treatments, so follow-up is important (Bodurka & Frumovitz, 2017).

Several types of vulvectomy procedures are used for CIS and invasive cancer. A *skinning vulvectomy* involves removal of the superficial vulvar skin; it is rarely performed.

A *simple vulvectomy* involves removal of all of the vulva (external genital organs, including the mons pubis, labia majora and minora, and possibly the clitoris). The clitoris usually can be saved if cancer is not present.

For invasive disease, a *partial* or *complete radical vulvectomy* is performed. A partial vulvectomy is the removal of part of the vulva and deep tissues. A complete vulvectomy includes the removal of the whole vulva, deep tissues, and the clitoris (Fig. 11.18). These procedures are not used often.

Skin grafts may be done if a large area of skin is removed during the vulvectomy; however, most wounds can be closed without grafts. If grafts are needed, a surgeon who performs reconstruction surgery may be consulted (ACS, 2019b).

The inguinal nodes may be removed through an inguinal (groin) node dissection. Usually only lymph nodes on the same side as the cancer are removed; however, nodes on both sides may be removed if the cancer is in the middle (see Fig. 11.18). Swelling of the leg often is a problem after this surgery.

A *sentinel node biopsy* may be done instead of the inguinal node dissection. This procedure involves injecting blue dye or radioactive material into the tumor site. A scan is performed to identify the sentinel (first) node to pick up the dye or radioactive material. The node is removed for microscopic study. If cancer cells are found, the rest of the lymph nodes are removed, but if cancer is not found, further lymph node removal is not done. This procedure continues to be studied for use with vulvar cancers (ACS, 2019b).

External radiation therapy can be used to shrink tumors before surgery, but it is not the primary treatment. Postoperative external radiation therapy can be used for women who are at risk for recurrence. Radiation treatment causes dermatitis and ulceration that are uncomfortable for the woman.

Chemotherapy has not been very effective as a treatment except for the topical application of 5-fluorouracil for VIN or CIS. This treatment

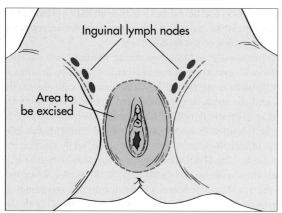

Fig. 11.18 Radical Vulvectomy. Note dotted lines denoting vulvectomy incision and inguinal groin incisions.

is painful and not used often. Chemotherapy continues to be investigated in combination with radiation as an adjunct to surgery in advanced cancer of the vulva (ACS, 2019b).

Nursing Interventions

Nursing care for the woman with vulvar cancer is similar to that for other gynecologic malignancies. Assessments include history of symptoms, physical examination, emotional status, and the woman's understanding of the surgical procedure.

Interventions for the woman treated with laser therapy include applying topical steroids to the area, administering sitz baths and drying the area with a hair dryer on the lowest setting, applying local anesthetics, or giving oral pain medication as needed. Women need to be informed that pain may get worse 3 to 4 days after the treatment.

Because there can be recurrences, information about vulvar self-examination and the need for follow-up with a health care provider is reinforced. Information about community support groups may be helpful.

A woman undergoing radical vulvectomy requires some special instructions in addition to routine postoperative care (see Teaching for Self-Management box: Care After Vulvectomy). She will need instruction about wound care and how to prevent infection. She should be told to report possible complications such as a change in her urine stream (may go to one side due to tissue removal around the urethral opening) and lymphedema (Herzog, 2018).

TEACHING FOR SELF-MANAGEMENT

Care After Vulvectomy

- Avoid sexual activity for 4-6 weeks or as your health care provider directs.
- Rest frequently.
- Avoid crossing your legs, sitting, or standing for long periods.
- Avoid tight, constricting clothing, and wear cotton underwear.
- Keep wound area clean and dry. Rinse area with warm water and pat dry after voiding.
- Continue wound care as prescribed (e.g., irrigate with solution of warm water; pack with gauze; dry using hair dryer on coolest setting). Report to your health care provider any swelling, redness, unusual tenderness, drainage, or foul odor of incision site.
- Report any temperature greater than 39°C (102.2°F).
- Eat a well-balanced diet to promote healing.
- Take all medications as prescribed.
- Elevate your legs periodically to prevent pelvic congestion.
- Call your health care provider or clinic if there are concerns or problems.

The woman is at high risk for sexual dysfunction related to the effects of the surgery. For example, she may have concerns that her partner will be repulsed by the scarring and loss of the vulva. She also may have concerns about reaching orgasm and vaginal numbness or painful vaginal penetration. Nursing actions that focus on minimizing these risks include the following:

- Encouraging verbalization of feelings
- Providing privacy for discussion
- Encouraging open communication between the woman and her partner
- Discussing when sexual activity can be safely resumed
- Discussing alternative methods to achieve sexual satisfaction
- Providing information about use of vaginal dilators and water-soluble lubricants for painful vaginal intercourse
- Providing resources for counseling if necessary

Cancer of the Vagina

Vaginal carcinomas account for 1% to 3% of gynecologic malignancies. More than 50% of cases occur between the ages of 70 and 90 years (Huang, Slomovitz, & Coleman, 2018).

Most lesions are squamous cell carcinomas and are secondary rather than primary carcinomas of the vagina. Vaginal intraepithelial neoplasia (VAIN) is uncommon. Clear-cell adenocarcinoma is even rarer. It is found primarily in young women (ages 15 to 30 years) and is related to intrauterine exposure to DES (Bodurka & Frumovitz, 2017).

The etiology is unknown, but vaginal cancer may be caused by chronic vaginal irritation, vaginal trauma, and genital viruses (e.g., HPV). Women with VAIN often have had cancer or currently have cancer of another part of the genital tract (Huang et al., 2018).

Vaginal lesions, usually seen in the upper third of the vagina, often extend into the bladder and the rectum in late stages. Metastasis can occur early because of the rich lymphatic drainage in the vaginal area.

Some women with vaginal cancer are asymptomatic. Diagnosis often comes after an abnormal Pap test. Symptoms associated with vaginal cancer include bleeding after coitus or examination, dyspareunia, and watery discharge. Bladder involvement results in urinary frequency or urgency; rectal extension causes painful defecation. A pelvic examination may reveal a single lesion, although multiple lesions are common (Huang et al., 2018).

Colposcopy examination and biopsy of Schiller-stained areas confirm the diagnosis. Therapy for vaginal cancer is directed by the extent of the lesion and the age and condition of the woman. Local excision is the preferred therapy for localized lesions. Topical application of 5-fluorouracil cream has been used with varying results. Laser surgery can be used to treat VAIN. Radical hysterectomy and removal of the upper vagina with dissection of the pelvic nodes or internal and external radiation are treatment options for invasive cancer. Radiation therapy is the usual treatment of choice (Huang et al., 2018).

If a vaginectomy is performed, sexual function will be lost without reconstructive surgery. Chemotherapy has not been effective in treating vaginal cancer, although studies are ongoing on the effectiveness of chemotherapy in combination with radiation. In early-stage cancer, 5-year survival rates are greater than 80%, with stage II survival rates in the 50% range (Huang et al., 2018).

Nursing care for the woman with vaginal cancer is similar to that for other gynecologic cancers. Women who are sexually active should be encouraged to continue sexual intercourse or to use a vaginal dilator to maintain vaginal patency (Huang et al., 2018). Sexual counseling or referral may be needed.

Cancer of the Uterine Tubes

Primary carcinoma of the uterine (fallopian) tube is one of the rarest cancers of the female genital tract, occurring in less than 1% of women. The peak incidence is between ages 50 and 60 years. The most common site is the distal third of the uterine tube (Hope, Maxwell, & Hamilton, 2018). The cause is unknown. Most women are asymptomatic in the early stages of tubal cancer. Vaginal bleeding is the most common symptom of tubal cancer, but clear vaginal discharge and lower abdominal pain also occur frequently. An enlarging unilateral pelvic mass or ascites may occur and is often misdiagnosed as ovarian or endometrial carcinoma. Differential diagnosis of tubal cancer is usually made postoperatively. Because uterine tube cancer is so rare, there is no established management plan.

Current therapy guidelines parallel those established for ovarian carcinoma; therefore, tumor-reducing surgery such as a TAH with BSO, omentectomy (removal of connective tissue covering the organs), and lymph node sampling are performed (Hope et al., 2018). Postoperative therapy consists of chemotherapy with cisplatin or other platinum-based drugs combined with paclitaxel, sometimes followed by second-look surgery to determine whether further treatment is needed. Radiation therapy is sometimes used if the disease is limited to the tube, ovary, and uterus, although reports of its effectiveness vary. The overall 5-year survival rate for all stages is 69%; the 5-year survival rates for stages I and II are approximately 80% (Hope et al., 2018).

Nursing care for the woman with uterine tube cancer is similar to that of the woman with ovarian cancer. Nursing care occurs within the context of an interprofessional team, with nurses as central health care providers in this team.

Cancer and Pregnancy

Cancer occurs with relative infrequency during the reproductive years. Approximately 1 of every 1000 pregnant women will have cancer (Salani, Eisenhauer, & Copeland, 2017). These malignancies may be responsible for up to one-third of maternal deaths. Although all forms of neoplasms have been documented in conjunction with pregnancy, the most frequently occurring types are breast cancer, cervical cancer, melanomas, ovarian cancer, leukemia and lymphomas, and thyroid cancers. Other cancers, including other gynecologic cancers, rarely are diagnosed in pregnancy (Salani et al., 2017). When pregnancy and cancer coincide, therapeutic issues are complex, and intense reactions occur in the woman, her family, and the health care team. Women are confronted with issues such as continuing or terminating the pregnancy. The selection and timing of therapies such as chemotherapy, radiation, and surgery are affected by the pregnancy. Add to this the conflicting feelings the woman has (i.e., the joy of pregnancy versus the fear and anxiety associated with cancer), and the task of providing comprehensive care for her and her family presents a formidable challenge to the health care team. A brief discussion of the most frequent types of cancers that occur during pregnancy and the current therapies associated with them follows.

Cancer of the Breast

Approximately 1% to 2% of women are pregnant or lactating at the time of diagnosis of cancer of the breast (Tewari, 2018). Breast cancer complicates about 1 in 3000 pregnancies. The survival rate for women who are diagnosed with breast cancer while pregnant may be as low as 15% to 20% because the disease is generally in the advanced stages when first diagnosed (Salani et al., 2017). Diagnosis is often delayed because breast engorgement may obscure the mass from palpation, and increased density of the tissue makes mammographic visualization more difficult. In addition, increased vascularity and lymphatic drainage in the breast of a pregnant woman may increase the speed of metastasis. Treatment is the same as for a nonpregnant woman,

although surgery is usually the treatment of choice for breast cancer in pregnancy (Tewari). If an invasive tumor is found, it must be determined whether the tissue is positive or negative for ERs. ER-negative tumors spread more rapidly than ER-positive tumors and are more common in pregnancy (Salani et al., 2017).

Maternal-fetal management involves consideration of the gestational age of the fetus, the extent of disease, the tumor growth potential, and the proposed treatment. Termination of the pregnancy in early stages of the disease appears to have no effect on survival. Therapeutic abortion may become an issue in the presence of advanced disease and may be deemed necessary to achieve effective palliation. In the first trimester, lumpectomy or partial mastectomy is the most commonly used surgical procedure, but radical mastectomy is tolerated well in these women. For advanced disease in the second or third trimester, alkylating agents, 5-fluorouracil, doxorubicin, and cyclophosphamide are relatively safe for the fetus. Radiation therapy is avoided if at all possible until after the birth, because even with careful shielding, the fetus may still receive sufficient radiation to produce detrimental effects (Salani et al., 2017; Tewari, 2018).

There is no agreement about whether a postpartum woman with breast cancer should breastfeed, although many surgeons recommend formula feeding. There are theoretic concerns that if one of the oncogenes for breast cancer is a virus, as many have postulated, the remaining breast may be contaminated, and the virus may be passed to the newborn, possibly acting as a latent inducer of breast carcinoma. Another reason is that lactation increases vascularity in the remaining breast, which may contain a neoplasm as well (Tewari, 2018).

Breastfeeding after lumpectomy is possible, but the site of the incision may interrupt the milk ducts or prevent the nipple from extending during feeding. Breastfeeding is contraindicated if the woman is receiving chemotherapy. Women receiving radiation have diminished ability to lactate in the irradiated breast (Salani et al., 2017; Tewari, 2018).

Pregnancy incidence after mastectomy is influenced by many factors, including prior treatment and duration of survival. In general, women with good prognoses (e.g., no positive nodes) are likely to be counseled to wait at least 2 years before attempting pregnancy (Tewari, 2018).

Cancer of the Cervix

The incidence of cervical cancer concurrent with pregnancy is reported to be about 1 in 2200 pregnancies, making it the most common reproductive tract cancer associated with pregnancy (Salani et al., 2017). The outcome for a woman with cervical cancer is roughly the same as that for a nonpregnant woman (Tewari, 2018).

Cervical abnormalities are diagnosed during pregnancy with an abnormal Pap test. If the report suggests that the pregnant woman has a squamous intraepithelial lesion, a colposcopy, possibly with directed biopsy, is done. If invasive disease is not found, treatment is delayed until after the woman gives birth. Colposcopy is often repeated every 6 to 8 weeks until the birth and again postpartum (Salani et al., 2017). Conization is not advised during pregnancy unless necessary to rule out invasive cancer because it is associated with bleeding, miscarriage, and preterm birth (Tewari, 2018).

The therapy of invasive carcinoma of the cervix during pregnancy is affected by many factors. The stage of the disease and the trimester in which the cancer is diagnosed are important. Equally important are the beliefs and desires of the woman and her family in terms of initiating therapy that can interrupt the pregnancy, as opposed to postponing the therapy until fetal viability is achieved. If the woman chooses not to continue the pregnancy, external radiation to the pelvis is done. Miscarriage usually occurs, and then internal radiation is done. If miscarriage does not occur, a modified radical hysterectomy may be performed. If the woman desires to continue the pregnancy, treatment of early-stage invasive cervical cancer can be delayed until 34 to 36 weeks, without harmful effects for the woman. Cesarean birth is usually performed after the mother has received antenatal steroids and fetal lung maturity is documented; radiation therapy is then initiated (Salani et al., 2017; Tewari, 2018).

Leukemia

The average age for pregnant women with acute leukemia is 28 years; incidence during pregnancy is about 1 in 75,000 (Tewari, 2018). Pregnancy seems to have no specific effect on the course of the disease, but vigorous therapy is detrimental to early gestation. Preterm labor and postpartum hemorrhage are associated with acute leukemia (Tewari, 2018). Acute myelocytic leukemia (60% of cases) has a more fulminant course and requires immediate therapy; in the presence of chronic myelocytic leukemia, therapy may be delayed. Some pregnant women with the chronic form of the disease who had chemotherapy and radiation therapy directed at the spleen have given birth to apparently healthy infants. The decision to terminate the pregnancy rests with the woman and her family; however, prompt, aggressive therapy is always advisable if remission is to be achieved. Decisions may be influenced by the aggressiveness of the disease.

Hodgkin Disease

Hodgkin disease is a malignant lymphoma that affects many younger people and complicates about 1 in 6000 pregnancies. Younger women (<40 years) have a better prognosis than women 40 years of age and older (Tewari, 2018).

Pregnancy appears to have no effect on the disease and vice versa, other than those effects resulting from therapy (Salani et al., 2017). Radiation therapy of the nodes and multiagent chemotherapy result in about a 90% cure rate. Unless gestation is well into the third trimester, delay in initiating therapy should be minimal, which brings up the dilemma of therapeutic abortion. Radiation therapy to diseased areas above the diaphragm can be initiated during the third trimester with proper shielding of the fetus (Salani et al., 2017). Chemotherapy is strongly contraindicated during the first trimester, but certain agents (antitumor antibiotics and antimicrotubule agents) appear safe to use in the second and third trimesters. Termination of the pregnancy during the course of the disease is not definitely indicated (Tewari, 2018).

Melanoma

Malignant melanoma may be one of the rare cancers that can be affected by pregnancy. This is suggested by some reports in which pregnancy has been shown to induce or exacerbate a melanoma. These suggestions are based on changes that occur naturally during pregnancy and include hyperpigmentation, an increase in melanocyte-stimulating hormone (MSH), and increased estrogen production. ERs have been identified in about half of all melanomas. Although pregnancy has been implicated in the more rapid metastases to regional lymph nodes, stage for stage there does not seem to be a significant difference in the survival of pregnant and nonpregnant women. As a result, most authorities recommend that women who have histories of malignant melanoma delay pregnancy for 2 to 3 years after surgical excision, because this is the period of highest risk for recurrence (Salani et al., 2017; Tewari, 2018).

Diagnosis is established by biopsy. Therapy consists of radical local excision. For most other malignancies, the placenta is resistant to invasion by maternal cancer. Although melanoma accounts for few cases of malignant disease during pregnancy, it is the most common cancer to metastasize to the placenta (Tewari, 2018).

Thyroid Cancer

The incidence of thyroid cancer in pregnancy is not established. Normally the thyroid gland enlarges during pregnancy, and an asymptomatic nodular mass is a common finding. Diagnosis is usually by cytologic testing of fine-needle aspirate. Thyroid suppression is the preferred treatment during pregnancy for a benign lesion. For a papillary or follicular malignancy found in the first or second trimester, the woman is advised to have a thyroidectomy in the second trimester followed by thyroid suppression. If a tumor is found in the third trimester, surgery can be delayed until after the birth. With other thyroid malignancies, treatment is individualized based on the wishes of the woman and her family (Tewari, 2018).

 MEDICATION ALERT

Radioactive iodine is contraindicated in pregnancy and lactation.

Colon Cancer

The incidence of colon cancer in pregnancy is approximately 1 in 13,000 (Tewari, 2018). The signs and symptoms such as constipation, hemorrhoids, and backache are often attributed to pregnancy, resulting in diagnosis at a more advanced stage. Colonoscopy and biopsy are usually not done in pregnancy because these procedures can cause placental abruption and fetal injury from maternal hypoxia or hypotension.

Management of the cancer is based on the weeks of gestation and tumor stage. In a woman who is less than 20 weeks of gestation, surgery may be performed to remove the tumor. If she is at more than 20 weeks of gestation, surgery may be delayed until after the birth. Chemotherapy and radiation are usually not used in pregnancy for colon cancer but may be used after the birth (Salani et al., 2017; Tewari, 2018).

Cancer Therapy and Pregnancy

Decisions about the type and timing of therapy for cancer in the pregnant woman evoke moral and philosophic dilemmas, as well as complex medical judgments and intense emotional responses.

Ethical considerations. When a pregnant woman has cancer and her survival is contingent on treatment that will harm the fetus, the interprofessional health care team must work with the woman and her significant others to make decisions about how to proceed with her care. If a one-client model of ethical decision making is used, the risk-benefit analysis is applied to the maternal-fetal unit. The pregnant woman decides what is best for her and the fetus. The woman may accept or refuse treatment. If a two-client model is used for decision making, more weight is given to fetal well-being, but the pregnant woman cannot be forced to accept harm to herself for the sake of the fetus. Thus she could elect to accept treatment.

The fetus is at risk with either chemotherapy or radiation therapy. The effect of cancer therapy on the fetus can include death, miscarriage, teratogenesis, alteration in growth and development, alterations in function, and genetic mutation. The long-term effects on the fetus are unknown. These theoretic dangers must be weighed against the potential detrimental effects to the mother if treatment is withheld (Terwari, 2018).

Timing of therapy. Timing of therapy is an important issue to discuss. Because most cancer therapy (except surgery) is geared toward having a differential and noxious effect on rapidly growing tissue, the fetus is most at risk during the first trimester, when organogenesis and rapid tissue growth occur. Surgery offers the least potential risk to the fetus; however, the risk of miscarriage and preterm labor may be increased. Surgery is usually scheduled in the second trimester and has been discussed in the previous sections on gynecologic cancers in nonpregnant women.

Chemotherapy is avoided in the first trimester if at all possible. Although use of most chemotherapeutic agents has had isolated reports of fetal abnormalities, data on the agents used after the first trimester have recorded few fetal abnormalities. The placenta may act as a barrier against the chemotherapeutic agents; therefore, although risk still exists, the judicious use of chemotherapy after the first trimester can result in live births with few congenital abnormalities. Acute drug toxicities may occur if treatment takes place just before birth. Breastfeeding by women who are taking chemotherapeutic drugs is not recommended because most of these drugs may be excreted in breast milk (Salani et al., 2017; Tewari, 2018).

Radiation therapy presents its own set of issues. During embryonic development, tissues are extremely radiosensitive. If cells are genetically altered or killed during this time, the child either fails to survive or has specific organ damage. From a radiologic stance, there are three significant periods in embryonic development (Tewari, 2018).

1. Preimplantation: If irradiation does not destroy the fertilized egg, it probably does not affect it significantly.
2. Critical period of organogenesis: During this period, especially between days 18 and 38, the organism is most vulnerable; microcephaly, anencephaly, eye damage, growth restriction, spina bifida, and foot damage may occur.
3. After day 40: Large doses may still cause observable malformation and damage to the central nervous system.

Radiation therapy should be delayed until the postpartum period if possible (Salani et al., 2017).

Pregnancy after cancer treatment. If cancer therapy has not included the removal of the uterus, ovaries, or uterine tubes, there is a possibility that the woman may still be able to become pregnant. Although her menstrual cycle may have resumed, pregnancy may be difficult to achieve. Therapy that has affected the pituitary or thyroid gland may make conception difficult. Radiation appears to have the most deleterious effects on the endocrine system. The use of chemotherapy may result in temporary or permanent sterility, depending on the drug, the dose, and the length of time since the therapy was completed. Rates of ovarian failure are increased with pelvic irradiation (Tewari, 2018).

Of growing concern is the increase in the number of childhood and adolescent cancer survivors. Long-term effects of therapy on fertility, including incidence of congenital anomalies, are not well known. Counseling issues to be discussed with the pregnant woman after cancer treatment include the risk of recurrence and the likely sites of recurrence, how the prior cancer treatment can affect fertility or reproductive outcome, and if a future pregnancy will adversely affect a tumor that is ER positive (Salani et al., 2017).

For recovery from the disease and treatment to be complete, a delay of at least 2 years from the end of therapy to conception often is advised (Tewari, 2018). Before conception, a woman who has had cancer should have a complete physical examination to rule out complications that may place her or a fetus in jeopardy. Cardiac, pulmonary, hematologic, neurologic, renal, or gonadal function can be impaired. The woman and the potential father (if partnered) may be referred for reproductive and genetic counseling as well.

Gestational Trophoblastic Neoplasia

Gestational trophoblastic disease (GTD) encompasses a spectrum of disorders arising from the placental trophoblast. It includes hydatidiform mole (see Chapter 28), invasive mole, and choriocarcinoma. *Gestational trophoblastic neoplasia (GTN)* refers to persistent trophoblastic tissue that is presumed to be malignant (Barber & Soper, 2018).

Table 11.2 describes the clinical classifications of GTN. For several reasons, GTN is recognized as the most curable gynecologic malignancy. There is a sensitive marker produced by the tumor (hCG); the

TABLE 11.2 Clinical Classification for Women With Malignant Gestational Trophoblastic Neoplasia

Classification	Criteria
Nonmetastatic disease	No evidence of disease outside uterus
Metastatic disease	Any disease outside uterus
Good prognosis metastatic disease	Short duration (<4 months)
	Low pretreatment hCG titer <40,000 milli-International Units/mL
	No prior term pregnancy
	No metastasis to brain or liver
	No prior chemotherapy
Poor prognosis metastatic disease	Any one risk factor:
	Long duration (>4 months)
	High pretreatment hCG titer >40,000 milli-International Units/mL
	Brain or liver metastasis
	Prior term pregnancy
	Prior chemotherapy

From Ko, E. M., & Soper, J. T. (2012). Gestational trophoblastic disease. In P. J. DiSaia, W. T. Creasman, R. S. Mannel, & D. S. Mutch (Eds.), *Clinical gynecologic oncology* (8th ed.). Philadelphia: Saunders.

tumor is extremely sensitive to various chemotherapeutic agents; high-risk factors in the disease process can be identified, allowing individualized therapy; and the aggressive use of multiple treatment methods is possible.

Malignant disease follows normal pregnancy in about 25% of cases and hydatidiform mole in about 50% of cases. Miscarriage or ectopic pregnancy or another gestational event precedes about 25% of cases (Barber & Soper, 2018). Metastasis occurs most often in the lungs, vagina, liver, and brain.

Continued bleeding after evacuation of a hydatidiform mole is usually the most suggestive symptom of GTN. Other clinical signs include abdominal pain and uterine and ovarian enlargement. Signs of metastasis include pulmonary symptoms (e.g., dyspnea, cough). The diagnosis is usually confirmed by increasing or plateauing hCG levels after evacuation of a molar pregnancy. Once diagnosis is confirmed, other clinical studies (e.g., CT scan of lungs and brain, chest x-ray, pelvic ultrasound, and liver scan) can determine the extent of the disease (Barber & Soper, 2018).

For women who wish to preserve their fertility and who have low-risk nonmetastatic or low-risk metastatic GTN, single-agent chemotherapy is chosen. Methotrexate has been the treatment of choice for years. High-dose methotrexate followed by folinic acid rescue within 24 hours also has shown excellent results and causes fewer toxic effects (Barber & Soper, 2018).

Dactinomycin has been used with equally good results and is used for women with liver or renal disease, both of which are contraindications for methotrexate. Hysterectomy with adjuvant chemotherapy is often the choice of treatment for nonmetastatic tumors in women who have completed their childbearing (Barber & Soper, 2018).

Women who have metastasis are classified as having either a good or poor prognosis, depending on the absence or presence of brain or liver metastasis, unsuccessful prior chemotherapy, symptoms lasting longer than 4 months, and elevation of serum B-hCG levels. Treatment progresses from single-agent chemotherapy in the good-prognosis metastatic GTN to multiple-agent chemotherapy and multiple methods of treatment for the poor-prognosis group. Cure rates for the good-prognosis group are almost as positive as for those with nonmetastatic disease, both approaching 100% (Barber & Soper, 2018).

Therapy is continued until negative hCG levels are obtained. After successful chemotherapy follow-up by serum hCG levels varies. One schedule is to obtain levels every 2 weeks for 3 months, every month for up to a year after completing therapy, and every 6 to 12 months up to 3 to 5 years (Barber & Soper, 2018; Bouchard-Fortier & Covens, 2017). Physical

examinations are done at least yearly as are chest x-rays if indicated. Contraception is needed until the woman has been in remission for 6 months to 1 year. OCs are preferred, but barrier methods are acceptable if OCs are contraindicated (Barber & Soper). During a subsequent pregnancy, pelvic ultrasonography is recommended because the woman is at higher risk (1% to 2%) to develop another molar pregnancy. Serum hCG levels should be obtained 6 weeks after the birth (Bouchard-Fortier & Covens, 2017).

■ KEY POINTS

- Gynecologic disorders diminish the quality of life for affected women and their families.
- Structural disorders of the uterus and vagina related to pelvic relaxation and urinary incontinence can be a delayed result of childbearing, but they can be seen in young or childless women.
- Bladder training and pelvic muscle exercises can significantly decrease or relieve mild to moderate urinary incontinence.
- The development of neoplasms, whether benign or malignant, can have a significant physical and emotional effect on a woman and her family.
- Abnormal uterine bleeding is the most common symptom of leiomyomas or fibroid tumors.
- Various alternatives to hysterectomy exist for structural and benign disorders of the uterus; women need to be informed about the risks and benefits to make an informed decision about treatment.
- Endometrial cancer is the most common reproductive system malignancy.
- Hysterectomy is the usual treatment for early-stage endometrial cancer.
- Human papillomavirus infection is the primary cause of cervical cancer and is linked to vulvar cancer in women younger than 50 years.

- The squamocolumnar junction is an important landmark identified with neoplastic changes of the cervix.
- Preinvasive cancer of the cervix may be treated with techniques such as electrosurgical excision, cryotherapy, and laser therapy to save the structure of the cervix, particularly in women who desire to retain childbearing ability.
- External and internal radiation therapy in combination is as successful as surgery in treating early stages of cancer of the cervix.
- A Pap test can detect approximately 90% of early cervical dysplasias.
- Cancer of the ovary causes more deaths than any other female genital tract cancer.
- Nurses can control their exposure to radiation by increasing the distance from the radiation source, by limiting the time of exposure, and by using lead shielding.
- Cancer is relatively infrequent during pregnancy, occurring in about 1 in 1000 pregnancies.
- Radiation or chemotherapy treatment of a pregnant woman who has cancer places the woman at risk for miscarriage and the fetus at risk for death, teratogenesis and alterations in growth and development.
- Gestational trophoblastic neoplasms are highly curable but require close monitoring of hCG levels after treatment.

REFERENCES

Agnihotri, S. (2016). Assessment and treatment of uterine fibroids. *Prescriber*, 27(6), 28–33.

American Cancer Society (ACS). (2019a). *Cancer facts and figures 2019.* Retrieved from: https://www.cancer.org/content/dam/cancer-org/research/cancer-facts-and-statistics/annual-cancer-facts-and-figures/2019/cancer-facts-and-figures-2019.pdf.

American Cancer Society (ACS). (2019b). *Vulvar cancer.* Retrieved from: https://www.cancer.org/cancer/vulvar-cancer.html.

American College of Obstetrics & Gynecology (ACOG). (2015). Practice bulletin no. 155: Urinary incontinence in women. *Obstetrics & Gynecology*, 126(5), e66–e81.

Barber, E. L., & Soper, J. T. (2018). Gestational trophoblastic disease. In P. J. Di Saia, W. T. Creasman, R. S. Mannel, D. S. McMeekin, & D. G. Mutch (Eds.), *Clinical gynecologic oncology* (9th ed.). Philadelphia: Elsevier.

Binkurian, N., Linnane, M., & Browne, F. (2015). Journal article review: Nursing care of a patient undergoing uterine artery embolization in the radiology department. *Journal of Radiology Nursing*, 34(3), 143–149.

Bodurka, D. C., & Frumovitz, M. (2017). Malignant diseases of the vagina. Intraepithelial neoplasia, carcinoma, sarcoma. In R. A. Lobo, D. M. Gershenson, G. M. Lentz, & F. A. Valea (Eds.), *Comprehensive gynecology* (7th ed.). Philadelphia: Elsevier.

Bouchard-Fortier, G., & Covens, A. (2017). Gestational trophoblastic disease: Hydatidiform mole, nonmetastatic and metastatic gestational trophoblastic tumor: Diagnosis and management. In R. A. Lobo, D. M. Gershenson, G. M. Lentz, & F. A. Valea (Eds.), *Comprehensive gynecology* (7th ed.). Philadelphia: Elsevier.

Bugge, C., Adams, E. J., Gopinath, D., & Reid, F. (2013). Pessaries (mechanical devices) for pelvic organ prolapsed in women. *The Cochrane Database of Systematic Reviews*, 2, CD004010.

Chu, C., & Rubin, S. (2018). Basic principles of chemotherapy. In P. J. Di Saia, W. T. Creasman, R. S. Mannel, et al. (Eds.), *Clinical gynecologic oncology* (9th ed.). Philadelphia: Elsevier.

Coleman, R., Ramirez, P., & Gershenson, D. (2017). Neoplastic diseases of the ovary. Screening, benign and malignant epithelial cell neoplasms, sex-cord stromal tumors. In R. A. Lobo, D. M. Gershenson, G. M. Lentz, & F. A. Valea (Eds.), *Comprehensive gynecology* (7th ed.). Philadelphia: Elsevier.

Creasman, W. T., & Miller, D. S. (2018). Adenocarcinoma of the uterine corpus. In P. J. Di Saia, W. T. Creasman, R. S. Mannel, et al. (Eds.), *Clinical gynecologic oncology* (9th ed.). Philadelphia: Elsevier.

Dolan, M. S., Hill, C., & Valea, F. A. (2017). Benign gynecologic lesions: Vulva, vagina, cervix, uterus, oviduct, ovary, ultrasound imaging of pelvic structures. In R. A. Lobo, D. M. Gershenson, G. M. Lentz, & F. A. Valea (Eds.), *Comprehensive gynecology* (7th ed.). Philadelphia: Elsevier.

Eisenhauer, E. L., Salani, R., & Copeland, L. J. (2018). Epithelial ovarian cancer. In P. J. Di Saia, W. T. Creasman, R. S., et al. (Eds.), *Clinical gynecologic oncology* (9th ed.). Philadelphia: Elsevier.

Fonseca, M. C. M., Castro, R., Machado, M., et al. (2017). Uterine artery embolization and surgical methods for the treatment of symptomatic uterine leiomyomas: A systemic review and meta-analysis followed by indirect treatment comparison. *Clinical Therapeutics*, 39(7), 1438–1455.

Gardella, C., Eckert, L. O., & Lentz, G. M. (2017). Genital tract infection: Vulva, vagina, cervix, Toxic shock syndrome, endometritis, and salpingitis. In R. A. Lobo, D. M. Gershenson, G. M. Lentz, & F. A. Valea (Eds.), *Comprehensive Gynecology* (7th ed.). Philadelphia: Elsevier.

Goodman, N., Cobin, R., Futterweit, W., et al. (2015). American Association of Clinical Endocrinologists, American College of Endocrinology, and Androgen Excess and PCOS Society disease state clinical review: Guide to the best practices in the evaluation and treatment of polycystic ovary syndrome-part 2. *Endocrine Practice, 21*(12), 1415–1426.

Herzog, T. J. (2018). Invasive cancer of the vulva. In P. J. Di Saia, W. T. Creasman, R. S. Mannel, et al. (Eds.), *Clinical gynecologic oncology* (9th ed.). Philadelphia: Elsevier.

Hope, E. R., Maxwell, G. L., & Hamilton, C. A. (2018). Fallopian tube cancer. In P. J. Di Saia, W. T. Creasman, R. S. Mannel, et al. (Eds.), *Clinical gynecologic oncology* (9th ed.). Philadelphia: Elsevier.

Huang, M., Slomovitz, B. M., & Coleman, R. L. (2018). Invasive cancer of the vagina. In P. J. Di Saia, W. T. Creasman, R. S. Mannel, et al. (Eds.), *Clinical gynecologic oncology* (9th ed.). Philadelphia: Elsevier.

Jayasena, C. N., & Franks, S. (2014). The management of patients with polycystic ovary syndrome. *Nature Reviews. Endocrinology, 10*(10), 624–636.

Kirby, A. C., & Lentz, G. M. (2017a). Anatomic defects of the abdominal wall and pelvic floor: Abdominal hernias, inguinal hernias, and pelvic organ prolapse: Diagnosis and management. In R. A. Lobo, D. M. Gershenson, G. M. Lentz, & F. A. Valea (Eds.), *Comprehensive gynecology* (7th ed.). Philadelphia: Elsevier.

Kirby, A. C., & Lentz, G. M. (2017b). Lower urinary tract function and disorders: Physiology of micturition, voiding dysfunction, urinary incontinence, urinary tract infections, and painful bladder syndrome. In R. A. Lobo, D. M. Gershenson, G. M. Lentz, & F. A. Valea (Eds.), *Comprehensive gynecology* (7th ed.). Philadelphia: Elsevier.

Lobo, R. A. (2017). Hyperandrogenism: and androgen excess: Physiology, etiology, differential diagnosis, management. In R. A. Lobo, D. M. Gershenson, G. M. Lentz, & F. A. Valea (Eds.), *Comprehensive gynecology* (7th ed.). Philadelphia: Elsevier.

Massad, L. S. (2018). Preinvasive disease of the cervix. In P. J. Di Saia, W. T. Creasman, R. S., et al. (Eds.), *Clinical gynecologic oncology* (9th ed.). Philadelphia: Elsevier.

Mayo Clinic. (2019). Vulvodynia. Retrieved from: https://www.mayoclinic.org/diseases-conditions/vulvodynia/diagnosis-treatment/drc-20353427.

Moyer, V. A., & U.S. Preventive Services Task Force. (2012). Screening for cervical cancer: U.S. Preventive Services Task Force recommendation statement. *Annals of Internal Medicine, 156*(12), 880–891.

Muth, C. C. (2017). Urinary incontinence in women. *JAMA, 318*(16), 1622.

National Cervical Cancer Coalition. (2019). Cervical cancer overview. Retrieved from: https://www.nccc-online.org/hpvcervical-cancer/cervical-cancer-overview/.

Parker, W. H., & Gambone, J. C. (2016). Benign conditions and congenital anomalies of the uterine corpus and cervix. In N. F. Hacker, J. C. Gambone, & C. J. Hobel (Eds.), *Hacker & Moore's essentials of obstetrics & gynecology* (5th ed.). Philadelphia: Elsevier.

Salani, R., Eisenhauer, E. L., & Copeland, L. J. (2017). Malignant disease and pregnancy. In S. G. Gabbe, J. R. Niebyl, J. L. Simpson, et al. (Eds.), *Obstetrics: Normal and problem pregnancies* (6th ed.). Philadelphia: Saunders.

Salcedo, M. P., Baker, E. S., & Schmeler, K. M. (2017). Intraepithelial neoplasia of the lower genital tract (cervix, vagina, vulva): Etiology, screening, diagnosis, management. comprehensive gynecology. In R. A. Lobo, D. M. Gershenson, G. M. Lentz, & F. A. Valea (Eds.), *Comprehensive gynecology* (7th ed.). Philadelphia: Elsevier.

Soliman, P. T., & Lu, K. H. (2017). Neoplastic diseases of the uterus. Endometrial hyperplasia, endometrial carcinoma, sarcoma: Diagnosis and management. In R. A. Lobo, D. M. Gershenson, G. M. Lentz, & F. A. Valea (Eds.), *Comprehensive gynecology* (7th ed.). Philadelphia: Elsevier.

Tewari, K. S. (2018). Cancer in pregnancy. In P. J. Di Saia, W. T. Creasman, R. S. Mannel, et al. (Eds.), *Clinical gynecologic oncology* (9th ed.). Philadelphia: Elsevier.

Tewari, K. S., & Monk, B. J. (2018). Invasive cervical cancer. In P. J. Di Saia, W. T. Creasman, R. S. Mannel, et al. (Eds.), *Clinical gynecologic oncology* (9th ed.). Philadelphia: Elsevier.

Viscosky, C., & Ponto, J. (2018). Care of patients with cancer. In D. D. Ignatavicius, M. L. Workman, C. R. Rebar, & N. M. Heimgartner (Eds.), *Medical-surgical nursing: Concepts for interprofessional collaborative care* (9th ed.). St. Louis: Elsevier.

Yashar, C. (2018). Basic principles of gynecologic radiotherapy. In P. J. Di Saia, W. T. Creasman, R. S. Mannel, et al. (Eds.), *Clinical gynecologic oncology* (9th ed.). Philadelphia: Elsevier.

12

Conception and Fetal Development

Jennie M. Wagner

LEARNING OBJECTIVES

- Summarize the process of fertilization and implantation.
- Identify the development, structure, and functions of the placenta.
- Explain the composition and functions of amniotic fluid.
- Distinguish the three organs or tissues arising from each of the three primary germ layers.
- Discuss the significant changes in growth and development of the embryo and fetus.
- Contrast the different types of multifetal pregnancies.
- Analyze the potential effects of teratogens during vulnerable periods of embryonic and fetal development.

This chapter presents an overview of the process of fertilization and the development of the normal embryo and fetus. This information is foundational to understanding pregnancy.

CONCEPTION

Conception, defined as the union of a single egg and sperm, marks the beginning of a pregnancy. Conception occurs not as an isolated event but as part of a sequential process, which includes gamete (egg and sperm) formation, ovulation (release of the egg), fertilization (union of the gametes), and implantation in the uterus. An explanation of cell division by mitosis and meiosis precedes discussion of gametogenesis.

Cell Division

Cells are reproduced by two different methods: mitosis and meiosis. In mitosis, body cells replace and repair themselves. The process supports the diploid number of 46 chromosomes, forming two daughter cells, each containing a single deoxyribonucleic acid (DNA) strand. The cells replicate to yield two cells with the same genetic makeup as the parent cell, unless a mutation occurs. First the cell makes a copy of its DNA, and then it divides. Each daughter cell receives one copy of the genetic material. Mitotic division facilitates growth and development or cell replacement.

Meiosis, the process by which germ cells divide and decrease their chromosomal number by half, from the diploid (46) to the haploid (23) number, produces gametes (eggs and sperm). Each homologous pair of chromosomes contains one chromosome received from the mother and one from the father; thus meiosis results in cells that contain one of each of the 23 pairs of chromosomes. Because these germ cells contain 23 single chromosomes, half of the genetic material of a normal somatic cell, they are called *haploid*. This halving of the genetic material is accomplished by replicating the DNA once and then dividing twice. When the female gamete (egg or ovum) and the male gamete (spermatozoon) unite to form the zygote, the diploid number of human chromosomes (46, or 23 pairs) is restored.

The process of DNA replication and cell division in meiosis allows different *alleles* (genes on corresponding loci that code for variations of the same trait) for genes to be distributed at random by each parent and then rearranged on the paired chromosomes. The chromosomes then separate and proceed to different gametes. Many combinations of genes are possible on each chromosome because parents have genotypes derived from four different grandparents. This random mixing of alleles accounts for the variation of traits seen in the offspring of the same two parents.

Gametogenesis

Oogenesis, the process of egg (ovum) formation, begins during fetal life in the female. All the cells that may undergo meiosis in a woman's lifetime are contained in her ovaries at birth and undergo a gradual degeneration process until menopause. The majority of the remaining 1 to 2 million (perhaps as few as 600,000 to 800,000) primary oocytes (the cells that undergo the first meiotic division) degenerate spontaneously (Blackburn, 2018). Only 400 to 500 ova will mature during the approximately 35 years of a woman's reproductive life. The primary oocytes begin the first meiotic division (i.e., they replicate their DNA) during fetal life, but they remain suspended at this stage until puberty (Fig. 12.1). After puberty the follicle-stimulating hormone (FSH) and luteinizing hormone (LH) from the pituitary gland promote an increase in the size of the oocyte. Then, usually monthly, one primary oocyte matures and completes the first meiotic division, yielding two unequal cells: the secondary oocyte and the first polar body, which degenerates. Both contain 22 autosomes and one X sex chromosome.

At ovulation the second meiotic division begins. However, the ovum does not complete the second meiotic division unless fertilization occurs. At fertilization, when the sperm is united with the mature ovum, a second polar body and the zygote (the united egg and sperm) are produced and the three polar bodies degenerate.

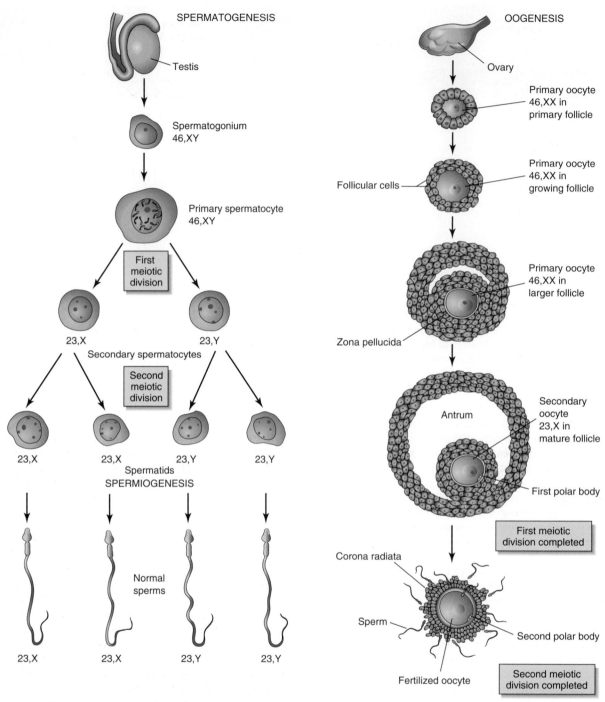

Fig. 12.1 Normal Gametogenesis: Conversion of Germ Cells into Gametes. The illustrations compare spermatogenesis and oogenesis. The chromosome complement of the germ cells is shown at each stage. The number designates the total number of chromosomes, including sex chromosome(s) (shown after the comma). Note: (1) After the two meiotic divisions, the diploid number of chromosomes, 46, is reduced to the haploid number, 23; (2) four sperms form from one primary spermatocyte, whereas only one secondary oocyte results from maturation of a primary oocyte; (3) the cytoplasm is conserved during oogenesis to form one large cell, the oocyte. (From Moore, K.L., Persaud, T.V.N., Torchia, M.G. [2016]. *Before we were born: Essentials of embryology and birth defects* [9th ed.]. Philadelphia: Elsevier.)

When a male reaches puberty, with the release of androgens his testes begin the process of spermatogenesis. The cells that undergo meiosis in the male are called *spermatocytes*. The primary spermatocyte, which undergoes the first meiotic division, contains the diploid number of chromosomes. The cell has already copied its DNA before division, so four alleles for each gene are present. The cell is still considered diploid because the copies are bound together (i.e., one allele plus its copy on each chromosome).

During the first meiotic division, two haploid secondary spermatocytes are formed. Each secondary spermatocyte contains 22 autosomes and one sex chromosome; one contains the X chromosome (plus its copy), and the other contains the Y chromosome (plus its copy). During the second meiotic division, the male produces two gametes with an X chromosome and two gametes with a Y chromosome, all of which will develop into viable sperm (see Fig. 12.1). When homologous

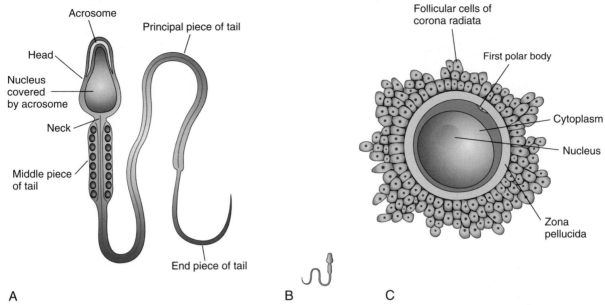

Fig. 12.2 Male and Female Gametes. (A) The parts of a human sperm (×1250). The head, composed mostly of the nucleus, is partly covered by the acrosome, an organelle containing enzymes. (B) A sperm drawn to approximately the same scale as the oocyte. (C) The human secondary oocyte (×200) is surrounded by the zona pellucida and corona radiata. (From Moore, K.L., Persaud, T.V.N., Torchia, M.G. [2016]. *Before we were born: Essentials of embryology and birth defects* [9th ed.]. Philadelphia: Elsevier.)

chromosomes fail to separate during gametogenesis (nondisjunction), some gametes have 24 chromosomes and others have 22. If a gamete with 24 chromosomes unites with a normal gamete with 23 chromosomes, the resulting zygote has 47 chromosomes. This produces a trisomy, as occurs in Down syndrome. When a gamete with 22 chromosomes unites with a normal gamete with 23 chromosomes, a zygote with 45 chromosomes results, producing a monosomy. Abnormal gametogenesis can occur in both sex chromosomes and in autosomes (Moore, Persaud, & Torchia, 2016). (See also Chapter 3.)

Ovum

Meiosis occurs in the female in the ovarian follicles and produces an egg, or ovum. Each month one ovum matures with a host of surrounding supportive cells. At ovulation the ovum is released from the ruptured ovarian follicle. High estrogen levels increase the motility of the uterine tubes so their cilia are able to capture the ovum and propel it through the tube toward the uterine cavity. An ovum cannot move by itself.

Two protective layers surround the ovum (Fig. 12.2). The inner layer is a thick, acellular layer, the *zona pellucida*. The outer layer, the *corona radiata,* is composed of elongated cells.

An ovum is considered fertile for approximately 24 hours after ovulation. If not fertilized by a sperm, the ovum degenerates and is resorbed.

Sperm

Ejaculation during sexual intercourse normally propels approximately 2 to 6 (mean of 3.5) mL of semen containing as many as 100 to 500 million sperm per milliliter, into the vagina. The sperm swim propelled by the flagellar movement of their tails, 2 to 3 mm per minute (Blackburn, 2018). Some sperm can reach the site of fertilization within 5 minutes, but average transit time is 4 to 6 hours. Sperm remain viable within the woman's reproductive system for an average of 2 to 3 days. Most sperm are lost in the vagina, within the cervical mucus, or in the endometrium, or they enter the uterine tube that contains no ovum. Despite the millions of sperm in the ejaculation, only 300 to 500 at a given point in time are found in the uterine (fallopian) tubes (Blackburn).

As the sperm travel through the female reproductive tract, enzymes are produced to aid in their capacitation. *Capacitation* is a physiologic change that removes the protective coating from the heads of the sperm. Small perforations then form in the acrosome (a cap on the sperm) and allow enzymes (e.g., hyaluronidase) to escape (see Fig. 12.2). These enzymes are necessary for the sperm to penetrate the protective layers of the ovum before fertilization.

Fertilization

Fertilization takes place in the ampulla (outer third) of the uterine (fallopian) tube. When a sperm successfully penetrates the membrane surrounding the ovum, both sperm and ovum are enclosed within the membrane, and the membrane becomes impenetrable to other sperm; this process is termed the *zonal reaction.* The second meiotic division of the secondary oocyte is then completed, and the nucleus of the ovum becomes the female pronucleus. The head of the sperm enlarges to become the male pronucleus, and the tail degenerates. The nuclei fuse, and the chromosomes combine, restoring the diploid number (46) (Fig. 12.3). Conception, the formation of the zygote (the first cell of the new unique individual), has been achieved.

Mitotic cellular replication, called *cleavage,* begins within 30 hours after fertilization and ends with the formation of the *blastocyst* (Blackburn, 2018). The zygote remains in the ampulla portion of the uterine tube for the first 24 hours and then is propelled by ciliary action, traveling through the uterine tube into the uterus. This transit takes 3 to 4 days. Because the fertilized egg divides rapidly with no increase in size, successively smaller cells called *blastomeres* are formed with each division. A 16-cell morula, a solid ball of cells, is produced within 3 days and is still surrounded by the protective *zona pellucida* (Fig. 12.4). Further development occurs as the morula floats freely within the uterus. Fluid passes through the zona pellucida into the intercellular spaces between the blastomeres, separating them into two parts, the trophoblast (which gives rise to the placenta) and the embryoblast (which gives rise to the embryo). A cavity forms within the cell mass as the spaces come together, forming a structure called the *blastocyst*

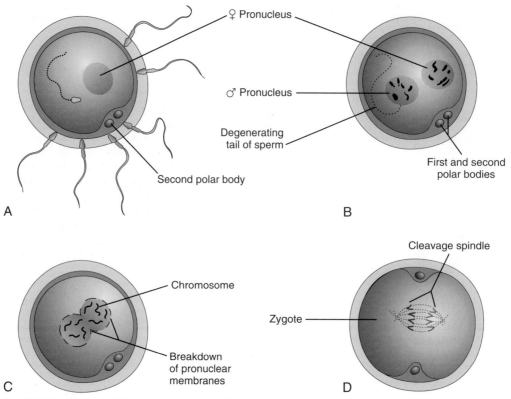

Fig. 12.3 Fertilization. (A) A sperm has entered the oocyte and the second meiotic division has occurred, resulting in the formation of a mature oocyte. The nucleus of the oocyte is now the female pronucleus. (B) The sperm head has enlarged to form the male pronucleus. (C) The pronuclei are fusing. (D) The zygote has formed; it contains 46 chromosomes. (From Moore, K.L., Persaud, T.V.N., Torchia, M.G. [2016]. *Before we were born: Essentials of embryology and birth defects* [9th ed.]. Philadelphia: Elsevier.)

cavity. When the cavity becomes recognizable, the whole structure of the developing embryo is known as the blastocyst. Stem cells are derived from the inner cell mass of the blastocyst. The outer layer of cells surrounding the blastocyst cavity is the trophoblast. The trophoblast differentiates into villous and extravillous trophoblast (Figs. 12.5 and 12.6).

Implantation

The zona pellucida degenerates, the trophoblast cells displace endometrial cells at the implantation site, and the blastocyst embeds in the endometrium, usually in the anterior or posterior fundal region. Between 6 and 10 days after conception, the trophoblast secretes enzymes that enable it to burrow into the endometrium until the entire blastocyst is covered. This is known as implantation. Endometrial blood vessels erode, and some women have slight implantation bleeding (slight spotting or bleeding at the time of the first missed menstrual period). Chorionic villi, fingerlike projections, develop out of the trophoblast and extend into the blood-filled spaces of the endometrium. These villi are vascular processes that obtain oxygen and nutrients from the maternal bloodstream and dispose of carbon dioxide and waste products into the maternal blood.

After implantation the endometrium is called the *decidua.* The portion directly under the blastocyst, where the chorionic villi tap into the maternal blood vessels, is the decidua basalis. The portion covering the blastocyst is the *decidua capsularis,* and the portion lining the rest of the uterus is the *decidua vera* (parietalis) (Fig. 12.7A). The decidua basalis forms the maternal portion of the placenta and stratum where separation of the placenta will occur after birth.

EMBRYO AND FETUS

Pregnancy lasts approximately 10 lunar months, 9 calendar months, 40 weeks, or 280 days. Length of pregnancy is computed from the first day of the last menstrual period (LMP) until the day of birth. However, conception occurs approximately 2 weeks after the first day of the LMP; thus the *postconception age* of the fetus is 2 weeks less, for a total of 266 days, or 38 weeks. Postconception age is used in the discussion of fetal development.

Intrauterine development is divided into three stages: ovum or preembryonic, embryo, and fetus (Fig. 12.8). The stage of the ovum lasts from conception until day 14. This period covers cellular replication, blastocyst formation, initial development of the embryonic membranes, and establishment of the primary germ layers.

Primary Germ Layers

During the third week after conception, the embryonic disk differentiates into three primary germ layers: the ectoderm, the mesoderm, and the endoderm (or entoderm) (see Fig. 12.5). All tissues and organs of the embryo develop from these three layers.

The upper layer of the embryonic disk, the *ectoderm,* gives rise to the epidermis, the glands (anterior pituitary, cutaneous, and mammary), the nails and hair, the central and peripheral nervous systems, the lens of the eye, the tooth enamel, and the floor of the amniotic cavity.

The middle layer, the *mesoderm,* develops into the bones and teeth, the muscles (skeletal, smooth, and cardiac), the dermis and connective tissue, the cardiovascular system and spleen, and the urogenital system.

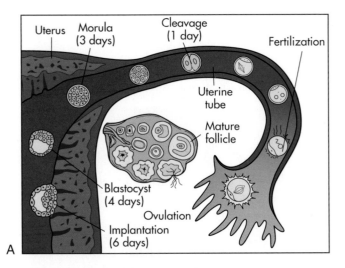

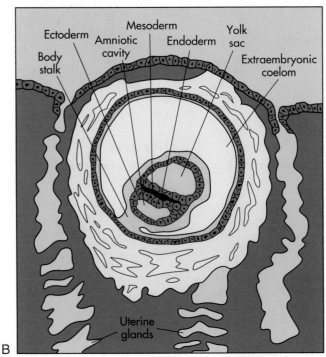

Fig. 12.4 First Weeks of Human Development. A, Follicular development in the ovary, ovulation, fertilization, and transport of the early embryo down the uterine tube and into the uterus, where implantation occurs. B, Blastocyst embedded in endometrium. Germ layers forming. (A, from Carlson, B. [2004]. *Human embryology and developmental biology* (3rd ed.). Philadelphia: Mosby; B, adapted from Langley, L. [1980]. *Dynamic anatomy and physiology.* [5th ed.]. New York: McGraw-Hill.)

The lower layer, the *endoderm,* gives rise to the epithelium lining the respiratory and digestive tracts, and the glandular cells of associated organs, including the oropharynx, the liver and pancreas, the urethra, the bladder, and the vagina. The endoderm forms the roof of the yolk sac.

Development of the Embryo

The stage of the embryo lasts from day 15 until approximately 8 weeks after conception. At the end of this stage the embryo measures approximately 3 cm from crown to rump. This embryonic stage is the period of organogenesis and the most critical time in the development of the organ systems and the main external features. Developing areas with rapid cell division are the most vulnerable to malformation caused by environmental teratogens (substances or exposure that causes abnormal development). At the end of the eighth week, all organ systems and external structures are present, and the embryo is unmistakably human (see Fig. 12.7).

Membranes

At the time of implantation, two fetal membranes that will surround the developing embryo begin to form. The chorion develops from the trophoblast and contains the chorionic villi on its surface. The villi burrow into the decidua basalis and increase in size and complexity as the vascular processes develop into the placenta. The chorion becomes the covering of the fetal side of the placenta. It contains the major umbilical blood vessels as they branch out over the surface of the placenta. As the embryo grows the decidua capsularis stretches. The chorionic villi on this side atrophy and degenerate, leaving a smooth chorionic membrane.

The inner cell membrane, the amnion, develops from the interior cells of the blastocyst. The cavity that develops between this inner cell mass and the outer layer of cells (trophoblast) is the amniotic cavity (see Fig. 12.5A). As it grows larger, the amnion forms on the side opposite the developing blastocyst (see Fig. 12.5B). The developing embryo draws the amnion around itself, forming a fluid-filled sac. The amnion becomes the covering of the umbilical cord and covers the chorion on the fetal surface of the placenta. As the embryo grows larger, the amnion enlarges to accommodate the embryo/fetus and the surrounding amniotic fluid. The amnion eventually comes into contact with the chorion surrounding the fetus.

Amniotic Fluid

During the first trimester of pregnancy the amniotic cavity initially derives its fluid primarily by diffusion from the maternal blood. Beginning in the second trimester, amniotic fluid is regulated by a balance between fetal fluid production (lung liquid and urine) and fluid resorption through fetal swallowing and flow across chorionic and amniotic membranes to the maternal uterus and the fetus. The volume of amniotic fluid increases weekly; there is less than 10 mL by 8 weeks' gestation, increasing to approximately 250 mL by 16 weeks' gestation, and 800 mL by 32 weeks, gestation. The volume remains fairly stable until 39 weeks, when there is 700 to 800 mL of amniotic fluid. The volume steadily decreases after term, with approximately 500 mL at 41 weeks (Ross & Beall, 2019; Ross & Ervin, 2017).

Amniotic fluid serves many functions, including helping to maintain a constant fetal body temperature, serving as a source of oral fluid and a repository for waste, and assisting in maintenance of fluid and electrolyte homeostasis. Amniotic fluid allows the fetus freedom of movement for musculoskeletal development and, with the uterine walls, provides the fetus with resistance to movements while being active. In addition, it cushions the fetus from trauma by outside forces allowing pressure to be distributed from one side to another with minimal exertion on the fetus. The weightless state allows the face and body of the fetus to develop symmetrically. Auditory stimulation is provided by the rhythmic sounds of the blood flow through the umbilical cord, and extrauterine sounds are transmitted in a muted form to the fetus. Amniotic fluid has antibacterial factors, including transferrin, fatty acids, immunoglobulins, and lysozyme, to protect the fetus from infection and, with adequate volume, facilitates normal fetal lung development (Blackburn, 2018). The fluid keeps the embryo from tangling with the membranes, facilitating symmetric growth. If the embryo does become tangled with the membranes, amputations of extremities or other deformities can occur from constricting amniotic bands.

The volume of amniotic fluid is an important factor in assessing fetal well-being throughout pregnancy. Having less than 300 mL of amniotic fluid (oligohydramnios) is associated with fetal renal abnormalities. Having more than 2 L of amniotic fluid (hydramnios or polyhydramnios) is associated with gastrointestinal and other malformations.

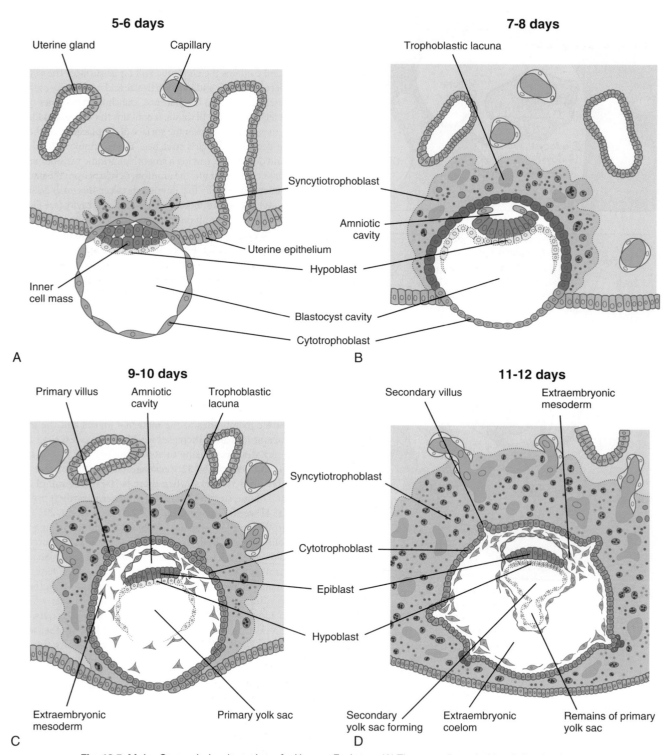

5-6 days

Uterine gland   Capillary

Syncytiotrophoblast

Uterine epithelium

Hypoblast

Inner
cell mass

Blastocyst cavity

Cytotrophoblast

A

7-8 days

Trophoblastic lacuna

Amniotic
cavity

B

9-10 days

Primary villus   Amniotic   Trophoblastic
cavity   lacuna

Syncytiotrophoblast

Cytotrophoblast

Epiblast

Hypoblast

Extraembryonic
mesoderm   Primary yolk sac

C

11-12 days

Secondary villus   Extraembryonic
mesoderm

Secondary   Extraembryonic   Remains of primary
yolk sac forming   coelom   yolk sac

D

Fig. 12.5 Major Stages in Implantation of a Human Embryo. (A) The syncytiotrophoblast is just beginning to invade the endometrial stroma. (B) Most of the embryo is embedded in the endometrium; there is early formation of the trophoblastic lacunae. The amniotic cavity and yolk sac are beginning to form. (C) Implantation is almost complete, primary villi are forming, and the extraembryonic mesoderm is appearing. (D) Implantation is complete; secondary villi are forming. (From Carlson, B.M. [2014]. *Human embryology and developmental biology* [5th ed.]. Philadelphia: Saunders.)

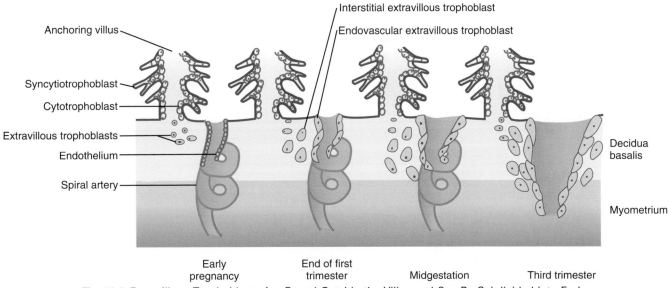

Fig. 12.6 Extravillous Trophoblasts Are Found Outside the Villus and Can Be Subdivided into Endovascular and Interstitial Categories. Endovascular trophoblasts invade and transform spiral arteries during pregnancy to create low-resistance blood flow that is characteristic of the placenta. Interstitial trophoblasts invade the decidua and surround spiral arteries. (From Cunningham, F., Leveno, K., Bloom, S., et al. [2018]. *Williams obstetrics* [25th ed.]. New York: McGraw-Hill.)

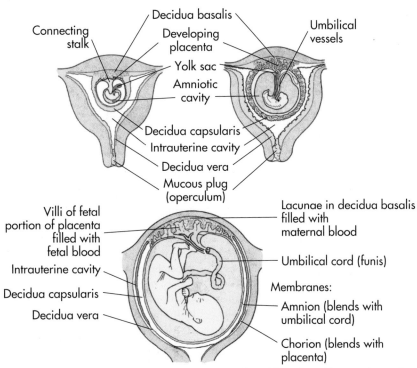

Fig. 12.7 Development of the Fetal Membranes. Note gradual obliteration of intrauterine cavity as decidua capsularis and decidua vera meet. Also note thinning of uterine wall. Chorionic and amniotic membranes are in apposition to each other but may be peeled apart.

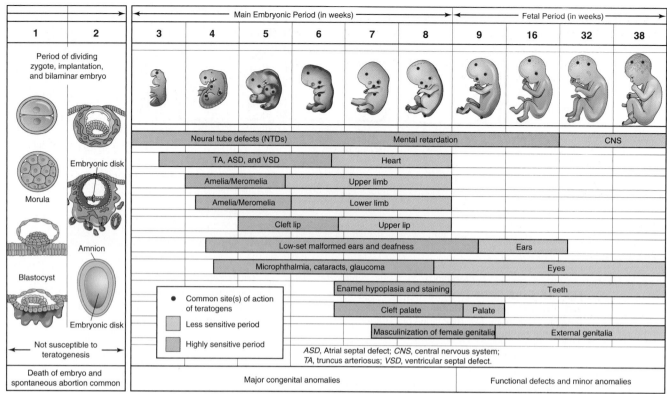

Fig. 12.8 Critical Periods in Human Prenatal Development. During the first 2 weeks, the embryo is not usually susceptible to teratogens. At this point, a teratogen damages all or most of the cells, resulting in death of the embryo, or damages only a few cells, allowing the conceptus to recover and the embryo to develop without birth defects. The purple areas denote highly sensitive periods, when major defects may be produced (e.g., amelia, absence of limbs). The green sections indicate stages that are less sensitive to teratogens, when minor birth defects may be induced. (From Moore, K.L., Persaud, T.V.N., Torchia, M.G. [2016]. *Before we were born: Essentials of embryology and birth defects* [9th ed.]. Philadelphia: Elsevier.)

Amniotic fluid is 98% to 99% water and contains albumin, urea, uric acid, creatinine, lecithin (L), sphingomyelin (S), bilirubin, fructose, fat, leukocytes, proteins, epithelial cells, enzymes, and lanugo hair. Study of fetal cells in amniotic fluid through amniocentesis yields important information about the fetus. Genetic studies (karyotyping) provide information about the sex and the number and structure of chromosomes (see Chapter 3). Other studies, such as the *lecithin/sphingomyelin* (L/S) ratio, determine the health or maturity of the fetus (see Chapter 26).

Yolk Sac

When the amniotic cavity and amnion are forming, another blastocyst cavity forms on the other side of the developing embryonic disk (see Fig. 12.5). This cavity becomes surrounded by a membrane, forming the *yolk sac*. The yolk sac aids in transferring maternal nutrients and oxygen that have diffused through the chorion, to the embryo. Blood vessels form to aid transport. Blood cells and plasma are manufactured in the yolk sac during the second and third weeks while uteroplacental circulation is being established and is forming primitive blood cells until hematopoietic activity begins. At the end of the third week the primitive heart begins to beat and circulate the blood through the embryo, the connecting stalk, the chorion, and the yolk sac.

The folding in of the embryo during the fourth week results in incorporation of part of the yolk sac into the embryo's body as the primitive digestive system. Primordial germ cells arise in the yolk sac and move into the embryo. The shrinking remains of the yolk sac degenerate. By the fifth or sixth week the remnant has separated from the embryo.

Umbilical Cord

By day 14 after conception, the embryonic disk, the amniotic sac, and the yolk sac are attached to the chorionic villi by the connecting stalk. During the third week the blood vessels develop to supply the embryo with maternal nutrients and oxygen. During the fifth week the embryo has curved inward on itself from both ends, bringing the connecting stalk to the ventral side of the embryo. The connecting stalk becomes compressed from both sides by the amnion and forms the narrower umbilical cord (see Fig. 12.7B). Two arteries carry blood from the embryo to the chorionic villi, and one vein returns blood to the embryo. Approximately 1% of umbilical cords contain only two vessels: one artery and one vein. This occurrence is sometimes associated with congenital malformations, specifically fetal cardiovascular, gastrointestinal (esophageal and anal atresia), and urinary tract anomalies (Blackburn, 2018).

The umbilical cord rapidly increases in length. At term the cord length averages from 40 to 70 cm (Cunningham et al., 2018). It spirals on itself and loops around the embryo/fetus. A true knot is rare (see Fig. 18.17), but false knots occur as folds or kinks in the cord and can jeopardize circulation to the fetus. Connective tissue called *Wharton's jelly* surrounds the vessels, preventing compression of the blood vessels and ensuring continued nourishment of the embryo or fetus. Compression can occur if the cord lies between the fetal head and the maternal pelvis or is twisted around the fetal body. When the cord is wrapped around the fetal neck, it is called a **nuchal cord**.

Because the placenta develops from the chorionic villi, the umbilical cord is usually located centrally and blood vessels are arrayed out from the center to all parts of the placenta. Variations of cord insertion into the placenta include *vasa previa* and *battledore* insertion; these increase the risk of fetal hemorrhage (see Chapter 28).

Placenta

Structure

The placenta begins to form at implantation. During the third week after conception the trophoblast cells of the chorionic villi continue to invade the decidua basalis. As the uterine capillaries are tapped, the endometrial spiral arteries fill with maternal blood. The chorionic villi grow into the spaces with two layers of cells: the outer syncytium and the inner cytotrophoblast. A third layer develops into anchoring septa, dividing the projecting decidua into separate areas called cotyledons. In each of the 15 to 20 cotyledons, the chorionic villi branch out, and a complex system of fetal blood vessels forms. Each cotyledon is a functional unit. The whole structure is the placenta (Fig. 12.9).

The maternal-placental-embryonic circulation is in place by day 17, when the embryonic heart starts beating. By the end of the third week, embryonic blood is circulating between the embryo and the chorionic villi. In the intervillous spaces, maternal blood supplies oxygen and nutrients to the embryonic capillaries in the villi (Fig. 12.10). Waste products and carbon dioxide diffuse into the maternal blood.

The placenta functions as a means of metabolic exchange. Exchange is minimal at this time because the two cell layers of the villous membrane are too thick. Permeability increases as the cytotrophoblast thins and disappears; by the fifth month, only the single layer of syncytium is left between the maternal blood and the fetal capillaries. The syncytium is the functional layer of the placenta. By the eighth week, genetic testing can be done on a sample of chorionic villi by aspiration biopsy; however, limb defects have been associated with chorionic villus sampling before 10 weeks. The structure of the placenta is complete by the 12th week. The placenta continues to grow wider until 20 weeks, when it covers approximately half of the uterine surface. It then continues to grow thicker. The branching villi continue to develop within the body of the placenta, increasing the functional surface area.

Functions

Endocrine gland function. One of the early functions of the placenta is as an endocrine gland that produces four hormones necessary to maintain the pregnancy and support the embryo and fetus. The hormones are produced in the syncytium.

The protein hormone human chorionic gonadotropin (hCG) can be detected in the maternal serum by 8 to 10 days after conception, shortly after implantation. This hormone is the basis for pregnancy tests (Chapter 13). The hCG preserves the function of the ovarian corpus luteum, ensuring the continued supply of estrogen and progesterone needed to maintain the pregnancy. Miscarriage occurs if the corpus luteum stops functioning before the placenta is producing sufficient estrogen and progesterone. The hCG reaches its maximum level at 60 to 70 days and then decreases to lowest levels at approximately 100 to 130 days as the placenta becomes the primary source of estrogen and progesterone (Liu, 2019).

The other protein hormone produced by the placenta is human placental lactogen (hPL), also known as chorionic somatotropin. This substance is similar to a growth hormone and stimulates the maternal metabolism to supply nutrients needed for fetal growth. hPL increases the resistance to insulin, facilitates glucose transport across the placental membrane, and stimulates breast development to prepare for lactation (Burton, Sibley, & Jauniaux, 2017) (Fig. 12.11).

During early pregnancy, progesterone is produced by the corpus luteum. As the placenta grows it gradually becomes the primary source

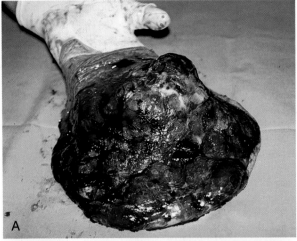

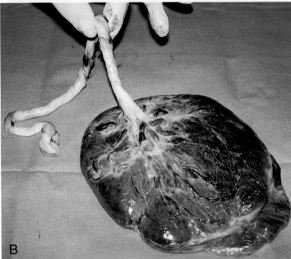

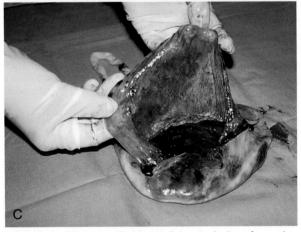

Fig. 12.9 Term Placenta. (A) Maternal (or uterine) surface, showing cotyledons and grooves. (B) Fetal (or amniotic) surface, showing blood vessels running under amnion and converging to form umbilical vessels at attachment of umbilical cord. (C) Amnion and smooth chorion are arranged to show that they are (1) fused and (2) continuous with margins of placenta. (Courtesy Marjorie Pyle, RNC, Lifecircle, Costa Mesa, CA.)

of this hormone. By 9 weeks, the corpus luteum regresses and no longer is needed to support the pregnancy (Burton, Sibley, & Jauniaux, et al., 2017). Progesterone maintains the endometrium, decreases the contractility of the uterus, and stimulates maternal metabolism and development of breast alveoli.

By 7 weeks of pregnancy the placenta is producing most of the maternal estrogens, which are steroid hormones. The major estrogen secreted by the placenta is estriol, whereas the ovaries produce mostly estradiol (Cunningham et al., 2018). Estriol levels may be measured to determine placental functioning. Estrogen stimulates uterine growth and uteroplacental blood flow. It causes a proliferation of the breast glandular tissue and stimulates myometrial contractility. Placental estrogen production increases greatly toward the end of pregnancy. One theory for the cause of the onset of labor is the decline in the ratio of circulating levels of progesterone to the increased levels of estrogen (Fig. 12.12).

Metabolic functions. The metabolic functions of the placenta are respiration, nutrition, excretion, and storage. Oxygen diffuses from the maternal blood across the placental membrane into the fetal blood, and carbon dioxide diffuses in the opposite direction. In this way the placenta functions as lungs for the fetus.

Carbohydrates, proteins, calcium, and iron are stored in the placenta for ready access to meet fetal needs. Water, inorganic salts, carbohydrates, proteins, fats, and vitamins pass from the maternal blood supply across the placental membrane into the fetal blood, supplying nutrition. Water and most

electrolytes with a molecular weight less than 500 readily diffuse through the membrane. Hydrostatic and osmotic pressures aid in the flow of water and some solutions. Facilitated diffusion and active transport assist in the transfer of glucose, amino acids, calcium, iron, and substances with higher molecular weights. Amino acids and calcium are transported against the concentration gradient between the maternal blood and fetal blood.

The fetal concentration of glucose is lower than the glucose level in the maternal blood because of its rapid metabolism by the fetus. Fetal demand for glucose is high, and it is transported from mother to fetus by facilitated diffusion.

Pinocytosis is a mechanism used for transferring large molecules, such as albumin and gamma globulins, across the placental membrane. This mechanism conveys the maternal immunoglobulins that provide early passive immunity to the fetus.

Metabolic waste products of the fetus cross the placental membrane from the fetal blood into the maternal blood for excretion by the maternal kidneys. Many viruses can cross the placental membrane and infect the fetus. Some bacteria and protozoa first infect the placenta and then the fetus (Box 12.1). The majority of medications cross the placenta through passive diffusion. Substances such as caffeine; alcohol; nicotine, carbon monoxide, and other toxic substances in cigarette smoke; and prescription and recreational drugs can cross the placental membrane and harm the fetus (see Box 12.1).

Although no direct link exists between the fetal blood in the vessels of the chorionic villi and the maternal blood in the intervillous spaces, only one cell layer separates the maternal and fetal blood. Breaks occasionally occur in the placental membrane. Fetal erythrocytes then leak into the maternal circulation, and the mother may develop antibodies to the fetal red blood cells, resulting in *isoimmunization*. This is what occurs when an Rh-negative mother becomes sensitized to the erythrocytes of her Rh-positive fetus (see Chapters 21 and 36).

Although the placenta and the fetus are analogous to living tissue transplants, they are not destroyed by the host mother (Mor & Abrahams, 2014). Either the placental hormones suppress the immunologic response or the tissue evokes no response.

Circulatory effects on placental function. Placental function depends on the maternal blood pressure supplying circulation. Maternal arterial blood, under pressure in the small uterine spiral arteries, spurts into the intervillous spaces (see Fig. 12.10). As long as rich arterial blood continues to be supplied, pressure is exerted on the blood already in the intervillous spaces, pushing it toward drainage by the low-pressure uterine veins. At term gestation, 10% of the maternal cardiac output goes to the uterus.

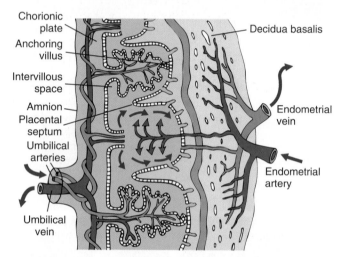

Fig. 12.10 Schematic Drawing of the Placenta Ilustrates How It Supplies Oxygen and Nutrition to the Embryo/Fetus and Removes Its Waste Products. Deoxygenated blood leaves the fetus through the umbilical arteries and enters the placenta, where it is oxygenated. Oxygenated blood leaves the placenta through the umbilical vein, which enters the fetus via the umbilical cord.

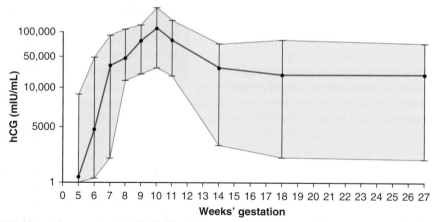

Fig. 12.11 Mean Concentration (95% CI) of Human Chorionic Gonadotropin (hCG) in Serum of Women Throughout Normal Pregnancy. (From Cunningham, F., Leveno, K., Bloom, S., et al. [2018]. *Williams obstetrics* [25th ed.]. New York: McGraw-Hill.)

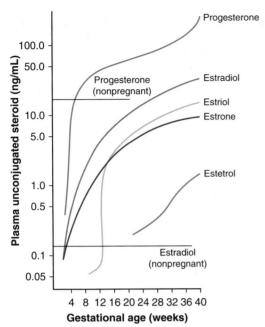

Fig. 12.12 Plasma Levels of Progesterone, Estradiol, Estrone, Estetrol, and Estriol in Women During the Course of Gestation. (From Cunningham, F., Leveno, K., Bloom, S., et al. [2018]. *Williams obstetrics* [25th ed.]. New York: McGraw-Hill.)

If there is interference with the circulation to the placenta, it is not adequately perfused and the placenta cannot supply the embryo or fetus. Vasoconstriction, such as that caused by hypertension and cocaine use, diminishes uterine blood flow. Decreased maternal blood pressure or cardiac output also diminishes uterine blood flow.

When a woman lies on her back with the pressure of the uterus compressing the vena cava, blood return to the right atrium is diminished (see discussion of supine hypotension in Chapter 19 and Fig. 19.6). Excessive maternal exercise that diverts blood to the muscles away from the uterus compromises placental circulation. Optimal circulation is achieved when the woman is lying at rest on her side. Decreased uterine circulation can lead to intrauterine growth restriction of the fetus and to infants who are small for gestational age.

Braxton Hicks contractions, painless contractions that occur intermittently after the first trimester, appear to enhance the movement of blood through the intervillous spaces, aiding placental circulation. However, prolonged contractions or too-short intervals between contractions during labor reduce blood flow to the placenta.

Fetal Maturation

The stage of the fetus lasts from 9 weeks (when the fetus becomes recognizable as a human being) until the pregnancy ends. Changes during the fetal period are not so dramatic, because refinement of structure and function is taking place. The fetus is less vulnerable to teratogens, except for those affecting functioning of the central nervous system (CNS).

Viability refers to the capability of the fetus to survive outside the uterus and is usually defined by fetal weight and pregnancy duration for statistical and legal purposes. A standard definition is 20 weeks' gestation and birth weight of 350, 400, or 500 g, but this varies by state. Nurses must be aware of the laws in their states. With modern technology and advancements in maternal and neonatal care, infants who are 22 to 25 weeks of gestation are on the threshold of viability (Cunningham, Leveno, Bloom, et al., 2018). The limitations on survival outside the uterus when an infant is born at this early stage are based on CNS function and the oxygenation capability of the lungs.

Table 12.1 summarizes embryonic and fetal development.

BOX 12.1   Chemical Teratogens During Embryonic and Fetal Development

Agent	Effects
Alcohol	Growth restriction, cognitive impairment, microcephaly, various malformations of face and trunk
Androgens	Masculinization of females, accelerated genital development in males
Anticoagulants (warfarin, dicumarol)	Skeletal abnormalities; broad hands with short fingers; nasal hypoplasia; anomalies of eye, neck, central nervous system
Antithyroid drugs (e.g., propylthiouracil, iodide)	Fetal goiter, hypothyroidism
Chemotherapeutic agents (methotrexate, aminopterin)	Variety of major anomalies throughout body
Cocaine	Cardiac and central nervous system anomalies, growth restriction
Diethylstilbestrol	Cervical and uterine abnormalities
Lead	Cognitive impairment, hearing deficits, growth restriction
Lithium	Heart anomalies
Organic mercury	Cognitive impairment, cerebral atrophy, spasticity, blindness
Phenytoin (Dilantin)	Cognitive impairment, poor growth, microcephaly, dysmorphic face, hypoplasia of digits and nails
Isotretinoin (Accutane)	Craniofacial defects, cleft palate, ear and eye deformities, nervous system defects
Streptomycin	Hearing loss, auditory nerve damage
Tetracycline	Hypoplasia and staining of tooth enamel, staining of bones
Thalidomide	Limb defects, ear defects, cardiovascular anomalies
Trimethadione and paramethadione	Cleft lip and palate, microcephaly, eye defects, cardiac defects, cognitive impairment
Valproic acid	Neural tube defects

Modified from Carlson, B.M. (2014). *Human embryology and developmental biology* (5th ed.). Philadelphia: Saunders.

Fetal Circulatory System

The cardiovascular system is the first organ system to function in the developing human. Blood vessel and blood cell formation begins in the third week and supplies the embryo with oxygen and nutrients from the mother. By the end of the third week the tubular heart begins to beat, and the primitive cardiovascular system links the embryo, connecting stalk, chorion, and yolk sac. During the fourth and fifth weeks the heart develops into a four-chambered organ. By the end of the embryonic stage, the heart is developmentally complete.

The fetal lungs do not function for respiratory gas exchange, so a special circulatory pathway, the ductus arteriosus, bypasses the lungs. Oxygen-rich blood from the placenta flows rapidly through the umbilical vein into the fetal abdomen (Fig. 12.13). When the umbilical vein reaches the liver, it divides into two branches; one branch circulates some oxygenated blood through the liver. Most of the blood passes through the ductus venosus into the inferior vena cava. There it mixes with the deoxygenated blood from the fetal legs and abdomen on its way to the right atrium. Most of this blood passes straight through the right atrium and through the foramen ovale, an opening into the left atrium. There it mixes with the deoxygenated blood returning from the fetal lungs through the pulmonary veins.

TABLE 12.1 Developmental Events During Embryonic and Fetal Periods

4 Weeks	8 Weeks	12 Weeks
External Appearance		
Body flexed, C-shaped; arm and leg buds present; head at right angles to body	Body fairly well formed; nose flat, eyes far apart; digits well formed; head elevating; tail almost disappeared; eyes, ears, nose, and mouth recognizable	Nails appearing; resembles a human; head erect but disproportionately large; skin pink, delicate
	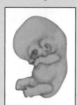	
Crown-to-Rump Measurement; Weight		
0.4–0.5 cm; 0.4 g	2.5–3 cm; 2 g	6–9 cm; 19 g
Gastrointestinal System		
Stomach at midline and fusiform; conspicuous liver; esophagus short; intestine a short tube	Intestinal villi developing; small intestines coil within umbilical cord; palatal folds present; liver very large	Bile secreted; palatal fusion complete; intestines have withdrawn from cord and assume characteristic positions
Musculoskeletal System		
All somites present	First indication of ossification—occiput, mandible, and humerus; fetus capable of some movement; definitive muscles of trunk, limbs, and head well represented	Some bones well outlined, ossification spreading; upper cervical to lower sacral arches and bodies ossify; smooth muscle layers indicated in hollow viscera
Circulatory System		
Heart develops, double chambers visible, begins to beat; aortic arch and major veins completed	Main blood vessels assume final plan; enucleated red cells predominate in blood	Blood forming in marrow
Respiratory System		
Primary lung buds appear	Pleural and pericardial cavities forming; branching bronchioles; nostrils closed by epithelial plugs	Lungs acquire definite shape; vocal cords appear
Renal System		
Rudimentary ureteral buds appear	Earliest secretory tubules differentiating; bladder-urethra separates from rectum	Kidney able to secrete urine; bladder expands as a sac
Nervous System		
Well-marked midbrain flexure; no hindbrain or cervical flexures; neural groove closed	Cerebral cortex begins to acquire typical cells; differentiation of cerebral cortex, meninges, ventricular foramina, cerebrospinal fluid circulation; spinal cord extends entire length of spine	Brain structural configuration almost complete; cord shows cervical and lumbar enlargements; fourth ventricle foramina are developed; sucking present
Sensory Organs		
Eye and ear appearing as optic vessel and otocyst	Primordial choroid plexuses develop; ventricles large relative to cortex; development progressing; eyes converging rapidly; internal ear developing; eyelids fuse	Earliest taste buds indicated; characteristic organization of eye attained
Genital System		
Genital ridge appears (fifth week)	Testes and ovaries distinguishable; external genitalia sexless but begin to differentiate	Sex recognizable; internal and external sex organs specific

TABLE 12.1 Developmental Events During Embryonic and Fetal Periods—cont'd

16 Weeks	20 Weeks	24 Weeks
External Appearance		
Head still dominant; face looks human; eyes, ears, and nose approach typical appearance on gross examination; arm/leg ratio proportionate; scalp hair appears	Vernix caseosa appears; lanugo appears; legs lengthen considerably; sebaceous glands appear	Body lean but fairly well proportioned; skin red and wrinkled; vernix caseosa present; sweat glands forming
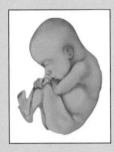	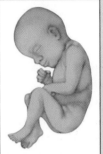	
Crown-to-Rump Measurement; Weight		
11.5–13.5 cm; 100 g	16–18.5 cm; 300 g	23 cm; 600 g
Gastrointestinal System		
Meconium in bowel; some enzyme secretion; anus open	Enamel and dentine depositing; ascending colon recognizable	
Musculoskeletal System		
Most bones distinctly indicated throughout body; joint cavities appear; muscular movements can be detected	Sternum ossifies; fetal movements strong enough for mother to feel	
Circulatory System		
Heart muscle well developed; blood formation active in spleen		Blood formation increases in bone marrow and decreases in liver
Respiratory System		
Elastic fibers appear in lungs; terminal and respiratory bronchioles appear	Nostrils reopen; primitive respiratory-like movements begin	Alveolar ducts and sacs present; lecithin begins to appear in amniotic fluid (weeks 26-27)
Renal System		
Kidney in position; attains typical shape and plan		
Nervous System		
Cerebral lobes delineated; cerebellum assumes some prominence	Brain grossly formed; cord myelination begins; spinal cord ends at level of first sacral vertebra (S1)	Cerebral cortex layered typically; neuronal proliferation in cerebral cortex ends
Sensory Organs		
General sense organs differentiated	Nose and ears ossify	Can hear
Genital System		
Testes in position for descent into scrotum: vagina open		Testes at inguinal ring in descent to scrotum

continued

TABLE 12.1   **Developmental Events During Embryonic and Fetal Periods—cont'd**

28 Weeks	30-31 Weeks	36-40 Weeks
External Appearance		
Lean body, less wrinkled and red; nails appear	Subcutaneous fat beginning to collect; more rounded appearance; skin pink and smooth; has assumed birth position	36 weeks: Skin pink, body rounded; general lanugo disappearing; body usually plump
		40 weeks: Skin smooth and pink; scant vernix caseosa; moderate to profuse hair; lanugo on shoulders and upper body only; nasal and alar cartilage apparent
Crown-to-Rump Measurement; Weight		
27 cm; 1100 g	31 cm; 1800–2100 g	36 weeks: 35 cm; 2200–2900 g; 40 weeks: 40 cm; 3200+ g
Musculoskeletal System		
Astragalus (talus, ankle bone) ossifies; weak, fleeting movements, minimum tone	Middle fourth phalanges ossify; permanent teeth primordia seen; can turn head to side	36 weeks: Distal femoral ossification centers present; sustained, definite movements; fair tone; can turn and elevate head
		40 weeks: Active, sustained movement; good tone; may lift head
Respiratory System		
Lecithin forming on alveolar surfaces	Lecithin/sphingomyelin (L/S) ratio = 1.2:1	36 weeks: lecithin/sphingomyelin (L/S) ratio > 2:1
		40 weeks: Pulmonary branching only two-thirds complete
Renal System		
		36 weeks: Formation of new nephrons ceases
Nervous System		
Appearance of cerebral fissures, convolutions rapidly appearing; indefinite sleep-wake cycle; cry weak or absent; weak suck reflex		36 weeks: End of spinal cord at level of third lumbar vertebra (L3); definite sleep-wake cycle
		40 weeks: Myelination of brain begins; patterned sleep-wake cycle with alert periods; strong suck reflex
Sensory Organs		
Eyelids reopen; retinal layers completed, light-receptive; pupils capable of reacting to light	Sense of taste present; aware of sounds outside mother's body	
Genital System		
	Testes descending to scrotum	40 weeks: Testes in scrotum; labia majora well developed

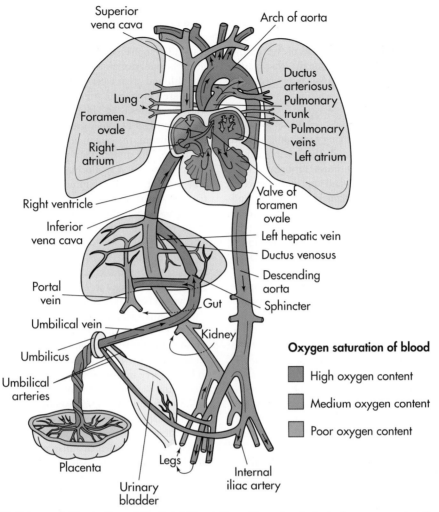

Fig. 12.13 Schematic Illustration of the Fetal Circulation. The colors indicate the oxygen saturation of the blood, and the *arrows* show the course of the blood from the placenta to the heart. The organs are not drawn to scale. A small amount of highly oxygenated blood from the inferior vena cava remains in the right atrium and mixes with poorly oxygenated blood from the superior vena cava. The medium-oxygenated blood then passes into the right ventricle. Observe that three shunts permit most of the blood to bypass the liver and lungs: (1) ductus venosus, (2) oval foramen, and (3) ductus arteriosus. The poorly oxygenated blood returns to the placenta for oxygen and nutrients through the umbilical arteries. (From Moore, K.L., Persaud, T.V.N., Torchia, M.G. [2016]. *Before we were born: Essentials of embryology and birth defects* [9th ed.]. Philadelphia: Elsevier.)

The blood flows into the left ventricle and is squeezed out into the aorta, where the arteries supplying the heart, head, neck, and arms receive most of the oxygen-rich blood. This pattern of supplying the highest levels of oxygen and nutrients to the head, neck, and arms enhances the *cephalocaudal* (head-to-rump) development of the embryo/fetus. Deoxygenated blood returning from the head and arms enters the right atrium through the superior vena cava. This blood is directed downward into the right ventricle, where it is squeezed into the pulmonary artery. A small amount of blood circulates through the resistant lung tissue, but the majority follows the path with less resistance through the ductus arteriosus into the aorta, distal to the point of exit of the arteries supplying the head and arms with oxygenated blood. The oxygen-poor blood flows through the abdominal aorta into the internal iliac arteries, where the umbilical arteries direct most of it back through the umbilical cord to the placenta. There the blood gives up its wastes and carbon dioxide in exchange for nutrients and oxygen. The blood remaining in the iliac arteries flows through the fetal abdomen and legs, ultimately returning through the inferior vena cava to the heart.

The following three special characteristics enable the fetus to obtain sufficient oxygen from the maternal blood:
- Fetal hemoglobin has a high affinity for oxygen and carries 20% to 30% more oxygen than maternal hemoglobin.
- The hemoglobin concentration of the fetus is approximately 50% greater than that of the mother.
- The fetal heart rate is 110 to 160 beats/min, making the cardiac output per unit of body weight higher than that of an adult.

Hematopoietic System

Hematopoiesis, the formation of blood, occurs in the yolk sac (see Fig. 12.1) beginning in the third week. Hematopoietic stem cells seed the fetal liver during the fifth week, and hematopoiesis begins there during the sixth week. This accounts for the relatively large size of the liver between the seventh and ninth weeks.

Stem cells seed the fetal bone marrow, spleen, thymus, and lymph nodes between weeks 8 and 11 (for more information about stem cells, see http://stemcells.nih.gov).

The antigenic factors that determine blood type are present in the erythrocytes soon after the sixth week. For this reason the Rh-negative woman is at risk for isoimmunization in any pregnancy that lasts longer than 6 weeks after fertilization.

Respiratory System

The respiratory system begins development during embryonic life and continues through fetal stages and into childhood. The development of the respiratory tract begins in week 4 and continues through week 17 with formation of the larynx, trachea, bronchi, and lung buds. Between 16 and 24 weeks the bronchi and terminal bronchioles enlarge, and vascular structures and primitive alveoli are formed. Between 24 weeks and term gestation, more alveoli form. Specialized alveolar cells, type I and type II cells, secrete pulmonary surfactants to line the interior of the alveoli. After 32 weeks, sufficient surfactant is present in developed alveoli to provide infants with a good chance of survival.

Pulmonary surfactants. The detection of the presence of pulmonary surfactants, surface-active phospholipids, in amniotic fluid is used to determine the degree of fetal lung maturity, or the ability of the lungs to function after birth. Lecithin is the most critical alveolar surfactant required for postnatal lung expansion. It is detectable at approximately 21 weeks and increases in amount after week 24. Another pulmonary phospholipid, sphingomyelin, remains constant in amount. Thus the measure of lecithin in relation to sphingomyelin, or the L/S ratio, is used to determine fetal lung maturity. When the L/S ratio reaches 2:1, the infant's lungs are considered to be mature. This occurs approximately in the middle of the third trimester (Mercer, 2019).

Certain maternal conditions that cause decreased maternal placental blood flow, such as maternal hypertension, placental dysfunction, infection, or corticosteroid use, can accelerate fetal lung maturity. This apparently is caused by the resulting fetal hypoxia, which stresses the fetus and increases the blood levels of corticosteroids that accelerate alveolar and surfactant development.

Conditions such as gestational diabetes and chronic glomerulonephritis can inhibit fetal lung maturity. Using intrabronchial synthetic surfactant to treat respiratory distress syndrome in the newborn has greatly improved the chances of preterm infant survival (see Chapter 34).

Fetal respiratory movements have been seen on ultrasound examination as early as week 11. These fetal respiratory movements can aid in development of the chest wall muscles and regulate lung fluid volume. The fetal lungs produce fluid that expands the air spaces in the lungs. The fluid drains into the amniotic fluid or is swallowed by the fetus.

Shortly before birth, secretion of lung fluid decreases. The lung fluid clearance at birth was originally attributed to the thoracic compression during vaginal delivery; current thinking is that the activity of clearing liquid from the lungs at birth is attributed to a complex process that begins well in advance of term birth. During labor, the lung fluid decreases and after birth, the remaining lung fluid is reabsorbed into the infant's bloodstream within a few hours. Neonates born by scheduled cesarean birth before 39 weeks' gestation without labor have an increased risk of transient tachypnea of the newborn and are likely to have crackles in their lungs for the first 24 to 48 hours (Plosa & Guttentag, 2018).

Gastrointestinal System

During the fourth week the shape of the embryo changes from being almost straight to a C shape, as both ends fold in toward the ventral surface. A portion of the yolk sac is incorporated into the body from head to tail as the primitive gut (digestive system).

The foregut produces the pharynx, part of the lower respiratory tract, the esophagus, the stomach, the first half of the duodenum, the liver, the pancreas, and the gallbladder. These structures evolve during the fifth and sixth weeks. The malformations that can occur in these areas are esophageal atresia, hypertrophic pyloric stenosis, duodenal stenosis or atresia, and biliary atresia (see Chapter 36).

The midgut becomes the distal half of the duodenum, the jejunum and the ileum, the cecum and the appendix, and the proximal half of the colon. The midgut loop projects into the umbilical cord between weeks 5 and 10. A malformation (omphalocele) results if the midgut fails to return to the abdominal cavity, causing the intestines to protrude from the umbilicus (see Fig. 36.8A). Meckel diverticulum is the most common malformation of the midgut. It occurs when a remnant of the yolk stalk that failed to degenerate attaches to the ileum, leaving a blind sac.

The hindgut develops into the distal half of the colon, the rectum and parts of the anal canal, the urinary bladder, and the urethra. Anorectal malformations are the most common abnormalities of the digestive system (see Chapter 36).

The fetus swallows amniotic fluid beginning in the fifth month. Gastric emptying and intestinal peristalsis occur. Fetal nutrition and elimination needs are taken care of by the placenta. As the fetus nears term, fetal waste products accumulate in the intestines as dark green to black, tarry meconium. Normally this substance is passed through the rectum within 24 hours of birth. Sometimes with a breech presentation or fetal hypoxia, meconium is passed in utero into the amniotic fluid. The failure to pass meconium after birth can indicate atresia somewhere in the digestive tract, an imperforate anus (see Fig. 36.9), or meconium ileus, in which a firm meconium plug blocks passage (seen in infants with cystic fibrosis).

The metabolic rate of the fetus is relatively low, but the fetus has great growth and development needs. Beginning in week 9 the fetus synthesizes glycogen for storage in the liver. Between 26 and 30 weeks the fetus begins to lay down stores of brown fat in preparation for extrauterine cold stress. Thermoregulation in the neonate requires increased metabolism and adequate oxygenation (see Chapter 23).

The gastrointestinal system is mature by 36 weeks. Digestive enzymes (except pancreatic amylase and lipase) are present in sufficient quantity to facilitate digestion.

Hepatic System

The liver and biliary tract develop from the foregut during the fourth week of gestation. The embryonic liver is prominent, occupying most of the abdominal cavity. Bile, a constituent of meconium, begins to form in the 12th week.

Glycogen is stored in the fetal liver beginning at week 9 or 10. At term, glycogen stores are twice those of the adult. Glycogen is the major source of energy for the fetus and neonate stressed by intrauterine hypoxia, extrauterine loss of the maternal glucose supply, the work of breathing, or cold.

Iron also is stored in the fetal liver. If the maternal intake is sufficient, the fetus can store enough iron to last 5 months after birth.

During fetal life the liver does not have to conjugate bilirubin for excretion because the unconjugated bilirubin is cleared by the placenta. Therefore the glucuronyl transferase enzyme needed for conjugation is present in the fetal liver in amounts less than those required after birth. This predisposes the neonate, especially the preterm infant, to hyperbilirubinemia (see Chapter 23).

Coagulation factors II, VII, IX, and X cannot be synthesized in the fetal liver because of the lack of vitamin K synthesis in the sterile fetal gut. This coagulation deficiency persists after birth for several days and is the rationale for the prophylactic administration of vitamin K to the newborn (see Chapter 24).

Renal System

The kidneys form during the fifth week and begin to function approximately 4 weeks later. Urine is excreted into the amniotic fluid and forms a major part of the amniotic fluid volume. Oligohydramnios is indicative of renal dysfunction. Because the placenta acts as the organ of excretion and maintains fetal water and electrolyte balance, the fetus does not need functioning kidneys while in utero. However, at birth, the kidneys are required immediately for excretory and acid-base regulatory functions.

A fetal renal malformation can be diagnosed in utero. Corrective or palliative fetal surgery may treat the malformation successfully, or plans can be made for treatment immediately after birth.

At term the fetus has fully developed kidneys. However, the glomerular filtration rate (GFR) is low, and the kidneys lack the ability to concentrate urine. This makes the newborn more susceptible to both overhydration and dehydration.

Most newborns void within 24 hours of birth. With the loss of the swallowed amniotic fluid and the metabolism of nutrients provided by the placenta, the amount voided for the first days of life is scanty until fluid intake increases.

Neurologic System

The nervous system originates from the ectoderm during the third week after fertilization. The open neural tube forms during the fourth week. It initially closes at what will be the junction of the brain and spinal cord, leaving both ends open. The embryo folds in on itself lengthwise at this time, forming a head fold in the neural tube at this junction. The cranial end of the neural tube closes, and then the caudal end closes. During week 5, different growth rates cause more flexures in the neural tube, delineating three brain areas: the forebrain, midbrain, and hindbrain.

The forebrain develops into the eyes (cranial nerve II) and the cerebral hemispheres. The development of all areas of the cerebral cortex continues throughout fetal life and into childhood. The olfactory system (cranial nerve I) and the thalamus also develop from the forebrain. Cranial nerves III and IV (oculomotor and trochlear) form from the midbrain. The hindbrain forms the medulla, the pons, the cerebellum, and the remainder of the cranial nerves. Brain waves can be recorded on an electroencephalogram by week 8.

The spinal cord develops from the long end of the neural tube. Another ectodermal structure, the neural crest, develops into the peripheral nervous system. By the eighth week, nerve fibers traverse throughout the body. At term the fetal brain is approximately one-fourth the size of an adult brain. Neurologic development continues. Stressors on the fetus and neonate (e.g., chronic poor nutrition or hypoxia, drugs, environmental toxins, trauma, disease) cause damage to the CNS long after the vulnerable embryonic time for malformations in other organ systems. Neurologic insult can result in cerebral palsy, neuromuscular impairment, intellectual disability, and learning disabilities.

Sensory awareness. Purposeful movements of the fetus have been demonstrated in response to a firm touch transmitted through the mother's abdomen. Because the fetus can feel pressure and pain, anesthesia is required for invasive procedures.

Fetuses respond to sound by 24 weeks. Different types of music evoke different movements. The fetus can be soothed by the sound of the mother's voice. Acoustic stimulation can be used to evoke a fetal heart rate response. The fetus becomes accustomed (i.e., habituates) to noises heard repeatedly. Hearing is fully developed at birth.

By 16 weeks, taste receptors are present and they increase to adult numbers by term gestation. The fetus swallows amniotic fluid, which varies in composition; flavors from the maternal diet are transferred to the fetus through amniotic fluid. By the fifth month, when the fetus is swallowing amniotic fluid, a sweetener added to the fluid causes the fetus to swallow faster, whereas a bitter substance results in decreased swallowing (Blackburn, 2018). The fetus also reacts to temperature changes. A cold solution placed into the amniotic fluid can cause fetal hiccups.

Eyelids are fused until 24 to 26 weeks, at which time the fetus can see. Eyes have both rods and cones in the retina by the seventh month. A bright light shone on the mother's abdomen in late pregnancy causes abrupt fetal movements. During sleep time, rapid eye movements have been observed similar to those occurring in children and adults while dreaming.

Endocrine System

The thyroid gland develops, along with structures in the head and neck, during the third and fourth weeks. The secretion of thyroxine begins during the eighth week. Maternal thyroxine does not readily cross the placenta; therefore the fetus who does not produce thyroid hormones will be born with congenital hypothyroidism. If untreated, hypothyroidism can result in severe intellectual disability. Hypothyroidism is included in routine newborn screening after birth (see Chapter 24).

The adrenal cortex is formed during the sixth week and produces hormones by the eighth or ninth week. As term approaches, the fetus produces more cortisol. This is believed to aid in initiation of labor by decreasing the maternal progesterone and stimulating production of prostaglandins.

The pancreas forms from the foregut during the fifth through eighth weeks. The islets of Langerhans develop during the 12th week. Insulin is produced by week 20. In fetuses of mothers with uncontrolled diabetes, maternal hyperglycemia produces fetal hyperglycemia, stimulating hyperinsulinemia and islet cell hyperplasia. This results in a macrosomic (large) fetus. The hyperinsulinemia also blocks lung maturation, placing the neonate at risk for respiratory distress (see Chapter 34) and hypoglycemia when the maternal glucose source is lost at birth (see Chapters 23 and 29). Control of the maternal glucose level before and during pregnancy minimizes problems for the fetus and infant.

Reproductive System

Sex differentiation begins in the embryo during the seventh week. Distinguishing characteristics of female and male genitalia appear around 9th week and are fully differentiated by the 12th week. When a Y chromosome is present, testes are formed. By the end of the embryonic period, testosterone is being secreted and causes formation of the male genitalia. By week 28 the testes begin descending into the scrotum. After birth, low levels of testosterone continue to be secreted until the pubertal surge.

The female, with two X chromosomes, forms ovaries and female external genitalia. By the 16th week, oogenesis has been established. At birth the ovaries contain the female's lifetime supply of ova. Most female hormone production is delayed until puberty. However, the fetal endometrium responds to maternal hormones, and withdrawal bleeding or vaginal discharge (*pseudomenstruation*) can occur at birth when these hormones are lost. The high level of maternal estrogen also stimulates mammary engorgement and secretion of fluid ("witch's milk") in newborn infants of both sexes.

Musculoskeletal System

Bones and muscles develop from the mesoderm by the fourth week of embryonic development. At that time the cardiac muscle is already beating. The mesoderm next to the neural tube forms the vertebral column and ribs. The parts of the vertebral column grow toward each other to enclose the developing spinal cord. Ossification, or bone formation, begins. If there is a defect in the bony fusion, various forms of spina bifida can occur (see Chapter 36). A large defect affecting several vertebrae may allow the membranes and spinal cord to pouch out from the back, producing neurologic deficits and skeletal deformity.

The flat bones of the skull develop during the embryonic period, and ossification continues throughout childhood. At birth, connective tissue sutures exist where the bones of the skull meet.

The areas where more than two bones meet (called *fontanels*) are especially prominent. The sutures and fontanels allow the bones of the skull to mold, or move during birth, enabling the head to pass through the birth canal (see Fig 23.14).

The bones of the shoulders, arms, hips, and legs appear in the sixth week as a continuous skeleton with no joints. Differentiation occurs, producing separate bones and joints. Ossification continues through childhood to allow growth. Beginning in the seventh week, muscles contract spontaneously. By week 11 or 12 the fetus makes respiratory movements, moves all extremities, and changes position in utero. The fetus can suck his or her thumb and swim in the amniotic fluid pool, turn somersaults, and occasionally tie a knot in the umbilical cord. Arm and leg movements are visible on ultrasound examination, although the mother does not perceive them until sometime between 16 and 20 weeks.

Integumentary System

The epidermis begins as a single layer of cells derived from the ectoderm at 4 weeks. By the seventh week, there are two layers of cells. The cells of the superficial layer are sloughed and become mixed with the sebaceous gland secretions to form the white, cheesy **vernix caseosa**, the material that protects fetal skin. The vernix is thick at 24 weeks but becomes scant by term.

The basal layer of the epidermis is the germinal layer, which replaces lost cells. Until 17 weeks the skin is thin and wrinkled, with blood vessels visible underneath. The skin thickens and all layers are present at term. After 32 weeks, as subcutaneous fat is deposited under the dermis, the skin becomes less wrinkled and red.

By 16 weeks the epidermal ridges are present on the palms of the hands, the fingers, the bottom of the feet, and the toes. Handprints and footprints are unique to each infant.

Hairs form from hair bulbs in the epidermis that project into the dermis. Cells in the hair bulb keratinize to form the hair shaft. As the cells at the base of the hair shaft proliferate, the hair grows to the surface of the epithelium. Very fine hairs, called **lanugo**, appear first at 12 weeks on the eyebrows and upper lip. By 20 weeks they cover the entire body. At this time the eyelashes, eyebrows, and scalp hair are beginning to grow. By 28 weeks the scalp hair is longer than the lanugo, which thins and may disappear by term gestation.

Fingernails and toenails develop from thickened epidermis at the tips of the digits beginning during the 10th week. They grow slowly. Fingernails usually reach the fingertips by 32 weeks, and toenails reach toe tips by 36 weeks.

Immune System

During the third trimester, albumin and globulin are present in the fetus. The only immunoglobulin that crosses the placenta, immunoglobulin G (IgG), provides passive acquired immunity to specific bacterial toxins. The fetus produces IgM by the end of the first trimester. These are produced in response to blood group antigens, gram-

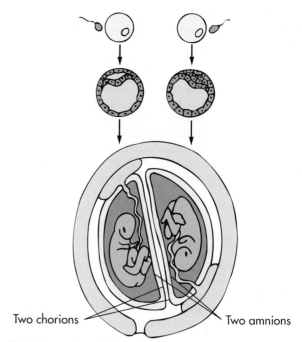

Fig. 12.14 Formation of Dizygotic Twins, With Fertilization of Two Ova, Two Implantations, Two Placentas, Two Chorions, and Two Amnions.

Two chorions   Two amnions

negative enteric organisms, and some viruses. IgA is not produced by the fetus; however, colostrum, the precursor to breast milk, contains large amounts of IgA and can provide passive immunity to the neonate who is breastfed.

The normal-term neonate can fight infection but not so effectively as an older child. The preterm infant is at much greater risk for infection.

Multifetal Pregnancy

Twins

Dizygotic twins. When multiple mature ova are produced in one ovarian cycle, usually due to increased levels of FSH, they have the potential to be fertilized by separate sperm. This often results in two zygotes, or **dizygotic twins** (Fig. 12.14). There are always two amnions, two chorions, and two placentas that may be fused (Fig. 12.15). These dizygotic, or fraternal, twins can be the same sex or different sexes and are genetically no more alike than siblings born at different times. Dizygotic twinning occurs in families, more often among African American women than among white women and least often among Asian women. Dizygotic twinning increases in frequency with maternal age, peaking at 37 years, with parity, and with the use of ART. There is an increased incidence of twinning following discontinuation of oral contraceptives as FSH levels rebound. Dizygotic twinning occurs in approximately 1% to 1.5% of natural conceptions (Newman & Unal, 2017). Maternal obesity may increase the rate of dizygotic twinning (Cunningham et al., 2018).

Monozygotic twins. Monozygotic twins develop from one fertilized ovum, which then divides (Fig. 12.16). They are the same sex. They are often referred to as *identical*, although genetically they are not exactly the same; the splitting of the one fertilized zygote does not necessarily cause equal sharing of genetic material. For example, one twin may have a genetic mutation that results in a congenital defect, whereas the other twin is normal. With monozygotic twinning, placentation (development of the placenta,

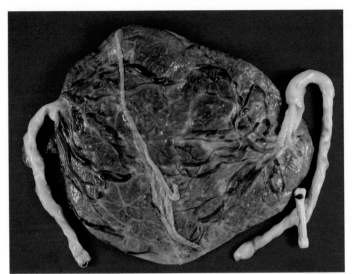

Fig. 12.15 Diamniotic-Monochorionic Twin Placenta. Overview showing thin intertwin membrane. Chorionic vessels are noted crossing the intertwin membrane. (From De Paepe, M.E. [2019]. Multiple gestation: The biology of twinning. In R. Resnik, C.J. Lockwood, T.R. Moore [Eds.]. *Creasy & Resnik's maternal-fetal medicine.* [8th ed.]. Philadelphia: Elsevier.)

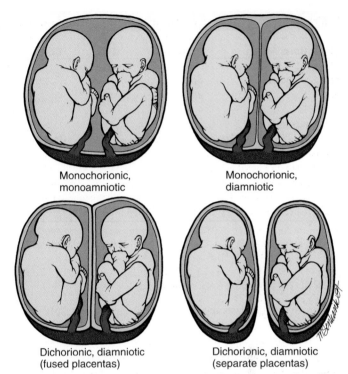

Monochorionic, monoamniotic

Monochorionic, diamniotic

Dichorionic, diamniotic (fused placentas)

Dichorionic, diamniotic (separate placentas)

Fig. 12.16 Placentation in Monozygotic Twin Pregnancies. (From Newman, R.B., & Unal, E.R. [2017]. Multiple gestations. In: S.G. Gabbe, J.R. Niebyl, J.R. Simpson, et al. [Eds.]. *Obstetrics: Normal and problem pregnancies.* [7th ed.]. Philadelphia: Elsevier.)

including chorionic and amniotic membranes) varies according to when zygotic division occurs. If division occurs soon after fertilization, two embryos, two amnions, two chorions, and two placentas that can be fused will develop. Most often, division occurs between 4 and 8 days after fertilization, and there are two embryos, two amnions, one chorion, and one placenta. Rarely, division occurs after the eighth day after fertilization. In this case, there are two embryos within a common amnion and a common chorion with one placenta. This often causes circulatory problems because the umbilical cords may tangle together, and one or both fetuses may die. *Conjoined,* or "Siamese," twins are a type of monozygotic twins in which cleavage is incomplete and occurs late (≥13 days post conception); this is a rare occurrence (Cunningham et al., 2018; Newman & Unal, 2017).

Monozygotic twinning occurs in approximately 0.4% of pregnancies. There is no association with race, heredity, maternal age, or parity. The use of ART increases the incidence of monozygotic twinning by more than tenfold. It is thought that injury to the zona pellucida with in vitro fertilization may predispose the zygote to split, resulting in monozygotic twinning (Cunningham et al., 2018; Newman & Unal, 2017).

Triplet and Higher-Order Births

Triplets can occur from the division of one zygote into two, with one of the two dividing again, producing identical triplets. Triplets also can be produced from two zygotes, one dividing into a set of monozygotic twins, and the second zygote developing as a single fraternal sibling, or from three zygotes. Quadruplets, quintuplets, sextuplets, and so on likewise have similar possible derivations.

FACTORS INFLUENCING FETAL GROWTH AND DEVELOPMENT

The growth, development, and well-being of the embryo and fetus are influenced by complex interactions between genetic and environmental factors. Fetal and parental genetics play a major role. For example,

many congenital anomalies and disorders are the result of chromosomal abnormalities (see Chapters 3 and 36).

Environmental influences on fetal development include the health of the placenta to provide adequate oxygen and nutrients; maternal health prior to and during pregnancy, especially nutritional status; maternal age; medications (prescription and over-the-counter), recreational drugs, chemicals, hormones, and viruses in the maternal system that are transferred to the fetus; and maternal stress. Environmental factors that can produce abnormalities in the embryo or fetus are known as **teratogens**. Many congenital anomalies are due to teratogens (see Chapter 36) (see Boxes 12.1 and 12.2).

The effect of environmental factors on embryonic and fetal development depends on the time in pregnancy that exposure occurs. Body systems and organs develop at varying speeds and proceed through predictable phases. Initially, there is a phase of rapid cell multiplication; this is followed by increase in cell size, along with further increase in number of cells; and finally, cell size continues to increase rapidly while cell division diminishes. The most critical period and time of greatest susceptibility to environmental influences is when both cell number and size are increasing. This means that the effect of environmental factors is largely dependent on the stage of development at which exposure occurs. The first 3 months of pregnancy are recognized as the most critical period for embryonic and fetal development. Within that period of time, teratogens have the greatest effect during the embryonic period from days 15 to 60. During the first 2 weeks of development, teratogens either have no effect or have effects so severe that they cause miscarriage. Brain growth and development continue during the fetal period, and teratogens can severely affect CNS development throughout gestation (see Fig. 12.8).

BOX 12.2 Infectious Diseases With Teratogenic Effects

Infectious Agent	Disease	Congenital Defects
Viruses		
Rubella virus	German measles	Cataracts, deafness, cardiovascular defects, fetal growth restriction
Cytomegalovirus	Cytomegalic inclusion disease	Microcephaly, microphthalmia, cerebral calcification, intrauterine growth restriction
Spirochetes		
Treponema pallidum (syphilis)	Syphilis	Dental anomalies, deafness, cognitive impairment, skin and bone lesions, meningitis
Protozoa		
Toxoplasma gondii	Toxoplasmosis	Microcephaly, hydrocephaly, cerebral calcification, microphthalmia, cognitive impairment, preterm birth
Zika	Zika virus infection	Microcephaly, ventriculomegaly, intracrebral calcifications

Data from Carlson, B.M. (2014). *Human embryology and developmental biology* (5th ed.). Philadelphia: Elsevier; Duff, P. (2019). Maternal and fetal infections. In R. Resnik, C.J. Lockwood, T.R. Moore (Eds.). *Creasy & Resnik's maternal-fetal medicine*. (8th ed.). Philadelphia: Elsevier.

KEY POINTS

- Human gestation lasts approximately 280 days after the LMP or 266 days after conception.
- Fertilization occurs in the uterine tube within 24 hours of ovulation. The zygote undergoes mitotic divisions, creating a 16-cell morula.
- Implantation begins 6 days after fertilization.
- The organ systems and external features develop during the embryonic period (i.e., the third to the eighth week after fertilization).
- Refinement of structure and function occurs during the fetal period, and the fetus becomes capable of extrauterine survival.
- During critical periods in human development, the embryo and fetus are vulnerable to environmental teratogens.
- Although twinning rates in the United States have stabilized, rates of triplets and higher-order births have steadily decreased, primarily due to advances in ART.

REFERENCES

Blackburn, S. T. (2018). *Maternal, fetal, & neonatal physiology. A clinical perspective* (5th ed.). St. Louis: Elsevier.

Burton, G. J., Sibley, C. P., & Jauniaux, E. R. (2017). Placental anatomy and physiology. In S. G. Gabbe, J. R. Niebyl, J. L. Simpson, et al. (Eds.), *Obstetrics: Normal and problem pregnancies* (7th ed.). Philadelphia: Elsevier.

Cunningham, F. G., Leveno, K. L., Bloom, S. L., et al. (2018). *Williams obstetrics* (25th ed.). New York: McGraw-Hill.

Liu, J. H. (2019). Endocrinology of pregnancy. In R. Resnik, C. J. Lockwood, T. R. Moore (Eds.), *Creasy & Resnik's maternal-fetal medicine* (8th ed.). Philadelphia: Elsevier.

Mercer, B. (2019). Assessment and induction of fetal pulmonary maturity. In R. Resnik, C. J. Lockwood, T. R. Moore, et al. (Eds.), *Creasy & Resnik's maternal-fetal medicine* (8th ed.). Philadelphia: Elsevier.

Moore, K. L., Persaud, T. V. N., & Torchia, M. G. (2016). *Before we were born: Essentials of embryology and birth defects* (9th ed.). Philadelphia: Saunders.

Mor, G., & Abrahams, V. (2019). Immunology of pregnancy. In R. Resnik, C. J. Lockwood, T. R. Moore, M. R. , et al. (Eds.), *Creasy & Resnik's maternal-fetal medicine: Principles and practice* (8th ed.). Philadelphia: Elsevier.

Newman, R. B., & Unal, E. R. (2017). Multiple gestations. In S. G. Gabbe, J. R. Niebyl, J. L. Simpson, et al. (Eds.), *Obstetrics: Normal and problem pregnancies* (7th ed.). Philadelphia: Elsevier.

Plosa, E., & Guttentag, S. H. (2018). Lung development. In C. A. Gleason, & S. E. Juul (Eds.), (2018). *Avery's diseases of the newborn* (10th ed.). Philadelphia: Elsevier.

Ross, M. G., & Beall, M. H. (2019). Amniotic fluid dynamics. In R. Resnik, C. J. Lockwood, T. R. Moore, et al. (Eds.), *Creasy & Resnik's maternal-fetal medicine: Principles and practice* (8th ed.). Philadelphia: Elsevier.

Ross, M. G., & Ervin, M. G. (2017). Fetal development and physiology. In S. G. Gabbe, J. R. Niebyl, J. L. Simpson, et al. (Eds.), *Obstetrics: Normal and problem pregnancies* (7th ed.). Philadelphia: Elsevier.

Sunderam, S., Kissin, D. M., Crawford, S. B., et al. (2017). Assisted reproductive technology surveillance—United States, 2014. *Morbidity and Mortality Weekly Report Surveillance Summaries*, 66(SS–6), 1–24.

13

Anatomy and Physiology of Pregnancy

Kathryn Rhodes Alden

ⓔ http://evolve.elsevier.com/Lowdermilk/MWHC/

LEARNING OBJECTIVES

- Describe the expected maternal anatomic and physiologic adaptations to pregnancy.
- Analyze the signs and symptoms of pregnancy in relation to the maternal anatomic and physiologic changes.
- Explore the types of pregnancy tests and their appropriate use.
- Categorize the signs and symptoms of pregnancy as presumptive, probable, or positive.

The goal of maternity care is a healthy pregnancy with a physically safe and emotionally satisfying outcome for mother, infant, and family. Consistent health supervision and surveillance are of utmost importance. Moreover, many maternal adaptations are unfamiliar to pregnant women and their families. Helping the pregnant woman recognize the relationship between her physical status and the plan for her care can enhance her ability to be an active participant in care management along with members of the interprofessional health care team.

ADAPTATIONS TO PREGNANCY

Maternal physiologic adaptations affect all body systems and are attributed to the hormones of pregnancy and to mechanical pressures arising from the enlarging uterus and other tissues. These adaptations protect the woman's normal physiologic functioning, meet the metabolic demands that pregnancy imposes on her body, and provide a nurturing environment for fetal development and growth. Although pregnancy is a normal phenomenon, problems can occur.

Reproductive System

Uterus

Changes in Size, Shape, and Position. High levels of estrogen and progesterone stimulate significant uterine growth in the first trimester. Early uterine enlargement results from increased vascularity and dilation of blood vessels, hyperplasia (production of new muscle fibers and fibroelastic tissue) and hypertrophy (enlargement of preexisting muscle fibers and fibroelastic tissue), and development of the decidua. Uterine weight increases dramatically from 4 g to 70 g in the nonpregnant state to 1200 g at term gestation. Volume increases from 10 mL before pregnancy to 5 L at term. By 7 weeks of gestation, the uterus is the size of a large hen's egg; by 10 weeks, it is the size of an orange (twice its nonpregnant size); and by 12 weeks, it is the size of a grapefruit. After the 3rd month, uterine enlargement is primarily the result of mechanical pressure of the growing fetus.

As the uterus enlarges, it also changes in shape and position. By 12 weeks the uterus changes from its nonpregnant pear shape to a more spherical or globular shape. Later, as the fetus grows, the uterus becomes larger and more ovoid. During the first trimester the uterus is a pelvic organ; by 12 weeks it rises out of the pelvis into the abdominal cavity.

The pregnancy may "show" after the 14th week, although this depends to some degree on the woman's height and weight. Abdominal enlargement may be less apparent in the nullipara with good abdominal muscle tone. Posture also influences the type and degree of abdominal enlargement that occurs. In normal pregnancies, the uterus enlarges at a predictable rate.

As the uterus grows, it can be palpated above the symphysis pubis sometime between the 12th and 14th weeks of pregnancy (Fig. 13.1). The uterus rises gradually to the level of the umbilicus by 20 to 22 weeks of gestation and nearly reaches the xiphoid process at term. Between weeks 38 and 40, fundal height decreases as the fetus begins to descend into the pelvis (lightening) in preparation for birth (see Fig. 13.1, *dashed line*). In general, lightening occurs in the nullipara approximately 2 weeks before the onset of labor and in the multipara at the start of labor.

As the uterus enlarges and rises in the abdomen, it rotates to the right, probably because of the presence of the rectosigmoid colon on the left side. There is increased tension on the broad and round ligaments as the uterus enlarges; some women experience discomfort as this occurs. Eventually the growing uterus touches the anterior abdominal wall and displaces the intestines to either side of the abdomen (Fig. 13.2). When a pregnant woman is standing, most of her uterus rests against the anterior abdominal wall and contributes to altering her center of gravity.

At approximately 6 weeks of gestation, softening and compressibility of the lower uterine segment (uterine isthmus) occurs (Hegar sign) (Fig. 13.3). This results in exaggerated uterine anteflexion during the first 3 months of pregnancy. In this position, the uterine fundus presses on the urinary bladder, causing the woman to have urinary frequency.

Changes in Contractility. Soon after the 4th month of pregnancy, intermittent uterine contractions may be felt through the abdominal wall.

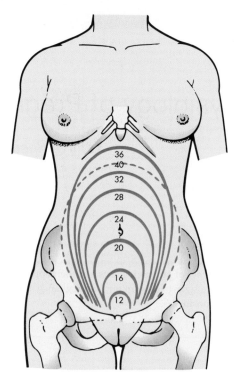

Fig. 13.1 Height of Fundus by Weeks of Normal Gestation With a Single Fetus. *Dashed line,* Height after lightening. (From Seidel, H.M., Ball, J.W., Dains J.E. et al. [2011]. *Mosby's guide to physical examination.* (7th ed). St. Louis: Mosby.)

These are referred to as Braxton Hicks contractions and are thought to enhance blood flow through the intervillous spaces. Braxton Hicks contractions are irregular and painless, although some women complain that they are annoying. After the 28th week, these contractions become more definite, but they usually cease with walking or exercise. Braxton Hicks contractions can be mistaken for true labor; however, they do not increase in intensity or duration or cause cervical dilation. Conversely, preterm labor contractions can be mistaken for Braxton Hicks contractions, which can lead to a delay in seeking treatment.

Uteroplacental Blood Flow. Placental perfusion depends on maternal blood flow to the uterus. Uterine blood flow increases 10-fold over the course of pregnancy as the uterus increases in size. In a normal term pregnancy, one-sixth of the total maternal blood volume is within the uterine vascular system. The rate of blood flow through the uterus averages 450 to 650 mL/min by term. Oxygen consumption of the gravid uterus increases to meet fetal needs, with the greatest consumption occurring during the last trimester when fetal growth is accelerated. Factors that decrease uterine blood flow are low maternal arterial pressure, uterine contractions, and maternal supine position. Estrogen stimulation can increase uterine blood flow. Doppler ultrasound examination may be used to measure uterine blood flow velocity, especially in pregnancies at risk because of conditions associated with decreased placental perfusion (e.g., hypertension, intrauterine growth restriction, diabetes mellitus, multiple gestation) (Blackburn, 2018).

By using an ultrasound device or a fetal stethoscope to auscultate fetal heart tones, the examiner may also hear the uterine souffle or bruit, a rushing or blowing sound of maternal blood flowing through uterine arteries to the placenta that is synchronous with the maternal pulse. The funic souffle, which is synchronous with the fetal heart rate and is caused by fetal blood coursing through the umbilical cord, may also be heard, as well as the fetus's actual heartbeat (see Fig. 14.5).

Changes Related to the Presence of the Fetus. Passive movement of the unengaged fetus is called ballottement and can be identified by the

examiner generally between the 16th and 18th weeks. Ballottement is a technique of palpating a floating structure by bouncing it gently and feeling it rebound. To palpate the fetus, the examiner places a finger within the vagina and taps gently upward on the cervix, causing the fetus to rise. The fetus then sinks, and a gentle tap is felt on the finger (Fig. 13.4).

Quickening is the first recognition of fetal movements, or "feeling life." It can be detected by the multiparous woman as early as 14 to 16 weeks of gestation. The nulliparous woman may not notice these sensations until the 18th week or later. Quickening is commonly described as a flutter and is difficult to distinguish from peristalsis. Fetal movements gradually increase in intensity and frequency as pregnancy progresses. The week in which quickening occurs provides a tentative clue in dating the duration of gestation.

Cervix

The cervix consists primarily of collagen-rich connective tissue and is responsive to hormonal changes of pregnancy. This results in the cervix being a firm, nondistensible, closed structure that maintains the pregnancy/fetus within the uterus and changing to a soft, highly elastic tissue that dilates and becomes almost indistinguishable during labor in preparation for birth.

In a normal, unscarred cervix, softening of the cervical tip can be observed about the beginning of the 6th week. This probable sign of pregnancy, Goodell sign, is due to increased vascularity, slight hypertrophy, and hyperplasia (increase in number of cells).

The glands near the external os proliferate beneath the stratified squamous epithelium, giving the cervix the velvety appearance characteristic of pregnancy. Friability (tissue is easily damaged) is increased and can result in slight bleeding after vaginal examination or after coitus with deep penetration.

Production of mucus by endocervical cells increases. The mucus fills the endocervical canal, resulting in the formation of the mucous plug (operculum) in early pregnancy (Fig. 13.5). The mucus is rich in immunoglobulins and acts as a barrier against bacterial invasion of the uterus.

Because of hormone-induced changes in basal cells and hyperplasia and hypersecretion of endocervical cells, the accuracy of Papanicolaou (Pap) tests during pregnancy can be complicated. However, Pap tests are a routine screening measure performed during prenatal care in an effort to detect cases of cervical cancer during pregnancy (Salani, Billingsley, & Crafton, 2014).

Ovaries

Ovulation does not occur during pregnancy due to suppression of follicle-stimulating hormone (FSH) and luteinizing hormone (LH) by estrogen and progesterone. The corpus luteum produces estrogen and progesterone for the first 6 to 10 weeks of pregnancy until the placenta becomes the primary source of these hormones.

Menstrual periods cease (amenorrhea) during pregnancy. Some women confuse menses with implantation bleeding that often occurs 6 to 12 days after conception, the time one might expect the menstrual period to begin.

Vagina and Vulva

Pregnancy hormones prepare the vagina for stretching during labor and birth by causing the vaginal mucosa to thicken, the connective tissue to loosen, the smooth muscle to hypertrophy, and the vaginal vault to lengthen. Increased vascularity results in the violet-blue color of the vaginal mucosa and cervix, known as Chadwick sign. This is evident at 6 to 8 weeks of pregnancy.

Vaginal discharge increases during pregnancy. Leukorrhea is a white or slightly gray mucoid vaginal discharge with a faint musty odor. This copious mucoid fluid occurs in response to cervical stimulation by estrogen and progesterone.

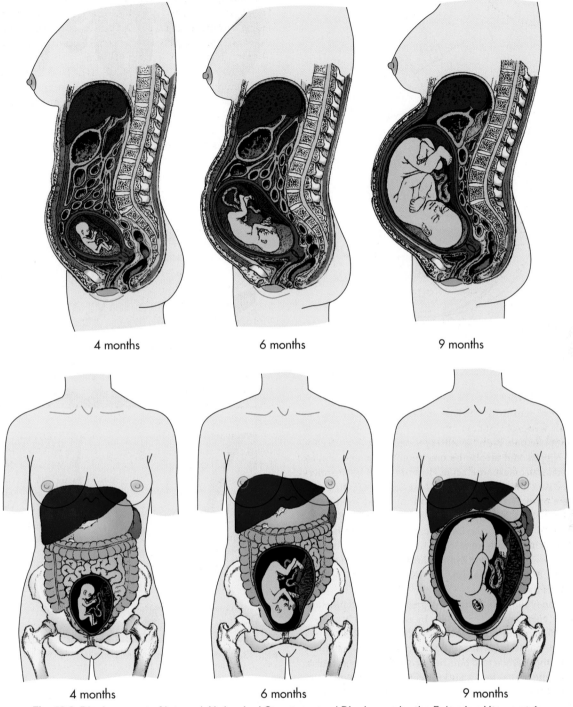

4 months   6 months   9 months

4 months   6 months   9 months

Fig. 13.2 Displacement of Internal Abdominal Structures and Diaphragm by the Enlarging Uterus at 4, 6, and 9 Months of Gestation.

The vaginal microbiome changes during pregnancy, with an increase in at least four species of *Lactobacillus* and a decrease in anaerobic bacteria. This results in a lower pH of vaginal secretions, ranging from approximately 3.5 to 6.0 (nonpregnant, 4.0 to 5.0). Alterations in the vaginal microbiome help to prevent ascending bacterial infections of the uterus that contribute to preterm labor and birth. However, because of the glycogen-rich environment of the vagina, the pregnant woman is more vulnerable to other infections such as candidiasis. Changes in the vaginal microbiome during pregnancy may be important in establishing the upper gastrointestinal microbiota of the neonate (Antony, Racusin, Aagaard, et al., 2017).

Blood flow to the pelvis increases during pregnancy. External structures of the perineum are enlarged during pregnancy because of increased vascularity, hypertrophy of the perineal body, and deposition of fat. Increased vascularity of the vagina and other pelvic viscera results in heightened sensitivity that can lead to a high degree of sexual interest and arousal, especially during the second trimester of pregnancy. The increased congestion, plus the relaxed walls of the blood vessels and the heavy uterus, can result in edema and varicosities of the vulva. The edema and varicosities usually resolve during the postpartum period.

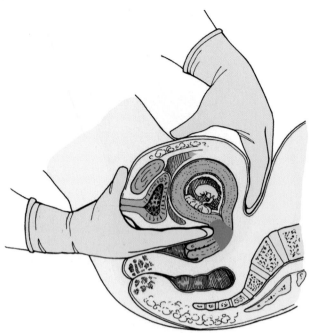

Fig. 13.3 Hegar Sign. Bimanual examination for assessing compressibility and softening of isthmus (lower uterine segment) while the cervix is still firm.

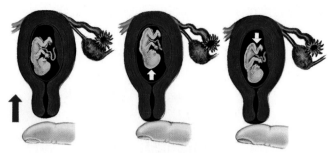

Fig. 13.4 Internal Ballottement (18 Weeks).

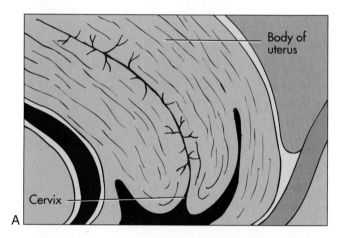

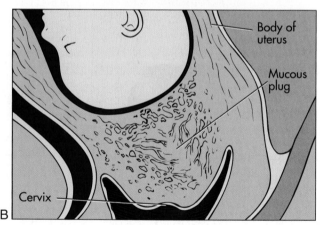

Fig. 13.5 Cervix. (A) In non pregnant woman (B) During pregnancy.

Breasts

Fullness, heightened sensitivity, tingling, and heaviness of the breasts begin in the early weeks of gestation in response to increased levels of estrogen and progesterone. Breast sensitivity varies from mild tingling to sharp pain. Nipples and areolae become more pigmented, areolae enlarge, and nipples become more erectile. Hypertrophy of Montgomery tubercles may be seen around the nipples. These sebaceous (oil) glands embedded in the primary areolae secrete lubricating and antiinfective substances to help protect the nipples and areolae during breastfeeding.

The richer blood supply to the breasts causes the vessels beneath the skin to dilate. Once barely noticeable, the blood vessels become visible, often appearing in an intertwining bluish network beneath the surface of the skin. Striae gravidarum, or stretch marks, can appear at the outer aspects of the breasts.

During pregnancy the breasts are being prepared for lactation and show progressive enlargement (Fig. 13.6). In early pregnancy, estrogen stimulates growth and proliferation of lactiferous (milk) ducts, while progesterone causes growth and development of the mammary lobes. Prolactin, progesterone, and human placental lactogen stimulate development and differentiation of alveolar epithelial cells into lactocytes that will produce colostrum. Prolactin, produced by the anterior pituitary gland, stimulates production of colostrum by the end of the first trimester. During the second trimester, human placental lactogen stimulates secretion of colostrum. This is known as lactogenesis stage I. Although development of the mammary glands is functionally complete by midpregnancy, lactation is inhibited until the progesterone level decreases after birth (Lawrence & Lawrence, 2016). See Chapter 25 for a discussion of lactation.

Cardiovascular System

Maternal adjustments to pregnancy involve extensive anatomic and physiologic changes in the cardiovascular system. Cardiovascular adaptations protect the woman's normal physiologic functioning, meet the metabolic demands pregnancy imposes on her body, and provide for fetal developmental and growth needs.

Blood Volume

Total blood volume (TBV) increases significantly during pregnancy by 40% to 50%. During the first half of pregnancy, TBV increases rapidly, peaks at approximately 28 to 34 weeks, and then stabilizes or decreases slightly by term. In a singleton pregnancy, plasma volume increases by approximately 1200 to 1500 mL, or 50% above prepregnancy levels by 30 weeks of gestation, decreasing slightly by term (Antony et al., 2017).

Increased blood volume is a protective mechanism. It is essential for meeting the blood volume needs of the hypertrophied vascular system of the enlarged uterus, for adequately hydrating fetal and maternal tissues when the woman assumes an erect or supine position, and for providing a fluid reserve to compensate for blood loss during birth and postpartum. Blood volume increases are greater with multiple gestation.

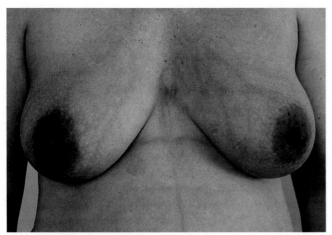

Fig. 13.6 Enlarged Breasts in Pregnancy With Venous Network and Darkened Areolae and Nipples. (From Ball, J.W., Dains, J.E., Flynn, J.A., et al. [2015]. *Mosby's guide to physical examination* [8th ed.]. St. Louis: Mosby.)

TABLE 13.1 Cardiovascular Changes in Pregnancy

Parameter	Change
Heart rate	Increases 15–20 beats/min
Blood pressure	
Systolic	Slight or no decrease from prepregnancy levels
Diastolic	Slight decrease to midpregnancy (24–32 weeks) and gradual return to prepregnancy levels by end of pregnancy
Blood volume	Increases by 1200–1500 mL or 40%–50% above prepregnancy level
Cardiac output	Increases 30%–50%

Data from Antony, K.M., Racusin, D.A., Aagaard, K., et al. (2017). Maternal physiology. In: S.G. Gabbe, J.R. Niebyl, J.L. Simpson, et al., (Eds.) *Obstetrics: Normal and problem pregnancies* (7th ed.). Philadelphia: Elsevier.

Cardiac Output

Cardiac output (CO) increases 30% to 50% during pregnancy, reaching a peak by 25 to 30 weeks and declining to approximately a 20% increase at 40 weeks of gestation. This elevated CO is largely a result of increased stroke volume and heart rate and occurs in response to increased tissue demands for oxygen (Mastrobattista & Monga, 2019). CO increases with any exertion such as labor and birth. Table 13.1 summarizes cardiovascular changes in pregnancy.

Blood Pressure

Blood pressure is influenced by two major factors: CO and systemic vascular resistance (SVR). Although CO increases significantly during pregnancy, maternal blood pressure remains the same or decreases slightly. This is due to reduced SVR caused primarily by the vasodilatory effects of progesterone, prostaglandins, and relaxin. The uteroplacental vascular system holds a large percentage of the maternal blood volume, which also contributes to decreased SVR (Mastrobattista & Monga, 2019). SVR is lowest at 16 to 34 weeks and increases gradually, approximating nonpregnant values by term. During the first trimester, systolic blood pressure usually remains the same as the prepregnancy level but can decrease slightly as pregnancy advances. Diastolic blood pressure begins to decrease in the first trimester, continues to drop

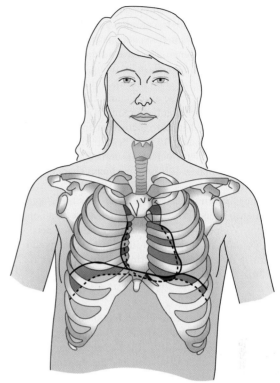

Fig. 13.7 Changes in Position of Heart in Pregnancy. *Broken line,* Nonpregnant state; *solid line,* change that occurs in pregnancy.

until 24 to 32 weeks, and gradually increases, returning to prepregnancy levels by term (Blackburn, 2018).

Various factors influence maternal blood pressure. These include age, activity level, presence of health problems, circadian rhythm, alcohol consumption, smoking, anxiety, and pain. Maternal position also affects blood pressure readings. Brachial blood pressure is highest when the woman is sitting; lowest when she is lying in the lateral recumbent position; and intermediate when she is supine, except for some women who experience hypotensive syndrome (see later discussion).

Some degree of compression of the vena cava occurs in any woman who lies on her back during the second half of pregnancy. CO is reduced by as much as 25% to 30% when a pregnant woman is turned from left lateral recumbent to supine position. Some women experience a fall of more than 30 mm Hg in their systolic pressure. After 4 to 5 minutes, a reflex bradycardia is noted, CO is reduced by half, and the woman feels faint. This condition is called *supine hypotensive syndrome* or *vena caval syndrome* (Mastrobattista & Monga, 2019) (see Fig. 19.5).

Compression of the iliac veins and inferior vena cava by the uterus causes increased venous pressure and reduced blood flow in the legs, except when the woman is in the lateral position. These alterations contribute to the dependent edema, varicose veins in the legs and vulva, and hemorrhoids that can develop in the latter part of term pregnancy and contributes to the increased risk for venous thromboembolism (VTE).

Structural Adaptations

Slight cardiac hypertrophy (enlargement) is probably secondary to increased blood volume and CO that occur in pregnancy. As the diaphragm is displaced upward by the enlarging uterus, the heart is elevated upward and rotated forward to the left (Fig. 13.7). The apical impulse, or point of maximal intensity (PMI), is shifted upward and laterally approximately 1 to 1.5 cm. The degree of shift depends on the duration of pregnancy and the size and position of the uterus.

The changes in heart size and position and the increases in blood volume and CO contribute to common auscultatory changes. By the end of the first trimester, there is audible splitting of S_1 and S_2. The majority of pregnant women also have a third heart sound (S_3) after midpregnancy due to rapid diastolic filling. Approximately 96% of women develop systolic ejection murmurs that are most audible over the left sternal border. These auscultatory changes are transient and usually disappear shortly after birth (Antony et al., 2017).

Maternal heart rate begins to increase at approximately 5 weeks of gestation, reaching a peak of 15 to 20 beats/min over the prepregnancy baseline by 32 weeks and persisting until term. This represents an increase of approximately 17% over the prepregnancy heart rate (Antony et al., 2017).

Pregnancy has limited effects on cardiac rhythm. Pregnant women may experience sinus dysrhythmia or premature atrial or ventricular contractions. Women with preexisting heart disease need close medical and obstetric supervision throughout pregnancy and may be at increased risk for arrhythmias during labor (Antony et al., 2017) (see Chapter 30).

Blood Components

By term, there is an increase in red blood cell (RBC) mass of 250 to 450 mL, or approximately 20% to 30% over prepregnancy values (Mastrobattista & Monga, 2019). The percentage of increase in RBCs depends on the amount of iron available. Because the plasma increase is greater than the increase in RBC production, there is a decrease in normal hemoglobin and hematocrit values (Table 13.2). This state of hemodilution is referred to as physiologic anemia of pregnancy. The decrease is more noticeable during the second trimester, when rapid expansion of blood volume occurs faster than RBC production. A pregnant woman is considered anemic if the hemoglobin is less than 11 g/dL or the hematocrit is less than 33% during the first or third trimester or if the hemoglobin is less than 10.5 g/dL or the hematocrit is less than 32% during the second trimester (West, Hark, & Catalano, 2017).

The total white blood cell count begins to increase as early as the 2nd month, then levels off in the second or third trimester (Blackburn, 2018). This increase is primarily in the granulocytes, nonclassic monocytes, and polymorphonuclear leukocytes; the lymphocyte count stays approximately the same throughout pregnancy (see Table 13.2) (Cunningham, Leveno, Bloom, et al., 2018).

Pregnancy is considered a hypercoagulable state in which women are at a fivefold to sixfold increased risk for thromboembolic disease (Antony et al., 2017). The circulation time decreases slightly by week 32 and returns to near normal by term. There is a greater tendency for blood to coagulate during pregnancy because of increases in various clotting factors (i.e., factors VII, VIII, IX, and X and fibrinogen) and decreases in factors that inhibit coagulation (e.g., protein S) (see Table 13.2). This tendency, combined with the fact that fibrinolytic activity (the splitting up or dissolving of a clot) is depressed during pregnancy and the postpartum period, provides a protective function to decrease the chance of bleeding but also makes the woman more vulnerable to thrombosis, especially after cesarean birth.

Respiratory System

Structural Adaptations

Structural and ventilatory adaptations occur during pregnancy to provide for maternal and fetal needs. Maternal oxygen consumption increases during pregnancy by 20% to 40% above nonpregnant levels. This increase is necessary to support the needs of the fetus, placenta, and changes in maternal organs (Antony et al., 2017). As pregnancy progresses, the enlarging uterus places upward pressure on the diaphragm causing the level of the diaphragm to rise by as much as 4 cm. The costal angle increases, and the lower rib cage appears to flare out. Ligaments of the rib cage relax due to the effects of progesterone, permitting increased chest expansion. The transverse diameter of the thoracic cage increases by approximately 2 cm and the circumference by 5 to 7 cm. Consequently, there is little change in total lung capacity.

With advancing pregnancy, chest breathing replaces abdominal breathing, and it becomes less possible for the diaphragm to descend with inspiration. Thoracic breathing is accomplished primarily by the diaphragm rather than by the costal muscles (Blackburn, 2018).

Pregnancy-related dyspnea is common, beginning in the first or second trimester. This physiologic dyspnea occurs with mild exertion or at rest. During late pregnancy, mechanical pressures can increase the dyspnea. It is important to differentiate physiologic from pathologic dyspnea, such as may be caused by cardiac decompensation (Blackburn, 2018).

Hormonal changes and increased blood volume contribute to capillary engorgement in the mucosa of the oropharynx and nasopharynx. As the capillaries become engorged, edema and hyperemia develop within the nose, pharynx, larynx, trachea, and bronchi. This congestion within the tissues of the respiratory tract gives rise to several conditions commonly seen during pregnancy, including nasal and sinus stuffiness, epistaxis (nosebleed), changes in the voice, and marked inflammatory response to even a mild upper respiratory infection (Antony et al., 2017). Increased vascularity of the upper respiratory tract also can cause the tympanic membranes and eustachian tubes to swell, giving rise to symptoms of impaired hearing, earache, or a sense of fullness in the ears.

Pulmonary Function

Tidal volume (the amount of air exchanged during normal inspiration and expiration) increases by 40% during pregnancy. Respiratory rate does not change during pregnancy, although minute ventilation (volume of gas expelled from the lungs per minute) increases by 30% to 50%. This is likely related to increased progesterone and increased basal metabolic rate (Mastrobattista & Monga, 2019).

Pregnancy is a state of chronic mild hyperventilation with reduced arterial carbon dioxide ($PaCO_2$) and increased oxygen (PaO_2) over nonpregnant levels. Respiratory changes in pregnancy are shown in Table 13.3. Progesterone may be responsible for increasing the sensitivity of the respiratory center receptors so that $PaCO_2$ decreases, the base excess (HCO_3, or bicarbonate) decreases, and pH increases slightly. These alterations in acid-base balance create a state of respiratory alkalosis (see Table 13.2). These changes also facilitate the transport of CO_2 from the fetus to the mother and O_2 release from the mother to the fetus.

Gastrointestinal System

Nausea and Vomiting

During pregnancy, a woman's appetite and food intake fluctuate. Up to 70% of pregnant women experience nausea with or without vomiting ("morning sickness") (Antony et al., 2017). Although the etiology of these symptoms is unknown, theories include high levels of human chorionic gonadotropin (hCG) and estradiol in early pregnancy, psychologic predisposition, and evolutionary adaptation to protect the fetus and woman from potentially dangerous foods. Nausea and vomiting of pregnancy (NVP) appears at approximately 4 to 6 weeks of gestation, peaks by 9 weeks, and usually subsides by the end of the first trimester (see Chapter 15). Severity varies from mild distaste for certain foods to more severe vomiting. The condition can be triggered by the sight or odor of various foods. By the end of the second trimester, the appetite increases in response to increasing metabolic needs. Rarely does NVP have harmful effects on the embryo, the fetus, or the woman.

TABLE 13.2 Laboratory Values for Pregnant and Nonpregnant Women

Values	Nonpregnant	Pregnant
Hematologic		
Complete Blood Count		
Hemoglobin, g/dL	12–16[a]	>11[a]
Hematocrit, packed cell volume, %	37–47	>33[a]
RBC count, million/mm³	4.2–5.4	5–6.25; 20%–30% increase
White blood cells, total per mm³	5,000–10,000	5,000–15,000
Neutrophils, %	55–70	60–85
Lymphocytes, %	20–40	15–40
Erythrocyte sedimentation rate, mm/h	20	Elevated in second and third trimesters
Mean corpuscular hemoglobin concentration (MCHC) (g/dL packed RBCs) g/dL packed RBCs	32–36	No change
Mean corpuscular hemoglobin (MCH) (pg), pg	27–31	No change
Mean corpuscular volume (MCV), per mm³	80–95	No change
Blood Coagulation and Fibrinolytic Activity[b]		
Factor VII	65–140	Increases in pregnancy, returns to normal in early puerperium
Factor VIII	55–145	Increases during pregnancy and immediately after birth
Factor IX	60–140	Same as factor VII
Factor X	45–155	Same as factor VII
Factor XI	65–135	Decreases in pregnancy
Factor XII	50–150	Same as factor VII
Prothrombin time (PT), sec	11–12.5	Decreases slightly in pregnancy
Partial thromboplastin time (PTT), sec	60–70	Decreases slightly in pregnancy and decreases during second and third stages of labor (indicates clotting at placental site)
Bleeding time, min	1–9 (Ivy method)	No appreciable change
Coagulation time, min	6–10 (Lee-White method)	No appreciable change
Platelets, per mm³	150,000–400,000	No significant change until 3–5 days after birth and then increases rapidly (may predispose woman to thrombosis) and gradually returns to normal
Fibrinolytic activity		Decreases in pregnancy and then abruptly returns to normal (protection against thromboembolism)
Fibrinogen, mg/dL	200–400	Levels increase late in pregnancy
Blood Glucose		
Fasting, mg/dL	70–105	60–90 before breakfast; 60–105 before lunch, dinner, bedtime snack
2-h postprandial, mg/dL	<140	<120
Acid-Base Values in Arterial Blood		
PO_2, mm Hg	80–100	104–108
PCO_2, mm Hg	35–45	27–32
Sodium bicarbonate (HCO_3), mEq/L	21–28	18–31
Blood pH	7.35–7.45	7.40–7.45 (slightly increased, more alkaline)
Hepatic		
Bilirubin, total, mg/dL	≤1	Unchanged
Serum cholesterol, mg/dL	120–200	Increases from 16 to 32 week of pregnancy; remains at this level until after birth
Serum alkaline phosphatase, units/L	30–120	Increases from week 12 of pregnancy to 6 weeks after birth
Serum albumin, g/dL	3.5–5	Increases 25% by term
Renal		
Bladder capacity, mL	1300	1500
Renal plasma flow, mL/min	490–700	Increases by 25%–30%

Continued

TABLE 13.2 Laboratory Values for Pregnant and Nonpregnant Women—cont'd		
Values	**Nonpregnant**	**Pregnant**
Glomerular filtration rate, mL/min	88–128	Increases by 30%–50%
Nonprotein nitrogen, mg/dL	25–40	Decreases
Blood urea nitrogen, mg/dL	10–20	Decreases
Serum creatinine, mg/dL	0.5–1.1	Decreases
Serum uric acid, mg/dL	2.7–7.3	Decreases but returns to prepregnancy level by end of pregnancy

[a]At sea level. Permanent residents of higher levels (e.g., Denver) require higher levels of hemoglobin.
[b]Pregnancy represents a hypercoagulable state.
pO_2, Partial pressure of oxygen; pCO_2, partial pressure of carbon dioxide; *pg*, picogram; *RBC*, red blood cell.
Data from Blackburn, S. [2018]. *Maternal, fetal, and neonatal physiology: A clinical perspective* [5th ed.]. St. Louis: Elsevier; Antony, K.M., Racusin, D.A., Aagaard, K., et al. [2017]. Maternal physiology. In: S.G. Gabbe, J.R. Niebyl, J.L. Simpson, et al., eds. *Obstetrics: Normal and problem pregnancies* [7th ed.]. Philadelphia: Elsevier; Landon, M.B., Catalano, P.J., Gabbe, S.G. [2017]. Diabetes mellitus complicating pregnancy. In: S.G. Gabbe, J.R. Niebyl, J.L. Simpson, et al., eds. *Obstetrics: Normal and problem pregnancies* [7th ed.]. Philadelphia: Elsevier; Pagana, K.D., Pagana, T.J., Pagana, T.N. [2017]. *Mosby's diagnostic and laboratory test reference* [13th ed.]. St. Louis: Mosby; and Samuels, P. [2017]. Hematologic complications of pregnancy. In: S.G. Gabbe, J.R. Niebyl, J.L. Simpson, et al., eds. *Obstetrics: Normal and problem pregnancies* [7th ed.] Philadelphia: Elsevier.

Whenever the vomiting is severe or persists beyond the first trimester or when it is accompanied by fever, pain, or weight loss, further evaluation is necessary and medical intervention is likely (see Chapter 29).

Women can have changes in their sense of taste, leading to cravings and changes in dietary intake. Some women have nonfood cravings (**pica**) such as for ice, clay, and laundry starch. Pica should be considered as a potential factor in cases of iron deficiency anemia or poor weight gain (Antony et al., 2017) (see Chapter 15 for a discussion of nutrition in pregnancy).

Mouth, Esophagus, Stomach, and Intestines

The gums can become hyperemic, spongy, and swollen during pregnancy. They tend to bleed easily because the increasing levels of estrogen cause selective increased vascularity and connective tissue proliferation (a nonspecific gingivitis). An **epulis** (gingival granuloma gravidarum) is a red, raised nodule on the gums that bleeds easily. This lesion may develop around the 3rd month and often continues to enlarge as pregnancy progresses. It is usually managed by avoiding trauma to the gums (e.g., using a soft toothbrush). An epulis commonly regresses spontaneously after birth.

Some pregnant women complain of **ptyalism** (excessive salivation), which can be caused by the unconscious decrease in swallowing by the woman when nauseated or caused by stimulation of salivary glands by eating starchy foods.

Increased progesterone causes decreased tone and motility of smooth muscles, resulting in esophageal regurgitation (reflux), slower emptying time of the stomach, and reverse peristalsis. As a result, the woman may experience acid indigestion, or heartburn (**pyrosis**), beginning as early as the first trimester and intensifying through the third trimester.

The incidence of hiatal hernia is increased during pregnancy as a result of the upward displacement of the stomach by the enlarging uterus, which causes a widening of the hiatus of the diaphragm. Hiatal hernia occurs more often in multiparas and older or obese women.

Smooth muscle relaxation and reduced peristalsis caused by increased progesterone result in an increase in water absorption from the colon and can cause constipation. Constipation can also result from food choices, lack of fluids, iron supplementation, side effects of antiemetic medications, decreased activity level, abdominal distention by the pregnant uterus, and displacement and compression of the intestines (Shin, Toto, & Schey, 2015). If the pregnant woman has

TABLE 13.3 Respiratory Changes in Pregnancy	
Parameter	**Change**
Respiratory rate	Unchanged or slightly increased
Tidal volume	Increased 40%
Vital capacity	Unchanged
Inspiratory capacity	Increased 6%
Expiratory reserve volume	Decreased 20%
Total lung capacity	Unchanged to slightly decreased
Minute ventilation	Increased 30%–50%
Oxygen consumption	Increased 20%–40%

Data from Mastrobattista, J.M., & Monga, M. (2019). Maternal cardiovascular, respiratory, and renal adaptation to pregnancy. In: R. Resnik, C.J. Lockwood, T.R. Moore, et al. (Eds.). *Creasy & Resnik's maternal fetal medicine: Principles and practice*. (8th ed.). Philadelphia: Elsevier.

hemorrhoids and is constipated, the hemorrhoids can evert or bleed during straining at stool.

The maternal gut microbiome changes during pregnancy. The bacterial diversity within the gut seems to decrease as pregnancy progresses. By the third trimester, there is an overall increase in *Proteobacteria* and a decrease in *Faecalibacterium*, which creates a gut microbiome that is similar to proinflammatory and prodiabetogenic states (Antony et al., 2017). Gestational changes in maternal vaginal and gut microbiomes seem to be adaptive responses that protect the fetus and contribute to establishing the neonatal microbiome (Mueller, Bakacs, Combellick, et al., 2015).

In response to increased needs during pregnancy, iron is absorbed more readily in the small intestine. Even when the woman is deficient in iron, it continues to be absorbed in sufficient amounts for the fetus to have a normal hemoglobin level.

Gallbladder and Liver

The gallbladder is often distended because of its decreased muscle tone during pregnancy. Increased emptying time and thickening of bile caused by prolonged retention are typical changes. These features, together with slight hypercholesterolemia from increased progesterone levels, can contribute to the development of gallstones during pregnancy (Blackburn, 2018).

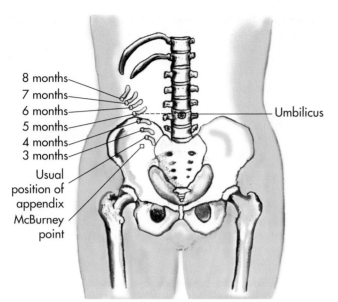

Fig. 13.8 Change in Position of Appendix in Pregnancy. Note the McBurney point.

Hepatic function is difficult to appraise during pregnancy. However, only minor changes in liver function develop. Liver size is unchanged during pregnancy. Serum albumin and total protein levels are reduced due to hemodilution. Serum alkaline phosphatase levels increase up to four times the nonpregnant level. Other liver function tests remain at nonpregnant levels (Antony et al., 2017).

Occasionally intrahepatic cholestasis (retention and accumulation of bile in the liver caused by factors within the liver) occurs late in pregnancy in response to placental steroids. It can result in severe itching with or without jaundice (Rapini, 2019).

Abdominal Discomfort

Intraabdominal alterations that can cause discomfort include pelvic heaviness or pressure, round ligament tension, flatulence, distention and bowel cramping, and uterine contractions. In addition to displacement of intestines, pressure from the expanding uterus causes an increase in venous pressure in the pelvic organs. Although most abdominal discomfort is a consequence of normal maternal alterations, the health care provider must be constantly alert to the possibility of disorders such as bowel obstruction or an inflammatory process.

Appendicitis can be difficult to diagnose in pregnancy because the appendix is displaced upward and laterally, high and to the right, away from the McBurney point (Fig. 13.8). See Chapter 30 for more information.

Urinary System

The kidneys are responsible for maintaining electrolyte and acid-base balance, regulating extracellular fluid volume, excreting waste products, and conserving essential nutrients.

Structural Adaptations

Changes in renal structure result from hormonal activity (estrogen and progesterone), pressure from an enlarging uterus, and an increase in blood volume. Kidneys enlarge during pregnancy. As early as the 10th week of pregnancy, the renal pelves and the ureters dilate. Dilation of the ureters is more pronounced above the pelvic brim, in part because they are compressed between the uterus and the pelvic brim. In most women, the ureters below the pelvic brim are normal size. The smooth-muscle walls of the ureters undergo hyperplasia and hypertrophy and muscle tone relaxation. The ureters elongate, become tortuous, and form single or double curves. In the latter part of pregnancy, the renal pelvis and ureter dilate more on the right side than on the left because the heavy uterus is displaced to the right by the sigmoid colon (Mastrobattista & Monga, 2019).

Because of these changes, a larger volume of urine is held in the pelves and ureters and urine flow rate is slowed, causing urinary stasis. Consequently, a lag occurs between the time urine is formed and when it reaches the bladder. Therefore clearance test results may reflect substances contained in glomerular filtrate several hours before. Because of the urinary stasis and potential stagnation, pregnant women are more susceptible to urinary tract infection.

Bladder irritability, nocturia, and urinary frequency and urgency (without dysuria) are commonly reported in early pregnancy and during the third trimester. Urinary frequency results initially from increased bladder sensitivity and later from compression of the bladder. In the second trimester, the bladder is pulled up out of the true pelvis into the abdomen. The urethra lengthens to 7.5 cm as the bladder is displaced upward. The pelvic congestion that occurs in pregnancy is reflected in hyperemia of the bladder and urethra. This increased vascularity causes the bladder mucosa to be easily traumatized. Bladder tone may decrease, which increases the bladder capacity to 1500 mL. At the same time, the bladder is compressed by the enlarging uterus, resulting in the urge to void even if the bladder contains only a small amount of urine.

Renal Function

In normal pregnancy renal function is altered considerably. Renal plasma flow (RPF) rises significantly from early in pregnancy, peaking by the end of the first trimester. RPF remains elevated above nonpregnant levels throughout pregnancy, although it begins to decrease after 34 weeks of gestation. The glomerular filtration rate (GFR) increases by 50% during the first trimester and remains elevated throughout pregnancy. These changes are caused by pregnancy hormones; an increase in blood volume; and the woman's posture, physical activity, and nutritional intake. The woman's kidneys must manage the increased metabolic and circulatory demands of the maternal body, as well as the excretion of fetal waste products. The increase in GFR results in increased creatinine clearance and a reduction in serum creatinine, blood urea nitrogen (BUN), and uric acid levels (Antony et al., 2017).

Renal function is most efficient when the woman lies in the lateral recumbent position and least efficient when the woman assumes a supine position. A side-lying position increases renal perfusion, which increases urine output and decreases edema. When the pregnant woman is lying supine, the heavy uterus compresses the vena cava and the aorta and CO decreases. As a result, blood flow to the brain and heart is continued at the expense of other organs, including the kidneys and uterus.

Fluid and Electrolyte Balance

By term gestation, there is an increase in total body water of 6.5 to 8.5 L. This additional water content can be attributed to expansion of maternal blood volume; water content of the fetus, placenta, and amniotic fluid; intracellular fluid in the uterus and breasts; extravascular fluid; and increase in adipose tissue (Antony et al., 2017).

Selective renal tubular reabsorption maintains sodium and water balance, regardless of changes in dietary intake and losses through sweat, vomitus, or diarrhea. To prevent excessive sodium depletion, the maternal kidneys undergo a significant adaptation by increasing tubular reabsorption. Because of the need for increased maternal intravascular and extracellular fluid volume, additional sodium is needed to expand fluid volume and maintain an isotonic state. Approximately 900 mEq of sodium is cumulatively retained during pregnancy, although maternal serum levels of sodium decrease by 3 to 4 mmol/L (Antony et al., 2017).

The capacity of the kidneys to excrete water is more efficient during the early weeks than later in pregnancy. As a result, some women feel thirsty in early pregnancy because of the greater amount of water loss. The pooling of fluid in the legs in the latter part of pregnancy decreases renal blood flow and GFR. This pooling is sometimes referred to as *physiologic* or *dependent edema* and requires no treatment. The normal diuretic response to the water load is triggered when the woman lies down, preferably on her side, and the pooled fluid reenters general circulation.

Normally the kidney reabsorbs almost all the glucose and other nutrients from the plasma filtrate. However, in pregnant women tubular reabsorption of glucose is impaired, causing glucosuria to occur at varying times and to varying degrees. Nonpregnant women excrete less than 100 mg/day, whereas pregnant women with normal blood glucose levels excrete 1 to 10 g of glucose each day (Antony et al., 2017). The mechanism by which this occurs is unclear, although it may be related to the increased GFR and tubular flow rate that exceeds the capacity for tubular reabsorption of glucose (Blackburn, 2018). Although glucosuria can be found in normal pregnancies (2+ levels can be seen with increased anxiety states), the possibility of diabetes mellitus and gestational diabetes must be considered.

During normal pregnancy, there is an increase in urinary excretion of protein and albumin, most notable after 20 weeks of gestation. This is due to increased GFR and impaired proximal tubular function. It is considered abnormal when proteinuria exceeds 300 mg/24 hours or albuminuria is greater than 30 mg/24 hours. The amount of protein excreted is not an indication of the severity of renal disease, nor does an increase in protein excretion in a pregnant woman with known renal disease necessarily indicate a progression in her disease. However, a pregnant woman with hypertension and proteinuria must be evaluated carefully because she may be at greater risk for adverse pregnancy outcomes (Antony et al., 2017).

Integumentary System

Alterations in hormone balance and mechanical stretching are responsible for several changes in the integumentary system during pregnancy. Hyperpigmentation is stimulated by the anterior pituitary hormone *melanotropin,* which is increased during pregnancy. Darkening of the nipples, areolae, axillae, and vulva occurs at approximately week 16 of gestation. Melasma (also called *chloasma* or *mask of pregnancy*) is a blotchy, brownish hyperpigmentation of the skin over the cheeks, nose, and forehead, especially in pregnant women with dark complexions. Melasma appears in 50% to 70% of pregnant women, beginning after the 16th week and increasing gradually until term. The sun intensifies this pigmentation in susceptible women. Melasma caused by normal pregnancy usually fades after birth but often recurs with oral contraceptive use or subsequent pregnancies (Wang & Kroumpouzos, 2017).

The linea nigra (Fig. 13.9) is a pigmented line extending from the symphysis pubis to the top of the fundus in the midline. This line is

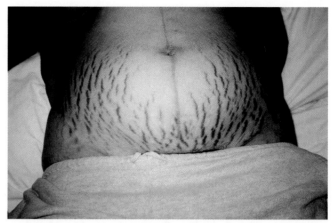

Fig. 13.9 Striae Gravidarum and Linea Nigra in a Dark-Skinned Person. (Courtesy Shannon Perry, Phoenix, AZ.)

known as the *linea alba* before hormone-induced pigmentation. In primigravidas, the extension of the linea nigra, beginning in the 3rd month, keeps pace with the rising height of the fundus; in multigravidas, the entire line often appears earlier than the 3rd month. Not all pregnant women develop linea nigra, and some women notice hair growth along the line with or without the change in pigmentation.

Striae gravidarum, or stretch marks (see Fig. 13.9), appear in 50% to 80% of pregnant women during the second half of pregnancy. Striae reflect separation within the underlying connective (collagen) tissue of the skin. These slightly depressed streaks tend to occur over areas of maximum stretch (the abdomen, thighs, and breasts). The stretching sometimes causes a sensation that resembles itching. The tendency to develop striae may be familial. After birth they usually fade, although they never disappear completely. No topical therapy has been shown to affect the course of striae, although pulsed laser therapy can reduce redness of early lesions (Rapini, 2019).

Angiomatas, commonly known as vascular spiders, are tiny star-shaped or branched, slightly raised, and pulsating end-arterioles usually found on the neck, thorax, face, and arms. Angiomatas appear during the 2nd to 5th months of pregnancy as a result of increased blood flow to the skin due to rising estrogen levels during pregnancy and usually disappear within the first 3 months postpartum (Wang & Kroumpouzos, 2017).

Pinkish red, diffusely mottled, or well-defined blotches are seen over the palmar surfaces of the hands in about 70% of Caucasian women and 30% of African American women during pregnancy (Wang & Kroumpouzos, 2017). These color changes, called palmar erythema, are related to increased estrogen levels.

Some dermatologic conditions have been identified as unique to pregnancy or as having an increased incidence during pregnancy. The most common dermatologic symptom during pregnancy is itching (pruritis). Mild pruritus, also known as pruritus gravidarum, usually occurs over the abdomen. Less than 2% of women have significant pruritus that requires further evaluation (Wang & Kroumpouzos, 2017). The problem usually resolves during the postpartum period.

The effect of pregnancy on acne is variable. In some women, the skin clears and looks radiant. Acne can worsen or occur for the first time during pregnancy or postpartum. Commonly used topical treatments for acne (e.g., benzoyl peroxide, topical antibiotics) are considered safe during pregnancy; topical retinoids should be avoided (Wang & Kroumpouzos, 2017).

Nail and hair growth may be accelerated. Some women notice thinning and softening of the nails. Hirsutism, the excessive growth of hair or growth of hair in unusual places, is commonly reported. An increase

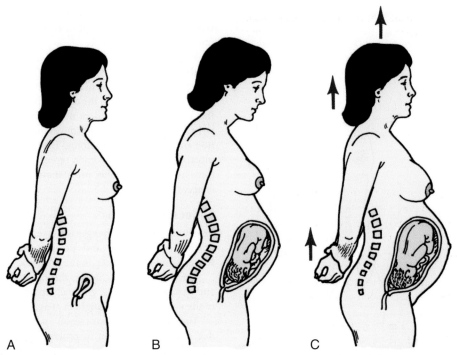

Fig. 13.10 Postural Changes During Pregnancy. (A) Nonpregnant. (B) Incorrect posture during pregnancy. (C) Correct posture during pregnancy.

in fine hair growth can occur but tends to disappear after pregnancy. However, growth of coarse or bristly hair does not usually disappear after pregnancy. The rate of scalp hair loss slows during pregnancy; increased hair loss may be noted in the postpartum period (Rapini, 2019).

Musculoskeletal System

The gradually changing body and increasing weight of pregnancy usually cause noticeable changes in a woman's posture (Fig. 13.10). Abdominal distention causes the pelvis to tilt forward, abdominal muscle tone decreases, and weight bearing increases; these changes require a realignment of the spinal curvatures. The woman's center of gravity shifts forward. An increase in the normal lumbosacral curve (lordosis) develops, and a compensatory curvature in the cervicodorsal region (exaggerated anterior flexion of the head) develops to help her maintain balance. Aching, numbness, and weakness of the upper extremities can result. Large breasts and a stoop-shouldered stance further accentuate the lumbar and dorsal curves. The ligamentous and muscular structures of the middle and lower spine can be severely stressed. These and related changes often cause musculoskeletal discomfort such as back pain, especially in older women or those with a back disorder or a faulty sense of balance.

During pregnancy there is increased mobility of the sacroiliac, sacrococcygeal, and pubic joints (Cunningham et al., 2018). By 28 to 32 weeks of gestation, the symphysis widens from approximately 3 to 4 mm to 7.7 to 7.9 mm. Separation of the symphysis pubis and the instability of the sacroiliac joints can cause pain and difficulty in walking. A waddling gait is common. Obesity or multifetal pregnancy tends to increase pelvic instability (Antony et al., 2017).

⚡ SAFETY ALERT

Pregnant women are at increased risk for falling due to the shifting center of gravity, impaired balance, and joint laxity.

The muscles of the abdominal wall stretch and ultimately lose some tone. During the third trimester, the rectus abdominis muscles can separate (**diastasis recti abdominis**) (Fig. 13.11), allowing abdominal contents to protrude at the midline. The umbilicus flattens or protrudes. After birth, the muscles gradually regain tone. However, separation of the muscles can persist.

Leg cramps are likely to occur during pregnancy as a result of changes in calcium and phosphorus metabolism. The cramps can also be caused by pressure of the enlarging uterus on pelvic blood vessels and nerves supplying the legs and feet. Restless legs syndrome is common during the third trimester of pregnancy (Blackburn, 2018).

Neurologic System

Changes in the neurologic system during pregnancy are subtle. Little is known about specific alterations in function of the neurologic system during pregnancy aside from hypothalamic-pituitary neurohormonal changes.

Pregnant women are prone to headaches resulting from muscular contraction, tension, or migraine without aura. Tension headaches are most often due to hormonal changes, eyestrain, emotional tension, nasal congestion, or fatigue.

⚡ SAFETY ALERT

Headache during pregnancy can be a symptom of a complication such as preeclampsia. Therefore all pregnant women complaining of headache should be carefully evaluated to rule out complications.

Lightheadedness, faintness, and even syncope (fainting) are common during early pregnancy. Vasomotor instability, postural hypotension, or hypoglycemia may be responsible.

Alterations in sleep are likely to occur. During the first trimester, most women experience fatigue; napping and total sleep time increase. During the second and third trimesters, alterations include difficulty falling asleep, awakening frequently, poorer sleep quality, and shorter periods of sleep (Blackburn, 2018).

Ocular changes during pregnancy are primarily increased edema and thickening of the cornea and decreased intraocular pressure. Corneal changes can result in problems with contact lenses (Antony et al., 2017).

The olfactory sense is altered during pregnancy. Many women report an enhanced sense of smell and sensitivity to certain odors that previously were benign.

Edema involving the peripheral nerves can result in carpal tunnel syndrome during the last trimester. The syndrome is characterized by paresthesia (abnormal sensation such as burning or tingling) and pain in the hand, radiating to the elbow. The sensations are caused by edema that compresses the median nerve beneath the carpal ligament of the wrist. Smoking and alcohol consumption can impair the microcirculation and worsen the symptoms. The dominant hand is usually affected most, although many women report symptoms in both hands. Symptoms usually regress after pregnancy. In some cases, surgical treatment is necessary.

Endocrine System

Profound endocrine changes are essential for pregnancy maintenance, normal fetal growth, and postpartum recovery. Hormones, their sources, and their effects on the pregnancy are presented in Table 13.4.

The thyroid gland enlarges during pregnancy. T3 and T4 levels rise and basal metabolic rate gradually increases up to 25% over the course of the pregnancy (Cunningham et al., 2014).

The pituitary gland increases in size during pregnancy primarily due to the proliferation of prolactin-producing cells in the anterior pituitary. Prolactin levels begin to rise about the 5th week of pregnancy and by term have increased 10-fold (Antony et al., 2017).

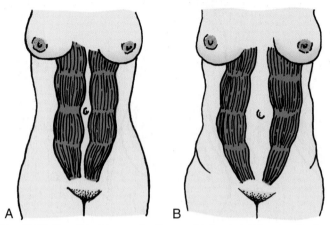

Fig. 13.11 Possible Change in Rectus Abdominis Muscles During Pregnancy. (A) Normal position in nonpregnant woman. (B) Diastasis recti abdominis in pregnant woman.

TABLE 13.4	Hormones and Effects of Changes During Pregnancy	
Hormone	**Source**	**Effects of Changes During Pregnancy**
Human chorionic gonadotropin (hCG)	Fertilized ovum and chorionic villi	Maintains corpus luteum production of estrogen and progesterone until placenta takes over the function
Progesterone	Corpus luteum until 6 to 10 weeks of gestation, then the placenta	Suppresses secretion of FSH and LH by the anterior pituitary gland; maintains pregnancy by relaxing smooth muscles, decreasing uterine contractility; causes fat to deposit in subcutaneous tissues over the maternal abdomen, back, and upper thighs; decreases mother's ability to use insulin
Estrogen	Corpus luteum until 6 to 10 weeks of gestation, then the placenta	Suppresses secretion of FSH and LH by the anterior pituitary gland; causes fat to deposit in subcutaneous tissues over the maternal abdomen, back, and upper thighs; promotes enlargement of genitals, uterus, and breasts; increases vascularity; relaxes pelvic ligaments and joints; interferes with folic acid metabolism; increases the level of total body proteins; promotes retention of sodium and water; decreases secretion of hydrochloric acid and pepsin; decreases mother's ability to use insulin
Serum prolactin	Anterior pituitary gland	Prepares breasts for lactation
Oxytocin	Posterior pituitary gland	Stimulates uterine contractions; stimulates milk ejection from breasts after birth
Human chorionic somatomammotropin (previously called *human placental lactogen*)	Placenta	Acts as a growth hormone; contributes to breast development; decreases maternal metabolism of glucose; increases the amount of fatty acids for metabolic needs
Thyroxine-binding globulin, thyroxine, triiodothyronine	Thyroid gland	With adequate iodine intake, little or no enlargement of thyroid gland. Total T3 and T4 levels are slightly increased, peak by midpregnancy; by term are 10%–15% lower than nonpregnant
Parathyroid	Parathyroid glands	Controls calcium and magnesium metabolism
Insulin	Pancreas	Increases production of insulin to compensate for insulin antagonism caused by placental hormones; effect of insulin antagonists is to decrease tissue sensitivity to insulin or ability to use insulin
Cortisol	Adrenal glands	Stimulates production of insulin; increases peripheral resistance to insulin
Aldosterone	Adrenal glands	Stimulates reabsorption of excess sodium from the renal tubules

FSH, Follicle-stimulating hormone; *LH,* luteinizing hormone.

After the first trimester, insulin needs increase during pregnancy (see Chapter 29). The hormones of pregnancy act as insulin antagonists to ensure adequate glucose supply for the fetus. The β cells in the islets of Langerhans in the pancreas undergo hypertrophy and hyperplasia to increase insulin production.

Immune System

The maternal immune system functions during pregnancy to protect the mother against infection while also preventing rejection of the genetically foreign fetus. Pregnancy is not a state of immunosuppression; instead, there is both activation and dampening of aspects of the maternal immune system. There is evidence that the placenta has an active role in regulating the differentiation and function of the immune cells of the mother to support the pregnancy while also protecting the fetus (Racicot, Kwon, Aldo, et al., 2017).

The maternal immune system is in flux during pregnancy. The first trimester and early second trimester represent a proinflammatory state to allow establishment of the pregnancy as implantation and placentation occur. The second trimester is predominantly an antiinflammatory state when there is rapid growth and development of the fetus. In the third trimester, the proinflammatory state returns when there is an influx of immune cells into the myometrium, contributing to the initiation of labor, cervical ripening, membrane rupture, and uterine contractions (Blackburn, 2018; Cunningham et al., 2018). The timing of immune changes appears to be important in maintaining pregnancy to term (Aghaeepour, Ganio, McIlwain, et al., 2017).

Changes in the maternal immune system cause some women with autoimmune disorders such as rheumatoid arthritis to experience improvement in their symptoms during pregnancy. However, when the pregnancy is over, there may be exacerbation of symptoms.

DIAGNOSIS OF PREGNANCY

Pregnancy Tests

Early detection of pregnancy allows for early initiation of prenatal care. hCG is the earliest biologic marker for pregnancy. Pregnancy tests are based on the recognition of hCG or a beta (β) subunit of hCG. Production of β-hCG begins as early as the day of implantation and can be detected in maternal serum or urine as soon as 7 to 8 days before the expected menses. hCG levels usually double approximately every 2 days for the first 4 weeks of pregnancy. The hCG level rises until it peaks at 60 to 70 days and then declines to lowest levels at approximately 100 to 130 days as the placenta becomes the primary source of estrogen and progesterone. Plasma levels of hCG remain at this lower level for the remainder of the pregnancy. Higher than normal levels of hCG are associated with abnormal gestation (e.g., fetus with Down syndrome, gestational trophoblastic disease) or multiple gestation. An abnormally slow increase in hCG or lower levels can indicate impending miscarriage or ectopic pregnancy (Liu, 2019).

Serum and urine pregnancy tests are performed in clinics, offices, women's health centers, and laboratory settings. Urine tests can also be done at home. Both serum and urine tests can provide accurate results.

Quantitative serum testing—the β-hCG test—has a high level of accuracy because it measures the exact amount of hCG in the blood and can detect even small amounts. hCG levels greater than 25 International Units/L are diagnostic for pregnancy. For serum testing, a 7- to 10-mL sample of venous blood is collected (Pagana, Pagana, & Pagana, 2017).

Sandwich-type immunoassay testing is the most popular method of testing for pregnancy and is the basis for most home pregnancy tests. It uses a specific monoclonal antibody (anti-hCG) with enzymes that bond with hCG in urine. Many different pregnancy tests are available (Fig. 13.12). With these one-step tests, the woman usually applies urine to a strip or absorbent-tipped applicator and reads the results. The test

kits come with directions for collection of the specimen, the testing procedure, and reading of results.

The accuracy of the results of home pregnancy testing is related to following the instructions correctly (see Community Activity box). However, instructions for some home pregnancy tests do not comply with the recommended guidelines for use of plain language, and many instructions are written at a seventh-grade reading level or above, which limits understanding by some users. A positive test result is indicated by a simple color change reaction or a digital reading. Most manufacturers of the kits provide a toll-free telephone number to call if users have concerns or questions about test procedures or results. A common error in performing home pregnancy tests is doing the test too early in pregnancy before a significant rise in hCG level; this can cause a false-negative result (Pagana et al., 2017) (see Clinical Reasoning Case Study).

> ### 🏠 COMMUNITY ACTIVITY
>
> **Home Pregnancy Tests**
> - Review web-based information about home pregnancy tests. Explore websites such as www.babycenter.com and www.parents.com. Assess the accuracy of information.
> - Visit a local pharmacy. How many different types of home pregnancy test kits are available, and what are the costs? Examine the packaging on three different home pregnancy test kits. Do the kits include supplies for more than one test? Are the directions printed in more than one language? After reading the directions, do you have questions about how to perform the test or how to interpret the results? If so, what does that say about the likelihood that the tests will be used correctly?

> ### ❓ CLINICAL REASONING CASE STUDY
> #### *Pregnancy Testing*
>
> When her menstrual period was 10 days late, Regine purchased a home pregnancy test on her way home from work and performed the test that evening. The result was negative. Regine and her partner have been trying to get pregnant so that the baby will be born when she is on summer break from her teaching job at the elementary school. She is disappointed that the test was negative, and she calls the clinic to ask the nurse if she should come in for a blood test to see if she is pregnant.
> 1. What is the priority concern or client need in this situation? Support your answer with data as stated in the case.
> 2. List other client needs/problems in this case.
> 3. Identify any additional information or assessment data that is needed by the nurse in planning care for this client.
> 4. What nursing actions are appropriate in this situation?
>   a. What is the priority nursing action?
>   b. Describe other nursing interventions that are important to providing optimal client care.
> 5. Describe the roles/responsibilities of the interprofessional health care team members (other than nurses) who may be involved in providing care for this client.

Interpreting the results of pregnancy tests requires some judgment. The type of pregnancy test and its degree of sensitivity (the ability to detect low levels of a substance) and specificity (the ability to discern the absence of a substance) must be considered in conjunction with the woman's history. This includes the date of her last normal menstrual period, her usual cycle length, and results of previous pregnancy tests. It is important to know about any medications or other substances she is taking. Medications such as anticonvulsants and tranquilizers can cause false-positive results, whereas diuretics and promethazine can cause false-negative results (Pagana et al. 2017). Improper collection of the specimen, hormone-producing tumors, and laboratory errors can also cause inaccurate results.

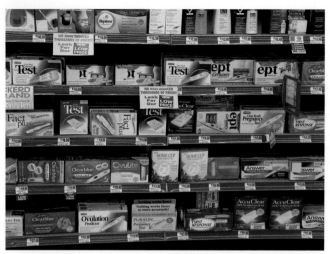

Fig. 13.12 Many Pregnancy Test Products Are Available Over the Counter. (Courtesy Dee Lowdermilk, Chapel Hill, NC.)

Women who use a home pregnancy test should be advised about the variations in accuracy and to use caution when interpreting results. Whenever there is any question, further evaluation or retesting may be appropriate (see Teaching for Self-Management box).

TEACHING FOR SELF-MANAGEMENT
Home Pregnancy Testing

1. Follow the manufacturer's instructions carefully. Do not omit steps.
2. Review the manufacturer's list of foods, medications, and other substances that can affect the test results.
3. Use a first-voided morning urine specimen.
4. If the test done at the time of your missed period is negative, repeat the test in 1 week if you still have not had a period.
5. If you have questions about the test, contact the manufacturer.
6. Contact your health care provider for follow-up if the test result is positive or if the test result is negative and you still have not had a period.

Signs of Pregnancy

Diagnosis of pregnancy involves assessment and evaluation of signs and symptoms of pregnancy (Table 13.5). These are commonly categorized as:

- Presumptive—subjective: changes experienced by the woman (e.g., fatigue, breast changes, quickening); these suggest the possibility of pregnancy but can also be caused by conditions other than pregnancy
- Probable—objective: changes observed/perceived by an examiner (e.g., positive pregnancy test, Hegar sign, Chadwick sign), strongly suggest pregnancy
- Positive—objective: changes observed/perceived by an examiner (e.g., fetal heart tones, ultrasound), indicate proof of pregnancy

TABLE 13.5 Signs of Pregnancy

Time of Occurrence (Gestational Age)	Sign	Other Possible Cause
Presumptive		
3–4 weeks	Breast changes	Premenstrual changes, oral contraceptives
4 weeks	Amenorrhea	Stress, vigorous exercise, early menopause, endocrine problems, malnutrition
4–14 weeks	Nausea, vomiting	Gastrointestinal virus, food poisoning
6–12 weeks	Urinary frequency	Infection, pelvic tumors
12 weeks	Fatigue	Stress, illness
16–20 weeks	Quickening	Gas, peristalsis
Probable		
5 weeks	Goodell sign	Pelvic congestion
6–8 weeks	Chadwick sign	Pelvic congestion
6–12 weeks	Hegar sign	Pelvic congestion
4–12 weeks	Positive pregnancy test (serum)	Hydatidiform mole, choriocarcinoma
6–12 weeks	Positive pregnancy test (urine)	False-positive result may be caused by pelvic infection, tumors
16 weeks	Braxton Hicks contractions	Myomas, other tumors
16–28 weeks	Ballottement	Tumors, cervical polyps
Positive		
5–6 weeks	Visualization of fetus by real-time ultrasound examination	No other causes
6 weeks	Fetal heart tones detected by ultrasound	No other causes
16 weeks	Visualization of fetus by radiographic study	No other causes
8–17 weeks	Fetal heart tones detected by Doppler ultrasound stethoscope	No other causes
17–19 weeks	Fetal heart tones detected by fetal stethoscope	No other causes
19–22 weeks	Fetal movements palpated by examiner	No other causes
Late pregnancy	Fetal movements visible to examiner	No other causes

KEY POINTS

- Maternal anatomic and physiologic adaptations to pregnancy affect all body systems and can be attributed to the hormones of pregnancy or to the mechanical pressures arising from the enlarging uterus and other tissues.
- Adaptations to pregnancy protect the woman's normal physiologic functioning, meet the metabolic demands that pregnancy imposes, and provide for fetal developmental and growth needs.

- Maternal blood volume increases by 40% to 45% during pregnancy and cardiac output increases up to 50%; however, blood pressure remains the same or decreases due to the effects of progesterone on system vascular resistance.
- Heart rate increases by 15 to 20 beats/min by 32 weeks and persists until term gestation.

- Physiologic anemia of pregnancy results from increase in plasma volume greater than the increase in red blood cell production.
- Pregnancy is a hypercoagulable state with increased risk for thromboembolic events.
- Respiratory rate is unchanged during pregnancy, although tidal volume and minute ventilation increase by 30% to 50%.
- Decreased muscle tone during pregnancy contributes to heartburn, reflux, and constipation.

- Dilation of renal pelves and ureters during pregnancy increases the risk of urinary tract infection.
- Endocrine changes are essential to maintaining pregnancy and promoting fetal growth.
- Accuracy of home pregnancy testing is dependent on following instructions correctly.
- Diagnosis of pregnancy is based on presumptive, probable, and positive signs of pregnancy.

REFERENCES

Aghaeepour, N., Ganio, E. A., McIlwain, D., et al. (2017). An immune clock of human pregnancy. *Science Immunology, 2*, eean2946, 1–11. Retrieved from: https://doi.org/10.1126/sciimmunol.aan2946.

Antony, K. M., Racusin, D. A., Aagaard, K., & Dildy, G. A. (2017). Maternal physiology. In S. G. Gabbe, J. R. Niebyl, J. L. Simpson, et al. (Eds.), *Obstetrics: Normal and problem pregnancies* (7th ed.). Philadelphia: Elsevier.

Blackburn, S. (2018). *Maternal, fetal, & neonatal physiology: A clinical perspective* (5th ed.). St. Louis, MO: Elsevier.

Cunningham, J. G., Leveno, K. J., Bloom, S. L., et al. (2018). *Williams' obstetrics* (25th ed.). New York: McGraw-Hill.

Lawrence, R. A., & Lawrence, R. M. (2016). *Breastfeeding: A guide for the medical profession* (8th ed.). Philadelphia: Elsevier.

Liu, J. H. (2019). Endocrinology of pregnancy. In R. Resnik, C. J. Lockwood, T. R. Moore, et al. (Eds.), *Creasy & Resnik's maternal-fetal medicine: Principles and practice* (8th ed.). Philadelphia: Elsevier.

Mastrobattista, J. M., & Monga, M. (2019). Maternal cardiovascular, respiratory, and renal adaptation to pregnancy. In R. Resnik, C. J. Lockwood, T. R. Moore, et al. (Eds.), *Creasy & Resnik's maternal-fetal medicine: Principles and practice* (8th ed.). Philadelphia: Elsevier.

Mueller, N. T., Bakacs, E., Combellick, J., et al. (2015). The infant microbiome development: Mom matters. *Trends in Molecular Medicine, 21*(2), 109–117.

Pagana, K. D., Pagana, T. J., & Pagana, T. N. (2017). *Mosby's diagnostic and laboratory test reference* (13th ed.). St. Louis: Elsevier.

Racicot, K., Kwon, J., Aldo, P., Silasi, M., & Mor, G., et al. (2014). Understanding the complexity of the immune system during pregnancy. *American Journal of Reproductive Immunology, 72*(2), 107–116.

Rapini, R. P. (2019). The skin and pregnancy. In R. Resnik, C. J. Lockwood, T. R. Moore, et al. (Eds.), *Creasy & Resnik's maternal-fetal medicine: Principles and practice* (8th ed.). Philadelphia: Elsevier.

Shin, G. H., Toto, E. L., & Schey, R. (2015). Pregnancy and postpartum bowel changes: Constipation and fecal incontinence. *American Journal of Gastroenterology, 110*(4), 521–529.

Wang, A. R., & Kroumpouzos, G. (2017). Skin disease and pregnancy. In S. G. Gabbe, J. R. Niebyl, J. L. Simpson, et al. (Eds.), *Obstetrics: Normal and problem pregnancies* (7th ed.). Philadelphia: Elsevier.

West, E. H., Hark, L., & Catalano, P. M. (2017). Nutrition during pregnancy. In S. G. Gabbe, J. R. Niebyl, J. L. Simpson, et al. (Eds.), *Obstetrics: Normal and Problem Pregnancies* (7th ed.). Philadelphia: Elsevier.

14

Nursing Care of the Family During Pregnancy

Denise G. Link

http://evolve.elsevier.com/lowdermilk/MWHC/

LEARNING OBJECTIVES

- Describe strategies for confirming pregnancy and estimating the date of birth.
- Summarize the physical, psychosocial, and behavioral changes that usually occur as the expectant mother and other family members adapt to pregnancy.
- Evaluate the benefits of prenatal care and issues of accessibility for some women.
- Outline the patterns of health care used to assess maternal and fetal health status at initial and follow-up visits during pregnancy.
- Select the typical nursing assessments, interventions, and methods of evaluation in providing care for the pregnant woman.

- Plan and provide education needed by pregnant women to understand and manage physical discomforts related to pregnancy and to recognize signs and symptoms of potential complications.
- Evaluate the effect of age, parity, and number of fetuses on the response of the family to the pregnancy and on the prenatal care provided.
- Analyze the effects of variations in childbearing choices, cultural beliefs, and practices on care of women during pregnancy.
- Compare the available options for expectant parents in selecting obstetric health care providers and birth settings.

The prenatal period is a time of physical and psychologic preparation for birth and parenthood. Becoming a parent is considered one of the maturational milestones of adult life. It is a time of intense learning for prospective parents and those close to them. The prenatal period provides a unique opportunity for nurses and other members of the interprofessional health care team to influence pregnancy outcome and family health. Health promotion interventions can affect the well-being of the woman, her unborn child, and the rest of her family for many years.

Regular prenatal visits, ideally beginning soon after the first missed menstrual period, offer opportunities to promote the health of the expectant mother and her infant. Prenatal health care enables discovery, diagnosis, and treatment of preexisting maternal disorders and any disorders that develop during the pregnancy. Prenatal care is designed to monitor the growth and development of the fetus and to identify abnormalities that will interfere with the course of normal labor and birth. Prenatal care also provides education and support for maternal self-care and parenting and should include the spouse, partner, or significant other.

Pregnancy, or gestation, lasts about 40 weeks or 280 days measured from the last menstrual period, or 266 days from conception. It is often described in terms of *trimesters*. The first trimester lasts from weeks 1 through 13; the second from weeks 14 through 26; and the third from weeks 27 through 40. A pregnancy is considered to be at term if it advances to 37 weeks or more. The focus of this chapter is on the health care needs of the expectant family over the course of pregnancy, which is known as the *prenatal period*.

DIAGNOSIS OF PREGNANCY

Women who are sexually active suspect pregnancy when they miss a menstrual period. Many women come to the first prenatal visit after a positive home pregnancy test; however, in some women the clinical diagnosis of pregnancy before the second missed period is difficult. Physical variations confound even the experienced examiner. Accuracy is important, however, because the emotional, social, health, or legal consequences of an inaccurate diagnosis, either positive or negative, can be serious.

Signs and Symptoms

The physical cues of pregnancy vary; therefore the diagnosis of pregnancy is uncertain for a time. Many of the indicators of pregnancy are clinically useful in the diagnosis of pregnancy and are classified as presumptive, probable, or positive (see Table 13.5).

Estimating Date of Birth

After the diagnosis of pregnancy, the woman's first question is usually when she will give birth. The estimated date of birth (EDB) is determined based on the date of the woman's last normal menstrual period (LMP) and the first accurate ultrasound examination. Accurate dating of pregnancy is vital to promoting a healthy outcome for the woman and fetus. The EDB is important for planning prenatal care, scheduling specific prenatal screening tests, assessing fetal growth, and making critical decisions for managing complications of pregnancy.

The most accurate assessment of the EDB is based on ultrasound measurement of the embryo or fetus during the first trimester of pregnancy (American College of Obstetricians and Gynecologists [ACOG], American Institute of Ultrasound in Medicine [AIUM], & the Society for Maternal-Fetal Medicine [SMFM], 2014).

The Naegele rule is a common method for calculating the EDB. It is based on the woman's accurate recall of her LMP. It assumes that the woman has a 28-day cycle and that fertilization occurred on the 14th day (Box 14.1). Only about 5% of women give birth spontaneously on the EDB as determined by the Naegele rule; most births occur 7 days before to 7 days after the EDB.

ADAPTATION TO PREGNANCY

Pregnancy affects all family members, and each must adapt to the pregnancy and interpret its meaning in light of his or her own needs. This process of family adaptation to pregnancy takes place within a cultural environment influenced by societal trends. Dramatic changes have occurred in Western society in recent years, and the nurse must be prepared to support all families in the childbearing experience, whether they are traditional families, single-parent families, same-sex couples, adoptive families, reconstituted families, and dual-career families.

The family is the best source of information about its beliefs, needs, and concerns. Through effective communication with each family, the nurse can assess its specific needs and use this information as the basis for the plan of care.

Maternal Adaptation

During the months of pregnancy women adapt to the maternal role, a complex process of social and cognitive learning. Early in pregnancy nothing seems to be happening, and a woman may spend much time sleeping due to the increased fatigue during this stage. With the perception of fetal movement in the second trimester, the woman turns her attention inward to her pregnancy and to relationships with her mother and/or other women who have been or who are pregnant.

Pregnancy is a maturational milestone that can be stressful but also rewarding as the woman prepares for a new level of caring and responsibility. Her self-concept changes in readiness for parenthood as she prepares for her new role. She moves gradually from being self-contained and independent to being committed to a lifelong concern for another human being. This growth requires the mastery of certain developmental tasks: accepting the pregnancy, identifying with the role of mother, reordering the relationships between herself and her mother or other significant female and between herself and her partner, establishing a relationship with the unborn child, and preparing for the birth experience. The partner's emotional support is an important factor in successfully accomplishing these developmental tasks. Single women with limited support can have difficulty making this adaptation.

Accepting the Pregnancy

The first step in adapting to the maternal role is accepting the idea of pregnancy and assimilating the pregnant state into the woman's way of life. Mercer (1995) described this process as *cognitive restructuring* and credited Rubin (1975, 1984) with having been the nurse theorist who pioneered our understanding of maternal role attainment. The degree of her acceptance is reflected in the woman's emotional responses. If the pregnancy was unintended, many women may initially be upset to discover that they are pregnant. Eventual acceptance of pregnancy parallels the growing acceptance of the reality of a child. However, nonacceptance of the pregnancy does not equate with rejection of the child, because a woman can dislike being pregnant yet still feel love for the child to be born.

Women who are happy and pleased about their pregnancy often view it as biologic fulfillment and part of their life plan. Despite a general feeling of well-being, many women are surprised to experience *emotional lability*—that is, rapid and unpredictable changes in mood. These swings in emotions and increased sensitivity to others are disconcerting to the expectant mother and those around her. Increased irritability and explosions of tears and anger can alternate with feelings of joy and cheerfulness, apparently with little or no provocation.

Profound hormonal changes that are part of the maternal response to pregnancy can be responsible for such mood changes. Other reasons, such as concerns about finances and changes in lifestyle, contribute to this seemingly erratic behavior.

Most women have ambivalent feelings during pregnancy, whether the pregnancy was intended or not. Ambivalence—having conflicting feelings simultaneously—is considered a normal response in people preparing for a new role. For example, during pregnancy some women feel pleased that they are fulfilling a lifelong dream, but they also feel regret that life as they have known it is ending.

Even women who are pleased to be pregnant can experience feelings of hostility toward the pregnancy or unborn child from time to time. Such incidents as a partner's chance remark about the attractiveness of a slim, nonpregnant woman or news of a colleague's promotion can give rise to ambivalent feelings. Body sensations, feelings of dependence, or the realization of the responsibilities of child care also can generate such feelings.

Intense feelings of ambivalence that persist through the third trimester can indicate an unresolved conflict with the motherhood role (Mercer, 1995). After the birth of a healthy child, memories of these ambivalent feelings are usually dismissed. If the child is born with a defect, however, a woman may look back at the times when she did not want the pregnancy and may believe that her ambivalence caused the birth defect. She will need assurance that her feelings were not responsible for the outcome.

Identifying With the Mother Role

The process of identifying with the mother role begins early in each woman's life when she is being mothered as a child. Her social group's perception of what constitutes the feminine role can subsequently influence her choice between motherhood or a career, being partnered or single, being independent rather than interdependent, or being able to manage multiple roles. Practicing roles—such as playing with dolls, babysitting, and taking care of siblings—can increase her understanding of what being a mother involves.

Many women have always wanted a baby, liked children, and looked forward to motherhood. Their high motivation to become a parent promotes acceptance of pregnancy and eventual prenatal and parental adaptation. Other women have not considered in any detail what motherhood means. During pregnancy these women must resolve conflicts such as not wanting the pregnancy as well as child- or career-related decisions.

Reordering Personal Relationships

Close relationships during pregnancy undergo change as a woman prepares emotionally for her new role as mother. As family members learn their new roles, periods of tension and conflict can arise. An understanding of the typical patterns of adjustment can help the nurse to reassure the pregnant woman that her experiences are normal and explore issues related to social support. Promoting effective communication patterns between the expectant mother and her own mother and between the expectant mother and her partner are common nursing interventions during the prenatal visits.

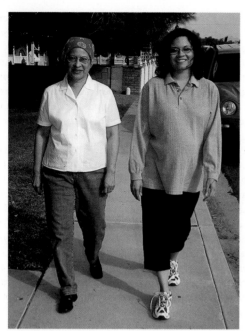

Fig. 14.1 A Pregnant Woman and Her Mother Enjoying a Walk Together. (Courtesy Michael S. Clement, MD, Mesa, AZ.)

The woman's relationship with her mother is significant in adaptation to pregnancy and motherhood. Important components in the pregnant woman's relationship with her mother are the mother's availability (past and present), her reactions to the daughter's pregnancy, respect for her daughter's autonomy, and willingness to reminisce (Mercer, 1995).

The mother's reaction to the daughter's pregnancy signifies her acceptance of the grandchild and of her daughter. If the mother is supportive, the daughter has an opportunity to discuss pregnancy and labor with her mother, who is likely knowledgeable and accepting (Fig. 14.1).

Although the woman's relationship with her mother is significant in considering her adaptation to pregnancy, the most important person to the pregnant woman is usually the father of her child (Fig. 14.2). With same-sex couples, the most important person is the partner. Women express two major needs within this relationship during pregnancy: feeling loved and valued and having the child accepted by the partner.

The marital or committed partner relationship is not static but evolves over time. The addition of a child changes forever the nature of the bond between partners. This can be a time when couples grow closer, and the pregnancy has a maturing effect on the partners' relationship as they assume new roles and discover new aspects of one another. Partners who trust and support each other are able to respond to mutual dependency needs (Mercer, 1995).

Sexual expression during pregnancy is highly individual. The sexual relationship is affected by physical, emotional, and interactional factors as well as the couple's knowledge about sexual activity during pregnancy. During the first trimester the woman's sexual desire usually decreases, especially if she has breast tenderness, nausea, or fatigue. As she progresses into the second trimester, however, her sense of well-being combined with the increased pelvic congestion that occurs at this time often increases her desire for sexual release. In the third trimester, somatic complaints and physical bulkiness can increase her physical discomfort and again diminish her interest in sex.

Partners need to feel free to discuss their sexual needs during pregnancy with one another. It is also important that they discuss their changing sexual responses during pregnancy with their health care provider (HCP) and nurses involved in their care (see later discussion).

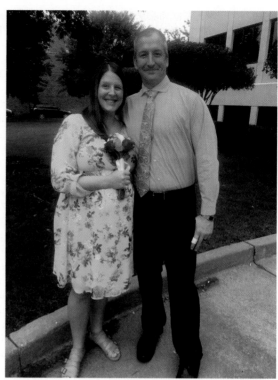

Fig. 14.2 A Pregnant Woman and Her Husband. (Courtesy Amber and Zack Gaynor, Apex, NC.)

Establishing a Relationship With the Fetus

Emotional attachment to the fetus—feelings of being bonded by affection or love—begins during the prenatal period as women use fantasizing and daydreaming to prepare themselves for motherhood (Rubin, 1975, 1984). They think of themselves as mothers and imagine maternal qualities they would like to possess. Expectant parents want to be warm, loving, and close to their child. They try to anticipate changes that the child will bring into their lives and wonder how they will react to noise, disorder, reduced freedom, and caregiving activities. According to Rubin (1975, 1984), the mother-child relationship progresses throughout pregnancy as a developmental process that unfolds in three phases:

- *Phase 1*: The woman accepts the biologic fact of pregnancy. She has to be able to state, "I am pregnant" and to incorporate the idea of a child into her body and self-image. The woman's thoughts center on herself and the reality of her pregnancy. The child is viewed as part of herself, not as a separate and unique person.
- *Phase 2*: The woman accepts the growing fetus as distinct from herself. This is usually accomplished by the 5th month. She can now say, "I am going to have a baby." This differentiation of the child from the woman's self marks the beginning of the mother-child relationship, which involves not only caring but also responsibility. Attachment of a mother to her child is enhanced by experiencing a planned or desired pregnancy, and it increases when ultrasound examination and quickening confirm the reality of the fetus. With acceptance of the reality of the child (hearing the heartbeat and feeling the fetus move) and an overall feeling of well-being, the woman enters a quiet period and becomes more introspective. A fantasy child becomes precious to her. As she seems to withdraw and concentrate her interest on the unborn child, her partner sometimes feels left out. If there are other children in the family, they can become more demanding in their efforts to redirect the mother's attention to themselves.

- *Phase 3*: At this point in the attachment process, the woman prepares realistically for the birth and parenting of the child. She expresses the thought, "I am going to be a mother" and defines the nature and characteristics of the child. She may, for example, speculate about the child's sex (if unknown) and personality traits based on patterns of fetal activity.

Although the mother alone experiences the child within her, both parents and siblings believe that the unborn child responds in a very individualized, personal manner. Family members may interact with the unborn child by talking to the fetus and stroking the mother's abdomen, especially when the fetus shifts position. The fetus may have a nickname used by family members.

Preparing for Birth

Many women actively prepare for birth by reading books and information on various websites, watching videos, attending parenting classes, and talking to other women. They seek advice, monitoring, and caring from the obstetric HCP. The multiparous woman has her own history of labor and birth, which influences her approach to this birth experience.

Anxiety can arise from concern about a safe passage for herself and her child during the birth process (Mercer, 1995; Rubin, 1975, 1984). Some women do not express this concern overtly, but they give cues to the nurse by making plans for care of the new baby and other children in case "anything should happen." Many women fear the pain of labor and birth because they do not understand anatomy and the birth process; they also may fear pain because they are not aware of their options to manage pain. Education by the nurse can alleviate many of these fears.

Toward the end of the third trimester, breathing becomes more difficult and fetal movements become vigorous enough to disturb the woman's sleep. Backaches, frequency and urgency of urination, constipation, and varicose veins can become troublesome. The bulkiness and awkwardness of her body may interfere with the woman's ability to care for other children, perform routine work-related duties, and assume a comfortable position for sleep and rest. By this time most women become impatient for labor to begin, whether the birth is anticipated with joy, dread, or a mixture of both. A strong desire to see the end of pregnancy, to be over and done with it, makes women at this stage ready to move on to birth.

Partner Adaptation

Fathers and nonpregnant partners in childbearing couples reflect on their future role as a parent and adapt to changes in the relationship as they prepare for the arrival of the child and the addition of a new family member. In opposite-sex couples, a father's beliefs and feelings about the ideal mother and father and his cultural expectations of appropriate behavior during pregnancy affect his response to his partner's need for him. One man may engage in nurturing behavior, whereas another may feel lonely and alienated as the woman becomes physically and emotionally engrossed in the unborn child. He may seek friends and relationships outside the home or become interested in a new hobby or involved with his work. Some men view pregnancy as proof of their masculinity and their dominant role. To others, pregnancy has no meaning in terms of responsibility to either mother or child. However, for most, pregnancy is a time of preparation for the parental role and for intense learning. These same kinds of feelings, positive and negative, can also exist in partners in lesbian and gay relationships and can be affected by a lack of recognition and acceptance of the partners' involvement with health care professionals and society in general.

Accepting the Pregnancy

The ways in which fathers adjust to the parental role has been the subject of considerable research. Changing cultural and professional attitudes have encouraged fathers' participation in the birth experience.

A man's emotional response to becoming a father, his concerns, and his informational needs change during pregnancy. May (1982) describes three phases characterizing the developmental tasks experienced by the expectant father:

- *Announcement phase*: The developmental task is to accept the biologic fact of pregnancy. The reaction to the confirmation of pregnancy depends on whether the pregnancy was desired, unplanned, or unwanted. Ambivalence in the early stages of pregnancy is common. Some men respond with joy, others find the alterations in their life plans difficult to accept. Battering may occur for the first time or increase in frequency (see Chapter 5 and later discussion in this chapter).
- *Moratorium phase*: The developmental task is to accept the reality of pregnancy. Men often become more introspective and engage in many discussions about their philosophy of life, religion, childbearing, and child-rearing practices and their relationships with family members, particularly with their own fathers.
- *Focusing phase*: The developmental task is to negotiate with his partner the role he is to play in labor and in preparing for parenthood. In this phase the man concentrates on his experience of the pregnancy and begins to think of himself as a father.

Identifying With the Parent Role

Partners bring to pregnancy attitudes that affect the way in which they adjust to the pregnancy and the parental role. Memories of the parenting they received, the experiences they have had with child care, and the perceptions of the parent role within their social group will guide their selection of the tasks and responsibilities they will assume. Some are highly motivated to nurture and love a child and are excited and pleased about the anticipated role of parent. Others are more detached or even hostile to the idea of parenthood.

Reordering Personal Relationships

The partner's main role in pregnancy is to nurture and respond to the pregnant woman's feelings of vulnerability. The partner also must deal with the reality of the pregnancy. The partner's support indicates involvement in the pregnancy and preparation for attachment to the child.

Some aspects of a partner's behavior can indicate rivalry, and this can be especially evident during sexual activity. However, feelings of rivalry are often unconscious and not verbalized but expressed in more subtle behaviors. The woman's increased introspection can cause her partner to feel uneasy as she becomes preoccupied with thoughts of the child and of her motherhood, her growing dependence on her HCP, and her reevaluation of the couple's relationship.

Establishing a Relationship With the Fetus

The nonpregnant partner's parent-child attachment can be as strong as the mother-child relationship; partners can be as competent as mothers at nurturing their infants. The parent-child attachment also begins during pregnancy. A partner may rub or kiss the maternal abdomen; try to listen, talk, or sing to the fetus; or play with the moving fetus. Calling the unborn child by name or nickname helps to confirm the reality of pregnancy and promotes attachment.

Partners prepare for parenting in many of the same ways as mothers do. Daydreaming about their role as parent is common in the last weeks before the birth, and they should be reassured that such daydreams are normal.

Nurses can help fathers and nonpregnant partners identify concerns and prepare for the reality of a baby by asking questions such as these:

- How do you expect the baby to look and act?
- How do you envision life as a parent?

- How will you be involved in helping to care for the baby?
- How will having a baby affect your relationship with your partner? As the birth date approaches, partners may have more questions about fetal and newborn behaviors. If an expectant partner can imagine only an older child and has difficulty visualizing or talking about an infant, this situation must be explored. The nurse can tell partners about the unborn child's ability to respond to light, sound, and touch and encourage them to feel and talk to the fetus. Discussions with other new parents, as in childbirth classes, may be welcomed.

Some partners become involved by choosing the child's name and anticipating the child's sex if it is not already known. Family tradition, religious customs, and the continuation of the parent's name or names of relatives or friends are important in the selection process.

Preparing for Birth

The days and weeks immediately before the expected day of birth are characterized by anticipation and anxiety. Boredom and restlessness are common as the couple focus on the birth process; however, during the last 2 months of pregnancy, many expectant parents experience a surge of creative energy at home and on the job. They tend to act on the need to alter the environment by remodeling or painting. This activity is their way of sharing in the childbearing experience. They can channel the anxiety and other feelings experienced during the final weeks before birth into productive activities. This behavior earns recognition and compliments from friends, relatives, and the expectant mother.

Major concerns for the father or nonpregnant partner are getting the mother to a health care facility in time for the birth and not appearing ignorant. Many partners want to be able to recognize labor and determine when it will be appropriate to leave for the hospital or call the health care provider.

Some prospective parents have questions about the labor suite's furniture and equipment, nursing staff, and location as well as the availability of the obstetric and anesthesia care providers. Others want to know what will be expected of them when their partners are in labor. The father or nonpregnant partner may also have fears concerning safe passage of the child and safety of the partner and the possible death or complications of the partner and child. It is important that there should be opportunities to verbalize these fears; otherwise the partner will not be able to help the mother deal with her spoken or unspoken apprehensions.

Adaptation to Pregnancy for Same-Sex Couples

Pregnancy is becoming increasingly more common among couples who are lesbian, gay, bisexual, transgender, or queer (LGBTQ). Health care professionals in maternity care are most likely to encounter lesbian couples where one of the women carries the pregnancy. There are several methods to achieve a pregnancy. One woman can be artificially inseminated and conceive a child who is genetically related to her. The fertilized egg of one partner can be implanted into the uterus of the other, who then carries the pregnancy. Alternatively, one woman can be implanted with the fertilized egg from a donor, so that the child is not biologically related to either partner (Bushe & Romero, 2017). In some cases, both women attempt conception to increase the couple's chances of a successful pregnancy (Carpinello, Jacob, Nulson, & Benadiva, 2016). The birth mother may be the one to carry the baby because of a greater desire to experience the pregnancy and birth and to be genetically related to the child. Other factors that influence the decision are age, health, infertility, and career considerations. Some lesbian couples who wish to become parents use a surrogate to carry the pregnancy, or they may adopt.

Same-sex couples who choose to be parents may also be gay men who partner with a surrogate to carry the pregnancy. In traditional surrogacy, the egg donor and the surrogate are the same woman. The egg donor and surrogate may be two different women or one woman who serves as both. Sperm from one or both male partners or from a sperm bank may be used. Conception may occur through artificial insemination or in vitro fertilization. Compensated surrogacy as a path to parenthood for gay couples is against the law in many states but changes are occurring. New laws are being enacted that protect both the parenting couple and the surrogate mothers. Still, legal challenges persist that must be considered, which adds additional stress to the adaptation process for these families.

There are other possibilities for pregnancy in a same-sex male couple. A transgender man in a gay couple may become pregnant. Alternatively, a lesbian and gay couple may collaborate to conceive and coparent a child (or children).

The same fears, questions, and concerns may affect birth partners who are not the biologic fathers or who are the nonpregnant partner in a same-sex couple. Much attention is paid to the needs of the pregnant partner, but the nonpregnant partner's needs receive less attention. For example, in lesbian couples, the nonpregnant female partner—who may be referred to as the "comother," "other mother," "nonbiologic mother," "coparent," or other term as desired by the couple—can feel excluded by the heterocentric and homophobic attitudes and actions of health care professionals (Gregg, 2018). Nonpregnant partners will be better prepared for the changes that come with pregnancy and parenting if they are included and considered in the process. In addition to dealing with their own feelings and the care of their partner or surrogate mother, nonpregnant partners in a lesbian or gay relationship are often not acknowledged or accepted as parents-to-be from within their own families and in society in general. Partners need to be kept informed, supported, and included in all activities in which the pregnant partner desires their participation (Bushe & Romero, 2017). Health care professionals can do much to promote pregnancy and birth as a family experience by providing the same quality of care they provide to heterosexual couples, establishing trusting relationships with the couple, and avoiding heteronormative attitudes (Cook, Gunter, & Lopez, 2017). They can provide information about resources for same-sex parents such as community and online support groups.

Sibling Adaptation

Sharing the spotlight with a new brother or sister can be the first major crisis for a child. Some of the factors that influence the child's response are age, the parents' attitudes, the roles of the parents, length of separation from the mother, the facility's visitation policy, and the way the child has been prepared for the new baby and the associated changes at home.

A mother with other children must devote time and effort to reorganizing her relationships with them. She has to prepare siblings for the baby's birth and begin the process of role transition in the family by including the children in the pregnancy and being sympathetic to older children's concerns about losing their places in the family hierarchy. Some parents take their children to sibling classes to help prepare them for the birth and the experience of visiting in the birth facility (Fig. 14.3). Siblings' responses to pregnancy vary with their age and dependency needs (Box 14.2). The 1-year-old infant seems largely unaware of the process, but the 2-year-old child notices the change in his or her mother's appearance. Toddlers' need for sameness in the environment makes children aware of any change. They can exhibit more clinging behavior and sometimes regress in toilet training or eating.

By 3 or 4 years of age, children like to be told the story of their own beginning and accept a comparison of their own development with that of the present pregnancy. They like to listen to the fetal heartbeat and feel the baby moving in utero (Fig. 14.4).

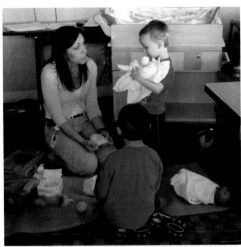

Fig. 14.3 A Preschooler in a Sibling Class Learns About Childbirth and Infant Care Using Dolls and a Bunny. (Courtesy Julie and Darren Nelson, Loveland, CO.)

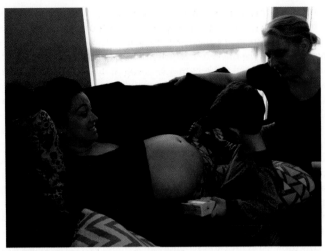

Fig. 14.4 Three-year old using doppler to hear fetal heart. (Courtesy Chelsea Lindblad, San Tan Valley, AZ.)

BOX 14.2   Sibling Adaptation: Tips for Sibling Preparation

Prenatal

- Take your child on a prenatal visit. Let the child listen to the fetal heartbeat and feel the baby move.
- Involve the child in preparations for the baby, such as helping decorate the baby's room.
- Move the child to a bed (if still sleeping in a crib) at least 2 months before the baby is due.
- Read books, show videos or DVDs, and/or take your child to sibling preparation classes, including a hospital tour.
- Answer your child's questions about the coming birth, what babies are like, and any other questions.
- Take your child to the homes of friends who have babies so that the child has realistic expectations of what babies are like.

During the Hospital Stay

- Have someone bring the child to the hospital to visit you and the baby (or plan to have the child attend the birth).
- When the child arrives, make sure your arms are open to embrace the child.
- Do not force interactions between the child and the baby. Often the child will be more interested in seeing you and being reassured of your love.
- Help the child explore the infant by showing how and where to touch the baby.
- Give the child a gift (from you, the father or your partner, and the baby).

Going Home

- Leave the child at home with a relative or babysitter or have someone such as the grandmother available to focus on the child during hospital discharge and on the trip home.
- Have someone else carry the baby from the car so that you can hug the child first.

Adjustment After the Baby Is Home

- Arrange for a special time for the child to be alone with each parent.
- Do not exclude the child during infant feeding times. The child can sit with you and the baby and feed a doll or drink juice or milk or sit quietly with a game. You can read aloud to the child while you are feeding the infant.
- Prepare small gifts for the child so that when the baby gets gifts, the sibling will not feel left out. The child can also help open the baby's gifts.
- Praise the child for acting appropriately for age (so that being a baby does not seem better than being older).

School-age children take a more clinical interest in their mother's pregnancy. They may want to know in more detail, "How did the baby get in there?" and "How will it get out?" Overall, they look forward to the new baby, see themselves as "mothers" or "fathers," and enjoy buying baby supplies and readying a place for the baby.

Early and middle adolescents preoccupied with the establishment of their own sexual identity can have difficulty accepting the overwhelming evidence of the sexual activity of their parents. Many pregnant women with teenage children will confess that the attitudes of their teenagers are the most difficult aspect of their current pregnancy.

Late adolescents do not appear to be unduly disturbed. They are busy making plans for their own lives and realize that they soon will be gone from home. Parents usually report that these older children are comforting and act more like other adults than as children.

Grandparent Adaptation

Most grandparents are delighted at the prospect of a new baby in the family. It reawakens the feelings of their own youth, the excitement of giving birth, and their delight in the behavior of the parents-to-be as infants themselves. They set up a memory store of the child's first smiles, first words, and first steps that they can use later for "claiming" the newborn as a member of the family. These behaviors provide a link between the past and present for the parents and grandparents-to-be.

In addition, the grandparent is the historian who transmits the family history, a resource person who shares knowledge based on experience; a role model; and a support person. The grandparent's presence and support can strengthen family systems by widening the circle of support and nurturance.

Unfortunately, not all grandparents are excited about their new role. For some expectant grandparents, a first pregnancy in a child is undeniable evidence that they are growing older. Many people think of a grandparent as old, white-haired, and becoming feeble of mind and body; however, some face grandparenthood while still in their 30s or 40s. Some individuals react negatively to the news that they will be grandparents, indicating that they are not ready for the new role. In some family units, expectant grandparents are nonsupportive and can inadvertently decrease the self-esteem of the parents-to-be.

CARE MANAGEMENT

Prenatal care occurs in physician or midwifery offices, public health or hospital clinics, or in the patient's home. Physicians, certified nurse- midwives (CNM), nurse practitioners, physician assistants, public health nurses, registered dieticians, childbirth educators, maternal-fetal medicine specialists, and other health care professionals may be part of the interprofessional health care team. Psychiatric care providers and social workers may be involved if the woman has mental health conditions such as a history of depression. The team works collaboratively to provide care that optimizes pregnancy outcomes (Gregory, Ramos, & Jauniaux, 2017).

The goal of prenatal care is to promote the health and well-being of the pregnant woman, her fetus, the newborn, and the family. It includes education about healthy lifestyle behaviors such as nutrition and physical activity, self-care for the common pregnancy discomforts, and information about changes in the mother and growth of the developing fetus. Routine screening is offered during pregnancy to help identify existing risk factors and potential problems so that efforts to reduce risk of harm to mother or baby and management of identified conditions can be initiated at the earliest opportunity. Major emphasis is placed on preventive aspects of care, primarily to support the pregnant woman in self-management between visits with health care professionals and to help her recognize and report changes that can signal problems early so that adverse effects for her or her fetus can be prevented or minimized. If health behaviors must be modified in early pregnancy, nurses must understand the psychosocial factors that can influence the woman. In holistic care, nurses provide information and guidance about the physical changes and psychosocial impact of pregnancy on the woman and members of her family. The goals of prenatal nursing care, therefore, are to foster a safe birth for the mother and infant and to promote satisfaction of the mother and family with the pregnancy and birth experience.

According to the National Center for Health Statistics, 77.3% of women in the United States in 2017 received pregnancy care in the first trimester and 6.3% began prenatal care in the third trimester or had no prenatal care at all. Women who were least likely to begin first-trimester prenatal care were non-Hispanic Native Hawaiian/Other Pacific Islanders (19.6%) (Martin, Hamilton, Osterman, et al., 2018).

Although women of middle or high socioeconomic status routinely seek prenatal care, women's reasons for delaying prenatal care include cost, lack of insurance, lack of child care, transportation barriers, or inability to take time off from work. Lack of culturally sensitive care providers, discrimination based on sexual orientation, and barriers to communication resulting from differences in language also interfere with access to care. Likewise, immigrant women who come from cultures in which prenatal care is not emphasized may not know that routine prenatal care is expected. Birth outcomes in these populations are less positive, with higher rates of maternal and fetal or newborn complications. Low birth weight (LBW; <2500 g) and infant mortality are associated with lack of adequate prenatal care.

The availability of CNMs as independent providers of care or in collaborative practice with physicians improves the availability and accessibility of prenatal care (American College of Nurse-Midwives [ACNM], 2012). A regular schedule of home visits by nurses helps in reducing barriers to care and contributes to improved maternal and infant outcomes (Meghea, You, Raffo, et al., 2015; Olds, Kitzman, Knudtson, et al., 2014; Roman, Raffo, Zhu, & Meghea, 2014).

The traditional model for provision of prenatal care has been used for more than a century. The initial visit usually occurs in the first trimester, with monthly visits through week 28 of pregnancy. Thereafter, visits are scheduled every 2 weeks until week 36 and then every week until birth. The trend is toward individualizing the schedule of care. Women with low-risk pregnancies may have fewer routine prenatal visits, whereas those at risk for complications may be seen more frequently than the traditional schedule would suggest (American Academy of Pediatrics [AAP] and ACOG, 2017) (Box 14.3).

BOX 14.3 Prenatal Visit Schedule

Traditional[a]	Centering Pregnancy[b]
• First visit within the first trimester (12 weeks)	• First visit within the first trimester (12 weeks)
• Monthly visits weeks 16 through 28	• Every 4 weeks—weeks 16 to 28
• Every 2 weeks from weeks 29 to 36	• Every 2 weeks—weeks 29 to 40
• Weekly visits week 36 to birth	

[a]Frequency of visits may be decreased in low-risk women and increased in women with high-risk pregnancies.
[b]Additional individual visits may be added as needed.
Data from Centering Healthcare Institute. (2016). *Centering Pregnancy.* Retrieved from: https://www.centeringhealthcare.org/what-we-do/centering-pregnancy.

Group prenatal care is an alternative model to traditional care during pregnancy. In group prenatal care, authority is shifted from the provider to the woman and other women who have similar due dates. The model creates an atmosphere that facilitates learning, encourages discussion, and develops mutual support. CenteringPregnancy (www.centeringhealthcare.org) is a well-known model of group prenatal care that involves three components: health care assessment, education, and peer support. Groups consist of 8 to 12 women at similar gestational ages who participate in 10 sessions lasting about 90 minutes each (see Box 14.3). At each meeting, the first 30 to 40 minutes consist of assessments (by the woman herself and by the HCP) and the remaining 60 to 75 minutes are spent in guided education and group discussion of specific issues such as the discomforts of pregnancy and preparation for labor and birth. Families and partners are encouraged to participate (Centering Healthcare Institute, 2019). Benefits associated with group prenatal care include improved birth outcomes such as lower rates of preterm birth, increased knowledge, improved satisfaction, and higher rates of breastfeeding initiation (Fiset, Hoffman, & Ehrenthal, 2016; Heberlein, Picklesimer, Billings, et al., 2016). Prenatal care is an interprofessional model in which nurses work with physicians, CNMs, registered dietitians, social workers, and others to provide holistic client-centered care. Maternity care coordination programs facilitate collaboration and shared decision making among the health care team, promoting continuity of care, providing maternal education, and making appropriate referrals. The nurse case manager is a key player in this model of care (Kroll-Desrosiers, Crawford, Moore Simas, et al., 2016)

In recent years the concept of preconception care has been recognized as an important contributor to positive pregnancy outcomes (see Chapter 4). If women can be taught healthy lifestyle behaviors and then practice them before conception—specifically good nutrition, entering pregnancy with as healthy a weight as possible, adequate intake of folic acid, avoidance of alcohol and other substances, and prevention of sexually transmitted infections (STIs) and other health hazards—the chance of having a healthier pregnancy is increased. Likewise, women who have chronic diseases such as diabetes mellitus can be counseled regarding their special needs with the intent of minimizing maternal and fetal complications.

Initial Visit

Once pregnancy has been confirmed and the woman's desire to continue the pregnancy has been validated, prenatal care begins. The assessment process begins at the initial prenatal visit and is continued throughout the pregnancy. Assessment techniques include the interview, physical examination, and laboratory tests. Because the initial visit and follow-up visits are distinctly different in content and process, they are described separately.

Prenatal Interview

The therapeutic relationship between the nurse and the woman is ideally established during the initial assessment interview. During this interview the nurse makes an effort to gain the woman's trust.

The pregnant woman and family members who are present should be told that the first prenatal visit is longer and more detailed than future visits. The initial evaluation includes a comprehensive health history emphasizing the current pregnancy, previous pregnancies, the family, a psychosocial profile, a physical assessment, diagnostic testing, and an overall risk assessment.

One or more family members often accompany the pregnant woman. With the woman's permission, the nurse includes those accompanying the woman in the initial prenatal interview. Observations and information about the woman's family is then included in the database. For example, if the woman has small children with her, the nurse can ask about plans for child care during the time of labor and birth. The nurse notes any special needs that are identified during this first interview (e.g., wheelchair access, assistance in getting on and off the examining table, difficulty speaking and/or understanding English, and cognitive deficits).

Reasons for seeking care. Although pregnant women are scheduled for routine prenatal visits, they often come to the HCP seeking information or reassurance about a concern. When the woman is asked a broad open-ended question such as, "How have you been feeling?" she may reveal problems that could otherwise be overlooked. The woman's chief concerns should be recorded in her own words to alert other personnel to the priority of needs as identified by her. At the initial visit the desire for information about what is normal during pregnancy is typical.

Current pregnancy. The signs of pregnancy, such as nausea and vomiting, can be of great concern to the woman. A review of symptoms she is experiencing and how she is coping with them helps establish a database to develop a plan of care. Some early teaching may be provided at this time.

Childbearing and female reproductive system history. Data are gathered on the woman's age at menarche, menstrual history, and contraceptive history; any infertility or reproductive system conditions; history of STIs; sexual history; and detailed history of all her pregnancies, including the present pregnancy, and their outcomes. The date of the last Papanicolaou (Pap) test and the result are noted. The date of her LMP is obtained to calculate the EDB.

Health history. The health history includes physical conditions or surgical procedures that can affect the pregnancy or that can be affected by the pregnancy. For example, a pregnant woman who has diabetes, hypertension, or epilepsy requires special care. A careful history of any allergies and the type of reaction, medication use, and immunizations must be included. Women may be anxious during the initial interview, the nurse may need to prompt the woman to recall allergies, chronic diseases, or medications (prescription and over-the-counter [OTC]) or herbal supplements being taken. In addition, the health history of the father of the baby is needed in an effort to identify conditions that can affect the fetus.

If a woman has undergone uterine surgery or extensive repair of the pelvic floor, a cesarean birth may be necessary; appendectomy rules out appendicitis as a cause of right lower quadrant pain in pregnancy; and spinal surgery may contraindicate the use of spinal or epidural anesthesia. Information about trauma involving the pelvis as from a motor vehicle accident or fall is relevant.

Women who have chronic or disabling conditions often forget to mention them during the initial assessment because they have become so adapted to them. The nurse asks about such conditions with sensitivity to obtain data that will enhance a comprehensive nursing care plan. Observations are vital components of the interview process because they prompt the nurse and woman to focus on the specific needs of the woman and her family.

Nutritional history. The woman's nutritional history is an important component of the prenatal history because her nutritional status has a direct effect on the growth and development of the fetus. A dietary assessment can reveal special dietary practices, food allergies, eating behaviors, the practice of pica (the consumption of nonfood substances, such as dirt or clay), and other factors related to her nutritional status that may place her or her fetus at risk (see Box 15.2). Body mass index (BMI) should be calculated on all women at the first prenatal visit to provide the basis for counseling about weight gain, physical activity, and healthy food choices (see Chapter 15). Referral to a registered dietitian is recommended for women with specific nutritional issues, including obesity, multiple gestation, inadequate weight gain, adolescent pregnancy, food allergies or intolerances, diabetes, eating disorders, history of LBW infants, and social factors such as poverty, which limit nutritional intake (West, Hark, & Catalano, 2017).

History of medication and herbal preparation use. The prenatal history includes past and current use of prescription and over-the-counter medications; vitamin supplements such as A, C, D, and E; herbal preparations; caffeine; alcohol; tobacco and other drugs (e.g., marijuana, cocaine, heroin). Many substances cross the placenta and can pose a risk to the developing fetus. See Chapter 31 for a discussion of substance use during pregnancy. Increasing numbers of individuals are using herbal preparations, and this includes pregnant women. Information about allergies to medications and the type of reaction should also be obtained and recorded in the health record.

The immunization record should be reviewed for vaccinations including rubella (German measles), varicella (chickenpox), seasonal influenza, hepatitis B, and pertussis (whooping cough) that can pose a risk to pregnant women or their infants during pregnancy and immediately following birth. Recommendations for vaccinations during the perinatal period are discussed later in this chapter.

Family history. The family history provides information about the woman's immediate family, including parents, siblings, and children. These data help identify familial or genetic disorders or conditions that could affect the health status of the woman or her fetus. The family history of the woman's partner (if the partner is the father of the baby) is important in identifying risk factors that can affect fetal well-being.

Social, experiential, and occupational history. Situational factors such as the family's ethnic and cultural background and socioeconomic status are assessed while the history is being obtained. The woman's perception of this pregnancy is explored by asking questions that focus on the following issues:

- Was this pregnancy planned or unintended? Is it desired or wanted?
- Is the woman pleased, displeased, accepting, or nonaccepting?
- Will any changes related to finances, career, or living accommodations occur because of the pregnancy?

The nurse assesses the family and social support system by asking the mother about the following areas:

- What primary support is available to her?
- What are the existing relationships among the mother, father or partner, siblings, and expectant grandparents?
- What preparations are being made for her care and that of dependent family members during labor and for the care of the infant after birth?
- Is financial, educational, or other support needed from the community?
- What are the woman's ideas about childbearing, her expectations of the infant's behavior, and her outlook on life and the maternal role?

Other questions can provide perspective on the woman's perceptions about becoming a mother. Examples of such questions to explore include these:

- What does the woman think it will be like to have a baby in the family?
- How is her life going to change by having a baby?
- How prepared does she feel for becoming a mother?

During interviews throughout the pregnancy, nurses should remain alert to the appearance of potential parenting problems, such as depression, lack of family support, and inadequate living conditions. Nurses assess the woman's attitude toward health care, particularly during childbearing, her expectations of HCPs, and her view of the relationship between herself and the nurse.

Early in the pregnancy the nurse should assess the woman's knowledge in various areas: pregnancy, maternal changes, fetal growth, and self-care. As pregnancy progresses the nurse explores the woman's concerns and desires related to labor and birth as well as her understanding of newborn care and parenting and her plan for infant feeding (breast or formula). It is important to ask about her attitudes toward unmedicated or medicated labor and birth and about her knowledge of the availability of parenting skills classes. Before planning for nursing care, the nurse will obtain information about the woman's decision-making abilities and lifestyle (i.e., exercise, sleep, diet, recreational interests, personal hygiene, and clothing). Common concerns that can be sources of stress during childbearing include the baby's welfare, the labor and birth process, behaviors of the newborn, the woman's relationships with her partner and her family, changes in body image, and physical symptoms.

The nurse explores attitudes concerning the range of safe sexual behavior during pregnancy by asking questions such as, "What have you been told about sex during pregnancy?" To gain insight into the woman's sexual self-concept, the nurse can ask questions such as, "How do you feel about the changes in your appearance? How does your partner feel about your body now? How do you feel about wearing maternity clothes?"

Women are questioned regarding their employment—past and present—because this can affect maternal and fetal health. For some women, heavy lifting and exposure to chemicals and radiation are part of their daily work. Standing for long periods at a retail checkout line or in front of a classroom is associated with orthostatic hypotension. For others, long hours of sitting at a desk working on a computer can contribute to carpal tunnel syndrome or circulatory stasis in the legs.

Mental health screening. As part of routine prenatal care, all women should be assessed and screened for mental health issues. Perinatal depression is the most common complication of pregnancy; if untreated, it can have serious adverse effects on the mother, her newborn, and her family. ACOG (2015b) recommends screening for depression and anxiety symptoms at least once during the perinatal period using a standardized, validated instrument such as the Patient Health Questionnaire 9 (PHQ-9) or the Edinburgh Postnatal Depression Scale. Appropriate follow-up and treatment, including referral to mental HCPs, is essential whenever there is a positive screen. Women are usually unlikely to initiate discussions with health care professionals related to mental health concerns, but they may be more willing to disclose issues and concerns when they are informed that the screening is part of routine prenatal care, when health care professionals are interested and sensitive, and when they are informed about the prevalence of mental health conditions during the perinatal period (Kingston, Austin, & Heaman, 2015). When mental health conditions are identified, appropriate referral and follow-up are needed. Risk factors for depression or anxiety during pregnancy include lack of support from partner, inadequate social support, history of intimate partner violence (IPV), personal history of mental illness, unintended pregnancy, pregnancy complications or loss, and stressful life events (Biaggi, Conroy, Pawlby, & Pariante, 2016).

History or risk of intimate partner violence. IPV—also known as battering, domestic abuse, or domestic violence—occurs in as many as 20% of pregnancies (AAP & ACOG, 2017) (see Chapter 5). Women are unlikely to initiate conversation with health care professionals about IPV; therefore it is critical that routine screening be done. ACOG recommends screening for IPV at the first prenatal visit, at least once every trimester, and at the postpartum visit (ACOG, 2012). It is essential that the screening be done in a safe, private setting with the woman alone (Association of Women's Health, Obstetric, and Neonatal Nurses [AWHONN], 2015). A simple and widely used tool is the Abuse Assessment Screen consisting of five items with a diagram for the abused woman to mark areas where she has been injured (McFarlane, Parker, & Bullock, 1992).

Nurses can ask the woman screening questions with routine assessments during pregnancy. Examples of questions that might be asked include the following:

- Are you with a spouse or partner who threatens or physically hurts you? If yes, who?
- Within the past year or in this pregnancy, has anyone hit, slapped, kicked, or otherwise hurt you? If yes, who? Are you currently with that person?
- Has anyone forced you to engage in sexual activities that made you uncomfortable? If yes, who? Are you currently with that person?

A pregnant woman is often accompanied by her partner to the prenatal appointment, especially if the woman does not speak English and the partner does. An interpreter is needed who is part of the staff or from a telecommunication service so that the woman can be interviewed alone.

If a woman discloses IPV, the first step is to assess for immediate danger and to act to protect the woman and her children if needed. A complete physical examination is needed to assess for injuries and to observe the woman's behaviors and verbal responses when asked about the various injuries (Bianchi, Cesario, & McFarlane, 2016). The next step is to provide the woman with resources to help her to formulate a safety plan (see Chapter 5).

Nurses should be aware that victims of human trafficking can be seen in prenatal settings because of unintended pregnancy. Like victims of IPV, these women may have signs of physical abuse or neglect such as scars, bruises, burns, unusual bald patches, or tattoos that can be a sign of branding. Such a woman may be accompanied by someone who never leaves her alone and speaks for her. She may not speak English and may lack identification documents. If the woman is alone, she may have her cell phone on and in speaker mode so that the person on the other end can hear everything that is said during the visit. Nurses and other HCPs must be creative in getting the woman alone for questioning. Strategies might include sending the other person to the front desk to fill out paperwork, interviewing the woman in the restroom, or telling her she needs to go for testing and cannot take her cell phone. With the consent of a suspected or confirmed victim of human trafficking, an intervention plan can be developed. An excellent resource is the National Human Trafficking Resource Center (https://polarisproject.org/get-assistance/national-human-trafficking-hotline; see Chapter 5).

Review of systems. During this portion of the interview the woman is asked to identify and describe current problems in any of her body systems, and her mental status is assessed. Pregnancy affects and is affected by all body systems; therefore information on the status of the body systems is important in planning care. For each symptom described, the following additional data should be obtained: onset, location, duration, characteristics, aggravating or relieving factors, treatments she has used and their effectiveness, and associated symptoms that occur with the primary symptom.

Physical Examination

The initial physical examination provides the baseline for assessing subsequent changes. The nurse should determine the woman's need for basic information regarding reproductive anatomy and provide this information, along with a demonstration of the equipment that may be used and an explanation of the procedure itself. The interaction requires an unhurried, sensitive, and gentle approach with a matter-of-fact attitude. Each examiner develops a routine for proceeding with the physical examination; most choose the head-to-toe progression. The nurse can coach the woman in breathing and relaxation techniques as needed. See Chapter 4 for a detailed description of the physical examination.

At each prenatal visit, blood pressure (BP) should be measured in the same arm and with the woman in a seated position with her back and arm supported. The upper arm should be at the level of the right atrium. The woman's position and that of the arm should be recorded along with the reading. If the BP is elevated, the woman should be given time to rest, after which the BP assessment can be repeated (Box 14.4).

Laboratory Tests

Laboratory data provide important information concerning the symptoms of pregnancy and the woman's health status. Urine, cervical, and blood samples are routinely obtained during the initial visit for a variety of recommended screening and diagnostic tests for infectious diseases and metabolic conditions that can affect the mother and/or developing fetus. (see Table 14.1.) Women should receive information about the various tests and the purpose of each and be given the opportunity to opt out of testing. Every pregnant woman should receive human immunodeficiency virus (HIV) risk-reduction counseling and be notified that she will be tested for antibody to HIV as part of routine prenatal testing unless she declines (AAP & ACOG, 2017; ACOG, 2015c; CDC, 2015) (Box 14.5). If the woman refuses testing for HIV, this should be documented. The Centers for Disease Control and Prevention recommend testing during the first prenatal visit for syphilis and hepatitis B. Screening for chlamydia and gonorrhea is done for women less than 25 years of age and those older than 25 years who are at risk (CDC). Screening for HIV, syphilis, chlamydia, and gonorrhea is repeated in the third trimester for women who are at high risk for contracting these infections. A Mantoux tuberculin skin test may be administered to assess exposure to tuberculosis in women who are high risk (AAP & ACOG). The urine is tested for protein, glucose, and leukocytes; urine culture may be done if indicated. A Pap test is performed during the pelvic exam if one is due based on current cervical cancer screening guidelines. In addition, pregnant couples with certain ancestry or a family history of various genetically linked disorders may choose to undergo genetic testing (see Chapter 3). Antenatal testing for risk factors in pregnancy is discussed in Chapter 26.

Follow-Up Visits

The timing of follow-up visits varies according to the model of care and the individual needs of the pregnant woman. The pattern of interviewing the woman first and then assessing physical changes and performing laboratory tests continues. Client education is part of every prenatal visit.

Interview

Follow-up visits are briefer and less intensive than the initial prenatal visit. At each follow-up visit, the woman is asked to summarize relevant events that have occurred since the previous visit. She is asked about her emotional and physical well-being and any concerns, problems, and questions she may have. Family needs are also identified and explored.

BOX 14.4 Procedure for Blood Pressure Measurement

- Measure BP with the woman seated comfortably with back and arm supported or in the lateral recumbent position, with the arm at heart level. If she is seated, the woman's feet should be planted on a firm surface and her legs uncrossed.
- Allow a period of rest (at least 5 min) before assessing BP.
- Use the right arm each time. Measure BP over the brachial artery whenever possible.
- Use the proper-size cuff. The ideal cuff has as bladder length that is 80% of the arm circumference and a width that is 40% of the arm circumference.
- Use both Korotkoff phase IV (muffling of sound) and phase V (disappearance of sound) for recording the diastolic value.
- Use measurement devices that have been validated and calibrated according to manufacturer guidelines.

BP, Blood pressure.
Data from Sibai, B. (2017). Preeclampsia and hypertensive disorders. In S.G. Gabbe, J.R. Niebyl, J.L. Simpson, et al. (Eds.). Obstetrics: Normal and problem pregnancies (7th ed.). Philadelphia: Elsevier; Witcher, P.M. (2017). Caring for the laboring woman with hypertensive disorders complicating pregnancy. In B.B. Kennedy & S.M. Baird (Eds.). Intrapartum management modules (5th ed.). Philadelphia: Wolters Kluwer.

Emotional changes are common during pregnancy; therefore it is reasonable to ask whether the woman has experienced any mood swings, reactions to changes in her body image, bad dreams, or worries. In addition, the nurse inquires about reactions of the partner and family members to the pregnancy.

During the third trimester it is important to assess current family situations and their effect on the woman as well as siblings' and grandparents' responses to the pregnancy and the coming child. This is a time to assess the woman and her family's knowledge of warning signs of emergencies, signs of preterm and term labor, the labor process and concerns about labor, and fetal development and methods to assess fetal well-being. The nurse should ask if the woman is planning to attend childbirth preparation classes and what she knows about the management of discomfort during labor.

A review of the woman's physical systems is appropriate at each prenatal visit, and any concerning symptoms are assessed in depth. The review of systems includes identifying any discomforts that may be related to adaptations to pregnancy. The nurse asks about success with self-care measures and outcomes of prescribed therapy.

Physical Examination

Reevaluation is a constant in a pregnant woman's care. Physiologic changes are documented as the pregnancy progresses and reviewed for possible deviations from normal progress. At each visit physical parameters are measured. The woman's BP and weight are assessed, and the appropriateness of the gestational weight gain is evaluated in relation to her BMI. Urine may be checked by dipstick, and the presence and degree of edema are noted. For examination of the abdomen, the woman lies on her back with her arms by her side and head supported by a pillow. A small wedge is placed under her right hip to tilt her slightly to the left. Abdominal inspection is followed by measurement of the height of the fundus (see Fig. 14.6 later in chapter). During each examination, the nurse must remain alert for supine hypotension—low BP that occurs while the woman is lying on her back (see Emergency box).

The information provided through the interview and the physical examination reflects the status of maternal adaptations. When any of the findings are outside the expected range, an in-depth examination is performed.

TABLE 14.1   Laboratory Tests in the Prenatal Period

Laboratory Test	Purpose
Hemoglobin, hematocrit, WBCs, differential	Detects anemia and infection
Hemoglobin electrophoresis	Identifies women with hemoglobinopathies (e.g., sickle cell anemia, thalassemia)
Blood type, Rh, and irregular antibody	Identifies women whose fetuses are at risk for developing erythroblastosis fetalis or hyperbilirubinemia in the neonatal period
Rubella titer	Determines immunity to rubella
Tuberculin skin testing; chest film after 20 weeks of gestation in women with reactive tuberculin tests	Screens for exposure to tuberculosis
Urinalysis, including microscopic examination of urinary sediment; pH, specific gravity, color, glucose, albumin, protein, RBCs, WBCs, casts, acetone; hCG	Identifies women with glycosuria, renal disease, hypertensive disease of pregnancy; infection; occult hematuria; hCG for confirmation of pregnancy
Urine culture	Identifies women with asymptomatic bacteriuria
Renal function tests: BUN, creatinine, electrolytes, creatinine clearance, total protein excretion	Evaluates level of possible renal compromise in women with a history of diabetes, hypertension, or renal disease
Pap test	Screens for cervical intraepithelial neoplasia; if a liquid-based test is used, may also screen for HPV
Cervical cultures for gonorrhea and chlamydia	Screens for asymptomatic infection at first visit
Vaginal/anal culture	GBS test done at 35–37 weeks for infection
RPR, VDRL, or FTA-ABS	Identifies women with untreated syphilis, done at first visit
HIV antibody, hepatitis B surface antigen, toxoplasmosis	Screens for the specific infections
1-h glucose tolerance	Screens for gestational diabetes; done at initial visit for women with risk factors; done at 24-28 weeks for pregnant women at risk whose initial screen was negative and for others who were not previously tested
3-h glucose tolerance	Tests for gestational diabetes in women with elevated glucose level after 1-h test; must have two elevated readings for diagnosis
Cardiac evaluation: ECG, chest x-ray, and echocardiogram	Evaluates cardiac function in women with a history of hypertension or cardiac disease

BUN, Blood urea nitrogen; *ECG,* electrocardiogram; *FTA-ABS,* fluorescent treponemal antibody absorption; *GBS,* group B streptococcus; *hCG,* human chorionic gonadotropin; *HIV,* human immunodeficiency virus; *HPV,* human papillomavirus; *RBCs,* red blood cells; *RPR,* rapid plasma reagin; *VDRL,* Venereal Disease Research Laboratory; *WBCs,* white blood cells.

✚ EMERGENCY

Supine Hypotension

Signs and Symptoms
- Pallor
- Dizziness, faintness, breathlessness
- Tachycardia
- Nausea
- Clammy (damp, cool) skin; sweating

Interventions
- Position woman on her side until her signs and symptoms subside and vital signs stabilize to within normal limits.

Fetal Assessment

Gestational age. In an uncomplicated pregnancy, fetal gestational age is estimated after the duration of pregnancy and the EDB have been determined. Fetal gestational age is determined from the menstrual history, contraceptive history, pregnancy test result, and the following findings obtained during the clinical evaluation:
- First uterine evaluation: date, size
- Fetal heart first heard: date, method (Doppler stethoscope)
- Date of first feelings of fetal movements (quickening)
- Current fundal height, estimated fetal weight (EFW)
- Current week of gestation by history of LMP and/or ultrasound examination

BOX 14.5   Human Immunodeficiency Virus Screening

- Pregnant women are ethically obligated to seek reasonable care during pregnancy and to avoid causing harm to the fetus. Women's health nurses should be advocates for the fetus while accepting of the pregnant woman's decision regarding testing and/or treatment for HIV.
- Without treatment, the incidence of perinatal transmission from an HIV-positive mother to her fetus is approximately 25%. Triple-drug antiviral or highly active antiretroviral therapy (HAART) during pregnancy decreases perinatal transmission to less than 1% (Centers for Disease Control and Prevention, 2017).
- The CDC (2017) recommends testing for HIV infections in all pregnant women as early as possible in pregnancy and a second test in the third trimester for women in certain geographic areas and those who are at high risk for HIV infection.
- Testing has the potential to identify HIV-positive women who can then be treated. HCPs have an obligation to ensure that pregnant women are well informed about HIV symptoms, testing, and methods of decreasing maternal-fetal transmission. The CDC (2017) and the American College of Obstetricians and Gynecologists (ACOG, 2016) recommend universal opt-out screening, which means that all pregnant women are offered HIV screening but have the opportunity to opt out if desired.

American College of Obstetricians and Gynecologists (2016). Committee opinion no. 418. Prenatal and perinatal human immunodeficiency virus testing—Expanded recommendations. Obstetrics & Gynecology, 105(5 Part 1), 1119–1124; Centers for Disease Control and Prevention. (2017). Reducing HIV transmission from mother-to-child: An opt-out approach to HIV screening. Retrieved from: https://www.cdc.gov/hiv/group/gender/pregnantwomen/opt-out.html.

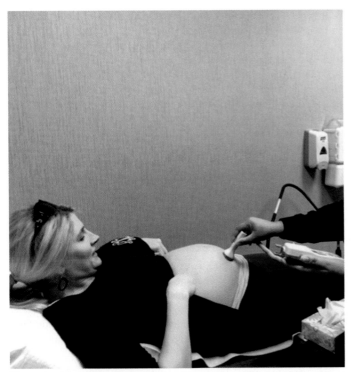

Fig. 14.5 Assessing the Fetal Heartbeat With a Doppler Ultrasound Stethoscope. (Courtesy Ashley Martin, Charlotte, NC.)

- Ultrasound examination: date, week of gestation, biparietal diameter (BPD)
- Reliability of dates

Quickening usually occurs between 16 and 20 weeks of gestation and is initially experienced as a fluttering sensation. The mother's report should be recorded. Multiparous women often perceive fetal movement earlier than primigravidas. Ultrasonography in early pregnancy is used to establish the duration of pregnancy. Ultrasound can detect a multiple gestation and provide information about the well-being of the fetus or fetuses (see Chapter 26 for further discussion).

Fetal heart tones. The fetal heart tones (FHTs) are assessed routinely at prenatal care visits. Early in pregnancy the fetal heartbeat can be detected during ultrasound examination. Late in the first trimester the heartbeat can be heard with a Doppler device that transmits FHTs through a speaker or attached earpieces (Fig. 14.5). Using the Doppler device allows the mother and others who are present to easily hear the fetal heartbeat. Identification of the fetus's position by the Leopold maneuvers (see Chapter 19) can help to position the Doppler optimally on the mother's abdomen. The heartbeat is counted for 1 minute; its quality and rhythm are noted. Once the heartbeat has been noted, its absence is cause for immediate investigation.

Health status. Assessment of the fetus's health status often includes consideration of fetal movement. Absence of fetal movement is correlated with fetal death; women who report decreased fetal movement have an increased risk for an adverse outcome (AAP & ACOG, 2017). The mother is instructed to note the extent and timing of fetal movements and to report immediately if the pattern changes or if movements decrease. See Chapter 26 for more information on maternal assessment of fetal movement.

Fetal health status is investigated intensively if any maternal or fetal complications arise (e.g., gestational hypertension, intrauterine growth restriction [IUGR], prelabor rupture of membranes [PROM], irregular or absent FHR, or decreased or absent fetal movements after quickening). Careful, precise, and concise recording of the woman's responses

and laboratory results provide the continuous and accurate supervision vital to promoting the well-being of both mother and fetus.

Fundal height. During the second trimester, the uterus becomes an abdominal organ. The fundal height (measurement of the height of the uterus above the symphysis pubis) is one indicator of fetal growth. The measurement also provides a gross estimate of the duration of pregnancy. From gestational weeks (GWs) 18 to 30, the height of the fundus in centimeters is approximately the same as the number of weeks of gestation (±2 GW) if the woman's bladder is empty at the time of measurement. As much as a 3-cm variation is possible if the bladder is full. The fundal height measurement can aid in identifying risk factors. A stable or decreased fundal height can indicate IUGR; an excessive increase can indicate the presence of a multiple gestation or polyhydramnios.

A disposable paper metric tape measure is preferred for measuring fundal height; plastic retractable tape measures should be cleaned after use and prior to retraction. Ideally the same person should examine the pregnant woman at each of her prenatal visits to increase the reliability of the measurement, but often this is not possible. All clinicians who examine a pregnant woman should be consistent in their measurement technique and a protocol should be established in which the measurement technique is explicitly set forth. Measurements obtained with the woman in various positions will differ, making it important to standardize the technique used to measure the fundal height. The protocol should specify the woman's position on the examining table, the measuring device, and the method of measurement. Conditions under which the measurements are taken can also be described in the woman's records, including whether the bladder was empty and whether the uterus was relaxed or contracted at the time of measurement. The tape can be placed in the middle of the woman's abdomen and the measurement made from the upper border of the symphysis pubis to the upper border of the fundus, with the tape measure held in contact with the skin for the entire length of the uterus (Fig. 14.6A). In another measurement technique, the upper curve of the fundus is not included in the measurement. Instead, one end of the tape measure is held at the upper border of the symphysis pubis with one hand while the other hand is placed at the upper border of the fundus. The tape is placed between the middle and index fingers of the other hand, and the point where these fingers intercept the tape measure is taken as the measurement (see Fig. 14.6B).

Laboratory Tests

The number of routine laboratory tests done during follow-up visits in pregnancy is limited. A clean-catch urine specimen is obtained to test for glucose, protein, nitrites, and leukocytes at each visit. Urine specimens for culture and sensitivity and cervical and vaginal smears and blood tests are repeated as necessary. ACOG (2013) recommends glucose screening for all pregnant women. Assessment for risk factors can be done through review of the health history, screening for clinical risk factors, or measurement of blood glucose levels. Risk factors that warrant early screening include obesity, history of gestational diabetes mellitus (GDM), or known impairment of glucose metabolism. If GDM is not diagnosed with early screening, blood glucose testing is repeated at 24 to 28 weeks. The standard screening test for GDM is a 1-hour 50-g oral glucose tolerance test (GTT). If the glucose level is elevated, further testing is done using a 3-hour 100-g GTT (see Chapter 29).

Group B streptococcus (GBS) testing is recommended between 35 and 37 weeks of gestation; cultures collected earlier will not accurately predict GBS status at time of birth. All pregnant women should have GBS testing, even those who are scheduled for a cesarean delivery, because labor can begin or membranes rupture prior to the routine administration of prophylactic antibiotics. Women with a history of

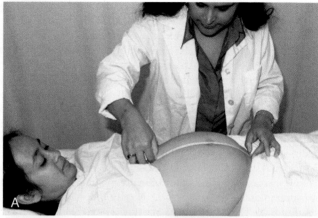

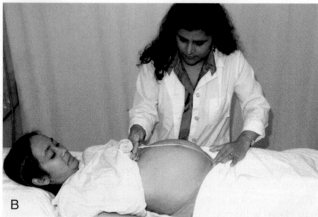

Fig. 14.6 Measurement of Fundal Height from Symphysis Pubis. (A) including the upper curve of the fundus and (B) not including the upper curve of the fundus. Note the position of the hands and measuring tape. (Courtesy Chris Rozales, San Francisco, CA.)

GBS in a previous pregnancy should be retested with each pregnancy (ACOG, 2015a).

Genetic Screening

Ideally, carrier screening and counseling is done in the preconception period to identify any risks for inherited medical conditions and genetic disorders. During pregnancy all women should be offered screening tests for chromosomal abnormalities based on factors such as age, previous obstetric history, family history, gestational age when prenatal care began, number of fetuses, availability of testing, and the desire for early results (AAP & ACOG, 2017).

Screening tests for fetal aneuploidy can detect Down syndrome and other trisomies (see Chapter 3). First-trimester screening can be done between 11 and 14 weeks using a sample of the maternal blood to measure biochemical markers, pregnancy-associated plasma protein A (PAPP-A) and human chorionic gonadotropin, and ultrasound examination for nuchal translucency. Noninvasive cell-free DNA (cfDNA) testing can be done as early as 10 weeks to test for common trisomies; this test can also identify the sex chromosome indicating the sex of the fetus (AAP & ACOG, 2017).

Women who begin prenatal care in the second trimester should be offered testing that includes quadruple screening (hCG, α-fetoprotein [AFP], unconjugated estriol, and dimeric inhibin), cfDNA screening, and ultrasound examination. Screening for neural tube defects and other open fetal defects in the second trimester is done by measuring the maternal serum AFP (MSAFP) level and by ultrasonography.

False-positive results are common and warrant further testing with amniocentesis (AAP & ACOG, 2017).

Some experts recommend performing both first- and second-trimester screening to increase the accuracy of results (ACOG & AAP, 2017; Driscoll, Simpson, Holzgreve, et al., 2017). *Integrated* screening includes both first- and second-trimester tests; it has high sensitivity and a low false-positive rate. Results are reported only after the second-trimester testing is complete. With *sequential* screening, if the woman's risk for aneuploidy is high based on the first-trimester screening, she is offered diagnostic testing (chorionic villus sampling, amniocentesis). If her risk is low or moderate, the second-trimester screening tests are done and a final adjusted risk is determined for trisomies 21 and 18 (Driscoll et al.).

Other diagnostic tests are available to assess the health status of the pregnant woman and her fetus. See Chapter 26 for more information.

Routine Fetal Ultrasound Examination

Routine ultrasound imaging is usually done in the first trimester to establish or confirm gestational age. In addition, unless there are indications for earlier testing, a fetal anatomy scan is done between 18 and 22 weeks. Ultrasonography can also detect the number of fetuses, fetal presentation, fetal biometry, location of the placenta, amniotic fluid volume, and cardiac activity (AAP & ACOG, 2017) (see Chapter 26).

Nursing Interventions

After obtaining information through the assessment process, the data are analyzed to identify deviations from expected values and to identify the unique needs of the pregnant woman and her family. The care of the woman and her fetus is optimized with a collaborative approach involving the obstetric care provider, nurse, other health care professionals, the woman herself, her partner, and her family.

The nurse-client relationship is critical in setting the tone for further interaction. The techniques of active listening with an attentive expression and using touch and eye contact (if culturally appropriate) have their place, as does recognizing the woman's feelings and her right to express these feelings. The interaction may occur in various formal or informal settings. A clinical setting, home visits, or telephone conversations all provide opportunities for contact and can be used effectively.

Education for Self-Management

The expectant mother needs information on many topics. The nurse who is observant, listens, and is familiar with typical concerns of expectant parents can anticipate the questions that will be asked and can encourage mothers and their partners to discuss their concerns. Printed literature can be given to supplement the individualized teaching the nurse provides. To be most effective, educational materials should be appropriate for the pregnant woman's or couple's ethnicity, culture, and literacy level and the agency's resources. Women often avidly read books, pamphlets, and web information related to their pregnancy experience. Nurses should be familiar with the educational materials that are distributed to expectant parents as well as popular web-based resources related to pregnancy. Nurses can direct pregnant women and their families to reliable websites that contain accurate information.

Because family members are common sources of health information, it is also important to include them in health education during pregnancy. This can enhance their ability to be supportive of the pregnant woman as she progresses through her term.

Pregnant women who receive conflicting advice or instruction are likely to grow increasingly frustrated with members of the health care team and the care provided. Several topics that can cause concerns in pregnant women are discussed in the following sections.

Expected maternal and fetal changes. Most expectant parents are curious about the growth and development of the fetus and the changes that occur in the mother's body during pregnancy. Mothers are often more tolerant of the discomforts related to the continuing pregnancy if they understand the underlying causes. Educational material that describes fetal and maternal changes can be used to explain changes as they occur. Couples can track the development of their growing fetus through apps for smartphones or on websites such as https://www.bab ycenter.com/pregnancy-week-by-week.

Nutrition. Good nutrition is important for the maintenance of maternal health during pregnancy and the provision of adequate nutrients for embryonic and fetal development. Assessing a woman's nutritional status and weight gain and providing ongoing education about nutrition are part of the nurse's responsibilities in providing prenatal care. Education for pregnant women includes recommendations about their daily intake of nutrients, calories, vitamins, and minerals. Based on the woman's BMI, the recommended weight gain during pregnancy is discussed. Additional information regarding nutrition during pregnancy may include mentioning foods high in iron, the importance of taking prenatal vitamins, and recommendations to avoid alcohol and to limit caffeine intake. Pregnant women are instructed about food safety and how to avoid food-borne illnesses such as listeriosis. At each visit the nurse assesses for the practice of pica. In some settings a registered dietitian counsels women individually or conducts classes for pregnant women about nutrition during pregnancy. Nurses can refer women to a registered dietitian if a need is identified during the nursing assessment. (For detailed information concerning maternal and fetal nutritional needs and related nursing care, see Chapter 15.)

Personal hygiene. During pregnancy the apocrine (sweat) glands are highly active because of hormonal influences, and women often perspire freely. They can be informed that the increase is normal and that their previous patterns of perspiration will return after the postpartum period. Baths and warm showers can be therapeutic because they relax tense, tired muscles; help counter insomnia; and make the pregnant woman feel fresh. Tub bathing is not restricted even in late pregnancy because little water enters the vagina unless it is under pressure. However, late in pregnancy, when the woman's center of gravity lowers, she is at risk for falling, making tub bathing risky. Tub bathing is contraindicated after rupture of the membranes.

Prevention of urinary tract infections. Because of physiologic changes that occur in the renal system during pregnancy (see Chapter 13), infections of the lower urinary tract (acute urethritis, acute cystitis) are common. *Escherichia coli* is the most common causative organism of urinary tract infection (UTI) in pregnant women (Duff & Birsner, 2017). Although UTIs can be asymptomatic, typical symptoms include frequency, urgency, dysuria, dribbling, and hesitancy; gross hematuria can occur. Women should be instructed to inform their HCP promptly if they experience these symptoms. UTIs pose a risk to the mother and fetus; thus their prevention or early treatment is essential. Oral antibiotics are commonly prescribed.

The nurse can assess the woman's understanding and use of appropriate hand hygiene techniques before and after urinating and the importance of wiping the perineum from front to back. Soft, absorbent toilet tissue, preferably white and unscented, should be used; harsh, scented, or printed toilet paper can cause irritation. Bubble bath or other bath oils should be avoided because these can irritate the urethra. Women should wear all-cotton undergarments and cotton-lined pantyhose and avoid wearing tight-fitting slacks or jeans for long periods of time; anything that allows a buildup of heat and moisture in the genital area can foster the growth of bacteria.

Some women do not consume enough fluids. The nurse should advise drinking at least 2.5 L of liquid (8 to 10 glasses of 8 oz each) daily, preferably water, to maintain an adequate fluid intake that ensures frequent urination. Pregnant women should not limit fluids to reduce the frequency of urination. Women need to know that if their urine appears dark (concentrated), they must increase their fluid intake.

The nurse should review healthy urination practices with the woman. Women are told not to ignore the urge to urinate because holding urine lengthens the time bacteria are in the bladder and allows them to multiply. Women should plan for when they are faced with situations that can require them to delay urination (e.g., a long car ride). They should always urinate before going to bed at night. Bacteria can be introduced during oral, anal, or vaginal sexual activity; therefore women are advised to urinate before and after sex and then drink a large glass of water to promote additional urination. Consumption of cranberry juice has been suggested as an intervention to prevent UTI based on the acidity of the juice. There appears to be greater benefit from cranberry supplements compared with cranberry juice. Recent evidence indicates that the value of using cranberry supplements is related to the component proanthocyanidins (PACs), which prevent bacteria from adhering to the bladder wall. Cranberry capsules are the best source of PACs, although it has been shown that there is high variability in the amount of PACs in commercially available products (Chughtai, Thomas, & Howell, 2016).

Kegel exercises. Kegel exercises (deliberate contraction and relaxation of the pubococcygeus muscle) strengthen the muscles around the reproductive organs and improve muscle tone. Many women are not aware of the muscles of the pelvic floor until it is pointed out that these are the muscles used during urination and sexual intercourse and that they can be consciously controlled. The muscles of the pelvic floor encircle the vaginal outlet and need to be exercised because an exercised muscle can then stretch and contract readily at the time of birth. Practice of pelvic muscle exercises during pregnancy also results in fewer complaints of urinary incontinence in late pregnancy and postpartum.

Several ways of performing Kegel exercises have been described. The method described in the box titled Teaching for Self-Management: Kegel Exercises, in Chapter 4, demonstrates evidence-based nursing care. Teaching has been effective if the woman reports an increased ability to control urine flow and greater muscular control during sexual intercourse.

Preparation for breastfeeding. During the first prenatal visit, the nurse asks if the woman is planning to breastfeed. A woman's decision about the method of infant feeding is usually made before pregnancy; thus it is essential to educate women of childbearing age about the benefits of breastfeeding. The woman and her partner are encouraged to decide which method of feeding is suitable for them; however, the benefits of breastfeeding should be emphasized. Once the couple has been given information about the advantages and disadvantages of breastfeeding and formula feeding, they can make an informed choice. Most women who choose to breastfeed do so because they are aware of the numerous benefits (see Chapter 25). Lack of knowledge about the benefits of breastfeeding and its perceived personal and social disadvantages can influence a woman not to breastfeed. Modesty issues, lack of support from the partner and family, incompatibility with lifestyle, and lack of confidence are among the reasons cited by women who decide to formula-feed their infants (Lawrence & Lawrence, 2016).

Assessment of a woman's breasts during the prenatal period can reveal potential concerns related to breastfeeding. Scars on the breast can indicate previous breast reduction surgery, which can affect milk production. The woman may have breast implants; this too may affect successful breastfeeding. Asymmetry of the breasts or tubular-shaped

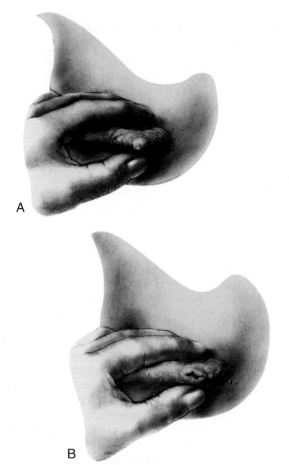

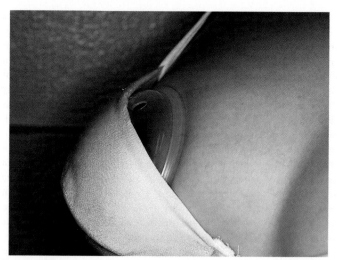

Fig. 14.8 Breast Shell in Place Inside Bra. Sometimes recommended for flat or inverted nipples. (Courtesy Michael S. Clement, MD, Mesa, AZ.)

Fig. 14.7 Test for Inverted Nipples. (A) Normal nipple everts with gentle pressure. (B) Inverted nipple inverts with gentle pressure. (Modified from Lawrence, R.A., & Lawrence, R.M. [2016]. Breastfeeding: A guide for the medical profession [8th ed.]. St. Louis: Mosby.)

breasts suggest a lack of glandular tissue and potential problems with adequate milk production. Examination of the breasts can reveal flat or inverted nipples, which can affect the baby's ability to latch onto the breast. To determine whether nipples are inverted, a woman can perform a test on her nipples to gauge their freedom to protrude (Fig. 14.7). The woman places her thumb and forefinger on her areola and presses inward gently. A normal nipple will evert or stand erect while an inverted nipple will appear to withdraw (Lawrence & Lawrence, 2016).

Exercises to break the adhesions that cause the nipple to invert do not work and can cause uterine contractions. Some clinicians recommend the use of breast shells (Fig. 14.8) during the last trimester for women with flat or inverted nipples, although evidence to support their effectiveness is lacking. They can be uncomfortable and cause irritation to the nipple or areola. Breast stimulation is contraindicated in women at risk for preterm labor; therefore the decision to suggest the use of breast shells to women with flat or inverted nipples must be made judiciously (Lawrence & Lawrence, 2016).

There is no special preparation of the nipples or breasts for breastfeeding. The woman is taught to cleanse the nipples with warm water to keep the ducts from being blocked with dried colostrum. Soap, ointments, alcohol, and tinctures should not be applied because they remove protective oils that keep the nipples supple. Breast pads with plastic liners should be avoided. Women with nipple piercings should be instructed to remove jewelry during pregnancy to allow the nipple to recover, which will help to prevent infection (Lawrence & Lawrence, 2016)

A bra that fits well and provides support promotes comfort as breasts increase in size during pregnancy. The woman who plans to breastfeed may want to purchase a nursing bra that will accommodate her increased breast size during the last few months of pregnancy and during lactation.

The nurse addresses the mother's questions and concerns related to breastfeeding and recommends sources of information, including books and websites. The mother may appreciate a list of local breastfeeding resources that includes prenatal breastfeeding classes as well as lactation consultants and the services they provide, such as inpatient and outpatient consultations, home visits, and breast pump rentals.

Umbilical cord blood banking. Parents may have read or heard about umbilical cord blood banking and ask for guidance on the subject. Umbilical cord blood has been found to contain hematopoietic stem cells (HSC); these cells are being studied for their potential in treating inborn errors of metabolism, certain types of leukemia, and disorders of the immune system as well as their use in regenerative procedures and in treating infectious disease. When used in treatment, the HSCs are transplanted into the patient. Parents should be provided with balanced and evidence-based information, including the conditions for which HSCs have been demonstrated to be most useful, the financial costs of collection and storage, and how to select a reputable vendor for this service (AAP & ACOG, 2017).

Oral health. Oral health during pregnancy is especially important because it can affect maternal health and pregnancy outcomes (Hartnett, Haber, Krainovich-Miller, et al.,2016). There is an increased incidence of gingivitis (swelling and inflammation of the gums) and periodontitis (infection of gums that can cause damage to soft tissues and bone) during pregnancy. Studies have shown an association between periodontal disease and preterm birth, LBW, very low birth weight (VLBW), preeclampsia, and gestational diabetes (Corbella, Taschieri, Del Fabbro, et al., 2016; Daalderop, Wieland, Tomsin, et al., 2018; Parihar, Katoch, Rajguru, et al., 2015).

HCPs should assess oral health at the initial prenatal visit and at intervals throughout pregnancy (ACOG, 2013/2017). It takes only 1 minute to complete an oral examination, so it can easily be incorporated into routine care. The provider or nurse should inquire about the woman's last dental visit. If it was more than 6 months earlier, she should schedule a dental examination soon. A high percentage of women do not have regular dental care, primarily due to financial barriers; those with insurance are more likely to visit the dentist.

Because calcium and phosphorus in the teeth are fixed in enamel, the adage "for every child a tooth" is not true. There is no evidence that filling teeth or the administration of local or nitrous oxide–oxygen anesthesia precipitates miscarriage or preterm labor. For deep gingival cleaning or oral surgery, antibacterial therapy should be considered to prevent sepsis, especially in pregnant women who have had rheumatic heart disease or nephritis. Diagnosis and treatment of oral health problems, including necessary dental x-rays and the use of local anesthetics or nitrous oxide–oxygen anesthesia, are considered safe during pregnancy. Dental care and nonemergent procedures are best scheduled during the second trimester, when the woman is past the stage of feeling nauseated and can sit comfortably in the chair. To avoid supine hypotension during dental procedures, the pregnant woman in her second or third trimester is positioned in the dental chair with a small pillow under one hip. Nurses can teach pregnant women about the importance of dental hygiene, including regular brushing and flossing. Women who experience nausea and vomiting episodes can prevent the erosion of tooth enamel by rinsing with a solution of baking soda after vomiting (ACOG, 2013/2017; American Dental Association, 2019).

Physical activity. Physical activity during pregnancy has minimal risks and promotes a feeling of well-being in pregnant women. It improves physical fitness and circulation, enhances physiologic well-being, promotes relaxation and rest, and counteracts boredom. Regular exercise helps with weight management and can reduce the risk of gestational diabetes, cesarean birth, and giving birth to an infant that is large for gestational age (ACOG, 2015d; Domenjoz, Kayser, & Boulvain, 2014). Detailed exercise tips for pregnancy are presented in the box Teaching for Self-Management: Exercise Tips for Pregnant Women (see also Clinical Reasoning Case Study).

Posture and body mechanics. Skeletal and musculature changes and hormonal changes in pregnancy can predispose the woman to backache and possible injury. As pregnancy progresses, the woman's center of

TEACHING FOR SELF-MANAGEMENT

Exercise Tips for Pregnant Women

- Consult your HCP to discuss your current exercise routine and exercises you would like to continue during pregnancy.
- Exercise regularly every day, if possible, to improve muscle tone and increase or maintain your stamina. Thirty minutes of moderate physical exercise is recommended. This activity can be broken up into shorter segments with rest in between.
- Consider decreasing jogging or running; substitute walking or non–weight-bearing activities such as swimming, cycling, or stretching.
- Consider decreasing your exercise intensity as your pregnancy progresses to adjust for normal changes in pregnancy that can reduce your exercise tolerance.
- Avoid risky activities such as contact sports, scuba diving, and sports that require precise balance and coordination. Avoid activities that require holding your breath and bearing down (Valsalva maneuver).
- You should be able to hold a conversation while exercising. If you cannot talk, you need to slow down.
- Avoid becoming overheated by limiting your activity to 30 minutes, especially in hot, humid weather. Do not use hot tubs and saunas.
- Perform warmup and stretching exercises to prepare your joints for exercise and lessen the likelihood of injury to your joints. After the 4th month of pregnancy, you should not perform exercises flat on your back.
- Include a cool-down period of mild activity involving your legs at the end of an exercise activity.
- Rest for 10 minutes after exercising, lying on your side, which helps to increase blood flow to your placenta and fetus. You should get up slowly from the floor to prevent dizziness or fainting.
- Drink water as needed during exercise and two or three 8-ounce glasses of water after you exercise to replace the body fluids lost through perspiration.
- Increase your food intake with healthy snacks to replace the calories burned during exercise and to provide the extra energy needs of pregnancy.

- Take your time. This is not the time to be competitive or train for activities requiring speed or long endurance.
- Wear a supportive bra. Your increased breast weight can cause changes in posture and put pressure on the ulnar nerve.
- Wear supportive shoes. As your uterus grows your center of gravity shifts making you feel off balance and more likely to fall.
- Stop exercising immediately and call your HCP if you experience shortness of breath, dizziness, numbness, tingling, pain of any kind, more than four uterine contractions per hour, decreased fetal activity, or vaginal bleeding.
- Recognize signs of danger, including vaginal bleeding; blurred vision; nausea; dizziness; fainting; breathlessness; heart palpitations; increased swelling in your hands, feet, and ankles; sharp pain in the abdomen and chest; and sudden change in body temperature.

? CLINICAL REASONING CASE STUDY

Exercise in Pregnancy

Lourdes is 27 years old and 14 weeks pregnant with her second child. In her first pregnancy 3 years ago she gained 50 pounds. To lose weight following that pregnancy and return to her prepregnant weight, she tried dieting and walking 3 days a week. She tried breastfeeding with the first baby but stopped at 6 weeks postpartum because "the baby wasn't getting enough milk." Lourdes has not exercised regularly for about a year. She wants to avoid gaining extra weight during this pregnancy and would like to start Zumba classes and follow a low-calorie diet. She was 8 weeks pregnant at her first prenatal visit; her BMI at that time was 31. She would also like to breastfeed this baby.

1. What is the priority concern or client need in this situation? Support your answer with data as stated in the case.
2. List other client needs/problems in this case.
3. Identify any additional information or assessment data needed by the nurse in planning care for this client.
   a. What is the priority nursing action?
   b. Describe other nursing interventions that are important to providing optimal care.
4. What nursing actions are appropriate in this situation?
5. Describe roles/responsibilities of the interprofessional health care team members (other than nurses) who may involved in providing care for this client.

gravity changes, pelvic joints soften and relax, and stress is placed on the abdominal musculature. Poor posture and body mechanics contribute to the discomfort and potential for injury. To minimize these problems, women can learn good body posture and body mechanics. Strategies to prevent or relieve backache are presented in the box Teaching for Self-Management: Posture and Body Mechanics. Exercises to help relieve low back pain during the second trimester are demonstrated in Fig. 14.9.

Rest and relaxation. Nurses can encourage women to plan regular rest periods, particularly as pregnancy advances. The side-lying position (Fig. 14.10) is recommended because it promotes uterine perfusion and fetoplacental oxygenation by eliminating pressure on the ascending vena cava and descending aorta, which can lead to supine hypotension.

The woman should be shown how to rise slowly from a side-lying position to prevent placing strain on the back and to minimize the orthostatic hypotension caused by rapid changes in position. To stretch and rest the woman's back muscles at home or work, the nurse can show her how to do the following exercises:

- Stand behind a chair. Support and balance yourself by using the back of the chair (Fig. 14.11). Squat for 30 seconds; stand for 15 seconds. Repeat six times several times a day as needed.
- While sitting in a chair, lower your head to your knees for 30 seconds. Raise your head. Repeat six times several times a day as needed.

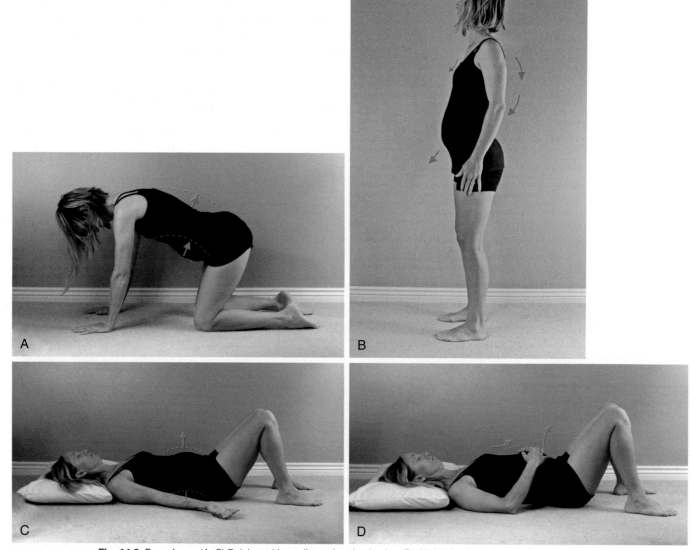

Fig. 14.9 Exercises. (A–C) Pelvic rocking relieves low backache. (D) Abdominal breathing aids relaxation and lifts abdominal wall from the uterus. (Courtesy, Julie Perry Nelson, Loveland, CO.)

TEACHING FOR SELF-MANAGEMENT

Posture and Body Mechanics

To Prevent or Relieve Backache
- Do a pelvic tilt: Fig. 14.9.
  - Pelvic tilt (rock) on hands and knees (see Fig. 14.9A) and while sitting in a straight-back chair.
  - Pelvic tilt (rock) in standing position against a wall or lying on the floor (see Fig. 14.9B and C).
  - Perform abdominal muscle contractions during pelvic tilt while standing, lying, or sitting to help strengthen rectus abdominis muscle (see Fig. 14.9D). Use good body mechanics.
- Use leg muscles to reach objects on or near the floor. Bend at the knees, not from the back. Knees are bent to lower the body to squatting position. Keep feet 12 to 18 inches apart to provide a solid base and maintain balance.

- Lift with the legs. To lift a heavy object (e.g., a young child), one foot is placed slightly in front of the other and kept flat while lowering the body to one knee. Lift the weight, holding it close to the body and never higher than the chest. To stand up or sit down, place one leg slightly behind the other while raising or lowering the body.

To Restrict the Lumbar Curve
- For prolonged standing (e.g., ironing, employment), place one foot on a low footstool or box; change position often.
- Move car seat forward so that your knees are bent and higher than your hips. If needed, use a small pillow to support the low back area.
- Sit in chairs low enough to allow both feet to rest on the floor, preferably with knees higher than hips.

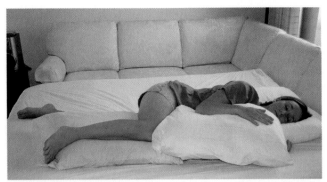

Fig. 14.10 Side-Lying Position for Rest and Relaxation. (Courtesy Julie Perry Nelson, Loveland, CO.)

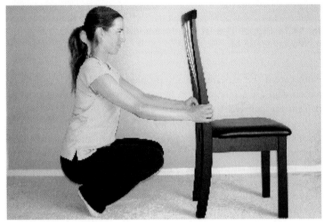

Fig. 14.11 Squatting for Muscle Relaxation and Strengthening and for Keeping Leg and Hip Joints Flexible. (Courtesy Julie Perry Nelson, Loveland, CO.)

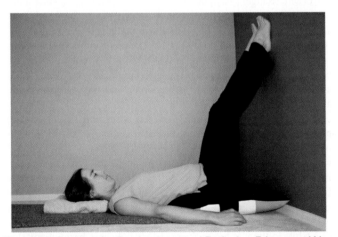

Fig. 14.12 Position for Resting Legs and Reducing Edema and Varicosities. Encourage the woman with vulvar varicosities to include a pillow under her hips. (Courtesy Julie Perry Nelson, Loveland, CO.)

Conscious relaxation is the process of releasing tension from the mind and body through deliberate effort and practice. The techniques for conscious relaxation are numerous and varied. The ability to relax consciously and intentionally is beneficial for the following reasons:

- It will relieve the normal discomforts related to pregnancy.
- It will reduce stress and therefore diminish pain perception during the childbearing cycle.
- It will heighten your self-awareness and trust in your ability to control physical responses and functions.
- It will help you to cope with stress in everyday life situations.

Employment. Employment of pregnant women usually has no adverse effects on pregnancy outcomes. Job discrimination that is based strictly on pregnancy is illegal. However, some job environments pose potential risks to the fetus (e.g., dry-cleaning plants, chemistry laboratories, parking garages). Excessive fatigue is usually the deciding factor in the termination of employment. Strategies to improve safety during pregnancy are described in the box Teaching for Self-Management: Safety During Pregnancy.

TEACHING FOR SELF-MANAGEMENT
Safety During Pregnancy

Changes in the body resulting from pregnancy include relaxation of the joints, alteration of the center of gravity, faintness, and discomforts. Problems with coordination and balance are common. Therefore the pregnant woman should follow these guidelines:

- Use correct body mechanics.
- Use safety features on tools and vehicles (e.g., seatbelts, shoulder harnesses, head rests, goggles, helmets) as specified.
- Avoid activities requiring coordination, balance, and concentration.
- Take rest periods; reschedule daily activities to meet your needs for rest and relaxation.

The developing fetus is vulnerable to environmental teratogens. Many potentially dangerous chemicals—cleaning agents, paints, sprays, herbicides, and pesticides—are present in the home, yard, and workplace. The soil and water supply may be unsafe. Therefore the pregnant woman should follow these guidelines:

- Read all labels for ingredients and proper use of a product.
- Ensure adequate ventilation with clean air.
- Dispose of wastes appropriately.
- Wear gloves when handling chemicals.
- Change job assignments or workplace as necessary.
- Avoid travel to high-altitude regions above 12,000 feet.

Women with sedentary jobs need to walk around at intervals to counter the usual sluggish circulation in the legs. They also should neither sit nor stand in one position for long periods, and they should avoid crossing their legs at the knees; all these activities can increase the risk of varices and thrombophlebitis. Standing for long periods also increases the risk of preterm labor. The pregnant woman's chair should provide adequate back support. Use of a footstool can prevent pressure on veins, relieve strain on varicosities, minimize edema of the feet, and prevent backache.

Clothing. Some women continue to wear their usual clothes during pregnancy if they fit and feel comfortable. If maternity clothing is needed, outfits can be purchased new or found in good condition at thrift shops or garage sales. Comfortable loose clothing is recommended. Tight bras and belts, stretch pants, garters, tight-top knee socks, panty girdles, and other constrictive clothing should be avoided because tight clothing over the perineum increases the risk of vaginitis and miliaria (heat rash), and impaired circulation in the legs can cause varicosities.

Maternity bras are constructed to accommodate the increased breast weight, chest circumference, and size of breast tail tissue (under the arm). A well-fitting support bra can help prevent neck ache and backache.

Maternal support hose provide considerable comfort and improve venous emptying in women with large varicose veins. Ideally, support stockings should be put on before getting out of bed in the morning. Fig. 14.12 demonstrates a position for resting the legs and reducing swelling and varicosities.

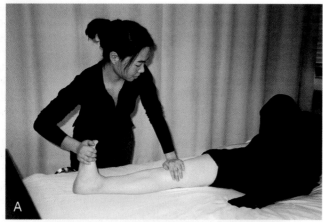

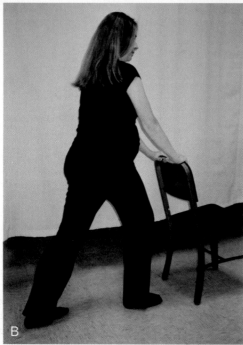

Fig. 14.13 Relief of Muscle Spasm (Leg Cramps). (A) Another person dorsiflexes the foot with the knee extended. (B) Woman stands and leans forward, thereby dorsiflexing the foot of the affected leg. (Courtesy Shannon Perry, Phoenix, AZ.)

Comfortable shoes that provide firm support and promote good posture and balance are advisable. Very high heels and platform shoes are not recommended because of the changes in the pregnant woman's center of gravity and softening of the pelvic joints in later pregnancy, which can cause her to lose her balance. In addition, in the third trimester, the woman's pelvis will tilt forward and her lumbar curve will increase. The resulting leg aches and cramps are aggravated by nonsupportive shoes. Exercises to relieve leg cramps are shown in Fig. 14.13.

Travel. Travel is not contraindicated in low-risk pregnant women; women with high-risk pregnancies are advised to avoid long-distance travel after fetal viability has been reached so as to avoid the consequences (economic and psychologic) of giving birth to a preterm infant far from home. Pregnant women should not travel to areas where health care is poor, water is untreated, or malaria or Zika are prevalent. Women who contemplate foreign travel should be aware that many health insurance carriers do not cover a birth in a foreign setting or even hospitalization for preterm labor. In addition, some vaccinations for foreign travel are contraindicated during pregnancy (e.g., bacille Calmette-Guérin [BCG] vaccine for tuberculosis). The woman should assess the availability of

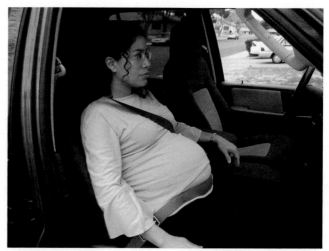

Fig. 14.14 Proper Use of Seatbelt and Head Rest. (Courtesy Brian and Mayannyn Sallee, Tucson, AZ.)

health care if she experiences any problems while traveling. Pregnant women who are accustomed to living and working abroad must seek advice from their HCPs (Morof & Carroll, 2018).

Pregnant women who travel for long distances should schedule periods of activity and rest. Prolonged periods of sitting during car or air travel increase the risk of venous stasis and thromboembolism. Six hours per day of sitting is the maximum amount of time for driving; the woman should stop at least every 2 hours to walk around for 10 minutes (Gregory et al., 2017). While sitting, the woman can practice deep breathing, foot circling, and alternately contracting and relaxing different muscle groups. She should avoid becoming fatigued.

A combination lap belt and shoulder harness is the most effective automobile restraint, and both should be used whether the mother is a driver or passenger seated in the front or back seats. The lap belt should be worn low across the pelvic bones as snugly as is comfortable. The shoulder harness should be worn above the gravid uterus and below the neck to prevent chafing (Fig. 14.14). The pregnant woman should sit upright. The head rest should be used to prevent whiplash injury. Airbags, if present, should remain engaged, but the steering wheel should be tilted upward, away from the abdomen and the seat moved back away from the steering wheel as much as possible.

Airline travel in large commercial jets poses little risk to a healthy pregnant woman. She is advised to inquire about restrictions or recommendations from her carrier. Most HCPs allow air travel up to 36 weeks of gestation for domestic travel and 32 to 35 weeks for international destinations for women without health- or pregnancy-related complications. Metal detectors used at airport security checkpoints emit low levels of radiation and should not pose an increased risk of harm to the fetus (Morof & Carroll, 2018). Exposure to cosmic radiation while in flight is below the dose that can cause harm at any stage of gestation (Health Physics Society, 2016). Women who fly frequently (e.g., flight attendants) should be aware of the increased exposure. The 8% humidity in the cabins of commercial airliners can result in water loss; fluid replacement with water is advised. The lower oxygen tension on commercial airliners does not create problems for women with uncomplicated pregnancies; however, those with severe anemia, sickle cell disease, or preexisting cardiovascular conditions may be affected. Sitting in the cramped seat of an airliner for prolonged periods can increase the risk of superficial and deep venous thrombosis; therefore the woman is encouraged to take a walk around the aircraft during each hour of travel and to wear graduated compression stockings to minimize this risk (Morof & Caroll).

Medications and herbal preparations. Although much has been learned in recent years about fetal drug toxicity, the possible teratogenicity of many medications, both prescription and OTC, is still unknown. This is especially true for new medications and combinations of drugs. Moreover, certain subclinical errors or deficiencies in intermediate metabolism in the fetus may cause an otherwise harmless drug to be converted into a hazardous one. The greatest danger of drug-caused developmental defects in the fetus extends from the time of fertilization through the first trimester, a time when the woman may not realize that she is pregnant. Self-treatment must be discouraged. The use of all drugs—including OTC medications, herbs, and vitamins—should be limited and a careful record kept of all therapeutic and nontherapeutic agents used.

The use of complementary and alternative modalities (CAMs) by pregnant women is widespread (Holden, Gardiner, Birdee, et al., 2015; Johnson, Kozhimannil, Jou, et al., 2016); as many as one-third of pregnant women admit to the use of CAMs. Actual use is likely higher, as some women do not disclose use of CAMs to their HCPs. There is limited research evidence about the safety of herbal preparations, especially during pregnancy. Although the use of CAMs is consistent with a holistic, woman-centered approach to care, caution is warranted in their use because of the lack of evidence of their safety and efficacy.

> **! NURSING ALERT**
>
> All pregnant women should be asked about the use of complementary and alternative modalities, including over-the-counter products (vitamins and herbal preparations). Nurses and obstetric care providers can discuss the safety of the modalities during pregnancy and caution women to avoid unsafe or potentially harmful practices.

Immunizations. Immunization with live or attenuated live viruses is contraindicated during pregnancy because of potential teratogenicity; recommended vaccination with these agents should be part of postpartum care. Live-virus vaccines include those for measles (rubeola and rubella), varicella (chickenpox), and mumps as well as the Sabin (oral) poliomyelitis vaccine (no longer used in the United States). Vaccines that can be administered during pregnancy include combined tetanus-diphtheria-acellular pertussis (Tdap), recombinant hepatitis B, and influenza (inactivated) vaccines (CDC, 2018a, 2018b).

Reported cases of pertussis (whooping cough) have increased significantly in the United States and Canada in recent years. Pertussis can cause serious and life-threatening complications in mothers and infants. To provide a maximal maternal antibody response and transfer passive immunity to the infant, Tdap should be administered between 27 and 36 weeks of gestation. Maternal antipertussis antibodies are short-lived and antibody levels drop significantly during the 1st year after vaccination. As a result, it is unlikely that a Tdap vaccination in one pregnancy will transfer passive immunity from mother to infant in a subsequent pregnancy. Therefore the recommendation is to administer Tdap to a pregnant woman during each pregnancy regardless of her prior vaccination history. If Tdap is not administered during pregnancy, it should be given immediately postpartum. Adolescents and adults (parents, grandparents, siblings, child care workers, and health care personnel) who will have close contact with an infant less than 12 months of age should receive a single dose of Tdap if they have not been vaccinated previously (CDC, 2018b). All women who are pregnant during the influenza season should be offered an influenza vaccination. The injectable inactivated influenza vaccine is safe throughout pregnancy. The intranasal influenza vaccine is contraindicated during pregnancy because it contains a live virus (ACOG, 2014).

Rh immune globulin. Testing to determine the pregnant woman's blood type is done at the first prenatal visit. Rh-negative women will also have an antibody screen in the first and third trimesters. Women with the Rh-negative (D-negative) blood type who are carrying an Rh-positive (D-positive) fetus can develop antibodies against the D antigen on the fetal red blood cell, causing lysis of the fetal red blood cells. This can lead to life-threatening hemolytic disease of the fetus and newborn (Aitken & Tichy, 2015).

Prophylactic Rh immune globulin can be administered to the Rh-negative (D-negative) pregnant woman to prevent the formation of antibodies (alloimmunization) by destroying any fetal red blood cells in the maternal circulation before her immune system recognizes the D-positive antigen and begins to produce antibodies (Blackburn, 2018). A dose of 300 µg of Rh immune globulin is routinely administered at 26 to 30 weeks to all Rh-negative women without evidence of anti-D alloimmunization. If she gives birth to an Rh-positive infant, the dose of Rh immune globulin is repeated within 72 hours after birth (see the Medication Guide in Chapter 21). Other indications for the administration of Rh immune globulin to Rh-negative women during pregnancy include chorionic villus sampling, amniocentesis, spontaneous or therapeutic abortion, ectopic pregnancy, external cephalic version, and abdominal trauma (Moise, 2017).

Substance use. Any drug or environmental agent that enters the pregnant woman's bloodstream has the potential to cross the placenta and harm the fetus. The nurse asks about the use of any substances at the initial prenatal visit and at all subsequent visits. See Chapter 4 for information on substance use during pregnancy.

Normal discomforts. Pregnant women have physical symptoms that would be considered abnormal in the nonpregnant state. They need explanations of the causes of the discomforts and advice on ways to relieve them. Information about the physiology, prevention, and self-management of discomforts experienced during the three trimesters of pregnancy is given in Table 14.2. Nurses can do much to allay a first-time mother's anxiety about such symptoms by telling her about them in advance and using terminology that the woman (or couple) can understand. Thus helping them to understand the rationale for treatment will promote their participation in care. Interventions should be individualized, with attention given to the woman's lifestyle and culture (see Nursing Care Plan).

Recognizing potential complications. One of the most important responsibilities of care providers is to alert the pregnant woman to signs and symptoms that indicate a potential complication of pregnancy. The woman must know how and to whom to report such warning signs. She and her family should receive a printed list of warning signs, written at the appropriate literacy level and in their language, that warrant a call to the HCP or clinic; phone numbers for the HCP or clinic should be listed.

The nurse answers questions as they arise during pregnancy. Pregnant women often have difficulty deciding when to report signs and symptoms. The mother is encouraged to refer to the printed list of potential complications (Table 14.3) and to listen to her body. If she senses that something is wrong, she should call her obstetric care provider. Several signs and symptoms must be discussed more extensively. These include vaginal bleeding, alteration in fetal movements, symptoms of preeclampsia, rupture of membranes, and preterm labor.

Sexual Counseling

Sexual counseling of expectant couples includes countering misinformation, providing reassurance of normality, and suggesting alternative behaviors. The uniqueness of each couple is considered within a biopsychosocial framework (see the box Teaching for Self-Management: Sexuality in Pregnancy). Nurses can initiate discussion about sexual adaptations during pregnancy, based on sound knowledge about the physical, social, and emotional responses to sex during pregnancy. Not all nurses are sufficiently knowledgeable or comfortable with discussing sexual concerns of their clients. Nurses should be aware of their personal strengths and limitations in dealing with sexual content and be prepared to make referrals if necessary.

◎ NURSING CARE PLAN

Discomforts of Pregnancy

Client Problem	Expected Outcome	Nursing Interventions	Rationales
First Trimester			
Risk for inadequate weight gain related to nausea and vomiting as evidenced by woman's report and weight loss	Woman: with normal prepregnancy BMI will gain 1 to 2.5 kg (2.2–5.5 lb) during first trimester.	Assess current weight, verify prepregnant weight and body mass index, and obtain diet history.	To plan realistic diet according to individual woman's nutritional needs and preferences and to identify current eating patterns and foods that may contribute to nausea, with referral to dietician as needed
		Teach woman about nutritional needs and recommended weight gain during pregnancy; suggest measures to alleviate or reduce nausea and vomiting.	To help her understand the importance of nutrition and to help her deal with the discomforts of nausea and vomiting
		Advise woman to call health care provider if vomiting is persistent and severe.	To prevent dehydration and excessive weight loss and to identify possible incidence of hyperemesis gravidarum
Fatigue related to effects of pregnancy hormones	Woman will report decreased fatigue and how she can adjust her lifestyle to enable her to get more rest.	Ask the woman to describe her fatigue in terms of severity, frequency, and what she has done to deal with it.	To determine how fatigue is affecting her body and her life
		Discuss use of support systems to help with responsibilities.	To decrease workload at work/home and decrease fatigue
		Explore with woman a variety of techniques to prioritize roles.	To decrease employer/family expectations
Second Trimester			
Constipation related to effect of progesterone on bowel motility as evidenced by woman's report of altered elimination pattern	Woman will report return to normal bowel elimination pattern after implementation of interventions.	Inquire about pattern of elimination and what she has done to treat constipation.	To gain understanding of the problem and what has helped or made it worse
		Help the woman to plan a diet that will promote regular bowel movements; oral fluid intake of least 8–10 glasses (2 L) of water daily, increase fiber in daily diet, and maintain a moderate exercise program.	To promote self-management care
		Advise woman that she should not use laxatives, stool softeners, or enemas without consulting her health care provider.	To prevent injury to woman or fetus
Third Trimester			
Interrupted sleep pattern related to discomforts of third trimester as evidenced by woman's report of inadequate rest	Woman will report improvement of quality and quantity of rest and sleep.	Assess pattern of sleep and factors that contribute to interruption.	To determine severity of problem and what she perceives as causing the interruption in sleep
		Suggest change of position to left side-lying with pillows between legs or to semi-Fowler position.	To increase support and decrease any problems with dyspnea or heartburn
		Discuss use of various sleep aids such as relaxation techniques, reading, and decreased activity before bedtime.	To reduce stimuli and establish a sleep routine before bedtime

TEACHING FOR SELF-MANAGEMENT

Sexuality in Pregnancy

- Be aware that maternal physiologic changes, such as breast enlargement and tenderness, nausea, fatigue, abdominal changes, perineal enlargement, leukorrhea, pelvic vasocongestion, and orgasmic responses can affect sexuality and sexual expression.
- Discuss concerns about sexuality during pregnancy with your partner.
- Keep in mind that cultural prescriptions ("do's") and proscriptions ("don'ts") can affect your attitudes and responses.
- Although your libido can be depressed during the first trimester, it often increases during the second trimester.
- Discuss and explore the following with your partner:
  - Alternative behaviors (e.g., mutual masturbation, foot massage, cuddling)
  - Alternative positions (e.g., pregnant woman in a superior position or side-lying)

- Various forms of vaginal penetration are safe provided that they are not uncomfortable. There is no correlation between vaginal stimulation or penetration and miscarriage, but observe the following precautions:
  - Abstain from vaginal penetration or orgasm if uterine cramping or vaginal bleeding occur; report these symptoms to your obstetric health care provider as soon as possible.
  - Abstain from any form of sexual activity that results in orgasm if you have a history of premature dilation of the cervix until otherwise advised by your obstetric HCP.
- Women at risk for acquiring or conveying STIs should use condoms during sexual intercourse throughout pregnancy.

TABLE 14.2 Discomforts Related to Pregnancy

Discomfort	Physiology	Education for Self-Management
First Trimester		
Breast changes: pain, tingling, tenderness, enlargement	Hypertrophy of mammary gland tissue and increased vascularization, pigmentation, and size and prominence of nipples and areolae caused by hormonal stimulation.	Wear supportive maternity bras with pads to absorb discharge, may be worn at night; wash with warm water and keep dry; breast tenderness may interfere with sexual expression or foreplay but is temporary.
Urgency and frequency of urination	Vascular engorgement and altered bladder function caused by hormones; bladder capacity reduced by enlarging uterus and fetal presenting part.	Empty bladder regularly; perform Kegel exercises; limit fluid intake before bedtime; avoid caffeine; wear perineal pad; report pain or burning sensation to obstetric care provider.
Languor and malaise; fatigue (most common in early pregnancy)	Unexplained; may be caused by increasing levels of estrogen, progesterone, and hCG or by elevated basal body temperature; psychologic response to pregnancy and its required physical and psychologic adaptations.	Rest as needed; eat well-balanced diet to prevent anemia
Nausea and vomiting, also known as morning sickness, occur in up to 70% of pregnant women; typically begins by 4-6 weeks of pregnancy, peaks by 9 weeks, and resolves by 12 weeks; can occur any time during day; fathers also may have symptoms.	Cause unknown; may result from hormonal changes, possibly hCG or estradiol; psychologic disposition; emotional response to pregnancy; evolutionary adaptation to protect mother and fetus	Avoid empty or overloaded stomach; maintain good posture—give stomach ample room; stop smoking; eat dry carbohydrate on awakening; remain in bed until feeling subsides, or alternate dry carbohydrate every other hour with fluids such as hot herbal decaffeinated tea, milk, or clear coffee until feeling subsides; eat five or six small meals per day; avoid fried, odorous, spicy, greasy, or gas-forming foods; wear acupressure bands used to treat motion sickness; ginger or acupuncture may be helpful; vitamin B_6 and doxylamine (Diclegis) may be ordered if weight loss occurs; consult primary health care provider if intractable vomiting occurs.
Ptyalism (excessive salivation) can occur starting 2-3 weeks after first missed period.	Possibly caused by elevated estrogen levels; may be related to reluctance to swallow because of nausea.	Use astringent mouthwash, chew gum and eat hard candy as comfort measures.
Gingivitis, hyperemia, hypertrophy, bleeding, tenderness of the gums.	Increased vascularity and proliferation of connective tissue from estrogen stimulation. May be due to inadequate dental care and chronic inflammation of the gums; can be associated with preterm labor and premature birth.	See dentist early in pregnancy, eat well-balanced diet with adequate protein and fresh fruits and vegetables; brush teeth gently with soft toothbrush and observe good dental hygiene.
Nasal stuffiness; epistaxis (nosebleed)	Hyperemia of mucous membranes related to increased estrogen levels.	Use humidifier; avoid trauma; normal saline nose drops or spray may be used.
Leukorrhea: often noted throughout pregnancy	Hormonally stimulated cervix becomes hypertrophic and hyperactive, producing an abundant amount of mucus.	Not preventable; do not douche; wear perineal pads; perform hygienic practices such as wiping front to back; report to obstetric care provider if accompanied by pruritus, foul odor, or change in character or color.
Emotional lability, mood swings	Hormonal and metabolic adaptations; feelings about female role, sexuality, timing of pregnancy, and resultant changes in life and lifestyle.	Participate in pregnancy support group; communicate concerns to partner, family, and health care provider; request referral for supportive services if needed (i.e., for financial assistance).
Second Trimester		
Pigmentation deepens: darkening of areola and vulva; linea negra; melasma (mask of pregnancy), acne, oily skin	Melanocyte-stimulating hormone (from anterior pituitary).	Not preventable; usually resolves during puerperium.
Spider nevi (angiomas) appear over neck, thorax, face, and arms during second or third trimester.	Focal networks of dilated arterioles (end arteries) from increased concentration of estrogens.	Not preventable; they fade slowly during late puerperium; rarely disappear completely.
Pruritus (noninflammatory)	Unknown cause; various types: nonpapular; closely aggregated pruritic papules. Increased excretory function of skin and stretching of skin possible factors.	Not preventable; contact obstetric care provider for diagnosis of cause; keep fingernails short; use comfort measures for symptoms; distraction; tepid baths with sodium bicarbonate or oatmeal added to water; lotions and oils; change of soaps or reduction in use of soap; loose clothing; oral or topical antihistamines or topical steroid cream if recommended by health care provider.

Continued

TABLE 14.2   Discomforts Related to Pregnancy—cont'd

Discomfort	Physiology	Education for Self-Management
Palpitations	Unknown; should not be accompanied by persistent cardiac irregularity.	Not preventable; contact primary health care provider if accompanied by symptoms of cardiac decompensation.
Supine hypotension (vena cava syndrome) and bradycardia	Caused by pressure of gravid uterus on ascending vena cava when woman is supine; reduces uteroplacental and renal perfusion.	Side-lying position or semisitting posture with knees slightly flexed (see Emergency: Supine Hypotension box).
Faintness and, rarely, syncope (orthostatic hypotension) may persist throughout pregnancy.	Vasomotor lability or postural hypotension from hormones; in late pregnancy may be caused by venous stasis in lower extremities.	Moderate exercise, deep breathing, vigorous leg movement; avoid sudden changes in position and warm crowded areas; move slowly and deliberately; keep environment cool; avoid hypoglycemia by eating five or six small meals per day; wear elastic hose; sit as necessary; if symptoms are serious, contact obstetric health care provider.
Food cravings	Cause unknown; craving influenced by culture or geographic area.	Not preventable; satisfy craving unless it interferes with well-balanced diet; report unusual cravings to obstetric health care provider.
Heartburn (acid indigestion): burning sensation, occasionally with burping and regurgitation of a little sour-tasting fluid	Progesterone slows gastrointestinal (GI) tract motility and digestion, reverses peristalsis, relaxes cardiac sphincter, and delays emptying time of stomach; stomach displaced upward and compressed by enlarging uterus.	Limit or avoid gas-producing or fatty foods and large meals; maintain good posture; sip milk for temporary relief; drink hot herbal tea; obstetric care provider may prescribe antacid between meals; contact health care provider for persistent symptoms.
Constipation	GI tract motility slowed because of progesterone, resulting in increased resorption of water and drying of stool; intestines compressed by enlarging uterus; predisposition to constipation because of oral iron supplementation.	Drink 2 L (8-10 glasses) of water per day; include high-fiber foods in diet; engage in moderate exercise; maintain regular schedule for bowel movements; use relaxation techniques and deep breathing; do not take stool softener, laxatives, mineral oil, other drugs, or enemas without first consulting obstetric care provider.
Flatulence with bloating and belching	Reduced GI motility because of progesterone, allowing time for bacterial action that produces gas; swallowing air.	Chew foods slowly and thoroughly; avoid gas-producing foods, fatty foods, large meals; maintain moderate exercise; maintain regular bowel habits.
Varicose veins (varicosities): can be associated with aching legs and tenderness; can be present in legs and vulva; hemorrhoids are varicosities in perianal area	Hereditary predisposition; relaxation of smooth muscle walls of veins because of hormones causing tortuous dilated veins in legs and pelvic vasocongestion; condition aggravated by enlarging uterus, gravity, and bearing down for bowel movements; thrombi from leg varices rare but can occur in hemorrhoids.	Avoid lengthy standing or sitting, constrictive clothing, and constipation or bearing down with bowel movements; moderate exercise; rest with legs and hips elevated (see Fig. 14.12); wear support hose; thrombosed hemorrhoid may be evacuated; relieve swelling and pain with warm sitz baths, local application of astringent compresses.
Headaches (through week 26)	Emotional tension (more common than vascular migraine headache); eye strain (refractory errors); vascular engorgement and congestion of sinuses resulting from hormone stimulation	Conscious relaxation; contact obstetric health care provider for constant or "worst ever" headache to assess for pre-eclampsia; OTC analgesics may be used if recommended by health care provider (e.g., acetaminophen)
Carpal tunnel syndrome (involves thumb, second, and third fingers, side of little finger)	Compression of median nerve resulting from changes in surrounding tissues; pain, numbness, tingling, burning; loss of skilled movements (e.g., typing); dropping of objects	Not preventable; elevate affected arms; splinting of affected hand may help; regresses after pregnancy; surgery is curative
Periodic numbness, tingling of fingers	Brachial plexus traction syndrome resulting from drooping of shoulders during pregnancy (occurs especially at night and early morning)	Maintain good posture; wear supportive maternity bra; condition will disappear after birth if lifting and carrying baby do not aggravate it
Round ligament pain (tenderness)	Stretching of ligament caused by enlarging uterus	Not preventable; rest, maintain good body mechanics to avoid overstretching ligament; relieve cramping by squatting or bringing knees to chest; sometimes heat helps
Joint pain, backache, and pelvic pressure; hypermobility of joints	Relaxation of symphyseal and sacroiliac joints because of hormones, resulting in unstable pelvis; exaggerated lumbar and cervicothoracic curves caused by change in center of gravity resulting from enlarging abdomen	Maintain good posture and body mechanics; avoid fatigue; wear low-heeled shoes; abdominal support may be useful; practice conscious relaxation; sleep on firm mattress; apply local heat or ice; get back massages; do pelvic tilt exercises; rest; condition will disappear 6-8 weeks after the birth

TABLE 14.2 Discomforts Related to Pregnancy—cont'd

Discomfort	Physiology	Education for Self-Management
Third Trimester		
Shortness of breath and dyspnea occur in 60% of pregnant women.	Expansion of diaphragm limited by enlarging uterus; diaphragm is elevated about 4 cm; some relief after lightening	Maintain good posture; sleep with extra pillows; avoid overloading stomach; stop smoking; contact health care provider if symptoms worsen to rule out anemia, emphysema, and asthma
Insomnia (later weeks of pregnancy)	Fetal movements, muscle cramping, urinary frequency, shortness of breath, or other discomforts	Reassurance; conscious relaxation; back massage or effleurage; support of body parts with pillows; warm milk or warm shower or bath before bedtime; no TV or other screen devices in the bedroom or 1 h before bedtime
Psychosocial responses: mood swings, mixed feelings, increased anxiety	Hormonal and metabolic adaptations; feelings about impending labor, birth, and parenthood	Reassurance and support from significant others and health care providers; improved communication with partner, family, and others
Urinary frequency and urgency return	Vascular engorgement and altered bladder function caused by hormones; bladder capacity reduced by enlarging uterus and fetal presenting part	Empty bladder regularly; Kegel exercises; limit fluid intake before bedtime; avoid caffeine; wear perineal pad; contact health care provider for pain or burning sensation
Perineal discomfort and pressure	Pressure from enlarging uterus, especially when standing or walking; worse with multiple gestation	Rest, conscious relaxation, and good posture; contact obstetric health care provider if pain is present
Braxton Hicks contractions	Intensification of uterine contractions in preparation for work of labor	Reassurance; rest; change of position; practice breathing techniques when contractions are bothersome; effleurage; differentiate from preterm labor
Leg cramps (gastrocnemius spasm), especially when reclining	Compression of nerves supplying lower extremities because of enlarging uterus; reduced level of diffusible serum calcium or elevation of serum phosphorus; aggravating factors: fatigue, poor peripheral circulation, pointing toes when stretching legs or when walking, drinking more than 1 L (1 qt) of milk per day	Dorsiflex foot until spasm relaxes (see Fig.14.13); stand on cold surface; oral supplementation with calcium carbonate or calcium lactate tablets; aluminum hydroxide gel, 30 mL, with each meal removes phosphorus by absorbing it (consult obstetric health care provider before taking these remedies)
Ankle edema (nonpitting) to lower extremities	Edema aggravated by prolonged standing, sitting, poor posture, lack of exercise, constrictive clothing, or hot weather	Ample fluid intake for natural diuretic effect; put on support stockings before arising; rest periodically with legs and hips elevated (see Fig. 14.12); exercise moderately; contact health care provider if generalized edema develops; diuretics are contraindicated

hCG, Human chorionic gonadotropin; *OTC,* over the counter.

Some women merely need permission to be sexually active during pregnancy. Others, however, need to be given information about the physiologic changes that occur during pregnancy, have the myths that are associated with sex during pregnancy dispelled, and participate in open discussions of positions for sexual activity that avoid pressure on the gravid abdomen. Counseling about sex practices for same- and opposite-sex couples is within the role of the nurse and should be an integral component of health care.

Some couples need to be referred for sex or family therapy. Couples with long-standing problems with sexual dysfunction that are intensified by pregnancy are candidates for sex therapy. Whenever a sexual problem is a symptom of a more serious relationship problem, family therapy can be beneficial.

Sexual history. The couple's sexual history provides a basis for counseling, but history taking also is an ongoing process. The couple's receptivity to changes in attitudes, body image, partner relationships, and physical status are relevant topics throughout pregnancy. The history reveals the woman's knowledge of female anatomy and physiology and her attitudes about sex during pregnancy as well as her perceptions of the pregnancy, the health status of the couple, and the quality of their relationship.

Countering misinformation. Many myths and much of the misinformation related to sex and pregnancy are masked by seemingly unrelated issues. For example, a discussion about the baby's ability to hear and see in utero can be prompted by questions about the baby being an "unseen observer" of the couple's sexual activities. The counselor must be extremely sensitive to the concerns behind such questions when counseling in this highly charged emotional area.

Safety and comfort during sexual activity. Pregnant women should be aware that they are likely to experience alterations in sexual desire and comfort during sexual activity. Uterine activity can increase with sexual intercourse; this can be related to breast stimulation, orgasm, or prostaglandins in male ejaculate. For most women, this is not a problem. However, a history of more than one miscarriage, a threatened miscarriage in the first trimester, impending miscarriage in the second trimester, and PROM, bleeding, or abdominal pain during the third trimester may warrant caution regarding sexual activity and orgasm.

Solitary and mutual masturbation and oral-genital intercourse may be used by couples as alternatives to penile-vaginal intercourse. Partners who enjoy cunnilingus (oral stimulation of the clitoris or vagina) can feel "turned off" by the normal increase in the amount and odor of vaginal discharge during pregnancy. Couples who practice cunnilingus

TABLE 14.3 Signs of Potential Complications: First, Second, and Third Trimesters

Signs and Symptoms	Possible Causes
First Trimester	
Severe vomiting	Hyperemesis gravidarum
Chills, fever	Infection
Burning on urination	Infection
Diarrhea	Infection
Abdominal cramping, vaginal bleeding	Miscarriage, ectopic pregnancy
Second and Third Trimesters	
Persistent severe vomiting	Hyperemesis gravidarum, hypertension, preeclampsia
Sudden discharge of fluid from vagina before 37 weeks	Prelabor premature rupture of membranes (PPROM)
Vaginal bleeding, severe abdominal pain	Miscarriage, placenta previa, abruptio placentae
Chills, fever, burning on urination, diarrhea	Infection
Severe backache or flank pain	Kidney infection or stones; preterm labor
Change in fetal movements: absence of fetal movements after quickening, any unusual change in pattern or amount of fetal movements	Fetal jeopardy or intrauterine fetal death
Absence of fetal heart rate	Intrauterine fetal death
Uterine contractions, pelvic pressure, cramping before 37 weeks	Preterm labor
Visual disturbances: blurring, double vision, or spots	Hypertensive conditions, preeclampsia
Swelling of face or fingers and over sacrum	Hypertensive conditions, preeclampsia
Headaches: severe, frequent, or continuous	Hypertensive conditions, preeclampsia
Muscular irritability or seizures	Hypertensive conditions, preeclampsia
Epigastric or abdominal pain (perceived as heartburn or severe stomachache)	Hypertensive conditions, preeclampsia; abruptio placentae
Glycosuria, positive glucose tolerance test reaction	Gestational diabetes mellitus

should be cautioned against the blowing of air into the vagina, particularly during the last few weeks of pregnancy when the cervix can be slightly open. An air embolism can occur if air is forced between the uterine wall and the fetal membranes and enters the maternal vascular system through the placenta.

For opposite-sex couples, the female-superior, side-by-side, rear-entry, and side-lying are possible alternatives to the traditional male-superior position. The woman astride (superior position) allows her to control the angle and depth of penetration as well as to protect her breasts and abdomen. During the third trimester, the side-by-side position or any position that places less pressure on the pregnant abdomen and requires less energy will likely be preferred.

Some women, especially multiparas, have significant breast tenderness in the first trimester. The nurse can recommend positions that avoid direct pressure on the breasts and decreased breast fondling during sexual activity. The woman also should be reassured that this condition is normal and temporary.

During the first and third trimesters, some women complain of lower abdominal cramping and backache after orgasm. A back rub can often relieve some of the discomfort and provide a pleasant experience. A tonic uterine contraction, often lasting up to a minute, replaces the rhythmic contractions of orgasm during the third trimester. Changes in the FHR without fetal distress have also been reported.

Risk-reduction measures against the acquisition and transmission of STIs (e.g., syphilis, gonorrhea, chlamydia, herpes simplex virus [HSV], HIV) are advised during sexual activity always, including during pregnancy. Because these diseases can be transmitted to the woman and her fetus, using male or female condoms is recommended throughout pregnancy if the woman is at risk for acquiring an STI (AAP & ACOG, 2017).

Psychosocial Support

Esteem, affection, trust, concern, consideration of cultural and religious beliefs and practices, and listening are all components of the emotional support given to the pregnant woman and her family. The woman's satisfaction with her relationships—partner and family—and their support, her feeling of competence, and her sense of being in control are important issues to be addressed in the third trimester. A discussion of fetal responses to stimuli, such as sound and light, as well as patterns of sleeping and waking, can be helpful. Other common concerns for the pregnant woman and her partner include fear of pain, loss of control, and possible birth of the infant before reaching the hospital; anxieties about parenthood; parental concerns about the safety of the mother and unborn child; siblings and their acceptance of the new baby; social and economic responsibilities; and issues arising from conflicts in cultural, religious, or personal value systems. In addition, the woman may have concerns about the father's or partner's commitment to the pregnancy and to the couple's relationship. Providing the prospective parents with an opportunity to discuss their concerns and validating the normality of their responses can meet their needs to varying degrees. Anticipatory guidance and health promotion strategies can help partners cope with their concerns. Nurses can facilitate and encourage open dialogue between the expectant mother and her partner.

VARIATIONS IN PRENATAL CARE

The course of prenatal care described thus far may seem to suggest that the experiences of childbearing women are similar and that nursing interventions are uniformly consistent across all populations. Although typical patterns of response to pregnancy are easily recognized and many aspects of prenatal care indeed are consistent, pregnant women and their families enter the health care system with unique concerns and needs. The nurse's ability to assess unique needs and to tailor interventions to the woman and her family is the hallmark of expertise in providing care. Variations that influence prenatal care include culture, maternal age, health and obstetric history, and number of fetuses.

Social and Cultural Influences

All health care professionals are responsible for providing safe, evidence-based care that helps people to attain and maintain their optimal state of health. Services that are offered in a way that respects people's social, cultural, and linguistic preferences have been demonstrated to improve the quality of health care and to reduce health disparities. The U.S. Department of Health and Human Services Office of Minority Health (2016) has developed standards for the delivery of socially, culturally, and linguistically appropriate health care; the standards can be accessed at https://minorityhealth.hhs.gov.

Prenatal care as we know it is a phenomenon of Western health practices. In the U.S. model of health care, women are encouraged to seek prenatal care as early as possible. This recommendation may be unfamiliar or seem strange to women of other cultures.

Many cultural variations are found in prenatal care. Even if the prenatal care described is familiar to a woman, some practices can conflict with the beliefs and practices of a subculture group to which she belongs. Because of these and other factors—such as lack of money, lack of transportation, and language barriers—women from diverse cultures may not seek prenatal care until late in pregnancy or they may not participate in the prenatal care system at all. A concern for modesty can be a deterrent to seeking prenatal care. For some women, exposing body parts, especially to a male, is considered a serious violation of their modesty. For many women, an invasive procedure such as a vaginal examination is so threatening that they cannot discuss it, even with their own partners. Many women prefer a female HCP. Too often, HCPs assume that women lose this modesty during pregnancy and labor, but most women value and appreciate efforts to maintain their modesty.

Because pregnancy is considered a normal process and the woman is in a state of good health, many cultural groups regard care from a health care professional to be necessary only in times of illness. Western medicine's view of problems in pregnancy can differ from that of members of other cultural groups.

Although pregnancy is considered normal by many, certain practices are expected of women of all cultures to promote a good outcome. Cultural prescriptions tell women what to do, and cultural proscriptions establish taboos. The purposes of these practices are to prevent maternal illness resulting from a pregnancy-induced imbalanced state and to protect the vulnerable fetus. Prescriptions and proscriptions regulate the woman's emotional response, clothing, activity, rest, sexual activity, and dietary practices. Exploring her beliefs, perceptions of the meaning of childbearing, and health care practices can help health care professionals foster the woman's self-actualization, promote attainment of the maternal role, and positively influence her relationship with her partner.

To provide culturally responsive care, nurses must be attuned to the existence of practices and customs; it is not possible to know about every culture or the many lifestyles that exist. It is important to learn about customs from the women and their families. The nurse can support and nurture those beliefs that promote physical or emotional adaptation. If potentially harmful beliefs or activities are identified, the nurse should sensitively provide education and partner with the woman to design modifications (see Community Activity box).

🏠 COMMUNITY ACTIVITY

Select an immigrant or other minority group in your community and identify childbearing-related beliefs and practices that are unique to that group. Are there stores in the area that sell items that meet that group's needs? Does the community center have activities or classes that are directed toward the group? Are perinatal education programs available that provide essential information while incorporating cultural patterns? Are classes available in languages other than English? What could you, as a nurse, contribute to the community that would help meet the needs of that group?

Emotional Response

Virtually all cultures emphasize the importance of maintaining a socially harmonious and agreeable environment for a pregnant woman. A lifestyle with minimal stress is important in promoting positive outcomes for the mother and baby. Harmony with other people must be fostered, and visits from extended family members may be required to demonstrate pleasant and noncontroversial relationships. If discord exists in a relationship, it is usually dealt with in culturally prescribed ways.

Some cultural proscriptions involve forms of magic. In some cultures, for example, a pregnant woman must not ridicule someone with an affliction for fear her child might be born with the same handicap. A folk belief widely held in many cultures is that the pregnant woman should refrain from raising her arms above her head because such movements can cause the umbilical cord to wrap around the baby's neck.

Physical Activity and Rest

Norms that regulate the physical activity of mothers during pregnancy vary tremendously. Some cultural groups encourage women to be active, to walk, and to engage in normal, although not strenuous, activities to ensure that the baby is healthy and not too large. Conversely, some groups believe that any activity is dangerous, and family members willingly take over the work of the pregnant woman, believing that this inactivity protects the mother and child. It is important for the nurse to identify how each pregnant woman views activity and rest.

Clothing

Although most cultural groups do not prescribe specific clothing to be worn during pregnancy, modesty is an expectation of many. Amulets, medals, and beads are worn by women from some cultures to promote health or protect the woman and fetus from danger (Fig. 14.15).

Sexual Activity

In most cultures sexual activity is not prohibited until the end of pregnancy. Some groups view sexual activity as necessary to keep the birth canal lubricated. Others may have definite proscriptions against sexual intercourse, requiring abstinence throughout the pregnancy because it is thought that sexual intercourse can harm the mother and fetus.

Diet

Nutritional information given by western HCPs can be a source of conflict for some cultural groups. Such a conflict commonly is not known by HCPs unless they understand the dietary beliefs and practices of the people for whom they are caring. For example, some religious groups have strict regulations regarding preparation of food, and if meat cannot be prepared as prescribed, they omit meats from their diets. Many cultures permit pregnant women to eat only warm foods.

Age Differences

The age of the childbearing couple can have a significant influence on their physical and psychosocial adaptation to pregnancy. Normal

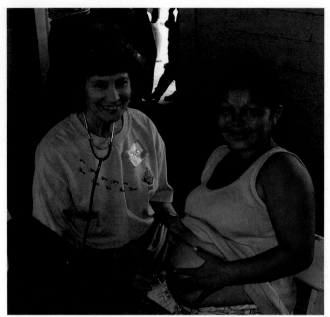

Fig. 14.15 A Young Woman from Honduras Wearing a Red Muñeco Given to Her by Her Mother to Ensure a Safe Birth. (Courtesy Dee Lowdermilk, Chapel Hill, NC.)

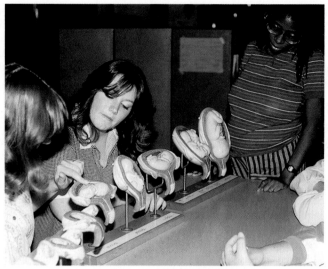

Fig. 14.16 Pregnant Adolescents Review Fetal Development. (Courtesy Marjorie Pyle, RNC, Lifecircle, Costa Mesa, CA.)

developmental processes that occur in both very young and older mothers are interrupted by pregnancy and require a different type of adaptation to pregnancy than that of the woman of typical childbearing age. Although the individuality of each pregnant woman is recognized, special needs of expectant mothers 15 years of age or younger or those 35 years of age or older are summarized.

Adolescents

Teenage pregnancy is a global concern. The United States has one of the highest teen birth rates among industrialized nations, although rates have steadily declined since the most recent peak in 1991. The birth rate in 2017 for teens 15 to 19 years of age decreased to the historic low of 18.8 births per 1000 women. Non-Hispanic American Indian/Alaska Native teens from 15 to 19 years of age had the highest birth rates at 32.9%, followed by Hispanic teens at 28.9%, and 27.5% for non-Hispanic black women (Martin et al., 2018).

Numerous adolescent pregnancy-prevention programs have had varying degrees of success. Characteristics of programs that make a difference are those that have sustained commitment to adolescents over a long time, involve the parents and other adults in the community, promote abstinence and personal responsibility, and assist adolescents to develop a clear strategy for reaching goals such as a college education or a career.

When adolescents become pregnant and decide to give birth, they are much less likely than older women to receive adequate prenatal care, often receiving no health care at all. These young women also are more likely to smoke and less likely to gain adequate weight during pregnancy. Infants born to adolescents are at increased risk of LBW and VLBW infants and infant death. Adolescents are at increased risk for maternal anemia, preterm birth, preeclampsia and/or HELLP syndrome, postpartum hemorrhage, and chorioamnionitis, but they do not have an increased likelihood of cesarean birth (Kawakita, Wilson, Grantz, et al., 2016; Torvie, Callegari, Schiff, & Debiec, 2015; World Health Organization, 2018).

Delayed entry into prenatal care can be the result of late recognition of pregnancy, denial of pregnancy, or confusion about the available

services. Such a delay in care can leave an inadequate time before birth to attend to correctable health problems. The very young pregnant adolescent is at higher risk for each of the variables associated with poor pregnancy outcomes (e.g., socioeconomic factors) and for those conditions associated with a first pregnancy, regardless of age (e.g., gestational hypertension).

The role of the nurse in reducing the risks and consequences of adolescent pregnancy is to encourage early and continued prenatal care; to provide early and ongoing education about pregnancy, birth, and parenting (Fig. 14.16); and to refer the adolescent, if necessary, for appropriate social support services, which can help decrease the effects of a negative socioeconomic environment (see Nursing Care Plan). Adolescents often see the nurse as trustworthy and someone who will maintain confidentiality, as well as provide them with accurate information. Therefore effective communication is essential in providing care to the pregnant adolescent (USDHHS Office of Adolescent Health, 2016).

Women Older Than 35 Years

Two groups of older parents have emerged in the population of women having a child late in their childbearing years. One group consists of multiparous women who intentionally or unintentionally become pregnant in the perimenopausal period. The other group consists of primigravidas: women who have deliberately delayed childbearing until their late 30s or early 40s and those who previously were unable to conceive due to fertility problems and became pregnant through assisted reproductive technology. These women may be referred to as being of "advanced maternal age."

In 2017, the birth rate for women ages 35 to 39 years was 52.3 per 1000 women; this is a slight decline from 52.7 in 2016, and the first decrease since 2010. Birth rates for women 40 to 44 years of age have risen steadily over the last 30 years to the 2017 rate of 11.6 births per 1000 women. Births to women 45 years of age and older have increased since 1997 to 0.9 per 1000 women (Martin et al., 2018).

As maternal age advances, there is a greater chance that the women will have preexisting conditions such as hypertension and diabetes (Gregory et al., 2017). Pregnancy for women older than 35 years of age is associated with increased risk for miscarriage, stillbirth, diabetes, hypertension, placenta previa, placental abruption, cesarean birth, and pregnancy-related mortality. These women are more likely than younger primiparas to have infants with chromosomal abnormalities, LBW

NURSING CARE PLAN

Adolescent Pregnancy

Client Problem	Expected Outcome	Interventions	Rationales
Nutritional intake insufficient to meet metabolic needs of fetus and adolescent client as evidenced by lack of weight gain	Adolescent will gain weight as prescribed by age and prepregnancy BMI.	Assess current diet history/intake.	To determine prescriptions for additions or changes in present dietary pattern
		Discuss her food preferences and teach her how to incorporate them into meal plans.	To engage in shared decision making to increase adherence to diet
		Include the person who purchases the groceries and prepares meals in the discussion.	To involve the person who plans and prepares family meals
Loneliness related to body image changes of pregnant adolescent as evidenced by client statements and concerns	Adolescent will identify support systems and report decreased feelings of isolation from her friends.	Establish a therapeutic relationship and encourage client to describe how she feels about her body.	To listen objectively and establish trust
		Discuss with client changes in relationships that have occurred as result of pregnancy.	To determine extent of isolation from family, peers, and baby's father
		Provide referrals and resources appropriate for the client's developmental stage.	To give information for client support
Potential for interruption of educational progress related to nonattendance at school	Adolescent will continue with studies and complete curriculum.	Discuss with client plans for career.	To create goals to increase chances that she will continue with schooling
		Initiate discussion of child care.	To assist the adolescent in problem solving for future needs
		Provide information on educational opportunities in her school and community.	To enhance knowledge and ability to solve problems

BMI, Body mass index.

infants, preterm birth, and multiple gestation (Creanga, Berg, Syverson, et al., 2015; Frederiksen, Ernst, Brix, et al., 2018; Mills & Lavender, 2014).

Multiparous women. For some multiparous women over the age of 35, pregnancy is desired. For others, it may be unplanned. Some multiparous women have never used contraceptives due to personal choice or lack of knowledge about contraceptives. Others may have used contraceptives successfully during the childbearing years; but as menopause approaches and they stop menstruating regularly, they stop using contraceptives and consequently become pregnant.

Pregnancy can bring feelings of joy as women consider continuing the maternal role and expanding the family. For some older multiparas, pregnancy can evoke feelings of isolation. Such a woman may feel that pregnancy separates her from her peer group and that her age is a hindrance to close associations with young mothers.

Primiparous women. Reasons for delaying pregnancy include a desire to obtain advanced education, career priorities, and use of effective contraceptive measures. Women with fertility issues may not delay pregnancy deliberately but may become pregnant at a later age using assisted reproductive techniques (ARTs). There is evidence of increased risk for preterm labor and preeclampsia for women older than 40 years of age who conceive through ART (Gregory et al., 2017).

Many primigravidas over the age of 35 deliberately choose parenthood. They often are successfully established in a career and a lifestyle with a partner that includes time for self-attention, the establishment of a home with accumulated possessions, and freedom to travel.

The dilemma of choice includes the recognition that being a parent will have positive and negative consequences. Couples should discuss the joys, responsibilities, and challenges of childbearing and childrearing before committing themselves to this lifelong venture.

First-time mothers older than 35 years select the "right time" for pregnancy; this time is influenced by their awareness of the increasing possibility of declining fertility or of genetic defects in infants of older women. Such women seek information about pregnancy from books, friends, and electronic resources. They actively try to prevent fetal disorders and are careful in searching for the best possible maternity care.

They identify sources of stress in their lives. They have concerns about having enough energy and stamina to meet the demands of parenting and their new roles and relationships.

When older women in a same-sex relationship or with a history of fertility problems become pregnant through ART, they can have ambivalent feelings about the pregnancy, the same as younger women who conceive intentionally. They may experience a multifetal pregnancy, which can create emotional and physical problems. Adjusting to parenting two or more infants requires adaptability and additional resources.

During pregnancy parents explore the possibilities and responsibilities of changing identities and new roles. They must prepare a safe and nurturing environment during pregnancy and after birth. They must integrate the child into an established family system and negotiate new roles (parent roles, sibling roles, grandparent roles) for family members.

Adverse perinatal outcomes are more common among older primiparas than younger women, even when they receive good prenatal care. The occurrence of these complications is quite stressful for the new parents, and nursing interventions that provide information and psychosocial support are needed, as well as care for physical needs.

Multifetal Pregnancy

Over the past 30 years, with the increased use of ART and more women over 35 giving birth, the incidence of multifetal pregnancy has increased, although more recently there has been a slight downward trend (Newman & Unal, 2017). In the United States, the twin birth rate for 2017 was 33.3 twins per 1000 births; this was slightly lower than the all-time high of 33.9 in 2014. The birth rate for triplets and higher-order multiples in 2017 was 101.6 per 100,000 live births; this is a slight increase from the 2016 rate of 101.4, which was the lowest level since 1992 (Martin et al., 2018).

A multifetal pregnancy places the mother and fetuses at increased risk for adverse outcomes. Maternal physiologic adaptation to pregnancy is more dramatic with multiple fetuses. Levels of pregnancy hormones, such as human chorionic gonadotropin, are significantly increased over a singleton pregnancy; this increases the risk for hyperemesis gravidarum. The maternal blood volume is increased beyond that of a singleton pregnancy, resulting in an increased strain on the maternal cardiovascular system. Anemia often develops because of a greater demand for iron by the fetuses. Marked uterine distention, increased pressure on the adjacent viscera and pelvic vasculature, and diastasis of the rectus abdominis muscles can occur (see Fig. 13.10). Multifetal gestation increases the risk for pregnancy complications, including miscarriage, gestational diabetes, hypertension, preeclampsia, placenta previa, and postpartum hemorrhage. Preterm birth is more likely with multifetal gestation; the risk rises as the number of fetuses increases. IUGR or discordant growth, LBW, VLBW, congenital abnormalities, neonatal death, and cerebral palsy are more common in multifetal gestation. There can be local shunting of blood between placentas (twin-to-twin transfusion); this causes the recipient twin to be larger and the donor twin to be small, pallid, dehydrated, malnourished, and hypovolemic. However, the larger twin can develop congestive heart failure during the first 24 hours after birth. The risk for death of one or more fetuses increases significantly with higher-order multiples (ACOG, 2016b; Newman & Unal, 2017).

If the presence of more than three fetuses is diagnosed, parents may receive counseling regarding selective reduction to reduce the incidence of premature birth and improve the opportunities for the remaining fetuses to grow to term gestation (ACOG, 2017). This situation poses an ethical dilemma for many couples, especially those who have worked hard to overcome problems with fertility and have strong values regarding right to life. Nurses can initiate discussions with couples to help them identify resources (e.g., a minister, priest, rabbi, or family counselor) to aid in the decision-making process.

The diagnosis of multifetal pregnancy comes as a shock to many expectant parents. They need additional support and education to help them cope with the changes they face.

The prenatal care for women with multifetal pregnancies includes changes in the pattern of care and modifications in other aspects. Prenatal visits are scheduled more frequently. Frequent ultrasound examinations, nonstress tests, and FHR monitoring will be performed. The mother needs information related to self-management of a multifetal pregnancy because guidelines differ in comparison with a singleton pregnancy. Specific instruction should be provided regarding nutrition, so that she consumes a well-balanced diet with adequate caloric intake and gains weight appropriately (Newman & Unal, 2017). Other pertinent information includes maternal adaptations during pregnancy, management of discomforts, and the risk of preterm labor and birth, including warning signs and when to call the provider. The uterine distention associated with multifetal pregnancy can cause the backache commonly experienced by pregnant women to be even worse. Maternal support hose may be worn to control leg varicosities. If risk factors such as premature dilation of the cervix or bleeding are present, abstinence from orgasm and nipple stimulation during the last trimester is recommended to help avert preterm labor (see Chapter 32).

Multiple newborns can place a strain on finances, space, workload, and coping capabilities for the woman and family. Lifestyle changes can be necessary. Parents need assistance in making realistic plans for the care of the infants. Parents should be referred to national organizations such as Multiples of America (http://www.multiplesofamerica.org/) and the La Leche League (https://www.llli.org/) for further support.

PERINATAL EDUCATION

The goal of perinatal education is to assist women and their family members to make informed, safe decisions about pregnancy, labor and birth, infant care, and early parenthood. Another goal is to assist them

to comprehend the long-lasting potential that empowering birth experiences have in the lives of women and that early experiences have on the development of children and the family.

Pregnant women consider maternity care providers and childbirth education classes as the most valuable sources of information about pregnancy and birth. However, time with providers for education during prenatal visits is limited, and only about half of pregnant women report having ever attended a childbirth education class. Attendance at formal childbirth classes has declined in recent years as women have been turning to electronic media for information. Many women seek information from online resources such as pregnancy websites, blogs, emails, apps, and social media as well as television shows about labor and birth (Declercq, Sakala, Corry, et al., 2013). Yet women do not typically discuss the information they retrieve from these sources with their HCPs. Many women are unable to differentiate between commercially sponsored and not-for-profit websites; they cannot assess the accuracy of the information they are reading or hearing. Nurses can help to fill the education gap by talking with pregnant women about the sources and types of information they are finding through the internet and other technology-based resources, offering to answer questions and directing women to sites that present reliable information about pregnancy, birth, newborn care, breastfeeding, parenting, and other issues of interest (Demirci, Cohen, Parker, et al., 2016).

Classes for Expectant Parents

The perinatal education program is an expansion of the earlier childbirth education movement that originally offered a set of classes in the third trimester of pregnancy to prepare parents for birth. Today perinatal education programs consist of a menu of class series and activities from preconception through the early months of parenting.

Expectant parents and their families have different interests and information needs as the pregnancy progresses. Parents may select a variety of classes such as the following:

- Early pregnancy classes that provide fundamental information including (1) early fetal development, (2) physiologic and emotional changes of pregnancy, (3) human sexuality, and (4) the nutritional needs of the mother and fetus. The classes often address environmental and workplace hazards. Exercises, nutrition, warning signs, drugs, and self-medication are also topics of interest and concern.
- Midpregnancy classes emphasize the woman's participation in self-management. Classes provide information on preparation for breastfeeding and formula feeding, infant care, basic hygiene, common discomforts and simple safe remedies, infant health, parenting, and planning for labor and birth.
- Late pregnancy classes emphasize different methods of coping with labor and birth, and these are often the basis for various prenatal classes. Because fear of pain in labor is a key issue for many women, childbirth preparation classes provide information on the management of discomfort during labor and birth and a tour of the birth facility. Topics include methods to reduce discomfort, such as relaxation and breathing techniques, imagery and visualization, and biofeedback. Pharmacologic interventions such as intravenous medications and epidural analgesia are also discussed. Including various pain management strategies helps couples manage the labor and birth with dignity and greater comfort.
- Perinatal education programs offer classes to meet specific learning needs. These include classes for adolescents, first-time mothers older than age 35, single women, same-sex couples that may involve a surrogate mother, adoptive parents, parents of multiples, or women with special needs such as those with visual or hearing impairments. In some agencies, classes are also offered in languages

other than English. Refresher classes for parents with children review coping techniques for labor and birth and help couples prepare for sibling reactions and adjustments to a new baby. Cesarean birth classes are available for couples who have this kind of birth scheduled because of breech presentation or other risk factors. Other classes focus on vaginal birth after cesarean (VBAC) because many women can successfully give birth vaginally after previous cesarean birth.

For the most part, the pregnant woman and support person of her choice attend perinatal education classes. There are also classes for grandparents and siblings to prepare them for their attendance at birth or the arrival of the baby. They learn to cope with changes that include a reduction in parental time and attention. Grandparents learn about current child care practices and how to help their adult children adapt to parenting in a supportive way.

Perinatal classes include discussion of support systems that people can use during pregnancy, labor and birth, and in the postpartum period. Such support systems help parents function independently and effectively. During all the classes the open expression of feelings and concerns about any aspect of pregnancy, birth, and parenting is welcomed. Perinatal education is focused on health promotion and emphasizes how a healthy body is best able to adapt to the changes that accompany pregnancy. Without this context of health, routine care and testing for risks can contribute to a mindset of families that pregnancy is a state of illness as opposed to a healthy mind-body-spirit event.

Some of the decisions the childbearing family must consider are the decision to have a baby, followed by choices of an HCP and type of care, the place for birth, the type of infant feeding, and infant care. If a woman has had a cesarean birth, she may consider having a vaginal birth if the reason for the previous operative birth is not present in the current pregnancy. Perinatal education can provide information to help childbearing families make informed decisions about these issues.

Previous pregnancy and childbirth experiences are important influences on current learning needs. The woman's (and support person's) age, sociocultural background, personal philosophy about labor and birth, socioeconomic status, spiritual beliefs, and learning styles are assessed to develop the best plan to help the woman meet her needs.

PERINATAL CARE CHOICES

Often the first decision the woman makes is to select her primary HCP for the pregnancy and birth. This decision usually affects where the birth will take place. The nurse can provide information about the different types of childbearing HCPs and the kind of care to expect from each one. Women are encouraged to ask potential care providers a series of pertinent questions (Box 14.6). Women report that the primary reasons for choosing a care provider or group are that they "accept my health insurance," they "are a good match for what I value/want," and they "attend births at a hospital I like" (Declercq et al., 2013).

Physicians

Doctors of medicine attended 84% of hospital births in the United States in 2015 (Martin, Hamilton, Osterman, et al., 2017). In general, family practice physicians provide care for primarily low-risk pregnant women and refer high-risk women to obstetricians. Obstetricians provide care for low- and high-risk pregnant women. High-risk pregnant women are often referred to maternal-fetal medicine specialists for part or all of their care. Care often includes pharmacologic management of problems and the use of technologic procedures.

> **BOX 14.6   Questions to Ask When Seeking a Maternity Care Provider**
>
> The Coalition for Improving Maternity Services, a group of more than 50 nursing and maternity care–oriented organizations, produced a document to assist women in selecting their perinatal care provider. After some explanation of choices, the nurse can encourage women to ask potential care providers the following questions:
> - Who can be with me during labor and birth?
> - What happens during a normal labor and birth in your setting?
> - How do you allow for differences in culture and beliefs?
> - May I walk and move around during labor? What position do you suggest for birth?
> - How do you make sure everything goes smoothly when my nurse, doctor, nurse-midwife, or agency work with one another?
> - What things do you normally do to a woman in labor?
> - How do you help mothers stay as comfortable as they can be? Besides drugs, how do you help mothers relieve the pain of labor?
> - What if my baby is born early or has special problems?
> - Do you circumcise babies?
> - How do you help mothers who want to breastfeed?

Modified from Coalition for Improving Maternity Services. Having a baby? 10 questions to ask; 2000. www.motherfriendly.org/Resources/Documents/Having_a_Baby-English.pdf.

Midwives

Increasing numbers of pregnant women are choosing CNMs and certified midwives (CMs) as their childbearing care providers. In 2015, some 8.1% of all hospital births and 32.3% of out-of-hospital births were attended by a CNM or other midwife (Martin et al., 2017).

The midwifery model of care emphasizes the natural ability of women to experience pregnancy, labor, and birth with minimal intervention. Midwifery care throughout pregnancy, labor, and birth is associated with benefits for mothers and babies. These include reduced use of epidurals and fewer episiotomies and instrument-assisted births. Midwifery care is associated with an increased likelihood of spontaneous vaginal birth (Sandall, Soltani, Gates, et al., 2016).

The services provided by midwives are dependent on their licensing and certification as well as the practice regulations in each state. Women who are interested in midwifery care should explore the various types of midwives, the care that is available, where they are allowed to practice and attend births, and reimbursement by insurance companies (see Evidence-Based Practice: Outcomes of Midwifery Care).

Certified Nurse-Midwives

CNMs are registered nurses with education in the two disciplines of nursing and midwifery. They are certified by the American College of Nurse Midwives (ACNM). Nurse midwifery programs are graduate level; since 2010, ACNM has mandated that entry into practice requires at least a master's degree. CNMs are educated to provide women's health care throughout the life span, not just during pregnancy and birth. Nurse-midwives care for women with low- and high-risk pregnancies; they practice collaboratively with physicians or independently with an arrangement for physician consultation based on the condition of the patient. Care is often noninterventionist, and the woman and her family are encouraged to be active participants in the care.

Direct-Entry Midwives

CMs and CPMs are trained in midwifery schools, colleges, or universities. A nursing degree is not required, although a bachelor's degree

EVIDENCE-BASED PRACTICE
Outcomes of Midwifery Care

Ask the Question

For pregnant women contemplating birth options, especially in rural settings, what are the differences between outcomes for births attended by midwives and physicians? What is the relative safety of home births compared with hospital births?

Search for the Evidence

Search Strategies: English research-based publications since 2013 on birth, midwife, home birth (or homebirth), and rural birth were included.

Databases Used: Cochrane Collaborative Database, National Guideline Clearinghouse (AHRQ), CINAHL, PubMed, UpToDate, PLoS ONE, and the professional websites for ACOG and AWHONN.

Critical Appraisal of the Evidence

Pregnant women who live in underserved rural areas or who desire alternatives to physician-attended hospital birth may choose midlevel HCPs, most commonly midwives. Midwives include masters-prepared certified nurse midwives (CNMs), and nonnurse certified professional midwives (CPMs) who have been prepared in programs that meet the International Confederation of Midwives (ICM) Global Standards of Midwife Education (ACOG, 2016).

- A systematic analysis of 15 randomized controlled trials noted that births attended by midwives were associated with less preterm birth, greater maternal satisfaction, and fewer interventions, including regional analgesia, instrumentation, amniotomy, and episiotomy than physician-led births. Cesarean births, adverse events, and intact perineum were similar between groups (Sandall, Soltani, Gates, et al., 2016). Studies that took place in countries where health care systems are highly coordinated between hospitals and various levels of HCPs may limit generalizability to the less well-integrated system in the United States (ACOG, 2016).

- Rural childbirth has its own challenges, including distance, few local health options, limited insurance, poverty, and care for other children that may increase the risk for mother and baby. CNMs attend about one in three rural births, and more in states that do not require the CNM to be supervised by a medical doctor (Kozhimannil, Hennings-Smith, & Hung, 2016).

- Less than 1% of U.S. births, or about 35,000 per year, occur at home, and about one-fourth of those are unplanned or unattended (ACOG). Pregnant women who inquire about home birth may seek to avoid interventions or prefer a noninstitutional setting. Although high-quality evidence is limited, observational studies suggest that home births are associated with fewer

interventions, perineal lacerations, and infections (ACOG). However, in over 1 million home births from 2006 to 2009, the risk for neonatal mortality was two to three times that of hospital births, with no significant difference between certified and uncertified midwives (Grunebaum, McCullough, Arabin, et al., 2016). In addition, the risk for neonatal seizures or neurologic dysfunction was triple for home births compared with medical settings (ACOG).

Apply the Evidence: Nursing Implications

- ACOG (2016) recommends the following to improve outcomes for home births: attendance by physician, CNM, or midwife prepared to ICM standards; access to consultation; and access to timely transport to the appropriate health care facility. In addition, fetal malpresentation, multiple gestation, and a history of cesarean birth are absolute contraindications to home birth.

- Interprofessional practice between physicians and CNMs improves health care coverage and options. State authority for CNMs to practice autonomously has been associated with increased access to care for rural pregnant women (Kozhimannil et al., 2016).

- Nurses can educate women as to safe practices and reasonable expectations for their birth and confidently recommend certified birth attendants in health care facilities for women examining their options.

- Health care facilities should smoothly coordinate the transfer in an attempted home birth, and provide compassionate care and welcome to the transferring patient, family, and attendant without judgment.

- Policy advocates can examine countries with highly coordinated and integrated birth systems, such as Canada and England, and seek to replicate their successful birth outcomes.

References

American College of Obstetrics and Gynecologists. (2016). Committee opinion #669: Planned home birth. *Obstetrics and Gynecology, 128*(2), e26–e31.

Grunebaum, A., McCullough, L. B., Arabin, B., et al. (2016). Neonatal mortality of planned home birth in the United States in relation to professional certification of birth attendants. *PLoS ONE, 11*(5), e0155721.

Kozhimannil, K. B., Henning-Smith, C., & Hung, P. (2016). The practice of midwifery in rural US hospitals. *Journal of Midwifery and Women's Health, 61*(4), 411–418.

Sandall, J., Soltani, H., Gates, S., et al. (2016). Midwife-led continuity models versus other models of care for childbearing women (review). *Cochrane Database of Systematic Reviews, 4,* CD004667.

Pat Mahaffee Gingrich

and specific health and science courses are required prior to entering a CM training program. CMs are credentialed by the ACNM based on a certification examination; a graduate degree is required for entry into practice.

Independent or *lay midwives* are also known as traditional or community-based midwives. These midwives are not certified. They are usually trained through self-study and apprenticeship. It is up to the woman seeking care from a lay midwife to assess the level of experience and expertise of such an individual. Lay midwives can legally practice and are licensed in some states, although there are specific requirements and guidelines that must be followed. Care by lay midwives is usually not covered by third-party payers.

Doulas

A labor doula is trained to provide physical, emotional, and informational support to women and their partners during labor and birth. The doula does not become involved with clinical tasks. There are

also postpartum doulas who provide support and care for women, newborns, and families during the first weeks after birth (Ahlemeyer & Mahon, 2015). Some doulas are certified by Doula International (DONA) or the Childbirth and Postpartum Professional Association (CAPPA), whereas others provide care without having certification.

While there is a lack of research comparing doula versus non-doula care, there is evidence that continuous labor support by trained (e.g., doulas) or untrained individuals has benefits over usual labor support that is provided in hospitals. These benefits include decreased need for pain medication, decreased use of epidural anesthesia, shorter labor, increased satisfaction with the birth experience, increased likelihood of a spontaneous vaginal birth, reduced risk of cesarean or instrument-assisted birth, and lower APGAR scores (Bohren, Hofmeyr, Sakala, et al., 2017). There are no known risks associated with labor support by a doula.

A doula typically meets with the woman and her spouse or partner before labor. At this meeting she ascertains the woman's expectations

BOX 14.7 Creating a Birth Plan

Topics for birth plan discussion and decision making may include any or all of the following:

Partner's participation: Attend prenatal visits? Childbirth and parent education classes? Present during labor? During birth? During cesarean birth?

Birth setting: Hospital birthing room (if available)? A birthing center? Home?

Labor management: Walk around during labor? Use a rocking chair? Use a shower? Use a whirlpool if available? Intermittent versus continuous use of an electronic fetal monitor? Have music or dimmed lighting? Have older children or other people present? Is telemetry monitoring available? Consider stimulation of labor? Consider medication—what kind?

Birth: Positions—Side-lying? On hands and knees, kneeling, or squatting? Use a birthing bed? Will you be photographing, videotaping, or recording any of the labor or birth? Who would you like to be present—partner, older siblings, other family members, or friends? What do you know about the use of forceps? Episiotomy? Will your partner want to cut the umbilical cord? Emergency considerations/contingencies (e.g., cesarean)?

Immediately after birth: Do you want to hold the baby skin-to-skin right away? Breastfeed immediately?

Postpartum care: What kind of care do you anticipate—labor, delivery, recovery, postpartum room; mother-baby couplet care? How long does your insurance company provide coverage for you to stay? Would you like to attend self-management classes or do you prefer to get such information from media sources? On which subjects?

---

and desires for the birth experience. The doula focuses her efforts on assisting the woman to achieve her goals. Doulas work collaboratively with nurses and other HCPs and the partner or other supportive individuals, but their primary goal is to assist the woman. Doulas who are also trained health interpreters can enhance the care of women with limited English proficiency.

Birth Plans

The birth plan is a natural evolution of a contemporary wellness-oriented lifestyle in which women assume a level of responsibility for their own health. The birth plan is a tool with which parents can explore their childbirth options and choose those that are most important to them. The plan must be viewed as tentative because the realities of what is feasible may change as the actual labor and birth unfold. It is understood to be a preference list based on a best-case scenario.

It is useful for the nurse in a prenatal practice setting to initiate a discussion of choices related to birth planning. Some maternity practices provide printed material describing available options and giving answers to commonly asked questions, and tours of the birth setting are offered by almost all birthing facilities. The nurse can provide couples with pertinent information and make them aware of the various options for care and the advantages and consequences of each, so that they can begin making informed decisions. Early plans can be modified as the couple learns more details in their childbirth classes. Topics for the expectant parents to consider when creating a birth plan are listed in Box 14.7.

Nurses can direct women and their partners to websites with information about creating a birth plan (http://americanpregnancy.org/labor-and-birth/birth-plan/). The birth plan can serve as a means of open communication between the pregnant woman and her partner and between the couple and the HCPs. An early introduction to the idea of a birth plan allows the couple time to think about events or situations that could make their childbearing experience more meaningful and those they would prefer to avoid.

Traditionally, birth plans are created prenatally and implemented on admission to the labor and birth unit. However, when women without predesigned birth plans are admitted, nurses can use a template with simple questions about preferences for care to help them develop a simple birth plan. This is in accordance with the AWHONN position statement on nursing support of laboring women, specifically creating individualized care plans for laboring women based on their needs, desires, and expectations (AWHONN, 2011).

Birth Setting Choices

The three primary options for birth settings are the hospital, free-standing birth center, and home. Women consider several factors in choosing a setting for birth, including the preference of their HCP, characteristics of the birthing unit, and reimbursement by third-party payers.

Although the majority of births occur in hospital settings, out-of-hospital births are gradually increasing. In 2015, some 1.5% of births occurred outside the hospital setting. Of those births, 63.1% were at home and 30.9% occurred in free-standing birth centers; the remainder took place in a HCP's office, clinic, or other location (Martin et al., 2017).

Hospital

The types of labor and birth services in hospital settings vary greatly, from the traditional labor and delivery rooms with separate postpartum and newborn units to in-hospital birthing centers where all or almost all care takes place in a single unit.

Labor, delivery, and recovery (LDR) and labor, delivery, recovery, and postpartum (LDRP) rooms offer families a comfortable, private space for labor and birth (Fig. 14.17). Women are admitted to LDR units, labor and give birth, and spend the first 1 to 2 hours postpartum there for immediate recovery and to allow time for their families to bond with the newborns. After this period, the mothers and newborns move to a postpartum unit and nursery or mother-baby unit for the duration of their stay.

In LDRP units, the same nursing staff usually provides total care from admission through postpartum discharge. The woman and her family may stay in this unit for 6 to 48 hours after giving birth. The units are furnished to provide a homelike atmosphere, as LDR units are, but they also have accommodations for family members to stay overnight. Both types of units have fetal monitors, emergency resuscitation equipment for mother and newborn, and heated cribs or warming units for the newborn. Often this equipment is out of sight in cabinets or closets when it is not being used.

Birth Centers

Free-standing birth centers are usually built in locations separate from the hospital but are often located nearby so that quick transfer of the woman or newborn can occur when needed. These birth centers offer families a safe and cost-effective alternative to hospital or home birth. The centers are usually staffed by CNMs or physicians who also have privileges at the local hospital. Only women at low risk for complications are accepted for care.

Birth centers typically have homelike accommodations, including a double bed for the couple and a crib for the newborn (Fig. 14.18). Emergency equipment and medications are usually in cabinets, out of view but easily accessible. Private bathroom facilities are incorporated into each birth unit. There may be an early labor lounge or a living room and small kitchen. The family is admitted to the birth center for labor and birth and will remain there until discharge, which often takes place within 6 hours of the birth. Services provided by the free-standing birth centers include those necessary for the safe management

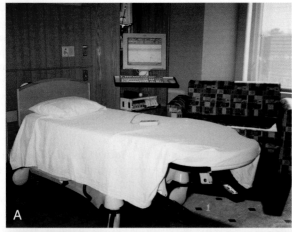

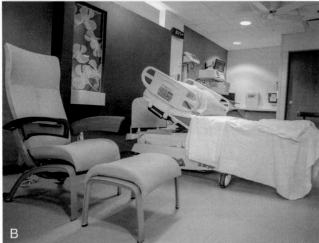

Fig. 14.17 Labor, Delivery, Recovery, and Postpartum Units. (A, Courtesy of Dee Lowdermilk, Chapel Hill, NC. B, Courtesy of Mercy Hospital, St. Louis, MO.)

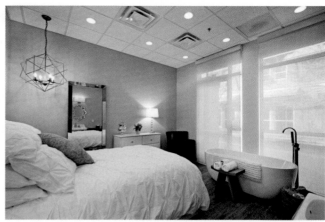

Fig. 14.18 Birth Center Birth Room With Large Queen Bed and Tub. (Courtesy Diane Ortega, CNM, Mesa, AZ. Photo location: Willow Midwife Center for Birth & Wellness, Mesa, AZ.)

of low-risk pregnant women during the childbearing cycle. Attendance at birthing and parenting classes is required of all clients. Expectant families develop birth plans. They must understand that some situations require transfer to a hospital, and they must agree to abide by those guidelines.

Birth centers and hospitals with comprehensive birthing programs usually provide resources for parents, such as a lending library that includes books, DVDs, supplies, and reference materials for childbirth educators. The centers may also have referrals for community resources that offer services relating to birth and early parenting, including support groups, genetic counseling, women's issues, and consumer action.

Ambulance service and emergency procedures must be readily available. Fees vary with the services provided by birthing centers but typically are less than or equal to those charged by local hospitals. Some base fees on the ability of the family to pay (a reduced-fee sliding scale). Several third-party payers, as well as Medicaid and the Civilian Health and Medical Programs of the Uniformed Services (TRICARE/CHAMPVA), recognize and reimburse these centers.

Home Birth

Home birth has always been popular in certain countries, such as the Netherlands. In developing countries, hospitals or adequate lying-in facilities are often unavailable to most pregnant women, making home birth a necessity. The number of planned home births in the United States is gradually increasing.

Home birth remains a controversial topic in American health care. According to ACOG (2016a), while women have the option of making an informed decision about where they will give birth, the safest setting for birth is a hospital or accredited birthing center. Women considering home birth must be informed about its risks and benefits; specifically, home birth is associated with fewer interventions, although it carries an increased risk for perinatal death and serious neurologic dysfunction in the infant. ACOG stresses the importance of appropriate selection of candidates for home birth (i.e., low-risk pregnancy) and identifies absolute contraindications to home birth (i.e., fetal malpresentation, multiple gestation, or prior cesarean birth). The woman should be attended by an obstetric physician, CNM, or other professional midwife with appropriate education and licensure. Safe and timely transport to a hospital and ready access to consultation should be available (ACOG).

Large-scale studies have documented the safety of planned home birth for healthy, low-risk women who are attended by CNMs and when there is a system in place for transfer to a hospital facility if need be (Cheyney, Boybjerg, Everson, et al., 2014; Rossi & Prefumo, 2018; McIntrye, 2012). The National Perinatal Association (2008) and the American College of Nurse Midwives (ACNM, 2011) support planned home birth for carefully selected low-risk women within a system that provides hospitalization as needed. The Association for Safe Alternatives in Childbirth (http://www.asac.ab.ca/) works to foster more humane childbearing practices at all levels, integrating the alternatives for childbirth to meet the needs of the total population.

There are advantages to a planned home birth. The family is in control of the experience. The birth may be more physiologically normal in familiar surroundings. The mother may be more relaxed than she would be in the hospital environment. Care providers who participate in home births tend to be more oriented toward support than toward intervention. The family can assist in and be a part of the happy event, and contact with the newborn is immediate and sustained. In addition, home birth may be less expensive than a hospital or birth-center birth. Serious infection may be less likely assuming that strict aseptic principles are followed because people generally are relatively immune to their own home bacteria.

KEY POINTS

- The prenatal period is a preparatory one both physically, in terms of fetal growth and parental adaptations, and psychologically, in terms of the anticipation of parenthood.
- Pregnancy affects partner and spouse relationships; and parent-child, sibling-child, and grandparent-child relationships.
- Discomforts and changes of pregnancy can cause anxiety for the woman and her family and require sensitive attention and a plan for teaching self-management measures.
- Education about safety during activity and exercise is essential given maternal anatomic and physiologic responses to pregnancy.
- Important components of the initial prenatal visit include detailed and carefully documented findings from the interview, a comprehensive physical examination, and selected laboratory tests.
- Follow-up visits are shorter than the initial visit and are important for monitoring the health of the mother and fetus and providing anticipatory guidance as needed.
- Even in normal pregnancy the nurse must remain alert to hazards such as supine hypotension, signs and symptoms of potential complications, and signs of family maladaptation.

- Blood pressure is evaluated based on absolute values and length of gestation and interpreted in light of modifying factors.
- Each pregnant woman needs to know how to recognize and report signs of potential complications such as preterm labor.
- The incidence of physical, mental, and verbal abuse is increased during pregnancy.
- Culture, age, parity, and multifetal pregnancy can have a significant effect on the course and outcome of the pregnancy.
- Nurses must ask pregnant women and their families about preferences, practices, and customs related to childbearing to provide culturally sensitive care.
- Childbirth education teaches tuning in to the body's inner wisdom and strategies that enhance women's ability to cope effectively with labor and birth.
- Perinatal education strives to promote healthier pregnancies and family lifestyles.
- Nurses can assist pregnant women and their families to make informed decisions about care providers, birth settings, and labor support.

REFERENCES

Ahlemeyer, J., & Mahon, S. (2015). Doulas for childbearing women. *American Journal of Maternal/Child Nursing, 40*(2), 122–127.

Aitken, S. L., & Tichy, E. M. (2015). Rh(O)D immune globulin products for prevention of alloimmunization during pregnancy. *American Journal of Health-System Pharmacy, 72*(4), 267–276.

American Academy of Pediatrics and American College of Obstetricians and Gynecologists Committee on Obstetric Practice. (2017). *Guidelines for perinatal care* (8th ed.). Washington, DC: Author.

American College of Nurse-Midwives. (2011). *Position statement: Home birth.* Silver Spring, MD: Author.

American College of Nurse-Midwives. (2012). *Midwifery: Evidence-based practice.* Silver Spring, MD: Author.

American College of Obstetricians and Gynecologists. (2012). Committee opinion no. 518: Intimate partner violence. *Obstetrics and Gynecology, 119*(2), 412–417.

American College of Obstetricians and Gynecologists. (2013, reaffirmed 2017). *Committee opinion no. 569: Oral health care during pregnancy and through the lifespan. Obstetrics and Gynecology, 122*(2 Pt 1), 417–422.

American College of Obstetricians and Gynecologists. (2013). Practice bulletin no. 137: Gestational diabetes mellitus. *Obstetrics and Gynecology, 122*(2 Pt 1), 406–416.

American College of Obstetricians and Gynecologists. (2014). Committee opinion no. 608: Influenza vaccination during pregnancy. *Obstetrics and Gynecology, 124*(3), 648–651.

American College of Obstetricians and Gynecologists. (2015a). Committee opinion no. 485: Prevention of early-onset group B streptococcal disease in newborns. *Obstetrics and Gynecology, 117*(4), 1019–1027.

American College of Obstetricians and Gynecologists. (2015b). Committee opinion no. 630: Screening for perinatal depression. *Obstetrics and Gynecology, 125*(5), 1268–1271.

American College of Obstetricians and Gynecologists. (2015c). Committee opinion No. 635: Prenatal and perinatal human immunodeficiency virus testing: expanded recommendations. *Obstetrics and Gynecology, 25*(6), 1544–1547.

American College of Obstetricians and Gynecologists. (2015d). Committee opinion no. 650: Physical activity and exercise during pregnancy and the postpartum period. *Obstetrics and Gynecology, 126*(6), e135–e142.

American College of Obstetricians and Gynecologists. (2016a). Committee opinion no. 669: Planned home birth. *Obstetrics and Gynecology, 128*(2), e26–e31.

American College of Obstetricians and Gynecologists. (2016b). Practice bulletin no. 169: Multifetal gestations: Twin, triplet, and higher-order multiples. *Obstetrics and Gynecology, 128*(4), e131–e146.

American College of Obstetricians and Gynecologists. (2017). Committee opinion no. 719: Multifetal pregnancy reduction. *Obstetrics and Gynecology, 130*(3), e158–e163.

American College of Obstetricians and Gynecologists. American Institute of Ultrasound in Medicine, & Society for Maternal-Fetal Medicine. (2014). Committee opinion no. 611: Method for estimating due date. *Obstetrics and Gynecology, 124*(4), 863–866.

American Dental Association. (2019). *Pregnancy.* Retrieved from: https://www.ada.org/en/member-center/oral-health-topics/pregnancy.

Association of Women's Health, Obstetric and Neonatal Nurses. (2011). Nursing support for laboring women. *Journal of Obstetric, Gynecologic and Neonatal Nursing, 40*(5), 665–666.

Association of Women's Health, Obstetric and Neonatal Nurses. (2015). AWHONN position statement: Intimate partner violence. *Journal of Obstetric, Gynecologic and Neonatal Nursing, 44*(3), 405–408.

Biaggi, A., Conroy, S., Pawlby, S., & Pariante, C. M. (2016). Identifying the women at risk of antenatal anxiety and depression: A systematic review. *Journal of Affective Disorders, 191*, 62–77.

Bianchi, A. L., Cesario, S. K., & McFarlane, J. (2016). Interrupting intimate partner violence during pregnancy with an effective screening and assessment program. *Journal of Obstetric, Gynecologic and Neonatal Nursing, 45*(4), 579–591.

Blackburn, S. (2018). *Maternal, fetal, and neonatal physiology* (4th ed.). St. Louis, MO: Elsevier.

Bohren, M. A., Hofmeyr, G. J., Sakala, C., et al. (2017). Continuous support for women during childbirth. *Cochrane Database of Systematic Reviews, 7,* CD003766.

Bushe, S., & Romero, I. L. (2017). Lesbian pregnancy: Care and considerations. *Seminars in Reproductive Medicine, 35*, 420–425.

Carpinello, O. J., Jacob, M. C., Nulsen, J., & Benadiva, C. (2016). Utilization of fertility treatment and reproductive choices by lesbian couples. *106*(7), 1709–1713.

Centering Healthcare Institute. (2019). *CenteringPregnancy.* Retrieved from: https://www.centeringhealthcare.org/what-we-do/centering-pregnancy.

Centers for Disease Control and Prevention. (2015). *Sexually transmitted diseases treatment guidelines: Screening recommendations and considerations referenced in treatment guidelines and original sources*, 2015. Retrieved from: https://www.cdc.gov/std/tg2015/screening-recommendations.htm.

Centers for Disease Control and Prevention. (2018a). *Information for adult patients: 2018 recommended immunizations for adults by health conditions.* Retrieved from: https://www.cdc.gov/vaccines/schedules/downloads/adult/adult-schedule-easy-read.pdf.

Centers for Disease Control and Prevention. (2018b). *Pregnancy and whooping cough: Vaccinating pregnant patients.* Retrieved from: https://www.cdc.gov/pertussis/pregnant/hcp/pregnant-patients.html.

Cheyney, M., Bovbjerg, M., Everson, C., et al. (2014). Outcomes of care for 16,924 planned home births in the United States: The Midwives Alliance of North America Statistics Project, 2004-2009. *Journal of Midwifery and Women's Health, 59*(1), 17–27.

Chughtai, B., Thomas, D., & Howell, A. (2016). Variability of commercial cranberry products for the prevention of uropathogenic bacterial adhesion. *American Journal of Obstetrics and Gynecology, 215*(1), 122–123.

Cook, S. C., Gunter, K. E., & Lopez, F. Y. (2017). Establishing effective health care partnerships with sexual and gender minority patients: Recommendations for obstetrician gynecologists. *Seminars in Reproductive Medicine, 35*(5), 397–407.

Corbella, S., Taschieri, S., Del Fabbro, M., et al. (2016). Adverse pregnancy outcomes and periodontitis: A systematic review and meta-analysis exploring potential association. *Quintessence International, 47*(3), 193–204.

Creanga, A. A., Berg, C. J., Syverson, C., et al. (2015). Pregnancy-related mortality in the United States, 2006-2010. *Obstetrics and Gynecology, 125*(1), 5–12.

Daalderop, L. A., Wieland, B. V., Tomsin, K., et al. (2018). Periodontal disease and pregnancy outcomes: Overview of systematic reviews. *Journal of Dental Research Clinical and Translational Research, 3*(1), 10–27.

Declercq, E. R., Sakala, C., Corry, M. P., et al. (2013). *Listening to mothers III: Pregnancy and birth.* New York, Childbirth Connection.

Demirci, J. R., Cohen, S. M., Parker, M., et al. (2016). Access, use, and preferences for technology-based perinatal and breastfeeding support among childbearing women. *Journal of Perinatal Education, 25*(1), 29–36.

Domenjoz, I., Kayser, B., & Boulvain, M. (2014). Effect of physical activity during pregnancy on mode of delivery. *American Journal of Obstetrics and Gynecology, 211*(4), 401.e1–401.e11.

Driscoll, D. A., Simpson, J. L., Holzgreve, W., et al. (2017). Genetic screening and prenatal genetic diagnosis. In S. G. Gabbe, J. R. Niebyl, J. L. Simpson, et al. (Eds.), *Obstetrics: Normal and problem pregnancies* (7th ed.). Philadelphia, Elsevier.

Duff, P., & Birsner, M. (2017). Maternal and perinatal infection-bacterial. In S. G. Gabbe, J. R. Niebyl, J. L. Simpson, et al. (Eds.), *Obstetrics: Normal and problem pregnancies* (7th ed.). Philadelphia, Elsevier.

Fiset, K. L., Hoffman, M. K., & Ehrenthal, D. B. (2016). Centering prenatal care: Can a care model impact preterm birth rates? *Obstetrics and Gynecology, 127*(Suppl 1), 1s–2s.

Frederiksen, L. E., Ernst, A., Brix, N., et al. (2018). Risk of adverse pregnancy outcomes at advanced maternal age. *Obstetrics and Gynecology, 131*(3), 457–463.

Gregg, I. (2018). The health care experiences of lesbian women becoming mothers. *Nursing for Women's Health, 22*(1), 40–50.

Gregory, K. D., Ramos, D. E., & Jauniaux, E. R. M. (2017). Preconception and prenatal care. In S. G. Gabbe, J. R. Niebyl, J. L. Simpson, et al. (Eds.), *Obstetrics: Normal and problem pregnancies* (7th ed.). Philadelphia, Elsevier.

Hartnett, E., Haber, J., Krainovich-Miller, B., et al. (2016). Oral health in pregnancy. *Journal of Obstetric, Gynecologic and Neonatal Nursing, 45*(4), 565–573.

Health Physics Society. (2016). *Pregnancy and flying.* Retrieved from: http://hps.org/publicinformation/ate/faqs/pregnancyandflying.html.

Heberlein, E. C., Picklesimer, A. H., Billings, D. L., et al. (2016). The comparative effects of group prenatal care on psychosocial outcomes. *Archives of Women's Mental Health, 19*(2), 259–269.

Holden, S. C., Gardiner, P., Birdee, G., et al. (2015). Complementary and alternative medicine use among women during pregnancy and childbearing years. *Birth, 42*(3), 261–269.

Johnson, P. J., Kozhimannil, K. B., Jou, J., et al. (2016). Complementary and alternative medicine use among women of reproductive age in the United States. *Women's Health Issues, 26*(1), 40–47.

Kawakita, T., Wilson, K., Grantz, K. L., et al. (2016). Adverse maternal and neonatal outcomes in adolescent pregnancy. *Journal of Pediatric and Adolescent Gynecology, 29*(2), 130–136.

Kingston, D., Austin, M., & Heaman, M. (2015). Barriers and facilitators of mental health screening in pregnancy. *Journal of Affective Disorders, 186*, 350–357.

Kroll-Desrosiers, A. R., Crawford, S. L., Moore Simas, T. A., et al. (2016). Improving pregnancy outcomes through maternity care coordination: A systematic review. *Women's Health Issues, 26*(1), 87–99.

Lawrence, R. A., & Lawrence, R. M. (2016). *Breastfeeding: A guide for the medical profession* (8th ed.). St. Louis, Elsevier.

Martin, J. A., Hamilton, B. E., Osterman, M. J., et al. (2017). *Births: Final data for 2015. National Vital Statistics Reports, 66*(1), 1–69. Hyattsville, MD: National Center for Health Statistics.

Martin, J. A., Hamilton, B. E., Osterman, M. J., et al. (2018). *Births: Final data for 2017. National Vital Statistics Reports, 67*(8), 1–49. Hyattsville, MD: National Center for Health Statistics.

May, K. (1982). Three phases of father involvement in pregnancy. *Nursing Research, 31*(6), 337–342.

McFarlane, J., Parker, B., & Bullock, L. (1992). Assessing for abuse during pregnancy: Severity and frequency of injuries and associated entry into prenatal care. *Journal of the American Medical Association, 267*(23), 3176–3178.

Meghea, C. I., You, Z., Raffo, J., et al. (2015). Statewide Medicaid enhanced prenatal care programs and infant mortality. *Pediatrics, 136*(2), 334–342.

Mercer, R. (1995). *Becoming a mother.* New York: Springer.

Mills, T. A., & Lavender, T. (2014). Advanced maternal age. *Obstetrics, Gynaecology, and Reproductive Medicine, 24*(2), 85–90.

Moise, K. J. (2017). Red cell alloimmunization. In S. G. Gabbe, J. R. Niebyl, J. L. Simpson, et al. (Eds.), *Obstetrics: Normal and problem pregnancies* (7th ed.). Philadelphia, Elsevier.

Morof, D. F., & Carroll, D. (2018). *Advising travelers with specific needs. Centers for Disease Control and Prevention. CDC health information for international travel 2018.* New York, Oxford University Press.

National Perinatal Association. (2008). *Position paper: Choice of birth setting.* Retrieved from: http://www.nationalperinatal.org/resources/Documents/Position%20Papers/Choice%20of%20Birth%20Setting%20pdf%20.pdf.

Newman, R., & Unal, E. R. (2017). Multiple gestations. In S. G. Gabbe, J. R. Niebyl, J. L. Simpson, et al. (Eds.), *Obstetrics: Normal and problem pregnancies* (7th ed.). Philadelphia, Elsevier.

Olds, D. L., Kitzman, H., Knudtson, M. D., et al. (2014). Effect of home visiting by nurses on maternal and child mortality. *JAMA Pediatrics, 168*(9), 800–806.

Parihar, A. S., Katoch, V., Rajguru, S. A., et al. (2015). Periodontal disease: A possible risk-factor for adverse pregnancy outcome. *Journal of International Oral Health, 7*(7), 137–142.

Roman, L., Raffo, J. E., Zhu, Q., & Meghea, C. I. (2014). A statewide Medicaid enhanced prenatal program: Impact on birth outcomes. *JAMA Pediatrics, 168*(3), 220–227.

Rossi, A. C., & Prefumo, F. (2018). Planned home birth versus planned hospital births in women at low-risk pregnancy: A systematic review with meta-analysis. *European Journal of Obstetrics and Gynecologic and Reproductive Biology, 222*, 102–108.

Rubin, R. (1975). Maternal tasks in pregnancy. *The Maternal and Child Nursing Journal, 4*(3), 143–153.

Rubin, R. (1984). *Maternal identity and the maternal experience.* New York: Springer.

Sandall, J., Soltani, H., Gates, S., et al. (2016). Midwife-led continuity models versus other models of care for childbearing women. *The Cochrane Database of Systematic Reviews, 4*, CD004667.

Torvie, A. J., Callegari, L. S., Schiff, M. A., & Debiec, K. E. (2015). Labor and delivery outcomes among young adolescents. *American Journal of Obstetrics and Gynecology, 213*(1), 95.e1–95.e8.

U.S. Department of Health and Human Services Office of Adolescent Health. (2016). *Teen pregnancy and childbearing.* Retrieved from: https://www.hhs.gov/ash/oah/adolescent-development/reproductive-health-and-teen-pregnancy/teen-pregnancy-and-childbearing/index.html.

U.S. Department of Health and Human Services Office of Minority Health. (2016). *National standards for culturally and linguistically appropriate services (CLAS) in health and health care.* Retrieved from https://minorityhealth.hhs.gov/omh/browse.aspx?lvl=2&lvlid=53World Health Organization. (2018). Adolescent pregnancy. Retrieved from www.whoint/mediacentre/factsheets/fs364/en/.

West, E. H, Hark, L., & Catalano, P. M. (2017). Nutrition during pregnancy. In S. G. Gabbe, J. R. Niebyl, J. L. Simpson, et al. (Eds.), *Obstetrics: Normal and problem pregnancies* (7th ed.). Philadelphia: Elsevier.

World Health Organization. (2018). *Adolescent pregnancy.* Retrieved from: https://www.who.int/en/news-room/fact-sheets/detail/adolescent-pregnancy.

15

Maternal and Fetal Nutrition

Kelly Ellington

http://evolve.elsevier.com/Lowdermilk/MWHC/

LEARNING OBJECTIVES

- Discuss recommendations for maternal weight gain during pregnancy.
- Compare the recommended level of intake of energy sources, protein, and key vitamins and minerals for the nonpregnant woman with recommendations during pregnancy and lactation.
- Give examples of the food sources that provide the nutrients required for optimal maternal nutrition during pregnancy and lactation.

- Examine the role of nutritional supplements during pregnancy.
- Discuss nutritional risk factors during pregnancy.
- Assess nutritional status during pregnancy.
- Integrate the woman's cultural beliefs and practices into dietary counseling during pregnancy.
- Discuss nutritional considerations for pregnant women who are obese and those who have had bariatric surgery.
- Describe food safety precautions for pregnant women.

A key component of preconception and prenatal care and counseling is maternal nutrition. The nutritional status of the pregnant woman influences the growth and development of her fetus, the outcome of her pregnancy, the future health of her offspring, and her own health and well-being. Nurses and other members of the interprofessional health care team who work with pregnant women need to be knowledgeable about nutritional needs and dietary recommendations for pregnancy and the postpartum period, including lactation. Nutrition care and counseling should be individualized for each woman, based on her current health status, prepregnancy height and weight, medical history, health habits, socioeconomic status and access to food, and cultural beliefs and practices.

Key components of nutrition care during the preconception period and pregnancy include the following:
- Nutrition assessment, including weight and height, and adequacy and quality of dietary intake and habits
- Recognition of nutrition-related problems or risk factors such as diabetes, phenylketonuria (PKU), obesity, bariatric surgery, eating disorders, and adolescent pregnancy
- Interventions based on an individual's dietary goals to promote appropriate weight gain, including ingesting a variety of foods, appropriate use of dietary supplements, and physical activity

This chapter focuses primarily on nutritional needs during pregnancy and care management to promote positive pregnancy outcomes. See Chapters 21 and 25 for information about nutritional needs during the postpartum period and for mothers who are lactating.

NUTRIENT NEEDS BEFORE CONCEPTION

The first trimester of pregnancy is crucial in terms of embryonic and fetal organ development. A healthy diet before conception and during pregnancy is the best way to ensure that adequate nutrients are available for the developing fetus. Folate or folic acid intake is of particular concern in the periconception period. *Folate (vitamin B9)* is the form in which this vitamin is found naturally in foods, and *folic acid* is the form used in fortification of grain products and other foods and in vitamin supplements. Neural tube defects (NTDs; e.g., spina bifida, anencephaly), resulting from failure in closure of the neural tube, are more common in infants of women with poor folic acid intake. Proper closure of the neural tube is required for normal formation of the spinal cord, and the neural tube begins to close within the first month of gestation, often before the woman realizes that she is pregnant. Therefore all adolescents and women who are capable of becoming pregnant should take 0.4 mg (400 mcg) of folic acid every day, in addition to consuming dietary sources of folate (Box 15.1). A woman who has had a pregnancy that resulted in the birth of a child with NTD should take 4 mg of folic acid daily, beginning at least 1 month before attempting to conceive and continuing through the first trimester of pregnancy (American College of Obstetricians and Gynecologists [ACOG], 2017a; Centers for Disease Control and Prevention [CDC], 2018).

Maternal and fetal risks in pregnancy are increased when the mother is significantly underweight or overweight when pregnancy begins (Deputy, Dub, Sharma, et al., 2018). Overweight and obese women who lose weight before pregnancy are likely to have healthier pregnancies. Counseling in regard to healthy diet and lifestyle practices, as well as behavioral modification techniques, should be available to women before they become pregnant. Ideally, all women will achieve their desirable body weight before conception (ACOG, 2013/2018; CDC, 2019).

NUTRIENT NEEDS DURING PREGNANCY

Nutrient needs are determined, at least in part, by the stage of gestation. The amount of fetal growth varies during the different stages

BOX 15.1 Food Sources of Folate

Foods Providing 500 mcg or More Per Serving
- Liver: chicken, turkey, goose (100 g [3.5 oz])

Foods Providing 200 mcg or More Per Serving
- Liver: lamb, beef, veal (100 g [3.5 oz])

Foods Providing 100 mcg or More Per Serving
- Legumes, cooked (½ cup)
  - Peas: black-eyed, chickpea (garbanzo)
  - Beans: black, kidney, pinto, red, navy
  - Lentils
- Vegetables (½ cup)
  - Asparagus
  - Spinach, cooked
- Papaya (1 medium)
- Breakfast cereal, ready-to-eat (½ to 1 cup)
- Wheat germ (¼ cup)

Foods Providing 50 mcg or More Per Serving
- Vegetables (½ cup)
  - Broccoli
  - Beans: lima beans, baked beans, or pork and beans
  - Greens: collards or mustard, cooked
  - Spinach, raw
- Fruits (½ cup)
  - Avocado
  - Orange or orange juice
- Pasta, cooked (1 cup)
- Rice, cooked (1 cup)

Foods Providing 20 mcg or More Per Serving
- Bread (1 slice)
- Egg (1 large)
- Corn (½ cup)

of pregnancy. During the first trimester, the synthesis of fetal tissues places relatively few demands on maternal nutrition. Therefore, during the first trimester, when the embryo or fetus is very small, the needs are only slightly increased over those before pregnancy. In contrast, the last trimester is a period of accelerated fetal growth when most of the fetal stores of energy sources and minerals are deposited. Thus, as fetal growth progresses during the second and third trimesters, the pregnant woman's need for some nutrients increases greatly. Factors that contribute to the increase in nutrient needs include the following:

- Development and growth of the uterine-placental-fetal unit
- Increase in maternal blood volume
- Maternal mammary development
- 25% increase in metabolic rate during pregnancy

Dietary Reference Intakes (DRIs) have been established for the people of the United States and Canada by the Institute of Medicine (IOM) and are updated regularly. The DRIs include recommendations for daily nutritional intakes that meet the needs of almost all of the healthy members of the population. They are different from the nutritional labeling on foods, which is based on Reference Daily Intakes (RDIs). The DRIs are divided into age, sex, and life-stage categories. There are specific recommendations for women during pregnancy and lactation and they can be used as goals in dietary planning (Table 15.1). The USDHHS and the U.S. Department of Agriculture (USDA, 2015) have developed guidelines for nutrition, with the most recent guidelines covering 2015 to 2020.

Energy Needs

The recommended energy (kcal) intake corresponds to the recommended pattern of gain. For a woman of normal prepregnancy weight with a singleton pregnancy, recommendations include 1800 kcal/day during the first trimester, 2200 kcal/day during the second trimester, and 2400 kcal/day during the third trimester (IOM, 2006). Energy needs are increased with multiple gestation. The amount of food providing the needed increase in energy is not large. The additional kcals needed during the second trimester can be provided by one additional serving from any one of the following groups: milk, yogurt, or cheese (all skim milk products); fruits; vegetables; and bread, cereal, rice, or pasta. In the third trimester, an additional one-third of a serving will provide the needed kilocalories.

Energy (kilocalories) needs are met by carbohydrate, fat, and protein in the diet. Longitudinal assessment of weight gain during pregnancy is the best way to determine whether the kilocalorie intake is adequate; very underweight or active women may require more than the recommended increase in kilocalories to sustain the desired rate of weight gain. Although protein can be used to supply energy, its primary role is to provide amino acids for the synthesis of new tissues (see discussion later in this chapter).

Weight Management

The desirable weight gain during pregnancy varies among women. The primary factor to consider in making a weight-gain recommendation is the appropriateness of the prepregnancy weight for the woman's height—that is, whether the woman's weight was normal before pregnancy or whether she was underweight or overweight. Whenever possible, the woman should achieve a weight in the normal range for her height before pregnancy. Maternal and fetal risks in pregnancy are increased when the mother is significantly underweight or overweight before pregnancy and when weight gain during pregnancy is either too low or too high. Severely underweight women are more likely to have preterm labor and to give birth to low birth weight (LBW) infants. Both normal-weight and underweight women with inadequate weight gain have an increased risk for giving birth to an infant with intrauterine growth restriction (IUGR). Greater than expected weight gain during pregnancy may occur for many reasons. It may also lead to several risks, noted in the "Excessive Weight Gain" section.

A commonly used method of evaluating the appropriateness of weight for height is the body mass index (BMI), which is calculated by the following formula:

$$BMI = Weight \div Height^2$$

in which the weight is in kilograms and height is in meters. Thus for a woman who weighed 51 kg (112 lb) before pregnancy and is 1.57 m (5 feet 2 inches) tall,

$$BMI = 51\ kg \div (1.57\ m)^2 = 20.7$$

Prepregnant BMI can be classified into the following categories: less than 18.5, underweight or low; 18.5 to 24.9, normal; 25 to 29.9, overweight or high; and 30 or greater, obese (CDC, 2017). The BMI can be calculated at http://www.nhlbi.nih.gov/guidelines/obesity/BMI/bmicalc.htm or https://www.choosemyplate.gov/pregnancy-weight-gain-calculator.

At the first prenatal visit, the pregnant woman should be helped to establish a weight-gain goal for pregnancy that is suited to her prepregnancy weight. Progress toward this goal should be monitored at each visit. Recommendations for weight gain during pregnancy are based on the prepregnant BMI (Table 15.2).

TABLE 15.1 Recommendations for Daily Dietary Allowances of Selected Nutrients During Pregnancy and Lactation

Nutrient (Units)	Recommendation for Nonpregnant Woman[a]	Recommendation for Pregnancy[a]	Recommendation for Lactation[a]	Role in Relation to Pregnancy and Lactation	Food Sources
Energy (kilocalories [kcal] or kilojoules [kJ][b])	Variable	First trimester, same as nonpregnant; second trimester, nonpregnant needs + 340 kcal (1424 kJ); third trimester, nonpregnant needs + 452 kcal (1892 kJ)	First 6 months, nonpregnant needs + 330 kcal (1382 kJ); second 6 months, nonpregnant needs + 400 kcal (1675 kJ)	Growth of fetal and maternal tissues; milk production	Carbohydrate, fat, and protein
Protein (g)	46	First trimester, same as nonpregnant; second and third trimesters, nonpregnant needs + 25 g[c]	Nonpregnant needs + 25 g	Synthesis of the products of conception; growth of maternal tissue and expansion of blood volume; secretion of milk protein during lactation	Meats, eggs, cheese, yogurt, legumes (dry beans and peas, peanuts), nuts, grains
Water (L) in food and beverages	2.7	3	3.8	Expansion of blood volume, excretion of wastes; milk secretion	Water and beverages made with water, milk, juices; all foods, especially frozen desserts, fruits, lettuce and other fresh vegetables
Fiber (g)	25	28	29	Promotes regular bowel elimination; reduces long-term risk for heart disease, diverticulosis, and diabetes	Whole grains, bran, vegetables, fruits, nuts and seeds
Minerals					
Calcium (mg)	1300/1000	1300/1000	1300/1000	Fetal skeleton and tooth formation; maintenance of maternal bone and tooth mineralization	Milk, cheese, yogurt, sardines or other fish eaten with bones left in, dark green leafy vegetables except spinach or Swiss chard, calcium-set tofu, baked beans, tortillas
Iron (mg)	15/18	27	10/9	Maternal hemoglobin formation, fetal liver iron storage	Liver, meats, whole grain or enriched breads and cereals, dark green leafy vegetables, legumes, dried fruits
Zinc (mg)	9/8	12/11	13/12	Component of numerous enzyme systems, possibly important in preventing congenital malformations	Liver, shellfish, meats, whole grains, milk
Iodine (mcg)	150	220	290	Increased maternal metabolic rate	Iodized salt, seafood, milk and milk products, commercial yeast breads, rolls, and donuts
Magnesium (mg)	360/310–320	400/350–360	360/310–320	Involved in energy and protein metabolism, tissue growth, muscle action	Nuts, legumes, cocoa, meats, whole grains

Continued

TABLE 15.1 Recommendations for Daily Dietary Allowances of Selected Nutrients During Pregnancy and Lactation—cont'd

Nutrient (Units)	Recommendation for Nonpregnant Woman[a]	Recommendation for Pregnancy[a]	Recommendation for Lactation[a]	Role in Relation to Pregnancy and Lactation	Food Sources
Fat-Soluble Vitamins					
A (mcg)	700	750/770	1200/1300	Essential for cell development, tooth bud formation, bone growth	Dark green leafy vegetables, dark yellow vegetables and fruits, liver, fortified margarine and butter
D (mcg)	15	15	15	Involved in absorption of calcium and phosphorus, improves mineralization	Fortified milk and breakfast cereals; salmon, tuna, and other oily fish; butter, liver
E (mg)	15	15	19	Antioxidant (protects cell membranes from damage), especially important for preventing breakdown of red blood cells (RBCs)	Vegetable oils, dark green leafy vegetables, whole grains, liver, nuts and seeds, cheese, fish
Water-Soluble Vitamins					
C (mg)	65/75	80/85	115/120	Tissue formation and integrity, formation of connective tissue, enhancement of iron absorption	Citrus fruits, strawberries, melons, broccoli, tomatoes, peppers, raw dark green leafy vegetables
Folate (mcg)	400	400[d]	500	Prevention of neural tube defects, increased maternal RBC formation	Fortified ready-to-eat cereals and other grain products, dark green leafy vegetables, oranges, broccoli, asparagus, artichokes, liver
B₆ or pyridoxine (mg)	1.2/1.3	1.9	2	Involved in protein metabolism	Meats, liver, dark green leafy vegetables, whole grains
B₁₂ (mcg)	2.4	2.6	2.8	Production of nucleic acids and proteins, especially important in formation of RBCs and neural functioning	Milk and milk products, eggs, meats, liver, fortified soy milk

[a]When two values appear, separated by a diagonal slash, the first is for females younger than 19 years and the second is for those 19 to 50 years of age.
[b]The international metric unit of energy measurement is the joule (J). 1 kcal = 4.184 kJ.
[c]Add an additional 25 g in twin pregnancies.
[d]4000 mcg daily if history of infant with neural tube defect.
Data from Institute of Medicine. (2011). *Dietary reference intakes for calcium and vitamin D*. Washington, DC: National Academies Press; Institute of Medicine. (2006). *Dietary reference intakes: The essential guide to nutrient requirements*. Washington, DC: National Academies Press.

Pattern of weight gain. The optimal rate of weight gain depends on the stage of pregnancy. During the first and second trimesters, growth takes place primarily in maternal tissues; during the third trimester, growth occurs primarily in fetal tissues. During the first trimester of singleton pregnancy, the recommended total weight gain is 2 to 4 lb (0.9 to 1.8 kg) for a woman of normal prepregnancy weight. Thereafter the recommended weight gain increases to approximately 1 lb (0.45

kg) per week for an underweight woman and a woman of normal weight. The recommended weekly weight gain during the second and third trimesters is 0.6 lb (0.3 kg) for overweight women and 0.5 lb (0.2 kg) for obese women (ACOG, 2013/2018; CDC, 2019; IOM, 2009; see Table 15.2).

The reasons for an inadequate weight gain should be evaluated thoroughly. Possible reasons for deviations from the expected rate of

TABLE 15.2 Recommended Weight Gain During Singleton Pregnancy

Category	BMI	Recommended Total Weight Gain (kg)	Recommended Rate of Weight Gain per Week in Second and Third Trimesters (kg)
Underweight or low	<18	12.7–18.1 (28–40 lb)	0.45–0.59 (1.0–1.3 lb)
Normal	18.5–24.9	11.5–16 (25–35 lb)	0.36–0.45 (0.8–1 lb)
Overweight or high	25–29.9	6.8–11.3 (15–25 lb)	0.23–0.32 (0.5–0.7 lb)
Obese	≥30	5.0–9.1 (11–20 lb)	0.18–0.27 (0.4–0.6 lb)

BMI, Body mass index.
Note: The IOM (2009) guideline includes a recommendation for twin pregnancy. The optimal weight gain recommendations for women with twin gestation have been made for all prepregnancy BMI categories except underweight. Twin pregnancy optimal weight gain: normal weight 16.8-24.5 kg (37-54 lb), overweight 14.1-22.7 kg (31-50 lb), obese 11.3-19.1 kg (25-42 lb) (ACOG, 2013/2018). The IOM (2009) recommendation recognizes research data to be insufficient for multifetal gestation (triplet or higher).
Data from American College of Obstetricians and Gynecologists. (2013, reaffirmed 2018). Practice bulletin no. 548: Weight gain during pregnancy; retrieved from https://www.acog.org/Clinical-Guidance-and-Publications/Committee-Opinions/Committee-on-Obstetric-Practice/Weight-Gain-During-Pregnancy; Centers for Disease Control and Prevention (2019). Weight gain during pregnancy; retrieved from https://www.cdc.gov/reproductive-health/maternalinfanthealth/pregnancy-weight-gain.htm; Institute of Medicine. (2009). *Weight gain during pregnancy: Reexamining the guidelines.* Washington, DC: National Academies Press.

weight gain, besides inadequate or excessive dietary intake, include measurement or recording errors or differences in weight of clothing or time of day. An exceptionally high gain is likely to be caused by an accumulation of fluids, and a gain of more than 6.6 lb (3 kg) in a month, especially after the 20th week of gestation, can be associated with the development of preeclampsia.

Low prepregnancy weight and inadequate weight gain. Low prepregnancy weight and inadequate weight gain during pregnancy increase the risk of preterm birth and small for gestational age infants (Goldstein, Abell, Ranasinha, et al., 2017).

An obsession with being thin and the practice of pervasive dieting in the North American culture can present challenges to healthy pregnancy outcomes. Figure-conscious women may find it difficult to make the transition from guarding against weight gain before pregnancy to valuing weight gain during pregnancy. In counseling these women, the nurse can emphasize the positive effects of good nutrition as well as the adverse effects of poor maternal nutrition (manifested by poor weight gain) on fetal growth and development. This counseling includes information on adequate weight gain during pregnancy (see Table 15.2) and the expected amount of weight loss that can be expected after birth. Because lactation can help reduce maternal energy stores gradually and promote weight loss, this provides an opportunity to promote breast-feeding (see Chapter 25).

While factors such as nausea and vomiting may inhibit food intake and limit weight gain or even result in weight loss during pregnancy, other influences to consider include access issues, such as lack of financial resources to purchase food. Low prepregnancy weight, failure to gain appropriate weight, or weight loss during pregnancy can be signs of a preexisting eating disorder (e.g., anorexia nervosa, bulimia) or its development during pregnancy. Some women are overly restrictive in their energy intake and/or exercise excessively to avoid weight gain during pregnancy (Kominiarek & Rajan, 2016).

Pregnancy is not a time for a weight-reduction diet. Even overweight or obese pregnant women need to gain at least enough weight to equal the weight of the products of conception (fetus, placenta, and amniotic fluid) (Table 15.3). If they limit their energy intake to prevent weight gain, they may also excessively limit their intake of important nutrients. Moreover, dietary restriction results in catabolism of fat stores, which in turn augments the production of ketones. The short- and long-term effects of ketonemia during pregnancy are unclear, but it may be associated with the occurrence of preterm labor. It should be stressed to obese women (and to all pregnant women) that the quality

TABLE 15.3 Components of Maternal Weight Gain at 40 Weeks of Gestation

Tissue	Kilograms	Pounds
Fetus	3.2–3.9	7–8.5
Placenta	0.9–1.1	2–2.5
Amniotic fluid	0.9	2
Increase in uterine tissue	0.9	2
Breast tissue	0.5–1.8	1–4
Increased blood volume	1.8–2.3	4–5
Increased tissue fluid	1.4–2.3	3–5
Increased stores (fat)	1.8–2.7	4–6

of the weight gain is important, with emphasis placed on the consumption of nutrient-dense foods and the avoidance of empty-calorie foods.

Obesity and excessive weight gain. Obesity increases the risk for adverse perinatal outcomes, including miscarriage, birth defects, stillbirth, abnormal fetal growth, and preterm birth. Maternal risks include gestational diabetes, hypertensive disorders, vacuum- and forceps-assisted birth, cesarean birth, surgical site infection, venous thromboembolism (VTE), and depression (Catalano & Kartik, 2017; Liu, Xu, Wang, et al., 2016; Marchi, Berg, Dencker, et al., 2015; Stang & Huffman, 2016). Excessive weight gained during pregnancy can be difficult to lose after pregnancy, thus contributing to chronic overweight or obesity—an etiologic factor in a host of chronic diseases, including hypertension, diabetes mellitus, and arteriosclerotic heart disease. In addition, the infant of a woman who is obese during pregnancy is more likely to be obese and to develop diabetes as an adult (Spencer, Hauk, MacDonald-Wicks, et al., 2015) (see Evidence-Based Practice box).

In the United States, 60% of women who give birth are overweight or obese; only 30% follow the weight gain recommendations for pregnancy, with most women gaining excessive amounts (CDC, 2019). Overweight and obese women are more likely to gain excessive amounts of weight during pregnancy compared with women of normal prepregnancy weight (Deputy et al., 2018). Weight gain is important, but pregnancy is not an excuse for uncontrolled dietary indulgence. The woman should place an emphasis on the quality of her food intake as she considers her needs and those of her fetus. During pregnancy, an emphasis on regular physical activity and a healthy dietary intake can help avert excessive weight gain (ACOG, 2015/2017) (see Clinical Reasoning Case Study).

EVIDENCE-BASED PRACTICE
Weight Management in Pregnancy

Ask the Question

For obese and overweight pregnant women, what weight management interventions are associated with improved outcomes?

Search for the Evidence

Search Strategies English research-based publications on pregnancy, obesity, weight gain, diet, and exercise were included.

Databases Used Cochrane Collaborative Database, National Guideline Clearinghouse (AHRQ), CINAHL, PubMed, UpToDate, Joanna Briggs Institute, and the professional websites for AWHONN and ACOG.

Critical Appraisal of the Evidence

- Half of all reproductive age women are overweight or obese (Spencer, Rollo, Hauck, et al., 2015) and are more likely to have gestational weight gain (GWG) in excess of recommendations (Jarman, Yuan, Pakseresht, et al., 2016). GWG in obese women tends to accelerate during the second trimester (Overcash, Hull, Moore, et al., 2015).
- Excessive GWG during pregnancy is associated with poor outcomes, due to gestational diabetes, gestational hypertension, fetal macrosomia (Stang & Huffman, 2016), stillbirth, and long-term maternal and childhood obesity (Spencer et al., 2015).
- Interventions promoting diet, exercise, or both resulted in significantly less gestational hypertension, and may lower the risk for cesarean birth, fetal macrosomia, and neonatal respiratory distress. Dietary interventions were associated with the best outcomes. Obese and overweight pregnant women benefited the most from interventions (Muktabhant, Lawrie, Lumbiganon et al., 2015).

Apply the Evidence: Nursing Implications

- Preconceptional counseling should include prevention of obesity, ideally from childhood. Prepregnancy weight loss improves fertility and decreases the risk of preterm birth, gestational diabetes, preeclampsia, assisted delivery, and fetal anomalies (Stang & Huffman, 2016).
- Nurses are frequently the main educators about nutrition and food choices. Successful interventions for pregnant women have utilized individual or group counseling, goal-setting, food diaries, and supportive emails or text messages, with follow-up lasting weeks or months (Spencer et al., 2015). Messages may need to be tailored to BMI categories (Jarman et al., 2016).
- Activity needs to be frequent, fun, and affordable. An excellent idea is encouraging the client to walk with other pregnant women, which provides social support and increased safety. Encourage this healthy habit in the postpartum period, to decrease weight retention and improve subsequent pregnancy outcomes. In addition, the nurse can advocate for low-cost indoor facilities in the community.

References

Jarman, M., Yuan, Y., Pakseresht, M., et al. (2016). Patterns and trajectories of gestational weight gain: A prospective cohort study. *CMAJ Open, 4*(2), E338–E345.

Muktabhant, B., Lawrie, T. A., Lumbiganon, P., et al. (2015). Diet or exercise, or both, for preventing excessive weight gain in pregnancy. *Cochrane Database of Systematic Reviews, 6*, CD007145.

Overcash, R. T., Hull, A. D., Moore, T. R., et al. (2015). Early second trimester weight gain in obese women predicts excessive gestational weight gain in pregnancy. *Maternal and Child Health Journal, 19*(11), 2412–2418.

Spencer, L., Rollo, M., Hauck, Y., et al. (2015). The effect of weight management interventions that include a diet component on weight-related outcomes in pregnant and postpartum women: A systematic review protocol. *JBI Database of Systematic Reviews and Implementation Reports, 13*(1), 88–98.

Stang, J., & Huffman, L. G. (2016). Position of the Academy of Nutrition and Dietetics: Obesity, reproduction, and pregnancy outcomes. *Journal of the Academy of Nutrition and Dietetics, 116*(4), 677–691.

Jennifer Taylor Alderman

❓ CLINICAL REASONING CASE STUDY
Nutrition and the Overweight Pregnant Woman

Rosa is a 27-year-old Hispanic woman who has missed her period for 2 consecutive months and suspects that she is pregnant. She comes for her initial appointment for diagnosis and care. She is married and cooks for her husband and her brother, who lives with her. She immigrated to the United States 2 years ago and speaks little English. She is overweight for her height (5 feet 2 inches [1.57 m] tall, 172 lb [78 kg]). Rosa tells you that this is the weight she has been for several years. When her pregnancy is confirmed, you are asked to plan a diet with Rosa that meets the minimum daily requirements and allows for growth of the pregnancy. You know that it is important to include consideration of personal preferences and cultural factors in your plan. With Rosa, identify barriers to implementing the plan.

1. What is the priority concern or client need in this situation? Support your answer with data as stated in the case.
2. List other client needs/problems in this case.
3. Identify any additional information or assessment data that is needed by the nurse in planning care for this client.
4. What nursing actions are appropriate at this time?
   a. What is the priority nursing action?
   b. Describe other nursing interventions that are important to providing optimal client care.
5. Describe the roles/responsibilities of the interprofessional health care team members (other than nurses) who would potentially be involved in providing care for this client.

Macronutrients
Protein

Protein, with its essential constituent *nitrogen*, is the nutritional element basic to growth. Adequate protein intake is essential to meet increasing demands in pregnancy.

These demands arise from the following:

- The rapid growth of the fetus
- The enlargement of the uterus and its supporting structures, the mammary glands, and the placenta
- The increase in the maternal circulating blood volume and the subsequent demand for increased amounts of plasma protein to maintain colloidal osmotic pressure
- The formation of amniotic fluid

Milk, meat, eggs, and cheese are *complete protein foods* with a high biologic value. Legumes (dried beans and peas), whole grains, and nuts are also valuable sources of protein. In addition, these protein-rich foods are a source of other nutrients, such as calcium, iron, and B vitamins. Plant sources of protein often provide needed dietary fiber. The recommended daily food plan (Table 15.4) is a guide to the amounts of these foods that would supply the quantities of protein needed. The recommendations provide for only a modest increase in protein intake daily over the prepregnant levels in adult women.

TABLE 15.4 Daily Food Guide for Pregnancy and Lactation

Food Group	Daily Amount of Food Recommended for Women[a]	Serving Size
Grains	6- to 8-oz equivalents At least half of grain servings should be whole grains. Whole grains are those that contain the entire grain kernel (bran, germ, endosperm) (e.g., whole wheat or cornmeal, oatmeal, and brown rice). Refined grains have been milled to remove the bran and germ (e.g., white flour, white bread, degermed cornmeal, white rice, and corn or flour tortillas).	1-ounce equivalent = 1 slice bread, 1 cup ready-to-eat cereal, or ½ cup cooked rice or pasta or cooked cereal
Vegetables Vary the vegetables consumed to take advantage of the different nutrients they offer	2½ to 3 cups Weekly intake should include at least the following: 3 cups dark green vegetables (e.g., spinach or greens, broccoli, bok choy, romaine lettuce); 2 cups orange vegetables (e.g., carrots; acorn, butternut, or Hubbard squash; sweet potatoes); 3 cups dry beans or peas (e.g., black, navy, or kidney beans; chickpeas; black-eyed peas; split peas; lentils; soybeans; tofu); 3 cups starchy vegetables (corn, green peas, potatoes); and 6½ cups of other vegetables (e.g., artichokes, asparagus, bean sprouts, green beans, cauliflower, cucumber, tomatoes, iceberg or head lettuce).	1 cup = 2 cups raw leafy greens; 1 cup of other vegetables, raw or cooked; or 1 cup of vegetable juice
Fruits	2 cups	1 cup = 1 cup raw, frozen, or canned fruit; 1 cup 100% juice; or ½ cup dried fruit
Milk, yogurt, and cheese (milk group)	3 cups Most milk group choices should be fat free or low fat.	1 cup = 1 cup milk or yogurt; 1½ ounces natural cheese; 2 ounces processed cheese (e.g., American); 2 cups cottage cheese; 1½ cups ice cream (choose fat-free or low-fat most often)
Meat, poultry, fish, dry beans, eggs, and nuts (meat and beans[b] groups)	5½- to 6½-oz equivalents Most meat and poultry choices should be lean or low fat. Fish, nuts, and seeds contain healthy oils, so choose these foods frequently instead of meat or poultry. (Note: Avoid shark, swordfish, king mackerel, or tilefish because they have too much mercury; white albacore tuna must be limited to 6 oz/week.)	1 ounce-equivalent = 1 ounce (30 g) meat, poultry, or fish; ¼ cup cooked dried beans[b]; 1 egg; 1 tablespoon (15 mL) peanut butter; ½ ounce nuts or seeds
Oils	6 teaspoons (30 mL) Choose oils rather than solid fats. Solid fats are fats that are solid at room temperature, such as butter, shortening, stick margarine, and pork, chicken, or beef fat. Read the label: choose products with no trans fats, limit intake of saturated fats, and choose oils high in monounsaturated and polyunsaturated fats.	1 teaspoon = 1 teaspoon liquid oil (e.g., olive, canola, sunflower, safflower, peanut, soybean, cottonseed) or soft margarine (tub or squeeze bottle); 1 tablespoon mayonnaise or Italian salad dressing; ¾ tablespoon thousand island salad dressing; 8 large olives; ⅙ medium avocado; ⅓ ounce dry roasted peanuts, mixed nuts, cashews, sunflower seeds[b]

[a]These are approximate amounts based on a relatively sedentary lifestyle and should be individualized. Intake may have to be increased for women with a more active lifestyle or multiple gestation, those who are underweight before pregnancy, or those exhibiting poor gestational weight gain. Needs during lactation may also be greater than these recommendations.
[b]Beans are also part of the vegetable group; avocados are also part of the fruit group, and nuts and seeds are part of the meat and beans group.
From US Department of Agriculture (2018). Making healthy choices in each food group; retrieved from https://www.choosemyplate.gov/moms-making-healthy-food-choices.

Protein intake in many people in the United States is relatively high; thus many women may not need to increase their protein intake at all during pregnancy. Three servings of milk, yogurt, or cheese (four for adolescents) and two servings (5 to 6 oz [140 to 168 g]) of meat, poultry, or fish would supply most of the recommended protein for a pregnant woman. Additional protein is provided by vegetables and breads, cereals, rice, or pasta. Pregnant adolescents, women from impoverished backgrounds, and women adhering to unusual diets such as a macrobiotic (highly restricted vegetarian) diet are those whose protein intake is most likely to be inadequate. High-protein supplements are not recommended because of potentially harmful effects on the fetus.

Fats

Fat intake during pregnancy should be no more than 20% to 35% of the daily calories (IOM, 2006), although recommendations for optimal types and quantities have not been established. Pregnant women should avoid the consumption of trans fatty acids, as they can have detrimental effects on fetal development (Garner, 2018).

The long-chain polyunsaturated fatty acids (LC-PUFAs) docosahexaenoic acid (DHA) and arachidonic acid (AA) are considered essential to fetal brain development and neurologic function. Supplementation of omega-3 ($n-3$) LC-PUFA during pregnancy has been associated with reduced risk for preterm birth and improved neurologic and visual development in the offspring (West, Hark, & Catalano, 2017). During pregnancy, DHA is recommended for healthy fetal brain and eye development. Many prenatal vitamins contain DHA; fish oil supplements are another source of DHA. Many providers recommend at least 300 mg/day of DHA for pregnant women. Women can get adequate amounts of DHA by eating 1 to 2 servings (8 to 12 oz) of seafood per week. Because of the risk for fetal neurotoxicity of methylmercury, pregnant women are cautioned to select fish species known to have lower levels of methylmercury.

> ### ⚡ SAFETY ALERT
>
> High levels of mercury can harm the developing nervous system of the fetus or young child, and certain fish are especially high in mercury. Women who may become pregnant, women who are pregnant or nursing, and young children need to follow some precautions: (1) Avoid eating shark, swordfish, king mackerel, and tilefish; (2) check local advisories about the safety of fish caught by family and friends in local bodies of water, but if no advisory is available, limit intake of these fish to 6 ounces and eat no other fish that week; and (3) eat as much as 12 ounces per week of a variety of commercially caught fish and shellfish low in mercury, such as shrimp, salmon, pollock, catfish, and canned light tuna (but limit intake of albacore or "white" tuna and tuna steaks, which contain more mercury, to 6 ounces per week.) (U.S. Food and Drug Administration [FDA], 2018b).

Carbohydrates

Carbohydrates are the primary source of energy. Carbohydrate needs increase during pregnancy to 175 g/day and carbohydrates should constitute no more than 45% to 64% of daily caloric intake. The ideal sources of carbohydrates are whole (fruits, vegetables, whole food grains) instead of processed foods. The diet should provide at least 28 g of fiber per day to help prevent or reduce constipation (IOM, 2006).

Micronutrients

In general, the nutrient needs of pregnant women, with perhaps the exception of folate and iron, can be met through dietary sources. Counseling about the need for a varied diet rich in vitamins and minerals should be a part of early prenatal care and should be reinforced throughout pregnancy (see the Community Activity box). Most health care providers recommend a multiple micronutrient (MMN) supplement (commonly referred to as a "prenatal vitamin") that includes vitamins and trace minerals before and during pregnancy; this is especially important during the first trimester when women are less likely to consume adequate folate and iron (West et al., 2017). Supplements are especially advisable for women with known nutritional risk factors (Box 15.2). It is important that the pregnant woman understand that the use of a vitamin-mineral supplement does not lessen the need to consume a nutritious, well-balanced diet.

> ### ⚡ SAFETY ALERT
>
> Nurses need to inquire about the use of self-prescribed vitamin, mineral, and herbal supplements during pregnancy. Combining other supplements with a multiple micronutrient supplement may cause vitamin and mineral toxicities, which can place the fetus at risk (Garner, 2018).
>
> Some women report that taking an MMN supplement worsens or causes nausea. Suggestions to ameliorate this discomfort include taking the supplement with food, such as after a meal or with a snack; taking the supplement in the evening or at bedtime instead of in the morning; and trying a different form of the MMN supplement such as a chewable ("gummie").

> ### 🏠 COMMUNITY ACTIVITY
>
> Visit a prenatal clinic. Identify sources of nutrition education that are evident in the waiting room. Does the clinic employ a nutritionist or dietitian? Who provides nutrition counseling in the clinic? Do all clinic clients receive nutrition counseling, in either individual or group settings? What ethnic and language groups are served by the clinic? Are print materials available in multiple languages? Are interpreters available? Are there sources for free materials on nutrition that could be placed in the clinic? Identify strengths and weaknesses of nutrition education in that setting. Develop a feasible plan for improving nutrition education in the clinic.

> ### BOX 15.2 Nondairy Calcium Sources
>
> Each of the following provides approximately the same amount of calcium as 1 cup of milk:
>
> **Fish**
> - 3-oz can of sardines
> - 4½-oz can of salmon (if bones are eaten)
>
> **Beans and Legumes**
> - 3 cups of cooked dried beans
> - 2½ cups of refried beans
> - 2 cups of baked beans with molasses
> - 1 cup of tofu (calcium added in processing)
>
> **Greens**
> - 1 cup of collards
> - 1½ cups of kale or turnip greens
>
> **Baked Products**
> - 3 pieces of cornbread
> - 3 English muffins
> - 4 slices of French toast
> - 2 (7-inch diameter) waffles
>
> **Fruits**
> - 11 dried figs
> - 1⅛ cups of orange juice with calcium added
>
> **Sauces**
> - 3 oz of creamy pesto sauce
> - 5 oz of cheese sauce

Vitamins

Fat-soluble vitamins. The fat-soluble vitamins include vitamins A, D, E, and K. Fat-soluble vitamins are stored in the body tissues; in the event of prolonged overdoses, these vitamins can reach toxic levels. Because of the high potential for toxicity, pregnant women are advised to take fat-soluble vitamin supplements only as prescribed. However, toxicity from dietary sources is very unlikely.

Vitamin A. Adequate intake of vitamin A is needed so that sufficient amounts of the vitamin can be stored in the fetus. Vitamin A is essential for cell differentiation and proliferation and for development of the heart, spine, eyes, and ears in the fetus. Vitamin A in excessive amounts is a known teratogen. Congenital malformations of the heart, lungs, skull, and eye have occurred in infants of mothers who took excessive amounts of vitamin A (from supplements) during pregnancy; thus supplements are not recommended routinely for pregnant women. Vitamin A is best obtained from dietary sources (National Institutes of Health Office of Dietary Supplements [NIHODS], 2018d; West et al., 2017).

A well-chosen diet, including adequate amounts of deep yellow and deep green vegetables and fruits such as leafy greens, broccoli, carrots, cantaloupe, and apricots, provides sufficient amounts of carotenes that can be converted in the body to vitamin A. Vitamin A analogs (e.g., isotretinoin [Accutane]), which are prescribed for the treatment of cystic acne, are a special concern. Isotretinoin use during early pregnancy has been associated with an increased incidence of heart malformations, facial abnormalities, cleft palate, hydrocephalus, and deafness and blindness in the infant, as well as an increased risk for miscarriage. Topical agents such as tretinoin (Retin-A) do not appear to enter the circulation in substantial amounts, but their safety in pregnancy has not been confirmed.

Vitamin D. Vitamin D plays an important role in absorption and metabolism of calcium. It is also important in immune function and in modulating cell growth. The main food sources of this vitamin are enriched or fortified foods such as milk and ready-to-eat cereals. Vitamin D is also produced in the skin by the action of ultraviolet light (in sunlight). A severe deficiency may lead to neonatal hypocalcemia and tetany, as well as to hypoplasia of the tooth enamel. Women with lactose intolerance and those who do not include milk in their diet for any reason are at risk for vitamin D deficiency. Other risk factors for deficiency are dark skin, with African American women being at high risk for deficiency; habitual use of clothing that covers most of the skin (e.g., Muslim women with extensive body covering); and living in northern latitudes where sunlight exposure is limited, especially during the winter (NIHODS, 2018h).

Vitamin E. Vitamin E is an antioxidant that helps protect against oxidative stress, and pregnancy is associated with increased oxidative stress. In addition, vitamin E is involved in anti-inflammatory processes, inhibition of platelet aggregation, and immune enhancement (NIHODS, 2018i). There is no evidence that supplementation with vitamin E during pregnancy improves outcomes; it does not prevent problems such as preeclampsia. In fact, there is evidence that supplementation may contribute to abdominal pain and increased risk for early rupture of membranes at term (Rumbold, Ota, Hori, et al., 2015). Vegetable oils and nuts are especially good sources of vitamin E, and whole grains and green leafy vegetables are moderately good sources.

Vitamin K. Vitamin K is needed for the synthesis of prothrombin and clotting factors VII, IX, and X. Small amounts are transported to the fetus during pregnancy. The DRI during pregnancy is the same as for nonpregnant women (IOM, 2006). Sources of vitamin K are broccoli, spinach, iceberg lettuce, and oils such as canola and soybean (NIHODS, 2018j).

Water-soluble vitamins. Body stores of water-soluble vitamins are much smaller than those of fat-soluble vitamins, and the water-soluble vitamins, in contrast to fat-soluble vitamins, are readily excreted in the urine. Therefore good sources of these vitamins must be consumed frequently. Toxicity with overdose is less likely than it is in people taking fat-soluble vitamins.

Folate. Folate is needed to reduce the risk of NTDs in the fetus; therefore, folic acid supplementation is recommended prior to and throughout pregnancy, most importantly during the first trimester. Because of the increase in RBC production during pregnancy, as well as the nutritional requirements of the rapidly growing cells in the fetus and placenta, pregnant women should consume 0.6 mg (600 mcg) of folic acid daily (ACOG, 2017a; CDC, 2016a). All women of

childbearing potential need careful counseling about including good sources of folate in their diets (see Box 15.1).

Pyridoxine (vitamin B$_6$). Pyridoxine, or vitamin B$_6$, is essential for carbohydrate, protein, and fat metabolism, and is involved in the synthesis of RBCs, antibodies, and neurotransmitters. Although the recommended intake during pregnancy is 1.9 mg/day, there is evidence that larger doses are effective for some women in reducing nausea and vomiting (NIHODS, 2018e; West et al., 2017).

Vitamin B$_{12}$. Vitamin B$_{12}$ is involved in production of nucleic acids and protein; it is especially important in the formation of RBCs and neural functioning. It is found in milk and milk products, eggs, meats, liver, and fortified soy milk. The recommended dietary allowance of vitamin B$_{12}$ for pregnant women is 2.6 mcg, and for lactating women, it is 2.8 mcg (NIHODS, 2018f).

Vitamin C. Vitamin C, or ascorbic acid, plays an important role in tissue formation and enhances the absorption of iron. The vitamin C needs of most women are readily met by a diet that includes at least one or two daily servings of citrus fruit or juice or another good source of the vitamin (see Table 15.1), but women who smoke and those who are exposed to secondhand smoke need more (NIHODS, 2018g).

Minerals

Iron. Iron is needed by the pregnant woman to allow transfer of adequate iron to the fetus and to permit expansion of the maternal RBC mass. Poor iron status, which can result in iron deficiency anemia, is relatively common among women in the childbearing years. This is not the same as the *physiologic anemia of pregnancy*, which is a normal occurrence as the maternal blood volume increases (see Chapter 13). A pregnant woman is considered anemic if the hemoglobin is less than 11 g/dL or the hematocrit is less than 33% during the first or third trimester, or if the hemoglobin is less than 10.5 g/dL or the hematocrit is less than 32% during the second trimester (West et al., 2017). Anemic women are poorly prepared to tolerate hemorrhage at the time of birth. Anemia increases the risk of maternal and fetal death, preterm birth, and low birth weight. In the United States, anemia is most common among adolescents, African American women, women of lower socioeconomic status and lower education, and women carrying more than one fetus (West et al.).

The recommended daily allowance for iron during pregnancy is 27 mg (IOM, 2006); this is the amount of elemental iron in most MMN supplements. Iron supplements may be poorly tolerated during the nausea prevalent in the first trimester, and starting the supplement after this point may improve tolerance. If maternal iron deficiency anemia is present (preferably diagnosed by measurement of serum ferritin, a storage form of iron), increased dosages may be required and must be discussed with the woman's health care provider. Certain foods taken with an iron supplement can promote or inhibit absorption of iron from the supplement. See the Teaching for Self-Management box: Iron Supplementation. Even when a woman is taking an iron supplement, she should also include good food sources of iron in her daily diet (see Table 15.1).

Calcium. There is no increase in the DRI of calcium during pregnancy and lactation compared with the recommendation for the nonpregnant woman (see Table 15.1). The normal amount for the nonpregnant woman appears to provide sufficient calcium for fetal bone and tooth development to proceed while maintaining maternal bone mass. Milk and yogurt are especially rich sources of calcium. Calcium-fortified juices and other beverages provide extra calcium. Nevertheless, many women do not consume these foods or do not consume adequate amounts to provide the recommended intake of calcium. One problem that can interfere with milk consumption is

lactose intolerance, the inability to digest milk sugar (lactose) caused by the lack of the lactase enzyme in the small intestine. It is relatively common in adults, particularly African Americans, Asians, Native Americans, and Inuits (Alaskan Natives). Milk consumption can cause abdominal cramping, bloating, and diarrhea in such people, although many lactose-intolerant individuals can tolerate small amounts of milk without symptoms. Yogurt, sweet acidophilus milk, buttermilk, cheese, chocolate milk, and cocoa may be tolerated even when fresh fluid milk is not. Commercial lactase supplements (e.g., Lactaid) are widely available to consume with milk, and many supermarkets stock lactase-treated milk. The lactase in these products hydrolyzes, or digests, the lactose in milk, making it possible for lactose-intolerant people to drink milk.

In some cultures it is uncommon for adults to drink milk. For example, Puerto Ricans and other Hispanic people may use milk only as an additive in coffee. Pregnant women from these cultures may need to consume nondairy sources of calcium (see Box 15.2). If calcium intake appears low and the woman does not change her dietary habits despite counseling, a calcium supplement may be needed daily, to be determined by her health care provider. Calcium supplements may also be recommended when a pregnant woman experiences leg cramps caused by an imbalance in the calcium-to-phosphorus ratio.

Magnesium. Magnesium is essential to numerous physiologic processes, including protein synthesis, muscle and nerve function, glycolysis, and regulation of blood pressure. Diets of women in the childbearing years are likely to be low in magnesium. Adolescents and low-income women are especially at risk. Dairy products, nuts, whole grains, and green leafy vegetables are good sources of magnesium (NIHODS, 2018b).

Zinc. Zinc is a constituent of numerous enzymes involved in major metabolic pathways. Zinc deficiency is associated with fetal malformations of the central nervous system. The recommended daily intake of zinc is 11 mg and may be higher for women on vegetarian diets. Sources of zinc include oysters and other seafood, red meat, poultry, dairy products, beans, nuts, whole grains, and fortified cereals (NIHODS, 2018k).

When large amounts of iron and folic acid are consumed, the absorption of zinc is inhibited and the serum zinc levels are reduced as a result. If a woman is taking more than 60 mg of elemental iron, she also needs a zinc supplement (West et al., 2017).

Choline. Choline is essential for fetal neural development and function; it is important for cell signaling and for integrity of cell membranes as well as for stem cell proliferation and apoptosis. Pregnant women should consume 450 mg/day. Good sources of choline include eggs, lean beef, tofu, brussels sprouts, cauliflower, navy beans, and peanut butter (NIHODS, 2018a; West et al., 2017).

Fluids and Electrolytes
Fluids

Water is the main substance of cells, blood, lymph, amniotic fluid, and other vital body fluids. It is essential during the exchange of nutrients and waste products across cell membranes. It also aids in maintaining body temperature. Adequate fluid intake promotes regular bowel function, which is sometimes a problem during pregnancy. The recommended daily intake is about 8 to 10 glasses (2.3 L) of fluid. Water, milk, and decaffeinated tea are good sources. Foods in the diet should supply an additional 700 mL or more of fluid for a total intake of 3 L/day (IOM, 2006). Dehydration may increase the risk for cramping, contractions, and preterm labor.

Sodium

During pregnancy, the need for sodium increases slightly, primarily because the body water is expanding (e.g., the expanding blood volume). Sodium is essential for maintaining body water balance. In the past, dietary sodium was routinely restricted in an effort to control the peripheral edema that commonly occurs during pregnancy. It is now recognized that moderate peripheral edema is normal in pregnancy, occurring as a response to the fluid-retaining effects of elevated levels of estrogen. Sodium is not routinely restricted in pregnancy, and restriction has not proved effective in preventing hypertensive disorders of pregnancy (e.g., preeclampsia) (ACOG, 2013). Severe sodium restriction may make it difficult for pregnant women to achieve an adequate diet. In general, sodium restriction is necessary only if the woman has a medical condition such as renal or liver failure or hypertension that warrants such a restriction.

Pregnancy is an opportune time to teach pregnant women that avoiding excessive salt intake is part of a healthy lifestyle. The recommended sodium intake for adults is less than 2300 mg/day (USDHHS & USDA, 2015). Table salt (sodium chloride) is the richest source of sodium, with approximately 2.3 g of sodium contained in 1 teaspoon (5 g) of salt. Most canned foods contain added salt, unless the label states otherwise. Large amounts of sodium are also found in many processed foods, including meats (e.g., smoked or cured meats, cold cuts, and corned beef), frozen entrees and meals, baked goods, mixes for casseroles or grain products, soups, and condiments. Products low in nutritive value and excessively high in sodium include pretzels, potato and other chips (except salt-free), pickles, ketchup, prepared mustard, steak and Worcestershire sauces, some soft drinks, and bouillon.

A moderate sodium intake can usually be achieved by salting food lightly during cooking; adding no additional salt at the table; and avoiding low-nutrient, high-sodium foods.

Potassium

Potassium is important in maintaining fluid and electrolyte balance, transmission of nerve impulses, muscle contraction, energy production, and regulation of blood pressure (NIHODS, 2018c).

Potassium has been identified as one of the nutrients most likely to be lacking in the diets of women of childbearing years. A diet including 8 to 10 servings of unprocessed fruits and vegetables daily, along with moderate amounts of low-fat meats and dairy products, has been effective in reducing sodium intake while providing adequate amounts of potassium.

Other Nutritional Considerations

Alcohol

Alcohol use is contraindicated throughout pregnancy. There is no safe amount or type of alcohol during pregnancy, and there is no time during pregnancy when alcohol consumption is without risk. Because alcohol is a teratogen, it can cause birth defects, impaired cognitive and psychomotor development, and emotional and behavioral problems. Fetal alcohol syndrome can result from maternal alcohol consumption; this severe disorder involves growth restriction, central nervous system abnormalities, and facial dysmorphia (see Chapter 35) (ACOG, 2017b).

Caffeine

Modest caffeine consumption of less than 200 mg daily has not been associated with miscarriage or preterm birth. The safety of caffeine use in pregnancy has been studied with some mixed results (ACOG, 2010/2016). Caffeine is found not only in coffee but also in tea, some soft drinks, chocolate, and energy drinks.

Artificial Sweeteners

Aspartame (NutraSweet, Equal), acesulfame potassium (Sunett), and sucralose (Splenda) are artificial sweeteners commonly used in low- or no-calorie beverages and low-calorie food products. They have not been found to have adverse effects on the mother or fetus and therefore are approved by the U.S. Food and Drug Administration (USFDA, 2018a) for use during pregnancy. However, aspartame, which contains phenylalanine, should be avoided by pregnant women with PKU. Stevia (stevioside) is a plant-based sweetener sold as a dietary supplement; no acceptable daily intake has been established for Stevia. Agave is another dietary supplement sweetener, but little is known about its safety or effects in pregnancy.

Pica and Food Cravings

Pica, which is the practice of consuming nonfood substances (e.g., clay, soil, and laundry starch) or excessive amounts of foodstuffs low in nutritional value (e.g., cornstarch, ice or freezer frost, baking powder, raw rice, flour), is often influenced by the woman's cultural background (Fig. 15.1). In the United States, it appears to be most common among African American and Hispanic women, women from rural areas, and women with a family history of pica. One problem with pica is that regular and heavy consumption of low-nutrient products may cause more nutritious foods to be displaced from the diet. In addition, the pica items consumed may interfere with the absorption of nutrients, especially minerals. Pica is strongly associated with iron deficiency during pregnancy, although the cause is unclear (Young & Cox, 2017).

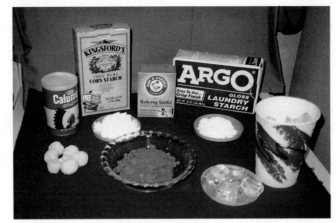

Fig. 15.1 Nonfood Substances Consumed in Pica: Baking Powder, Cornstarch, Baking Soda, Laundry Starch, Ice, Nzu from Nigeria, and red clay from Georgia. Some individuals practice poly-pica, consuming more than one of these or other nonfood substances. (Courtesy Shannon Perry, Phoenix, AZ.)

Moreover, there is a risk that nonfood items are contaminated with heavy metals or other toxic substances. Among Hispanic and Latino women, consumption of *"tierra"* includes both soil and pulverized Mexican pottery. Lead contamination of soils and soil-based products has caused high levels of lead in pregnant women and their newborns. Questions about regular household use of Mexican pottery in cooking or serving food or ingestion of ground pottery must be included in interviews or questionnaires regarding the nutrition intake of pregnant women.

Screening for pica should occur at the first prenatal visit, every trimester, and anytime anemia is present (Young & Cox, 2017). The practice of pica, as well as details of the types and amounts of products ingested, is likely to be discovered only by the sensitive interviewer who has developed a relationship of trust with the woman. In a nonjudgmental manner, the interviewer may ask questions such as "Have you had any cravings? "Have you had cravings for things that are not food, such as ice, clay, or dirt?" "How much of these things have you eaten and how often?" (Young & Cox).

Many women experience food cravings during pregnancy. In general, consuming foods to satisfy the cravings is not harmful. However, there is some concern that it can lead to dietary imbalances, especially if the cravings involve pica. The nurse can suggest choosing healthy alternatives for cravings, eating small amounts of the craved foods (buying single servings), eating regularly and including healthy snacks to avoid drops in blood glucose levels, and using distraction to curb the craving (take a walk or make a call to a friend).

Vegetarian Diets

Vegetarian diets represent a dietary modification that is most often by personal choice. Vegetarian diets can vary widely. Foods basic to almost all vegetarian diets are vegetables, fruits, legumes, nuts, seeds, and grains, but with many variations. Lacto-vegetarian diets include milk products. Lacto-ovovegetarians consume eggs and dairy products in addition to plant products. Strict vegetarians, or vegans, consume only plant products. All of these types of vegetarian diets, if they are well planned, can be nutritionally adequate for pregnant and lactating women. In general, vegetarian diets, if not well planned, are likely to be deficient in iron; zinc; vitamins D, E, and B$_{12}$; choline; calcium; and essential fatty acids (Garner, 2018).

Well-balanced vegetarian diets provide adequate protein. Plant proteins tend to be "incomplete," in that they lack one or more amino acids required for growth and the maintenance of body tissues. However, the daily consumption of a variety of different plant proteins—grains, dried beans and peas, nuts, and seeds—can provide all of the essential amino acids (Garner, 2018).

> ## ! NURSING ALERT
>
> All pregnant women who consume vegan diets should be referred to a dietician for nutritional counseling (West et al., 2017). This should ideally be done in the preconception period, or as early as possible during pregnancy.

Gluten-Free Diets

Increasingly, women are eliminating gluten from their diets based on health benefits popularized by the lay press. However, there is little evidence to support such benefits, except in women with celiac disease or gluten sensitivity. Gluten-free diets are usually deficient in folate, thiamin, niacin, riboflavin, and iron. The deficiencies can be reduced through substitution of whole grain foods that do not contain gluten (Garner, 2018).

CARE MANAGEMENT

During pregnancy, nutrition plays a key role in optimizing perinatal outcomes. Interest in achieving and maintaining a healthy lifestyle and the desire to comply with dietary recommendations may be enhanced during pregnancy because parents want to "do what is best for the baby." Optimal nutrition cannot eliminate all problems that may arise during pregnancy, but it does establish a good foundation for supporting the needs of the mother and the fetus.

Assessment

Ideally a nutritional assessment is performed before conception so that any recommended changes in diet, lifestyle, and weight can be initiated before the woman becomes pregnant. Information on nutrition and diet is obtained from an interview and review of the woman's health records, physical examination, and laboratory results. A nutritional assessment is also completed at the first prenatal visit. In follow-up prenatal care visits throughout the pregnancy, the nurse or health care provider monitors the woman's nutritional status and related needs and concerns.

Health History

A thorough health history completed at the first prenatal visit provides data related to nutritional needs and concerns. The woman's nutritional status may be affected by chronic maternal illnesses or disorders such as diabetes mellitus, renal disease, liver disease, cystic fibrosis, or other malabsorptive disorders (e.g., Crohn disease), seizure disorders and the use of anticonvulsant agents, hypertension, PKU, and eating disorders. Bariatric surgery has serious implications for nutritional health during pregnancy. Information about current medications (prescription and over the counter) and the use of alcohol, tobacco, other drugs, and herbal supplements should be part of the health history.

Review of the obstetric and gynecologic history may reveal nutritional concerns. Nutrition reserves may be depleted in the multiparous woman or one who has had frequent pregnancies (especially three pregnancies within 2 years). A history of preterm birth or the birth of an LBW or small for gestational age (SGA) infant may indicate inadequate dietary intake. Birth of a large for gestational age (LGA) infant often indicates the existence of maternal diabetes mellitus.

Contraceptive methods also may affect reproductive health. Increased menstrual blood loss often occurs during the first 3 to 6 months after placement of an intrauterine contraceptive device; consequently, the user may have low iron stores or even iron deficiency anemia. Oral contraceptive agents are associated with decreased menstrual losses and increased iron stores; however, oral contraceptives may interfere with folic acid metabolism.

It is important to note if the pregnant woman is an adolescent and whether this is a singleton pregnancy or multiple gestation. Adolescent pregnancy and multiple gestation have implications for nutritional care and counseling.

Usual Maternal Diet

Assessment includes collecting information about the woman's usual food and beverage intake. A self-administered questionnaire can be used to gain information about the woman's typical diet (Box 15.3). In addition, a nutritional assessment includes the adequacy of her income and other resources to meet her nutritional needs; any dietary modifications, food allergies, and intolerances; all medications and nutrition supplements being taken; and unusual cravings, pica, and cultural dietary practices. In addition, the presence and severity of nutrition-related discomforts of pregnancy such as nausea and vomiting, constipation, and pyrosis (heartburn) should be determined. The nurse should be alert to any evidence of eating disorders, such as anorexia nervosa, bulimia, or frequent and rigorous dieting before or during pregnancy.

The effect of food allergies and intolerances on nutritional status varies. Lactose intolerance is of special concern in pregnant and lactating women because no other food group equals milk and milk products in terms of calcium content. If a woman has lactose intolerance, the interviewer should explore her intake of other calcium sources (Box 15.4).

The assessment must include an evaluation of the woman's financial status and her knowledge of sound dietary practices. The quality of the diet improves with increasing socioeconomic status and educational level. Poor women may not have access to adequate refrigeration and cooking facilities and may find it difficult to obtain adequate nutritious food. Foodborne illnesses may cause adverse effects in pregnancy, and the woman's understanding of safe food-handling practices should be assessed. When potential problems are identified, they should be followed up with specific questions.

Physical Examination

Anthropometric (body) measurements provide short- and long-term information on a woman's nutritional status and are thus essential to the assessment. At a minimum, the woman's height and weight must be determined at the time of her first prenatal visit, and her weight should be measured at each subsequent visit (see earlier discussion of BMI). The BMI is used to determine the appropriate weight gain recommendations during pregnancy (see Table 15.2).

A careful physical examination can reveal objective signs of poor nutrition (Table 15.5). It is important to note, however, that some of these signs are nonspecific and that the physiologic changes of pregnancy may complicate the interpretation of physical findings. For example, lower-extremity edema often occurs when kilocalorie and protein deficiencies are present, but it may also be a normal finding in the third trimester of pregnancy. The interpretation of physical findings is made easier by a thorough health history and by laboratory testing if indicated.

Laboratory Testing

The only nutrition-related laboratory testing needed by most pregnant women is a hematocrit or hemoglobin measurement to screen for

BOX 15.3 Food Intake Questionnaire

Which of the following did you eat or drink yesterday? If the way you ate yesterday wasn't the way you usually eat, choose a recent day that was typical for you.

Food or Drink	Number of Servings
Beer, wine, other alcoholic drinks	_____
Tea	_____
Coffee	_____
Caffeinated	_____
Decaffeinated	_____
Fruit drink	_____
Water	_____
Cheese	_____
Macaroni and cheese	_____
Other foods with cheese (e.g., lasagna, enchiladas, cheeseburgers)	_____
Orange or grapefruit	_____
Bananas	_____
Peaches or apricots	_____
Green salad	_____
Spinach or greens	_____
Green peas	_____
Sweet potatoes	_____
Carrots	_____
Meat	_____
Fish	_____
Peanut butter	_____
Dried beans or peas	_____
Bacon or sausage	_____
Bread	_____
Rice	_____
Spaghetti or other pasta	_____
Tortillas	_____
French fries	_____
Orange or grapefruit juice	_____
Fruit juice other than orange or grapefruit	_____
Soft drinks	_____
Milk	_____
Cereal with milk	_____
Yogurt	_____
Pizza	_____
Melon (e.g., watermelon, cantaloupe, honeydew)	_____
Berries (kind)	_____
Apples	_____
Other fruit	_____
Broccoli	_____
Green beans	_____
Potatoes (other than fried)	_____
Corn	_____
Other vegetables	_____

Food or Drink	Number of Servings
Chicken or turkey	_____
Egg	_____
Nuts	_____
Hot dog	_____
Cold cuts (e.g., bologna)	_____
Roll/bagel	_____
Noodles	_____
Chips	_____
Cake	_____
Donut or pastry	_____
Cookie	_____
Pie	_____

Are you often bothered by any of the following? (Circle all that apply.)
Nausea Vomiting Heartburn Constipation

Are you on a special diet? No _______ Yes _______
If yes, what kind?
____
____

Do you try to limit the amount or kind of food you eat to control your weight?
No _______ Yes _______

Do you avoid any foods for health or religious reasons?
No _______ Yes _______
If yes, what foods?
____
____

Do you take any prescribed drugs or medications? No _______ Yes _______
If yes, what are they?
____
____

Do you take any over-the-counter medications (e.g., vitamins, aspirin, cold medicines, acetaminophen [Tylenol])? No _______ Yes _______
If yes, what are they?
____
____

Do you take any herbal supplements? No _______ Yes _______
If yes, what are they?
____
____

Do you ever have trouble affording the food you need?
No _______ Yes _______

Do you have any help getting the food you need? No _______ Yes _______
If yes, what kind? SNAP (Food stamps) _____ WIC _____ School lunch or breakfast _____ Food pantry, soup kitchen, or food bank _____

BOX 15.4   Indicators of Nutritional Risk in Pregnancy

- Adolescence or less than 2 years postmenarche
- Frequent pregnancies: three within 2 years
- Poor fetal outcome in a previous pregnancy
- Poverty/food insecurity
- Poor dietary habits with resistance to change
- Use of tobacco, alcohol, or other substances
- Weight at conception under or over normal weight
- Problems with weight gain
- Any weight loss
- Weight gain of less than 2.2 lb (1 kg)/month after the first trimester
- Weight gain of more than 6.6 lb (3 kg)/month after the first trimester
- Multifetal pregnancy
- Low hemoglobin and/or hematocrit values
- Diabetes
- Chronic illness, including an eating disorder, that affects intake, absorption, or metabolism of nutrients

anemia (see previous content under "Iron"). This is typically done at the first prenatal visit and again in the late second trimester or early third trimester.

A woman's history or physical findings may indicate the need for additional testing. These tests might include a complete blood cell count with a differential to identify megaloblastic or macrocytic anemia and measurement of levels of specific vitamins or minerals believed to be lacking in the diet.

Nutrition Care and Education

For many women with uncomplicated pregnancies, the nurse serves as the primary source of nutrition education provided through individual and/or group instruction. The registered dietitian, who has specialized education in diet evaluation and planning, nutritional needs during illness, ethnic and cultural food patterns, as well as translating nutrient needs into food patterns, frequently serves as a consultant. Pregnant women with serious nutritional problems, those with concurrent illnesses such as diabetes (either preexisting or gestational), and any others requiring in-depth dietary counseling should be referred to the dietitian. Nutrition care involves an interprofessional team, including the nurse, dietitian, obstetric care provider, other specialists as needed, and social worker, who collaborate in helping the woman achieve nutrition-related expected outcomes. Nutritional care and teaching generally involve the following concepts (Garner, 2018):

- Nutritional needs during pregnancy
- Appropriate weight gain based on her BMI and risks of excessive or inadequate weight gain
- Dietary planning to provide recommended calories and nutrients while conforming to her personal, family, cultural, financial, and health circumstances
- Strategies for coping with nutrition-related discomforts of pregnancy
- Appropriate use of nutrition supplements
- Avoiding alcohol, tobacco, and other harmful substances
- Safe food preparation and handling

If the assessment reveals that the woman lacks the financial resources to purchase healthy foods, the nurse can refer her to a social worker who may be able to help her find sources of assistance. Two programs that provide nutrition services are the Supplemental Nutrition Assistance Program (SNAP [i.e., food stamps]) and the Special Supplemental Nutrition Program for Women, Infants and Children (WIC), which provides vouchers for selected foods for pregnant and lactating women as well as for infants and children at nutritional risk. WIC foods include items such as eggs, milk (or cheese, soy milk, or tofu), juice, fortified cereals, legumes, and peanut butter. WIC participants receive nutrition counseling, and the program encourages breastfeeding (see Nursing Care Plan).

Dietary Planning

The foundation for adherence to dietary recommendations is for the woman to understand why and how maternal nutrition influences pregnancy outcomes (Lucas, Charlton, & Yeatman, 2014). The nurse should emphasize the importance of choosing a varied diet composed primarily of whole, unprocessed foods. General dietary guidelines for healthy eating patterns for adults can be incorporated into nutritional education (USDHHS & USDA, 2015), recognizing that absolutely no alcohol should be consumed during pregnancy.

The daily food guide (see Table 15.3) can be used in educating women about nutritional needs during pregnancy and lactation. This food plan is general enough to be used by women from a wide variety of cultures, including those who follow a vegetarian diet. One of the more helpful teaching strategies is to help the woman plan daily menus that follow the food plan and are affordable, have realistic preparation times, and are compatible with personal preferences and cultural practices. Information regarding cultural food patterns is provided later in this chapter. Women can find information about nutrition and meal planning using the web-based program, MyPlate, provided by the USDA at https://www.choosemyplate.gov.

Cultural Influences

Consideration of a woman's cultural food preferences enhances communication and provides a greater opportunity for following the agreed-on pattern of intake. Women in most cultures are encouraged to eat a diet typical for them. The nurse needs to be aware of what constitutes a typical diet for each cultural or ethnic group present in her patient population. However, several variations may occur within one cultural group. Thus a careful exploration of individual preferences is needed. Although ethnic and cultural food beliefs may seem at first glance to conflict with the dietary instruction provided by health care providers, nurses, and dietitians, it is often possible for the health care professional to identify cultural beliefs that are congruent with the modern understanding of pregnancy and fetal development. Many cultural food practices have some merit or the culture would not have survived. Food cravings during pregnancy are considered normal by many cultures, but the kinds of cravings often are culturally specific. Cultural influences on food intake usually lessen if the woman and her family become more integrated into the dominant culture. Nutritional beliefs and the practices of selected cultural groups are summarized in Table 15.6.

Weight Management

The pregnant woman must understand what adequate weight gain during pregnancy means, recognize the reasons for its importance, and be able to evaluate her own gain in terms of the desirable pattern. Many women, particularly those who have worked hard to control their weight before pregnancy, may find it difficult to understand why the weight-gain goal is so high when a newborn infant is so small. The nurse can explain that maternal weight gain consists of increases in the weight of many tissues, not just the growing fetus (see Table 15.3).

Dietary overindulgence, which may result in excessive fat stores that persist after giving birth, should be discouraged. Nevertheless, it is best not to focus unduly on weight gain because this could result in feelings of stress and guilt in the woman who does not follow the preferred pattern of gain. Teaching regarding weight gain during pregnancy is summarized in Table 15.2.

NURSING CARE PLAN

Nutrition During Pregnancy

Client Problem	Expected Outcomes	Nursing Interventions	Rationales
Lack of understanding related to nutritional requirements during pregnancy	Client will describe nutritional requirements and exhibit evidence of incorporating requirements into her diet.	At the initial prenatal visit, assess current diet history/intake and understanding of a healthy diet during pregnancy.	To determine need for additions or changes in present dietary pattern and to identify gaps in knowledge
	Client will eat a balanced, healthy diet and take multiple micronutrient supplement as prescribed.	Teach basic nutritional requirements for a healthy diet by using recommended dietary guidelines, emphasizing appropriate weight gain based on her body mass index.	To provide knowledge baseline for discussion and to set dietary goals
	Client will exhibit an appropriate weight gain and will maintain normal hemoglobin and hematocrit.	Assist client with diet planning, based on nutritional recommendations, food preferences, financial resources, cultural eating patterns or beliefs, prepregnancy eating patterns, and lifestyle.	To promote maternal well-being and normal fetal growth and development
Nausea and vomiting related to physiologic alterations of first trimester of pregnancy	Nausea and vomiting will not be so severe that it interferes with adequate nutrient intake.	Assess state of hydration, current weight, pattern of weight gain or loss during pregnancy, and recent history of food and fluid intake.	To ensure that client does not have a deficient fluid volume; to ensure that nausea is not preventing adequate energy intake
	Nausea and vomiting will not substantially reduce quality of life.	Teach history of nausea and vomiting (i.e., frequency of episodes of nausea, likelihood of nausea progressing to vomiting, factors precipitating or associated with nausea, and any relief measure that client has tried).	To determine severity of problem and to begin to identify effective and ineffective measures for coping with nausea and vomiting
	Client will maintain adequate fluid intake.	Teach measures for prevention or relief of nausea and vomiting.	To ensure that client is knowledgeable about measures that are often effective in alleviating these discomforts
		Teach client signs of dehydration and fluid and electrolyte imbalance, and when to notify the health care provider.	To prevent complications
Poor nutrition related to inadequate intake of needed calories and nutrients	Client will verbalize nutritional requirements to support fetal growth and development.	Review recent diet history (including food aversions) using self-administered questionnaire; review activity and exercise patterns, and factors or reasons that lead to decreased food intake	To identify dietary inadequacies contributing to insufficient weight gain, and to identify energy expenditure, and lifestyle factors related to nutrition
	Client will demonstrate ability to plan and follow a diet that meets requirements and supports adequate weight gain.	Review optimal weight gain guidelines and their rationale.	To ensure that client is knowledgeable about healthful weight gain rates
	Weekly weight gain will be increased to appropriate rate using her body mass index and recommended weight gain ranges as guidelines.	Set target weight gains for remaining weeks of pregnancy and monitor weight with each prenatal visit.	To establish set, measurable goals, and to monitor progress toward meeting goals

Food Safety

While safe preparation and handling of food is important for the health and well-being of all persons, it is especially relevant during pregnancy to prevent food-borne illnesses that may impact the fetus such as *E. coli*, salmonella, listeriosis, toxoplasmosis, and brucellosis (Garner, 2018). Hormonal changes of pregnancy increase susceptibility of the woman and her fetus to food-borne illness. The U.S. Food and Drug Administration (USFDA, 2018c) program *Food Safety for Moms-to-Be* (http://www.fda.gov/pregnancyfoodsafety) targets pregnant women and provides simple instructions for safe food practices. These include careful hand hygiene; cleansing food preparation surfaces and utensils frequently; avoiding contact between raw meat, fish, or poultry and other foods that will not be cooked before consumption; washing of fruits and vegetables; and storing foods properly. Meat, poultry, eggs, and fish should be cooked to a safe internal temperature. Pregnant women should not consume raw fish that is part of sushi or sashimi.

TABLE 15.5 Physical Assessment of Nutritional Status

Signs of Good Nutrition	Signs of Poor Nutrition
General Appearance	
Alert, responsive, energetic, good endurance	Listless, apathetic, cachectic, easily fatigued, appears tired
Muscles	
Well developed, firm, good tone, some fat under skin	Flaccid, poor tone, tender, "wasted" appearance
Gastrointestinal Function	
Good appetite and digestion, normal regular elimination, no palpable organs or masses	Anorexia, indigestion, constipation or diarrhea, liver or spleen enlargement
Cardiovascular Function	
Normal heart rate and rhythm, no murmurs, normal blood pressure for age	Rapid heart rate, enlarged heart, abnormal rhythm, elevated blood pressure
Hair	
Shiny, lustrous, firm, not easily plucked, healthy scalp	Stringy, dull, brittle, dry, thin and sparse, depigmented, can be easily plucked
Skin (General)	
Smooth, slightly moist, good color	Rough, dry, scaly, pale, irritated, easily bruised, petechiae
Face and Neck	
Skin color uniform, smooth, pink, healthy appearance; no enlargement of thyroid gland; lips not chapped or swollen	Scaly, swollen, skin dark over cheeks and under eyes, lumpiness or flakiness of skin around nose and mouth; thyroid enlarged; lips swollen, angular lesions or fissures at corners of mouth
Oral Cavity	
Reddish pink mucous membranes and gums; no swelling or bleeding of gums; tongue healthy pink or deep reddish in appearance, not swollen or smooth, surface papillae present; teeth bright and clean, no cavities, no pain, no discoloration	Gums spongy, bleed easily, inflamed or receding; tongue swollen, scarlet and raw, magenta color, beefy, hyperemic and hypertrophic papillae, atrophic papillae; teeth with unfilled caries, absent teeth, worn surfaces, mottled
Eyes	
Bright, clear, shiny, no sores at corners of eyelids, membranes moist and healthy pink color, no prominent blood vessels or mound of tissue (Bitot spots) on sclera, no fatigue circles beneath	Eye membranes pale, redness of membrane, dryness, signs of infection, redness and fissuring of eyelid corners, dryness of eye membrane, dull appearance of cornea, blue sclerae
Extremities	
No tenderness, weakness, or swelling; nails firm and pink	Edema, tender calves, tingling, weakness; nails spoon-shaped, brittle
Skeleton	
No malformations	Bowlegs, knock-knees, chest deformity at diaphragm, beaded ribs, prominent scapulae

Coping With Nutrition-Related Discomforts of Pregnancy

The most common nutrition-related discomforts of pregnancy are nausea and vomiting (or "morning sickness"), constipation, and pyrosis.

Nausea and vomiting. Nausea and vomiting of pregnancy (NVP) are most common during the first trimester. Usually, NVP causes only mild to moderate problems nutritionally, although it may be a source of substantial discomfort. Antiemetic medications, vitamin B_6, ginger, and P6 acupressure may be effective in reducing the severity of nausea, although the evidence supporting them is not strong (ACOG, 2015/2018). Suggestions for alleviating NVP are listed in the Teaching for Self-Management box: Managing Nausea and Vomiting During Pregnancy.

Hyperemesis gravidarum, or severe and persistent vomiting causing weight loss, dehydration, and electrolyte abnormalities, occurs in up to 1% of pregnant women (see Chapter 29). Intravenous fluid and electrolyte replacement, enteral tube feeding, and rarely total parenteral nutrition have been used to nourish women with hyperemesis gravidarum. There is very limited evidence that acupressure and ginger might provide some relief.

TEACHING FOR SELF-MANAGEMENT
Managing Nausea and Vomiting During Pregnancy

- Eat dry, starchy foods such as dry toast, melba toast, or crackers on awakening in the morning and at other times when nausea occurs.
- Avoid consuming excessive amounts of fluids early in the day or when nauseated (but compensate by drinking fluids at other times).
- Eat small amounts frequently (every 2-3 h), and avoid large meals that distend the stomach.
- Avoid skipping meals and thus becoming extremely hungry, which may worsen nausea. Have a snack such as cereal with milk, a small sandwich, or yogurt before bedtime.
- Avoid sudden movements. Get out of bed slowly.
- Decrease intake of fried and other fatty foods. Try high-carbohydrate foods such as toast, rice, or potatoes. Some women find high-protein meals or snacks helpful.
- Breathe fresh air to help relieve nausea. Keep the environment well ventilated (e.g., open a window), go for a walk outside, or decrease cooking odors by using an exhaust fan.
- Eat foods served at cool temperatures and foods that give off little aroma. Avoid spicy foods.
- Avoid brushing teeth immediately after eating.
- Try salty and tart foods (e.g., potato chips and lemonade) during periods of nausea. Sucking a lemon slice may help.
- Try herbal teas such as those made with raspberry leaf or peppermint to decrease nausea.
- Try some form of ginger: ginger ale, candied ginger, add fresh ginger to tea, or boil fresh ginger in water with a small amount of sugar.
- Wear motion sickness wristbands.
- Vitamin B_6 or a medication such as Diclegis (made of vitamin B_6 and doxylamine) may be recommended by the health care provider.

TABLE 15.6 **Popular Foods of Various Cultural and Ethnic Groups**

Cultural or Ethnic Group or Eating Pattern	FOOD GROUPS				
	Grains	Vegetable	Fruit	Dairy	Protein
Mexican	Tortilla Taco shell Posole (corn soup) Rice Postres (pastries)[a]	*Other vegetables:* Chayote (Mexican squash) Jicama (root vegetable) Nopales (cactus leaves) Tomato Corn	Avocado Mango Papaya Plátano (cooking banana) Zapote (sweet, yellowish fruit)	Queso blanco (white Mexican cheese) Custard (1 cup = 1 cup milk serving) Leche (milk)	Chorizo (sausage)[a] Chicken, beef, goat, or pork Beans, dried, cooked
African American soul food (Southern-style cooking)	Biscuit Cornbread Grits, rice, macaroni, or noodles Hominy Crackers Hush puppies	*Dark green:* Collard, kale, mustard, or turnip greens *Orange:* Sweet potatoes *Other:* Okra Snap, pole (green), lima, and butter beans Turnips Summer squash (yellow or zucchini) Coleslaw	Blackberries Melons Muscadines (grapes) Peaches	Buttermilk	Pork (cured ham and uncured cuts), chicken, beef, fish Peas or beans (black-eyed, crowder, pur-ple-hull, or cream)
Vegetarian	Whole-grain bread Cereal, cooked or ready-to-eat Brown rice Whole-grain pasta Bagel	All	All	Milk and cheese (lacto-vegetarians) Soy milk, calcium-fortified Soy cheese	Cooked dried beans or peas Tofu (soybean curd) or tempeh (fermented soy) Nuts or seeds Peanut butter Egg (ovo-vegetarians)
Italian	Breadsticks, breads Gnocchi Polenta Risotto Pastas	*Dark green:* Spinach *Other:* Artichoke Eggplant Mushrooms Marinara sauce	Berries Figs Pomegranate	Cheeses (e.g., moz-zarella, Parmesan, Romano, ricotta) Gelato (Italian ice cream)	Veal or beef Fish Sausage[a] Luncheon meats[a] Lentils Squid Almonds, pistachios
Chinese	Rice or millet Rice vermicelli Cellophane noodles (bean thread) Steamed rolls Rice congee (soup) Rice sticks	*Other:* Pea pods Yard-long beans Baby corn Bamboo shoots Straw mushrooms Eggplant Bitter melon	Guava Lychee Persimmon Pummelo Kumquat Star fruit	Soy milk	Pork, fish, chicken Shrimp, crab, lobster Tofu or tempeh
Indian (South Asia)	Breads: roti (chapati), naan, paratha, batura, puris, dosa, idli Rice or rice pilau Pooha, upma, sabudana	*Dark green:* Saag (mixed greens and potatoes) Spinach *Other:* Green peppers Cabbage Eggplant Green beans Methi (fenugreek leaves) Cucumbers Chutney or vegetable pickles	Mango Dates Raisins Melons Figs Fruit juices and nectars	Yogurt	Dal (lentils, mung beans, other dried beans) Beef, chicken (some are vegetarian)
Native American[b]	Bread Fry bread Wild rice or oats Popcorn Tortilla Mush (cooked cereal)	*Orange:* Winter squash (hard outer shell) *Starchy:* Potato Corn *Other:* Rhubarb	Berries Cherries Plums Apples Peaches		Wild game (deer, rabbit, elk, beaver) Lamb Salmon and other fish Clams, mussels Crab Duck or quail

continued

TABLE 15.6   Popular Foods of Various Cultural and Ethnic Groups—cont'd

Cultural or Ethnic Group or Eating Pattern	FOOD GROUPS				
	Grains	**Vegetable**	**Fruit**	**Dairy**	**Protein**
Middle Eastern	Rice or bulgur (cracked wheat)	*Yellow:*	Apricots	Yogurt	Lamb, goat, fish
	Couscous	Pumpkin or winter squash (butternut)	Grapes		Almonds
	Bread	*Other:*	Melons		Pistachio nuts
	Pita	Peppers	Dried fruits: dates, raisins, apricots		Dried beans and peas, lentils
		Tomatoes			Eggs
		Grape leaves			
		Cucumbers			
		Fava beans			
		Eggplant			

[a]High fat, use sparingly.
[b]Varies widely, depending on tribal grouping and locale.

Constipation. Improved bowel function generally results from increasing the intake of fiber (e.g., bran and whole-wheat products, popcorn, and raw or lightly steamed vegetables) in the diet. Fiber helps create a bulky stool that stimulates intestinal peristalsis; the recommended daily allowance is 28 g (IOM, 2006). An adequate fluid intake helps hydrate the fiber and increase the bulk of the stool. Making a habit of regular physical activity that uses large muscle groups (walking, swimming, water aerobics) also helps stimulate bowel motility.

Pyrosis. *Pyrosis*, or heartburn, is usually caused by reflux of gastric contents into the esophagus. This condition can be minimized by eating small, frequent meals rather than two or three larger meals daily. Because fluids increase the distention of the stomach, they should not be consumed with foods. The woman needs to drink adequate amounts between meals. Avoiding spicy foods may help alleviate the problem. Reflux can be exacerbated by lying down immediately after eating and wearing clothing that is tight across the abdomen.

Dietary Modifications

Because of medical need, there may be dietary modifications before, during, and after pregnancy. For example, pregnant adolescents have unique nutritional needs because of their own physical immaturity. Women with pregestational or gestational diabetes need to adhere to a dietary plan that helps maintain desired glucose levels (see Chapter 29); women with food allergies and sensitivities follow dietary plans that eliminate specific foods (e.g., lactose intolerance, gluten sensitivity or allergy). Women who have had bariatric surgery have special nutritional needs.

Nurses need to be aware of any dietary modifications that are recommended by the health care provider, assess the woman's understanding of the dietary plan and her ability to follow it, and refer the woman for nutritional counseling by a registered dietician with knowledge and experience in maternity care. Members of the interprofessional health care team are often involved in nutrition therapy for medical needs.

Adolescent pregnancy. Many adolescent females have diets that provide less than the recommended intakes of key nutrients, including calcium and iron. Pregnant adolescents and their infants are at increased risk for complications during pregnancy and parturition. Growth of the pelvis is delayed in comparison with growth in stature, and this helps explain why cephalopelvic disproportion and other mechanical problems associated with labor are common among young adolescents. Competition for nutrients between the growing adolescent and the fetus may also contribute to some of the poor outcomes apparent in teen pregnancies. Recommended weight-gain goals are not different from those of adult women. Pregnant adolescents are encouraged to choose a weight-gain goal at the upper end of the range for their BMI. BMI is calculated the same as for adult women rather than by using the adolescent BMI growth charts (CDC, 2017). Adolescent females who have given birth have greater percentages of total fat and visceral fat (associated with the metabolic syndrome and cardiovascular disease) than those who have never given birth (Ramö, Kjølhede, & Blomberg, 2017); thus the adolescent mother needs careful teaching regarding nutritional intake and physical activity to control body weight in the postpartum period.

Efforts to improve the nutritional health of pregnant adolescents focus on the following:
- Improving the nutrition knowledge, meal planning, and selection and food preparation skills of young women
- Promoting access to prenatal care
- Developing nutrition interventions and educational programs that are effective with adolescents
- Striving to understand the factors that create barriers to change in the adolescent population

Pregnancy after bariatric surgery. Women who have had bariatric surgery face nutritional challenges during pregnancy because the surgical procedures result in deficiencies of macro- and micronutrients. The specific deficiencies that are most common after bariatric surgery include folate, vitamin B_{12}, iron, calcium, and vitamin D (Carreau, Nadeau, Marceau, et al., 2017). Malabsorptive procedures such as Roux-en-y gastric bypass and biliopancreatic diversion carry a high risk for nutritional deficits; however, even restrictive-type procedures such as laparoscopic adjustable gastric banding are associated with nutritional problems. All women with a history of bariatric surgery should be screened for nutritional deficiencies throughout pregnancy, monitored for appropriate weight gain, and provided nutritional supplementation as needed. Iron deficiency can be a long-term problem after bariatric surgery, so iron levels should be carefully monitored. Infants born to mothers with a history of bariatric surgery are at increased risk for prematurity, small for gestational age, and NICU admission; the risk is greater if the time between the surgery and birth is less than 2 years (Carreau et al., 2017; Parent, Martopullo, Weiss, et al., 2017).

KEY POINTS

- A woman's nutritional status before, during, and after pregnancy contributes significantly to her well-being and that of her developing fetus and newborn.
- Many physiologic changes occurring during pregnancy influence the need for additional nutrients and the efficiency with which the body uses them.
- Both the total maternal weight gain and the pattern of weight gain are important determinants of the outcome of pregnancy.
- The appropriateness of the woman's prepregnancy weight for height (BMI) is a major determinant of her recommended weight gain during pregnancy.
- Nutritional risk factors include adolescent pregnancy; use of tobacco, alcohol, or drugs; underweight or overweight/obesity; short interpregnancy spacing; eating disorders; poverty; and history of bariatric surgery.

- Iron supplementation is usually routinely recommended during pregnancy, with a multiple micronutrient supplement (prenatal vitamin) containing adequate amounts for most women.
- Pregnant women with anemia need additional iron and should be instructed about how best to prevent and manage side effects.
- Food safety is important for pregnant women to prevent adverse maternal and fetal effects.
- Seafood consumed by pregnant women should be low in methylmercury.
- The nurse and the woman are influenced by cultural and personal values and beliefs during nutrition counseling.
- Pregnancy complications that can be nutrition-related include anemia, gestational hypertension, gestational diabetes, preterm birth, and IUGR.
- Dietary modifications can be effective interventions for some of the common discomforts of pregnancy, including nausea and vomiting, constipation, and heartburn.

REFERENCES

American College of Obstetricians and Gynecologists. (2010, reaffirmed 2016). *Committee opinion no. 462: Moderate caffeine consumption during pregnancy.* Retrieved from: www.acog.org/Resources-And-Publications/Committee-Opinions/Committee-on-Obstetric-Practice/Moderate-Caffeine-Consumption-During-Pregnancy.

American College of Obstetricians and Gynecologists. (2013). Hypertension in pregnancy: Executive summary. *Obstetrics and Gynecology, 122*(5), 1122–1131.

American College of Obstetricians and Gynecologists. (2013, reaffirmed 2018). *Practice bulletin no. 548: Weight gain during pregnancy.* Retrieved from: https://www.acog.org/Clinical-Guidance-and-Publications/Committee-Opinions/Committee-on-Obstetric-Practice/Weight-Gain-During-Pregnancy.

American College of Obstetricians and Gynecologists. (2015, reaffirmed 2017). *Physical activity and exercise during pregnancy and the postpartum period.* Retrieved from: http://www.acog.org/Resources-And-Publications/Committee-Opinions/Committee-on-Obstetric-Practice/Physical-Activity-and-Exercise-During-Pregnancy-and-the-Postpartum-Period.

American College of Obstetricians and Gynecologists. (2015, reaffirmed 2018). Practice bulletin no. 153: Nausea and vomiting of pregnancy. *Obstetrics and Gynecology, 126*(3), e12–e24.

American College of Obstetricians and Gynecologists. (2017a). Practice bulletin no. 187: Neural tube defects. *Obstetrics and Gynecology, 130*(6), 1395–1396.

American College of Obstetricians and Gynecologists. (2017b). *Tobacco, alcohol, drugs and pregnancy.* Retrieved from: https://www.acog.org/Patients/FAQs/Tobacco-Alcohol-Drugs-and-Pregnancy.

Carreau, A. M., Nadeau, M., & Marceau, S. (2017). Pregnancy after bariatric surgery. *Canadian Journal of Diabetes, 41*(4), 432–438.

Catalano, P. M., & Kartik, S. (2017). Obesity and pregnancy: Mechanisms of short term and long term adverse consequences for mother and child. *British Medical Journal, 356*, j1.

Centers for Disease Control and Prevention. (2017). *About BMI.* Retrieved from: https://www.cdc.gov/healthyweight/assessing/bmi/adult_bmi/index.html.

Centers for Disease Control and Prevention. (2018). *Recommendations: Women and folic acid.* Retrieved from https://www.cdc.gov/ncbddd/folicacid/recommendations.html.

Centers for Disease Control and Prevention. (2019). *Weight gain during pregnancy.* Retrieved from: https://www.cdc.gov/reproductivehealth/maternalinfanthealth/pregnancy-weight-gain.htm.

Deputy, N. P., Dub, B., Sharma, A. J., et al. (2018). Prevalence and trends in prepregnancy normal weight — 48 states, New York City, and District of Columbia, 2011–2015. *Morbidity and Mortality Weekly Report, 66*(5152), 1402–1407.

Garner, C. D. (2018). Nutrition in pregnancy. In C. J. Lockwood (Ed.), *UptoDate.* Retrieved from: https://www-uptodate-com.

Goldstein, R. F., Abell, S. K., Ranasinha, S., et al. (2017). Association of gestational weight gain with maternal and infant outcomes: A systematic review and meta-analysis. *Journal of the American Medical Association, 317*(21), 2207–2225.

Institute of Medicine. (2006). *Dietary reference intakes: The essential guide to nutrient requirements.* Washington, D.C.: National Academies Press.

Institute of Medicine. (2009). *Weight gain during pregnancy: Reexamining the guidelines.* Washington, DC: National Academies Press.

Kominiarek, M. A., & Rajan, P. (2016). Nutritional recommendations in pregnancy and lactation. *Medical Clinics of North America, 100*(6), 1199–1215.

Liu, P., Xu, L., Wang, Y., et al. (2016). Association between perinatal outcomes and maternal pre-pregnancy body mass index. *Obesity Reviews, 17*(11), 1091–1102.

Lucas, C., Charlton, K. E., & Yeatman, H. (2014). Nutrition advice during pregnancy: Do women receive it and can health professionals provide it? *Maternal Child Health Journal, 18*(10), 2465–2478.

Marchi, J., Berg, M., Dencker, A., et al. (2015). Risks associated with obesity in pregnancy, for the mother and baby: A systematic review of reviews. *Obesity Reviews, 16*(8), 621–638.

National Institutes of Health Office of Dietary Supplements. (2018a). *Choline: Fact sheet for health professionals.* Retrieved from: https://ods.od.nih.gov/factsheets/Choline-HealthProfessional/.

National Institutes of Health Office of Dietary Supplements. (2018b). *Magnesium: Fact sheet for health professionals.* Retrieved from: https://ods.od.nih.gov/factsheets/Magnesium-HealthProfessional/.

National Institutes of Health Office of Dietary Supplements. (2018c). *Potassium: Fact sheet for health professionals.* Retrieved from: https://ods.od.nih.gov/factsheets/Potassium-HealthProfessional/.

National Institutes of Health Office of Dietary Supplements. (2018d). *Vitamin A: Fact sheet for health professionals.* Retrieved from https://ods.od.nih.gov/factsheets/VitaminA-HealthProfessional/.

National Institutes of Health Office of Dietary Supplements. (2018e). *Vitamin B6: Dietary supplement fact sheet.* Retrieved from: https://ods.od.nih.gov/factsheets/VitaminB6-HealthProfessional/.

National Institutes of Health Office of Dietary Supplements. (2018f). *Vitamin B12: Dietary supplement fact sheet.* Retrieved from: https://ods.od.nih.gov/factsheets/VitaminB12-HealthProfessional/.

National Institutes of Health Office of Dietary Supplements. (2018g). *Vitamin C: Dietary supplement fact sheet.* Retrieved from: https://ods.od.nih.gov-/factsheets/VitaminC-HealthProfessional/#en1.

National Institutes of Health Office of Dietary Supplements. (2018h). *Vitamin D: Dietary supplement fact sheet.* Retrieved from: https://ods.od.nih.gov-/factsheets/VitaminD-HealthProfessional/#en1.

National Institutes of Health Office of Dietary Supplements. (2018i). *Vitamin E: Dietary supplement fact sheet.* Retrieved from: https://ods.od.nih.gov-/factsheets/VitaminE-HealthProfessional/#en1.

National Institutes of Health Office of Dietary Supplements. (2018j). *Vitamin K: Dietary supplement fact sheet.* Retrieved from: https://ods.od.nih.gov-/factsheets/VitaminK-HealthProfessional/#en1.

National Institutes of Health Office of Dietary Supplements. (2018k). *Zinc: Fact sheet for health professionals.* https://ods.od.nih.gov/factsheets/Zinc-HealthProfessional/.

Parent, B., Martopullo, I., Weiss, N. S., et al. (2017). Bariatric surgery in women of childbearing age, timing between an operation and birth, and associated perinatal complications. *Journal of the American Medical Association Surgery, 152*(2), 128–135.

Ramö, A., Kjølhede, P., & Blomberg, M. (2017). Obstetric outcomes in adolescents related to body mass index and compared with low-risk adult women. *Journal of Women's Health, 26*(5), 426–434.

Rumbold, A., Ota, E., Hori, H., et al. (2015). Vitamin E supplementation in pregnancy. *Cochrane Database of Systematic Reviews, 9,* CD004069.

Spencer, L., Hauk, R. M., MacDonald-Wicks, L., et al. (2015). The effect of weight management interventions that include a diet component on weight-related outcomes in pregnant and postpartum women: A systematic review protocol. *JBI Database of Systematic Review and Implementation Reports, 13*(1), 88–98.

Stang, J., & Huffman, L. G. (2016). Position of the academy of nutrition and dietetics: Obesity, reproduction, and pregnancy outcomes. *Journal of the Academy of Nutrition and Dietetics, 116*(4), 677–691.

US Department of Health and Human Services and U.S. Department of Agriculture (2015). *2015 – 2020 dietary guidelines for Americans* (8th ed.). Retrieved from: http://health.gov/dietaryguidelines/2015/guidelines/.

US Food and Drug Administration. (2018a). *Additional information about high-intensity sweeteners permitted for use in food in the United States.* Retrieved from: https://www.fda.gov/Food/IngredientsPackagingLabeling/FoodAdditivesIngredients/ucm397725.htm.

US Food and Drug Administration. (2018b). *Eating fish: What pregnant women and parents should know.* Retrieved from: www.fda.gov/Food/ResourcesForYou/Consumers/ucm393070.htm.

US Food and Drug Administration. (2018c). *Food safety for moms-to-be.* Retrieved from: https://www.fda.gov/Food/FoodborneIllnessContaminants/PeopleAtRisk/ucm081785.htm.

US Food and Drug Administration. (2019). *Food safety for moms-to-be: While you're pregnant—Listeria.* Retrieved from: http://www.fda.gov/Food/ResourcesForYou/HealthEducators/ucm083320.htm.

West, E. H., Hark, L., & Catalano, P. M. (2017). Nutrition during pregnancy. In S. G. Gabbe, J. R. Niebyl, J. L. Simpson, et al. (Eds.), *Obstetrics: Normal and problem pregnancies* (7th ed.). Philadelphia: Elsevier.

Young, S., & Cox, T. J. (2017). Pica in pregnancy. In V. Berghella (Ed.), *UpToDate.* Retrieved from: http://www.uptodate.com/home.

16

Labor and Birth Processes

Kitty Cashion

http://evolve.elsevier.com/Lowdermilk/MWHC/

LEARNING OBJECTIVES

- Explain the five major factors that affect the labor process.
- Describe the anatomic structure of the bony pelvis.
- Identify the normal measurements of the diameters of the pelvic inlet, cavity, and outlet.
- Explain the significance of the size and position of the fetal head during labor and birth.
- Summarize the cardinal movements of the mechanism of labor for a vertex presentation.
- Examine the maternal anatomic and physiologic adaptations to labor.
- Describe factors thought to contribute to the onset of labor.
- Describe fetal adaptations to labor.

During late pregnancy, the woman and fetus prepare for the labor process, a series of events by which the fetus is expelled from the uterus. The fetus has grown and developed in preparation for extrauterine life. The woman has undergone various physiologic adaptations during pregnancy that prepare her for giving birth and for motherhood. Labor and birth represent the end of pregnancy, the beginning of extrauterine life for the newborn, and a change in the lives of the family. This chapter discusses the factors affecting labor, the processes involved, the normal progression of events, and the adaptations made by both the woman and fetus.

FACTORS AFFECTING LABOR

At least five factors affect the process of labor and birth. These are easily remembered as the five *P*'s: *passengers* (fetus and placenta), *passageway* (birth canal), *powers* (contractions), *position* of the mother, and *psychologic response*. The first four factors are presented here as the basis for understanding the physiologic process of labor. The fifth factor is discussed in Chapter 19. Other factors can influence the woman's labor and birth experience, including place of birth, preparation, type of provider (e.g., obstetrician or family medicine physician, nurse-midwife), nursing care, and procedures. These factors are discussed generally in Chapter 19, as they relate to nursing care during labor.

Passenger

The way the passenger, or fetus, moves through the birth canal is determined by several interacting factors: the size of the fetal head, fetal presentation, fetal lie, fetal attitude, and fetal position. Because the placenta also must pass through the birth canal, it can be considered a passenger along with the fetus; however, the placenta rarely interferes with the process of labor in a normal vaginal birth. An exception is the case of placenta previa (see Chapter 28).

Size of the Fetal Head

Because of its size and relative rigidity, the fetal head has a major effect on the birth process. The fetal skull is composed of two parietal bones, two temporal bones, the frontal bone, and the occipital bone (Fig. 16.1A). These bones are united by connective tissue *sutures:* sagittal, lambdoidal, coronal, and frontal (see Fig. 16.1B). The areas where more than two bones meet are called *fontanels.* During labor after rupture of membranes, palpation of fontanels and sutures during vaginal examination reveals fetal presentation, position, and attitude (see Fig.16.1B). The larger of these, the anterior fontanel, is diamond shaped approximately 3 cm by 2 cm, and lies at the junction of the sagittal, coronal, and frontal sutures. It closes by 18 months after birth. The posterior fontanel lies at the junction of the sutures of the two parietal bones and the occipital bone, is triangular, and is approximately 1 cm by 2 cm. It closes 6 to 8 weeks after birth.

Sutures and fontanels make the skull flexible to accommodate the infant brain, which continues to grow for some time after birth. However, because the bones are not firmly united, slight overlapping or *molding* of the shape of the head occurs during labor. This capacity of the bones to slide over one another also permits adaptation to the various diameters of the maternal pelvis. Molding can be extensive, but the heads of most newborns assume their normal shape within 3 days after birth (see Fig. 23.14).

Although the size of the fetal shoulders may affect passage, their position can be altered relatively easily during labor, so one shoulder may occupy a lower level than the other. This creates a shoulder diameter that is smaller than the skull, facilitating passage through the birth canal. After the birth of the head and shoulders, the rest of the body usually emerges quickly.

Fetal Presentation

Presentation refers to the part of the fetus that enters the pelvic inlet first and leads through the birth canal during labor at term. The three main presentations are *cephalic presentation* (head first), occurring in approximately 97% of births (Fig. 16.2); *breech presentation* (buttocks, feet, or both first), occurring in approximately 3% of births (Fig. 16.3A to C); and *shoulder*

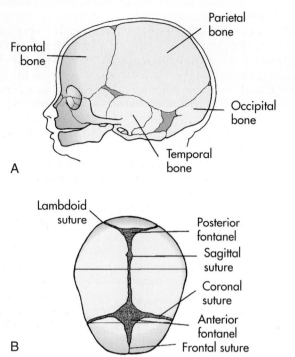

A

B

Fig. 16.1 Fetal Head at Term. (A) Bones. (B) Sutures and fontanels.

presentation, seen in fewer than 1% of births (see Fig. 16.3D) (Cunningham, Leveno, Bloom, et al., 2018). The presenting part is that part of the fetus that lies closest to the internal os of the cervix. It is the part of the fetal body first felt by the examining finger during a vaginal examination. In a cephalic presentation, the presenting part is usually the occiput; in a breech presentation, it is the sacrum; in the shoulder presentation, it is the scapula. When the presenting part is the occiput, the presentation is noted as *vertex* (see Fig. 16.2). Factors that determine the presenting part include fetal lie, fetal attitude, and extension or flexion of the fetal head.

Fetal Lie

Lie is the relation of the long axis (spine) of the fetus to the long axis (spine) of the mother. The two primary lies are longitudinal, or vertical, in which the long axis of the fetus is parallel with the long axis of the mother (see Fig. 16.2); and transverse, horizontal, or oblique, in which the long axis of the fetus is at a right angle diagonal to the long axis of the mother (see Fig. 16.3D). Longitudinal lies are either cephalic or breech presentations, depending on the fetal structure that first enters the mother's pelvis. Vaginal birth cannot occur when the fetus stays in a transverse lie. An oblique lie, one in which the long axis of the fetus is lying at an angle to the long axis of the mother, is less common and usually converts to a longitudinal or transverse lie during labor (Cunningham et al., 2018).

Fetal Attitude

Attitude is the relation of the fetal body parts to one another. The fetus assumes a characteristic posture (attitude) in utero partly because of

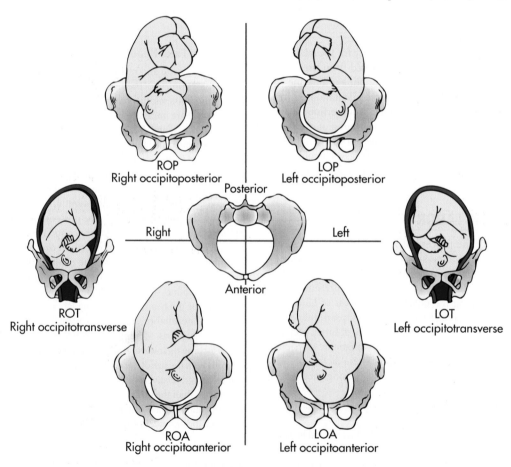

Lie: Longitudinal or vertical
Presentation: Vertex
Reference point: Occiput
Attitude: General flexion

Fig. 16.2 Examples of fetal vertex (occiput) presentations in relation to front, back, or side of maternal pelvis.

the mode of fetal growth and partly because of the way the fetus conforms to the shape of the uterine cavity. Normally the back of the fetus is rounded so that the chin is flexed on the chest, the thighs are flexed on the abdomen, and the legs are flexed at the knees. The arms are crossed over the thorax, and the umbilical cord lies between the arms and the legs. This attitude is termed *general flexion* (see Fig. 16.2).

Deviations from the normal attitude may cause difficulties in childbirth. For example, in a cephalic presentation, the fetal head may be extended or flexed in a manner that presents a head diameter that exceeds the limits of the maternal pelvis, leading to prolonged labor, forceps- or vacuum-assisted birth, or cesarean birth.

Certain critical diameters of the fetal head can be measured by ultrasound. The biparietal diameter, which is about 9.25 cm at term, is the largest transverse diameter and an important indicator of fetal head size (Fig. 16.4B). In a well-flexed cephalic presentation, the biparietal diameter is the widest part of the head entering the pelvic inlet. Of the several anteroposterior diameters, the smallest and the most critical one is the suboccipitobregmatic diameter (about 9.5 cm at term). When the head is in complete flexion, this diameter allows the fetal head to pass through the true pelvis easily (Fig. 16.5A; see Fig. 16.4A). As the head is more extended, the anteroposterior diameter widens, and the head may not be able to enter the true pelvis (see Fig. 16.5).

Fetal Position

The presentation, or presenting part, indicates that portion of the fetus that overlies the pelvic inlet. **Position** is the relationship of a reference point on the presenting part (occiput, sacrum, mentum [chin], or sinciput [deflexed vertex]) to the four quadrants of the mother's pelvis (see Fig. 16.2). Position is denoted by a three-part abbreviation. The first letter of the abbreviation denotes the location of the presenting part in the right (*R*) or left (*L*) side of the mother's pelvis. The middle letter stands for the specific presenting part of the fetus (*O* for occiput, *S* for sacrum, *M* for mentum [chin], and *Sc* for scapula [shoulder]). The final letter stands for the location of the presenting part in relation to the anterior (*A*), posterior (*P*), or transverse (*T*) portion of the maternal pelvis. For example, ROA means that the occiput is the presenting part and is located in the right anterior quadrant of the maternal pelvis (see Fig. 16.2 ROA). LSP means that the sacrum is the presenting part and is located in the left posterior quadrant of the maternal pelvis (see Fig. 16.3 A or C).

Station is the relationship of the presenting fetal part to an imaginary line drawn between the maternal ischial spines and is a measure of the degree of descent of the presenting part of the fetus through the birth canal. The placement of the presenting part is measured in centimeters above or below the ischial spines (Fig. 16.6). For

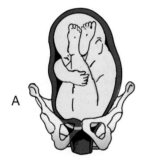

A

Frank breech

Lie: Longitudinal or vertical
Presentation: Breech (incomplete)
Presenting part: Sacrum
Attitude: Flexion, except for legs at knees

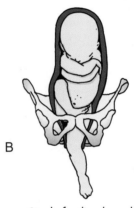

B

Single footling breech

Lie: Longitudinal or vertical
Presentation: Breech (incomplete)
Presenting part: Sacrum
Attitude: Flexion, except for one leg extended at hip and knee

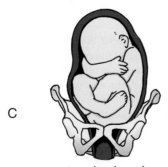

C

Complete breech

Lie: Longitudinal or vertical
Presentation: Breech (sacrum and feet presenting)
Presenting part: Sacrum (with feet)
Attitude: General flexion

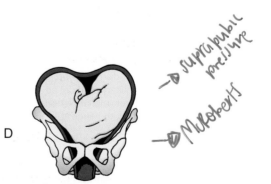

D

Shoulder presentation

Lie: Transverse or horizontal
Presentation: Shoulder
Presenting part: Scapula
Attitude: Flexion

Fig. 16.3 Fetal Presentations. (A to C) Breech (sacral) presentations. (D) Shoulder presentation.

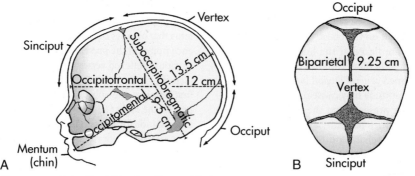

Fig. 16.4 Diameters of the Fetal Head at Term. (A) Cephalic presentations: occiput, vertex, and sinciput; and cephalic diameters: suboccipitobregmatic, occipitofrontal, and occipitomental. (B) Biparietal diameter.

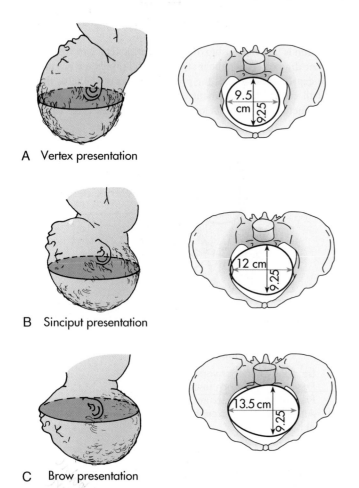

Fig. 16.5 Head Entering Pelvis. Biparietal diameter is indicated with shading (9.25 cm). (A) Suboccipitobregmatic diameter: complete flexion of head on chest so that smallest diameter enters. (B) Occipitofrontal diameter: moderate extension (military attitude) so that large diameter enters. (C) Occipitomental diameter: marked extension (deflection), so that the largest diameter, which is too large to permit head to enter pelvis, is presenting.

example, when the lowermost portion of the presenting part is 1 cm above the spines, it is noted as being minus (−) 1. At the level of the spines, the station is referred to as 0 (zero). When the presenting part is 1 cm below the spines, the station is said to be plus (+) 1. Birth is imminent when the presenting part is at +4 to +5 cm. The station of the presenting part should be determined when labor begins, so that the rate of descent of the fetus during labor can be assessed accurately.

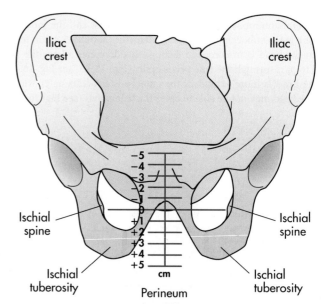

Fig. 16.6 Stations of Presenting Part, or Degree of Descent. The lowermost portion of the presenting part is at the level of the ischial spines, station 0.

Engagement is the term used to indicate that the largest transverse diameter of the presenting part (usually the biparietal diameter) has passed through the maternal pelvic brim or inlet into the true pelvis and usually corresponds to station 0. It often occurs in the weeks just before labor begins in nulliparas and may occur before or during labor in multiparas. Engagement can be determined by abdominal or vaginal examination.

Passageway

The passageway, or birth canal, is composed of the mother's rigid bony pelvis and the soft tissues of the cervix, the pelvic floor, the vagina, and the introitus (the external opening to the vagina). Although the soft tissues, particularly the muscular layers of the pelvic floor, contribute to vaginal birth of the fetus, the maternal pelvis plays a far greater role in the labor process because the fetus must successfully accommodate itself to this relatively rigid passageway. The size and shape of the pelvis can be determined at the initial prenatal visit or on admission in labor. This information can then be used in the assessment of labor progress (Thorp and Grantz, 2019).

Bony Pelvis

The anatomy of the bony pelvis is described in Chapter 4. The following discussion focuses on the importance of pelvic configurations as they relate to the labor process. (It may be helpful to refer to Fig. 4.4.)

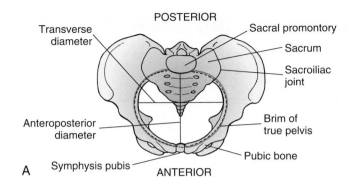

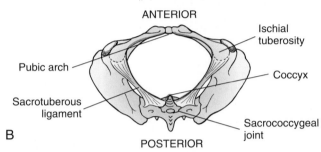

Fig. 16.7 Female Pelvis. (A) Pelvic brim from above. (B) Pelvic outlet from below, as seen by health care provider when the woman is lying supine.

The bony pelvis is formed by the fusion of the ilium, ischium, pubis, and sacral bones. The four pelvic joints are the symphysis pubis, the right and left sacroiliac joints (Fig. 16.7A), and the sacrococcygeal joint (see Fig. 16.7B). The bony pelvis is separated by the brim, or inlet, into two parts: the false and the true pelves. The false pelvis is the part above the brim and plays no part in childbearing. The true pelvis, the part involved in birth, is divided into three planes: the inlet, or brim; the midpelvis, or cavity; and the outlet.

The pelvic inlet, which is the upper border of the true pelvis, is formed anteriorly by the upper margins of the pubic bone, laterally by the iliopectineal lines along the innominate bones, and posteriorly by the anterior upper margin of the sacrum and the sacral promontory.

The pelvic cavity, or midpelvis, is a curved passage with a short anterior wall and a much longer concave posterior wall. It is bounded by the posterior aspect of the symphysis pubis, the ischium, a portion of the ilium, the sacrum, and the coccyx.

The pelvic outlet is the lower border of the true pelvis. Viewed from below it is ovoid, somewhat diamond shaped, and bounded by the pubic arch anteriorly, the ischial tuberosities laterally, and the tip of the coccyx posteriorly (see Fig. 16.7B). In the latter part of pregnancy, the coccyx is movable (unless it has been previously fractured and has fused to the sacrum during healing).

The pelvic canal varies in size and shape at various levels. The diameters at the plane of the pelvic inlet, midpelvis, and outlet, plus the axis of the birth canal (Fig. 16.8), determine whether vaginal birth is possible and the manner by which the fetus may pass down the birth canal.

The subpubic angle, which determines the type of pubic arch, together with the length of the pubic rami and the intertuberous diameter, is of great importance. Because the fetus must first pass beneath the pubic arch, a narrow subpubic angle is less accommodating than a rounded wide arch. The method of measurement of the subpubic arch is shown in Fig. 16.9. A summary of obstetric measurements is given in Table 16.1.

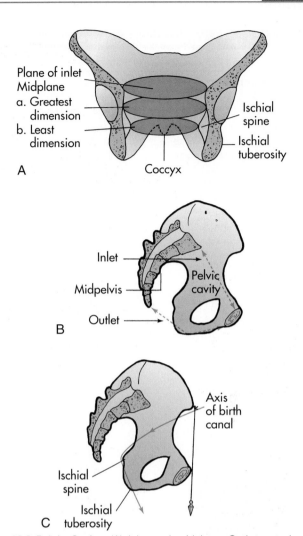

Fig. 16.8 Pelvic Cavity. (A) Inlet and midplane. Outlet not shown. (B) Cavity of true pelvis. (C) Note curve of sacrum and axis of birth canal.

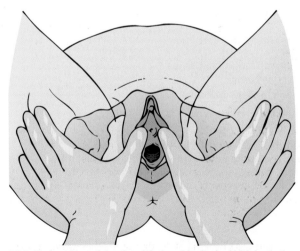

Fig. 16.9 Estimation of Angle of Subpubic Arch. With both thumbs, examiner externally traces descending rami down to tuberosities. (From Barkauskas, V., Baumann, L., Darling-Fisher, C. [2002]. *Health and physical assessment* [3rd ed.]. St. Louis: Mosby.)

TABLE 16.1 Obstetric Measurements

Plane	Diameter	Measurements
Inlet (superior strait) Conjugates Diagonal Obstetric: measurement that determines whether presenting part can engage or enter superior strait True (vera) (anteroposterior)	12.5–13 cm 1.5–2 cm less than diagonal (radiographic) ≥11 cm (12.5) (radiographic)	Length of diagonal conjugate *(solid colored line)*, obstetric conjugate *(broken colored line)*, and true conjugate *(blue line)**
Midplane Transverse diameter (interspinous diameter) The midplane of the pelvis normally is its largest plane and the one of greatest diameter	10.5 cm	Measurement of interspinous diameter[a]
Outlet Transverse diameter (intertuberous diameter) (biischial) The outlet presents the smallest plane of the pelvic canal	≥8 cm	Use of Thom pelvimeter to measure intertuberous diameter*

[a]From Seidel, H., Ball, J., Dains, J., et al. (2011). *Mosby's guide to physical examination* (7th ed.). St. Louis: Mosby.

TABLE 16.2   Comparison of Pelvic Types

	Gynecoid (50% of Women)	Android (23% of Women)	Anthropoid (24% of Women)	Platypelloid (3% of Women)
Brim	Slightly ovoid or transversely rounded	Heart shaped, angulated	Oval, wider anteroposteriorly	Flattened anteroposteriorly, wide transversely
Shape	Round	Heart	Oval	Flat
Depth	Moderate	Deep	Deep	Shallow
Side walls	Straight	Convergent	Straight	Straight
Ischial spines	Blunt, somewhat widely separated	Prominent, narrow interspinous diameter	Prominent, often with narrow interspinous diameter	Blunted, widely separated
Sacrum	Deep, curved	Slightly curved, terminal portion often beaked	Slightly curved	Slightly curved
Subpubic arch	Wide	Narrow	Narrow	Wide
Effects on labor/birth[a]	Classic female shape; associated with birth in the OA position	In theory, has an increased risk of CPD	More often associated with birth in the OP position	In theory, increases the likelihood of a transverse arrest

[a]Data from Kilpatrick, S. & Garrison, E. (2017). Normal labor and delivery. In: Gabbe, S.G., Niebyl, J.R., Simpson, J.L., et al., (Eds.). *Obstetrics: Normal and problem pregnancies* (7th ed.). Philadelphia: Elsevier.
CPD, Cephalopelvic disproportion; *OA,* occipitoanterior; *OP,* occipitoposterior.

The four basic types of pelvis are classified as follows:
1. *Gynecoid* (the classic female type)
2. *Android* (resembling the male pelvis)
3. *Anthropoid* (oval shaped, with a wider anteroposterior diameter)
4. *Platypelloid* (the flat pelvis)

The gynecoid pelvis is the most common, with major gynecoid pelvic features present in approximately 50% of all women. Anthropoid and android features are less common, and platypelloid pelvic features are the least common. Mixed types of pelves are more common than are pure types (Cunningham et al., 2018). Examples of pelvic variations and their effects on mode of birth are given in Table 16.2.

Assessment of the bony pelvis can be performed during the first prenatal evaluation and need not be repeated if the pelvis is of adequate size and suitable shape. In the third trimester of pregnancy, the examination of the bony pelvis may be more thorough and the results more accurate because there is relaxation and increased mobility of the pelvic joints and ligaments as a result of hormonal influences. Widening of the joint of the symphysis pubis and the resulting instability may cause pain in any or all of the pelvic joints.

Because the examiner does not have direct access to the bony structures and because the bones are covered with varying amounts of soft tissue, estimates of size and shape are approximate. Precise bony pelvis measurements can be determined by the use of radiographic computed tomography (CT) or magnetic resonance imaging (MRI). However, these procedures are rarely performed for this purpose because evidence is lacking that they are beneficial. Indeed, some data show possible harm associated with their use because of an increase in cesarean birth rates (Kilpatrick & Garrison, 2017). Even precise measurements do not always predict a woman's ability to give birth vaginally because of the many ways the fetus can negotiate the pelvis and the accommodation of maternal soft tissues. Therefore pelvimetry results rarely contraindicate a trial of labor.

Soft Tissues

The soft tissues of the passageway include the distensible lower uterine segment, the cervix, the pelvic floor muscles, the vagina, and the introitus. Before labor begins, the uterus is composed of the uterine body (corpus) and the cervix (neck). After labor has begun, uterine contractions cause the uterine body to have a thick and muscular upper segment and a thin-walled, passive, muscular lower segment. A *physiologic retraction ring* separates the two segments (Fig. 16.10). The lower uterine segment gradually distends to accommodate the intrauterine contents as the wall of the upper segment thickens and its accommodating capacity is reduced. The contractions of the uterine body thus exert downward pressure on the fetus, pushing it against the cervix.

The cervix effaces (thins) and dilates (opens) sufficiently to allow the first fetal portion to descend into the vagina. As the fetus descends, the cervix is actually drawn upward and over this first portion.

The pelvic floor is a muscular layer that separates the pelvic cavity above from the perineal space below. This structure helps the fetus rotate anteriorly as it passes through the birth canal. Chapter 13 describes changes in the vagina that occur during pregnancy. At term the vagina can dilate to accommodate the fetus and permit its passage to the external world.

Powers

Involuntary and voluntary powers combine to expel the fetus and placenta from the uterus. Involuntary uterine contractions, called the *primary powers*, signal the beginning of labor. Once the cervix has dilated, voluntary bearing-down efforts by the woman, called the *secondary powers*, augment the force of the involuntary contractions.

Primary Powers

The involuntary contractions originate at certain pacemaker points in the thickened muscle layers of the upper uterine segment. From the pacemaker points, contractions move downward over the uterus in waves, separated by short rest periods. Terms used to describe these involuntary contractions include *frequency* (the time from the beginning of one contraction to the beginning of the next), *duration* (length of contraction), and *intensity* (strength of contraction at its peak).

The primary powers are responsible for the effacement and dilation of the cervix and descent of the fetus. Effacement of the cervix means the shortening and thinning of the cervix during the first stage of labor. The cervix, normally 2 to 3 cm long and approximately 1 cm thick, is obliterated or "taken up" by a shortening of the uterine muscle bundles during the thinning of the lower uterine segment that occurs in advancing labor.

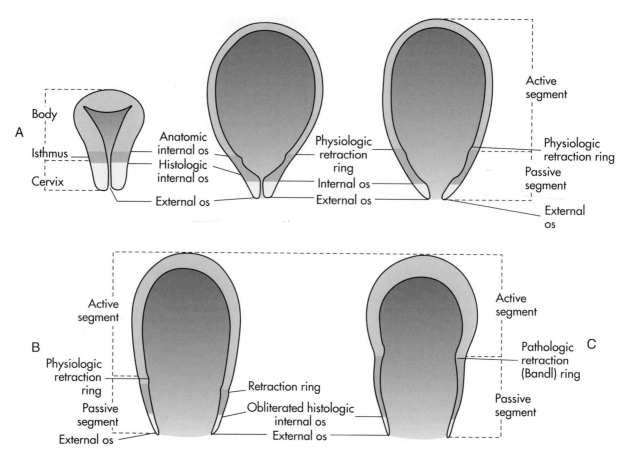

Fig. 16.10 (A) Uterus in normal labor in early first stage and (B) in second stage. Passive segment is derived from lower uterine segment (isthmus) and cervix, and physiologic retraction ring is derived from anatomic internal os. (C) Uterus in abnormal labor in second-stage dystocia. Pathologic retraction (Bandl) ring that forms under abnormal conditions develops from the physiologic ring.

Only a thin edge of the cervix can be palpated by an examiner when effacement is complete. Effacement generally progresses significantly in first-time term pregnancy before more than slight dilation occurs. In subsequent pregnancies, effacement and dilation of the cervix tend to progress together. Degree of effacement is expressed in percentages from 0% to 100% (e.g., a cervix is 50% effaced; Fig. 16.11A to C).

Dilation of the cervix is the enlargement or widening of the cervical opening and the cervical canal that normally occurs once labor has begun. The diameter of the cervix increases from less than 1 cm to full dilation (approximately 10 cm) to allow birth of a term fetus. When the cervix is fully dilated (and completely retracted), it can no longer be palpated by an examiner (see Fig. 16.11D). Full cervical dilation marks the end of the first stage of labor.

Dilation of the cervix occurs by the drawing upward of the musculofibrous components of the cervix, caused by strong uterine contractions. Pressure exerted by the amniotic fluid while the membranes are intact or by the force applied by the presenting part can promote cervical dilation. Scarring of the cervix as a result of prior infection or surgery may slow cervical dilation.

In the first and second stages of labor, increased intrauterine pressure caused by contractions exerts pressure on the descending fetus and the cervix. When the presenting part of the fetus reaches the perineal floor, mechanical stretching of the cervix occurs. Stretch receptors in the posterior vagina cause release of endogenous oxytocin that triggers the maternal urge to bear down, or the *Ferguson reflex.*

Uterine contractions are usually independent of external forces. For example, laboring women who are paralyzed because of spinal cord lesions above the 12th thoracic vertebra have normal but painless uterine contractions. In addition, use of epidural analgesia during labor does not decrease the frequency or intensity of contractions (Cunningham et al., 2018).

Secondary Powers

As soon as the presenting part reaches the pelvic floor, the contractions change in character and become expulsive. The laboring woman experiences an involuntary urge to push. She uses secondary powers (bearing-down efforts) to aid in expulsion of the fetus as she contracts her diaphragm and abdominal muscles and pushes. These bearing-down efforts result in increased intraabdominal pressure that compresses the uterus on all sides and adds to the power of the expulsive forces.

The secondary powers have no effect on cervical dilation, but they are of considerable importance in the expulsion of the infant from the uterus and vagina after the cervix is fully dilated. When and how a woman pushes in the second stage of labor are much-debated topics. Continued study is needed to determine the effectiveness and appropriateness of strategies used by nurses to teach pushing techniques, the suitability and effectiveness of various pushing techniques related to abnormal fetal heart patterns, and the standards for length of pushing in terms of maternal and fetal outcomes. See Chapter 19 for further discussion regarding pushing during the second stage of labor.

Position of the Laboring Woman

Position affects the woman's anatomic and physiologic adaptations to labor. Frequent changes in position reduce fatigue, increase comfort,

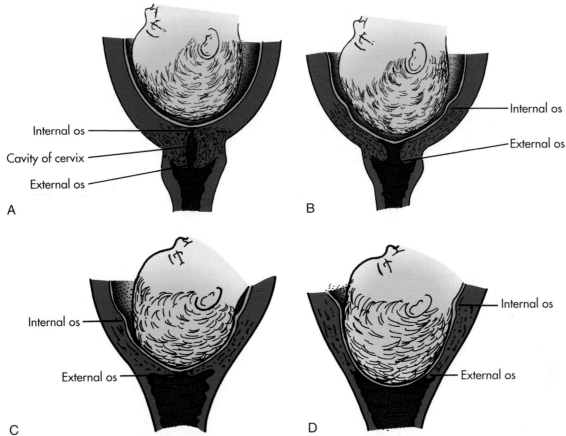

Fig. 16.11 Cervical Effacement and Dilation. Note how cervix is drawn up around presenting part (internal os). Membranes are intact, and head is not well applied to cervix. (A) Before labor. (B) Early effacement. (C) Complete effacement (100%). Head is well applied to cervix. (D) Complete dilation (10 cm). Cranial bones overlap somewhat, and membranes are still intact.

and improve circulation. Therefore a laboring woman should be encouraged to find positions that are most comfortable to her.

Positioning for second-stage labor may be determined by the woman's preference, but choices are limited by her condition or that of the fetus, the environment, and the health care provider's confidence in assisting in a birth in a specific position. See Chapter 19 for further discussion of positioning during labor and birth.

PROCESS OF LABOR

The term *labor* refers to the process of moving the fetus, placenta, and membranes out of the uterus and through the birth canal. Various changes take place in the woman's reproductive system in the days and weeks before labor begins. Labor itself can be discussed in terms of the mechanisms involved in the process and the stages through which the woman moves.

Signs Preceding Labor

In first-time pregnancies, the uterus sinks downward and forward about 2 weeks before term, when the presenting part of the fetus (usually the fetal head) descends into the true pelvis. This settling is called *lightening*, or *dropping*, and usually happens gradually. After lightening, women feel less pressure below the ribcage and breathe more easily, but usually more bladder pressure results from this shift. Consequently, a return of urinary frequency occurs. In a multiparous woman, lightening may not take place until after uterine contractions are established and true labor is in progress.

The woman may complain of persistent low backache and sacroiliac distress as a result of relaxation of the pelvic joints. She may

> ### BOX 16.1 Signs Preceding Labor
>
> - Lightening
> - Return of urinary frequency
> - Backache
> - Stronger Braxton Hicks contractions
> - Weight loss of 0.5–1.5 kg (approximately 1–3.5 lb)
> - Surge of energy
> - Increased vaginal discharge; bloody show
> - Cervical ripening
> - Possible rupture of membranes

identify strong, frequent, but irregular uterine (Braxton Hicks) contractions.

The vaginal mucus becomes more profuse in response to the extreme congestion of the vaginal mucous membranes. Brownish or blood-tinged cervical mucus may be passed *(bloody show)*. The cervix becomes soft (ripens) and partially effaced and may begin to dilate. The membranes may rupture spontaneously.

Other phenomena are common in the days preceding labor: (1) weight loss of 0.5 to 1.5 kg (approximately 1 to 3.5 lb), caused by water loss resulting from electrolyte shifts that in turn are produced by changes in estrogen and progesterone levels; and (2) a surge of energy. The woman may have a burst of energy that allows her to do whatever activities she feels will help her to prepare for labor. Less commonly, some women have diarrhea, nausea, vomiting, and indigestion. Box 16.1 lists signs that may precede labor (see the Clinical Reasoning Case Study).

"I Think I'm in Labor"

Erica is a 15-year-old G 1 P 0 at 39 weeks gestation. She presents by ambulance to the triage area in your labor and birth unit and announces, "I'm here to have my baby. I think I'm in labor." Erica reports that she saw a thick brownish red vaginal discharge several days ago and noticed bright red vaginal spotting when wiping after urinating earlier today. She states that she has lower abdominal cramping ("It feels like the cramps I have with my periods") but denies leakage of vaginal fluid. Erica also reports active fetal movement. When asked to rate her pain, she replies that her current pain level is 8 on a scale of 1 to 10, while alternating between texting on her phone and chatting with her mother, who accompanied her to the hospital.

1. What is the priority concern or client need in this situation? Support your answer with data as stated in the case.
2. List other client needs/problems in this case.
3. Identify any additional information or assessment data that is needed by the nurse in planning care for this client.
4. What nursing actions are appropriate in this situation?
   a. What is the priority nursing action? (What should the nurse do first?)
   b. Describe other nursing interventions that are important to providing optimal client care.
5. Describe the roles/responsibilities of the interprofessional health care team members (other than nurses) who may be involved in providing care for this client.

Onset of Labor

The onset of true labor cannot be ascribed to a single cause. Many factors, including changes in the maternal uterus, cervix, and pituitary gland, are involved. Hormones produced by the normal fetal hypothalamus, pituitary gland, and adrenal cortex probably contribute to the onset of labor. Progressive uterine distention and increasing intrauterine pressure seem to be associated with increasing myometrial irritability. This is a result of increased concentrations of estrogen, oxytocin, and prostaglandins and decreasing progesterone levels. The mutually coordinated effects of these factors result in the occurrence of strong, regular, rhythmic uterine contractions (Blackburn, 2018; Kilpatrick & Garrison, 2017). The outcome of these factors working together is normally the birth of the fetus and the expulsion of the placenta.

Stages of Labor

The course of labor at or near term gestation in a woman without complications and a fetus in vertex presentation consists of (1) regular progression of uterine contractions, (2) progressive effacement and dilation of the cervix, and (3) progress in descent of the presenting part. Four stages of labor are recognized. (These stages are discussed in greater detail, along with nursing care for the laboring woman and family, in Chapter 19.)

The *first stage of labor* is considered to last from the onset of regular uterine contractions to full dilation of the cervix. Commonly the onset of labor is difficult to establish, because the woman may be admitted to the labor unit just before birth and the beginning of labor may be only an estimate. The first stage is much longer than the second and third combined. However, great variability is the rule, depending on the factors discussed previously in this chapter. The first stage of labor has traditionally been divided into three phases: a latent (early) phase, an active phase, and a transition phase. In women who labor with epidural anesthesia, however, a separate transition phase may not always be identified based on maternal physical sensations and behavior (Simpson & O'Brien-Abel, 2014). Therefore the first stage of labor is now divided into only two phases: latent (early) and active (Kilpatrick & Garrison, 2017). During the latent phase, there is more progress in effacement of the cervix and little increase in descent. During the active phase, there is more rapid dilation of the cervix and increased rate of descent of the presenting part.

The *second stage of labor* lasts from the time the cervix is fully dilated to the birth of the infant. It is composed of two phases: the latent (passive fetal descent) phase and the active pushing phase. During the latent phase, the fetus continues to descend passively through the birth canal and rotate to an anterior position as a result of ongoing uterine contractions. The urge to bear down during this phase is not strong, and some women do not experience it at all. During the active pushing phase, the woman has strong urges to bear down as the presenting part of the fetus descends and presses on the stretch receptors of the pelvic floor.

The *third stage of labor* lasts from the birth of the infant until the placenta is delivered. The placenta normally separates from the uterine wall with the third or fourth strong uterine contraction after the infant has been born. After it has separated, the placenta can be expelled with the next uterine contraction.

The *fourth stage of labor* begins with the delivery of the placenta and includes at least the first 2 hours after birth. During this stage, the woman begins to recover physically from birth, so it is an important time to observe for complications, such as abnormal bleeding (see Chapter 33).

Mechanism of Labor

As already discussed, the female pelvis has varied contours and diameters at different levels, and the presenting part of the passenger is large in proportion to the passage. Therefore, for vaginal birth to occur, the fetus must adapt to the birth canal during the descent. The turns and other adjustments necessary in the human birth process are termed the *mechanism of labor* (Fig. 16.12). The seven cardinal movements of the mechanism of labor that occur in a vertex presentation are *engagement, descent, flexion, internal rotation, extension, external rotation (restitution),* and *birth by expulsion*. Although these movements are discussed separately, in actuality, a combination of movements occurs simultaneously. For example, engagement involves both descent and flexion.

Engagement

When the biparietal diameter of the head passes the pelvic inlet, the head is said to be engaged in the pelvic inlet (see Fig. 16.12A). In most nulliparous pregnancies, this occurs before the onset of active labor because the firmer abdominal muscles direct the presenting part into the pelvis. In multiparous pregnancies in which the abdominal musculature is more relaxed, the head often remains freely movable above the pelvic brim until labor is established.

Asynclitism. The head usually engages in the pelvis in a synclitic position (i.e., one that is parallel to the anteroposterior plane of the pelvis). Frequently asynclitism occurs (the head is deflected anteriorly or posteriorly in the pelvis), which can facilitate descent because the head is being positioned to accommodate to the pelvic cavity (Fig. 16.13). Extreme asynclitism can cause cephalopelvic disproportion, even in a normal-size pelvis, because the fetal head is positioned so that it cannot descend through the maternal pelvis (see Chapter 32).

Descent

Descent refers to the progress of the presenting part through the pelvis. It depends on at least four forces: (1) pressure exerted by the amniotic fluid, (2) direct pressure exerted by the contracting fundus on the fetus, (3) force of the contraction of the maternal diaphragm and abdominal muscles in the second stage of labor, and (4) extension and straightening of the fetal

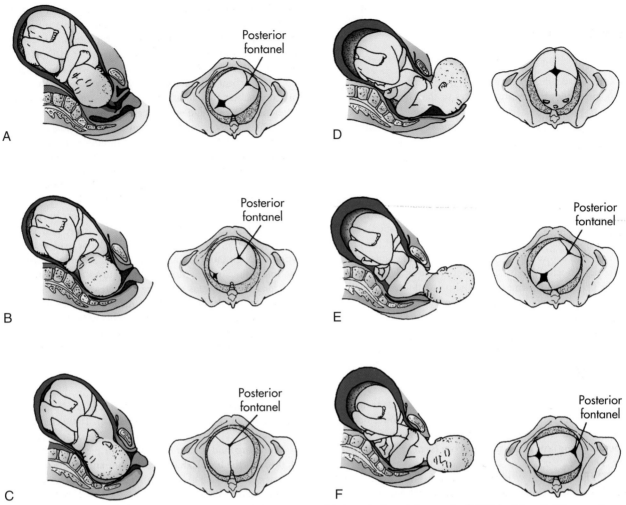

Fig. 16.12 Cardinal Movements of the Mechanism of Labor. Left occipitoanterior (LOA) position. Pelvic figures show the position of the fetal head, as seen by the birth attendant. (A) Engagement and descent. (B) Flexion. (C) Internal rotation to occipitoanterior position (OA). (D) Extension. (E) External rotation beginning (restitution). (F) External rotation.

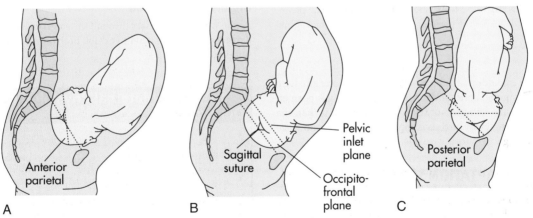

Fig. 16.13 Synclitism and Asynclitism. (A) Anterior asynclitism. (B) Normal synclitism. (C) Posterior asynclitism.

body. The effects of these forces are modified by the size and shape of the maternal pelvic planes and the size of the fetal head and its capacity to mold.

The degree of descent is measured by the station of the presenting part (see Fig. 16.6). As mentioned, little descent occurs during the latent phase of the first stage of labor. Descent accelerates in the active phase when the cervix has dilated to 5 to 6 cm. It is especially apparent when the membranes have ruptured.

During first-time labor and birth, descent is usually slow but steady; in subsequent pregnancies, descent may be rapid. Progress in descent of the presenting part is assessed by abdominal palpation and vaginal examination until the presenting part can be seen at the introitus (see Chapter 19).

Flexion

As soon as the descending head meets resistance from the cervix, pelvic wall, or pelvic floor, it normally flexes so that the chin is brought into closer contact with the fetal chest (see Fig. 16.12B). Flexion permits the smaller suboccipitobregmatic diameter (9.5 cm) rather than the larger diameters to present to the outlet.

Internal Rotation

The maternal pelvic inlet is widest in the transverse diameter; therefore the fetal head passes the inlet into the true pelvis in the occipitotransverse position. The outlet is widest in the anteroposterior diameter; for the fetus to exit, the head must rotate. Internal rotation begins at the level of the ischial spines but is not completed until the presenting part reaches the lower pelvis. As the occiput rotates anteriorly, the face rotates posteriorly. With each contraction the fetal head is guided by the bony pelvis and the muscles of the pelvic floor. Eventually the occiput will be in the midline beneath the pubic arch. The head is almost always rotated by the time it reaches the pelvic floor (see Fig. 16.12C). Both the levator ani muscles and the bony pelvis are important for achieving anterior rotation. A previous birth injury or regional anesthesia may compromise the function of the levator sling.

Extension

When the fetal head reaches the perineum for birth, it is deflected anteriorly by the perineum. The occiput passes under the lower border of the symphysis pubis first, and then the head emerges by extension: first the occiput, then the face, and finally the chin (see Fig. 16.12D).

Restitution and External Rotation

After the head is born, it rotates briefly to the position it occupied when it was engaged in the inlet. This movement is referred to as restitution (see Fig. 16.12E). The 45-degree turn realigns the infant's head with the back and shoulders. The head can then be seen to rotate further. This external rotation occurs as the shoulders engage and descend in maneuvers similar to those of the head (see Fig. 16.12F). As noted, the anterior shoulder descends first. When it reaches the outlet, it rotates to the midline and is delivered from under the pubic arch. The posterior shoulder is guided over the perineum until it is free of the vaginal introitus.

Expulsion

After birth of the shoulders, the head and shoulders are lifted up toward the mother's pubic bone, and the trunk of the baby is born by flexing it laterally in the direction of the symphysis pubis. When the baby has emerged completely, birth is complete, and the second stage of labor ends.

PHYSIOLOGIC ADAPTATION TO LABOR

In addition to the maternal and fetal anatomic adaptations that occur during birth, physiologic adaptations must occur. Accurate assessment of the laboring woman and fetus requires knowledge of these expected adaptations.

Fetal Adaptation

Several important physiologic adaptations occur in the fetus. These changes occur in fetal heart rate (FHR), fetal circulation, respiratory movements, and other behaviors.

Fetal Heart Rate

FHR monitoring provides reliable and predictive information about the condition of the fetus related to oxygenation. The average FHR at term is 140 beats/minute; the normal range is 110 to 160 beats/minute. Earlier in gestation, the FHR is higher, with an average of approximately 160 beats/minute at 20 weeks of gestation. The rate decreases progressively as the maturing fetus reaches term. However, temporary accelerations and slight early decelerations of the FHR can be expected in response to spontaneous fetal movement, vaginal examination, fundal pressure, uterine contractions, abdominal palpation, and fetal head compression. Stresses to the uterofetoplacental unit result in characteristic FHR patterns (see Chapter 18 for further discussion).

Fetal Circulation

Fetal circulation can be affected by many factors, including maternal position, uterine contractions, blood pressure, and umbilical cord blood flow. Uterine contractions during labor tend to decrease circulation through the spiral arterioles and subsequent perfusion through the intervillous space. Most healthy fetuses are well able to compensate for this stress and exposure to increased pressure while moving passively through the birth canal during labor. Usually the umbilical cord moves freely in the amniotic fluid. However, it can be compressed during uterine contractions (Blackburn, 2018; Miller, Miller, & Cypher, 2017).

Fetal Respiration

Certain changes stimulate chemoreceptors in the aorta and carotid bodies to prepare the fetus for initiating respirations immediately after birth (Blackburn, 2018; Fraser, 2014). These changes include the following:

- Fetal lung fluid is cleared from the air passages as the infant passes through the birth canal during labor and (vaginal) birth. The process of labor itself also contributes to the absorption of some of the lung fluid before birth.
- Fetal oxygen pressure (Po_2) decreases.
- Arterial carbon dioxide pressure (Pco_2) increases.
- Arterial pH decreases.
- Bicarbonate level decreases.
- Fetal respiratory movements decrease during labor.

Maternal Adaptation

As the woman progresses through the stages of labor, various body system adaptations cause her to exhibit both objective signs and subjective symptoms (Box 16.2).

BOX 16.2 Maternal Physiologic Changes During Labor

- Cardiac output increases 10%–15% in first stage, 30%–50% in second stage.
- Heart rate increases slightly in first and second stages.
- Blood pressure (both systolic and diastolic) increases during contractions and returns to baseline levels between contractions. Systolic values increase more than diastolic values.
- White blood cell (WBC) count increases.
- Respiratory rate increases.
- Temperature may be slightly elevated.
- Proteinuria may occur.
- Gastric motility and absorption of solid food are decreased; nausea and vomiting may occur during transition to second stage labor.
- Blood glucose level decreases.

Cardiovascular Changes

During each contraction an average of 300 to 500 mL of blood is shunted from the uterus into the maternal vascular system. By the end of the first stage of labor, cardiac output during contractions is increased by 51% above baseline pregnancy values at term. Cardiac output peaks about 10 to 30 minutes after both vaginal and cesarean birth and returns to its prelabor baseline within the first postpartum hour. A drop in maternal heart rate accompanies this increase in cardiac output (Antony, Racusin, Aagaard, & Dildy, 2017).

Changes in blood pressure also occur. In general, both systolic and diastolic pressures increase during contractions and return to baseline levels between contractions. Systolic values increase more than diastolic values (Blackburn, 2018).

Supine hypotension (see Fig. 19.5) occurs when the ascending vena cava and descending aorta are compressed. The laboring woman is at greater risk for supine hypotension if the uterus is particularly large because of a larger than usual fetus multifetal pregnancy or polyhydramnios or if she is obese, dehydrated, or hypovolemic. In addition, some medications can cause hypotension.

panting (or hehhh)

! NURSING ALERT

The woman should be discouraged from using the Valsalva maneuver (holding one's breath and tightening abdominal muscles) for pushing during the second stage. This activity increases intrathoracic pressure, reduces venous return, and increases venous pressure. Cardiac output and blood pressure increase, and the pulse slows temporarily. During the Valsalva maneuver, fetal hypoxia may occur. The process is reversed when the woman takes a breath.

The white blood cell (WBC) count increases during labor (Blackburn, 2018). Although the mechanism leading to this increase in WBCs is unknown, it may be secondary to physical or emotional stress or to tissue trauma. Labor is strenuous, and physical exercise alone can increase the WBC count. Some peripheral vascular changes occur, perhaps in response to cervical dilation or compression of maternal vessels by the fetus passing through the birth canal. Flushed cheeks, hot or cold feet, and eversion of hemorrhoids may result.

Respiratory Changes

Increased physical activity with greater oxygen consumption is reflected in an increase in the respiratory rate. Hyperventilation may cause respiratory alkalosis (an increase in pH), hypoxia, and hypocapnia (decrease in carbon dioxide). In the unmedicated woman in the second stage of labor, oxygen consumption almost doubles. Anxiety also increases oxygen consumption.

Renal Changes

During labor, spontaneous voiding may be difficult for various reasons such as tissue edema caused by pressure from the presenting part, discomfort, analgesia, and embarrassment. Proteinuria of 1+ is a normal finding because it can occur in response to the breakdown of muscle tissue from the physical work of labor.

Integumentary Changes

The integumentary system changes are evident, especially in the great distensibility (stretching) in the area of the vaginal introitus. The degree of distensibility varies with the individual. Despite this ability to stretch, even in the absence of episiotomy or lacerations, minute tears in the skin around the vaginal introitus do occur.

Musculoskeletal Changes

The musculoskeletal system is stressed during labor. Diaphoresis, fatigue, proteinuria (1+), and possibly an increased temperature accompany the marked increase in muscle activity. Backache and joint aches (unrelated to fetal position) occur as a result of increased joint laxity at term. The labor process itself and the woman's pointing her toes can cause leg cramps.

Neurologic Changes

Sensorial changes occur as the woman moves through the phases of the first stage of labor and from one stage to the next. Initially she may be euphoric. Euphoria gives way to increased seriousness, then to amnesia between contractions during the second stage, and finally to elation or fatigue after giving birth. Endogenous endorphins (morphine-like chemicals produced naturally by the body) raise the pain threshold and produce sedation. In addition, physiologic anesthesia of perineal tissues caused by pressure of the presenting part decreases the perception of pain.

Gastrointestinal Changes

During labor, gastrointestinal motility and absorption of solid foods are decreased, and stomach-emptying time is slowed. Nausea and vomiting of undigested food eaten after the onset of labor are common. Nausea and belching also occur as a reflex response to full cervical dilation. The woman may state that diarrhea accompanied the onset of labor, or the nurse may palpate the presence of hard or impacted stool in the rectum.

Endocrine Changes

The onset of labor may be triggered by decreasing levels of progesterone and increasing levels of estrogen, prostaglandins, and oxytocin (Simpson & O'Brien-Abel, 2014). Metabolism increases, and blood glucose levels may decrease with the work of labor.

■ KEY POINTS

- Labor and birth are affected by the five Ps: *p*assengers, *p*assageway, *p*owers, *p*osition of the woman, and *p*sychologic response.
- Because of its size and relative rigidity, the fetal head is a major factor in determining the course of birth.
- The diameters at the plane of the pelvic inlet, the midpelvis, and the outlet plus the axis of the birth canal determine whether vaginal birth is possible and the manner in which the fetus passes down the birth canal.
- Involuntary uterine contractions act to expel the fetus and placenta during the first stage of labor; these are augmented by voluntary bearing-down efforts during the second stage.

- The first stage of labor lasts from the onset of regular uterine contractions to full dilation of the cervix.
- The second stage of labor lasts from the time of full cervical dilation to the birth of the infant.
- The third stage of labor lasts from the infant's birth to the expulsion of the placenta.
- The fourth stage of labor begins with the delivery of the placenta and includes at least the first 2 hours after birth.

- The cardinal movements of the mechanism of labor are engagement, descent, flexion, internal rotation, extension, restitution and external rotation, and expulsion of the infant.
- Although the events precipitating the onset of labor are unknown, many factors, including changes in the maternal uterus, cervix, and pituitary gland, are thought to be involved.

- A healthy fetus with an adequate uterofetoplacental circulation is able to compensate for the stress of uterine contractions.
- As the woman progresses through labor, various body systems adapt to the birth process.

REFERENCES

Antony, K. M., Racusin, D. A., Aagaard, K., & Dildy, G. A. (2017). Maternal physiology. In S. G. Gabbe, J. R. Niebyl, J. L. Simpson, et al. (Eds.), *Obstetrics: Normal and problem pregnancies* (7th ed.). Philadelphia: Elsevier.

Blackburn, S. T. (2018). *Maternal, fetal, and neonatal physiology: A clinical perspective* (5th ed.). St. Louis: Elsevier.

Cunningham, F., Leveno, K., Bloom, S., et al. (2018). *Williams obstetrics* (25th ed.). New York: McGraw-Hill Education.

Fraser, D. (2014). Newborn adaptation to extrauterine life. In K. R. Simpson, & P. Creehan (Eds.), *AWHONN's perinatal nursing* (4th ed.). Philadelphia: Lippincott Wil1liams & Wilkins.

Kilpatrick, S., & Garrison, E. (2017). Normal labor and delivery. In S. G. Gabbe, J. R. Niebyl, J. L. Simpson, et al. (Eds.), *Obstetrics: Normal and problem pregnancies* (7th ed.). Philadelphia: Elsevier.

Miller, L., Miller, D., & Cypher, R. (2017). *Mosby's pocket guide to fetal monitoring: A multidisciplinary approach* (8th ed.). St. Louis: Elsevier.

Simpson, K., & O'Brien-Abel, N. (2014). Labor and birth. In K. R. Simpson, & P. Creehan (Eds.), *AWHONN's perinatal nursing* (4th ed.). Philadelphia: Lippincott.

Thorp, J. M., & Grantz, K. L. (2019). Clinical aspects of normal and abnormal labor. In R. Resnik, C. J. Lockwood, T. R. Moore, et al. (Eds.), *Creasy & Resnik's maternal-fetal medicine: Principles and practice* (8th ed.). Philadelphia: Elsevier.

17

Maximizing Comfort for the Laboring Woman

Rebecca Bagley

http://evolve.elsevier.com/Lowdermilk/MWHC/

LEARNING OBJECTIVES

- Describe nonpharmacologic strategies used to enhance relaxation and promote comfort during labor and birth.
- Compare pharmacologic methods used to relieve discomfort in different stages of labor and for vaginal or cesarean birth.
- Discuss the effects of medication management for the mother and its effect on the newborn both during and after birth.
- Construct an evidence-based plan to manage the discomfort that a woman experiences during childbirth.
- Explain the nurse's role and responsibilities while providing care for a woman receiving analgesia or anesthesia during labor.
- Describe the nurse's role in promoting comfort and safety throughout the labor and birth process.

Although labor and birth are considered to be natural processes, laboring women experience a significant amount of discomfort and pain as well as a variety of other challenging sensations. Pain is a highly individualized phenomenon with sensory and emotional components. Even though most women experience discomfort or pain during labor and birth, it is the intensity of the discomfort and the response to the discomfort that is unique to the individual. Pregnant women are generally concerned about the discomfort and pain they will experience during labor and birth and about how they will respond and cope. A variety of nonpharmacologic and pharmacologic methods are available to help the woman and her partner maximize her comfort during the labor and birth process. The methods that are recommended for use by members of the interprofessional health care team depend on the situation, the availability of these methods, and the preferences of the woman and her health care providers. This chapter discusses sources of intrapartum discomfort and pain and factors that affect women's responses. It also describes nonpharmacologic and pharmacologic methods commonly used to maximize comfort during labor and birth.

PAIN DURING LABOR AND BIRTH

Neurologic Origins

The pain and discomfort of labor have two origins—visceral and somatic. During the first stage of labor, uterine contractions cause cervical dilation and effacement. Uterine ischemia (decreased blood flow and therefore local oxygen deficit) results from compression of the arteries supplying the myometrium during uterine contractions. Pain impulses during the first stage of labor are transmitted via the T10 to T12 and L1 spinal nerve segments and accessory lower thoracic and upper lumbar sympathetic nerves. These nerves originate in the uterine body and cervix (Blackburn, 2018).

The pain from distention of the lower uterine segment, stretching of cervical tissue as it effaces and dilates, pressure and traction on adjacent structures (e.g., uterine tubes, ovaries, ligaments) and nerves, and uterine ischemia during the first stage of labor is visceral pain. It is located over the lower portion of the abdomen. Referred pain occurs when pain that originates in the uterus radiates to the abdominal wall, lumbosacral area of the back, iliac areas, gluteal area, thighs, and lower back (Blackburn, 2018) (Fig. 17.1).

During most of the first stage of labor, the woman usually has discomfort only during contractions and is free from pain between contractions. Some women, especially those whose fetuses are in a posterior position, experience continuous contraction-related lower back pain even in the interval between contractions. As labor progresses and the pain becomes more intense and persistent, women become fatigued and discouraged, often experiencing difficulty in coping with contractions (Blackburn, 2018; Burke, 2014; Lowe, Openshaw, & King, 2017).

During the end of first stage labor and in the second stage of labor, the woman has somatic pain, which is often described as intense, sharp, burning, and well localized. This pain results from the following:

- Distention and traction on the peritoneum and uterocervical supports during contractions
- Pressure against the bladder and rectum
- Stretching and distention of perineal tissues and the pelvic floor to allow passage of the fetus
- Lacerations of soft tissue (e.g., cervix, vagina, and perineum)

As women concentrate on the work of bearing down to give birth, they may report a decrease in pain intensity. However, some will have increased pain during this stage (Blackburn, 2018; Burke, 2014; Lowe et al., 2017). Pain impulses during the second stage of labor are transmitted via the pudendal nerve through spinal nerve segments S2 to S4 and the parasympathetic system (see Fig. 17.1) (Blackburn).

Perception of Pain

The physiologic causes of pain during labor are the same for all women. However, pain is a subjective experience and is defined completely by the person who is experiencing it. Therefore women vary in how they

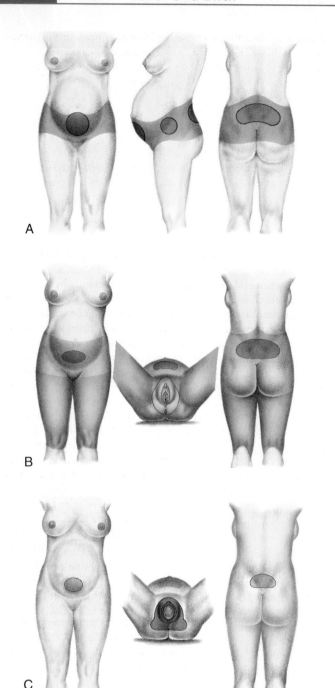

Fig. 17.1 Pain During Labor. (A) Distribution of labor pain during first stage. (B) Distribution of labor pain during active phase of first stage and early phase of second stage. (C) Distribution of pain during the late second stage and actual birth. (*Gray areas* indicate mild discomfort; *light pink areas* indicate moderate discomfort; *dark red areas* indicate intense discomfort.)

perceive and cope with labor pain. Factors that influence the way in which a woman deals with pain include her culture; age; previous personal experience with pain; parity; and the physical, psychologic, and emotional support available to her (Collins, 2017) (see Community Activity box: Dealing With Pain During Labor and Birth). The perception of pain is related to the woman's psychologic state. If she accepts the pain as natural, she is more likely to cope with it. If she associates it with suffering, she is likely to become distressed and lose control. The pain is not the issue. The issue is whether or not the woman is able to cope with the pain (Simkin, Hanson, & Ancheta, 2017).

Expression of Pain

Pain is expressed by both physiologic and sensory or emotional (affective) reactions. During labor and birth, the pain or discomfort experienced gives rise to identifiable physiologic effects. Sympathetic nervous system activity is stimulated in response to anxiety, stress, and intensifying pain, resulting in increased catecholamine levels. Blood pressure and heart rate increase. Maternal respiratory patterns change in response to an increase in oxygen consumption. Hyperventilation, sometimes accompanied by respiratory alkalosis, can occur as pain intensifies. Placental perfusion may decrease and uterine activity may diminish, potentially prolonging labor and affecting fetal well-being (Burke, 2014).

Certain emotional (affective) expressions of pain are often seen. Such changes include increasing anxiety with lessened perceptual field, writhing, crying, groaning, gesturing (hand clenching and wringing), and excessive muscular excitability throughout the body. In assessing how a woman is coping with labor, she should be asked what she felt during her last contraction instead of the level of her pain on a scale (Simkin et al., 2017).

FACTORS INFLUENCING PAIN RESPONSE

Physiologic Factors

A variety of physiologic factors can affect the intensity of pain during labor and birth. Fatigue can decrease a woman's ability to cope effectively with contraction pain (Burke, 2014). The interval and duration of contractions, fetal size, rapidity of fetal descent, maternal position, and maternal mobility during labor also affect a woman's perception of discomfort during labor and birth.

β-endorphins are endogenous opioids secreted by the pituitary gland that act on the central and peripheral nervous systems to reduce pain. The level of β-endorphins increases during pregnancy and labor and birth in humans. β-endorphins are associated with feelings of euphoria and analgesia. The pain threshold may rise as β-endorphin levels increase, enabling women in labor to tolerate acute pain (Blackburn, 2018).

Culture

The population of pregnant women reflects the increasingly multicultural nature of society in the United States. As nurses care for women and families from a variety of cultural backgrounds, they must have knowledge and understanding of how culture mediates the response to pain. Although all women expect to experience at least some pain and discomfort during labor and birth, their cultural and religious belief systems may determine how they perceive, interpret, respond to, and manage the pain. Cultural influences may impose certain expectations regarding acceptable and unacceptable behavior when experiencing pain (Lauderdale, 2016). A woman's cultural background may cause her to express pain vocally or to be more stoic.

An understanding of the beliefs, values, expectations, and practices of the woman's background narrows the cultural gap and helps the nurse assess the laboring woman's pain experience more accurately. The nurse can then provide appropriate, culturally sensitive care by using pain relief measures that preserve the woman's sense of control and self-confidence (see Cultural Considerations box: Some Cultural Beliefs About Pain).

Although a woman's behavior in response to pain may vary according to her cultural background, it may not accurately reflect the intensity of the pain she is experiencing (Lauderdale, 2016). It is the nurse's role to assess the woman for the physiologic effects of pain and listen to the words she uses to describe the sensory and affective qualities of her pain.

🌐 CULTURAL CONSIDERATIONS

Some Cultural Beliefs About Pain

> The following examples demonstrate how women of different cultural backgrounds may react to pain. Because they are generalizations, the nurse must assess each woman's experience of her pain related to labor and birth.
> - Chinese women may not exhibit reactions to pain, although exhibiting pain during labor and birth is acceptable. They consider accepting something when it is first offered as impolite; therefore pain interventions must be offered more than once. Acupuncture may be used for pain relief.
> - Arab or Middle Eastern women may be vocal in response to labor pain. They may prefer medication for pain relief.
> - Japanese women may be stoic in response to labor pain, but they may request medication when pain becomes severe.
> - Southeast Asian women may endure severe pain before requesting relief.
> - Hispanic women may be stoic until late in labor, when they may become vocal and request pain relief.
> - African American women may express pain openly. Their response to being offered medication for pain relief varies.

Anxiety

Anxiety is commonly associated with increased pain. Mild anxiety is considered normal for a woman during labor and birth. Excessive anxiety and fear, however, cause more catecholamine secretion, which increases the stimuli to the brain from the pelvis because of decreased blood flow and increased muscle tension. This action, in turn, magnifies pain perception. Thus, as anxiety and fear heighten, muscle tension increases, the effectiveness of uterine contractions decreases, the experience of discomfort increases, and a cycle of increased fear and anxiety begins (Blackburn, 2018). Ultimately this cycle will slow the progress of labor. The woman's confidence in her ability to cope with pain will be diminished, potentially resulting in reduced effectiveness of the pain relief measures being used.

Previous Experience

Previous experience with pain during labor and birth may affect a woman's description of her pain and her ability to cope with it. For a healthy young woman, labor and birth may be her first experience with significant pain; as a result, she may not have developed effective strategies for coping with it. She may describe the intensity of even early labor pain as pain "as bad as it can be." The nature of previous birth experiences may also affect a woman's responses to pain. For women who had a difficult and painful previous birth experience, anxiety and fear from this past experience may lead to increased pain perception.

Parity may affect the perception of labor pain because nulliparous women often have longer labors and therefore greater fatigue. Fatigue magnifies pain, thus causing many women to have an increased perception of the intensity of pain during labor.

❗ NURSING ALERT

> Survivors of sexual abuse are at an increased risk for being retraumatized during labor; they must therefore be treated with respect and compassion. Pelvic exams, being connected to a fetal monitor, and experiencing pain in the pelvic region may trigger increased pain and anxiety in women with a history of sexual abuse (Simkin et al., 2017).

Gate-Control Theory of Pain

Intense pain stimuli can at times be ignored. This is possible because certain nerve cell groupings within the spinal cord, brain stem, and cerebral cortex have the ability to modulate the pain impulse through a blocking mechanism. The gate-control theory of pain helps to explain the way hypnosis and the pain relief techniques taught in labor and birth preparation classes work to relieve the pain of labor. According to this theory, pain sensations travel along sensory nerve pathways to the brain, but only a limited number of sensations, or messages, can travel through these nerve pathways at one time. Using distraction techniques reduces or completely blocks the capacity of nerve pathways to transmit pain. These distractions are thought to work by closing down a hypothetical gate in the spinal cord, thus preventing pain signals from reaching the brain. The perception of pain is thereby diminished (Blackburn, 2018). Obstetric pain management techniques utilizing distraction include massage, aromatherapy, hypnosis, music, and guided imagery. Research into immersion virtual reality (VR) in pain management shows promise for adaptation to management of pain in labor.

When the laboring woman engages in neuromuscular and motor activity, activity within the spinal cord itself further modifies the transmission of pain. Cognitive work involving concentration on breathing and relaxation requires selective and directed cortical activity that activates and closes the gating mechanism as well. As labor intensifies, more complex cognitive techniques are required to maintain effectiveness. The main impetus behind the gate-control theory as it relates to pain is to introduce the brain to a positive stimulus by using all of the five senses. The brain then begins to accept the more positive stimulus while paying less attention to negative stimuli such as discomfort or pain. Stimulating the senses will not create a pain-free environment, but it can help to decrease the discomforts of labor.

Comfort

Although the predominant medical approach to labor is that it is painful and the pain must be reduced or eliminated, an alternative view is that labor is a natural process and that women can transcend the discomfort or pain, culminating in the joyful moment of birth. Having their needs and desires met promotes a feeling of comfort. The most helpful interventions in enhancing comfort are a caring nursing approach and a supportive presence. The provision of positive feedback, encouragement, and reminders that labor and birth are normal processes is an extremely beneficial intervention.

Support

A woman's satisfaction with her labor and birth experience is determined by how well her personal expectations of labor and birth are met and the quality of support and interaction she receives from her caregivers (Box 17.1). In addition, satisfaction is influenced by the degree to which she is able to stay in control of her labor and to participate in decision making regarding it, including the pain relief measures to be used (Collins, 2017).

BOX 17.1   Suggested Measures for Supporting a Woman in Labor

- Provide companionship and reassurance.
- Offer positive reinforcement and praise for her efforts.
- Encourage participation in distracting activities and nonpharmacologic measures for comfort.
- Give nourishment (if allowed by obstetric health care provider).
- Assist with personal hygiene.
- Offer information and advice.
- Involve the woman in decision making regarding her care.
- Interpret the woman's wishes to other health care providers and to her support group.
- Create a relaxing environment.
- Use a calm and confident approach.
- Support and encourage the woman's support people by role-modeling labor support measures and providing time for breaks.

The value of the continuous supportive presence of a person (e.g., partner, family member, friend, nurse, doula, midwife) during labor who provides physical and emotional comfort facilitates communication and offers information and guidance to the woman in labor has long been known. Emotional support is demonstrated by giving praise and reassurance and conveying a positive, calm, and confident demeanor in caring for the woman in labor (Simkin et al., 2017). Women who have continuous support beginning early in labor are less likely to use pain medications or epidural analgesia or anesthesia and are more likely to experience a spontaneous vaginal birth and to express satisfaction with their labor and birth experience. Interestingly, research findings have concluded that a more positive effect was achieved when continuous support was provided by people other than hospital staff members (Simpson & O'Brien Abel, 2014; Steel, Frawley, Adams, & Diezel, 2015).

Environment

When the laboring woman experiences discomfort, the quality of her environment can help her to view her experience more positively. The woman's environment includes the individuals present (e.g., how they communicate; their philosophy of care, including a belief in the value of nonpharmacologic pain relief measures and in the woman's specific birth plan; practice policies; and quality of support) and the physical space in which the labor occurs. Women who are in a supportive environment feel more in control and therefore are more likely to have a better labor and birth experience.

Women usually prefer to be cared for by familiar caregivers in a comfortable, homelike setting. The environment should be safe and private, allowing the woman to feel free to be herself as she tries out different comfort measures. Stimuli such as light, noise, and temperature should be adjusted according to her preferences. The environment should have space for movement and equipment such as birth balls, squatting bars, and birth chairs. Comfortable chairs, tubs, and showers should be readily available to facilitate the woman's participation in a variety of nonpharmacologic pain-relief measures. The familiarity of the environment can be enhanced by bringing items from home, such as pillows, objects to serve as focal points, and music (Simkin et al., 2015).

NONPHARMACOLOGIC PAIN MANAGEMENT

Relieving or reducing pain is important. Commonly it is not the amount of pain the woman experiences but whether she meets the goals she set for herself to cope with the pain that influences her perception of the birth experience as good or bad. The observant nurse looks for clues to the woman's desired level of control and her goals in the management of pain.

The labor and birth nurse can use a variety of nonpharmacologic methods for pain relief while providing support and encouragement to the laboring woman and her partner. Nonpharmacologic measures are often simple and safe; they have few if any major adverse reactions; are relatively inexpensive; and can be used throughout labor. Additionally, they provide the woman with a sense of control as she makes choices about the measures that are best for her. During the prenatal period, she should explore a variety of nonpharmacologic measures. Techniques she usually finds helpful in relieving stress and enhancing relaxation (e.g., music, meditation, massage, warm baths) may be very effective as components of a plan for managing labor pain. The woman should be encouraged to communicate to her health care providers her preferences for relaxation and pain relief measures and for active participation in their implementation.

Many of the nonpharmacologic methods for relief of discomfort are taught in different types of prenatal preparation classes, or the woman or her partner may have searched the internet or read various books and articles on the subject in advance. Many of these methods require practice for best results (e.g., hypnosis, patterned breathing and controlled relaxation techniques, focal point, distraction), although the nurse may use some of them successfully without the woman or her partner having prior knowledge of them (e.g., slow-paced breathing, massage and touch, effleurage, counterpressure, relaxation, music, hot or cold packs, movement or positioning). Women should be encouraged to try a variety of methods and to seek alternatives, including pharmacologic methods, when the measure being used is no longer effective (American College of Obstetricians and Gynecologists [ACOG], 2017).

Because of the increased use of epidural analgesia or anesthesia, nurses may be less likely to encourage women to use nonpharmacologic measures, in part because these methods may be viewed as more complex and time consuming than monitoring a woman receiving an epidural. In addition, new nurses may not have had the opportunity to develop skill in the implementation of these methods. It is imperative that perinatal nurses develop a commitment to and expertise in using a variety of nonpharmacologic pain-relief strategies in order for women in labor to feel comfortable in using them. Although research evidence to support the effectiveness of many of these nonpharmacologic measures is limited, there are sufficient reports of their benefits from women and health care providers to recommend that nurses encourage their use. The analgesic effect of many nonpharmacologic measures is comparable to or even superior to that of opioids administered parenterally (Box 17.2).

Methods of Preparing for Labor and Birth

The childbirth education movement began in the 1950s. Historically, popular childbirth methods taught in the United States were the Dick-Read method, the Lamaze (psychoprophylaxis) method, and the Bradley (husband-coached childbirth) method. Although the organizations that founded these methods continue to exist, they are now less focused on a "method" approach. Rather, women are helped to develop their birth philosophy and inner knowledge and then to choose from a variety of skills they can use to cope with the labor process.

Childbirth education has moved away from these traditional models to hospital-based classes taught by staff members. Also growing in popularity are methods developed and promoted by groups such as Birthing from Within (www.birthingfromwithin.com), Birthworks International (www.birthworks.org), the Childbirth and Postpartum Professional Association (CAPPA) (www.cappa.net), and HypnoBirthing (www.hypnobirthing.com). These organizations offer classes and other services that focus on fostering a woman's confidence in her innate ability to give

BOX 17.2 Nonpharmacologic Strategies to Promote Relaxation and Reduce Pain

Cutaneous Stimulation Strategies
- Counterpressure
- Effleurage (light massage)
- Therapeutic touch and massage
- Walking
- Rocking
- Changing positions
- Application of heat or cold
- Transcutaneous electrical nerve stimulation (TENS)
- Acupressure
- Water therapy (showers, baths, whirlpool baths)
- Intradermal water block

Sensory Stimulation Strategies
- Aromatherapy
- Breathing techniques
- Music
- Imagery
- Use of focal points

Cognitive Strategies
- Childbirth education
- Hypnosis

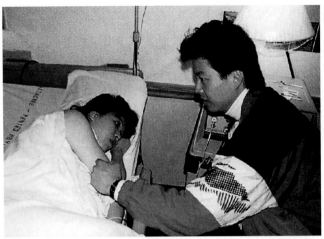

Fig. 17.2 A Laboring Woman Using Focusing and Breathing Techniques During a Uterine Contraction With Coaching from Her Partner. (Courtesy Marjorie Pyle, RNC, Lifecircle, Costa Mesa, CA.)

Drinking herbal tea can have the additional benefit of maintaining fluid balance. Some hospitals prohibit the use of oral intake during labor due to a fear of maternal aspiration. However, studies have demonstrated this risk to be extremely low (American College of Nurse-Midwives [ACNM], 2016).

The nurse can assist the woman by providing a quiet and relaxed environment, offering cues as needed, and recognizing signs of tension (e.g., frowning, change in tone of voice, clenching of fists). A relaxed environment for labor is created by controlling sensory stimuli (e.g., light, noise, temperature), and reducing interruptions. Nurses should remain calm and unhurried in their approach and sit rather than stand at the bedside whenever possible (Burke, 2014).

Breathing Techniques

Conscious breathing helps the laboring woman focus on something other than the contractions. In the past, Lamaze classes taught patterned breathing that was done a specific way during the different phases of labor. It has been found that women will find their own style of breathing and rhythm as the labor progresses. It is recommended that women start with slow breathing in early labor, as it takes less concentration, and later, when labor becomes more active and intense, to move to quick breathing (Lothian & De Vries, 2016). Different approaches to labor and birth preparation stress varying breathing techniques to provide distraction, thereby reducing the perception of pain and helping the woman maintain control throughout contractions. In the first stage of labor, such breathing techniques can promote relaxation of the abdominal muscles and thereby increase the size of the abdominal cavity. This lessens discomfort generated by friction between the uterus and abdominal wall during contractions. Because the muscles of the genital area also become more relaxed, they do not interfere with fetal descent. In the second stage, breathing is used to increase abdominal pressure and thereby assist in expelling the fetus. Breathing can also be used to relax the pudendal muscles to prevent precipitate expulsion of the fetal head (Fig. 17.3).

For women (and their partners) who have prepared for labor by practicing relaxing and breathing techniques, a simple review with occasional reminders may be all that is necessary to help them along. For those who have had no preparation, instruction and practice in simple breathing and relaxation techniques can be given early in labor and are often surprisingly successful. Nurses can also model breathing techniques and breathe in synchrony with the woman and her partner. Motivation is high and readiness to learn is enhanced by the reality of labor (see Clinical Reasoning Case Study: Laboring Without an Epidural).

birth. The woman or her partner are helped to recognize the uniqueness of their pregnancy and labor and birth experience.

Attendance at childbirth education classes has declined in recent years. Increasing numbers of women are utilizing online childbirth education rather than attending traditional classes because it is less expensive and more convenient for many working women and their partners. It has been demonstrated that childbirth education of some sort combined with making a birth plan decreases the risk of cesarean births (Afshar, Wang, Mei, et al., 2017).

Relaxation and Breathing Techniques
Focusing and Relaxation Techniques

Focusing and relaxation techniques reduce tension and stress, allowing the woman to rest and conserve energy in preparation for giving birth. The woman may focus on a still object in the room while performing her relaxation techniques to keep her from becoming distracted and losing control. Using *imagery*, the woman focuses her thoughts on a pleasant scene, a place where she feels relaxed, or an activity she enjoys. She might imagine walking through a restful garden or breathing in light, energy, and a healing color and breathing out worries and tension. Choosing the subject for the imagery and practicing the technique during pregnancy can enhance its effectiveness during labor.

During labor and birth preparation classes, the partner can learn how to palpate a woman's body to detect tense and contracted muscles. The woman then learns how to relax the tense muscle in response to the gentle stroking of the muscle by the partner (Fig. 17.2). In a common feedback mechanism, the woman and her partner say the word *relax* at the onset of each contraction and throughout it as needed. With practice, the partner can effectively use support, feedback, and touch to facilitate the woman's relaxation and thereby reduce tension and stress, thus enhancing the progress of labor (Burke, 2014).

Women may find that drinking herbal tea during labor can help them to relax (e.g., chamomile); it is also useful in reducing nausea (e.g., lemon balm, peppermint), and enhancing energy (e.g., ginger, ginsing).

🔅 CLINICAL REASONING CASE STUDY

Laboring Without an Epidural

Ellen is a 24-year-old G1P0 who has been admitted for induction of labor at 41 weeks gestation. She and her husband were not able to attend childbirth education classes owing to their schedules. Ellen read some information online and wants to labor without an epidural because she is afraid of the needle in her back. She will accept intravenous analgesia if indicated but prefers a "natural labor" without medications. On admission her cervix was 2-cm dilated, 80% effaced, and the presenting part was cephalic at a –1 station. Ellen was started on oxytocin an hour ago and is now experiencing contractions every 2-3 min. Her husband came to the nursing station to ask for help because Ellen was experiencing a lot of discomfort with the contractions. She was found in a supine position, crying, and states that she does not think that she will be able to do this without an epidural.

1. What is the priority concern or client need in this situation?
2. List other client needs/problems in this case.
3. Identify any additional information or assessment data that is needed by the nurse in planning care for this client.
4. What nursing actions are appropriate in this situation?
   a. What is the priority nursing action? (What should the nurse do first?)
   b. Describe other nursing interventions that are important to providing optimal client care.
5. Describe the roles/responsibilities of the interprofessional health care team (other than nurses) who may be involved in providing care for this client.

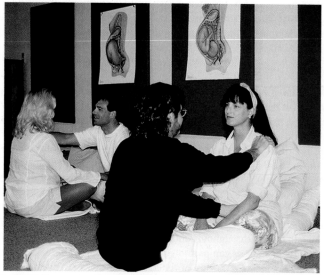

Fig. 17.3 Expectant Parents Learning Relaxation Techniques. (Courtesy Marjorie Pyle, RNC, Lifecircle, Costa Mesa, CA.)

Two types of breathing techniques can be used for controlling pain during contractions: slow breathing and quick breathing (Box 17.3). The nurse must determine what if any techniques the laboring couple know before giving them instruction. The woman should be allowed to perform any breathing pattern that works for her. Simple patterns are more easily learned. Slow breathing is performed in early labor when the contractions are more tolerable. She will transition to quick breathing when labor becomes more intense. Each labor is different, and nursing support includes helping couples to adapt the breathing techniques to their individual labor experience (Simkin, 2017).

The most difficult time to maintain control during contractions comes during the latter part of the active phase of the first stage of

BOX 17.3   Paced Breathing Techniques

Cleansing Breath
- Relaxed breath in through nose and out through mouth. Used at the beginning and end of each contraction.

Slow-Paced Breathing (Approximately 6-8 Breaths/Min)
- Performed at approximately half the normal breathing rate (number of breaths per minute divided by 2)
- IN-2-3-4/OUT-2-3-4/IN-2-3-4/OUT-2-3-4…

Modified-Paced Breathing (Approximately 32–40 Breaths/Min)
- Performed at about twice the normal breathing rate (number of breaths per minute multiplied by 2, according to the woman's comfort)
- IN-OUT/IN-OUT/IN-OUT/IN-OUT…
- For more flexibility and variety, the woman may combine the slow and modified breathing by using the slow breathing for beginnings and ends of contractions and modified breathing for more intense peaks. This technique conserves energy, lessens fatigue, and reduces risk for hyperventilation.

Patterned-Paced or Pant-Blow Breathing (Same Rate as Modified)
- Enhances concentration
- 3:1 Patterned breathing IN-OUT/IN-OUT/IN-OUT/IN-BLOW (repeat through contraction)
- 4:1 Patterned breathing IN-OUT/IN-OUT/IN-OUT/IN-OUT/IN-BLOW (repeat through contraction)

Modified from Nichols, F. (2000). Paced breathing techniques. In F. H. Nichols & S. S. Humenick (Eds.), *Childbirth education: Practice, research, and theory* (2nd ed.). Philadelphia: Saunders.

labor, when the cervix dilates from 8 to 10 cm. Even for the woman who has prepared for labor, concentration on breathing techniques then becomes difficult to maintain. *Quick breathing* is suggested during this time. It is performed at the same rate as modified-paced breathing and consists of panting breaths combined with soft blowing breaths at regular intervals. The patterns may vary (i.e., *pant, pant, pant, pant, blow* [4:1 pattern] or *pant, pant, pant, blow* [3:1 pattern]). An undesirable reaction to this type of breathing is hyperventilation.

⚡ SAFETY ALERT

The woman and her support person must be aware of and watch for symptoms of respiratory alkalosis, which can result from hyperventilation: light-headedness, dizziness, tingling of the fingers, or numbness around the mouth.

Having the woman breathe into a paper bag held tightly around her mouth and nose may eliminate respiratory alkalosis. This enables her to rebreathe carbon dioxide and replace the bicarbonate ions. The woman can also breathe into her cupped hands if no bag is available. Maintaining a breathing rate that is no more than twice her normal rate will lessen chances of hyperventilation. The partner can help the woman maintain her breathing rate with visual, tactile, or auditory cues.

As the fetal head reaches the pelvic floor, the woman may feel the urge to push and may automatically begin to exert downward pressure by contracting her abdominal muscles. During second-stage pushing, the woman should find a breathing pattern that is relaxing and feels good to her and is safe for her baby. Any regular or rhythmic breathing that avoids prolonged breath holding during pushing should maintain a good oxygen flow to the fetus.

The woman can control the urge to push by taking panting breaths or by slowly exhaling through pursed lips (as though she were blowing out a candle or blowing up a balloon). This type of breathing can be used to overcome the urge to push when the cervix is not fully prepared (e.g., less than 8 cm dilated, not retracting) and to facilitate a slow birth of the fetal head.

Effleurage and Counterpressure

Effleurage (light massage) and counterpressure have brought relief to many women during the first stage of labor. The gate-control theory may supply the reason for the effectiveness of these measures. Effleurage is light stroking, usually of the abdomen, in rhythm with breathing during contractions. It is used to distract the laboring woman and has been found to decrease the sensation of pain (Cherian & Peter, 2016). Often the presence of electronic fetal monitor belts makes it difficult to perform effleurage on the abdomen; therefore a thigh or the chest may be used instead. As labor progresses, hyperesthesia (hypersensitivity to touch) may make effleurage uncomfortable and thus less effective.

Counterpressure is steady pressure applied by a support person to the sacral area with a firm object (e.g., tennis ball) or the fist or heel of the hand. Pressure can also be applied to both hips (double hip squeeze) or to the knees (Burke, 2014). Application of counterpressure helps the woman cope with the sensations of internal pressure and pain in the lower back. It is especially helpful when back pain is caused by pressure of the occiput against spinal nerves when the fetal head is in a posterior position. Counterpressure lifts the occiput off these nerves, thereby providing pain relief. The support person will have to be relieved occasionally because the application of counterpressure is hard work.

Touch and Massage

Touch and massage have been an integral part of the traditional care process for women in labor. Both of these techniques are described in this section.

Touch can be as simple as holding the woman's hand, stroking her body, and embracing her. When touch is being used to communicate caring, reassurance, and concern, it is important that the woman's preferences for touch (e.g., who can touch her, where they can touch her, and how they can touch her) and responses to touch be determined. A woman with a history of sexual abuse or certain cultural beliefs may be uncomfortable with touch. Touch may not be desired or appreciated by some women in labor, as it may break their concentration if they are using certain prepared childbirth methods (Collins, 2017). Touch also can involve very specialized techniques that require manipulation of the human energy field.

Head, hand, back, and foot massage may be very effective in reducing tension and enhancing comfort. Back massage has been shown to be safe and effective in decreasing pain and anxiety during labor. Hand and foot massage may be especially relaxing in advanced labor when hyperesthesia limits a woman's tolerance for touch on other parts of her body (Bala, Babu, & Rastogi, 2017). Combining massage with aromatherapy oil or lotion enhances relaxation both during and between contractions, thus decreasing pain scores (Janula & Mahipal, 2015). The woman and her partner should be encouraged to experiment with different types of massage during pregnancy to determine which might feel best and be most relaxing during labor.

Application of Heat and Cold

Warmed blankets, warm compresses, heated rice bags, a warm bath or shower, or a moist heating pad can enhance relaxation and reduce pain during labor. Heat relieves muscle ischemia and increases blood flow to the area of discomfort. Heat application is effective in reducing back pain caused by a posterior presentation or general backache from fatigue. During second-stage labor, the application of warm, moist compresses to the perineum relieves the burning sensation women often feel when the fetal head crowns (Collins, 2017).

Cold application such as cold cloths, frozen gel packs, or ice packs applied to the back, the chest, and/or the face during labor may be effective in increasing comfort when the woman feels warm. These cold applications also may be applied to areas of musculoskeletal pain. Cooling relieves pain by reducing the muscle temperature and relieving muscle spasms (Burke, 2014). However, a woman's culture may make the use of cold during labor unacceptable.

> ## ⚡ SAFETY ALERT
>
> Heat and cold may be used alternately for a greater effect. Neither heat nor cold should be applied over ischemic or anesthetized areas because tissues can be damaged (Collins, 2017). One or two layers of cloth should be placed between the skin and a hot or cold pack to prevent damage to the underlying integument.

Acupressure and Acupuncture

Acupressure and acupuncture can be used in pregnancy, labor, and postpartum to relieve pain and other discomforts. A licensed acupuncturist is required to perform acupuncture, but acupressure can be administered by a trained health care professional in any setting (Schlaeger, Gabzdyl, Bussell, et al., 2017). Acupuncture points, stimulated with the insertion of fine needles, have an increased density of neuroreceptors and increased electrical conductivity. The insertion of these needles into specific areas of the body restores the flow of *qi* (energy) and decreases pain, which is thought to obstruct the flow of energy. Effectiveness may be attributed to the alteration of chemical neurotransmitter levels in the body or to the release of endorphins as a result of hypothalamic activation (Schlaeger et al.).

Acupressure is said to promote circulation of blood, the harmony of yin and yang, and the secretion of neurotransmitters, thus maintaining normal body functions and enhancing well-being. Acupressure is best applied over the skin without using lubricants. Pressure is usually applied with the thumbs, fingertips, or knuckles (Fig. 17.4). Pressure is applied with contractions intermittently for a period of 20 minutes (Schlaeger et al., 2017). Synchronized breathing by the caregiver and the woman is suggested for greater effectiveness. Acupressure points are found on the neck, the shoulders, the wrists, the lower back including sacral points, the hips, the area below the kneecaps, the ankles, the nails on the small toes, and the soles of the feet. Research indicates that women may experience pain relief with the use of acupressure or acupuncture (Collins, 2017; Schlaeger et al.).

Transcutaneous Electrical Nerve Stimulation

Transcutaneous electrical nerve stimulation (TENS) involves the placing of two pairs of flat electrodes on either side of the woman's thoracic and sacral spine (Fig. 17.5). These electrodes provide continuous low-intensity electrical impulses or stimuli from a battery-operated device. During a contraction, the woman increases the stimulation from low to high intensity by turning control knobs on the device. High intensity should be maintained for at least 1 minute to facilitate release of endorphins. Women describe the resulting sensation as a tingling or buzzing. TENS is most useful for lower back pain during the early first stage of labor. Women tend to rate the device as helpful, although its use does not decrease pain. It appears that the electrical impulses or stimuli somehow make the pain less disturbing. Because women maintain control of the TENS device, this element of autonomy may increase their satisfaction with the method. No serious safety concerns are associated with the use of TENS (Collins, 2017; Hawkins & Bucklin, 2017).

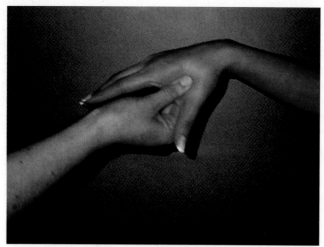

Fig. 17.4 Hoku Acupressure Point (Back of Hand Where Thumb and Index Finger Come Together) Used to Enhance Uterine Contractions Without Increasing Pain. (Courtesy Julie Perry Nelson, Loveland, CO.)

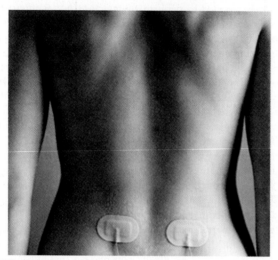

Fig. 17.5 Placement of Transcutaneous Electrical Nerve Stimulation Electrodes on Back for Relief of Labor Pain.

Water Therapy (Hydrotherapy)

Bathing, showering, and jet hydrotherapy (whirlpool baths) with warm water are nonpharmacologic measures that can promote comfort and relaxation during labor (Figs. 17.6A and B). Water immersion is a specific form of hydrotherapy that involves immersion of the laboring woman in water deep enough to completely cover her abdomen. The water increases buoyancy and provides a sense of weightlessness and freedom of movement. (See Community Activity box.) In a systematic review of hydrotherapy research, women who labored in water reported less anxiety and pain and greater satisfaction with their birth experience. Water immersion has not been associated with increases in adverse maternal, fetal, or neonatal outcomes (Brickhouse, Isaacs, Batten, & Price, 2015; Shaw-Battista, 2017).

> ### 🏠 COMMUNITY ACTIVITY
>
> Interview several women who have given birth and explore the positions they used while in labor. Which positions were most helpful, and why? Which did they find least helpful? Did any of the women use hydrotherapy? Share your findings with your fellow students.

Tub hydrotherapy may be contraindicated for some women. Women who require continuous electronic fetal heart rate (FHR) monitoring are not candidates for hydrotherapy unless waterproof monitors are available. Women with fever (≥38°C/100.4°F), infectious diseases (e.g., HIV positivity, active herpes simplex virus), and vaginal bleeding greater than a normal bloody show should not be offered water immersion. Additionally, tub hydrotherapy is contraindicated for women in preterm labor (gestational age <37 weeks) (Collins, 2017). Hydrotherapy using a shower provides comfort through the application of heat as the handheld shower head is directed to areas of discomfort (see Fig.17.6B). The partner can participate in this comfort measure by holding and directing the shower head.

> ### ⚡ SAFETY ALERT
>
> Because warm water can cause dizziness, a shower stool should be used and the woman should be helped when getting into and out of the tub.

Women must never be left alone while using hydrotherapy. Another person should always be present to assist the woman with getting out of the tub or shower quickly if necessary. The water temperature should be maintained above 35°C (95°F) and no higher than 37.8°C (100°F). Tubs must be thoroughly cleaned after each use to prevent bacterial growth and cross-contamination between women (Brickhouse et al., 2015; Collins, 2017).

ACOG has expressed concerns about actual birthing in water (water birth) because insufficient data are available from which to draw conclusions about its relative risks and benefits. There are concerns that water birth may predispose babies to potentially serious neonatal complications such as infection, water aspiration, and umbilical cord avulsion. Therefore, until sufficient data are available, ACOG recommends against the use of water birth (ACOG, 2016).

However, a recent study using data collected from the Midwives Alliance of North America Statistics Project reported water birth outcomes from a large number of midwife-attended births occurring at home and in birthing centers in the United States. They found no evidence of any subsequent neonatal risk for adverse outcome (5-minute Apgar score <7, neonatal transfer to the hospital, and any hospital admission, including to the neonatal intensive care unit, during the first 6 weeks of life) in neonates born under water. The researchers concluded that water birth does not confer additional risks to neonates (Bovbjerg, Cheyney, & Everson, 2016).

Intradermal Water Block

An intradermal water block involves the injection of small amounts of sterile water (e.g., 0.05 to 0.1 mL) using a fine-gauge (e.g., 25-gauge) needle into four locations on the lower back to relieve lower back pain (Fig. 17.7). It is a simple procedure to perform, and there is evidence that it is effective, perhaps because of the gate-control mechanism (Collins, 2017). Other possible explanations for the effectiveness of the intradermal water block are the mechanism of counterirritation (i.e., reducing localized pain in one area by irritating the skin in an area nearby) or an increase in the level of endogenous opioids (endorphins) produced by the injections. Intense stinging will occur for about 30 seconds after injection, but relief of back pain for up to 90 minutes has been reported. The pain from the injections may be decreased if two health professionals inject at the same time (Simkin et al., 2017). A qualitative study on laboring women's experience with sterile water injections demonstrated that women would ask for the procedure again (Lee, Kildea, & Stapleton, 2017). Although the effectiveness of this technique is largely unproven, no serious safety concerns are associated with its use (Hawkins & Bucklin, 2017).

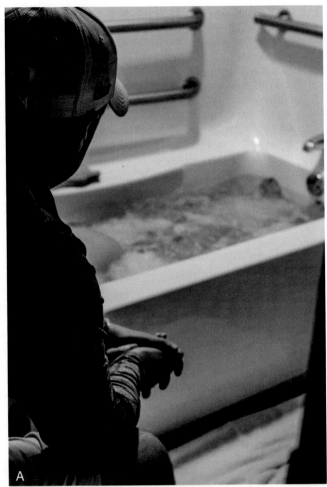

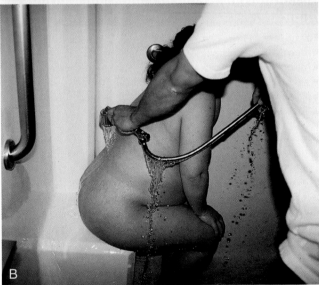

Fig. 17.6 Water Therapy During Labor. (A) Laboring woman relaxes in a tub. (B) Woman experiencing back labor relaxes as partner sprays warm water on her back. ([A] Courtesy Shannon Keller, CNM, UNC Midwives, Chapel Hill, NC; [B] Courtesy Marjorie Pyle, RNC, Lifecircle, Costa Mesa, CA.)

Aromatherapy

Aromatherapy uses oils distilled from plants, flowers, herbs, and trees to promote health and to treat and balance the mind, body, and spirit. These essential oils are highly concentrated, complex essences and are mixed with lotions or creams before they are applied to the skin (e.g.,

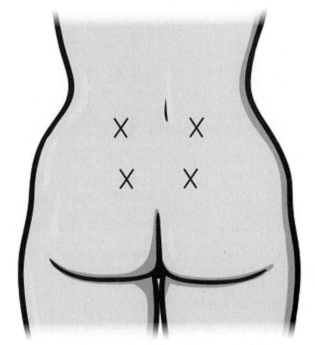

Fig. 17.7 Intradermal Injections of 0.1 mL of Sterile Water in the Treatment of Women With Back Pain During Labor. Sterile water is injected into four locations on the lower back, two over each posterior superior iliac spine (PSIS), and two 3 cm below and 1 cm medial to the PSIS. The injections should raise a bleb on the skin. Simultaneous injections administered by two clinicians will decrease the pain of the injections. (From Jaynes A.C., & Scott, K.E. (2012). Intrapartum care the midwifery way: A review. *Primary Care: Clinics in Office Practice. 38*(1), 189–206.)

for a back massage). Jasmine, geranium, rose, clary sage, neroli, ylang ylang, and lavender have been reported to provide good relief when used in labor. Because these oils contain medicinal properties, they should be used in the smallest amount that provides relief (Collins, 2017). Oils may also be used by adding a few drops to a warm bath, to warm water used for soaking compresses that can be applied to the body, or to an aromatherapy lamp to vaporize a room. Drops of essential oils can be put on a pillow or on a woman's brow or palms or used as an ingredient in creating massage oil. They can be used with a diffuser that disperses the oils into the air. Aromatherapy is inexpensive, easy to administer, pleasing to women, and does no harm (Janula & Mahipal, 2015).

Music

Music, recorded or live, can provide distraction, enhance relaxation, and lift spirits during labor, thereby reducing the woman's level of stress, anxiety, and perception of pain. It can be used to promote relaxation in early labor and to stimulate movement as labor progresses. Music can help create a more relaxed atmosphere in the labor and birth room, leading to a more relaxed approach by the health care team. Women should be encouraged to prepare their musical preferences in advance and to bring an electronic musical device to the hospital or birthing center. They should choose familiar music that is associated with pleasant memories, which can also facilitate the process of guided imagery and cause the release of endorphins, thus altering the perception of pain (Burke, 2014; Collins, 2017). Use of a headset or earphones may increase the effectiveness of the music because other sounds will be shut out. Live music provided at the bedside by a support person may be very helpful in transmitting energy that decreases tension and elevates mood. Changing the tempo of the music to coincide with the rate and rhythm of each breathing technique may facilitate proper pacing. There is evidence that supports the effectiveness of music as a method for reducing pain and anxiety during labor (John & Angeline, 2017; Karkal, Kharde, & Dhumale, 2017).

Hypnosis

Hypnosis is a form of deep relaxation, similar to daydreaming or meditation (see www.hypnobirthing.com). While under hypnosis, women are in a state of focused concentration and the subconscious mind can be more easily accessed. Women who attend certain childbirth preparation classes may be taught to perform self-hypnosis. Hypnosis techniques used for labor and birth place an emphasis on enhancing relaxation and diminishing fear, anxiety, and perception of pain. A few negative effects of hypnosis have been reported, including mild dizziness, nausea, and headache. These negative effects seem to be associated with failure to dehypnotize the woman properly. Although some initial small studies found hypnosis to be beneficial, a Cochrane systematic review showed no difference between women who were hypnotized and those who were not in regard to their use of pain medication during labor or their satisfaction with pain relief or the overall birth experience. However, it was noted that more research is needed (Madden, Middleton, Cyna, et al., 2016).

PHARMACOLOGIC PAIN MANAGEMENT

Pharmacologic measures for pain management should be implemented before pain becomes so severe that catecholamines increase and labor is prolonged. It is unacceptable for women in labor to endure severe pain when safe and effective relief measures are available (ACOG, 2017). Pharmacologic and nonpharmacologic measures, when used together, increase the level of pain relief and create a more positive labor experience for the woman and her family. Nonpharmacologic measures can be used for relaxation and pain relief, especially in early labor. Pharmacologic measures can be implemented as labor becomes more active and discomfort and pain intensify. Less pharmacologic intervention often is required because nonpharmacologic measures enhance relaxation and potentiate the analgesic effect. However, women in the United States are increasingly using pharmacologic measures, especially epidural analgesia, to relieve their pain during labor and birth. Of these women, increased rates of epidural use are seen among those with higher levels of education (ACOG, 2017). Pharmacologic measures for pain management are generally used in hospital settings rather than in birthing centers or in home births.

> ### ⚡ SAFETY ALERT
>
> Whenever medications are administered, nurses must remain alert for adverse reactions (e.g., difficulty breathing) and be prepared to administer antidotes or summon assistance if necessary. It is important to remember that adverse reactions can occur even if the woman has received the same medication in the past without problems.

Sedatives

Sedatives relieve anxiety and induce sleep. They may be given to a woman experiencing a prolonged early phase of labor when there is a need to decrease anxiety or promote sleep. They may also be given to augment analgesics and reduce nausea when an opioid is used.

Barbiturates such as secobarbital sodium (Seconal) easily cross the placenta and have a long half-life. They can cause undesirable side effects, including respiratory and vasomotor depression, affecting both the woman and her fetus. Because of the potential for neonatal central nervous system (CNS) depression, barbiturates should be avoided if birth is anticipated within 12 to 24 hours. As a result of these disadvantages, barbiturates are seldom used in obstetrics (Lowe et al., 2017).

Phenothiazines (e.g., promethazine [Phenergan]) do not relieve pain. In the past, promethazine was often given with opioids to enhance their analgesic effects as well as to decrease anxiety and apprehension, increase sedation, and reduce nausea and vomiting. However, there is no research evidence to support this practice. Metoclopramide (Reglan), an antiemetic, has been found to effectively potentiate the effects of analgesics. Therefore it may be a better choice than promethazine (Burke, 2014; Hawkins & Bucklin, 2017).

Benzodiazepines (e.g., diazepam [Valium], lorazepam [Ativan]), when given with an opioid analgesic, seem to enhance pain relief and reduce nausea and vomiting. Because benzodiazepines cause significant maternal amnesia, however, their use should be avoided during labor. A major disadvantage of diazepam is that it disrupts thermoregulation in newborns, making them less able to maintain body temperature. Flumazenil (Romazicon) is a specific benzodiazepine antagonist that can be administered if necessary to effectively reverse benzodiazepine-induced sedation and respiratory depression (Hawkins & Bucklin, 2017).

Analgesia and Anesthesia

Nursing management of obstetric analgesia and anesthesia combines the nurse's expertise in maternity care with a knowledge and understanding of anatomy and physiology and of medications and their therapeutic effects, adverse reactions, and methods of administration.

Anesthesia encompasses analgesia, amnesia, relaxation, and reflex activity. Anesthesia abolishes pain perception by interrupting the nerve impulses to the brain. The loss of sensation may be partial or complete, sometimes with the loss of consciousness. The term *analgesia* refers to the alleviation of the sensation of pain or the raising of the threshold for pain perception without loss of consciousness. The type of anesthetic or analgesic chosen is determined in part by the stage of labor of the woman and by the method of birth planned (Box 17.4).

> ### BOX 17.4 Pharmacologic Control of Discomfort by Stage of Labor and Method of Birth
>
> **First Stage**
> - Opioid agonist analgesics
> - Opioid agonist-antagonist analgesics
> - Epidural (block) analgesia
> - Combined spinal-epidural (CSE) analgesia
> - Nitrous oxide
>
> **Second Stage**
> - Nerve block analgesia and anesthesia
>   - Local infiltration anesthesia
>   - Pudendal block
>   - Spinal (block) anesthesia
>   - Epidural (block) analgesia
>   - CSE analgesia
> - Nitrous oxide
>
> **Vaginal Birth**
> - Local infiltration anesthesia
> - Pudendal block
> - Epidural (block) analgesia and anesthesia
> - Spinal (block) anesthesia
> - CSE analgesia and anesthesia
> - Nitrous oxide
>
> **Cesarean Birth**
> - Spinal (block) anesthesia
> - Epidural (block) anesthesia
> - General anesthesia

Systemic Analgesia

Systemic analgesics (opioids) can be administered as intermittent intravenous (IV) or intramuscular (IM) doses by health care professionals or by the woman herself using patient-controlled analgesia (PCA). With PCA, the woman self-administers small doses of an opioid analgesic by using a pump programmed for dose and frequency. Overall, a lower total amount of analgesic is used. Women appreciate the sense of autonomy provided by this method of pain relief as well as the elimination of treatment delays while the nurse obtains and administers the medication (Hawkins & Bucklin, 2017).

Opioids provide sedation and euphoria, but their analgesic effect in labor is limited. The pain relief they provide is incomplete, temporary, and more effective in the early part of active labor. All opioids cause side effects, the most serious of which is respiratory depression. Other undesirable opioid side effects include sedation, nausea and vomiting, dizziness, altered mental status, euphoria, decreased gastric motility, delayed gastric emptying, and urinary retention (Hawkins & Bucklin, 2017; Swart & Kelly, 2017). Prolonged gastric emptying time increases the risk for aspiration if general anesthesia becomes necessary in a woman who has received opioids (Hawkins & Bucklin). Bladder and bowel elimination can be inhibited. Because heart rate (e.g., bradycardia), blood pressure (e.g., hypotension), and respiratory effort (e.g., depression) can be adversely affected, opioid analgesics should be used cautiously in women with respiratory and cardiovascular disorders. Safety precautions should be taken after opioid administration, because several opioid side effects increase the risk for injury due to falls.

⚡ SAFETY ALERT

Opioids decrease maternal heart and respiratory rates as well as blood pressure and fetal oxygenation. Therefore maternal vital signs as well as the FHR and pattern must be assessed and documented before and after administration of opioids for pain relief.

Opioids readily cross the placenta. Effects on the fetus and newborn can be profound, including absent or minimal FHR variability during labor and significant neonatal respiratory depression requiring treatment after birth (Hawkins & Bucklin, 2017; Swart & Kelly, 2017).

Classifications of analgesic drugs used to relieve the pain of childbirth include opioid (narcotic) agonists and opioid (narcotic) agonist-antagonists. Choice of which medication to use often depends on the obstetric health care provider's preferences and the situation of the laboring woman, including factors such as her preferences, physical condition, and current medications. The type of systemic analgesics used therefore often varies among obstetric units. There is insufficient evidence to recommend the use of one opioid over another (Burke, 2014; Collins, 2017; Swart & Kelly, 2017). The opioids commonly used currently in obstetrics are meperidine, fentanyl, remifentanil, and nalbuphine (Hawkins & Bucklin, 2017).

Opioid agonist analgesics. Meperidine, fentanyl, and remifentanil are opioid (narcotic) agonist analgesics. As pure opioid agonists, they stimulate major opioid receptors, μ and κ. They have no amnesic effect but create a feeling of well-being or euphoria and enhance a woman's ability to rest between contractions. Because opioids can inhibit uterine contractions, they should not be administered until labor is well established unless they are being used to enhance therapeutic rest during a prolonged early phase of labor (Burke, 2014).

Meperidine (Demerol) is a synthetic opioid that has frequently been used worldwide as a systemic medication for labor pain (Cunningham et al., 2018; Lowe et al., 2017). Its widespread use is probably related to its low cost, the fact that care providers are quite familiar

with the drug, and studies (done many years ago) which found that it caused less respiratory depression than morphine (see the Meperidine Hydrochloride [Demerol] Medication Guide). However, its use during labor is becoming more controversial because of undesirable side effects, particularly in the neonate (Lowe et al., 2017). Both meperidine and normeperidine, an active metabolite of meperidine, cross the placenta and cause prolonged neonatal sedation and neurobehavioral changes. These metabolite-related effects cannot be reversed with naloxone (ACOG, 2019). Because meperidine and normeperidine have long half-lives, the neonatal effects can persist for the first 2 to 3 days of life (Hawkins & Bucklin, 2017).

MEDICATION GUIDE

Meperidine Hydrochloride (Demerol)

Classification
Opioid agonist analgesic

Action
Synthetic opioid agonist analgesic that stimulates both μ and κ opioid receptors to decrease the transmission of pain impulses. Meperidine 100 mg is roughly equivalent in analgesic effect to morphine 10 mg, but it is reported to cause less maternal respiratory depression. Onset of action begins almost immediately after administration and lasts approximately 1.5-2 h.

Indication
Moderate to severe labor pain and postoperative pain after cesarean birth

Dosage and Route
IV: 25-50 mg every 1-2 h
PCA pump: 15 mg every 10 min as needed until birth

Adverse Effects
Tachycardia, sedation, nausea and vomiting, dizziness, altered mental status, euphoria, decreased gastric motility, delayed gastric emptying, and urinary retention

Nursing Considerations
Implement safety measures as appropriate, including the use of side rails and assistance with ambulation; continue use of nonpharmacologic pain relief measures. Do not give if birth is expected to occur within 1-4 h after administration because infants born to women who received meperidine during labor may have respiratory depression, peaking at 2-3 h after administration of the drug. Respiratory depression caused by normeperidine, an active metabolite of meperidine, cannot be reversed with naloxone. Both meperidine and normeperidine have long half-lives. Therefore neonates whose mothers received meperidine during labor can exhibit sedation and neurobehavioral changes for the first 2-3 days of life.

Data from Anderson, D. (2011). A review of systemic opioids commonly used for labor pain relief. *Journal of Midwifery & Women's Health, 56*(3), 222–239: Hawkins, J. L., & Bucklin, B. A. (2017). Obstetric anesthesia. In S. G. Gabbe, J. R. Niebyl, J. L. Simpson, et al. (Eds.), *Obstetrics: Normal and problem pregnancies* (7th ed.). Philadelphia: Elsevier.

Fentanyl (Sublimaze) is a potent short-acting synthetic opioid agonist analgesic (see the Fentanyl Citrate [Sublimaze] Medication Guide). It rapidly crosses the placenta so is present in fetal blood within 1 minute after intravenous maternal administration. As compared with meperidine, fentanyl provides equivalent analgesia with fewer neonatal effects and less maternal sedation and nausea. Fentanyl is used as a labor analgesic because of its rapid onset of action, short half-life, and lack of a metabolite (Anderson, 2011; Hawkins & Bucklin, 2017). A disadvantage of fentanyl is that more frequent dosing is required because of its relatively short duration of action (Hawkins & Bucklin). As a result, this medication is most commonly administered by PCA pump, although it is also administered intrathecally or epidurally alone or in combination with a local anesthetic agent.

MEDICATION GUIDE
Fentanyl Citrate (Sublimaze)

Classification
Opioid agonist analgesic

Action
Opioid agonist analgesic that stimulates both μ and κ opioid receptors to decrease the transmission of pain impulses. Has a rapid onset of action with a short duration (0.5-1 h IV; 1-2 h IM).

Indication
Moderate to severe labor pain and postoperative pain after cesarean birth

Dosage and Route
IV: 50-100 μg every hour
IM: 50-100 μg every hour
PCA pump: (sample setting) 50-μg incremental dose with a 10-min lockout and no basal rate

Adverse Effects
Sedation, respiratory depression, nausea, and vomiting

Nursing Considerations
Assess for respiratory depression; naloxone should be available as an antidote. Implement safety measures as appropriate, including use of side rails and assistance with ambulation; continue use of nonpharmacologic pain-relief measures. Because of its short duration of action, frequent dosing will be necessary when fentanyl is given intravenously. Maximal total dose for labor is usually 500-600 μg.

Data from Anderson, D. (2011). A review of systemic opioids commonly used for labor pain relief. *Journal of Midwifery & Women's Health, 56*(3), 222–239; Cunningham, F., Leveno, K., Bloom, S., et al. (2018). *Williams obstetrics* (25th ed.). New York: McGraw-Hill Education; Hawkins, J. L., & Bucklin, B. A. (2017). Obstetric anesthesia. In S. G. Gabbe, J. R. Niebyl, J. L. Simpson, et al. (Eds.), *Obstetrics: Normal and problem pregnancies* (7th ed.). Philadelphia: Elsevier.

Remifentanil (Ultiva) has an even faster onset; it is a shorter-acting synthetic opioid agonist with no active metabolites (see Remifentanil Hydrochloride [Ultiva] in Medication Guide). Its time to onset of action is approximately 1 minute. Remifentanil does cross the placenta but is metabolized rapidly in the fetus, so that it does not cause neonatal depression. Because remifentanil is metabolized by plasma esterases, it is not affected by impaired renal or hepatic function. Remifentanil should be administered only by PCA pump because of its short (only 3-minute) half-life. Sedation and hypoventilation with oxygen desaturations occur more frequently with remifentanil than with other opioids, so respiratory monitoring is required with its use (Burke, 2014; Hawkins & Bucklin, 2017).

Opioid (narcotic) agonist-antagonist analgesics. An **agonist** is an agent that activates or stimulates a receptor to act; an **antagonist** is an agent that blocks a receptor or a medication designed to activate a receptor. Nalbuphine (Nubain) is a commonly used opioid (narcotic) agonist-antagonist analgesic (Hawkins & Bucklin, 2017).

MEDICATION GUIDE
Remifentanil Hydrochloride (Ultiva)

Classification
Opioid agonist analgesic

Action
Fast-onset, short-acting synthetic opioid with no active metabolites. Has a rapid onset of action (approximately 1 min). Because of its very short half-life (only 3 min), remifentanil should be administered only by PCA pump.

Indication
Moderate to severe first-stage labor pain

Dosage and Route
PCA pump (sample setting, as the ideal dosing regimen has not been determined): 0.5 μg/kg every 2-3 min with no basal rate

Adverse Effects
Sedation and hypoventilation with oxygen desaturations

Nursing Considerations
Close maternal monitoring (suggested 1:1 nurse/patient ratio) and continuous oxygen saturation monitoring are required. Administer through a dedicated intravenous line. Implement safety measures as appropriate; continue use of nonpharmacologic pain relief measures. Can be given to patients with impaired renal or hepatic function.

Data from Burke, C. (2014). Pain in labor: Nonpharmacologic and pharmacologic management. In K. R. Simpson & P. Creehan (Eds.), *AWHONN's perinatal nursing* (4th ed.). Philadelphia: Lippincott Williams & Wilkins; and Hawkins, J. L., & Bucklin, B. A. (2017). Obstetric anesthesia. In S. G. Gabbe, J. R. Niebyl, J. L. Simpson, et al. (Eds.), *Obstetrics: Normal and problem pregnancies* (7th ed.). Philadelphia: Elsevier.

Opioid agonist-antagonist analgesics are agonists at κ opioid receptors and either antagonists or weak agonists at μ opioid receptors. In the doses used during labor, these mixed opioids provide adequate analgesia without causing significant respiratory depression in the mother or neonate. Their major advantage is their ceiling effect for respiratory depression; higher doses do not produce additional respiratory depression. They are less likely to cause nausea and vomiting, but sedation may be as great or greater when compared with pure opioid agonists (Anderson, 2011; Hawkins & Bucklin, 2017).

Nalbuphine use also has some disadvantages. Its antagonist activity may limit the amount of analgesia it can produce. Also, it is not suitable for use in women with an opioid dependence, because the antagonist activity could precipitate withdrawal symptoms (abstinence syndrome) in both the mother and her newborn (Hawkins & Bucklin, 2017) (see the Medication Guide: Nalbuphine Hydrochloride [Nubain] and the Signs of Potential Complications box: Maternal Opioid Abstinence Syndrome [Opioid/Narcotic Withdrawal]).

Opioid (narcotic) antagonists. Opioids such as meperidine and fentanyl can cause excessive CNS depression in the mother, the newborn, or both, although the current practice of giving lower doses of opioids intravenously has reduced the incidence and severity of opioid-induced CNS depression. **Opioid (narcotic) antagonists** such as naloxone (Narcan) can promptly reverse the CNS depressant effects, especially respiratory depression, in most situations. As stated earlier, however, naloxone cannot reverse the effects of normeperidine, an

MEDICATION GUIDE

Nalbuphine Hydrochloride (Nubain)

Classification
Opioid agonist-antagonist analgesic

Action
Mixed agonist-antagonist analgesic that stimulates κ opioid receptors and blocks or weakly stimulates μ opioid receptors, resulting in good analgesia but with less respiratory depression and nausea and vomiting when compared with opioid agonist analgesics. Nalbuphine's analgesic effect is similar to morphine, on a milligram-to-milligram basis. Produces a maternal ceiling effect on pain relief and respiratory depression after 30 mg of the drug has been administered. Duration of action is 2-4 h when given intravenously and 4-6 h when given intramuscularly.

Indication
Moderate to severe labor pain and postoperative pain after cesarean birth; may be used to treat pruritus associated with epidural opioids

Dosage and Route
IV: 5-10 mg every 3 h as needed
IM: 10 mg every 3 h as needed

Adverse Effects
Sedation, drowsiness, nausea, vomiting, dizziness, respiratory depression, temporary absent or minimal fetal heart rate (FHR) variability

Nursing Considerations
May precipitate withdrawal symptoms in opioid-dependent women and their newborns. Assess maternal vital signs, degree of pain, FHR, and uterine activity before and after administration. Observe for maternal respiratory depression, notifying obstetric health care provider if maternal respirations are 12 breaths/min or less. Encourage voiding every 2 h and palpate for bladder distention. If birth occurs within 1-4 h of dose administration, observe newborn for respiratory depression. Implement safety measures as appropriate, including use of side rails and assistance with ambulation. Continue use of nonpharmacologic pain relief measures.

Data from Anderson, D. (2011). A review of systemic opioids commonly used for labor pain relief. *Journal of Midwifery & Women's Health, 56*(3), 222–239; Cunningham, F., Leveno, K., Bloom, S., et al. (2018). *Williams obstetrics* (25th ed.). New York: McGraw-Hill Education; and Hawkins, J. L., & Bucklin, B. A. (2017). Obstetric anesthesia. In S. G. Gabbe, J. R. Niebyl, J. L. Simpson, et al. (Eds.), *Obstetrics: Normal and problem pregnancies* (7th ed.). Philadelphia: Elsevier.

SIGNS OF POTENTIAL COMPLICATIONS

Maternal Opioid Abstinence Syndrome (Opioid/Narcotic Withdrawal)

- Yawning, rhinorrhea (runny nose), sweating, lacrimation (tearing), mydriasis (dilation of pupils)
- Anorexia
- Irritability, restlessness, generalized anxiety
- Tremors
- Chills and hot flashes
- Piloerection ("gooseflesh" or "chill bumps")
- Violent sneezing
- Weakness, fatigue, and drowsiness
- Nausea and vomiting
- Diarrhea, abdominal cramps
- Bone and muscle pain, muscle spasms, kicking movements

active metabolite of meperidine. In addition, the antagonist counters the effect of the stress-induced levels of endorphins. An opioid antagonist is especially valuable if labor is more rapid than expected and birth occurs when the opioid is at its peak effect. The antagonist may be given intravenously, or it can be administered intramuscularly (see the Naloxone Hydrochloride [Narcan] Medication Guide). The woman should be told that the pain that was relieved with the use of the opioid analgesic will return with the administration of the opioid antagonist.

MEDICATION GUIDE

Naloxone Hydrochloride (Narcan)

Classification
Opioid antagonist

Action
Blocks both μ and κ opioid receptors from the effects of opioid agonists

Indication
Reverses opioid-induced respiratory depression in woman or newborn; may be used to reverse pruritus from epidural opioids

Dosage and Route
Adult
Opioid overdose: 0.4-2 mg IV, may repeat at 2- to 3-min intervals until a maximum of 10 mg has been given; if the intravenous route is unavailable, intramuscular or subcutaneous administration may be used.

Newborn
Although naloxone has been used in newborns, there is insufficient evidence to evaluate the safety and efficacy of this practice. Animal studies and case reports have raised concerns about complications from naloxone, including pulmonary edema, cardiac arrest, and seizures.

Adverse Effects
Maternal hypotension or hypertension, tachycardia, hyperventilation, nausea and vomiting, sweating, and tremulousness

Nursing Considerations
The woman should delay breastfeeding until the medication is out of her system (approximately 2 h after the last dose has been given). Do not give this medication to the woman or the newborn if the woman is opioid dependent as that may cause abrupt withdrawal in both the woman and newborn. If given to the woman for reversal of respiratory depression caused by an opioid analgesic, pain will return suddenly. The duration of action of naloxone is shorter than that of most opioids. Therefore the woman must be monitored closely for the return of opioid depression when the effects of naloxone are gone. Additional doses of naloxone may be necessary to maintain reversal.

Data on newborn administration from American Academy of Pediatrics & American Heart Association. (2016). *Textbook of neonatal resuscitation* (7th ed.). Elk Grove Village, IL.

MEDICATION ALERT

An opioid antagonist (e.g., naloxone [Narcan]) is contraindicated for opioid-dependent women because it may precipitate abstinence syndrome (withdrawal symptoms). For the same reason, opioid agonist-antagonist analgesics such as nalbuphine (Nubain) should not be given to opioid-dependent women (see Signs of Potential Complications box: Maternal Opioid Abstinence Syndrome [Opioid/Narcotic Withdrawal]).

Nerve Block Analgesia and Anesthesia

Several different methods, referred to as *neuraxial analgesic and anesthetic techniques,* are used in obstetrics to produce sensory blockade and various degrees of motor blockade over a specific region of the body (Hawkins & Bucklin, 2017). A variety of local anesthetic agents are used in these techniques to produce regional analgesia (some pain relief and motor block) and regional anesthesia (complete pain relief and motor block). Most of these agents are related chemically to cocaine and end with the suffix *-caine.* This helps identify a local anesthetic.

The principal pharmacologic effect of local anesthetics is the temporary interruption of the conduction of nerve impulses, notably pain. Examples of common agents given are bupivacaine (Marcaine), chloroprocaine (Nesacaine), and lidocaine (Xylocaine). Rarely, people are sensitive (allergic) to one or more local anesthetics. Such a reaction may include respiratory depression, hypotension, and other serious adverse effects. Epinephrine, antihistamines, oxygen, and supportive measures should reverse these effects. Administering minute amounts of the drug to test for an allergic reaction may identify sensitivity.

Local perineal infiltration anesthesia. Local perineal infiltration anesthesia may be used when an episiotomy is to be performed or when lacerations must be sutured after birth in a woman who does not have regional anesthesia. Rapid anesthesia is produced by injecting approximately 10 to 20 mL of 1% lidocaine or 2% chloroprocaine into the skin and then subcutaneously into the region to be anesthetized. Epinephrine often is added to the solution to localize and intensify the effect of the anesthesia in a region and to prevent excessive bleeding and systemic absorption by constricting local blood vessels. Injections can be repeated to keep the woman comfortable while repairs following birth are completed.

Pudendal nerve block. Pudendal nerve block, administered late in the second stage of labor, is useful if an episiotomy is to be performed or if forceps or a vacuum extractor are to be used to facilitate birth. It can also be administered during the third stage of labor if an episiotomy or lacerations must be repaired (Hawkins & Bucklin, 2017). A pudendal nerve block is a relatively safe and simple method of providing pain relief for spontaneous vaginal birth (Cunningham, Leveno, Bloom, et al., 2018; Hawkins & Bucklin, 2017). Although a pudendal nerve block does not relieve the pain from uterine contractions, it does relieve pain in the lower vagina, vulva, and perineum (Fig. 17.8A). A pudendal nerve block should be administered 10 to 20 minutes before perineal anesthesia is needed.

The pudendal nerve traverses the sacrosciatic notch just medial to the tip of the ischial spine on each side. Injection of an anesthetic solution at or near these points anesthetizes the pudendal nerves peripherally (Fig. 17.9). The transvaginal approach is generally used because it is less painful for the woman, has a higher rate of success in blocking pain, and tends to cause fewer fetal complications. Pudendal block does not change maternal hemodynamic or respiratory functions, vital signs, or the FHR. However, the bearing-down reflex is lessened or lost completely.

Spinal anesthesia. In spinal anesthesia (block), an anesthetic solution containing a local anesthetic alone or in combination with an opioid agonist analgesic is injected through the third, fourth, or fifth lumbar interspace into the subarachnoid space (Figs. 17.10A and B), where the anesthetic solution mixes with cerebrospinal fluid (CSF). Low spinal anesthesia (block) may be used for vaginal birth, but it is not suitable for labor. Spinal anesthesia (block) used for cesarean birth provides anesthesia from the nipple (T6) to the feet. If it is used for

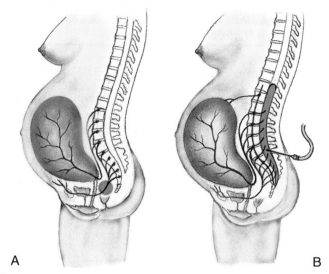

Fig. 17.8 Pain Pathways and Sites of Pharmacologic Nerve Blocks. (A) Pudendal nerve block: suitable during second and third stages of labor and for repair of episiotomy or lacerations. (B) Epidural block: suitable for all stages of labor and types of birth and for repair of episiotomy and lacerations.

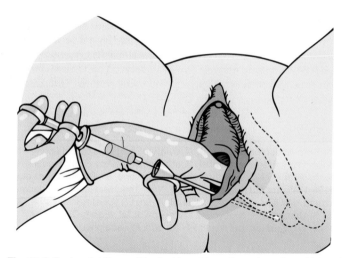

Fig. 17.9 Pudendal Nerve Block. Use of introducer (needle guide) and Luer-Lok syringe to inject medication.

vaginal birth, the anesthesia level is from the hips (T10) to the feet (see Fig. 17.10C).

For spinal anesthesia (block), the woman sits or lies on her side (e.g., modified Sims position) with her back curved to widen the intervertebral space; this position facilitates insertion of a small-gauge spinal needle and injection of the anesthetic solution into the spinal canal (Fig. 17.11). The nurse supports the woman and encourages her to use breathing and relaxation techniques because she must remain still during the placement of the spinal needle. The needle is inserted and the anesthetic injected between contractions. After the anesthetic solution has been injected, the woman may be positioned upright to allow the anesthetic solution to flow downward to obtain the lower level of anesthesia suitable for a vaginal birth. To obtain

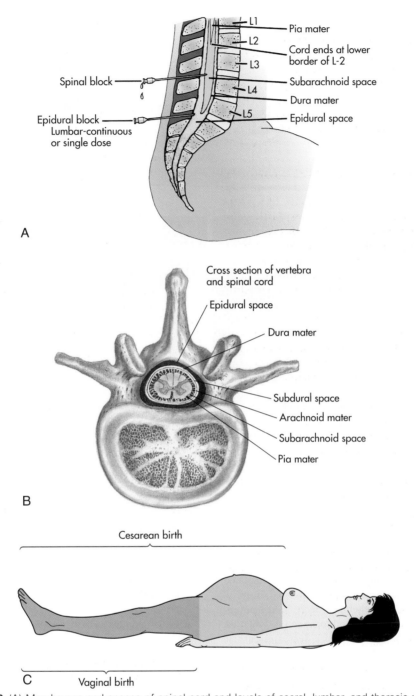

Fig. 17.10 (A) Membranes and spaces of spinal cord and levels of sacral, lumbar, and thoracic nerves. (B) Cross section of vertebra and spinal cord. (C) Level of anesthesia necessary for cesarean birth and vaginal birth.

the higher level of anesthesia desired for cesarean birth, she will be positioned supine with head and shoulders slightly elevated. To prevent supine hypotensive syndrome, the uterus is displaced laterally by tilting the operating table or placing a wedge under one of the woman's hips. Usually the level of the block will be complete and fixed within 5 to 10 minutes after the anesthetic solution is injected, but it can continue to creep upward for 20 minutes or longer. The anesthetic effect will last 1 to 3 hours, depending on the type and amount of agent used.

> ### ⚡ SAFETY ALERT
>
> To reduce the risk of transmitting pathogens, the woman's back is cleansed before the procedure. Before the induction of spinal and epidural anesthesia or analgesia, anesthesia care providers remove their jewelry and wash their hands; during the procedure, they wear sterile gloves and fresh face masks (Hawkins & Bucklin, 2017). Also, spinal or epidural anesthesia or analgesia should not be initiated in a woman who has a tattoo at the site where the needle would be inserted.

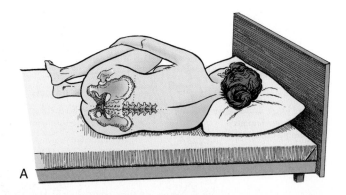

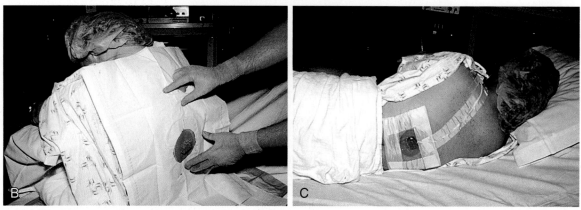

Fig. 17.11 Positioning for Spinal and Epidural Blocks. (A) Lateral position. (B) Upright position. (C) Catheter for epidural is taped to woman's back with port segment located near her shoulder. ([B and C] Courtesy Michael S. Clement, MD, Mesa, AZ.)

Marked hypotension, impaired placental perfusion, and an ineffective breathing pattern may occur during spinal anesthesia. Before induction of the spinal anesthetic, maternal vital signs are assessed and a 20- to 30-minute electronic fetal monitoring (EFM) strip is obtained and evaluated. In addition, the woman's fluid balance is assessed. A bolus of IV fluid (usually 500 to 1000 mL of lactated Ringers or normal saline solution) may be administered 15 to 30 minutes before induction of the anesthetic to decrease the potential for hypotension caused by sympathetic blockade (vasodilation with pooling of blood in the lower extremities decreases cardiac output). The practice guidelines published by the American Society of Anesthesiologists in 2016 state that IV fluid preloading may be used to reduce the frequency of maternal hypotension after spinal anesthesia for cesarean birth. However, the initiation of spinal anesthesia should not be delayed in order to deliver a fixed volume of fluid (American Society of Anesthesiologists Task Force on Obstetric Anesthesia & Society for Obstetric Anesthesia and Perinatology, 2016). Fluid that is used for the bolus should not contain dextrose, which could contribute to neonatal hypoglycemia (Hawkins & Bucklin, 2017).

After administration of the anesthetic, maternal blood pressure, pulse, and respirations as well as FHR and pattern must be assessed and documented every 5 to 10 minutes. If signs of serious maternal hypotension (e.g., a drop in systolic blood pressure to 100 mm Hg or less or below 20% of the baseline blood pressure) or fetal distress (e.g., bradycardia, minimal or absent variability, late decelerations) develops, emergency care must be given (Burke, 2014) (see Emergency Treatment box: Maternal Hypotension With Decreased Placental Perfusion).

✚ EMERGENCY

Maternal Hypotension With Decreased Placental Perfusion

Signs and Symptoms

Maternal hypotension (20% decrease from preblock baseline level or ≤100 mm Hg systolic)

Fetal bradycardia

Absent or minimal fetal heart rate (FHR) variability

Interventions

Turn the woman to lateral position or place pillow or wedge under one hip to displace uterus.

Maintain intravenous (IV) infusion at rate specified, or increase rate of flow per hospital protocol.

Administer oxygen by nonrebreather face mask at 10-12 L/min or per protocol.

Elevate the woman's legs.

Notify the obstetric and anesthesia health care providers.

Administer IV vasopressor (e.g., ephedrine 5-10 mg or phenylephrine 50-100 μg) per protocol if previous measures have been ineffective.

Remain with the woman; continue to monitor maternal blood pressure and FHR every 5 min until her condition is stable or per obstetric health care provider's order.

Because the woman is unable to sense her contractions, she must be instructed when to bear down during a vaginal birth. Using a combination of a local anesthetic agent and an opioid reduces the degree of motor function loss, enhancing a woman's ability to push effectively. If the

BOX 17.5   Side Effects of Neuraxial Anesthesia

- Hypotension
- Local anesthetic toxicity
  - Light-headedness
  - Dizziness
  - Tinnitus (ringing in the ears)
  - Metallic taste
  - Numbness of the tongue and mouth
  - Bizarre behavior
  - Slurred speech
  - Convulsions
  - Loss of consciousness
- Fever
- Urinary retention
- Pruritus (itching)
- Limited movement
- Longer second-stage labor
- Increased use of oxytocin
- Increased likelihood of forceps- or vacuum-assisted birth
- High or total spinal anesthesia

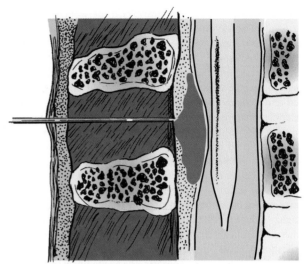

Fig. 17.12 Blood-patch Therapy for Spinal Headache.

birth occurs in a delivery room (rather than a labor-delivery-recovery room), the woman will need assistance in the transfer to a recovery bed after expulsion of the placenta and perineal repair, if required.

The advantages of spinal anesthesia include ease of administration and absence of fetal hypoxia with maintenance of maternal blood pressure within a normal range. Maternal consciousness is maintained, excellent muscular relaxation is achieved, and blood loss is not excessive.

Disadvantages of spinal anesthesia include possible medication reactions (e.g., allergy), hypotension, and impaired breathing; cardiopulmonary resuscitation may be needed. When a spinal anesthetic is given, operative birth (e.g., episiotomy, forceps-assisted birth, or vacuum-assisted birth) tends to become more likely because the woman's voluntary expulsive efforts are reduced or eliminated. After birth, the incidence of bladder and uterine atony as well as post–dural puncture headache (PDPH) is higher (Box 17.5).

Leakage of CSF from the site of puncture of the dura mater (membranous covering of the spinal cord) is thought to be the major causative factor in PDPH, commonly referred to as a *spinal headache*. This is much more likely to occur when the dura is accidentally punctured during the process of administering an epidural block. The needle used for an epidural block has a much larger gauge than the one used for spinal anesthesia and thus creates a bigger opening in the dura, resulting in a greater loss of CSF (i.e., "wet tap"). Presumably postural changes cause the diminished volume of CSF to exert traction on pain-sensitive CNS structures. Characteristically, assuming an upright position triggers or intensifies the headache, whereas assuming a supine position achieves relief (Hawkins & Bucklin, 2017). The headache, auditory problems (e.g., tinnitus), and visual problems (e.g., blurred vision, photophobia) resulting from CSF leakage begin within 2 days of the puncture and may persist for days or weeks.

The likelihood of headache after dural puncture can be reduced if the anesthesia care provider uses a small-gauge pencil-point spinal needle. Passing an epidural catheter through the dural opening at the time of puncture to provide continuous spinal anesthesia, with removal of the catheter 24 hours later, may help to prevent spinal headache. Hydration and bed rest in the prone position have been recommended as preventive measures but have proven to be of little value (Hawkins & Bucklin, 2017).

Conservative management for a PDPH includes administration of oral analgesics and methylxanthines (e.g., caffeine). Methylxanthines cause constriction of the cerebral blood vessels and may provide symptomatic relief. An autologous epidural blood patch is the most rapid, reliable, and beneficial relief measure for PDPH. The woman's blood (i.e., 20 mL) is injected slowly into the lumbar epidural space, creating a clot that patches the tear or hole in the dura mater. Treatment with a blood patch is considered if the headache is severe or debilitating or does not resolve after conservative management. The blood patch is remarkably effective and is nearly free of complications (Hawkins & Bucklin, 2017) (Fig. 17.12).

The woman should be observed for alterations in vital signs, pallor, clammy skin, and leakage of CSF for 1 hour after the blood patch has been placed. If no complications occur, she may then resume normal activity. She should, however, be instructed to avoid coughing or straining for the first day after placement of the blood patch (Hawkins & Bucklin, 2017).

Epidural anesthesia or analgesia (block). Relief from the pain of uterine contractions and birth (vaginal and cesarean) can be achieved by injecting a suitable local anesthetic agent (e.g., bupivacaine, ropivacaine), an opioid analgesic (e.g., fentanyl, sufentanil), or both into the epidural (peridural) space. Injection is made between the fourth and fifth lumbar vertebrae for a lumbar epidural block (see Figs. 17.8B and 17.10A). Depending on the type, amount, and number of medications used, an anesthetic or analgesic effect will occur, with varying degrees of motor impairment. The combination of an opioid with the local anesthetic agent reduces the dose of anesthetic required, thereby preserving a greater degree of motor function.

Epidural anesthesia and analgesia are the most effective pharmacologic pain relief methods available for labor. As a result, it is used by the majority of women in the United States (Hawkins & Bucklin, 2017). For relieving the discomfort of labor and vaginal birth, a block from T10 to S5 is required. For cesarean birth, a block from at least T8 to S1 is essential. The diffusion of epidural anesthesia depends on the location of the catheter tip, the dose and volume of the anesthetic agent used, and the woman's position (e.g., horizontal or head up). The woman must cooperate and maintain her position without moving during insertion of the epidural catheter in order to prevent misplacement, neurologic injury, or hematoma formation.

> **! NURSING ALERT**
>
> Epidural anesthesia effectively relieves the pain caused by uterine contractions. For most women, however, it does not completely remove the pressure sensations that occur as the fetus descends in the pelvis.

For the induction of an epidural block, the woman is positioned as for a spinal block. She may sit with her back curved or assume a modified Sims position with her shoulders parallel, legs slightly flexed, and back arched (see Fig. 17.11). A large-bore (16-, 17-, or 18-gauge) needle is inserted into the epidural space. A catheter is then threaded through the needle until its tip rests in the epidural space. The needle is then removed, and the catheter is taped in place. After the epidural catheter has been inserted and secured, a small amount of medication, called a *test dose,* is injected to make sure that the catheter has not been accidentally placed in the subarachnoid (spinal) space or in a blood vessel (Hawkins & Bucklin, 2017).

Initiating neuraxial anesthesia may be difficult when the woman is obese. Early initiation may be considered, both for comfort and to decrease oxygen consumption in labor. Early initiation of neuraxial anesthesia may reduce potential problems associated with intubation during an emergent cesarean birth, since obese women are at risk for airway complications (Baird, Kennedy, & Dalton, 2017). Catheter placement can present technical challenges, however. The woman may find it harder to assume a position necessary for catheter placement. In addition, excess adipose tissue can obscure the anatomic landmarks used to identify the location of the appropriate insertion site. Up to 75% of women weighing more than 300 pounds may require more than one attempt at catheter placement, and there is a high risk for placement failure. Although it was inserted in the correct location, the catheter may later become dislodged with movement. Despite these potential difficulties, epidural anesthesia presents less risk for the obese woman than does general anesthesia (American Society of Anesthesiologists Task Force, 2016).

After the epidural has been initiated, the woman is positioned preferably on her side; this is done so that the uterus does not compress the ascending vena cava and descending aorta, which can impair venous return, reduce cardiac output and blood pressure, and decrease placental perfusion. Her position should be alternated from side to side every hour. Upright positions and ambulation may be possible depending on the degree of motor impairment. Oxygen should be available if hypotension occurs despite maintenance of hydration with IV intravenous fluid and displacement of the uterus to the side. Ephedrine or phenylephrine (vasopressors used to increase maternal blood pressure) and increased IV fluid infusion may be needed (see Emergency box: Maternal Hypotension With Decreased Placental Perfusion). The FHR and pattern, contraction pattern, and progress in labor must be monitored carefully because the woman may not be aware of changes in the strength of the uterine contractions or the descent of the presenting part.

Several methods can be used for an epidural block. The most common method is the continuous infusion epidural (CIE), achieved by using a pump to infuse the anesthetic solution through an indwelling plastic catheter. Some providers prefer to use CIE with opioids because it decreases the motor block, allowing the laboring woman more mobility in bed. Patient-controlled epidural analgesia (PCEA) is another method; it uses an indwelling catheter and a programmed pump that allows the woman to control the dosing. PCEA has been found to provide optimal analgesia with higher maternal satisfaction and enhanced sense of control during labor while decreasing the total amount of medication, including local anesthetic, used (American Society of Anesthesiologists Task Force, 2016).

There are several advantages of an epidural block in laboring women:
- The most effective form of pain relief is provided.
- Good relaxation is achieved.
- Airway reflexes remain intact.
- Only partial motor paralysis develops.

Fetal complications are rare but may occur in the event of rapid absorption of the medication or marked maternal hypotension. The dose, volume, type, and number of medications used can be modified to (1) allow the woman to push, to assume upright positions, and even to walk; (2) produce perineal anesthesia; and (3) permit forceps-assisted, vacuum-assisted, or cesarean birth if required.

There are also a number of disadvantages of epidural block. The woman's ability to move freely and to maintain control of her labor is limited, related to the use of numerous medical interventions (e.g., an IV infusion and electronic monitoring) and the occurrence of orthostatic hypotension and dizziness, sedation, and weakness of the legs. CNS effects (see Box 17.5) can occur if a solution containing a local anesthetic agent is accidentally injected into a blood vessel or if excessive amounts of local anesthetic are given. High spinal or "total spinal" anesthesia, resulting in respiratory arrest, can occur if the relatively high dosage used with an epidural block is accidentally injected into the subarachnoid space. Women who receive an epidural have a higher rate of fever (i.e., intrapartum temperature of 38°C [100.4°F] or higher), especially when labor lasts longer than 12 hours; the temperature elevation most likely is related to thermoregulatory changes, although infection cannot be ruled out. The elevation in temperature can result in fetal tachycardia and the need for neonatal workup for sepsis, whether or not signs of infection are present (see Box 17.5).

Hypotension as a result of sympathetic blockade can occur in about 5% to 30% of women who receive regional (spinal or epidural) analgesia during labor (Witcher & Scott, 2019) (see Emergency box: Maternal Hypotension With Decreased Placental Perfusion). Hypotension can result in a significant decrease in uteroplacental perfusion and oxygen delivery to the fetus. Urinary retention and stress incontinence can occur in the immediate postpartum period. This temporary difficulty in urinary elimination could be related not only to the effects of the epidural block and the need for catheterization but also to the increased duration of labor and need for forceps- or vacuum-assisted birth associated with the block. Pruritus (itching) is a side effect that often occurs with the use of an opioid, especially fentanyl. A relationship between epidural analgesia and increased use of oxytocin and forceps- or vacuum-assisted birth has been documented (Cunningham et al., 2018; Hawkins & Bucklin, 2017). Epidural analgesia does not, however, increase the risk for cesarean birth (Cunningham et al.; Hawkins & Bucklin). For some women, the epidural block is not effective and a second form of analgesia is required to establish effective pain relief. When women progress rapidly in labor, pain relief may not be obtained before birth occurs.

Combined spinal-epidural analgesia. In the combined spinal-epidural (CSE) analgesia technique, sometimes referred to as a *walking epidural,* an epidural needle is inserted into the epidural space. Before the epidural catheter is placed, a smaller-gauge spinal needle is inserted through the bore of the epidural needle into the subarachnoid space. A small amount of opioid or combination of opioid and local anesthetic is then injected intrathecally to rapidly provide analgesia. Afterward the epidural catheter is inserted as usual. The CSE technique is an increasingly popular approach that can be used to block pain transmission without compromising motor function. The concentration of opioid receptors is high along the pain pathway in the spinal cord, brain stem, and thalamus. Because these receptors are highly sensitive to opioids, a small quantity of an opioid agonist analgesic produces marked pain relief lasting for several hours. If additional pain relief is needed, medication can be injected through the epidural catheter (see Fig. 17.10A). The most common side effects of opioids administered intrathecally are pruritus and nausea, which are usually mild and easily treated (Hawkins & Bucklin, 2017). CSE analgesia is also associated with a greater incidence of FHR abnormalities than is epidural analgesia alone, necessitating close assessment of FHR and pattern (Cunningham et al., 2018).

Although women can walk (hence the term *walking epidural*), they often choose not to do so because of sedation, fatigue, abnormal sensations in and weakness of the legs, and a feeling of insecurity. Often health care professionals are reluctant to encourage or assist women to ambulate for fear of injury. However, women can be helped to change position and use an upright position during labor and birth.

Epidural and intrathecal (spinal) opioids. Opioids can also be used alone, entirely eliminating the need for a local anesthetic. The use of epidural or intrathecal opioids without the addition of a local anesthetic agent during labor has several advantages. Opioids administered in this manner do not cause maternal hypotension or affect vital signs. The woman feels contractions but not pain. Her ability to bear down during the second stage of labor is preserved because the pushing reflex is not lost and her motor power remains intact.

Fentanyl, sufentanil, or preservative-free morphine can be used. Fentanyl and sufentanil produce short-acting analgesia while morphine can provide pain relief for a longer period of time (Cunningham et al., 2018). Using short-acting opioids with multiparous women and morphine with nulliparous women or women with a history of long labors is appropriate. Because opioids alone usually do not provide adequate analgesia, however, they are most often given in combination with a local anesthetic.

A more common indication for the administration of epidural or intrathecal analgesics is the relief of postoperative pain. For example, a woman who gives birth by cesarean can receive fentanyl or morphine through a catheter. The catheter can then be removed, and the woman is usually free from pain for 24 hours. Occasionally the catheter is left in place in the epidural space in case another dose is needed.

Women receiving epidurally administered morphine after a cesarean birth can ambulate sooner than women who do not. The early ambulation and freedom from pain also facilitate bladder emptying; they also enhance peristalsis and prevent clot formation (e.g., thrombophlebitis) in the lower extremities. Women may require additional medication for breakthrough pain during the first 24 hours after surgery. If so, they will usually be given an nonsteroidal antiinflammatory drug (NSAID) such as ketorolac (Toradol), indomethacin (Indocin), or ibuprofen (Motrin) rather than an opioid.

Side effects of opioids administered by the epidural and intrathecal routes include nausea, vomiting, diminished peristalsis, pruritus, urinary retention, and delayed respiratory depression. These effects are more common when morphine is administered. Antiemetics, antipruritics, and opioid antagonists are used to relieve these symptoms. For example, naloxone or metoclopramide may be administered. Hospital protocols or detailed health care provider orders should provide specific instructions for the treatment of these side effects. Use of epidural opioids is not without risk. Respiratory depression is a serious concern; for this reason the woman's respiratory status should be assessed and documented every hour for 24 hours or as designated by hospital protocol.

> **! NURSING ALERT**
>
> Naloxone should be readily available for use if the respiratory rate decreases to less than 12 breaths/min or if the oxygen saturation rate decreases to less than 89%. Administration of oxygen by nonrebreather face mask can also be initiated, and the anesthesia care provider should be notified.

Contraindications to subarachnoid (spinal) and epidural blocks. Contraindications to spinal and epidural analgesia (Burke, 2014; Cunningham et al., 2018; Hawkins & Bucklin, 2017) include the following:

- Active or anticipated serious maternal hemorrhage. Acute hypovolemia leads to increased sympathetic tone to maintain the blood pressure. Any anesthetic technique that blocks the sympathetic fibers can produce significant hypotension that can endanger the mother and fetus.

EVIDENCE-BASED PRACTICE

Nitrous Oxide: Laughing Gas for Labor

Ask the Question
Is nitrous oxide a safe and effective form of pain relief that can be recommended for laboring women?

Search for the Evidence
Search Strategies English language research-based publications since 2011 on nitrous oxide, laughing gas, labor pain relief were included.

Databases Used Cochrane Collaborative Database, National Guideline Clearinghouse (AHRQ), CINAHL, PubMed, UpToDate, and the professional websites for ACOG and AWHONN.

Critical Appraisal of the Evidence
Nitrous oxide is a patient-controlled analgesia/anesthesia used for pain relief since the 1880s. It has been commonly used for labor analgesia in Canada and the United Kingdom for decades. It is delivered via mask, which the laboring woman holds to her face during contractions. Its recent introduction into practice in the United States is limited by the supply of equipment to blend the mixture of 50/50 nitrous oxide and oxygen (Likis, Andrews, Collins, et al., 2014).

- Nitrous oxide increases endorphin and dopamine levels, diminishing pain and anxiety.
- Systematic analyses comparing epidural to nitrous oxide have not shown a difference between the Apgar scores or special care admission rates between the two groups (Likis et al., 2014). Further research is needed for long-term effects.
- When compared with nitrous oxide, epidurals were associated with more hypotension, fever, motor blockade, urinary retention, and instrumental and cesarean births for fetal distress, although there was no difference in cesarean rates overall (Anim-Somuah, Smyth, Cyna, & Cuthbert, 2018).

- Although nitrous oxide does not relieve pain as well as an epidural, it does provide other benefits: it is inexpensive, less invasive than epidural, requires less intensive monitoring, and does not limit mobility (Likis et al., 2014).
- The most common side effects of nitrous oxide are nausea, vomiting, dizziness, and drowsiness (Likis et al., 2014).

Apply the Evidence: Nursing Implications
1. Some women will want the maximum pain relief of epidurals, while others may be willing to trade that for the benefits of sense of control, mobility, and limited monitoring of nitrous oxide (Anim-Somuahet al., 2018).
2. Because nitrous has a rapid onset and clearance, it can be an excellent choice for women who want to wait for an epidural, whose epidural is not effective, or who come in too late for an epidural (Likis et al., 2014).
3. Nitrous oxide has a rapid onset (Likis et al., 2014). Women can start with nitrous oxide and easily move to another pain relief method, as needed.
4. Health care providers are exposed to ambient gas vapors in close settings. The effects of this are unknown. Appropriate ventilation greatly diminishes this exposure (Likis et al., 2014).
5. Because nitrous oxide produces euphoria and dissociation with pain, future research on women's satisfaction with the method may be a better measure than "pain relief" (Likis et al., 2014).

References
Anim-Somuah, M., Smyth, R., Cyna, A. M., & Cuthbert, A. (2018). Epidural versus non-epidural or no analgesia for pain management in labour. *Cochrane Database of Systematic Reviews* (5), CD000331.

Likis, F. E., Andrews, J. C., Collins, M. R., et al. (2014). Nitrous oxide for the management of labor pain: A systematic review. *Anesthesia & Analgesia, 118*(1), 153–168.

Jennifer Taylor Alderman

- Maternal hypotension.
- Coagulopathy. If a woman is receiving anticoagulant therapy (e.g., last dose of low-molecular-weight heparin within 12 hours) or has a bleeding disorder, injury to a blood vessel may cause the formation of a hematoma that may compress the cauda equina or the spinal cord and lead to serious CNS complications.
- Infection at the needle insertion site. Infection can be spread through the peridural or subarachnoid spaces if the needle traverses an infected area.
- Increased intracranial pressure caused by a mass lesion.
- Allergy to the anesthetic drug.
- Maternal refusal or inability to cooperate.
- Some types of maternal cardiac conditions.

Effects of epidural block on the newborn. Analgesia or anesthesia during labor and birth has little or no lasting effect on the physiologic status of the newborn. There is no evidence that the administration of maternal analgesic or anesthetic agents during labor and birth has a significant effect on the child's later mental or neurologic development (AAP & ACOG, 2017).

Nitrous Oxide for Analgesia

Nitrous oxide, commonly called *laughing gas,* is an inhaled anesthetic gas. It was used more widely for labor analgesia in the United States in the past but never as extensively as in other countries. Recently, however, interest in using nitrous oxide during labor has increased in the United States. See the Evidence-Based Practice box: Nitrous Oxide: Laughing Gas for Labor.

Nitrous oxide is administered in a 50:50 mix with oxygen using a blender device and a mask held by the woman (Fig. 17.13). Women report that nitrous oxide does not completely relieve pain but reduces their perception of pain. It causes a feeling of euphoria and decreases anxiety.

The main side effects of nitrous oxide are nausea and dizziness. Nitrous oxide is safe for both mother and fetus and does not affect uterine activity. Other advantages of nitrous oxide use include rapid onset of action, quick clearance through exhalation without accumulation in maternal or fetal tissues, and the fact that the woman can self-administer the gas while remaining awake, alert, and completely able to function. Nitrous oxide can also be used during short, painful intrapartum procedures such as perineal repair and manual removal of the placenta (Collins, 2017; Hawkins & Bucklin, 2017).

A face mask is used to self-administer the gas. The woman places the mask over her mouth and nose as soon as a contraction begins. The nurse teaches the woman how to position the face mask correctly to create a seal. When the woman inhales, a valve opens and the gas is released. When inhalation stops, the valve closes, which prevents accidental overdosing. The woman is the *only* person allowed to hold the mask. Special equipment collects the woman's exhalations to protect health care workers from repetitive occupational exposure to nitrous oxide (AAP & ACOG, 2017; Collins, 2017; Hawkins & Bucklin, 2017).

General Anesthesia

General anesthesia is rarely used for uncomplicated vaginal births. It is used for only about 10% of cesarean births in the United States (Hawkins & Bucklin, 2017). General anesthesia may be necessary if a spinal or epidural block is contraindicated or if circumstances necessitate rapid birth (vaginal or emergent cesarean) without sufficient time or available personnel to perform a regional block (AAP & ACOG, 2017; Witcher & Scott, 2019). In addition, being awake and aware during major surgery may be unacceptable to some women having a cesarean birth. The major risks associated with

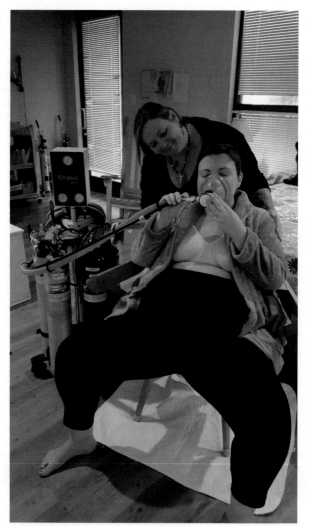

Fig. 17.13 Use of Nitrous Oxide in a Birthing Center. (Courtesy Women's Birth & Wellness Center, Chapel Hill, NC.)

general anesthesia are difficulty with or inability to intubate and aspiration of gastric contents (Cunningham et al., 2018; Hawkins & Bucklin, 2017). Anesthesia care providers are more likely to encounter difficulty with intubating obese patients, especially in an emergency situation, than women of normal weight (Hawkins & Bucklin; Witcher & Scott).

If general anesthesia is being considered, an IV infusion is started using an 18-gauge catheter, and the woman is given nothing by mouth. If time allows, the woman is premedicated with a nonparticulate (clear) oral antacid (e.g., sodium citrate/citric acid [Bicitra]) to neutralize the acidic contents of the stomach. Aspiration of highly acidic gastric contents will damage lung tissue. Some anesthesia care providers also order the administration of a histamine (H_2)-receptor blocker such as famotidine (Pepcid) or ranitidine (Zantac) to decrease the production of gastric acid and metoclopramide (Reglan) to accelerate gastric emptying (American Society of Anesthesiologists, 2016; Cunningham et al., 2018; Hawkins & Bucklin, 2017). Before the anesthesia is given, a wedge should be placed under one of the woman's hips to displace the uterus. Uterine displacement prevents compression of the aorta and vena cava, which maintains cardiac output and placental perfusion (Cunningham et al.; Hawkins & Bucklin).

Prior to anesthesia induction, the woman is preoxygenated with 100% oxygen by nonrebreather face mask for 2 to 3 minutes. This is especially important in pregnant women, who are more likely than other adults to rapidly become hypoxemic if there is a delay in successful intubation. Next, propofol (Diprivan), etomidate (Amidate), or ketamine (Ketalar) is administered intravenously to induce anesthesia by rendering the woman unconscious. After that, succinylcholine (Anectine), a muscle relaxer, is administered to facilitate passage of an endotracheal tube (Cunningham et al., 2018; Hawkins & Bucklin, 2017). Sometimes the nurse is asked to assist by applying cricoid pressure before intubation as the woman begins to lose consciousness. This maneuver blocks the esophagus and prevents aspiration should the woman vomit or regurgitate (Fig. 17.14). Pressure is released once the endotracheal tube is securely in place.

After the woman is intubated, nitrous oxide and oxygen in a 50:50 mixture are administered. A low concentration of a volatile halogenated agent (e.g., desflurane or sevoflurane) also may be administered to provide amnesia. These inhalational anesthetic agents, most commonly used in the United States, produce a faster onset of action than more traditional gases, such as isofluane (Cunningham et al., 2018). In low concentrations, inhalational anesthetics do not relax the uterus, so bleeding should not increase because of their use (Hawkins & Bucklin, 2017). In higher concentrations, desflurane, sevoflurane, isoflurane or methoxyflurane relax the uterus quickly and facilitate intrauterine manipulation, version, and extraction. However, at higher concentrations, these agents cross the placenta readily and can produce narcosis in the fetus and could reduce uterine tone after birth, increasing the risk for hemorrhage. Because of the risk for neonatal narcosis, it is critical that the baby is delivered as soon as possible after inducing anesthesia to reduce the degree of fetal exposure to the anesthetic agents and the CNS depressants administered to the mother (Cunningham et al.; Hawkins & Bucklin).

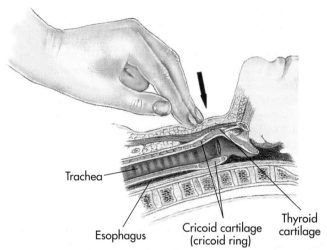

Fig. 17.14 Technique of Applying Pressure on the Cricoid Cartilage to Occlude the Esophagus and Prevent Aspiration of Gastric Contents During Induction of General Anesthesia.

Priorities for postanesthesia care are to maintain an open airway and cardiopulmonary function and to prevent postpartum hemorrhage. Women who had surgery under general anesthesia will require pain medication soon after regaining consciousness. Routine postpartum care is organized to facilitate parent-infant attachment as soon as possible and to answer the mother's questions. When appropriate, the nurse assesses the mother's readiness to see her baby as well as her response to the anesthesia and to the event that necessitated general anesthesia (e.g., emergency cesarean birth when vaginal birth was anticipated). (See Chapter 32 for more information regarding cesarean birth.)

◎ NURSING CARE PLAN

Nonpharmacologic Pain Management

Client Problem	Expected Outcome	Interventions	Rationales
Lack of knowledge about pain management during labor and birth	The client will participate in planning care for labor	Assess the client's birth plan and knowledge about the birth process	To identify gaps in knowledge as a basis for client teaching
		Provide information about the process of labor and birth	To correct any misconceptions
		Teach different methods to manage pain from contractions	To provide more options for coping strategies
Pain related to labor	The client will express a decrease in labor pain	Assess maternal vital signs, fetal heart rate, contraction pattern, loss of amniotic fluid, vaginal bleeding, and location and type of pain	To determine labor progress
		Review the birth plan created by the client and her support person	To plan supportive strategies that address specific needs
		Teach the woman and support person different positions and the use of pillows	To reduce stiffness, aid circulation, and promote comfort
Decreased ability to cope	The client will demonstrate increased ability to cope with the contractions	Assess client behaviors/actions during contractions	To determine if strategies other than those she is currently using might better help her cope with contractions
		Demonstrate focusing, relaxation and breathing techniques, effleurage, and sacral pressure (if client complains of back pain)	To enhance chances of success in using these techniques
		Teach the support person how to assist the laboring woman	To provide continuous support and increase the likelihood of a positive response to comfort measures

CARE MANAGEMENT

Pain Assessment During Labor and Birth

A pain scale, where 0 represents no pain and 10 represents pain as bad as it could possibly be, is often used to evaluate a woman's pain before and after pain relief interventions are implemented. By comparing the woman's answers, the effectiveness of pain-relief interventions can be evaluated objectively. Sometimes a coping scale rather than a pain scale is used to evaluate how well the woman is dealing with the discomfort of labor (Simkin et al., 2017).

The choice of pain-relief interventions depends on a combination of factors, including the woman's special needs and wishes, the availability of the desired method or methods, the knowledge and expertise in nonpharmacologic and pharmacologic methods of the health care team involved in the woman's care, and the stage and phase of labor.

Nonpharmacologic Interventions

The nurse supports and assists the woman as she uses nonpharmacologic interventions for pain relief and relaxation. During labor, the nurse evaluates the effectiveness of the specific pain management techniques used. Appropriate interventions can then be planned or continued for effective care, such as trying other nonpharmacologic methods or combining nonpharmacologic methods with medications (see Nursing Care Plan: Nonpharmacologic Pain Management).

Pharmacologic Interventions

Informed Consent

Pregnant women have the right to be active participants in determining the best pain-management approach to use during labor and birth. The obstetric care provider and anesthesia care provider are responsible for fully informing women of the alternative methods of pharmacologic pain relief available in the birth setting. A description of the various anesthetic techniques and what they entail is essential to informed consent, even if the woman received information about analgesia and anesthesia earlier in her pregnancy. The initial discussion of pain-management options ideally should take place in the third trimester, so that the woman has time to consider alternatives. Nurses play a part in obtaining informed consent by clarifying and describing procedures or by acting as the woman's advocate and asking the obstetric or anesthesia health care providers for further explanations. The three essential components of an informed consent are as follows:

- First, the procedure and its advantages and disadvantages must be thoroughly explained in a manner the woman can understand.
- Second, the woman must agree with the plan of pain management as explained to her.
- Third, her consent must be given freely without coercion or manipulation from her health care provider.

(ACOG, 2009/2015)

Timing of Administration

Nonpharmacologic measures can be used to relieve pain and stress and enhance progress at any time during labor. Timing for implementing is determined by the nurse's assessment and the woman's willingness to try the suggested measure.

It is often the nurse who notifies the obstetric health care provider that the woman is in need of pharmacologic measures to relieve her pain and discomfort. Orders are often written for the administration of pain medication as needed by the woman and based on the nurse's clinical judgment. In the past, pharmacologic measures for pain

---

> **LEGAL TIP**
>
> **Informed Consent for Anesthesia**
>
> The woman receives (in an understandable language and manner) the following:
> - Explanation of available methods of anesthesia and analgesia
> - Description of the anesthetic, including its effects and the procedure for its administration
> - Description of the benefits, discomforts, risks, and consequences for the mother, the fetus, and the newborn
> - Explanation of how complications can be treated
> - Information that the anesthetic is not always effective
> - Indication that the woman may withdraw consent at any time
> - Opportunity to have any questions answered
> - Opportunity to have components of the consent explained in the woman's own words
>
> The consent form will:
> - Be written or explained in the woman's primary language
> - Have the woman's signature
> - Have the date of consent
> - Carry the signature of the anesthetic care provider, certifying that the woman has received and expresses understanding of the explanation

---

> **! NURSING ALERT**
>
> In some cultures, a husband is expected to consent to procedures performed on his wife. Although in the United States the woman is the person who gives consent and signs any necessary forms, she may not be willing to do so unless her husband or partner also approves.

---

relief, particularly epidural anesthesia, were usually not implemented until cervical dilation reached approximately 4 to 5 cm so as to avoid suppressing the progress of labor. However, it is now known that epidural anesthesia in early labor does not increase the rate of cesarean birth. Whereas it may shorten the duration of first-stage labor in some women, epidural anesthesia lengthens it in others (Hawkins & Bucklin, 2017). It is no longer recommended that women in labor reach a certain level of cervical dilation or fetal station before receiving epidural anesthesia (AAP & ACOG, 2017; American Society of Anesthesiologists Task Force, 2016; Cunningham et al., 2018).

Preparation for Procedures

The methods of pain relief available to the woman are reviewed and information is clarified as necessary. The procedure and what will be expected of the woman (e.g., to maintain a flexed position during insertion of the epidural needle) must be explained.

The woman can also benefit from knowing the method through which the medication is to be given, the interval before the medication takes effect, and the expected pain relief from the medication. Skin-preparation measures are described, and an explanation is given for the need to empty the bladder before the analgesic or anesthetic is administered and the reason for keeping the bladder empty. When an indwelling catheter is to be threaded into the epidural space, the woman should be told that she may have a momentary twinge down her leg, hip, or back and that this feeling is not a sign of injury.

Administration of Medication

Accurate monitoring of the progress of labor forms the basis for the nurse's judgment that a woman needs pharmacologic control of her pain. Knowledge of the medications used during childbirth is essential. The most effective route of administration is selected for each woman; then the medication is prepared and administered.

Any medication can cause a minor or severe allergic reaction. As part of the assessment for such allergic reactions, the nurse should monitor the woman's vital signs, respiratory effort, cardiovascular status, integument, and platelet and white blood cell counts. The woman is observed for side effects of drug therapy, especially drowsiness and dyspnea. Minor reactions can consist of rash, rhinitis, fever, shortness of breath, or pruritus. Management of the less acute allergic response is not an emergency.

Severe allergic reactions (anaphylaxis) may occur suddenly and lead to shock or death. The most dramatic form of anaphylaxis is sudden severe bronchospasm, upper airway obstruction, and hypotension (Brasted & Ruppel, 2016). Signs of anaphylaxis are largely caused by contraction of smooth muscles and may begin with irritability, extreme weakness, nausea, and vomiting. This may lead to dyspnea, cyanosis, convulsions, and cardiac arrest. Anaphylaxis must be diagnosed and treated immediately. Initial treatment usually consists of placing the woman in a supine position, injecting epinephrine intramuscularly, administering fluid intravenously, supporting the airway with ventilation if necessary, and giving oxygen. If the response to these measures is inadequate, IV epinephrine should be given (Brasted & Ruppel). Cardiopulmonary resuscitation may be necessary (see Chapter 30).

Intravenous route. The preferred route of administration of medications such as meperidine, fentanyl, remifentanil, or nalbuphine is through IV tubing, administered into the port nearest the point of insertion of the infusion (proximal port). The medication is given slowly, in small amounts, during a contraction. It may be given over a period of three to five consecutive contractions if needed to complete the dose. It is given during contractions to decrease fetal exposure to the medication because uterine blood vessels are constricted during contractions and the medication stays within the maternal vascular system for several seconds before the uterine blood vessels reopen. The IV infusion is then restarted slowly to prevent a bolus of medication from being administered. With this method of injection, the amount of medication crossing the placenta to the fetus is minimized. With decreased placental transfer, the mother's degree of pain relief is maximized. The IV route has the following advantages:

- Onset of pain relief is rapid and more predictable.
- Pain relief is obtained with small doses of the drug.
- Duration of effect is more predictable.

Intramuscular route. Although analgesics are still sometimes given intramuscularly, it is not the preferred route of administration for the woman in labor. The advantages of using the IM route are quick administration and no need to start an IV line.

Disadvantages of the IM route include the following:

- Onset of pain relief is delayed.
- Higher doses of medication are required.
- Medication is released at an unpredictable rate from the muscle tissue and is available for transfer across the placenta to the fetus.

The maternal medication levels (after IM injections) are unequal because of uneven distribution (maternal uptake) and metabolism. If neuraxial anesthesia is planned later in labor, the deltoid muscle is the preferred site. The autonomic blockade from the neuraxial anesthesia increases blood flow to the gluteal region and accelerates absorption of medication that may be sequestered there. Administration of opioids subcutaneously in the upper arm avoids this risk and, as a result, is often used as an alternative to IM injection.

Regional (epidural or spinal) anesthesia. According to professional standards (Association of Women's Health, Obstetric and Neonatal Nurses [AWHONN], 2015):

The nonanesthetist registered nurse is permitted to do the following:

- Monitor the status of the woman receiving regional anesthesia, the fetus, and the progress of labor

- Replace empty infusion syringes or bags with the same medication and concentration
- Stop the infusion if there is a safety concern or the woman has given birth
- Remove the catheter if properly educated to do so
- Initiate emergency measures if the need arises
- Communicate clinical assessments and changes in client status to obstetric and anesthesia care providers

Only qualified, licensed anesthesia care providers should perform the following procedures:

- Insertion, initial injection, bolus injection, additional bolus injection, or initiation of a continuous infusion of catheters for analgesia and anesthesia
- Preparation and programming the medication and infusion devices
- Verification of correct catheter placement
- Increasing or decreasing the rate of a continuous infusion and program doses for PCEA administration

> ### ⚡ SAFETY ALERT
>
> Safe regional or neuraxial anesthesia administration requires specialized education, experience, and competence. A potential for significant maternal and/or fetal morbidity and mortality is associated with some obstetric anesthesia complications. Therefore a licensed, credentialed anesthesia care provider should manage neuraxial anesthesia and analgesia during labor and birth and be readily available to manage obstetric anesthesia–related emergencies (AWHONN, 2015).

Because spinal nerve blocks can reduce bladder sensation, resulting in difficulty voiding, the woman should empty her bladder before the induction of the block and should be encouraged to void at least every 2 hours thereafter. The nurse should palpate for bladder distention and measure urinary output to ensure that the bladder is being completely emptied. A distended bladder can inhibit uterine contractions and fetal descent, resulting in a slowing of the progress of labor. For this reason, an indwelling urinary (Foley) catheter is often routinely inserted immediately after epidural or spinal anesthesia is initiated and left in place for the remainder of the first stage of labor.

The status of the maternal-fetal unit and the progress of labor must be established before the block is initiated. The nurse must assist the woman to assume and maintain the correct position for induction of epidural and spinal anesthesia (see Figs. 17.11A and B).

Depending on the level of motor blockade, the woman should be assisted to remain as mobile as possible. When in bed, her position should be alternated from side to side every hour to ensure adequate distribution of the anesthetic solution and to maintain circulation to the uterus and placenta.

> ### ⚡ SAFETY ALERT
>
> After receiving a neuraxial block or opioid intravenously for pain, the woman should not be allowed to ambulate alone. She must either remain in bed or request assistance before attempting to get out of bed. The nurse must assess the woman for signs of orthostatic hypotension and return of sensation and motor function of the lower extremities prior to ambulation.

There is conflicting information regarding whether epidurals increase the length of labor (Wong, 2017). However, health care providers should be aware that effective epidural anesthesia may prolong the second stage of labor by 30 minutes (Antonakou & Papoutsis, 2016). A delay in the second stage of labor does not negatively affect

---

BOX 17.6   Nursing Interventions for the Woman Receiving Neuraxial Anesthesia

Prior to the Block
- Assist obstetric care provider and/or anesthesia care provider with explaining the procedure and obtaining the woman's informed consent.
- Assess maternal vital signs, level of hydration, labor progress, and fetal heart rate (FHR) and pattern.
- Start an intravenous (IV) line, and infuse a bolus of fluid (lactated Ringers solution or normal saline) if ordered (e.g., 500-1000 mL 15-30 min before induction of the anesthesia).
- Obtain laboratory results (hematocrit or hemoglobin level, other tests as ordered).
- Assess the woman's level of pain using a pain scale (from 0 [no pain] to 10 [pain as bad as it could possibly be]).
- Assist the woman to void.

During Initiation of the Block
- Assist the woman to assume and maintain the proper position.
- Verbally guide the woman through the procedure, explaining sounds and sensations as she experiences them.
- Assist the anesthesia care provider with documentation of vital signs, time and amount of medications given, etc.
- Monitor maternal vital signs (especially blood pressure) and FHR as ordered.
- Have oxygen and suction readily available.
- Monitor for signs of local anesthetic toxicity (see Box 17.5) as the test dose of medication is administered.

While the Block Is in Effect
- Continue to monitor maternal vital signs and FHR as ordered (continuous monitoring of maternal heart rate [electrocardiogram] and blood pressure may be ordered to monitor for accidental IV injection of medication).

- Continue to assess the woman's level of pain with every check of vital signs using a pain scale (from 0 [no pain] to 10 [pain as bad as it could possibly be]).
- Monitor for bladder distention:
  - Assist with spontaneous voiding on bedpan or toilet.
  - Insert a urinary catheter if necessary.
- Encourage or assist the woman to change positions from side to side every hour.
- Promote safety:
  - Keep the side rails up on the bed.
  - Place the telephone and call light within easy reach.
  - Instruct the woman not to get out of bed without help.
  - Make sure there is no prolonged pressure on anesthetized body parts.
- Keep the insertion site for the epidural catheter clean and dry.
- Continue to monitor for anesthetic side effects (see Box 17.5).

While the Block Is Wearing Off After Birth
- Assess regularly for the return of sensory and motor function.
- Continue to monitor maternal vital signs as ordered.
- Monitor for bladder distention:
  - Assist with spontaneous voiding on bedpan or toilet.
  - Insert a urinary catheter if necessary.
- Promote safety:
  - Keep the side rails up on the bed.
  - Place the telephone and call light within easy reach.
  - Instruct the woman not to get out of bed without help.
  - Make sure there is no prolonged pressure on anesthetized body parts.
- Keep the epidural catheter insertion site clean and dry.
- Continue to monitor for anesthetic side effects (see Box 17.5).

---

maternal or fetal outcome as long as the FHR tracing is normal, maternal hydration and analgesia are adequate, and there is ongoing progress in the descent of the fetal head. Therefore operative interventions (e.g., the use of forceps or vacuum) to hasten the birth solely because the second stage is prolonged are unnecessary. Reducing the density of the epidural block during the second stage of labor, delaying pushing until the woman feels the urge to do so, and avoiding arbitrary definitions for the "normal" duration of second-stage labor are suggested as interventions to decrease the risk for operative vaginal birth (Hawkins & Bucklin, 2017) (see Chapter 19 for a full discussion of second-stage labor management). Box 17.6 summarizes the nursing interventions for women receiving neuraxial (epidural or spinal) anesthesia.

Nursing Care

The nurse monitors and records the woman's response to nonpharmacologic pain relief methods and to medications. This includes the degree of pain relief, the level of apprehension, the return of sensations and perception of pain, and allergic or adverse reactions (e.g., hypotension, respiratory depression, fever, pruritus, and nausea and

vomiting). The nurse continues to monitor maternal vital signs, FHR, the strength and frequency of uterine contractions, changes in the cervix and station of the presenting part, the presence and quality of the bearing-down reflex, bladder filling, and state of hydration. Determining the fetal response after administration of analgesia or anesthesia is vital. The woman is asked if she, her partner, or other support people have any questions. The nurse also assesses the woman's and her support people's understanding of the need for ensuring her safety (e.g., making sure the call light and phone are within easy reach, calling for assistance as needed, keeping side rails up, monitoring the temperature of tub water, ambulating after analgesia or anesthesia).

The time that elapses between the administration of an opioid and the baby's birth is documented. Medications given to the newborn to reverse opioid effects are recorded. After birth, the woman who has had spinal, epidural, or general anesthesia is assessed for return of sensory and motor function in addition to the usual postpartum assessments. Both the nurse and the anesthesia care provider are responsible for documenting assessments and care in relation to neuraxial (epidural or spinal) anesthesia.

▎ KEY POINTS

- Nonpharmacologic pain and stress-management strategies are valuable for managing labor discomfort alone or in combination with pharmacologic methods.
- The gate-control theory of pain and the stress response are the bases for many of the nonpharmacologic methods of pain relief.

- The type of analgesic or anesthetic to be used is determined by maternal and health care provider preference, the stage of labor, and the method of birth.
- Sedatives may be appropriate for women in prolonged early labor when there is a need to decrease anxiety or promote sleep or therapeutic rest.

- Naloxone (Narcan) is an opioid (narcotic) antagonist that can, in most cases, reverse narcotic effects, especially respiratory depression.
- Pharmacologic control of pain during labor requires collaboration among the health care providers and the laboring woman.
- The nurse must understand medications, their expected effects, potential side effects, and methods of administration.
- Maintenance of maternal fluid balance is essential during spinal and epidural nerve blocks.
- Maternal analgesia or anesthesia potentially affects neonatal neurobehavioral response.

- The use of opioid agonist-antagonist analgesics in women with preexisting opioid dependence may cause symptoms of abstinence syndrome (opioid withdrawal).
- Epidural anesthesia and analgesia is the most effective available pharmacologic pain relief method for labor. It is used by the majority of women in the United States.
- General anesthesia is rarely used for vaginal birth but may be used for cesarean birth or whenever rapid anesthesia is needed in an emergency childbirth situation.

REFERENCES

Afshar, Y., Wang, E., Mei, J., et al. (2017). Childbirth education class and birth plans are associated with a vaginal delivery. *Birth, 44*(1), 29–34.

American Academy of Pediatrics & American College of Obstetricians and Gynecologists. (2017). *Guidelines for perinatal care* (8th ed.). Washington, DC: American College of Obstetricians and Gynecologists.

American College of Nurse-Midwives. (2016). Providing oral nutrition to women in labor. *Journal of Midwifery & Women's Health, 61*(4), 528–534.

American College of Obstetricians and Gynecologists. (2009, reaffirmed 2015). Committee opinion no. 439: Informed consent. *Obstetrics & Gynecology, 114*(2 Part 1), 401–408.

American College of Obstetricians and Gynecologists. (2016). Committee opinion no. 679: Immersion in water during labor and delivery. *Obstetrics & Gynecology, 128*(5), e231–e236.

American College of Obstetricians and Gynecologists. (2019). Practice bulletin no. 209: Obstetric analgesia and anesthesia. *Obstetrics & Gynecology, 133*(3), e208–e225.

American Society of Anesthesiologists Task Force on Obstetric Anesthesia & Society for Obstetric Anesthesia and Perinatology. (2016). Practice guidelines for obstetric anesthesia: An updated report. *Anesthesiology, 124*(2), 270–300.

Anderson, D. (2011). A review of systemic opioids commonly used for labor pain relief. *Journal of Midwifery & Women's Health, 56*(3), 222–239.

Antonakou, A., & Papoutsis, D. (2016). The effect of epidural analgesia on the delivery outcome of induced labour: A retrospective case series. *Obstetrics and Gynecology International*, Article ID 5740534.

Association of Women's Health, Obstetric and Neonatal Nurses. (2015). Role of the registered nurse in the care of the pregnant woman receiving analgesia and anesthesia by catheter techniques. *Journal of Obstetric, Gynecologic & Neonatal Nursing, 44*(1), 151–154.

Bala, I., Babu, M., & Rastogi, S. (2017). Effectiveness of back massage versus ambulation during first stage of labour among primigravida mothers in terms of pain and anxiety. *International Journal of Nursing Education, 9*(3), 28–32.

Baird, S. M., Kennedy, B. B., & Dalton, J. (2017). Special considerations for individualized care of the laboring woman. In B. B. Kennedy, & S. M. Baird (Eds.), *Intrapartum management modules: A perinatal education program* (5th ed.). Philadelphia: Wolters Kluwer.

Blackburn, S. T. (2018). *Maternal, fetal, and neonatal physiology: A clinical perspective* (5th ed.). St. Louis: Elsevier.

Bovbjerg, M. L., Cheyney, M., & Everson, C. (2016). Maternal and newborn outcomes following waterbirth: The midwives alliance of North America statistics project, 2004 to 2009 cohort. *Journal of Midwifery & Women's Health, 61*(1), 11–20.

Brasted, I., & Ruppel, M. (2016). Anaphylaxis and its treatment. *Emergency Services World, 45*(9), 31–37.

Brickhouse, B., Isaacs, C., Batten, M., & Price, A. (2015). Strategies for providing low-cost water immersion therapy with limited resources. *Nursing for Women's Health, 19*(6), 526–532.

Burke, C. (2014). Pain in labor: Nonpharmacologic and pharmacologic management. In K. R. Simpson, & P. Creehan (Eds.), *AWHONN's perinatal nursing* (4th ed.). Philadelphia: Lippincott Williams & Wilkins.

Cherian, A., & Peter, L. (2016). Effectiveness of abdominal effleurage versus pharmacological intervention on labour pain among primi parturients admitted in labour room. *International Journal of Nursing Education, 8*(3), 93–98.

Collins, M. R. (2017). Pain in labor and nonpharmacologic modes of relief. In B. B. Kennedy, & S. M. Baird (Eds.), *Intrapartum management modules: A perinatal education program* (5th ed.). Philadelphia: Wolters Kluwer.

Cunningham, F., Leveno, K., Bloom, S., et al. (2018). *Williams obstetrics* (25th ed.). New York: McGraw-Hill Education.

Hawkins, J. L., & Bucklin, B. A. (2017). Obstetric anesthesia. In S. G. Gabbe, J. R. Niebyl, J. L. Simpson, et al. (Eds.), *Obstetrics: Normal and problem pregnancies* (7th ed.). Philadelphia: Elsevier.

Janula, R., & Mahipal, S. (2015). Effectiveness of aromatherapy and biofeedback in promotion of labour outcome during childbirth among primigravidas. *Health Science Journal, 9*(1:9), 1–5.

John, N., & Angeline, A. (2017). Effectiveness of music therapy on anxiety and pain among mothers during first stage of labour in selected hospitals at Kollam. *International Journal of Nursing Education, 9*(2), 24–29.

Karkal, E., Kharde, S., & Dhumale, H. (2017). Effectiveness of music therapy in reducing pain and anxiety among primigravid women during active phase of first stage of labor. *International Journal of Nursing Education, 9*(2), 57–60.

Lauderdale, J. (2016). Transcultural perspectives in childbearing. In M. M. Andrews & J. S. Boyle (Eds.), *Transcultural concepts in nursing care* (7th ed.). Philadelphia: Wolters Kluwer.

Lee, N., Kildea, S., & Stapleton, H. (2017). "No pain, no gain": The experience of women using sterile water injections. *Women and Birth, 30*, 153–158.

Lowe, N. K., Openshaw, M., & King, T. L. (2017). Labor. In M. Brucker, & T. L. King (Eds.), *Pharmacology for women's health* (2nd ed.). Burlington, MA: Jones & Bartlett.

Madden, K., Middleton, P., Cyna, A. M., et al. (2016). Hypnosis for pain management during labour and childbirth. *Cochrane Database of Systematic Reviews* (5), CD009356.

Schlaeger, J., Gabzdyl, E., Bussell, J., et al. (2017). Acupuncture and acupressure in labor. *Journal of Midwifery & Women's Health, 62*(1), 12–28.

Shaw-Battista, J. (2017). Systematic review of hydrotherapy research. *Journal of Perinatal & Neonatal Nursing, 31*(4), 303–316.

Simkin, P. (2015). *Lamaze International for parents: 10 labor tips*. Retrieved from: http://www.lamaze.org/10LaborTips.

Simkin, P., Hanson, L., & Ancheta, R. (2017). *The labor progress handbook: Early interventions to prevent and treat dystocia* (4th ed.). Hoboken, NJ: Wiley & Sons.

Simpson, K., & O'Brien-Abel, N. (2014). Labor and birth. In K. R. Simpson, & P. Creehan (Eds.), *AWHONN's perinatal nursing* (4th ed.). Philadelphia: Lippincott Williams & Wilkins.

Steel, A., Frawley, J., Adams, J., & Diezel, H. (2015). Trained or professional doulas in the support and care of pregnant and birthing women: A critical integrative review. *Health and Social Care in the Community, 23*(3), 225–241.

Swart, S. C., & Kelly, F. C. (2017). Pharmacologic management of labor pain. In B. B. Kennedy, & S. M. Baird (Eds.), *Intrapartum management modules: A perinatal education program* (5th ed.). Philadelphia: Wolters Kluwer.

Witcher, P. M., & Scott, J. C. (2019). Anesthesia emergencies in the obstetric setting. In N. H. Troiano, P. M. Witcher, & S. M. Baird (Eds.), *AWHONN's High risk and critical care obstetrics* (4th ed.). Philadelphia: Wolters Kluwer.

Wong, C. (2017). Epidural labor analgesia: Whence come our patients' misconceptions? *Journal of Clinical Anesthesia, 42*(2017), 84–85.

18

Fetal Assessment During Labor

Kitty Cashion

http://evolve.elsevier.com/Lowdermilk/MWHC/

LEARNING OBJECTIVES

- Interpret typical signs of normal and abnormal fetal heart rate (FHR) patterns.
- Compare FHR monitoring performed by intermittent auscultation with external and internal electronic methods.
- Explain the baseline FHR and evaluate periodic changes.
- Describe nursing measures that can be used to maintain FHR patterns within normal limits.

- Differentiate among the nursing interventions used for managing specific FHR patterns, including tachycardia and bradycardia, absent or minimal variability, and late and variable decelerations.
- Review the documentation of the monitoring process necessary during labor.

The ability to assess the fetus by auscultation of the fetal heart was initially described more than 300 years ago. With the advent of the fetoscope and stethoscope after the turn of the 20th century, the listener could hear clearly enough to count the fetal heart rate (FHR). When electronic FHR monitoring made its debut for clinical use in the early 1970s, the anticipation was that its use would result in less long-term neurologic impairment in the form of cerebral palsy (Miller, 2017). However, research has not been able to show that intrapartum FHR monitoring leads to a significant decrease in neonatal neurologic morbidity (Miller, Miller, & Cypher, 2017).

Still, electronic fetal monitoring (EFM) is a useful tool for visualizing FHR and uterine contraction (UC) patterns on a monitor screen or printed tracing. A majority of the women who give birth each year in the United States will have EFM during some or all of their labor (Miller et al., 2017). Pregnant women should be informed about the equipment and procedures used and the risks, benefits, and limitations of intermittent auscultation (IA) and EFM. This chapter discusses the basis for intrapartum fetal monitoring, the types of monitoring, and nursing assessment and management of abnormal FHR and UC patterns.

BASIS FOR MONITORING

Fetal Response

Because labor is a period of physiologic stress for the fetus, frequent monitoring of fetal status is part of the nursing care during labor. The fetal oxygen supply must be maintained during labor to prevent fetal compromise and promote newborn health after birth. The fetal oxygen supply can decrease in a number of ways:

- Reduction of blood flow through the maternal vessels as a result of maternal hypertension (chronic hypertension, preeclampsia, or gestational hypertension), hypotension (caused by supine maternal position, hemorrhage, or epidural anesthesia), or hypovolemia (caused by hemorrhage)

- Reduction of the oxygen content in the maternal blood as a result of hemorrhage or severe anemia
- Alterations in fetal circulation occurring with compression of the umbilical cord (transient, during UCs, or prolonged, resulting from cord prolapse), partial placental separation or complete abruption, or head compression (head compression causes increased intracranial pressure and vagal nerve stimulation with an accompanying decrease in FHR)
- Reduction in blood flow to the intervillous space in the placenta secondary to uterine hypertonus (generally caused by excessive exogenous oxytocin) or secondary to deterioration of the placental vasculature associated with maternal disorders such as hypertension or diabetes mellitus

Fetal well-being during labor can be measured by the response of the FHR to UCs. Since 2008, a group of fetal monitoring experts, including the National Institute for Child Health and Human Development (NICHD), the American College of Obstetricians and Gynecologists (ACOG), and the Society for Maternal Fetal Medicine (SMFM) have recommended that FHR tracings demonstrating certain reassuring characteristics be described as *normal* (category I) (Macones, Hankins, Spong, et al., 2008) (Box 18.1).

Uterine Activity

Likewise, uterine activity (UA) can be identified as normal or abnormal. Table 18.1 describes normal UA during labor.

Fetal Compromise

The goals of intrapartum FHR monitoring are to identify and differentiate the normal (reassuring) patterns from the abnormal (nonreassuring) patterns, which can indicate fetal compromise. Although both the 2008 NICHD workshop (Macones, et al., 2008) and ACOG (2009/2017) recommend use of the terms *normal* and *abnormal* to describe FHR tracings, the terms *reassuring* and *nonreassuring* are still frequently used clinically.

BOX 18.1 Three-Tier Fetal Heart Rate Classification System

Category I

Category I FHR tracings include all of the following:

- Baseline rate 110-160 beats/min (bpm)
- Baseline FHR variability: moderate
- Late or variable decelerations: absent
- Early decelerations: either present or absent
- Accelerations: either present or absent

Category II

Category II FHR tracings include all FHR tracings not categorized as category I or category III. Examples of category II tracings include any of the following:

- Baseline rate
  - Bradycardia not accompanied by absent baseline variability
  - Tachycardia
- Baseline FHR variability
  - Minimal baseline variability
  - Absent baseline variability not accompanied by recurrent decelerations
  - Marked baseline variability
- Accelerations
  - No acceleration produced in response to fetal stimulation
- Periodic or episodic decelerations
  - Recurrent variable decelerations accompanied by minimal or moderate baseline variability
  - Prolonged decelerations (≥2 min but <10 min)
  - Recurrent late decelerations with moderate baseline variability
  - Variable decelerations with other characteristics, such as slow return to baseline, "overshoots," or "shoulders"

Category III

Category III FHR tracings include the following:

- Absent baseline variability and any of the following:
  - Recurrent late decelerations
  - Recurrent variable decelerations
  - Bradycardia
- Sinusoidal pattern

FHR, Fetal heart rate.
Data from Macones, G., Hankins, G., Spong, C., et al. (2008). The 2008 National Institute of Child Health and Human Development workshop report on electronic fetal monitoring: Update on definitions, interpretation, and research guidelines. *Journal of Obstetric, Gynecologic & Neonatal Nursing, 37*(5), 510–515.

TABLE 18.1 Normal Uterine Activity During Labor

Characteristic	Description
Frequency	Contraction frequency overall generally ranges from two to five per 10 min during labor, with lower frequencies seen in first stage of labor and higher frequencies (up to five contractions in 10 min) seen in second stage.
Duration	Contraction duration remains fairly stable throughout first and second stages, ranging from 45 to 80 seconds, not generally exceeding 90 seconds.
Strength	Uterine contractions generally range from peaking at 40-70 mm Hg in first stage labor to over 80 mm Hg in second stage. Contractions palpated as "mild" would likely peak at less than 50 mm Hg if measured internally, whereas contractions palpated as "moderate" or "strong" would likely peak at 50 mm Hg or greater if measured internally.
Resting tone	Average resting tone during labor is 10 mm Hg; if using palpation, should palpate as "soft" (i.e., easily indented, no palpable resistance).
Relaxation time	Relaxation time is commonly 60 seconds or more in first stage and 45 seconds or more in second stage.
Montevideo units	MVUs usually range from 100 to 250 in first stage; may rise to 300-400 in second stage. Contraction intensities of 40 mm Hg or more and MVUs of 80-120 are generally sufficient to initiate spontaneous labor. MVUs are used only with internal monitoring of contractions.

Data from Macones, G. A., Hankins, G. D., Spong, C. Y., et al. (2008). The 2008 National Institute of Child Health and Human Development Workshop Report on Electronic Fetal Monitoring: Update on definitions, interpretation, and research guidelines. *Journal of Obstetric, Gynecologic & Neonatal Nursing, 37*(5), 510–515; Miller, L., Miller, D., & Cypher, R. (2017). *Mosby's pocket guide to fetal monitoring: A multidisciplinary approach* (8th ed.). St. Louis: Elsevier.

Abnormal FHR patterns are those associated with fetal **hypoxemia**, which is a deficiency of oxygen in the blood. If uncorrected, hypoxemia can deteriorate to severe fetal **hypoxia**, an inadequate supply of oxygen at the cellular level that can cause metabolic acidosis. Metabolic acidosis, in turn, can lead to **acidemia**, or increased hydrogen ion content (decreased pH) in the blood. Metabolic acidemia may be a marker of clinically significant interruption of fetal oxygenation (Miller, 2017). See Box 18.1 for examples of abnormal (category III) FHR tracings.

MONITORING TECHNIQUES

The ideal method of fetal assessment during labor, IA or EFM, continues to be debated (see Evidence-Based Practice box: Fetal Cardiac Assessment During Labor: How Are You Doing In There?). Some clinicians prefer the use of IA in low-risk women because it promotes mobility during labor, may be used with hydrotherapy, and provides a more natural birthing experience (Miller et al., 2017). ACOG (2009/2017) suggests continuous EFM during labor for women with high-risk conditions because the safety of IA use in high-risk pregnancies remains uncertain. The continued reliance on EFM in the United States is most likely because of staffing patterns, staffing mix, and the increased use of defensive practices in a litigious environment (Miller et al.).

Intermittent Auscultation

Intermittent auscultation involves listening to fetal heart sounds at periodic intervals to assess the FHR. IA of the fetal heart can be performed with a Doppler ultrasound (Fig. 18.1A), an ultrasound stethoscope (see Fig. 18.1B), or a DeLee-Hillis fetoscope (see Fig. 18.1C). Doppler ultrasound and ultrasound stethoscopes transmit ultra–high-frequency sound waves, reflecting movement of the fetal heart, and convert these sounds into an electronic signal that can be counted. Box 18.2 describes how to perform IA.

IA is easy to use, inexpensive, and less invasive than EFM. It is often more comfortable for the woman and gives her more freedom of movement. Other care measures, such as ambulation and

EVIDENCE-BASED PRACTICE

Fetal Cardiac Assessment During Labor: How Are You Doing in There?

Ask the Question

For low-risk women, which assessments of fetal cardiac function during labor provide better outcomes?

Search for the Evidence

Search Strategies: English research-based publications on fetal assessment, monitoring, labor, labour, cardiotocography, fetal electrocardiography, auscultation, pulse oximetry, electrocardiogram, scalp pH, and scalp lactate were included. Exclusions included preterm, postterm, and high risk.

Databases Used: Cochrane Collaborative Database, Joanna Briggs Institute, National Guideline Clearinghouse (AHRQ), CINAHL, PubMed, and the professional websites for AWHONN and SOGC.

Critical Appraisal of the Evidence

Intermittent auscultation utilizes regular assessment of the fetal heart rate using a handheld Doppler device or special stethoscope. It is appropriate and recommended for low-risk women (Lewis, Downe, & FIGO Intrapartum Fetal Monitoring Expert Consensus Panel, 2015).

EFM uses ultrasound to monitor fetal heartbeats.

- As a tool, EFM has high sensitivity, meaning that the reassuring combined presence of moderate variability and accelerations nearly always mean a well-oxygenated fetus. However, it has a low specificity (many false positives), meaning that suspicious patterns may or may not indicate actual distress (Visser, Ayres-de-Campo, & FIGO Intrapartum Fetal Monitoring Expert Consensus Panel, 2015).
- Fetal electrocardiography (fECG) analyzes the fetal heart tracing, on the theory that hypoxia and acidemia would show up as abnormal ECG patterns. Electrodes attach invasively to the fetal scalp, or newer noninvasive models utilize electrodes attached to the maternal abdomen, and can be used concurrently with EFM (Neilson, 2015).
- In all outcomes, fECG plus EFM is not more beneficial than EFM alone (Saccone, Schuit, Amer-Wahlin, et al., 2016). In the presence of maternal obesity, the fECG provides more accurate and reliable fetal monitoring than EFM (Cohen & Hayes-Gill, 2014).
- To address differences between practitioners in EFM interpretation, computer analysis has been developed to alert staff to patterns predictive of hypoxia and acidemia (Visser et al., 2015).

Apply the Evidence: Nursing Implications

- Even though it is not supported by strong evidence of significantly improved outcomes, EFM use has been widespread in hospitals for more than a generation. As a screening tool for possible fetal distress, every member of the health care team should have appropriate training and regular updates in its interpretation.
- Overtreatment, such as unnecessary cesarean births, may be a result of fear of litigation, and create additional risks and costs. New evidence of client safety with intermittent auscultation should reassure caregivers and low-risk laboring women. Evaluating and communicating the evidence becomes paramount for changing long-term institutional habits.
- For obese clients, fECG offers more accurate fetal assessment than EFM. However, the cost of the single-use fECG electrodes is much greater than EFM, whose transducers are reusable.
- Both scalp fECG and scalp blood sampling require rupture of membranes. If this does not occur spontaneously, there is debate about the benefits versus risks of artificially rupturing membranes (increased maternal contraction pain, fetal infection, fetal distress). It falls to nurses to maintain perineal hygiene, including minimizing cervical examinations and documenting invasive procedures.

References

Cohen, W. R., & Hayes-Gill, B. (2014). Influence of maternal body mass index on accuracy and reliability of external fetal monitoring techniques. *Obstetricia et Gynecologica Scandinavica, 93*(6), 590–595.

Lewis, D., Downe, S., & International Federation of Gynecology and Obstetrics Intrapartum Fetal Monitoring Expert Consensus Panel. (2015). FIGO consensus guidelines on intrapartum fetal monitoring: Intermittent auscultation. *International Journal of Gynecology & Obstetrics, 131*(1), 9–12.

Neilson, J. P. (2015). Fetal electrocardiogram (ECG) for fetal monitoring during labour. *Cochrane Database of Systematic Reviews, 5*, CD000116.

Saccone, G., Schuit, E., Amer-Wahlin, I., et al. (2016). Electrocardiogram ST analysis during labor: A systemic review and meta-analysis of randomized controlled trials. *Obstetrics & Gynecology, 127*(1), 127–135.

Visser, G. H., Ayres-de-Campo, D., & FIGO Intrapartum Fetal Monitoring Expert Consensus Panel. (2015). FIGO consensus guidelines on intrapartum fetal monitoring: Adjunct technologies. *International Journal of Gynecology & Obstetrics, 131*(1), 25–29.

Jennifer Taylor Alderman

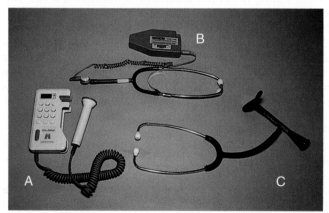

Fig. 18.1 Intermittent Auscultation. (A) Ultrasound Doppler. (B) Ultrasound stethoscope. (C) DeLee-Hillis fetoscope. (Courtesy Michael S. Clement, MD, Mesa, AZ.)

the use of baths or showers, are easier to carry out when IA is used. However, it may be difficult to perform transabdominally in women who are obese. A transvaginal fetal Doppler probe is available that provides closer proximity to the uterus, making it easier to auscultate the FHR when the woman is obese or early in gestation (Miller et al., 2017). Because IA is intermittent, significant events may occur during a time when the FHR is not being auscultated. In addition, IA does not provide a permanent documented visual record of the FHR and cannot be used to assess visual patterns of the FHR variability or periodic changes. When using IA the nurse can assess the baseline FHR, rhythm, and increases and decreases from baseline (Miller et al.).

There is a lack of literature to recommend the optimal intervals for FHR auscultation during latent- and active-phase labor. Therefore, several professional organizations have provided general guidelines for frequency of assessment for low- and high-risk clients during the intrapartum period. These organizations include the Association of Women's Health, Obstetric and Neonatal Nurses (AWHONN), the American Academy of Pediatrics (AAP), ACOG, the National Institute for Health and Care Excellence (NICE), and the Society of Obstetricians and Gynaecologists of Canada (SOGC). The suggested frequencies are generally based on protocols reported in research clinical trials in which investigators compared clinical outcomes associated with IA and EFM (AWHONN, 2015a).

BOX 18.2 Procedure for Intermittent Auscultation of the Fetal Heart Rate

1. Perform Leopold maneuvers by palpating the maternal abdomen to identify fetal presentation and position (see Box 19.5).
2. Apply ultrasonic gel to device if using Doppler ultrasound. Place listening device (see Fig. 18.1A) over area of maximal intensity and clarity of fetal heart sounds to obtain clearest and loudest sound, which is easiest to count. This location is usually over the fetal back. If using fetoscope, firm pressure may be needed.
3. Count maternal radial pulse while listening to FHR to differentiate it from fetal rate.
4. Palpate abdomen for presence or absence of UA to count FHR between contractions.
5. Count FHR for 30-60 seconds after a uterine contraction to identify auscultated baseline rate and changes (increases or decreases) in it.
6. Auscultate FHR before, during, and after contraction to identify FHR during the contraction or as a response to the contraction and to assess for absence or presence of increases or decreases in FHR.
7. When distinct discrepancies in FHR are noted during listening periods, auscultate for longer period during, after, and between contractions to identify significant changes that may indicate need for another mode of FHR monitoring.

FHR, Fetal heart rate; *UA,* uterine activity.
From Miller, L., Miller, D., & Cypher, R. (2017). *Mosby's pocket guide to fetal monitoring: A multidisciplinary approach* (8th ed.). St. Louis: Elsevier.

! NURSING ALERT

When the FHR is auscultated and documented it is inappropriate to use the descriptive terms associated with EFM (e.g., *moderate variability, variable deceleration*) because most of the terms are visual descriptions of the patterns produced on the monitor tracing. However, terms that are numerically defined such as *bradycardia* and *tachycardia* can be used. When FHR is auscultated, it should be described as a baseline number or range and as having a regular or irregular rhythm. The presence of abrupt or gradual increases or decreases in FHR before, during, and immediately after contractions should also be noted (AWHONN, 2015b; Miller et al., 2017).

AWHONN recommends the following IA frequencies for low-risk women who are not receiving oxytocin: latent phase (<4 cm) at least hourly; latent phase (4 to 5 cm) every 15 to 30 minutes; active phase (≥6 cm) every 15 to 30 minutes; second stage, passive fetal descent every 15 minutes; and second stage, active pushing every 5 to 15 minutes (AWHONN, 2015a).

Every effort should be made to use the method of fetal assessment the woman desires if possible. However, auscultation of the FHR in accordance with the frequency guidelines suggested earlier may be difficult in today's busy labor and birth units. When used as the primary method of fetal assessment, auscultation requires a one-to-one nurse-to-client staffing ratio. If acuity and census change so that auscultation standards are no longer met, the nurse must inform the physician or nurse-midwife that continuous EFM will be used until staffing can be arranged to meet the standards.

The woman can become anxious if the examiner cannot readily count the fetal heart sounds. It often takes time for the inexperienced listener to locate the heartbeat and find the area of maximal intensity. To allay the woman's concerns, she can be told that the nurse is "finding the spot where the sounds are loudest." If it takes considerable time to locate the fetal heartbeat, the examiner can reassure the woman by offering her an opportunity to listen. If the examiner cannot locate the fetal heartbeat, assistance should be requested. In some cases, ultrasound can be used to help locate the fetal heartbeat. Seeing the FHR on the ultrasound screen is reassuring to the woman if there was initial difficulty in locating the best area for auscultation.

TABLE 18.2 External and Internal Modes of Monitoring

External Mode	Internal Mode
Fetal Heart Rate	
Ultrasound transducer: High-frequency sound waves reflect mechanical action of the fetal heart. Noninvasive. Does not require rupture of membranes or cervical dilation. Used during both the antepartum and intrapartum periods.	*Spiral electrode:* Converts the fetal electrocardiogram as obtained from the presenting part to the fetal heart rate via a cardiotachometer. Can be used only when membranes are ruptured and the cervix is sufficiently dilated during the intrapartum period. Electrode penetrates into the fetal presenting part by 1.5 mm and must be attached securely to ensure a good signal.
Uterine Activity	
Toco transducer: Monitors frequency and duration of contractions by means of a pressure-sensing device applied to the maternal abdomen. Used during both the antepartum and intrapartum periods.	*IUPC:* Monitors the frequency, duration, and intensity of contractions. The two types of IUPCs are a fluid-filled system and a solid catheter. Both measure intrauterine pressure at the catheter tip and convert the pressure into millimeters of mercury on the uterine activity panel of the strip chart. Both types can be used only when membranes are ruptured and the cervix is sufficiently dilated during the intrapartum period.

IUPC, Intrauterine pressure catheter.

When using IA, UA is assessed by palpation. The examiner should keep his or her fingertips placed over the fundus before, during, and after contractions. The contraction intensity is usually described as mild, moderate, or strong. The contraction duration is measured in seconds, from the beginning to the end of the contraction. The frequency of contractions is measured in minutes, from the beginning of one contraction to the beginning of the next. The examiner should keep his or her hand on the fundus after the contraction is over to evaluate uterine resting tone or relaxation between contractions. Resting tone between contractions is usually described as soft or hard (Lyndon, O'Brien-Abel, & Simpson, 2014).

Accurate and complete documentation of fetal status and UA is especially important when IA and palpation are being used because no paper tracing record or computer storage of these assessments is provided as is the case with continuous EFM. Labor flow records or computer charting systems that prompt notations of all assessments are useful for ensuring such comprehensive documentation.

Electronic Fetal Monitoring

The purpose of EFM is to assess the adequacy of fetal oxygenation during labor. If the monitor demonstrates evidence of interruption, further evaluation can be initiated, or interventions implemented to improve fetal oxygenation. If these actions are not successful, the monitor can provide information to assist in making decisions regarding the optimal timing and method of birth to avoid the potential consequences of fetal hypoxia (Miller, 2017). The two modes of EFM are the external mode, which uses external transducers placed on the maternal abdomen to assess FHR and UA, and the internal mode, which uses a spiral electrode applied to the fetal presenting part to assess the FHR and an intrauterine pressure catheter (IUPC) to assess UA and uterine resting tone. The differences between the external and internal modes of EFM are summarized in Table 18.2.

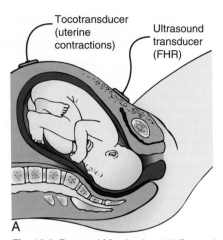
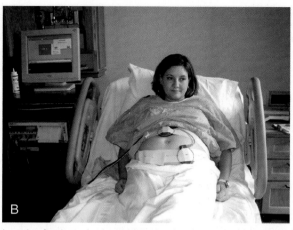

Tocotransducer
(uterine
contractions)

Ultrasound
transducer
(FHR)

A

B

Fig. 18.2 External Monitoring. (A) External noninvasive fetal monitoring with toco transducer and ultrasound transducer. (B) Ultrasound transducer is placed over the area where fetal heart rate is best heard, usually below the umbilicus, and toco transducer is placed on the uterine fundus. *FHR*, Fetal heart rate. (B, Courtesy Julie Perry Nelson, Loveland, CO.)

External Monitoring

Separate transducers are used to monitor the FHR and UCs (Fig. 18.2A). The **ultrasound transducer** works by reflecting high-frequency sound waves off a moving interface: in this case, the fetal heart and valves. It is sometimes difficult to reproduce a continuous and precise record of the FHR because of artifact introduced by fetal and maternal movement. Maternal obesity, occiput posterior position of the fetus, and anterior attachment of the placenta can cause weak or absent signals (AWHONN, 2015b). The FHR is printed on specially formatted monitor paper. The standard paper speed used in the United States is 3 cm/min. Once the area of maximal intensity of the FHR has been located, conductive gel is applied to the surface of the ultrasound transducer, and the transducer is then positioned over this area and held securely in place using an elastic belt.

The **toco transducer** (tocodynamometer) measures UA transabdominally. The device is placed over the fundus above the umbilicus and held securely in place using an elastic belt (see Fig. 18.2B). UCs or fetal movements depress a pressure-sensitive surface on the side next to the abdomen. The toco transducer can measure and record the frequency and approximate duration of UCs but not their intensity. This method is especially valuable for measuring UA during the first stage of labor in women with intact membranes or for antepartum testing. If the woman is obese, the toco transducer may be unable to detect the exact frequency and duration of UA.

Because the toco transducer of most electronic fetal monitors is designed for assessing UA in a term pregnancy, it may not be sensitive enough to detect preterm UA. When monitoring the woman in preterm labor, the fundus may be located below the level of the umbilicus. The nurse may need to rely on the woman to indicate when UA is occurring and to use palpation as an additional way of assessing contraction frequency and validating the monitor tracing.

The external transducers are applied easily by the nurse but often must be readjusted as the woman or fetus changes position. The woman is asked to assume the semi-Fowler or lateral position. Use of external transducers confines the woman to bed or chair.

Portable telemetry monitors allow observation of the FHR and UC patterns by means of centrally located electronic display stations. These portable units permit the woman to walk around during electronic monitoring.

Use of another type of external monitor, which uses an integrated system of abdominally obtained electronic impulses to concurrently monitor both maternal heart rate and FHR and UA, is becoming increasingly

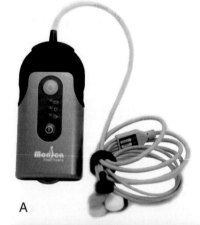

A

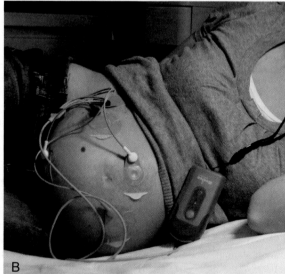

B

Fig. 18.3 Wireless External Monitoring. (A) The Monica AN24 is a wireless and beltless device that can be used with existing monitors to obtain fetal heart rate via abdominal electrocardiogram (ECG). (B) Electrodes placed on maternal abdomen monitor ECG from fetal and maternal heart and electromyogram from uterine muscle. (Courtesy Monica Healthcare Ltd., Nottingham, UK.)

popular (Fig. 18.3A and B). The monitor uses five electrodes placed on the woman's abdomen to directly monitor the electrocardiogram from the maternal and fetal hearts and the electromyogram from the uterine muscle. This information is transmitted wirelessly, via Bluetooth technology, to an interface device that allows the FHR and UA data to print or display on a standard fetal monitor (Miller et al., 2017). Another version of this monitoring system, in which a single-use patch replaces the five electrodes placed on the woman's abdomen, is now available.

This integrated monitoring system eliminates much of the problem caused by signal loss resulting from maternal or fetal movement or maternal obesity that often occurs with traditional external monitors. The monitor also more accurately measures the frequency, occurrence of peak, and duration of UCs than does the traditional toco transducer, although it does not provide actual intensity measurement in millimeters of mercury (mm Hg) as an IUPC does. Other advantages of the device are that it eliminates the need for abdominal belts and frequent readjustment of the toco transducer and ultrasound transducer and provides some client mobility. The woman may move up to 50 feet away from the interface device without signal loss. This type of monitor may not be readily available for use in all labor and birth settings (Miller et al., 2017). Also, in the United States, the device is only approved for use in monitoring singleton pregnancies at term (see Clinical Reasoning Case Study: Monitoring the Fetus of an Obese Woman) (AWHONN, 2015b).

❓ CLINICAL REASONING CASE STUDY

Monitoring the Fetus of an Obese Woman

Tameka is a 23-year-old G 4 P 2 0 1 2 at 35 weeks of gestation. She has had chronic hypertension since she was 16 years of age and is morbidly obese. Today she weighs 305 pounds and has a body mass index (BMI) of 41.8. Tameka was sent from the antepartum testing area to the labor and birth unit for prolonged monitoring because she had a nonreactive nonstress test (NST) and her blood pressure (BP) was elevated at her appointment today. You are Tameka's nurse. After spending half an hour admitting her to the unit you walk out to the nurses' station and announce to your colleagues, "I am *so* frustrated! No matter what I do, I just can't keep that baby on the monitor!"

1. What is the priority concern or client need in this situation? Support your answer with data as stated in the case.
2. List other client needs/problems in this case.
3. Identify any additional information or assessment data that is needed by the nurse in planning care for this client.
4. What nursing actions are appropriate in this situation?
   a. What is the priority nursing action? (What should the nurse do first?)
   b. Describe other nursing interventions that are important to providing optimal client care.
5. Describe the roles/responsibilities of the interprofessional health care team members (other than nurses) who may be involved in providing care for this client.

Internal Monitoring

The technique of continuous internal FHR or UA monitoring provides a more accurate appraisal of fetal well-being during labor than external monitoring because it is not interrupted by fetal or maternal movement or affected by maternal size (Fig. 18.4). For this type of monitoring, the membranes must be ruptured, the cervix sufficiently dilated (at least 2 to 3 cm), and the presenting part, which is usually the fetal head, low enough to allow placement of the spiral electrode or IUPC, or both. Internal and external modes of monitoring may be combined (i.e., internal FHR with external UA or external FHR with internal UA) without difficulty.

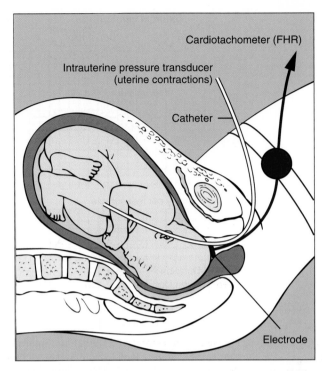

Fig. 18.4 Internal Monitoring. Diagrammatic representation of internal invasive fetal monitoring with intrauterine pressure catheter and spiral electrode in place (membranes ruptured and cervix dilated). *FHR,* Fetal heart rate.

Internal monitoring of the FHR is accomplished by attaching a small spiral electrode to the presenting part. For UA to be monitored internally, an IUPC is introduced into the uterine cavity. The catheter has a pressure-sensitive tip that measures changes in intrauterine pressure. As the catheter is compressed during a contraction, pressure is placed on the pressure transducer. This pressure is then converted into a pressure reading in millimeters of mercury. The IUPC can objectively measure the frequency, duration, and intensity of UCs, and uterine resting tone.

Because it can measure the intensity of individual UCs precisely, the IUPC can be used to evaluate the adequacy of UA for achieving progress in labor. **Montevideo units (MVUs)** are calculated by subtracting the baseline uterine pressure from the peak contraction pressure for each contraction that occurs in a 10-minute window and then adding together the pressures generated by each contraction that occurs during that period of time. Spontaneous labor usually begins when MVUs are between 80 and 120 (see Table 18.1) (Cunningham, Leveno, Bloom, et al., 2018; Miller et al., 2017).

Display

The FHR and UA are displayed on the monitor paper or computer screen, with the FHR in the upper section and UA in the lower section. Fig. 18.5 contrasts the internal and external modes of electronic monitoring. Note that each small square on the monitor paper or screen represents 10 seconds; each larger box of six squares equals 1 minute (when paper is moving through the monitor at the rate of 3 cm/min).

FETAL HEART RATE PATTERNS

Characteristic FHR patterns are associated with fetal and maternal physiologic processes and have been identified for many years. Because EFM was introduced into clinical practice before consensus was reached in regard to standardized terminology, however, variations in the description and interpretation of common fetal heart rate patterns were often great. In 1997 the NICHD published a proposed nomenclature system for EFM

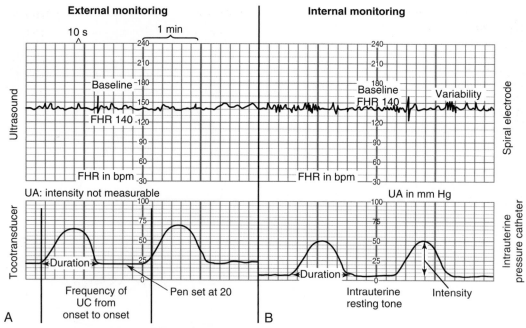

Fig. 18.5 Comparison of External and Internal Monitoring. Display of fetal heart rate *(FHR)* and uterine contractions *(UC)* as seen using the external mode of monitoring (A) as compared to the internal mode of monitoring (B). *UA,* Uterine activity. (From Miller, L., Miller, D., & Cypher, R. [2017]. *Mosby's pocket guide to fetal monitoring: A multidisciplinary approach* [8th ed.]. St. Louis: Elsevier.)

interpretation with standardized definitions for FHR monitoring (NICHD, 1997). Currently ACOG, the American College of Nurse-Midwives (ACNM), and AWHONN all support the use of standardized terminology (Miller et al., 2017). All three organizations cited concerns regarding client safety and the need for improved communication among caregivers as reasons for using standard EFM definitions in clinical practice.

In April 2008 the NICHD, ACOG, and SMFM partnered to sponsor another workshop to revisit the FHR definitions recommended by the NICHD in 1997. The 1997 FHR definitions were reaffirmed at this workshop. In addition, new definitions related to UA were recommended, as well as a three-tier system of FHR pattern interpretation and categorization (see Box 18.1) (Macones et al., 2008).

Baseline Fetal Heart Rate

The intrinsic rhythmicity of the fetal heart, the central nervous system (CNS), and the fetal autonomic nervous system control the FHR. An increase in sympathetic response results in acceleration of the FHR, whereas an increase in parasympathetic response produces a slowing of the FHR. Usually a balanced increase of sympathetic and parasympathetic response occurs during contractions, with no observable change in the baseline FHR.

The baseline fetal heart rate is the average rate during a 10-minute segment that excludes periodic or episodic changes, periods of marked variability, and segments of the baseline that differ by more than 25 beats/min. There must be at least 2 minutes of interpretable baseline data in a 10-minute segment of tracing in order to determine the baseline FHR (Macones et al., 2008). After 10 minutes of tracing is observed, the approximate mean rate is rounded to the closest 5 beats/min interval (AWHONN, 2015b). For example, if the FHR varies between 130 and 140 beats/min over a 10-minute period, the baseline is recorded as 135 beats/min. The normal FHR range is 110 to 160 beats/min.

Variability

Variability of the FHR can be described as irregular waves or fluctuations in the baseline FHR of two cycles per minute or greater (Macones

et al., 2008). It is a characteristic of the baseline FHR and does not include accelerations or decelerations of the FHR. Variability is quantified in beats per minute and is measured from the peak to the trough of a single cycle. Four possible categories of variability have been identified: absent, minimal, moderate, and marked (Fig. 18.6). In the past, variability was described as either long term or short term (beat to beat). The NICHD definitions do not distinguish between long- and short-term variability, however, because in actual practice they are visually determined as a unit (NICHD, 1997).

Absent variability (see Fig. 18.6A) is defined as an amplitude range of the FHR fluctuations that is not detectable to the unaided eye. Minimal variability (see Fig. 18.6B) has an amplitude range that is detectable to the unaided eye, but is less than 5 beats/min (Miller et al., 2017). Depending on other characteristics of the FHR tracing, absent or minimal variability is classified as either abnormal or indeterminate (Macones et al., 2008). It can result from fetal hypoxemia and metabolic acidemia. Other possible causes of absent or minimal variability include fetal sleep cycles, fetal tachycardia, extreme prematurity, medications that cause CNS depression, congenital anomalies, and preexisting neurologic injury (Miller et al.).

Moderate variability, with an amplitude range of 6 to 25 bpm, is considered normal (see Fig. 18.6C). Its presence reliably predicts a normal fetal acid–base balance (absence of fetal metabolic acidemia). Moderate variability indicates that FHR regulation is not significantly affected by fetal sleep cycles, tachycardia, prematurity, congenital anomalies, preexisting neurologic injury, or CNS depressant medications (Macones et al., 2008; Miller et al., 2017).

The significance of marked variability, with an amplitude range ≥ 25 bpm, (see Fig. 18.6D) is unclear (Macones et al., 2008). In many cases, it likely represents a normal variant (Miller et al., 2017).

A sinusoidal pattern (i.e., a regular smooth, undulating wavelike pattern) is not included in the definition of FHR variability. This uncommon pattern classically occurs with severe fetal anemia (Fig. 18.7). Variations of the sinusoidal pattern have been described in association with chorioamnionitis, fetal sepsis, and administration of opioid analgesics (Miller et al., 2017).

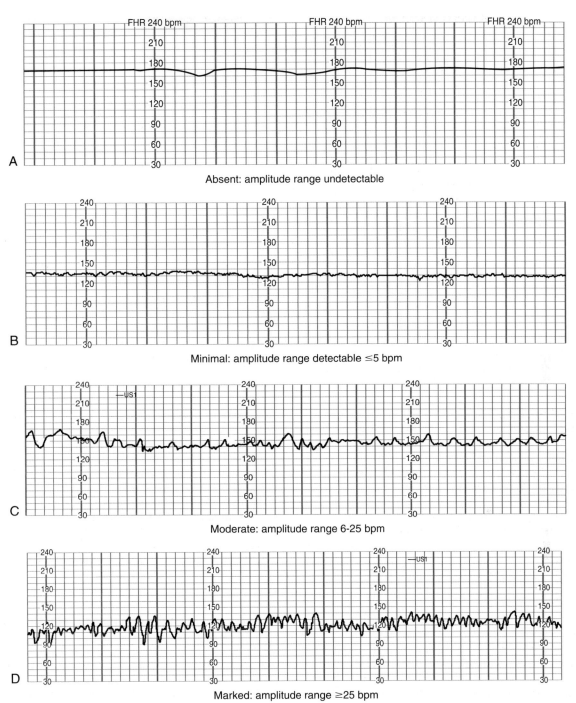

Fig. 18.6 Classification of Fetal Heart Rate Variability. (A) Absent. (B) Minimal. (C) Moderate. (D) Marked. *FHR,* Fetal heart rate. (From Miller, L., Miller, D., & Cypher, R. [2017]. *Mosby's pocket guide to fetal monitoring: A multidisciplinary approach* [8th ed.]. St. Louis: Elsevier.)

Tachycardia

Tachycardia is a baseline FHR greater than 160 beats/min for 10 minutes or longer (Fig. 18.8). It can be considered an early sign of fetal hypoxemia, especially when associated with late decelerations and minimal or absent variability. Fetal tachycardia can result from many other causes not directly related to fetal oxygenation. For example, tachycardia can be caused by maternal or fetal infection; by maternal hyperthyroidism or fetal anemia; or in response to medications such as atropine, hydroxyzine (Vistaril), terbutaline (Brethine), or illicit drugs such as cocaine or methamphetamines. Tachycardia can also be caused

by abnormalities involving fetal cardiac pacemakers and/or the cardiac conduction system (Miller et al., 2017). Table 18.3 lists causes, clinical significance, and nursing interventions for tachycardia.

Bradycardia

Bradycardia is a baseline FHR less than 110 beats/min for 10 minutes or longer (Fig. 18.9). True bradycardia occurs rarely and is not specifically related to fetal oxygenation. It must be distinguished from a prolonged deceleration because the causes and management of these two conditions are very different. Bradycardia is often caused by some

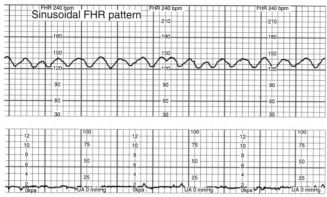

Fig. 18.7 Sinusoidal Pattern. *FHR*, Fetal heart rate. (From Miller, L., Miller, D., & Cypher, R. [2017]. *Mosby's pocket guide to fetal monitoring: A multidisciplinary approach.* [8th ed.]. St. Louis: Elsevier.)

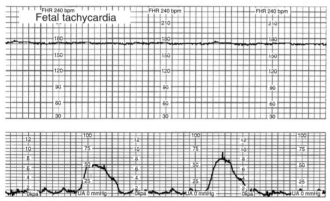

Fig. 18.8 Fetal Tachycardia. Fetal heart rate (FHR) above 160 beats/min. (From Miller, L., Miller, D., & Cypher, R. [2017]. *Mosby's pocket guide to fetal monitoring: A multidisciplinary approach* [8th ed.]. St. Louis: Elsevier.)

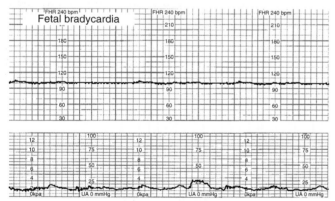

Fig. 18.9 Fetal Bradycardia. Fetal heart rate (FHR) below 110 beats/min. (From Miller, L., Miller, D., & Cypher, R. [2017]. *Mosby's Pocket Guide to Fetal Monitoring: A Multidisciplinary Approach* [8th ed.]. St. Louis: Elsevier.)

type of fetal cardiac problem such as structural defects involving the pacemakers or conduction system or fetal heart failure. Other causes of bradycardia include viral infections (e.g., cytomegalovirus), maternal hypoglycemia, and maternal hypothermia. Medications do not commonly cause bradycardia (Miller et al., 2017). (See Table 18.3 for a list of causes, clinical significance, and nursing interventions for bradycardia.)

TABLE 18.3 Tachycardia and Bradycardia

Tachycardia	Bradycardia
Definition	
FHR >160 beats/min lasting >10 min	FHR <110 beats/min lasting >10 min
Possible Causes	
Early fetal hypoxemia	Atrioventricular dissociation (heart block)
Fetal cardiac arrhythmias	Structural defects
Maternal fever	Viral infections (e.g., cytomegalovirus)
Infection (including chorioamnionitis)	Medications
Parasympatholytic drugs (atropine, hydroxyzine)	Fetal heart failure
Beta-sympathomimetic drugs (terbutaline)	Maternal hypoglycemia
Maternal hyperthyroidism	Maternal hypothermia
Fetal anemia	
Drugs (caffeine, cocaine, methamphetamines)	
Clinical Significance	
Persistent tachycardia in absence of periodic changes does not appear serious in terms of neonatal outcome (especially true if tachycardia is associated with maternal fever); tachycardia is abnormal when associated with late decelerations, severe variable decelerations, or absent variability.	Baseline bradycardia alone is not specifically related to fetal oxygenation. The clinical significance of bradycardia depends on the underlying cause and the accompanying FHR patterns, including variability, accelerations, or decelerations.
Nursing Interventions	
Dependent on cause; reduce maternal fever with antipyretics and cooling measures as ordered; oxygen at 10 L/min by nonrebreather face mask may be of some value; carry out health care provider's orders based on alleviating cause	Dependent on cause

FHR, Fetal heart rate.

Periodic and Episodic Changes in Fetal Heart Rate

Changes in FHR from the baseline are categorized as periodic or episodic. **Periodic changes** are those that occur with UCs. **Episodic changes** are those that are not associated with UCs. These patterns include both accelerations and decelerations (Macones et al., 2008).

Accelerations

Acceleration of the FHR is defined as a visually apparent, abrupt (onset to peak less than 30 seconds) increase in FHR above the baseline rate (Fig. 18.10). The peak is at least 15 beats/min above the baseline, and the acceleration lasts 15 seconds or more, with the return to baseline less than 2 minutes from the beginning of the acceleration. Before 32 weeks of gestation, the definition of an acceleration is a peak of 10 beats/min or more above the baseline and a duration of at least 10 seconds. Acceleration of the FHR for more than 10 minutes is considered a change in baseline rate (Miller et al., 2017).

Accelerations can be either periodic or episodic. They may occur in association with fetal movement or spontaneously. If accelerations do not occur spontaneously, they can be elicited by fetal scalp or vibroacoustic stimulation. Another possible cause of accelerations is transient compression of the umbilical vein, resulting in decreased fetal venous return and a reflex rise in heart rate. Similar to moderate variability, accelerations are considered an indication of fetal well-being. Their presence is highly predictive of a normal fetal acid–base balance (absence of fetal metabolic acidemia) (Miller et al., 2017). Box 18.3 lists causes and clinical significance for accelerations.

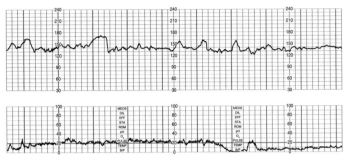

Fig. 18.10 Accelerations of Fetal Heart Rate in a Term Pregnancy. Note that the 15 beats/min peak and 15-second duration criteria are met. (Courtesy Miller, L., Miller, D. & Cypher, R. [2017]. *Mosby's pocket guide to fetal monitoring: A multidisciplinary approach* [8th ed.]. St. Louis: Elsevier.)

BOX 18.3   Accelerations

Causes
- Spontaneous fetal movement
- Vaginal examination
- Electrode application
- Fetal scalp stimulation
- Fetal reaction to external sounds
- Breech presentation
- Occiput posterior position
- Uterine contractions
- Fundal pressure
- Abdominal palpation

Clinical Significance
Normal pattern. Acceleration with fetal movement signifies fetal well-being representing fetal alertness or arousal states.

Nursing Interventions
None required

Decelerations

A *deceleration* (caused by dominance of a parasympathetic response) may be benign or abnormal. FHR decelerations are categorized as early, late, variable, or prolonged. They are described by their visual relation to the onset and end of a contraction and by their shape.

Early decelerations. Early deceleration of the FHR is a visually apparent, gradual (onset to lowest point ≥30 seconds) decrease in and return to baseline FHR associated with UCs. It is thought to be caused by transient fetal head compression and is considered a normal and benign finding (Macones et al., 2008; Miller et al., 2017). Generally the onset, *nadir* (lowest point), and recovery of the deceleration correspond to the beginning, peak, and end of the contraction (Figs. 18.11 and 18.12). For this reason, an early deceleration is sometimes called the *mirror image* of a contraction.

Early decelerations may occur during UCs, during vaginal examinations, as a result of fundal pressure, and during placement of the internal mode of fetal monitoring. They have no known relationship to fetal oxygenation. Instead, they are thought to represent a fetal autonomic response to changes in intracranial pressure and/or cerebral blood flow caused by fetal head compression (Miller et al., 2017). When present, they usually occur during the first stage of labor when the cervix is dilated 4 to 7 cm. However, they are sometimes seen during the second stage when the woman is pushing.

Because early decelerations are considered to be benign, interventions are not necessary. The value in identifying them is so they can be distinguished from late or variable decelerations, which can be abnormal and for which interventions are appropriate. Box 18.4 lists causes and clinical significance for early decelerations.

Late decelerations. Late deceleration of the FHR is a visually apparent, gradual (onset to lowest point >30 seconds) decrease in and return to baseline FHR associated with UCs (Macones et al., 2008). The deceleration begins after the contraction has started, and the lowest point of the deceleration occurs after the peak of the contraction. The deceleration usually does not return to baseline until after the contraction is over (Figs. 18.13 and 18.14).

Late decelerations are caused by a reflex fetal response to transient hypoxemia during a UC that reduces the delivery of oxygenated blood to the intervillous space of the placenta (Miller et al., 2017). A number of conditions can cause disruption of oxygen transfer from the environment to the fetus. Common causes include maternal hypotension and uterine hypertonus. If interruption of fetal oxygenation results in metabolic acidemia, late decelerations may result from direct hypoxic

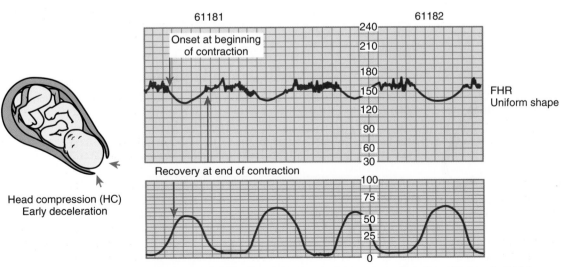

Fig. 18.11 Line Drawing Illustrating Early Decelerations. *FHR,* Fetal heart rate. (From Tucker, S. [2004]. *Pocket guide to fetal monitoring and assessment* [5th ed.]. St. Louis: Mosby.)

myocardial depression during a contraction (Miller, 2017). The clinical significance and nursing interventions for late decelerations are described in Box 18.5.

Variable decelerations. Variable deceleration of the FHR is defined as a visually abrupt (onset to lowest point less than 30 seconds) and apparent decrease in FHR below the baseline. The decrease is at least 15 beats/min or more below the baseline, lasts at least 15 seconds, and returns to baseline in less than 2 minutes from the time of onset (Macones et al., 2008). Variable decelerations are caused by compression of the vessels in the umbilical cord and can occur with or without UCs (Miller, 2017) (Figs. 18.15 to 18.17).

The appearance of variable decelerations differs from those of early and late decelerations, which closely approximate the shape of the corresponding UC. Instead, variable decelerations have a U, V, or W shape, characterized by a rapid descent and ascent to and from the nadir of the deceleration (see Figs. 18.15 and 18.16). Some variable decelerations are preceded and followed by brief accelerations of the FHR known as *shoulders,* which is an appropriate compensatory response to compression of the umbilical vein.

Occasional variables have little clinical significance. Recurrent variable decelerations, however, indicate repetitive disruption in the oxygen supply of the fetus. This can result in hypoxemia, hypoxia, metabolic acidosis, and, eventually, metabolic acidemia. Variable decelerations may also be caused by a fetal vagal response to umbilical cord stretching as the fetus descends in the pelvis during labor (Miller et al., 2017). Box 18.6 lists causes, clinical significance, and nursing interventions for variable decelerations.

Prolonged decelerations. A prolonged deceleration is a visually apparent decrease (may be either gradual or abrupt) in FHR of at least 15 beats/min below the baseline and lasting more than 2 minutes but less than 10 minutes. A deceleration lasting more than 10 minutes is considered a baseline change (Macones et al., 2008) (Fig. 18.18).

Prolonged decelerations are caused when the mechanisms responsible for late or variable decelerations last for an extended period (more than 2 minutes). Conditions that can cause an interruption in the fetal oxygen supply long enough to produce a prolonged deceleration can occur anywhere along the oxygen pathway. For example, at the level of the maternal lungs, a prolonged deceleration may result from maternal apnea during an eclamptic seizure. At the level of the umbilical cord, cord compression, stretch, or prolapse can result in a prolonged deceleration (Miller, 2017).

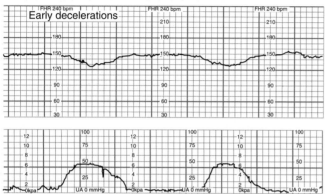

Fig. 18.12 Electronic Fetal Monitor Tracing Showing Early Decelerations. *FHR,* Fetal heart rate; *UA,* uterine activity. (From Miller, L., Miller, D., & Cypher, R. [2017]. *Mosby's pocket guide to fetal monitoring: A multidisciplinary approach* [8th ed.]. St. Louis: Elsevier.)

BOX 18.4   Early Decelerations

Causes

Head compression resulting from the following:
- Uterine contractions
- Vaginal examination
- Fundal pressure
- Placement of internal mode of monitoring

Clinical Significance

Normal pattern; not associated with fetal hypoxemia, acidemia, or low Apgar scores

Nursing Interventions

None required

! NURSING ALERT

Nurses should notify the physician or nurse-midwife immediately and initiate appropriate treatment of abnormal patterns when they see a prolonged deceleration.

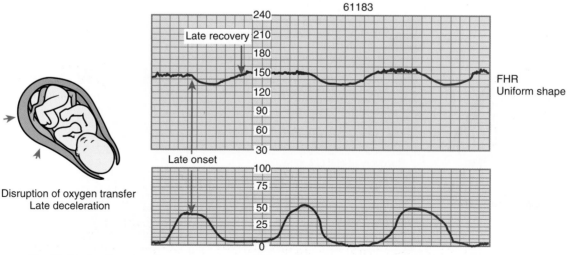

Disruption of oxygen transfer
Late deceleration

Fig. 18.13 Line Drawing Illustrating Late Decelerations. *FHR,* Fetal heart rate. (Modified from Tucker, S. [2004]. *Pocket guide to fetal monitoring and assessment* [5th ed.]. St. Louis: Mosby.)

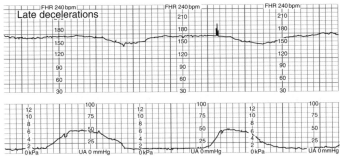

Fig. 18.14 Electronic Fetal Monitor Tracing Showing Late Decelerations. *FHR,* Fetal heart rate; *UA,* uterine activity. (From Miller, L., Miller, D., & Cypher, R. [2017]. *Mosby's pocket guide to fetal monitoring: A multidisciplinary approach* [8th ed.]. St. Louis: Elsevier.)

CARE MANAGEMENT

Care of the woman receiving EFM in labor begins with evaluation of the EFM equipment. The nurse must ensure that the monitor is recording FHR and UA accurately and that the tracing is interpretable. If external monitoring is not adequate, changing to a fetal spiral electrode or IUPC may be necessary. A checklist for fetal monitoring equipment can be used to evaluate the equipment functions (Box 18.7).

After ensuring that the monitor is recording properly, the FHR and UA tracings are evaluated regularly throughout labor. *Guidelines for Perinatal Care,* published jointly by AAP and ACOG (2017), recommends that the FHR tracing be evaluated every 30 minutes during the active phase of the first stage of labor and at least every 15 minutes during the second stage of labor in low-risk women. If risk factors are present, the FHR tracing should be evaluated more frequently: at least every 15 minutes in the active phase of the first stage of labor and at least every 5 minutes in the second stage of labor (AAP/ACOG).

BOX 18.5 Late Decelerations

Causes

Disruption of oxygen transfer from environment to fetus, resulting in transient fetal hypoxemia. Late decelerations are caused by the following:

- Uterine tachysystole
- Maternal supine hypotension
- Epidural or spinal anesthesia
- Placenta previa
- Placental abruption
- Hypertensive disorders
- Postterm gestation
- Intrauterine growth restriction
- Diabetes mellitus
- Chorioamnionitis

Clinical Significance

Abnormal pattern associated with fetal hypoxemia, acidemia, and low Apgar scores; considered ominous if persistent and uncorrected, especially when associated with absent or minimal baseline variability

Nursing Interventions

The usual priority is as follows:

1. Discontinue oxytocin if infusing.
2. Assist woman to lateral (side-lying) position.
3. Administer oxygen at 10 L/min by nonrebreather face mask.
4. Correct maternal hypotension by elevating legs.
5. Increase rate of maintenance intravenous solution.
6. Palpate uterus to assess for tachysystole.
7. Notify physician or nurse-midwife.
8. Consider internal monitoring for more accurate fetal and uterine assessment.
9. Assist with birth (vaginal-assisted or cesarean) if pattern cannot be corrected.

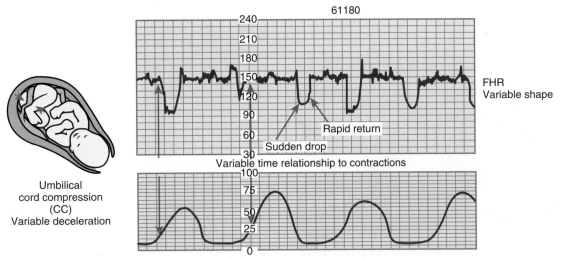

Fig. 18.15 Line Drawing Illustrating Variable Decelerations. *FHR,* Fetal heart rate. (From Tucker, S. [2004]. *Pocket guide to fetal monitoring and assessment* [5th ed.]. St. Louis: Mosby.)

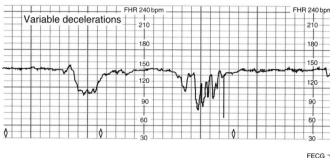

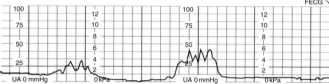

Fig. 18.16 Electronic Fetal Monitor Tracing Showing Variable Decelerations. *FHR*, Fetal heart rate; *FECG*, Fetal electrocardiogram. (From Miller, L., Miller, D., & Cypher, R. [2017]. *Mosby's pocket guide to fetal monitoring: A multidisciplinary approach* [8th ed.]. St. Louis: Elsevier.)

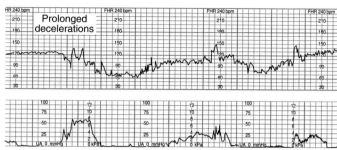

Fig. 18.18 Prolonged Decelerations. *FHR*, Fetal heart rate; *UA*, uterine activity. (From Miller, L., Miller, D., & Cypher, R. [2017]. *Mosby's pocket guide to fetal monitoring: A multidisciplinary approach* [8th ed.]. St. Louis: Elsevier.)

BOX 18.6 Variable Decelerations

Causes

Umbilical cord compression caused by the following:
- Maternal position with cord between fetus and maternal pelvis
- Cord around fetal neck, arm, leg, or other body part
- Short cord
- Knot in cord (see Fig. 18.17)
- Prolapsed cord

Clinical Significance

Variable decelerations occur in approximately 50% of all labors and usually are transient and correctable

Nursing Interventions

The usual priority is as follows:
1. Discontinue oxytocin if infusing.
2. Change maternal position (side to side, knee chest).
3. Administer oxygen at 10 L/min by nonrebreather face mask.
4. Notify physician or nurse-midwife.
5. Assist with vaginal or speculum examination to assess for cord prolapse.
6. Assist with amnioinfusion if ordered.
7. Assist with birth (vaginal-assisted or cesarean) if pattern cannot be corrected.

BOX 18.7 Checklist for Fetal Monitoring Equipment

Preparation of Monitor
1. Is paper inserted correctly (if using paper)?
2. Are transducer cables plugged securely into appropriate port on monitor?
3. Is paper speed set to 3 cm/min (in North America)?
4. Were monitor date and time verified (when using electronic documentation)?

Ultrasound Transducer
1. Has ultrasound transmission gel been applied to the transducer?
2. Was FHR tested and noted on monitor strip?
3. Was FHR compared with maternal pulse and noted?
4. Does a signal light flash or an audible beep occur with each heartbeat?
5. Is belt secure and snug but comfortable for the laboring woman?

Toco transducer
1. Is toco transducer firmly positioned at site of least maternal tissue?
2. Has it been applied without gel or paste?
3. Was UA baseline adjusted between contractions to print at the 20 mm Hg line?
4. Is belt secure and snug but comfortable for the laboring woman?

Spiral Electrode
1. Is connector attached firmly to electrode pad (on leg plate or abdomen)?
2. Is spiral electrode attached to presenting part of fetus?
3. Is inner surface of electrode pad pre-gelled or covered with electrode gel?
4. Is electrode pad properly secured to woman's thigh or abdomen?

Internal Catheter or Strain Gauge
1. Is length line on catheter visible at introitus?
2. Is it noted on monitor paper that UA test or calibration was performed?
3. Has monitor been set to zero according to manufacturer's instructions?
4. Is intrauterine pressure catheter properly secured to woman?
5. Is baseline resting tone of uterus documented?

FHR, Fetal heart rate; *UA*, uterine activity.
From Miller, L., Miller, D., & Cypher, R. (2017). *Mosby's pocket guide to fetal monitoring: A multidisciplinary approach* (8th ed.). St. Louis: Elsevier.

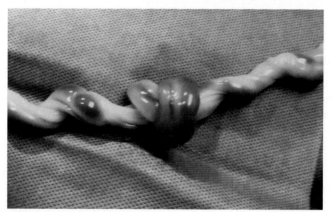

Fig. 18.17 Umbilical Cord Containing a True Knot. (Courtesy Carshawna Knighton, Memphis, TN.)

The nurse providing care to a woman in labor has many important responsibilities. These include assessing FHR and UA patterns, implementing independent nursing interventions, documenting observations and actions according to established standards of care, and reporting abnormal patterns to the obstetric care provider (e.g., physician or certified nurse-midwife).

Current technology has made access to and communication regarding electronic FHR tracings much more convenient for health care

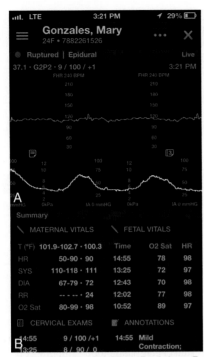

Fig. 18.19 Providers Can Access Near Real-time Fetal Heart Rate (FHR) Tracings and Review Client Data Using Their Mobile Phones. (A) FHR tracing, including MHR. (B) Client listing. (© 2017 AirStrip Technologies. All rights reserved. iPhone is a registered trademark of Apple Inc.)

BOX 18.8 Management of Abnormal Fetal Heart Rate Patterns

Basic Interventions
- Administer oxygen by nonrebreather face mask at a rate of 10 L/min for approximately 15-30 min.
- Assist woman to a side-lying (lateral) position.
- Increase maternal blood volume by increasing rate of primary IV infusion.

Interventions for Specific Problems
- Maternal hypotension
  - Increase rate of primary IV infusion.
  - Change to lateral or Trendelenburg positioning.
  - Administer ephedrine or phenylephrine if other measures are unsuccessful in increasing blood pressure.
- Uterine tachysystole
  - Reduce or discontinue dose of any uterine stimulants in use (e.g., oxytocin [Pitocin]).
  - Administer uterine relaxant (tocolytic) (e.g., terbutaline [Brethine]).
- Abnormal fetal heart rate pattern during second stage of labor
  - Use open-glottis pushing.
  - Use fewer pushing efforts during each contraction.
  - Make individual pushing efforts shorter.
  - Push only with every other or every third contraction.
  - Push only with a perceived urge to push (in women with regional anesthesia).

IV, Intravenous.

---

providers. Many hospitals use central monitor displays, which provide the opportunity to view the tracings of several women at the same time at the nurses' station or in other locations on the nursing unit. Health care providers can also access the FHR tracings of one woman or several clients from remote locations, including office and home. It is even possible to access FHR tracings and other client data using mobile phones (Fig. 18.19) (Miller et al., 2017).

Electronic Fetal Monitoring Pattern Recognition and Interpretation

Nurses must evaluate many factors to determine whether an FHR pattern is normal or abnormal. They evaluate these factors based on the presence of other obstetric complications, progress in labor, and use of analgesia or anesthesia. They also must consider the estimated time interval until birth. Therefore, interventions are based on clinical judgment of a complex, integrated process. Several different organizations offer EFM courses for nurses and other health care professionals. It is also possible to earn certification in EFM.

LEGAL TIP

Fetal Monitoring Standards

Nurses who care for women during labor and birth are legally responsible for correctly interpreting FHR patterns, initiating appropriate nursing interventions based on those patterns, and documenting the outcomes of those interventions. Perinatal nurses are responsible for the timely notification of the physician or nurse-midwife in the event of abnormal FHR patterns. They also are responsible for initiating the institutional chain of command should differences in opinion arise among health care providers concerning the interpretation of the FHR pattern and the intervention required.

Categorizing Fetal Heart Rate Tracings

As previously mentioned, a three-tier system of categorizing FHR tracings is recommended (see Box 18.1). Category I FHR tracings are normal and strongly predictive of normal fetal acid-base status at the time of observation. These tracings may be followed in a routine manner and do not require any specific action. Category II FHR tracings are indeterminate. This category includes all tracings that do not meet category I or category III criteria. Category II tracings require continued observation and evaluation. Category III FHR tracings are abnormal. Immediate evaluation and prompt intervention are required when these patterns are identified (Macones et al., 2008).

Nursing Management of Abnormal Patterns

The five essential components of the FHR tracing that must be evaluated regularly are baseline rate, baseline variability, accelerations, decelerations, and changes or trends over time. Whenever one of these five essential components is assessed as abnormal, corrective measures must be taken immediately. The purpose of these actions is to improve fetal oxygenation (Miller et al., 2017). The term *intrauterine resuscitation* is sometimes used to refer to specific interventions initiated when an abnormal FHR pattern is noted. Basic corrective measures include providing supplemental oxygen, instituting maternal position changes, and increasing intravenous (IV) fluid administration. These interventions are implemented to improve uterine and intervillous space blood flow and increase maternal oxygenation and cardiac output (Miller et al.). Box 18.8 lists basic interventions to improve maternal and fetal oxygenation status.

Depending on the underlying cause of the abnormal FHR pattern, other interventions such as correcting maternal hypotension, reducing UA, and altering second-stage pushing techniques also may be instituted (Miller et al., 2017). Box 18.8 lists interventions for these specific problems. Some of the items listed are not independent nursing interventions. Any medications administered, for example, must be authorized either through inclusion in a specific unit protocol or by a written or verbal order. Some interventions are specific to the FHR pattern. (See Table 18.3 and Boxes 18.5 and 18.6 for nursing interventions for tachycardia, late decelerations, and variable decelerations.) Based on the FHR response to these interventions, the obstetric health care provider decides whether additional interventions should be instituted or whether immediate vaginal or cesarean birth should be performed.

Other Methods of Assessment and Intervention

A major shortcoming of EFM is its high rate of false-positive results. Even the most abnormal patterns are poorly predictive of neonatal morbidity. Therefore, other methods of assessment have been developed to evaluate fetal status. Fetal scalp stimulation, vibroacoustic stimulation, and umbilical cord acid-base determination are frequently performed assessments. Fetal scalp blood sampling is another available assessment technique. Amnioinfusion and tocolytic therapy are interventions often used in an attempt to improve abnormal FHR patterns.

Assessment Techniques

Fetal scalp stimulation and vibroacoustic stimulation. Studies have shown that an FHR acceleration in response to digital or vibroacoustic stimulation was highly predictive of a normal scalp blood pH. The two methods of fetal stimulation used most often in clinical practice are scalp stimulation (using digital pressure during a vaginal examination) and vibroacoustic stimulation (using an artificial larynx or fetal acoustic stimulation device on the maternal abdomen over the fetal head continuously for 1 to 5 seconds). The desired result of these stimulation methods is an acceleration in the FHR of at least 15 beats/min for at least 15 seconds (Miller et al., 2017). A FHR acceleration indicates the absence of metabolic acidemia. If the fetus does not respond to stimulation with an acceleration, fetal compromise is not necessarily indicated; however, further evaluation of fetal well-being is needed. Fetal stimulation should be performed at times when the FHR is at baseline. Neither fetal scalp nor vibroacoustic stimulation should be instituted if FHR decelerations or bradycardia are present (Miller et al.).

Umbilical cord blood acid-base determination. In assessing the immediate condition of the newborn after birth, a sample of cord blood is a useful adjunct to the Apgar score, especially if there has been an abnormal or confusing FHR tracing during labor or neonatal depression at birth. Generally the procedure is performed by withdrawing blood from both the umbilical artery and the umbilical vein. Both samples are then tested for pH, carbon dioxide pressure (Pco_2), oxygen pressure (Po_2), and base deficit or base excess. Umbilical arterial values reflect fetal condition, whereas umbilical vein values indicate placental function (Miller et al., 2017).

ACOG and AAP (2015/2019) suggest obtaining umbilical artery cord blood values when a newborn has an Apgar score of 5 or above at 5 minutes of age. Normal umbilical artery and vein cord blood values are listed in Table 18.4. Normal findings preclude the presence of acidemia at or immediately before birth. If acidemia is present (e.g., pH <7.20), the type of acidemia is determined (respiratory, metabolic, or mixed) by analyzing the blood gas values (Table 18.5) (Miller et al., 2017).

Fetal scalp blood sampling. Fetal scalp blood sampling is performed by obtaining a blood sample from the fetal scalp through the dilated cervix after the membranes have ruptured. Its use is limited by many factors, including the requirement for cervical dilation and membrane rupture, technical difficulty of the procedure, need for repetitive

TABLE 18.4 Approximate Normal Values for Cord Blood

Vessel	pH	Pco_2	Po_2	Base Deficit
Artery	7.2-7.3	45-55	15-25	<12
Vein	7.3-7.4	35-45	25-35	<12

From Miller, L., Miller, D., & Cypher, R. (2017). *Mosby's pocket guide to fetal monitoring: A multidisciplinary approach* (8th ed.). St. Louis: Elsevier.

TABLE 18.5 Types of Acidemia

Value	Respiratory	Metabolic	Mixed
pH	<7.20	<7.20	<7.20
Pco_2	Elevated	Normal	Elevated
Base deficit	<12 mmol/L	≥12 mmol/L	≥12 mmol/L

From Miller, L., Miller, D., & Cypher, R. (2017). *Mosby's pocket guide to fetal monitoring: A multidisciplinary approach* (8th ed.). St. Louis: Elsevier.

pH determinations, and uncertainty regarding interpretation and application of results. Fetal scalp blood sampling is now seldom used in the United States but remains a common practice in many other countries (Miller et al., 2017).

Interventions

Amnioinfusion. Amnioinfusion is infusion of room-temperature isotonic fluid (usually normal saline or lactated Ringer solution) into the uterine cavity if the volume of amniotic fluid is low. Without the buffer of amniotic fluid, the umbilical cord can easily become compressed during contractions or fetal movement, diminishing the flow of blood between the placenta and fetus. The purpose of amnioinfusion is to relieve intermittent umbilical cord compression that results in variable decelerations and transient fetal hypoxemia by restoring the amniotic fluid volume to a normal or near-normal level. Amnioinfusion has no known effect on late decelerations and is no longer recommended as a means to dilute meconium-stained amniotic fluid (Miller et al., 2017). Women with an abnormally small amount of amniotic fluid (oligohydramnios) or no amniotic fluid (anhydramnios) are candidates for this procedure. Conditions that can result in oligohydramnios or anhydramnios include uteroplacental insufficiency and prelabor rupture of membranes.

Risks of amnioinfusion are overdistention of the uterine cavity and increased uterine tone. Fluid is administered through an IUPC by either gravity flow or an infusion pump. Usually a bolus of fluid is administered over 20 to 30 minutes; then the infusion is slowed to a maintenance rate. Likely no more than 1000 mL of fluid will need to be administered. The fluid can be warmed for the preterm fetus by infusing it through a blood warmer (Miller et al., 2017).

Intensity and frequency of UCs should be continually assessed during the procedure. The recorded uterine resting tone during amnioinfusion appears higher than normal because of resistance to outflow and turbulence at the end of the catheter. Uterine resting tone should not exceed 40 mm Hg during the procedure. The amount of vaginal fluid return must be estimated and documented during amnioinfusion to prevent overdistention of the uterus. The volume of fluid returned should be approximately the same as the amount infused (Miller et al., 2017).

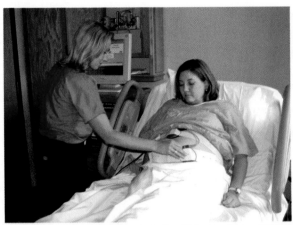

Fig. 18.20 Nurse Explains Electronic Fetal Monitoring as Ultrasound Transducer Monitors the Fetal Heart Rate. (Courtesy Julie Perry Nelson, Loveland, CO.)

Tocolytic therapy. Tocolysis (relaxation of the uterus) can be achieved through the administration of medications that inhibit UCs. This therapy can be used along with other interventions because excessive UA is a common cause of interrupted fetal oxygenation. Tocolysis improves blood flow through the placenta by inhibiting UCs. It may be ordered by the obstetric health care provider when other interventions to reduce UA, such as maternal position change and discontinuance of an oxytocin infusion, have not diminished the UCs effectively. Tocolytics are often administered when women are having excessive UCs spontaneously. They are also frequently administered after a decision for cesarean birth has been made while preparations for surgery are under way. A commonly used tocolytic in these situations is terbutaline (Brethine) (Miller et al., 2017). If the FHR and UC patterns improve, the woman may be allowed to continue labor; if no improvement is seen, immediate cesarean birth may be needed.

CLIENT AND FAMILY TEACHING

Although the use of EFM can be reassuring to many parents, it can be a source of anxiety to some. Therefore, the nurse must be particularly sensitive and respond appropriately to the emotional, informational, and comfort needs of the woman in labor and those of her family (Fig. 18.20 and Box 18.9).

Part of the nurse's role includes partnering with other members of the interprofessional health care team, the woman, and her family to achieve an optimal birthing experience. The nurse provides education and support for the woman and her family regarding the labor and birth process, use of equipment, breathing and relaxation techniques, and pain management options.

The nurse can help with two factors that have an effect on fetal status: positioning and pushing. The nurse should enlist the woman's cooperation in avoiding the supine position because it can cause hypotension, which impairs placental perfusion and fetal oxygenation. Instead, the woman should be encouraged to maintain the side-lying or semi-Fowler position with a lateral tilt to the uterus. In addition, the nurse should instruct the woman to keep her mouth and glottis open and to let air escape from her lungs as she pushes. Both of these interventions help to improve fetal oxygenation. See Chapter 19 for further discussion of maternal positioning and pushing techniques.

DOCUMENTATION

Clear and accurate documentation in the woman's medical record is essential. Each FHR and UA assessment must be documented completely. More and more hospitals are moving to use of the electronic medical record and computerized charting. With computerized charting, each required component usually appears on the screen so it will be addressed routinely. Computerized charting often includes forced choices that greatly increase the use of standardized FHR terminology by all members of the health care team. In the past, nurses were often encouraged to chart both on the monitor strip and in the medical record. However, charting directly on the monitor strip is unnecessary when an electronic medical record is used (Fig. 18.21). Any information that is handwritten on the monitor strip will not be recorded in the computer record. Furthermore, given that the EFM tracing is stored on a computer, the paper strips are destroyed after the woman is discharged. No permanent record of the handwritten charting exists.

In institutions that still use a paper chart, documentation on the woman's monitor strip is started before initiating monitoring and consists of identifying information plus other relevant data. This documentation is continued and updated according to institutional protocol as monitoring continues and labor progresses.

In some institutions, observations noted and interventions implemented are recorded on the monitor strip to produce a

Fetal Monitor Integration

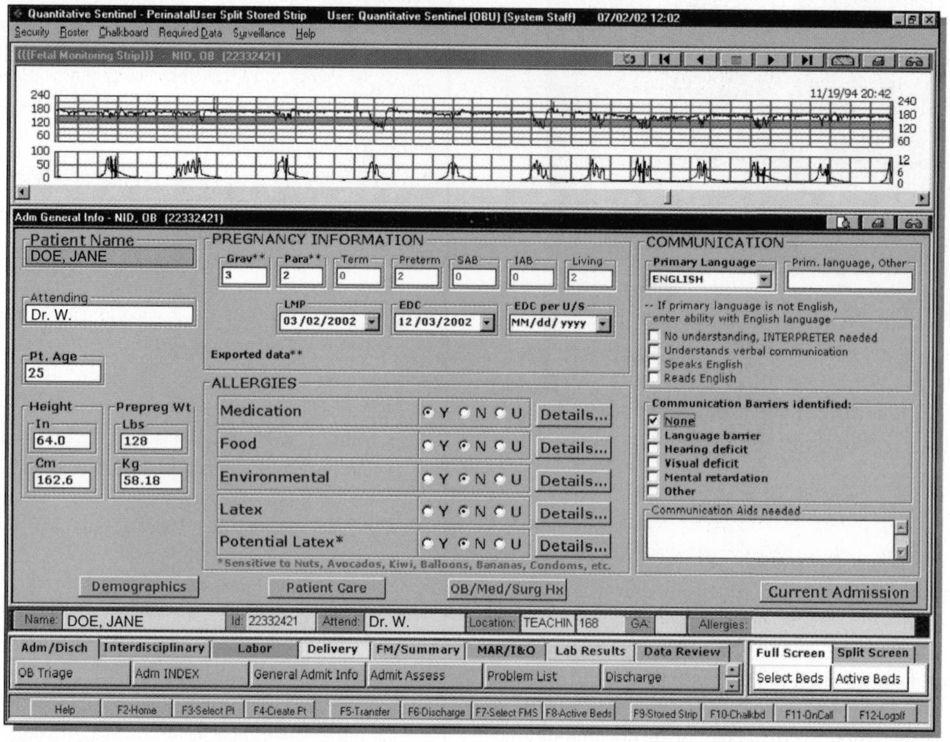

Fig. 18.21 With Integration of the Fetal Monitor Tracing into the Electronic Medical Record, the Nurse Can View the Fetal Tracing While Charting. (Courtesy General Electric Healthcare Technologies, Barrington, IL.)

comprehensive document that chronicles the course of labor and the care rendered. In other institutions this documentation is confined to the labor flow record. Advocates of documenting on both the medical record and the EFM strip cite as advantages of this approach the ease of writing directly on the strip while at the bedside and the improved accuracy in documenting critical events and the interventions implemented. Others believe that charting on the EFM strip constitutes duplicate documentation of the same information noted in the medical record and thus it is unnecessary additional paperwork for the nurse.

A disadvantage of documenting on both the EFM strip and the medical record is that the times noted for events and interventions on the EFM strip frequently do not correlate with what is later documented in the medical record. These inaccuracies can lead people involved in the retrospective review process carried out during litigation to infer that documentation errors have occurred. Therefore, if institutional policy mandates documentation both on the monitor strip and in the medical record, the nurse must make sure the times and notations of events and interventions recorded in each place correspond with one another..

KEY POINTS

- Fetal well-being during labor is gauged by the response of the FHR to UCs.
- Standardized definitions for many common FHR patterns have been adopted for use in clinical practice by the ACNM, ACOG, and AWHONN.
- The five essential components of the FHR tracing are baseline rate, baseline variability, accelerations, decelerations, and changes or trends over time.
- The monitoring of fetal well-being includes FHR and UA assessment, and assessment of maternal vital signs.
- The FHR can be monitored by either IA or EFM. The FHR and UA can be assessed by EFM using either the external or internal monitoring mode.

- Assessing FHR and UA patterns, implementing independent nursing interventions, and reporting abnormal patterns to the physician or nurse-midwife are the nurse's responsibilities.
- AWHONN and ACOG have established and published health care professional standards and guidelines for FHR monitoring.
- The emotional, informational, and comfort needs of the woman and her family must be addressed when the mother and her fetus are being monitored.
- Documentation of fetal assessment is initiated and updated according to institutional protocol.

REFERENCES

American Academy of Pediatrics and American College of Obstetricians and Gynecologists. (2017). *Guidelines for perinatal care* (8th ed.). Washington, DC: American College of Obstetricians and Gynecologists.

American College of Obstetricians and Gynecologists. (2009, reaffirmed 2017). Practice bulletin no. 106: Intrapartum fetal heart rate monitoring: Nomenclature, interpretation, and general management principles. *Obstetrics & Gynecology*, 114(1), 192–202.

American College of Obstetricians and Gynecologists and American Academy of Pediatrics. (2015, reaffirmed 2019). Committee opinion no. 644: The Apgar score. *Obstetrics & Gynecology*, 126(4), e52–e55.

Association of Women's Health, Obstetric and Neonatal Nurses. (2015a). AWHONN position statement: Fetal heart monitoring. *Journal of Obstetric, Gynecologic & Neonatal Nursing*, 44(5), 683–686.

Association of Women's Health, Obstetric and Neonatal Nurses. (2015b). *Fetal heart monitoring principles and practice* (5th ed.). Dubuque, IA: Kendall/Hunt.

Cunningham, F., Leveno, K., Bloom, S., et al. (2018). *Williams obstetrics* (25th ed.). New York: McGraw Hill Education.

Lyndon, A., O'Brien-Abel, N., & Simpson, K. (2014). Fetal assessment during labor. In K. R. Simpson, & P. Creehan (Eds.), *AWHONN's perinatal nursing* (4th ed.). Philadelphia, PA: Lippincott Williams & Wilkins.

Macones, G., Hankins, G., Spong, C., et al. (2008). The 2008 National Institute of Child Health and Human Development workshop report on electronic fetal monitoring: Update on definitions, interpretation, and research guidelines. *Journal of Obstetric, Gynecologic & Neonatal Nursing*, 37(5), 510–515.

Miller, D. (2017). Intrapartum fetal evaluation. In S. G. Gabbe, J. R. Niebyl, J. L. Simpson, et al. (Eds.), *Obstetrics: Normal and problem pregnancies* (7th ed.). Philadelphia: Elsevier.

Miller, L., Miller, D., & Cypher, R. (2017). *Mosby's pocket guide to fetal monitoring: A multidisciplinary approach* (8th ed.). St. Louis: Elsevier.

National Institute of Child Health and Human Development Research Planning Workshop. (1997). Electronic fetal heart rate monitoring: Research guidelines for interpretation. *American Journal of Obstetrics & Gynecology*, 177(6), 1385–1390.

19

Nursing Care of the Family During Labor and Birth

Renee Oakley Spain

 http://evolve.elsevier.com/Lowdermilk/MWHC/

LEARNING OBJECTIVES

- Review the data included in the initial assessment of the woman in labor.
- Describe the ongoing assessment of maternal progress during the first, second, third, and fourth stages of labor.
- Interpret the physical and psychosocial findings indicative of maternal progress during labor.
- Describe fetal assessment during labor.
- Identify signs of developing complications during labor and birth.
- Incorporate evidence-based nursing interventions into a plan of care relevant to each stage of labor.

- Recognize the importance of support (partner, family member, friend, nurse, doula) in fostering maternal confidence and facilitating the progress of labor and birth.
- Analyze the influence of cultural and religious beliefs and practices on labor and birth.
- Describe the roles and responsibilities of the nurse during emergency birth.
- Evaluate the effect of perineal trauma on the woman's reproductive and sexual health.

The labor and birth processes are natural phenomena. The American College of Nurse-Midwives (ACNM) defines normal physiologic birth as "one that is powered by the innate human capacity of the woman and fetus" (ACNM, 2012, p. 2). Physiologic labor and birth have positive long- and short-term health implications for both mother and baby. Even in the event of complications, support of physiologic labor and birth has the potential to enhance positive outcomes (ACNM). This is an exciting and potentially anxious time for the woman, her partner, and significant others. In a relatively short period of time, they experience profound changes in their lives. Birth may take place in the hospital, birth center, or home setting or unexpectedly at any number of locations. The woman and her significant others may be cared for by an interprofessional team of caregivers, including nurses, doulas, nurse-midwives, and physicians. During labor and birth, nurses provide comprehensive care for women and families by using evidence-based knowledge of physiologic and psychosocial processes and selected pharmacologic and nonpharmacologic measures (see the Community Activity box).

For most women labor begins with regular uterine contractions, continues with hours of hard work during cervical dilation and birth, and ends as the woman begins to recover physically from birth as she and her significant others begin the attachment process with the newborn. Nursing care management focuses on assessment and support of the woman and her partner throughout labor and birth as well as assessment of fetal well-being and response to labor. The goal of nursing care is to ensure the best possible outcome for all involved. The focus of this chapter is on nursing care that facilitates the normal birth process.

🏠 COMMUNITY ACTIVITY

- Compare and contrast childbirth education classes offered by various groups in the community (hospital, birth center, practice groups, independent practitioners). Visit the website of a hospital that offers childbirth education classes in your community. Review the client information about the childbirth classes. If you are not able to find this information on their website, contact one of the instructors. What is the philosophy of the class? Is a specific childbirth method taught? Are the classes offered by nurses, nurse-midwives, physicians, or someone else? How long are the classes—one class versus a series of classes? What information is covered? Are significant others welcome to attend? Is breastfeeding information given? Is skin-to-skin contact immediately following birth discussed? How much of the information relates to hospital policies and practices rather than to childbirth coping strategies and newborn care? Are women encouraged to develop a birth plan?
- Visit the website of a community group or birth center offering childbirth education classes in your city or state that teaches a specific method, such as Lamaze or Bradley. If you cannot find the information on the website, contact one of the instructors. What is the philosophy of the method? What are the credentials and education of the instructor? Are the classes offered as a series or as one-time events only? Are significant others and children welcome? Where do women/families attending these classes plan to give birth? Are women encouraged to develop a birth plan?

FIRST STAGE OF LABOR

The **first stage of labor** begins with the onset of regular uterine contractions and ends with complete cervical effacement and dilation. Traditionally the first stage of labor was considered to comprise three phases: the *latent phase* (through 3 cm of dilation), the *active phase* (4 to 7 cm of dilation), and the *transition phase* (8 to 10 cm of dilation). However, these definitions have changed on the basis of research findings. After studying the labors of thousands of contemporary women, researchers have concluded that they differ in several characteristics from the women who gave birth more than half a century ago, when E. A. Friedman published his findings regarding the length of "normal" labor. Contemporary women tend to be older and heavier than their earlier counterparts. They progress more slowly during the active phase of labor than was previously believed and experience longer labors. Active labor begins at 6 cm for both nulliparous and multiparous women. During the early phase of first-stage labor, nulliparous and multiparous women progress at similar rates. After reaching a cervical dilation of 6 cm, however, multiparous women progress more rapidly (Hanson & VandeVusse, 2014; Kelly, Swart, & Baird, 2017; Kilpatrick & Garrison, 2017).

Therefore the first stage of labor is now divided into only two phases. The **latent phase** extends from the onset of labor—characterized by regular, painful uterine contractions that cause cervical change—to the beginning of the active phase, when cervical dilation occurs more rapidly. The **active phase** is defined as the period during which the greatest rate of cervical dilation occurs, which begins at 6 cm and ends with complete cervical dilation at 10 cm (Kelly et al., 2017; Kilpatrick & Garrison, 2017).

CARE MANAGEMENT

Many nulliparous women planning to give birth in a hospital or birth center may seek admission in the latent (early) phase because they have not experienced labor before and are unsure of the "right" time to come in. Multiparous women may not present to the birth center or hospital until they are in the active phase of the first stage of labor. Even though no two labors are identical, women who have given birth before are often less anxious about the process unless their previous experience was negative. Women who have received group prenatal care (vs standard prenatal care) are more likely to present to the birth setting in the active phase of the first stage of labor regardless of parity (Tilden, Emeis, Caughey, et al., 2016).

Assessment

Assessment begins at the first contact with the woman, whether by telephone or in person. Some women may call the hospital or birth center first for validation as to whether they should come in for evaluation or admission or whether they should remain at home. Many hospitals, however, discourage the nurse from giving advice by telephone regarding what to do because of legal liability. Nurses are often instructed to tell women who call with questions to call their nurse-midwife or physician or to come to the hospital if they feel the need to be checked. Telephone triage should be done per agency policy. A pregnant woman may first call her nurse-midwife or physician or go to the hospital or birth center while in false labor or early in the latent phase of the first stage of labor. Often,

TEACHING FOR SELF-MANAGEMENT
How to Distinguish True Labor From False Labor

True Labor
Contractions
- Occur regularly, becoming stronger, lasting longer, and occurring closer together
- Become more intense with walking
- Are usually felt in the lower back, radiating to the lower portion of the abdomen
- Continue despite use of comfort measures

False Labor
Contractions
- Occur irregularly or become regular only temporarily
- Often stop with walking or position change
- Can be felt in the back or the abdomen above the umbilicus
- Can often be stopped through the use of comfort measures

when women have presented to the labor and birth unit and are found not to be in active labor, they are reluctant to go home (Mikolajczyk, Zhang, Grewal, et al., 2016; Neal, Lamp, Buck, et al., 2014). Teaching regarding the stages of labor and the signs indicating its onset should occur during the third trimester of pregnancy. (See the Teaching for Self-Management box: How to Distinguish True Labor From False Labor.)

If the woman lives near the hospital or birth center and has adequate support and transportation, she may be encouraged to stay at home or return home to allow labor to progress (e.g., until the uterine contractions are more frequent and intense). The ideal setting at this time for the woman at low risk for obstetric complications is usually the familiar environment of her home, where she can move around freely and eat and drink at will. However, the woman who lives at a considerable distance from the hospital or birth center who lacks adequate support and transportation or has a history of rapid labors may be admitted in latent labor. The same measures used by the woman at home should be offered to the woman admitted in early labor. Nonpharmacologic strategies can help the woman rest and even sleep, especially if false or early labor is occurring at night. Ambulation, showers, mindful meditation, acupressure, partner support, massage, and nutrition have all been studied as strategies for early labor management (Paul, Yount, Breman, et al., 2017). One innovative approach is an early-labor lounge, a room for women who are in early labor and wish to remain on site. Women utilizing the early-labor lounge remain there as outpatients until they are admitted or discharged (Paul, et al.).

When the woman arrives at the birth center or hospital perinatal unit, assessment is the top priority (Fig. 19.1). The nurse first performs a screening assessment by using the techniques of interview and physical assessment and reviews the laboratory and diagnostic test findings to determine the health status of the woman and her fetus and the progress of her labor. The nurse also notifies the nurse-midwife or physician of his or her findings. If the woman is admitted, a detailed systems assessment is done.

When the woman is admitted to a hospital, she is usually moved from an observation or triage area to a labor room; a labor, delivery, and recovery (LDR) room; or a labor, delivery, recovery, and postpartum (LDRP) room. If the woman wishes, the nurse can include her partner, family member, or other support person in the assessment and

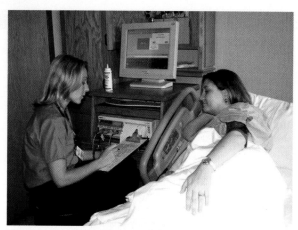

Fig. 19.1 Woman Being Assessed for Admission to the Labor and Birth Unit. (Courtesy Julie Perry Nelson, Loveland, CO.)

admission process. The nurse can direct significant others not participating in this process to the appropriate waiting area. In the hospital setting the woman undresses and puts on her own gown or a hospital gown. The nurse places an identification band on the woman's wrist. Her personal belongings are put away safely or given to family members, according to agency policy. Women who have participated in expectant parents' classes often bring a birth bag with them. The nurse then shows the woman and her partner the layout and operation of the unit and room, how to use the call light and telephone system, how to adjust lighting in the room, and the different bed positions.

The nurse assures the woman that she is in competent, caring hands and that she and those to whom she gives permission can ask questions related to her care and status and that of her fetus at any time during labor. The nurse can minimize the woman's anxiety by explaining terms commonly used during labor. The woman's interest, response, and prior experience will guide the depth and breadth of these explanations.

Most hospitals have specific forms, whether paper or electronic, used to obtain important assessment information when a woman in labor is being evaluated or admitted (Fig. 19.2A and B). More and more hospitals now use an electronic medical record; almost all charting is done by computer. Sources of data include the prenatal record, initial interview, physical examination to determine baseline physiologic parameters (e.g., vital signs), laboratory and diagnostic test results, select psychosocial and cultural factors, and clinical evaluation of labor status.

Prenatal Data

The nurse reviews the prenatal record to identify the woman's individual needs and risks. Copies of prenatal records are generally filed in the hospital's perinatal unit at some time during the woman's pregnancy (usually in the third trimester) or accessed by computer so that they will be readily available on admission. If the woman has had no prenatal care or her prenatal records are unavailable, the nurse must obtain certain baseline information. If the woman is having discomfort, the nurse should ask questions between contractions when the woman can concentrate more fully on her answers. At times the partner or support person or persons may have to be secondary sources of essential information. According to the Health

Insurance Portability and Accountability Act (HIPAA), the woman must give permission for other individuals to be involved in the exchange of information regarding her care. Ideally, this permission should be obtained during pregnancy and the signed form included in her health records.

Knowing the woman's age is important so that the nurse can individualize care to the needs of her age group. For example, a 14-year-old adolescent and a 40-year-old woman have different but specific needs, and their ages place them at risk for different problems. Accurate height and weight measurements are also important. Other factors to consider are the woman's general health status, current medical conditions or allergies, respiratory status, and previous surgical procedures.

The nurse should carefully review the woman's prenatal records, taking note of her obstetric history, including gravidity, parity, and problems such as history of vaginal bleeding, gestational hypertension, anemia, pregestational or gestational diabetes, infections (e.g., bacterial, viral, sexually transmitted) and immunodeficiency status. In addition, the expected date of birth (EDB) should be confirmed. Other important data found in the prenatal record include patterns of maternal weight gain; physiologic measurements such as maternal vital signs (blood pressure, temperature, pulse, respirations); fundal height; baseline fetal heart rate (FHR); and laboratory and diagnostic test results. See Table 14.1 for a list of common prenatal laboratory tests. Common diagnostic and fetal assessment tests performed prenatally include amniocentesis, nonstress testing (NST), biophysical profile (BPP), and ultrasound examination. See Chapter 26 for more information.

If this labor and birth experience is not the woman's first, the nurse must note the characteristics of her previous experiences. This information includes the duration of previous labors; the types of pain relief measures, including anesthesia used; the type of birth (e.g., spontaneous vaginal, forceps-assisted, vacuum-assisted, or cesarean birth); and the condition of the newborn. The nurse must explore the woman's perception of her previous labor and birth experiences because this perception may influence her attitude toward her current experience.

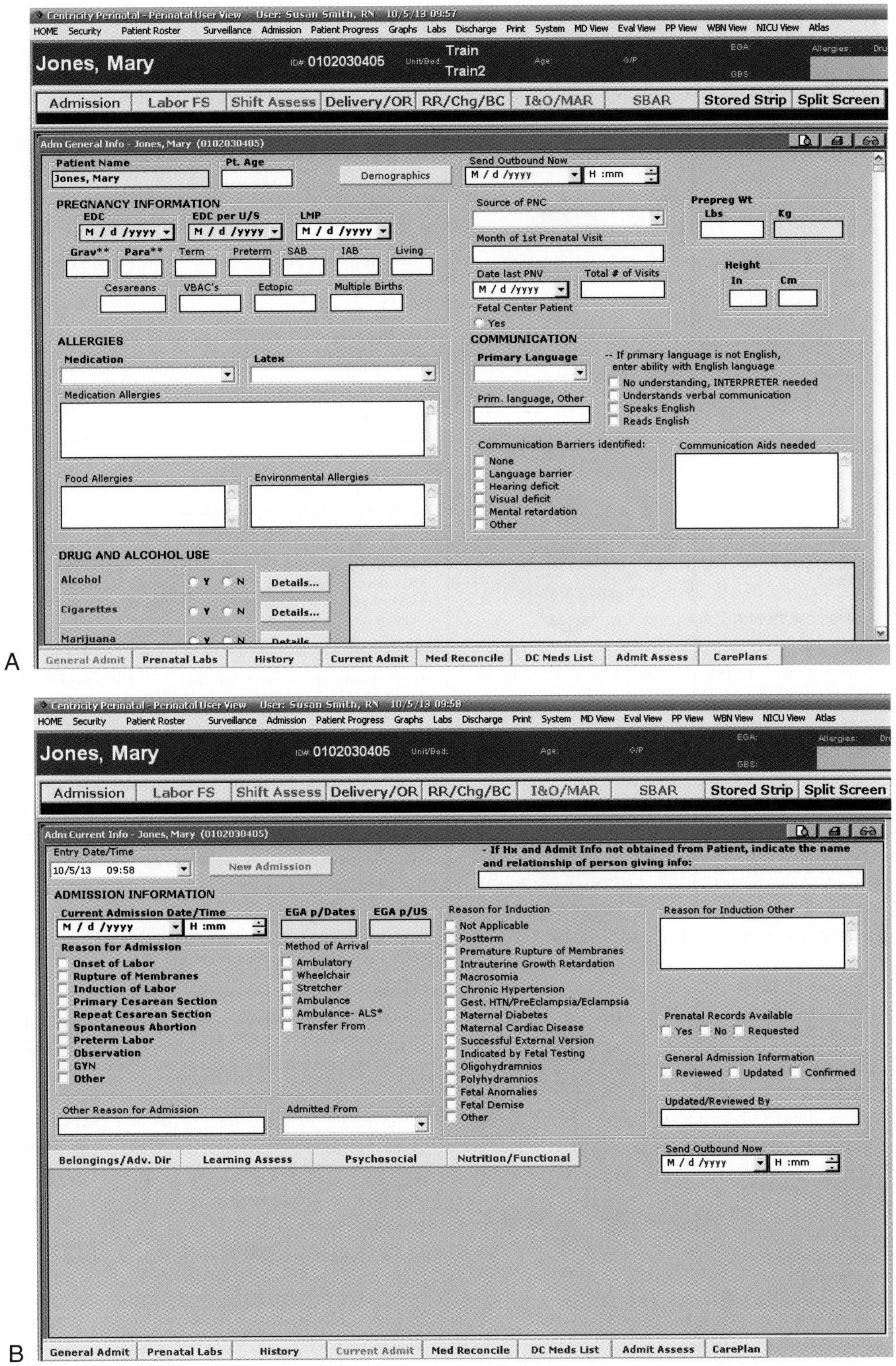

Fig. 19.2 Admission Screens in an Electronic Health Record. (A) General admission screen. (B) Current admission screen. (Courtesy Kitty Cashion, RN-BC, MSN, Memphis, TN.)

Interview

The woman's primary reason for coming to the hospital is determined in the interview. Her primary reason may be, for example, suspicion of ruptured membranes or desire for a period of observation because she is unsure about the onset of labor. Labor triage units offer time without official hospital admission to evaluate for labor or other concerns

(Paul et al., 2017). Fig 19.3 shows the Maternal Fetal Triage Index developed by the Association of Women's Health, Obstetric and Neonatal Nurses (AWHONN), a tool for screening pregnant women who present to a hospital for care (Ruhl, Scheich, Onokpise, & Bingham, 2015).

During the triage process, the nurse must determine the status of the woman's amniotic membranes. If the woman has noticed a gush or

Maternal Fetal Triage Index (MFTI)

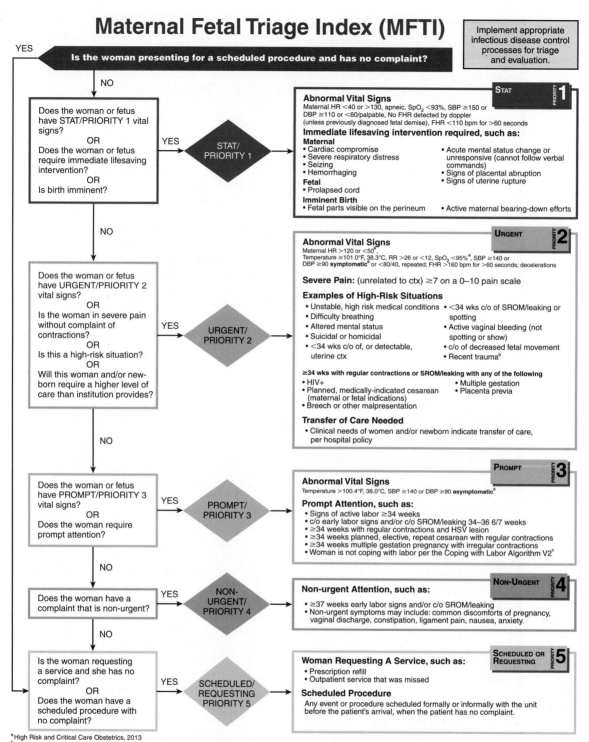

Fig. 19.3 Maternal Fetal Triage Index (MFTI). (From Ruhl, C., Scheich, B., Onokpise, B., & Bingham, D. (2015). Interrater reliability of testing the maternal triage index. *Journal of Obstetric, Gynecologic, and Neonatal Nursing, 46*(6), 710–716.)

leakage of fluid, the membranes may have ruptured (spontaneous rupture of membranes [SROM]). If there has been a discharge that may be amniotic fluid, in many instances a sterile speculum examination and Nitrazine (pH) and *fern tests* can determine whether the membranes have ruptured (Box 19.1).

Bloody show is distinguished from vaginal bleeding by the fact that it is pink and feels sticky because of its mucoid nature. There is very little bloody show in the beginning, but the amount increases with effacement and dilation of the cervix. A woman may report a small amount of brownish-to-bloody discharge that may be attributed to

BOX 19.1 Procedure: Tests for Rupture of Membranes

Nitrazine Test for pH
- Explain procedure to the woman or couple.

Procedure
- Perform hand hygiene and put on sterile gloves.
- Use a cotton-tipped applicator impregnated with Nitrazine dye for determining pH (differentiates amniotic fluid, which is slightly alkaline, from urine and purulent material [pus], which are acidic).
- Dip the cotton-tipped applicator deep into the vagina to sample fluid (this procedure may be performed during speculum examination).

Read Results
- Membranes probably intact: identifies vaginal and most body fluids that are acidic:

Yellow	pH 5.0
Olive-yellow	pH 5.5
Olive-green	pH 6.0

- Membranes probably ruptured: identifies amniotic fluid that is alkaline:

Blue-green	pH 6.5
Blue-gray	pH 7.0
Deep blue	pH 7.5

- Realize that false test results are possible because of presence of bloody show or semen, or insufficient amount of amniotic fluid.
- Provide pericare as needed.
- Remove gloves and perform hand hygiene.

Document Results
- Results are reported as positive or negative.

Test for Ferning or Fern Pattern
- Explain the procedure to the woman or couple.

Procedure
- Perform hand hygiene and put on sterile gloves, obtain a sample of fluid (usually during a sterile speculum examination).
- Spread a drop of fluid from the vagina on clean glass slide with a sterile cotton-tipped applicator.
- Allow the fluid to dry.
- Examine the slide under the microscope; observe for the appearance of ferning (a frond-like crystalline pattern). Do not confuse this with the cervical mucus test, when high levels of estrogen also cause ferning.
- Observe for absence of ferning (alerts staff to possibility that amount of specimen was inadequate or that specimen was urine, vaginal discharge, or blood).
- Provide continuing care as needed.
- Remove gloves and perform hand hygiene.

Document Results
- Results are reported as positive or negative.

---

cervical trauma resulting from vaginal examination or coitus (intercourse) within the preceding 48 hours.

Assessing the woman's respiratory status is important in case general anesthesia is needed in an emergency. The nurse determines this status by auscultating the lung fields and asking the woman if she has a "cold" or related symptoms (e.g., stuffy nose, sore throat, or cough). History of respiratory illnesses such as asthma should also be noted. The status of allergies, including allergies to latex and tape, and medications routinely used in obstetrics such as opioids (e.g., meperidine [Demerol], fentanyl [Sublimaze], remifentanil [Ultiva], and nalbuphine [Nubain]), local anesthetic agents (e.g., bupivacaine, lidocaine, ropivacaine), and antiseptics (Betadine) is reviewed. Some allergic responses cause swelling of the mucous membranes of the respiratory tract, which could interfere with breathing and the administration of inhalation anesthesia. Because vomiting and subsequent aspiration into the respiratory tract can complicate an otherwise normal labor, the nurse records the time and type of the woman's most recent solid and liquid intake.

The nurse obtains any information not found in the prenatal record during the admission assessment. Pertinent data include the birth plan (Box 19.2), the type of pain management (including nonpharmacologic comfort measures) preferred, the choice of infant feeding method, and the name of the pediatric health care provider. The nurse inquires about the woman's preparation for childbirth, the support person or family members whose presence is desired during labor and birth and their availability, and cultural expectations and needs. The nurse also asks about the woman's use of alcohol, drugs, and tobacco before or during pregnancy. The nurse reviews the birth plan. If there is no written plan, the nurse helps the woman to formulate a birth plan by describing the options available and determining the woman's wishes and preferences. As caregiver and advocate, the nurse integrates the woman's desires into the nursing care plan while explaining what may or may not be possible to meet all her expectations given the birthing facility's policies. The nurse also prepares

BOX 19.2 The Birth Plan

The birth plan should include the woman's or couple's preferences related to
- Presence of birth companions such as the partner, older children, parents, friends, and doula, and the role each will play
- Presence of other people such as students, male attendants, and interpreters
- Clothing to be worn
- Environmental modifications such as lighting, music, privacy, focal point, and items from home such as pillows
- Labor activities such as preferred positions for labor and for birth, ambulation, birth balls, showers and whirlpool baths, oral food and fluid intake
- List of comfort and relaxation measures
- Labor and birth medical interventions such as pharmacologic pain relief measures, intravenous therapy, electronic monitoring, induction or augmentation measures, and episiotomy
- Care and handling of the newborn immediately after birth, such as immediate skin-to-skin contact, cutting of the cord, eye care, and breastfeeding
- Cultural and religious requirements related to the care of the mother, newborn, and placenta

There are several websites that can provide couples with an interactive birth plan along with examples of birth plans and descriptions of the options that can be included.

the woman for the possibility that her plan may change as labor progresses and assures her that the staff will provide information so she can make informed decisions. Choices for birth will vary by setting. For example, what is available as a choice in a birth center may not be available as a choice in a hospital setting.

The nurse should discuss with the woman and her partner their plans for preserving birth memories through the use of photography and videotaping. Information should be provided about the agency's policies regarding these practices and under what circumstances they are allowed. Protection of privacy and safety and infection control are major concerns

TABLE 19.1   Expected Maternal Progress in First Stage of Labor

Criterion	Early Phase 0–5 cm	Active Phase 6–10 cm
Duration[a,b]	Nulliparous and multiparous women progress at similar rates	Multiparous women progress more rapidly than nulliparous women
Contractions		
Strength[c]	Mild to moderate by palpation	Moderate to strong by palpation
Frequency[c]	2–30 min apart; may be irregular	1.5–5 min apart
Duration[c]	30–40 sec	40–90 sec
Descent		
Station of presenting part[a]		Nulliparous women 0 by 6 cm Multiparous women −1 by 6 cm
Show		
Color	Brownish discharge, mucus plug, or pale pink mucus	Pink-to-bloody mucus
Amount	Scant	Moderate to copious
Behavior and appearance[d]	Excited; thoughts center on self, labor, and baby; able to walk or talk through most contractions; may be talkative or silent, calm or tense; some apprehension; pain controlled fairly well; alert, follows directions readily; open to instructions	Becomes more serious, doubtful of pain control, more apprehensive; desires companionship and encouragement; attention more inwardly directed; has some difficulty following directions As active labor continues: Pain may be described as severe; backache is common; frustration, fear of loss of control, and irritability may be voiced; expresses doubt about ability to continue; nausea and vomiting, especially if hyperventilating; perspiration of forehead and upper lip; shaking tremor of thighs; feeling of need to defecate, pressure on anus

[a]Data from Kennedy, B.B. & Baird, S.M. (2017). *Intrapartum management modules: A perinatal education program* (5th ed.). Philadelphia: Wolters Kluwer.
[b]Duration of each phase is influenced by such factors as parity; maternal emotions; position; level of activity; and fetal size, presentation, and position.
[c]Data from Simpson, K.R. & Creehan P. (2014). *AWHONN's perinatal nursing* (4th ed.). Philadelphia: Lippincott.
[d]Women who have epidural analgesia for pain relief may not demonstrate some of these behaviors.

for the expectant parents and the agency. To avoid future embarrassment and distress, the nurse should clarify with the woman exactly what parts of her labor and birth she wishes to have photographed and the degree of detail. The nurse reminds women and their families that photographs or videos should not be posted on social media sites without the knowledge and consent of *every* person who appears in the picture.

LEGAL TIP

Recording of Birth

The woman's record should reflect that the birth was recorded. Some hospitals and health care providers do not allow videotaping of the birth because of concerns related to legal liability.

Psychosocial Factors

The woman's general appearance and behavior (and that of her partner, family member, or other support person) provide valuable clues to the type of supportive care she will need. However, keep in mind that general appearance and behavior may vary depending on the stage and phase of labor (Table 19.1 and Box 19.3).

Women with a history of sexual abuse. Labor can trigger memories of sexual abuse, especially during intrusive procedures such as vaginal examinations. It is often difficult to identify those women who have been victims of sexual abuse and assault or rape. Therefore a universal approach to care is best (Parker, 2015). Respectful care includes asking permission prior to touching the woman. This is especially important for procedures that may trigger memories of the event. The nurse should allow the woman as much choice as possible while maintaining

the safety of the birth. Flexibility allows the woman to have a sense of control over the situation. Limiting the number of people who interact with the woman and maintaining continuity of care providers are also important interventions (Parker). As an example, in an academic hospital, it is preferable to choose a specific resident physician or nurse-midwife to care for the woman and to avoid having multiple students involved in her care.

The nurse can help the abuse survivor associate the sensations she is experiencing with the process of labor and birth and not with her past abuse and maintain her sense of control by explaining all procedures and why they are needed, validating her needs, and paying close attention to her requests. The nurse should avoid using words and phrases that can cause the woman to recall the words of her abuser (e.g., "open your legs," "relax and it won't hurt so much"). As much as possible, health care professionals should limit the number of procedures that invade the woman's body (e.g., vaginal examinations, urinary catheter, internal monitor, forceps, or vacuum extractor). Another suggested intervention is encouraging the woman to choose a person (e.g., doula, friend, family member) to be with her during labor to provide continuous support and comfort and to act as her advocate. Careful attention to these care measures can help a woman perceive her labor and birth experience in positive terms.

Stress in Labor

The way in which women and their partners or family members approach labor is related to the manner in which they have been prepared for and socialized to childbearing as well as how they deal with other stressors in their lives. Their reactions reflect their life experiences regarding labor and birth—physical, social, cultural, and religious. Society communicates its expectations regarding

BOX 19.3 Psychosocial Assessment of the Laboring Woman

Verbal Interactions
- Does the woman ask questions?
- Can she ask for what she needs?
- Does she talk to her support person or persons?
- Does she talk freely with the nurse or respond only to questions?

Body Language
- Does she change positions or lie rigidly still?
- What is her anxiety level?
- How does she react to being touched by the nurse or support person?
- Does she avoid eye contact?
- Does she look tired? If she appears tired, ask her how much rest she has had in the past 24 hrs.

Perceptual Ability
- Is there a language barrier?
- Are repeated explanations necessary because her anxiety level interferes with her ability to comprehend?
- Can she repeat what she has been told or otherwise demonstrate her understanding?

Discomfort Level
- To what degree does the woman describe what she is experiencing, including her pain experience?
- How does she react to a contraction?
- How does she react to assessment and care measures?
- Are any nonverbal pain messages noted?
- Can she ask for comfort measures?

acceptable and unacceptable maternal behaviors during labor and birth. These expectations may be used by some women as the basis for evaluating their own actions. An idealized perception of labor and birth may be a source of guilt and cause a sense of failure if the woman finds the process less than joyous, especially when the pregnancy is unplanned or is the product of a dysfunctional or terminated relationship. Often women have heard horror stories or have seen friends or relatives going through labors that were difficult and painful. Multiparous women often base their expectations of the current labor on their previous labor and birth experiences.

The nurse encourages the woman to express her feelings about the pregnancy and her concerns and fears related to labor and birth. This discussion is especially important if the woman is a primigravida who has not attended birthing classes but has obtained information on labor and birth from the internet or reality television shows about birth or is a multiparous woman who has had a previous negative birth experience. Women in labor usually have a variety of concerns that they will voice if asked but may not volunteer. Major fears and concerns relate to the process and effects of labor and birth maternal and fetal well-being, and the attitude and actions of the health care staff. Every effort should be made to provide support and encourage those with her to be supportive. Women who have continuous labor support are more likely to have a spontaneous vaginal birth and are less likely to have intrapartum analgesia or anesthesia, a cesarean or an operative vaginal birth, a baby with a low 5-minute Apgar score, or to report dissatisfaction with their labor and birth experiences (American College of Obstetricians and Gynecologists [ACOG], 2019a).

The partner, coach, or significant other also experiences stress during labor. The nurse can assist and support these individuals by identifying their needs and expectations, helping to make sure these are met, and interpreting events that are occurring. The degree of involvement and participation in labor support varies; therefore, it is important for the nurse to determine the intended role of the support person and whether or not that person is prepared to fulfill the role. For example, has the support person attended birth preparation classes? Does the support person appear anxious? What is the interaction between the support person and the laboring woman? Is the support person actively involved in labor support or sitting quietly at the bedside? If the support person is touching the woman, what is the character of the touch? Is the person watching TV or engaged in computer or smart phone activities? Does the support person display an aggressive or hostile attitude or behavior? The nurse must demonstrate sensitivity to the needs of support people, and provide teaching and support as appropriate. In many instances the support these people provide to the laboring woman may be in direct proportion to the support they receive from the nurses and other health care professionals.

Cultural Factors

As the population becomes more diverse, it is increasingly important to note the woman's ethnic or cultural and religious values, beliefs, and practices in order to anticipate nursing interventions to add or eliminate from an individualized, mutually acceptable plan of care that provides a feeling of safety and control (Fig. 19.4). Nurses should be committed to providing culturally sensitive care and developing an appreciation and respect for cultural diversity (Callister, 2014). The nurse encourages the woman to request specific caregiving behaviors and practices that are important to her. If a special request contradicts usual practices in the given setting, the woman or the nurse can ask the woman's nurse-midwife or physician to write an order to accommodate the special request. For example, in many cultures it is unacceptable to have a male caregiver examine a pregnant woman. In some cultures, it is traditional to take the placenta home; in others, the woman may receive only certain nourishments during labor. Some women believe that cutting the body, as with an episiotomy, allows her spirit to leave her body and that rupturing the membranes prolongs rather than shortens labor. It is always important to listen respectfully and to carefully explain the rationale for recommended care measures (see the Cultural Considerations box: Examples of Birth Practices and Behaviors in Different Cultures).

🌐 CULTURAL CONSIDERATIONS

Examples of Birth Practices and Behaviors in Different Cultures

Somalia: Because Somalis in general do not like to show any sign of weakness, these women are extremely stoic during labor and birth

Japan: Natural childbirth methods practiced, women may labor silently and may eat during labor, father may be present

China: Stoic response to pain, father not usually present, side-lying position preferred for labor and birth because this position is thought to reduce infant trauma

India: Natural childbirth methods preferred, father not usually present, female relatives usually present

Iran: Father not present, female support and female caregivers preferred

Mexico: Women may be stoic about discomfort until the second stage and then may request pain relief; father and female relatives may be present

Laos: May use squatting position for birth, father may or may not be present, female attendants preferred

Data from D'Avanzo, C. (2008). *Mosby's pocket guide to cultural health assessment* (4th ed.). St. Louis: Mosby.

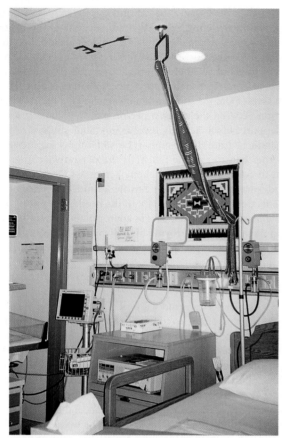

Fig. 19.4 Birthing Room Specific to a Native American Population. Note the arrow pointing east, the rug on the wall, and the rope or sash belt hanging from the ceiling. (Courtesy Patricia Hess, San Francisco, CA; Chinle Comprehensive Health Care Center, Chinle, AZ.)

Within cultures, women may have an idea of the "right" way to behave in labor and may react to the pain experienced in that way. These behaviors can range from total silence to moaning or screaming, but they do not necessarily indicate the degree of pain being experienced. A woman who moans with contractions may not be in as much physical pain as a woman who is silent but winces during contractions. Some women believe that screaming or crying out in pain is shameful if a man is present. If the woman's support person is her mother, she may perceive the need to "behave" more strongly than if her support person is the father of the baby. She may perceive herself as failing or succeeding based on her ability to follow these "standards" of behavior. Conversely, a woman's behavior in response to pain may influence the support received from significant others. In some cultures, women who lose control and cry out in pain may be scolded, whereas in others the support persons will become more helpful.

Culture and partner participation. A partner or companion is an important source of support, encouragement, and comfort for women during childbirth. The woman's cultural and religious background influences her choice of birth companion, as do trends in the society in which she lives. For example, in Western societies the father of the baby is often viewed as the ideal birth companion. For many years, European American couples traditionally attended childbirth classes together as an expected activity, although this is not as common today. Laotian (Hmong) husbands also traditionally participate actively in the labor process. In some other cultures the

father may be available but his presence in the labor room with the mother may not be considered appropriate, or he may be present but resist active involvement in the mother's care. Such behavior could be perceived by the nursing staff to indicate a lack of concern, caring, or interest. Women from many cultures prefer female caregivers and want to have at least one female companion present during labor and birth. They are also usually very concerned about modesty. If couples from these cultures immigrate to the United States or Canada, their roles may change. The nurse must talk to the woman and her support people to determine the roles they will assume.

The Non–English-Speaking Woman in Labor

A woman's level of anxiety in labor increases when she does not understand what is happening to her or what is being said. Non–English-speaking women often feel a complete loss of control over their situation if no health care professional is present who speaks their language. They can panic and withdraw or become physically abusive when someone tries to do something they perceive might harm them or their babies. A support person is sometimes able to serve as an interpreter. However, caution is warranted because the interpreter may not be able to convey exactly what the nurse or others are saying or what the woman is saying, which can increase the woman's stress level even more. Additionally, agency policy may prohibit the use of family members as interpreters.

Ideally, a bilingual or bicultural nurse will care for the woman. Alternatively, a hospital employee or volunteer interpreter may be contacted for assistance (see Box 2.2). For some women, a female is more acceptable than a male interpreter. If no one in the facility can interpret, an interpreter may be accessed by telephone or electronic media. Even when the nurse has limited ability to communicate verbally with the woman, in most instances the woman appreciates his or her efforts to do so. Speaking slowly, avoiding complex words and medical terms, and using gestures can help a woman and her partner understand. Often the woman understands English much better than she speaks it. Interpretation should be done according to agency policy.

Physical Examination

The initial physical examination includes a general systems assessment and an assessment of fetal status. During the examination, uterine contractions are assessed and a vaginal examination is performed. Findings of the admission physical examination serve as a baseline for assessing the woman's progress in labor from that point. The information obtained from a complete and accurate assessment during the initial examination serves as the basis for determining whether the woman should be admitted and what her ongoing care should be (see Clinical Reasoning Case Study: Initial Assessment of the Laboring Woman). Expected maternal progress and minimal assessment guidelines during the first stage of labor are presented in Tables 19.1 and 19.2.

Birth is a time when nurses, nurse-midwives, physicians, and other staff members are exposed to a great deal of maternal and newborn blood and body fluids. Therefore standard precautions should guide all assessment and care measures (Box 19.4). Hand hygiene (e.g., washing hands with soap or application of an alcohol-based antiseptic rub) before and after assessing the woman and providing care is a critical step in the prevention of infection transmission. The nurse should explain assessment findings to the woman and her partner whenever possible. Throughout labor, accurate documentation following agency policy is done as soon as possible after a procedure has been performed (Fig. 19.5).

CLINICAL REASONING CASE STUDY

Initial Assessment of the Laboring Woman

Sharnell is a 20-year-old single African American female who presents to the labor triage unit at 38 weeks and 5 days of gestation. She is a G2 with one early spontaneous pregnancy loss. Sharnell reports that she felt a "large gush of fluid like I peed on myself" several hours earlier. Now Sharnell is having abdominal pain that she is unable to talk through and having some pink vaginal discharge. Sharnell states that she does not know whether she has felt the baby move since experiencing the gush of fluid.

1. What is the priority concern or client need in this situation? Support your answer with data as stated in the case.
2. List other client needs/problems in this case.
3. Identify any additional information or assessment data that is needed by the nurse in planning care for this client.
4. What nursing actions are appropriate in this situation?
   a. What is the priority nursing action? (What should the nurse do first?)
   b. Describe other nursing interventions that are important to providing optimal client care.
5. Describe the roles/responsibilities of the professional health care team members (other than nurses) who may be involved in providing care for this client.

BOX 19.4 Standard Precautions During Childbirth

- Perform hand hygiene by washing hands before and after putting on gloves and performing procedures; cleansing alcohol rubs can be used if hands are not visibly soiled.
- Wear gloves (clean or sterile, as appropriate) when you are performing procedures that require contact with the woman's genitalia and body fluids, including bloody show (e.g., during vaginal examination, amniotomy, hygienic care of the perineum, insertion of an internal scalp electrode and intrauterine pressure monitor, and urinary catheterization).
- Wear a mask that has a shield or protective eyewear and cover your gown when you are assisting with the birth. Cap and shoe covers are worn for cesarean birth but are optional for vaginal birth in a birthing room. Gowns worn by the nurse-midwife or physician who is attending the birth should have a waterproof front and sleeves and should be sterile. A mask should also be worn during a spinal puncture or insertion of an epidural catheter.
- Drape the woman with sterile towels and sheets as appropriate. Explain to the woman what can and cannot be touched.
- Help the woman's partner put on appropriate coverings for the type of birth, such as cap, mask, gown, and shoe covers. Show the partner where to stand and what can and cannot be touched.
- Wear gloves and a gown when you are handling the newborn immediately after birth.
- Use an appropriate method to suction the newborn's airway, such as a bulb syringe or mechanical wall suction.

TABLE 19.2 Nursing Assessments in First-Stage Labor

Labor Phase	Time Frame	Specific Assessments
Early	Every 30-60 min	Maternal blood pressure, pulse, and respirations
		Uterine activity[a]
		Fetal heart rate (FHR) and pattern[a]
		Presence of bloody show
	Every 30 min	Changes in maternal appearance, mood, affect, energy level, and involvement of partner or coach
	Every 2-4 hrs	Temperature (every 4 hrs until membranes rupture, then every 2 hrs)
	As needed	Vaginal examination to identify progress in labor
Active	Every 15-30 min	Maternal blood pressure, pulse, and respirations
	Every 15-30 min	FHR and pattern[a]
		Uterine activity[a]
		Presence of bloody show
	Every 5-15 min	Changes in maternal appearance, mood, affect, energy level, and involvement of partner or coach
	Every 2-4 hrs	Temperature (every 4 hrs until membranes rupture, then every 2 hrs)
	As needed	Vaginal examination to identify progress in labor

[a]Kennedy, B. B., & Baird, S. M. (2017). *Intrapartum management modules: A perinatal education program* (5th ed.). Philadelphia: Wolters Kluwer.

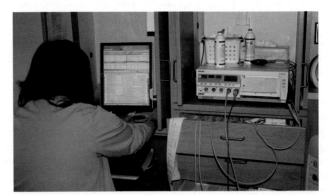

Fig. 19.5 Nurse Documenting Assessment Findings on a Computer in a Labor, Delivery, Recovery, Postpartum Room. (Courtesy Shannon Perry, Phoenix, AZ.)

General systems assessment. On admission, the nurse should perform a general systems assessment. This includes an assessment of the heart, lungs, and skin, and an examination to determine the presence and extent of edema of the face, hands, sacrum, and legs. It also includes testing of deep tendon reflexes and for clonus if indicated. The woman's weight is measured and recorded. Increasing numbers of women are overweight or obese. Excessive size can make nursing care during labor and birth more difficult and places the woman at risk for complications such as operative birth, infection, and venous thromboembolism. See Chapter 32 for further information.

Vital signs. The nurse assesses vital signs (temperature, pulse, respirations, and blood pressure using a cuff of the correct size) on admission. The initial values are used as the baseline for comparison with all future measurements. If the blood pressure is elevated, it should be reassessed 30 minutes later or per agency policy between contractions to obtain a reading after the woman has relaxed. The woman is encouraged to lie on her side to prevent supine

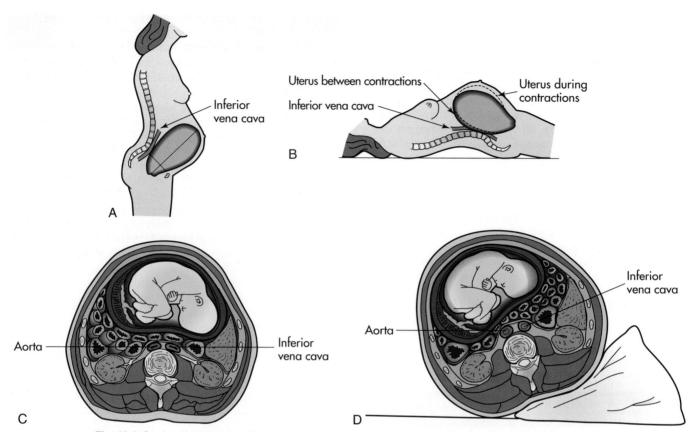

Fig. 19.6 Supine Hypotension. Note relation of pregnant uterus to ascending vena cava in standing position (A), and in the supine position (B). (C) Compression of aorta and inferior vena cava with woman in supine position. (D) Compression of these vessels is relieved by placement of a wedge pillow under the woman's side.

hypotension and the resulting fetal hypoxemia (Fig. 19.6). Body temperature is monitored in an effort to identify signs of infection or a fluid deficit (e.g., dehydration associated with inadequate fluid intake).

Leopold maneuvers. Leopold maneuvers are performed using abdominal palpation (Box 19.5). These maneuvers help to answer three important questions: (1) Which fetal part is in the uterine fundus? (2) Where is the fetal back located? (3) What is the presenting fetal part? Leopold maneuvers can also be used to estimate fetal size.

Assessment of fetal heart rate and pattern. The point of maximal intensity (PMI) of the FHR is the location on the maternal abdomen at which the FHR is heard the loudest. It is usually directly over the fetal back. In a vertex presentation the FHR can usually be heard below the mother's umbilicus in either the right or the left lower quadrant of the abdomen. In a breech presentation the FHR is most easily heard above the mother's umbilicus. The PMI is where the nurse places the ultrasound transducer when the electronic fetal monitor is used to assess the FHR. Table 19.2 summarizes assessments recommended for determining fetal status during the first stage of labor. In addition, it is essential to assess the FHR after ROM because this is the most common time for the umbilical cord to prolapse, after any change in the contraction pattern or maternal status, and before and after the woman receives medication or a procedure is performed.

Assessment of uterine contractions. A general characteristic of effective labor is regular uterine activity (i.e., contractions becoming more frequent with increased duration and intensity), but uterine activity is not directly related to labor progress. Uterine contractions represent the primary force that acts involuntarily to expel the fetus and placenta from the uterus. Several methods can be used to evaluate uterine contractions, including the woman's subjective description, palpation and timing of contractions by the nurse or another health care professional, and electronic monitoring.

Each contraction exhibits a wave-like pattern. It begins with a slow increment (the increasing intensity of a contraction from its onset), gradually reaches a peak, and then diminishes rapidly (decrement, the decreasing intensity of the contraction). An interval of rest ends when the next contraction begins. The outward appearance of the woman's abdomen during and between contractions and the pattern of a typical uterine contraction are shown in Fig. 19.7.

A uterine contraction is described in terms of the following characteristics:

- *Frequency:* How often uterine contractions occur; the time that passes from the beginning of one contraction to the beginning of the next contraction
- *Intensity:* The strength of a contraction at its peak
- *Duration:* The time that passes between the onset and the end of a contraction
- *Resting tone:* The tension in the uterine muscle between contractions; relaxation of the uterus

Uterine contractions are assessed by palpation or by using external or internal electronic monitors (see Chapter 18 for further discussion). Frequency and duration can be measured by all three methods of uterine activity monitoring. The accuracy of determining intensity and resting tone varies by the method used. The woman's description and examiner's palpation are more subjective and less precise ways of determining the intensity of uterine contractions and resting tone than

BOX 19.5   Procedure: Leopold Maneuvers

- Perform hand hygiene.
- Ask the woman to empty her bladder.
- Position the woman supine with one pillow under her head and her knees slightly flexed.
- Place a small rolled towel under the woman's right or left hip to displace the uterus off major blood vessels (prevents supine hypotensive syndrome; see Fig. 19.6D).
- If you are right-handed, stand on the woman's right, facing her (if you are left-handed, stand on the woman's left):
  - Identify the fetal part that occupies the fundus. The head feels round, firm, and freely movable; the breech feels less regular and softer. This maneuver identifies fetal lie (longitudinal or transverse) and presentation (cephalic or breech) (Fig. A).
  - Using the palmar surface of one hand, locate and palpate the smooth convex contour of the fetal back and the irregularities that identify the small parts (feet, hands, knees, elbows). This maneuver helps to identify fetal presentation (Fig. B).

- With your right hand, determine which fetal part is presenting over the inlet to the true pelvis. Gently grasp the lower pole of the uterus between your thumb and fingers, pressing in slightly (Fig. C). If the head is presenting and not engaged, determine the attitude of the head (flexed or extended).
- Turn to face the woman's feet. Using both hands, outline the fetal head (Fig. D) with the palmar surface of your fingertips. When the presenting part has descended deeply, only a small portion of it may be outlined. Palpation of the cephalic prominence helps identify the attitude of the head. If the cephalic prominence is found on the same side as the small parts, this means that the head must be flexed and the vertex is presenting (see Fig. D). If the cephalic prominence is on the same side as the back, this indicates that the presenting head is extended and the face is presenting.
- Document fetal presentation, position, and lie and whether the presenting part is flexed or extended, engaged, or free-floating. Use agency protocol for documentation (e.g., "Vtx, LOA, floating").

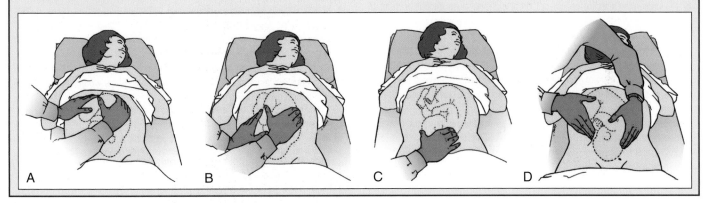

A   B   C   D

are the external or internal electronic monitors. The following terms describe contractions based on what is felt on palpation:

- *Mild:* Slightly tense fundus that is easy to indent with the fingertips (feels like pressing a finger to the tip of the nose)
- *Moderate:* Firm fundus that is difficult to indent with the fingertips (feels like pressing a finger to the chin)
- *Strong:* Rigid, board-like fundus that is almost impossible to indent with the fingertips (feels like pressing a finger to the forehead)

Women in labor tend to describe the pain of contractions in terms of the sensations they are experiencing in the lower abdomen or back, which is sometimes unrelated to the firmness of the uterine fundus. Therefore a woman's assessment of the strength of her contractions may be less accurate than that of the nurse health care provider, although the amount of discomfort reported is valid.

External electronic monitoring provides some information about the strength of uterine contractions when the appearance of contractions on admission is compared with those that occur later in labor. However, internal electronic monitoring with an intrauterine pressure catheter is the most accurate way of assessing the intensity of uterine contractions and the resting tone of the uterus.

On admission to a hospital, uterine contractions and FHR and pattern are usually monitored electronically for at least a 20- to 30-minute period as a baseline; however, monitoring should always be done per hospital policy. In birth centers monitoring is done intermittently for both uterine contractions and assessment of the FHR. The minimal times for assessing uterine activity during

the phases of stage one labor are listed in Table 19.2. The findings expected as the first stage of labor progresses are summarized in Table 19.1.

⚡ SAFETY ALERT

If the nurse observes that the characteristics of contractions are abnormal, either exceeding or falling below what is considered acceptable in terms of the standard characteristics, this finding must be promptly reported to the nurse-midwife or physician.

The nurse considers uterine activity in the context of its effect on cervical effacement and dilation and on the degree of descent of the presenting part (see Chapter 16). It is also important to consider the effect of uterine activity on the fetus. Often the progress of labor is evaluated using graphic charts (also called *partograms* or *labor graphs*) on which cervical dilation is plotted as labor progresses. This type of graphic charting facilitates the early identification of deviations from expected labor patterns. Fig. 19.8 provides examples of a modern labor graph and partogram that incorporate new knowledge regarding the labor process in contemporary women. Hospitals and birth centers may develop their own assessment graphs, which may include data not only on dilation and descent but also on maternal vital signs, FHR, and uterine activity. These

EVIDENCE-BASED PRACTICE

Correcting Fetal Malpresentations: Version and Moxibustion

Ask the Question

For women near term with noncephalic fetal presentation, what are the options to maximize the chance of a vaginal birth?

Search for the Evidence

Search strategies English language research–based publications since 2014 on external cephalic version, moxibustion, postural, obesity, and tocolytics were included.

Databases used Cochrane Collaborative Database, National Guideline Clearinghouse (AHRQ), CINAHL, PubMed, UpToDate, and the professional websites for ACOG and AWHONN

Critical Appraisal of the Evidence

Noncephalic presentation (breech or transverse) makes vaginal birth risky or impossible and is a common reason for scheduled cesarean birth. Malpresentations can sometimes be corrected. Ideally correction occurs before engagement of the presenting part in the pelvis ("dropping") yet close enough to term to maintain the position until birth and minimize the risk of preterm birth.

External cephalic version (ECV) is an ultrasound-guided hands-on procedure to externally manipulate the fetus into a cephalic lie. It is done at 36 to 37 weeks' gestation in the hospital setting. Hutton and colleagues (2015), in a Cochrane systematic review, found that ECV performed between 34 and 36 weeks' gestation significantly increased the chance of a cephalic presentation at birth.

- Beta stimulants to relax the uterus, such as terbutaline, have the best evidence for premedication (Morris, Geraghty, & Sundin, 2018).
- Successful outcome of a vaginal birth is most likely for multiparous women with adequate amniotic fluid (Hutton, Hofmeyr, & Dowswell, 2015).
- The risk of a negative outcome from undergoing an ECV is small and the cesarean rate is significantly lower among women who have experienced a successful ECV. All women near a term gestational age with breech presentations should be offered an ECV if there are no contraindications (American College of Obstetricians and Gynecologists, 2016/2018).

Postural management, the practice of positioning women with their pelvis elevated, does not have sufficient evidence to support it as an effective corrective technique (Hutton et al., 2015).

Moxibustion, the Chinese practice of burning mugwort close to acupuncture point 67, the tip of the fifth toe, has some promising evidence (Morris et al., 2018).

Apply the Evidence: Nursing Implications

Promoting cephalic vaginal birth is protective against the complications of cesarean birth, which include a high risk for future cesarean births.

- Even with tocolytics (uterine relaxers) ECV is very uncomfortable or painful and carries its own risks for placental abruption, cord accident, and emergent cesarean birth. Women benefit from having a support person present (Morris et al., 2018).
- Moxibustion is a welcome noninvasive technique that shows promise and does no harm. Proper training is required to avoid burns and respiratory reaction. Lack of familiarity probably impedes its uptake. More research is needed to determine the efficacy of moxibustion (Morris et al., 2018).

Women with fetal malposition need to understand the mechanics of vaginal birth and the risk factors associated with all options. Some women may prefer a cesarean birth even with its increased risks.

References

American College of Obstetricians and Gynecologists. (2016, reaffirmed 2018). Practice bulletin no. 161: External cephalic version. *Obstetrics and Gynecology, 127*(2), e54–e61.

Hutton, E. K., Hofmeyr, G. J., & Dowswell, T. (2015). External cephalic version for breech presentation before term. *Cochrane Database of Systematic Reviews, 7,* CD 000084.

Morris, S., Geraghty, S., & Sundin, D. (2018). Moxibustion: An alternative option for breech presentation. *British Journal of Midwifery, 26*(7), 440–447.

Jennifer Taylor Alderman

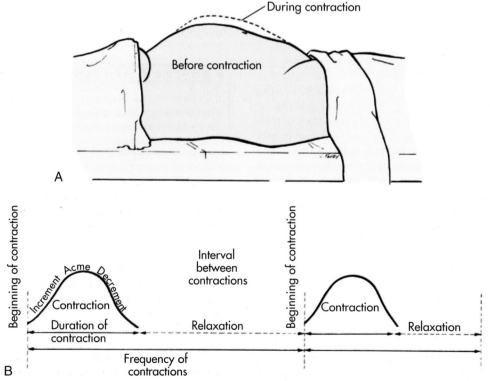

Fig. 19.7 Assessment of Uterine Contractions. (A) Abdominal contour before and during uterine contraction. (B) Wavelike pattern of contractile activity.

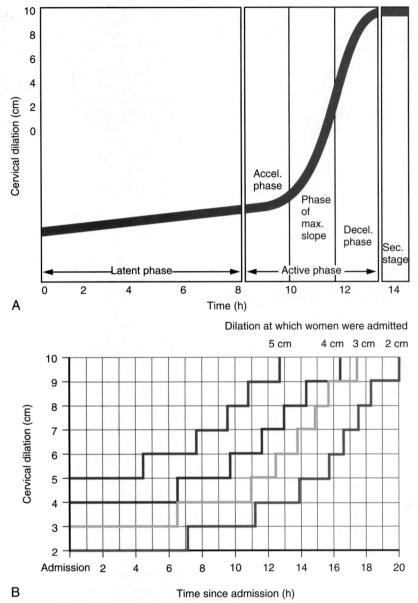

Fig. 19.8 Use of Graphic Charts to Evaluate Labor Progress. (A) Modern labor graph. Characteristics of the average cervical dilation curve for nulliparous labor. (B) Zhang labor partogram. The 95th percentiles of cumulative duration of labor from admission among singleton-term nulliparous women with spontaneous onset of labor. (From Gabbe, S. G., Niebyl, J. R., Simpson, J. L., et al. (Eds.). (2017). *Obstetrics: Normal and problem pregnancies* (7th ed.). Philadelphia: Elsevier.)

⚡ SAFETY ALERT

The nurse should recognize that active labor can actually last longer than the expected labor patterns because each woman is different. This finding is not a cause for concern unless the maternal-fetal unit exhibits signs of stress (e.g., abnormal FHR patterns, maternal fever).

---

may be included in the electronic health record and should be completed per agency policy.

Vaginal examination. The vaginal examination reveals whether the woman is in true labor and enables the examiner to determine whether the membranes have ruptured (Fig. 19.9). Because this examination is often stressful and uncomfortable for the woman and may introduce microorganisms into the vagina if

the membranes are ruptured, it is performed only when indicated by the status of the woman and her fetus. For example, a vaginal examination is performed on admission, prior to administering medications (e.g., analgesics, oxytocin infusion), when significant change has occurred in uterine activity, on maternal request or perception of perineal pressure or the urge to bear down, when membranes rupture, or when variable decelerations of the FHR are noted. A full explanation of the examination and support of the woman are important in reducing the stress and discomfort associated with the examination (Simpson & O'Brien-Abel, 2014) (Box 19.6).

Laboratory and Diagnostic Tests

Urinalysis. A clean-catch urine specimen may be obtained to gather further data about the pregnant woman's health. Analysis

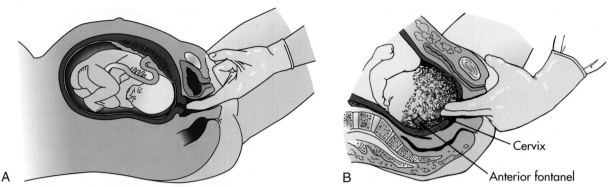

Fig. 19.9 Vaginal Examination. (A) Undilated uneffaced cervix; membranes intact. (B) Palpation of sagittal suture line. Cervix effaced and partially dilated.

BOX 19.6   Procedure: Vaginal Examination of the Laboring Woman

- Use a sterile glove and antiseptic solution or soluble gel for lubrication.
- Position the woman to prevent supine hypotension. Drape to ensure privacy.
- Cleanse the perineum and vulva if needed.
- After obtaining the woman's permission to touch her, gently insert your index and middle fingers into the woman's vagina.
- Determine
  - Cervical dilation, effacement, and position (e.g., posterior, middle, anterior).
  - Presenting part, position, and station; molding of the head with development of caput succedaneum (may affect accuracy of determination of station).
  - Status of membranes (intact, bulging, or ruptured).
  - Characteristics of amniotic fluid (e.g., color, clarity, and odor) if membranes are ruptured.
- Explain the findings of the examination to the woman.
- Document your findings and report them to the nurse-midwife or physician.

---

of the specimen is a convenient and simple procedure that can provide information about her hydration status (e.g., specific gravity, color, amount); nutritional status (e.g., ketones); infection status (e.g., leukocytes); or the status of possible complications such as preeclampsia (e.g., proteinuria). In many hospitals this test must be done in the laboratory rather than at the bedside even if a urine dipstick is used.

Blood tests. The blood tests performed vary with agency protocol and the woman's health status. Currently almost all blood tests must be performed in the hospital laboratory rather than on the perinatal unit. Often blood samples are obtained from the hub of the catheter when an intravenous line is started or a saline lock inserted. A hematocrit or complete blood count (CBC) will likely be ordered. The CBC measures hematocrit as well as other parameters including white blood cell count, red blood cell count, hemoglobin level, and platelet count. A CBC may be ordered for women with a history of infection, anemia, gestational hypertension, or other disorders. Many hospitals require that a CBC be done before epidural anesthesia is initiated. Any woman whose human immunodeficiency virus (HIV) status is undocumented at the time of labor should be screened with a rapid HIV test unless she declines (opts out of) testing (ACOG, 2018; Centers for Disease Control and Prevention [CDC], 2016).

Most hospitals require that a "type and screen" or "clot to hold"—to determine the woman's blood type, Rh status, and antibody—be performed on admission. Even if these tests have already been performed during pregnancy, the hospital's laboratory or transfusion services department (blood bank) must verify the results in house. If the woman had no prenatal care or if her prenatal records are not available, blood for a prenatal screen will likely be drawn on admission. The prenatal screen includes laboratory tests that would normally have been drawn at the initial prenatal visit (see Table 14.1).

Other tests. If the woman's group B streptococcus status is not known, a rapid test may be done on admission. The rapid test results are usually available within an hour or so and will determine if the woman must be given antibiotics during labor.

Assessment of amniotic membranes and fluid. Labor is initiated at term by SROM in approximately 25% of pregnant women. A lag period, rarely exceeding 24 hours, may precede the onset of labor. Membrane rupture can also occur at any time during labor but most commonly in the active phase of the first stage of labor. Box 19.1 explains how to determine if membranes are ruptured. If the membranes do not rupture spontaneously, artificial rupture of membranes (AROM), called an *amniotomy*, may be attempted by the physician or nurse-midwife using a plastic AmniHook or a surgical clamp during labor. However, this practice is discouraged if there is no medical reason for it because it can increase the laboring woman's sensation of pressure and pain and is not necessary for a normal birth to occur. Whether the membranes rupture spontaneously or artificially, the time of rupture should be recorded. Other necessary documentation includes information regarding the FHR immediately before and after rupture, the color (clear or meconium-stained), estimated amount, and odor of the fluid. (See Chapter 32 for additional information.)

⚡ SAFETY ALERT

The umbilical cord may prolapse when the membranes rupture. The FHR and pattern should be monitored closely for several minutes immediately after ROM to determine fetal well-being, and the findings should be documented.

Infection. When membranes rupture, microorganisms from the vagina can then ascend into the amniotic sac, causing chorioamnionitis and placentitis to develop. For this reason vaginal examinations must be limited and maternal temperature and vaginal discharge monitored frequently (at least every 2 hours) to quickly identify signs of infection. Even when membranes are intact, however, microorganisms can ascend and cause infection.

SIGNS OF POTENTIAL COMPLICATIONS

Complications of Labor

- Intrauterine pressure equal to or greater than 80 mm Hg or resting tone equal to or greater than 20 mm Hg (both determined by internal monitoring with intrauterine pressure catheter [IUPC])
- Contractions lasting equal to or greater than 90 sec
- More than five contractions in a 10-minute period (contractions that occur more frequently than every 2 min)
- Relaxation between contractions lasting less than 30 sec
- Fetal bradycardia or tachycardia; absent or minimal variability not associated with fetal sleep cycle or temporary effects of central nervous system (CNS)-depressant drugs given to the woman; late, variable, or prolonged fetal heart rate (FHR) decelerations
- Irregular FHR; suspected fetal arrhythmias
- Appearance of meconium-stained or bloody fluid from the vagina
- Arrest in progress of cervical dilation or effacement, descent of the fetus, or both
- Maternal temperature equal to or greater than 38°C (100.4°F)
- Foul-smelling vaginal discharge
- Persistent bright or dark red vaginal bleeding.

Assessment findings serve as a baseline for evaluating the woman's subsequent progress during labor. Although some problems can be anticipated, others may appear unexpectedly during the clinical course of labor (see box Signs of Potential Complications).

Nursing Interventions

The nursing process provides the framework for the nursing care management of women in labor. The nursing care given to a woman in labor is an essential component of her management. The current emphasis on evidence-based practice supports the management of care by using this approach to enhance the safety, effectiveness, and acceptability of the physical care measures chosen to support the woman during labor and birth (Box 19.7). The various physical needs, the necessary nursing actions, and the rationale for care are presented in Table 19.3 and the Nursing Care Plan.

General Hygiene

In general, women in labor may use showers or warm-water baths, if available, to enhance the feeling of well-being and minimize the discomfort of contractions. Water immersion during active labor is associated with a decrease in the use of analgesia and reports of less maternal pain (Arendt & Tessmer-Tuck, 2013; Shaw-Battista, 2017). Both the ACNM and ACOG endorse the use of water immersion in labor for low-risk women at term (ACOG, 2016; Shaw-Battista).

◎ NURSING CARE PLAN

The Woman in Labor

Client Problem	Expected Outcome	Interventions	Rationales
Anxiety related to labor and the birthing process	Woman reports decreased anxiety level using an anxiety scale (from 0 [no anxiety] to 10 [anxiety as bad as it could possibly be])	Assess woman's knowledge, experience, and expectations of labor; identify specific source(s) of anxiety	To establish a baseline for care and better target interventions
		Teach the expected progression of labor and describe what to expect during the process. Answer all questions asked by the woman or her support person	To decrease anxiety associated with the unknown
		Actively involve the woman in care decisions during labor, interpret sights and sounds of the environment (monitor sights and sounds, unit activities), and share information on the progress of labor (e.g., cervical dilation and effacement, fetal station)	To increase her sense of control and lessen fears
Acute pain related to increasing frequency and intensity of contractions	Woman reports decreased pain level using a pain scale (from 0 [no pain] to 10 [pain as bad as it could possibly be])	Assess woman's level of pain and strategies that she has used to cope with it	To establish baseline for intervention
		Teach the woman and support person to use specific nonpharmacologic pain relief measures such as conscious relaxation, breathing techniques, imagery, and touch	To increase relaxation, help the woman cope with the intensity of contractions and promote the use of controlled thought and direction of energy
		Administer analgesics or assist with regional anesthesia (e.g., epidural) as ordered or desired	To provide effective pain relief during labor and birth
Urinary retention related to sensory impairment secondary to labor	Woman's bladder is emptied at least every 2 hrs either by spontaneous voiding or urinary catheter	Palpate bladder superior to symphysis frequently (at least every 2 hrs)	To detect a full bladder that occurs from increased fluid intake and inability to feel the urge to void
		Encourage frequent voiding (at least every 2 hrs) by helping the woman to the bathroom to void if appropriate and providing privacy. Catheterize if necessary	To avoid bladder distention by facilitating bladder emptying (a distended bladder impedes progress of the fetus down the birth canal and may result in trauma to bladder)
		Teach the woman techniques to stimulate spontaneous voiding such as listening to the sound of running water or placing her hands in warm water	To facilitate spontaneous voiding

---

BOX 19.7 Evidence-Based Care Practices Designed to Promote, Protect, and Support Normal Labor and Birth

- Allow labor to begin on its own: encourage spontaneous labor rather than fostering elective labor inductions.
- Encourage freedom of movement throughout labor to facilitate the progress of labor and enhance maternal comfort and control of the labor process.
- Provide support beginning early in labor and continuing throughout the process of childbirth to relieve maternal anxiety and stress and decrease the use of epidural anesthesia and the likelihood of cesarean birth; support should be provided by someone not employed by the hospital (e.g., doula).
- Avoid routine implementation of interventions (e.g., intravenous fluids, oral intake restrictions, continuous electronic fetal monitoring, labor augmentation measures [e.g., amniotomy, oxytocin administration], and epidural anesthesia).
- Support the practice of spontaneous nondirected pushing in nonsupine positions (e.g., lateral, squatting, standing, kneeling, and semi-sitting) to facilitate the progress of fetal descent and shorten the second stage of labor.
- After birth, avoid separation of the mother from her healthy baby by encouraging skin-to-skin contact of mother and baby to keep the newborn warm, prevent neonatal infection, enhance the newborn's physiologic adjustment to extrauterine life, and foster early breastfeeding.

Data from American College of Obstetricians and Gynecologists. (2019a). Committee opinion no. 766: Approaches to limit intervention during labor and birth. *Obstetrics & Gynecology, 133*(2), e164–e173; Association of Women's Health, Obstetric and Neonatal Nurses. (2018). Continuous Labor Support for Every Woman. *Journal of Obstetric, Gynecologic & Neonatal Nursing, 47*(1), 73–74.

Women should be encouraged to wash their hands or use cleansing foam after voiding and performing self-hygiene measures. Linens are changed whenever they are wet or soiled; linen savers (e.g., Chux) placed underneath the woman can be changed frequently to help maintain cleanliness and comfort.

Nutrient and Fluid Intake

Oral intake. Before the 1940s, women were allowed to eat and drink during labor to maintain the energy required to sustain labor and the stamina required to give birth. When concern arose regarding the risk of anesthesia complications and their secondary effects, if general anesthesia were required in an emergency, this practice changed, allowing the laboring woman only clear liquids or ice chips or nothing by mouth during the active phase of labor. The feared secondary effects include the aspiration of gastric contents and resultant compromise of oxygen perfusion, which could endanger the lives of both mother and fetus (Collins, 2017; Simpson & O'Brien-Abel, 2014; Tillett & Hill, 2016). There have been few randomized trials evaluating the ingestion of solid foods during labor; therefore current management is based mostly on expert opinion. For example, ACOG, the American Society of Anesthesiologists (ASA), and the Canadian Anesthesiologists' Society recommend avoiding solid food during labor (Simpson & O'Brien-Abel; Ciardulli, Saccone, Anatasio, & Berghella, 2017). This practice is being challenged by many health care providers, however, because regional anesthesia is used more often than general anesthesia, even for emergency cesarean births. Women are awake during regional anesthesia and are able to participate in their own care and protect their airways (Collins). The ACNM supports

self-determination regarding the intake of food and drink during labor (ACNM, 2016).

An adequate intake of fluids and calories is required to meet the energy demands and compensate for fluid losses associated with labor and birth. The progress of labor slows, with a more rapid development of hypoglycemia and ketosis, if these demands are not met and fat is metabolized. Reduced energy for bearing-down efforts (pushing) increases the risk for a forceps- or vacuum-assisted birth. This is most likely to occur in women who begin to labor early in the morning after a night without caloric intake. When women are permitted to consume fluid and food freely, they typically regulate their own oral intake, eating light foods (e.g., eggs, yogurt, ice cream, dry toast and jelly, fruit), drinking fluids during early labor and tapering off to the intake of clear fluids and sips of water or ice chips as labor intensifies and the second stage approaches (ACNM, 2016).

Common hospital practice is to allow clear liquids during labor. ACOG (2019a) now supports the oral intake of moderate amounts of clear liquids by laboring women who do not have complications. The ASA recommends that laboring women at low risk for cesarean birth be allowed to have clear liquids during labor (Tillett & Hill, 2016). Clear fluids recommended for labor include water, fruit juices without pulp, carbonated beverages, clear teas and coffee, flavored gelatin, fruit ices, popsicles, and broth (Collins, 2017). Herbal teas can provide not only hydration but also other beneficial effects and are commonly used in birth centers. However, there is no consensus in hospital policies regarding oral intake in labor. A woman's culture may influence what she will eat and drink during labor. In addition, women who use nonpharmacologic pain relief measures and labor at home or in birth centers are more likely to eat and drink during labor. The amount of solid and liquid carbohydrates to offer a woman in labor is still unclear. The energy requirements of labor are thought to be similar to those of continuous moderate aerobic exercise. However, there is no published research that specifically addresses this need. Although no causal relationship has been demonstrated, an association exists between ketone production and prolonged labor (ACNM, 2016).

A Cochrane database review of this topic concluded that there is no justification for restricting food or fluid intake during labor in women at low risk for complications (Ciardulli et al., 2017). Nurses should follow the orders of the woman's obstetric health care provider when offering the woman food or fluid during labor. However, as advocates, nurses can facilitate change by informing others of the current research findings that support the safety and effectiveness of the oral intake of food and fluid during labor and initiating such research themselves.

Intravenous intake. If the woman is not permitted oral intake during labor, fluids are administered intravenously to maintain hydration and meet her increased energy needs. Traditionally, 125 mL/h of intravenous fluid has been infused. However, this may not be enough to meet the fluid needs of the laboring woman, and the resulting dehydration may affect the progress of labor negatively. It may be more appropriate to infuse 250 mL/h to ensure proper hydration (Kelly et al., 2017; King & Pinger, 2014). Although it is somewhat controversial, some practitioners infuse intravenous fluids containing 5% dextrose in a balanced salt solution in order to meet the woman's energy needs

---

⚡ SAFETY ALERT

Nurses should carefully monitor the intake and output of laboring women receiving intravenous fluids because they face an increased danger of hypervolemia related to the fluid retention that occurs during pregnancy.

TABLE 19.3   Physical Nursing Care During First- and Second-Stage Labor

Need	Nursing Actions	Rationale
General Hygiene		
Showers, bed baths, tub baths, or whirlpool baths	Assess for progress in labor	Determines appropriateness of the activity
	Supervise showers or baths closely if woman is in true labor	Prevents injury from fall; labor may be accelerated
	Suggest allowing warm water to flow over back	Aids relaxation; increases comfort
Perineum	Cleanse frequently, especially after rupture of membranes and when show increases	Enhances comfort and reduces risk for infection
Oral hygiene	Offer toothbrush or mouthwash or wash teeth with ice-cold wet washcloth as needed	Refreshes mouth; helps counteract dry, thirsty feeling
Hair	Brush, braid per woman's wishes	Improves morale; increases comfort
Handwashing	Offer washcloths or cleansing foam before and after voiding and as needed	Maintains cleanliness; prevents infection
Face	Offer cool washcloth	Provides relief from diaphoresis; cools and refreshes
Gowns and linens	Change as needed	Improves comfort; enhances relaxation
Nutrient and Fluid Intake		
Oral	Offer fluids and solid foods as ordered by nurse-midwife or physician and desired by laboring woman	Provides hydration and calories; enhances positive emotional experience and maternal control
Intravenous	Establish and maintain intravenous line as ordered	Maintains hydration; provides venous access for medications or blood products, if needed
Elimination		
Voiding	Encourage voiding at least every 2 hrs	A full bladder may impede descent of presenting part; overdistention may cause bladder atony and injury as well as postpartum voiding difficulty
Ambulatory woman	Allow ambulation to bathroom according to orders of nurse-midwife or physician *if*	
	the presenting part is engaged	Reinforces normal process of urination
	the membranes are not ruptured	Precautionary measure to protect against prolapse of umbilical cord
	the woman is not medicated	Precautionary measure to protect against injury from a fall
Woman on bed rest	Offer bedpan	Prevents complications of bladder distention and ambulation
	Encourage upright position on bedpan, allow tap water to run; place woman's hands in warm water; pour warm water over vulva; give positive suggestion	Encourages voiding
	Provide privacy	Shows respect for woman
	Put up side rails on bed	Prevents injury from a fall
	Place call bell and telephone within reach	Reinforces safe care
	Offer washcloth or cleansing foam for hands	Maintains cleanliness; prevents infection
	Cleanse vulvar area	Maintains cleanliness; enhances comfort; prevents infection
Urinary catheterization	Catheterize according to orders of nurse-midwife or physician or hospital protocol if measures to facilitate spontaneous voiding are ineffective	Prevents complications of bladder distention
	Insert catheter between contractions	Minimizes discomfort
	Avoid force if obstacle to insertion is noted	"Obstacle" may be caused by compression of urethra by presenting part
Bowel elimination—sensation of rectal pressure	Perform vaginal examination.	Prevents misinterpretation of rectal pressure from presenting part as need to defecate
		Determines degree of descent of presenting part
	Help the woman ambulate to the bathroom or offer bedpan if rectal pressure is not from presenting part	Reinforces normal process of bowel elimination and safe care
	Cleanse perineum immediately after passage of stool	Reduces risk for infection and sense of embarrassment

during labor as well as to ensure hydration. To help prevent maternal and fetal hyperglycemia, glucose-containing solutions should not be administered as fluid boluses in situations such as preloading before the initiation of regional anesthesia or for intrauterine resuscitation (Kelly et al.).

Elimination

Voiding. The laboring woman should be encouraged to void every 2 hours (Simkin, Hanson, & Ancheta, 2017). A distended bladder can impede descent of the presenting part, slow or stop uterine contractions, and lead to decreased bladder tone or uterine atony after birth. Women who receive epidural analgesia or anesthesia are especially at risk for the retention of urine. Therefore the need to void should be assessed more frequently with them.

The nurse helps the woman to the bathroom to void unless any of the following apply: The nurse-midwife or physician has ordered bed rest, the woman is receiving epidural analgesia or anesthesia, internal monitoring is being used, or ambulation will compromise the status of the laboring woman or her fetus. External monitoring can usually be interrupted long enough for the woman to go to the bathroom.

If the use of a bedpan is necessary, spontaneous voiding is encouraged by providing privacy and having the woman sit upright (as she would on a toilet). Other interventions to encourage urination, either in the bathroom or on the bedpan, are having the woman listen to the sound of water slowly running from a faucet, placing her hands in warm water, having her blow bubbles into a glass of water using a straw, or pouring warm water over the vulva and perineum using a plastic perineal care bottle.

Catheterization. If the woman is unable to void and her bladder is distended, she may have to be catheterized. Many hospitals have protocols or standing orders that rely on the nurse's judgment concerning the need for catheterization. Before performing the catheterization, the vulva and perineum should be cleansed because vaginal show and amniotic fluid may be present. If an obstacle prevents advancement of the catheter, it is most likely the fetal presenting part. If the catheter cannot be advanced, it is withdrawn, the procedure is stopped, and the nurse-midwife or physician is notified.

Bowel elimination. Most women do not have bowel movements during labor because of decreased intestinal motility. Stool that has formed in the large intestine often moves downward toward the anorectal area as a result of pressure exerted by the fetal presenting part as it descends. This stool is often expelled during second-stage pushing and birth. However, the passage of stool with bearing-down efforts increases the risk of infection and may embarrass the woman, thereby reducing the effectiveness of her pushing efforts. To prevent these problems, the nurse should immediately cleanse the perineal area to remove any stool while reassuring the woman that the passage of stool at this time is a normal and expected event because the same muscles used to expel the baby also expel stool. When the presenting part is deep in the pelvis, even in the absence of stool in the anorectal area, the woman may feel rectal pressure and think that she needs to defecate.

> **! NURSING ALERT**
>
> If the woman expresses the urge to defecate, the nurse should perform a vaginal examination to assess cervical dilation and station. When a multiparous woman experiences the urge to defecate, it often means that birth will follow quickly.

Ambulation and Positioning

For laboring women, upright positions and mobility may be more pleasant than lying in bed. These practices have also been associated with improved uterine contraction intensity and shorter labors, less need for pain medications, a reduced rate of operative birth (e.g., cesarean birth, forceps- and vacuum-assisted birth), increased maternal autonomy and control, distraction from the discomforts of labor, and an opportunity for close interaction with the woman's partner and care provider as they help her assume upright

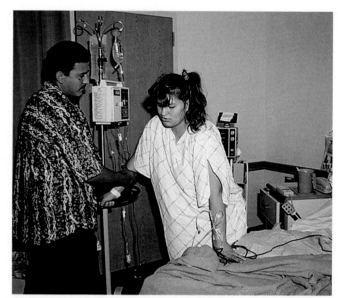

Fig. 19.10 Woman Preparing to Walk With Partner. (Courtesy Marjorie Pyle, RNC, Lifecircle, Costa Mesa, CA.)

positions and remain mobile (ACOG, 2019a; Kilpatrick & Garrison, 2017; King & Pinger, 2014; Simpson & O'Brien-Abel, 2014). No harmful effects have been observed from maternal activity and position changes. However, confinement to bed is the norm for laboring women in U.S. hospitals. The increased use of epidurals during labor and birth accompanied by multiple medical interventions (e.g., electronic fetal monitors, intravenous infusions) and reduced motor control contribute to this practice, thereby interfering with a woman's freedom of movement and potentially slowing the progress of labor.

It is important to encourage ambulation if the membranes are intact, after ROM if the fetal presenting part is engaged, and if the woman has not received medication for pain (Fig. 19.10). The woman also may find it comfortable to stand and lean forward on her partner, doula, or nurse for support at times during labor (Fig. 19.11A). Use of birth balls and chairs may provide comfort to women in labor. In some circumstances ambulation may be contraindicated because of maternal or fetal status.

When the woman lies in bed, she usually changes her position spontaneously as labor progresses. If she does not change position every 30 to 60 minutes, the nurse helps her to do so. The side-lying (lateral) position is preferred because it promotes optimal uteroplacental and renal blood flow and increases fetal oxygen saturation (Fig. 19.12B). If the woman wants to lie supine, the nurse should place a pillow under one hip as a wedge to prevent the uterus from compressing the aorta and vena cava (see Fig. 19.6). Sitting is not contraindicated unless it adversely affects fetal status, which can be determined by checking the FHR and pattern. If the fetus is in the occiput posterior position, it may be helpful to encourage the woman to squat during contractions because this position increases the pelvic diameter, allowing the head to rotate to a more anterior position (see Fig. 19.12A). A position on hands and knees during contractions (see Fig. 19.11B) or a lateral position (see Fig. 19.12B) on the same side as the fetal spine may also be recommended to facilitate rotation of the fetal occiput from a posterior to an anterior position as gravity pulls the fetal back forward. These positions also provide access to the back for application of counterpressure by the partner, doula, or nurse (Simkin et al., 2017; Simpson & O'Brien-Abel, 2014)

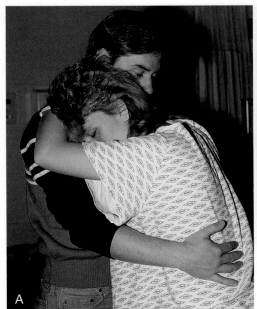
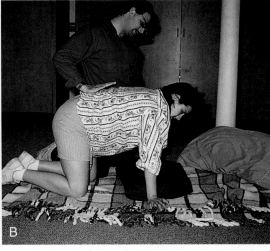

Fig. 19.11 Various Labor Positions. (A) Woman standing and leaning forward with support. (B) Woman in hands-and-knees position. (Courtesy Marjorie Pyle, RNC, Lifecircle, Costa Mesa, CA.)

(see Fig. 19.12B). Women with epidural anesthesia may not be able to squat or assume a hands-and-knees position depending on the degree of motor involvement resulting from the epidural. Much research continues to focus on acquiring a better understanding of the physiologic and psychologic effects of maternal positioning in labor. Box 19.8 describes a variety of positions that are commonly used and recommended.

The woman can use a birth ball (gymnastic ball, physical therapy ball) to support her body as she assumes a variety of labor and birth positions (Fig. 19.13). She can sit on the ball while leaning over the bed or lean over the ball to support her upper body and reduce stress on her arms and hands when she assumes a hands-and-knees position. The birth ball can encourage pelvic mobility and pelvic and perineal relaxation when the woman sits on the firm yet pliable ball and rocks in rhythmic movements. Warm compresses applied to the perineum and lower back can maximize the effect of relaxation and comfort. The birth ball should be large enough that, when the woman sits, her knees are bent at a 90-degree angle and her feet are flat on the floor and approximately 2 feet apart.

For women receiving epidural anesthesia, use of a peanut ball may be beneficial. Epidural anesthesia is associated with prolonged second-stage labor and increased frequency of instrument-assisted birth. A study by Tussey, Botsios, Gerkin, et al. (2015) found that positioning with a peanut ball shortened the second stage of labor and resulted in fewer cesarean births in women with epidural anesthesia. The peanut-shaped ball is placed between the woman's legs with a pillow behind her back for support (Fig. 19.14). The woman should be turned side to side every 1 to 2 hours.

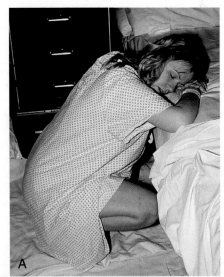
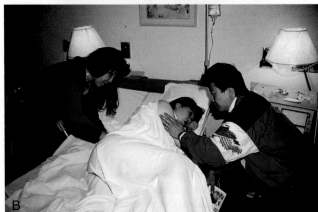

Fig. 19.12 Maternal Positions for Labor. (A) Squatting. (B) Lateral position. Support person is applying sacral pressure while partner provides encouragement. (Courtesy Marjorie Pyle, RNC, Lifecircle, Costa Mesa, CA.)

⚡ **SAFETY ALERT**

A woman may experience dizziness as she changes upright positions during labor. It is essential that the nurse or support person be present to provide assistance should dizziness occur.

BOX 19.8   Common Maternal Positions[a] During Labor and Birth

Semirecumbent Position (See Figs. 19.16B and 19.17B)

With the woman sitting with her upper body elevated to at least a 30-degree angle, place a wedge or small pillow under her hip to prevent vena cava compression and reduce the likelihood of supine hypotension (see Fig. 19.6).

- The greater the angle of elevation, the more gravity or pressure is exerted that promotes fetal descent, the progress of contractions, and the widening of pelvic dimensions.
- This position is convenient for providing care measures and for external fetal monitoring.

Lateral Position (See Figs. 19.12B and 19.16A)

Have the woman alternate between a left and right side-lying position, and provide abdominal and back support as needed for comfort.

- Removes pressure from the vena cava and back, enhances uteroplacental perfusion, and relieves backache
- Facilitates internal rotation of fetus in a posterior position to an anterior position (woman should lie on same side as fetal spine)
- Makes it easier to perform back massage or counterpressure
- Associated with less frequent, but more intense, contractions
- May be more difficult to obtain good quality external fetal monitor tracings
- May be used as a birthing position
- Takes pressure off perineum, allowing it to stretch gradually
- Reduces risk for perineal trauma

Upright Position

The gravity effect enhances the contraction cycle and fetal descent. The weight of the fetus places increasing pressure on the cervix; the cervix is pulled upward, facilitating effacement and dilation; impulses from the cervix to the pituitary gland increase, causing more oxytocin to be secreted; and contractions are intensified, thereby applying more forceful downward pressure on the fetus, but they are less painful.

- Fetus is aligned with pelvis, and pelvic diameters are widened slightly
- Effective upright positions include:
  - Ambulation (see Fig. 19.10)
  - Standing and leaning forward with support provided by coach (see Fig. 19.11A), end of bed, back of chair, or birth ball; relieves backache and facilitates application of counterpressure or back massage
  - Sitting up in bed, in chair, in birthing chair, on toilet, or on bedside commode (see Fig. 19.16B)
  - Squatting (see Figs. 19.12A and 19.17E)

Hands-and-Knees Position—Position for Posterior Positions of the Presenting Part (See Figs. 19.11B and 19.13)

Assume an "all fours" position or lean over an object (e.g., birth ball) while on the knees in bed or on a covered floor; can also place knees on seat section of bed while leaning up over back of raised head of bed; allows for pelvic rocking.

- Relieves backache characteristic of "back labor"
- Facilitates internal rotation of the fetus by increasing mobility of the coccyx, increasing the pelvic diameters, and using gravity to turn the fetal back and rotate the head (**NOTE:** A side-lying position, double hip squeeze, or knee squeeze also can facilitate internal rotation.)

[a]Assess the effect of each position on the laboring woman's comfort and anxiety level, progress of labor, and fetal heart rate and pattern. Alternate positions every 30 to 60 min, allowing the woman to take control of her position changes.

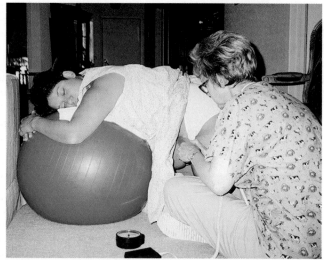

Fig. 19.13 Woman Laboring Using Birth Ball. (Courtesy Polly Perez, Cutting Edge Press, Johnson, VT.)

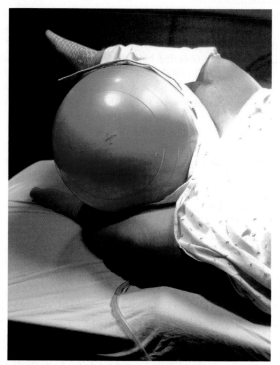

Fig. 19.14 Use of the Peanut Ball for Positioning During Labor. (Courtesy Shanika Mayfield, Joiner, AR.)

Supportive Care During Labor and Birth

Support during labor and birth involves emotional support, physical care and comfort measures, and advice and information. The value of the continuous supportive presence of a person (e.g., partner, family member, friend, nurse, doula) during labor has long been known. Women who have continuous support beginning in early labor are less likely to use pain medication or epidurals and are more likely to have a spontaneous vaginal birth and increased satisfaction with their birth experience. No harmful effects from continuous labor support have been identified. To the contrary, there is good evidence that labor support improves important health outcomes (AWHONN, 2018; Strauss, Giessler, & McAllister, 2015). Continuous labor support is associated with greater benefits when the provider of that support is not a hospital staff member (Simpson & O'Brien-Abel, 2014).

Labor rooms should be airy, clean, and homelike. The laboring woman should feel safe in this environment and free to be herself and use the comfort and relaxation measures she prefers. To enhance relaxation, the use of bright overhead lights is avoided and noise and intrusions are kept to a minimum. The room's temperature is adjusted to ensure the laboring woman's comfort. The room should be large enough to accommodate a comfortable chair for the woman's partner, the monitoring equipment, and hospital personnel. Some women bring their own pillows to make the hospital surroundings more homelike and facilitate position changes. Environmental modifications should reflect the preferences of the woman, including the number of visitors and availability of a telephone, television, electronic devices (e.g., computer, smartphone), and music.

Labor support by the nurse. Supportive nursing care for a woman in labor includes the following:

- Helping her to maintain control and participate to the extent she wishes in the birth of her infant
- Providing continuity of care by the same nurse throughout the shift
- Providing care that is nonjudgmental and respectful of her cultural and religious values and beliefs
- Helping the woman meet her expected outcomes for her labor
- Listening to her concerns and encouraging her to express her feelings
- Acting as her advocate, supporting her decisions and respecting her choices as appropriate, and relating her wishes as needed to other health care providers
- Helping her conserve her energy and cope effectively with her pain and discomfort by using a variety of comfort measures that are acceptable to her
- Acknowledging her efforts during labor, including her strength and courage and those of her partner, and providing positive reinforcement
- Protecting her privacy, modesty, and dignity

Women who have attended childbirth education classes will know something about the labor process, coaching techniques, and comfort measures. The nurse plays a supportive role and keeps the woman and her partner informed of the labor progress. If necessary, the nurse reviews the methods learned in class and practiced at home because it may be difficult for the woman to effectively use these methods and techniques now that she is in labor and in an unfamiliar setting.

Even when a laboring woman has not attended childbirth classes, the nurse can teach her simple breathing and relaxation techniques during the early phase of labor. In this case, the nurse provides coaching and supportive care until the support person feels ready to take on a more active coaching role (see Chapter 17). The nurse can demonstrate comfort measures while encouraging the support person to assist and the laboring woman to express her needs and feelings. Observing the comforting approaches of the nurse can help the partner learn effective comfort measures.

Comfort measures vary with the situation (Fig. 19.15). The nurse can draw on the woman's list of comfort measures and relaxation techniques learned during the pregnancy and through life experiences. Such measures include maintaining a comfortable, calm, supportive atmosphere in the labor and birth area; using touch therapeutically (e.g., heat or cold applied to the lower back in the event of back labor, a cool cloth applied to the forehead, massage); providing nonpharmacologic measures to relieve discomfort (e.g., hydrotherapy); and, most importantly just being there (see Table 19.3). See Chapter 17 for a full discussion of pharmacologic and nonpharmacologic comfort measures.

Most women in labor respond positively to touch; the nurse should obtain permission before using any touching measures. Women

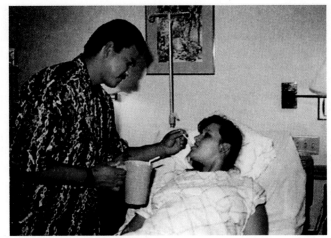

Fig. 19.15 Partner Providing Comfort Measures. (Courtesy Marjorie Pyle, RNC, Lifecircle, Costa Mesa, CA.)

appreciate gentle handling by staff members. Back massage and counterpressure may be offered, especially if the woman is experiencing back labor. The nurse can teach the support person to exert counterpressure against the woman's sacrum over the occiput of the head of a fetus in a posterior position (see Fig. 19.12B). Double hip or knee squeezes can also be helpful in reducing back pain. The back pain is caused by the occiput pressing on spinal nerves; counterpressure lifts the occiput off these nerves, providing some pain relief. The partner needs to be relieved after a while, however, because exerting counterpressure is hard work. Hand and foot massage can also be soothing and relaxing.

The woman's perception of the soothing qualities of touch may change as labor progresses. Many women become more sensitive to touch (hyperesthesia) as labor progresses. This is a typical response during the active phase. They may tell their coach to leave them alone or not to touch them. The partner who is unprepared for this normal response may feel rejected and react by withdrawing active support. The nurse can reassure him or her that this response is a positive indication that the first stage is ending and the second stage is approaching. Women with increased sensitivity to touch may tolerate it better on surfaces of the body where hair does not grow, such as the forehead, the palms of the hands, and the soles of the feet.

Labor support by the partner. The father of the baby is usually the primary support person for the laboring woman, although a same-sex partner, family member, or friend may assume that role. The partner is often able to provide the comfort measures and touch that the laboring woman needs. When the woman becomes focused on her pain, sometimes the partner can persuade her to try nonpharmacologic variations of comfort measures. In addition, the partner is usually able to interpret the woman's needs and desires for staff members.

The emotions and responses of a first-time father change as labor progresses. Although he is often calm at the onset of labor, feelings of fear and helplessness begin to dominate as labor becomes more active and the father realizes that the process is more stressful than he had anticipated. Indeed, first-time fathers experience a wide range of emotions from wonder at new life to shock, anxiety, and worry (Poh, Koh, Seow, & He, 2014). A study of Chinese fathers found that the men perceived their presence as beneficial to the partner by providing emotional support (He, Vehviläinen-Julkunen, Qian, et al., 2015).

BOX 19.9   Guidelines for Supporting the Father or Partner

- Orient him to the labor room and the unit; explain location of the cafeteria, toilet, waiting room, and nursery; give information about visiting hours; introduce personnel by name and describe their functions.
- Inform him of sights and smells he can expect; encourage him to leave the room if necessary.
- Respect his or the couple's decision about the degree of his involvement. Offer them freedom to make decisions.
- Tell him when his presence has been helpful, and continue to reinforce this throughout labor.
- Offer to teach him comfort measures; demonstrate or role-play these measures.
- Inform him frequently of the progress of the labor and the woman's needs. Keep him informed about procedures to be performed.
- Prepare him for changes in the woman's behavior and physical appearance.
- Remind him to eat; offer him snacks and fluids if possible.
- Relieve him of the job of support person as necessary. Offer him blankets if he is to sleep in a chair by the bedside.
- Acknowledge the stress experienced by each partner during labor and birth, and identify normal responses.
- Attempt to modify or eliminate unsettling stimuli, such as extra noise and extra light; create a relaxing and calm environment.

These guidelines are appropriate for any support person.

Staff members should assure the father or partner that his/her presence is helpful and encourage him/her to be involved in the care of the woman to the extent that is comfortable for him/her and his/her partner. He/she should be reassured that he/she is not assuming the responsibility for observation and management of his/her partner's labor but that his/her responsibility is to support her as the labor progresses. The nurse can suggest alternative comfort measures when those he/she is using are no longer helpful or are rejected by his/her partner.

The first-time father or partner may feel excluded as birth preparations begin during the active phase. Once the second stage begins and birth nears, the partner's focus shifts toward the baby about to be born, and he/she will be exposed to many new sights and smells. Therefore the nurse must tell him/her what to expect and make him/her feel comfortable about leaving the room to regain his/her composure, should he/she feel the need, but must also make sure that someone else is available to support the woman during his/her absence.

Nursing actions that support the father or partner convey several important concepts: first, he/she is a person of value; second, he/she can be a partner in the woman's care; and third, childbearing is a team effort. Box 19.9 suggests ways in which the nurse can support the father or partner. A well-informed father or partner can make an important contribution to the health and well-being of the mother and child, their family relationship, and his/her self-esteem.

Labor support by doulas. Continuity of care has been cited by women as a critical component of a satisfying labor and birth experience. A specially trained, experienced female labor attendant called a doula can meet this need. The doula is a professional or lay labor support person who is present during labor in addition to the labor and birth nurse (Burke, 2014). The primary role of the doula is to focus on the laboring woman and provide physical and emotional support by using soft, reassuring words of praise and encouragement, touching, stroking, and hugging. The doula also administers comfort measures to reduce pain and enhance relaxation and coping, walks with the woman, helps her to change positions, and coaches her bearing-down efforts. Doulas provide information about the progress of labor and explain procedures and events. They advocate for the woman's right to participate actively in managing her labor.

The doula also supports the woman's partner, who may feel overwhelmed or unqualified to be the sole labor support; he or she may find it difficult to watch the woman when she is experiencing pain. The doula can encourage and praise the partner's efforts, create a partnership as caregivers and provide respite care. Doulas also facilitate communication between the laboring woman and her partner as well as between the couple and the health care team (Simkin, 2014).

Doula support during labor is associated with decreased use of analgesia, fewer operative births, more spontaneous vaginal births, and greater maternal satisfaction with the labor and birth experience (Kilpatrick & Garrison, 2017; Simkin, 2014).

The roles of the nurse and the doula are complementary. They should work together as a team, recognizing and respecting the role each plays in supporting and caring for the woman and her partner during the labor and birth process. Both the nurse and the doula provide supportive care. The nurse also focuses on monitoring the status of the maternal-fetal unit, implementing clinical care protocols (including pharmacologic interventions), and documenting assessment findings, actions, and responses (Simkin, 2014).

Labor support by grandparents. When a grandparent (usually the mother of the laboring woman) is the primary support person during labor, it is especially important to support and treat her or him with respect. Grandparents may have ways of dealing with pain based on their experience. They should be encouraged to help as long as their actions do not compromise the status of the mother or the fetus. The nurse treats grandparents with dignity and respect by acknowledging the value of their contributions to parental support and recognizing the difficulty parents have in witnessing the woman's discomfort or crisis. Depending on their previous experiences with birth, the nurse may need to provide grandparents with explanations of what is happening. Many of the activities used to support fathers or partners also are appropriate for grandparents (see Box 19.9).

Siblings During Labor and Birth

Preparing siblings for acceptance of the new child helps to promote the attachment process and may help older children accept this change. According to parents' preferences and agency policy, children may be allowed in the labor room. Older children sometimes become active participants in the birthing process. Rehearsal for the event before labor is essential.

The ages and developmental levels of children influence their responses; therefore preparation to be present during labor is adjusted to meet each child's needs. The child younger than 2 years of age shows little interest in pregnancy and labor. However, for the older child, such preparation may reduce fears and misconceptions. Parents must be prepared for labor and birth themselves and feel comfortable about the process and the presence of their children. Most parents have a "feel" for their children's maturational level and their physical and emotional ability to observe and cope with the events of the labor and birth process. Preparation can include a description of the anticipated sights, events (e.g., ROM, monitors, intravenous infusions), smells, and sounds; a labor and birth demonstration; a tour of the birthing unit; sibling classes (see Fig. 14.3); and an opportunity to be around a real newborn. Storybooks about the birth process can be read to or by children to prepare them for the event. Videos are available for preparing preschool and school-age children to participate in the labor and birth experience. Children must learn that their mother will be working hard during labor and birth. She will not be able to talk to them during contractions. She may groan, scream, grunt, and pant at times and say things she would not say otherwise (e.g., "I can't take this anymore," "Take this baby out of me," or "This pain is killing me"). You can tell them that labor is uncomfortable but that their mother's body is made for giving birth.

Most agencies require that a specific person be designated to watch over the children who are participating in their mother's labor and birth experience to provide them with support, explanations, diversions, and comfort as needed. Health care providers involved in attending women during birth must be comfortable with the presence of children and the unpredictability of their questions, comments, and behaviors.

Emergency Interventions

Although rare, emergency conditions that require immediate nursing intervention can arise with startling speed. See Chapter 18 for information on management of an abnormal FHR. Management of other emergency situations—including meconium-stained amniotic fluid, shoulder dystocia, prolapsed umbilical cord, ruptured uterus, and amniotic fluid embolus—is discussed in Chapter 32.

SECOND STAGE OF LABOR

The second stage of labor is the stage at which the infant is born. It begins with full cervical dilation (10 cm) and complete effacement (100%) and ends with the baby's birth (Kelly et al., 2017). The force exerted by uterine contractions, gravity, and maternal bearing-down efforts facilitates the achievement of a spontaneous, uncomplicated vaginal birth. The length of second-stage labor varies considerably among women and is affected by parity and the use of epidural anesthesia. As is true for first-stage labor, researchers have discovered that second-stage labor lasts longer than had been believed in the past (Kopas, 2014). Other factors that influence the length of second-stage labor include the woman's age, body mass index (BMI), emotional state and adequacy of support, and level of fatigue; fetal size, position, and sometimes presentation also play a role (Kelly et al., 2017; Kilpatrick & Garrison, 2017).

Both ACOG and the Society for Maternal Fetal Medicine (SMFM) have endorsed the use of the Ottawa Hospital Protocol as the standard for evaluating the second stage of labor. The Ottawa Hospital Protocol defines the limits of the second stage based upon parity and use of epidural anesthesia. For primiparous women without an epidural, upper limits are set at 3 hours and with an epidural 4 hours. In multiparous women, the limits are set at 2 hours without an epidural and 3 hours with an epidural. These limits allow the woman to progress through the second stage of labor more slowly and potentially decrease rates of cesarean birth. Evidence supports this approach as long as the mother and baby are tolerating the labor process (Simkin et al., 2017). A prolonged second stage is diagnosed once these time limits have been exceeded. The second stage of labor comprises two phases: the latent phase and the active pushing phase. Maternal verbal and nonverbal behaviors, uterine activity, the urge to bear down, and fetal descent characterize these phases.

The latent phase, sometimes referred to as *delayed pushing, laboring down*, or *passive descent*, is a period of rest and relative calm. During this phase the fetus continues to descend passively through the birth canal and rotate to an anterior position as a result of ongoing uterine contractions. The woman is quiet and often relaxes with her eyes closed between contractions. The urge to bear down is not strong, and some women do not experience it at all or only during the acme (peak) of a contraction. Delayed pushing has been shown to result in significant increases in the duration of second-stage labor but significant decreases in pushing time and a reduction in the number of operative vaginal births. On the other hand, no differences in the number of cesarean births, perineal lacerations or episiotomies, or fetal complications have been linked to delayed pushing (Simkin et al., 2017).

Based on research evidence, however, ACOG recommends that nulliparous women with regional anesthesia begin pushing at the start of second stage labor. In these women, delayed pushing has not been shown to improve the chance of vaginal birth. It does, however, increase the risk of hemorrhage and infection (ACOG, 2019a).

Careful monitoring with assurance of normal fetal status should be used during delayed pushing. If descent is slow and the woman becomes anxious, she should be encouraged to change positions frequently or to stand by the bedside to use the advantages of gravity and movement to facilitate descent and progress to the active pushing phase signaled by a perception of the need to bear down.

During the active pushing (descent) phase the woman has strong urges to bear down, as the Ferguson reflex is activated when the presenting part presses on the stretch receptors of the pelvic floor. This stimulation causes the release of oxytocin from the posterior pituitary gland, which provokes stronger expulsive uterine contractions. The woman becomes more focused on bearing-down efforts, which become rhythmic. She changes positions frequently to find a more comfortable pushing position. The woman often announces the onset of contractions and becomes more vocal as she bears down. The urge to bear down intensifies as descent progresses and the presenting part reaches the perineum. The woman may be more verbal about the pain she is experiencing.

The nurse encourages the woman to "listen" to her body as she progresses through the phases of the second stage of labor. When a woman listens to her body to tell her when to bear down, she is using an internal locus of control and often feels more satisfied with her efforts to give birth to her baby. This enhances her sense of self-esteem and accomplishment and her efforts become more effective. The woman's trust in her own body and her ability to give birth to her baby should always be encouraged. Her experience of pressure, stretching, and straining should be validated as normal and a signal that the descent of the fetus is progressing and that her body is capable of withstanding birth. The nurse should honestly explain what is happening and describe the progress being made.

CARE MANAGEMENT

Box 19.10 lists several signs that suggest the onset of second-stage labor and describes nursing care during the second stage of labor. The only certain objective sign that the second stage of labor has begun is the inability to feel the cervix during vaginal examination, indicating that it is fully dilated and effaced. The precise moment that this occurs is not easily determined because it depends on when a vaginal examination is performed to validate full dilation and effacement. This makes timing of the actual duration of the second stage difficult. These signs commonly appear at the time the cervix reaches full dilation. However, they can appear earlier in labor. Women with an epidural block may not exhibit such signs.

Women who are laboring without regional anesthesia can experience an irresistible urge to bear down before full cervical dilation. For some this occurs as early as 5 cm of dilation. This is most often related to the station of the presenting part below the level of the ischial spines of the maternal pelvis. It creates a conflict between the woman, whose body is telling her to push, and her health care providers, who may believe that pushing the fetal presenting part against an incompletely dilated cervix will result in cervical edema and lacerations and also slow the progress of labor. The premature urge to bear down may be a sign of labor progress, possibly indicating the onset of the second stage. If the woman's cervix is not yet completely dilated, encouraging her to breathe through her contractions using shallow, frequent panting or puffing breaths (as though she were blowing out a candle) and to assume a side-lying or hands-and-knees position may be beneficial in helping her to avoid pushing (Kelly et al., 2017).

BOX 19.10 Nursing Care in Second-Stage Labor

Assessment
Signs That Suggest the Onset of the Second Stage
Increase in frequency and intensity of uterine contractions
Urge to push or feeling need to have a bowel movement
An episode of vomiting
Increased bloody show
Uncontrolled shivering
Verbalizations of being out of control or unable to cope
Involuntary bearing-down efforts

Physical Assessment
Perform every 5 to 30 min: maternal blood pressure, pulse, and respirations.
Assess every 5 to 15 min, depending on risk status: fetal heart rate and pattern.
Assess every 10 to 15 min: vaginal show, signs of fetal descent, and changes in maternal appearance, mood, affect, energy level, and involvement of partner/coach.
Assess every contraction and bearing-down effort.

Interventions
Latent Phase
Help the woman to rest in a position of comfort; encourage relaxation to conserve energy.
Promote progress of fetal descent and onset of urge to bear down by encouraging position changes, pelvic rock, ambulation, showering.

Active Pushing Phase
- Provide 1:1 nursing care (1 labor nurse to 1 laboring woman). Do not leave the woman alone.
- Help the woman to change position, and encourage spontaneous bearing-down efforts.
- Help the woman to relax and conserve energy between contractions.
- Provide comfort and pain-relief measures as needed.
- Cleanse the perineum promptly if fecal material is expelled.
- Coach the woman to pant during contractions and to gently push between contractions when head is emerging.
- Provide emotional support, encouragement, and positive reinforcement of efforts.
- Keep the woman informed regarding progress.
- Create a calm and supportive environment.
- Offer a mirror to watch birth.
- Encourage the woman to touch the fetal head when it is visible at the perineum.

Data from Kennedy, B. B., & Baird, S. M. (2017). *Intrapartum management modules: A perinatal education program* (5th ed.). Philadelphia: Wolters Kluwer; American Academy of Pediatrics & American College of Obstetricians and Gynecologists. (2017). *Guidelines for perinatal care* (8th ed.). Washington, DC: American College of Obstetricians and Gynecologists.

Assessment

Assessment continues during the second stage of labor. Professional standards and agency policy determine the specific type and timing of assessments, as well as the way in which findings are documented (see Box 19.10). Signs and symptoms of impending birth (Table 19.4) may appear unexpectedly, requiring immediate action by the nurse (Box 19.11).

The nurse continues to monitor maternal-fetal status and events of the second stage and to provide comfort measures for the mother.

This includes physical care measures (see Table 19.3 and Box 19.10) as well as keeping unnecessary noise, conversation, and other distractions (e.g., laughing, conversations of attending personnel in or outside the labor area) to a minimum. The woman is encouraged to indicate other support measures she would like (see Table 19.3; Nursing Care Plan).

In the hospital, birth may occur in an LDR, LDRP, or delivery room. If the mother is to be transferred to the delivery room for birth, it is best to perform the transfer early enough to avoid rushing her. The birth area is also readied (see later discussion).

Preparing for Birth
Maternal Position
No single ideal position for labor and birth exists. Labor is a dynamic, interactive process involving the woman's uterus, pelvis, and voluntary muscles. In addition, angles between the fetus and the woman's pelvis constantly change as the fetus turns and flexes down the birth canal. The woman may want to assume various positions for labor and birth. She should be encouraged to change positions frequently and helped to attain and maintain her positions of choice (Figs. 19.16 and 19.17). Supine, semirecumbent, or lithotomy positions are still widely used in western societies despite evidence that an upright position shortens labor (Desseauve, Fradet, Lacouture, & Pierre, 2017).

Birth attendants play a major role in influencing a woman's choice of positions for birth, with nurse-midwives tending to suggest non-lithotomy positions (e.g., upright, lateral) for the second stage of labor. An upright position (walking, sitting, kneeling, or squatting) has a number of advantages. Gravity can promote the descent of the fetus. Uterine contractions are generally stronger and more efficient in effacing and dilating the cervix, resulting in shorter labor (Blackburn, 2018; Desseauve et al., 2017). An upright position is also beneficial to the mother's cardiac output, thereby increasing perfusion of the uterus. The use of upright and lateral positions is also associated with less pain and perineal damage, fewer episiotomies and abnormal FHR patterns, and fewer operative vaginal births (Desseauve et al., 2017).

Squatting is highly effective in facilitating the descent and birth of the fetus. It is one of the best and most natural positions for second-stage labor and has been associated with the same benefits as other upright and lateral positions A firm surface is required for this position, and the woman will need side support (see Fig. 19.12A). In a birthing bed, a squat bar is available that she can use to support herself (Fig. 19.17E). A birth ball can also help a woman maintain the squatting position. The fetus will be aligned with the birth canal, and pelvic and perineal relaxation is facilitated as she sits on the ball or holds it in front of her for support as she squats (see Box 19.8).

When a woman uses the supported standing position for bearing down, her weight is borne on both femoral heads, allowing the pressure in the acetabulum to cause the transverse diameter of the pelvic outlet to increase by up to 1 cm. This can be helpful if descent of the head is delayed because the occiput has not rotated from the lateral (transverse diameter of pelvis) to the anterior position. Birthing chairs or rocking chairs may be used to provide a position that will enhance bearing-down efforts (see Box 19.8), although some women may feel restricted by a chair. The upright position also provides a potential psychologic advantage in that it allows the mother to see the birth as it occurs and to maintain eye contact with the attendant.

Oversized beanbag chairs and large floor pillows can be used for both labor and birth. They can mold around and support the mother in whichever position she selects. These chairs are of value for mothers who wish to be actively involved in the birth process. Birthing stools can be used to support the woman in an upright position similar to squatting. Some women may feel more comfortable sitting on a toilet or commode during pushing because they are concerned about stool incontinence

TABLE 19.4   Expected Maternal Progress in the Second Stage of Labor

Criterion	Latent Phase	Active Pushing Phase (Average Duration Varies)[a]
Contractions		
Intensity	Period of physiologic lull for all criteria; period of peace and rest; passive descent occurs	Significant increase becoming overwhelmingly strong and expulsive; strong by palpation
Frequency		Every 2-3 min progressing to every 1-2 min
Duration		90 sec
Descent, station	0-2 or more	2-4 or more; rate of descent increases and Ferguson reflex[b] is activated; fetal head becomes visible at introitus and birth occurs
Show: color and amount		Significant increase in dark red bloody show; bloody show accompanies emergence of head
Spontaneous bearing down efforts	Slight to absent, except at peak of strongest contractions	Increased urge to bear down; becomes stronger as fetus descends to vaginal introitus and reaches perineum
Vocalization	Quiet	Grunting sounds or expiratory vocalizations; announces contractions; may scream or swear
Maternal behavior	Experiences sense of relief that transition to second stage is finished	Senses increased urge to push and describes increasing pain; describes *ring of fire* (burning sensation of acute pain as vagina stretches and fetal head crowns)
	Feels fatigued and sleepy	Expresses feeling of powerlessness
	Feels a sense of accomplishment and optimism because the "worst is over"	Shows decreased ability to listen to or concentrate on anything but giving birth
	Feels in control	Alters respiratory pattern: has short 4- to 5-sec breath holds with regular breaths in between 5 and 7 times per contraction
		Frequent repositioning
		Often shows excitement immediately after birth of head

[a]Duration of descent phase can vary depending on maternal parity, effectiveness of bearing-down efforts, and presence of spinal anesthesia or epidural analgesia.

[b]Pressure of presenting part on stretch receptors of pelvic floor stimulates release of oxytocin from posterior pituitary gland, resulting in more intense uterine contractions.

Data from Kopas, M. L. (2014). A review of evidence–based practices for management of the second stage of labor. *Journal of Midwifery & Women's Health, 59*(3), 264–276; Association of Women's Health, Obstetric and Neonatal Nurses. (2008). *Nursing care and management of the second stage of labor: Evidence-based clinical practice guideline* (2nd ed.). Washington, DC; Simkin, P., Hanson, L., & Ancheta, R. (2017). *The labor progress handbook: Early interventions to prevent and treat dystocia* (4th ed.). Hoboken, NJ: John Wiley & Sons Inc.

during this stage. They should be encouraged to empty their bladder to avoid the effects of a distended bladder. The nurse must closely monitor these women, however, and ask them to move from the toilet before birth becomes imminent. Because sitting on chairs, stools, toilets, or commodes can increase perineal edema and blood loss, it is important to help the woman change her position frequently (e.g., every 10 to 15 minutes).

The side-lying, or lateral, position, with the upper part of the woman's leg held by the nurse or coach or placed on a pillow, is an effective position for the second stage of labor (see Fig. 19.16A and Box 19.8). Some women prefer a semisitting (semirecumbent) position instead (see Fig. 19.17B and Box 19.8). If the semirecumbent position is used, the woman's legs are not forced against her abdomen as she bears down. Because this position increases perineal stretching and the risk for perineal trauma as well as spinal and lower extremity neurologic injuries, it is physiologically inappropriate and should not be used (Simpson & O'Brien-Abel, 2014). The hands-and-knees position is yet another effective position for birth, especially if the fetal position is posterior, because it can facilitate rotation (Kelly et al., 2017) (see Fig. 19.11B and Box 19.8).

The birthing bed can be set for different positions according to the woman's needs (see Fig. 19.17; Fig. 19.18). The woman can squat, kneel, sit, recline, or lie on her side, choosing the position most comfortable for her without having to climb into bed for the birth. At the same time, the birthing bed provides excellent access and visualization for the birth attendant to perform examinations, place electrodes, and assist the woman giving birth. The bed can be positioned for the administration of anesthesia and is ideal for the woman receiving an epidural, helping her to assume different positions. The bed can also be used to transport the woman to the operating room if a cesarean birth should become necessary. The woman can use squat bars, over-the-bed tables, birth balls, and pillows for support.

Bearing-Down Efforts

As the fetal head reaches the pelvic floor, most women experience the urge to bear down. Reflexively the woman will begin to exert downward pressure by contracting her abdominal muscles while relaxing her pelvic floor. This bearing down is an involuntary response to the Ferguson reflex. A strong expiratory grunt or groan (vocalization) often accompanies pushing when the woman exhales as she pushes. This natural vocalization by women during open-glottis bearing-down efforts should not be discouraged.

When a woman is being coached to push, she is encouraged to push as she feels the urge to do so (instinctive, spontaneous pushing) rather than to give a prolonged push on command (directed, closed-glottis pushing). Prolonged breath-holding, or sustained, directed bearing down is still a common practice, often beginning at 10-cm dilation and before the urge to bear down is perceived. The woman is coached to hold her breath, closing her glottis, and to push while the nurse or partner counts to 10. This method of bearing down is strongly discouraged because it may trigger the Valsalva maneuver, which occurs when the woman closes her glottis (closed-glottis pushing), causing an increase in intrathoracic and cardiovascular pressure, thus reducing cardiac output and

BOX 19.11 Guidelines for Assistance at the Emergency Birth of a Fetus in the Vertex Presentation

1. The woman usually assumes the position most comfortable for her. A lateral position is often recommended to facilitate a controlled birth of the head, thereby minimizing the risk for perineal trauma and neonatal head injury.
2. Reassure the woman that birth is usually uncomplicated in these situations. Use eye-to-eye contact and a calm, relaxed manner. If there is someone else available, such as the partner, that person can help support the woman in the position, assist with coaching, and provide positive reinforcement and praise of her efforts.
3. Perform hand hygiene; wash your hands or use hand sanitizer; put on gloves, if available.
4. Place under the woman's buttocks whatever clean material is available.
5. Avoid touching the vaginal area to decrease the possibility of infection.
6. As the head begins to crown, you should perform the following tasks:
   a. Tear the amniotic membranes if they are still intact.
   b. Instruct the woman to pant or pant-blow, thus minimizing the urge to push.
   c. Place the flat side of your hand on the exposed fetal head and apply *gentle* pressure toward the vagina to prevent the head from "popping out." The mother may participate by placing her hand under yours on the emerging head. CAUTION: Rapid birth of the fetal head must be prevented because a rapid change of pressure within the molded fetal skull follows, which may result in dural or subdural tears. Rapid birth also may cause vaginal or perineal lacerations.
7. After the birth of the head, check to see if the umbilical cord is around the baby's neck. If it is, *gently* try to slip it over the baby's head or pull it *gently* to get some slack so that you can slip it over the shoulders.
8. Support the baby's head as external rotation occurs. Then with one hand on each side of the baby's head, exert *gentle* pressure downward so that the anterior shoulder emerges under the symphysis pubis and acts as a fulcrum; then, as *gentle* pressure is exerted upward, the posterior shoulder, which has passed over the sacrum and coccyx, emerges.
9. Be alert! Hold the baby securely because the rest of the body may emerge quickly. The baby will be slippery!
10. Cradle the baby's head and back in one hand and the buttocks in the other. Keep the baby's head down to drain away the mucus. Use a bulb syringe, if needed, to remove mucus from the baby's mouth and then from the nose.
11. Immediately place the baby skin-to-skin on the mother's abdomen. Dry the baby quickly to prevent rapid heat loss. Keep the baby at the same level as the mother's uterus until the cord stops pulsating. **NOTE:** The baby should be kept at the same level as the mother's uterus to prevent the baby's blood from flowing to or from the placenta and resulting in hypovolemia or hypervolemia. Also, do not "milk" the cord.
12. With the baby on the mother's abdomen, cover the baby (remember to keep the head warm, too) with a warmed blanket or the mother's clothing, and have her cuddle the baby. Compliment her (them) on a job well done, and on the baby, if appropriate.
13. Wait for the placenta to separate. *Do not* tug on the cord. **NOTE:** Inappropriate traction may tear the cord, separate the placenta, or invert the uterus. Signs of placental separation include a slight gush of dark blood from the introitus, lengthening of the cord, and change in the uterine contour from a discoid to globular shape.
14. Instruct the mother to push to deliver the separated placenta. Gently ease out the placental membranes using an up-and-down motion until the membranes are removed. If birth occurs outside a hospital setting, to minimize complications do not cut the cord without proper clamps and a sterile cutting tool. Inspect the placenta for intactness. Place the baby on the placenta and wrap the two together for additional warmth.
15. Check the firmness of the uterus. Gently massage the fundus and demonstrate to the mother how she can massage her own fundus properly.
16. If supplies are available, clean the mother's perineal area and apply a peripad.
17. In addition to gentle massage of the fundus, the following measures can be taken to prevent or minimize hemorrhage:
    a. Put the baby to the mother's breast as soon as possible. Sucking or nuzzling and licking the nipple stimulates the release of oxytocin from the posterior pituitary gland. **NOTE:** If the baby does not or cannot nurse, manually stimulate the mother's nipples.
    b. Do not allow the mother's bladder to become distended. Assess the bladder for fullness and encourage her to void if fullness is found.
    c. Expel any clots from the mother's uterus after ensuring that the fundus is firm.
18. Comfort or reassure the mother and her family or friends. Keep the mother and the baby warm. Give her fluids if available and tolerated.
19. If there is more than one baby, identify the infants in order of birth (using letters *A, B,* and so on).
20. Make notations regarding the following aspects of the birth:
    a. Fetal presentation and position
    b. Presence of cord around neck (nuchal cord) or other parts and number of times cord encircled part
    c. Color, character, and estimated amount of amniotic fluid, if rupture of membranes occurred immediately before birth
    d. Time of birth
    e. Estimated time of determination of Apgar score (e.g., 1 and 5 min after birth), resuscitation efforts implemented, and ultimate condition of baby
    f. Gender of baby
    g. Time of placental expulsion, as well as the appearance and completeness of the placenta
    h. Maternal condition: affect, behavior, and demeanor, amount of bleeding, and status of uterine tonicity
    i. Any unusual occurrences during the birth (e.g., maternal or paternal response, verbalizations, or gestures in response to birth of baby).

---

decreasing perfusion of the uterus and placenta. Adverse effects associated with prolonged breath-holding and forceful pushing include fetal hypoxia and subsequent acidosis and increased risk for pelvic floor damage (structural and neurogenic) and perineal trauma (Blackburn, 2018; Kopas, 2014; Simkin, et al., 2017; Simpson & O'Brien-Abel, 2014). The benefits of spontaneous pushing efforts rather than sustained Valsalva pushes include less fatigue and enhanced comfort. In addition, these more effective bearing-down efforts result in less time spent actively pushing (Blackburn; Simpson & O'Brien-Abel). Based on this evidence, it is essential that labor and birth nurses advocate for the practice of delayed and spontaneous bearing-down efforts with the woman in an upright or lateral position (Kopas; Simkin et al.).

Spontaneous open-glottis pushing (bearing down while exhaling) for 6 to 8 seconds at a time is encouraged. The nurse or support person reminds the woman to take a cleansing breath after each contraction. Open-glottis pushing and taking breaths between bearing-down efforts help to maintain adequate oxygen levels for the mother and fetus, thus enhancing fetal well-being. The active pushing phase of the second stage of labor is considered the most physiologically stressful part of labor. Therefore, every effort should be made to ensure that women

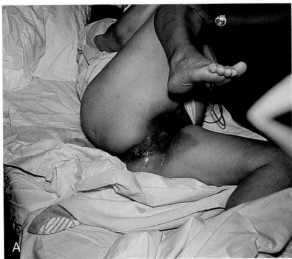
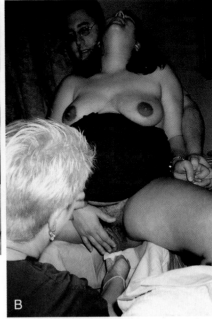

Fig. 19.16 Birth. (A) Pushing, side-lying position. Perineal bulging can be seen. (B) Pushing, semi-sitting position. Nurse-midwife helps mother to feel top of fetal head. (A, Courtesy Michael S. Clement, MD, Mesa, AZ. B, Courtesy Roni Wernik, Palo Alto, CA.)

use nondirected spontaneous pushing to conserve energy and maximize the effect of each bearing-down effort. Laboring women should be allowed time to figure out the best position and method for pushing (Kopas, 2014).

A woman may reach the second stage of labor and then experience a lack of readiness to complete the process and give birth to her baby. She may have doubts about her readiness to be a mother or insist on waiting for her support person or nurse-midwife or physician to arrive. Fear, anxiety, or embarrassment regarding unfamiliar or painful sensations and behaviors during pushing (e.g., sounds made, passage of stool) may be other inhibiting factors. Fear that the baby will be in danger once it emerges from the protective intrauterine environment may also be present. By recognizing that a woman may feel the need to hold back the birth of her baby, the nurse can address her concerns and effectively coach her during this stage of labor.

To ensure the slow birth of the fetal head, the woman is encouraged to control the urge to bear down by coaching her to take panting breaths or exhale slowly through pursed lips as the baby's head crowns. At this point the woman needs simple, clear directions from one person. Amnesia between contractions often occurs in the second stage of labor; therefore the nurse may have to rouse the woman to get her to cooperate in the bearing-down process. Couples who have attended childbirth education classes may have devised a set of verbal cues for the laboring woman to follow.

Fetal Heart Rate and Pattern

The nurse must check the FHR regularly (see Chapter 18 for further discussion). If the baseline rate begins to slow, if absent or minimal variability occurs, or if abnormal (e.g., late, variable, or prolonged) deceleration patterns develop, interventions are initiated promptly. The first action is to turn the woman onto her side to reduce the pressure of the uterus against the ascending vena cava and descending aorta (see Fig. 19.6). Oxygen can be administered by nonrebreather mask at 10 L/min (Miller et al., 2017). These interventions are often all that is necessary to restore a normal pattern. If the FHR and pattern do not become

normal immediately, the next step is to notify the nurse-midwife or physician because the woman may need medical intervention to give birth. See Chapter 18 for more interventions related to abnormal FHR.

LEGAL TIP

Documentation

The course of labor and the maternal-fetal response may change without warning. Documentation of all observations (e.g., maternal vital signs, fetal heart rate and pattern, progress of labor) and nursing interventions, including the woman's response, must be accurate, complete, timely, and according to agency policy.

Support of the Partner

During the second stage the woman needs continuous support and coaching (see Table 19.4 and Box 19.10). Because the coaching process is often physically and emotionally tiring for support people, the nurse may offer nourishment and fluids and encourage short breaks as needed (see Box 19.9). If birth occurs in an LDR or LDRP room, the support person usually wears street clothes. The support person who attends the birth in a delivery or operating room may be asked to put on a cover gown or scrub clothes, mask, cap, and shoe covers if required by agency policy. The nurse also specifies support measures that can be used for the laboring woman and points out areas of the room in which the partner can move freely.

The nurse encourages partners to be present at the birth of their infants if doing so is in keeping with their cultural and personal expectations and beliefs. The presence of partners maintains the psychologic closeness of the family unit, and the partner can continue to provide the supportive care given during labor. The woman and her partner must have equal opportunities to initiate the attachment process with the baby.

Supplies, Instruments, and Equipment

Necessary supplies, instruments, and equipment should be gathered and prepared for use well before the anticipated time of birth. To prepare for

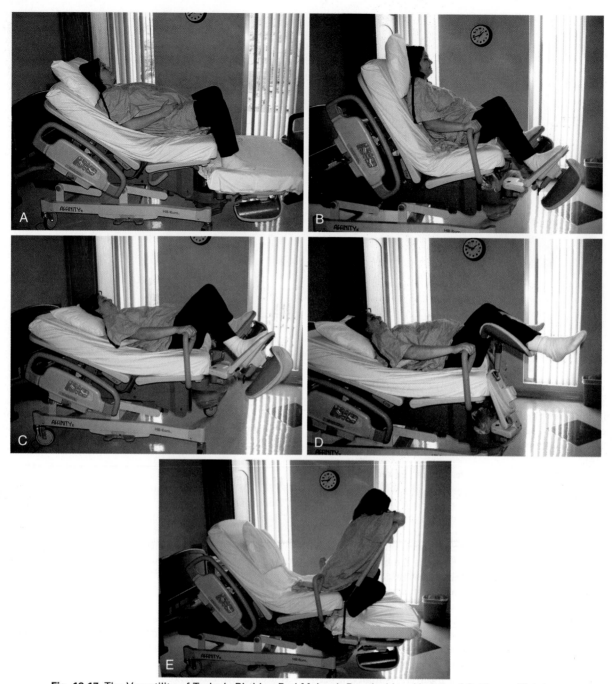

Fig. 19.17 The Versatility of Today's Birthing Bed Makes It Practical in a Variety of Settings. (A) Labor bed. (B) Birth chair. (C) Birth bed with support provided by foot rests. (D) Birth bed with legs supported by stirrups. (E) Squatting with use of birth bar. (Courtesy Julie Perry Nelson, Loveland, CO.)

birth in any setting, the instrument table or delivery cart is usually set up late in the active phase of first-stage labor for nulliparous women and earlier in that phase for multiparous women. Instruments are arranged according to agency protocol (Fig. 19.19). The health care team follows standard procedures for gloving, identifying and opening sterile packages, adding sterile supplies to the instrument table, unwrapping sterile instruments, and handing them to the nurse-midwife or physician. The crib or radiant warmer and equipment for the support and stabilization of the newborn are placed for ready access (Fig. 19.20). In some agencies this may be done by the surgical technician or the nursing assistant. The items used at a birth may vary from one facility to another; this may be clarified by consulting the facility's procedure manual to determine its

particular protocols. Additionally, providers may have personal preferences regarding what equipment is to be used at the birth.

The nurse estimates the time until the birth will occur and notifies the nurse-midwife or physician if he or she is not in the woman's room. Even the most experienced nurse can err in estimating the time left before birth occurs; therefore every nurse who attends a woman in labor must be prepared to assist with an emergency birth if the physician or nurse-midwife is not present (see Box 19.11).

Birth in a Delivery Room or Birthing Room

Currently women most often give birth vaginally in a birthing room, in the same bed where they have labored, rather than in a delivery room.

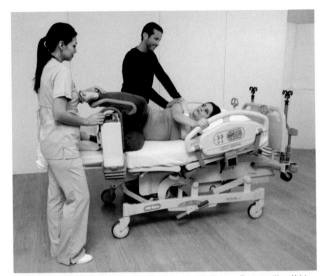

Fig. 19.18 Birthing Bed. (Courtesy Hill-Rom, Batesville, IN.)

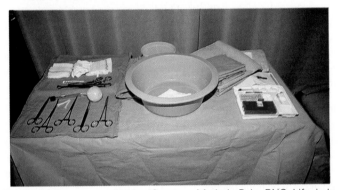

Fig. 19.19 Instrument Table. (Courtesy Marjorie Pyle, RNC, Lifecircle, Costa Mesa, CA.)

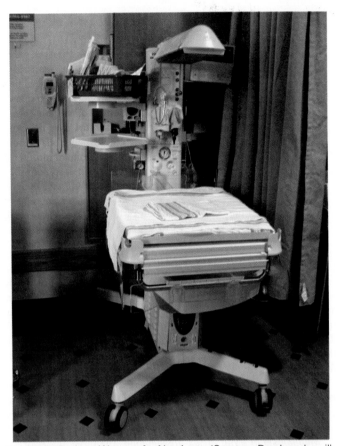

Fig. 19.20 Radiant Warmer for Newborn. (Courtesy Dee Lowdermilk, Chapel Hill, NC.)

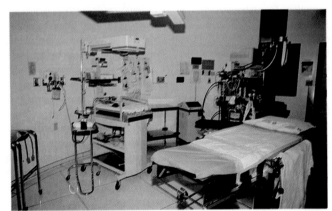

Fig. 19.21 Delivery Room. (Courtesy Michael S. Clement, MD, Mesa, AZ.)

The maternal position for birth in a birthing room varies from a lithotomy position with the woman's feet in stirrups or resting on foot rests or with her legs held and supported by the nurse or support person, to one in which her feet rest on footrests while she holds on to a squat bar, to a side-lying position with the woman's upper leg supported by the coach, nurse, or squat bar. Once the woman is positioned, the foot of the bed may be removed so that the nurse-midwife or physician attending the birth can gain better perineal access for performing an episiotomy, delivering a large baby, using forceps or a vacuum extractor, or getting access to the emerging head to facilitate suctioning. Alternatively, the foot of the bed can be left in place and lowered slightly to form a ledge that allows access for birth and serves as a place to lay the newborn (see Fig. 19.17A).

The woman will need assistance if she must move from the labor bed to the delivery table (Fig. 19.21). The positions assumed for birth in a delivery room are the Sims or lateral position, in which the attendant supports the upper part of the woman's leg, the dorsal position (supine position with one hip elevated), and the lithotomy position.

The lithotomy position makes dealing with some complications that arise more convenient for the nurse-midwife or physician (see Fig. 19.17D). For this position, the nurse brings the woman's buttocks to the edge of the bed or table and places the legs in stirrups. The nurse pads the stirrups, carefully raises and places both legs simultaneously, and then adjusts the shanks of the stirrups so the calves of the legs are supported. No pressure should be placed on the popliteal space. Stirrups that are not the same height will strain ligaments in the woman's back as she bears down,

leading to considerable discomfort in the postpartum period. The lower portion of the table may be dropped down and rolled back under the table.

Once the woman is positioned for birth either in a birthing room or delivery room, the vulva and perineum are cleansed. Hospital or birthing center protocols and the preferences of nurse-midwives or physicians for cleansing may vary.

The nurse continues to coach and encourage the woman and monitor the fetal status (see Box 19.10), keeping the nurse midwife or physician informed of the FHR and pattern. The nurse obtains or prepares an oxytocic medication such as oxytocin (Pitocin) so that it is ready to be administered immediately after expulsion of the baby or the placenta. Standard precautions are always followed throughout the process of labor and birth (see Box 19.4).

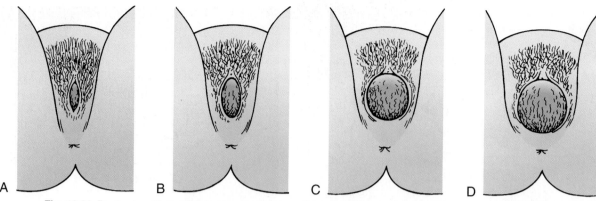

Fig. 19.22 Beginning Birth With Vertex Presenting. (A) Anteroposterior slit. (B) Oval opening. (C) Circular shape. (D) Crowning.

In the hospital delivery room, the nurse-midwife or physician may put on a cap, a mask that has a shield or protective eyewear, and shoe covers. After performing hand hygiene, the provider puts on a sterile gown (with waterproof front and sleeves) and sterile gloves. Nurses attending the birth may also have to wear caps, protective eyewear, masks, gowns, and gloves. The woman may then be draped with sterile drapes. In the birthing room, standard precautions are observed, but the amount and type of protective covering worn by those in attendance may vary.

During the birth process, the nurse maintains contact with the parents by touching, verbally comforting them, describing the progress, explaining the reasons for the ongoing care, and sharing in the parents' joy at the birth of their baby.

Mechanism of birth: vertex presentation. The three phases of the spontaneous birth of a fetus in a vertex presentation are (1) birth of the head, (2) birth of the shoulders, and (3) birth of the body and extremities (see Chapter 16).

With voluntary bearing-down efforts, the head appears at the introitus (Fig. 19.22A–D). Crowning occurs when the widest part of the head (the biparietal diameter) distends the vulva just before birth. Immediately before birth, the perineal musculature becomes greatly distended. If an episiotomy (incision into the perineum to enlarge the vaginal outlet) is necessary, it is done at this time to minimize soft-tissue damage. A local anesthetic may be administered if necessary before performing an episiotomy. Box 19.12 shows the process of normal vaginal birth in a series of photographs.

The physician or nurse-midwife may use a hands-on approach to control the birth of the head, believing that guarding the perineum results in a gradual birth that will prevent fetal intracranial injury, protect maternal tissues, and reduce postpartum perineal pain. This approach involves (1) applying pressure against the rectum, drawing it downward to aid in flexing the head as the back of the neck catches under the symphysis pubis; (2) applying upward pressure from the coccygeal region (modified *Ritgen maneuver*) (Fig. 19.23) to extend the head during the actual birth, thereby protecting the musculature of the perineum; and (3) assisting the mother with voluntary control of the bearing-down efforts by coaching her to pant while letting uterine forces expel the fetus.

Some health care providers use a hands-poised (hands-off) approach when they are attending a birth. In this approach, the hands are prepared to place light pressure on the fetal head to prevent rapid expulsion. The provider does not place his or her hands on the perineum or use them to assist with birth of the shoulders and body.

The hands-on and hands-poised approaches have similar results in terms of perineal and vaginal tears, but the hands-on technique is associated with a higher incidence of episiotomies. Laceration rates are similar between the two groups (Kopas, 2014).

The umbilical cord may encircle the neck (*nuchal cord*) but rarely so tightly as to cause hypoxia. After the head is born, gentle palpation is used to feel for the cord. If present, the health care provider slips the cord gently over the head if possible. If the loop is tight or there is a second loop, he or she will probably clamp the cord twice, cut between the clamps, and unwind the cord from around the neck before the birth is allowed to continue. Suctioning immediately following birth should be done only for those infants with respiratory obstruction or those requiring positive pressure ventilation. Avoiding unnecessary suctioning of the nasopharynx avoids inducing bradycardia (Reed, 2017).

Immediate Assessments and Care of the Newborn

The time of birth is the precise time when the entire body is out of the mother and must be recorded. In the case of multiple births, each birth is noted in the same way. If the mother's and newborn's conditions allow, immediate skin-to-skin contact and delayed cord clamping are likely to be implemented.

Skin-to-skin contact is recommended for the healthy term newborn immediately after vaginal birth and as soon as possible following cesarean birth. The baby is placed prone on the woman's bare abdomen or chest and dried. Next, a cap is placed on his or her head. The wet blankets are removed, and baby and woman are covered with fresh warm blankets (Fig. 19.24). Immediate skin-to-skin contact has been shown to positively affect maternal-infant bonding, breastfeeding duration, cardiorespiratory stability, and body temperature. Blood glucose levels during the first 2 hours of life are higher in these babies compared with newborns who did not receive immediate skin-to-skin contact (Kilpatrick & Garrison, 2017; Stewart & Rodgers, 2017). It is recommended that immediate skin-to-skin contact be considered the standard of care because this practice conveys many benefits and has no adverse effects. Routine assessments and procedures can be completed with the newborn on the woman's abdomen/chest (King & Pinger, 2014).

It is now recommended that the umbilical cord not be clamped until 1 to 5 minutes after birth, or until after the cord stops pulsating, to allow physiologic transfer of blood to the newborn. The optimal duration of delayed cord clamping appears to be up to 3 minutes unless the cord stops pulsating sooner. Delayed cord clamping allows for a placental transfusion of up to 30% of the total fetal-placental blood volume. This transfusion includes many types of stem cells, RBCs, and whole blood. It is recommended that delayed cord clamping be considered the standard of care because it improves both the short- and long-term hematologic status of the newborn and has no clinically significant adverse effects (King & Pinger, 2014). At the appropriate time, the nurse-midwife or physician may ask if the woman's partner would like to cut the cord. If so, the partner is given a pair of sterile scissors and instructed to cut the cord approximately 2.5 cm above the clamp.

BOX 19.12 Normal Vaginal Birth

First Stage

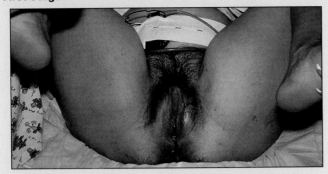

Anteroposterior slit. Vertex visible during contraction.

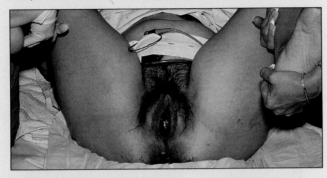

Oval opening. Vertex presenting. **NOTE:** Nurse *(on left)* is wearing gloves, but support person *(on right)* is not.

Second Stage

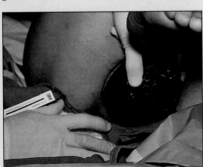

Crowning.

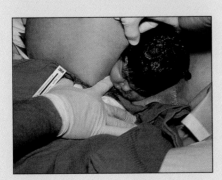

Nurse-midwife using Ritgen maneuver as head is born by extension.

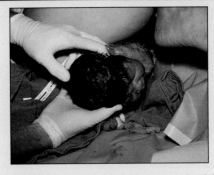

After nurse-midwife checks for nuchal cord, she supports head during external rotation and restitution.

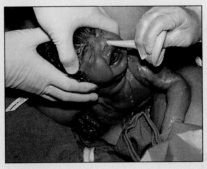

Use of bulb syringe to suction mucus.

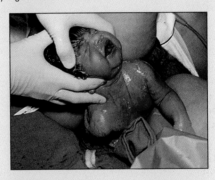

Birth of posterior shoulder.

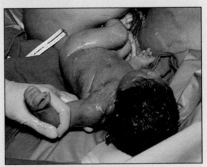

Birth of newborn by slow expulsion.

BOX 19.12   Normal Vaginal birth—cont'd

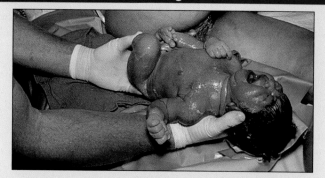

Second stage complete. Note that newborn is not completely pink yet.

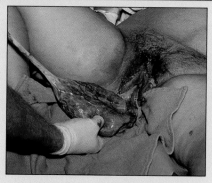

Expulsion is complete, marking the end of the third stage.

Third Stage

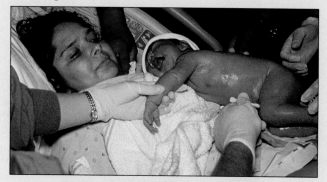

Newborn placed on mother's abdomen while cord is clamped and cut.

The Newborn

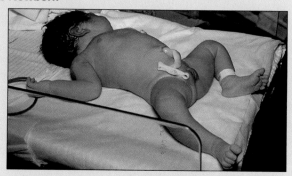

Newborn awaiting assessment. Note that color is almost completely pink.

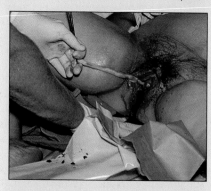

Note increased bleeding as placenta separates.

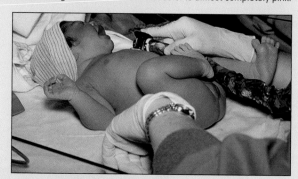

Newborn assessment under radiant warmer.

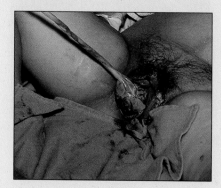

Expulsion of placenta.

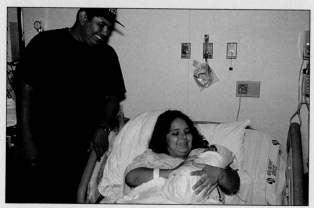

Parents admiring their newborn.

(Photos courtesy of Michael S. Clement, MD; Mesa, AZ.)

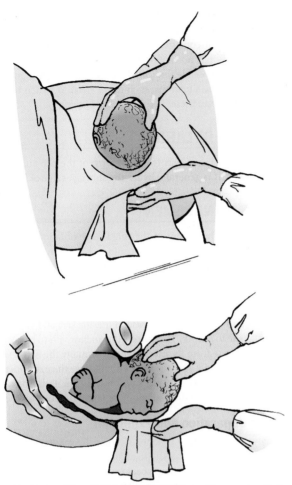

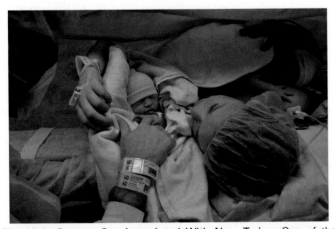

Fig. 19.23 Birth of Head With Modified Ritgen Maneuver. Note control to prevent too-rapid birth of head.

Fig. 19.24 Parents Get Acquainted With New Twins. One of the newborns is enjoying skin-to-skin contact with mom. (Courtesy of Emily and Kevin Jones, Holly Springs, NC.)

In another approach, referred to as *lotus birth*, the cord is not clamped and cut at all. Instead, the cord and placenta remain attached to the baby until the cord naturally separates from the baby several days after birth (Zinsser, 2018).

The care given immediately after the birth focuses on assessing and stabilizing the newborn. The Neonatal Resuscitation Program (NRP) (Reed, 2015) and AWHONN (2010) recommend that at least two nurses be present for each birth. One nurse is responsible for care

of the newborn while the other helps the nurse-midwife or physician with delivery of the placenta and care of the mother. The "baby nurse" must observe the infant for any signs of distress and initiate appropriate interventions. AWHONN and NRP also recommend that, in cases of multiple births, each baby has his or her own nurse.

The nurse performs a brief assessment of the newborn immediately even while skin-to-skin contact is being performed. This assessment includes assigning Apgar scores at 1 and 5 minutes after birth (see Table 24.1). Major priorities for immediate newborn care include maintaining a patent airway, supporting respiratory effort, and preventing cold stress by drying and preferably covering the newborn with a warmed blanket while on his or her mother's abdomen/chest or, less optimally, placing him or her under a radiant warmer. If the newborn appears to be stable, further examination, identification procedures, and care can be postponed until later in the third stage of labor or early in the fourth stage.

Perineal Trauma Related to Childbirth

Most acute injuries and lacerations of the perineum, vagina, uterus, and their support tissues occur during childbirth. Interventions such as application of warm compresses and gentle perineal massage and stretching have been suggested as measures to decrease perineal lacerations and trauma. Perineal massage during the last month of pregnancy has clear benefits of reducing perineal trauma during birth and pain afterward for women who have not previously given birth vaginally (Kopas, 2014). A Cochrane review found that massage and warm compresses during the second stage of labor may be beneficial in reducing the incidence of third- and fourth-degree lacerations (Aasheim, Nilsen, Reinar, & Lukasse, 2017).

Some degree of trauma to the soft tissues of the birth canal and adjacent structures occurs during every birth. The tendency to sustain lacerations varies with each woman; that is, the soft tissue in some women may be less distensible. Damage usually is more pronounced in nulliparous women because the tissues are firmer and more resistant than those in multiparous women. Heredity is also a factor. For example, the tissue of light-skinned women, especially those with reddish hair, is not as readily distensible as that of darker-skinned women, and healing may be less efficient. Other risk factors associated with perineal trauma include maternal nutritional status, birth position, pelvic anatomy (e.g., narrow subpubic arch with a constricted outlet), fetal malpresentation and position (e.g., breech, occiput posterior position), large (macrosomic) infants, use of forceps or vacuum to facilitate birth, prolonged second-stage labor, and rapid labor in which there is insufficient time for the perineum to stretch.

Some injuries to the supporting tissues, whether they are acute or nonacute or are repaired or not, may lead to genitourinary and sexual problems later in life (e.g., pelvic relaxation, uterine prolapse, cystocele, rectocele, dyspareunia, and urinary and bowel dysfunction) (see Chapter 11). Performing Kegel exercises in the prenatal and postpartum periods improves and restores the tone and strength of the perineal muscles (see box Teaching for Self-Management: Kegel Exercises in Chapter 4). Proper health practices, including good nutrition and appropriate hygienic measures, help to maintain the integrity and suppleness of the perineal tissues, enhance healing, and prevent infection.

Perineal lacerations. Perineal lacerations may occur as the fetal head is being born. The extent of the laceration is defined in terms of its depth (Cunningham, Leveno, Bloom, et al., 2018; Kilpatrick & Garrison, 2017) as follows:

First degree: Laceration that extends through the skin and structures superficial to muscles

Second degree: Laceration that extends through muscles of the perineal body

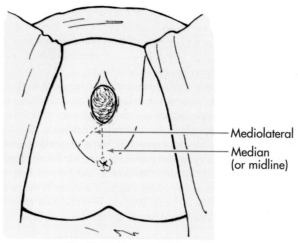

Fig. 19.25 Types of Episiotomies.

Third degree: Laceration that continues through the external anal sphincter muscle

Fourth degree: Laceration that extends completely through the anal sphincter and the rectal mucosa

Perineal injury is often accompanied by small lacerations on the medial surfaces of the labia minora below the pubic rami and to the sides of the urethra (periurethral) and clitoris. Lacerations in this highly vascular area often result in profuse bleeding. Third- and fourth-degree lacerations must be carefully repaired so that the woman will retain fecal continence. Simple perineal injuries usually heal without permanent disability regardless of whether they are repaired. However, repairing a new perineal injury to prevent future complications is easier than correcting long-term damage.

Vaginal and urethral lacerations. Vaginal lacerations often occur in conjunction with perineal lacerations. Vaginal lacerations tend to extend up the lateral walls (sulci) and, if deep enough, involve the levator ani muscle. Additional injury may occur high in the vaginal vault near the level of the ischial spines. Vaginal vault lacerations are often circular and may result from use of forceps to rotate the fetal head, rapid fetal descent, or precipitous birth.

Cervical injuries. Cervical injuries occur at the lateral angles of the external os when the cervix retracts over the advancing fetal head. Most lacerations are shallow and bleeding is minimal. Larger lacerations may extend to the vaginal vault or beyond it into the lower uterine segment; serious bleeding may occur. Extensive lacerations may follow hasty attempts to enlarge the cervical opening artificially or to deliver the fetus before full cervical dilation is achieved. Injuries to the cervix can have adverse effects on future pregnancies and births.

Episiotomy. An episiotomy is an incision made in the perineum to enlarge the vaginal outlet (Fig. 19.25). Its use has steadily declined in recent years due to a lack of sound, rigorous research to support its benefits. Episiotomies are performed in approximately 10% of births in the United States (Simpson & O'Brien-Abel, 2014). This practice is even less common in Europe and Canada, probably because of the more routine use in those countries of the side-lying position for birth. This position places less tension on the perineum, making possible its gradual stretching with fewer indications for episiotomy. Whenever possible, giving birth over an intact perineum provides the best outcome (e.g., less blood loss, less risk for infection, and less postpartum pain).

Different types of episiotomies may be performed, classified by the site and direction of the incision (see Fig. 19.25). Both types have advantages and disadvantages, and it is unclear which, if either, is a better choice (Kilpatrick & Garrison, 2017). Midline episiotomies are associated with a

higher incidence of third- and fourth-degree lacerations, whereas mediolateral episiotomies may be more painful (Cunningham et al., 2018). Based on the lack of consistent evidence that episiotomy is beneficial, *routine* episiotomy has no role in modern obstetric care and should be avoided whenever possible. *Indicated* episiotomy, however, may still be performed in specific situations, such as the need to hasten birth when FHR abnormalities are present (Kilpatrick & Garrison).

THIRD STAGE OF LABOR

The third stage of labor lasts from the birth of the baby until the placenta is expelled. It is generally by far the shortest stage of labor.

📋 CARE MANAGEMENT

The goal in the management of the third stage of labor is the prompt separation and expulsion of the placenta, achieved in the easiest, safest manner. Under normal circumstances the placenta is attached to the decidual layer of the basal plate's thin endometrium by numerous fibrous anchor villi—much in the same way a postage stamp is attached to a sheet of postage stamps. After the birth of the fetus, strong uterine contractions and the sudden decrease in uterine size and volume cause the placental site to shrink. This causes the anchor villi to break and the placenta to separate from its attachments. Normally the first few strong contractions that occur after the baby's birth cause the placenta to shear away from the basal plate. A placenta cannot detach itself from a flaccid (relaxed) uterus because the placental site is not reduced in size.

Placental Separation and Expulsion

Historically, the third stage of labor was usually managed passively or expectantly in the United States, with no interventions implemented until spontaneous separation of the placenta occurred. Passive management involves patiently watching for signs that the placenta has separated from the uterine wall spontaneously and monitoring for spontaneous expulsion. Signs of placental separation include lengthening of the umbilical cord and a gush of blood from the vagina (Fig. 19.26). After separation occurs, the woman is instructed to push to aid in expelling the placenta. When passive management is practiced, the placenta is usually expelled within 15 minutes after the birth of the baby. As soon as the placenta is expelled, the uterine fundus is massaged and medication to contract the uterus (usually oxytocin [Pitocin]) is administered (Box 19.13).

More recent research, however, has led to the recommendation for active management of the third stage of labor (AMTSL). When AMTSL is practiced, oxytocic medication (usually oxytocin) is administered immediately after the baby is born but before the placenta is expelled. Gentle continuous controlled umbilical cord traction and counterpressure are used to support the uterus until the placenta separates and is expelled. Immediately after the placenta is expelled, the uterine fundus is massaged (Kilpatrick & Garrison, 2017). Benefits of AMTSL include a shorter duration of third-stage labor, less risk for postpartum hemorrhage, and decreased risk for anemia for both the woman and the newborn (Kelly et al., 2017; Schorn, Dietrich, Donaghey, & Minnick, 2017). AMTSL is currently practiced in many countries around the world.

After the placenta and the amniotic membranes emerge, the nurse-midwife or physician examines them for intactness to ensure that no portion remains in the uterine cavity (i.e., no fragments of the placenta or membranes are retained) (Fig. 19.27). At this time the nurse will obtain a sample of blood from the umbilical cord to be used for determining the baby's blood type and Rh status. Some parents will also have arranged to have blood from the cord collected for storage and possible future use.

Blood from the umbilical cord contains hematopoietic stem cells, which, when transplanted, offer several advantages over bone marrow

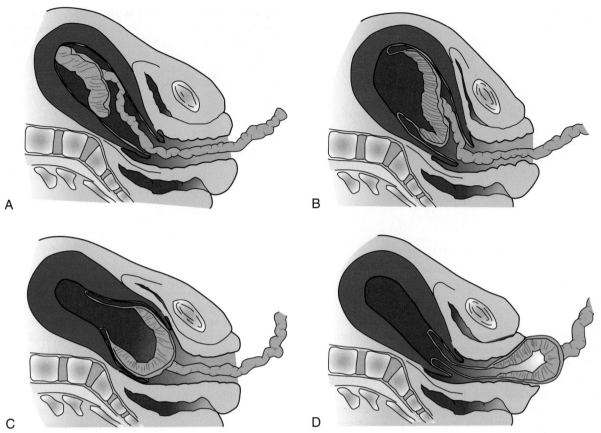

Fig. 19.26 Third Stage of Labor. (A) Placenta begins to separate in central portion, accompanied by retroplacental bleeding. Uterus changes from discoid to globular shape. (B) Placenta completes separation and enters lower uterine segment. Uterus has globular shape. (C) Placenta enters vagina, cord is seen to lengthen, and there may be an increase in bleeding. (D) Expulsion (delivery) of placenta and completion of third stage.

BOX 19.13   Nursing Care in Third-Stage Labor

Assessment

Signs That Suggest the Onset of the Third Stage

- A firmly contracting fundus
- A change in the uterus from a discoid to a globular ovoid shape as the placenta moves into the lower uterine segment
- A sudden gush of dark blood from the introitus
- Apparent lengthening of the umbilical cord as the placenta descends to the introitus
- The finding of vaginal fullness (the placenta) on vaginal or rectal examination or of fetal membranes at the introitus

Physical Assessment

- Perform every 15 min: maternal blood pressure, pulse, and respirations.
- Assess for signs of placental separation and amount of bleeding.
- Assist with determination of Apgar score at 1 and 5 min after birth (see Table 24.1).
- Assess maternal and partner response to completion of birth process and their reaction to the newborn.

Interventions

- Assist mother to bear down to facilitate expulsion of the separated placenta.
- Administer an oxytocic medication as ordered to ensure adequate contraction of the uterus, thereby preventing hemorrhage.
- Provide nonpharmacologic and pharmacologic comfort and pain relief measures.
- Perform hygienic cleansing measures.
- Keep mother/partner informed of progress of placental separation and expulsion and perineal repair if appropriate.
- Explain purpose of medications administered.
- If mother's and baby's conditions permit, encourage immediate skin-to-skin contact and delayed cord clamping.
- Introduce parents to their baby and facilitate the attachment process by delaying eye prophylaxis.
- Provide private time for parents to bond with new baby; help them create memories.
- Encourage breastfeeding if desired.

---

or stem cells obtained from other locations. Current recommendations for cord blood transplant are limited to certain genetic, hematologic, and malignant disorders, however, and it is very unlikely that the child or another family member will develop a condition that could be treated with a transfusion of autologous umbilical cord blood. Umbilical cord blood banking is not part of routine obstetric care and is not medically indicated. Cord blood collection should not interfere with delayed cord

clamping. Circumstances may arise during the birth process that prevent the collection of an adequate amount of cord blood. If the parents still want this to be done, blood can be collected from the umbilical cord either before or after the placenta is expelled (ACOG, 2019b).

When the third stage of labor has been completed, the nurse-midwife or physician examines the woman for any perineal, vaginal, or cervical lacerations requiring repair. The nurse may have to assist by

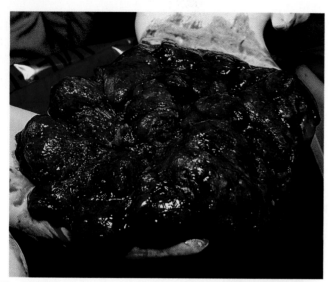

Fig. 19.27 Examination of the Placenta. (Courtesy Michael S. Clement, MD, Mesa, AZ.)

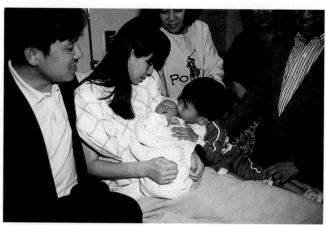

Fig. 19.28 Big Brother Becomes Acquainted With New Baby Sister. (Courtesy Marjorie Pyle, RNC, Lifecircle, Costa Mesa, CA.)

providing adequate lighting or exposure of the woman's perineum and vagina so that a thorough examination can be performed. If an episiotomy was performed, it will be sutured. Immediate repair promotes healing, limits residual damage, and decreases the possibility of infection. The woman usually feels some discomfort while the nurse-midwife or physician carries out the postbirth vaginal examination. The nurse helps the woman to use breathing and relaxation or distraction techniques to assist her in dealing with the discomfort. During this time the "baby nurse" performs a quick assessment of the newborn's physical condition and places matching identification bands on baby and mother. Weighing the baby and administering eye prophylaxis and a vitamin K injection can be delayed until after the initial bonding time with the parents (see Chapter 24).

After any necessary repairs have been completed, the nurse cleanses the vulvar area gently with warm water or normal saline and applies a perineal pad or an ice pack to the perineum. The next step is to reposition the birthing bed or table and lower the woman's legs simultaneously from the stirrups if she gave birth in a lithotomy position. After removing any drapes, the nurse places dry linen under the woman's buttocks and provides her with a clean gown and a blanket, which is warmed if needed. Some women and their families have culturally based beliefs regarding the care of the placenta and the manner of its disposal after birth, viewing the care and disposal of the placenta as a way of protecting the newborn from bad luck and illness. In Spanish the placenta is referred to as *el compañero* or "the companion" of the child (Callister, 2014). A request by the woman to take the placenta home and dispose of it according to her customs sometimes conflicts with health care agency or local government policies, especially those related to infection control and the disposal of biologic wastes. Many cultures follow specific rules regarding the disposal of the placenta in terms of method (burning, drying, burying, eating), site for disposal (in or near the home), and timing of disposal (immediately after birth, time of day, astrologic signs). Disposal rituals may vary according to the gender of the child and the length of time before another child is desired. Some cultures believe that eating the placenta is a means of restoring a woman's well-being after birth or ensuring high-quality breast milk. Health care providers can offer culturally sensitive health care by encouraging women and their families to express their wishes regarding the care and disposal of the placenta and by establishing a policy to fulfill these requests (Baergen, Thaker, & Heller, 2013).

FOURTH STAGE OF LABOR

The **fourth stage of labor** begins with the expulsion of the placenta and lasts until the woman is stable in the immediate postpartum period, usually within the first hour after birth (Simpson & O'Brien-Abel, 2014). The immediate postpartum recovery period lasts longer. It usually includes at least the first 2 hours after birth, based on maternal status (American Academy of Pediatrics [AAP] & ACOG, 2017). This is a crucial time for mother and newborn. Both are not only recovering from the physical process of birth but are also becoming acquainted with one another and additional family members. During this time maternal organs undergo their initial readjustment to the nonpregnant state, and the functions of body systems begin to stabilize.

CARE MANAGEMENT

In most hospitals the mother remains in the labor and birth area during the immediate postpartum recovery period. In an institution where LDR rooms are used, the woman stays in the same room where she gave birth. In traditional settings, women are taken from the delivery room to a separate recovery area for observation. Arrangements for care of the newborn vary during the immediate postpartum recovery period. In many settings the baby remains with the mother, and the labor or birth nurse cares for both of them. In other institutions the baby is taken to the nursery for several hours of observation after an initial bonding period with the parents, siblings, and perhaps other family members (Fig. 19.28).

Assessment

If the recovery nurse has not previously cared for the new mother, he or she begins with an oral report from the nurse who attended the woman during labor and birth and a review of the prenatal, labor, and birth records. Of primary importance are conditions that could predispose the mother to hemorrhage, such as precipitous labor, a large baby, grand multiparity (i.e., having given birth to five or more viable infants), or induced labor. For healthy women, hemorrhage is the most dangerous potential complication during the fourth stage of labor.

During the fourth stage of labor the mother is assessed frequently (Box 19.14). The AAP and ACOG recommend that blood pressure and pulse be assessed at least every 15 minutes for the first 2 hours after birth. Temperature should be assessed every 4 hours for the first 8 hours after birth and then at least every 8 hours (AAP & ACOG, 2017).

BOX 19.14   Assessment During the Fourth Stage of Labor

Blood Pressure

- Assess every 15 min for the first 2 hrs.[a]

Pulse

- Assess rate and regularity. Assess every 15 min for the first 2 hrs.[a]

Temperature

- Assess at the beginning of the recovery period. Temperature should then be assessed every 4 hrs for the first 8 hrs after birth and then at least every 8 hrs.[a]

Fundus

- Position the woman with knees flexed and head flat.
- Just below umbilicus, cup your hand and press it firmly into the woman's abdomen. At the same time, stabilize the uterus at the symphysis with the opposite hand (see Fig. 20.1).
- If the fundus is firm (and bladder is empty), with uterus in midline, measure its position relative to the woman's umbilicus. Lay your fingers flat on the woman's abdomen under the umbilicus; measure how many fingerbreadths (fb) or centimeters (cm) fit between the umbilicus and the top of the fundus. Fundal height is documented according to agency guidelines. For example, if the fundus is 1 fb or 1 cm above the umbilicus, fundal height may be recorded as either +1, u+1, or 1/u. If the fundus is 1 fb or 1 cm below the umbilicus, fundal height may be recorded as either −1, u−1, or u/1.
- If the fundus is not firm, massage it gently to contract and expel any clots before measuring the distance from the umbilicus.
- Place your hands appropriately; massage gently only until the fundus is firm.
- Expel clots while keeping your hands placed as in Fig. 20.1. With your upper hand, firmly apply pressure downward toward the vagina; observe the perineum for the amount and size of expelled clots.

Bladder

- Assess its distention by noting the location and firmness of the uterine fundus and by observing and palpating the bladder. A distended bladder is seen as a suprapubic rounded bulge that is dull to percussion and fluctuates like a water-filled balloon. When the bladder is distended, the uterus is usually boggy in consistency, well above the umbilicus, and to the woman's right side.
- Assist woman to void spontaneously. Measure and record the amount of urine voided.
- Catheterize as necessary.
- Reassess after voiding or catheterization to make sure the bladder is not palpable and the fundus is firm and in the midline.

Lochia

- Observe the lochia on perineal pads and on the linen under the mother's buttocks. Determine its amount and color; note the size and number of clots; note the odor.
- Observe the perineum for sources of bleeding (e.g., episiotomy, lacerations).

Perineum

- Ask or assist the woman to turn onto her side and flex her upper leg on her hip.
- Lift her upper buttock.
- Observe the perineum in good lighting.
- Assess the episiotomy or laceration repair for redness (erythema), edema, ecchymosis (bruising), drainage, and approximation (REEDA).
- Assess for the presence of hemorrhoids.

[a]Data from American Academy of Pediatrics & American College of Obstetricians and Gynecologists. (2017). *Guidelines for perinatal care* (8th ed.). Washington, DC: American College of Obstetricians and Gynecologists.

Postanesthesia Recovery

The woman who has given birth by cesarean or has received regional anesthesia for a vaginal birth requires special attention during the recovery period. Obstetric recovery areas are held to the same standard of care that would be expected of any other postanesthesia recovery (PAR) unit (AAP & ACOG, 2017). A PAR score is determined for each woman on arrival and is updated as part of every 15-minute assessment. Components of the PAR score include activity, respirations, blood pressure, level of consciousness, and color.

If the woman received general anesthesia, she should be awake and alert and oriented to time, place, and person. Her respiratory rate should be within normal limits, and her oxygen saturation level at least 95%, as measured by a pulse oximeter.

If the woman received epidural or spinal anesthesia, she should be able to raise her legs, extended at the knees, off the bed, or flex her knees, place her feet flat on the bed, and raise her buttocks well off the bed. The numb or tingling, prickly sensation should be entirely gone from her legs. The length of time required to recover from regional anesthesia varies greatly. Often it takes several hours for these anesthetic effects to disappear completely.

⚡ SAFETY ALERT

Regardless of her obstetric status, no woman should be discharged from the recovery area until she has completely recovered from the effects of anesthesia.

Nursing Interventions

Care of the New Mother

If food and fluids were restricted, especially if excessive fluid loss (blood, perspiration, or emesis) occurred during the birth, the woman will be very hungry and thirsty soon after the birth. In the absence of complications, a woman who has given birth vaginally may have fluids and a regular diet as soon as she likes (AAP & ACOG, 2017). In the immediate postpartum period, women who give birth by cesarean are usually restricted to clear liquids and ice chips.

As soon as they have had a chance to bond with the baby and eat, most new mothers are ready for a nap or at least a quiet period of rest. Following this rest period, the woman may want to shower and change clothes. Most new mothers are capable of self-care or are assisted in these activities by family members or support people.

Care of the Family

Most parents enjoy being able to hold, explore, and examine the baby immediately after birth. Both parents can assist with thoroughly drying the infant. Skin-to-skin contact is encouraged. The nurse places the unwrapped infant on the woman's chest or abdomen and then covers the baby and mother with a warm blanket. Holding the newborn next to her skin helps the mother maintain the baby's body heat. Stockinette caps are often used to keep the newborn's head warm and prevent heat loss (see Fig. 19.24). Before being held by the partner, the newborn is wrapped snugly in a receiving blanket.

Many women wish to begin breastfeeding their newborns immediately after birth to take advantage of the infant's alert state (*first period of reactivity*) and to stimulate the production of oxytocin, which promotes contraction of the uterus and prevents hemorrhage. In hospitals with Baby-Friendly designation, breastfeeding is initiated within the first hour after birth, and any unnecessary separation of mother and baby is strongly discouraged. However, some women prefer to wait to breastfeed until they have had time to rest. In some cultures breastfeeding is not acceptable to some women until the milk comes in. For some women of Hispanic background, for example, the colostrum is thought to be bad or old milk (Callister, 2014). They typically wait until 3 or 4 days after birth to begin breastfeeding, when their "milk is in" (onset of lactogenesis II) (see Chapter 25).

Family-Newborn Relationships

Maternal exhaustion can affect her response to the newborn. The woman's reaction to the sight of her newborn may range from excited outbursts of laughing, talking, and even crying to apparent apathy. A polite smile and nod may be her only acknowledgment of the comments from nurses and the nurse-midwife or physician. Occasionally the reaction is one of anger or indifference; the woman turns away from the baby, concentrates on her own pain, and sometimes makes hostile comments. These varied reactions can arise from pleasure, exhaustion, or deep disappointment. When the nurse is evaluating parent-newborn interactions after birth, he or she should consider the cultural characteristics of the woman and her family and the expected behaviors of that culture. In some cultures the birth of a male child is preferred and women may grieve when a female child is born (Callister, 2014).

Whatever the reaction and its cause, the woman needs continuing acceptance and support from members of the health care team.

Appropriate nursing actions include making a notation in the recovery record regarding the parents' reaction to the newborn; assessing this reaction by asking questions such as, "What do the parents say?" and "What do they do?" Thereafter further assessments of the parent-newborn relationship may be conducted during the recovery and postpartum period. These assessments are especially important if warning signs (e.g., passive or hostile reactions to the newborn, disappointment with the gender or appearance of the newborn, absence of eye contact, or limited interaction of parents with each other) are noted immediately after birth. Nurses should discuss any warning signs with the woman's nurse-midwife or physician.

Siblings, who may have appeared only remotely interested in the final phases of the second stage, tend to experience renewed interest and excitement when the newborn appears. With supervision, they can be encouraged to hold the baby (see Fig. 19.28).

Parents usually respond to praise of their newborn. Many need to be reassured that the dusky appearance of their baby's hands and feet immediately after birth is normal until circulation is well established. If appropriate, the nurse explains the reason for the molding of the newborn's head. The nurse communicates information about hospital routine, recognizing, however, that the cultural background of the parents may influence their expectations regarding the care and handling of their newborn immediately after birth. For example, Korean mothers may believe that the head should not be touched because it is the most sacred part of a person's body. Hispanic mothers may believe that the "evil eye" or too much praise of the baby will cause illness, restlessness, or excessive crying (Callister, 2014). Members of the interprofessional health care team, by their interest and concern, can provide the environment for making this a satisfying experience for parents, family, and significant others.

KEY POINTS

- The onset of labor may be difficult to determine for both nulliparous and multiparous women.
- The familiar environment of her home is most often the ideal place for a woman during the latent phase of the first stage of labor.
- The nurse assumes much of the responsibility for assessing the progress of labor and for keeping the nurse-midwife or physician informed about that progress and deviations from expected findings.
- The fetal heart rate and pattern reveal the fetal response to the stress of the labor process.
- Assessing the laboring woman's urinary output and bladder is critical to ensure labor progress and to prevent bladder injury.
- Regardless of the actual labor and birth experience, the woman's or couple's perception of the birth experience is most likely to be positive when events and performances are consistent with expectations, especially in terms of maintaining control and the adequacy of pain relief.
- The woman's level of anxiety may increase when she does not understand what is being said to her about her labor because of the medical terminology used or because of a language barrier.
- Coaching, emotional support, and comfort measures assist the woman to use her energy constructively in relaxing and working with the contractions.
- The progress of labor is enhanced when a woman changes her position frequently during the first stage of labor.
- Doulas provide a continuous, supportive presence during labor that can have a positive effect on the process of labor and birth and its outcome.

- The cultural beliefs and practices of a woman and her significant others, including her partner, can have a profound influence on their approach to labor and birth.
- Siblings present for labor and birth need preparation and support for the event.
- Women with a history of sexual abuse often experience profound stress and anxiety during labor and birth.
- Inability to palpate the cervix during vaginal examination indicates that complete effacement and full dilation have occurred and is the only certain, objective sign that the second stage of labor has begun.
- Women may have an urge to bear down at various times during labor; for some it may be before the cervix is fully dilated and for others it may not occur until the active phase of the second stage of labor.
- When encouraged to respond to the rhythmic nature of the second stage of labor, the woman normally changes body positions, bears down spontaneously, and vocalizes (open-glottis pushing) when she perceives the urge to push (Ferguson reflex).
- Women should bear down several times during a contraction using the open-glottis pushing method. They should avoid sustained closed-glottis pushing because this will decrease oxygen transport to the fetus.
- Nurses can use the role of advocate to prevent the routine use of episiotomy and reduce the incidence of lacerations by empowering women to take an active role in giving birth and by educating health care providers about approaches to managing labor and birth that reduce the incidence of perineal trauma.

- Objective signs indicate that the placenta has separated and is ready to be expelled; excessive traction (pulling) on the umbilical cord before the placenta has separated can result in maternal injury.

- During the fourth stage of labor, the woman's fundal tone, lochial flow, and vital signs should be assessed frequently to ensure that she is recovering well after giving birth.
- Most parents and families enjoy being able to hold, explore, and examine the baby immediately after the birth.

REFERENCES

Aasheim, V., Nilsen, A. B. V., Reinar, L. M., & Lukasse, M. (2017). Perineal techniques during the second stage of labour for reducing perineal trauma. *Cochrane Database of Systematic Reviews*, 6, CD006672.

American Academy of Pediatrics & American College of Obstetricians and Gynecologists. (2017). *Guidelines for perinatal care* (8th ed.). Washington, DC: American College of Obstetricians and Gynecologists.

American College of Nurse-Midwives. (2012). *Supporting healthy and normal physiologic childbirth: A consensus statement by ACNM, MANA, and NACPM*. Retrieved from: http://www.midwife.org/ACNM/files/ACNMLibraryData/UPLOADFILENAME/000000000272/Physiological%20Birth%-20Consensus%20Statement-%20FINAL%20May%202012%20FINAL.pdf.

American College of Nurse-Midwives. (2016). Providing oral nutrition to women in labor. *Journal of Midwifery & Women's Health*, 61(4), 528–534.

American College of Obstetricians and Gynecologists. (2016). Committee opinion no. 679: Immersion in water during labor and delivery. *Obstetrics & Gynecology*, 128(5), 1198–1199.

American College of Obstetricians and Gynecologists. (2018). Committee opinion no. 752: Prenatal and perinatal human immunodeficiency virus testing. *Obstetrics & Gynecology*, 132(3), e138–e142.

American College of Obstetricians and Gynecologists. (2019a). Committee opinion no. 766: Approaches to limit intervention during labor and birth. *Obstetrics & Gynecology*, 133(2), e164–e173.

American College of Obstetricians and Gynecologists. (2019b). Committee opinion no. 771: Umbilical cord blood banking. *Obstetrics & Gynecology*, 133(3), e249–e253.

Arendt, K. W., & Tessmer-Tuck, J. A. (2013). Nonpharmacologic labor analgesia. *Clinics in Perinatology*, 40(3), 351–371.

Association of Women's Health, Obstetric and Neonatal Nurses. (2010). *Guidelines for professional registered nurse staffing for perinatal units*. Washington, DC: Association of Women's Health, Obstetric and Neonatal Nurses.

Association of Women's Health, Obstetric and Neonatal Nurses. (2018). Continuous labor support for every woman. *Journal of Obstetric, Gynecologic & Neonatal Nursing*, 47(1), 73–74.

Baergen, R. N., Thaker, H. M., & Heller, D. S. (2013). Placental release or disposal? Experiences of perinatal pathologists. *Pediatric and Developmental Pathology*, 16(5), 327–330.

Blackburn, S. T. (2018). *Maternal, fetal, and neonatal physiology: A clinical perspective* (5th ed.). St. Louis: Elsevier.

Burke, C. (2014). Pain in labor: Nonpharmacologic and pharmacologic management. In K. R. Simpson, & P. Creehan (Eds.), *AWHONN's perinatal nursing* (4th ed.). Philadelphia: Lippincott Williams & Wilkins.

Callister, L. C. (2014). Integrating cultural beliefs and practices when caring for childbearing women and families. In K. R. Simpson, & P. Creehan (Eds.), *AWHONN's perinatal nursing* (4th ed.). Philadelphia: Lippincott Williams & Wilkins.

Centers for Disease Control and Prevention. (2016). *Rapid HIV testing of women in labor and delivery*. Retrieved from: http://www.cdc.gov/hiv/testing/clinical/women.html.

Ciardulli, A., Saccone, G., Anastasio, H., & Berghella, V. (2017). Less-restrictive food intake during labor in low-risk singleton pregnancies: A systematic review and meta-analysis. *Obstetrics & Gynecology*, 129(3), 473–480.

Collins, M. R. (2017). Pain in labor and nonpharmacologic modes of relief. In B. B. Kennedy, & S. M. Baird (Eds.), *Intrapartum management modules: A perinatal education program* (5th ed.). Philadelphia: Wolters Kluwer.

Cunningham, F., Leveno, K., Bloom, S., et al. (2018). *Williams obstetrics* (25th ed.). New York: McGraw-Hill Education.

Desseauve, D., Fradet, L., Lacouture, P., & Pierre, F. (2017). Position for labor and birth: State of knowledge and biomechanical perspectives. *European Journal of Obstetrics & Gynecology and Reproductive Biology*, 208, 46–54.

Hanson, L., & VandeVusse, L. (2014). Supporting labor progress toward physiologic birth. *Journal of Perinatal & Neonatal Nursing*, 28(2), 101–107.

He, H., Vehviläinen–Julkunen, K., Qian, X., et al. (2015). Fathers' feelings related to their partners' childbirth and views on their presence during labour and childbirth: A descriptive quantitative study. *International Journal of Nursing Practice*, 21(S2), 71–79.

Kelly, F. C., Swart, S. C., & Baird, S. M. (2017). Caring for the laboring woman. In B. B. Kennedy, & S. M. Baird (Eds.), *Intrapartum management modules: A perinatal education program* (5th ed.). Philadelphia: Wolters Kluwer.

Kilpatrick, S., & Garrison, E. (2017). Normal labor and delivery. In S. G. Gabbe, J. R. Niebyl, J. L. Simpson, et al. (Eds.), *Obstetrics: Normal and problem pregnancies* (7th ed.). Philadelphia: Elsevier.

King, T. L., & Pinger, W. (2014). Evidence-based practice for intrapartum care: The pearls of midwifery. *Journal of Midwifery & Women's Health*, 59(6), 572–585.

Kopas, M. L. (2014). A review of evidence–based practices for management of the second stage of labor. *Journal of Midwifery & Women's Health*, 59(3), 264–276.

Mikolajczyk, R. T., Zhang, J., Grewal, J., et al. (2016). Early versus late admission to labor affects labor progression and risk of cesarean section in nulliparous women. *Frontiers in Medicine*, 3(26).

Miller, L. A., Miller, D. A., & Cypher, R. L. (2017). *Mosby's pocket guide to fetal monitoring: A multidisciplinary approach* (8th ed.). St. Louis: Elsevier.

Neal, J. L., Lamp, J. M., Buck, J. S., et al. (2014). Outcomes of nulliparous women with spontaneous labor onset admitted to hospitals in preactive versus active labor. *Journal of Midwifery & Women's Health*, 59(1), 28–34.

Parker, C. (2015). An innovative nursing approach to caring for an obstetric patient with rape trauma syndrome. *Journal of Obstetric, Gynecologic & Neonatal Nursing*, 44(3), 397–404.

Paul, J. A., Yount, S. M., Breman, R. B., et al. (2017). Use of an early labor lounge to promote admission in active labor. *Journal of Midwifery & Women's Health*, 62(2), 204–209.

Poh, H. L., Koh, S. S. L., Seow, H. C. L., & He, H. (2014). First-time fathers' experiences and needs during pregnancy and childbirth: a descriptive qualitative study. *Midwifery*, 30(6), 779–787.

Reed, C. (2015). *Neonatal resuscitation program, 2015* (7th ed.). Elk Grove Village, IL: American Academy of Pediatrics.

Ruhl, C., Scheich, B., Onokpise, B., & Bingham, D. (2015). Interrater reliability of testing the maternal triage index. *Journal of Obstetric, Gynecologic and Neonatal Nursing*, 46(6), 710–716.

Schorn, M. N., Dietrich, M. S., Donaghey, B., & Minnick, A. F. (2017). U.S. physician and midwife adherence to active management of the third stage of labor international recommendations. *Journal of Midwifery & Women's Health*, 62(1), 58–67.

Shaw-Battista, J. (2017). Systematic review of hydrotherapy research: Does a warm bath in labor promote normal physiologic childbirth? *Journal of Perinatal & Neonatal Nursing*, 31(4), 303–316.

Simkin, P. (2014). Preventing primary cesareans: Implications for laboring women, their partners, nurses, educators, and doulas. *Birth*, 41(3), 220–222.

Simkin, P., Hanson, L., & Ancheta, R. (2017). *The labor progress handbook: Early interventions to prevent and treat dystocia* (4th ed.). Hoboken, NJ: John Wiley & Sons Inc.

Simpson, K., & O'Brien-Abel, N. (2014). Labor and birth. In K. R. Simpson, & P. Creehan (Eds.), *AWHONN's perinatal nursing* (4th ed.). Philadelphia: Lippincott Williams & Wilkins.

Stewart, L. S., & Rodgers, E. (2017). Assessment and care of the term newborn transitioning to extrauterine life. In B. B. Kennedy, & S. M. Baird (Eds.), *Intrapartum management modules: A perinatal education program* (5th ed.). Philadelphia: Wolters Kluwer.

Strauss, N., Giessler, K., & McAllister, E. (2015). How doula care can advance the goals of the affordable care act: A snapshot from New York City. *Journal of Perinatal Education, 24*(1), 8.

Tilden, E. L., Emeis, C. L., Caughey, A. B., et al. (2016). The influence of group versus individual prenatal care on phase of labor at hospital admission. *Journal of Midwifery & Women's Health, 61*(4), 427–434.

Tillett, J., & Hill, C. (2016). Eating and drinking in labor: Reexamining the evidence. *Journal of Perinatal & Neonatal Nursing, 30*(2), 85–87.

Tussey, C. M., Botsios, E., Gerkin, R. D., et al. (2015). Reducing length of labor and cesarean surgery rate using a peanut ball for women laboring with an epidural. *Journal of Perinatal Education, 24*(1), 16–24.

Wilson-Griffin, J. (2014). Maternal-fetal transport. In K. R. Simpson, & P. Creehan (Eds.), *AWHONN's perinatal nursing* (4th ed.). Philadelphia: Lippincott Williams & Wilkins.

Zinsser, L. (2018). Lotus birth: A holistic approach on physiological cord clamping. *Women and Birth, 31*, e73-e76-e78.

Postpartum Physiologic Changes

Kathryn Rhodes Alden

ⓔ http://evolve.elsevier.com/Lowdermilk/MWHC/

LEARNING OBJECTIVES

- Describe the anatomic and physiologic changes that occur in the reproductive system during the postpartum period.
- Discuss the anatomic and physiologic changes that occur in other body systems during the postpartum period.

- Identify expected values for postpartum vital signs and possible causes for deviations from normal findings.

The **postpartum period** is the interval between birth and the return of the reproductive organs to their normal nonpregnant state. This period is sometimes referred to as the *puerperium,* or fourth trimester of pregnancy. Although the puerperium has traditionally been considered to last 6 weeks, this time frame varies among women. The physiologic changes that occur during the reversal of the processes of pregnancy are distinctive, but they are normal. To provide care during the recovery period that is beneficial to the mother, her infant, and her family, the nurse must synthesize knowledge of maternal anatomy and physiology of the recovery period, the newborn's physical and behavioral characteristics, infant care activities, and the family's response to the birth. This chapter focuses on anatomic and physiologic changes that occur in the mother during the postpartum period.

REPRODUCTIVE SYSTEM AND ASSOCIATED STRUCTURES

Uterus

Involution

The return of the uterus to a nonpregnant state after birth is called **involution**. This process begins immediately after expulsion of the placenta with contraction of the uterine smooth muscle.

At the end of the third stage of labor, the uterus is in the midline, approximately 2 cm below the level of the umbilicus, with the fundus resting on the sacral promontory. At this time, the uterus weighs approximately 1000 g (Isley & Katz, 2017).

Within 12 hours, the fundus can rise to approximately 1 cm above the umbilicus (Fig. 20.1). By 24 hours after birth, the uterus is about the same size as it was at 20 weeks of gestation. Involution progresses rapidly during the next few days. The fundus descends 1 to 2 cm every 24 hours. By the sixth postpartum day, the fundus is normally located halfway between the umbilicus and the symphysis pubis. The uterus should not

be palpable abdominally after 2 weeks and should have returned to its nonpregnant location by 6 weeks after birth (Blackburn, 2018).

The uterus, which at full term weighs approximately 11 times its prepregnancy weight, involutes to approximately 500 g by 1 week after birth and to 300 g by 2 weeks after birth. By 4 weeks postpartum, it weighs approximately 100 g, which is the nonpregnant size (Cunningham, Leveno, Bloom, et al., 2019).

Increased estrogen and progesterone levels are responsible for stimulating the massive growth of the uterus during pregnancy. Uterine growth results from both hyperplasia (an increase in the number of muscle cells) and hypertrophy (an enlargement of the existing cells). After birth, the decrease in these hormones causes **autolysis**—the self-destruction of excess hypertrophied tissue. The additional cells laid down during pregnancy remain and account for the slight increase in uterine size after each pregnancy.

Subinvolution is the failure of the uterus to return to a nonpregnant state due to ineffective uterine contractions. The most common causes of subinvolution are retained placental fragments and infection (see Chapter 33).

Contractions

Postpartum hemostasis is achieved primarily by compression of intramyometrial blood vessels as the uterine muscle contracts rather than by platelet aggregation and clot formation. The hormone oxytocin, released from the pituitary gland, strengthens and coordinates these uterine contractions, which compress blood vessels and promote hemostasis. During the first 1 to 2 postpartum hours, uterine contractions can decrease in intensity and become uncoordinated. Because it is vital that the uterus remains firm and well contracted, exogenous oxytocin (Pitocin) is usually administered intravenously or intramuscularly immediately after expulsion of the placenta (some health care providers order oxytocin [Pitocin] after the birth of the baby to shorten the third stage of labor and to decrease blood loss). The uterus is very

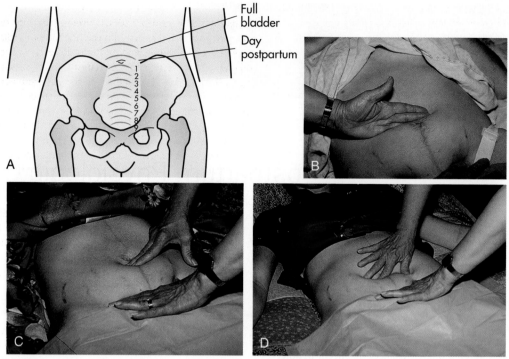

Fig. 20.1 Assessment of Involution of Uterus After Birth. (A) Normal progress, days 1 to 9. (B) Size and position of uterus 2 hours after birth. (C) Two days after birth. (D) Four days after birth. Note linea nigra and striae gravidarum ("stretch marks") in B–D. ([B–D] Courtesy Marjorie Pyle, RNC, Lifecircle, Costa Mesa, CA.)

sensitive to oxytocin during the first week or so after birth. Breastfeeding immediately after birth and in the early days postpartum increases the release of oxytocin, which promotes uterine contractions, therefore decreasing blood loss and reducing the risk for postpartum hemorrhage (Lawrence & Lawrence, 2016).

In primiparous women, uterine tone is good, the fundus generally remains firm, and the woman usually perceives only mild uterine cramping. Periodic relaxation and vigorous contractions are more common in subsequent pregnancies and can cause uncomfortable cramping called afterpains (afterbirth pains), which typically resolve in 3 to 7 days. Afterpains are more noticeable after births in which the uterus was overdistended (e.g., large infant, multifetal gestation, polyhydramnios). Breastfeeding and exogenous oxytocic medication usually intensify afterpains because both stimulate uterine contractions.

Placental Site

Immediately after the placenta and membranes are expelled, vascular constriction and thromboses reduce the placental site to an irregular nodular and elevated area averaging 4 to 5 cm in diameter. Upward growth of the endometrium causes sloughing of necrotic tissue and prevents the scar formation characteristic of normal wound healing. This unique healing process enables the endometrium to resume its usual cycle of changes and to allow implantation and placentation in future pregnancies. Endometrial regeneration begins within 3 days after birth and is completed by the third week; regeneration at the placental site is complete by the sixth week (Blackburn, 2018).

Lochia

The characteristics of postbirth uterine discharge, known as lochia, correlate with uterine involution and changes in the endometrium. Most women experience lochia for 4 to 6 weeks after birth. For the first 2 hours after birth, the amount of uterine discharge should be about that of a heavy menstrual period. After that time, the lochial flow will steadily decrease in amount and the characteristic appearance of the lochia will change (Table 20.1)

TABLE 20.1	Characteristics of Lochia		
Type of Lochia	Appearance	Timing After Birth	Contents
Rubra	Bright red	1-3 days	Blood from placental site; trophoblastic tissue debris, vernix, lanugo, meconium
Serosa	Pinkish-brown	4-10 days	Blood, wound exudate, RBCs, WBCs, trophoblastic tissue debris, cervical mucus, microorganisms
Alba	Whitish-yellow	10-14 days, can last 3-6 weeks	WBCs, trophoblastic tissue debris

RBCs, Red blood cells; *WBCs,* white blood cells.

If the woman receives an oxytocic medication, regardless of the route of administration, the flow of lochia is often scant until the effects of the medication wear off. The amount of lochia is usually less after a cesarean birth because the surgeon suctions the blood and fluids from the uterus or wipes the uterine lining before closing the incision. Flow of lochia usually increases with ambulation and breastfeeding. Lochia tends to pool in the vagina when the woman is lying in bed; the woman then can experience a gush of blood when she stands. This gush should not be confused with hemorrhage.

Persistence of lochia rubra in the postpartum period suggests continued bleeding as a result of retained fragments of the placenta or membranes. It is not uncommon for women to experience a sudden, but brief, increase in bleeding 7 to 14 days after birth when sloughing of eschar over the placental site occurs. If this increase in bleeding does not subside within 1 to 2 hours, the woman needs to be evaluated for possible retained placental fragments (Isley & Katz, 2017).

About 10% to 15% of women still have normal lochia serosa discharge at their 6-week postpartum examination (Isley & Katz, 2017).

However, the continued flow of lochia serosa or lochia alba by 3 to 4 weeks after birth can indicate endometritis, particularly if the woman has fever, pain, or abdominal tenderness. Lochia should smell like normal menstrual flow; an offensive odor usually indicates infection.

Not all postpartal vaginal bleeding is lochia; vaginal bleeding after birth can be caused by unrepaired vaginal or cervical lacerations. Box 20.1 distinguishes between lochial and nonlochial bleeding.

Cervix

The cervix is soft immediately after birth. After vaginal birth, the cervix protrudes into the vagina and appears bruised, edematous, and may have some small lacerations, creating optimal conditions for the development of infection. Over the next 12 to 18 hours, the cervix shortens and becomes firmer. Within 2 to 3 days postpartum, the cervix has shortened, become firm, and regained its form. The cervix up to the lower uterine segment remains edematous, thin, and fragile for several days after birth. The cervical os, which dilated to 10 cm during labor, closes gradually. By the second or third postpartum day, the cervical dilation has decreased to 2 to 3 cm, and by 1 week after birth, it is approximately 1 cm dilated (Blackburn, 2018). The external cervical os never regains its prepregnancy appearance; it no longer has a circular shape but, instead, appears as a jagged slit often described as a "fish mouth." Lactation delays the production of cervical and other estrogen-influenced mucus and affects mucosal characteristics.

Ovaries

Lactating and nonlactating women differ in the timing of their first ovulation and resumption of menstruation. Ovulation occurs as early as 27 days after birth in nonlactating women, with a mean time of about 7 to 9 weeks. About 70% of nonlactating women resume menstruating by 12 weeks after birth. The mean time to ovulation in women who breastfeed is about 6 months (Isley & Katz, 2017). The persistence of elevated serum prolactin levels in lactating women appears to be responsible for suppressing ovulation; the resumption of ovulation and the return of menses are determined in large part by breastfeeding patterns. For example, ovulation is delayed longer in women who breastfeed exclusively compared with women who breastfeed and offer supplemental infant formula to their infants. Because of the uncertainty about the return of ovulation and menstruation, discussion of contraceptive options early in the postpartum period is necessary. The first menstrual flow after birth is usually heavier than normal. Within three or four cycles, the amount of menstrual flow returns to the prepregnancy volume.

Vagina and Perineum

Postpartum estrogen deprivation is responsible for the thinness of the vaginal mucosa and the absence of rugae. The smooth-walled vagina that was greatly distended during birth gradually decreases in size and regains tone, although it does not completely return to its prepregnancy state. Rugae reappear within 3 weeks, but they are never as prominent as in the nulliparous woman. Most rugae are permanently flattened. The mucosa remains atrophic in the lactating woman, at least until menstruation resumes. Thickening of the vaginal mucosa occurs with the return of ovarian function. Estrogen deficiency is responsible for a decreased amount of vaginal lubrication; vaginal dryness is more prevalent among breastfeeding mothers. Localized dryness and coital discomfort (dyspareunia) can persist until ovarian function returns and menstruation resumes. The use of a water-soluble lubricant during sexual intercourse is usually recommended.

Immediately after vaginal birth, the introitus is erythematous and edematous, especially in the area of an episiotomy or laceration repair. It is barely distinguishable from that of a nulliparous woman if lacerations or an episiotomy have been carefully repaired, hematomas are prevented or treated early, and the woman practices good hygiene during the first 2 weeks after birth.

Most episiotomies and laceration repairs are visible only if the woman is lying on her side with her upper buttock raised or if she is placed in the lithotomy position. A good light source is essential for visualization of some repairs. Healing of an episiotomy or laceration is the same as any surgical incision. Signs of infection (pain, redness, warmth, swelling, or discharge) or lack of approximation (separation of the edges of the incision) can occur. Initial healing occurs within 2 to 3 weeks, but 4 to 6 months can be required for the repair to heal completely (Blackburn, 2018). If vacuum or forceps were used for the birth, the woman may have experienced vaginal or cervical lacerations or hematomas of the pelvic soft tissues (see Chapter 32).

Hemorrhoids (anal varicosities) are common. Hemorrhoids often develop during pregnancy, and internal hemorrhoids can evert while the woman is pushing during birth. Women often experience associated symptoms such as itching, discomfort, and bright red bleeding with defecation. Hemorrhoids usually decrease in size within 6 weeks of birth and eventually regress.

Pelvic Muscular Support

The supporting structure (muscles and ligaments) of the uterus and vagina can be injured during birth; this can contribute to later gynecologic problems. Supportive tissues of the pelvic floor that are torn or stretched during birth can require up to 6 months to regain tone. Kegel exercises, which help strengthen perineal muscles and encourage healing, are recommended after birth (see Patient Teaching box: Kegel Exercises, Chapter 4). Later in life, women can experience pelvic relaxation—the lengthening and weakening of the fascial supports of pelvic structures. These structures include the uterus, upper posterior vaginal wall, urethra, bladder, and rectum. Although relaxation can occur in any woman, it is commonly a direct but delayed complication of birth.

Breasts

Promptly after birth, a decrease occurs in the concentrations of hormones (i.e., estrogen, progesterone, hCG, prolactin, cortisol, and insulin) that stimulated breast development during pregnancy. The time required for these hormones to return to prepregnancy levels is determined in part by whether or not the mother breastfeeds her infant.

Breastfeeding Mothers

During the first 24 hours after birth, there is little if any change in the breast tissue. Colostrum, or early milk, a clear yellow fluid, can be expressed from the breasts. The breasts gradually become fuller and heavier as the colostrum transitions to mature milk by about 72 to 96

TABLE 20.2 Vital Signs After Birth

Normal Findings	Deviations from Normal Findings and Probable Causes
Temperature	
During first 24 h temperature can increase to 38°C (100.4°F) as a result of dehydrating effects of labor. After 24 h, the woman should be afebrile.	A diagnosis of puerperal sepsis is suggested if an increase in maternal temperature to 38°C (100.4°F) or higher is noted after the first 24 h after birth and recurs or persists for 2 days. Other possible causes are mastitis, endometritis, urinary tract infection, or other systemic infection.
Pulse	
Pulse, along with stroke volume and cardiac output, remains elevated for the first hour or so after birth. It gradually decreases over the first 48 h postpartum. Puerperal bradycardia (40-50 beats/min) is common.	A rapid pulse rate or one that is increasing can indicate hypovolemia due to hemorrhage.
Respirations	
The respiratory rate, which was unchanged or slightly increased during pregnancy, should be within the woman's normal prepregnancy range soon after birth.	Hypoventilation (respiratory depression) can occur after an unusually high subarachnoid (spinal) block or epidural opioid medication after a cesarean birth.
Blood Pressure	
Blood pressure shows a transient increase of approximately 5% over the first few days after birth, returning to prepregnancy levels over weeks or months. Orthostatic hypotension, as indicated by feelings of faintness or dizziness immediately after standing up, can develop in the first 48 h as a result of the splanchnic engorgement that can occur after birth.	A low or decreasing blood pressure can indicate hypovolemia secondary to hemorrhage; however, it is a late sign, and other symptoms of hemorrhage usually are present. An increased reading can result from excessive use of vasopressor or oxytocic medications. Elevated BP (>140/90 on two occasions 4 h apart) can be a sign of gestational hypertension or preeclampsia and should be evaluated.

hours after birth; this is often referred to as the "milk coming in," or lactogenesis II. The breasts can feel warm, firm, and somewhat tender. Bluish white milk with a skim-milk appearance (true milk) can be expressed from the nipples. As milk glands and milk ducts fill with milk, breast tissue can feel somewhat nodular or lumpy. Unlike the lumps associated with fibrocystic breast changes or cancer (which can be palpated consistently in the same location), the nodularity associated with milk production tends to shift in position. Some women experience engorgement at this time due to an increase in blood and lymphatic fluid as milk production increases. Engorged breasts are hard and uncomfortable and mild temperature elevation can occur; the fullness of the nipple tissue can make it difficult for the infant to latch on and feed. With frequent breastfeeding and proper care, engorgement is a temporary condition that typically lasts only 24 to 48 hours (see Chapter 25).

Nonbreastfeeding Mothers

The breasts generally feel nodular in contrast to the granular feel of breasts in nonpregnant women. The nodularity is bilateral and diffuse. Prolactin levels drop rapidly. Colostrum is present for the first few days after birth. Palpation of the breasts on the second or third day as milk production begins can reveal tissue tenderness in some women. On the third or fourth postpartum day, engorgement can occur. The breasts are distended (swollen), firm, tender, and warm to the touch. Breast distention is caused primarily by the temporary congestion of veins and lymphatics rather than by an accumulation of milk. Milk is present but should not be expressed. Axillary breast tissue (the tail of Spence) and any accessory breast or nipple tissue along the milk line can be involved. Engorgement resolves spontaneously, and discomfort decreases usually within 24 to 36 hours (see Chapter 21) and lactation ceases within a few days to 1 week.

CARDIOVASCULAR SYSTEM

Blood Volume

Changes in blood volume after birth depend on several factors, such as blood loss during birth and the amount of extravascular water

(physiologic edema) mobilized and excreted. Pregnancy-induced hypervolemia (an increase in blood volume of 40% to 45% above nonpregnancy levels) allows most women to tolerate considerable blood loss during birth. The average blood loss for a vaginal birth of a single fetus ranges from 300 to 500 mL (10% of blood volume). The typical blood loss for women who give birth by cesarean is 500 to 1000 mL (15% to 30% of blood volume). During the first few days after birth, the plasma volume decreases further as a result of diuresis (Blackburn, 2018).

Maternal physiologic changes in the puerperium enable the woman to cope with the blood loss that normally occurs during birth by increasing her circulating blood volume. These changes are (1) elimination of uteroplacental circulation that reduces the size of the maternal vascular bed by 10% to 15%, (2) loss of placental endocrine function that removes the stimulus for vasodilation, and (3) mobilization of extravascular water stored during pregnancy. By the third postpartum day, the plasma volume has been replenished as extravascular fluid returns to the intravascular space (Isley & Katz, 2017).

Cardiac Output

Pulse rate, stroke volume, and cardiac output increase throughout pregnancy. Dramatic changes in maternal hemodynamic status occur with birth of the newborn and delivery of the placenta. The immediate blood loss reduces plasma volume without reducing cardiac output. This is due to the compensatory influx of nearly 500 mL of blood into the maternal system from the uteroplacental bed, a rapid decrease in uterine blood flow, and mobilization of extracellular fluid. Typically, cardiac output is increased immediately after birth by 60% to 80% over prelabor values; it returns to prelabor values within 1 hour. By 2 weeks after birth, cardiac output decreases by 30% and gradually decreases to prepregnant levels by 6 to 8 weeks postpartum in the majority of women (Blackburn, 2018).

Vital Signs

Few alterations in vital signs are seen under normal circumstances (Table 20.2). Heart rate is increased immediately after birth and can remain elevated for the first hour. Puerperal bradycardia is common, with heart rate decreasing to 40 to 50 beats/min (James, 2014).

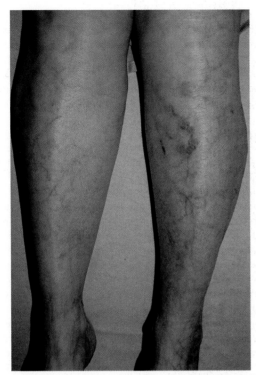

Fig. 20.2 Varicosities in Legs. (Courtesy Cheryl Briggs, RNC, Annapolis, MD.)

There is a transient increase in blood pressure of approximately 5% during the first few days after birth (Isley & Katz, 2017). It can take weeks or months for pulse and blood pressure to return to prepregnancy levels. Increase in blood pressure greater than 140/90 when measured on two or more occasions at least 4 hours apart can indicate gestational hypertension or preeclampsia.

Respiratory function rapidly returns to nonpregnant levels after birth. After the uterus is emptied, the diaphragm descends, the normal cardiac axis is restored, and the point of maximal impulse and the electrocardiogram are normalized.

Low-grade fever is not uncommon during the first 24 hours after birth. However, temperature elevation of 38°C (100.4°F) or higher during the first 10 days postpartum can indicate infection and should be evaluated (Berens, 2018).

As many as 50% of women experience shivering episodes during the first few minutes up to the first hour after birth. The exact cause is unknown, and usually no treatment is needed; if the shivering is related to the effects of anesthesia, pharmacologic treatment may be needed (Berens, 2018).

Varicosities

Varicosities (varices) of the legs (Fig. 20.2) and around the anus (hemorrhoids) are common during pregnancy. All varices, even the less common vulvar varices, regress rapidly immediately after birth. Total or nearly total regression of varicosities is expected in the postpartum period.

Blood Components

In women with an average blood loss during birth, the hematocrit level drops moderately for 3 to 4 days, then begins to increase, and reaches nonpregnant levels by 8 weeks postpartum (Isley & Katz, 2017). A postpartum hematocrit can be lower than normal if the blood loss was increased or if the hypervolemia of pregnancy was less than normal.

During and after labor the white blood cell (WBC) count may rise to 30,000/mm³. Leukocytosis, coupled with the increase in erythrocyte sedimentation rate that normally occurs, can obscure the diagnosis of acute infection (Antony, Racusin, Aagaard, et al., 2017).

Clotting factors and fibrinogen are normally increased during pregnancy and remain elevated in the immediate puerperium. When combined with vessel damage and immobility, this hypercoagulability causes an increased risk for venous thromboembolism, especially after a cesarean birth. Fibrinolytic activity also increases during the first few days after birth (Isley & Katz, 2017). Factors I, II, VIII, IX, and X decrease to nonpregnant levels within a few days. Fibrin split products, probably released from the placental site, can be found in maternal blood.

RESPIRATORY SYSTEM

With birth there is an immediate decrease in intraabdominal pressure, which allows for greater excursion of the diaphragm. With decreased pressure on the diaphragm and reduced pulmonary blood flow, chest wall compliance increases. Rib cage elasticity can take months to return to a prepregnancy state. The costal angle that was increased during pregnancy may not completely return to the prepregnancy level. The decline in progesterone that occurs with loss of the placenta causes the partial pressure of carbon dioxide ($PaCO_2$) levels to rise (Blackburn, 2018).

ENDOCRINE SYSTEM

Placental Hormones

Significant hormonal changes occur during the postpartum period. Expulsion of the placenta results in dramatic decreases in the hormones produced by that organ.

Estrogen and progesterone levels drop markedly after birth and reach their lowest levels 1 week after birth. Decreased estrogen levels are associated with the diuresis of excess extracellular fluid accumulated during pregnancy. In nonlactating women, estrogen levels begin to increase by 2 weeks after birth and by postpartum day 17 are higher than in women who breastfeed (Isley & Katz, 2017).

HCG disappears fairly quickly from maternal circulation. However, because removing hCG from the extravascular and intracellular spaces takes additional time, the hormone can be detected in the maternal system for 3 to 4 weeks after birth (Blackburn, 2018).

Pituitary Hormones

After birth, the fall in progesterone triggers a rise in prolactin. Prolactin, produced by the anterior pituitary, is the hormone that stimulates milk production. In a woman who breastfeeds, prolactin levels are highest during the first month after birth and remain elevated above nonpregnant levels as long as she is breastfeeding. Serum prolactin levels are influenced by the frequency of breastfeeding, the duration of each feeding, and use of supplementary feedings. Individual differences in the strength of an infant's sucking stimulus also affect prolactin levels. In nonbreastfeeding women, prolactin levels decline after birth and reach the prepregnant range by the third postpartum week (Isley & Katz, 2017).

The posterior pituitary produces oxytocin in response to infant suckling or nipple stimulation with milk expression. Oxytocin triggers the milk ejection or let-down reflex which releases the milk to the nipple from the alveoli in the breasts where it is produced (see Chapter 25).

Metabolic Changes

Decreases in human placental lactogen, estrogens, cortisol, and the placental enzyme insulinase reverse the diabetogenic effects of pregnancy, resulting in significantly lower blood glucose levels in the immediate postpartum period. Mothers with type 1 diabetes will likely require much less insulin for several days after birth, especially if they are breastfeeding. Because these normal hormonal changes make the puerperium a transitional period for carbohydrate metabolism, it is more difficult to interpret results of glucose tolerance tests at this time.

The thyroid gland gradually returns to normal by 3 months after birth. Levels of thyroxine and triiodothyronine decrease to prepregnant levels within 4 weeks. There is an increased risk for transient autoimmune thyroiditis in the postpartum period (Isley & Katz, 2017).

The basal metabolic rate remains elevated for the first 1 to 2 weeks after birth (James, 2014). It gradually returns to prepregnancy levels.

URINARY SYSTEM

Renal Function

The hormonal changes of pregnancy (i.e., high steroid levels) contribute to an increase in renal function; diminishing steroid levels after birth may partly explain the reduced renal function that occurs during the puerperium. Renal function returns to normal by 8 weeks after birth. About 6 weeks are required for the pregnancy-induced hypotonia and dilation of the ureters and renal pelves to return to the nonpregnant state. In a small percentage of women, dilation of the urinary tract can persist for 3 months or longer, increasing the risk of urinary tract infection (Isley & Katz, 2017).

Renal glycosuria induced by pregnancy disappears by 1 week postpartum, but lactosuria can occur in lactating women. The blood urea nitrogen level increases during the puerperium as autolysis of the involuting uterus occurs. Plasma creatinine levels return to normal by 6 weeks postpartum. Pregnancy-associated proteinuria resolves by 6 weeks after birth (Blackburn, 2018). Ketonuria can occur in women with an uncomplicated birth or after a prolonged labor with dehydration.

Fluid Loss

Within 12 hours of birth, women begin to lose excess tissue fluid accumulated during pregnancy. Postpartal diuresis caused by decreased estrogen levels, removal of increased venous pressure in the lower extremities, and loss of the remaining pregnancy-induced increase in blood volume aids the body in ridding itself of excess fluid. Urine output of 3000 mL or more each day during the first 2 to 3 days after birth is common. Profuse diaphoresis often occurs, especially at night, for the first 2 to 3 days after birth. Fluid loss through perspiration and increased urinary output accounts for a weight loss of 2 to 3 kg (5 to 6.6 lb) during the early puerperium (Cunningham et al., 2019).

Urethra and Bladder

Birth-induced trauma, increased bladder capacity after birth, and the effects of conduction (e.g., epidural or spinal) anesthesia can result in a decreased urge to void. In addition, pelvic soreness caused by the forces of labor, vaginal or perineal lacerations, or episiotomy can reduce or alter the voiding reflex. Decreased voiding combined with postpartal diuresis can result in bladder distention.

Immediately after birth, excessive bleeding can occur if the bladder becomes distended because it pushes the uterus up and to the side and prevents it from contracting firmly. Later in the puerperium, overdistention can make the bladder more susceptible to infection and impede the resumption of normal voiding. With adequate bladder emptying, bladder tone is usually restored by 5 to 7 days after birth.

Some women experience *stress incontinence* during the postpartum period. This is more likely to occur after vaginal than cesarean birth. Stress incontinence can be related to tissue trauma to the pelvic floor occurring with maternal expulsive efforts and increased size of the neonate. Coached pushing versus uncoached (non-Valsalva) pushing during the second stage of labor can increase the risk for damage to the pelvic floor and subsequent stress incontinence (James, 2014).

GASTROINTESTINAL SYSTEM

Most new mothers are very hungry after full recovery from analgesia, anesthesia, and fatigue. Requests for extra portions of food and frequent snacks are common.

A spontaneous bowel evacuation may not occur for 2 to 3 days after birth. This delay can be explained by slowed peristalsis related to decreased muscle tone in the intestines during labor and the immediate postpartum period, prelabor diarrhea, lack of food, dehydration, or the effects of opioid analgesics. Some women anticipate discomfort related to perineal tenderness as a result of an episiotomy, lacerations, or hemorrhoids and resist the urge to defecate. Regular bowel habits should be reestablished when bowel tone returns.

Third- and fourth-degree perineal lacerations that involve the anal sphincter are associated with an increased risk for postpartum anal incontinence. Women with this problem are more often incontinent of flatus than of stool. If anal incontinence lasts more than 6 months, diagnostic studies should be conducted to determine the specific cause and appropriate treatment (Isley & Katz, 2017).

INTEGUMENTARY SYSTEM

Melasma (chloasma or "mask of pregnancy") usually disappears in the postpartum period but persists in about 30% of women (Wang & Kroumpouzos, 2017). Hyperpigmentation of the areolae and *linea nigra* may not regress completely after birth. Some women will have permanent darker pigmentation of those areas. *Striae gravidarum* (stretch marks) on the breasts, abdomen, hips, and thighs may fade but usually do not disappear completely.

Vascular abnormalities such as *angiomatas* (vascular spiders) and palmar erythema generally regress in response to the rapid decline in estrogens after birth. For some women, vascular spiders persist indefinitely.

For the first 3 months after birth, women often report hair loss when they brush or comb their hair. The abundance of fine hair seen during pregnancy usually disappears after giving birth; however, any coarse or bristly hair that appears during pregnancy usually remains. Fingernails return to their prepregnancy consistency and strength.

MUSCULOSKELETAL SYSTEM

When the woman stands during the first days after birth, her abdomen protrudes and gives her a still-pregnant appearance. During the first 2 weeks after birth, the abdominal wall is relaxed. It takes about 6 weeks for the abdominal wall to return almost to its prepregnancy state (Fig. 20.3). The return of muscle tone depends on previous tone, proper exercise, and the amount of adipose tissue. Occasionally, with or without overdistention because of a large fetus or multiple fetuses, the abdominal wall muscles separate, a condition termed *diastasis recti abdominis* (Fig. 20.4). Persistence of this separation can be disturbing to the woman, but surgical correction rarely is necessary. With time, the separation becomes less apparent.

Other adaptations of the mother's musculoskeletal system that occur during pregnancy are reversed in the puerperium. These adaptations include the relaxation and subsequent hypermobility of the joints and the change in the mother's center of gravity in response to the enlarging uterus. Back pain usually resolves in a few weeks or months following birth.

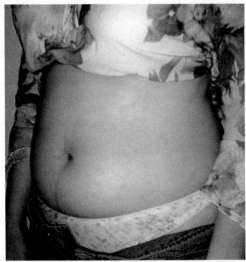

Fig. 20.3 Abdominal Wall 6 Weeks After Vaginal Birth Is Almost Back to Prepregnancy Appearance. Note that the linea nigra is still visible. (Courtesy Jodi Brackett, Phoenix, AZ.)

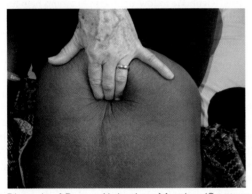

Fig. 20.4 Diastasis of Rectus Abdominus Muscles. (Courtesy Shannon Perry, Phoenix, AZ.)

The joints are completely stabilized by 6 to 8 weeks after birth. Although all other joints return to their normal prepregnancy state, those in the parous woman's feet do not. The new mother may notice a permanent increase in her shoe size.

NEUROLOGIC SYSTEM

Neurologic changes during the puerperium result from a reversal of maternal adaptations to pregnancy and from trauma during labor and birth.

Headaches are common in the first postpartum week; they are usually bilateral and frontal (Blackburn, 2018). However, headache requires careful assessment. Postpartum headaches can be caused by various conditions, including postpartum-onset preeclampsia, stress, and leakage of cerebrospinal fluid into the extradural space during placement of the needle for administration of epidural or spinal anesthesia.

Pregnancy-induced neurologic discomforts disappear after birth. Elimination of physiologic edema through the diuresis that follows birth relieves carpal tunnel syndrome by easing compression of the median nerve. The periodic numbness and tingling of fingers usually disappear after the birth unless lifting and carrying the baby aggravate the condition. Nasal stuffiness, tinnitus, and laryngeal changes resolve within a few days postpartum.

IMMUNE SYSTEM

The exact timeline for the maternal immune system to return to normal after birth is unclear (Blackburn, 2018). The rebound of the immune system can trigger exacerbation of autoimmune conditions such as multiple sclerosis or lupus erythematosus (Isley & Katz, 2017).

◼ KEY POINTS

- The rapid decrease in estrogen and progesterone levels after expulsion of the placenta triggers many of the anatomic and physiologic changes in the puerperium.
- Within 6 weeks after birth, the majority of physiologic changes that occurred during pregnancy have reverted to their nonpregnant state.
- Fundal height and lochia are indicators of progression of uterine involution.
- The uterus involutes rapidly and returns to the true pelvis by 2 weeks after birth.
- The return of ovulation and menses is determined in part by whether or not the woman is lactating (breastfeeding).
- Few alterations in postpartum vital signs are seen under normal circumstances.
- Rapid or increasing pulse rate and low or decreasing blood pressure can indicate hypovolemia secondary to hemorrhage.
- Hypercoagulability, vessel damage, and immobility predispose the woman to venous thromboembolism.
- Marked diuresis, decreased bladder sensitivity and overdistention of the bladder can lead to problems with urinary elimination.

REFERENCES

Antony, K. M., Racusin, D. A., Aagaard, K., & Dildy, G. A. (2017). Maternal physiology. In S. G. Gabbe, J. R. Niebyl, J. L. Simpson, et al. (Eds.), *Obstetrics: normal and problem pregnancies* (7th ed.). Philadelphia: Elsevier.

Berens, P. (2018). Overview of postpartum care. In C. J. Lockwood (Ed.), *UpToDate*. Retrieved from: http://www.uptodate.com/home.

Blackburn, S. T. (2018). *Maternal, fetal, and neonatal physiology* (5th ed.). St. Louis: Elsevier.

Cunningham, F. G., Leveno, K., Bloom, S. L., et al. (2019). *Williams obstetrics* (25th ed.). New York: McGraw Hill.

Isley, M. M., & Katz, V. L. (2017). Postpartum care and long-term considerations. In S. G. Gabbe, J. R. Niebyl, J. L. Simpson, et al. (Eds.), *Obstetrics: Normal and problem pregnancies* (7th ed.). Philadelphia: Elsevier.

James, D. C. (2014). Postpartum care. In K. R. Simpson, & P. A. Creehan (Eds.), *Perinatal nursing* (4th ed.). Philadelphia: Lippincott Williams & Wilkins.

Lawrence, R. M., & Lawrence, R. A. (2016). *Breastfeeding: A guide for the medical profession* (8th ed.). St. Louis: Elsevier.

Wang, A. R., & Kroumpouzos, G. (2017). Skin disease and pregnancy. In S. G. Gabbe, J. R. Niebyl, J. L. Simpson, et al. (Eds.), *Obstetrics: Normal and problem pregnancies* (7th ed.). Philadelphia: Elsevier.

21

Nursing Care of the Family During the Postpartum Period

Jennifer T. Alderman

 http://evolve.elsevier.com/Lowdermilk/MWHC/

LEARNING OUTCOMES

- Describe components of a systematic postpartum assessment.
- Recognize signs of potential complications in the postpartum woman.
- Formulate a nursing care plan for a woman and her family in the postpartum period.
- Explain the influence of cultural beliefs and practices on postpartum care.
- Identify psychosocial needs of the woman and family in the early postpartum period.
- Prepare a plan for postpartum teaching for self-management.
- Describe the nurse's role in these postpartum follow-up strategies: home visits, telephone follow-up, warm lines and help lines, support groups, and referrals to community resources.

At no other time is family-centered maternity care more important than in the postpartum period. Nursing care is provided in the context of the family unit and focuses on assessment and support of the woman's physiologic and emotional adaptation after birth. During the early postpartum period, components of nursing care include assisting the mother with rest and recovery from labor and birth, assessing physiologic and psychologic adaptation after birth, preventing complications, educating regarding self-management and infant care, and supporting the mother and her partner during the initial transition to parenthood. In addition, the nurse considers the needs of other family members and includes strategies in the nursing care plan to assist the family in adjusting to the new baby.

Care of women after birth is wellness oriented and is best provided by an interprofessional health care team that often includes an obstetric care provider, a primary care provider, a pediatric care provider, nurses in the birthing facility and outpatient facilities, lactation consultants, a case manager or care coordinator, a social worker, home care staff, and, as needed, consultants such as maternal-fetal medicine or internal medicine specialists (American College of Obstetricians and Gynecologists [ACOG], 2016).

In the United States, most women remain hospitalized no more than 1 or 2 days after vaginal birth and some as few as 6 hours. Because so much important information needs to be shared with these women in a very short time, their care must be thoughtfully planned and provided. Ideally, discharge planning and education begins during pregnancy (ACOG, 2016). This chapter discusses nursing care of the woman and her family in the postpartum period extending into the *fourth trimester*—the first 3 months after birth. Care of the woman after cesarean birth is discussed in Chapter 32.

TRANSFER FROM THE RECOVERY AREA

After the initial recovery period has been completed (see Chapter 19), and provided that her condition is stable, the woman may be transferred to a postpartum room in the same or another nursing unit. In facilities with labor, delivery, recovery, postpartum (LDRP) rooms, the woman is not moved and the nurse who provides care during the recovery period usually continues caring for the woman. In many settings, women who have received general or regional anesthesia must be cleared for transfer from the recovery area by a member of the anesthesia care team. In other settings, a nurse makes the determination.

In preparing the transfer report or "hand-off," the labor and birth or postanesthesia care nurse uses information from the records of admission, birth, and recovery. Information that must be communicated to the postpartum nurse includes the woman's name, age, identity of the health care provider; gravidity and parity; anesthetic used; any medications given; duration of labor and time of rupture of membranes; whether labor was induced or augmented; mode of birth (vaginal or cesarean); perineal repair or type of cesarean incision; blood type and Rh status; group B streptococcus (GBS) status; status of rubella immunity; human immunodeficiency virus (HIV), hepatitis B, and syphilis serology test results; other infections identified during pregnancy (e.g., gonorrhea, chlamydia) and whether these were treated; type and amount of intravenous fluids; physiologic status since birth; description of fundus, lochia, bladder, and perineum; gender and weight of infant; time of birth; name of pediatric care provider; chosen method of feeding; any abnormalities noted; and assessment of initial parent-infant interaction. In addition, specific information should be provided regarding the newborn's Apgar scores (see Chapter 24), weight, voiding, stooling, skin-to-skin care, feeding since birth, eye prophylaxis, and vitamin K injection.

In recent years, many inpatient nursing units, including perinatal care areas, have a bedside report. Bedside reporting is increasingly being used instead of the traditional report given at the nurses' station. Bedside reporting has been shown to improve client safety and satisfaction. Clients feel more involved in their plan of care, which increases their satisfaction. In addition, holding reports at the bedside has enabled many nurses to both visualize and communicate with the client at the time of report, which improves client safety (Groves, Manges, & Scott-Cawiezell, 2016).

PLANNING FOR DISCHARGE

From their initial contact with the postpartum woman, nurses prepare the new mother for her return to home. Planning for discharge begins with the first interaction among the nurse, the woman, and her family and continues until they leave the hospital or birthing facility.

The length of hospital stay after giving birth depends on many factors. These include the physical condition of the mother and the newborn, mental and emotional status of the mother, social support at home, client education needs for self-care and infant care, and financial constraints.

Women who give birth in birthing centers may be discharged within a few hours, after the woman's and infant's conditions are stable. Mothers and newborns who are at low risk for complications may be discharged from the hospital within 24 to 36 hours after vaginal birth. The typical stay in the hospital after vaginal birth is approximately 48 hours.

The American Academy of Pediatrics (AAP, 2015) recommends that the hospital stay for a mother with a healthy term newborn should be of sufficient length to identify early problems and determine that the mother and family are prepared and able to care for the newborn at home. The health of the mother and her newborn should be stable, the mother should be able and confident to provide care for her infant, and there should be adequate support systems in place and access to follow-up care.

It is essential that nurses consider the individual needs of the woman and her newborn and provide care that is intentionally planned to meet these needs. As members of the interprofessional health care team, hospital-based maternity nurses continue to play key roles as caregivers, teachers, and advocates for mothers, newborns, and families in developing and implementing effective home-care strategies. Postpartum order sets and maternal-newborn teaching checklists that address the mother's learning needs can be used to accomplish client care tasks and educational outcomes.

CARE MANAGEMENT: PHYSICAL NEEDS

The nursing plan of care includes the postpartum woman, her newborn, and her family. Most birth facilities use the couplet or mother/baby model of care (Association of Women's Health, Obstetric and Neonatal Nurses [AWHONN], 2010). Nurses in these settings have been educated in both mother and infant care and function as primary nurses for both mother and infant, even if the infant is kept in the nursery. This approach is a variation of rooming-in, in which the mother and infant room together and mother and nurse share in the infant's care. The organization of the mother's care must take the newborn's feeding and care needs into consideration.

Ongoing Physical Assessment

Ongoing assessments are performed throughout hospitalization. In addition to vital signs, physical assessment of the postpartum woman focuses on evaluation of the breasts, uterine fundus, lochia, perineum, bladder and bowel function, and lower extremities (Table 21.1).

Routine Laboratory Tests

Several laboratory tests may be performed in the immediate postpartum period. Hemoglobin and hematocrit values are often evaluated on the first postpartum day to assess blood loss during birth, especially after cesarean birth. In some hospitals, a clean-catch or catheterized urine specimen is obtained and sent for routine urinalysis or culture and sensitivity, especially if an indwelling urinary catheter was inserted during the intrapartum period. In addition, if the woman's rubella immunity and Rh status are unknown, tests to determine her status and need for possible treatment should be performed at this time.

Nursing Interventions

Based on the available data (e.g., medical record) and assessment findings, the nurse plans with the woman which nursing measures are appropriate and which are to be given priority. The nursing care plan includes periodic assessments to detect variations from normal physical changes, measures to relieve discomfort or pain, safety measures to prevent injury and infection, and education and counseling measures designed to promote the woman's feelings of competence in self-management and infant care. The nurse evaluates continually and is ready to change the plan if indicated. Almost all hospitals use standardized care plans as a base. Nurses individualize care of the postpartum woman and neonate according to their specific needs (see the Nursing Care Plan). Signs of potential problems that may be identified during the assessment process are listed in Table 21.1.

Nurses assume many roles while implementing the nursing care plan. They provide direct physical care, educate new mothers and their families, and provide anticipatory guidance and counseling. Perhaps most important, they nurture the woman by providing encouragement and support as she begins to assume the many tasks of motherhood. Nurses who take the time to "mother the mother" do much to increase feelings of self-confidence in new mothers. Nurses are careful to include the woman's spouse or partner and other primary support persons in education and counseling.

The first step in providing client-centered care is to confirm the woman's identity by checking her wristband. At the same time, the infant's identification number is matched with the corresponding band on the mother's wrist and in some instances the father's or partner's wrist. The nurse determines how the mother wishes to be addressed and notes her preference in her medical record and her nursing care plan. The nurse orients the woman and her family to their surroundings. Familiarity with the unit, routines, resources, and personnel reduces one potential source of anxiety—the unknown. The mother is reassured through knowing whom and how she can call for assistance and what she can expect in the way of supplies and services. If the woman's usual daily routine before admission differs from the routine of the facility, the nurse works with the woman to develop a mutually acceptable routine. Nurses discuss infant security precautions with the mother and her family (see Chapter 24).

Preventing Excessive Bleeding

All women who have given birth are at risk for excessive bleeding that can progress to postpartum hemorrhage (see Chapter 33). The most frequent cause of excessive bleeding after birth is *uterine atony* (i.e., failure of the uterine muscle to contract firmly). The two most important interventions for preventing excessive bleeding are maintaining good uterine tone and preventing bladder distention. If uterine atony occurs, the relaxed uterus distends with blood and clots, blood vessels in the placental site are not clamped off, and excessive bleeding results. Although the cause of uterine atony is not always clear, it often results from retained placental fragments.

⊚ NURSING CARE PLAN

Postpartum Care—Vaginal Birth

Client Problem	Expected Outcomes	Nursing Interventions	Rationales
Potential for excessive bleeding related to uterine atony	Fundus is firm and midline. Lochia is moderate. There is no evidence of hemorrhage.	Monitor lochia (color, amount, consistency), and count or weigh sanitary pads if lochia is heavy.	To evaluate amount of bleeding
		Monitor and palpate fundus for location and tone to determine status of uterus and dictate further interventions.	Because uterine atony is the most common cause of postpartum hemorrhage
		If fundus is boggy, apply gentle massage, express clots, and assess tone response.	To promote uterine contractions and increase uterine tone. (Do not overstimulate because doing so can cause fundal relaxation.)
		Explain process of involution, and teach client to assess and massage fundus and report any persistent bogginess.	To involve her in self-management and increase sense of self-control
Acute pain related to perineal trauma during vaginal birth	Discomfort will be decreased within one hour after interventions.	Assess location, type, and quality of pain.	To direct intervention
	Woman will describe and implement appropriate interventions for pain relief.	Explain to woman about the source and reason for pain, its expected duration, and treatments.	To decrease anxiety and increase sense of control
	Vital signs remain within normal limits.	Administer prescribed pain medication and evaluate effectiveness within 1 h.	To provide pain relief
		Use nonpharmacologic pain relief techniques such as ice packs in first 24 h; after 24 h, warm sitz bath.	To reduce edema and vulvar irritation and reduce discomfort
Potential for difficult urination related to perineal trauma and fear of discomfort	Woman will void within 3-4 h after birth and empty bladder completely.	Assess woman's ability to urinate, and assess position and character of uterine fundus and bladder.	To ascertain if any further interventions are indicated because of displacement of fundus or distention of bladder
	Woman will verbalize and demonstrate understanding of measures to promote urination.	Instruct woman in interventions to promote urination such as increasing fluid intake, pouring warm water over perineum, running water in sink, and providing privacy.	To encourage voiding
	Woman will have adequate oral intake and adequate urinary output.	Encourage oral fluid intake and monitor intake and output.	To assess adequacy of fluid intake and urine output; a full or distended bladder increases the risk for uterine atony
		Administer analgesics as indicated.	To reduce perineal discomfort

Excessive blood loss after birth can also be caused by vaginal or vulvar hematomas or unrepaired lacerations of the vagina or cervix. These potential sources might be suspected if excessive vaginal bleeding occurs in the presence of a firmly contracted uterine fundus.

> ⚠ **NURSING ALERT**
>
> A perineal pad saturated in 15 minutes or less and pooling of blood under the buttocks are indications of excessive blood loss, requiring immediate assessment, intervention, and notification of the obstetric health care provider.

Accurate visual estimation of blood loss is an important nursing responsibility. Blood loss is usually described subjectively as scant, light, moderate, or heavy (profuse). Fig. 21.1 shows examples of perineal pad saturation corresponding to each of these descriptions.

Although postpartum blood loss can be estimated by observing the amount of drainage on a perineal pad, judging the amount of lochia is difficult if based only on observation of perineal pads. Quantification of blood loss by weighing clots and items saturated with blood (1 mL equals 1 g) is recommended as the most accurate way to objectively determine blood loss.

Any estimation of lochial flow is inaccurate and incomplete without considering the time factor. The woman who saturates a perineal pad in 1 hour or less is bleeding much more heavily than the woman who saturates one perineal pad in 8 hours. When assessing blood loss, the nurse asks the woman how long it has been since her perineal pad was changed.

Nurses in general tend to overestimate rather than underestimate blood loss. Different brands of perineal pads vary in their saturation volume and soaking appearance. For example, blood placed on some brands tends to soak down into the pad, whereas on other brands it tends to spread outward. A perineal pad with an enclosed cold pack lacks absorbency. Nurses should determine saturation volume and

TABLE 21.1   Postpartum Assessment and Signs of Potential Complications

Assessment	Normal Findings	Signs of Potential Complications
Blood pressure (BP)	Consistent with BP baseline during pregnancy; transient increase of 5% first few days after birth; can have orthostatic hypotension for 48 h	Hypertension: anxiety, preeclampsia, essential hypertension Hypotension: hemorrhage
Temperature	36.2°C-38°C (97.2°F-100.4°F)	>38°C (100.4°F) after 24 h: infection
Pulse	50-90 beats/min	Tachycardia: pain, fever, dehydration, hemorrhage
Respirations	16-20 breaths/min	Bradypnea: effects of opioid medications Tachypnea: anxiety; may be sign of respiratory disease
Breath sounds	Clear to auscultation	Crackles: possible fluid overload
Breasts	Days 1-2: soft Days 2-3: filling Days 3-5: full, soften with breastfeeding (milk is "in")	Firmness, heat, pain: engorgement
Nipples	Skin intact; no soreness reported	Redness, bruising, cracks, fissures, abrasions, blisters: usually associated with latching problems
Uterus (fundus)	Firm, midline; first 24 h at level of umbilicus; involutes ≈1 cm (1 fingerbreadth)/day	Soft, boggy, higher than expected level: uterine atony Lateral deviation: distended bladder
Lochia	Days 1-3: rubra (dark red) Days 4-10: serosa (brownish red or pink) After 10 days: alba (yellowish white) Amount: scant to moderate Few clots Fleshy odor	Large amount of lochia, large clots: uterine atony, vaginal or cervical laceration Foul odor: infection
Perineum	Minimal edema	Pronounced edema, bruising, hematoma
	Laceration or episiotomy: edges approximated	Redness, warmth, drainage: infection
	Pain minimal to moderate: controlled by analgesics, nonpharmacologic techniques, or both	Excessive discomfort first 1-2 days: hematoma; after day 3: infection
Rectal area	No hemorrhoids; if hemorrhoids are present, soft and pink	Discolored hemorrhoidal tissue, severe pain: thrombosed hemorrhoid
Bladder	Able to void spontaneously; no distention; able to empty completely; no dysuria	Overdistended bladder possibly causing uterine atony, excessive lochia
	Diuresis begins ≈12 h after birth; can void 3000 mL/day	Dysuria, frequency, urgency, burning: infection
Abdomen and bowels	Abdomen soft, active bowel sounds in all quadrants	
	Bowel movement by day 2 or 3 after birth	No bowel movement by day 3 or 4: constipation; diarrhea
	Cesarean: incision dressing clean and dry; suture line intact	Abdominal incision—redness, edema, warmth, drainage: infection
Legs	Deep tendon reflexes (DTRs) 1+ to 2+	DTRs ≥3+: preeclampsia
	Peripheral edema possibly present	
	Homan sign[a] negative	Redness, tenderness, pain, thrombophlebitis
Energy level	Able to care for self and infant; able to sleep	Lethargy, extreme fatigue, difficulty sleeping: postpartum depression
Emotional status	Excited, happy, interested or involved in infant care	Sad, tearful, disinterested in infant care: postpartum blues or depression

[a]Homan sign was traditionally included in routine postpartum assessments; however, it is no longer common practice due to concern about its limited sensitivity and specificity in diagnosing venous thromboembolism and the potential risk for dislodging a clot when the test is performed.

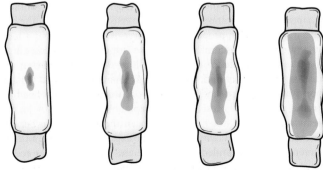

Fig. 21.1 Blood loss after birth is assessed by the extent of perineal pad saturation as *(left to right)* scant (<2.5 cm), light (<10 cm), moderate (>10 cm), or heavy (one pad saturated within 2 hours).

soaking appearance for the brands used in their institution so that they can improve accuracy of blood loss estimation.

⚡ SAFETY ALERT

The nurse always checks for blood under the mother's buttocks, as well as on the perineal pad. Although the amount on the perineal pad can appear to be small, blood can flow between the buttocks onto the linens under the mother. When this happens, excessive bleeding can go undetected.

When excessive bleeding occurs, vital signs are monitored closely. Blood pressure is not a reliable indicator of impending shock from early postpartum hemorrhage because compensatory mechanisms prevent a significant drop in blood pressure until the woman has lost

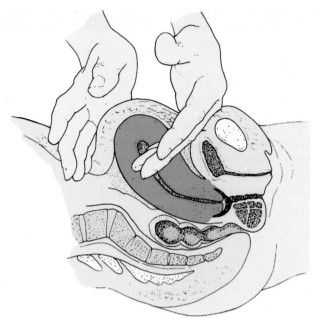

Fig. 21.2 Fundal Massage. Note that upper hand is cupped over fundus; lower hand dips in above symphysis pubis and supports uterus while it is massaged gently.

30% to 40% of her blood volume (see Chapter 33). Respirations, pulse, skin condition, urinary output, and level of consciousness are more sensitive indicators of hypovolemic shock (see Chapter 33). The frequent physical assessments performed during the fourth stage of labor are designed to provide prompt identification of excessive bleeding. Nurses maintain vigilance for excessive bleeding throughout the hospital stay as they perform periodic assessments of the uterine fundus and lochia.

Maintaining Uterine Tone

A major intervention to alleviate uterine atony and restore uterine muscle tone is stimulation by gently massaging the fundus until firm (Fig. 21.2). Fundal massage can cause a temporary increase in the amount of vaginal bleeding seen as pooled blood leaves the uterus. Clots can also be expelled. The uterus can remain boggy even after massage and clot expulsion.

Fundal massage can be a very uncomfortable procedure. If the nurse explains the purpose of fundal massage and the causes and dangers of uterine atony and assists her with breathing and relaxation techniques, the woman will likely be more cooperative. Teaching the woman to massage her own fundus enables her to maintain some control and decreases her anxiety.

When uterine atony and excessive bleeding occur, additional interventions likely to be used are administration of intravenous fluids and oxytocic medications (drugs that stimulate contraction of the uterine smooth muscle) (see Medication Guide: Uterotonic Drugs to Manage Postpartum Hemorrhage in Chapter 33 for information about common oxytocic medications).

Preventing Bladder Distention

Uterine atony and excessive bleeding after birth can be the result of bladder distention. A full bladder causes the uterus to be displaced above the umbilicus and well to one side of midline in the abdomen. It also prevents the uterus from contracting normally.

Women can be at risk for bladder distention resulting from urinary retention based on intrapartum factors, including epidural anesthesia, episiotomy, extensive vaginal or perineal lacerations, vacuum- or

forceps-assisted birth, or prolonged labor. Women who have had indwelling catheters, such as with cesarean birth, can experience some difficulty as they initially attempt to void after the catheter is removed. Nurses who are aware of these risk factors can be proactive in preventing complications.

Nursing interventions for a postpartum woman focus on helping the woman to empty her bladder spontaneously as soon as possible. The first priority is to assist the woman to the bathroom or onto a bedpan if she is unable to ambulate. Having the woman listen to running water, placing her hands in warm water, or pouring water from a squeeze bottle over her perineum may stimulate voiding. Other techniques include assisting the woman into the shower or sitz bath and encouraging her to void; relaxation techniques can also be helpful. Administering analgesics, if ordered, may be indicated because some women fear voiding because of anticipated pain. If these measures are unsuccessful, a sterile catheter may be inserted to drain the urine.

Preventing Infection

Nurses in the postpartum setting are acutely aware of the importance of preventing infection. One important means of preventing infection is by maintaining a clean environment. Bed linens should be changed as needed. Disposable pads and draw sheets are changed frequently. Women should wear slippers when walking about to prevent contamination of the linens when they return to bed. Personnel must be conscientious about their hand hygiene to prevent cross-infection. Standard precautions must be practiced. Staff members with colds, coughs, or skin infections (e.g., a cold sore [herpes simplex virus lesion] on the lip) must follow hospital protocol when in contact with postpartum women. In many hospitals, staff members with open herpetic lesions, strep throat, conjunctivitis, upper respiratory infections, or diarrhea are encouraged to avoid contact with mothers and infants by staying home until the condition is no longer contagious. Visitors with signs of illness are not permitted to enter the postpartum unit.

Perineal lacerations and episiotomies can increase the risk for infection as a result of interruption in skin integrity. Proper perineal care helps to prevent infection in the genitourinary area and aids the healing process. Educating the woman to wipe from front to back (urethra to anus) after voiding or defecating is a simple first step. In many hospitals, a squeeze bottle filled with warm water or an antiseptic solution is used after each voiding to cleanse the perineal area. The woman should change her perineal pad from front to back each time she voids or defecates and wash her hands thoroughly before and after doing so (Box 21.1).

Promoting Comfort

Most women experience some degree of discomfort during the postpartum period. Common causes of discomfort include pain from uterine contractions (*afterpains*), perineal lacerations or episiotomy, hemorrhoids, sore nipples, and breast engorgement. The woman's description of the location, type, and severity of her pain is the best guide in choosing appropriate interventions. To confirm the location and extent of discomfort, the nurse inspects and palpates areas of pain as appropriate for redness, swelling, discharge, and heat and observes for body tension, guarded movements, and facial tension. Blood pressure, pulse, and respirations can be elevated in response to acute pain. Diaphoresis can accompany severe pain. A lack of objective signs does not necessarily mean there is no pain because there can be a cultural component to the expression of pain. Nursing interventions are intended to eliminate the pain entirely or reduce it to a tolerable level that allows the woman to care for herself and her newborn. Nurses may use nonpharmacologic and pharmacologic interventions to promote comfort. Pain relief is enhanced by using more than one method or route.

BOX 21.1   Interventions for Perineal Lacerations, Episiotomy, and Hemorrhoids

Explain procedure and rationale before implementation.

Cleansing
- Perform hand hygiene before and after cleansing perineum and changing pads.
- Wash perineum with mild soap and warm water at least once daily.
- Cleanse from symphysis pubis to anal area.
- Apply peripad from front to back, protecting inner surface of pad from contamination.
- Wrap soiled pad, and place in covered waste container.
- Change pad with each void or defecation or at least four times per day.
- Assess amount and character of lochia with each pad change.

Ice Pack
- Apply a covered ice pack or perineal pad with enclosed ice pack to perineum from front to back:
  - During first 24 h following birth to decrease edema formation and increase comfort
  - After first 24 h following birth as needed to provide anesthetic effect

Squeeze Bottle
- Fill bottle with tap water warmed to approximately 38°C (100.4°F) (comfortably warm on wrist).
- Instruct woman to position nozzle between her legs so squirts of water reach perineum as she sits on toilet seat. Explain that it will take the entire bottle of water to cleanse the perineum.
- Remind her to blot dry with toilet paper or clean wipes.
- Remind her to avoid contamination from anal area by wiping "front to back."
- Apply clean pad.

Sitz Bath
Built-in Type
- Prepare bath by thoroughly scrubbing with cleaning agent and rinsing.
- Pad with towel before filling.
- Fill one-third to one-half full with water of correct temperature, 38°C-40.6°C (100.4°F-105.1°F). Some women prefer cool sitz baths. Add ice to water to lower temperature to a comfortable level.
- Encourage woman to use at least twice a day for 20 min.
- Place call bell within easy reach.
- Teach woman to enter bath by tightening gluteal muscles and keeping them tightened and then relaxing them after she is in bath.
- Place dry towels within reach.
- Ensure privacy.
- Check woman in 15 min.

Disposable Type
- Clamp tubing and fill bag with warm water.
- Raise toilet seat; place bath in bowl with overflow opening directed toward back of toilet.
- Place bag above toilet bowl.
- Attach tube into groove at front of bath.
- Loosen tube clamp to regulate rate of flow; fill bath to about one-half full; continue as for built-in sitz bath.

Topical Applications
- Apply anesthetic cream or spray after cleansing perineal area: use sparingly three or four times per day.
- Apply witch hazel pads after cleansing perineum.
- Apply hemorrhoidal cream, as ordered, to anal area after cleansing.

⚡ SAFETY ALERT

If a postpartum woman complains of extreme perineal pain, especially after having received pain medication, the first action by the nurse should be to assess the perineum. There may be a hematoma or perineal infection that is causing the pain. Although rare, an unusual degree of pain can be a sign of serious complications, including perineal cellulitis, necrotizing fasciitis, or angioedema (Isley & Katz, 2017).

Nonpharmacologic interventions. Various nonpharmacologic measures are used to reduce postpartum discomfort. These include distraction, imagery, touch, relaxation, acupressure, aromatherapy, hydrotherapy, massage therapy, music therapy, and transcutaneous electrical nerve stimulation (TENS). See Chapter 17 for more information on these techniques.

For women who are experiencing discomfort associated with uterine contractions, application of warmth (e.g., heating pad) or lying prone can be helpful. Interaction with the infant can also provide distraction and decrease this discomfort. Because afterpains are more severe during and after breastfeeding, interventions are planned to provide the most timely and effective relief. A simple intervention that can decrease the discomfort associated with an episiotomy or perineal lacerations is to encourage the woman to lie on her side whenever possible. Other interventions include application of an ice pack; topical application (if ordered) of anesthetic spray or cream; cleansing with water from a squeeze bottle; and a cleansing shower, tub bath, or sitz bath. Many of these interventions are also effective for hemorrhoids, especially ice packs, sitz baths, and topical applications (such as witch hazel pads). Box 21.1 gives additional specific information about these interventions.

Sore nipples in breastfeeding mothers are most likely related to ineffective latch technique. Assessment and assistance with feeding can help to alleviate the cause. To ease discomfort associated with sore nipples, the mother may apply topical preparations or hydrogel pads (see Chapter 25).

Breast engorgement can occur whether the woman is breastfeeding or formula feeding. The discomfort associated with engorged breasts may be reduced by applying ice packs or cabbage leaves (or both) to the breasts (Fig. 25.17) and wearing a well-fitted support bra. Antiinflammatory medications such as ibuprofen can also be helpful in relieving some of the discomfort. Decisions about specific interventions for engorgement are based on whether the woman chooses breastfeeding or formula feeding. For example, breastfeeding mothers can feed frequently and use hand expression or a breast pump to reduce engorgement and promote comfort (see Chapter 25). Formula-feeding mothers with engorged breasts should not express breast milk as it can stimulate milk production and worsen engorgement.

Pharmacologic interventions. Pharmacologic interventions are commonly used to relieve or reduce postpartum discomfort. Most health care providers routinely order a variety of analgesics to be administered as needed, including both opioid and nonopioid (e.g., nonsteroidal antiinflammatory drugs [NSAIDs]). NSAIDs commonly used are ibuprofen or naproxen. These medications provide better relief from uterine cramping and perineal pain than acetaminophen or propoxyphene. Ibuprofen is preferred for breastfeeding women because it has a low milk/maternal plasma drug concentration ratio and a short-half life (Isley & Katz, 2017). In some hospitals, NSAIDs are administered on a scheduled basis, especially if the woman had perineal repair. Topical application of antiseptic or anesthetic ointment or spray can be used for perineal pain. Patient-controlled analgesia (PCA) pumps and epidural analgesia are commonly used to provide pain relief after cesarean birth.

Many women want to participate in decisions about analgesia. However, severe pain can interfere with active participation in choosing pain relief measures. If an analgesic is needed, the nurse uses clinical reasoning skills to select and administer the appropriate medication from the health provider's orders. The woman is informed of the prescribed analgesic and its common side effects; this teaching is documented.

Breastfeeding mothers often have concerns about the effects of an analgesic on the infant. Although nearly all drugs present in maternal circulation are also found in breast milk, many analgesics commonly used during the postpartum period are considered relatively safe for breastfeeding mothers and infants. Often the timing of medications can be adjusted to minimize infant exposure. A mother may be given pain medication immediately after breastfeeding so that the interval between medication administration and the next breastfeeding session is as long as possible. The decision to administer medications of any kind to a breastfeeding mother must always be made by carefully weighing the woman's need against actual or potential risks to the infant. Resources are readily accessible for nurses and health care providers to examine the safety of medications for breastfeeding mothers (e.g., LactMed [https://toxnet.nlm.nih.gov/newtoxnet/lactmed.htm]).

If acceptable pain relief has not been obtained in 1 hour, the nurse should reassess the woman and may need to contact the obstetric care provider for additional pain relief orders or further directions. Unrelieved pain results in fatigue, anxiety, and a worsening perception of the pain. It might also indicate the presence of a previously unidentified or untreated problem.

Promoting Rest

Lack of sleep and fatigue are common complaints of new parents. Sleep loss, feeling stressed, and physical exhaustion have been reported as the top three problems women experience within the first 2 months after giving birth (Declercq, Sakala, Corry, et al., 2014). The early postpartum period is the time that new parents experience the greatest disruption to their lives as they try to adjust to the nearly constant demands of a newborn (Krawczak, Minuzzi, Hidalgo, & Frey, 2016). Other factors that contribute to physical fatigue or exhaustion include long labor or cesarean birth, hospital routines that interrupt periods of sleep and rest, physical discomfort, and visitors. Fatigue can also be associated with anemia, infection, or thyroid dysfunction. The excitement and exhilaration experienced after the birth of the infant makes resting difficult. Disrupted sleep and fatigue in the postpartum woman may contribute to the development of postpartum depressive symptoms and increase the risk for postpartum depression (PPD) (Bhati & Richards, 2015; Doering, Sims, & Miller, 2017; Okun, 2015, 2016).

Fatigue is likely to worsen over the first 6 weeks after birth, often because of situational factors. After discharge from the hospital, fatigue increases as the woman provides care and feeding for the newborn in combination with other family and household responsibilities such as caring for other children, preparing meals, and doing laundry. Many women have partners, family members, or friends to provide much-needed assistance, whereas others can be without any help at all. The nurse needs to inquire about resources available to the woman after discharge and help her to plan accordingly. It is important to remember that the partner is also prone to fatigue if he or she is helping the new mother with infant care and attending to other children and household tasks. Partners can also develop PPD (see Chapter 31).

Interventions are planned to meet the woman's individual needs for sleep and rest while she is in the hospital. Comfort measures and medications to promote sleep may be necessary. The side-lying position for breastfeeding minimizes fatigue in nursing mothers. Support and encouragement of mothering behaviors help to reduce anxiety. Hospital and nursing care routines can be adjusted to meet the needs of individual mothers. In addition, the nurse can help the family to limit visitors and provide a comfortable chair or bed for the partner or other family member who is staying with the new mother.

Because postpartum fatigue can be very debilitating, follow-up after hospital discharge is important. Assessment for fatigue can be done with a nurse-initiated telephone call within the first two weeks after discharge as well as at the routine follow-up visit with the health care provider. Nurses in the pediatric care provider's office or clinic should also be alert for signs of maternal fatigue. The infant will be seen within the first few days after birth—before the woman sees her obstetric care provider.

Promoting Ambulation

Early ambulation is associated with a reduced incidence of venous thromboembolism (VTE) (see Chapter 33); it also promotes the return of strength. Free movement is encouraged once anesthesia wears off unless an opioid analgesic has been administered. After the initial recovery period, the mother is encouraged to ambulate frequently.

In the early postpartum period, some women feel lightheaded or dizzy when standing. The rapid decrease in intraabdominal pressure after birth results in a dilation of blood vessels supplying the intestines (splanchnic engorgement) and causes blood to pool in the viscera. This condition contributes to the development of orthostatic hypotension when the woman who has recently given birth sits or stands up, first ambulates, or takes a warm shower or sitz bath. When assisting a woman to ambulate, the nurse needs to consider the baseline blood pressure; amount of blood loss; and type, amount, and timing of analgesic or anesthetic medications administered.

Women who have had regional (epidural or spinal) anesthesia can experience slow return of sensory and motor function in their lower extremities, increasing the risk for falls with early ambulation. Careful assessment by the postpartum nurse can prevent falls. Factors that the nurse should consider are the time lapse since epidural or spinal medication was given; the woman's ability to bend both knees, place both feet flat on the bed, and lift buttocks off the bed without assistance; medications since birth; vital signs; and estimated blood loss with birth. Before allowing the woman to ambulate, the nurse assesses the ability of the woman to stand unassisted beside her bed, simultaneously bending both knees slightly, and then standing with knees locked. If the woman is unable to balance herself, she can be safely eased back into bed without injury (Gaffey, 2015).

Preventing VTE is important. Blood is hypercoagulable in the postpartum period, especially during the first 48 hours after birth (Isley & Katz, 2017). Women who must remain in bed after giving birth are at increased risk for this complication. Antiembolic stockings (TED hose) or a sequential compression device (SCD boots) may be ordered prophylactically. If a woman remains in bed longer than 8 hours (e.g., for postpartum magnesium sulfate therapy for preeclampsia), exercise to promote circulation in the legs is indicated, using the following routine:

- Alternate flexion and extension of the feet.
- Rotate the ankles in a circular motion.

- Alternate flexion and extension of the legs.
- Press the back of the knees to the bed surface; relax.

If the woman is susceptible to VTE, she is encouraged to walk about actively for true ambulation and is discouraged from sitting immobile in a chair. Women with varicosities are encouraged to wear support hose. If a thrombus is suspected, as evidenced by warmth, redness, or tenderness in the suspected leg, the obstetric health care provider should be notified. Meanwhile the woman should be confined to bed, with the affected limb elevated on pillows.

Promoting Exercise

Postpartum exercise can begin soon after birth, although the woman should be encouraged to start with simple exercises and gradually progress to more strenuous ones. Fig. 21.3 illustrates a number of exercises appropriate for the new mother. Abdominal exercises are postponed until approximately 4 to 6 weeks after cesarean birth.

Promoting Nutrition

During the hospital stay, most women have a good appetite and eat well. They may request that family members bring favorite or culturally appropriate foods. Cultural dietary preferences must be respected. This interest in food presents an ideal opportunity for nutritional counseling on dietary needs after pregnancy, with specific information related to breastfeeding, preventing constipation and anemia, promoting weight loss, and promoting healing and well-being (see Chapter 15).

A well-balanced diet helps to promote healing and health in the postpartum period. The recommended caloric intake for the moderately active, nonlactating postpartum woman is 1800 to 2200 kcal/day. Lactating women need an additional 450 to 500 kcal/day, which can usually be met with simple adjustments in a normally balanced diet. Women who are underweight, exercise excessively, or are breastfeeding more than one infant need additional calories. Dietary intake for lactating women should include 200 to 300 mg of the omega-3 long-chain polyunsaturated fatty acid (docosahexaenoic acid [DHA]) so that there is adequate DHA in the breast milk. The addition of one or two weekly portions of fish with low mercury content provides the additional DHA. Women on selected vegan diets and those who are poorly nourished may need to take DHA and multivitamin supplements (AAP Section on Breastfeeding, 2012).

Prenatal vitamins may be continued until 6 weeks after birth or until the supply has been depleted. Iron supplements may be prescribed for women with low hemoglobin and hematocrit levels.

Promoting Normal Bladder and Bowel Patterns

Bladder function. The mother should void spontaneously within 6 to 8 hours after giving birth. The first several voidings should be measured to document adequate emptying of the bladder. A volume of at least 150 mL is expected for each voiding. Some women experience difficulty in emptying the bladder, possibly as a result of diminished bladder tone, edema from trauma, or fear of discomfort. Nursing interventions for inability to void and bladder distention are discussed in the "Preventing Bladder Distention" section earlier in the chapter.

Urinary incontinence is not uncommon, especially if there was significant perineal trauma with birth. Pelvic floor muscle training, also known as Kegel exercises, helps to strengthen muscle tone, particularly after vaginal birth. Kegel exercises help women to regain the muscle tone that is often lost as pelvic tissues are stretched and torn during pregnancy and birth. Women who maintain muscle strength benefit years later by retaining urinary continence. Women must learn to perform Kegel exercises correctly (see Guidelines box: Kegel Exercises in Chapter 4). Some women perform the exercises incorrectly and can increase the risk for incontinence, which can occur when inadvertently bearing down on the pelvic floor muscles, thrusting the perineum outward. The health care provider can assess the woman's technique during the pelvic examination at her follow-up visit by inserting two fingers intravaginally and noting whether the pelvic floor muscles correctly contract and relax.

Bowel function. After birth, women can be at risk for constipation related to side effects of medications (opioid analgesics, iron supplements, magnesium sulfate), dehydration, immobility, or the presence of episiotomy, perineal lacerations, or hemorrhoids. The woman can be fearful of pain with the first bowel movement.

Nursing interventions to promote normal bowel elimination include educating the woman about measures to prevent constipation, such as ambulation and increasing the intake of fluids and fiber. Alerting the woman to side effects of medications such as opioid analgesics (e.g., decreased gastrointestinal tract motility) can encourage her to implement measures to reduce the risk for constipation. Stool softeners or laxatives may be necessary during the early postpartum period. These are used only at the direction of the health care provider.

⚡ SAFETY ALERT

Rectal suppositories and enemas should not be administered to women with third- or fourth-degree perineal lacerations. These measures to treat constipation can be very uncomfortable and can cause hemorrhage or damage to the suture line. They can also predispose the woman to infection.

Some mothers experience gas pains; this is more common following cesarean birth. Ambulation or rocking in a rocking chair can stimulate passage of flatus and provide relief. Antiflatulent medications may be ordered. The mother can avoid foods (e.g., legumes, beans, broccoli) that tend to produce gas.

Promoting breastfeeding. The ideal time to initiate breastfeeding is within the first 1 to 2 hours after birth. Newborns should be placed in skin-to-skin contact with their mothers as soon as possible after birth and remain there for at least 1 hour. Nurses can encourage mothers to observe their babies for signs that they are ready to breastfeed and then assist the mothers as needed to initiate breastfeeding. During this first hour, most infants are alert and ready to nurse. Breastfeeding aids in contracting the uterus and preventing maternal hemorrhage. This initial breastfeeding session allows the nurse to assess the mother's basic knowledge of breastfeeding and the physical appearance of the breasts and nipples. Throughout the hospital stay, nurses provide education and assistance for the breastfeeding mother, making appropriate referrals to lactation consultants as needed. Nurses also provide information about community breastfeeding support groups (see Community Activity box and Chapter 25 for more information on assisting the breastfeeding woman).

🏠 COMMUNITY ACTIVITY

Breastfeeding Support

Women breastfeed longer if they feel supported in their breastfeeding efforts. Nurses and lactation consultants provide support during inpatient stays after birth. Women can find support in the community in various groups. Social support interventions that include peer support are successful in increasing the duration of exclusive breastfeeding and satisfaction with breastfeeding. In their discharge planning, nurses can refer breastfeeding mothers to community groups such as the La Leche League for support. Community and home health care nurses can facilitate breastfeeding efforts through organizing or facilitating support groups. Mothers experienced in breastfeeding can facilitate these efforts.

Identify sources of breastfeeding support in your community. Who offers the support? Is it through hospitals, nonprofit groups, health departments, or other sources? What resources are available to low-income mothers?

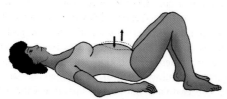

Abdominal Breathing. Lie on back with knees bent. Inhale deeply through nose. Keep ribs stationary and allow abdomen to expand upward. Exhale slowly but forcefully while contracting the abdominal muscles; hold for 3-5 s while exhaling. Relax.

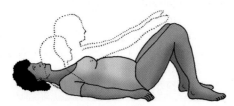

Reach for the Knees. Lie on back with knees bent. While inhaling, deeply lower chin onto chest. While exhaling, raise head and shoulders slowly and smoothly and reach for knees with arms outstretched. The body should rise only as far as the back will naturally bend while waist remains on floor or bed (about 6-8 inches). Slowly and smoothly lower head and shoulders back to starting position. Relax.

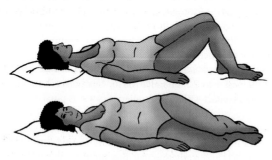

Double Knee Roll. Lie on back with knees bent. Keeping shoulders flat and feet stationary, slowly and smoothly roll knees over to the left to touch floor or bed. Maintaining a smooth motion, roll knees back over to the right until they touch floor or bed. Return to starting position and relax.

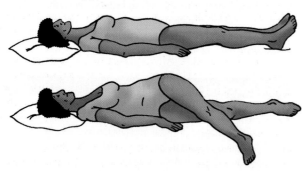

Leg Roll. Lie on back with legs straight. Keeping shoulders flat and legs straight, slowly and smoothly lift left leg and roll it over to touch the right side of floor or bed and return to starting position. Repeat, rolling right leg over to touch left side of floor or bed. Relax.

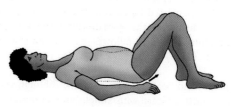

Combined Abdominal Breathing and Supine Pelvic Tilt (Pelvic Rock). Lie on back with knees bent. While inhaling deeply, roll pelvis back by flattening lower back on floor or bed. Exhale slowly but forcefully while contracting abdominal muscles and tightening buttocks. Hold for 3-5 s while exhaling. Relax.

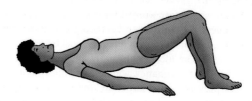

Buttocks Lift. Lie on back with arms at sides, knees bent, and feet flat. Slowly raise buttocks and arch back. Return slowly to starting position.

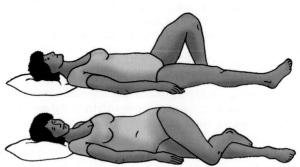

Single Knee Roll. Lie on back with right leg straight and left leg bent at the knee. Keeping shoulders flat, slowly and smoothly roll left knee over to the right to touch floor or bed and then back to starting position. Reverse position of legs. Roll right knee over to the left to touch floor or bed and return to starting position. Relax.

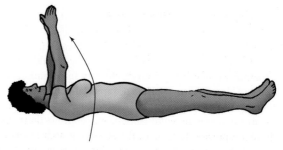

Arm Raises. Lie on back with arms extended at 90-degree angle from body. Raise arms so they are perpendicular and hands touch. Lower slowly.

Fig. 21.3 Postpartum Exercise Should Begin As Soon As Possible. The woman should start with simple exercises and gradually progress to more strenuous ones.

Lactation suppression. Lactation suppression is necessary when a woman has decided not to breastfeed or in the case of neonatal death. The woman wears a well-fitted support bra continuously for at least the first 72 hours after giving birth. She should avoid breast stimulation, including running warm water over the breasts, newborn suckling, or expressing milk. Some nonbreastfeeding mothers experience severe breast engorgement (swelling of breast tissue caused by increased blood and lymph supply to the breasts as the body produces milk, occurring about 72 to 96 hours after birth). Breast engorgement can usually be managed satisfactorily with nonpharmacologic interventions.

Periodic application of ice packs to the breasts can help to decrease the discomfort associated with engorgement. Although there is lack of scientific evidence to support effectiveness, cabbage leaves are often recommended to help relieve engorgement; formula-feeding mothers may be told to place fresh green cabbage leaves over their breasts and to replace the leaves when they are wilted (Fig. 25.17). A mild analgesic or antiinflammatory medication can reduce discomfort associated with engorgement. Medications that were once prescribed for lactation suppression (e.g., estrogen, estrogen and testosterone, and bromocriptine) are no longer used.

Health Promotion for Future Pregnancies

Rubella vaccination. For women who have not had rubella or who are serologically nonimmune (titer of 1:8 or less or enzyme immunoassay level <0.8), a subcutaneous injection of rubella vaccine is recommended in the postpartum period prior to hospital discharge to prevent the possibility of contracting rubella in future pregnancies; this is given as the measles, mumps, rubella (MMR) vaccine. Women are cautioned to avoid becoming pregnant for 28 days after receiving the rubella vaccine because of the potential teratogenic risk to the fetus. The live attenuated rubella virus is not communicable in breast milk; therefore breastfeeding mothers can be vaccinated. However, because the virus is shed in urine and other body fluids, the vaccine should not be given if the mother or other household members are immunocompromised. Fever, transient arthralgia, rash, and lymphadenopathy are common side effects of the rubella vaccine (Centers for Disease Control and Prevention [CDC], 2015a).

Varicella vaccination. The CDC recommends that varicella vaccine be administered before discharge in postpartum women who have no immunity. A second dose is given at the postpartum follow-up visit (4 to 8 weeks after the first dose) (CDC, 2015b).

LEGAL TIP: Rubella and Varicella Vaccination

Informed consent for rubella and varicella vaccination in the postpartum period includes information about possible side effects and the risk for teratogenic effects on the fetus. Women must understand that they should not become pregnant for 28 days after being vaccinated (CDC, 2015a,b).

Tetanus-diphtheria-acellular pertussis vaccine. Tetanus-diphtheria-acellular pertussis (Tdap) vaccine is recommended for postpartum women who have not previously received the vaccine; it is given before discharge from the hospital or as early as possible in the postpartum period to protect women from pertussis and to decrease the risk for infant exposure to pertussis. Women should be advised that other adults and children who will be around the newborn should be vaccinated with Tdap if they have not previously received the vaccine. This vaccination should occur at least 2 weeks before contact with the infant in order to allow time for immunity to be established. Women who receive the vaccine can continue to breastfeed (Liang, Tiwari, Moro, et al., 2018).

Preventing Rh isoimmunization. Injection of Rh immune globulin (a solution of γ globulin that contains Rh antibodies) within 72 hours after birth prevents sensitization in the Rh-negative woman who has had a fetomaternal transfusion of Rh-positive fetal red blood cells (RBCs) (see the Medication Guide). Rh immune globulin promotes lysis of fetal Rh-positive blood cells before the mother forms her own antibodies against them (Aitken & Tichy, 2015). Administration of Rh immune globulin is intended to prevent problems in future pregnancies should the Rh-negative woman have an Rh-positive fetus.

MEDICATION GUIDE

Rh Immune Globulin, RhoGAM, Gamulin Rh, HypRho-D, Rhophylac

Action
Suppression of immune response in nonsensitized women with Rh-negative blood who receive Rh-positive blood cells because of fetomaternal hemorrhage, transfusion, or accident

Indications
Routine antepartum prevention at 28 weeks of gestation in women with Rh-negative blood; suppress antibody formation after birth, miscarriage, pregnancy termination, abdominal trauma, ectopic pregnancy, amniocentesis, version, or chorionic villus sampling

Dosage and Route
Standard dose: 1 vial (300 mcg) IM in deltoid or gluteal muscle; microdose: 1 vial (50 mcg) IM in deltoid muscle; Rh_o(D) immune globulin (Rhophylac) can be given IM or IV (available in prefilled syringes).

Adverse Effects
Myalgia, lethargy, localized tenderness and stiffness at injection site, mild and transient fever, malaise, headache; rarely nausea, vomiting, hypotension, tachycardia, possible allergic response

Nursing Considerations
- Give standard dose to mother at 28 weeks of gestation as prophylaxis or after an incident or exposure risk that occurs after 28 weeks of gestation (e.g., amniocentesis, second-trimester miscarriage or abortion, and after external version).
- Give standard dose within 72 h after birth if neonate is Rh-positive.
- Give microdose for first-trimester miscarriage or abortion, ectopic pregnancy, chorionic villus sampling.
- Verify that the woman is Rh-negative and has not been sensitized, if postpartum that Coombs test is negative, and that baby is Rh-positive. Provide explanation to the woman about the procedure, including the purpose, possible side effects, and effect on future pregnancies. Have the woman sign a consent form if required by agency. Verify correct dosage and confirm lot number and woman's identity before giving injection (verify with another registered nurse or by other procedure per agency policy); document administration per agency policy. Observe client for at least 20 min after administration for allergic response.
- Document lot number and expiration date in the client record.
- The medication is made from human plasma (a consideration if woman is a Jehovah Witness). The risk for transmitting infectious agents, including viruses, cannot be eliminated completely.

IM, Intramuscular; *IV,* intravenous.
Data from Aitken, S. L., & Tichy, E. M. (2015). Rh(O)D immune globulin products for prevention of alloimmunization during pregnancy. *American Journal of Health-System Pharmacists, 72*(4), 267–276; Kedron Biopharma Inc. (2018). *Rho(D) immune globulin (human).* Melville, NY: Biopharma Inc. Retrieved from http://www.rhogam.com/hcp/hcp-home/.

A dose of 300 mcg (1 vial) of Rh immune globulin is usually sufficient to prevent maternal sensitization. However, if a large fetomaternal transfusion is suspected, the dosage needed should be determined by performing a Kleihauer-Betke test, which detects the amount of fetal blood in the maternal circulation. If more than 30 mL of fetal blood is present in the maternal circulation, the dosage of Rh immune globulin must be increased (AAP & ACOG, 2017).

There is some disagreement about whether Rh immune globulin should be considered a blood product. Health care providers need to discuss the most current information about this issue with women whose religious beliefs conflict with having blood products administered to them (e.g., Jehovah Witnesses).

⚡ SAFETY ALERT

Rh immune globulin suppresses the immune response. Therefore the woman who receives both Rh immune globulin and a live virus immunization such as rubella must be tested in 3 months to see if she has developed rubella immunity. If not, she will need another dose of the vaccine.

CARE MANAGEMENT: PSYCHOSOCIAL NEEDS

Meeting the psychosocial needs of new parents involves assessing their reactions to the birth experience, feelings about themselves, and interactions with the new baby (Fig. 21.4) and other family members. Specific interventions are planned to increase the parents' knowledge and self-confidence as they assume the care and responsibility of the new baby and integrate this new member into their existing family structure in a way that meets their cultural expectations (see Chapters 22 and 24).

Careful assessment of the woman's current psychological and emotional status is foundational to planning effective care. Through review of the woman's medical record and through interactions with the woman and her family, the nurse may identify risk factors for psychosocial problems. For example, a history of preconception or prenatal depression increases the risk for PPD (see Chapter 31). Social concerns such as lack of financial resources may also be identified. Observations of interactions between the woman and her partner may suggest the possibility of intimate partner violence (see Chapter 5).

Taking time to assess maternal emotional needs and to address concerns before discharge can promote better psychologic health and adjustment to parenting. Ongoing support for postpartum women is needed. Even though issues such as fatigue are often evident during the hospital stay, they are likely to worsen after discharge, making support for the woman an even greater need as she is providing care for the newborn, herself, and other family members. Postpartum support is especially beneficial to at-risk populations such as low-income primiparas, those at risk for family dysfunction and child abuse, and those at risk for PPD. Home visitation programs for postpartum women and their families promote better outcomes.

Sometimes the psychosocial assessment indicates serious actual or potential problems that must be addressed. Box 21.2 identifies psychosocial characteristics and behaviors that warrant ongoing evaluation after hospital discharge. The nurse should notify the obstetric health care provider if signs of actual or potential problems are present. Further assessment and care management are best accomplished through interprofessional care that may include the obstetrician or nurse midwife, nursing staff, a psychiatrist or psychiatric nurse practitioner, and social worker.

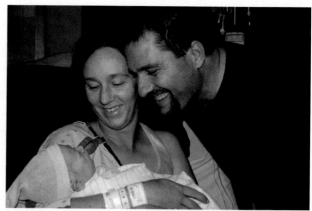

Fig. 21.4 Parents Getting Acquainted With Their New Son. (Courtesy Julie and Darren Nelson, Loveland, CO.)

BOX 21.2 Signs of Potential Complications: Postpartum Psychosocial Concerns

The following signs suggest potentially serious complications and should be reported to the health care provider or clinic (these may be noticed by the partner or other family members):

- Unable or unwilling to discuss labor and birth experience
- Refers to self as ugly and useless
- Excessively preoccupied with self (body image)
- Markedly depressed
- Lacks a support system
- Partner or other family members react negatively to the baby
- Refuses to interact with or care for baby; for example, does not name baby, does not want to hold or feed baby, is upset by vomiting and wet or soiled diapers (cultural appropriateness of actions must be considered)
- Expresses disappointment over baby's sex
- Sees baby as messy or unattractive
- Baby reminds mother of family member or friend she does not like
- Has difficulty sleeping
- Experiences loss of appetite

Nurses need to be knowledgeable about perinatal mood disorders, especially PPD, and should provide information to the woman and her family about signs of PPD, differences between postpartum blues and depressive symptoms, and the need to report symptoms promptly to the health care provider. In some facilities routine screening for PPD is done prior to discharge using a tool such as the Edinburgh Postnatal Depression Scale (see Chapter 31). Screening for PPD should also be done after discharge (see Chapter 31). The AAP recommends that pediatric care providers routinely perform maternal screening for PPD during infant follow-up visits at 1, 2, and 4 months (American Academy of Pediatrics, 2010) (see Clinical Reasoning Case Study).

Effect of the Birth Experience

Many women need to review and reflect on their labor and birth experience. Their partners may have similar needs. If their birth experience was different from their birth plan (e.g., induction, epidural anesthesia, cesarean birth), both partners may need to mourn the loss of their expectations before they can adjust to the reality of their actual birth experience. Inviting them to review the events and describe how they feel helps the nurse to assess how well they understand what happened and how well they have been able to put their birth experience into perspective.

Adaptation to Parenthood and Parent-Infant Interactions

The psychosocial assessment includes assessment of adaptation to parenthood as evidenced by the parents' reactions to and interactions with the new baby. Clues indicating successful adaptation begin to appear early in the postbirth period as parents react positively to the newborn infant and continue the process of establishing a relationship with their child.

Parents are adapting well to their new roles when they exhibit a realistic perception and acceptance of their newborn's needs and limited abilities, immature social responses, and helplessness. Examples of positive parent-infant interactions include taking pleasure in the infant and in providing care, responding appropriately to infant cues, and providing comfort. If these indicators are missing, the nurse needs to investigate further in an attempt to identify what is hindering the normal adaptation process (see Chapter 22).

? CLINICAL REASONING CASE STUDY

Potential for Postpartum Depression

Elisabeth, a 38-year-old multipara, has just given birth to her fourth baby. The ages of her other children are 8, 4, and 2. During the morning nursing assessment, Elisabeth was noted to be tearful and stated that she was feeling "overwhelmed" and "very unsure" of herself and how to take care of the new baby, although she has three previous children. She shared that her mother was diagnosed with cancer 2 months ago and is undergoing treatment. Her husband will be starting a much-needed new job next week and will not be able to get any time off for a while. Other family members do not live close by except for her sister, who is out of town often due to her job responsibilities. Elisabeth is concerned about how she will manage taking care of her newborn and three other children with a seemingly depleted support system.

1. What is the priority concern or client need in this situation? Support your answer with data as stated in the case.
2. List other client needs/problems in this case.
3. Identify any additional information or assessment data that is needed by the nurse in planning care for this client.
4. What nursing actions are appropriate in this situation?
   a. What is the priority nursing action?
   b. Describe other nursing interventions that are important to providing optimal client care.
5. Describe roles/responsibilities of the interprofessional health care team members (other than nurses) who may be involved in providing care for this client.

Family Structure and Functioning

A woman's adjustment to her role as mother is affected greatly by her relationships with her partner, her mother and other relatives, and any other children (Fig. 21.5). Nurses can help to ease the new mother's return home by identifying possible conflicts among family members and by helping the woman plan strategies for dealing with these problems before discharge. Such a conflict can arise when couples have very different ideas about parenting. Dealing with the stresses of sibling rivalry and unsolicited grandparent advice also can affect the woman's transition to motherhood. Only by asking about other nuclear and extended family members can the nurse discover potential problems in such relationships and help plan workable solutions for them.

Effect of Cultural Beliefs and Practices

The final component of a complete psychosocial assessment is the woman's cultural beliefs, values, and practices. Cultural beliefs and traditions strongly influence the behaviors of the woman and her family during the postpartum period. Nurses are likely to come into contact with women from many different countries and cultures. All cultures have developed safe and satisfying methods of caring for new mothers and babies. The nurse can identify some cultural beliefs and practices through observation and interaction with the mother and her family. Only by understanding and respecting the values and beliefs of each woman can the nurse design a plan of care to meet the individual's needs.

To identify cultural beliefs and practices when planning and implementing care, the nurse conducts a cultural assessment. This can be accomplished most easily through conversation with the woman and her partner. Some hospitals have assessment tools designed to identify cultural beliefs and practices that can influence care. Components of the cultural assessment include the ability to read and write English, primary language spoken, family involvement and support, dietary preferences, infant care, attachment, religious or cultural beliefs, folk medicine practices, nonverbal communication, and personal space preferences.

Postpartum care occurs within a sociocultural context. Rest, seclusion, dietary constraints, and ceremonies honoring the mother are common traditional practices that are followed for the promotion of the health and well-being of the mother and baby. In some cultures, the postpartum period is considered a time of increased vulnerability for the mother. To protect her, there are restrictions on activity, diet, bathing, and infant caretaking. The postpartum period is seen by some cultures as a time of impurity for the mother. For as many days or weeks as she has lochial flow, she is considered "impure" and has limited contact with others. Sexual activity is prohibited during this time (see Cultural Considerations box).

The nurse should not assume that a mother desires to use traditional health practices that represent a particular cultural group merely because she is a member of that culture. Many young women who are first- or second-generation Americans follow their cultural traditions only when older family members are present or not at all.

It is important that nurses consider all cultural aspects when planning care and not use their own cultural beliefs as the framework for that care. Although the beliefs and behaviors of other cultures can seem different or strange, they should be encouraged as long as the mother wants to conform to them and she and the baby have no ill effects.

⚡ SAFETY ALERT

The nurse needs to determine whether a woman is using any complementary or alternative therapies (i.e., "folk medicine") during the postpartum period because active ingredients in some herbal preparations can have adverse physiologic effects when used in combination with prescribed medicines.

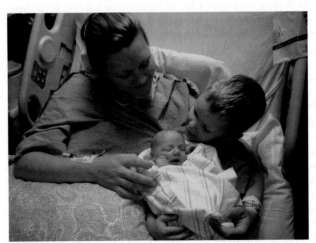

Fig. 21.5 Older Sibling Cuddles With Mother and New Baby. (Courtesy Jennifer Hobgood, Creedmoor, NC.)

⊕ CULTURAL CONSIDERATIONS

Examples of Cultural Beliefs and Practices in the Postpartum Period

Asian Culture

The practice of "doing the month" is common in many Asian cultures. The mother is confined to home while she and the newborn are cared for by family members. The balance between yin and yang (cold and hot) is necessary for balance and harmony with the environment. Postpartum practices focus on helping the mother achieve this balance. Pregnancy is considered a "hot" condition. It is believed that birth depletes the mother's body of heat through loss of blood and inner energy; this places her in a "cold" state for approximately 40 days until her womb is healed. The woman consumes only "hot" foods and beverages; for example, rice, eggs, beef, and chicken soup. Seaweed soup is thought to increase milk production and help to rid the body of lochia. Family members often bring in foods from home. To help prevent the loss of heat from the body, the mother does not bathe or shower for several days or weeks; however, there is attention to perineal care and hygiene. The temperature of the hospital room is warmer than usual. The mother likely spends most of the time in bed to prevent cold air from entering the body, and she has minimal contact with the infant.

Hispanic and Latino Culture

Many Hispanic and Latino women often observe the period of 40 days (6 weeks) after birth as *la cuarentena*. During this period of confinement, the woman's body is perceived to be "open" and vulnerable to drafts; la cuarentena is about "closing the body." Traditional practices associated with la cuarentena include a liquid diet of nutritious drinks, soups, and broths in the early postpartum period; avoiding spicy and heavy foods; binding the abdomen with a cloth known as a *faja*; avoiding cool air; covering her head and neck with garments; not washing hair; and maintaining sexual abstinence. Activity is restricted, and the mother stays at home where she and the infant are cared for by family members.

Data from Callister, L. C. (2014). Integrating cultural beliefs and practices when caring for childbearing women and families. In K. R. Simpson, & P. A. Creehan (Eds.), *Perinatal nursing* (4th ed.). Philadelphia: Lippincott Williams & Wilkins; Fok, D., Aris, I. M., & Ho, J. (2016). A comparison of practices during the confinement period among Chinese, Malay, and Indian mothers in Singapore. *Birth, 43*(3), 247–254; Waugh, L. J. (2011). Beliefs associated with Mexican immigrant families' practice of la cuarentena during postpartum recovery. *Journal of Obstetric, Gynecologic and Neonatal Nursing, 40*(6), 732–741.

DISCHARGE TEACHING

Self-Care and Signs of Complications

Discharge planning begins at the time of admission to the unit and should be reflected in the nursing care plan developed for each woman. For example, a great deal of time during the hospital stay is usually spent in teaching about maternal self-management and care of the newborn because the goal is for all women to be capable of providing basic care for themselves and their infants at the time of discharge. In addition, every woman must be taught to recognize physical and psychological signs and symptoms that might indicate problems and how to obtain advice and assistance quickly if these signs appear. Table 21.1 and Box 21.2 list several common indications of maternal physical and psychosocial problems in the postpartum period (see Chapter 33 for more information on postpartum complications). Before discharge, women need basic instruction regarding a variety of self-management topics such as nutrition, exercise, family planning, the resumption of sexual intercourse, medications, and routine mother-baby follow-up care.

Because of the limited time available for teaching, nurses must target their teaching on expressed needs of the woman. Giving the woman a list of topics and asking her to indicate her learning needs help the nurse to maximize teaching efforts and can increase retention of information. Providing written materials on postpartum self-management, breastfeeding, and infant care that the woman can consult after discharge is helpful. Nurses can direct women to online resources; some hospitals and birth centers provide information for new parents on their websites.

Just before the time of discharge, the nurse reviews the woman's records to see that laboratory reports, medications, signatures, and other items are in order. Some facilities have a checklist to use before the woman's discharge. The nurse verifies that medications, if ordered, have arrived on the unit; that any valuables kept secured during the woman's stay have been returned to her and that she has signed a receipt for them; and that the infant is ready to be discharged. The woman's and the baby's identification bands are checked carefully.

In many birthing facilities, new mothers (breastfeeding and formula feeding) are routinely presented with gift bags that contain samples of infant formula. This practice is not consistent with the Baby-Friendly (BF) Hospital Initiative and is contrary to the International Code of Marketing of Breast-Milk Substitutes (World Health Organization, 2017). Prepackaged formula should not be given to mothers who are breastfeeding. Such "gifts" are associated with earlier cessation of breastfeeding.

⚡ SAFETY ALERT

No medication that can cause drowsiness should be administered to the mother before discharge if she is the one who will be holding the baby when they leave the hospital. In most instances, the woman is seated in a wheelchair and given the baby to hold. Some families leave unescorted and ambulatory, depending on hospital protocol. The newborn must be secured in a car seat for the drive home.

Sexual Activity and Contraception

Discussing sexual activity with women and their partners before they leave the hospital is important because many couples resume sexual activity before the postpartum follow-up visit with the health care provider after birth. For most women, the risk for hemorrhage or infection is minimal by approximately 2 weeks postpartum. Couples may be anxious about the topic but uncomfortable and unwilling to bring it up. The nurse needs to discuss the physical and psychological effects that giving birth can have on sexual activity (see Teaching for Self-Management box: Resuming Sexual Activity After Birth).

Many factors can influence the timing and quality of sexual activity after birth. Postpartum perineal pain and dyspareunia (painful intercourse) are common among women with perineal lacerations or episiotomy; the discomfort may last for weeks or months. Discomfort is more severe and lasts longer with third- and fourth-degree lacerations (see Evidence-Based Practice box: Perineal Trauma and Postpartum Sexual Function.

Breastfeeding mothers often experience vaginal dryness related to high prolactin levels and low estrogen levels. Changes in family structure and altered sleep patterns can make it difficult for a couple to find time for privacy and intimacy. PPD is associated with decreased sexual desire; medication used to treat PPD can reduce sexual desire and inhibit orgasm.

TEACHING FOR SELF-MANAGEMENT

Resuming Sexual Activity After Birth

- Unless your health care provider indicates otherwise, you can safely resume sexual activity (intercourse) by the second to fourth week after birth, when bleeding has stopped and the perineum is healed. Most women resume sexual activity by 5 to 6 weeks after birth, although this varies and is often related to perineal discomfort. Perineal lacerations or episiotomy increase the chances of discomfort with intercourse. For the first 6 weeks to 6 months, vaginal lubrication might be decreased, especially among breast-feeding women. Your physiologic reactions to sexual stimulation for the first 3 months after birth may be slower and less intense. The strength of the orgasm may be reduced.

- A water-soluble gel or contraceptive cream or jelly might be recommended for lubrication. If some vaginal tenderness is present, your partner can be instructed to insert one or more clean, lubricated fingers into the vagina and rotate them to help the vagina relax and identify possible areas of discomfort. A position in which you have control of the depth of the insertion of the penis also is useful. The side-by-side or female-on-top position may be most comfortable.

- The presence of the baby influences sexual activity and enjoyment. Parents hear every sound made by the baby; conversely you may be concerned that the baby hears every sound you make. In either case, any phase of the sexual response cycle can be interrupted by hearing the baby cry or move, leaving both of you frustrated and unsatisfied. In addition, the amount of psychologic energy expended by you in child-care activities can lead to fatigue. Newborns require a great deal of attention and time.

- Some women have reported feeling sexual stimulation and orgasms when breastfeeding their babies. This is not abnormal. Breastfeeding mothers often are interested in returning to sexual activity before nonbreastfeeding mothers.

- You should be instructed to perform the Kegel exercises correctly to strengthen your pubococcygeal muscle. This muscle is associated with bowel and bladder function and vaginal feeling during intercourse.

Contraceptive options should also be discussed with women (and their partners, if present) before discharge so that they can make informed decisions about fertility management before resuming sexual activity. Waiting to discuss contraception at the 6-week follow-up visit can be too late. Ovulation can occur as soon as 1 month after birth, particularly in women who formula-feed their infants. Breastfeeding mothers should be informed that breastfeeding is not a reliable means of contraception and that other methods should be used; nonhormonal methods are best because oral contraceptives can interfere with milk production. Women who are undecided about contraception at the time of discharge need information about using condoms with spermicidal foam or creams until the first postpartum checkup. Contraceptive options are discussed in detail in Chapter 8.

Medications

Women routinely continue to take their prenatal vitamins during the postpartum period. Breastfeeding mothers may continue prenatal vitamins for the duration of breastfeeding. Supplemental iron may be prescribed for mothers with lower than normal hemoglobin levels. Women with perineal lacerations or episiotomies are usually prescribed stool softeners to take at home. Pain medications (opioid and nonopioid) may be prescribed, especially for women who had cesarean births. The nurse should make certain that the woman knows the route, dosage, frequency, and common side effects of all medications that she will be taking at home. Written information about the medications is usually included in the discharge instructions.

Follow-Up After Discharge

Routine Schedule of Care

There has been a recent paradigm shift in recommendations for postpartum care in the United States. The traditional postpartum follow-up visit to the obstetric care provider at 6 weeks after birth is no longer the standard of practice. ACOG (2018) recommends that postpartum care should not be a one-time encounter, but instead, an ongoing process in which each woman's individual needs determine the services and support she receives.

Within the first 3 weeks after birth, all women should have contact with their obstetric care provider. At this time, an initial assessment is done to identify any current problems or concerns (e.g., pain, excessive fatigue, breastfeeding problems, signs of postpartum depression). This may be as a follow-up visit to the provider's office or clinic, or as a telephone call. Early follow-up is warranted for women who experienced complications such as hypertensive disorders of pregnancy, those with chronic health conditions, women at high risk for depression, and breastfeeding mothers who are experiencing feeding problems (ACOG, 2018).

Follow-up to the initial contact should occur no later than 12 weeks postpartum in the form of a comprehensive well-woman evaluation by the obstetric health care provider. The comprehensive evaluation should address physical, social, and psychological aspects of the woman's health. Specific assessment topics include physical recovery from birth, sleep and fatigue, mood and emotional well-being, infant feeding and care, sexuality, birth spacing, and contraception. Women with chronic diseases such as hypertension and diabetes should be counseled about the importance of ongoing follow-up care. Health maintenance includes review and update of vaccinations. Well-woman screening (Pap test, pelvic examination) is also performed. Recommended follow-up care is documented in the medical record, communicated to the woman, and to appropriate health team members, including her primary care provider (ACOG, 2018).

Early initial follow-up is warranted for women who experienced complications such as hypertensive disorders of pregnancy, those with chronic health conditions, women at high risk for depression, and breastfeeding mothers who are experiencing lactation problems (ACOG, 2018). The nurse should explain the importance of follow-up care. The date and time for the follow-up appointment should be included in the discharge instructions. If an appointment has not been made before the woman leaves the hospital, she should be encouraged to call the health care provider's office or clinic to schedule one.

As many as 40% of new mothers forego the postpartum visit (ACOG, 2018). There are a variety of reasons for this, including thinking that they are feeling fine and do not need to follow-up, believing that their maternity care was already completed, difficulty getting to an appointment, and lack of insurance (Declercq et al., 2014). In an effort to increase compliance with postpartum visits, discussions related to discharge planning should begin during pregnancy with providers and nurses emphasizing the importance of follow-up care (ACOG). A postpartum plan of care can be developed during pregnancy in collaboration with the woman and her partner, considering the mother's physical and mental health, individual and family needs and desires, support system, and available resources. The plan of care should be reviewed after birth, prior to hospital discharge, and revised as needed at the postpartum follow-up visit. An interprofessional team for postpartum care may include the obstetric and pediatric health care providers, lactation consultants, home visitation nurses or peer counselors, public health nurses, nutritionists,

EVIDENCE-BASED PRACTICE
Perineal Trauma and Postpartum Sexual Function

Ask the Question

Which perinatal interventions for perineal trauma minimize pain and prevent sexual dysfunction?

Search for the Evidence

Search Strategies: English language research-based publications on perineal trauma, birth, postpartum, and sexual function were included.

Databases Used: Cochrane Collaborative Database, National Guideline Clearinghouse (AHRQ), CINAHL, PubMed, and UpToDate

Critical Appraisal of the Evidence

- Sexual dysfunction affects approximately 40% of women (Yeniel & Petri, 2014). One major cause is dyspareunia (painful intercourse) after perineal trauma, especially third- and fourth-degree lacerations requiring repair. Other causes may include decreased libido and lower estrogen levels resulting from breastfeeding, postpartum depression, and fatigue (Leeman, Rogers, Borders, et al., 2016; Yeniel & Petri). Studies have estimated that 0.6% to 0.9% of women will experience severe trauma to the perineum during birth (Van Limbeek, Davis, Currie, et al., 2016).
- Women who experience second-degree lacerations during birth are not at increased risk for dysfunction of the pelvic floor other than increased pain, and slightly decreased sexual function scores at 6 months postpartum (Leeman et al., 2016).
- Routine episiotomy during birth is not recommended (Van Limbeek et al., 2016).
- Warm compresses and perineal massage during first- and second-stage labor significantly decrease third- and fourth-degree tears (Aasheim, Nilsen, Reinar, & Lukasse, et al., 2017).
- Evidence is still mixed for whether to suture or not suture first- and second-degree lacerations. Nonsuturing or the use of skin adhesives are associated with less pain (Seijmonsbergen-Schermers, Sahami, Lucas, et al., 2015).

Apply the Evidence: Nursing Implications

Women may be embarrassed to discuss sexual function with their partners and/or with health care professionals. Nurses are ideally placed to initiate and keep the dialog going throughout childbearing. The following guidelines are recommended for assessing and preventing postpartum sexual dysfunction:

- Discussion of anatomy, physiology, and sexual function should begin in early pregnancy and continue throughout the postpartum period, including a brief, valid, and reliable sexual function survey (Khajehei & Doherty, 2018).
- Antenatal perineal massage should be taught to minimize perineal damage (Ugwu, Iferikigwe, Obi, et al., 2018; Vieira, Guimarães, Souza, et al., 2018).
- Vacuum- or forceps-assisted birth and episiotomy should be avoided when possible. Careful repair of anal sphincter lacerations should be performed using synthetic, absorbable sutures. (Van Limbeek et al., 2016).
- Before hospital discharge discussions should be initiated with women and their partners regarding pain, dyspareunia, resumption of intercourse, and contraception. Women should know the hypoestrogenic and sensitivity changes that they can experience as a result of breastfeeding and the need for additional vaginal lubrication (Khajehei & Doherty, 2018).
- Postpartum follow-up visits should include assessment of urine, bowel, and sexual function; inspection of the perineum; and discussion of mood and intimacy challenges such as fatigue and timing issues (Alligood-Percoco, Kjerulf, & Repke, 2016; Seehusen, Baird, & Bode, 2014).

References

Aasheim, V., Nilsen, A. B., Reinar, L., & Lukasse, M. (2017). Perineal techniques during the second stage of labour for reducing perineal trauma. *The Cochrane Database of Systematic Reviews, 6,* CD006672.

Alligood-Percoco, N. R., Kjerulff, K. H., & Repke, J. T. (2016). Risk factors for dyspareunia after first childbirth. *Obstetrics & Gynecology, 128*(3), 512–518.

Khajehei, M., & Doherty, M. (2018). Women's experience of their sexual function during pregnancy and after childbirth: A qualitative study. *British Journal of Midwifery, 26*(5), 318–328.

Leeman, L., Rogers, R., Borders, N., et al. (2016). The effect of perineal lacerations on pelvic floor function and anatomy at 6 months postpartum in a prospective cohort of nulliparous women. *Birth: Issues in Perinatal Care, 43*(4), 293–302.

Seehusen, D. A., Baird, D. C., & Bode, D. V. (2014). Dyspareunia in women. *American Family Physician, 90*(7), 465–470.

Seijmonsbergen-Schermers, A. E., Sahami, S., Lucas, C., & Jonge, Ad. (2015). Nonsuturing or skin adhesives versus suturing of the perineal skin after childbirth: A systematic review. *Birth: Issues in Perinatal Care, 42*(2), 100–115.

Ugwu, E. O., Iferikigwe, E. S., Obi, S. N., et al. (2018). Effectiveness of antenatal perineal massage in reducing perineal trauma and postpartum morbidities: A randomized controlled trial. *Journal of Obstetrical and Gynaecological Research, 44*(7), 1252–1258.

Van Limbeek, S., Davis, D., Currie, M., & Wong, N. (2016). Non-surgical intrapartum practices for the prevention of severe perineal trauma: A systematic review protocol. *Joanna Briggs Database of Systematic Reviews and Implementation Reports, 14*(4), 30–40.

Vieira, F., Guimarães, J. V., Souza, M. C., et al. (2018). Scientific evidence on perineal trauma during labor: An integrative review. *European Journal of Obstetrics and Gynecology and Reproductive Biology, 223,* 18–25.

Yeniel, A. O., & Petri, E. (2014). Pregnancy, childbirth, and sexual function: Perceptions and facts. *International Urogynecology Journal, 25*(1), 5–14.

Jennifer Taylor Alderman

---

mental health care providers, and other specialists based on the specific needs of the mother and infant.

Prior to discharge from the birthing facility, the nurse emphasizes the need for follow-up care for the newborn. Breastfeeding infants are routinely seen by the pediatric health care provider or clinic within 3 to 5 days after birth or 48 to 72 hours after hospital discharge and again at approximately 2 weeks of age (AAP Section on Breastfeeding, 2012). Early follow-up is important for breastfed infants to assess feeding adequacy and weight loss. Formula-feeding infants may be seen for the first time at 2 weeks of age. If an appointment was not scheduled for the infant's follow-up visit before leaving the hospital, the parents should be encouraged to call the office or clinic soon after their arrival home. This visit is essential for evaluating the status of the infant and provides an opportunity for assessing the mother for PPD, even before she returns to her obstetric health care provider.

Home Visits

Home visits to mothers and babies within a few days of discharge can help to bridge the gap between hospital care and routine visits to health care providers. In the United States, home visitation programs often target special populations such as low-income, first-time mothers; women who were discharged early from the birthing facility; women with special needs related to complications during pregnancy or birth; victims of intimate partner violence; or families with preterm infants. Nurses can assess the mother, infant, family, and home environment; answer questions and provide education and emotional support; and make referrals to community resources if necessary. The support provided by nurses and other trained community health care workers such as peer counselors can enhance parent-infant interaction and parenting skills; home visits also help to promote mutual support between the mother and her partner. Breastfeeding outcomes can be enhanced through home visitation programs.

Home nursing care may not be available, even if needed, because no agencies are available to provide the service or no coverage is in place for payment by third-party payers. If care is available, a referral form containing information about the mother and baby should be completed at discharge from the birthing facility and sent immediately to the home care agency.

The home visit is most commonly scheduled on the woman's second day home from the hospital, but it can be scheduled on any of the first 4 days at home, depending on the individual family's situation and needs. Additional visits are planned throughout the first week, as needed. The home visits may be extended beyond that time if the family's needs warrant it and if a home visit is the most appropriate option for carrying out the follow-up care required to meet the specific needs identified.

During the home visit, the nurse conducts a systematic assessment of mother and newborn to determine physiologic adjustment and identify any existing complications. The assessment also focuses on the mother's emotional adjustment and her knowledge of self-management and infant care. Conducting the assessment in a private area of the home provides an opportunity for the mother to ask questions on potentially sensitive topics such as breast care, constipation, sexual activity, or family planning. The nurse assesses family adjustment to the newborn and addresses any concerns during the home visit. See Chapter 2 for more information on home visits.

During the newborn assessment, the nurse can demonstrate and explain normal newborn behavior and capabilities and encourage the mother and family to ask questions or express concerns they have. The home care nurse verifies if the blood sample for newborn screening has been drawn (see Chapter 24). If the baby was discharged from the hospital before 24 hours of age, a blood sample for the newborn screen may be drawn by the home care nurse, or the family will need to take the infant to the health care provider's office or clinic to have the blood sample drawn.

Telephone Follow-Up

In addition to or instead of a home visit, postpartum telephone follow-up calls are sometimes used for assessment, health teaching, and identification of complications to facilitate timely intervention and referrals. Telephone follow-up may be offered by hospitals, private physicians, clinics, or private agencies. It may be either a separate service or combined with other strategies for extending postpartum care. Telephone nursing assessments are frequently used as follow-up to postpartum home visits to reassess a woman's knowledge about the signs and symptoms of adequate intake by the breastfeeding infant or, after initiating home phototherapy, to assess the caregiver's knowledge regarding equipment complications. There is evidence that phone support for new mothers during the postpartum period is beneficial; it can contribute to improved breastfeeding outcomes, reduced depression scores, and increased client satisfaction (Miller, Dane, Thompson, 2014).

Warm Lines

The warm line is another type of telephone link between the new family and concerned caregivers or experienced parent volunteers. A warm line is a help line or consultation service, not a crisis intervention line. The warm line is appropriately used for dealing with less extreme concerns that seem urgent at the time the call is placed but are not actual emergencies. Calls to warm lines commonly relate to infant feeding, prolonged crying, or sibling rivalry. Families are encouraged to call when concerns arise. Telephone numbers for warm lines should be given to parents before hospital discharge.

Support Groups

The woman adjusting to motherhood may desire interaction and conversation with other women who are having similar experiences. Postpartum women who have met earlier in prenatal clinics or on the hospital unit can begin to associate for mutual support. Members of childbirth classes who attend a postpartum reunion may decide to extend their relationship during the fourth trimester. Fathers or partners also benefit from participation in support groups.

A postpartum support group enables mothers and partners/fathers to share experiences and concerns and support one another as they adjust to parenting. Many new parents find it reassuring to discover that they are not alone in their feelings of confusion and uncertainty. An experienced parent can often impart concrete information that is valuable to other group members. Inexperienced parents can imitate the behavior of others in the group whom they perceive as particularly capable. There are local support groups for a variety of postpartum topics and concerns. For example, women can find breastfeeding support through local meetings of La Leche League (http://www.llli.org/webus.html).

Internet technology can help women to connect with support groups. Women can find support through groups on social media. They can participate in virtual meetings while in the comfort of their own homes, and they can participate in forums on specific topics. One example of an online support group is through Postpartum Support International. This organization provides weekly online support group meetings for women with PPD and other mental health issues (http://www.postpartum.net/psi-online-support-meetings/).

Referral to Community Resources

To develop an effective referral system, the nurse should have an understanding of the needs of the woman and family and of the organization and community resources available for meeting those needs. Locating and compiling information about available community services contributes to the development of a referral system. The nurse also needs to develop his or her own resource file of local and national services that are frequently useful to postpartum families. This list should be updated regularly as services and/or providers change frequently.

▌ KEY POINTS

- Postpartum care is family centered and modeled on the concept of health.
- Cultural beliefs and practices affect the maternal and family response to the postpartum period.
- The nursing care plan includes assessments to detect variations from normal, comfort measures to relieve discomfort or pain, and safety measures to prevent injury or infection.
- Common nursing interventions in the postpartum period focus on preventing excessive bleeding, bladder distention, and infection; providing nonpharmacologic and pharmacologic relief of discomfort associated with the episiotomy, lacerations, or breastfeeding; and instituting measures to promote or suppress lactation.
- Teaching and counseling measures are designed to promote the woman's feelings of competence in self-management and infant care.
- Meeting the psychosocial needs of new mothers involves taking into consideration the composition and functioning of the entire family.
- Early discharge classes, telephone follow-up, home visits, warm lines, and support groups are effective means of facilitating physiologic and psychologic adjustments in the postpartum period.

REFERENCES

Aitken, S. L., & Tichy, E. M. (2015). RhO (D) immune globulin products for prevention of alloimmunization during pregnancy. *American Journal of Health-System Pharmacy, 72*(4), 267–276.

American Academy of Pediatrics. (2010). Incorporating recognition and management of perinatal and postpartum depression into pediatric practice. *Pediatrics, 126*(5), 1032–1039.

American Academy of Pediatrics. (2015). Hospital stay for healthy term newborn infants. *Pediatrics, 135*(5), 948–953.

American Academy of Pediatrics & American College of Obstetricians and Gynecologists. (2017). *Guidelines for perinatal care* (8th ed.). Washington, DC: Author.

American Academy of Pediatrics Section on Breastfeeding. (2012). Breastfeeding and the use of human milk. *Pediatrics, 129*(3), e827–e841.

American College of Obstetricians and Gynecologists. (2018). Optimizing postpartum care. *Obstetrics and Gynecology, 131*(5), e140–e150.

Association of Women's Health, Obstetric and Neonatal Nurses. (2010). *Guidelines for professional registered nurse staffing for perinatal units.* Washington, DC: Author.

Bhati, S., & Richards, K. (2015). A systematic review of the relationship between postpartum sleep disturbance and postpartum depression. *Journal of Obstetric, Gynecologic and Neonatal Nursing, 44*(3), 350–357.

Centers for Disease Control and Prevention. (2015a). Rubella. In J. Hamborsky, A. Kroger, & S. Wolfe (Eds.), *Epidemiology and prevention of vaccine-preventable diseases* (13th ed.). Washington, DC: Public Health Foundation.

Centers for Disease Control and Prevention. (2015b). Varicella. In J. Hamborsky, A. Kroger, & S. Wolfe (Eds.), *Epidemiology and prevention of vaccine-preventable diseases* (13th ed.). Washington, DC: Public Health Foundation.

Declercq, R., Sakala, C., Corry, M. P., et al. (2014). Major survey findings of Listening to Mothers III: New mothers speak out. *Journal of Perinatal Education, 23*(1), 17–24.

Doering, J. J., Sims, D. A., & Miller, D. D. (2017). How postpartum women with depressive symptoms manage sleep disruption and fatigue. *Research in Nursing and Health, 40*(2), 132–142.

Gaffey, A. D. (2015). Fall prevention in our healthiest patients: Assessing risk and preventing injury for moms and babies. *Journal of Healthcare Risk Management, 34*(3), 37–40.

Groves, P. S., Manges, K. A., & Scott-Cawiezell, J. (2016). Handing off safety at the bedside. *Clinical Nursing Research, 25*(5), 473–493.

Isley, M. M., & Katz, V. L. (2017). Postpartum care and long-term health considerations. In S. G. Gabbe, J. R. Niebyl, J. L. Simpson, et al. (Eds.), *Obstetrics: Normal and problem pregnancies* (7th ed.). Philadelphia: Elsevier.

Krawczak, E. M., Minuzzi, L., Hidalgo, M. P., & Frey, B. N. (2016). Do changes in subjective sleep and biological rhythms predict worsening in postpartum depressive symptoms? A prospective study across the perinatal period. *Archives of Women's Mental Health, 19*(4), 591–598.

Liang, J. L., Tiwari, T., Moro, P., et al. (2018). Prevention of pertussis, tetanus, and diphtheria with vaccines in the United States: Recommendations of the Advisory Committee on Immunization Practices (ACIP). *Morbidity and Mortality Weekly Report, 67*(2), 1–44.

Miller, Y. D., Dane, A. C., & Thompson, R. (2014). A call for better care: The impact of postnatal contact services on women's parenting confidence and experiences of postpartum care in Queensland, Australia. *BMC Health Services Research, 14*(1), 1–13.

Okun, M. L. (2016). Disturbed sleep and postpartum depression. *Current Psychiatry Reports, 18*(66), 1–7.

Okun, M. L. (2015). Sleep and postpartum depression. *Current Opinion in Psychiatry, 28*(6), 490–496.

World Health Organization. (1981). *International code of marketing breast-milk substitutes: Frequently asked questions, 2017 update.* Geneva Switzerland: Author. Retrieved from: https://apps.who.int/iris/bitstream/handle/10665/254911/WHO-NMH-NHD-17.1-eng.pdf;jsessionid=65FC-796CA5F43D91DF7FABEBB764F2B6?sequence=1.

World Health Organization. (2018). *Protecting, promoting, and supporting breastfeeding in facilities providing maternity and newborn services: The revised Baby-Friendly Hospital Initiative.* Geneva Switzerland: Author. Retrieved from: https://www.who.int/nutrition/publications/infantfeeding/bfhi-implementation-2018.pdf.

22

Transition to Parenthood

Nicole Lyn Letourneau

http://evolve.elsevier.com/Lowdermilk/MWHC/

LEARNING OBJECTIVES

- Describe parent and infant behaviors that either facilitate or inhibit the parent-child relationship, especially bonding and attachment.
- Describe sensual responses that strengthen the parent-child relationship.
- Examine the process of becoming a mother and becoming a father.
- Compare maternal adjustment and paternal adjustment to parenthood.
- Describe nursing interventions that facilitate parent-infant relationships and adjustment.

- Examine the effects of the following on parenting responses and behavior: parental age (i.e., adolescence and older than 35 years), social support, culture, same-sex parenting, socioeconomic conditions, personal aspirations, and sensory impairment.
- Describe sibling adjustment.
- Discuss grandparent adaptation.

Becoming a parent brings great joy and amazement to most people. The transition to parenthood involves change and adaptation as the family adjusts to life with a new baby. During the first months of having a child the parents define their parental roles and adjust to parenthood. This can be a period of instability, determined by whether parenthood is biologic or adoptive and whether the parents are married husband-wife couples, cohabiting couples, single mothers, single fathers, or same sex couples. Parenting is a process of role attainment and role transition. The transition is an ongoing process as parents and infants develop and change while establishing their lifelong relationships with each other.

PARENT-INFANT RELATIONSHIPS, BONDING, AND ATTACHMENT

A good-quality parent-infant relationship is essential to a child's development, and the earliest experiences are crucial to establish this early foundation for success (Barnard, Hammond, Booth, et al., 1989; Center on the Developing Child at Harvard University, 2016). The mother-infant bond—or formation of an intense emotional connection between a mother and her infant—is understood to lead to more positive parenting behavior as well as more optimal child development in the cognitive, linguistic, and behavioral domains. In their bonding theory, Klaus and Kennell (1976) proposed that there is a sensitive period during the first few minutes or hours after birth when mothers and fathers must have close contact with their infants to optimize their child's later development. Klaus and Kennell (1982) later revised their theory of parent-infant bonding, modifying their claim of the critical nature of immediate contact with the infant after birth. They acknowledged the adaptability of human parents, stating that more than minutes or hours are needed for parents to form an emotional relationship with their infants.

The term bonding has been confused with the term attachment; however, the terms refer to related but different processes. Bonding occurs through mutually satisfying experiences. For example, a mother

commented on her son's grasp reflex, "I put my finger in his hand, and he grabbed right on. It is just a reflex, I know, but it felt good anyway" (Fig. 22.1). Attachment theory was first described by Bowlby (1969) and then elaborated by Ainsworth and colleagues (1978). Bonding and attachment, as essential processes in healthy parent-child relationships, both describe the importance of interaction and proximity (staying close) to the infant. Bonding refers to earlier processes, through which the parent becomes acquainted with the infant, identifies the infant as an individual, and claims the infant as a member of the family. Over time, positive interactions between the parent and the infant through social, verbal, and nonverbal responses (whether real or perceived) facilitates the development of secure parent-infant attachment. For an infant to attain a secure attachment to his or her parent, the parent must be able to provide a secure base for the infant's exploration and a safe haven in the face of distressing stimuli. This means that insofar as is reasonable, the parent maintains proximity to the infant and responds consistently to the infant's bids for attention that indicate needs.

Healthy parent-infant relationships also include mutuality; that is, the infant's behaviors and characteristics elicit a corresponding set of parental behaviors and characteristics. The infant displays signaling behaviors such as crying, smiling, and cooing that initiate the contact and bring the caregiver to the child. These behaviors are followed by executive behaviors such as rooting, grasping, and postural adjustments that maintain the contact. Most caregivers are attracted to an alert, responsive, cuddly infant but find it less desirable to interact with an irritable, apparently disinterested infant. Healthy parent-infant relationships occur more readily with the infant whose temperament, social capabilities, appearance, and sex fit the parent's expectations. If the infant does not meet these expectations, the parent's disappointment can delay bonding and affect the quality of subsequent parent-infant attachment. Table 22.1 presents a comprehensive list of classic infant behaviors affecting parent-child relationships; Table 22.2 presents a corresponding list of parental behaviors.

An important part of parent-infant relationships is acquaintance. Parents use eye contact (Fig. 22.2), touching, talking, and exploring to become acquainted with their infant during the immediate postpartum period. Adoptive parents undergo the same process when they first meet their new child. During this period families engage in the claiming process, which is the identification of the new baby (Fig. 22.3). The child is first identified in terms of "likeness" to other family members, then in terms of "differences," and finally in terms of "uniqueness." The unique newcomer is thus incorporated into the family. Mothers and fathers examine their infant carefully and point out characteristics that the child shares with other family members and that are indicative of a relationship between them. Maternal comments such as the following reveal the claiming process: "Everyone says, 'He's the image of his father,' but I found one part like me—his toes are shaped like mine."

On the other hand, some mothers react negatively. They "claim" the infant in terms of the discomfort or pain the baby causes. The mother interprets the infant's normal responses as being negative toward her and reacts to her child with dislike or indifference. She does not hold the child close or touch the child in a comforting way. For example,

"The nurse put the baby into Lydia's arms. She promptly laid him across her knees and glanced up at the television. 'Stay still until I finish watching; you've been enough trouble already.'"

Nursing interventions related to the promotion of parent-infant attachment are numerous and varied (Letourneau, Tryphonopoulos, Giesbrecht, et al., 2015) (Table 22.3). They can enhance positive parent-infant contacts by heightening parental awareness of an infant's responses and ability to communicate. As the parent attempts to become competent and loving in that role, nurses can bolster the parent's self-confidence and ego. Nurses can identify actual and potential problems and collaborate with other health care professionals who will provide care for the parents after discharge. Nursing considerations for fostering maternal-infant bonding among special populations can vary (see the Cultural Considerations box).

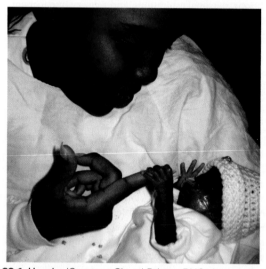

Fig. 22.1 Hands. (Courtesy Cheryl Briggs, RNC, Annapolis, MD.)

⊕ CULTURAL CONSIDERATIONS

Fostering Healthy Parent-Infant Relationships in Women From Varying Ethnic and Cultural Groups

The childbearing practices and rituals of other cultures are not always congruent with standard practices associated with bonding in the Anglo-American culture. For example, Chinese families traditionally use extended family members to care for the newborn so that the mother can rest and recover, especially after a cesarean birth. Some Native American, Asian, and Hispanic women do not initiate breastfeeding until their breast milk comes in. Haitian families name their babies after the 40-day confinement period following birth. The amount of eye contact varies among cultures as well. Yup'ik Eskimo mothers almost always position their babies so that they can make eye contact.

Nurses should become knowledgeable about the childbearing beliefs and practices of diverse cultural and ethnic groups. Because individual cultural variations exist within groups, nurses need to clarify with the client and family members or friends what cultural norms they follow. Incorrect judgments can be made about parent-infant bonding and relationships if nurses do not practice culturally sensitive care.

Modified from D'Avanzo, C. (2008). *Mosby's pocket guide to cultural health assessment* (4th ed.). St. Louis: Mosby.

TABLE 22.1 Infant Behaviors Affecting Parental Attachment

Facilitating Behaviors	Inhibiting Behaviors
Visually alert; eye-to-eye contact; tracking, or following parent's face	Sleepy; eyes closed most of the time; gaze aversion
Appealing facial appearance; randomness of body movements reflecting helplessness	Resemblance to person parent dislikes; hyperirritability or jerky body movements when touched
Smiles	Bland facial expression; infrequent smiles
Vocalization; crying only when hungry or wet	Crying for hours on end; colicky
Grasp reflex	Exaggerated motor reflex
Anticipatory approach behaviors for feedings, sucks well, feeds easily	Feeds poorly; regurgitates; vomits often
Enjoys being cuddled and held	Resists holding and cuddling by crying, stiffening body
Easily consolable	Inconsolable; unresponsive to parenting, caretaking tasks
Activity and regularity somewhat predictable	Unpredictable feeding and sleeping schedule
Attention span sufficient to focus on parents	Inability to attend to parent's face or offered stimulation
Differential crying, smiling, and vocalizing; recognizes and prefers parents	Shows no preference for parents over others
Approaches through locomotion	Unresponsive to parent's approaches
Clings to parent; puts arms around parent's neck	Seeks attention from any adult in room
Lifts arms to parents in greeting	Ignores parents

Modified from Gerson, E. (1973). *Infant behavior in the first year of life.* New York: Raven Press.

TABLE 22.2 Parental Behaviors Affecting Infant Attachment

Facilitating Behaviors	Inhibiting Behaviors
Looks; gazes; takes in physical characteristics of infant; assumes en face position; eye contact	Turns away from infant, ignores infant's presence
Hovers; maintains proximity; directs attention to infant and points to infant	Avoids infant, does not seek proximity, refuses to hold infant when given the opportunity
Identifies infant as unique individual	Identifies infant with someone parent dislikes fails to recognize infant's unique features
Claims infant as family member, names infant	Fails to place infant in family context or identify infant with family member, has difficulty naming infant
Touches, progresses from fingertip to fingers to palms to encompassing contact	Fails to move from fingertip touch to palmar contact and holding
Smiles at infant	Maintains bland countenance or frowns at infant
Talks, coos, or sings to infant	Wakes infant when infant is sleeping, handles infant roughly, hurries feeding by moving nipple continually
Expresses pride in infant	Expresses disappointment, displeasure in infant
Relates infant's behavior to familiar events	Does not incorporate infant into life
Assigns meaning to infant's actions and sensitively interprets infant's needs	Makes no effort to interpret infant's actions or needs
Views infant's behaviors and appearance in positive light	Views infant's behavior as exploiting, deliberately uncooperative; views infant's appearance as distasteful or ugly

Modified from Mercer, R. (1983). Parent-infant attachment. In L. Sonstegard, K. Kowalski, & B. Jennings (Eds.), *Women's health* (vol. 2). New York: Grune & Stratton.

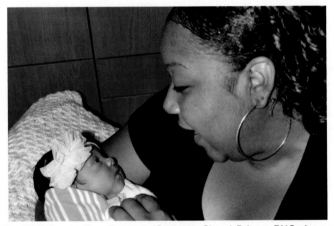

Fig. 22.2 Eye-to-Eye Contact. (Courtesy Cheryl Briggs, RNC, Annapolis, MD.)

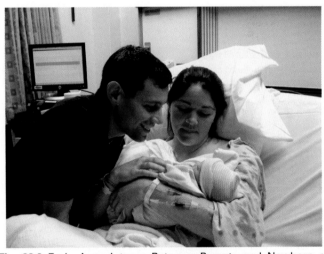

Fig. 22.3 Early Acquaintance Between Parents and Newborn as Mother Holds Infant in En Face Position. (Courtesy Allison and Matt Wyatt, Eagle, CO.)

Assessment of the Quality of the Parent-Child Relationship

One of the most important areas of assessment is careful observation of specific behaviors thought to indicate the formation of emotional bonds between the newborn and the family, especially the mother. Unlike physical assessment of the neonate, which has concrete guidelines to follow, assessment of parent-infant relationship quality relies more on skillful observation and interviewing. Rooming-in of mother and infant and liberal visiting privileges for the father or partner, siblings, and grandparents provide nurses with excellent opportunities to observe interactions and identify behaviors that demonstrate positive or negative connection. Parent-infant relationship quality can be easily observed during infant feeding sessions. Box 22.1 presents guidelines for assessment of parent-child relationship quality.

During pregnancy and often even before conception occurs, parents develop an image of the "ideal" or "fantasy" infant. At birth the fantasy infant becomes the real infant. How closely the dream child resembles the real child influences the bonding process. Assessing such expectations during pregnancy and at the time of the infant's birth allows identification of discrepancies in the parents' view of the fantasy child versus the real child.

Labor and birth significantly affect the immediate attachment of mothers to their newborn infants. Factors such as a long labor, feeling tired or "drugged" after birth, preterm or complicated birth, cesarean birth, problems with breastfeeding, and being separated from the infant at birth can delay the development of initial positive feelings toward the newborn.

PARENT-INFANT CONTACT

Early Contact

Early close contact can facilitate the attachment process between parent and child. Although a delay in contact does not necessarily mean that bonding or the establishment of healthy parent-infant relationships will

TABLE 22.3 Examples of Parent-Infant Attachment Interventions

Intervention Label and Definition	Activities
Attachment Promotion Facilitation of development of parent-infant relationship	Provide opportunity for parent or parents to see, hold, and examine newborn immediately after birth. Encourage parent or parents to hold infant skin-to-skin. Assist parent or parents to participate in infant care. Provide rooming-in while in hospital.
Environmental Management: Attachment Process Manipulation of individuals' surroundings to facilitate development of parent-infant relationship	Create environment that fosters privacy. Individualize daily routine to meet parents' needs. Encourage father or significant other to sleep in room with mother. Develop policies that encourage presence of significant others as much as desired.
Family Integrity Promotion: Childbearing Family Facilitation of growth of individuals or families who are adding infant to family unit	Prepare parent or parents for expected role changes involved in becoming a parent. Prepare parent or parents for responsibilities of parenthood. Monitor effects of newborn on family structure. Reinforce positive parenting behaviors.
Lactation Counseling Use of interactive helping process to assist in achieving and maintaining successful breastfeeding	Correct misconceptions, misinformation, and inaccuracies about breastfeeding. Assess feeding techniques and assist as needed. Evaluate parents' understanding of infant's feeding cues (e.g., rooting, sucking, alertness). Determine frequency of feedings in relation to infant's needs. Demonstrate breast massage and discuss its advantages to increasing milk supply. Provide education, encouragement, and support.
Parent Education: Infant Instruction on nurturing and physical care needed during first year of life	Determine parents' knowledge, readiness, and ability to learn about infant care. Provide anticipatory guidance about developmental changes during first year of life. Teach parent or parents skills needed to care for newborn. Demonstrate ways in which parent or parents can stimulate infant's development. Discuss infant's capabilities for interaction. Demonstrate quieting techniques.
Risk Identification: Childbearing Family Identification of individual or family likely to experience difficulties in parenting; prioritization of strategies to prevent parenting problems	Determine developmental stage of parent or parents. Review prenatal history for factors that predispose individuals or family to complications. Ascertain understanding of English or other language used in community. Monitor behavior that may indicate problem with attachment. Plan for risk-reduction activities in collaboration with individual or family.

Modified from Butcher, H.K., Bulechek, G.M., Dochterman, J.M., Wagner, C.M. (2018). *Nursing interventions classification (NIC)* (7th ed.). St. Louis: Mosby.

be inhibited, additional psychologic energy can be necessary to achieve the same effect. To date, no scientific evidence has demonstrated that immediate contact after birth is essential for the human parent-child relationship.

Early skin-to-skin contact between the mother and newborn immediately after birth and during the first hour facilitates maternal affectionate and connective behaviors (Kilpatrick & Garrison, 2017; King & Pinger, 2014; Stewart & Rodgers, 2017). The newborn is placed in the prone position on the mother's bare chest; the baby and mother are covered with a warm blanket, and a cap is placed on the infant's head to prevent heat loss. This practice promotes early and effective breastfeeding and increases breastfeeding duration (Moore, Bergman, Anderson, et al., 2016). It is also associated with less infant crying, improved thermoregulation (especially in low-birth-weight infants), and improved cardiorespiratory stability in late-preterm infants (Kilpatrick & Garrison, 2017; Stewart & Rodgers, 2017).

Parents who are unable to have early contact with their newborns (e.g., when an infant has been transferred to the intensive care nursery) can be reassured that such contact is not essential for healthy parent-infant relationships. This reassurance is especially important for adoptive parents who may not have been present at the birth, but are capable of forming strong, affectionate ties with their infant. Nurses must stress that the parent-infant relationship is a process that occurs over time.

Extended Contact

Rooming-in is common in family-centered care. With this practice the infant stays in the room with the mother. In some facilities the newborn never leaves the mother's presence; nurses perform the initial assessment and care in the room with the parents. In other hospitals the infant is transferred to the postpartum or mother-baby unit from

BOX 22.1   Assessing Attachment Behavior

- When the infant is brought to the parents, do they reach out for the infant and call the infant by name? (Recognize that in some cultures parents may not name the infant in the early newborn period.)
- Do the parents speak about the infant in terms of identification—whom the infant resembles and what appears special about their infant over other infants?
- When parents are holding the infant, what kind of body contact is seen—do parents feel at ease in changing the infant's position, are fingertips or whole hands used, do they avoid touching parts of the infant's body or do they investigate and scrutinize particular areas?
- When the infant is awake, what kinds of stimulation do the parents provide—do they talk to the infant, to each other, or to no one, and how do they look at the infant—direct visual contact, avoiding eye contact, or looking at other people or objects?
- How comfortable do the parents appear in terms of caring for the infant? Do they express any concern regarding their ability to deal with certain activities, such as changing diapers?
- What type of affection do they demonstrate to the newborn, such as smiling, stroking, kissing, or rocking?
- If the infant is fussy, what kinds of comforting techniques do the parents use, such as rocking, swaddling, talking, or stroking?

the transitional nursery (if the facility uses one) after showing satisfactory extrauterine adjustment. Nurses encourage the father or partner to actively participate in caring for the infant. They can also encourage siblings and grandparents to visit and become acquainted with the infant. Whether the method of family-centered care is rooming-in, mother-baby or couplet care, or a family birth unit; mothers, their partners, and family members are integral parts of the developing family.

Extended contact with the infant should be available for all parents but especially for those at risk for parenting inadequacies, such as adolescents and low-income women. Postpartum nurses must consider and encourage activities that optimize family-centered care (Davidson, Aslakson, Long, et al., 2017). Attaining baby-friendly status for a hospital is one means to promote family-centered care. Baby-friendly hospitals originated through the Baby-Friendly Hospital Initiative (BFHI), which encouraged hospitals to create spaces that are conducive to the forming of bonds between new mothers and their babies and to be supportive of breastfeeding (Pérez-Escamilla, Martinez, & Segura-Pérez, 2016).

COMMUNICATION BETWEEN PARENT AND INFANT

The parent-infant relationship is strengthened through the use of sensual responses and abilities by both partners in the interaction. The nurse should keep in mind that cultural variations are often seen in these interactive behaviors.

The Senses
Touch
Touch, or the tactile sense, is used extensively by parents as a means of becoming acquainted with their newborns. Many mothers reach out for their infants as soon as they are born. Mothers lift their infants to their breasts, enfold them in their arms, and cradle them. Once the infant is close, the mother begins the exploration process with her fingertips, one of the most touch-sensitive areas of the body. Within a short time she uses her palm to caress the baby's trunk and eventually enfolds the infant. A similar progression of touching is demonstrated by fathers,

partners, and other caregivers. Gentle stroking motions are used to soothe and quiet the infant; patting or gently rubbing the infant's back is a comfort after feedings. Infants also pat the mother's breast as they nurse. Both seem to enjoy sharing each other's body warmth. Parents seem to have an innate desire to touch, pick up, and hold their infants. They comment on the softness of the baby's skin and note details of the baby's appearance. Parents become increasingly sensitive to the infant's preferences for different types of touch.

Touching behaviors by mothers vary in different cultural groups. For example, minimal touching and cuddling is a traditional Southeast Asian practice thought to protect the infant from evil spirits. Because of tradition and spiritual beliefs, women in India and Bali have practiced infant massage since ancient times. Field (2017) described the benefits of the worldwide practice of infant massage, which may be used to mitigate painful procedures like heel sticks.

Eye Contact
Parents repeatedly demonstrate interest in having eye contact with their babies. Some mothers remark that once their babies have looked at them, they feel much closer to them. Parents are intent on getting their babies to open their eyes and look at them. In North American culture, eye contact appears to reinforce the development of a trusting relationship and is an important factor in human relationships at all ages. In other cultures, eye contact is perceived differently. For example, in Mexican culture, sustained direct eye contact is considered to be rude, immodest, and dangerous by some. This danger can arise from the *mal de ojo* (evil eye), resulting from excessive admiration. Women and children are thought to be more susceptible to *mal de ojo*.

As newborns become functionally able to sustain eye contact with their parents, they spend time in mutual gazing, often in the en face position, in which the parent's and infant's faces are approximately 30 cm (12 inches) apart and on the same plane (see Fig. 22.2). Nurses, physicians, or nurse midwives can facilitate eye contact immediately after birth by positioning the infant on the mother's abdomen or chest with the mother's and the infant's faces on the same plane. Dimming the lights encourages the infant's eyes to open. To promote eye contact, instillation of prophylactic antibiotic ointment in the infant's eyes can be delayed until the infant and parents have had some time together in the first hour after birth.

Voice
The shared response of parents and infants to each other's voices is remarkable. Parents wait tensely for the first cry. Once that cry has reassured them of the baby's health, they begin comforting behaviors. As the parents speak, the infant is alerted and turns toward them. Infants respond to higher-pitched voices and can distinguish their mother's voice from others soon after birth.

Scent
Another behavior shared by parents and infants is a response to each other's scent. Mothers comment on the smell of their babies when first born and have noted that each infant has a unique scent. Infants learn rapidly to distinguish the scent of their mother's breast milk.

Entrainment
Newborns move in time with the structure of adult speech, which is termed entrainment. They wave their arms, lift their heads, and kick their legs, seemingly "dancing in tune" to a parent's voice. Culturally determined rhythms of speech are ingrained in the infant long before he or she uses spoken language to communicate. This shared rhythm also gives the parent positive feedback and establishes a positive setting for effective communication.

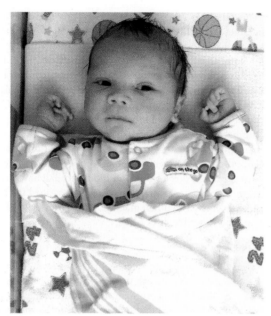

Fig. 22.4 Infant in Alert State. (Courtesy Cheryl Briggs, RNC, Annapolis, MD.)

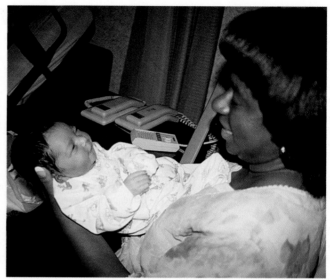

Fig. 22.5 Sharing a Smile: An Example of Synchrony. (Courtesy Marjorie Pyle, RNC, Lifecircle, Costa Mesa, CA.)

Biorhythmicity

Biorhythmicity refers to the infant being in tune with the mother's natural rhythms. The mother's heartbeat or a recording of a heartbeat can soothe a crying infant. One of the newborn's tasks is to establish a personal biorhythm. Parents can help in this process by giving consistent loving care and using their infant's alert state to develop responsive behavior and increase social interactions and opportunities for learning (Fig. 22.4).

Reciprocity and Synchrony

Reciprocity is a type of body movement or behavior that provides the observer with cues. The observer or receiver interprets those cues and responds to them. Reciprocity often takes several weeks to develop with a new baby. For example, when the newborn fusses and cries, the mother responds by picking up and cradling the infant, the baby becomes quiet and alert and establishes eye contact, and the mother verbalizes, sings, and coos while the baby maintains eye contact. The baby then averts its eyes and yawns as the mother decreases her active response. If the parent continues to stimulate the infant, the baby can become fussy.

The term synchrony refers to the "fit" between the infant's cues and the parent's response. When parent and infant experience a synchronous interaction, it is mutually rewarding (Fig. 22.5). Parents need time to interpret the infant's cues correctly. For example, the infant develops a specific cry in response to different situations such as boredom, loneliness, hunger, and discomfort. The parent may need assistance in interpreting these cries, along with trial-and-error interventions, before synchrony develops.

TRANSITION TO PARENTHOOD

Adapting to the role of parent is a developmental transition in which parents come to terms with commitments, demonstrate growing competence in child-care activities, and become increasingly more attuned to the infant's behavior. It can be a time of disorder and disequilibrium as well as satisfaction and joy for mothers and their partners. Usual methods of coping often seem ineffective during

this time. Some parents are so distressed that they are unable to be supportive of each other. Because men typically identify their spouses or partners as their primary or only source of support, the transition can be comparatively harder for the fathers. They often feel deprived when the mothers, who are also experiencing stress, cannot provide their usual level of support. Many parents are unprepared for the strong emotions—such as helplessness, inadequacy, and anger—that arise in the course of dealing with a crying infant. However, the parental role allows adults to develop and display a selfless, warm, and caring side of themselves that may not otherwise be expressed.

For the majority of mothers and their partners, the transition to parenthood is an opportunity rather than a time of crisis. Parents try new coping strategies as they work to master their new roles and reach new developmental levels. As they work through the transition, they often develop new personal strength and resourcefulness.

Parental Tasks and Responsibilities

Parents must reconcile the actual child with their fantasy or dream child. This process means coming to terms with the infant's physical appearance, gender, innate temperament, and physical status. If the real child differs greatly from the fantasy child, some parents will delay acceptance of the child. In other cases they never accept the child.

Many parents know the sex of the infant before birth through prenatal testing. For those who do not have this information, disappointment over the baby's sex can take time to resolve. The parents may provide adequate physical care but have difficulty in being sincerely involved with the infant until this internal conflict has been resolved. As one mother remarked, "I really wanted a boy. I know it is silly and irrational, but when they said, 'She's a lovely little girl,' I was so disappointed and angry—yes, angry—I could hardly look at her. Oh, I looked after her okay, her feedings and baths and things, but I couldn't feel excited. To tell the truth, I felt like a monster not liking my child. Then one day, she was lying there and she turned her head and looked right at me. I felt a flooding of love for her come over me, and we looked at each other a long time. It's okay now. I wouldn't change her for all the boys in the world."

The normal appearance of the neonate—size, color, molding of the head, or bowed appearance of the legs—is startling for some parents. Nurses can encourage parents to examine their babies and to ask questions about newborn characteristics.

Parents must become adept in the care of the infant, including caregiving activities, noting the communication cues given by the infant to indicate needs, and responding appropriately to the infant's needs. The more quickly parents become competent in child care activities, the more quickly they can direct their psychologic energy toward observing and responding to these communication cues. Self-esteem grows with competence. Breastfeeding helps mothers believe that they are contributing in a unique way to the welfare of their infant. The parent may interpret the infant's response to the parental care and attention as a comment on the quality of that care. Infant behaviors that parents interpret as positive responses to their care include being consoled easily, enjoying being cuddled, and making eye contact. Spitting up frequently after feedings, crying, and being unpredictable are often perceived as negative responses to parental care. Continuation of these infant responses that parents view as negative can result in alienation of parent and infant.

Some people view assistance, including advice by spouses, partners, wives, mothers, mothers-in-law, and health care professionals, as supportive. Others view advice as criticism or an indication of how inept these people judge the new parents to be. Criticism, real or imagined, of the new parents' ability to provide adequate physical care, nutrition, and social stimulation for the infant can be devastating. By providing encouragement and praise for parenting efforts, nurses can enhance the new parents' confidence.

Parents must establish a place for the newborn within the family group. Whether the infant is the firstborn or the last born, all family members must adjust their roles to accommodate the newcomer.

Becoming a Mother

Rubin (1961) identified three phases of maternal role attainment in which the mother adjusts to her parental role. These phases extend over the first several weeks and are characterized by dependent behavior, dependent-independent behavior, and interdependent behavior (Table 22.4).

Mercer (2004) suggested that the concept of *maternal role attainment* be replaced with *becoming a mother* to signify the transformation and growth of the mother's identity. Becoming a mother implies more than attaining a role. It includes learning new skills and increasing her confidence in herself as she meets new challenges in caring for her child or children.

Mercer and Walker (2006) identified four stages in the process of becoming a mother: "(a) commitment, connection to the unborn baby, and preparation for delivery and motherhood during pregnancy; (b) acquaintance to the infant, learning to care for the infant, and physical restoration during the first 2 to 6 weeks following birth; (c) moving toward a new normal; and (d) achievement of a maternal identity through redefining self to incorporate motherhood (around 4 months)" (pp. 568–569). The time of achievement of the stages is variable and the stages can overlap. Achievement is influenced by maternal and infant variables and the social environment.

Maternal sensitivity or maternal responsiveness is an important determinant of the maternal-infant relationship. It can be defined as the quality of a mother's sensitive behaviors that are based on her awareness, perception, and responsiveness to infant cues and behaviors. Maternal sensitivity significantly influences the infant's physical, psychologic, and cognitive development. Maternal qualities inherent to this sensitivity include awareness and responsiveness to infant cues, affect, timing, flexibility, acceptance, and conflict negotiation. Maternal sensitivity develops over time in a reciprocal give-and-take relationship with the infant (Cassibba, Castoro, Costantino, et al., 2015).

TABLE 22.4 Phases of Maternal Postpartum Adjustment

Phase	Characteristics
Dependent: taking-in phase	First 24 hours (range, 1-2 days)
	Focus on self and meeting of basic needs:
	Reliance on others to meet needs for comfort, rest, closeness, and nourishment
	Excited and talkative
	Desire to review birth experience
Dependent-independent: taking-hold phase	Starts second or third day; lasts 10 days to several weeks
	Focus on care of baby and competent mothering:
	Desire to take charge
	Still has need for nurturing and acceptance by others
	Eagerness to learn and practice—optimal period for teaching by nurses
	Handling of physical discomforts and emotional changes
	Possible experience with "blues"
Interdependent: letting-go phase	Focus on forward movement of family as unit with interacting members:
	Reassertion of relationship with partner
	Resumption of sexual intimacy
	Resolution of individual roles

Data from Rubin, R. (1961). Basic maternal behavior. *Nursing Outlook, 9*(11), 683–686.

The transition to motherhood requires adjustment for the mother and her family. Not all mothers experience the transition to motherhood in the same way. Circumstances such as problems in postpartum recovery or giving birth to a high-risk infant add to the disruption. For some women, becoming a mother entails multiple losses. For example, for a single woman, loss of the family of origin can occur when the family does not accept her decision to have the child. There can be loss of a relationship with the father of the baby, with friends, and with her own sense of self. Some women describe a loss of dreams that includes loss of job, financial security, and a future profession. Accompanying these losses is a loss of support.

Reality-based perinatal education programs help to prepare mothers and decrease their anxiety. Live classes allow time for questions to be answered and for mothers to lend support to one another. Mothers need to know that it is common to feel overwhelmed and insecure and to experience physical and mental fatigue during the first months of parenthood. They need to be assured that this situation is temporary and that it can take 3 to 6 months to become comfortable in caregiving and in being a mother. Maternal support by professionals should not end with hospital discharge but instead should extend over the next 4 to 6 months. Nurses can advocate for the extension of support services well into the postpartum period (Letourneau, Secco, Colpitts, et al., 2015).

During pregnancy and after birth, nurses can discuss the usual postpartum concerns that mothers experience. They can provide anticipatory guidance on coping strategies, such as resting when the infant sleeps and planning with an extended family member or friend to do the housework for the first week or two after the baby is born. Once a mother is home, periodic telephone calls from a nurse who cared for her in the birth setting can provide the mother with an opportunity to vent her concerns and get support and advice from "her" nurse. Nurses should plan additional supportive counseling for first-time mothers inexperienced in child care, women whose careers had provided outside stimulation, women who lack friends or family members with whom to share delights and concerns, and adolescent mothers. When possible, home visits should be included in the postpartum care.

Postpartum "Blues"

The "pink" period surrounding the first day or two after birth, characterized by heightened joy and feelings of well-being, is often followed by a "blue" period. Approximately 50% to 80% of women of all ethnic and racial groups experience the postpartum blues, or "baby blues." During the blues, women are emotionally labile and often cry easily for no apparent reason. This lability seems to peak around the fifth day and subsides by the tenth day. Other symptoms of postpartum blues include depressed mood, a let-down feeling, restlessness, fatigue, insomnia, headache, anxiety, sadness, and anger. Biochemical, psychologic, social, and cultural factors have been explored as possible causes of postpartum blues; however, the cause remains unknown.

Whatever the cause, the early postpartum period appears to be one of emotional and physical vulnerability for new mothers, who are often psychologically overwhelmed by the reality of parental responsibilities. Mothers feel deprived of the supportive care they received from family members and friends during pregnancy. Some mothers regret the loss of the mother–unborn child relationship and mourn its passing. Still others experience a let-down feeling when labor and birth are complete.

The majority of women experience fatigue after birth, which is compounded by the around-the-clock demands of the new baby. Postpartum fatigue increases the risk of postpartum depressive symptoms (Tomfohr, Buliga, Letourneau, et al., 2015) and can have a negative effect on maternal role attainment (Meighan, 2017). During the postpartum period, it is common for women to experience disrupted sleep. Although breastfeeding mothers may be awake more frequently during the night to breastfeed compared with mothers who formula-feed, there is evidence to suggest that breastfeeding, which enhances maternal role attainment, can also help to improve maternal sleep (Shaver, 2015).

A few questions on a discharge checklist can help mothers to assess their level of blues and decide when to seek advice from their nurse, nurse-midwife, or physician. Home visits and telephone follow-up calls by a nurse are important to assess the mother's pattern of blue feelings and behavior over time. To help mothers cope with postpartum blues, nurses can suggest various strategies (see the Teaching for Self-Management box).

Although the postpartum blues are usually mild and short-lived, approximately 8% to 20% of women experience a more severe disorder termed *postpartum depression* (PPD) (Isley & Katz, 2017). It is likely, however, that the actual occurrence of PPD is greater than the reported numbers because it is often unrecognized and undiagnosed (American College of Obstetricians and Gynecologists [ACOG], 2018). Symptoms of PPD can range from mild to severe, with women having good days and bad days. Fathers can also experience PPD, and screening for PPD should be performed with both mothers and fathers. PPD can go undetected because new parents —out of embarrassment, guilt, or fear—generally do not voluntarily admit to this kind of emotional distress. Nurses must include teaching about how to differentiate symptoms of the blues and PPD and,

---

TEACHING FOR SELF-MANAGEMENT
Coping With Postpartum Blues

- Remember that the blues are normal and that both the mother and father or partner can experience them.
- Get plenty of rest; nap when the baby does if possible. Go to bed early and let friends and family know when to visit and how they can help. (Remember, you are not Supermom.)
- Use relaxation techniques learned in birthing classes (or ask the nurse to teach you and your partner some techniques).
- Do something for yourself. Take advantage of the time your partner or family members care for the baby—soak in the tub (a 20-minute soak can be the equivalent of a 2-hour nap), or go for a walk.
- Plan a day out of the house—go to the mall with the baby, being sure to take a stroller or carriage, or go out to eat with friends without the baby. Many communities have churches or other agencies that provide child care programs such as Mothers' Morning Out.
- Talk to your partner about the way you feel—for example, about feeling tied down, to what extent the birth met your expectations, and things that might help you (do not be afraid to ask for specifics).
- If you are breastfeeding, give yourself and your baby time to learn.
- Seek out and use community resources such as La Leche League or community mental health centers. One nationally recognized resource is

Postpartum Support International
927 North Kellogg Ave.
Santa Barbara, CA 93111
(805) 967-7636
https://www.postpartum.net/

---

if they occur, urge parents to report depressive symptoms promptly (see Chapter 31).

Becoming a Father

For many men, fatherhood begins at the moment of birth, whereas women are more likely to begin the journey toward motherhood when the pregnancy is confirmed. Most fathers expect to have an immediate emotional bond with their newborns; they want immediate physical contact soon after birth, and look forward to being involved in caring for the infant. Involvement in the labor and birth process by doing things like cutting the umbilical cord can enhance the partner's feelings of connection with the newborn. The father's involvement with the infant is somewhat dependent on the mother in terms of what she will allow the father to do and on the support he receives from her (Scism & Cobb. 2017).

The realities of the first few weeks at home with a newborn cause fathers to change their expectations, set new priorities, and redefine their roles. They develop strategies for balancing work, their own needs, and the needs of their partner and infant. Men become increasingly more comfortable with infant care. During this time they may struggle for recognition and positive feedback from their partner, the infant, and others. They begin to develop strategies for balancing work with their own needs and the needs of their partner and infant. Fathers can feel excluded from support and attention by health care providers (Garfield, 2015) (Table 22.5).

Research on paternal adjustment to parenthood suggests that men go through predictable phases during their transition to parenthood as they seek to become involved fathers (Goodman, 2005). In the first phase men enter parenthood with intentions of being an emotionally involved father with deep connections to the infant. They consider how they were parented by their own fathers. Many want to parent

TABLE 22.5	Early Development of the Involved Father Role
Phases	**Characteristics**
Expectations and intentions	Desire for emotional involvement and deep connection with infant
Confronting reality	Dealing with unrealistic expectations, frustration, disappointment, feelings of guilt, helplessness, and inadequacy
Creating the role of involved father	Altering expectations, establishing new priorities, redefining role, negotiating changes with partner, learning to care for infant, increasing interaction with infant, struggling for recognition
Reaping rewards	Infant smile, sense of meaning, completeness, and immortality

From Goodman, J. (2005). Becoming an involved father of an infant. *Journal of Obstetric, Gynecologic and Neonatal Nursing, 34*(2), 190–200.

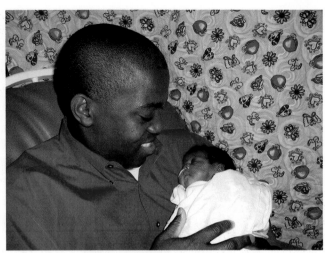

Fig. 22.6 Father Interacts With His Newborn Son. (Courtesy Cheryl Briggs, RNC, Annapolis, MD.)

differently, whereas others plan to adopt the parenting style of their fathers (Chin, Hall, & Daiches, 2011).

The second phase is a time of confronting reality, when men realize that their expectations were inconsistent with the realities of life with a newborn during the first few weeks. During this period fathers experience intense emotions. Many acknowledge that their expectations were of limited value once they were immersed in the reality of parenthood. Feelings that often accompany this reality are sadness, ambivalence, jealousy, frustration, and an overwhelming desire to be more involved. Some men are surprised that establishing a relationship with the infant is more gradual than expected. Fathers often feel alone, having no one with whom to discuss their feelings during this time because the mothers are often preoccupied with infant care and their own transition to parenting.

The third phase is working to create the role of involved father. Men strive to become increasingly more comfortable with infant care. Uncertainty about their child care skills can lead to feelings of anxiety (Goodman, 2005). Communicating with other new fathers about their experiences can help alleviate some of this anxiety (Chin et al., 2011). During this time they may struggle for recognition and positive feedback from their partner, the infant, and others and may feel excluded from support and attention by health care providers. Leaving their partner and the newborn to return to work after the birth can be difficult for fathers; many find it challenging to balance their time between work and spending time with their families. Some men reprioritize their activities or negotiate work hours to allow them to be at home more often (Chin et al.).

The final phase of becoming an involved father is one of reaping rewards, the most significant being reciprocity from the infant, such as a smile. This phase typically occurs around 6 weeks to 2 months. Increased sociability of the infant enhances this father-infant relationship (Goodman, 2005).

Newborns often have a powerful effect on their fathers, who become intensely involved with their babies. The term used for the father's absorption, preoccupation, and interest in the infant is **engrossment**. Characteristics of engrossment include some of the sensual responses relating to touch and eye-to-eye contact that were discussed earlier and the father's keen awareness of features both unique and similar to himself that validate his claim to the infant. The father feels a strong attraction to the newborn. This relationship between a father and his newborn is beneficial to both. Fathers spend considerable time interacting with the infant and taking delight in the infant's responses to them (Fig. 22.6). Fathers experience increased self-esteem and a sense of being proud, bigger, more mature, and older after seeing their baby for the first time.

Fathers receive less interpersonal and professional support compared with mothers and can feel excluded from prenatal appointments and perinatal classes (Shorey, Dennis, Bridge, et al., 2017). They need information and encouragement related to infant care, parenting, and relationship changes during pregnancy and in the postpartum period. New fathers are at risk for PPD and should receive information about risks, symptoms, and resources for help (Garfield, 2015). During the postpartum hospital stay, nurses can arrange to teach infant care when the father is present and provide anticipatory guidance for fathers about the transition to parenthood. Separate prenatal and parenting classes and parenting support groups for fathers can provide them with an opportunity to discuss their concerns and have some of their needs met. To prepare fathers for the transition to parenthood, perinatal education should include information about role changes associated with parenting, the importance of parenting "teamwork," and the increased risk of mental distress and depression. Fathers also need information about providing support to the mother, interpreting and responding to infant behaviors, and dealing with infant crying (Widarsson, Engstrom, Tyden, et al., 2015). Postpartum telephone calls and home visits by the nurse should include time for assessment of the father's adjustment and needs. Health interventions that engage fathers can have positive effects on the couple's communication and decision making about maternal and newborn health and can improve caretaking and home care practices (Tokhi, Comrie-Thomson, Davis, et al., 2018).

Adjustment for the Couple

The transition to parenthood brings about changes in the relationship between the mother and her partner. A strong healthy marriage or couple relationship is the best foundation for parenthood, although even the best relationships are often shaken by the addition of a new baby. During the first few weeks after birth, parents experience many emotions. Even though they may feel an overwhelming love toward their newborn and a sense of amazement, they can also feel a strong

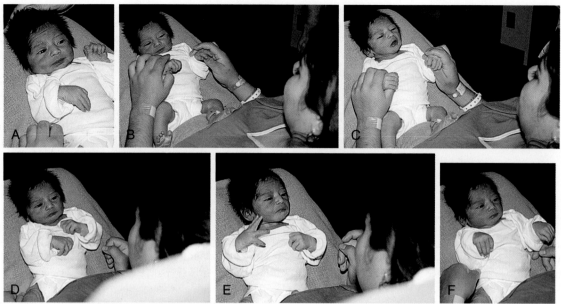

Fig. 22.7 Mother Interacts With Her Daughter, 6 Hours Old. (A) Infant is quiet and alert. (B) Mother begins talking to daughter. (C) Infant responds, opens mouth like her mother. (D) Infant gazes at her mother. (E) Infant waves hand. (F) Infant glances away, resting; hands relax. (Courtesy Marjorie Pyle, RNC, Lifecircle, Costa Mesa, CA.)

sense of responsibility. Even if the mother and her partner have been to prenatal classes, read books, consulted internet sources, or sought advice from family or friends, they are usually surprised by the realities of life with a new baby and the changes in their relationship. Because men and women experience pregnancy and birth differently, the expectation is that they will also vary in their transition to parenthood.

Common issues that couples face as they become parents include changes in their relationship with one another, sexual intimacy, division of household and infant care responsibilities, financial concerns, balancing work and parental responsibilities, and social activities (Feinberg, Jones, Hostetler, et al., 2016). To help new parents in their transition, nurses can encourage them during pregnancy and in the postpartum period to share personal expectations with each other and to assess their relationship periodically. Couples must schedule time in their busy lives for one-on-one conversation and try to have regular "dates" or time apart from the infant. The mother and her partner need to express appreciation for one another and their baby. Support from family, friends, and community health professionals should be identified early and used as needed during pregnancy, in the postpartum period, and beyond. The couple who are willing to experiment with new approaches to their lifestyle and habits will find the transition to parenthood less difficult.

Nurses can provide opportunities for parents to discuss concerns and ask questions about resuming sexual intimacy (see Chapter 21). Sexual intimacy enhances the adult aspect of the family, and the adult pair share a closeness denied to other family members. Changes in a woman's sexual desire after birth are related to hormonal shifts, increased breast size, uneasiness with a body that has yet to return to a prepregnant size, chronic fatigue related to sleep deprivation, and physical exhaustion. Partners can feel alienated when they observe the intimate mother-infant relationship, and some are frank in expressing feelings of jealousy toward the infant. The resumption of sexual intimacy seems to bring the parents' relationship back into focus. Before and after birth, nurses should review with new parents their plans for other pregnancies and their preferences for contraception. (See the box Teaching for Self-Management: Resuming Sexual Intimacy in Chapter 21.)

Infant-Parent Adjustment

It has long been recognized that newborns participate actively in shaping their parents' reaction to them. Behavioral characteristics of the infant influence parenting behaviors. The infant and the parent each have unique rhythms, behaviors, and response styles that are brought to every interaction. Infant-parent interactions can be facilitated in any of the following three ways: (1) modulation of rhythm, (2) modification of behavioral repertoires, and (3) mutual responsivity. Nurses can teach parents about these three aspects of infant-parent interaction through discussions, written materials, and media resources describing infant capabilities. A creative approach is to make a video recording of the parent-infant pair during an interaction and then use that recording to discuss the pair's rhythm, behavioral repertoire, and responsivity.

Rhythm

To modulate rhythm, both parent and infant must be able to interact. The alert state (Fig. 22.7) occurs most often during a feeding or in face-to-face play. Holding the infant approximately 12 to 18 inches away (the distance at which most newborns can focus), the parent interacts with the infant until the infant displays signs of overstimulation or shutting down (e.g., looking away, color change, changes in movement).

Mothers learn to reserve stimulation for pauses in sucking activity and not to talk or smile excessively while the infant is sucking because the infant will stop feeding to interact with her. With maturity the infant can sustain longer interactions by modulating activity rhythms, that is, limb movement, sucking, gaze alternation, and habituation. Meanwhile, the parent becomes more attuned to the infant's rhythms and learns to modulate the rhythms, facilitating a rhythmic turn-taking interaction.

Behavioral Repertoires

Both the infant and the parent have a repertoire of behaviors they can use to facilitate interactions. Fathers and mothers engage in these behaviors depending on the extent of contact and caregiving of the infant. Nurses can teach parents to recognize, interpret, and respond to infant behaviors. An innovative program called HUG Your Baby (Help, Understanding and

Guidance for Young Families: www.hugyourbaby.org) is designed to prepare health care professionals to teach parents how to understand their newborns and prevent problems related to crying, sleeping, eating, attachment, and bonding (see Chapter 24: Teaching for Self-Management: Helping Parents Recognize, Interpret, and Respond to Newborn Behaviors).

The infant's behavioral repertoire includes gazing, vocalizing, facial expression, and body gestures (movements). From birth the infant is able to focus, follow the human face, and alternate its gaze voluntarily, looking away from the parent's face when understimulated or overstimulated. One of the key responses for the parents to learn is to be sensitive to the infant's capacity for attention and inattention. Developing this sensitivity is especially important when one is interacting with preterm infants.

Body gestures form a part of the infant's "early language." An infant can raise an eyebrow or soften facial expression to elicit loving attention. Game playing can stimulate them to smile or laugh. Pouting or crying, arching of the back, and general squirming usually signal the end of an interaction.

The parents' repertoire includes various types of interactive behaviors such as constantly looking at the infant and noting the response. New parents often remark that they are exhausted from looking at the baby and smiling. Adults also "infantilize" their speech to help the infant "listen." They do this by slowing the tempo, speaking loudly and rhythmically, and emphasizing key words. Phrases are repeated frequently. Infantilizing does not mean using "baby talk," which involves distorting sounds.

To communicate emotions to the infant, parents often use facial expressions such as slow and exaggerated looks of surprise, happiness, and confusion. Games such as peek-a-boo and imitation of the infant's behaviors are other means of interaction. For example, if the baby smiles, so does the parent; if the baby frowns, the parent responds in kind.

Responsivity

Contingent responses (responsivity) are those that occur within a specific time frame and are similar in form to a stimulus behavior. The adult has the feeling of having an influence on the interaction. Infant behaviors such as smiling, cooing, and sustained eye contact, usually in the en face position, are viewed as contingent responses. The infant's responses act as rewards to the initiator and encourage the adult to continue with the game when the infant responds positively. When the adult imitates the infant, the infant appears to enjoy it. A progression occurs in the types of behaviors that parents present for the baby to imitate; for example, in early interactions, the parent will grimace rather than laugh, which is in keeping with the infant's developmental level. Such "turnabout" behaviors sustain interactions and promote harmony in the relationship.

INFLUENCES ON TRANSITION TO PARENTHOOD

Various factors—including age, social networks, socioeconomic conditions, and personal aspirations for the future—influence how parents respond and adapt to the birth of a child. Cultural beliefs and practices also affect parenting behaviors. Factors that are recognized to increase the incidence of parenting problems include age (adolescent mothers or those older than 35 years), same-sex parenting, lack of social support, culture, unfavorable socioeconomic conditions, and conflicts between parenting and personal aspirations. Sensory impairments—such as difficulties with vision or hearing—can also affect the transition to parenthood.

Age

Maternal age has a definite effect on the transition to parenting. The mother, fetus, and newborn are at highest risk when the mother is an adolescent or older than 35 years.

Adolescence

Adolescent pregnancy is a global issue that occurs predominantly in marginalized communities and is often associated with lack of education, poverty, and lack of employment (WHO, 2018). In most cases the pregnancy is unplanned or unintended, although some adolescents do desire and plan pregnancy and childbirth (Macutkiewicz & MacBeth, 2017). Pregnancy may be the result of sexual coercion, with the adolescent being forced to give birth. The emotional needs of adolescent mothers often exceed those of other women (WHO).

The adolescent mother and father face immediate developmental tasks that include completing the developmental tasks of adolescence, making a transition to parenthood, and sometimes adapting to marriage. At the same time they are also dealing with a variety of other stressors. They may face stigma or rejection by their families and peers. Pregnancy and parenthood may force adolescents to drop out of school. Relationships between adolescent mothers and fathers tend to be less stable than those among adults, and they often deteriorate or dissolve soon after birth.

As adolescent parents move through the transition to parenthood, they can feel "different" from their peers, excluded from "fun" activities, and prematurely forced to adopt an adult social role. The conflict between their own desires and the infant's demands, in addition to the low tolerance for frustration that is typical of adolescence, further contribute to the normal psychosocial stress of birth and parenting. Maintaining a relationship with the baby's father is often beneficial for the teen mother and her infant, although in adolescent pregnancy it is often found that the young father departs from the relationship.

Adolescent mothers. Adolescent mothers and their infants are at risk for adverse outcomes. There is increased risk for preeclampsia, postpartum endometritis, and systemic infections. Anemia is common among pregnant teens. Teens are more likely to give birth to preterm and/or low-birth-weight infants and infants with serious neonatal conditions (Jeha, Usta, Ghulmiyyah, & Nassar, 2015; WHO, 2018). There is an increased risk for PPD, substance abuse, posttraumatic stress disorder, intimate partner violence, and repeat pregnancy (Hodgkinson, Beers, Southammakosane, & Lewin, 2014; WHO). Children of adolescent parents are more prone to growth and development issues, specifically language, speech, and cognitive delays, and they have an increased risk of neglect and accidental injury (Bartlett & Easterbrooks, 2015; Thompson & Canadian Paediatric Society [CPS], 2016).

Even with these increased risks, the majority of teen mothers have positive outcomes that are comparable to those of their peers who bear children later in life, especially when they have strong social and functional support (Hodgkinson et al., 2014). In some families or communities, adolescent parenthood is considered a normal or positive life event. Even so, adolescent pregnancy and parenting are important public health concerns.

Anticipatory guidance through developmentally appropriate education is needed to prepare adolescents for parenting. Specific topics include infant nutrition, growth and development, sleep, infant safety, and immunizations (Thompson & CPS, 2016). A medical home model of care is recommended for adolescent parents and their offspring. Through this model, an interprofessional approach to care can address the full spectrum of needs (Pinzon, Jones, Committee on Adolescence, & Committee on Early Childhood, 2012).

Adolescent mothers provide warm and attentive physical care; however, they use less verbal interaction than older parents, tend to be less responsive, and interact less positively with their infants than older mothers. Interventions emphasizing verbal and nonverbal communication skills between mother and infant are important. Such intervention strategies must be concrete and specific because of the cognitive and developmental level of adolescents. In comparison with older mothers, teenage mothers have limited knowledge of child development. They tend to expect too much of their infants too soon and often characterize their infants as being fussy. This limited knowledge can cause teenagers to respond to their infants inappropriately.

Many young mothers pattern their maternal role on what they experienced with their own mothers. Therefore nurses must determine the type of support that people close to the young mother are able and prepared to give as well as the kinds of community assistance available to supplement this support. Many teen mothers can identify a source of social support, with the predominant source being their own mothers.

Community-based programs for pregnant adolescents and adolescent parents improve access to health care, education, and other support services. Home visiting programs are beneficial, especially for low-income adolescents (Easterbrooks, Kotake, Raskin, & Bumgarner, 2016; Hodgkinson et al., 2014). Many school-based programs include a parenting and life skills curriculum as well as pregnancy prevention strategies. Serious problems can be prevented through outreach programs concerned with self-management, parent-child interactions, infant development, and child safety. As the adolescent performs her mothering role within the framework of her family, she may need to address issues of dependence versus independence. The adolescent's family members also need help adapting to their new roles. Some mothers and fathers of adolescents may feel they are too young to be grandparents and unprepared for that role (see Clinical Reasoning Case Study).

? CLINICAL REASONING CASE STUDY

Transition to Parenthood for the Adolescent Couple

You are the mother/baby nurse caring for Sherika, a 16-year-old who, a day ago, gave birth at 39 weeks' gestation to a 6-lb, 5-oz (2863-g) baby girl by an uncomplicated vaginal delivery. According to the hand-off report from the night shift RN, Jeremy, the baby's father, is Sherika's 17-year-old "on again, off again" boyfriend who has visited once since the baby was born, but only for a couple of hours. At that time he held the baby briefly but appeared uncomfortable and admitted that he has never been around babies. Sherika's mother was with her for the birth but had to go home to care for her own 8-year-old twins. The nurse reports that Sherika has had little interaction with the baby. Sherika says she wants to breastfeed her baby, but the baby has been sleepy and feeding attempts have not been successful. When you enter the room for the morning assessment, you see that Sherika is texting on her phone; the baby is in the bassinet crying.

1. What is the priority concern or client need in this situation? Support your answer with data as stated in the case.
2. List other client needs/problems in this case.
3. Identify any additional information or assessment data that are needed by the nurse in planning care for this client.
4. What nursing actions are appropriate in this situation?
   a. What is the priority nursing action? (What should the nurse do first?)
   b. Describe other nursing interventions that are important to providing optimal client care.
5. Describe the roles/responsibilities of the interprofessional health care team members (other than nurses) who may be involved in providing care for this client.

Adolescent fathers. The vast majority of adolescent fathers do not live with the mother and infant, although many visit on a regular basis. They are often living in poverty, have limited education, and—owing to tenuous employment—have little ability to offer financial help in caring for the infant (Thompson & CPS, 2016).

The involvement of the father with the infant is dependent on his relationship with the mother, who also controls his access to the infant. The father's involvement can have a positive influence on breastfeeding, maternal mental health, parenting practices, and family functioning as well as the child's well-being, cognitive development, and behavioral outcomes (Thompson & CPS, 2016).

Health care professionals should actively include adolescent fathers in care management, beginning as early as possible during pregnancy and continuing into the postpartum period and beyond (Thompson & CPS, 2016). The nurse can initiate interaction with the adolescent father during prenatal visits, labor and birth, and the postpartum hospitalization. The nurse can assess the relationship between the two adolescents and encourage them to discuss their plans for the father's involvement with the mother and infant after birth. During the hospital stay, the nurse can include the adolescent father in teaching sessions about infant care and parenting. The nurse can ask him to be present during postpartum home visits and to accompany the mother and baby to well-baby follow-up visits at the clinic or pediatrician's office. With the adolescent mother's approval, the nurse may contact the father directly.

Adolescent fathers need support to discuss their emotional responses to the pregnancy, birth, and fatherhood. The nurse must be aware of the father's feelings of guilt, powerlessness, or bravado because these feelings can have negative consequences for both the parents and the child. Counseling of adolescent fathers must be reality-oriented and should include topics such as finances, child care, parenting skills, and the father's role in the parenting experience. Teenage fathers also need to know about reproductive physiology and birth control options as well as sexual practices that lower the risk of pregnancy and sexually transmitted infections.

The adolescent father may continue to be involved in an ongoing relationship with the young mother and his baby. In those instances he plays an important role in decisions about child care and raising the child. He may need help to develop realistic perceptions of his role as "father to a child" and is encouraged to use coping mechanisms that are not harmful to his own, his partner's, or his child's well-being. The nurse may enlist support systems, parents, and professional agencies on his behalf.

Advanced Maternal Age

By definition, advanced maternal age refers to women who give birth after the age of 35. Women above that age have continued their childbearing either by choice or because of the lack or failure of contraception during the perimenopausal years. Added to this group are women who have postponed pregnancy because of their careers or for other reasons as well as women of infertile couples who finally become pregnant with the aid of assisted reproductive technology.

Support from partners aids in the adjustment of older mothers to changes involved in becoming a parent and seeing themselves as competent. Support from other family members and friends is also important for a positive self-evaluation of parenting, a sense of well-being and satisfaction, and help in dealing with stress. Women of advanced maternal age can experience social isolation. Older mothers may have less family and social support than younger mothers. They are less likely to live near family, and their own parents may be unable to provide assistance or support because of their age or health issues. Mothers of advanced maternal age are often caught in the "sandwich generation," taking on responsibility for the care of aging parents while also parenting young children. Social support can be lacking because their peers are probably busy with their careers and have limited time to help. Their friends are likely to have older children and have less in common with the new mother.

Changes in the sexual aspect of a relationship can create stress for new midlife parents. Mothers report that it is difficult to find the time and energy for a romantic rendezvous. They attribute much of this difficulty to the reality of caring for an infant, but the decreasing libido that normally accompanies getting older also contributes.

Work and career issues are sources of conflict for older mothers. Conflicts emerge over being disinterested in work, worrying about giving enough attention to work with the distractions of a new baby, and anticipating what returning to work will entail. Child care is a major factor in causing stress about work.

Another major issue for older mothers with careers is the perception of loss of control. Older mothers as compared with younger mothers are at a different stage in their careers, having attained high levels of education, career, and income. The loss of control experienced in going from the consistency of a work role to the inconsistency of the parent role comes as a surprise to many older women. It is essential to help the older mother have realistic expectations of herself and of parenthood.

New mothers who are also perimenopausal can experience difficulty distinguishing fatigue, loss of sleep, decreased libido, or other physiologic symptoms as the causes of the change in their sex lives. Although many women view menopause as a natural stage of life, for midlife mothers, the cessation of menstruation coincides with the state of parenthood. The changes of midlife and menopause can add more emotional and physical stress to older mothers' lives because of the time- and energy-consuming aspects of raising a young child.

Same-Sex Couples

Although same-sex couples experience many of the same adjustments and challenges of parenting as heterosexual couples, the transition to parenting for same-sex couples can present unique issues and concerns. Whether the couple consists of two women or two men, issues such as a lack of family acceptance and support, public ignorance, and social and legal invisibility influence their ability to adapt as new parents. They are likely to encounter stressors related to identity transformation as they become parents. Same-sex couples deal with minority status as lesbian women or gay men within a heterosexual parenting community and as parents within the lesbian, bisexual, gay, transgender, queer (LGBTQ) community; if the couple is also an ethnic minority, there can be additional stress. Expectations and pressures from within these communities can cause anxiety and stress and lead to feelings of isolation, alienation, and discrimination (Cao, Mills-Koonce, Wood, & Fine, 2016; Farr & Tornello, 2016).

Attitudes of health care professionals can either positively or negatively affect the care provided to same-sex couples (Cook, Gunter, & Lopez, 2017; Farr & Tornello, 2016). Same-sex couples may be concerned about confidentiality and disclosure, discriminatory attitudes and treatment, and limited access to care.

Lesbian Couples

The transition to parenting for many lesbian couples is unique in that there are two women with maternal status, one who gave birth and the other who may be referred to as "the other mother," "nonbiologic mother," "co-parent," "co-mother," or another term preferred by the couple (Fig. 22.8). It is important for health care providers to determine the couple's preference about how they wish to be identified.

Health care providers demonstrate a variety of reactions to lesbian couples, ranging from rejection and exclusion to complete acceptance and inclusion. Judgmental attitudes, confusion, or lack of understanding can affect the quality of care provided to these families (Cook et al., 2017). ACOG (2012/2018) endorses equitable treatment for lesbian couples and their families for direct and indirect health care needs. Although the traditional roles of the mother and father in heterosexual relationships are well recognized, the role of the lesbian co-parent can be questioned, misunderstood, and ignored by society and by health care providers. Intentionally or accidentally, health care providers can exclude partners or fail to acknowledge their roles in pregnancy, birth, and parenting.

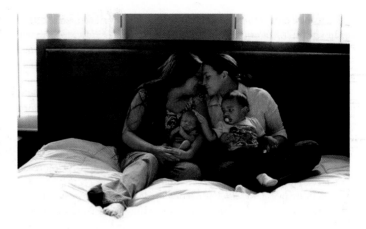

Fig. 22.8 Co-Mothers With Newborn and Older Sibling. (Courtesy Diane Ortega, CNM, Mesa, AZ.)

Integration of the co-parent into care includes offering the opportunities afforded male partners of heterosexual women, such as "cutting the cord" and rooming in with the mother and baby during hospitalization. An option not available to male partners is to actually breastfeed the infant. For couples who select to co-nurse, the female co-partner can stimulate milk production through induced lactation involving medications and regular pumping. A supplemental feeding device containing expressed breast milk or formula can be used to provide additional milk to the breastfeeding infant (see Fig. 25.8). Women who choose not to induce lactation yet desire to have the breastfeeding experience can put the baby to a breast by using a supplemental feeding device. Health care professionals must be aware of protocols for inducing lactation; this process for the female co-parent should be initiated weeks or months in advance of the birth. The same protocols can be used to induce lactation in adoptive mothers (Lawrence & Lawrence, 2016).

Similar to heterosexual parents, lesbian couples face challenges in adjusting to life with a new baby. They experience the same sleep deprivation and changes in relationship quality that having a newborn brings. The division of household and child care responsibilities may be challenging. The birth mother may be the one most responsible for child care because she is likely to be working fewer hours than her partner. Tensions can arise between the partners in relation to their roles. This can be compounded by the lack of a formal, recognized relationship between the co-parent and the infant and the issues surrounding her legal rights in relation to her partner and the infant (Farr & Tornello, 2016; Cao et al., 2016).

Lesbian couples face strong social sanctions regarding pregnancy and parenting. Their families may not have resolved their initial dismay and guilt over learning of their daughters' homosexuality, or they may disagree with the lesbian couple's decision to conceive and be parents. Lesbian parents deal with public ignorance, social and legal invisibility, and the lack of biologic connection to the child by using various techniques. These techniques include carefully planning and accomplishing their transition to parenthood, displaying public acts of equal mothering, sharing parenting at home, establishing a distinct parenting role within the family, and supporting each partner's sense of identity as a mother. In situations in which family support is limited or absent, the nurse can help lesbian couples to locate supportive social groups, lesbian or heterosexual.

Gay Couples

Some men in same-sex relationships, or gay couples, choose to become parents by adoption or through assisted reproduction, in which a gestational carrier (surrogate) is impregnated by artificial insemination or in vitro fertilization. Female-to-male transgender individuals in gay relationships have been known to become pregnant. Same-sex male couples face the same social sanctions regarding pregnancy and parenting that lesbian couples encounter (Farr & Tornello, 2016).

Nurses are likely to encounter gay couples in the hospital setting if they are present for birth by a surrogate or if they are adopting a newborn and visit the hospital to spend time with the neonate and learn about infant care. Nurses can help these men to locate support groups that will address their needs. They must ensure that these families receive effective health care. Data on gay parenting are limited and focus more on the developmental outcomes of the children than on parenting styles or parental caregiving. Research is needed to identify the needs of gay parents and ways to support them in their parenting endeavors.

Social Support

Social support is strongly related to positive adaptation by new parents during the transition to parenthood. Social support is multidimensional and includes the number of members in a person's social network, types of support, perceived general support, actual support received, and satisfaction with support available and received. Partner support in pregnancy has a positive influence on adaptation in the postpartum period (Thomas, Letourneau, Bryce, et al., 2017).

Across cultural groups, families and friends of new parents form an important dimension of the parent's social network. By seeking help within the social network, new mothers learn culturally valued practices and develop role competency.

Social networks provide a support system on which parents can rely for assistance, but they also can be a source of conflict. Sometimes a large network can cause problems because it results in conflicting advice that comes from numerous people. Grandparents or in-laws are most appreciated when they assist with household responsibilities and do not intrude into the parents' privacy or judge them critically.

Because of the extent of restructuring and reorganization that occurs in a family with the birth of another child, the mother's moods and fatigue in the postpartum period can be helped more by situation-specific support from family and friends than by general support. Situation-specific support relates to practical concerns such as physical needs and child care. For example, the practical support of a grandparent bathing the infant can help lessen a second-time mother's feelings of loss by giving her time to be with her firstborn child. General support addresses the feelings of being loved, supported, and valued.

Culture

Cultural beliefs and practices are important determinants of parenting behaviors. Culture influences the interactions with the baby as well as the parents' or the family's caregiving style.

All cultures place importance on desiring and valuing children. Knowledge of cultural beliefs can help the nurse make more accurate assessments and analyses of observed parenting behaviors. For example, nurses can become concerned when they observe cultural practices that appear to reflect poor maternal-infant bonding. Algerian mothers may not unwrap and explore their infants as part of the acquaintance process because in Algeria, babies are wrapped tightly in swaddling clothes to protect them physically and psychologically. The nurse may observe a Vietnamese woman who gives minimal care to her infant but refuses to cuddle or further interact with her baby. This apparent lack of interest in the newborn is this cultural group's attempt to ward off "evil spirits" and actually reflects an intense love and concern for the infant (Galanti, 2015). An Asian mother might be criticized for almost immediately relinquishing the care of the infant to the grandmother and not even attempting to hold her baby when it is brought to her room. However, in Asian extended families, members show their support for a new mother's rest and recuperation by assisting with the care of the baby. Contrary to the guidance that is sometimes given to mothers in the United States about exclusive breastfeeding, a mix of breastfeeding and bottle feeding is standard practice for Japanese mothers. This tradition is related to concern for the mother's rest during the first 2 to 3 months and does not usually lead to problems with lactation; breastfeeding is widespread and successful among Japanese women.

Cultural beliefs and values give perspective to the meaning of childbirth for a new mother. Nurses can provide an opportunity for a new mother to talk about her perception of the meaning of childbearing. In helping new families adjust to parenthood, nurses must provide culturally sensitive care by following principles that facilitate nursing practice within transcultural situations.

Socioeconomic Conditions

Socioeconomic conditions often determine access to available resources. Parents whose economic condition is made worse with the birth of each child and who are unable to use an effective method of fertility management can find birth complicated by concern for their own health and a sense of helplessness. Mothers who are single, separated, or divorced from their husbands or without a partner, family, and friends can view the birth of a child with dread. Serious financial problems can negatively affect mothering behaviors. Similarly, fathers who are overwhelmed with financial stresses may lack effective parenting skills and behaviors.

Personal Aspirations

For some women parenthood interferes with or blocks plans for personal freedom or career advancement. Unresolved resentment affects caregiving activities and adjustment to parenting. This situation can result in indifference and neglect of the infant or in excessive concerns; the mother may set impossibly high standards for her own behavior or the child's performance.

Nursing interventions include providing opportunities for mothers to express their feelings freely to an objective listener, to discuss measures to permit personal growth, and to learn about the care of their infant. Referring the woman to a support group of other mothers "in the same situation" may also be helpful.

Nurses can be proactive in influencing changes in work policies related to maternity and paternity leaves, varying models of work sharing and family-friendly work environments. Some corporations already structure their worksites to support new mothers (e.g., by providing on-site day care facilities and lactation rooms).

Parental Sensory Impairment

In early interactions between the parent and child, each one uses all senses—sight, hearing, touch, taste, and smell—to initiate and sustain the process of establishing a healthy parent-infant relationship. A parent who has an impairment of one or more of the senses needs to maximize use of the remaining senses. Mothers with disabilities tend to value the importance of performing parenting tasks in the perceived culturally usual way.

Visually Impaired Parent

Visual impairment alone does not seem to have a negative effect on early parenting experiences. These parents, just like sighted parents, express the wonders of parenthood and encourage other visually impaired people to become parents.

Although visually impaired parents can initially feel pressure to conform to traditional, sighted ways of parenting, they soon adapt and develop methods better suited to them. Examples of activities that visually impaired parents perform differently include preparation of the infant's nursery, clothes, and supplies. Some parents put an entire clothing outfit together and hang it in the closet rather than keeping items separate in drawers. Some develop a labeling system for the infant's clothing and place diapering, bathing, and other care supplies where they will be easy to locate.

BOX 22.2 Working With Visually Impaired Parents

- A visually impaired parent needs an orientation to the hospital room that allows him or her to move about the room independently. For example, "Go to the left of the bed and trail the wall until you feel the first door. That is the bathroom."
- Parents who are visually impaired need explanations of routines.
- Parents who are visually impaired need to feel devices (e.g., portable sitz bath equipment, breast pump) and to hear descriptions of the devices.
- Visually impaired parents need a chance to ask questions.
- Visually impaired parents need the opportunity to hold and touch the newborn after birth.
- Nurses need to demonstrate infant care by touch and to follow with, "Now show me how you would do it."
- Nurses need to give instructions such as, "I'm going to give you the baby. The head is to your left side."

BOX 22.3 Working With Hearing-Impaired Parents

- Before initiating communication, the nurse must be aware of the parents' preferences and capabilities: Does either or do both wear hearing aids? Do they read lips? Do they wish to have an interpreter?
- The nurse should make certain that the parent or parents see the nurse approaching to avoid startling them.
- Before speaking, the nurse must be directly in front of the parent and should have his or her full attention.
- When speaking, the nurse should face the parent directly and should be at the same level.
- It is best to avoid standing in front of a light or a window while speaking with the parent.
- Keep your hands away from your face while speaking to minimize distractions.
- If the parent relies on lip reading, the nurse should sit close enough that the parent can easily see his or her lip movements.
- The nurse should speak clearly with a regular voice volume and lip movements while also maintaining eye contact.
- The nurse should speak in short, simple sentences to facilitate understanding.
- If the parent does not understand something, it is better to find a different way to say what needs to be communicated rather than repeating the same words over and over.
- Written messages aid in communication. A small white or black erasable board can be useful.
- Educational materials should be given to hearing-impaired parents and they should be asked to read the materials prior to a teaching session. They can also refer to the materials after discharge.
- Visual aids such as pictures, diagrams, or other devices should be used during client teaching.
- When the nurse is doing parent teaching, it is helpful for a hearing person (partner or family member) to be present.
- The nurse should allow ample time to communicate with the hearing-impaired parent; being in a rush can evoke stress and create barriers to effective communication.

A strength that visually impaired parents have is a heightened sensitivity to other sensory outputs. Visually impaired parents can tell when their infant is facing them because they notice the baby's breath on their faces.

One of the major difficulties that visually impaired parents experience is the skepticism, open or hidden, of health care professionals. Visually impaired people may sense reluctance on the part of others to acknowledge that they have a right to be parents. All too often nurses and physicians lack the experience to deal with the childbearing and childrearing needs of visually impaired parents as well as parents with other disabilities, such as those who are hearing impaired or physically or mentally challenged. The nurse's best approach is to assess the parents' capabilities and to use that information as a basis for making plans to assist them, often in much the same way as for parents without impairments. Visually impaired mothers have made suggestions about providing care for women such as themselves during childbearing (Box 22.2). Such approaches can help avoid a sense of increased vulnerability on the parent's part. Materials for perinatal education are available in Braille.

Eye contact is important in most western cultures. With a parent who is visually impaired, this critical factor in the process of establishing and maintaining a healthy parent-child relationship is obviously missing. However, the blind parent, who may never have experienced this method of strengthening relationships, does not miss it. The infant will need other sensory input from that parent. An infant looking into the eyes of a parent who is blind can be unaware that the eyes are unseeing. Other people in the newborn's environment can also participate in active eye-to-eye contact to supply this need. A problem may arise, however, if the visually impaired parent has little facial expression. The infant, after making repeated unsuccessful attempts to engage in face play with the mother, will abandon that behavior and intensify it with the father or other people in the household. Nurses can provide anticipatory guidance regarding this situation and help the mother learn to nod and smile while talking and cooing to the infant.

Hearing Impaired Parent

A parent who has a hearing impairment faces challenges in caregiving and parenting, particularly if the deafness dates from birth or early childhood. Whether one or both parents are hearing impaired, they are likely to have established an independent household. Devices that transform sound into light flashes can be placed in the infant's room to permit immediate detection of crying. Even if the parent is not speech trained, vocalizing can serve as both a stimulus and a response to the infant's early vocalizing. Deaf parents can provide additional vocal training by use of recordings and television so that from birth the child is aware of the full range of the human voice. Young children acquire sign language readily, and the first sign used is as varied as the first word.

Section 504 of the Rehabilitation Act of 1973 requires that hospitals and other institutions receiving funds from the U.S. Department of Health and Human Services use various communication techniques and resources with the deaf, including having staff members or certified interpreters who are proficient in sign language. For example, provision of written materials with demonstrations and having nurses stand where the parent can read their lips (if the parent practices lip reading) are two techniques that can be used. A creative approach is for the nursing unit to develop videos in which information on postpartum care, infant care, and parenting issues is signed by an interpreter and spoken by a nurse. A video recording in which a nurse signs while speaking is ideal. With the advent of the Internet, many resources are available to deaf parents. Box 22.3 lists suggestions for working with hearing-impaired parents.

SIBLING ADAPTATION

Because the family is an interactive, open unit, the addition of a new family member affects everyone in the family. Siblings have to assume new positions within the family hierarchy. Parents often face the task of caring for the neonate while also attending to the needs of other children and attempting to distribute their attention equitably. When the newborn is preterm or has special needs, this task can be difficult.

Reactions of siblings result from temporary separation from the mother, changes in the mother's or father's behavior, or the infant coming home. Positive behavioral changes of siblings include interest in and concern for the baby and increased independence. Regression in toileting and sleep habits, aggression toward the baby, and increased seeking of attention and whining are examples of negative behaviors.

The parents' attitudes toward the arrival of the baby can set the stage for the other children's reactions. Because the baby absorbs the time and attention of the important people in the other children's lives, jealousy (**sibling rivalry**) is common once the initial excitement of having a new baby in the home is over.

Parents, especially mothers, spend much time and energy promoting sibling acceptance of a new baby. Sibling preparation classes can help children adjust. Older children may be actively involved in preparing for the infant, and this involvement can intensify after the birth. Parents have to manage the feeling of guilt that the older children are being deprived of parental time and attention and monitor the behavior of older children toward the more vulnerable infant and divert aggressive behavior. The Teaching for Self-Management box: Strategies for Facilitating Sibling Acceptance of a New Baby presents strategies that parents have used to facilitate sibling acceptance of a new baby.

TEACHING FOR SELF-MANAGEMENT

Strategies for Facilitating Sibling Acceptance of a New Baby

- Take your older child (or children) on a tour of your hospital room and point out similarities between this birth and his or her birth. "This is like the room I was in with you, and the baby is in the same kind of bassinet that you were in."
- Have a small gift from the baby to give to your older child each day he or she visits in the hospital.
- Give the older child a T-shirt that says "I'm a big brother" [or "sister"].
- Arrange for your children to be among the first to see the newborn. Let them hold the baby in the hospital.
- When the older child visits for the first time, make sure you are not holding the new baby. Your arms need to be open and available for the older child. Instruct the person accompanying the older child to call ahead or give a warning knock to give you time to lay the baby down or have someone else hold the baby.
- Plan individual time with each child. The father or partner can spend time with the older siblings while the mother is taking care of the baby and vice versa. Siblings like to have time and attention from both parents.
- Give preschool and early school-age siblings a newborn doll as "their baby." Give the sibling a photograph of the new baby to take to school to show off "his" or "her" baby. Older siblings may enjoy the responsibility of helping care for the newborn, such as learning how to give the baby a bottle or change a diaper. Remember to supervise interactions between the siblings and new baby.

Siblings demonstrate acquaintance behaviors with the newborn. The acquaintance process depends on the information given to the child before the baby is born and on the child's cognitive and developmental levels. At the first meeting, siblings typically begin by gazing at the newborn, and progress to touching as they feel comfortable (Fig. 22.9). The initial adjustment of older children to a newborn takes time, and parents should allow children to interact at their own pace rather than forcing them to interact. To expect a young child to accept and love a rival for the parents' affection assumes an unrealistic level of maturity. Sibling love grows as does other love, that

is, by being with another person and sharing experiences. The bond between siblings involves a secure base in which one child provides support for the other, is missed when absent, and is looked to for comfort and security.

GRANDPARENT ADAPTATION

Becoming a grandparent or a great-grandparent is most often associated with great joy and happiness (Fig. 22.10). Yet it is a time of transition as roles and relationships change and new opportunities arise. Emotions are varied and can change from day to day; feelings of joy, anticipation, and excitement are often intermingled with some degree of anxiety and uncertainty. Circumstances surrounding the pregnancy and birth influence the feelings, reactions, and responses of grandparents.

Pregnancy and birth necessitate redefining intergenerational roles and relationships within the family. A primary role of the grandparents is to support, nurture, and empower their children in the parenting role. Grandparents must acknowledge that things have changed since

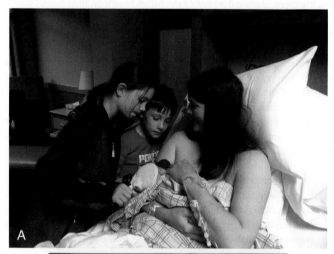

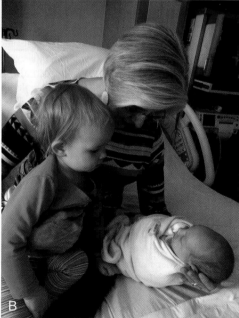

Fig. 22.9 First Meeting. (A) School-age sister and brother visit their mother and newborn brother soon after birth. (B) Younger (2-year-old) sister examines newborn with grandmother's help. (Courtesy Allison and Matthew Wyatt, Eagle, CO.)

they first became parents as they deal with changes in practices and attitudes toward pregnancy, birth, childrearing, and men's and women's roles at home and in the workplace. The degree to which grandparents understand and accept current practices can influence how supportive they are to their adult children.

At the same time that they are adjusting to grandparenthood, many grandparents are experiencing typical life transitions and events, such as retirement and a move to smaller housing, and they may need support from their adult children. Some may feel regret about their limited involvement because of poor health or geographic distance.

The extent of grandparent involvement in the care of the newborn depends on many factors such as the willingness to become involved, the proximity of the grandparents, and cultural expectations of the grandparents' role. For example, if the new parents live in the United States, Asian grandparents will typically come to the United States to care for the baby and the mother after birth and to care for the children once the parents return to work.

Relationships between grandparents and parents can change with the birth of a new baby. For first-time parents, pregnancy and parenthood can reawaken old issues related to dependence versus independence. Couples often do not plan on their parents' help immediately after the baby arrives. They want time "to be a family," implying a couple-baby unit, not the intergenerational family network. Contrary to their expectations, however, new parents do call on their parents for help, especially the maternal grandmother. Many grandparents are aware of their adult children's wishes for autonomy, respect these wishes, and remain available to help when asked.

Grandparenting classes can be used to bridge the generation gap and to help the grandparents understand their adult children's parenting concepts. The classes include information on up-to-date childbearing practices; family-centered care; infant care, feeding, and safety (car seats); and exploration of roles that grandparents play in the family unit.

Increasing numbers of grandparents are providing permanent care for their grandchildren as a result of divorce, substance abuse, child abuse or neglect, abandonment, teenage pregnancy, death, human immunodeficiency virus and acquired immunodeficiency syndrome, unemployment, incarceration, and mental health problems. This emerging trend requires the nurse to evaluate the role of the grandparent in parenting the infant. Educational and financial considerations must be addressed and available support systems identified for these families.

CARE MANAGEMENT

Numerous changes occur during the first weeks of parenthood. As parents prepare for discharge from the birth facility (Fig. 22.11), nursing care management should be directed toward helping parents cope with infant care, role changes, altered lifestyle, and change in family structure resulting from the addition of a new baby. Developing skill and confidence in caring for an infant can be anxiety-provoking. Anticipatory guidance can help prevent a shock of reality in the transition from hospital or birthing center to home that might negate the parents' joy or cause them undue stress.

Through education, support, and encouragement, nurses are instrumental in assisting mothers and their partners in the transition to parenthood, whether they are first-time parents or the parents of several other children. Early and ongoing assessment and intervention promotes positive outcomes for parents, infants, and family members (see Nursing Care Plan).

In collaboration with the family, incorporating their priorities and preferences to meet their specific needs, nurses can:

- Talk about opportunities for parent-infant interaction in the daily routine—feeding, bathing, diaper changing, putting in the car seat, etc.
- Implement strategies to facilitate sibling acceptance of the infant (see Teaching for Self-Management box: Strategies for Facilitating Sibling Acceptance of a New Baby).
- Provide practical suggestions for infant care (see Chapter 24).
- Provide anticipatory guidance on what to expect as the infant grows and develops including sleep-wake cycles, interpretation of infant behaviors, quieting techniques, infant developmental milestones, sensory enrichment/infant stimulation, recognizing signs of illness, well-baby follow-up and immunizations.
- Provide positive reinforcement for loving and nurturing behaviors with the infant.
- Closely monitor parents who interact in inappropriate or abusive ways with their infants, and notify an appropriate mental health practitioner or professional social worker.

While the nurse may be able to evaluate the effectiveness of some interventions before the mother and infant are discharged from the hospital, ongoing evaluation is needed. This is likely to be done by the infant's primary health care provider in follow-up visits.

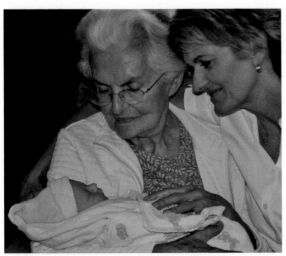

Fig. 22.10 Great-Grandmother and Grandmother get Acquainted with Newborn. (Courtesy Barbara Wilson, West Jordan, UT.)

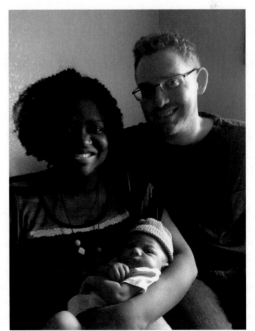

Fig. 22.11 A New Mother and Father Ready to Take Their Newborn Home. (Courtesy Diane Ortega, CNM, Mesa, AZ.)

NURSING CARE PLAN

Transition to Parenthood

Client Problem	Expected Outcome	Interventions	Rationales
Lack of knowledge about infant care related to inexperience	Parents provide safe and adequate care, and infant appears healthy.	Observe infant care routines (bathing, diapering, feeding, play).	To evaluate parental ease with care and adequacy of techniques
		Observe infant's appearance (height-weight ratio, head circumference, fontanels, skin tone and turgor), and assess vital signs, overall tone, reflexes, and age-appropriate developmental skills.	To evaluate for signs indicative of inadequate care
		Explore available support systems for infant care.	To determine adequacy of existing system
		Provide ongoing follow-up and referrals as needed.	To ensure that identified potential and actual care deficits are addressed and resolved
Lack of sleep related to infant demands and environmental interruptions	Woman sleeps for uninterrupted periods and states that she feels rested upon waking.	Assess sleeping patterns, and identify factors that interfere with sleep.	To determine scope of problem and direct interventions
		Explore ways woman and significant others can make environment more conducive to sleep (e.g., privacy, darkness, quiet, back rubs, soothing music, warm milk); teach use of guided imagery and relaxation techniques; eliminate factors or routines that can interfere with sleep (e.g., caffeine, foods that induce heartburn, strenuous mental or physical activity); limit visitors; mother should sleep when the baby sleeps.	To promote optimal conditions for sleep
		Help family to identify persons such as family members or friends who can help with household tasks, infant care, and care of other children.	To allow mother more time to rest
Risk for difficulty incorporating newborn into current family situation	Family members adapt satisfactorily to having newborn in the home.	Explore with family ways that birth and neonate have changed family structure and function.	To evaluate functional and role adjustment
		Observe family's interaction with newborn, and note degree of bonding, evidence of sibling rivalry, and involvement in newborn care.	To evaluate acceptance of newest family member
		Clarify identified misinformation and misconceptions and assist family in exploring options for solutions to identified problems.	To promote clear communication and effective problem resolution
		If needed, make referrals to appropriate social services or community agencies.	To ensure ongoing support and care

COMMUNITY ACTIVITY

- Visit the website of a hospital that provides maternity services in your community. Does the hospital offer prepared childbirth, parenting, sibling or infant/child cardiorespiratory resuscitation (CPR) classes? Are group tours of the birthing center provided for expectant parents?
- Visit the website babycenter.com. Review the information about postpartum emotional health, causes and treatments of baby blues, and baby blues versus PPD. Examine the same topics on the National Institute of Mental Health website: https://www.nimh.nih.gov/health/publications/postpartum-depression-facts/index-.shtml. Compare the information on the two sites.

KEY POINTS

- The birth of a child necessitates changes in the existing interactional structure of a family.
- Good-quality parent-infant relationship is essential to children's development, and the earliest experiences are crucial to establish this early foundation for success.
- The parent-infant bond is the formation of an intense emotional connection between a mother and her infant.
- Security of parent-infant attachment is strengthened through a parent's establishment of a secure base and safe haven from distress for the infant.
- Women go through predictable stages in becoming a mother.
- Many mothers exhibit signs of postpartum blues (baby blues).
- Fathers experience emotions and adjustments during the transition to parenthood that are similar to and also distinctly different from those of mothers.

KEY POINTS—CONT'D

- Modulation of rhythm, modification of behavioral repertoires, and mutual responsivity facilitate infant-parent adjustment.
- Examples of factors that influence adaptation to parenthood include age, culture, socioeconomic level, and expectations of what the child will be like.
- A parent who has a sensory impairment must maximize use of the remaining senses.

- Sibling adjustment to a new baby requires creative parental interventions.
- Grandparents can have a positive influence on the postpartum family.
- Nurses play a major role in educating and supporting new parents in the transition to parenthood.

REFERENCES

Ainsworth, M., Blehar, M., Waters, B., & Wall, S. (1978). *Patterns of attachment: A psychological study of the strange situation*. Hillsdale, N.J.: Lawrence Erlbaum Associates.

American College of Obstetricians and Gynecologists. (2012, reaffirmed 2018). Committee opinion no. 525: Health care for lesbians and bisexual women. *Obstetrics & Gynecology*, 119(5), 1077–1080.

American College of Obstetricians and Gynecologists. (2018). Committee opinion no. 757: Screening for perinatal depression. *Obstetrics & Gynecology*, 132(5), e208–e212.

Barnard, K., Hammond, M., Booth, C., et al. (1989). *Measurement and meaning of parent-child interaction*. San Diego, CA: In Academic Press.

Bartlett, J. D., & Easterbrooks, M. A. (2015). The moderating effect of relationships on intergenerational risk for infant neglect by young mothers. *Child Abuse and Neglect, 45*, 21–34.

Bowlby, J. (1969). *Attachment and loss* (Vol. 1). New York: Basic Books.

Cao, H., Mills-Koonce, W. R., Wood, C., & Fine, M. A. (2016). Identity transformation during the transition to parenthood among same-sex couples: An ecological, stress-strategy-adaptation perspective. *Journal of Family Theory and Review, 8*, 30–59.

Cassibba, R., Castoro, G., Costantino, E., et al. (2015). Enhancing maternal sensitivity and infant attachment security with video feedback: An exploratory study in Italy. *Infant Mental Health Journal, 36*(1), 53–61.

Center on the Developing Child at Harvard University. (2016). *From best practices to breakthrough impacts: A science-based approach to building a more promising future for young children and families*. Boston, MA: Harvard University. Retrieved from http://www.developingchild.harvard.edu.

Chin, R., Hall, P., & Daiches, A. (2011). Fathers' experiences of their transition to fatherhood: A metasynthesis. *Journal of Reproductive & Infant Psychology, 29*(1), 4–18.

Cook, S. C., Gunter, K. E., & Lopez, F. Y. (2017). Establishing effective health care partnerships with sexual and gender minority patients: Recommendations for obstetrician gynecologists. *Seminars in Reproductive Medicine, 35*(5), 397–407.

Davidson, J. E., Aslakson, R. A., Long, A. C., et al. (2017). Guidelines for family-centered care in the neonatal, pediatric, and adult ICU. *Critical Care Medicine, 45*(1), 103–128.

Easterbrooks, M., Kotake, A., Raskin, C., & Bumgarner, M. (2016). Patterns of depression among adolescent mothers: Resilience related to father support and home visiting program. *American Journal of Orthopsychiatry, 86*(1), 61–68.

Farr, R. H., & Tornello, S. L. (2016). The transition to parenthood and early child development in families with same-sex parents. *Journal of Birth and Parent Education, 3*(3), 9–14.

Feinberg, M. E., Jones, D. E., Hostetler, M. L., et al. (2016). Couple-focused prevention at the transition to parenthood, a randomized trial: Effects on coparenting, parenting, family violence, and parent and child adjustment. *Prevention Science, 17*(6), 751–764.

Field, T. (2017). Newborn massage therapy. *International Journal of Pediatrics and Neonatal Health, 1*(2), 54–64.

Galanti, C. A. (2015). *Caring for patients from different cultures* (5th ed.). Philadelphia: University of Pennsylvania Press.

Garfield, C. F. (2015). Supporting fatherhood before and after it happens. *Pediatrics, 135*(2), e528–e530.

Goodman, J. (2005). Becoming an involved father of an infant. *Journal of Obstetric, Gynecologic and Neonatal Nursing, 34*(2), 190–200.

Hodgkinson, S., Beers, L., Southammakosane, C., & Lewin, A. (2014). Addressing the mental health needs of pregnant and pareanting adolescents. *Pediatrics, 133*(1), 114–122.

Isley, M. M., & Katz, V. L. (2017). Postpartum care and long-term health considerations. In S. G. Gabbe, J. R. Neibyl, J. L. Simpson, et al. (Eds.), *Obstetrics: Normal and problem pregnancies* (7th ed.). Philadelphia: Elsevier.

Jeha, D., Usta, I., Ghulmiyyah, L., & Nassar, A. (2015). A review of the risks and consequences of adolescent pregnancy. *Journal of Neonatal and Perinatal Medicine, 8*(1), 1–8.

Kilpatrick, S., & Garrison, E. (2017). Normal labor and delivery. In S. G. Gabbe, J. R. Niebyl, J. L. Simpson, et al. (Eds.), *Obstetrics: Normal and problem pregnancies* (7th ed.). Philadelphia: Elsevier.

King, T. L., & Pinger, W. (2014). Evidence-based practice for intrapartum care: The pearls of midwifery. *Journal of Midwifery and Women's Health, 59*(6), 572–585.

Klaus, M., & Kennell, J. (1976). *Maternal-infant bonding*. St. Louis: Mosby.

Klaus, M., & Kennell, J. (1982). *Parent-infant bonding* (2nd ed.). St. Louis: Mosby.

Lawrence, R. M., & Lawrence, R. A. (2016). *Breastfeeding: A guide for the medical profession* (8th ed.). St. Louis: Elsevier.

Letourneau, N., Secco, L., Colpitts, J., et al. (2015). Quasi–experimental evaluation of a telephone–based peer support intervention for maternal depression. *Journal of Advanced Nursing, 71*(7), 1587–1599.

Letourneau, N., Tryphonopoulos, P., Giesbrecht, G., et al. (2015). Narrative and meta-analytic review of interventions aiming to improve maternal-child attachment security. *Infant Mental Health Journal, 36*(4), 366–387.

Macutkiewicz, J., & MacBeth, A. (2017). Intended adolescent pregnancy: A systematic review of qualitative studies. *Adolescent Research Reviews, 2*, 113–119.

Meighan, M. (2017). *Maternal role attainment—Becoming a mother*. Nursing Theorists and Their Work-E-Book, 432.

Mercer, R. (2004). Becoming a mother versus maternal role attainment. *Journal of Nursing Scholarship, 36*(3), 226–232.

Mercer, R., & Walker, L. (2006). A review of nursing interventions to foster becoming a mother. *Journal of Obstetric, Gynecologic and Neonatal Nursing, 35*(5), 568–582.

Moore, E. R., Bergman, N., Anderson, G. C., & Medley, N. (2016). Early skin-to-skin contact for mothers and their healthy newborn infants. *Cochrane Database of Systematic Reviews, 11*, CD003519.

Pérez–Escamilla, R., Martinez, J. L., & Segura–Pérez, S. (2016). Impact of the Baby–friendly Hospital Initiative on breastfeeding and child health outcomes: a systematic review. *Maternal & Child Nutrition, 12*(3), 402–417.

Pinzon, J. L., Jones, V. F., Committee on Adolescence, & Committee on Early Childhood. (2012). Care of adolescent parents and their children. *Pediatrics, 130*(6), e1743–e1756.

Rubin, R. (1961). Basic maternal behavior. *Nursing Outlook, 9*(11), 683–686.

Scism, A. R., & Cobb, R. L. (2017). Integrative review of factors and interventions that influence early father-infant bonding. *Journal of Obstetric, Gynecologic and Neonatal Nursing, 46*(2), 163–170.

Shaver, J. L. F. (2015). Promoting healthy sleep. In E. F. Olshansky (Ed.), *Women's health and wellness across the lifespan*. Philadelphia: Wolters Kluwer.

Shorey, S., Dennis, C. L., Bridge, S., et al. (2017). First–time fathers' postnatal experiences and support needs: A descriptive qualitative study. *Journal of Advanced Nursing, 73*(12), 2987–2996.

Stewart, L. S., & Rodgers, E. (2017). Assessment and care of the term newborn transitioning to extrauterine life. In B. B. Kennedy, & S. M. Baird (Eds.), *Intrapartum management modules: A perinatal education program* (5th ed.). Philadelphia, Wolters Kluwer.

Thomas, J. C., Letourneau, N., Bryce, C. I., et al. (2017). Biological embedding of perinatal social relationships in infant stress reactivity. *Developmental Psychobiology, 59*(4), 425–435.

Thompson, G., & Canadian Paediatric Society. (2016). *Meeting the needs of adolescent parents and their children Paediatric and Child Health, 21*(5), 273.

Tokhi, M., Comrie-Thomson, L., Davis, J., et al. (2018). Involving men to improve maternal and newborn health: A systematic review of the effectiveness of interventions. *PLoS One, 13*(1), e0191620.

Tomfohr, L. M., Buliga, E., Letourneau, N. L., et al. (2015). Trajectories of sleep quality and associations with mood during the perinatal period. *Sleep, 38*(8), 1237–1245.

Widarsson, M., Engström, G., Tydén, T., et al. (2015). 'Paddling upstream': Fathers' involvement during pregnancy as described by expectant fathers and mothers. *Journal of Clinical Nursing, 24*(7-8), 1059–1068.

World Health Organization. (2018). *Adolescent pregnancy*. Retrieved from: www.whoint/mediacentre/factsheets/fs364/en/.

Physiologic and Behavioral Adaptations of the Newborn

Kathryn Rhodes Alden

LEARNING OBJECTIVES

- Analyze the physiologic adaptations the neonate must make to successfully transition to the extrauterine environment.
- Describe behavioral adaptations that are characteristic of the newborn during the transition period.
- Explain mechanisms of thermoregulation in the neonate and potential consequences of hypothermia and hyperthermia.
- Describe newborn reflexes and differentiate normal from abnormal responses.
- Discuss the sensory and perceptual functioning of the neonate.
- Interpret signs in each body system that indicate that the neonate may be at risk.

The neonatal period includes the time from birth through day 28 of life. During this time, the neonate or newborn must make many physiologic and behavioral adaptations to extrauterine life. Physiologic adjustment tasks are those that involve: (1) establishing and maintaining respirations; (2) adjusting to circulatory changes; (3) regulating temperature; (4) ingesting, retaining, and digesting nutrients; (5) eliminating waste; and (6) regulating weight. Behavioral tasks include: (1) establishing a regulated behavioral tempo independent of the mother, which involves self-regulating arousal, self-monitoring changes in state, and patterning sleep; (2) processing, storing, and organizing multiple stimuli; and (3) establishing a relationship with caregivers and the environment. The term infant usually makes these adjustments with little or no difficulty. This chapter describes the physiologic and behavioral adaptations required by the neonate for transition to extrauterine life.

STAGES OF TRANSITION TO EXTRAUTERINE LIFE

The major adaptations associated with transition from intrauterine to extrauterine life occur during the first 6 to 8 hours after birth. The predictable series of events during transition are mediated by the sympathetic nervous system and result in changes that involve heart rate, respirations, temperature, and gastrointestinal (GI) function. This transition period represents a time of vulnerability for the newborn and warrants careful observation. To detect disorders in adaptation soon after birth, nurses must be aware of normal features of the transition period.

In their classic work on newborn adaptation to extrauterine life, Desmond, Rudolph, and Phitaksphraiwan (1966) proposed three stages of newborn transition. The stages are still considered valid. The first stage of the transition period lasts up to 30 minutes after birth and is called the *first period of reactivity*. The newborn's heart rate increases rapidly to 160 to 180 beats/min but gradually falls after 30 minutes or so to a baseline rate of 100 to 120 beats/min. Respirations are irregular, with a rate between 60 and 80 breaths/min. Fine crackles can be heard on auscultation. Audible grunting, nasal flaring, and retractions of the chest also can be present, but these should cease within the first hour after birth. The infant is alert and may have spontaneous startles, tremors, crying, and head movement from side to side. Bowel sounds are audible, and meconium may be passed.

After the first period of reactivity, the newborn either sleeps or has a marked decrease in motor activity. This *period of decreased responsiveness* lasts from 60 to 100 minutes. During this time the infant is pink, and respirations are rapid (up to 60 breaths/min) and shallow but unlabored. Bowel sounds are audible, and peristaltic waves may be noted over the rounded abdomen.

The *second period of reactivity* occurs approximately between 2 and 8 hours after birth and lasts from 10 minutes to several hours. Brief periods of tachycardia and tachypnea occur, associated with increased muscle tone, changes in skin color, and mucus production. Meconium is commonly passed at this time. Most healthy newborns experience this transition, regardless of gestational age or type of birth; very preterm infants do not because of physiologic immaturity.

PHYSIOLOGIC ADAPTATIONS

Respiratory System

As the infant emerges from the intrauterine environment and the umbilical cord is clamped and severed, profound adaptations are necessary for survival. The most critical of these is the establishment of effective respirations. Most newborns breathe spontaneously after birth and are able to maintain adequate oxygenation. Preterm infants often encounter respiratory difficulties related to their immature lungs.

Initiation of Breathing

During intrauterine life, oxygenation of the fetus occurs through transplacental gas exchange. At birth, the lungs must be established as the site of gas exchange. In utero, fetal blood was shunted away from the lungs, but when birth occurs the pulmonary vasculature must be fully perfused for this purpose. Clamping the umbilical cord causes a rise in blood pressure (BP), which increases circulation and lung perfusion.

There is no single trigger for newborn respiratory function. The initiation of respirations in the neonate is the result of a combination of chemical, mechanical, thermal, and sensory factors (Blackburn, 2018).

Chemical factors. The activation of chemoreceptors in the carotid arteries and aorta results from the relative state of hypoxia associated with labor. With each labor contraction there is a temporary decrease in uterine blood flow and transplacental gas exchange, resulting in transient fetal hypoxia and hypercarbia. Although the fetus is able to recover between contractions, there appears to be a cumulative effect that results in progressive decline in PO_2, increased PCO_2, and lowered blood pH. Decreased levels of oxygen and increased levels of carbon dioxide seem to have a cumulative effect that is involved in initiating neonatal breathing by stimulating the respiratory center in the medulla. Another chemical factor may also play a role; it is thought that as a result of clamping the cord, there is a drop in levels of a prostaglandin that can inhibit respirations.

Mechanical factors. Respirations in the newborn can be stimulated by changes in intrathoracic pressure resulting from compression of the chest during vaginal birth. As the infant passes through the birth canal, the chest is compressed. With birth this pressure on the chest is released, and the negative intrathoracic pressure helps to draw air into the lungs. Crying increases the distribution of air in the lungs and promotes expansion of the alveoli. The positive pressure created by crying helps to keep the alveoli open.

Thermal factors. With birth the newborn enters the extrauterine environment in which the temperature is significantly lower. The profound change in environmental temperature stimulates receptors in the skin, resulting in stimulation of the respiratory center in the medulla.

Sensory factors. Sensory stimulation occurs in a variety of ways at birth. Some of these include handling by the obstetric health care provider, suctioning the mouth and nose, and drying by the nurses. Environmental factors (lights, sounds, smells) stimulate the respiratory center.

Establishing Respiration

At term the lungs hold approximately 20 mL of fluid per kilogram. Air must be substituted for the fluid that filled the fetal respiratory tract. Traditionally it had been thought that the thoracic squeeze occurring during normal vaginal birth resulted in significant clearance of lung fluid. However, it appears that this event plays a minor role. In the days preceding labor, there is reduced production of fetal lung fluid and concomitant decreased alveolar fluid volume. Shortly before the onset of labor, there is a catecholamine surge that seems to promote fluid clearance from the lungs, which continues during labor. The movement of lung fluid from the air spaces occurs through active transport into the interstitium, with drainage occurring through the pulmonary circulation and lymphatic system. Retention of lung fluid can interfere with the infant's ability to maintain adequate oxygenation, especially if other factors that compromise respirations (e.g., meconium aspiration, congenital diaphragmatic hernia, esophageal atresia with fistula, choanal atresia, congenital cardiac defect, immature alveoli) are present. Infants born by cesarean in which labor did not occur before birth can experience some lung fluid retention, although it typically clears without harmful effects on the infant. These infants are also more likely to develop transient tachypnea of the newborn (TTN) (Fraser, 2015).

The alveoli of the term infant's lungs are lined with **surfactant**, a lipoprotein manufactured in type II lung cells. Lung expansion depends largely on chest wall contraction and adequate surfactant secretion. Surfactant lowers surface tension, therefore reducing the pressure required to keep the alveoli open with inspiration, and prevents total alveolar collapse on exhalation, thereby maintaining alveolar stability. The decreased surface tension results in increased lung compliance, helping to establish the functional residual capacity of the lungs (Blackburn, 2018). With absent or decreased surfactant, more pressure must be generated for inspiration, which can soon tire or exhaust preterm or sick term infants.

Breathing movements that began in utero as intermittent become continuous after birth, although the mechanism for this is not well understood. Once respirations are established, breaths are shallow and irregular, ranging from 30 to 60 breaths/min, with periods of breathing that include pauses in respirations lasting less than 20 seconds. These episodes of periodic breathing occur most often during the active (rapid eye movement [REM]) sleep cycle and decrease in frequency and duration with age. Apneic periods longer than 20 seconds are abnormal and should be evaluated.

Newborn infants are by preference nose breathers, which enhances the ability to coordinate sucking, swallowing, and breathing. The reflex response to nasal obstruction is to open the mouth to maintain an airway. This response is not present in most infants until 3 weeks after birth; therefore cyanosis or asphyxia can occur with nasal blockage.

In most newborns, auscultation of the chest reveals loud, clear breath sounds that seem very near because little chest tissue intervenes. Breath sounds should be clear and equal bilaterally, although fine rales for the first few hours are not unusual. The ribs of the infant articulate with the spine at a horizontal rather than a downward slope; consequently, the rib cage cannot expand with inspiration as readily as that of an adult. Because neonatal respiratory function is largely a matter of diaphragmatic contraction, abdominal breathing is characteristic of newborns. The newborn infant's chest and abdomen rise simultaneously with inspiration.

Signs of Respiratory Distress

Signs of respiratory distress can include nasal flaring, intercostal or subcostal retractions (in-drawing of tissue between the ribs or below the rib cage), or grunting with respirations. Suprasternal or subclavicular retractions with stridor or gasping most often represent an upper airway obstruction. Seesaw or paradoxic respirations (exaggerated rise in abdomen with respiration as the chest falls) instead of abdominal respirations are abnormal and should be reported. A respiratory rate of less than 30 or greater than 60 breaths/min with the infant at rest must be evaluated. The respiratory rate of the infant can be slowed, depressed, or absent as a result of the effects of analgesics or anesthetics administered to the mother during labor and birth. Apneic episodes can be related to events such as rapid increase in body temperature, hypothermia, hypoglycemia, or sepsis. Tachypnea can result from inadequate clearance of lung fluid, or it can be an indication of respiratory distress syndrome (RDS). Tachypnea can be the first sign of respiratory, cardiac, metabolic, or infectious illnesses (Gardner, Enzman-Hines, & Nyp, 2016).

Changes in the infant's color can indicate respiratory distress. Normally, within the first 3 to 5 minutes after birth, the newborn's color changes from blue to pink. **Acrocyanosis**, the bluish discoloration of hands and feet, is a normal finding in the first 24 hours after birth. Transient periods of duskiness while crying are common immediately after birth; however, central cyanosis is abnormal and signifies hypoxemia. With central cyanosis, the lips and mucous membranes are bluish (*circumoral cyanosis*). It can be the result of inadequate delivery of oxygen to the alveoli, poor perfusion of the lungs that inhibits gas exchange, or cardiac dysfunction. Because central cyanosis is a late sign of distress, newborns usually have significant hypoxemia when cyanosis appears.

Infants who experience mild TTN often have signs of respiratory distress during the first 1 to 2 hours after birth as they transition to extrauterine life. Tachypnea with rates up to 100 breaths/min can be present along with intermittent grunting, nasal flaring, and mild retractions. Supplemental oxygen may be needed. TTN usually resolves in 48 to 72 hours (Blackburn, 2018).

In neonates with more serious respiratory problems, symptoms of distress are more pronounced and tend to last beyond the first 2 hours after birth. Respiratory rates can exceed 120 breaths/min. Moderate to severe retractions, grunting, pallor, and central cyanosis can occur. The respiratory symptoms can be accompanied by hypotension, temperature instability, hypoglycemia, acidosis, and signs of cardiac problems. Common respiratory complications affecting neonates include RDS, meconium aspiration, pneumonia, and persistent pulmonary hypertension of the newborn (PPHN). Congenital defects such as anomalies of the great vessels, diaphragmatic hernia, or chest wall defects can cause severe respiratory problems. Blood incompatibilities such as hydrops fetalis can result in respiratory compromise (Gardner, Enzman-Hines, & Nyp, 2016) (see Chapter 36).

Cardiovascular System

The cardiovascular system changes significantly after birth. The infant's first breaths, combined with increased alveolar capillary distention, inflate the lungs and reduce pulmonary vascular resistance to pulmonary blood flow from the pulmonary arteries. Pulmonary artery pressure drops, and pressure in the right atrium declines. Increased pulmonary blood flow from the left side of the heart increases pressure in the left atrium, which causes a functional closure of the foramen ovale. During the first few days of life, crying can temporarily reverse the flow through the foramen ovale and lead to mild cyanosis. Soon after birth, cardiac output nearly doubles and blood flow increases to the lungs, heart, kidneys, and GI tract.

In utero, fetal PO_2 is 20 to 30 mm Hg. After birth, when the PO_2 level in the arterial blood approximates 50 mm Hg, the ductus arteriosus constricts in response to increased oxygenation. Circulating prostaglandin E_2 (PGE_2) levels also have an important role in closing the ductus arteriosus. In term infants, it functionally closes within the first 24 hours after birth; permanent (anatomic) closure usually occurs within 2 to 3 months, and the ductus arteriosus becomes a ligament. The ductus arteriosus can reopen in response to low oxygen levels in association with hypoxia, asphyxia, prolonged crying, or pathologic problems. With auscultation of the chest, a patent ductus arteriosus can be detected as a heart murmur (Blackburn, 2018).

When the cord is clamped and severed, the umbilical arteries, umbilical vein, and ductus venosus are functionally closed; they are converted into ligaments within 2 to 3 months. The hypogastric arteries also occlude and become ligaments.

Heart Rate and Sounds

The heart rate for a term newborn ranges from 120 to 160 beats/min, with brief fluctuations greater and less than these values usually noted during sleeping and waking states. The range of the heart rate in the term infant is approximately 80 to 100 beats/min during deep sleep and can increase to 180 beats/min or higher when the infant cries. A heart rate that is either high (more than 160 beats/min) or low (fewer than 100 beats/min) should be reevaluated within 30 minutes to 1 hour or when the activity of the infant changes.

The apical impulse (point of maximal impulse [PMI]) in the newborn is at the fourth intercostal space and to the left of the midclavicular line. The PMI is often visible and easily palpable because of the thin chest wall; this is also called *precordial activity*.

Irregular heart rate or sinus dysrhythmia is common in the first few hours of life but thereafter may need to be evaluated. Heart sounds during the neonatal period are of higher pitch, shorter duration, and greater intensity than during adult life. The first sound (S_1) is typically louder and duller than the second sound (S_2), which is sharp. The third and fourth heart sounds are not audible in newborns. Most heart murmurs heard during the neonatal period have no pathologic significance, and more than one-half of the murmurs disappear by 6 months of age. However, the presence of a murmur and accompanying signs such as poor feeding, apnea, cyanosis, or pallor is considered abnormal and should be investigated. There can be significant cardiac defects without a murmur or other symptoms. This reinforces the importance of ongoing assessment.

Blood Pressure

The primary factors affecting BP are gestational age, postconceptional age, and birth weight (Flynn, 2017). BP values rise as these variables increase. Cuff size, state of alertness, and movement also affect BP measurement. Hospitals and health care providers can compare infant BP measurements with available nomograms and tables to determine if values are within expected parameters. The mean arterial pressure (MAP) should be nearly equivalent to the weeks of gestation. For example, an infant born at 40 weeks of gestation should have a MAP of at least 40. The BP increases predictably over the first 5 days of life and then levels off, with minor variations noted during the first month of life. A drop in systolic BP (approximately 15 mm Hg) in the first hour of life is common. Expected values for BP (systolic/diastolic) in a term infant are (www.fpnotebook.com):

At birth: 75–95/37–55

12 hours: 50–70/25–45

96 hours: 60–90/20–60

Blood Volume

Blood volume in the term newborn ranges from 80 to 100 mL/kg of body weight. In the preterm infant, the range is 90 to 105 mL/kg (Diehl-Jones & Fraser, 2015). The preterm infant has a relatively greater blood volume than the term newborn. This occurs because the preterm infant has a proportionately greater plasma volume, not a greater red blood cell (RBC) mass.

Delayed clamping of the umbilical cord changes the circulatory dynamics of the newborn. Delayed cord clamping (DCC) expands the blood volume from the so-called *placental transfusion* of blood to the newborn by as much as 100 mL, depending on the length of time to cord clamping and cutting. DCC has been associated with increased blood volume and BP and reduced risk for intraventricular hemorrhage and necrotizing enterocolitis (Perlman, Wyllie, Kattwinkel, et al., 2015). These benefits are most important for preterm infants. Polycythemia that occurs with delayed clamping is usually not harmful, although there can be an increased risk for hyperbilirubinemia that requires phototherapy. The American College of Obstetricians and Gynecologists (ACOG, 2018) and the American Academy of Pediatrics (AAP, 2017) recommend that DCC is practiced whenever possible. DCC is reasonable for term and preterm newborns who do not need resuscitation; there is a lack of evidence regarding DCC for neonates who require immediate resuscitation (Perlman et al.).

Signs of Cardiovascular Problems

Variations in vital signs can be indicative of cardiovascular problems. Persistent tachycardia (more than 160 beats/min) can be associated with anemia, hypovolemia, hyperthermia, or sepsis. Persistent bradycardia (less than 80 beats/min) can be a sign of a congenital heart block or hypoxemia. Unequal or absent pulses, bounding pulses, and decreased or elevated BP can indicate cardiovascular problems (Verklan, 2015).

The newborn's skin color can reflect cardiovascular problems. Pallor in the immediate postbirth period is often a sign of underlying problems such as anemia or marked peripheral vasoconstriction as a result of intrapartum asphyxia or sepsis. Cyanosis other than in the hands or feet, with or without increased work of breathing, can indicate respiratory and/or cardiac problems. The presence of jaundice can indicate ABO or Rh factor incompatibility problems (see Chapter 36).

Congenital heart defects are the most common types of congenital malformations (Centers for Disease Control and Prevention [CDC], 2018) (see Chapter 36). Although the more serious defects such as tetralogy of Fallot are likely to have clinical manifestations such as cyanosis, dyspnea, and hypoxia, others such as small ventricular septal defects can be asymptomatic. The prenatal history can provide information regarding risk factors for congenital heart defects so the nurse knows to be more alert for symptoms. Maternal illness such as rubella, metabolic disease such as diabetes, and maternal drug ingestion are associated with an increased risk for cardiac defects.

Hematologic System

Red Blood Cells

Because fetal circulation is less efficient at oxygen exchange than the lungs, the fetus needs additional RBCs for transport of oxygen in utero. Therefore at birth the average levels of RBCs, hemoglobin, and hematocrit are higher than those in the adult; these levels fall slowly over the first month. At birth, the RBC count ranges from 4.6 to 5.2 million/mm^3 (Blackburn, 2018). The term newborn can have a hemoglobin concentration of 14 to 24 g/dL at birth, decreasing gradually to 12 to 20 g/dL during the first 2 weeks (Pagana, Pagana, & Pagana, 2017). Hematocrit at birth ranges from 51% to 56%, increases slightly in the first few hours or days as fluid shifts from intravascular to interstitial spaces (Blackburn, 2018), and by 8 weeks is between 39% and 59% (Pagana et al.). Polycythemia (central venous hematocrit greater than 65%) can occur in term and preterm infants as a result of DCC, maternal hypertension or diabetes, or intrauterine growth restriction.

The source of the sample is a significant factor in levels of RBCs, hemoglobin, and hematocrit. Capillary blood yields higher values than venous blood.

The timing of blood sampling is also significant; the slight rise in RBCs after birth is followed by a substantial drop. At birth the infant's blood contains an average of 70% fetal hemoglobin; however, because of the shorter life span of the cells containing fetal hemoglobin, the percentage falls rapidly, so that by the age of 6 to 12 months there is only a trace of fetal hemoglobin remaining (Christensen & Ohls, 2016). Iron stores generally are sufficient to sustain normal RBC production for approximately 4 months in the term infant, at which time a transient physiologic anemia can occur.

Leukocytes

Leukocytosis, with a white blood cell (WBC) count ranging from 9000 to 30,000/mm^3, is normal at birth (Pagana et al., 2017). The number of WBCs increases up to 24,000/mm^3 during the first day after birth. The initial high WBC count of the newborn decreases rapidly, and a stable level of 12,000/mm^3 is normally maintained during the neonatal period (Blackburn, 2018). Newborns are susceptible to infection. Leukocytes, especially the polymorphonuclear neutrophils, are limited in their ability to recognize foreign protein and localize and fight infection early in life (Benjamin, Mezu-Ndubuisi, & Maheshwari, 2015). Sepsis can

be accompanied by a concomitant rise in neutrophils; however, some infants initially have clinical signs of sepsis without a significant elevation in WBCs. In addition, events other than infection (i.e., prolonged crying, maternal hypertension, asymptomatic hypoglycemia, hemolytic disease, meconium aspiration syndrome, labor induction with oxytocin, surgery, difficult labor, high altitude, and maternal fever) can cause neutrophilia in the newborn.

Platelets

Platelets appear to be activated during the birth process and demonstrate improved aggregation in the first hours after birth. The platelet count ranges between 150,000 and 300,000/mm^3 and is essentially the same in newborns as in adults. Levels of vitamin K–dependent clotting factors II, VII, IX, and X increase slowly after birth and reach adult levels by 6 months of age (Monagle, 2017).

Blood Groups

The infant's blood group is determined genetically and established early in fetal life. However, during the neonatal period the strength of the agglutinogens present in the RBC membrane gradually increases. Cord blood samples can be used to identify the infant's blood type and Rh status.

Thermogenic System

Next to establishing respirations and effective extrauterine circulation, heat regulation is most critical to the newborn's survival. During the first 12 hours after birth, the neonate attempts to achieve thermal balance in adjusting to the extrauterine environmental temperature. Thermoregulation is the maintenance of balance between heat loss and heat production. Newborns attempt to stabilize their core body temperatures within a narrow range. Hypothermia from excessive heat loss is a common and potentially serious problem.

Anatomic and physiologic characteristics of neonates place them at risk for heat loss. Newborns have a thin layer of subcutaneous fat. The blood vessels are close to the surface of the skin. Newborns have larger body surface–to–body weight (mass) ratios than children and adults. Changes in environmental temperature alter the temperature of the blood, thereby influencing temperature regulation centers in the hypothalamus (Blackburn, 2018).

Heat Loss

The body temperature of newborn infants depends on the heat transfer between the infant and the external environment. Factors that influence heat loss to the environment include the temperature and humidity of the air, the flow and velocity of the air, and the temperature of surfaces in contact with and around the infant. The goal of care is to provide a neutral thermal environment for the newborn in which heat balance is maintained. The neutral thermal environment is the ideal environmental temperature that allows the newborn to maintain a normal body temperature to minimize oxygen and glucose consumption. Heat loss in the newborn occurs by four modes:

1. *Convection* is the flow of heat from the body surface to cooler ambient air. Because of heat loss by convection, the ambient temperature in newborn care areas should range between 22°C and 26°C (72°F to 78°F) and the humidity between 30% and 60% (AAP & ACOG, 2017). Newborns in open bassinets are wrapped to protect them from the cold. A cap may be worn to decrease heat loss from the infant's head.

2. *Radiation* is the loss of heat from the body surface to a cooler solid surface not in direct contact but in relative proximity. To prevent this type of loss, bassinets and examining tables are placed away from outside windows, and care is taken to avoid direct air drafts.

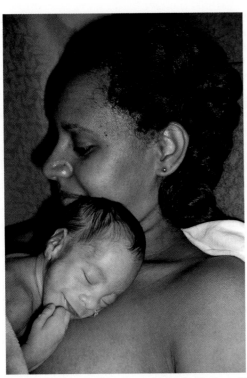

Fig. 23.1 Infant in Skin-to-Skin Contact With Mother. Note infant smile. (Courtesy Cheryl Briggs, RNC, Annapolis, MD.)

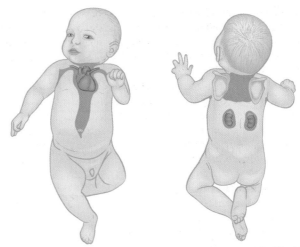

Fig. 23.2 Distribution of Brown Fat in the Newborn. (Modified from Murray, S. S., & McKinney, E. S. [2010]. *Foundations of maternal-newborn and women's health nursing* [6th ed.]. St. Louis: Elsevier.)

3. *Evaporation* is the loss of heat that occurs when a liquid is converted to a vapor. In the newborn, heat loss by evaporation occurs as a result of moisture vaporization from the skin. This heat loss is intensified by failing to completely dry the newborn after birth or with bathing. Evaporative heat loss, as a component of insensible water loss, is the most significant cause of heat loss in the first few days of life.

4. *Conduction* is the loss of heat from the body surface to cooler surfaces in direct contact. During the initial assessment, the newborn is placed on a prewarmed bed under a radiant warmer to minimize heat loss. The scales used for weighing the newborn should have a protective cover to minimize conductive heat loss.

Heat loss must be controlled to protect the infant. Control of such modes of heat loss is the basis of caregiving policies and techniques. Drying the infant quickly after birth is essential to prevent hypothermia. Skin-to-skin contact with the mother is an effective means of reducing conductive and radiant heat loss and enhancing newborn temperature control and maternal-infant interaction. The naked newborn is placed on the mother's bare chest and covered with a warm blanket; a cap may be placed on the infant's head to help conserve heat (Fig. 23.1). Alternatively, the neonate is placed under a radiant warmer to reduce heat loss and promote thermoregulation.

Thermogenesis

In response to cold, the neonate attempts to generate heat (**thermogenesis**) by increasing muscle activity. Cold infants may cry and appear restless. Because of vasoconstriction the skin can feel cool to touch, and acrocyanosis can be present. There is an increase in cellular metabolic activity, primarily in the brain, heart, and liver; this also increases oxygen and glucose consumption.

In an effort to conserve heat, term newborns assume a position of flexion that helps to guard against heat loss because it diminishes the amount of body surface exposed to the environment. Infants also can reduce the loss of internal heat through the body surface by constricting peripheral blood vessels.

Adults are able to produce heat through shivering; however, the shivering mechanism of heat production is rarely operable in the newborn unless there is prolonged cold exposure (Blackburn, 2018). Newborns produce heat through **nonshivering thermogenesis**. This is accomplished primarily by metabolism of **brown fat**, which is unique to the newborn; and secondarily by increased metabolic activity in the brain, heart, and liver. Brown fat is located in superficial deposits in the interscapular region and axillae and in deep deposits at the thoracic inlet, along the vertebral column, and around the kidneys (Fig. 23.2). Brown fat has a richer vascular and nerve supply than ordinary fat. Heat produced by intense lipid metabolic activity in brown fat can warm the newborn by increasing heat production as much as 100%. Reserves of brown fat, usually present for several weeks after birth, are rapidly depleted with cold stress. The amount of brown fat reserve increases with the weeks of gestation. A full-term newborn has greater stores than a preterm infant.

Hypothermia and Cold Stress

When the neonate's temperature drops, vasoconstriction occurs as a mechanism to conserve heat. The infant can appear pale and mottled; the skin feels cool, especially on the extremities. If the hypothermia is not corrected, it will progress to cold stress, which imposes metabolic and physiologic demands on all infants, regardless of gestational age and condition. The respiratory rate increases in response to the increased need for oxygen. In the cold-stressed infant, oxygen consumption and energy are diverted from maintaining normal brain and cardiac function and growth to thermogenesis for survival. If the infant cannot maintain an adequate oxygen tension, vasoconstriction follows and jeopardizes pulmonary perfusion. As a consequence, the PO_2 is decreased and the blood pH drops. Surfactant synthesis can be altered. These changes can prompt a transient respiratory distress or aggravate existing RDS. Moreover, decreased pulmonary perfusion and oxygen tension can maintain or reopen the right-to-left shunt across the ductus arteriosus.

The basal metabolic rate increases with cold stress. If cold stress is protracted, anaerobic glycolysis occurs, resulting in increased production of acids. Metabolic acidosis develops, and, if a defect in respiratory function is present, respiratory acidosis also develops (Fig. 23.3). Excessive fatty acids can displace the bilirubin from the albumin-binding sites and exacerbate hyperbilirubinemia. Hypoglycemia is another metabolic consequence of cold stress. The process of anaerobic glycolysis

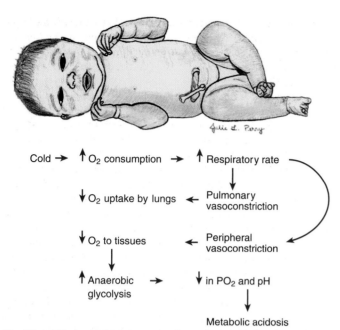

Cold → ↑O₂ consumption → ↑Respiratory rate

↓O₂ uptake by lungs ← Pulmonary vasoconstriction

↓O₂ to tissues ← Peripheral vasoconstriction

↑Anaerobic glycolysis → ↓in PO₂ and pH

↓

Metabolic acidosis

Fig. 23.3 Effects of Cold Stress. When an infant is stressed by cold, oxygen consumption increases, and pulmonary and peripheral vasoconstriction occur, thereby decreasing oxygen uptake by the lungs and oxygen to the tissues; anaerobic glycolysis increases, and there is a decrease in PO₂ and pH, leading to metabolic acidosis. (Modified from Murray, S. S., & McKinney, E. S. [2010]. *Foundations of maternal-newborn and women's health nursing* [6th ed.]. St. Louis: Elsevier.)

can deplete existing stores. If the infant is sufficiently stressed and low glucose stores are not replaced, hypoglycemia, which can be asymptomatic in the newborn, can develop (Gardner & Hernández, 2016).

Hyperthermia

Although less frequently than hypothermia, hyperthermia can occur and must be corrected. A body temperature greater than 37.5°C (99.5°F) is considered to be abnormally high and is typically caused by excess heat production related to sepsis or a decrease in heat loss. Hyperthermia can result from the inappropriate use of external heat sources such as radiant warmers, phototherapy, sunlight, increased environmental temperature, and the use of excessive clothing or blankets. The clinical appearance of the infant who is hyperthermic often indicates the causative mechanism. Infants who are overheated because of environmental factors such as being swaddled in too many blankets exhibit signs of heat-losing mechanisms: skin vessels dilate, skin appears flushed, hands and feet are warm to touch, and the infant assumes a posture of extension. The newborn who is hyperthermic because of sepsis appears stressed: vessels in the skin are constricted, color is pale, and hands and feet are cool. Hyperthermia develops more rapidly in a newborn than in an adult because of the relatively larger surface area of an infant. Sweat glands do not function well. Hyperthermia can cause neurologic injury and increased risk for seizures; severe cases can result in heat stroke and death (Gardner & Hernández, 2016).

Renal System

At term, the kidneys occupy a large portion of the posterior abdominal wall. The bladder lies close to the anterior abdominal wall and is both an abdominal and a pelvic organ. In the newborn, almost all palpable masses in the abdomen are renal in origin.

At birth, a small quantity (approximately 40 mL) of urine is usually present in the bladder of a full-term infant. Many newborns void at the time of birth, although this is easily missed and may not be recorded. During the first few days, term infants generally excrete 15 to 60 mL/

kg/day of urine; output gradually increases over the first month (Blackburn, 2018). The frequency of voiding varies from 2 to 6 times per day during the first and second days of life and increases during the subsequent 24 hours. After day 4, approximately six to eight voidings per day of pale straw-colored urine indicate adequate fluid intake.

> ### ⚠ NURSING ALERT
>
> Noting and recording the first voiding are important. An infant who has not voided by 24 hours should be assessed for adequacy of fluid intake, bladder distention, restlessness, and signs of discomfort. The neonatal health care provider should be notified.

Full-term newborns have limited capacity to concentrate urine; therefore the specific gravity is usually low (less than 1.004) (Cadnapaphornchai, Schoenbein, Woloschuk, et al., 2016). The ability to concentrate urine fully is attained by approximately 3 months of age. After the first voiding, the infant's urine can appear cloudy (because of mucus content) and have a much higher specific gravity. This decreases as fluid intake increases. Normal urine during early infancy is usually straw colored and almost odorless. Sometimes pink-tinged uric acid crystals or "brick dust" appear on the diaper. Uric acid crystals are normal during the first week but thereafter can be a sign of inadequate intake (Janke, 2014). Loss of fluid through urine, feces, lungs, increased metabolic rate, and limited fluid intake can result in a 5% to 10% loss of the birth weight over the first 3 to 5 days. Excessive weight loss can be related to feeding difficulties or other issues. The neonate should regain the birth weight within 10 to 14 days, depending on the feeding method (breastfeeding, breast milk feeding, or infant formula).

Fluid and Electrolyte Balance

In the term neonate, approximately 75% of body weight consists of total body water (extracellular and intracellular). A reduction in extracellular fluid occurs with diuresis during the first few days after birth. The weight loss experienced by most newborns during the first few days after birth is caused primarily by extracellular water loss (Cadnapaphornchai et al., 2016).

The daily fluid requirement for neonates weighing more than 1500 g is 60 to 80 mL/kg during the first 2 days of life. From 3 to 7 days the requirement is 100 to 150 mL/kg/day, and from 8 to 30 days it is 120 to 180 mL/kg/day (Dell, 2015).

At birth, the glomerular filtration rate (GFR) of a newborn is significantly lower than in the adult. This results in a decreased ability to remove nitrogenous and other waste products from the blood. The GFR rapidly increases during the 2 to 4 weeks after birth as a result of postnatal physiologic changes, including decreased renal vascular resistance, increased renal blood flow, and increased filtration pressure. The GFR gradually rises to adult levels by 2 years of age (Blackburn, 2018; Vogt & Dell, 2015).

Sodium reabsorption is decreased as a result of a lowered sodium- or potassium-activated adenosine triphosphatase activity. The decreased ability to excrete excess sodium results in hypotonic urine compared with plasma, leading to a higher concentration of sodium, phosphates, chloride, and organic acids and a lower concentration of bicarbonate ions. The infant has a higher renal threshold for glucose than adults.

Tubular reabsorption of glucose in the term neonate is similar to that of an adult. Although the renal threshold for glucose is lower, newborns do not typically exhibit glycosuria.

Because of a lower renal threshold for bicarbonate and a limited capacity for reabsorption, the neonate's serum bicarbonate and plasma pH levels are lower. Buffering capacity is decreased. This reduces the newborn's ability to cope with events (e.g., cold stress) that produce acidosis (Blackburn, 2018).

Signs of Renal System Problems

The renal system has a wide range of functions. Dysfunction resulting from physiologic abnormalities can range from the lack of a steady stream of urine to gross anomalies such as hypospadias and exstrophy of the bladder, which can be identified easily at birth. Enlarged or cystic kidneys can be identified as masses during abdominal palpation. Some kidney anomalies also can be detected by ultrasound examination during pregnancy (see Chapter 36).

Gastrointestinal System

The full-term newborn is capable of swallowing, digesting, metabolizing, and absorbing proteins and simple carbohydrates and emulsifying fats. With the exception of pancreatic amylase, the characteristic digestive enzymes are present even in low-birth-weight neonates.

In the adequately hydrated infant, the mucous membrane of the mouth is moist and pink; the hard and soft palates are intact. The presence of moderate to large amounts of mucus is common in the first few hours after birth. Small whitish areas (Epstein pearls) may be found on the gum margins and at the juncture of the hard and soft palates. The cheeks are full because of well-developed sucking pads. These, like the labial tubercles (sucking calluses) on the upper lip, disappear at approximately 12 months of age when the sucking period is over.

Feeding behavior is related to gestational age and is influenced by neuromuscular maturity, maternal medications during labor and birth, and the type of initial feeding. Feeding requires that the neonate is able to coordinate sucking, swallowing, and breathing. Sucking is a reflex behavior that begins in utero as early as 15 to 16 weeks. By 28 weeks, some infants can coordinate sucking and swallowing. By 32 to 34 weeks, most are able to coordinate sucking, swallowing, and breathing; these abilities are well developed by 36 to 38 weeks (Blackburn, 2018). Sucking takes place in small bursts of 3 or 4 and up to 8 to 10 sucks at a time, with a brief pause between bursts. The neonate is unable to move food from the lips to the pharynx; therefore placing the nipple (breast or bottle) well inside the baby's mouth is necessary. Peristaltic activity in the esophagus is uncoordinated in the first few days of life. It quickly becomes a coordinated pattern in healthy full-term infants, and they swallow easily.

Teeth begin developing in utero, with enamel formation continuing until approximately 10 years of age. Tooth development is influenced by neonatal or infant illnesses and medications and by maternal illnesses or medications taken by the mother during pregnancy. The fluoride level in the water supply also influences tooth development. Occasionally an infant may be born with one or more teeth. These natal teeth have poorly formed roots and, as they loosen, place the infant at risk for aspiration. Therefore they are usually extracted.

The mucosal barrier in the intestines is not fully mature until 4 to 6 months of age, which allows antigens and other macromolecules such as bacteria to be transported across the intestinal wall into the systemic circulation. This increases the risk for allergies and infection (Blackburn, 2018).

Intestinal flora, or gut microbiota, are established within the first week after birth; and normal intestinal flora help to synthesize vitamin K, folate, and biotin. Traditionally it was thought that the fetus grows and develops in a sterile environment. Research on the human microbiome suggests that the pregnant woman and the developing fetus coexist with a variety of commensal and symbiotic microbes that have important influences on the health of both the mother and her infant. Research evidence of microbial presence in amniotic fluid, placenta, and meconium indicates that the fetus is exposed to microbes during pregnancy. The mode of birth (vaginal or cesarean) seems to play a major role in the microbial colonization of the neonate. Infants born vaginally appear to be initially colonized by the maternal vaginal microbes, whereas infants born by cesarean section are first colonized by maternal skin microbes. This initial colonization plays a major role in establishing intestinal flora; research is ongoing to identify the implications for the child's future health. The microbiome of the infant is also influenced by diet, antibiotics, and environmental factors (Bäckhed, Roswall, Peng, et al., 2015; Mueller, Bakacs, Combellick, et al., 2015; Neu, 2017).

Breastfeeding is important in establishing the intestinal microbiome of the newborn. Human milk contains a variety of microbes that appear to originate in the mother's GI tract. Oligosaccharides in human milk may have a prebiotic function that facilitates the growth of beneficial bacteria in the neonatal GI tract (Neu, 2017).

The capacity of the newborn stomach varies widely, depending on the size of the infant, from less than 10 mL on day 1 to nearly 30 mL on day 3 and expanding to 60 mL on day 7. After birth, the newborn stomach becomes increasingly more compliant and relaxed to accommodate larger volumes. Several factors such as time and volume of feedings or type and temperature of food can affect the emptying time.

The normal intermittent relaxation of the lower esophageal sphincter results in involuntary backflow of stomach contents into the esophagus, known as gastroesophageal reflux (GER). As a result, newborns are prone to regurgitation, "spitting," and vomiting, especially during the first 3 months. GER can be minimized by avoiding overfeeding, burping, and positioning the infant with the head slightly elevated.

In some infants, GER is severe enough to cause dysphagia, esophagitis, and aspiration. This is known as gastroesophageal reflux disease (GERD). Treatment may include medications to reduce gastric acidity such as antacids, histamine-blocking agents, or proton pump inhibitors; and medication to increase gastric motility. In severe cases, surgical treatment may be considered (Richards & Goldin, 2018).

Digestion

The infant's ability to digest carbohydrates, fats, and proteins is regulated by the presence of certain enzymes. Most of these enzymes are functional at birth except for pancreatic amylase and lipase. Amylase is produced by the salivary glands after approximately 3 months of age and by the pancreas at approximately 6 months of age. This enzyme is necessary to convert starch into maltose and occurs in high amounts in colostrum. The other exception is lipase, also secreted by the pancreas; it is necessary for the digestion of fat. Therefore the normal newborn is capable of digesting simple carbohydrates and proteins but has a limited ability to digest fats. Mammary lipase in human milk aids in digestion of fats by the neonate.

Lactase levels in newborns are higher than in older infants. This enzyme is necessary for digestion of lactose, the major carbohydrate in human milk and commercial infant formula.

Stools

Meconium fills the lower intestine at birth. It is formed during fetal life from the amniotic fluid and its constituents, intestinal secretions (including bilirubin), and cells (shed from the mucosa). Meconium is greenish black and viscous and contains occult blood. Most healthy term infants pass meconium within the first 12 to 24 hours of life, and almost all do so by 48 hours (Fig. 23.4). The number of stools passed varies during the first week, being most numerous between the third and sixth days. Newborns fed early pass stools sooner. The colostrum consumed by breastfed neonates during the first 2 to 3 days after birth promotes stooling. Progressive changes in the stooling pattern indicate a properly functioning GI tract (Box 23.1).

Feeding Behaviors

Variations occur among infants regarding interest in food, signs of hunger, and amount ingested at one time. The amount the infant consumes at any feeding depends on gestational and chronologic age, weight, hunger level, and alertness. When put to breast, some infants feed

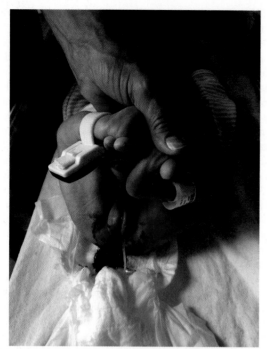

Fig. 23.4 Meconium Stool in 24-Hour-Old Newborn; Mucous Discharge From Vagina. (Courtesy Kathryn Alden, Apex, NC.)

BOX 23.1 Changes in Stooling Patterns of Newborns

Meconium
- First stool: composed of amniotic fluid and its constituents, intestinal secretions, shed mucosal cells, and possibly blood (ingested maternal blood or minor bleeding of alimentary tract vessels).
- Passage of meconium should occur within the first 24-48 h, although it can be delayed up to 7 days in very low birthweight infants. Passage of meconium can occur in utero and can be a sign of fetal distress.

Transitional Stools
- Usually appear by third day after initiation of feeding
- Greenish brown to yellowish brown; thin and less sticky than meconium; can contain some milk curds

Milk Stool
- Usually appears by the fourth day
- *Breastmilk:* yellow to golden, pasty in consistency; resemble a mixture of mustard and cottage cheese, with an odor similar to sour milk
- *Commercial infant formula:* Stools pale yellow to light brown, firmer consistency, stronger odor than breast milk stools

---

immediately, whereas others require a longer learning period. Random hand-to-mouth movement and sucking of fingers are well developed at birth and intensify when the infant is hungry. Caregivers should be alert and responsive to these hunger cues (Lawrence & Lawrence, 2016).

Signs of Gastrointestinal Problems

The time, color, and character of the infant's first stool should be noted. Failure to pass meconium can indicate bowel obstruction related to conditions such as an inborn error of metabolism (e.g., cystic fibrosis) or a congenital disorder (e.g., Hirschsprung disease or an imperforate anus). An active rectal "wink" reflex (contraction of the anal sphincter muscle in response to touch) is a sign of good sphincter tone. Passage of meconium from the vagina or urinary meatus is a sign of a possible fistulous tract from the rectum.

Fullness of the abdomen above the umbilicus can be caused by hepatomegaly, duodenal atresia, or distention. Abdominal distention at birth usually indicates a serious disorder such as a ruptured viscus (from abdominal wall defects) or tumors. Distention that occurs later can be the result of overfeeding or can be a sign of a GI disorder. A scaphoid (sunken) abdomen, with bowel sounds heard in the chest and signs of respiratory distress, indicates a diaphragmatic hernia. Fullness below the umbilicus can indicate a distended bladder.

Some infants are intolerant of certain commercial infant formulas. If an infant is allergic or unable to digest a formula, the stools can become very soft with a high water content that is signaled by a distinct water ring around the stool on the diaper. Forceful ejection of stool and a water ring around the stool are signs of diarrhea. Care must be taken to avoid misinterpreting transitional stools for diarrhea. The loss of fluid in diarrhea can rapidly lead to fluid and electrolyte imbalance.

The amount and frequency of regurgitation, "spitting," or vomiting after feedings should be documented. Color change, gagging, and projectile (very forceful) vomiting occur in association with esophageal and tracheoesophageal anomalies. Vomiting in large amounts, especially if it is projectile, can be a sign of pyloric stenosis. Bilious (green) emesis is suggestive of intestinal obstruction or malrotation of the bowel.

Hepatic System

In the newborn, the liver can be palpated approximately 1 to 2 cm below the right costal margin because it is enlarged and occupies approximately 40% of the abdominal cavity. The infant's liver plays an important role in iron storage, glucose and fatty acid metabolism, bilirubin synthesis, and coagulation. Although the liver is relatively immature at birth, healthy term infants do not typically experience problems.

Iron Storage

The fetal liver, which serves as the site for production of hemoglobin after birth, begins storing iron in utero. The infant's iron store is proportional to total body hemoglobin content and length of gestation. At birth, the term infant has an iron store sufficient to last approximately 4 months. Iron stores of preterm and small-for-gestational-age infants are often lower and are depleted sooner than in healthy term infants. Although both breast milk and cow's milk contain iron, the bioavailability of iron in breast milk (lactoferrin) is far superior.

Glucose Homeostasis

The liver is responsible for regulation of blood glucose levels. In utero, the glucose concentration in the umbilical vein is approximately 70% of the maternal level. At birth, the newborn is removed from the maternal glucose supply resulting in an initial drop in blood glucose from fetal levels of 70 to 90 mg/dL to levels of 55 to 60 mg/dL between 30 and 90 minutes after birth. During this time, glucagon levels increase while insulin levels decrease and the limited hepatic glycogen stores are mobilized. The initiation of feedings helps to stabilize blood glucose levels as milk lactose is metabolized. Glucose production also occurs through glycogenolysis and gluconeogenesis. Glucose levels rise gradually and stabilize by the second or third day at levels greater than 70 mg/dL (Hawkes & Stanley, 2017).

Glucose levels are not routinely assessed in newborns unless there are risk factors or symptoms of hypoglycemia. Risk factors include small or large for gestational age, preterm, and infant of a diabetic mother. The hypoglycemic infant can be asymptomatic or can display the classic symptoms of jitteriness, lethargy, apnea, feeding problems, or seizures. Hypoglycemia in the initial newborn period is most often transient and easily corrected through feeding. Persistent or recurrent hypoglycemia necessitates intravenous glucose therapy and possible pharmacologic intervention.

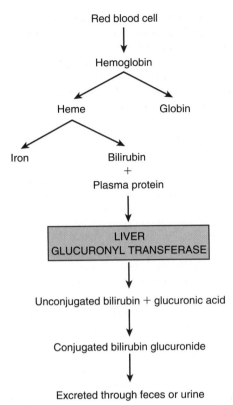

Red blood cell

Hemoglobin

Heme — Globin

Iron — Bilirubin + Plasma protein

LIVER GLUCURONYL TRANSFERASE

Unconjugated bilirubin + glucuronic acid

Conjugated bilirubin glucuronide

Excreted through feces or urine

Fig. 23.5 Formation and Excretion of Bilirubin.

Fatty Acid Metabolism

Fatty acid metabolism is an additional source of energy for the neonate in the initial hours after birth. Catecholamine release increases the rate of lipolysis, which produces fatty acids for oxidation and ketone body synthesis. Hepatic ketogenesis is increased in term newborns for the first 3 days.

Bilirubin Synthesis

The liver is responsible for the conjugation of bilirubin, which results from the breakdown of RBCs. When RBCs reach the end of their life span, their membranes rupture, and hemoglobin is released. The hemoglobin is phagocytosed by macrophages; it then splits into heme and globin. The heme is broken down by the reticuloendothelial cells, converted to bilirubin, and released in an unconjugated form. The unconjugated (indirect) bilirubin is relatively insoluble and almost entirely bound to circulating albumin, a plasma protein. Bilirubin that is not bound to albumin, or free bilirubin, can easily cross the blood-brain barrier and cause neurotoxicity (acute bilirubin encephalopathy or kernicterus [see later discussion]).

The unconjugated bilirubin must be conjugated so it becomes soluble and excretable. In the liver, the unbound bilirubin is conjugated with glucuronic acid in the presence of the enzyme glucuronyl transferase. The conjugated form of bilirubin (direct bilirubin) is soluble and excreted from liver cells as a constituent of bile. Along with other components of bile, direct bilirubin is excreted into the biliary tract system that carries the bile into the duodenum. Bilirubin is converted to urobilinogen and stercobilinogen within the duodenum through the action of the bacterial flora. Urobilinogen is excreted in urine and feces; stercobilinogen is excreted in the feces. The effectiveness of bilirubin excretion through the feces depends on the stooling pattern of the newborn and the substances in the intestine that break down conjugated bilirubin. In the newborn intestine, the enzyme β-glucuronidase is able to convert conjugated bilirubin into the unconjugated form, which is subsequently reabsorbed by the intestinal mucosa and transported to the liver; this is called *enterohepatic circulation*. Feeding is important in reducing serum bilirubin levels because it stimulates peristalsis and produces more rapid passage of meconium, thus diminishing the amount of reabsorption of unconjugated bilirubin. Feeding also introduces bacteria to aid in the reduction of bilirubin to urobilinogen. Colostrum, a natural laxative, facilitates the passage of meconium in breastfed infants (Fig. 23.5).

When levels of unconjugated bilirubin exceed the ability of the liver to conjugate it, plasma levels of bilirubin increase and jaundice appears. Jaundice, the visible yellowish color of the skin and sclera, is likely to appear when the total serum bilirubin (TSB) level exceeds 6 to 7 mg/dL. Jaundice is generally noticeable first in the head, especially in the sclera and mucous membranes, and progresses gradually to the thorax, abdomen, and extremities. The degree of jaundice is determined by serum total bilirubin measurements (Kamath-Rayne, Thilo, Deacon, et al., 2016).

The newborn is at risk for hyperbilirubinemia because of distinctive aspects of normal neonatal physiology. The higher RBC mass at birth and shorter life span of neonatal RBCs create the need for greater bilirubin synthesis. The ability of the liver to conjugate bilirubin is reduced during the first few days after birth; it can metabolize and excrete only approximately two-thirds of the circulating bilirubin. In addition, there are fewer bilirubin binding sites because newborns have lower serum albumin levels. In the intestines, conjugated bilirubin becomes unconjugated and recirculated through the enterohepatic circulation, which increases serum bilirubin levels.

Traditionally, newborn jaundice has been categorized as either *physiologic* or *pathologic* (nonphysiologic), depending primarily on the time it appears and on serum bilirubin levels. Controversy surrounds the definitions of normal or physiologic ranges of TSB. TSB levels in newborns are affected by variables such as gestational age, chronologic age, weight, race, nutritional status, mode of feeding, and presence of extravasated blood (e.g., cephalhematoma or severe bruising) (Blackburn, 2018). The time of onset of jaundice is a key factor in evaluating its cause and determining if treatment is needed.

Among the factors that increase the risk for hyperbilirubinemia, preterm birth is the most significant. Prematurity affects liver and brain metabolism and albumin binding sites, placing preterm and late preterm infants at greater risk for hyperbilirubinemia. Infants of Asian, Native-American, and Eskimo ethnicity have higher bilirubin levels. Breastfeeding infants are at greater risk for hyperbilirubinemia (see later discussion) (Watchko, 2018). Risk factors for severe hyperbilirubinemia are listed in Box 23.2.

Physiologic jaundice. Physiologic or nonpathologic jaundice (unconjugated hyperbilirubinemia) occurs in approximately 60% of term newborns. It appears after 24 hours of age and usually resolves without treatment.

In normal full-term newborns, TSB levels progressively increase from 2 mg/dL in cord blood to an average peak of 5 to 6 mg/dL by 72 to 96 hours of life. From that point, TSB levels gradually decrease to a plateau of approximately 3 mg/dL by 1 week of age, reaching normal adult levels of 2 mg/dL or less by 2 weeks of age. This pattern varies according to racial group, method of feeding (breast vs. formula), and gestational age (Kamath-Rayne et al., 2016).

> ### ⚡ SAFETY ALERT
>
> The appearance of jaundice during the first 24 hours of life or persistence beyond the ages previously delineated usually indicates a potential pathologic process that requires investigation.

Pathologic jaundice. Bilirubin can accumulate to hazardous levels and lead to a pathologic condition. Pathologic or nonphysiologic jaundice is unconjugated hyperbilirubinemia that is either pathologic in origin or severe enough to warrant further evaluation and treatment. Jaundice is usually considered pathologic or nonphysiologic if it appears within 24 hours after birth, TSB levels increase by more than 0.2 mg/dL per hour, TSB is greater than the 95th percentile for age in hours, direct serum bilirubin levels exceed 1.5 to 2 mg/dL, or clinical jaundice lasts for more than 2 weeks (Kamath-Rayne et al., 2016). High levels of unconjugated bilirubin are usually caused by excessive production of bilirubin through hemolysis; the most frequent cause is hemolytic disease of the newborn due to maternal/newborn blood group incompatibility (Rh, ABO, or minor blood groups). Other factors contributing to increased hemolysis include enclosed hemorrhage (e.g., cephalhematoma, excessive bruising), polycythemia, delayed passage of meconium, and delayed feeding. It can also be caused by glucose-6-phosphate dehydrogenase (G6PD) deficiency, a genetic disorder that is most prevalent among infants with genetic heritage from Asia, Africa, the Middle East, and the Mediterranean region (Watchko, 2018). Unconjugated hyperbilirubinemia can be the result of altered hepatic clearance of bilirubin related to immaturity, metabolic disorders such as Crigler-Najjar disease, asphyxia, sepsis, and congenital anomalies such as biliary atresia (Blackburn, 2018; Watchko).

If increased levels of unconjugated bilirubin are left untreated, neurotoxicity can result as bilirubin is transferred into the brain cells. Acute bilirubin encephalopathy refers to the acute manifestations of bilirubin toxicity that occur during the first weeks after birth. This can include a range of symptoms such as lethargy, hypotonia, irritability, seizures, coma, and death. Kernicterus refers to the irreversible, long-term consequences of bilirubin toxicity such as hypotonia, delayed motor skills, hearing loss, cerebral palsy, and gaze abnormalities (Blackburn, 2018) (see Chapter 36).

Jaundice related to breastfeeding. Two forms of breastfeeding-related jaundice are recognized: breastfeeding-associated jaundice and breast milk jaundice. These typically occur in otherwise healthy infants. Both types can occur in the same infant and are not easily differentiated (Kamath-Rayne et al., 2016).

Breastfeeding-associated jaundice (early-onset jaundice) begins at 2 to 5 days of age. Breastfeeding does not cause the jaundice; rather it is a lack of effective breastfeeding that contributes to the hyperbilirubinemia. If the infant is not feeding effectively, there is less caloric and fluid intake and possible dehydration. Hepatic clearance of bilirubin is reduced. With less intake, there are fewer stools. As a result, bilirubin is reabsorbed from the intestine back into the bloodstream and must be conjugated again so it can be excreted (Blackburn, 2018; Lawrence & Lawrence, 2016).

Breast milk jaundice (late-onset jaundice) usually occurs at 5 to 10 days of age. Infants are typically feeding well and gaining weight appropriately. Rising levels of unconjugated bilirubin peak during the second week and gradually diminish. Despite high levels of bilirubin that can persist for 3 to 12 weeks, these infants have no signs of hemolysis or liver dysfunction. The etiology of breast milk jaundice is uncertain. However, it seems to be related to factors in the breast milk (e.g., pregnanediol, fatty acids, and β-glucuronidase) that either inhibit the conjugation of bilirubin or decrease the excretion of bilirubin (Blackburn, 2018). (See Chapter 25 for a discussion of these conditions in relation to newborn nutrition.)

Coagulation

The liver plays an important role in blood coagulation. Coagulation factors, which are synthesized in the liver, are activated by vitamin K. The lack of intestinal bacteria needed to synthesize vitamin K results in transient blood coagulation deficiency between the second and fifth days of life. The levels of coagulation factors slowly increase to reach adult levels by 9 months of age. The administration of intramuscular vitamin K shortly after birth helps to prevent vitamin K deficiency bleeding (VKDB) which can occur suddenly and can be catastrophic (Shearer, 2017). Any bleeding problems noted in the newborn should be reported immediately and tests for clotting ordered.

Drug Metabolism

The immaturity of the liver and depressed liver enzyme systems at birth result in slower biotransformation and elimination of drugs. This can result in slower drug clearance, increased serum levels, and longer half-lives (Blackburn, 2018).

Signs of Hepatic System Problems

Hypoglycemia and hyperbilirubinemia are the most common liver-related problems experienced by newborns. In most cases the problems are transient and require little, if any treatment. Preterm infants are at increased risk for hepatic system problems because of the immaturity of the liver.

The hematologic status of all newborns should be assessed for anemia. For the first week of life, neonates are at risk for bleeding until the coagulation factors are well established. Male newborns who are circumcised prior to discharge from the birth facility must be monitored carefully for bleeding.

Immune System

Beginning early in gestation, the immune system of the fetus is developing the capacity to respond to foreign antigens. The development of the immune system is necessary to equip the neonate to meet the numerous environmental challenges (e.g., microorganisms) associated with life in the extrauterine world. Compared with adults, the immune response at birth is reduced, leading to increased susceptibility to pathogens.

Neonatal levels of circulating immunoglobins are low in comparison with adult levels. Most of the circulating antibodies in the newborn are immunoglobulin G (IgG) antibodies that were transported across the placenta from the maternal circulation. This transfer of antibodies from the mother begins as early as 14 weeks of gestation and is greatest during the third trimester. By term, the IgG levels in the cord blood of the infant are higher than those in maternal blood. The passive immunity afforded the infant through the placental transfer of IgG usually provides sufficient antimicrobial protection during the first 3 months of life. Production of adult concentrations of IgG is reached by 4 to 6 years of age (Benjamin et al., 2015).

The fetus is capable of producing IgM by the eighth week of gestation, and low levels (less than 10% of adult levels) are present at term. IgM is important for immunity to blood-borne infections and is the major immunoglobulin synthesized during the first month. By 2 years of age, IgM reaches adult levels. The production of IgA, IgD, and IgE is much more gradual, and maximal levels are not attained until early childhood (Benjamin et al., 2015).

The membrane-protective IgA is missing from the respiratory and urinary tracts, and, unless the newborn is breastfed, it also is absent from the GI tract. The secretory IgA in human milk acts locally in the intestines to neutralize bacterial and viral pathogens. It can also lessen the risk for allergy and food intolerance through modulation of exposure to foreign milk protein antigens (Turfkruyer & Verhasselt, 2015).

Other components of breast milk strengthen the neonate's immune system. Antimicrobial factors such as oligosaccharides, lysozyme, and lactoferrin aid in microbial clearance. Infants who are breastfed have enhanced antibody responses to vaccines. Long-term effects of breastmilk on the immune system are demonstrated by lower risk for immune-mediated conditions such as allergies, inflammatory bowel disease, and type I diabetes mellitus (Turfkruyer & Verhasselt, 2015).

The WBCs of the newborn display a delayed response to invading bacteria. Neutrophil levels are low, and therefore their key functions of phagocytosis, chemotaxis, and intracellular killing are limited. The influx of phagocytic cells to areas of inflammation is somewhat slowed, although the ability of these cells to attack and destroy bacteria is equivalent to that of adults. B cells and T cells are present in the newborn, although their function is immature (Benjamin et al., 2015).

Risk for Infection

All newborns, and preterm newborns especially, are at high risk for infection during the first several months of life. During this period, infection is one of the leading causes of morbidity and mortality. The newborn cannot limit the invading pathogen to the portal of entry because of the generalized hypofunctioning of the inflammatory and immune mechanisms.

Early signs of infection must be recognized so prompt diagnosis and treatment can occur. Temperature instability or hypothermia can be symptomatic of serious infection; newborns do not typically exhibit fever, although hyperthermia can occur (temperature greater than 38°C [100.4°F]). Lethargy, irritability, poor feeding, vomiting or diarrhea, decreased reflexes, and pale or mottled skin color are some of the clinical signs that suggest infection. Respiratory symptoms such as apnea, tachypnea, grunting, or retracting can be associated with infection such as pneumonia (Bodin, 2014). Any unusual discharge from the infant's eyes, nose, mouth, or other orifice must be investigated. If a rash appears, it must be evaluated closely; many normal rashes in the newborn are not associated with any infection. Infants must be protected from infections by the use of proper hand hygiene.

The greatest risk factor for neonatal infection is prematurity, because of immaturity of the immune system. Other risk factors include premature rupture of membranes, chorioamnionitis, maternal fever, antenatal or intrapartal asphyxia, invasive procedures, stress, and congenital anomalies.

Integumentary System

All skin structures are present at birth. The epidermis and dermis are loosely bound and extremely thin. After 35 weeks of gestation, the skin is covered by vernix caseosa (a cheeselike, whitish substance) that is fused with the epidermis and serves as a protective covering. Vernix caseosa is a complex substance that contains sebaceous gland secretions. It has emollient and antimicrobial properties and prevents fluid loss through the skin; it also has antioxidant properties. Removal of the vernix is followed by desquamation of the epidermis in most infants. There is evidence that leaving residual vernix intact after birth has positive benefits for neonatal skin such as decreasing the skin pH,

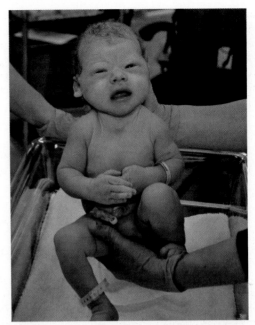

Fig. 23.6 Newborn Infant With Acrocyanosis of Upper and Lower Extremities. (Courtesy Barbara Wilson, West Jordan, UT.)

decreasing skin erythema, and improving skin hydration (Association of Women's Health, Obstetric, and Neonatal Nurses [AWHONN], 2018; Visscher, Adam, Brink, et al., 2015).

The skin of a term infant is erythematous (red) for a few hours after birth, and then it fades to its normal color. The skin often appears blotchy or mottled, especially over the extremities. The hands and feet appear slightly cyanotic (acrocyanosis); this is caused by vasomotor instability and capillary stasis. Acrocyanosis is common during the first 48 hours and appears intermittently over the first 7 to 10 days, especially with exposure to cold (Fig. 23.6).

The healthy term infant usually has a plump appearance because of large amounts of subcutaneous tissue and extracellular water content. Subcutaneous fat accumulated during the last trimester acts as insulation. Fine lanugo hair may be noted over the face, shoulders, and back. Edema of the face and ecchymosis (bruising) or petechiae may be noted as a result of face presentation, forceps-assisted birth, or vacuum extraction.

Creases are located on the palms of the hands and the soles of the feet. The simian line, a single palmar crease, is often seen in Asian infants and infants with Down syndrome. The soles of the feet should be inspected for the number of creases during the first few hours after birth; as the skin dries, more creases appear. More creases correlate with a greater maturity rating. Preterm newborns have few, if any, creases.

Sweat Glands

Distended, small, white sebaceous glands noticeable on the newborn face are known as milia (Fig. 23.7). Although sweat glands are present at birth, term infants usually do not sweat for the first 24 hours. By day 3, sweating begins on the face, then progresses to the palms. Infants can sweat as a function of body or environmental temperature; there can also be emotional sweating from crying or pain (Hoath & Narendran, 2015).

Desquamation

Desquamation (peeling) of the skin of the term infant does not occur until a few days after birth. Large generalized areas of skin desquamation present at birth can be an indication of postmaturity.

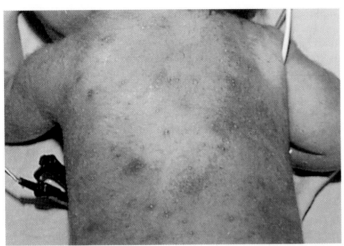

Fig. 23.10 Erythema Toxicum. (Kliegman, R., Stanton, B., St. Geme, J., Schor, N. [2015]. *Nelson textbook of pediatrics* [20th ed.]. Philadelphia: Elsevier.)

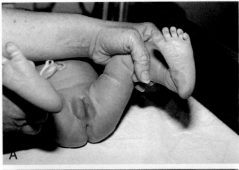

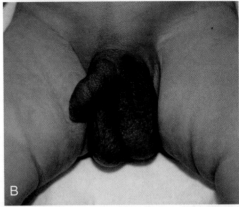

Fig. 23.11 External Genitalia. (A) Genitalia in female term infant. (B) Genitalia in uncircumcised male infant. Rugae cover scrotum, indicating term gestation. (Courtesy Marjorie Pyle, RNC, Lifecircle, Costa Mesa, CA.)

hemangiomas, although experts deem that term inappropriate. Most lesions reach maximum growth in approximately 6 months and then begin a slow process of involution that can take 5 to 10 years (Martin, 2016).

Erythema Toxicum

Erythema toxicum, a transient rash, is also called *erythema neonatorum, newborn rash,* or *flea bite dermatitis.* It first appears in term neonates during the first 24 to 72 hours after birth and can last up to 3 weeks of age (Blackburn, 2018). It has lesions in different stages: erythematous macules, papules, and small vesicles (Fig. 23.10). The lesions can appear suddenly anywhere on the body. The rash is thought to be an inflammatory response. Eosinophils, which help to decrease inflammation, are found in the vesicles. Although the appearance is alarming, the rash has no clinical significance and requires no treatment.

Signs of Integumentary Problems

Close observation of the newborn's skin color can lead to early detection of potential problems. Any pallor, plethora (deep purplish color from increased circulating RBCs), petechiae, central cyanosis, or jaundice should be noted and documented. The skin should be examined for signs of birth injuries such as forceps marks and lesions related to fetal monitoring. Bruises or petechiae can be present on the head, neck, and face of an infant born with a nuchal cord (cord around the neck) or who had a face presentation at birth. Bruising can increase the risk for hyperbilirubinemia. Petechiae can be present if increased pressure was applied to an area. Petechiae scattered over the infant's body should be reported to the health care provider because petechiae can indicate underlying problems such as low platelet count or infection.

Unilateral or bilateral periauricular papillomas (skin tags) occur fairly frequently. Their occurrence is usually a family trait and of no consequence.

Reproductive System

Female

An increase in estrogen during pregnancy followed by a drop after birth causes female newborns to have mucoid vaginal discharge (see Fig. 23.4) and even some slight bloody spotting (pseudomenstruation). External genitalia (i.e., labia majora and minora) are usually edematous

with increased pigmentation. In term neonates, the labia majora and minora cover the vestibule (Fig. 23.11A). In preterm infants, the clitoris is prominent and the labia majora are small and widely separated. Vaginal or hymenal tags are common findings and have no clinical significance. Vernix caseosa can be present between the labia and should not be forcibly removed during bathing.

If the girl was born in the breech position, the labia can be edematous and bruised. The edema and bruising resolve in a few days; no treatment is necessary.

Male

In the uncircumcised newborn, the foreskin or prepuce completely covers the glans. The foreskin adheres to the glans and is not fully retractable for 3 to 4 years. The position of the urethra should be at the tip of the penis. With *hypospadias,* the urethral opening is located in an abnormal position, at any point on the ventral surface of the penis surface from the glans to the perineum. If the urethral opening is located on the dorsal surface of the penis, it is known as *epispadias;* this is less common and is often associated with extrophy of the bladder (Elder, 2016). A common finding in newborn males is small, white, firm lesions called *epithelial pearls* at the tip of the prepuce.

By 28 to 36 weeks of gestation, the testes can be palpated in the inguinal canal and a few rugae appear on the scrotum. At 36 to 40 weeks of gestation, the testes are palpable in the upper scrotum and rugae appear on the anterior portion. After 40 weeks, the testes can be palpated in the scrotum and rugae cover the scrotal sac. The postterm neonate has deep rugae and a pendulous scrotum. Undescended testes (cryptorchidism) occur in approximately 4% of term newborn males;

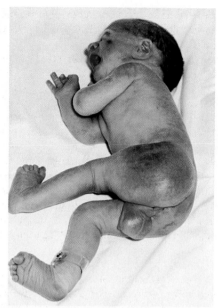

Fig. 23.12 Swelling of the Genitals and Bruising of the Buttocks After a Breech Birth. (From O'Doherty, N. [1986]. *Neonatology: Micro atlas of the newborn.* Nutley, NJ: Hoffman-LaRoche.)

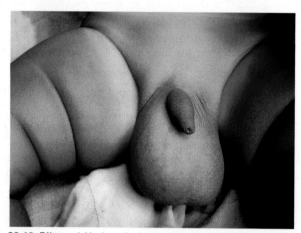

Fig. 23.13 Bilateral Hydrocele in the Newborn. The scrotum is distended by fluid; note jaundice of skin. (From Poenaru, D. [2012]. Abdominal wall problems. In C.A. Gleason, & S.U. Devaskar, [Eds.], *Avery's diseases of the newborn* [9th ed.]. Philadelphia: Saunders.)

in most cases the testes gradually descend without intervention (Lissauer, 2015). The primary risk factors for cryptorchidism are preterm birth and low birthweight (Lee, 2017).

The scrotum is usually more deeply pigmented than the rest of the skin (see Fig. 23.11B), particularly in darker-skinned infants. A bluish discoloration of the scrotum suggests testicular torsion, which needs immediate attention. If the male infant is born in a breech presentation, the scrotum can be very edematous and bruised (Fig. 23.12). The swelling and discoloration subside within a few days.

Hydrocele, caused by an accumulation of fluid around the testes, can be present. Hydroceles can be easily transilluminated with a light and usually resolve without treatment (Fig. 23.13).

Swelling of Breast Tissue

Swelling of the breast tissue in term infants of both sexes is caused by the hyperestrogenism of pregnancy. In a few infants a thin discharge ("witch's milk") can be seen. This finding has no clinical significance, requires no treatment, and subsides within a few days as the maternal hormones are eliminated from the infant's body.

The nipples should be symmetric on the chest. Breast tissue and areola size increase with gestation. The areola appears slightly elevated at 34 weeks of gestation. By 36 weeks, a breast bud of 1 to 2 mm is palpable; this increases to 12 mm by 42 weeks.

Signs of Reproductive System Problems

The infant must be inspected closely for ambiguous genitalia and other abnormalities. Normally in a female infant the urethral opening is located behind the clitoris. Any deviation from this can incorrectly suggest that the clitoris is a small penis, which can occur in conditions such as adrenal hyperplasia. Nearly all female infants are born with hymenal tags; absence of such tags can indicate vaginal agenesis. Fecal discharge from the vagina indicates a rectovaginal fistula. Any of these findings must be reported to the neonatal or pediatric health care provider for further evaluation.

Hypospadias, undescended testes, or other abnormalities of the male genitalia must be reported. Circumcision is contraindicated in the presence of hypospadias because the foreskin is used in repair of this anomaly.

Inguinal hernias can be present and become more obvious when the infant cries. They are common, especially in African-American neonates, and usually require no treatment because they resolve with time.

Skeletal System

The infant's skeletal system undergoes rapid development during the first year of life. At birth, more cartilage is present than ossified bone.

Head and Skull

Because of cephalocaudal (head-to-rump) development, the newborn looks somewhat out of proportion. The head at term is approximately one-fourth of the total body length. The arms are slightly longer than the legs. In the newborn, the legs are approximately one-third of the total body length. As growth proceeds, the midpoint in head-to-toe measurements gradually descends from the level of the umbilicus at birth to the level of the symphysis pubis at maturity.

The face appears small in relation to the skull. The skull appears large and heavy. Cranial size and shape can be distorted by molding (the shaping of the fetal head by overlapping of the cranial bones to facilitate movement through the birth canal during labor) (Fig. 23.14).

Caput succedaneum is a generalized, easily identifiable edematous area of the scalp, most often on the occiput (Fig. 23.15A). With vertex presentation, the sustained pressure of the presenting part against the cervix results in compression of local vessels, slowing venous return. The slower venous return causes an increase in tissue fluids within the skin of the scalp, and edema develops. This edematous area, present at birth, extends across suture lines of the skull and usually disappears spontaneously within 3 to 4 days. Infants who are born with the assistance of vacuum extraction usually have a caput in the area where the cup was applied. Bruising of the scalp is often seen in the presence of caput succedaneum.

Cephalhematoma is a collection of blood between a skull bone and its periosteum. Therefore a cephalhematoma does not cross a cranial suture line (see Fig. 23.15B). A cephalhematoma is firmer and better defined than a caput. Often caput succedaneum and cephalhematoma occur simultaneously. A cephalhematoma usually resolves in 2 to 8 weeks. As the hematoma resolves, hemolysis of RBCs occurs, and hyperbilirubinemia can result.

Subgaleal hemorrhage is bleeding into the subgaleal compartment (see Fig. 23.15C). The subgaleal compartment is a potential space that contains loosely arranged connective tissue; it is located beneath the galea aponeurosis, the tendinous sheath that connects the frontal and occipital muscles and forms the inner surface of the scalp. Subgaleal hemorrhage is the result of traction or application of shearing forces to the scalp, commonly associated with difficult operative vaginal birth, especially vacuum extraction. The scalp is pulled away from the bony calvarium; the vessels are torn, and blood collects in the subgaleal space. Blood loss can be severe, resulting in hypovolemic shock, disseminated intravascular coagulation (DIC), and death (Mangurten, Puppala, & Prazad, 2015).

Early detection of the hemorrhage is vital; serial head circumference measurements and inspection of the back of the neck for increasing edema and a firm mass are essential. A boggy scalp, pallor, tachycardia, and increasing head circumference can be early signs of a subgaleal hemorrhage. Computed tomography or magnetic resonance imaging is useful in confirming the diagnosis. Replacement of lost blood and clotting factors is required in acute cases of hemorrhage. Another possible early sign of subgaleal hemorrhage is a forward and lateral positioning of the newborn's ears because the hematoma extends posteriorly. Monitoring the infant for changes in level of consciousness and decreases in hematocrit is also key to early recognition and management. An increase in serum bilirubin level may be seen as a result of the degradation of blood cells within the hematoma (Mangurten et al., 2015).

Spine

The bones in the vertebral column of the newborn form two primary curvatures—one in the thoracic region and one in the sacral region. Both are forward, concave curvatures. As the infant gains head control at approximately 3 months of age, a secondary curvature appears in the cervical region. The newborn's spine appears straight and can be flexed easily. The newborn can lift the head and turn it from side to side when prone. The vertebrae should appear straight and flat. If a pilonidal dimple is noted, further inspection is required to determine whether a sinus is present. A pilonidal dimple, especially with a sinus and nevus pilosis (hairy nevus), can be associated with spina bifida.

Extremities

The infant's extremities should be symmetric and of equal length. Fingers and toes should be equal in number (five fingers on each hand and five toes on each foot) and should have nails present. Digits may be missing (*oligodactyly*). Extra digits (*polydactyly*) are sometimes found on the hands or feet. Fingers or toes may be fused (*syndactyly*).

The infant is examined for developmental dysplasia of the hips (DDH). In newborns with DDH, the affected hip is unlikely to be dislocated at birth; instead it is easily dislocatable. Postnatal factors determine whether the hip dislocates, subluxates, or remains stable. DDH occurs more often in breech presentations (Fig. 23.16), first-born infants, female infants, and in infants with a family history of DDH (Son-Hing & Thompson, 2015; White, Bouchard, & Goldberg, 2018).

Signs of DDH are asymmetric gluteal and thigh skinfolds, uneven knee levels, a positive Ortolani test, and a positive Barlow test. The

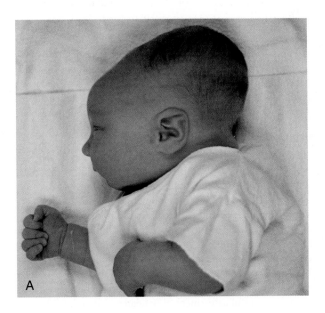

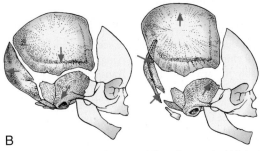

Fig. 23.14 Molding. (A) Significant molding after vaginal birth. (B) Schematic of bones of skull when molding is present. (A, Courtesy Kim Molloy, Knoxville, IA.)

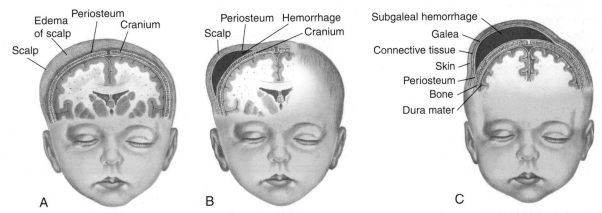

Fig. 23.15 Injuries to the Newborn Head due to Birth Trauma. (A) Caput succedaneum. (B) Cephalhematoma. (C) Subgaleal hemorrhage. (A and B, From Seidel, H., Ball, J., Dains, J., & Benedict, G. [2006]. *Mosby's guide to physical examination* [6th ed.]. St. Louis: Mosby.)

hips are inspected for symmetry. Gluteal and thigh skinfolds should be equal and symmetric, and legs should be of equal length (Fig. 23.17A). The level of the knees in flexion should be equal (see Fig. 23.17C). Hip integrity is assessed by using the Barlow test and the Ortolani maneuver. For the Barlow test, the examiner places the middle finger over the greater trochanter and the thumb along the midthigh. The hip is flexed to 90 degrees and adducted, followed by gentle downward pushing of the femoral head. If the hip can be dislocated with this maneuver, the femoral head moves out of the acetabulum, and the examiner feels a "clunk." The hip is then checked to determine if the femoral head can be returned into the acetabulum using the Ortolani maneuver. As the hip is abducted and upward leverage is applied, a dislocated hip returns to the acetabulum with a clunk that is felt by the examiner (see Fig. 23.17B and D).

⚡ SAFETY ALERT

Only expert examiners (e.g., physicians, nurse practitioners) should perform the Barlow test and Ortolani maneuver to assess for DDH. An unskilled examiner can cause injury to the newborn.

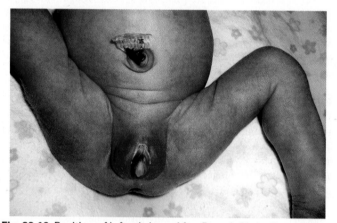

Fig. 23.16 Position of Infant's Legs After Breech Birth. Note preterm genitalia and vaginal discharge. (Courtesy Cheryl Briggs, RNC, Annapolis, MD.)

Signs of Skeletal Problems

Abnormalities of the skeletal system can be congenital, developmental, drug induced, or the result of intrapartum or postnatal factors. Signs of DDH, additional digits or webbing of digits, and any other abnormality should be documented and reported to the neonatal or pediatric health care provider.

A fractured clavicle often occurs in large infants and in those who had a difficult birth (e.g., shoulder dystocia). Unequal movement of the upper extremities or crepitus over the clavicular area can indicate fracture.

The newborn's feet can appear to be abnormally positioned. This can indicate congenital deformity or can be related to fetal positioning in utero. For example, clubfoot (talipes equinovarus), a deformity in which the foot turns inward and is fixed in a plantar-flexion position, is a congenital condition that warrants attention. If the foot is turned inward in the plantar-flexion position but can be moved into the normal position, it is likely caused by fetal positioning and should gradually resolve.

Neuromuscular System

The neuromuscular system is almost completely developed at birth. The term newborn is a responsive and reactive being with remarkable capacity for social interaction and self-organization.

Growth of the brain after birth follows a predictable pattern of rapid growth during infancy and early childhood; it becomes more gradual during the remainder of the first decade and minimal during adolescence. By the end of the first year, the cerebellum ends its growth spurt, which began at approximately 30 weeks of gestation.

The brain requires glucose as a source of energy and a relatively large supply of oxygen for adequate metabolism. The necessity for glucose requires careful assessment of neonates who are at risk for hypoglycemia (e.g., infants of mothers who have diabetes; infants who are macrosomic or small for gestational age; and newborns who experienced prolonged birth, hypoxia, or preterm birth).

Spontaneous motor activity can be seen as transient tremors of the mouth and chin, especially during crying episodes, and of the extremities, notably the arms and hands. Transient tremors are normal and can be observed in nearly every newborn. They most often involve the mouth and chin or the arms and hands. These tremors should not be present when the infant is quiet and should not persist beyond 1 month of age. Persistent tremors or tremors involving the total body can indicate

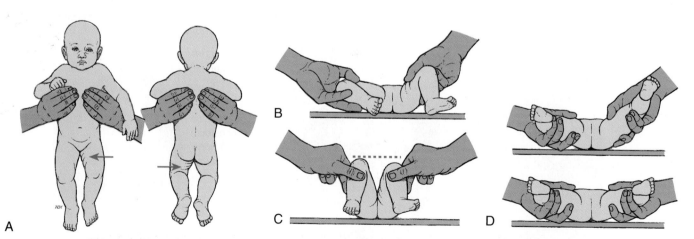

Fig. 23.17 Signs of Developmental Dysplasia of the Hip. (A) Asymmetry of gluteal and thigh folds with shortening of the thigh (Galeazzi sign). (B) Limited hip abduction, as seen in flexion (Ortolani test). (C) Apparent shortening of the femur, as indicated by the level of the knees in flexion (Allis sign). (D) Ortolani maneuver with femoral head moving in and out of acetabulum (in infants 1 to 2 months of age). (From Hockenberry, M. J., Wilson, D., & Rodgers, C. C. [2017]. *Wong's essentials of pediatric nursing* [10th ed.]. St. Louis: Elsevier.)

pathologic conditions. Normal tremors, tremors (jitteriness) of hypoglycemia, and seizure activity must be differentiated so corrective care can be instituted as necessary (Ditzenberger & Blackburn, 2014).

To differentiate between tremors or jitteriness and seizure activity, the nurse can consider the following signs (Ditzenberger & Blackburn, 2014):

- Tremors or jitteriness are easily elicited by motions or voice and cease with gentle restraint of the body part, whereas seizure activity continues.
- Passive flexion and repositioning of the tremulous extremity reduces or stops the movement.
- Seizure activity is associated with ocular changes (eyes deviating or staring) and autonomic changes (apnea, tachycardia, pupil changes, increased salivation); these signs are not associated with jitteriness or tremors.

The posture of the term newborn demonstrates flexion of the arms at the elbows and the legs at the knees. Hips are abducted and partially flexed. Intermittent fisting of the hands is common.

Muscle tone and strength are directly related. The infant with normal tone and strength exhibits some resistance to passive movement such as when being pulled to sit or when the arm or leg is extended by the examiner. The hypotonic neonate shows little resistance and can feel like a "rag doll." Hypertonia is evidenced by increased resistance to passive movement.

Although neuromuscular control is very limited, it can be noted. If newborns are placed face down on a firm surface, they will turn their heads to the side. They attempt to hold their heads in line with their bodies if they are raised by their arms. Various reflexes serve to promote safety and adequate food intake.

Newborn Reflexes

The newborn has many primitive reflexes. The times at which these reflexes appear and disappear reflect the maturity and intactness of the developing nervous system. The most common reflexes found in the normal term newborn are described in Table 23.1.

TABLE 23.1 Assessment of Newborn Reflexes

Reflex	Eliciting the Reflex	Characteristic Response	Comments
Rooting and sucking	Touch infant's lip, cheek, or corner of mouth with nipple or finger.	Infant turns head toward stimulus and opens mouth in search of sucking source (e.g., nipple, finger); begins to suck when nipple or examiner's finger is inserted into mouth.	Response is difficult if not impossible to elicit after infant has been fed; if response is weak or absent, consider preterm birth or neurologic defect. Parental guidance: Avoid trying to turn head toward breast or nipple; allow infant to root; response disappears after 3-4[a] months but can persist up to 1 year.
Swallowing	Feed infant; swallowing usually follows sucking and obtaining fluids.	Swallowing is usually coordinated with sucking and breathing and usually occurs without gagging, coughing, apnea, or vomiting.	If response is weak or absent, it can indicate preterm birth, effects of maternal analgesics or anesthetics, or illness that needs investigation. Sucking, swallowing, and breathing are often uncoordinated in preterm infant.
Grasp			
Palmar	Place finger in palm of hand.	Infant's fingers curl around examiner's finger.	Palmar response lessens by 3-4 months; parents enjoy this contact with infant.
Plantar	Place finger at base of toes.	Toes curl downward around examiner's finger.	Plantar response lessens by 8 months.

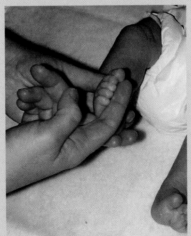

Plantar Grasp Reflex. (From Zitelli, B. J., & Davis, H. W. [2007]. *Atlas of pediatric physical diagnosis* [5th ed.]. St. Louis: Mosby.)

Continued

TABLE 23.1   Assessment of Newborn Reflexes—cont'd

Reflex	Eliciting the Reflex	Characteristic Response	Comments
Extrusion	Touch or depress tip of tongue.	Newborn forces tongue outward.	Response disappears by about 4-5 months.
Glabellar (Myerson)	Tap over forehead, bridge of nose, or maxilla of newborn whose eyes are open.	Newborn blinks for first four or five taps.	Continued blinking with repeated taps is consistent with extrapyramidal signs.
Tonic neck or "fencing"	With infant in supine neutral position, turn head quickly to one side.	With infant facing left side, arm and leg on that side extend; opposite arm and leg flex (turn head to right, and extremities assume opposite postures).	Responses in leg are more consistent. Complete response disappears by 3-4 months; incomplete response may be seen until 3-4 years. After 6 weeks, persistent response is sign of possible cerebral palsy.

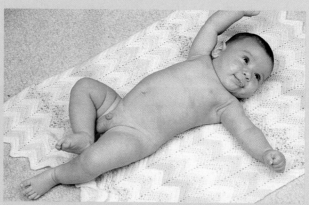

Classic Pose in Tonic Neck Reflex. (Courtesy Marjorie Pyle, RNC, Lifecircle, Costa Mesa, CA.)

Moro	Hold infant in semisitting position, allow head and trunk to fall backward to angle of at least 30 degrees (with support). OR Place infant supine on flat surface; perform sharp hand clap.	Symmetric abduction and extension of arms are seen; fingers fan out and form a *C* with thumb and forefinger; slight tremor may be noted; arms are adducted in embracing motion and return to relaxed flexion and movement. A cry may accompany or follow motor movement. Legs may follow similar pattern of response. Preterm infant does not complete "embrace"; instead arms fall backward because of weakness.	Response is present at birth; complete response may be seen until 8 weeks; body jerk is seen only between 8 and 18 weeks; response is absent by 6 months if neurologic maturation is not delayed; response may be incomplete if infant is in deep sleep state; give parental guidance about normal response. Asymmetric response can indicate injury to brachial plexus, clavicle, or humerus. Persistent response after 6 months indicates possible neurologic abnormality.

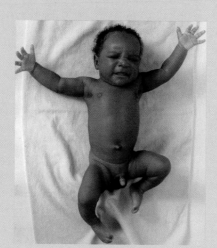

Moro Reflex. (Courtesy Paul Vincent Kuntz, Texas Children's Hospital, Houston, TX.)

TABLE 23.1   Assessment of Newborn Reflexes—cont'd

Reflex	Eliciting the Reflex	Characteristic Response	Comments
Stepping or "walking"	Hold infant vertically under arms or on trunk, allowing one foot to touch table surface.	Infant will simulate walking, alternating flexion and extension of feet; term infants walk on soles of their feet, and preterm infants walk on their toes.	Response is normally present for 3-4 weeks.

Stepping Reflex. (From Dickason, E. J., Silverman, B. L., & Kaplan, J. A. [1998]. *Maternal-infant nursing care* [3rd ed.]. St. Louis: Mosby.)

Reflex	Eliciting the Reflex	Characteristic Response	Comments
Crawling	Place newborn on abdomen.	Newborn makes crawling movements with arms and legs.	Response should disappear by about 6 weeks of age.

Crawling Reflex. (Courtesy Paul Vincent Kuntz, Texas Children's Hospital, Houston, TX.)

Reflex	Eliciting the Reflex	Characteristic Response	Comments
Deep tendon	Use finger instead of percussion hammer to elicit patellar, or knee-jerk, reflex; newborn must be relaxed.	Reflex jerk is present; even with newborn relaxed, nonselective overall reaction may occur.	It is usually more difficult to elicit upper extremity reflexes than lower extremity reflexes.
Crossed extension	With infant in supine position, examiner extends one leg of infant and presses down knee. Stimulation of sole of foot of fixated limb should cause free leg to flex, adduct, and extend as if attempting to push away stimulating agent.	Opposite leg flexes, adducts, and then extends.	This reflex should be present during newborn period.

Continued

TABLE 23.1 Assessment of Newborn Reflexes—cont'd

Reflex	Eliciting the Reflex	Characteristic Response	Comments

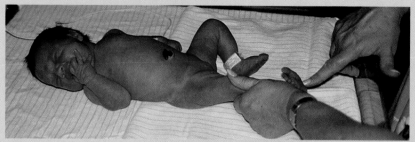

Crossed Extension Reflex. (Courtesy Marjorie Pyle, RNC, Lifecircle, Costa Mesa, CA.)

Reflex	Eliciting the Reflex	Characteristic Response	Comments
Babinski (plantar)	On sole of foot, beginning at heel, stroke upward along lateral aspect of sole; then move finger across ball of foot.	All toes hyperextend, with dorsiflexion of big toe—recorded as a positive sign.	Absence requires neurologic evaluation; should disappear after 1 year of age. Response depends on infant's general muscle tone, maturity, and condition.

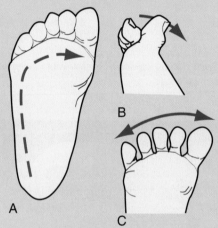

Babinski Reflex. (A) Direction of stroke. (B) Dorsiflexion of big toe. (C) Fanning of toes. (From Hockenberry, M. J., Wilson, D., & Rodgers, C. C. [2017]. *Wong's nursing care of infants and children* [10th ed.]. St. Louis: Elsevier.)

Reflex	Eliciting the Reflex	Characteristic Response	Comments
Pull-to-sit (traction response); postural tone	Pull infant up by wrists from supine position with head in midline.	Head lags until infant is in upright position; then head is held in same plane with chest and shoulder momentarily before falling forward; infant attempts to right head.	Response depends on general muscle tone and maturity and condition of infant.
Truncal incurvation (Galant)	Place infant prone on flat surface; run finger down back approximately 4-5 cm lateral to spine, first on one side and then down the other.	Trunk is flexed, and pelvis is swung toward stimulated side.	Response disappears by 4 weeks. Response varies but should be exhibited in all infants, including preterm. Absence suggests general depression of nervous system. With transverse lesions of cord, no response below level of lesion is present.

TABLE 23.1 Assessment of Newborn Reflexes—cont'd

Reflex	Eliciting the Reflex	Characteristic Response	Comments

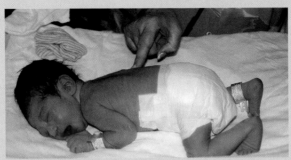

Trunk Incurvation Reflex. (Courtesy Marjorie Pyle, RNC, Lifecircle, Costa Mesa, CA.)

| Magnet | Place infant in supine position, partially flex both lower extremities, and apply light pressure with fingers to soles of feet (Fig. A). Normally, while examiner's fingers maintain contact with soles of feet, lower limbs extend. | Both lower limbs should extend against examiner's pressure (Fig. B). | Absence suggests damage to central nervous system. Weak reflex may be seen after breech presentation *without* extended legs or may indicate sciatic nerve stretch syndrome. Breech presentation *with* extended legs may evoke exaggerated response. |

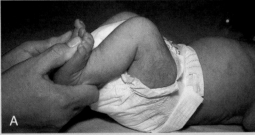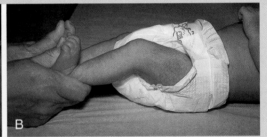

Magnet Reflex. (Courtesy Michael S. Clement, MD, Mesa, AZ.)

| Additional newborn responses: yawn, stretch, burp, hiccup, sneeze | These are spontaneous behaviors. | Responses can be slightly depressed temporarily because of maternal analgesia or anesthesia, fetal hypoxia, or infection. | Parental guidance: Most of these behaviors are pleasurable to parents.
Parents need to be assured that behaviors are normal.
Sneeze is usually a response to mucus in the nose and not an indicator of upper respiratory infection.
No treatment is needed for hiccups; sucking may help. In a preterm infant, these are signs of neurodevelopmental immaturity and physiologic stress. |

[a]All durations for persistence of reflexes are based on time elapsed after 40 weeks of gestation (i.e., if newborn was born at 36 weeks of gestation, add 1 month to all time limits given).

BEHAVIORAL ADAPTATIONS

The healthy infant must accomplish behavioral and biologic tasks to develop normally. Behavioral characteristics form the basis of the social capabilities of the infant. Newborns progress through a hierarchy of developmental challenges as they adapt to their environment and caregivers. They must first be able to regulate their physiologic or autonomic system, including involuntary physiologic functions such as heart rate, respiration, and temperature. The next level is motor organization, in which infants regulate or control their motor behavior.

This includes controlling random movements, improving muscle tone, and reducing excessive activity. The third level of behavior is *state regulation,* which refers to the ability to modulate the state of consciousness. The infant develops predictable sleep and wake states and is able to react to stress through self-regulation or communicating with the caregiver by crying and then being consoled. Finally, the infant reaches the fourth level of attention and social interaction. He or she is able to attend to visual and auditory stimulation, stay alert for long periods, and engage in social interaction (Brazelton & Nugent, 2011).

BOX 23.3 Clusters of Neonatal Behaviors in Brazelton Neonatal Behavioral Assessment Scale

- Habituation—Ability to respond to and then inhibit responding to discrete stimulus (e.g., light, rattle, bell, pinprick) while asleep
- Orientation—Quality of alert states and ability to attend to visual and auditory stimuli while alert
- Motor performance—Quality of movement and tone
- Range of state—Measure of general arousal level or arousability of infant
- Regulation of state—How infant responds when aroused
- Autonomic stability—Signs of stress (e.g., tremors, startles, skin color) related to homeostatic (self-regulator) adjustment of the nervous system
- Reflexes—Assessment of several neonatal reflexes

From Brazelton, T., & Nugent, J. (2011). *Neonatal behavioral assessment scale* (4th ed.). London. UK: MacKeith.

This progression in behavior is the basis for the Brazelton Neonatal Behavioral Assessment Scale (NBAS) (Brazelton & Nugent, 2011). The NBAS is an interactive examination that assesses the infant's response to 28 areas organized according to the clusters in Box 23.3. It is generally used as a research or diagnostic tool and requires special training. The NBAS helps the practitioner to identify where the infant falls along the continuum of behaviors and determine the type of support needed.

Sleep-wake States

Healthy newborns differ in their activity levels, feeding patterns, sleeping patterns, and responsiveness. Parents' reactions to their newborns are often determined by these differences. Showing parents the unique characteristics of their infant helps them to develop a more positive perception of the infant and promotes increased interaction between infant and parent. Infant responses to environmental stimuli and to their caregivers depend on the infant's state or state of consciousness.

In the early newborn period, infants tend to alternate periods of sleep and wakefulness that resemble their fetal inactivity and activity patterns. Variations in the state of consciousness of infants are called sleep-wake states. The six states form a continuum from deep sleep to extreme irritability (Fig. 23.18): two sleep states (deep sleep and light sleep) and four wake states (drowsy, quiet alert, active alert, and crying) (Brazelton & Nugent, 2011). Each state has specific characteristics and state-related behaviors. The optimal state of arousal is the quiet alert state. During this state, infants smile, vocalize, move in synchrony with speech, watch their parents' faces, and respond to people talking to them. They respond to internal and external environmental factors by controlling sensory input and regulating the sleep-wake states; the ability to make smooth transitions between states is called *state modulation*. The ability to regulate sleep-wake states is essential in the infant's neurobehavioral development. Term infants are better able than preterm infants to cope with external or internal factors that affect the sleep-wake patterns.

Infants use purposeful behavior to maintain the optimal arousal state as follows: (1) actively withdrawing by increasing physical distance, (2) rejecting by pushing away with hands and feet, (3) decreasing sensitivity by falling asleep or breaking eye contact by turning the head, or (4) using signaling behaviors such as fussing and crying. These behaviors permit infants to quiet themselves and reinstate readiness to interact.

The first 6 weeks of life involve a steady decrease in the proportion of active REM sleep to total sleep. A steady increase in the proportion of quiet sleep to total sleep also occurs. Periods of wakefulness increase. For the first few weeks, the wakeful periods seem dictated by hunger,

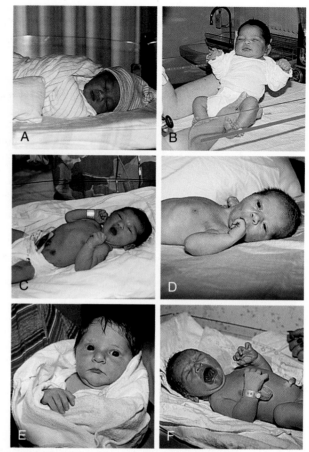

Fig. 23.18 Newborn Sleep-Wake States. (A) Deep sleep. (B) Light sleep. (C) Drowsy. (D) Quiet alert. (E) Active alert. (F) Crying. (Courtesy Marjorie Pyle, RNC, Lifecircle, Costa Mesa, CA.)

but soon a need for socializing appears. The newborn sleeps approximately 16 to 19 hours per day, with periods of wakefulness gradually increasing. By the fourth week of life, some infants stay awake from one feeding to the next (Gardner, Goldson, & Hernández, 2016).

Infants demonstrate neurobehavioral cues that can guide parents and other caregivers in providing care and social interaction. Cues that indicate stability and engagement include alertness, eye-to-eye contact, facial gaze, smiling, vocalization, smooth movements, and flexion of arms and legs. Signs of distress or disengagement include facial grimace or worried expression, splaying of fingers, gaze aversion, staring, regurgitation or vomiting, and jitteriness (Blackburn, 2018).

Other Factors Influencing Newborn Behavior

Gestational Age

Gestational age and level of central nervous system (CNS) maturity affect infant behavior. In the preterm neonate with an immature CNS, the entire body responds to a pinprick of the foot, although the response may not be observed by an untrained observer. The more mature infant withdraws only the foot. CNS immaturity is reflected in reflex development, sleep-wake states, and ability (or lack thereof) to regulate or modulate a smooth transition between different states. Preterm infants have brief periods of alertness but have difficulty maintaining alertness without becoming overstimulated, which leads to autonomic instability unless intervention is implemented. Premature or sick infants show signs of fatigue or physiologic stress sooner than full-term healthy infants.

Time

The time elapsed since birth affects the behavior of infants as they attempt to become organized initially. Time elapsed since the previous feeding and time of day also can influence infants' responses.

Stimuli

Environmental events and stimuli affect the infant's behavioral responses. The newborn responds to animate and inanimate stimuli. Nurses in intensive care nurseries observe that infants respond to loud noises, bright lights, monitor alarms, and tension in the unit. If a mother is tense, nervous, or uncomfortable while feeding her infant, the infant may sense her tension and demonstrate difficulty feeding.

Medication

No conclusive evidence exists regarding the effects of maternal analgesia or anesthesia during labor on neonatal behavior. Researchers who have studied the effects of epidural medications on breastfeeding behaviors have been unable to show a cause-and-effect relationship (Hoyt & Pages-Arroyo, 2015).

Sensory Behaviors

From birth, infants possess sensory capabilities that indicate a state of readiness for social interaction. They effectively use behavioral responses in establishing their first dialogues. These responses, coupled with the newborns' "baby appearance" (e.g., facial proportions of forehead, eyes larger than the lower portion of the face) and their small size and helplessness, rouse feelings of wanting to hold, protect, and interact with them.

Vision

At birth the eye is structurally incomplete, and the muscles are immature. The process of accommodation is not present but improves over the first 3 months of life. The pupils react to light, the blink reflex is stimulated easily, and the corneal reflex is activated by light touch. Term newborns can see objects as far away as 50 cm (2.5 feet). The clearest visual distance is 17 to 20 cm (8 to 12 inches), which is approximately the distance between the mother's and infant's faces during breastfeeding or cuddling. Newborns seem to have a preference for faces and can recognize the mother's face. This facilitates interaction and promotes bonding. They will engage the mother or caregiver with eye contact. Newborns can imitate facial expressions and motions such as protruding the tongue (Gardner, Goldson, & Hernández, 2016). Newborns prefer complex patterns over non-patterned stimuli. They prefer black and white, possibly because of the greater contrast. By 2 months, color vision is present (Kaufman, Miller, & Gupta, 2015).

Hearing

Term newborns can hear and differentiate among various sounds. They will turn toward a sound and attempt to locate the source. The neonate recognizes and responds readily to the mother's voice and shows a preference for high-pitched intonation. Newborns respond to rhythmic sounds. They are accustomed to hearing the regular rhythm of the mother's heartbeat, which was a constant sound during intrauterine life. As a result, they respond by relaxing and ceasing to fuss and cry if a regular heartbeat simulator is placed nearby; a lullaby can have the same effect. Hearing is integral to bonding and attachment and may be more important than vision (Gardner, Goldson, & Hernández, 2016).

Routine hearing screening is recommended for all newborns before hospital discharge. See Chapter 24 and Fig. 24.11 for a discussion about newborn hearing screening.

Smell

Newborns have a highly developed sense of smell and can detect and discriminate distinct odors. It has been shown that preterm infants as early as 28 weeks are capable of reacting to odors. They react to strong odors such as alcohol or vinegar by turning their heads away but are attracted to sweet smells. By the fifth day of life, newborn infants can recognize their mother's smell. Breastfed infants are able to smell breast milk and can differentiate their mothers from other lactating women (Lawrence & Lawrence, 2016).

Taste

Young infants are particularly oriented toward the use of their mouths, both for meeting their nutritional needs for rapid growth and for releasing tension through sucking. The early development of circumoral sensation, muscle activity, and taste would seem to be preparation for survival in the extrauterine environment. The newborn can distinguish among tastes and has a preference for sweet solutions (Gardner, Goldson, & Hernández, 2016).

Touch

The infant is responsive to touch on all parts of the body. The face (especially the mouth), hands, and soles of the feet seem to be the most sensitive. Reflexes can be elicited by stroking the infant. The newborn's responses to touch suggest that this sensory system is well prepared to receive and process tactile messages (Gardner, Goldson, & Hernández, 2016). Early skin-to-skin contact with the mother promotes tactile interaction and stimulation. Touch and motion are essential to normal growth and development. However, each infant is unique, and variations can be seen in newborns' responses to touch. Birth trauma or stress and depressant drugs taken by the mother can decrease the infant's sensitivity to touch or painful stimuli.

Response to Environmental Stimuli

Temperament

Each neonate has a unique repertoire of behaviors that are influenced by various factors including temperament, sensory threshold, ability to habituate, and consolability. Temperament refers to individual variations in the reaction pattern of newborns. Newborns possess individual characteristics that affect selective responses to various stimuli present in the internal and external environments. Some infants appear to be quiet by nature and can remain still for extended periods. Their movements may be smooth and relaxed most of the time, and they have little difficulty settling down for feeding. Other infants are more active and seem to be in constant motion; they seem to be excited and interested in exploring the faces and sounds around them. These infants often need help to settle; containment (swaddling), physical contact, and boundaries surrounding the infant in the crib can facilitate a quiet alert state.

Habituation

Habituation is a protective mechanism that allows the infant to become accustomed to environmental stimuli. It is a psychologic and physiologic phenomenon in which the response to a constant or repetitive stimulus is decreased. In the term newborn, this can be demonstrated in several ways. Shining a bright light into a newborn's eyes causes a startle or squinting the first two or three times. The third or fourth flash elicits a diminished response, and by the fifth or sixth flash the infant ceases to respond (Brazelton & Nugent, 2011). The same response pattern holds true for the sounds of a rattle or stroking the bottom of the foot.

The ability to habituate allows the healthy term newborn to select stimuli that promote continued learning about the social world, thus avoiding overload. The intrauterine environment seems to have programmed the newborn to be especially responsive to human voices, soft lights, soft sounds, and sweet tastes.

The newborn quickly learns the sounds in the home environment and is able to sleep in their midst. The selective responses of the newborn indicate cerebral organization capable of memory and making choices. The ability to habituate depends on the state of consciousness, hunger, fatigue, and temperament. These factors also affect consolability, cuddliness, irritability, and crying.

Consolability

Newborns vary in the ability to console themselves or be consoled. In the crying state, most newborns initiate one of several ways to reduce their distress. Hand-to-mouth movements with or without sucking and being alert to voices, noises, or visual stimuli are common. Some infants are consoled only if they are held and rocked (Brazelton & Nugent, 2011).

Cuddliness

Cuddliness is especially important to parents because they often gauge their ability to care for the child by the child's responses to their actions. The degree to which newborns relax and mold into the contours of the person holding them varies. One extreme is the infant who always resists being held with thrashing and stiffening of the body. This is in contrast to the infant who immediately relaxes when held and molds to the body of the person. Less extreme behavior is demonstrated by infants who are passive when held and those who gradually mold after being held for a while (Brazelton & Nugent, 2011).

Irritability

Some newborns cry longer and harder than others. For some, the sensory threshold seems low. They are easily upset by unusual noises, hunger, wetness, or new experiences and thus respond intensely. Others with a high sensory threshold require a great deal more stimulation and variation to reach the active, alert state.

Crying

Crying is the language an infant uses most often to communicate needs. It can signal hunger, discomfort, pain, desire for attention, or fussiness. Infants may cry in response to environmental stimuli such as cold, being overstimulated, or being held by multiple persons. Responsiveness of the caregiver to the crying creates trust as the infant learns to associate the caregiver with comfort.

The amount and tone of crying vary based on gestational age, weight, and the reason for the cry (e.g., hunger, pain). A high-pitched cry can be a sign of a neurologic disorder. Some mothers state that they learn to distinguish among the cries. The breastfeeding mother's body responds physiologically to infant crying by stimulating the milk-ejection reflex ("let-down").

The duration of crying also varies greatly in each infant; newborns may cry for as little as 5 minutes or as much as 2 hours or more per day. The amount of crying peaks in the second month and then decreases. There is a diurnal rhythm of crying, with more crying occurring in the evening hours.

KEY POINTS

- By term gestation, the neonate's anatomic and physiologic systems have reached a level of development and functioning to allow physical existence apart from the mother.
- The neonate's most critical adaptation to extrauterine life is to establish effective respirations.
- Heat loss in the healthy term newborn can exceed the ability to produce heat, leading to hypothermia, cold stress, and metabolic and respiratory complications.
- Physiologic jaundice occurs in 60% of term infants.
- Jaundice is considered pathologic if it appears within the first 24 hours of life, if serum bilirubin levels increase by more than 6 mg/dL in 24 hours, or if serum bilirubin exceeds 15 mg/dL at any time.
- Some reflex behaviors are important for the newborn's survival.
- The healthy term newborn has sensory abilities that indicate a state of readiness for social interaction.
- Sleep-wake states and other factors influence newborn behavior.
- Newborn behavior progresses from self-regulation of autonomic processes to social interaction.
- Each term newborn has a predisposed capacity to handle the multitude of stimuli in the external world.

REFERENCES

American Academy of Pediatrics. (2017). Statement of endorsement: Delayed umbilical cord clamping after birth. *Pediatrics, 139*(6), e20170957.

American Academy of Pediatrics and American College of Obstetricians and Gynecologists. (2017). *Guidelines for perinatal care* (8th ed.). Washington, DC: Author.

American College of Obstetricians and Gynecologists.(2017, reaffirmed 2018). Committee opinion no. 684: Timing of umbilical cord clamping after birth. *Obstetrics & Gynecology, 129*, e5–e10.

Association of Women's Health, Obstetric and Neonatal Nurses. (2018). *Neonatal Skin Care* (4th ed.). Washington, DC: Author.

Bäckhed, F., Roswall, J., Peng, Y., et al. (2015). Dynamics and stabilization of the human gut microbiome during the first year of life. *Cell Host and Microbe, 17*(5), 690–703.

Benjamin, J. T., Mezu-Ndubuisi, O. J., & Maheshwari, A. (2015). Developmental immunology. In R. J. Martin, A. A. Fanaroff, & M. C. Walsh (Eds.), *Fanaroff & Martin's neonatal-perinatal medicine* (10th ed.). Philadelphia: Saunders.

Blackburn, S. T. (2018). *Maternal, fetal, and neonatal physiology* (5th ed.). St. Louis: Elsevier.

Bodin, M. B. (2014). Immune system. In C. Kenner, & J. W. Lott (Eds.), *Comprehensive neonatal nursing care* (5th ed.). New York: Springer.

Brazelton, T., & Nugent, J. (2011). *Neonatal behavioral assessment scale* (4th ed.). London, UK: MacKeith.

Cadnapaphornchai, M. A., Schoenbein, M. B., Woloschuk, R., et al. (2016). Neonatal nephrology. In S. L. Gardner, B. S. Carter, M. Enzman-Hines, et al. (Eds.), *Merenstein & Gardner's handbook of neonatal intensive care* (8th ed.). St. Louis: Elsevier.

Centers for Disease Control and Prevention. (2018). *Congenital heart defects: Data and statistics.* Retrieved from: http://www.cdc.gov/ncbddd/heartdefects/data.html.

Christensen, R. D., & Ohls, R. K. (2016). Development of the hematopoietic system. In R. M. Kliegman, B. F. Stanton, J. W. St Geme, et al. (Eds.), *Nelson textbook of pediatrics* (20th ed.). Philadelphia: Elsevier.

Dell, K. M. (2015). Fluids, electrolytes, and acid-base homeostasis. In R. J. Martin, A. A. Fanaroff, & M. C. Walsh (Eds.), *Fanaroff & Martin's neonatal-perinatal medicine* (10th ed.). St. Louis: Saunders.

Desmond, M., Rudolph, A., & Phitaksphraiwan, P. (1966). The transitional care nursery: A mechanism for preventive medicine in the newborn. *Pediatric Clinics of North America, 13*(3), 651–668.

Diehl-Jones, W., & Fraser, D. (2015). Hematologic disorders. In M. T. Verklan, & M. Walden (Eds.), *Core curriculum for neonatal intensive care nursing* (5th ed.). St. Louis: Elsevier.

Ditzenberger, G. R., & Blackburn, S. T. (2014). Neurologic system. In C. Kenner, & J. W. Lott (Eds.), *Comprehensive neonatal nursing care* (5th ed.). New York: Springer.

Elder, J. S. (2016). Anomalies of the penis and urethra. In R. M. Kliegman, B. F. Stanton, J. W. St.Geme, et al. (Eds.), *Nelson textbook of pediatrics* (20th ed.). Philadelphia: Elsevier.

Flynn, J. G. (2017). Etiology, clinical features, and diagnosis of neonatal hypertension. In J. A. Garcia-Prats, & T. K. Mattoo (Eds.), *UpToDate*. Retrieved from: http://www.uptodate.com/home.

Fraser, D. (2015). Respiratory distress. In M. T. Verklan, & M. Walden (Eds.), *Core curriculum for neonatal intensive care nursing* (5th ed.). St. Louis: Elsevier.

Gardner, S. L., Enzman Hines, M., & Nyp, M. (2016). Respiratory diseases. In S. L. Gardner, B. S. Carter, M. Enzman-Hines, et al. (Eds.), *Merenstein & Gardner's handbook of neonatal intensive care* (8th ed.). St. Louis: Elsevier.

Gardner, S. L., Goldson, E., & Hernández, J. A. (2016). The neonate and the environment: Impact on development. In S. L. Gardner, B. S. Carter, M. Enzman-Hines, et al. (Eds.), *Merenstein & Gardner's handbook of neonatal intensive care* (8th ed.). St. Louis: Elsevier.

Gardner, S. L., & Hernández, J. A. (2016). Heat balance. In S. L. Gardner, B. S. Carter, M. Enzman-Hines, et al. (Eds.), *Merenstein & Gardner's handbook of neonatal intensive care* (8th ed.). St. Louis: Elsevier.

Hawkes, C. P., & Stanley, C. A. (2017). Pathophysiology of neonatal hypoglycemia. In R. A. Polin, S. H. Abman, D. H. Rowitch, et al. (Eds.), *Fetal and neonatal physiology* (5th ed.). Philadelphia: Elsevier.

Hoath, S. B., & Narendran, V. (2015). The skin of the neonate. In R. J. Martin, A. A. Fanaroff, & M. C. Walsh (Eds.), *Fanaroff & Martin's neonatal-perinatal medicine* (10th ed.). Philadelphia: Saunders.

Hoyt, M. R., & Pages-Arroyo, E. M. (2015). Anesthesia for labor and delivery. In R. J. Martin, A. A. Fanaroff, & M. C. Walsh (Eds.), *Fanaroff & Martin's neonatal-perinatal medicine* (10th ed.). Philadelphia: Saunders.

Janke, J. (2014). Newborn nutrition. In K. R. Simpson, & P. A. Creehan (Eds.), *Perinatal nursing* (4th ed.). Philadelphia: Lippincott Williams & Wilkins.

Kamath-Rayne, B. D., Thilo, E. H., Deacon, J., et al. (2016). Neonatal hyperbilirubinemia. In S. L. Gardner, B. S. Carter, M. Enzman-Hines, et al. (Eds.), *Merenstein & Gardner's handbook of neonatal intensive care* (8th ed.). St. Louis: Elsevier.

Kaufman, L. M., Miller, M. T., & Gupta, B. K. (2015). The eye. In R. J. Martin, A. A. Fanaroff, & M. C. Walsh (Eds.), *Fanaroff & Martin's neonatal-perinatal medicine* (10th ed.). Philadelphia: Saunders.

Lawrence, R. A., & Lawrence, R. M. (2016). *Breastfeeding: A guide for the medical profession* (8th ed.). St. Louis: Mosby.

Lee, M. M. (2017). Testicular development and descent. In R. A. Polin, S. H. Abman, D. H. Rowitch, et al. (Eds.), *Fetal and neonatal physiology* (5th ed.). Philadelphia: Elsevier.

Lissauer, T. (2015). Physical examination of the newborn. In R. J. Martin, A. A. Fanaroff, & M. C. Walsh (Eds.), *Fanaroff & Martin's neonatal-perinatal medicine* (10th ed.). Philadelphia: Saunders.

Mangurten, H. H., Puppala, B. L., & Prazad, R. A. (2015). Birth injuries. In R. J. Martin, A. A. Fanaroff, & M. C. Walsh (Eds.), *Fanaroff & Martin's neonatal-perinatal medicine* (10th ed.). Philadelphia: Saunders.

Martin, K. L. (2016). Vascular disorders. In R. M. Kliegman, B. F. Stanton, J. W. St.Geme, et al. (Eds.), *Nelson textbook of pediatrics* (20th ed.). Philadelphia: Elsevier.

Monagle, P. (2017). Developmental hemostasis. In R. A. Polin, S. H. Abman, D. H. Rowitch, et al. (Eds.), *Fetal and neonatal physiology* (5th ed.). Philadelphia: Elsevier.

Mueller, N. T., Bakacs, E., Combellick, J., et al. (2015). The infant microbiome development: Mom matters. *Trends in Molecular Medicine, 21*(2), 109–117.

Neu, J. (2017). The developing microbiome of the fetus and newborn. In R. A. Polin, S. H. Abman, D. H. Rowitch, et al. (Eds.), *Fetal and neonatal physiology* (5th ed.). Philadelphia: Elsevier.

Pagana, K. D., Pagana, T. J., & Pagana, T. N. (2017). *Mosby's diagnostic and laboratory test reference* (13th ed.). St. Louis: Elsevier.

Perlman, J. M., Wyllie, J., Kattwinkel, J., et al. (2015). Part 7: Neonatal resuscitation: 2015 international consensus on cardiopulmonary resuscitation and emergency cardiovascular care science with treatment recommendations. *Circulation, 132*(16 Suppl. 1), S204–S241.

Richards, M. K., & Goldin, A. B. (2018). Neonatal gastroesophageal reflux. In C. A. Gleason, & S. E. Juul (Eds.), *Avery's diseases of the newborn* (10th ed.). Philadelphia: Elsevier.

Shearer, M. J. (2017). Vitamin K metabolism in the fetus and neonate. In R. A. Polin, S. H. Abman, D. H. Rowitch, et al. (Eds.), *Fetal and neonatal physiology* (5th ed.). Philadelphia: Elsevier.

Son-Hing, J. P., & Thompson, G. H. (2015). Congenital abnormalities of the upper and lower extremities and spine. In R. J. Martin, A. A. Fanaroff, & M. C. Walsh (Eds.), *Fanaroff & Martin's neonatal-perinatal medicine* (10th ed.). Philadelphia: Saunders.

Turfkruyer, M., & Verhasselt, V. (2015). Breast milk and its impact on the maturation of the neonatal immune system. *Current Opinions in Infectious Diseases, 28*(3), 199–206.

Verklan, M. T. (2015). Adaptation to extrauterine life. In M. T. Verklan, & M. Walden (Eds.), *Core curriculum for neonatal intensive care nursing* (5th ed.). St. Louis: Elsevier.

Visscher, M. O., Adam, R., Brink, S., et al. (2015). Newborn infant skin: Physiology, development. *Clinics in Dermatology, 33*(3), 271–280.

Vogt, B. A., & Dell, K. M. (2015). The kidney and urinary tract of the neonate. In R. J. Martin, A. A. Fanaroff, & M. C. Walsh (Eds.), *Fanaroff & Martin's neonatal-perinatal medicine* (10th ed.). Philadelphia: Saunders.

Watchko, J. F. (2018). Neonatal indirect hyperbilirubinemia and kernicterus. In C. A. Gleason, & S. E. Juul (Eds.), *Avery's diseases of the newborn* (10th ed.). Philadelphia: Elsevier.

White, K. K., Bouchard, M., & Goldberg, M. J. (2018). Common neonatal orthopedic conditions. In C. A. Gleason, & S. E. Juul (Eds.), *Avery's diseases of the newborn* (10th ed.). Philadelphia: Elsevier.

24

Nursing Care of the Newborn and Family

Patricia A. Scott

LEARNING OBJECTIVES

- Explain the purpose and components of the Apgar score.
- Describe how to perform a physical assessment of a newborn.
- Describe the process for assessing gestational age of a newborn.
- Compare characteristics of the preterm, late preterm, early term, term, and postterm neonate.
- Provide nursing care to assist the newborn in transitioning to the extrauterine environment.
- Explain the components of a safe environment.
- Discuss phototherapy and guidelines for instructing parents about this treatment.

- Explain the purposes and methods for newborn male circumcision (NMC), postoperative care, and parent teaching.
- Describe procedures for administering an intramuscular (IM) injection and for performing a heelstick and venipuncture.
- Evaluate pain in the newborn based on physiologic changes and behavioral observations.
- Discuss pharmacologic and nonpharmacologic interventions to reduce neonatal pain.
- Review anticipatory guidance provided by nurses for new parents regarding newborn care.

Although most newborns make the necessary biopsychosocial adjustments to extrauterine life without great difficulty, their well-being depends on the care they receive. This chapter describes the assessment and care of the newborn immediately after birth until discharge from the birth setting, as well as important anticipatory guidance for parents related to ongoing infant care.

CARE MANAGEMENT: BIRTH THROUGH THE FIRST 2 HOURS

Care begins immediately after birth and focuses on assessing and stabilizing the newborn's condition. Interprofessional care is key to optimizing outcomes for newborns. While the obstetric health care provider is focused on the mother, the labor and birth nurse is responsible for care of the neonate immediately after birth. There may be a second labor and birth nurse who is available for newborn care. In some hospitals, a "stork nurse" from the newborn nursery is assigned to do newborn care and administer medications. The nurse must be alert for any signs of distress or unusual physical characteristics and initiate appropriate interventions as needed.

When risk factors or birth events are likely to affect the well-being of the newborn, the labor and birth nurse notifies the neonatal or pediatric care team to request their attendance at the birth, or may call for them once the infant is born. Depending on the status of the newborn, additional health team members from other professions such as respiratory therapy and pharmacy may be needed.

The foundation for providing comprehensive, family-centered newborn care is awareness of the mother's preconception and prenatal history as well as intrapartal events. Recognition of risk factors (Box 24.1) enables the nurse to make astute observations, accurate assessments, and to identify early signs of complications. This allows for earlier intervention and promotes positive outcomes.

> ### ⚡ SAFETY ALERT
>
> With the possibility of transmission of viruses such as hepatitis B virus (HBV), hepatitis C virus, and human immunodeficiency virus (HIV) through maternal blood and blood-stained amniotic fluid, the newborn must be considered a potential contamination source until proven otherwise. As part of Standard Precautions, the nurse should wear gloves when handling the newborn until blood and amniotic fluid are removed by the initial bath.

Immediate Care After Birth

The primary goal of care in the first moments after birth is to assist the newborn to successfully transition to extrauterine life. The first priority is to establish effective respirations. If the newborn is at term, has good muscle tone, and is crying or breathing, routine care is all that is required (Weiner & Zaichkin, 2016). Routine care includes placing the newborn skin-to-skin on the mother's chest or abdomen. Drying the infant with gentle rubbing removes the moisture, which helps minimize evaporative heat loss. Wet linens should be removed, and the mother and baby should be covered with a warm blanket. After drying the newborn's head, a cap should be applied. Nasal and oral secretions are wiped away; the bulb syringe may be used if secretions appear to be blocking the airway. The nurse begins ongoing assessment of the neonate's breathing, color, and activity (Weiner & Zaichkin; Wyckoff, Aziz, Escobedo, et al., 2015).

A newborn who is not term, has poor muscle tone, or is not crying or breathing is placed immediately under a radiant warmer. Assessments and interventions are accomplished under the warmer until the infant is stable and can be safely placed skin-to-skin with the mother or transported to a nursery or neonatal intensive care (NICU) setting (Wyckoff et al., 2015).

BOX 24.1   Assessment of Preconception, Prenatal, and Intrapartum Risk Factors

Preconception

- Age
- Preexisting medical conditions: diabetes, hypertension, cardiac disease, anemia, thyroid disorder, renal disease, obesity
- Genetic factors: family history
- Obstetric history: gravidity, parity, number of living children and their ages, history of stillbirth, previous infant with congenital anomalies, history of miscarriages, use of assisted reproductive technology, interpregnancy spacing
- Blood type and Rh status

Prenatal

- Prenatal care: when started
- Nutrition: weight gain, diet, obesity, eating disorders
- Health-compromising behaviors: smoking, alcohol use, substance abuse
- Blood group or Rh sensitization
- Medications: prescription, over-the-counter, and complementary and alternative medications
- History of infection: sexually transmitted infections, TORCH[a] infections, group B streptococcus status, hepatitis B or C status

Intrapartum

- Length of gestation: preterm, late preterm, early term, term, or postterm
- First stage of labor: length, electronic fetal monitoring—internal or external, rupture of membranes (time, presence of meconium), signs of fetal distress (decelerations)
- Group B streptococcus status: treatment during labor
- Second stage of labor: length, vaginal or cesarean, birth, forceps- or vacuum-assisted birth, complications (shoulder dystocia, bleeding [abruptio placentae or placenta previa]), cord prolapse, maternal analgesia and/or anesthesia

[a]TORCH is the collective name for toxoplasmosis, other infections (e.g., hepatitis), rubella virus, cytomegalovirus (CMV), and herpes simplex virus.
Modified from Hurst, H.M. (2015). Antepartum-intrapartum complications. In: M.T. Verklan & M. Walden (Eds.), *Core curriculum for neonatal intensive care nursing* (5th ed.). St. Louis, MO: Elsevier.

The newborn should be breathing spontaneously. The trunk and lips should be pink; bluish discoloration of the hands and feet *(acrocyanosis)* is a normal finding (see Fig. 23.6). If the newborn is apneic or has gasping respirations, the newborn should be placed on the radiant warmer and positive pressure ventilation should be initiated (Weiner & Zaichkin, 2016). It may take a term newborn several minutes to "pink up." Visual inspection of cyanosis is not reliable; therefore, when central cyanosis persists, a pulse oximeter should be applied to the newborn's right hand (Weiner & Zaichkin). The oxygen saturation value as compared to the newborn's age in minutes helps guide the use of supplemental oxygen immediately after birth (Fig. 24.1).

The heart rate is quickly assessed by grasping the base of the cord or by auscultating the chest with a stethoscope. The nurse counts for 6 seconds and multiplies by 10 to calculate the heart rate. It should be greater than 100 beats/min. If the newborn requires respiratory or circulatory support, the nurse and other members of the health care team (e.g., neonatologist, respiratory therapist) should follow the most recent guidelines of the Neonatal Resuscitation Program, published by the American Heart Association (AHA) and the American Academy

of Pediatrics (AAP) (Wyckoff et al., 2015). The neonatal resuscitation algorithm directs the care (Fig. 24.1).

As soon as possible after birth, the nurse places identically numbered bands on the newborn's wrist and ankle, on the mother, and in some birth settings, on the father or significant other. These identification bands should be placed prior to the newborn being separated from the mother. An electronic infant security tag or abduction system alarm should be placed on all newborns to help protect against infant abduction. The infant is footprinted with ink or a scanning device within 2 hours of birth (see Preventing Infant Abduction section later in the chapter). Some facilities also take color photographs of the infant for identification.

Initial Assessment and Apgar Scoring

The initial assessment of the neonate is performed immediately after birth as the nurse conducts a brief physical examination (Table 24.1) and assigns an Apgar score (Table 24.2). A more comprehensive physical assessment and a gestational age assessment (Fig. 24.3 and Box 24.2) are completed within the first few hours of life; this is usually outlined by facility policy (Tappero & Honeyfield, 2015).

Initial Physical Assessment

The initial examination of the newborn (Table 24.1) may be accomplished while the infant is lying on the mother's abdomen or chest or in her arms immediately after birth (Fig. 24.2), or alternatively while the newborn is lying on the radiant warmer bed. Efforts should be directed toward minimizing interference during the first few minutes of life, allowing time for the parents to become acquainted with their newborn. If the newborn is breathing effectively, is pink, and has no apparent life-threatening anomalies or risk factors requiring immediate attention, further examination may be delayed until after the parents have had an opportunity to interact with the infant. Ideally, the newborn remains skin-to-skin with the mother for at least the first 1 to 2 hours after birth, and breastfeeding is initiated during that time. Routine procedures and the admission process can be carried out in the mother's room or in a separate nursery.

Apgar Score

The Apgar score is a routine rapid assessment of the newborn's overall status and response to resuscitation (AAP & American College of Obstetricians and Gynecologists [ACOG], 2017). This assessment is based on five signs that indicate the physiologic state of the neonate: (1) heart rate, based on auscultation with a stethoscope or palpation of the umbilical cord; (2) respiratory effort, based on observed movement of the chest wall; (3) muscle tone, based on degree of flexion and movement of the extremities; (4) reflex irritability, based on presence of a grimace, crying, or active withdrawal; and (5) generalized skin color, described as pallid, cyanotic, or pink (see Table 24.2). Evaluations can be completed by the nurse or birth attendant, depending on facility policy. Apgar scores of 0 to 3 indicate severe distress, scores of 4 to 6 indicate moderate difficulty, and scores of 7 to 10 indicate that the newborn is having minimal or no difficulty adjusting to extrauterine life. An Apgar score is assigned at 1 and 5 minutes after birth. For scores less than 7 at 5 minutes, the assessment should be repeated every 5 minutes for up to 20 minutes. Apgar scores do not predict future neurologic outcome for the newborn but are useful in describing the newborn's transition to the extrauterine environment and response to resuscitative efforts, if needed. If resuscitation is required, it should be initiated before the 1-minute Apgar score is determined (AAP & ACOG, 2017).

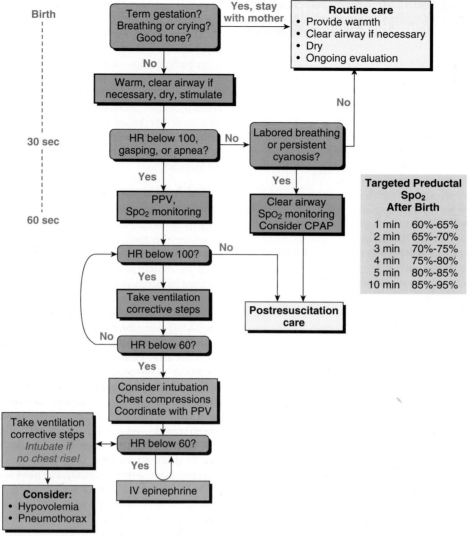

Fig. 24.1 Neonatal Resuscitation Algorithm. *CPAP,* Continuous positive airway pressure; *HR,* heart rate; *IV,* intravenous; *PPV,* positive-pressure ventilation; *Spo₂,* blood oxygen saturation. (From Wyckoff, M. H., Aziz, K., Escobedo, M. B., et al. [2015]. Part 13: Neonatal resuscitation: 2015 American Heart Association guidelines update for cardiopulmonary resuscitation and emergency cardiovascular care. *Circulation, 132*[18, suppl 2], S543–S560. Reprinted with permission from the American Heart Association.)

Physical Assessment

Although the initial assessment after birth can reveal significant anomalies, birth injuries, and cardiopulmonary problems that have immediate implications, a more detailed, thorough physical examination (Table 24.3) should follow within the first few hours of life, according to facility policy. The parents' presence during this and other examinations encourages discussion of their concerns and actively involves them in the health care of their infant from birth. It also gives the nurse an opportunity to observe parental interactions with the infant. The findings provide data for planning nursing care of the newborn and education for the parents. Ongoing assessments are made throughout the infant's stay in the facility.

General Appearance

Features to assess in the general survey include color, posture, activity, any obvious signs of anomalies that can cause initial distress, presence of bruising or other birth trauma, and state of alertness. The neonate's maturity level can be determined by assessing general appearance. The normal resting position of the term newborn is one of general flexion.

Vital Signs

The temperature, heart rate, and respiratory rate are assessed. Blood pressure (BP) is not routinely measured unless cardiac problems are suspected. Abnormalities in the heart rate, an abnormal heart rhythm, or the presence of a heart murmur can indicate the need for further evaluation of the newborn's circulatory status, including BP measurement.

The axillary temperature is a safe, accurate measurement of temperature. Electronic thermometers have expedited this task and provide a reading within 1 minute. Taking an infant's temperature can cause the infant to cry and struggle against the placement of the thermometer in the axilla. Before assessing the temperature, the examiner should determine the apical heart rate and respiratory rate while the infant is quiet and at rest. The desired range for axillary temperature is 36.5° to 37.5°C (97.7° to 99.5°F).

⚡ SAFETY ALERT

Rectal temperatures should not routinely be performed on a newborn because of the risk for perforation and vagal stimulation.

TABLE 24.1 Initial Physical Assessment of the Newborn: Normal Findings

General appearance	☐ Color pink
	☐ Acrocyanosis present
	☐ Flexed posture
	☐ Alert
	☐ Active
Respiratory system	☐ Airway patent
	☐ No upper airway congestion
	☐ No retractions or nasal flaring
	☐ Respiratory rate, 30-60 breaths/min
	☐ Lungs clear to auscultation bilaterally
	☐ Chest expansion symmetric
Cardiovascular system	☐ Heart rate >100 beats/min; strong and regular
	☐ No murmurs heard
	☐ Pulses strong and equal bilaterally
Neurologic system	☐ Moves extremities
	☐ Normotonic
	☐ Symmetric features, movement
	☐ Reflexes present:
	☐ Sucking
	☐ Rooting
	☐ Moro
	☐ Grasp
	☐ Anterior fontanel soft and flat
Gastrointestinal system	☐ Abdomen soft, no distention
	☐ Cord attached and clamped
	☐ Anus appears patent
Eyes, nose, mouth	☐ Eyes clear
	☐ Palate intact
	☐ Nares patent
Skin	☐ No signs of birth trauma
	☐ No lesions or abrasions
Genitourinary system	☐ Normal genitalia

Comments:

_____

_____

_____

_____

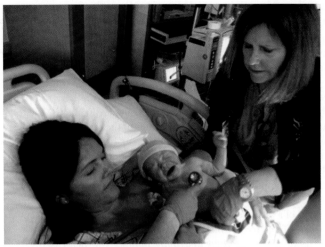

Fig. 24.2 Initial Assessment During Skin-To-Skin Time with Mother. (Courtesy Allison and Matthew Wyatt, Eagle, CO)

The respiratory rate varies with the state of alertness and activity after birth. Respirations are abdominal in nature and can be counted by observing or lightly feeling the rise and fall of the abdomen. Newborn respirations are shallow and irregular; this irregularity is called *periodic breathing*, and is a normal finding in the newborn. Because of the normal irregularity, respirations should be counted for a full minute. The nurse also observes for symmetry of chest movement. The normal range for newborn respirations is 30 to 60 breaths/min; the respiratory rate can exceed 60 breaths/min if the newborn is very active or crying. A consistent respiratory rate greater than 60 breaths/min can be a sign of distress and should be evaluated.

An apical pulse rate should be obtained on all newborns. Auscultation is done for a full minute, preferably when the infant is asleep or in a quiet alert state. The newborn may need to be held and comforted during assessment. The normal heart rate ranges from 120 to 160 beats/min when the infant is awake (Benjamin & Furdon, 2015). It is common to detect brief irregularities in the heart rate. The heart rate varies with the newborn's behavioral state. Bradycardia is a heart rate less than 80 beats/min. However, a term newborn in deep sleep can have a heart rate in the 70s to 90s; the rate should increase when the newborn awakens. Tachycardia is a heart rate exceeding 180 to 200 beats/min. It is not unusual for a crying infant to have a heart rate greater than 180; the heart rate should decrease when the crying ceases (Tappero & Honeyfield, 2015).

Assessment of newborn BP is based on facility policy. If BP is measured, an oscillometric monitor calibrated for neonatal pressures is preferred. An appropriate-size cuff (width-to-arm or width-to-calf ratio of 0.45 to 0.70) is essential for accuracy. To ensure that the correct size is being used, many neonatal BP cuffs have the appropriate extremity circumference printed on the cuff. Newborn BP usually is highest immediately after birth, decreasing over the next 3 hours, and then rising steadily until it reaches a plateau between 4 and 6 days after birth. This measurement is usually equal to that of the immediate postbirth BP. The BP varies with the newborn's activity; accurate measurement is best obtained while the newborn is at rest. BP varies with gestational age, chronologic age, and birth weight. Refer to Chapter 23 for information on normal BP values in the newborn. According to facility protocol, four extremity BPs may be assessed routinely or only when a murmur is auscultated. Normally, the BP is higher in the lower extremities. If the upper extremity systolic pressures are more than 20 mm Hg greater than those in the lower extremities, the infant may have a cardiac defect such as coarctation of the aorta (Gardner & Hernández, 2016b). Peripheral pulses are also palpated as part of the assessment in any infant with a heart murmur. In addition, if a murmur is present, oxygen saturation is usually measured using pulse oximetry.

TABLE 24.2 Apgar Score

	SCORE		
Sign	**0**	**1**	**2**
Heart rate	Absent	Slow (<100/min)	≥100/min
Respiratory effort	Absent	Slow, weak cry	Good cry
Muscle tone	Flaccid	Some flexion of extremities	Well flexed
Reflex irritability	No response	Grimace	Cry
Color	Blue, pale	Body pink, extremities blue	Completely pink

Baseline Measurements of Physical Growth

Baseline measurements are done and recorded to help assess the progress and determine the growth patterns of the infant. These measurements may be recorded on growth charts. The following measurements are made when the newborn is assessed.

Weight. The newborn is weighed soon after birth. This assessment is performed in the labor and birthing area, the mother's room, or in the nursery. The nurse ensures that the scales are balanced. The totally unclothed neonate is placed in the center of the scale, which is covered with a disposable pad or cloth to prevent heat loss via conduction and to prevent cross-infection. The nurse should place one hand over (but not touching) the newborn to be prepared to prevent the infant from falling off the scale. Ideally, during the hospital stay the infant is weighed at the same time each day and with the same scale. Birth weight of a term newborn is typically in the range of 2700 to 4000 g (6 to 9 lb) (Tappero & Honeyfield, 2015).

Head circumference and body length. The head is measured at the widest part, which is the occipitofrontal diameter. The tape measure is placed around the head just above the infant's eyebrows. The term neonate's head circumference typically ranges from 32.5 to 37.5 cm (12.5 to 14.5 in.) (Tappero & Honeyfield, 2015). Accuracy of the head circumference can be altered by temporary swelling due to pressure on the head during labor and birth or by overlapping of the cranial bones (*molding*) (Gardner & Hernández, 2016b; see Fig. 23.13).

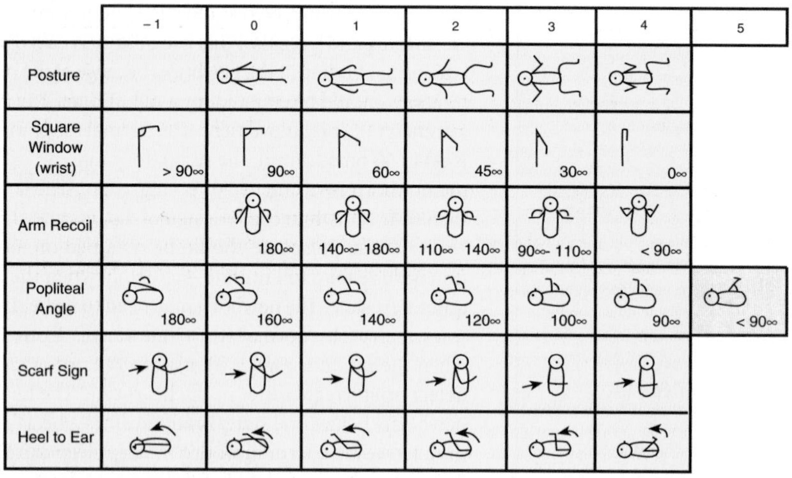

Length can be difficult to measure accurately because of the flexed posture of the newborn. The nurse places the newborn on a flat surface and extends the leg until the knee is flat against the surface. Placing the head against a perpendicular surface and extending the leg can assist with obtaining this measurement. In the term newborn, head-to-heel length is typically in the range of 48 to 53 cm (19 to 21 in.) (Tappero & Honeyfield, 2015).

Neurologic Assessment

The physical examination includes a neurologic assessment of newborn reflexes (see Table 23.1). This assessment provides useful

Fig. 24.3 Estimation of Gestational Age. (A) New Ballard score for newborn maturity rating. Expanded scale includes extremely premature infants and has been refined to improve accuracy in more mature infants.

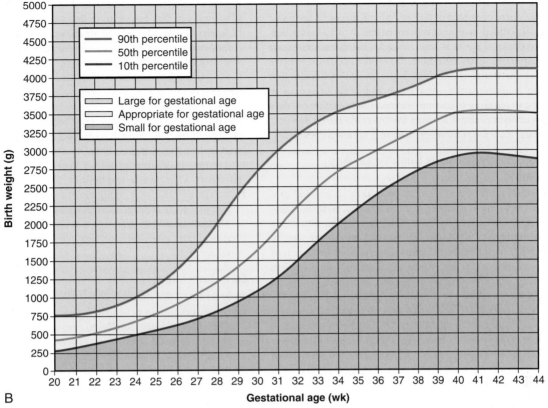

B
Gestational age (wk)

Fig. 24.3, cont'd (B) Intrauterine growth: birth weight percentiles based on live single births at gestational ages 20 to 44 weeks. (A, From Ballard, J.L., Khoury, J.C., Wedig, K., et al. [1991]. New Ballard score, expanded to include extremely premature infants. *Journal of Pediatrics, 119*[3], 417–423; B, Data from Alexander, G.R., Himes, J.H., Kaufman, R.B., et al. [1996]. A United States national reference for fetal growth. *Obstetrics and Gynecology,* 87[2], 163-168.)

BOX 24.2 Maneuvers Used in Assessing Gestational Age

Posture

With infant quiet and in supine position, observe degree of flexion in arms and legs. Muscle tone and degree of flexion increase with maturity. Full flexion of the arms and legs = score 4.[a]

Square Window

With thumb supporting back of arm below wrist, apply gentle pressure with index and third fingers on dorsum of hand without rotating infant's wrist. Measure angle between base of thumb and forearm. Full flexion (hand lies flat on ventral surface of forearm) = score 4.[a]

Arm Recoil

With infant supine, fully flex both forearms on upper arms and hold for 5 s; pull down on hands to extend fully, and rapidly release arms. Observe rapidity and intensity of recoil to a state of flexion. A brisk return to full flexion = score 4.[a]

Popliteal Angle

With infant supine and pelvis flat on a firm surface, flex lower leg on thigh and then flex thigh on abdomen. While holding knee with thumb and index finger, extend lower leg with index finger of other hand. Measure degree of angle behind knee (popliteal angle). An angle of less than 90 degrees = score 5.[a]

Scarf Sign

With infant supine, support head in midline with one hand; use other hand to pull infant's arm across the shoulder so that infant's hand touches shoulder. Determine location of elbow in relation to midline. Elbow does not reach midline = score 4.[a]

Heel to Ear

With infant supine and pelvis flat on a firm surface, pull foot as far as possible (without using force) up toward ear on same side. Measure distance of foot from ear and degree of knee flexion (same as popliteal angle). Knees flexed with a popliteal angle of less than 10 degrees = score 4.[a]

[a]See Fig. 24.3 for scale and interpretation of scores
From Hockenberry, M.J., & Wilson D. (2015). *Wong's nursing care of infants and children* (10th ed..) St. Louis, MO: Mosby.

---

information about the newborn's nervous system and state of neurologic maturation. Many reflex behaviors (e.g., sucking, rooting) are important for proper development. Other reflexes such as gagging and sneezing act as primitive safety mechanisms. The assessment needs to be carried out as soon as possible after birth because abnormalities may require further investigation before the newborn is discharged home.

Gestational Age Assessment

Assessment of gestational age is important because perinatal morbidity and mortality rates are related to gestational age and birth weight. A frequently used method of determining gestational age is the New Ballard Score, which can be used to measure gestational ages of infants as young as 20 weeks (see Fig. 24.3A). It assesses six external physical and six neuromuscular signs. Each sign has a numeric score, and the cumulative score correlates with a maturity rating (gestational age). The examination of infants with a gestational age of 26 weeks or less should be performed at a postnatal age of less than 12 hours. For infants with a gestational age of at least 26 weeks, the examination can be performed up to 96 hours after birth. To ensure accuracy, experts recommend that the initial examination is performed within the first 48 hours of life. Neuromuscular adjustments after birth in extremely immature neonates require a follow-up examination to further validate neuromuscular criteria (Ballard, Khoury, Wedig, et al., 1991). Box 24.2 highlights specific maneuvers used in gestational age assessment.

Classification of Newborns by Gestational Age and Birth Weight

The classification of newborns at birth by both birth weight and gestational age provides a more accurate method for predicting mortality risks and providing guidelines for care management than estimating gestational age or birth weight alone. The newborn's birth weight, length, and head circumference are plotted on standardized graphs that identify normal values for gestational age. A normal range of birth weights exists for each gestational week (see Fig. 24.3B).

The infant whose weight is appropriate for gestational age (AGA) (birth weight between the 10th and 90th percentiles) can be presumed to have grown at a normal rate regardless of the length of gestation—preterm, term, or postterm. The infant who is large for gestational age (LGA) (birth weight >90th percentile) can be presumed to have grown at an accelerated rate during intrauterine life; the small for gestational age (SGA) infant (birth weight <10th percentile) can be presumed to have grown at a restricted rate during intrauterine life. When gestational age is determined according to the New Ballard Score, the newborn will fall into one of the following nine possible categories for birth weight and gestational age: AGA—term, preterm, postterm; SGA—term, preterm, postterm; or LGA—term, preterm, postterm. Birth weight influences mortality: The lower the birth weight, the higher the mortality (Gardner & Hernández, 2016b).

Infants may also be classified in the following ways according to gestational age. The use of "term" has been discouraged by ACOG and the Society for Maternal-Fetal Medicine (SMFM) (2013/2017) because it does not account for the increased mortality and morbidity associated with birth prior to 39 weeks or after 42 weeks gestation. They recommend that newborns be classified in the following ways:

Preterm, or premature—born before 37 0/7 weeks of gestation, regardless of birth weight

Late preterm—34 0/7 through 36 6/7 weeks

Early term—37 0/7 through 38 6/7 weeks

Full term—39 0/7 through 40 6/7 weeks

Late term—41 0/7 through 41 6/7 weeks

Postterm—42 0/7 weeks and beyond

Postmature—born after completion of week 42 of gestation and showing the effects of progressive placental insufficiency

The gestational age of an infant at birth is an important predictor of survival. Infant morbidity and mortality are inversely related to gestational age.

Early-Term Infant

Early term (37 0/7 through 38 6/7 weeks) is a recent addition to the categories describing newborns according to gestational age. In 2016, 25.47% of births were considered early term; this is an increase of 2% from 2015 (Martin, Hamilton, Osterman, et al., 2018). Compared with full-term infants, early-term infants are at increased risk for morbidity and mortality. Early-term birth is associated with higher risk for hypoglycemia, respiratory problems such as respiratory distress syndrome and transient tachypnea of the newborn (TTN), and a greater likelihood of NICU admission (ACOG & SMFM, 2013/2017; Kardatzke, Rose, & Engle, 2017; Parikh, Reddy, Männistö, et al., 2014). Currently there is a lack of evidence about the long-term effects of early term birth. Nurses and other health care providers need to be aware of the vulnerability of this population of neonates and monitor them closely.

Text continued on p. 503.

TABLE 24.3   Physical Assessment of Newborn

Area Assessed and Appraisal Procedure	NORMAL FINDINGS		Deviations From Normal Range: Possible Problems (Etiology)
	Expected Findings	Normal Variations	
Posture			
Inspect newborn before disturbing for assessment. Refer to maternal chart for fetal presentation, position, and type of birth (vaginal, cesarean), given that newborn readily assumes in utero position.	Vertex: arms, legs in moderate flexion; fists clenched Resistance to having extremities extended for examination or measurement, crying possible when attempted Cessation of crying when allowed to resume curled-up fetal position (lateral) Normal spontaneous movement bilaterally asynchronous (legs moving in bicycle fashion) but equal extension in all extremities	Frank breech: legs straighter and stiff, hips may be flexed allowing legs to point toward the newborn's head, newborn assuming intrauterine position in repose for a few days Prenatal pressure on limb or shoulder possibly causing temporary facial asymmetry or resistance to extension of extremities	Hypotonia, relaxed posture while awake (preterm or hypoxia in utero, maternal medications, neuromuscular disorder such as spinal muscular atrophy) Hypertonia (chemical dependence, central nervous system [CNS] disorder) Limitation of motion in any extremity
Vital Signs			
Heart rate and pulses			
Thorax (chest)			
Inspection	Visible pulsations in left midclavicular line, fifth intercostal space		
Palpation	Apical pulse, fourth intercostal space 120-160 beats/min when awake	80-100 beats/min (sleeping) to 160 beats/min (crying); possibly irregular for brief periods, especially after crying	Tachycardia: persistent, ≥180 beats/min (respiratory distress syndrome [RDS]; pneumonia) Bradycardia: persistent, ≤80 beats/min (congenital heart block, maternal lupus)

TABLE 24.3   Physical Assessment of Newborn—cont'd

Area Assessed and Appraisal Procedure	NORMAL FINDINGS		Deviations From Normal Range: Possible Problems (Etiology)
	Expected Findings	Normal Variations	

Auscultation
  Apex: mitral valve
  Second interspace, left of sternum: pulmonic valve
  Second interspace, right of sternum: aortic valve
  Junction of xiphoid process and sternum: tricuspid valve
	Quality: first sound (closure of mitral and tricuspid valves) and second sound (closure of aortic and pulmonic valves) sharp and clear	Murmur, especially over base or at left sternal border in interspace 3 or 4 (foramen ovale anatomically closing at approximately 1 year of age)	Murmur (possibly functional)
			Dysrhythmias: irregular rate
			Sounds:
			  Distant (pneumopericardium)
			  Poor quality
			  Extra
			Heart on right side of chest (dextrocardia, often accompanied by reversal of intestines)

Peripheral pulses: femoral, brachial, popliteal, posterior tibial	Peripheral pulses equal and strong		Weak or absent peripheral pulses (decreased cardiac output, thrombus, possible coarctation of aorta if pulses not equal from side to side or upper to lower, bounding)
Temperature Axillary: method of choice Temporal and intraauricular thermometers not effective in measuring newborn temperature	Axillary: 37°C (98.6°F) Temperature stabilized by 8-10 h of age	36.5-37.5°C (97.7-99.5°F) Heat loss: from evaporation, conduction, convection, radiation	Subnormal (preterm birth, infection, low environmental temperature, inadequate clothing, dehydration) Increased (infection, high environmental temperature, excessive clothing, proximity to heating unit or in direct sunshine, chemical dependence, diarrhea and dehydration) Temperature not stabilized by 6-8 h after birth (if mother received magnesium sulfate, newborn less able to conserve heat by vasoconstriction; maternal analgesics possibly reducing thermal stability in newborn)
Respirations Observe respirations when infant is at rest. Observe respiratory effort. Count respirations for full minute.	30-60/min Tendency to be shallow and irregular in rate, rhythm, and depth when infant is awake	First period (reactivity): 50-60/min Second period: 50-70/min Stabilization (1-2 days): 30-40/min	Apneic episodes: >20 s (preterm infant: rapid warming or cooling of infant; CNS or blood glucose instability) Bradypnea: <30/min (maternal narcosis from analgesics or anesthetics, birth trauma) Tachypnea: >60/min (RDS, transient tachypnea of the newborn, congenital diaphragmatic hernia)
Auscultate breath sounds. Listen for sounds audible without stethoscope.	Crackles may be heard after birth No adventitious sounds audible on inspiration and expiration Breath sounds: bronchial; loud, clear	Short periodic breathing episodes and no evidence of respiratory distress or apnea (>20 s); periodic breathing Crackles (fine)	Breath sounds: Crackles (coarse), rhonchi, wheezing Expiratory grunt (narrowing of bronchi) Distress evidenced by nasal flaring, grunting, retractions, labored breathing Stridor (upper airway occlusion)
Blood Pressure (BP) (Usually Not Assessed in Normal Term Infant With No Signs of Concern)			

Check oscillometric monitor BP cuff: BP cuff width affects readings, use appropriate-size cuff, and palpate brachial, popliteal, or posterior tibial pulse (depending on measurement site).	Depends on gestational age and weight; term newborn of average weight 60-80/40-50 mm Hg (approximate ranges)
	At birth
	  Systolic: 60-80 mm Hg
	  Diastolic: 40-50 mm Hg
	At 2 weeks
	  Systolic: 68-88 mm Hg
	  Diastolic: 40-60 mm Hg
		Variation with change in activity level: awake, crying, sleeping	Difference between upper and lower extremity pressures (coarctation of aorta)
			Hypotension (sepsis, hypovolemia)
			Hypertension (coarctation of aorta, renal involvement, thrombus)

Continued

TABLE 24.3 Physical Assessment of Newborn—cont'd

Area Assessed and Appraisal Procedure	NORMAL FINDINGS		Deviations From Normal Range: Possible Problems (Etiology)
	Expected Findings	**Normal Variations**	
Weight Put cloth or paper protective liner in place, and adjust scale to 0 g or pounds and ounces. Weigh at same time each day. Protect newborn from heat loss.	Female: 3400 g (7.5 lb) Male: 3500 g (7.7 lb) Regaining of birth weight within first 2 weeks	2700-4000 g (6-9 lb) Acceptable weight loss: 5%-10% or less in first 3-5 days	Weight ≤2700 g (preterm, small for gestational age, rubella syndrome) Weight ≥4000 g (large for gestational age, maternal diabetes, heredity—normal for these parents) Weight loss more than 10% (growth failure, breastfeeding difficulty, dehydration)

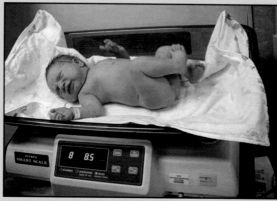

Weighing the Infant. The nurse never leaves the infant alone on a scale. The scale is covered to protect against cross-infection. (Courtesy Wendy and Marwood Larson-Harris, Roanoke, VA.)

Length Measure length from top of head to heel; measuring is difficult in term infant because of presence of molding, incomplete extension of knees.	50.5 cm (20 in.)	48-53 cm (19-21 in.)	<48 cm (17.7 in.) or >53 cm (21.7 in.) (chromosomal abnormality, heredity—normal for these parents); some syndromes present shorter than average limb length (skeletal dysplasias, achondroplasia)

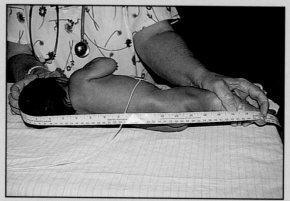

Measuring Length Crown to Heel. To determine total length, include length of legs. If measurements are taken before the infant's initial bath, wear gloves. (Courtesy Marjorie Pyle, RNC, Lifecircle, Costa Mesa, CA.)

Head Circumference Measure head at greatest diameter: occipitofrontal circumference May need to remeasure on second or third day after resolution of molding and caput succedaneum	35 cm (13.5 in.) Circumference of head and chest approximately the same for first 1 or 2 days after birth Chest rarely measured on routine basis	32.5-37.5 cm (12.5-14.5 in.)	Microcephaly, head ≤32 cm (maternal rubella, toxoplasmosis, cytomegalovirus, fused cranial sutures [craniosynostosis]) Hydrocephaly: sutures widely separated, circumference ≥4 cm more than chest circumference (infection) Increased intracranial pressure (hemorrhage, space-occupying lesion)

TABLE 24.3 Physical Assessment of Newborn—cont'd

Area Assessed and Appraisal Procedure	NORMAL FINDINGS		Deviations From Normal Range: Possible Problems (Etiology)
	Expected Findings	Normal Variations	

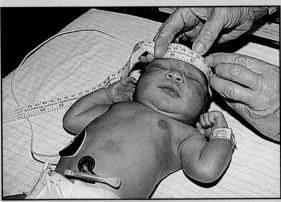

Measuring Head Circumference. (Courtesy Marjorie Pyle, RNC, Lifecircle, Costa Mesa, CA.)

Area Assessed and Appraisal Procedure	Expected Findings	Normal Variations	Deviations From Normal Range: Possible Problems (Etiology)
Chest Circumference Measure at nipple line	2-3 cm (0.8-1.2 in.) less than head circumference; average 30-33 cm (11.8-13 in.)	≤30 cm	Prematurity

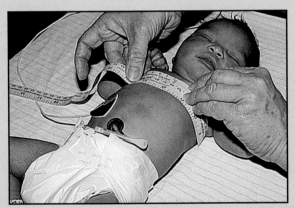

Measuring Chest Circumference. (Courtesy Marjorie Pyle, RNC, Lifecircle, Costa Mesa, CA.)

Area Assessed and Appraisal Procedure	Expected Findings	Normal Variations	Deviations From Normal Range: Possible Problems (Etiology)
Skin Check color: Inspect and palpate. Inspect seminaked newborn in well-lighted, warm area without drafts; natural daylight best. Inspect newborn when quiet and alert.	Generally pink Varies with ethnic origin, skin pigmentation beginning to deepen right after birth in basal layer of epidermis Acrocyanosis common for the first 48 h after birth	Mottling Harlequin sign Plethora Nevus simplex (telangiectatic nevi, "stork bites") (Fig. 23.9A) Erythema toxicum/neonatorum ("newborn rash") (see Fig. 23.10) Milia (see Fig. 23.7) Petechiae over presenting part Ecchymoses from forceps in vertex births or over buttocks, genitalia, and legs in breech births (see Fig. 23.12)	Dark red (preterm, polycythemia) Gray (hypotension, poor perfusion) Pallor (cardiovascular problem, CNS damage, blood dyscrasia, blood loss, twin-to-twin transfusion syndrome, infection) Cyanosis (hypothermia, infection, hypoglycemia, cardiopulmonary diseases, neurologic or respiratory malformations) Generalized petechiae (clotting factor deficiency, infection) Generalized ecchymoses (hemorrhagic disease)
Observe for jaundice.	None in the first 24 h of life	Physiologic jaundice in up to 60% of term infants in first week of life	Jaundice within first 24 h (increased hemolysis, Rh isoimmunization, ABO incompatibility)

Continued

TABLE 24.3   Physical Assessment of Newborn—cont'd

Area Assessed and Appraisal Procedure	NORMAL FINDINGS		Deviations From Normal Range: Possible Problems (Etiology)
	Expected Findings	Normal Variations	
Observe for birthmarks or bruises: Inspect and palpate for location, size, distribution, characteristics, color, if obstructing airway or oral cavity.		Mongolian spot (see Fig. 23.8) in infants of African American, Asian, Native American, and (rarely) Caucasian origin	Nevus flammeus (port-wine stain) Infantile hemangioma
Check skin condition			
Inspect and palpate skin for intactness, smoothness, texture, edema, pressure points if ill or immobilized.	Edema confined to eyelid (result of eye prophylaxis) Opacity: few large blood vessels visible indistinctly over abdomen	Slightly thick; superficial cracking, peeling, especially of hands, feet No visible blood vessels, a few large vessels clearly visible over abdomen Some fingernail scratches	Edema on hands, feet; pitting over tibia; periorbital (overhydration; hydrops) Texture thin, smooth, or of medium thickness; rash or superficial peeling visible (preterm, postterm) Numerous vessels visible over abdomen (preterm) Texture thick, parchment-like; cracking, peeling (postterm) Skin tags, webbing Papules, pustules, vesicles, ulcers, maceration (impetigo, candidiasis, herpes, diaper dermatitis)
Gently pinch skin between thumb and forefinger over abdomen and inner thigh to check for turgor.	After pinch released, skin returns to original state immediately.		Loose, wrinkled skin (prematurity, postmaturity, dehydration: fold of skin persisting after release of pinch) Tense, tight, shiny skin (edema, extreme cold, shock, infection)
Note presence of subcutaneous fat deposits (adipose pads) over cheeks, buttocks.		Variation in amount of subcutaneous fat	Lack of subcutaneous fat, prominence of clavicle or ribs (preterm, malnutrition)
Check for vernix caseosa: Observe color, amount, and odor before bath.	Whitish, cheesy, odorless	Usually more found in creases, folds	Absent or minimal (postmature) Abundant (preterm) Green color (possible in utero release of meconium or presence of bilirubin) Odor (possible intrauterine infection)
Assess lanugo: Inspect for this fine, downy hair, amount and distribution.	Over shoulders, pinnae of ears, forehead	Variation in amount	Absent (postmature) Abundant (preterm, especially if lanugo abundant, long, and thick over back)
Head			
Palpate skin.	(See "Skin")	Caput succedaneum, possibly showing some ecchymosis (see Fig. 23.15A)	Cephalhematoma (see Fig. 23.15B) Subgaleal hemorrhage (see Fig. 23.15C)
Inspect shape, size.	Making up one-fourth of body length Molding (see Fig. 23.14)	Slight asymmetry from intrauterine position Lack of molding (preterm, breech presentation, cesarean birth)	Severe molding (birth trauma) Indentation (fracture from trauma)
Palpate, inspect, and note size and status of fontanels (open vs. closed).	Anterior fontanel 5-cm diamond, increasing as molding resolves Posterior fontanel triangle, smaller than anterior	Variation in fontanel size with degree of molding Difficulty in feeling fontanels possible because of molding	Fontanels: Full, bulging (tumor, hemorrhage, infection) Large, flat, soft (malnutrition, hydrocephaly, delayed bone age, hypothyroidism) Depressed (dehydration)
Palpate sutures.	Palpable and separated sutures	Possible overlap of sutures with molding	Sutures: Widely spaced (hydrocephaly) Premature closure (fused) (craniosynostosis)
Inspect pattern, distribution, amount of hair; feel texture.	Silky, single strands lying flat; growth pattern toward face and neck	Variation in amount	Fine, wooly (preterm) Unusual swirls, patterns, or hairline; or coarse, brittle (endocrine or genetic disorders)

TABLE 24.3   Physical Assessment of Newborn—cont'd

Area Assessed and Appraisal Procedure	NORMAL FINDINGS		Deviations From Normal Range: Possible Problems (Etiology)
	Expected Findings	Normal Variations	
Eyes Check placement on face.	Eyes and space between eyes each one-third the distance from inner to outer canthus	Epicanthal folds: characteristic in some ethnicities	Epicanthal folds when present with other signs (chromosomal disorders such as Down, cri du chat syndromes)

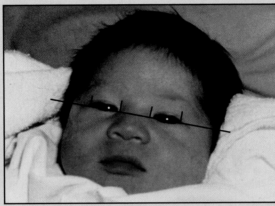

Eyes. In pseudostrabismus, inner epicanthal folds cause the eyes to appear misaligned; however, corneal light reflexes are perfectly symmetric. Eyes are symmetric in size and shape and are well placed.

Area Assessed and Appraisal Procedure	Expected Findings	Normal Variations	Deviations From Normal Range: Possible Problems (Etiology)
Check for symmetry in size, shape.	Symmetric in size, shape		
Check eyelids for size, movement, blink.	Blink reflex	Edema if eye prophylaxis drops or ointment instilled	
Assess for discharge.	None No tears	Occasional presence of tears	Discharge: purulent (infection) Chemical conjunctivitis from eye medication is common—requires no treatment
Evaluate eyeballs for presence, size, shape.	Both present and of equal size, both round, firm	Subconjunctival hemorrhage	Agenesis or absence of one or both eyeballs Lens opacity or absence of red reflex (congenital cataracts, possibly from rubella, retinoblastoma [cat's-eye reflex]) Lesions: coloboma, absence of part of iris (congenital) Pink color of iris (albinism) Jaundiced sclera (hyperbilirubinemia)
Check pupils.	Present, equal in size, reactive to light		Pupils: unequal, constricted, dilated, fixed (intracranial pressure, medications, tumor)
Evaluate eyeball movement.	Random, jerky, uneven, focus possible briefly, following to midline	Transient strabismus or nystagmus until third or fourth month	Persistent strabismus Doll eyes (increased intracranial pressure) Sunset (increased intracranial pressure)
Assess eyebrows: amount of hair, pattern.	Distinct (not connected in midline)		Connection in midline (Cornelia de Lange syndrome)
Nose Observe shape, placement, patency, configuration.	Midline Some mucus but no drainage Preferential nose breather Sneezing to clear nose	Slight deformity (flat or deviated to one side) from in utero positioning or passage through birth canal	Copious drainage (rarely congenital syphilis); membranous or bony blockage with cyanosis at rest and return of pink color with crying (choanal atresia) Malformed (congenital syphilis, chromosomal disorder) Flaring of nares (respiratory distress)

Continued

TABLE 24.3   Physical Assessment of Newborn—cont'd

Area Assessed and Appraisal Procedure	NORMAL FINDINGS		Deviations From Normal Range: Possible Problems (Etiology)
	Expected Findings	Normal Variations	
Ears			
Observe size, placement on head, amount of cartilage, open auditory canal.	Correct placement line drawn through inner and outer canthi of eyes reaching to top notch of ears (at junction with scalp) Well-formed, firm cartilage	Size: small, large, floppy Darwin tubercle (nodule on posterior helix)	Agenesis Lack of cartilage (preterm) Low placement (chromosomal disorder, intellectual disability, kidney disorder) Preauricular tag or sinus Size: possibly overly prominent or protruding ears

Placement of Ears on the Head in Relation to a Line Drawn from the Inner to the Outer Canthus of the Eye. (A) Normal position. (B) Abnormally angled ear. (C) True low-set ear. (Courtesy Mead Johnson Nutritionals, Evansville, IN.)

Area Assessed and Appraisal Procedure	Expected Findings	Normal Variations	Deviations From Normal Range: Possible Problems (Etiology)
Assess hearing	Responds to voice and other sounds	State (e.g., alert, asleep) influencing response	Lack of response to loud noise should not imply deafness
Perform universal newborn hearing screening to identify deficits (see Fig. 24.11).	Both ears pass		One or both ears fail
Facies			
Observe overall appearance and symmetry of face.	Rounded and symmetric; influenced by birth type, molding, or both	Positional deformities	Usually accompanied by other features such as low-set ears, other structural disorders (hereditary, chromosomal aberration)
Mouth			

Inspect and palpate.
Assess buccal mucosa:
  Dry or moist
  Pink
  Status intact
Assess lips for color, configuration, movement.
	Symmetry of lip movement	Transient circumoral cyanosis	Gross anomalies in placement, size, shape (cleft lip or palate [or both], gums)
			Cyanosis, circumoral pallor (respiratory distress, hypothermia)
			Asymmetry in movement of lips (seventh cranial nerve paralysis)

Check gums.	Pink gums	Inclusion cysts (Epstein pearls—Bohn nodules, whitish, hard nodules on gums or roof of mouth)	Teeth: predeciduous or deciduous (hereditary)
Assess tongue for color, mobility, movement, size.	Tongue not protruding, freely movable, symmetric in shape, movement Sucking pads inside cheeks	Short lingual frenulum (ankyloglossia)	Macroglossia (preterm, chromosomal disorder) Thrush: white plaques on cheeks or tongue that bleed if touched (*Candida albicans*)

Assess palate (soft, hard):
  Arch
  Uvula
	Soft and hard palates intact
	Uvula in midline
		Anatomic groove in palate to accommodate nipple, disappearance by 3-4 years of age
		Epstein pearls
			Cleft of hard or soft palate

TABLE 24.3 Physical Assessment of Newborn—cont'd

Area Assessed and Appraisal Procedure	NORMAL FINDINGS		Deviations From Normal Range: Possible Problems (Etiology)
	Expected Findings	Normal Variations	
Assess chin.	Distinct chin		Micrognathia—recessed chin with prominent overbite (Pierre Robin or other syndrome)
Evaluate saliva for amount, character.	Mouth moist, pink		Excessive salivation and choking or turning blue (esophageal atresia, tracheoesophageal fistula)
Check reflexes: Rooting Sucking Tongue extrusion	Reflexes present	Reflex response dependent on state of wakefulness and hunger	Absent (preterm)
Neck			
Inspect and palpate for movement, flexibility, masses, bruising.	Short, thick, surrounded by skin folds; no webbing		Webbing (Turner syndrome or other genetic syndrome)
Check sternocleidomastoid muscles, movement and position of head.	Head held in midline (sternocleidomastoid muscles equal), no masses Freedom of movement from side to side and flexion and extension, no movement of chin past shoulder	Transient positional deformity apparent when newborn is at rest: passive movement of head possible	Restricted movement, holding of head at angle (torticollis [wryneck], opisthotonos) Absence of head control (preterm birth, Down syndrome, hypotonia [spinal muscular atrophy])
Assess trachea for position and thyroid gland.	Thyroid not palpable		Masses (enlarged thyroid) Distended veins (cardiopulmonary disorder) Skin tags
Chest			
Inspect and palpate shape.	Almost circular, barrel shaped	Tip of sternum (xiphoid process) possibly prominent	Bulging of chest, unequal movement (pneumothorax, pneumomediastinum) Malformation (funnel chest—pectus excavatum)
Observe respiratory movements.	Symmetric chest movements, chest and abdominal movements synchronized during respirations	Occasional retractions, especially when crying	Retractions with or without respiratory distress (preterm, respiratory distress syndrome [RDS]) Paradoxic breathing
Evaluate clavicles.	Clavicles intact		Fracture of clavicle (trauma); crepitus
Assess ribs.	Rib cage symmetric, intact; moves with respirations		Poor development of rib cage and musculature (preterm)
Assess nipples for size, placement, number.	Nipples prominent, well formed; symmetrically placed		Nipples Supernumerary, along nipple line Malpositioned or widely spaced
Check breast tissue.	Breast nodule: approximately 6 mm in term infant	Breast nodule: 3-10 mm Secretion of "witch's milk"	Lack of breast tissue (preterm)
Auscultate: Heart sounds and rate and breath sounds (see "Vital Signs")			Sounds: bowel sounds audible in chest: diaphragmatic hernia (see "Abdomen")
Abdomen			
Inspect and palpate umbilical cord.	Two arteries, one vein (vein is larger with thinner wall, arteries are whitish in color and constricted) Whitish gray Definite demarcation between cord and skin, no intestinal structures within cord Dry around base, drying Odorless Cord clamp in place for 24-48 h	Reducible umbilical hernia	One artery (renal anomaly) Meconium stained (intrauterine distress) Bleeding or oozing around cord (hemorrhagic disease) Redness or drainage around cord (infection, possible persistence of urachus) Hernia: herniation of abdominal contents through cord opening (e.g., omphalocele); defect covered with thin, friable membrane, possibly extensive

Continued

TABLE 24.3   Physical Assessment of Newborn—cont'd

Area Assessed and Appraisal Procedure	NORMAL FINDINGS		Deviations From Normal Range: Possible Problems (Etiology)
	Expected Findings	Normal Variations	
Inspect size of abdomen and palpate contour.	Rounded, prominent, dome shaped because abdominal musculature not fully developed Liver possibly palpable 1-2 cm (0.4-0.8 in.) below right costal margin No other masses palpable No distention Few visible veins on abdominal surface	Some diastasis recti (separation) of abdominal musculature	Gastroschisis: herniation of abdominal contents to the side or above the cord, contents not covered by membranous tissue and may include liver Distention at birth: ruptured viscus, genitourinary masses or malformations: hydronephrosis, teratomas, abdominal tumors Mild (overfeeding, high gastrointestinal tract obstruction) Marked (lower gastrointestinal tract obstruction, anorectal malformation, anal stenosis), often with bilious emesis Intermittent or transient (overfeeding) Partial intestinal obstruction (stenosis of bowel) Visible peristalsis (obstruction) Malrotation of bowel or adhesions Sepsis (infection)
Auscultate bowel sounds, and note number, amount, and character of stools.	Sounds present within minutes after birth in healthy term infant Meconium stool passing within 24-48 h after birth		Scaphoid, with bowel sounds in chest and severe respiratory distress (diaphragmatic hernia)
Assess color.		Linea nigra possibly apparent due to maternal hormone influence during pregnancy	
Observe movement with respiration.	Respirations primarily diaphragmatic, abdominal and chest movement synchronous		Decreased or absent abdominal movement with breathing (phrenic nerve palsy, diaphragmatic hernia)
Genitalia **Female (see Fig. 23.11A)** Inspect and palpate:			
General appearance		Increased pigmentation caused by pregnancy hormones	Ambiguous genitalia—wide variation (small phallus not well distinguished from enlarged clitoris)
Clitoris	Usually edematous		Virilized female—extremely large clitoris (congenital adrenal hyperplasia)
Labia majora	Usually edematous, covering labia minora in term newborns	Edema and ecchymosis after breech birth Some vernix caseosa between labia possible	
Labia minora	Possible protrusion over labia majora		Enlarged clitoris with urinary meatus on tip, absent scrotum, micropenis, fused labia Stenosed meatus Labia majora widely separated and labia minora prominent (preterm)
Discharge	Smegma	Blood-tinged discharge from pseudomenstruation caused by pregnancy hormones	Fecal discharge (fistula)
Vagina	Open orifice Mucoid discharge Hymenal/vaginal tag		Absence of vaginal orifice
Urinary meatus	Beneath clitoris, difficult to see		Bladder exstrophy (bladder outside abdominal cavity)

TABLE 24.3 Physical Assessment of Newborn—cont'd

Area Assessed and Appraisal Procedure	NORMAL FINDINGS		Deviations From Normal Range: Possible Problems (Etiology)
	Expected Findings	Normal Variations	
Urination	Void within 24 h; voiding 2-6 times per 24 h for first 1-2 days; voiding 6-8 times per 24 h by day 4 or 5	Rust-stained urine (uric acid crystals)	No void within first 24 h (renal agenesis [Potter syndrome])
Male (see Fig. 23.11B) Inspect and palpate:			
General appearance		Increased size and pigmentation caused by pregnancy hormones (wide variation in size of genitalia)	Ambiguous genitalia Micropenis
Penis			
Urinary meatus appearance	Foreskin covers glans (if uncircumcised), meatus at tip of penis		Urinary meatus not on tip of glans penis (hypospadias, epispadias, foreskin may be retracted or absent)
Prepuce (foreskin)—do not forcibly retract foreskin if uncircumcised	Prepuce covering glans penis and not retractable	Prepuce removed if circumcised	Round meatal opening
Scrotum: Rugae (wrinkles)	Large, edematous, pendulous in term infant; covered with rugae	Scrotal edema and ecchymosis if breech birth Hydrocele, small, noncommunicating	Scrotum smooth and testes undescended (preterm, cryptorchidism) Bifid scrotum Hydrocele Inguinal hernia
Testes	Palpable on each side	Bulge palpable in inguinal canal	Undescended (preterm)
Urination	Voiding within 24 h, stream adequate; voiding 2-6 times per 24 h for first 1-2 days; voiding 6-8 times per 24 h by day 4 or 5	Rust-stained urine (uric acid crystals)	No void in first 24 h (renal agenesis [Potter syndrome])
Check reflexes:			
Cremasteric	Testes retracted, especially when newborn is chilled		
Extremities			
General appearance: Inspect and palpate Degree of flexion Range of motion Symmetry of motion Muscle tone	Assuming of position maintained in utero Attitude of general flexion Full range of motion, spontaneous movements	Transient positional deformities	Limited motion (malformations) Poor muscle tone (preterm, maternal medications, CNS anomalies)
Check arms and hands: Inspect and palpate: Color Intactness Appropriate placement	Longer than legs in newborn period Contours and movements symmetric	Slight tremors sometimes apparent Some acrocyanosis	Asymmetry of movement (fracture/crepitus, brachial nerve trauma, malformations) Asymmetry of contour (malformations, fracture) Amelia or phocomelia (teratogens) Palmar creases Simian line with short, incurved little fingers (Down syndrome)
Count number of fingers.	Five on each hand Fist often clenched with thumb under fingers		Webbing of fingers: syndactyly Absence of finger Extra finger (polydactyly) Strong, rigid flexion; persistent fists; positioning of fists in front of mouth constantly (CNS disorder) Yellowed nailbeds (meconium staining)
Evaluate joints: Shoulders Elbows Wrists Fingers	Full range of motion, symmetric contour		Increased tonicity, clonus, prolonged tremors (CNS disorder)

Continued

TABLE 24.3   Physical Assessment of Newborn—cont'd

Area Assessed and Appraisal Procedure	NORMAL FINDINGS		Deviations From Normal Range: Possible Problems (Etiology)
	Expected Findings	Normal Variations	
Check reflexes (see Table 23.1)			
Palmar grasp	Infant's fingers tightly flex around examiner's finger when palm is stimulated	May occur spontaneously when sucking	Weak or absent reflexes can indicate CNS depression
Check legs and feet:			
Inspect and palpate Color Intactness Length in relation to arms and body and to each other	Appearance of bowing because lateral muscles more developed than medial muscles	Feet appearing to turn in but can be easily rotated externally, positional defects tending to correct while infant is crying Acrocyanosis	Amelia, phocomelia (chromosomal defect, teratogenic effect) Temperature of one leg differing from that of the other (circulatory deficiency, CNS disorder)
Number of toes	Five on each foot		Webbing, syndactyly (chromosomal defect) Absence or excess of digits (chromosomal defect, familial trait)
Femur Head of femur as legs are flexed and abducted, placement in acetabulum (see Fig. 23.17)	Intact femur		Femoral fracture (difficult breech birth) Developmental dysplasia of the hip (DDH)
Major gluteal folds	Major gluteal folds even		Gluteal folds uneven: DDH
Soles of feet	Soles well lined (or wrinkled) over two-thirds of foot in term infants Plantar fat pad giving flat-footed effect		Soles of feet: Few creases (preterm) Covered with creases (postmature) Congenital clubfoot
Evaluate joints: Hips Knees Ankles Toes	Full range of motion, symmetric contour		Hypermobility of joints (Down syndrome)
Check reflexes (see Table 23.1)			Asymmetric movement (trauma, CNS disorder)
Plantar grasp	Infant's toes flex and curl around examiner's finger when sole of foot at base of toes is stimulated		
Back Assess anatomy: General Appearance Inspect and palpate		Temporary minor positional deformities, correction with passive manipulation	Limitation of movement (fusion or deformity of vertebra) Spina bifida cystica (meningocele, myelomeningocele)
Spine	Spine straight and easily flexed Infant able to raise and support head momentarily when prone		Pigmented nevus with tuft of hair, location anywhere along the spine often associated with spina bifida occulta
Base of spine—pilonidal dimple or sinus			Sinus (opening to spinal cord)
Shoulders Scapulae Iliac crests	Shoulders, scapulae, and iliac crests line up in same plane		
Check reflexes (spinal related).			
Trunk incurvation reflex.	Trunk flexed and pelvis swings to stimulated side	May not be apparent in first few days but is usually present in 5-6 days	If transverse lesion is present, no response below lesion; absence of response: CNS abnormality or CNS depression
Magnet reflex.	Lower limbs extend as pressure applied to feet with legs in semi-flexed position	Weak or exaggerated response with breech presentation	Absence: suggestive of CNS damage or malformation

TABLE 24.3 Physical Assessment of Newborn—cont'd

Area Assessed and Appraisal Procedure	NORMAL FINDINGS		Deviations From Normal Range: Possible Problems (Etiology)
	Expected Findings	Normal Variations	
Anus Inspect and palpate: Placement Patency Test for sphincter response (active "wink" reflex) Observe for the following: Abdominal distention Passage of meconium from anal opening Fecal drainage from perineum, penis, vagina	One anus with good sphincter tone Passage of meconium within 24 h after birth Anal "wink" present, anal opening patent	Passage of meconium within 48 h of birth	Imperforate anus without fistula Rectal atresia and stenosis Absence of anal opening; drainage of fecal material from vagina in female or urinary meatus in male (rectal fistula) or along perineal raphe (midline area between base of penis and anus)—anorectal malformation
Stools Observe frequency, color, consistency.	Meconium followed by transitional and soft yellow stool		No stool (obstruction) Frequent watery stools (infection, phototherapy)

Late-Preterm Infant

The rate of preterm birth in the United States was 9.85% in 2016; this is an increase of 2% from 2015. The majority of preterm births are considered late preterm, occurring from 34 0/7 through 36 6/7 weeks of gestation. These late-preterm infants account for 7.09% of all births and approximately 75% of preterm births (Martin et al., 2018). Elective vaginal and cesarean births before 39 weeks have contributed significantly to late-preterm birth rates in the United States.

Late-preterm infants have been called "the great impostors" because they are often the size and weight of term infants and, unfortunately, are often treated as term newborns. Late-preterm infants are at increased risk for respiratory distress, temperature instability, hypoglycemia, apnea, feeding difficulties, and hyperbilirubinemia (Kardatzke et al., 2017). Nurses and health care providers must be aware of these possible complications and be continually vigilant for the development of problems related to the infant's immaturity. In an effort to identify these infants, a gestational age assessment should be performed on all newborns soon after birth. The late-preterm infant's care is further addressed in Chapter 34.

Postterm or Postmature Infant

Infants born at 42 0/7 weeks of gestation or beyond are considered postterm, regardless of birth weight. Some infants are AGA but show characteristics of progressive placental insufficiency. These infants are labeled as postmature and are likely to have little if any vernix caseosa, absence of lanugo, abundant scalp hair, and long fingernails. The skin is often cracked, parchment-like, and peeling. A common finding in postmature infants is a wasted physical appearance that reflects placental insufficiency. Depletion of subcutaneous fat gives them a thin, elongated appearance. The scant amounts of vernix caseosa that remain in the skinfolds may be stained deep yellow or green, which is usually an indication of meconium in the amniotic fluid.

There is a significant increase in fetal and neonatal mortality in postmature infants compared with those born at term. They are especially prone to fetal distress associated with placental insufficiency, macrosomia, and meconium aspiration syndrome.

Immediate Interventions

Changes can occur quickly in newborns immediately after birth. Assessment must be followed by prompt implementation of appropriate care.

Airway Maintenance

In general, the healthy term infant born vaginally has little difficulty clearing the airway. Most secretions are moved by gravity and brought by the cough reflex to the oropharynx to be drained, swallowed, or wiped away. If the airway is obstructed, then the mouth and nasal passages can be gently suctioned with a bulb syringe (see the Teaching for Self-Management box: Suctioning With a Bulb Syringe, and Fig. 24.4). Vigorous suctioning should be avoided; it can cause trauma to fragile tissues. Routine chest percussion and suctioning of healthy term or late-preterm infants should be avoided; evidence is insufficient to support anything other than gentle nasopharyngeal and oropharyngeal suctioning to clear secretions from an obstructed airway. The nurse should auscultate the infant's chest with a stethoscope to assess for abnormal breath sounds or inspiratory stridor. Fine crackles may be auscultated for several hours after birth, especially in neonates born by cesarean. If the bulb syringe does not clear mucus interfering with respiratory effort, deeper mechanical suction may be needed to remove mucus from the newborn's nasopharynx or posterior oropharynx. However, this type of suctioning should be performed only after an assessment of the associated risks, such as bradycardia (Weiner & Zaichkin, 2016).

TEACHING FOR SELF-MANAGEMENT
Suctioning with a Bulb Syringe

- Keep the bulb syringe easily accessible and visible (e.g., in the newborn's crib). It is to be used when there is concern that the airway is obstructed. This suctioning can cause swelling and trauma to the nasal mucosa.
- Suction the mouth before the nose to prevent the infant from inhaling pharyngeal secretions by gasping as the nares are touched.
- Compress the bulb (see Fig. 24.4), and insert the tip into one side of the mouth. Avoid the center of the infant's mouth because the gag reflex can be stimulated.
- Gently suction nasal passages one nostril at a time.
- When the airway is no longer obstructed, suctioning should be stopped.
- After each use, clean bulb syringe with warm soapy water and rinse thoroughly.

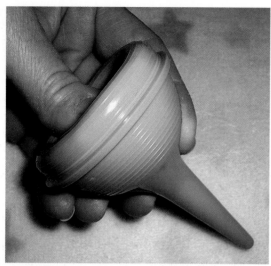

Fig. 24.4 Bulb Syringe. Bulb is compressed before inserting tip into mouth. (Courtesy Cheryl Briggs, RNC, Annapolis, MD.)

BOX 24.3 Signs of Potential Complications

Abnormal Newborn Breathing
- Bradypnea (<30 respirations/min)
- Tachypnea (>60 respirations/min)
- Abnormal breath sounds: coarse or fine crackles, wheezes
- Audible expiratory grunt
- Respiratory distress: nasal flaring, retractions, stridor, gasping, chin tug
- Seesaw or paradoxical respirations
- Skin color: central cyanosis, mottling
- Pulse oximetry value: <95%

Data from Gardner, S.L., & Hernández, J.A. (2016). Initial nursery care. In S.L. Gardner, B.S. Carter, M. Enzman-Hines, & J.A. Hernández (Eds.). Merenstein & Gardner's handbook of neonatal intensive care (8th ed.). St. Louis: Elsevier.

If the newborn has an obstruction that is not cleared with suctioning, the neonatal or pediatric care provider should be notified. Further investigation may be needed to determine if a mechanical defect (e.g., tracheoesophageal fistula or choanal atresia [see Chapter 36]) is causing the obstruction.

Maintaining an Adequate Oxygen Supply

Four conditions are essential for maintaining an adequate oxygen supply:
- A clear airway
- Effective establishment of respirations
- Adequate circulation, adequate perfusion, and effective cardiac function
- Adequate thermoregulation

Newborns who encounter respiratory problems are likely to exhibit signs and symptoms that indicate some degree of distress (Box 24.3). Preterm infants are at greatest risk for respiratory distress (see Chapter 34).

Maintaining Body Temperature

Effective newborn care includes maintenance of a neutral thermal environment (see Chapter 23). Cold stress increases the need for oxygen and can deplete glucose stores. The infant can react to exposure to cold by increasing the respiratory rate and can become cyanotic.

The ideal method for promoting warmth and maintaining neonatal body temperature is early skin-to-skin care (SSC) (see Fig. 19.24).

The unclothed newborn is placed prone directly on the mother's chest; both mother and infant are then covered with a warm blanket, and a cap is placed on the infant's head. SSC in the first hour of life increases neonatal blood glucose concentrations, improves temperature stability, and improves breastfeeding initiation and duration (AAP & ACOG, 2017; Cleveland, Hill, Pulse, et al., 2017; Moore, Bergman, Anderson, et al., 2016). In addition, SSC and breastfeeding at birth can reduce the risk for postpartum hemorrhage (Saxton, Fahy, Rolfe, et al., 2015). Other interventions to promote warmth include drying and wrapping the newborn in warm blankets immediately after birth, keeping the head well covered, and keeping the ambient temperature of the nursery or mother's room at 22° to 26°C (72°F to 78°F) (AAP & ACOG, 2017).

If the newborn does not remain skin-to-skin with the mother during the first 1 to 2 hours after birth, the nurse places the thoroughly dried infant under a radiant warmer or in a warm incubator until the body temperature stabilizes. The infant's skin temperature is used as the point of control in a warmer with a servo-controlled mechanism. The control panel is usually set between 36° and 37°C (96.8° and 98.6°F) to maintain the healthy term newborn's skin temperature at approximately 36.5° to 37°C (97.7° to 98.6°F). A thermistor probe (automatic sensor) is usually placed on the upper quadrant of the abdomen immediately below the right or left costal margin (never over a bone); the probe is covered with a reflector adhesive patch. This probe is designed to detect minor temperature changes resulting from external environmental factors or neonatal factors (peripheral vasoconstriction, vasodilation, or increased metabolism) before a dramatic change in core body temperature develops. The servo controller adjusts the temperature of the warmer to maintain the infant's skin temperature within the preset range.

⚡ SAFETY ALERT

The thermistor probe should be checked periodically to make sure it is securely attached to the infant's skin. If it becomes loose, the radiant heating device will increase heat output, potentially overheating the newborn. Using the manual control mode on the radiant warmer can have the same effect on the newborn; the radiant warmer will continue to increase heat output, potentially overheating the newborn. Therefore radiant warmers should only be used in the servo-controlled setting.

The nurse assesses the axillary temperature of the newborn every hour (or more often as needed) until the newborn's temperature stabilizes. The length of time to stabilize and maintain body temperature varies; therefore care should be individualized so that each newborn is allowed to achieve thermoregulation.

During all procedures, heat loss must be avoided or minimized for the newborn; therefore examinations and activities are performed in a way to minimize heat loss. The initial bath for an uncompromised term infant should be postponed for at least 6 hours and until the newborn's skin temperature is stable as indicated by two consecutive axillary temperatures at or above 36.8°C (98.2°F). The bath time should be limited to 5 minutes (Association for Women's Health, Obstetric and Neonatal Nurses [AWHONN], 2018).

Even a healthy term infant can become hypothermic. Inadequate drying and wrapping immediately after birth, being left on wet linens, a cold birthing room, or birth in a car on the way to the birthing facility can cause the newborn's temperature to fall below the normal range (hypothermia). The hypothermic infant should be warmed gradually because rapid warming can cause apneic spells, hypovolemia, and acidosis. Therefore the warming process should be carefully monitored and allowed to progress slowly, depending on the infant's clinical status (Gardner & Hernández, 2016a; Karlsen, 2012).

Eye Prophylaxis

The American Academy of Pediatrics (AAP Committee on Infectious Diseases, 2018) and the U.S. Preventive Services Task Force (USPSTF, 2011) recommend instilling a prophylactic agent in the eyes of all newborns to prevent ophthalmia neonatorum or neonatal conjunctivitis, which is an inflammation caused by sexually transmitted bacteria acquired during passage through the mother's birth canal. Because ascending infection can occur, eye prophylaxis is recommended for all newborns, including those born by cesarean. The Canadian Paediatric Society (CPS) no longer recommends routine eye prophylaxis for newborns, although some jurisdictions still require it (Moore, MacDonald, & CPS Infectious Diseases and Immunization Committee, 2015/2018).

In the United States, erythromycin 0.5% ophthalmic ointment is the recommended prophylactic medication to prevent infection from *Neisseria gonorrhoeae* (see Medication Guide: Eye Prophylaxis: Erythromycin Ophthalmic Ointment, 0.5%). Without prompt treatment, this infection can lead to blindness. Eye prophylaxis is usually administered within the first hour after birth. It may be delayed up to 2 hours until after the first breastfeeding so that eye contact and parent-infant attachment and bonding are facilitated (Fig. 24.5). Eye prophylaxis for every newborn is mandated by law in the majority of U.S. states without regard to the mode of birth. In some states, parents may refuse eye prophylaxis by signing a form that becomes part of the newborn record (AAP Committee on Infectious Diseases, 2018).

MEDICATION GUIDE

Eye Prophylaxis: Erythromycin Ophthalmic Ointment, 0.5%

Action
Bacteriostatic and bactericidal for *N. gonorrhoeae*.

Indication
To prevent ophthalmia neonatorum in newborns of mothers who are infected with *N. gonorrhoeae*. Eye prophylaxis for ophthalmia neonatorum is required by law in most U.S. states and in some Canadian provinces.

Neonatal Dosage
Apply a 1- to 2-cm ribbon of ointment to the lower conjunctival sac of each eye.

Adverse Reactions
Can cause chemical conjunctivitis that lasts 24-48 h; vision can be blurred temporarily

Nursing Considerations
Administer within 1-2 h of birth. Wear gloves. Use a sterile cotton ball to wipe each eyelid prior to administering the ointment. Open the eyes by putting a thumb and finger at the corner of each lid and gently pressing on the periorbital ridges. Squeeze the tube, and spread the ointment from the inner canthus of the eye to the outer canthus. Do not touch the tube to the eye. Gently massage the closed eyelids to disperse the ointment. After 1 min, excess ointment may be wiped away. Observe eyes for irritation. Explain the treatment to the parents.

Data from American Academy of Pediatrics Committee on Infectious Diseases. (2018). Section 5: Antimicrobial prophylaxis. In D. W. Kimberlin, M. T. Brady, M. A. Jackson, et al. (Eds.), *Red book: 2018-2021 report of the Committee on Infectious Diseases* (31st ed.). Itasca, IL: Author.

Topical antibiotics such as erythromycin are not effective in preventing chlamydial conjunctivitis. Oral erythromycin or azithromycin is used to treat chlamydial conjunctivitis (AAP Committee on Infectious Diseases, 2018).

Vitamin K Prophylaxis

At birth, neonates have low vitamin K levels related to limited transplacental transfer of vitamin K and the lack of normal intestinal flora necessary for vitamin K synthesis. The establishment of normal intestinal flora begins with early feedings, and by 7 days of age, healthy newborns are able to produce their own vitamin K.

AAP and ACOG (2017) recommend that every newborn receive a single dose of phytonadione 0.5 to 1 mg to prevent vitamin K–dependent hemorrhagic disease of the newborn. Administration of this injection should be delayed to allow for the infant to spend some skin-to-skin time with the parents and for the first breastfeeding. CPS concurs with the AAP/ACOG on this position (Ng, Loewy, & Fetus and Newborn Committee, 2018). Oral administration of vitamin K is not as effective in the prevention of late hemorrhagic disease.

MEDICATION GUIDE

Vitamin K: Phytonadione (AquaMEPHYTON, Konakion)

Action
Provides vitamin K because the newborn does not have the intestinal flora to produce this vitamin for approximately 1 week after birth. It also promotes formation of clotting factors (II, VII, IX, X) in the liver.

Indication
To prevent vitamin K deficiency bleeding (hemorrhagic disease) of the newborn.

Neonatal Dosage
Administer a 0.5-mg (0.25-mL) dose to newborns weighing ≤1500 g and a 1-mg (0.5-mL) dose to newborns weighing >1500 g intramuscularly soon after birth; the injection can be delayed until after initial breastfeeding.[a] In rare cases, vitamin K may be given by the intravenous (IV) route for the prevention of hemorrhagic disease of the newborn when the patient is a preterm infant who has little to no muscle mass. In such instances, the medication is diluted and given over 10-15 min while closely monitoring the infant with a cardiorespiratory monitor. Rapid IV administration of vitamin K can cause cardiac arrest.

Adverse Reactions
Edema, erythema, and pain at the injection site occur rarely; hemolysis, jaundice, and hyperbilirubinemia have been reported, particularly in preterm infants.

Nursing Considerations
Follow the procedure for IM injection (see Fig. 24.16). Encourage parents to use comfort measures for neonate such as SSC before, during, and after injection.

[a]Administration may be delayed for up to 6 h in Canada.
Data from American Academy of Pediatrics Committee on Fetus and Newborn. (2003, reaffirmed 2014). Controversies concerning vitamin K and the newborn. *Pediatrics, 112*(1), 191–192; Ng, E., Loewy, A.D., & Fetus and Newborn Committee. (2018). Guidelines for vitamin K prophylaxis in newborns. *Paediatrics and Child Health, 23*(6), 394-397.

Increasingly, parents are refusing vitamin K injections, related to concerns about synthetic or toxic ingredients, excessive dose, side effects, and pain with administration (Hamrick, Gable, Freeman et al., 2016). Neonatal or pediatric care providers should explain benefits versus risks related to vitamin K administration. Providers and nurses can encourage parents to use comfort measures such as SSC before, during, and after the injection.

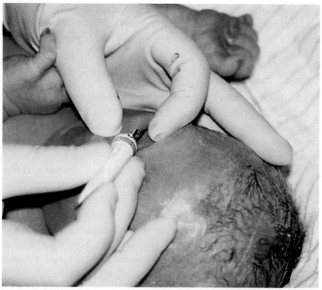

Fig. 24.5 Instillation of Medication Into Eye of Newborn. Thumb and forefinger are used to open the eye; medication is placed in the lower conjunctiva from the inner to the outer canthus. (Courtesy Marjorie Pyle, Lifecircle, Costa Mesa, CA.)

Promoting Parent-Infant Interaction

Contemporary birthing practices are family centered. Parents generally desire to share in the birth process and have early and continuous contact with their newborn. SSC with the mother beginning immediately after birth and breastfeeding within the first 1 to 2 hours after birth are important in promoting maternal-infant attachment. Early mother-infant contact produces physiologic benefits for the neonate and the mother. SSC promotes physiologic stability of the newborn. Maternal levels of oxytocin and prolactin rise with SSC and early breastfeeding. Rooming-in after birth until discharge from the birthing facility promotes parent-infant interaction.

CARE MANAGEMENT: FROM 2 HOURS AFTER BIRTH UNTIL DISCHARGE

Depending on the model of care delivery, the mother-baby nurse or newborn nursery nurse is responsible for ongoing assessment and care of the newborn. Accurate assessment skills and appropriate interventions promote positive outcomes, especially for newborns who experience any problems before going home. Newborn care is family centered—the nurse provides education and support for the new parents throughout the stay in the birthing facility and assists them in preparing for discharge (see the Nursing Care Plan).

◎ NURSING CARE PLAN

The Normal Newborn

Actual or Potential Problem	Expected Outcome	Nursing Interventions	Rationales
Risk for obstructed airway related to excess mucus production or improper positioning	Newborn's airway is patent. Breath sounds are clear. Abnormal breath sounds, such as crackles, rhonchi, and wheezes or stridor, are absent. No respiratory distress is evident. Oxygen saturation level is within the normal range.	Assess the newborn for signs of an obstructed airway and auscultate lung sounds. Position infant on back when sleeping. Teach parents that gagging and sneezing are normal neonatal responses and how and when to use bulb syringe and how to relieve airway obstruction.	The newborn's airway must be patent and the lungs clear so that air exchange and oxygenation can occur. To prevent suffocation and aspiration. To help parents understand what is normal and to enable parents to clear airway safely.
Risk for hypothermia related to larger body surface relative to body mass.	Temperature remains in range of 36.5°-37.5°C (97.7°-99.5°F). Parents verbalize understanding of infant thermoregulation.	Monitor axillary temperature frequently. Keep newborn skin-to-skin for the first 1-2 h after birth. Bathe after 6 h of age, when temperature is stable, using warm water, drying carefully, and avoiding exposure to drafts. Teach parents principles of thermoregulation, how to prevent heat loss when bathing, how to dress newborn appropriately for the ambient temperature.	To identify any changes promptly and to prevent hyperthermia or hypothermia and cold stress. To provide warmth and avoid heat loss. To avoid heat loss from evaporation and convection. To prevent hypothermia and overheating.
Risk for developing infection related to immature immune system and environmental exposure.	Vital signs are within normal range. Newborn is alert and active. Newborn is free from signs of infection. Umbilical cord will heal properly and remain free from infection. Family members demonstrate hand hygiene technique before handling newborn.	Review maternal record for evidence of any risk factors. Have all care providers, including parents, perform proper hand hygiene before handling newborn. Teach parents to keep newborn away from crowds and environmental irritants, such as tobacco smoke. Teach parents signs of infection and when to notify health care provider.	To ascertain whether neonate is predisposed to infection. To protect newborn from infection. To reduce potential sources of infection. To identify early signs of infection for prompt treatment.

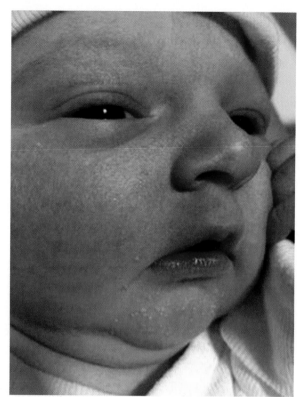

Fig. 23.7 Milia. (Courtesy Ashley and Andrew Martin, Charlotte, NC.)

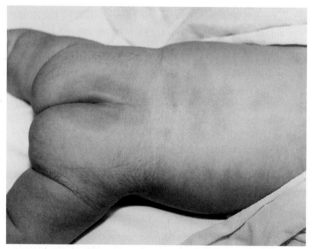

Fig. 23.8 Mongolian Spot.

Mongolian Spots

Mongolian spots, bluish black areas of pigmentation, can appear over any part of the exterior surface of the body, including the extremities. They are most common on the back and buttocks (Fig. 23.8). These pigmented areas occur most frequently in newborns whose ethnic origins are Latin America, Asia, Africa, or the Mediterranean area. They are more common in dark-skinned individuals but can occur in 5% to 13% of Caucasians (Blackburn, 2018). Mongolian spots fade gradually over months or years.

The presence of Mongolian spots on the newborn should be documented carefully in the medical record. These normal skin pigmentations can be mistaken for bruises once the infant is discharged, and this can raise suspicion of physical abuse.

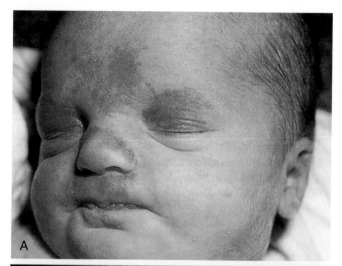

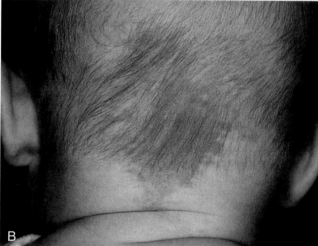

Fig. 23.9 Nevus Simplex. (A) Forehead, eyelids, nose, below nose. (B) Nape of neck. (From Eichenfield, L. F., Frieden, I. J., & Esterly, N. B. [Eds]. [2008]. *Neonatal dermatology* [2nd ed.]. Philadelphia: Saunders.)

Nevi

Nevus simplex, also known as salmon patches, telangiectatic nevi, "stork bites," or "angel kisses," is the result of a superficial capillary defect and occur in up to 80% of newborns. They are usually small, flat, and pink and are easily blanched (Fig. 23.9). The most common sites are the upper eyelids, nose, upper lip, and nape of the neck. They have no clinical significance and require no treatment. Facial lesions usually fade between the first and second years of life, whereas neck lesions can be visible into adulthood (Hoath & Narendran, 2015).

A port-wine stain, or **nevus flammeus**, is usually visible at birth and is due to an asymmetric postcapillary venule malformation. It is usually pink and flat at birth but darkens with time, becoming red or purple and pebbly in consistency. True port-wine stains do not blanch on pressure or disappear. They are found most commonly on the face and neck (Hoath & Narendran, 2015).

Infantile Hemangioma

Infantile hemangiomas consist of dilated newly formed capillaries occupying the entire dermal and subdermal layers with associated connective tissue hypertrophy. The typical lesion is a raised, sharply demarcated, bright or dark red rough-surfaced swelling that may be present at birth or may appear during the early weeks after birth. Common sites are the scalp, face, back, and anterior chest. These lesions are sometimes called *strawberry*

Common Newborn Problems

Birth Injuries

Birth trauma includes any physical injury sustained by a newborn during labor and birth. Although most injuries are minor and resolve during the neonatal period without treatment, some types of trauma require intervention; a few are serious enough to be fatal (see Chapter 35 for more information on birth injuries).

Retinal and subconjunctival hemorrhages result from rupture of capillaries caused by increased pressure during birth. These hemorrhages usually clear within 7 to 10 days and present no further problems. Parents need explanation and reassurance that these injuries are harmless.

Erythema, ecchymoses, petechiae, abrasions, lacerations, or edema of the buttocks and extremities can be present. Localized discoloration can appear over the presenting part as a result of forceps- or vacuum-assisted birth. Ecchymoses and edema can appear anywhere on the body. Petechiae (pinpoint hemorrhagic areas) acquired during birth can extend over the upper trunk and face. These lesions are benign if they disappear within 2 or 3 days of birth and no new lesions appear. Ecchymoses and petechiae can be signs of a more serious disorder, such as thrombocytopenic purpura. To differentiate hemorrhagic areas from a skin rash or discolorations, the nurse attempts to blanch the skin by pressing with two fingers, lifting the fingers off the skin, and waiting for the return of blood. Petechiae and ecchymoses will not blanch because extravasated blood remains within the tissues, whereas skin rashes and discolorations will blanch.

Trauma to the presenting fetal part can occur during labor and birth. Caput succedaneum and cephalhematoma are discussed in Chapter 23 (see Fig. 23.15). Forceps injury and bruising from the vacuum cup occur at the site of application of the instruments. A forceps injury commonly produces a linear mark across both sides of the face in the shape of forceps blades. If the skin is broken, then the affected areas should be kept clean to minimize the risk for infection. These injuries usually resolve spontaneously within several days with no further intervention.

Bruises over the face can be the result of face presentation (Fig. 24.6). In a breech presentation, bruising and swelling may be seen over the buttocks or genitalia (see Fig. 23.12). The skin over the entire head can be ecchymotic and covered with petechiae caused by a tight nuchal cord. If the hemorrhagic areas do not disappear spontaneously in 2 days or if the infant's condition changes, the primary health care provider is notified.

Accidental lacerations can be inflicted with a scalpel during a cesarean birth. These cuts can occur on any part of the body but are most often found on the scalp, buttocks, and thighs. They are usually superficial and need only to be kept clean. If skin closure is needed, an adhesive substance or strips may be applied. Sutures are rarely needed.

Physiologic Problems

Hyperbilirubinemia

Assessment and screening. The majority of newborn infants experience some level of jaundice, most of which is benign. In most cases, this is *physiologic jaundice*, caused by increased levels of unconjugated bilirubin; physiologic jaundice is usually self-limiting and requires no treatment. This type of jaundice occurs after 24 hours of age, peaks at about 3 to 5 days in term infants, and resolves after 1 to 2 weeks. In some cases, phototherapy is needed to lower bilirubin levels to within an acceptable range. Physiologic jaundice must be differentiated from pathologic jaundice, which is associated with higher levels of unconjugated bilirubin (see Chapter 23). Jaundice can also be associated with breastfeeding (see Chapters 23 and 25).

Every newborn should be assessed for jaundice at least every 8 to 12 hours; this can be easily done when vital signs are assessed. To differentiate cutaneous jaundice from normal skin color, the nurse applies pressure with a finger over a bony area (e.g., the nose, forehead, sternum) for several seconds to empty all the capillaries in that spot, then releases the pressure by lifting the finger. If jaundice is present, the blanched area will appear yellowish before the capillaries refill. The conjunctival sacs and buccal mucosa also are assessed, especially in darker-skinned infants. Assessing for jaundice in natural light is recommended because artificial lighting and reflection from walls can distort the actual skin color.

Visual assessment of jaundice alone does not provide an accurate assessment of hyperbilirubinemia, especially in dark-skinned newborns (Tappero & Honeyfield, 2015). AAP recommends universal predischarge bilirubin screening to prevent severe hyperbilirubinemia and the neurologic complications of acute bilirubin encephalopathy and kernicterus. This can be accomplished by measuring the total serum bilirubin (TSB) level or the transcutaneous bilirubin (TcB) level (Fig 24.7). In general, if the TcB level is greater than 12 to 15 mg/dL, a serum bilirubin check is performed as a confirmatory test. Recent developments in transcutaneous bilirubin technology have increased the accuracy of TcB measurement in dark-skinned neonates (Kamath-Rayne, Thilo, Deacon, et al., 2016). TcB monitors can be used to screen for clinically significant jaundice and decrease the need for serum bilirubin measurements (Kamath-Rayne et al.).

The second way to assess for hyperbilirubinemia is to draw a serum bilirubin value. The levels, TcB or TSB, are interpreted by plotting them on an hour-specific nomogram to determine the infant's risk for hyperbilirubinemia. Repeat testing is based on the risk level (low, intermediate, or high), the age of the neonate, and the progression of jaundice (AAP Subcommittee on Hyperbilirubinemia, Pediatrics 2004; Barrington, Sankaran, & CPS Fetus and Newborn Committee, 2007/2018). Many providers use a bilirubin

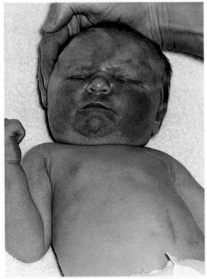

Fig. 24.6 Marked Bruising on the Entire Face of an Infant Born Vaginally After Face Presentation. Less severe ecchymoses were present on the extremities. Phototherapy was required for treatment of jaundice resulting from the breakdown of accumulated blood. (From O'Doherty, N. [1986]. *Neonatology: Micro atlas of the newborn.* Nutley, NJ: Hoffman-La Roche.)

tool (www.bilitool.org) that facilitates calculating the risk for neonatal hyperbilirubinemia.

Infants in the low-risk category are less likely to develop hyperbilirubinemia. However, the AAP warns that all infants should be considered as being at potential risk for hyperbilirubinemia, even if they were identified as being in the low-risk category. This means that all newborns should be followed after discharge from the birthing facility for the development of unexpected jaundice, and that parents should be given printed and oral information about newborn jaundice (AAP & ACOG, 2017).

Adequate feeding is essential in preventing hyperbilirubinemia. Newborns should breastfeed early (within 1–2 hours after birth) and often (at least 8–12 times/24 hours) (AAP Section on Breastfeeding, 2012; AAP Subcommittee on Hyperbilirubinemia, 2004). Frequent feedings help decrease the risk of hyperbilirubinemia. Colostrum acts as a laxative to promote stooling, which helps rid the body of bilirubin. Formula-fed infants should be fed within the first hour of life and then at least every 8 to 12 times every 24 hours.

Newborns should be assessed for risk factors for severe hyperbilirubinemia. The most common risk factor is gestational age less than 35 to 36 weeks.

Close follow-up of infants at risk for hyperbilirubinemia is essential; parents should be educated and encouraged to follow postdischarge recommendations (AAP Subcommittee on Hyperbilirubinemia, 2004). Follow-up should occur 48 to 72 hours after discharge from the birthing facility, or sooner based on the length of stay and presence of risk factors for hyperbilirubinemia (AAP & ACOG, 2017).

If an infant appears jaundiced in the first 24 hours of life, a TcB or TSB level should be measured and results interpreted based on the newborn's age in hours according to the hour-specific nomogram for infants born at 35 weeks of gestation or later (AAP Subcommittee on Hyperbilirubinemia, 2004). This type of jaundice is called *pathologic*. Repeat testing is based on the risk level (low, intermediate, or high), the age of the newborn, and the progression of jaundice. Additional labs may also be ordered for this newborn.

Therapy for hyperbilirubinemia. The decision to treat an infant for hyperbilirubinemia is based on TSB levels, the infant's gestational age, and the presence of risk factors. Using a nomogram that plots bilirubin levels according to the infant's age in hours at the time the specimen was drawn, the provider determines the appropriate management plan. The AAP established guidelines that provide direction for health care providers in determining the need for phototherapy or exchange transfusion (AAP Committee on Hyperbilirubinemia, 2004).

The goal of treatment of hyperbilirubinemia is to reduce the newborn's serum levels of unconjugated bilirubin. There are two ways to reduce unconjugated bilirubin levels: phototherapy and exchange blood transfusion. Phototherapy is the most common treatment. Exchange transfusion is used to treat those infants whose serum bilirubin levels are rising rapidly despite the use of intensive phototherapy.

Phototherapy. Phototherapy uses light energy to change the shape and structure of unconjugated bilirubin, converting it into a conjugated form that can be excreted through urine and stool. Phototherapy can be delivered by a lamp, blanket, pad, or cover-body devices. The severity of the newborn's hyperbilirubinemia determines the type of phototherapy device and strength of light, duration of treatment, and location of treatment (hospital or home). The newborn's response to phototherapy depends on the bilirubin level, the effectiveness of the phototherapy device, and the infant's ability to excrete the bilirubin (Bhutani & Committee on Fetus and Newborn, 2011).

The dose and effectiveness of phototherapy are affected by the source of light. Phototherapy units vary in the spectrum of light they deliver and in the filters used. The most effective therapy is achieved with special blue fluorescent tubes or a specially designed light-emitting diode (LED). Phototherapy lights do not emit significant ultraviolet radiation; the small amount that is emitted does not cause erythema. Most of the ultraviolet light is absorbed by the glass wall of the fluorescent tube and by the plastic cover of the light (Bhutani & Committee on Fetus and Newborn, 2011; Kamath-Rayne et al., 2016). Phototherapy is usually effective in treating hyperbilirubinemia that has not reached levels associated with acute bilirubin encephalopathy or kernicterus.

The effectiveness of phototherapy is related to the distance between the light and the neonate and to the surface area of skin that is exposed. To maximize skin exposure, multiple devices may be used simultaneously. For example, a neonate may be placed under a phototherapy lamp while also lying on a fiberoptic pad or LED mattress (Bhutani & Committee on Fetus and Newborn, 2011).

During phototherapy using a lamp, the neonate, wearing only a diaper, is placed under a bank of lights approximately 45 to 50 cm from the light source. Phototherapy can be used for the infant in an incubator (Fig. 24.8) or in an open crib. The distance varies according to unit protocol and type of light used. The irradiance of the light is monitored routinely with a radiometer, with measurements at several sites over

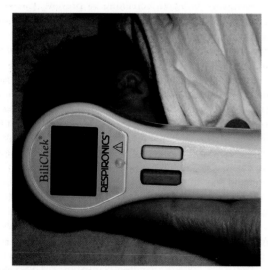

Fig. 24.7 Transcutaneous Monitoring of Bilirubin With a Transcutaneous Bilirubinometry Monitor. (Courtesy Cheryl Briggs, RNC, Annapolis, MD.)

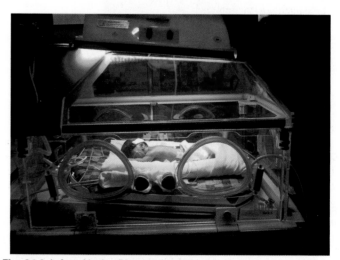

Fig. 24.8 Infant Under Phototherapy Lights While in an Incubator. (Courtesy Cheryl Briggs, RNC, Annapolis, MD.)

the neonate's body surface during treatment to ensure efficacy of therapy (Bhutani & Committee on Fetus and Newborn, 2011).

If phototherapy is effective, the bilirubin level should begin to decrease within 4 to 6 hours after phototherapy is initiated and within 24 hours should decrease by 30% to 40% (Kamath-Rayne et al., 2016). Phototherapy is used until the infant's serum bilirubin level decreases to within an acceptable range. The decision to discontinue therapy is based on the observation of a definite downward trend in the bilirubin values and the age of the newborn.

> ### ⚡ SAFETY ALERT
>
> When a phototherapy lamp is used, the infant's eyes must be protected by a special opaque mask that is designed to prevent retinal damage. The eye shield should cover the eyes completely but not occlude the nares. Before the mask is applied, the infant's eyes should be closed gently to prevent excoriation of the corneas. The mask should be removed periodically and during infant feedings so that the eyes can be assessed and cleansed with water and the parents can have visual contact with the infant (Kamath-Rayne et al., 2016).

Phototherapy can cause changes in the infant's temperature, depending partially on the bed used—bassinet, incubator, or radiant warmer. The infant's temperature should be closely monitored for hypothermia and hyperthermia.

Phototherapy lights, especially if the newborn is low birth weight or under a radiant warmer, can increase the rate of insensible water loss, which contributes to fluid loss and dehydration. Therefore the infant must be adequately hydrated. Hydration maintenance in the healthy newborn is accomplished through breastfeeding, pasteurized donor milk, or infant formula. Feedings of glucose water or plain water should not be used because these liquids do not promote excretion of bilirubin in the stools.

The nurse closely monitors urinary output as an indicator of hydration status while the infant is receiving phototherapy. Urine output can be decreased or unaltered; the urine can have a dark gold or brown appearance.

The number and consistency of stools are monitored. Bilirubin is excreted primarily through the stool, so it is important that the infant is having bowel movements. Bilirubin breakdown increases gastric motility, which can result in loose stools that can cause skin excoriation and breakdown. The infant's buttocks must be cleaned after each stool to help maintain skin integrity.

> ### ⚡ SAFETY ALERT
>
> When phototherapy lights are used, no ointments, creams, or lotions should be applied to the newborn's skin because they can absorb heat and cause burns.

Infants under phototherapy lights need to be repositioned at least every 2 to 3 hours to maximize skin exposure. Transient skin rashes or tanning of the skin can occur during phototherapy. In rare instances, there can be bullous eruptions or the development of bronze baby syndrome in which the skin appears grayish brown (Kamath-Rayne et al., 2016). There is a lack of evidence regarding the long-term effects of phototherapy (Bhutani & Committee on Fetus and Newborn, 2011).

In addition to phototherapy lights, other systems are used for phototherapy. A bassinet system provides special blue light above and beneath the infant. Another phototherapy device is a fiberoptic

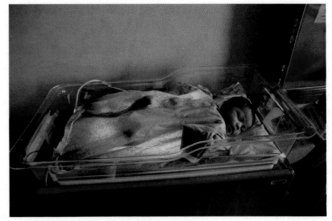

Fig. 24.9 Infant Receiving Phototherapy Using a Bilirubin Bed. (Courtesy Cheryl Briggs, RNC, Annapolis, MD.)

blanket that is connected to a light source. The blanket is flexible and can be placed around the infant's torso or underneath the infant in the bassinet. There are also bilirubin beds with LED lights in a pad that covers the surface of the bassinet (Fig. 24.9). The LEDs do not produce heat and can be used with radiant warmers. These devices are usually less effective when used alone as compared with conventional phototherapy lights. They can be very useful in combination with overhead phototherapy lights. In certain instances, the infant's bilirubin levels increase rapidly and intensive phototherapy is required; this situation involves the use of a combination of conventional lights and fiberoptic blankets to maximize bilirubin reduction. Although fiberoptic lights do not produce heat as do conventional lights, staff should ensure that a covering pad is placed between the infant's skin and the fiberoptic device to prevent skin burns, especially in preterm infants. The newborn can remain in the mother's room in an open crib or in her arms during treatment. The use of eye patches depends on whether the devices are used alone or in combination with phototherapy lights.

The use of home phototherapy should be reserved for healthy term infants with bilirubin levels in the "optional phototherapy" range according to the nomogram. The concern is that home phototherapy units do not provide the same level of irradiance or body surface coverage as phototherapy devices used in the hospital (AAP Committee on Hyperbilirubinemia, 2004). The use of home phototherapy is also dependent on the newborn's insurance coverage; many companies do not cover this therapy.

Phototherapy treatment is associated with concerns related to psychobehavioral issues, including parent-infant separation, potential social isolation, decreased sensorineural stimulation, altered biologic rhythms, altered feeding patterns, and activity changes. Parental anxiety can be greatly increased, particularly at the sight of the newborn with eyes covered and under special lights. The interruption of breastfeeding for phototherapy is a potential deterrent to successful maternal-infant attachment and interaction. Although there are conflicting opinions about continuous versus intermittent phototherapy, for most infants phototherapy can safely be interrupted for feedings, parental interaction, assessments, and obtaining blood samples for testing (Kamath-Rayne et al., 2016).

Close follow-up is needed for infants who have been treated for hyperbilirubinemia. Repeat testing of serum bilirubin levels and follow-up visits with the pediatric health care provider are expected. In some cases, a nurse may conduct a home visit to evaluate the infant's condition, draw blood for bilirubin testing, and monitor the mother's health. In some cases, parents take the newborn to an outpatient clinic or physician's office to be evaluated. This specimen is usually obtained via heelstick.

Exchange transfusion. When phototherapy is not effective in reducing serum bilirubin levels or with severe hyperbilirubinemia such as in hemolytic disease, or for treatment of acute bilirubin encephalopathy, exchange transfusion may be needed. This procedure is done in a neonatal intensive care (NICU) setting and can reduce bilirubin levels by 45% to 85%. A portion of the infant's blood is replaced with donor blood (Kamath-Rayne et al., 2016) (see Chapter 36).

Hypoglycemia. Hypoglycemia in a term infant during the early newborn period is defined as a blood glucose concentration inadequate to support neurologic, organ, and tissue function; however, there is a lack of consensus among experts regarding the precise glucose level at which harm can occur. Similarly, there is no consensus about when to screen for hypoglycemia or the level at which treatment should be instituted (Adamkin, 2017; AAP & ACOG, 2017). The lower limit for normal plasma glucose levels during the first 72 hours after birth is often cited as 40 to 45 mg/dL. There is concern about neurologic injury as a result of severe or prolonged hypoglycemia, especially in combination with ischemia (Rozance, McGowan, Price-Douglas, et al., 2016).

At birth, the maternal source of glucose is eliminated when the umbilical cord is clamped. Most healthy term newborns experience a transient decrease in glucose levels to as low as 30 mg/dL during the first 1 to 2 hours after birth, with a subsequent mobilization of free fatty acids and ketones to help maintain adequate glucose levels (Blackburn, 2018). Early and regular feeding promotes normoglycemia. There is no need to routinely assess glucose levels of healthy term infants.

Infants considered to be at risk for hypoglycemia should be screened during the first several hours of life. Infants at risk include those who are preterm or late preterm; SGA or LGA; low birth weight; infants of mothers with diabetes; and infants who experienced perinatal stress such as asphyxia, cold stress, or respiratory distress (AAP & ACOG, 2017; Wight, Marinelli, & Academy of Breastfeeding Medicine, 2014).

Screening and treatment protocols vary across institutions. Glucose levels should be measured in all newborns with risk factors for hypoglycemia and in any newborn with clinical manifestations of hypoglycemia. The frequency of glucose testing is determined by the risk factors for each individual newborn. According to the AAP, late preterm and term SGA, infants of mothers with diabetes/LGA neonates are at risk for hypoglycemia and should be fed within the first hour, with glucose testing done 30 minutes after feeding. For at least the first 24 hours after birth, these infants should be fed every 2 to 3 hours, with glucose levels measured before each feeding. Further testing is based on glucose levels and feeding skills (Adamkin & Committee on Fetus and Newborn, 2011). Early, frequent breastfeeding and SSC with the mother for as long as possible after birth promote thermoregulation and stabilization of glucose levels (Wight et al., 2014).

Nurses should observe all newborns for signs of hypoglycemia. Glucose testing should be done on any infant with clinical signs of hypoglycemia. These signs can be transient or recurrent and include jitteriness, lethargy, poor feeding, abnormal cry, hypotonia, temperature instability (hypothermia), respiratory distress, apnea, and seizures (Rozance et al., 2016). It is important to remember that hypoglycemia can be present in the absence of clinical manifestations.

Bedside glucose monitoring is performed using reagent test strips with or without a reflectance colorimeter. Because of variations in devices and operator techniques, it is recommended that any level less than 45 mg/dL should be confirmed with a stat serum glucose level, depending on facility policy. However, treatment of hypoglycemia should not be delayed while awaiting serum glucose results (Rozance et al., 2016; Wight et al., 2014). Protocols for treatment of hypoglycemia vary and change frequently based on new evidence. In general, for newborns who are clinically stable and well appearing, early and frequent oral feedings are suggested. Infants who are at an increased risk for aspiration, who have poor perfusion, or are thought to have a bowel obstruction are not enterally fed and will need intravenous fluids to normalize and maintain their blood glucose levels (Karlsen, 2012). (See Chapters 23 and 34 for more information on hypoglycemia.)

> **! NURSING ALERT**
>
> A heel warmer should be applied prior to every glucose assessment via heelstick. If the extremity is cool, the test result can be falsely low.

Laboratory and Diagnostic Tests

Because newborns experience many transitional events in the first 28 days of life, blood samples are often collected to determine adequate physiologic adaptation and to identify disorders that can adversely affect the child's life beyond the neonatal period. Blood samples for most laboratory tests can be obtained from the newborn with a heel puncture, also known as a *heelstick*. Tests commonly performed other than blood glucose and bilirubin levels include newborn screening tests and serum drug levels. Standard laboratory values for a term newborn are listed in Table 24.4.

Universal Newborn Screening

Mandated by U.S. law, newborn screening is an important public health program aimed at early detection of genetic diseases that result in severe health problems if not treated early. The universal screening program is state based and involves a variety of components, including education, screening, follow-up, treatment, and a system for monitoring and evaluation. The Health Resources and Services Administration Committee on Heritable Disorders in Newborns and Children (2018) recommends screening for 35 core disorders and 26 secondary disorders. The core disorders include hemoglobinopathies (e.g., sickle cell disease), inborn errors of metabolism (e.g., phenylketonuria [PKU], galactosemia), severe combined immunodeficiency, hearing loss, and critical congenital heart disease (CCHD). The majority of disorders included in the screening are not symptomatic at birth. Individual states select additional disorders to include in the screening.

In Canada, universal newborn screening policies and practices are varied. Individual provinces in Canada determine the disorders included in newborn screening; however, all provinces screen for PKU and congenital hypothyroidism (Canadian Organization for Rare Disorders, 2015). Capillary blood samples are obtained using a heelstick; blood is collected on a special filter paper and sent to a designated state laboratory for analysis (Fig. 24.10). Samples are usually collected in the hospital after 24 hours of age and before discharge; testing may be delayed for sick or preterm infants or those born outside the hospital. The screening test may need to be repeated if the initial specimen was obtained prior to 24 hours of age, after a blood transfusion was given, or if the infant's birth weight was less than 1500 g.

The American College of Medical Genetics (2009) recommends that states retain the residual dried blood filter spots. These blood samples are useful for future testing and research purposes. However,

TABLE 24.4 Standard Laboratory Values in a Term Neonate

Hematology	Values
Hemoglobin (g/dL)	15-24
Hematocrit (%)	44-70
Red blood cells (RBCs)/µL	4.8×10^6 to 7.1×10^6
Reticulocytes (%)	1.8-4.6
Fetal hemoglobin (% of total)	50-70
Platelet count/mm³	
≤1week	84,000-478,000
>1week	150,000-300,000
White blood cells (WBCs)/µL	9000-30,000
Bilirubin, total (mg/dL)[a]	
24 h	2-6
48 h	6-7
3-5 days	4-6
Serum glucose (mg/dL)	
<1 day	40-60
>1 day	50-90
Arterial blood gases	
pH	7.35-7.45
P_{CO_2}	35-45 mm Hg
P_{O_2}	60-80 mm Hg
HCO_3	18-26 mEq/L
Base excess	(−5) to (+5)
O_2 saturation	92%-94%

dL, Deciliter; *µL,* microliter; *P_{CO_2},* partial pressure of carbon dioxide; *P_{O_2},* partial pressure of oxygen.

[a]Bilirubin levels should be interpreted according to the hour-specific nomogram (AAP Subcommittee on Hyperbilirubinemia, 2004).
American Academy of Pediatrics [AAP] Subcommittee on Hyperbilirubinemia. (2004). Clinical practice guideline: Management of hyperbilirubinemia in the newborn infant 35 or more weeks of gestation. *Pediatrics, 114*(1), 297–316; Blackburn, S.T. (2018). *Maternal, fetal, and neonatal physiology* (5th ed.). St. Louis: Elsevier; Kliegman, R.M., Stanton, B.F., St. Geme III, et al. (Eds.), (2016). *Nelson textbook of pediatrics* (20th ed.), Philadelphia, PA: Elsevier; Pagana, K.D., & Pagana, T.J. (2014). *Mosby's manual of diagnostic and laboratory tests* (5th ed.). St. Louis: Elsevier; Barry, J.S., Deacon, J., Hernández, C., et al. (2016). Acid-base homeostasis and oxygenation. In: S.L. Gardner, Carter, B.S., Enzman-Hines, M., et al., (Eds.), *Merenstein & Gardner's handbook of neonatal intensive care* (8th ed.). St. Louis: Elsevier.

ethical concerns are related to the need for parental consent to retain blood samples and use them for biomedical research. Nurses need to be aware of policies and procedures in the state and facility where they practice so they are able to provide information to parents (AWHONN, 2016).

Families should be educated about universal newborn screening during the prenatal period (ACOG Committee on Genetics, 2015). However, this is not common practice; newborn screening is not usually discussed with parents prior to birth. This may be related to the fact that in the majority of states informed consent is not required for newborn screening. In many cases, discussion about newborn screening occurs in the birth facility at the time of blood sample collection. Nurses can provide education for parents regarding the purpose of the screening, the procedure for blood sampling, when to expect results, and the importance of follow-up (AWHONN, 2016) (see the Community Activity box).

🏠 COMMUNITY ACTIVITY

Newborn Screening

> Visit the National Newborn Screening and Genetics Resource Center (NNSGRC) website (http://genes-r-us.uthscsa.edu). Review the information for parents and family about resources, disorders tested, and screening programs.
>
> At the NNSGRC website, visit the newborn screening program site for your state. What types of disorders are included in newborn screening? Does your state require newborn hearing screening? Review the information for parents about diagnostic testing and community support services.

Newborn hearing screening. The Recommended Uniform Screening Panel includes the dried bloodspot specimen and two point-of-care conditions for newborn screening: hearing loss and CCHD. Early detection of newborn hearing loss allows the opportunity for early intervention and treatment. It is estimated that permanent hearing loss affects approximately 1.6 out of every 1000 infants born in the United States (Williams, Alam, & Gaffney, 2015). The Joint Committee on Infant Hearing (2007) recommends routine hearing screening for all newborns before hospital discharge or no later than 1 month of age. The CPS recommends hearing screening for all newborns (Patel, Feldman, & CPS Community Paediatrics Committee, 2011/2016). Through early hearing detection and intervention programs, the outcome for infants who are deaf or hard of hearing can be maximized.

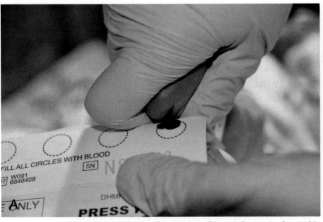
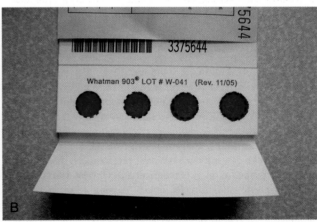

Fig. 24.10 Nurse Obtaining Blood Sample from Newborn's Heel for Universal Screening. (A) Sample is applied to filter paper. (B) All circles on the filter paper must be filled in completely. (Courtesy Cheryl Briggs, RNC, Annapolis, MD.)

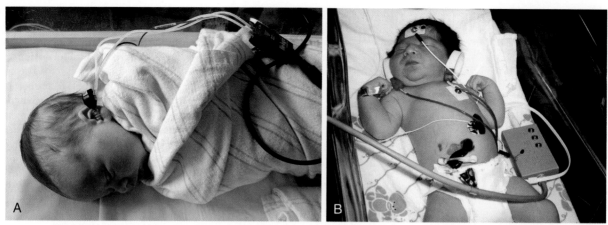

Fig. 24.11 Newborn Hearing Screening. (A) Evoked otoacoustic emissions test. (B) Auditory brain response test. (A, Courtesy Julie and Darren Nelson, Loveland, CO. B, Courtesy Dee Lowdermilk, Chapel Hill, NC.)

Using noninvasive technology, newborn hearing screening provides information about the pathways from the external ear to the cerebral cortex. Screening should be performed using the evoked optoacoustic emissions (EOAE) test, the auditory brainstem response (ABR), or a combination of the two (AAP & ACOG, 2017). Neither test is definitive in diagnosing hearing loss; they are used to determine whether further, more accurate hearing testing is needed through audiologic evaluation. For the EOAE test, a soft rubber earpiece that makes a soft clicking noise is placed in the baby's outer ear (Fig. 24.11A). A healthy ear will "echo" the click sound back to a microphone inside the earpiece. The ABR test is performed by attaching sensors to the baby's forehead and behind each ear. An earphone is placed in the baby's outer ear and sends a series of quiet sounds into the sleeping baby's ear (see Fig. 24.11B). The sensors measure the responses of the baby's acoustic nerve. The responses are recorded and stored in a computer.

Newborns who do not pass the initial hearing screening test should have the test repeated as part of follow-up care. If the infant still does not pass, a comprehensive audiologic evaluation should be done by 3 months of age by a pediatric audiologist. Regardless of the outcome of hearing testing, all infants should have regular and ongoing surveillance of developmental, hearing, and speech-language skills through regular well-child visits beginning at 2 months of age so that any hearing loss can be promptly identified and treated (AAP & ACOG, 2017; Joint Committee on Infant Hearing, 2007).

Screening for critical congenital heart disease. CCHD represents some of the most serious types of heart defects, requiring surgery or cardiac catheterization in the first year of life. It has been estimated that 6 of 10,000 apparently healthy term or late-preterm infants will have critical congenital cardiac disease (Plana, Zamora, Suresh, et al., 2018). CCHD was added to the uniform screening panel in the United States in 2011 and is endorsed by the AAP (AAP Section on Cardiology and Cardiac Surgery Executive Committee, 2012). The noninvasive screening test is performed using pulse oximetry to measure oxygen saturation for the purpose of detecting hypoxemia. Pulse oximetry testing can detect some critical congenital heart defects that present with hypoxemia in the absence of other physical symptoms. Hypoxemia can be the first sign that a congenital heart defect is present, and other symptoms can develop once the newborn has been discharged. Screening is performed at 24 to 48 hours of age. Oxygen saturation is measured in the right hand and one foot. A "passing" result is oxygen saturation of greater than 95% in either extremity, with a less than 3% absolute difference between the upper and lower extremity readings. Immediate evaluation is needed if the oxygen saturation is less than

90%. The baby is evaluated for hemodynamic stability and hypoxemia; an echocardiogram is usually performed (AAP Section on Cardiology and Cardiac Surgery Executive Committee).

Collection of Specimens

Ongoing evaluation and screening of a newborn often requires obtaining blood by heelstick or venipuncture or the collection of a urine specimen. Laboratory tests may be ordered routinely (e.g., newborn screening) or for a specific purpose as directed by the health care provider.

Heelstick. Blood samples may be drawn by laboratory technicians or bedside caregivers, depending on facility policies. These specimens may be used for glucose monitoring, newborn screening, or other tests. A heelstick is usually considered appropriate when the volume of blood required is less than 1 mL.

Blood samples should be collected in a manner that minimizes pain and trauma to the infant and maximizes the accuracy of test results. If a laboratory technician is collecting the specimen, the nurse assists as needed to maximize safety and infant comfort.

It is helpful to warm the heel before the sample is taken; application of heat for 5 to 10 minutes helps dilate the vessels in the area. A cloth soaked with warm water and wrapped loosely around the foot provides effective warming (Fig. 24.12A). Disposable heel warmers are available from a variety of companies but should be used with care to prevent burns. Nurses should wear gloves when collecting any specimen. The nurse cleanses the area with an appropriate skin antiseptic, restrains the infant's foot with a free hand, and then punctures the site. A spring-loaded automatic puncture device causes less pain and requires fewer punctures than a manual lance blade.

The most serious complication of an infant heelstick is necrotizing osteochondritis resulting from lancet penetration of the bone. To prevent this complication, the puncture is made at the outer aspect of the heel and penetrates no deeper than 2.4 mm in a term infant. To identify the appropriate puncture site, the nurse draws an imaginary line from between the fourth and fifth toes and parallel to the lateral aspect of the foot to the heel, where the puncture is made; a second line can be drawn from the great toe to the medial aspect of the heel (see Fig. 24.12B). Repeated trauma to the walking surface of the heel can cause fibrosis and scarring that can lead to problems with walking later in life.

After the specimen has been collected, gentle pressure is applied with a dry gauze pad. No further skin cleanser or alcohol should be applied because it will cause the site to continue to bleed. The site is then covered with an adhesive bandage or gauze secured with paper

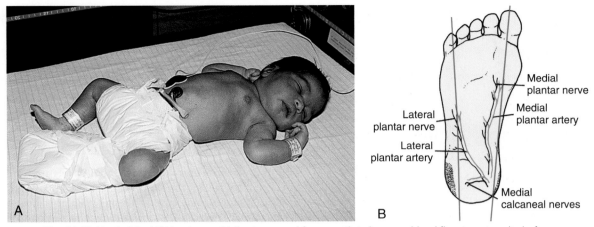

Fig. 24.12 Heelstick. (A) Newborn with foot wrapped for warmth to increase blood flow to extremity before heelstick. (B) Heelstick sites *(shaded areas)* on infant's foot for obtaining samples of capillary blood. (A, Courtesy Marjorie Pyle, RNC, Lifecircle, Costa Mesa, CA.)

tape. The nurse safely disposes of equipment used, reviews the laboratory requisition for correct identification, and checks the specimen for accurate labeling and routing.

A heelstick is traumatic for the infant and causes pain. After several heelsticks, infants have been observed to withdraw their feet when they are touched. Evidence-based interventions that have been found to minimize the pain associated with heelsticks include offering a pacifier with sucrose, swaddling, containment, facilitated tucking, breastfeeding, and SSC with the mother (Peng, Yin, Yang et al., 2018; Walden, 2015; Witt, Coynor, Edwards, et al., 2016) (see the "Neonatal Pain" section later in the chapter). To reassure the infant and promote feelings of safety, the neonate should be cuddled and comforted when the procedure is complete, and appropriate management measures should be taken to minimize the pain.

Venipuncture. Occasionally laboratory tests are ordered that require larger samples of blood than can be collected with a heelstick. Venous blood samples can be drawn from antecubital, saphenous, superficial wrist, and rarely, scalp veins. When venipuncture is required, positioning of the needle is extremely important. A 23- or 25-gauge butterfly needle or hypodermic needle with a syringe is used (Fig. 24.13). Patience is required during the procedure because the blood return in small veins is slow, and consequently the small needle must remain in place longer than a larger needle. A tourniquet is optional but can help increase blood flow with venipuncture. The infant is carefully restrained during the procedure to prevent injury. If venipuncture or arterial puncture is performed for blood gas studies, crying, fear, and agitation will affect the values; therefore, every effort must be made to keep the infant quiet during the procedure. Central veins and arteries should only be punctured by health care professionals who are competent and skilled in this procedure. Pressure must be maintained over these sites with a dry gauze square for 3 to 5 minutes to prevent bleeding from the site.

For 1 hour after any venipuncture, the nurse observes the infant frequently for evidence of bleeding or hematoma formation at the puncture site. The infant is cuddled and comforted when the procedure is completed, and appropriate pain management measures are taken. The nurse assesses and documents the infant's tolerance of the procedure.

Urine specimens. Analysis of urine is a valuable laboratory tool for infant assessment; the way in which the specimen is collected can influence the results. The most common reason that a urine specimen is needed for a newly born infant is to evaluate for in utero drug exposure. The urine sample should be fresh and analyzed within 1 hour of collection; ideally, the specimen is the infant's first urine after birth. A urine collection bag is often used to obtain a specimen.

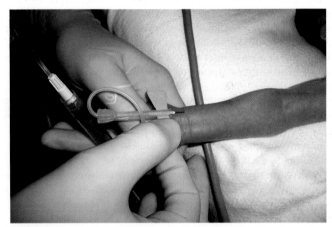

Fig. 24.13 Venipuncture Using a Butterfly Needle. (Courtesy Cheryl Briggs, RNC, Annapolis, MD.)

Interventions
Protective Environment

The provision of a protective environment is basic to the care of the newborn. The construction, maintenance, and operation of nurseries in accredited hospitals are monitored by national professional organizations such as the AAP, The Joint Commission (TJC), the Occupational Safety and Health Administration (OSHA), and local or state governing bodies. In addition, hospital personnel develop their own policies and procedures for protecting the newborns under their care. Prescribed standards cover areas such as environmental factors, measures to control infection, and safety factors.

Current health care trends and the focus on nonseparation of mothers and babies (rooming-in) have prompted many hospitals to abandon having a separate newborn nursery. In the mother-baby model of care, the infant stays in the mother's room, which reduces the need for a separate nursery.

Environmental factors. Environmental factors include provision of adequate space, appropriate lighting, elimination of potential fire hazards, safety of electrical appliances, adequate ventilation, and controlled temperature and humidity (AAP & ACOG, 2017).

Infection-control factors. Preventing and limiting the spread of infection is an important responsibility for the facility and for all of the staff involved in patient care. Measures to control infection in newborn nurseries include adequate floor space to permit the positioning of

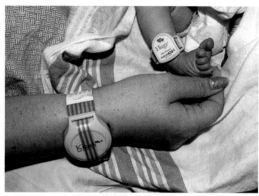

Fig. 24.14 Mother and Infant Wear Electronic Bracelets as Part of an Infant Security System. (Courtesy Shannon Perry, Phoenix, AZ.)

bassinets at least 3 feet apart in all directions, the practice of hand hygiene, appropriate cleaning and decontamination of the physical environment, promotion of breastfeeding, limiting the number of visitors, cohorting infants who are colonized with the same pathogen, and limiting the number of invasive procedures (AAP & ACOG, 2017). Only specified personnel directly involved in the care of mothers and infants are allowed in these areas, thereby reducing the opportunities for the transmission of pathogenic organisms.

> ### ⚡ SAFETY ALERT
>
> Proper hand hygiene is essential to prevent the spread of health care–associated infection. Personnel should wash hands with soap and water or use an alcohol-based hand rub in accordance with hospital infection-control policies. Hand hygiene should be performed before and after touching the infant, before an invasive procedure or medication administration, after contact with potentially contaminated objects (e.g., computer keyboards, telephone, countertop surfaces), and after removing sterile or non-sterile gloves (World Health Organization [WHO], 2009).

As part of Standard Precautions, all health care workers should wear gloves when handling infants until blood and amniotic fluid have been removed by the initial bath. Gloves should also be worn any time the nurse is drawing blood or handling urine, stool, or bloody drainage, as might occur when changing a circumcision dressing.

Visitors such as siblings and grandparents are expected to perform hand hygiene before having contact with infants or equipment. Individuals with infectious conditions are excluded from contact with newborns or must take special precautions when working with infants. This group includes people with upper respiratory tract infections, gastrointestinal tract infections, and infectious skin conditions.

Preventing infant abduction. Nurses discuss infant security precautions with the mother and her family because infant abductions are an ongoing concern. Many birthing facilities have special limited-entry systems. Nurses teach mothers and their families to check the identity of any person who comes to remove the newborn from their room. Families are also encouraged to question why and where their infant is being taken. Personnel should wear picture identification badges. On some units, all staff members wear matching scrubs or special badges. Other units use closed-circuit television, computer monitoring systems, fingerprint identification pads, or infant bracelet security systems (Fig. 24.14) that alarm if the newborn is separated from the mother or is taken outside the boundaries of the unit. Nurses and new parents must work together to ensure the safety of newborns in the hospital environment (AAP & ACOG, 2017).

> ### ⚡ SAFETY ALERT
>
> Nurses play a critical role in educating parents about measures to prevent infant abduction. Parents should be instructed how to identify legitimate hospital personnel and to request a second staff member to verify the identity of any questionable person who wants to take the baby from the mother's room. Parents should never leave the newborn in the birthing facility room without direct supervision. Parents should be instructed to use caution when posting photos of the new baby on the internet and publishing public notices about the birth (AAP & ACOG, 2017).

Preventing newborn injury. Newborn infants are at risk for injury as a result of falling. The Joint Commission (2018) defines a newborn *fall* as "a sudden, unintentional descent, with or without injury to the patient that results in the patient coming to rest on the floor on or against another surface, on another person or object." This is differentiated from a newborn *drop*, defined by The Joint Commission (2018) as "a fall in which a baby being held or carried by a health care professional, parent, family member, or visitor falls or slips from that person's hands, arms, lap, etc." Infants who experience a fall or drop, even from low-level surfaces such as beds or chairs, are at risk for sustaining head injury that can include skull fracture. Parents may hesitate to report falls due to feelings of guilt and fear of reproach from staff members (Ainsworth, Summerlin-Long, & Mog, 2016).

Newborn falls is a relatively new topic of concern, and consequently there are limited publications related to the incidence of newborn falls. Kahn, Fisher, and Hertzler (2017) reported that in a period of 40 months, the newborn fall rate averaged 5.9 times per 10,000 hospital births in their hospital system. This translates to an annual rate of approximately 2500 newborn falls in the United States, significantly higher than the previously reported rate of 600 to 1600 falls each year in U.S. hospitals (Helsey, McDonald, & Stewart, 2010). Factors that have been identified as possible contributors to this type of injury include maternal medications (e.g., opioids), exhaustion in parents, light-headedness, incoordination, or other factors (Feldman-Winter, Goldsmith, Committee on Fetus and Newborn, et al., 2016). Nurses can help prevent newborn falls by identifying these risk factors and implementing appropriate precautions. For example, if the mother becomes sleepy while holding her newborn, she should be instructed to call for help or place her newborn in the supine position in the bassinet. Parents need to be educated that bed-sharing is not a safe sleep practice and should be made aware of the potential risks related to this practice. Some hospitals ask parents and staff to sign an infant safety pledge to promote safety; staff members may conduct more frequent rounds to monitor for fall risks. Newborns are always transported in their bassinets and are never carried in arms outside the mother's room. One hospital developed a debriefing form to be used after a fall. This tool, completed by staff and parents, is used to identify factors that may have contributed to the fall. The parents are approached in a way that reduces their grief and guilt, also encouraging them to speak freely (Ainsworth et al., 2016). Some facilities have developed scripts to use for these parent discussions (Kahn et al., 2017). Currently there is no standardized system for reporting newborn falls, and furthermore, there is no standardized tool for assessing newborn fall risk (Ainsworth et al.).

Another concern is related to *sudden unexpected postnatal collapse* (SUPC). This term describes any condition that results in temporary or permanent cessation of respirations or cardiorespiratory failure. By definition, SUPC occurs during the first week of life in any term or near-term infant who is well at birth; collapses suddenly to the point of needing intermittent positive-pressure ventilation; and dies, requires intensive care, or develops encephalopathy. The vast majority of SUPC cases occur during the first 2 hours after birth and appear to be related to suffocation or entrapment. SUPC has occurred when newborns are held prone on the mother's chest or abdomen during SSC, and when mothers are not paying close attention to the infant as they are breastfeeding or holding the infant (Feldman-Winter et al., 2016).

> ### ⚡ SAFETY ALERT
>
> Nurses need to closely observe mothers and newborns during SSC, especially during the first few hours after birth (Box 24.4).

Therapeutic and Surgical Procedures

Intramuscular injection. Newborns routinely receive IM injections before discharge. A single dose of vitamin K is administered shortly after birth, and hepatitis B (HepB) vaccine is often administered before discharge. Under specific circumstances, other IM injections may be ordered, such as a dose of HepB immune globulin for infants born to mothers who are positive for hepatitis B (see Medication Guide).

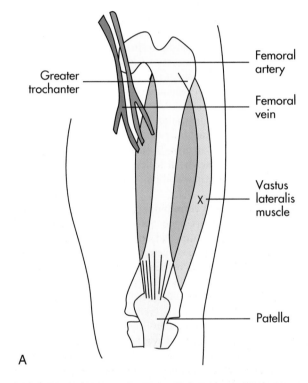

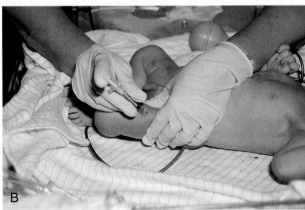

Fig. 24.15 Intramuscular Injection. (A) Acceptable intramuscular injection site for newborn infant. *X,* injection site. (B) Infant's leg stabilized for intramuscular injection. Nurse is wearing gloves to give injection. (B, Courtesy Marjorie Pyle, Lifecircle, Costa Mesa, CA.)

Selection of the appropriate equipment and site for IM injection is important. In most cases, a 25-gauge, ⅝-inch needle is used. Injections must be given in muscles large enough to accommodate the medication, and major nerves and blood vessels must be avoided. The muscles of newborns may not tolerate more than 0.5 to 1.0 mL per IM injection. The preferred injection site for newborns is the vastus lateralis (Fig. 24.15A). The dorsogluteal muscle is very small, poorly developed, and dangerously close to the sciatic nerve, which occupies a proportionately larger area in infants than in older children. Therefore it is not recommended as an injection site in small children. The deltoid muscle has inadequate muscle mass for IM administration. A key factor in preventing and minimizing local reaction to IM injections is adequate deposition of the medication deep within the muscle; therefore muscle size, needle length, and amount of medication injected should be carefully considered.

The nurse wears gloves when administering an injection. The neonate's leg should be stabilized. The nurse cleanses the injection site with an appropriate skin antiseptic, allows the antiseptic to dry, and then stabilizes the vastus lateralis muscle between the thumb and forefinger (Fig. 24.15B). The needle is inserted into the vastus lateralis at a 90-degree angle. The medication is injected slowly. After the medication is injected, the nurse withdraws the needle quickly and places a dry gauze pad over the site, applying gentle pressure to minimize pain and bleeding.

The nurse discards equipment properly. Needles are never recapped but are properly discarded in an appropriate safety container. The name of the medication, date and time, amount, route, and site of injection are documented in the newborn's record.

Nonpharmacologic techniques should be used to decrease the newborn's pain response during the injection. This may include administering the injection while the mother is holding the infant skin-to-skin. Oral sucrose administered prior to the injection and/or nonnutritive sucking (NNS) during the procedure can reduce discomfort. Comfort measures should be used to calm and comfort the newborn after the injection.

Immunizations

Hepatitis B (HepB) vaccine is recommended for all newborns before discharge from the birth facility (see Medication Guide: Hepatitis B Vaccine). Prior to administering the vaccine, the nurse confirms the mother's HepB status and obtains parental consent. Infants at highest risk for contracting HepB are those born to women who have HepB or those whose HepB status is unknown. If the mother is positive

> ### BOX 24.4 Safe Skin-to-Skin Positioning
>
> - The newborn's face is visible.
> - The newborn's nose and mouth are uncovered.
> - The newborn's neck is straight and the head is turned to one side, in "sniffing position."
> - The newborn's chest and shoulders face the mother.
> - The newborn's legs are flexed.
> - The newborn's back is covered with blankets.
> - Labor and birth nursing staff continuously monitor the mother and newborn in skin-to-skin contact after birth.
> - Postpartum or mother-baby nurses provide regular monitoring of mothers and newborns in skin-to-skin contact.
> - When the mother is finished with skin-to-skin contact, a staff member or support person who is awake and alert places the newborn in the bassinet.
>
> Data from Feldman-Winter, L., Goldsmith, J. P., & Committee on Fetus and Newborn, and Task Force on Sudden Infant Death Syndrome. (2016). Safe sleep and skin-to-skin care in the neonatal period for healthy term newborns. *Pediatrics, 138*(3), e1–e10.; Ludington-Hoe, S., & Morgan, K. (2014). Infant assessment and reduction of sudden unexpected postnatal collapse risk during skin-to-skin contact. *Newborn and Infant Nursing Reviews, 14*(1),28–33.

MEDICATION GUIDE

Hepatitis B Vaccine (Recombivax HB, Engerix-B)

Action

Hepatitis B (HepB) vaccine induces protective antihepatitis B antibodies in 95%-99% of healthy infants who receive the recommended three doses. The duration of protection of the vaccine is unknown.

Indication

HepB vaccine is for immunizing against infection caused by all known subtypes of HBV.

Neonatal Dosage

The usual dosage is Recombivax HB 5 mcg/0.5 mL or Engerix-B 10 mcg/0.5 mL intramuscularly within 24 h after birth, at 1-2 months, and at 6-18 months.

Adverse Reactions

Common adverse reactions are rash, fever, erythema, swelling, and pain at the injection site.

Nursing Considerations

- Obtain parental consent.
- Follow proper procedure for administration of IM injection (see Fig. 24.15). If the infant also needs hepatitis B immune globulin (HBIG), use separate sites for the two injections.
- Use nonpharmacologic measures to decrease the newborn's pain response during the injection.
- For infants born to mothers with negative HepB status, as routine universal prophylaxis:
  - For medically stable infants with birth weight ≥2000 g, administer HepB vaccine within first 24 h.
  - For infants <2000 g, administer HepB vaccine at 1 month of age or at hospital discharge, whichever comes first.
- For infants born to hepatitis B surface antigen (HBsAg)–positive mothers, administer HepB vaccine and HBIG within 12 h after birth, regardless of any previous antiviral therapy during pregnancy. Note: administer HepB vaccine and HBIG in separate sites (one in each vastus lateralis).
- For infants born to mothers whose HepB status is unknown (test mother immediately after admission to birthing facility):
  - For infants with birth weight ≥2000 g: administer HepB vaccine within 12 h; if mother's HepB results are positive or remain unknown, give HBIG by 7 days of age or by discharge from the birthing facility, whichever comes first.
  - For infants with birth weight <2000 g: administer HepB vaccine within 12 h after birth unless the mother tests negative for HepB before that time.
- Document the date, time, and site of injection; according to facility policy, document the lot number and expiration date of the vaccine.

Data from AAP Committee on Infectious Diseases and Committee on Fetus and Newborn. (2017). Elimination of perinatal hepatitis B: Providing the first vaccine dose within 24 hours of birth. *Pediatrics, 140*(3), e20171870; Schillie, S., Vellozzi, C., Reingold, A., et al. (2018). Prevention of hepatitis b virus infection in the United States: Recommendations of the Advisory Committee on Immunization Practices. *Morbidity and Mortality Weekly Report, 67*(1), 1–31.

for HepB, the newborn should receive the HepB vaccine and HepB immune globulin (HBIG) within 12 hours after birth (Schillie, Vellozzi, Reingold, et al., 2018).

Newborn Male Circumcision (NMC)

Policies and recommendations. **Circumcision** is the removal of the foreskin (prepuce) of the penis, exposing the glans. Usually it is performed during the first few days of life but is sometimes done at a later time for preterm or ill neonates or for religious or cultural reasons.

The most recent data from the CDC indicates that rates of newborn circumcision performed in U.S. hospitals peaked at 64.5% in 1981, dropping to a low of 55.4% in 2007. Rates increased slightly to 58.3% in 2010 (Owings, Uddin, & Williams, 2013).

Changes in recommendations from the AAP regarding NMC have likely influenced U.S. circumcision rates. The AAP policy on circumcision that was issued in 1999 and reaffirmed in 2005 recognized potential benefits of NMC, although the AAP did not deem them sufficient to recommend routine newborn circumcision (AAP Task Force on Circumcision, 2005). In 2012, the AAP issued a new policy statement regarding NMC. The policy states that "evaluation of current evidence indicates that the health benefits of NMC outweigh the risks and that the procedure's benefits justify access to this procedure for families who choose it" (AAP Task Force on Circumcision, 2012, p. 585). The health benefits of NMC cited by the AAP include prevention of urinary tract infection in male infants younger than 1 year of age, reduced risk for penile cancer, and reduced risk for heterosexual acquisition of sexually transmitted infections, particularly HIV (AAP Task Force on Circumcision, 2012). In spite of the new evidence, the AAP does not recommend the practice of routine newborn circumcision. Similarly, the CPS revised the policy on newborn circumcision in 2015; while recognizing the potential benefits to certain at-risk populations, the CPS does not recommend routine newborn circumcision (Sorokan, Finlay, Jefferies, et al., 2015).

The World Health Organization (WHO) (2012) recognizes male circumcision as an important intervention in reducing the risk for heterosexually acquired HIV in men. The organization recommends early infant circumcision for newborn males weighing more than 2500 g and without medical contraindication (World Health Organization & Jhpiego, 2010).

Ethical and legal issues surrounding NMC create ongoing controversy about this procedure. Opponents of circumcision feel that newborn circumcision is unnatural and unnecessary, and that it violates basic human rights. They cite concerns about acute pain; risks related to acute complications such as hemorrhage, infection, and penile injury (removal of excessive skin, damage to the meatus or glans); and long-term implications such as adverse effects on sexual function and pleasure.

Parental decision. Circumcision is a matter of personal parental choice. Parents usually decide to have their newborn circumcised for one or more of the following reasons: hygiene, religious conviction, tradition, culture, or social norms. Cost and insurance coverage are considerations in the parents' decision-making process. Parents need to make an informed choice regarding newborn circumcision based on the most current evidence and recommendations. Health care providers and nurses who care for childbearing families can help parents make an informed choice about newborn circumcision by providing factual, unbiased, evidence-based information. They can provide opportunities for discussion about the benefits and risks of the procedure.

Expectant parents need to begin learning about circumcision during the prenatal period, but circumcision often is not discussed with the parents. An excellent resource for parents can be found at www.acog/org/Patients/FAQs/Newborn-Male-Circumcision. In many instances, it is only when the mother is being admitted to the hospital or birthing unit that she is first confronted with the decision regarding circumcision. Because the stress of the intrapartum period makes this a difficult time for parental decision making, this is not an ideal time to broach the topic of circumcision and expect a well-informed decision.

Procedure. Circumcision is not performed immediately after birth because of the danger of cold stress and decreased clotting factors but is usually done in the hospital before discharge. The circumcision of a Jewish male infant is commonly performed on the eighth day after birth at home in a ceremony called a *bris*. This timing is logical from a physiologic standpoint because clotting factors decrease somewhat immediately after birth and do not return to prebirth levels until the end of the first week.

Feedings may be withheld up to 2 to 3 hours before the circumcision to prevent vomiting and aspiration, although in some hospitals, infants are allowed to breastfeed until they are taken to the nursery for the procedure. To prepare the infant for the circumcision, he is positioned on a plastic restraint form (Fig. 24.16), and the penis is cleansed

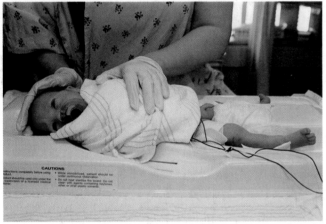

Fig. 24.16 Positioning of Infant for Circumcision in Immobilizer Device. Note swaddling of upper body and use of pacifier as measures to reduce discomfort. (Courtesy Paul Vincent Kuntz, Texas Children's Hospital, Houston, TX.)

with an antiseptic solution such as povidone-iodine. The infant is draped to provide warmth and a sterile field, and the sterile equipment is readied for use.

In the hospital setting, newborn circumcision is usually performed using the Gomco (Yellen) or Mogen clamp or the Plasti-Bell device. The technique is usually based on health care provider training and preference. The procedure takes only a few minutes to perform. Use of the Gomco or Mogen clamp involves surgical removal of the foreskin. The clamp technique minimizes blood loss (Fig. 24.17). After the circumcision is completed, a small petrolatum gauze dressing is applied to the penis for the first 24 hours; thereafter, parents are instructed to apply petrolatum with each diaper change for 7 to 10 days to keep the penis from adhering to the diaper (AWHONN, 2018).

With the PlastiBell technique, the plastic bell is first fitted over the glans, a suture is tied around the rim of the bell, and excess foreskin is cut away. The plastic rim remains in place for about 1 week; it falls off after healing has taken place, usually within 5 to 7 days (Fig. 24.18). Petrolatum or dressings are usually not applied to the penis following circumcision with the PlastiBell (AWHONN, 2018).

Procedural pain management. Circumcision is painful. The pain is characterized by both physiologic and behavioral changes in the infant (see discussion that follows). Commonly used anesthetics for circumcision include dorsal penile nerve block (DPNB), ring block, and topical anesthetic cream such as eutectic mixture of local anesthetic (EMLA) (prilocaine-lidocaine) or LMX4 (4% lidocaine). In addition to these anesthetics, nonpharmacologic methods such as concentrated oral sucrose, NNS, and swaddling can also be used to enhance pain management.

A DPNB consists of subcutaneous injections of buffered lidocaine at the 2 o'clock and 10 o'clock positions on the dorsum of the penis. Alternatively, buffered lidocaine may be administered using a ring block with injections around the base of the penis. To ensure adequate anesthesia, circumcision should not be performed for at least 5 to 8 minutes after these injections (Gardner, Enzman-Hines, & Agarwal, 2016).

EMLA cream is applied to the penis at least 1 hour before the circumcision. The area where the prepuce attaches to the glans is well coated with 1 g of the cream and then covered with a transparent occlusive dressing or finger cot. Just before the procedure, the cream is removed. Blanching or redness of the skin can occur (Gardner et al., 2016).

After the circumcision, the infant is comforted until he is quiet. If the parents were not present during the procedure, the infant is

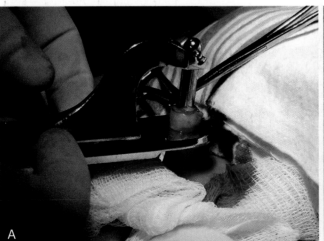
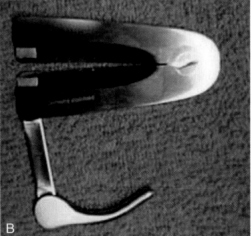

Fig. 24.17 Circumcision. (A) Gomco (Yellen) clamp. After hemostasis occurs, the foreskin (over the metal dome) is cut away. B, The Mogen clamp. (A, Courtesy Cheryl Briggs, RNC, Annapolis, MD. B, Courtesy Patricia A. Scott, Nashville, TN.)

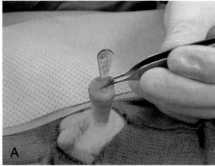
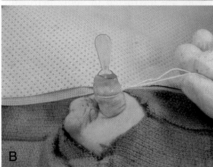

Fig. 24.18 The PlastiBell Technique. (A) The PlastiBell is placed over the glans inside the prepuce. (B) A string is then tied around the prepuce and positioned in the groove of the bell. The excess foreskin is trimmed, and the handle is broken off the bell. The foreskin remnant and bell are expected to slough in 1 to 2 weeks. (From Holcomb, G.W., Murphy, J.P., Ostlie, D.J. [2014]. *Ashcraft's pediatric surgery* [6th ed.]. Philadelphia: Elsevier.)

returned to them. The infant can be fussy for several hours and can have disturbed sleep-wake states and disorganized feeding behaviors. Some infants will go into a deep sleep after circumcision until they are awakened for feeding. Liquid acetaminophen may be administered orally after the procedure and repeated every 6 hours for the first 24 hours as ordered by the health care provider (Gardner et al., 2016).

Care of the newly circumcised infant. Postcircumcision protocols vary. In many settings, the circumcision site is assessed for bleeding every 15 to 30 minutes for the first hour and then hourly for the next 4 to 6 hours. The nurse monitors the infant's urinary output, noting the time and amount of the first voiding after the circumcision.

If bleeding occurs from the circumcision site, the nurse applies gentle pressure with a folded sterile gauze pad. A hemostatic agent such as Gelfoam powder or sponge can be applied to help control bleeding. If bleeding is not easily controlled, a blood vessel may need to be ligated. In this event, one nurse notifies the health care provider and prepares the necessary equipment (i.e., circumcision tray and suture material) while another nurse maintains intermittent pressure until the provider arrives.

Nurses provide education for parents related to care of the circumcised infant, which includes observing for complications such as bleeding or infection (see the Teaching for Self-Management box: Care of the Circumcised Newborn at Home). Parents need support and encouragement as they perform postcircumcision care. Newborns typically cry when the diaper is changed and when petrolatum gauze is removed and reapplied. This can make new parents feel anxious because they do not want to inflict pain on the infant. Nurses can inform parents that the discomfort is usually temporary and will soon subside. In addition, nurses can teach parents a variety of nonpharmacologic comfort measures.

TEACHING FOR SELF-MANAGEMENT

Care of the Circumcised Newborn at Home

Wash hands or use a waterless hand cleaner before touching the newly circumcised penis.

Check for Bleeding
- Check circumcision site for bleeding with each diaper change.
- If bleeding occurs, apply gentle pressure with a folded sterile gauze square. If bleeding does not stop with pressure, notify the pediatric health care provider.

Observe for Urination
- Check to see that the infant urinates after being circumcised.
- Infant should have a wet diaper 2-6 times per 24 h the first 1-2 days after birth and then at least 6-8 times per 24 h after 3-4 days.

Keep Area Clean
- Change the diaper often. Inspect the circumcision with each diaper change.
- For the first 3-4 days cleanse the penis gently with water only. Do not use baby wipes.
- For 4-7 days apply petrolatum to the glans with each diaper change (petrolatum is usually not used after PlastiBell circumcision).
- If a PlastiBell was used:
  - With diaper changes inspect the position of the plastic ring. Notify the pediatric care provider if the ring moves onto the shaft of the penis.
  - The plastic ring should fall off after 1 week. If it is still in place after 8 days, notify the pediatric care provider.
- Apply the diaper loosely over the penis to prevent pressure on the circumcised area.
- Use sponge bathing for the first week, until the circumcision is healed.

Check for Infection
- The glans of the penis is dark red after circumcision and then becomes covered with yellow exudate in 24-48 h, which is normal and will persist for 2-3 days. Do not attempt to remove this exudate; this is granulation tissue and is part of the healing process.
- Redness, swelling, discharge, or odor indicates infection. Notify the pediatric health care provider if you think the circumcision area is infected.

Provide Comfort
- Circumcision is painful. Handle the area gently.
- Provide comfort measures such as holding the baby skin to skin, breastfeeding, cuddling, swaddling, or rocking.

Data from American Association of Pediatrics. (2016). *How to care for your baby's penis.* Retrieved from https://www.healthychildren.org/English/ages-stages/baby/bathing-skin-care/Pages/Caring-For-Your-Sons-Penis.aspx; Association of Women's Health, Obstetric and Neonatal Nurses. (2018). *Neonatal skin care: Evidence-based clinical practice guideline* (4th ed.). Washington, DC: Author; World Health Organization & Jhpiego. (2010). *Manual for early infant male circumcision under local anesthesia.* Geneva, Switzerland: WHO Press.

Neonatal Pain

Neonatal responses to pain. There is clear evidence that neonates can feel pain, despite previous thinking that the immaturity of the nervous system prevented or blunted pain sensation and that neonates were incapable of remembering painful experiences. Pain in the neonate and pain in later life can be qualitatively different, but research has substantiated that newborns do experience pain (Blackburn, 2018).

Pain has physiologic and behavioral components. The central nervous system is well developed as early as 24 weeks of gestation.

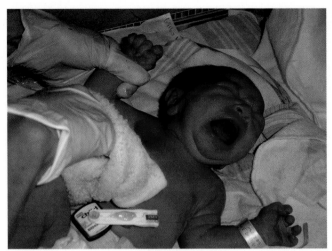

Fig. 24.19 Signs of Discomfort. Note eye squeeze, brow bulge, nasolabial furrow, and wide-spread mouth. (Courtesy Kathryn Alden, Apex, NC.)

The peripheral and spinal structures that transmit pain information are present and functional between the first and second trimesters. The pituitary-adrenal axis is also well developed at this time, and a fight-or-flight reaction is observed in response to the catecholamines released in response to stress.

The physiologic response to pain in neonates can be life threatening. Pain response can decrease tidal volume, increase demands on the cardiovascular system, increase metabolism, and cause neuroendocrine imbalance. The hormonal-metabolic response to pain in a term infant has greater magnitude and shorter duration than in adults. The newborn's sympathetic response to pain is less mature and therefore less predictable than an adult's response.

Pain response is influenced by a variety of factors, including characteristics of the painful stimulus, gestational age, biologic factors, and behavioral state. The source, location, and timing of the pain affect the response; newborns respond differently to acute pain than to prolonged or recurrent pain. There can be genetic differences in pain responses related to the amounts and types of neurotransmitters and receptors available to mediate pain. The behavioral state of the neonate also affects the pain response. Those who are more awake tend to have more robust pain responses than those in sleep states (Gardner et al., 2016).

The most common behavioral sign of pain is a vocalization or crying, ranging from a whimper to a distinctive high-pitched, shrill cry. Facial expressions include grimacing, eye squeeze, brow contraction, deepened nasolabial furrows, a taut and quivering tongue, and an open mouth (Fig. 24.19; Box 24.5). The infant will flex and adduct the upper body and lower limbs in an attempt to withdraw from the painful stimulus. The preterm infant has a lower than normal threshold for initiation of this response (Gardner et al., 2016).

Pain can result in significant changes in heart rate, BP (increased or decreased), intracranial pressure, vagal tone, respiratory rate, and oxygen saturation. Neonates respond to painful stimuli with release of epinephrine, norepinephrine, glucagon, corticosterone, cortisol, 11-deoxycorticosterone, lactate, pyruvate, and glucose (Blackburn, 2018).

Assessment of neonatal pain. In assessing pain, the nurse needs to consider the health of the neonate, the type and duration of the painful stimulus, environmental factors, and the infant's state of alertness. For example, severely compromised or preterm neonates may be unable to generate a pain response, although they are, in fact, experiencing pain.

BOX 24.5 Manifestations of Acute Pain in the Neonate

Physiologic Responses
- Vital signs
  - Increased heart rate
  - Increased blood pressure
  - Rapid, shallow respirations
- Oxygenation
  - Decreased transcutaneous oxygen saturation
  - Decreased arterial oxygen saturation
- Skin
  - Pallor or flushing
  - Diaphoresis
  - Palmar sweating
- Laboratory evidence of metabolic or endocrine changes
  - Hyperglycemia
  - Lowered pH
  - Elevated corticosteroids
- Other observations
  - Increased muscle tone
  - Dilated pupils
  - Decreased vagal nerve tone
  - Increased intracranial pressure

Behavioral Responses
- Vocalizations
  - Crying
  - Whimpering
  - Groaning
- Facial expression
  - Grimace
  - Brow furrowed
  - Chin quivering
  - Eyes tightly closed
  - Mouth open and squarish
- Body movements and posture
  - Limb withdrawal
  - Thrashing
  - Rigidity
  - Flaccidity
  - Fist clenching
- Changes in state
  - Changes in sleep-wake cycles
  - Changes in feeding behavior
  - Changes in activity level
  - Fussiness, irritability
  - Listlessness

Data from Blackburn, S. T. (2018). *Maternal, fetal, and neonatal physiology: A clinical perspective* (5th ed.). St. Louis, MO: Elsevier; Gardner, S. L., Enzman-Hines, M., & Agarwal, R. (2016). Pain and pain relief. In S. L. Gardner, B. S. Carter, M. Enzman-Hines, et al. (Eds.), *Merenstein & Gardner's handbook of neonatal intensive care* (8th ed.). St. Louis, MO: Elsevier.

Every neonate should have an initial pain assessment as well as a pain management plan. Pain should be assessed and documented on a regular basis. The National Association of Neonatal Nurses (NANN) developed practice guidelines stating that all nurses who care for newborns should have education and competency validation in pain assessment (Walden, 2015; Walden & Gibbins, 2012).

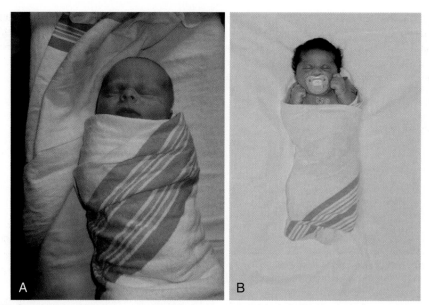

Fig. 24.20 Swaddling. (A) Newborn is swaddled with arms extended. (B) Newborn is swaddled with arms flexed. (A, Courtesy Jennifer and Travis Alderman, Durham, NC. (B) Courtesy Cheryl Briggs, RNC, Annapolis, MD.)

Pain assessment tools include the following:

- Neonatal Infant Pain Scale (NIPS) (Lawrence, Alcock, McGrath, et al., 1993)
- Premature Infant Pain Profile (PIPP) (Stevens, Johnston, Petryshen, et al., 1996)
- Neonatal Pain Agitation and Sedation Scale (NPASS) (Hummel, Puchalski, Creech, et al., 2008)
- CRIES (Krechel & Bildner, 1995)

Healthy term newborns are exposed to fewer sources of pain than preterm infants in an NICU where painful procedures are inherent to care management. Even in low-risk newborns, nurses need to assess for signs of discomfort as part of routine assessments and especially during and after routine procedures such as heelsticks, injections, and circumcisions (Walden, 2015).

Management of neonatal pain. The goals of pain management are to (1) minimize the intensity, duration, and physiologic cost of the pain; and (2) maximize the neonate's ability to cope with and recover from the pain. Nonpharmacologic and pharmacologic strategies are used. It is important to note that despite research evidence, policies, and standards of practice focused on assessing and managing pain in newborns, acute infant pain remains undermanaged and, in some cases, unmanaged (Gardner et al., 2016).

Nonpharmacologic management. A variety of nonpharmacologic pain management techniques are used with neonates. Combining two or more nonpharmacologic methods can result in more effective pain reduction. Nonpharmacologic strategies include swaddling, containment and positioning, breastfeeding/breastmilk, NNS, skin-to-skin care during the painful event, and the use of sucrose for procedural pain (Witt et al., 2016).

One of the most commonly used measures is swaddling or snugly wrapping the infant with a blanket. Swaddling limits the neonate's boundaries, aids in self-regulation, and reduces physiologic and behavioral stress resulting from acute pain. Swaddling is popular among nurses and parents as a comfort measure for calming a fussy baby and for promoting sleep. However, it is important that it is done properly. Safe swaddling involves wrapping the infant snugly in a lightweight blanket with the arms extended, legs flexed, and hips in neutral position without rotation (Fig. 24.20A) (AAP & ACOG, 2017). In the early newborn period, nurses often swaddle infants with the arms flexed (see Fig. 24.20B).

> ### ⚡ SAFETY ALERT
>
> Swaddling an infant tightly with legs extended is associated with increased risk for hip dislocation (developmental dysplasia of the hip [DDH]). The correct way to swaddle an infant is with the hips in slight flexion and abducted, allowing freedom of movement of the knees. It is important that the blanket is not wrapped too tightly as it can cause overheating or respiratory compromise. There should be space for two to three adult fingers between the infant's chest and the swaddle. A swaddled infant should be lying on his or her back. Swaddling is not recommended after approximately 2 months of age, when the infant is capable of rolling over (AAP, 2017).
>
> Facilitated tucking is another nonpharmacologic pain relief measure used by nurses and parents. Facilitated tucking, a hand-swaddling technique in which the care provider holds the neonate in a flexed, side-lying position, is effective for reducing pain and distress in preterm infants (Witt et al., 2016).

NNS on a pacifier is a common comfort measure used with newborns. A single dose of 0.05 to 2 mL of a 12% to 25% sucrose solution has been shown to reduce newborn pain. When using oral sucrose, the best results are obtained when it is given approximately 2 minutes prior to the painful procedure and if the baby is also given an opportunity for nonnutritive sucking when the sucrose is given. The use of sucrose as an analgesic for minor procedures has been demonstrated to be effective as evidenced by a decrease in pain scores and crying (Liu, Huang, Luo, et al., 2017; Stevens, Yamada, Ohlsson, et al., 2016; Witt et al., 2016).

SSC with the mother who holds the infant prone on her chest, also known as *kangaroo care,* during a painful procedure can help reduce pain (Johnston, Campbell-Yeo, Disher, et al., 2017; Peng et al., 2017; Witt et al., 2016). Breastfeeding or breast milk helps reduce pain during heel lancing and blood collection (Peng et al., 2017; Witt et al., 2016).

Distraction with visual, oral, auditory, or tactile stimulation can be helpful in term neonates or older infants (see the Evidence-Based Practice box: Nonpharmacologic Pain Relief for Newborns). Sensorial stimulation uses multiple senses to diminish minor pain. This technique involves speaking softly to the infant, massaging the face, and providing oral sucrose solution on the tongue (Locatelli & Bellieni, 2017). Other nonpharmacologic measures for reducing pain in newborns include touch, massage, rocking, holding, and environmental modification (e.g., low noise and lighting).

EVIDENCE-BASED PRACTICE

Nonpharmacologic Pain Relief for Newborns

Ask the Question

For term newborns, what complementary or alternative pain relief is effective for minor painful procedures, such as heelstick?

Search for the Evidence

Search Strategies

English language research-based publications on newborn, pain, kangaroo care, SSC, breastfeeding, heelstick, and sucrose were included.

Databases Used

Cochrane Collaborative Database, National Guidelines Clearinghouse (AHRQ), CINAHL, and PubMed.

Critical Appraisal of the Evidence

Pain scales in newborns are used to assess physical and behavioral changes to determine pain levels. Physical measures typically include heart rate, respiratory rate, and peripheral oxygen saturation. Other physiologic measures include gas exchange across skin, skin sensitivity measures, and electroencephalogram (EEG). Ways to measure behavioral changes include various scales utilizing breathing patterns, states of arousal, facial tension, leg movement, activity, cry, and consolability.

Cochrane Database systematic analyses revealed the following:

- Sucrose is effective at decreasing pain response for single painful procedures, especially when paired with sucking (Stevens, Yamada, & Ohlsson, 2016).
- SSC is safe to use during a single painful procedure, such as heelstick, and is effective in reducing pain as measured by behavioral and physiologic indicators. Combining SSC with other measures such as breastfeeding or oral sucrose may enhance pain reduction, but there is a lack of firm evidence; more studies are needed to examine the synergistic effects of SSC with other measures (Johnston, Campbell-Yeo, Disher, et al., 2017).
- For preterm infants until 3 years of age, pain reactivity and immediate pain regulation were significantly improved with NNS, swaddling, and holding/rocking (Pillai, Riddell, Racine, Gennis, et al., 2015).

A randomized controlled study of 102 newborns found that the smells of lavender and breast milk decreased both physiologic and behavioral responses to pain during heelstick more than control (Akcan & Polat, 2016).

Another randomized controlled study showed that music therapy with sucrose administration was more effective for pain relief in newborns than sucrose or music therapy alone (Shah, Kadage, & Sinn, 2017).

Apply the Evidence: Nursing Implications

- For newborns who experienced a painful stimuli, subsequent painful procedures caused increased response (Gokulu, Bilgen, Ozdemir, et al., 2016). This has implications for decreasing the initial pain response as much as possible, especially in the neonatal critical care setting where multiple painful stimuli may be necessary.
- Nonpharmacologic pain relief methods for newborns utilize the gate-control theory to distract the newborn's attention by using strong single or multi-sensorial stimulation. Warmth, touch, sensory attention, swaddling, rocking, sucking a sweet solution, and smells decrease pain scores.
- During single painful procedures such as heelstick, venipuncture, or injection, use of SSC alone or in combination with other measures such as breastfeeding or oral sucrose may reduce the infant's pain response (Johnston et al., 2017).
- Parents who are taught these techniques become active participants in their newborn's procedural care. However, they need clear education that using sucrose is not an appropriate long-term strategy for use at home.
- Comfort measures may work best when initiated a few minutes prior to the procedure, to allow the newborn time to relax and reorganize.

References

Akcan, E., & Polat, S. (2016). Comparative effect of the smells of amniotic fluid, breast milk, and lavender on newborns' pain during heel lance. *Breastfeeding Medicine, 11*(6), 309–314.
Gokulu, G., Bilgen, H., Ozdemir, H., et al. (2016). Comparative heelstick study showed that newborn infants who had undergone repeated painful procedures showed increased short-term pain responses. *Acta Paediatrica, 105*(11), e520–e525.
Johnston, C., Campbell-Yeo, M., Disher, T., et al. (2017). Skin-to-skin care for procedural pain in neonates. *Cochrane Database of Systematic Reviews, 2*, CD008435.
Pillai Riddell, R. R., Racine, N. M., Gennis, H. G., et al. (2015). Non-pharmacological management of infant and young child procedural pain. *Cochrane Database of Systematic Reviews, 12*, CD006275.
Shah, S. R., Kadage, S., & Sinn, J. (2017). Trial of music, sucrose, and combination therapy for pain relief during heel prick procedures in neonates. *Journal of Pediatrics, 190*, 153–158, e2.
Stevens, B., Yamada, J., Ohlsson, A., et al. (2016). Sucrose for analgesia in newborn infants undergoing painful procedures. *Cochrane Database of Systematic Reviews, 7*, CD001069.

Jennifer Taylor Alderman

Pharmacologic management. Pharmacologic agents are used to alleviate pain associated with procedures. Local anesthesia is routinely used during procedures such as circumcision. Topical anesthesia is used for circumcision, lumbar puncture, venipuncture, and heelsticks. Nonopioid analgesia (oral liquid acetaminophen) is effective for mild to moderate pain from inflammatory conditions. Morphine and fentanyl are the most widely used opioid analgesics for pharmacologic management of moderate to severe neonatal pain. Continuous or bolus IV infusion of opioids provides effective and safe pain control. Neonates requiring this degree of pain relief are closely monitored for signs of respiratory depression. Other methods for managing neonatal pain are epidural infusion, local and regional nerve blocks, and intradermal or topical anesthetics (Gardner et al., 2016).

Promoting Parent-Infant Interaction

Nurses play an important role in promoting early social interaction between parents and their newborn infant. From birth throughout the hospital stay, nurses assess attachment behaviors (see Chapter 22) and provide support and education to parents as they become acquainted with the neonate. Nurses working in outpatient settings or home care provide follow-up assessments and care related to parent-child interactions. By teaching parents to recognize infant cues and respond appropriately, the nurse facilitates development of the parents' confidence in meeting the needs of their newborn (see the Teaching for Self-Management box: Helping Parents Recognize, Interpret, and Respond to Newborn Behaviors).

TEACHING FOR SELF-MANAGEMENT

Helping Parents Recognize, Interpret, and Respond to Newborn Behaviors

Learning to read a baby's body language can enable parents to be more effective in preventing and solving problems around the infant's sleeping, eating, and crying, and enhances parent-infant interaction. Nurses can teach new parents the following:

1. Identify three newborn "zones" (traditionally referred to as *newborn states*).
   - "Resting zone": also known as *sleep states*
     - *Still/deep sleep:* Baby is completely still. Breathing is regular. No spontaneous activity. No movement of eyes, and eyelids stay shut. No vocalizing. Muscles are totally relaxed.
     - *Active/light sleep:* Baby may wiggle or vocalize. Eyes may flash open. Baby may make sucking movements—but still be asleep.
   - "Ready zone": also known as *alert state*
     - Baby's eyes are bright. Baby can focus on an object or person. Baby reacts to stimulation. Motor activity is minimal.
   - "Rebooting zone": also known as *fussy/crying state*
     - Baby's motor activity increases and is jerky. Baby is less responsive and moves from fussing to crying.
2. Identify signs of stress.
   - When babies are stressed or overstimulated, they show changes in their body and behavior. These changes are called *SOSs* (Signs of Over-Stimulation), traditionally referred to as a baby's *stress response.*
     - *Body SOSs:* changes in color (becoming more red or pale); changes in breathing (becoming more irregular or choppy); changes in movement (becoming jerky or having more tremors)
     - *Behavioral SOSs:* "spacing out" (going from an alert state to a drowsy state); "switching off" (gaze aversion, or looking away from parent); "shutting down" (going from drowsy to a sleep state)
   - When baby shows an SOS, parents should *decrease* stimulation and *increase* support by doing one or several of the following:
     - Quiet one's voice.
     - Glance away from baby.
     - Encourage baby to suck a finger or mother's breast.
     - Swaddle baby.
     - Place baby skin to skin.

3. Help baby sleep well.
   - Distinguish active/light sleep from still/deep sleep.
   - Parent's care:
     - *Prepare baby to sleep:* swaddling may help; feed in quiet, dark room at night and active, light environment during day.
     - *Get baby to sleep:* put baby down for sleep while he or she is still awake.
     - *Help baby stay asleep:* don't pick up during active/light sleep.
     - After breastfeeding is well established, notice when sleeping baby moves into active/light sleep. Wait and see if baby will transition from active/light sleep back to deep/still sleep—and sleep a bit longer.
4. Help baby eat well.
   - Recognize early signs of hunger during the first few weeks: wiggling, making sucking movements, bringing hand to mouth.
   - Notice if a fragile baby "spaces out" or "shuts down" when trying to eat. Bring this baby skin to skin and decrease stimulation before resuming feeding.
   - If a parent needs to wake a fragile or small baby to eat, do so from active/light sleep, not from still/deep sleep.
5. Help crying baby: consider what "TO DO."
   - **T:** *Talk* quietly to baby in sing-song voice.
   - **O:** *Observe* to see if baby takes self-calming actions: brings his or her hand to his or her mouth, making sucking movements, or moves into the fencing reflex position.
   - **DO:** *Bring* baby's hands to his or her chest; encourage sucking; make gentle "shooshing" sounds; swaddle baby; and/or bring baby skin to skin.
6. Play with baby so he or she can learn and grow.
   - Demonstrate baby's ability to look at a parent's face, watch a toy move, or turn to parent's voice.
   - Watch for an SOS during play. If an SOS occurs, decrease stimulation and increase support as described previously.
   - Observe baby's developing process of interaction: first, getting quiet and still; second, turning toward parent; third, turning toward and looking at parent.
   - Reinforce benefits of sensitive, face-to-face parent interaction with baby.

Data from Tedder, J.L. (2008). Give them the HUG: An innovative approach to helping parents understand the language of their newborn. *Journal of Perinatal Education,17*(2),14–20; Tedder, J.L. (2019). H.U.G.: Help-understanding-guidance for young families, www.hugyourbaby.org.

The sensitivity of the parent to the social responses of the infant is basic to the development of a mutually satisfying parent-child relationship. Sensitivity increases over time as parents become more aware of their infant's social capabilities. In supporting parents, nurses need to consider cultural beliefs and traditions that influence parenting behaviors and infant care practices (see Cultural Considerations box: Cultural Beliefs and Practices Related to Infant Care).

The activities of daily care during the neonatal period are ideal for infant and family interactions. While caring for their newborn, the mother and father (or other family member) can talk or sing to their infant, play baby games, caress and cuddle the baby, and perhaps use infant massage. Feeding is an optimal time for interaction because the infant is usually awake and alert, at least at the beginning of the feeding. Too much stimulation should be avoided after feeding and before a sleep period.

Discharge Planning and Parent Education

Infant care activities can cause anxiety for new parents. Support from nurses can influence whether new parents seek and accept help in the future. It is best for the nurse to avoid trying to cover all the content about newborn care at one time because the parents can be overwhelmed by too much information and become more anxious. Instead, parent education should occur throughout the stay in the birthing facility. Printed materials about newborn care are usually given to parents to augment the teaching done by the mother-baby or postpartum nurses. Some birthing facilities provide information about newborn care on their websites (e.g., www.mombaby.org). Nurses can direct parents to reliable websites for information on infant care (e.g., www.healthychildren.org). Some facilities have around-the-clock television programming on topics related to newborn and postpartum care. Postpartum and newborn home visitation programs may be available; the home visit nurse assesses the parents' learning needs and provides appropriate information.

To set priorities for teaching, the nurse follows parental cues. Knowledge deficits or gaps should be identified before beginning to teach. Normal growth and development and the changing needs of the infant (e.g., for personal interaction and stimulation, growth milestones, exercise, injury prevention, and social contacts), as well as the topics that follow, should be included during discharge planning with parents.

Temperature

Parents need to understand practical information related to thermoregulation. The nurse explains causes for change in body temperature such as overwrapping and cold stress, and the body's response to extremes in environmental temperatures. Instructions about promoting normal

🌐 CULTURAL CONSIDERATIONS

Cultural Beliefs and Practices Related to Infant Care

Nurses working with childbearing families from other cultures and ethnic groups must be aware of cultural beliefs and practices that are important to individual families. People with a strong sense of heritage may hold on to traditional health beliefs long after adopting other U.S. lifestyle practices. These health beliefs can involve practices regarding the newborn. For example, some Asians, Hispanics, Eastern Europeans, and Native Americans delay breastfeeding until the mother's milk is "in" (day 3 or 4) because they believe that colostrum is "bad." Some Hispanics and African Americans place a belly band over the infant's umbilicus. In some Hispanic cultures, infants wear a special bracelet to help protect them from the evil eye (*mal de ojo*; see photo). The birth of a male child is generally preferred by Asians and Eastern Indians, and some Asians and Haitians delay naming their infants. Families of Hindu heritage name the baby on the 11th day during a "cradle ceremony." Some women from India keep the cord of a male infant as a good omen that will ward off evil and will bring them more male infants in the future. The practice of SSC after birth may conflict with cultural beliefs about thermoregulation; some women from Africa prefer that the newborn is wrapped prior to being placed on the mother's chest. On the other hand, women from Mexico are wrapped in warm blankets after birth and wrap the newborn inside their blankets. Cultural beliefs influence when the newborn is taken out of the house, such as after the cord falls off, or after the mother's confinement period is over (approximately 30 days after birth). Weighing the infant can raise concerns for some women such as those from rural India, who may believe that frequent weighing will slow the infant's growth.

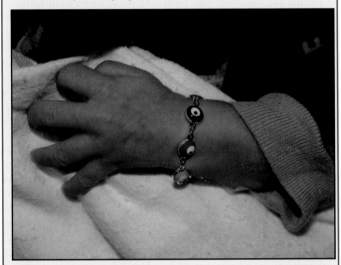

Newborn Wearing "Evil-Eye" Bracelet. (Courtesy Cheryl Briggs, RNC, Annapolis, MD.)

Data from Giger, J.N. (2013). *Transcultural nursing* (6th ed.). St. Louis, MO: Mosby; Purnell, L.D. (2014). *Culturally competent health care* (3rd ed.). Philadelphia, PA: F.A. Davis.

body temperature include dressing the infant appropriately for the environmental temperature and protecting the skin from exposure to direct sunlight. Parents need to understand how to assess the infant's temperature using an axillary thermometer and should be aware of the normal temperature range. They should notify the pediatric health care provider for high or low temperatures with accompanying fussiness, lethargy, irritability, poor feeding, and excessive crying.

Respirations

The nurse provides information to parents regarding the normal characteristics of newborn respirations, emergency procedures (e.g., choking, use of bulb syringe), and measures to protect the infant such as avoiding contact with persons with respiratory illnesses (see the Teaching

for Self-Management box: Safe Sleep). It is helpful to discuss signs of respiratory infection and when to call the pediatric health care provider.

Feeding

Nurses instruct parents about infant feeding and provide assistance based on whether they have chosen breastfeeding, expressed milk feeding, formula feeding, or a combination. Infant feeding is discussed in Chapter 25.

Elimination

Awareness of the normal elimination patterns of newborns helps parents recognize problems related to voiding or stooling. The desired urine output for a newborn is at least two to six voidings per 24 hours for the first 1 to 3 days; then a minimum of six to eight voidings per 24 hours thereafter. Urine should be pale yellow (like lemonade). Newborn stools should gradually transition from meconium to yellow (see Box 23.1). Breastfed infants should have at least three stools every 24 hours for the first few weeks. Formula-fed infants may stool less.

Sleeping, Positioning, and Holding

Infants should be placed in the supine position for sleep during the first year of life to reduce the incidence of sudden infant death syndrome (SIDS) (see the Teaching for Self-Management box: Safe Sleep) (AAP Task Force on SIDS, 2016; National Institute of Child Health and Human Development [NICHD], 2014).

TEACHING FOR SELF-MANAGEMENT

Safe Sleep

- Always lay the baby flat in bed (in the bassinet or crib) on his or her back for sleep, for naps, and at night. Do not place your infant on the abdomen for sleep.
- Room-sharing, but not bed-sharing, is recommended for the first year; this is most important for the first 6 months.
- Never put your baby on a cushion, pillow, beanbag, or waterbed to sleep. Your baby may suffocate.
- Avoid soft bedding, including bumper pads, blankets, pillows, stuffed toys, or other soft objects in the baby's crib because of the risk for suffocation.
- Do not cover the baby with blankets or quilts; dress the baby in light sleep clothing such as a sleep sack or one-piece sleeper.
- Check your baby's crib for safety. Slats should be no more than 2.25 inches apart. The space between the mattress and sides should be less than two finger widths. The bedposts should have no decorative knobs.
- The crib mattress should be firm and should fit snugly against the crib rails.
- Do not use a crib with drop rails.
- Cover the mattress with a tight-fitting sheet.
- Supervised, awake tummy time is recommended each day to facilitate motor development.
- Do not use home monitors or devices that are marketed to decrease the risk of sudden infant death syndrome (SIDS) (e.g., wedges or positioners).
- Offer a pacifier at nap and bedtime.
- Do not tie anything around your baby's neck. For example, a pacifier tied around the neck with a ribbon or string can strangle your baby.
- Avoid exposing your baby to cigarette or cigar smoke in your home or other places. Passive exposure to tobacco smoke greatly increases the likelihood that your infant will have respiratory symptoms and illnesses. It also increases the risk for SIDS.
- Avoid exposing the baby to alcohol and illicit drugs.

Data from American Academy of Pediatrics Task Force on Sudden Infant Death Syndrome. (2016). SIDS and other sleep-related infant deaths: Updated 2016 recommendations for a safe infant sleeping environment. *Pediatrics, 138*(5), e1–e12; Feldman-Winter, L., Goldsmith, J.P., Committee on Fetus and Newborn, et al. (2016). Safe sleep and skin-to-skin care in the neonatal period for healthy term newborns. *Pediatrics, 138*(3), e1–e10.

Parent education prior to hospital discharge should include specific information about safe sleep practices. The *Safe to Sleep* campaign from the National Institute of Child Health and Human Development provides materials for health care professionals and parents (http://safetosleep.nichd.nih.gov). The educational resources are designed to reach culturally diverse audiences with messages about promoting a safe sleep environment and preventing SIDS. (See Clinical Reasoning Case Study: Safe Infant Sleep Practices.)

❓ CLINICAL REASONING CASE STUDY
Safe Infant Sleep Practices

The mother-baby nurse is providing care to the Scott family in room 202. The parents, Brett and Mary, have a 12-year-old son and, now, a newborn daughter named Caroline. The parents admit that it has been a very long time since they cared for a newborn; they are eager to learn about current infant care practices. They enjoyed bed-sharing when their older child was born and verbalized that they would be practicing this again with their newborn.

1. What is the priority concern or client need in this situation?
2. List other client needs/problems in this case.
3. Identify any additional information or assessment data that is needed by the nurse in planning care for this client.
4. What nursing actions are appropriate in this situation?
   a. What is the priority nursing action?
   b. Describe other nursing interventions that are important to providing optimal client care.
5. Describe the roles/responsibilities of the interprofessional health care team members (other than nurses) who may be involved in providing care for this client.

Anatomically, the infant's shape—a barrel chest and flat, curveless spine—facilitates the infant to roll from the side to the prone position; therefore the side-lying position for sleep is not recommended. When the infant is awake, "tummy time" can be provided under parental supervision so the infant can begin to develop appropriate muscle tone for eventual crawling; placing the infant prone at intervals when awake aids in preventing a misshapen head (**positional plagiocephaly**) (AAP Task Force on SIDS, 2016).

Care must be taken to prevent the infant from rolling off flat, unguarded surfaces. When an infant is on such a surface, the parent or nurse who must turn away from the infant even for a moment should always keep one hand placed securely on the infant.

The infant is always held securely with the head supported because newborns are unable to maintain an erect head posture for more than a few moments. Fig. 24.21A and B illustrate various positions for holding an infant with adequate support.

Rashes

Diaper rash. Many infants develop a diaper rash at some time. This is usually irritant contact dermatitis or skin inflammation appearing as redness, scaling, blisters, or papules. Various factors can contribute to diaper rash, including infrequent diaper changes, diarrhea, use of plastic pants to cover the diaper, a change in the infant's diet such as when solid foods are added, antibiotics, or when breastfeeding mothers eat certain foods (AWHONN, 2018).

Parents are instructed in measures to help prevent diaper rash. Diapers should be checked often and changed as soon as the infant voids or stools. Plain water with mild soap, if needed, is used to cleanse the diaper area; if baby wipes are used, they should be unscented and contain no alcohol. The infant's skin should be allowed to dry completely before applying another diaper.

When diaper rash occurs, it is helpful to use emollients, creams, or other protectants such as zinc oxide ointment to restore skin integrity while providing some protection from the irritants of urine and stool (Visscher, Adam, Brink, et al., 2015). Although diaper rash can be alarming to parents and annoying to babies, most cases resolve within a few days with simple home treatments. There are instances, however, when diaper rash is more serious and requires medical treatment.

The warm, moist atmosphere in the diaper area provides an optimal environment for *Candida albicans* growth; this type of dermatitis can appear in the perianal area, inguinal folds, and lower abdomen. The affected area is intensely erythematous with a sharply demarcated, scalloped edge, often with numerous satellite lesions that extend beyond the larger lesion (AWHONN, 2018). Therapy consists of applications of an anticandidal ointment, such as clotrimazole or miconazole, with each diaper change. Sometimes the infant is given an oral antifungal preparation such as nystatin or fluconazole to eliminate any gastrointestinal source of infection.

Other rashes. A rash on the cheeks can result from the infant's scratching with long unclipped fingernails or from rubbing the face against the crib sheets, particularly if regurgitated stomach contents are not washed off promptly. The newborn's skin begins a natural process of peeling and sloughing after birth. Dry skin may be treated with an emollient applied at least once daily (AWHONN, 2018). Newborn rash, *erythema toxicum*, is a common finding (see Fig. 23.9) and needs no treatment.

Clothing

Parents commonly ask how warmly they should dress their infant. A simple suggestion is to dress the child for the environment as they dress themselves, adding no more than one layer more than they would be wearing as adults. Overheating should be avoided (AAP Task Force on SIDS, 2016). A cap or bonnet is needed to protect the scalp and minimize heat loss if the weather is cool or to protect against sunburn. Overdressing in warm temperatures can cause discomfort, as can underdressing in cold weather. Parents are encouraged to dress the infant at all times in flame-retardant clothing. The eyes should be shaded if it is sunny and hot. Infant sunglasses are available to protect the infant's eyes when outdoors (Fig. 24.22).

For sleep, infants can be placed in a safe sleeping bag or sleep sack with fitted neck and arm openings and no hood. Some hospitals use sleep sacks for all newborns (Fig. 24.23). A safe sleep sack prevents the infant from rolling over on the abdomen and keeps the legs contained so they do not go through the crib rails. For additional warmth, the infant can be dressed in fitted clothing in layers as needed prior to being placed in the sleep sack.

For the first 2 to 3 months until the infant is able to roll over, safe swaddling for sleep can be done using a lightweight blanket or wrap (not in combination with a sleep sack). The head, neck, and chin are not covered, and the wrap should not be tight around the chest or legs.

Car Seat Safety

Infants and toddlers to the age of 2 years should travel only in federally approved rear-facing safety seats secured in the rear seat using the vehicle safety belt or an anchor and tether system (Fig. 24.24). A car safety seat that faces the rear gives the best protection for

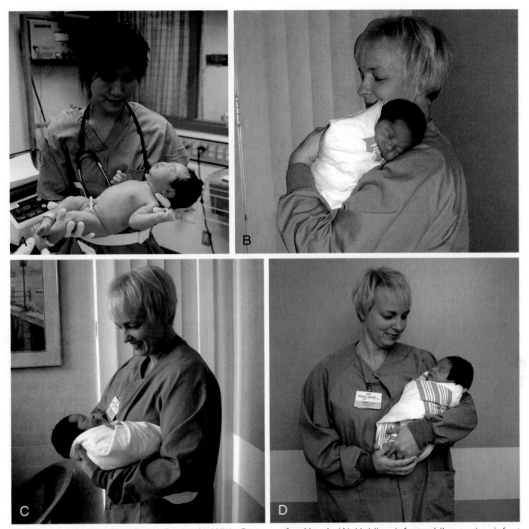

Fig. 24.21 Holding The Baby Securely With Support for Head. (A) Holding infant while moving infant from scale to bassinet. Baby is undressed to show posture. (B) Holding baby upright in "burping" position. (C) "Football" (under the arm) hold. (D) Cradling hold. (A, Courtesy Kim Molloy, Knoxville. B, C, and D, Courtesy Julie Perry Nelson, Loveland, CO.)

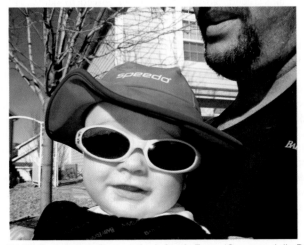

Fig. 24.22 Sunglasses Protect the Infant's Eyes. (Courtesy Julie Perry Nelson, Loveland, CO.)

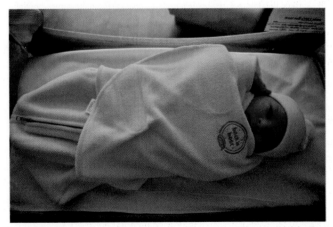

Fig. 24.23 Newborn in Sleep Sack. (Courtesy Allison and Matthew Wyatt, Eagle, CO.)

TEACHING FOR SELF-MANAGEMENT

Key Points About Car Seat Safety

General

- Always place your baby in an approved car safety seat when traveling in a motor vehicle (car, truck, bus, van), train, or airplane.
- Your baby should be in a rear-facing infant car safety seat from birth for as long as possible until exceeding the car seat's limits for height and weight. The car safety seat should be in the back seat of the car (see Fig. 24.24).
- Before purchasing an infant car seat, investigate which car seat is the most appropriate based on the infant's size and the type of vehicle in which the car seat will be installed (https://www.nhtsa.gov/equipment/car-seats-and-booster-seats).
- For help with proper installation of the car seat, go to a car seat safety station in your community (https://cert.safekids.org/get-car-seat-checked).
- The car seat should have a five-point safety harness that goes over both shoulders and both hips, and buckles at the crotch.
- Shoulder harnesses are placed in the slots at or below the level of the infant's shoulders. The harness should be snug, and the retainer clip should be placed at the level of the infant's armpits, not on the abdomen or neck area.
- Position infant at a 45-degree angle in the car seat to prevent slumping and airway obstruction; a tightly rolled blanket may be placed on either side of infant if needed.
- Avoid bulky clothing on the infant; this could cause the harness to loosen and increase the risk of infant injury.
- Blankets on top of the infant may be added for warmth.
- An infant car seat challenge is recommended by the AAP for infants who are born at less than 37 weeks' gestation. This test is performed for at least 90-120 min or a period of time equal to the length of the car ride home. The infant is monitored for apnea, bradycardia, and a decrease in oxygen saturation. If the infant exhibits any of these clinical signs, travel home should be in an approved car bed.

Cars with front air bags

- Rear-facing infant seats should never be placed in the front seat, because if the air bag deploys it can be dangerous, even fatal, for the infant.
- If the infant must ride in the front seat, the air bag must be turned off.

Cars with side air bags

- Parents need to read the vehicle owner's manual for information about car seat placement.

Data from American Academy of Pediatrics. (2018). *Rear facing car seats for infants and toddlers*. Itasca, IL: Author. Retrieved from https://www.healthychildren.org/English/safety-prevention/on-the-go/Pages/Rear-Facing-Car-Seats-for-Infants-Toddlers.aspx; American Academy of Pediatrics & American College of Obstetricians and Gynecologists. (2017). *Guidelines for perinatal care* (8th ed.). Elk Grove Village, IL: Author; Bull, M.J.; Engle, W. A.; Committee on Injury, Violence, and Poison Prevention; and Committee on Fetus and Newborn. (2009). Safe transportation of preterm and low birth weight infants at hospital discharge. *Pediatrics, 123*(5), 1424–1429.

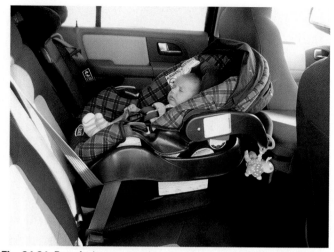

Fig. 24.24 Rear-facing car seat in rear seat of car. Infant is placed in seat when going home from the hospital. (Courtesy Brian and Mayannyn Sallee, Tucson, AZ.)

⚡ SAFETY ALERT

If the parents do not have a car safety seat, arrangements should be made to make an appropriate seat available for purchase, loan, or donation. Parents need to be cautioned about purchasing a secondhand car safety seat without knowing its history. They should never use a car seat that was involved in a moderate to severe crash, is too old, has visible cracks, does not have a label with the model number and manufacture date, does not come with instructions, is missing parts, or was recalled (AAP, 2018).

Pacifiers

Sucking provides pleasure for infants. However, sucking needs may not be satisfied by breastfeeding or bottle-feeding alone, and infants may suck on their fingers or a pacifier. There is compelling evidence that pacifiers help prevent SIDS. The AAP Task Force on SIDS (2016) suggests that parents consider offering a pacifier for naps and bedtime. The pacifier should be used when the infant is placed supine for sleep, and it should not be reinserted once the infant falls asleep. No infant should be forced to take a pacifier. Pacifiers must be cleaned often and replaced regularly and should not be coated with any type of sweet solution. Pacifier use for breastfeeding infants should be delayed until breastfeeding is well established.

Problems arise when parents are concerned about the sucking of fingers, thumb, or pacifier and try to restrain this natural tendency. Before giving advice, nurses should investigate the parents' feelings and base the guidance they give on the information solicited. For example, some parents see no problem with the infant sucking on a thumb or finger but find the use of a pacifier objectionable. In general, either practice need not be restrained unless thumb-sucking or pacifier use persists past 4 years of age or past the time when the permanent teeth erupt. Parents are advised to consult with their pediatric health care provider or pediatric dentist about this topic.

A parent's excessive use of the pacifier to calm the infant should also be explored, however. Placing a pacifier in the infant's mouth as soon as the infant begins to cry can reinforce a pattern of distress and relief.

---

an infant's disproportionately weak neck and heavy head. In this position, the force of a frontal crash is spread over the head, neck, and back; the back of the car safety seat supports the spine (AAP, 2018). Additional information related to car seat safety is located in the Teaching for Self-Management box: Key Points About Car Seat Safety.

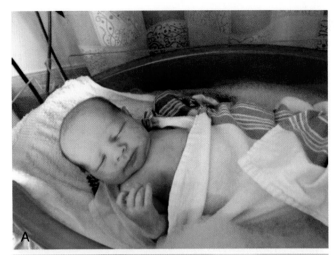

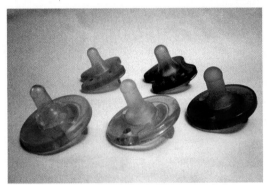

Fig. 24.25 Safe Pacifiers for Term and Preterm Infants. Note one-piece construction, easily grasped handle, and large shield with ventilation holes. (Courtesy Julie Perry Nelson, Loveland, CO.)

Bathing and Umbilical Cord Care

Bathing. Bathing serves several purposes. It provides opportunities for (1) cleansing the skin, (2) completing a thorough physical assessment, (3) promoting comfort, and (4) parent-infant-family interaction.

An important consideration in skin cleansing is the preservation of the skin's acid mantle, which is formed from the uppermost horny layer of the epidermis, sweat, superficial fat, metabolic products, and external substances such as amniotic fluid and microorganisms. To protect the newborn's skin, it is best to use a cleanser with a neutral pH and preferably without preservatives or with preservatives recognized as safe and well tolerated in neonates. Antimicrobial cleansers should not be used (AWHONN, 2018).

Neonatal skin care guidelines from AWHONN (2018) indicate that bathing should be performed according to facility protocols using immersion bathing, swaddled immersion, or sponge bathing. Practices vary across institutions. Some health care providers recommend waiting until the umbilical cord falls off and the umbilicus is healed before using an immersion bath. Parents need to be taught the techniques of sponge bathing and immersion bathing. There are also important safety tips that need to shared with parents (see the Teaching for Self-Management box: Home Care: Bathing, Cord Care, Skin Care, and Nail Care).

For immersion bathing, the water should be warm (38°C [100.4°F]) and deep enough to cover the shoulders, but not the head and neck (Lund & Durand, 2016) (Fig. 24.26A and B). Bathing by immersion has been found to allow less heat loss and provoke less crying. It has not been shown to increase the risk for bacterial colonization of the cord. Swaddled bathing is a type of immersion bathing in which the newborn is swaddled in a blanket or towel and immersed in a tub of warm water. One body part at a time is unwrapped and washed (AWHONN, 2018).

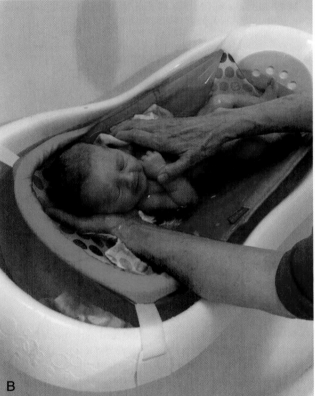

Fig. 24.26 Newborn Bath. (A) Initial newborn bath by swaddled immersion. (B) Immersion bath at home. (A, Courtesy Allison and Matthew Wyatt, Eagle, CO.; B, Courtesy Ashley and Andrew Martin, Charlotte, NC.)

A daily bath is not necessary for achieving cleanliness and can do harm by disrupting the integrity of the newborn's skin. Cleansing the perineum after a soiled diaper and daily cleansing of the face are usually sufficient. In general, infants should not be bathed more frequently than every other day; the hair should be shampooed once or twice a week (AWHONN, 2018).

Bath time is an ideal time for parent-infant social interaction (Fig. 24.27). While bathing the baby, parents can talk to the infant, caress and cuddle the infant, and engage in arousal and imitation of facial expressions and smiling.

Umbilical cord care. The goal of cord care is to prevent or decrease the risk for hemorrhage and infection. The umbilical cord stump is an excellent medium for bacterial growth and can easily become infected. Facility protocol determines the technique for routine cord care.

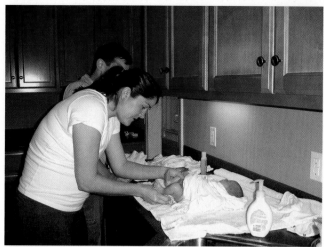

Fig. 24.27 Mother and Father Giving Newborn a Sponge Bath at Home. (Courtesy Allison and Matthew Wyatt, Eagle, CO.)

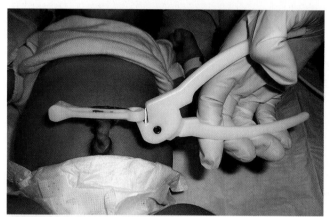

Fig. 24.28 Cord Clamp Removal. With special tool, nurse removes clamp after cord dries (approximately 24 to 48 hours after birth). (Courtesy Cheryl Briggs, RNC, Annapolis, MD.)

AWHONN (2018) recommendations for cord care include cleaning the cord with water (using cleanser sparingly if needed to remove debris) during the initial bath and with routine bathing. Evidence does not support the routine use of antiseptic or antimicrobial preparations for cord care. However, the AAP recognizes the benefit of applying selected antimicrobial agents to the umbilical cords of infants born at home in resource-limited countries, for births occurring outside of hospitals or birth centers, and in resource-limited populations such as Native American communities (Stewart, Benitz, & Committee on Fetus and Newborn, 2016).

The plastic cord clamp that was applied at birth is removed once the stump has dried (Fig. 24.28), typically in 24 to 48 hours. The stump and base of the cord should be assessed for edema, redness, and purulent drainage with each diaper change. The area should be kept clean and dry and open to air or loosely covered with clothing. If soiled, the area is cleansed with plain water and dried thoroughly. The diaper is folded down and away from the stump (AWHONN, 2018). The umbilical cord begins to dry, shrivel, and blacken by the second or third day of life. Cord separation time is influenced by several factors, including type of cord care, type of birth, and other perinatal events. The average cord separation time is 10 to 14 days, although it can take up to 3 weeks. Some dried blood may be seen

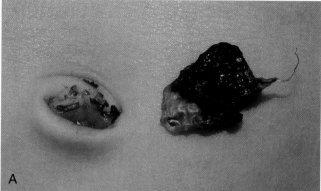

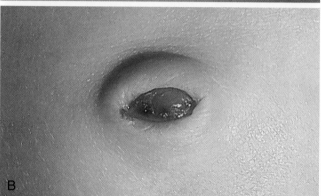

Fig. 24.29 Cord Separation. (A) Cord separated with some dried blood still in the umbilicus. (B) Umbilicus cleansed and beginning to heal. (Courtesy Cheryl Briggs, RNC, Annapolis, MD.)

in the umbilicus at separation (Fig. 24.29). Parents are instructed in appropriate home cord care (per pediatric health care practitioner or institution protocol) and the expected time of cord separation (see the Teaching for Self-Management box: Home Care: Bathing, Cord Care, Skin Care, and Nail Care).

Infant Follow-Up Care

Follow-up care after discharge from the birthing facility usually occurs within 48 to 72 hours at the pediatric clinic or health care provider's office. This is especially important for breastfed newborns for monitoring their weight and hydration status. When infants are discharged at less than 48 hours of age, the follow-up visit may be the day after discharge. For some families, follow-up is done by a home care nurse.

Cardiopulmonary Resuscitation

Parents should receive instruction in relieving airway obstruction and CPR. Classes are often offered in hospitals and clinics during the prenatal period or to parents of newborns. Such instruction is especially important for parents whose infants were preterm or have a history of cardiac or respiratory problems. It is important that all caregivers such as grandparents and babysitters understand the basics of CPR and relieving airway obstruction.

Practical Suggestions for the First Weeks at Home

Numerous changes occur during the first weeks of parenthood. Care management should be directed toward helping parents cope with infant care, role changes, altered lifestyle, and changes in family structure resulting from the addition of a new baby.

Parents must be helped to anticipate events during the transition from birthing facility to home. This is especially important for

Timing
- Newborns do not need a bath every day. Three times a week is often enough.
- Give a bath at any time convenient to you but not immediately after a feeding period because the increased handling can cause regurgitation. Bathing before bedtime can promote sleep.

Prevent Heat Loss
- The temperature of the room should be 26°-27°C (79°-81°F), and the bathing area should be free of drafts (close the door in the room where the bath is performed).
- The water temperature should be 38°-40°C (100°- <104°F). A water thermometer is useful for determining appropriate water temperature.
- Control heat loss during the bath to conserve the infant's energy. Bathe the infant quickly; with a sponge bath, expose only a portion of the body at a time; and dry thoroughly.

Gather Supplies and Clothing Before Starting
- Tub for bathing in a safe place on a sturdy surface
- Towels for drying the infant and a clean washcloth
- Mild cleanser with a neutral pH and preferably with no preservatives
- Diaper
- Clothing suitable for wearing indoors: shirt; stretch suit or nightgown optional
- Cotton balls
- Lightweight blanket

Bathe the Baby
- Take the infant to the bathing area when all supplies are ready.
- Never leave the infant alone on bath table or in the bathwater, not even for a second! If you have to leave, take the infant with you or place the infant back into the crib.
- Test the temperature of the water. Do not hold the infant under running water—the water temperature can change, and the infant can be scalded or chilled rapidly. For immersion bathing (tub bath), carefully lower the infant into the tub; the head and neck should be above the water. The tub should be filled with enough water to keep the baby's shoulders covered; this helps reduce heat loss. First wash the baby's face with a soft washcloth and plain water. Then proceed to wash the rest of the body, going from top to bottom.
- If sponge bathing, undress the baby and wrap in a towel with the head exposed. Uncover and gently wash one part of the body at a time, taking care to keep the rest of the baby covered as much as possible to prevent heat loss.
- Begin by washing the baby's face with water; do not use soap on the face. Cleanse the eyes from the inner canthus outward using separate parts of a clean washcloth for each eye. For the first 2-3 days, a discharge can result from the reaction of the conjunctiva to the substance (erythromycin) used as a prophylactic measure against infection. After 2-3 days of age, any discharge should be considered abnormal and reported to the pediatric health care provider.
- Cleanse the ears and nose with twists of moistened cotton or a corner of the washcloth. Do not use cotton-tipped swabs because they can cause injury. The areas behind the ears also need cleansing.
- Wash between the skinfolds. Place your hand under the baby's shoulders and lift gently to expose the neck, lift the chin, and wash the neck, taking care to cleanse between the skinfolds.
- Wash the genital area last.
- If the hair is to be washed, begin by wrapping the infant in a towel with the head exposed. Hold the infant in a football position (under the arm) with one hand, using the other hand to wash the hair. Wash the scalp with water and shampoo that is mild for the eyes and safe for babies. Massage the scalp gently, rinse well, and dry thoroughly. Never use a blow dryer on an infant because even on the lowest setting the temperature is too hot for a baby's skin.
- Wash hair with baby wrapped to limit heat loss.

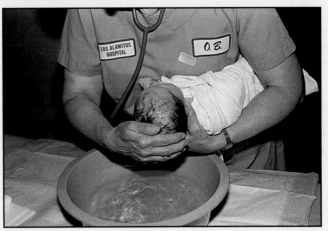

(Courtesy Marjorie Pyle, RNC, Lifecircle, Costa Mesa, CA.)

Skin Care
- If the skin appears dry or cracking, apply an emollient (lotion) at least once daily. Check with your pediatric health care provider about the type of emollient to use.
- The fragile skin can be injured by too vigorous cleansing. If stool or other debris has dried and caked on the skin, soak the area to remove it. Do not attempt to rub it off because abrasion can result. Cleanse gently using a mild cleanser, and pat dry.

Cord Care
- Cleanse with plain water around base of the cord where it joins the skin. Notify the pediatric health care provider of any odor, discharge, or redness of the skin around the cord. The clamp is removed by the nurse when the cord is dry (approximately 24-48 h after birth). Keep the diaper folded down so that it does not cover the cord. A wet or soiled diaper will slow or prevent drying of the cord and foster infection. When the cord drops off after 10-14 days, a few small drops of blood may be seen. If there is active bleeding, notify the pediatric health care provider.

Nail Care
- Do not cut fingernails and toenails immediately after birth. The nails have to grow out far enough from the skin so that the skin is not cut by mistake. If the baby scratches himself or herself, apply loosely fitted mitts over each of the baby's hands. Do so as a last resort, however, because it interferes with the baby's ability for self-consolation sucking on thumb or finger. When the nails have grown, the fingernails and toenails can be trimmed with manicure scissors or clippers; nails should be cut straight across. The ideal time to trim the nails is when the infant is sleeping. Soft emery boards may be used to file the nails. Nails should be kept short.

Genital Care
- Cleanse the genitalia of infants after voiding or stooling using disposable diaper wipes (not containing alcohol) or soft cloths and water (with gentle cleanser if needed). For girls, the genitalia are cleansed by gently separating the labia and gently washing from the pubic area to the anus. For uncircumcised boys, wash and rinse the penis with soap and warm water. Do not attempt to retract the foreskin. The health care provider will inform you when the foreskin can safely be retracted. By 3 years of age in the majority of boys, the foreskin can be retracted easily without causing pain or trauma. For others, the foreskin is not retractable until adolescence. As soon as the foreskin is partly retractable and the child is old enough, he can be taught self-care. Once healed, the circumcised penis does not require any special care other than cleansing with diaper changes.
- The infant's skin should be allowed to dry completely before applying another diaper.
- Exposing the buttocks to air can help resolve diaper rash. Because bacteria thrive in moist dark areas, exposing the skin to dry air decreases bacterial proliferation. Zinc oxide ointments can be used to protect the infant's skin from moisture and further excoriation.

Data from American Academy of Pediatrics. (2009). Bathing your newborn. https://www.healthychildren.org/English/ages-stages/baby/bathing-skin-care/Pages/Bathing-Your-Newborn.aspx; Association of Women's Health, Obstetric and Neonatal Nurses. (2018). *Neonatal skin care* (4th ed.). Washington, DC: Author.

first-time parents. Even the simplest strategies can provide enormous support. Printed materials reinforcing education topics are helpful, as is a list of available community resources and websites that provide reliable information about child care. Classes in the prenatal period or during the postpartum stay are helpful. Instructions for the first days at home include relevant topics such as activities of daily living, dealing with visitors, and activity and rest.

Interpretation of crying and use of quieting techniques. Crying is an infant's first social communication. Some babies cry more than others, but all babies cry. They cry to communicate that they are hungry, uncomfortable, wet, ill, or bored, and sometimes for no apparent reason at all. The longer parents are around their infants, the easier it becomes to interpret the meaning of infant cries and to respond appropriately. Many infants have a fussy period during the day, often in the late afternoon or early evening when everyone is naturally tired. Environmental tension adds to the length and intensity of crying spells. Babies also have periods of vigorous crying when no comforting can help. These periods of crying can last for long stretches until the infants seem to cry themselves to sleep. The nurse should educate new parents that time and infant maturation will take care of these types of cries. Parents need to understand what to do when crying episodes occur. If parents have a greater understanding of infant crying, they may be less likely to inflict harm, such as occurs with shaken-baby syndrome. For parent education, many facilities utilize the "The Period of Purple Crying" program from the National Center for Shaken Baby Syndrome (http://www.purplecrying.info/what-is-the-period-of-purple-crying.php).

Nurses should instruct new parents about strategies to calm a crying or fussy baby. Certain types of sensory stimulation can calm and quiet infants and help them get to sleep. Important characteristics of this sensory stimulation—whether tactile, vestibular, auditory, or visual—appear to be that the stimulation is mild, slow, rhythmic, and consistently and regularly presented. Tactile stimulation can include SSC, warmth, patting, and back massage. Swaddling provides widespread and constant tactile stimulation and a sense of security. Vestibular stimulation is especially effective and can be accomplished by mild rhythmic movement such as rocking or by holding the infant upright, as on the parent's shoulder. Some infants respond to being held in a body carrier (see Fig. 25.9). Rhythmic sounds can provide auditory stimulation; parents can use devices that provide white noise or sounds resembling the mother's heartbeat.

Recognizing signs of illness. In addition to explaining the need for well-baby follow-up visits, the nurse should discuss with parents the signs of illness in newborns (see the Teaching for Self-Management box: Signs of Illness). Of particular importance is the parents' assessment of jaundice in newborns discharged early. Parents should be advised to call their pediatric care provider immediately if they notice increasing jaundice or signs of illness.

TEACHING FOR SELF-MANAGEMENT
Signs of Illness

Notify the pediatric health care provider if any of the following signs occur:
- Fever: temperature greater than 38°C (100.4°F) axillary; also a continual rise in temperature (Note: Tympanic [ear] thermometers are not recommended for infants <3 mo of age.)
- Hypothermia: temperature less than 36.5°C (97.7°F) axillary
- Poor feeding or little interest in food: refusing two feedings in a row
- Vomiting: more than one episode of forceful vomiting or frequent vomiting (over a 6-h period)
- Bilious (bright green in color) emesis: this can be a sign of bowel obstruction and should be reported to the pediatric health care provider immediately.
- Diarrhea: two consecutive green, watery stools (Note: Stools of breastfed infants are normally looser than stools of formula-fed infants. Diarrhea leaves a water ring around the stool, whereas breastfed stools do not.)
- Decreased bowel movement: in a breastfed infant, fewer than three stools per day; in a formula-fed infant, less than one stool every other day
- Decreased urination: fewer than six to eight wet diapers per day after 3 to 4 days of age
- Breathing difficulties: labored breathing with flared nostrils or absence of breathing for more than 15 sec (Note: A newborn's breathing is normally irregular and between 30 and 60 breaths/min. Count the breaths for a full minute.)
- Cyanosis (bluish skin color), whether accompanying a feeding or not
- Lethargy: sleepiness, difficulty waking, or periods of sleep longer than 6 h (Most newborns sleep for short periods, usually 1-4 h, and wake to be fed.)
- Inconsolable crying (attempts to quiet not effective) or continuous high-pitched cry
- Bleeding or purulent (yellowish) drainage from umbilical cord or circumcision; foul odor or redness at the site
- Drainage from the eyes

KEY POINTS

- Assessment of the newborn requires data from the prenatal, intrapartal, and postnatal periods.
- The immediate assessment of the newborn after birth includes Apgar scoring and a general evaluation of physical status.
- Knowledge of biologic and behavioral characteristics is essential for guiding assessment and interpreting data.
- Gestational age assessment provides important information for predicting risks and guiding care management.
- Nursing care immediately after birth includes maintaining a patent airway, preventing heat loss, and promoting parent-infant interaction.
- Providing a protective environment includes careful identification procedures, support of physiologic functions, prevention of infection, and prevention of newborn falls or other injury.
- The newborn has social and physical needs.
- Nurses caring for newborns should be aware of physiologic and behavioral manifestations of pain.
- Nonpharmacologic and pharmacologic measures are used to reduce neonatal pain.
- Before hospital discharge, nurses provide anticipatory guidance for parents regarding feeding and elimination patterns; positioning and holding; safe sleep practices; comfort measures; infant safety, including the use of car seats; bathing, skin care, cord care, and nail care; and signs of illness.
- All parents should have instruction in infant CPR.

REFERENCES

Adamkin, D. H. (2017). Neonatal hypoglycemia. *Seminars in Fetal & Neonatal Medicine, 22*(1), 36–41.

Adamkin, D. H., & Committee on Fetus and Newborn. (2011). Clinical report—Postnatal glucose homeostasis in late-preterm and term infants. *Pediatrics, 127*(3), 575–579.

Ainsworth, R. M., Summerlin-Long, S., & Mog, C. (2016). A comprehensive initiative to prevent falls among newborns. *Nursing for Women's Health, 20*(3), 247–257.

American Academy of Pediatrics. (2017). *Swaddling: is it safe?* Elk Grove Village, IL: Author. Retrieved from: https://www.healthychildren.org/English/ages-stages/baby/diapers-clothing/Pages/Swaddling-Is-it-Safe.aspx.

American Academy of Pediatrics. (2018). *Rear-facing care seats for infants and toddlers.* Itasca, IL: Author. Retrieved from: https://www.healthychildren.org/English/safety-prevention/on-the-go/Pages/Rear-Facing-Car-Seats-for-Infants-Toddlers.aspx.

American Academy of Pediatrics & American College of Obstetricians and Gynecologists. (2017). *Guidelines for perinatal care* (8th ed.). Elk Grove Village, IL: Author.

American Academy of Pediatrics Committee on Infectious Diseases. (2018). Section 5: Antimicrobial prophylaxis. In D. W. Kimberlin, M. T. Brady, M. A. Jackson, et al. (Eds.), *Red book: 2018-2021 report of the Committee on Infectious Diseases* (31st ed.). Itasca, IL: Author.

American Academy of Pediatrics Section on Breastfeeding. (2012). Breastfeeding and the use of human milk—Policy statement. *Pediatrics, 129*(3), e827–e841.

American Academy of Pediatrics Section on Cardiology and Cardiac Surgery Executive Committee. (2012). Endorsement of health and human services recommendation for pulse oximetry screening for critical congenital heart disease. *Pediatrics, 129*(1), 190–192.

American Academy of Pediatrics Subcommittee on Hyperbilirubinemia. (2004). Clinical practice guideline: Management of hyperbilirubinemia in the newborn infant 35 or more weeks of gestation. *Pediatrics, 114*(1), 297–316.

American Academy of Pediatrics Task Force on Circumcision. (1999, reaffirmed 2005). Circumcision policy statement. *Pediatrics, 103*(3), 686–693.

American Academy of Pediatrics Task Force on Circumcision. (2012). Circumcision policy statement. *Pediatrics, 130*(3), 585–586.

American Academy of Pediatrics Task Force on Sudden Infant Death Syndrome. (2016). SIDS and other sleep-related infant deaths: Updated 2016 recommendations for a safe infant sleeping environment. *Pediatrics, 138*(5), e1–e12.

American College of Medical Genetics. (2009). *Position statement on importance of residual newborn screening dried blood spots.* Retrieved from: https://www.acmg.net/PDFLibrary/NBS-Blood-Spot-Retention.pdf.

American College of Obstetricians and Gynecologists & Society for Maternal-Fetal Medicine. (2013, reaffirmed 2017). Definition of term pregnancy. *Obstetrics and Gynecology, 122*(5), 1139–1140.

American College of Obstetricians and Gynecologists Committee on Genetics. (2015). Committee opinion no. 616: Newborn screening and the role of the obstetrician-gynceologist. *Obstetrics and Gynecology, 125*(1), 256–260.

Association of Women's Health, Obstetric and Neonatal Nurses. (2016). AWHONN position statement: Newborn screening. *Journal of Obstetric, Gynecologic and Neonatal Nursing, 45*(1), 135–136.

Association of Women's Health, Obstetric and Neonatal Nurses. (2018). *Neonatal skin care: evidence-based clinical practice guideline* (4th ed.). Washington, DC: Author.

Ballard, J. L., Khoury, J. C., Wedig, K., et al. (1991). New Ballard score, expanded to include extremely premature infants. *Journal of Pediatrics, 119*(3), 417–423.

Barrington, K. J., Sankaran, K., & Canadian Paediatric Society Fetus and Newborn Committee. (2007, reaffirmed 2018). Guidelines for detection, management, and prevention of hyperbilirubinemia in term and late preterm newborn infants. *Paediatrics & Child Health, 12*(B Suppl), 1B–12B.

Benjamin, K., & Furdon, S. A. (2015). Physical assessment. In M. T. Verklan, & M. Walden (Eds.), *Core curriculum for neonatal intensive care nursing* (5th ed.). St. Louis, MO: Elsevier.

Bhutani, V. K., & Committee on Fetus and Newborn. (2011). Phototherapy to prevent severe neonatal hyperbilirubinemia in the newborn infant 35 or more weeks of gestation. *Pediatrics, 128*(4), e1046–e1052.

Blackburn, S. T. (2018). *Maternal, fetal, and neonatal physiology: A clinical perspective* (5th ed.). St. Louis: Elsevier.

Bull, M. J., Engle, W. A., & Committee on Injury, Violence, and Poison Prevention; and Committee on Fetus and Newborn (2009). Safe transportation of preterm and low birth weight infants at hospital discharge. *Pediatrics, 123*(5), 1424–1429.

Canadian Organization for Rare Disorders. (2015). Newborn screening in Canada status report. Retrieved from: https://www.raredisorders.ca/content/uploads/Canada-NBS-status-updated-Sept.-3-2015.pdf.

Cleveland, L., Hill, C. M., Pulse, W. S., et al. (2017). Systematic review of skin-to-skin care for full-term, healthy newborns. *Journal of Obstetric, Gynecologic and Neonatal Nursing, 46*(6), 857–869.

Feldman-Winter, L., Goldsmith, J. P., & Committee on Fetus and Newborn., et al. (2016). Safe sleep and skin-to-skin care in the neonatal period for healthy term newborns. *Pediatrics, 138*(3), e1–e10.

Gardner, S. L., Enzman-Hines, M., & Agarwal, R. (2016). Pain and pain relief. In S. L. Gardner, B. S. Carter, M. Enzman-Hines, et al. (Eds.), *Merenstein & Gardner's handbook of neonatal intensive care* (8th ed.). St. Louis: Elsevier.

Gardner, S. L., & Hernández, J. A. (2016a). Heat balance. In S. L. Gardner, B. S. Carter, M. Enzman-Hines, et al. (Eds.), *Merenstein & Gardner's handbook of neonatal intensive care* (8th ed.). St. Louis: Elsevier.

Gardner, S. L., & Hernández, J. A. (2016b). Initial nursery care. In S. L. Gardner, B. S. Carter, M. Enzman-Hines, et al. (Eds.), *Merenstein & Gardner's handbook of neonatal intensive care* (8th ed.). St. Louis: Elsevier.

Gokulu, G., Bilgen, H., Ozdemir, H., et al. (2016). Comparative heel stick study showed that newborn infants who had undergone repeated painful procedures showed increased short-term pain responses. *Acta Paediatrica, 105*(11), e520–e525.

Hamrick, H. J., Gable, E. K., Freeman, E. H., et al. (2016). Reasons for refusal of newborn vitamin K prophylaxis: Implications for management and education. *Hospital Pediatrics, 6*(1), 15–21.

Health Resources and Services Administration Advisory Committee on Heritable Disorders in Newborns and Children. (2018). *Recommended uniform screening panel.* Retrieved from: https://www.hrsa.gov/advisory-committees/heritable-disorders/index.html.

Helsey, L., McDonald, J. V., & Stewart, V. T. (2010). Addressing in-hospital "falls" of newborn infants. *Joint Commission Journal on Quality and Patient Safety, 36*(7), 327–333.

Hummel, P., Puchalski, M., Creech, S. D., et al. (2008). Clinical reliability and validity of the N-PASS: Neonatal pain, agitation and sedation scale with prolonged pain. *Journal of Perinatology, 28*(1), 55–60.

Johnston, C., Campbell-Yeo, M., Disher, T., et al. (2017). Skin-to-skin care for procedural pain in neonates. *Cochrane Database of Systematic Reviews, 2,* CD008435.

Joint Committee on Infant Hearing. (2007). Year 2007 position statement: Principles and guidelines for early hearing detection and intervention programs. *Pediatrics, 120*(4), 898–921.

Kahn, D. J., Fisher, P. D., & Hertzler, D. A. (2017). Variation in management of in-hospital newborn falls: A single center experience. *Journal of Neurosurgical Pediatrics, 20*(2), 176–182.

Kamath-Rayne, B. D., Thilo, E. H., Deacon, J., et al. (2016). Neonatal hyperbilirubinemia. In S. L. Gardner, B. S. Carter, M. Enzman-Hines, et al. (Eds.), *Merenstein & Gardner's handbook of neonatal intensive care* (8th ed.). St. Louis: Elsevier.

Kardatzke, M. A., Rose, R. S., & Engle, W. A. (2017). Late preterm and early term birth: At-risk populations and targets for reducing such early births. *NeoReviews, 18*(5), e265–e276.

Karlsen, K. (2012). *S.T.A.B.L.E. The program: pre-transport / post-resuscitation stabilization care of sick infants* (6th ed.). Park City, UT: The S.T.A.B.L.E. Program.

Krechel, S. W., & Bildner, J. (1995). CRIES: A new neonatal postoperative pain measurement score—Initial testing of validity and reliability. *Paediatric Anaesthesia, 5*(1), 53–61.

Lawrence, J., Alcock, D., McGrath, P., et al. (1993). The development of a tool to assess neonatal pain. *Neonatal Network, 12*(6), 59–66.

Liu, Y., Huang, X., Luo, B., et al. (2017). Effects of combined oral sucrose and nonnutritive sucking (NNS) on procedural pain of NICU newborns, 2001-2016: A PRISMA-compliant systematic review and meta-analysis. *Medicine, 96*(6), e6108.

Locatelli, C., & Bellieni, C. V. (2017). Sensorial saturation and neonatal pain: A review. *Journal of Maternal-Fetal & Neonatal Medicine, 31*(23), 3209–3213.

Lund, C. H., & Durand, D. J. (2016). Skin and skin care. In S. L. Gardner, B. S. Carter, M. Enzman-Hines, et al. (Eds.), *Merenstein & Gardner's handbook of neonatal intensive care* (8th ed.). St. Louis: Elsevier.

Martin, J. A., Hamilton, B. E., Osterman, M. J. K., et al. (2018). Births: Final data for 2016. *National Vital Statistics Reports, 67*(1), 1–55.

Moore, D. L., MacDonald, N. E., & Canadian Paediatric Society Infectious Diseases and Immunization Committee. (2015, reaffirmed 2018). Position statement: Preventing ophthalmia neonatorum. *Paediatrics & Child Health, 20*(2), 93–96.

Moore, E. R., Bergman, N., Anderson, G. C., et al. (2016). Early skin-to-skin contact for mothers and their healthy newborn infants. *Cochrane Database of Systematic Reviews, 11*, CD003519.

National Institute of Child Health and Human Development. (2014). *Sudden unexplained infant death (sids) and other sleep-related causes of infant death: Questions and answers for health care providers.* Rockville, MD: Author.

Ng, E., Loewy, A. D., Fetus, & Newborn Committee. (2018). Guidelines for vitamin K prophylaxis in newborns. *Paediatrics and Child Health, 23*(6), 394–397.

Owings, M., Uddin, S., & Williams, S. (2013). *Trends in circumcision for male newborns in US hospitals: 1979-2010.* Health E-Stats. Retrieved from: www.cdc.gov/nchs/data/hestat/circumcision_2013/circumcision_2013.htm.

Parikh, L. I., Reddy, U. M., Männistö, T., et al. (2014). Neonatal outcomes of early term birth. *American Journal of Obstetrics and Gynecology, 211*(3), e1–e265.

Patel, H., Feldman, M., & Canadian Paediatric Society Community Paediatrics Committee. (2011, reaffirmed 2016). Universal newborn hearing screening. *Paediatrics & Child Health, 16*(5), 301–305.

Peng, H. F., Yin, T., Yang, L., et al. (2018). Non-nutritive sucking, oral breast milk, and facilitated tucking relieve preterm infant pain during heel-stick procedures: A prospective, randomized controlled trial. *International Journal of Nursing, 77*, 162–170.

Plana, M. N., Zamora, J., Suresh, G., et al. (2018). Pulse oximetry screening for critical congenital heart defects. *Cochrane Database of Systematic Reviews, 3*, CD011912.

Rozance, P. J., McGowan, J. E., Price-Douglas, W., et al. (2016). Glucose homeostasis. In S. L. Gardner, B. S. Carter, M. Enzman-Hines, et al. (Eds.), *Merenstein & Gardner's handbook of neonatal intensive care* (8th ed.). St. Louis: Elsevier.

Saxton, A., Fahy, K., Rolfe, M., et al. (2015). Does skin-to-skin and breastfeeding at birth affect the rate of primary postpartum haemorrhage: Results of a cohort study. *Midwifery, 31*(11), 1110–1117.

Schillie, S., Vellozzi, C., Reingold, A., et al. (2018). Prevention of hepatitis b virus infection in the United States: Recommendations of the Advisory Committee on Immunization Practices. *Morbidity and Mortality Weekly Report, 67*(1), 1–31.

Sorokan, S. T., Finlay, J. C., Jefferies, A. L., et al. (2015). Newborn male circumcision. *Paediatrics & Child Health, 20*(6), 311–315.

Stevens, B., Johnston, C., Petryshen, P., et al. (1996). Premature infant pain profile: Development and initial validation. *Clinical Journal of Pain, 12*(1), 13–22.

Stevens, B., Yamada, J., Ohlsson, A., et al. (2016). Sucrose for analgesia in newborn infants undergoing painful procedures. *Cochrane Database of Systematic Reviews, 7*, CD001069.

Stewart, D., Benitz, W., & Committee on Fetus and Newborn. (2016). Umbilical cord care in the newborn infant. *Pediatrics, 138*(3), e1–e5.

Tappero, E. P., & Honeyfield, M. E. (2015). *Physical assessment of the newborn* (5th ed.). Petaluma, CA: NICU Ink.

The Joint Commission. (2018). Preventing newborn falls and drops. *Quick Safety, 40*, 1–2.

United States Preventive Services Task Force. (2011). *Ocular prophylaxis for gonococcal ophthalmia neonatorum: Preventive Medication.* Retrieved from: www.uspreventiveservicestaskforce.org/uspstf10/gonoculproph/gonocupsum.htm.

Visscher, M. O., Adam, R., Brink, S., et al. (2015). Newborn infant skin care: Physiology, development, and care. *Clinics in Dermatology, 33*(3), 271–280.

Walden, M. (2015). Pain assessment and management. In M. T. Verklan, & M. Walden (Eds.), *Core curriculum for neonatal intensive care nursing* (5th ed.). St. Louis: Elsevier.

Walden, M., & Gibbins, S. (2012). *Newborn pain assessment and management guideline for practice* (3rd ed.). Chicago, IL: National Association of Neonatal Nurses.

Weiner, G. M., & Zaichkin, J. (Eds.). (2016). *Textbook of neonatal resuscitation* (7th ed.) Elk Grove Village, IL: American Academy of Pediatrics and American Heart Association.

Wight, N., Marinelli, K. A., & Academy of Breastfeeding Medicine (2014). ABM protocol no. 1: Guidelines for blood glucose monitoring and treatment of hypoglycemia in term and late preterm neonates, revised 2014. *Breastfeeding Medicine, 9*(4), 173–179.

Williams, T. R., Alam, S., & Gaffney, M. (2015). Progress in identifying infants with hearing loss—United States, 2006-2012. *Morbidity and Mortality Weekly Report, 64*(13), 351–356.

Witt, N., Coynor, S., Edwards, C., et al. (2016). A guide to pain assessment and management in the neonate. *Current Emergency and Hospital Medicine Reports, 4*, 1–10.

World Health Organization. (2009). *WHO guidelines on hand hygiene in health care.* Geneva, Switzerland: WHO Press.

World Health Organization. (2012). *Voluntary medical male circumcision for HIV prevention.* Retrieved from: www.who.int/hiv/topics/malecircumcision/fact_sheet/en/.

World Health Organization & Jhpiego. (2010). *Manual for early infant male circumcision under local anesthesia.* Geneva, Switzerland: WHO Press.

Wyckoff, M. H., Aziz, K., Escobedo, M. B., et al. (2015). Part 13: Neonatal resuscitation: 2015 American Heart Association guidelines update for cardiopulmonary resuscitation and emergency cardiovascular care. *Circulation, 132*(18, Suppl 2), S543–S560.

25

Newborn Nutrition and Feeding

Valerie Coleman

http://evolve.elsevier.com/Lowdermilk/MWHC/

LEARNING OBJECTIVES

- Describe current recommendations for infant feeding.
- Explain the nurse's role in helping families select an infant feeding method.
- Discuss benefits of breastfeeding for infants, mothers, families, and society.
- Describe nutritional needs of infants.
- Describe anatomic and physiologic aspects of human lactation.
- Recognize newborn feeding cues.

- Explain maternal and infant indicators of effective breastfeeding.
- Examine nursing interventions to facilitate and promote successful breastfeeding.
- Analyze common problems associated with breastfeeding and interventions to resolve them.
- Compare powdered, concentrated, and ready-to-use forms of commercial infant formula.
- Develop a teaching plan for the formula feeding family.

Good nutrition in infancy fosters optimal growth and development. Infant feeding is more than providing nutrition; it is an opportunity for social, psychologic, and even educational interaction between parent and infant. It can establish a basis for developing good eating habits that last a lifetime.

Through preconception and prenatal education and counseling, nurses play an instrumental role in helping parents make an informed decision about infant feeding. Scientific evidence is clear that human milk provides the best nutrition for infants, and parents should be strongly encouraged to choose breastfeeding (American Academy of Pediatrics [AAP] Section on Breastfeeding, 2012). Although many consider commercial infant formula to be equivalent to breast milk, this belief is erroneous. Human milk is the gold standard for infant nutrition. It is species-specific, uniquely designed to meet the needs of human infants. The composition of human milk changes to meet the nutritional needs of growing infants. It is highly complex, with anti-infective and nutritional components combined with growth factors, enzymes that aid in digestion and absorption of nutrients, and fatty acids that promote brain growth and development. Commercial infant formulas are usually adequate in providing nutrition to maintain infant growth and development within normal limits, but they are not equivalent to human milk.

Breastfeeding is defined as the transfer of human milk from the mother to the infant; the infant receives milk directly from the mother's breast. *Exclusive breastfeeding* means that the infant receives no other liquid or solid food (AAP Section on Breastfeeding, 2012). If the infant is fed expressed breast milk from the mother or a donor milk bank, it is called *human milk feeding*.

Whether the parents choose breastfeeding, human milk feeding, or formula-feeding, nurses provide support and ongoing education. It is essential that parent education and care management are based on current research findings and standards of practice. Nurses and lactation consultants provide education, assistance, and support for mothers, infants, and families prior to discharge from the birthing facility. After discharge, nurses and lactation consultants in primary care and community health settings provide ongoing support and assistance to promote optimal feeding practices and positive health outcomes.

This chapter focuses on meeting nutritional needs for normal growth and development from birth to 6 months of age, emphasizing the neonatal period when feeding practices and patterns are established. Breastfeeding and formula-feeding are addressed. Information on breastfeeding is focused on the direct transfer of milk from mother to infant.

RECOMMENDED INFANT NUTRITION

The AAP recommends exclusive breastfeeding for the first 6 months of life and that breastfeeding continues as complementary foods are introduced. Breastfeeding should continue for 1 year and thereafter as desired by the mother and her infant (AAP Section on Breastfeeding, 2012). According to the World Health Organization (WHO, 2016), infants should be exclusively breastfed for 6 months, receive safe and nutritionally adequate complementary foods beginning at 6 months, and continue breastfeeding until 2 years of age or beyond.

Exclusive breastfeeding for the first 6 months of life is also recommended by other professional health care organizations such as the American College of Nurse-Midwives (ACNM, 2016), American Academy of Family Physicians (AAFP, 2012), Academy of Breastfeeding Medicine (Chantry, Eglash, & Labbok, 2015), the American College of Obstetricians and Gynecologists (ACOG, 2018), and the American Dietetic Association (ADA, 2009). The Association of Women's Health, Obstetric, and Neonatal Nurses (AWHONN, 2014; 2015) actively supports breastfeeding as the ideal form of infant nutrition and provides guidelines for nurses in promoting breastfeeding and supporting breastfeeding families.

Breastfeeding Rates

Breastfeeding rates in the United States have risen steadily over the past decade. The Centers for Disease Control and Prevention (CDC, 2018b) reported that the U.S. breastfeeding initiation rate (ever breastfed) for

TABLE 25.1 Benefits of Breastfeeding

Benefits for the Infant/Child	Benefits for the Mother	Benefits for Families and Society

• Reduced infant and child mortality
• Reduced risk for:
  • Nonspecific gastrointestinal infections
  • Celiac disease
  • Childhood inflammatory bowel disease
  • Necrotizing enterocolitis in preterm infants
  • Asthma
  • Atopic dermatitis
  • Lower respiratory tract infection
  • Otitis media
  • SIDS
  • Obesity in childhood, adolescence, and adulthood
  • Type 2 diabetes
  • Acute lymphocytic and myeloid leukemia
  • Dental malocclusions
  • Enhanced neurodevelopmental outcomes, including higher intelligence
	• Decreased postpartum bleeding and more rapid uterine involution
	• Reduced risk for:
	  • Ovarian cancer and breast cancer
	  • Type 2 diabetes
	  • Hypertension, hypercholesterolemia, and cardiovascular disease
	  • Rheumatoid arthritis
	• More rapid postpartum weight loss
	• Delayed return of menses
	• Unique bonding experience
	• Increased maternal role attainment
		• Convenient; ready to feed
		• No bottles or other necessary equipment
		• Less expensive than infant formula
		• Reduced annual health care costs
		• Less parental absence from work because of ill infant
		• Reduced environmental burden related to disposal of formula packaging and equipment

SIDS, Sudden infant death syndrome.
Data from American Academy of Pediatrics Section on Breastfeeding. (2012). Breastfeeding and the use of human milk—Policy statement. *Pediatrics, 129*(3), e827–e841; Chowdhury, R., Sinha, B., Sankar, M. J., et al. (2015). Breastfeeding and maternal health outcomes: A systematic review and meta-analysis. *Acta Paediatrica, 104*(S467), 96–113; Grummer-Strawn, L. M., & Rollins, N. (2015). Summarising the health benefits of breastfeeding. *Acta Paediatrica, 104*(S467), 1–2; Horta, B. L., de Mola, C. L., & Victora, C. G. (2015). Breastfeeding and intelligence: A systematic review and meta-analysis. *Acta Paediatrica, 104*(S467), 14–19; Sankar, M. J., Sinha, B., Chowdhury, R., et al. (2015). Optimal breastfeeding practices and infant and child mortality: A systematic review and meta-analysis. *Acta Paediatrica, 104*(S467), 3–13; Victora, C. G., Bahl, R., Barros, A. J., et al. (2016). Breastfeeding in the 21st century: Epidemiology, mechanisms, and lifelong effect. *Lancet, 387*(10017), 473–490.

infants born in 2015 was 83.2%, which is the highest ever reported. The 6-month breastfeeding rate was 57.6%, and the 12-month rate was 35.9%. The rate of exclusive breastfeeding at 3 months was 46.9% and at 6 months, 24.9%. Commercial infant formula was fed to approximately 1 in 6 (17.2%) breastfed newborns during the first 2 days of life. Factors contributing to the increase in breastfeeding rates are the rise in the percentage of births occurring at Baby-Friendly hospitals and the increased breastfeeding support from employers (CDC).

The United States has exceeded the Healthy People 2020 goal of 81.9% of infants ever breastfed, as well as the goal of exclusive breastfeeding through 3 months (46.2%). However, the U.S. continues to fall short of meeting Healthy People goal of breastfeeding at 6 months (60.6%) and the goal of exclusive breastfeeding through 6 months (25.5%) (CDC, 2018b; Office of Disease Prevention and Health Promotion [ODPHP], 2018).

Despite increases in national breastfeeding rates, ongoing disparities exist. The lowest breastfeeding rates continue to be among non-Hispanic black infants and among lower income families and those living in rural areas. Younger women (ages 20 to 29) are less likely to breastfeed than those who are 30 years of age or older (CDC, 2018a). Historically, women participating in the Special Supplemental Nutrition Program for Women, Infants, and Children (WIC) have had lower breastfeeding rates than those who were eligible but did not participate and those who were ineligible. In recent years, breastfeeding rates (ever breastfed) among WIC participants have been rising; in 2015, the breastfeeding (ever breastfed) rate among WIC participants was 76.9% (CDC).

Benefits of Breastfeeding

Extensive evidence exists concerning the health benefits of breastfeeding and human milk for infants, with some of the benefits extending into adulthood (Table 25.1). For example, breastfed infants have a decreased incidence of respiratory tract infections, otitis media,

gastrointestinal (GI) infections, and sudden infant death syndrome (SIDS). Benefits are optimized when infants are breastfed exclusively and when the duration of breastfeeding is increased (AAP Section on Breastfeeding, 2012; Grummer-Strawn & Rollins, 2015; Sankar, Sinha, Chowdhury et al., 2015; Victora, Bahl, Barros, et al., 2016).

Breastfeeding is associated with health benefits for mothers, such as reduced risk of breast cancer and ovarian cancer (AAP Section on Breastfeeding, 2012; Chowdhury, Sinha, Sankar, et al., 2015). The benefits are increased with the number of children who were breastfed and the total length of time of lactation.

The psychologic benefits for mothers include enhanced bonding and attachment. For many women, breastfeeding is associated with a sense of empowerment in the ability to provide nutrition for the infant.

Breastfeeding is convenient. The milk is ready to feed and at the proper temperature. In most cases, there is no need for bottles or other equipment unless mother and infant are separated due to work, school or other events,

The economic benefits of breastfeeding affect families, employers, insurers, and the entire nation. Because infant formula is expensive, breastfeeding presents significant savings for families. It reduces health care costs because breastfed infants are ill less often and need fewer prescriptions and visits to their health care providers. Breastfeeding decreases employee absenteeism because parents miss fewer days staying home to care for ill infants.

Breastfeeding has environmental benefits. It reduces the waste that is deposited in landfills, including formula packaging, bottles, nipples, and other equipment. There is no need for fuel to prepare or transport human milk, which saves energy resources.

Infant Feeding Decision-Making

The majority of women make the infant feeding decision either before or during pregnancy. Women tend to select the same method of infant feeding for each of their children. If the first child was breastfed, subsequent children will likely also be breastfed.

The choice of infant feeding method is influenced by a variety of personal and sociocultural factors. The decision may not be as simple as choosing whether to breastfeed or formula-feed; it often is about weighing the positive and negative aspects of breastfeeding (Roll & Cheater, 2016). The evidence supporting breastfeeding as the ideal form of infant nutrition is so strong that health care professionals may need to present information about it from two perspectives: benefits of breastfeeding and risks of not breastfeeding.

For some women, there is a clear choice to either breastfeed or formula-feed. In some cases, women decide to combine breastfeeding and formula-feeding. However, this practice can be associated with a shorter duration of breastfeeding. Some women want their infants to receive breast milk but prefer not to feed directly from their breasts. These women express their milk and bottle-feed it to their infants.

Women most often choose to breastfeed because they are aware of the benefits to the infant. Evidence of the effectiveness of health promotion efforts and activities have raised public awareness of the benefits of breastfeeding for infants, mothers, and families (Roll & Cheater, 2016).

The concept of the maternal role is important in the decision to breastfeed. Women who decide to breastfeed are likely to view breastfeeding as a natural extension of pregnancy and childbirth; it is much more than simply a means of supplying nutrition. Many women seek the unique bonding experience between mother and infant that is characteristic of breastfeeding (Kanhadilok & McGrath, 2015; Roll & Cheater, 2016).

Partner and family support is a major factor in the mother's decision to breastfeed. Women who perceive their partners and family members (especially the maternal grandmother) to prefer breastfeeding are more likely to breastfeed. Women are more likely to breastfeed successfully when partners and family members provide encouragement and support (Kanhadilok & McGrath, 2015; Mueffelmann, Racine, Warren-Findlow, et al., 2015; Odom, Li, Scanlon, et al., 2014; Roll & Cheater, 2016).

Female role models and their transfer of information and sharing of experiences about breastfeeding, either positive or negative, influence the mother's infant feeding decision. Mothers who have observed others breastfeeding may be more likely to breastfeed (Roll & Cheater, 2016).

Cultural factors influence infant feeding decisions. For example, in the Hispanic culture breastfeeding is the norm, whereas formula-feeding is more common among African American families (see the "Cultural Influences on Infant Feeding" section later in the chapter).

For some women and their partners, perceptions of breast function influence the decision to formula-feed. The breast may be seen as a sexual object. There can be modesty issues; women fear embarrassment when having to breastfeed in public. Some women fear pain related to breastfeeding or worry that they will not produce sufficient milk for their infants.

The mother's perception of the practical aspects of feeding influence her decision. Some view breastfeeding as more convenient, while others choose to formula-feed because people other than the mother can bottle-feed the infant. They may think that breastfeeding is time-consuming. They consider formula-feeding as imposing fewer restrictions on family and social life.

Some women initiate breastfeeding in response to pressure from family members, health care professionals, or their own perception of being a "good mother." These women may say they plan to "try breastfeeding," while lacking commitment and determination. They benefit from care by nurses who will help them explore their feelings and concerns and will provide evidenced-based information, support, and assistance.

There appears to be a relationship between maternal weight and infant feeding decisions. Women who are overweight or obese are less likely to breastfeed than women who are underweight or of average weight (Turcksin, Bel, Galjaard, et al., 2014).

Other factors influence decisions about infant nutrition. The widespread marketing by infant formula companies, including free samples through the mail, can encourage women to formula-feed. In addition, there is a lack of prenatal breastfeeding education for expectant parents and insufficient training and education of health care professionals about breastfeeding. In some institutions, the policies and practices do not support exclusive breastfeeding.

A major obstacle to breastfeeding for some women is employment and the need to return to work after birth. Access to breast pumps, pumping facilities, and time for pumping impact a mother's ability to continue breastfeeding when she returns to work or to school. This is especially problematic for women employed in lower-income jobs such as waitressing. More employers are acknowledging the value of providing space and time for the pumping and storage of breastmilk, recognizing that employee absenteeism is reduced among breastfeeding mothers.

Awareness of the availability of breastfeeding resources can influence a mother's decision to breastfeed. For example, women who participate in the WIC program may benefit from information about in-hospital breastfeeding support, peer counseling programs, and breast pump programs.

Health care professionals are influential in the infant feeding decision. Strategies that promote breastfeeding decisions in the prenatal setting include a breastfeeding-friendly office or clinic environment; intentional promotion, education, and support for breastfeeding throughout prenatal care; and discussion of breastfeeding at each prenatal visit (Rosen-Carole, Hartman, & the Academy of Breastfeeding Medicine [ABM], 2015). Because of their significant influence on the mother's decision to breastfeed, partners and family members should be included in discussions about breastfeeding. Through the education, support, and encouragement of health care professionals during the prenatal period, women and their families can make informed decisions about infant feeding (ACOG, 2018; AWHONN, 2015).

Contraindications to Breastfeeding

Breastfeeding is contraindicated in a few circumstances. Newborns who have galactosemia should not receive human milk. Breastfeeding is contraindicated for mothers who are positive for human T-cell lymphotropic virus types I or II and those with untreated brucellosis. Women should not breastfeed if they have active tuberculosis (TB) or if they have active herpes simplex lesions on the breasts. However, neither of these conditions precludes a mother from expressing milk for her infant. Women with active TB can breastfeed when they have been treated for at least 2 weeks and are deemed noninfectious. Varicella that occurs 5 days before or 2 days after birth and acute H1N1 infection require temporary separation of mother and infant. In both instances, it is safe for infants to receive expressed milk (AAP Section on Breastfeeding, 2012).

In the United States, maternal human immunodeficiency virus (HIV) infection is considered a contraindication for breastfeeding (AAP Section on Breastfeeding, 2012). However, this is not true in other countries. In developing countries where HIV is prevalent, the benefits of breastfeeding for infants outweigh the risk of contracting HIV from infected mothers (WHO, 2013).

CULTURAL INFLUENCES ON INFANT FEEDING

Cultural beliefs and practices are significant influences on infant feeding methods. Although recognized cultural norms exist, one cannot assume that generalized observations about any cultural group hold true for all members of that group. Many regional and ethnic cultures are found within the United States. Dealing effectively with these groups requires that nurses are knowledgeable and sensitive to the cultural factors influencing infant feeding practices.

Breastfeeding beliefs and practices vary across cultures. For example, among the Muslim culture, breastfeeding for 24 months is customary. Before the first feeding, rubbing a small piece of softened date on the newborn's palate is a ritual. Because of the cultural emphasis on privacy and modesty, Muslim women may choose to bottle-feed formula or expressed breast milk while in the hospital.

Because of beliefs about the harmful nature or inadequacy of colostrum, some cultures apply restrictions on breastfeeding for a period of days after birth. Such is the case for many cultures in southern Asia, the Pacific Islands, and parts of sub-Saharan Africa. Before the mother's milk is deemed to be "in," babies are fed prelacteal food such as honey or clarified butter in the belief that these substances will help clear out meconium. Other cultures begin breastfeeding immediately and offer the breast each time the infant cries.

A common practice among Mexican women is *las dos cosas* ("both things"). This refers to combining breastfeeding and commercial infant formula. It is based on the belief that by combining the two methods, the mother and infant receive the benefits of breastfeeding, and the infant receives the additional vitamins from infant formula. This practice can result in problems with milk supply and babies refusing to latch on to the breast, which can lead to early termination of breastfeeding.

Cultural expectations influence breastfeeding patterns and behaviors. In many Western cultures, women are more likely to try to "schedule" feeding sessions. This is in contrast to more frequent breastfeeding in some developing countries where mothers "wear" their babies close against their bodies as they go about daily activities. Those babies have constant or frequent access to the breast to feed on demand.

Some cultures have specific beliefs and practices related to the mother's intake of foods that foster milk production. Korean mothers often eat seaweed soup and rice to enhance milk production. Hmong women believe that boiled chicken, rice, and hot water are the only appropriate nourishments during the first postpartum month. The balance between energy forces, hot and cold, or yin and yang is integral to the diet of the lactating mother. Hispanics, Vietnamese, Chinese, East Indians, and Arabs often use this belief in choosing foods. "Hot" foods are considered best for new mothers. This belief does not necessarily relate to the temperature or spiciness of foods. For example, chicken and broccoli are considered "hot," whereas many fresh fruits and vegetables are considered "cold." Families often bring desired foods into the health care setting.

Lactation and Lesbian, Gay, Bisexual, Transgender, Queer/Questioning Families

Increasingly, members of the lesbian, gay, bisexual, transgender, queer/questioning (LGBTQ) community are becoming parents and providing human milk to their infants through a variety of methods. There is a lack of research, clinical papers, and commentaries in the literature on the topic of lactation and the LGBTQ community. These families face lactation and family adjustment issues similar to those of heterosexual mothers, while also dealing with unique challenges (Farrow, 2015). For example, in lesbian couples who become parents, one woman may give birth and breastfeed, and the co-parent may choose to induce lactation so that she can also nurse the baby. Induction of lactation involves frequent pumping and may involve medications. The co-parent may decide to breastfeed using a supplemental feeding device with expressed milk from the mother who gave birth. Transgender men may give birth and provide human milk through breastfeeding (also known as *chest feeding*) (Wolfe-Roubatis & Spatz,

2015); the female partner may also breastfeed by induced lactation or the use of a supplementary feeding device. Same-sex mothers may adopt a newborn who was born to a surrogate; the surrogate may provide expressed milk, and the two adoptive mothers may also breastfeed or feed expressed milk from induced lactation (Wilson, Perrin, Fogleman, et al., 2015). Nurses, lactation consultants, and other health care professionals who care for LGBTQ families can provide more effective care if they are familiar with needs of these parents. Information on resources about lactation and LGBTQ families can be found at http://dianawest.com/lgbtqia-resources/.

NUTRIENT NEEDS

Fluids

During the first 2 days of life, the fluid requirement for healthy infants (more than 1500 g) is 60 to 80 mL/kg of body weight per day. From day 3 to day 7, the requirement is 100 to 150 mL/kg/day; from day 8 to day 30, it is 120 to 180 mL/kg/day (Dell, 2015).

⚡ **SAFETY ALERT**

In general, neither breastfed nor formula-fed infants need to be given water, not even those living in very hot climates. Breast milk contains 87% water, which easily meets daily fluid requirements. Feeding water to infants can decrease caloric consumption at a time when they are growing rapidly. Inappropriate water consumption may also result in hyponatremia, which can subsequently cause seizures.

Infants have room for little fluctuation in fluid balance and should be monitored closely for fluid intake and water loss. They lose water through excretion of urine and insensibly through respiration. Under normal circumstances, they are born with some fluid reserve, and some of the weight loss during the first few days is related to fluid loss. However, in some cases they do not have this fluid reserve, possibly because of inadequate maternal hydration during labor or birth.

Energy

Infants require adequate caloric intake to provide energy for growth, digestion, physical activity, and maintenance of organ metabolic function. Energy needs vary according to age, maturity level, thermal environment, growth rate, health status, and activity level. For the first 3 months, the infant needs 110 kcal/kg/day. From 3 months to 6 months, the requirement is 100 kcal/kg/day. This level decreases slightly to 95 kcal/kg/day from 6 months to 9 months and increases to 100 kcal/kg/day from 9 months to 1 year (AAP Committee on Nutrition, 2014).

Human milk provides an average of 67 kcal/100 mL or 20 kcal/oz. The fat portion of the milk provides the greatest amount of energy. Infant formulas simulate the caloric content of human milk. Usually standard commercial infant formula contains 19 to 20 kcal/oz, although the composition differs among brands.

Carbohydrate

According to the Institute of Medicine (IOM, 2005), the recommended adequate intake (AI) for carbohydrate in the first 6 months of life is 60 g/day and 95 g/day for the second 6 months. Because newborns have only small hepatic glycogen stores, carbohydrates should provide at least 40% to 50% of the total calories in the diet. Moreover, newborns may have a limited ability to carry out gluconeogenesis (the formation of glucose from amino acids and other substrates) and ketogenesis (the formation of ketone bodies from fat), the mechanisms that provide alternative sources of energy.

As the primary carbohydrate in human milk and commercial infant formula, lactose is the most abundant carbohydrate in the diet of infants up to 6 months of age. Lactose provides calories in an easily available form. Its slow breakdown and absorption also increase calcium absorption. Corn syrup solids or glucose polymers are added to infant formulas to supplement the lactose in the cow's milk and thereby provide sufficient carbohydrates.

Oligosaccharides, another form of carbohydrate found in breast milk, are critical in the development of microflora in the intestinal tract of the newborn. These prebiotics promote an acidic environment in the intestines, preventing the growth of gram-negative and other pathogenic bacteria, thus increasing the infant's resistance to GI illness.

Fat

Fats provide a major energy source for infants, supplying as much as 50% of the calories in breast milk and formula. The recommended AI of fat for infants younger than 6 months of age is 31 g/day (IOM, 2005). The fat content of human milk is composed of lipids, triglycerides, and cholesterol; cholesterol is an essential element for brain growth. Human milk contains the essential fatty acids (EFAs) linoleic acid and linolenic acid and the long-chain polyunsaturated fatty acids arachidonic acid (ARA) and docosahexaenoic acid (DHA). Fatty acids are important for growth, neurologic development, and visual function. Cow's milk contains fewer of the EFAs and no polyunsaturated fatty acids. Most formula companies add DHA to their products, although there is a lack of evidence supporting the benefit (Lawrence & Lawrence, 2016). Modified cow's milk is used in most infant formulas, but the milk fat is removed, and another fat source such as corn oil, which the infant can digest and absorb, is added in its place. If whole milk or evaporated milk without added carbohydrate is fed to infants, the resulting fecal loss of fat (and therefore loss of energy) can be excessive because the milk moves through the infant's intestines too quickly for adequate absorption to take place. This can lead to poor weight gain.

Protein

High-quality protein from breast milk, infant formula, or other complementary foods is necessary for infant growth. The protein requirement per unit of body weight is greater in the newborn period than at any other time of life. For infants younger than 6 months of age, the recommended AI for protein is 9.1 g/day (IOM, 2005).

Human milk contains the two proteins whey and casein in a ratio of approximately 70:30 compared with the ratio of 20:80 in some cow's milk–based formulas. This whey-to-casein ratio in human milk makes it more easily digestible and produces the soft stools seen in breastfed infants. The primary whey protein in human milk is α-lactalbumin; this protein is high in the essential amino acids needed for growth. The whey protein lactoferrin in human milk has iron-binding capabilities and bacteriostatic properties, particularly against gram-positive and gram-negative aerobes, anaerobes, and yeasts. The casein in human milk enhances the absorption of iron, thus preventing iron-dependent bacteria from proliferating in the GI tract (Lawrence & Lawrence, 2016). The amino acid components of human milk are uniquely suited to the newborn's metabolic capabilities. For example, cystine and taurine levels are high, whereas phenylalanine and methionine levels are low.

Vitamins

With the exception of vitamin D, human milk contains all of the vitamins required for infant nutrition, with individual variations based on maternal diet and genetic differences. Vitamins are added to cow's milk–based formulas to resemble levels found in breast milk. Although cow's milk contains adequate amounts of vitamins A and B complex, vitamin C (ascorbic acid), vitamin E, and vitamin D must be added.

Vitamin D facilitates intestinal absorption of calcium and phosphorus, bone mineralization, and calcium resorption from bone. According to the AAP and the ABM, all infants who are breastfed should receive 400 to 800 International Units of vitamin D daily, beginning the first few days of life. There is evidence that maternal intake of 6400 IU/day may provide adequate vitamin D for her breastfeeding infant (Taylor & the ABM, 2018; Wagner, Grier, & AAP Section on Breastfeeding and Committee on Nutrition, 2008). Nonbreastfeeding infants and older children who consume less than 1 quart/day of vitamin D–fortified milk should also receive 400 International Units of vitamin D each day (Wagner, et al.).

Vitamin K, required for blood coagulation, is produced by intestinal bacteria. However, the gut is sterile at birth, and a few days are required for intestinal flora to become established and produce vitamin K. To prevent hemorrhagic problems in the newborn, an injection of vitamin K is given at birth to all newborns in the United States and Canada, regardless of feeding method (AAP Section on Breastfeeding, 2012; McMillan & Canadian Paediatric Society Fetus and Newborn Committee, 1997/2016). (See the Medication Guide: Vitamin K: Phytonandione [AquaMEPHYTON, Konakion] in Chapter 24.)

The breastfed infant's vitamin B_{12} intake depends on the mother's dietary intake and stores. Mothers who are on strict vegetarian (vegan) diets and those who consume few dairy products, eggs, or meat are at risk for vitamin B_{12} deficiency. Mothers who have had bariatric surgery are also at risk for vitamin B_{12} deficiency. Breastfeeding infants may need vitamin B_{12} supplements in these instances.

Minerals

The mineral content of commercial infant formula is designed to reflect that of breast milk. Unmodified cow's milk is much higher in mineral content than human milk, which also makes it unsuitable for infants during the first year of life. Minerals are typically highest in human milk during the first few days after birth and decrease slightly throughout lactation.

The ratio of calcium to phosphorus in human milk is 2:1, an optimal proportion for bone mineralization. Although cow's milk is high in calcium, the calcium-to-phosphorus ratio is low, resulting in decreased calcium absorption. Consequently, young infants fed unmodified cow's milk are at risk for hypocalcemia, seizures, and tetany. The calcium-to-phosphorus ratio in commercial infant formula is between that of human milk and cow's milk.

Iron levels are low in all types of milk; however, iron from human milk is better absorbed than iron from cow's milk, iron-fortified formula, or infant cereals. Breastfed infants draw on iron reserves deposited in utero and benefit from the high lactose and vitamin C levels in human milk that facilitate iron absorption. Full-term infants have enough iron stores from the mother to last for the first 4 to 5 months. After 4 months of age, infants who are exclusively breastfed are at risk for iron deficiency. The AAP recommends giving exclusively breastfed infants an iron supplement (1 mg/kg/day) beginning at 4 months and continuing until the infant is consuming iron-containing complementary foods such as iron-fortified cereals. Infants who are partially breastfed should receive the same iron supplement if more than half of their daily feedings consist of human milk and they are not consuming iron-rich foods. Formula-feeding infants should receive an iron-fortified commercial infant formula until 12 months of age. Infants younger than 1 year of age should never be fed whole milk (Baker, Greer, & AAP Committee on Nutrition, 2010).

Fluoride levels in human milk and commercial formulas are low. This mineral, which is important in preventing dental caries, can cause spotting of the permanent teeth (fluorosis) in excess amounts. Experts recommend that no fluoride supplements are given to infants younger than 6 months of age. From 6 months to 3 years of age, fluoride supplements are based on the concentration of fluoride in the water supply (AAP Section on Breastfeeding, 2012).

ANATOMY AND PHYSIOLOGY OF LACTATION

Anatomy of the Lactating Breast

Each female breast is composed of approximately 15 to 20 segments (lobes) embedded in fat and connective tissues and well supplied with blood vessels, lymphatic vessels, and nerves (Fig. 25.1). Within each lobe is glandular tissue consisting of alveoli, the milk-producing cells, surrounded by myoepithelial cells that contract to send the milk forward to the nipple during milk ejection. Each nipple has multiple pores that transfer milk to the suckling infant. The ratio of glandular to adipose tissue in the lactating breast is approximately 2:1 compared with a 1:1 ratio in the nonlactating breast. Within each breast is a complex, intertwining network of milk ducts that transport milk from the alveoli to the nipple. The milk ducts dilate and expand with milk ejection (Fig. 25.2).

The size and shape of the breast are not accurate indicators of its ability to produce milk. Although nearly every woman can lactate, a small number have insufficient mammary gland development to breastfeed their infants exclusively. Typically, these women experience few breast changes during puberty or early pregnancy. In some cases, they are still able to produce some breast milk, although the quantity is not likely to be sufficient to meet the nutritional needs of the infant. These mothers can offer supplemental nutrition to support optimal infant growth.

Because of the effects of estrogen, progesterone, human placental lactogen, and other hormones of pregnancy, changes occur in the breasts in preparation for lactation. Breasts increase in size due to growth of glandular and adipose tissue. Blood flow to the breasts nearly doubles during pregnancy. Sensitivity of the breasts increases, and veins become more prominent. The nipples become more erect, and the areolae darken. Nipples and areola enlarge. At around week 16 of gestation, the alveoli begin producing prepartum milk, or colostrum. Montgomery glands on the areola enlarge. The oily substance secreted by these sebaceous glands helps to protect the nipples against the mechanical stress of sucking and invasion by pathogens. The odor of the secretions can be a means of communication with the infant.

Lactogenesis

After the mother gives birth, a precipitous fall in progesterone triggers the release of prolactin from the anterior pituitary gland. During pregnancy, prolactin prepares the breasts to secrete milk and during lactation to synthesize and secrete milk. Prolactin levels are highest during the first 10 days after birth, gradually declining over time but remaining above baseline levels for the duration of lactation. Prolactin is produced in response to infant suckling and emptying of the breasts (Fig. 25.3A). Milk production is a supply-meets-demand system (i.e., as milk is removed from the breast, more is produced). Incomplete removal of milk from the breasts can lead to decreased milk supply.

Oxytocin is essential to lactation. As the nipple is stimulated by the suckling infant, the posterior pituitary gland is prompted by the hypothalamus to produce oxytocin. This hormone is responsible for the milk ejection reflex (MER), or let-down reflex (see Fig. 25.3B). The myoepithelial cells surrounding the alveoli respond to oxytocin by contracting and sending the milk forward through the ducts to the nipple. The MER is triggered multiple times during a feeding session. Thoughts, sights, sounds, or odors that the mother associates with her baby (or other babies), such as hearing the baby cry, can trigger the MER. Many women report a tingling "pins and needles" sensation in

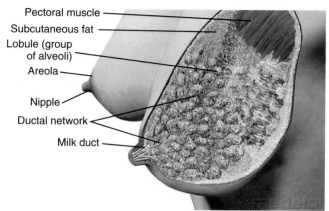

Fig. 25.1 Anatomy of the Lactating Breast. (Copyright 2017 by Medela LLC.)

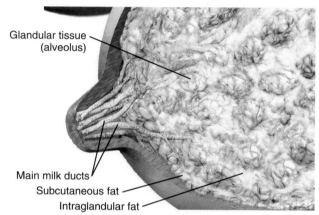

Fig. 25.2 Enhanced View of Milk Glands and Ducts. (Copyright 2017 by Medela LLC.)

the breasts as milk ejection occurs, although some mothers can detect milk ejection only by observing the sucking and swallowing of the infant. The MER also can occur during sexual activity because oxytocin is released during orgasm. The reflex can be inhibited by fear, stress, and alcohol consumption.

Oxytocin is the same hormone that stimulates uterine contractions during labor. Consequently, the MER can be triggered during labor, as evidenced by leakage of colostrum. This reflex readies the breasts for immediate feeding by the infant after birth. Oxytocin has the important function of contracting the mother's uterus after birth to control postpartum bleeding and promote uterine involution. Thus mothers who breastfeed are at decreased risk for postpartum hemorrhage. Uterine contractions that occur with breastfeeding are often painful during and after feeding for the first 3 to 5 days. These after pains are more common in multiparas and tend to resolve completely within 1 week after birth.

Prolactin and oxytocin have been called the "mothering hormones" because they affect the postpartum woman's emotions and her physical state. Many women report feeling thirsty or very relaxed during breastfeeding, probably as a result of these hormones.

The nipple-erection reflex is an important part of lactation. When the infant cries, suckles, or rubs against the breast, the nipple becomes erect, which aids in the propulsion of milk through the ducts to the nipple pores. Nipple sizes, shapes, and ability to become erect vary with individuals. Some women have flat or inverted nipples that do not become erect with stimulation; these women likely need assistance

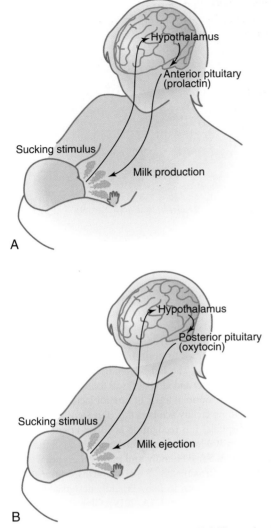

Fig. 25.3 Maternal Breastfeeding Reflexes. (A) Milk production. (B) Milk ejection (let-down).

with effective latch. Their infants should not be offered bottles or pacifiers until breastfeeding is well established.

Uniqueness of Human Milk

Human milk is the ideal food for human infants. It is a dynamic substance with a composition that changes to meet the changing nutritional and immunologic needs of the growing infant. Breast milk is specific to the needs of each infant; for example, the milk produced by mothers of preterm infants differs in composition from that of mothers who give birth at term.

Human milk contains immunologically active components that provide some protection against a broad spectrum of bacterial, viral, and protozoal infections. The major immunoglobulin (Ig) in human milk is secretory IgA; IgG, IgM, IgD, and IgE are also present. Human milk also contains T lymphocytes and B lymphocytes, epidermal growth factor, cytokines, interleukins, bifidus factor, complement (C3 and C4), and lactoferrin, all of which have a specific role in preventing localized and systemic bacterial and viral infections (Lawrence & Lawrence, 2016).

Breast milk promotes colonization and maturation of the infant's intestinal microbiome, which is essential to development of the immune system. The bacteria in human milk vary according to the stage of lactogenesis and gestational age of the infant. Maternal health

status and mode of birth affect breast milk microbiota. The predominant flora of breastfed infants are *L. bifidus* and *Bifidobacterium* spp., which metabolize milk saccharides and lower the pH of infant stool; this limits the growth of pathogenic bacteria such as *E. coli*, *Bacteroides*, and *Staphylococcus*. In contrast, the gut microbiota of the formula-fed infant are predominantly gram-negative bacteria, especially *Bacteroides Clostridium*, *Enterobacter*, and *Enterococcus* (Lawrence & Lawrence, 2016; Mueller, Bakacs, Combellick, et al., 2015). Antibiotics, cesarean birth, and formula-feeding can alter the gut microbiome and may be causally associated with development of autoimmune and metabolic diseases (Mueller et al.).

Human milk composition and volumes vary according to the stage of lactation. In lactogenesis stage I, beginning at approximately 16 to 18 weeks of pregnancy, the breasts prepare for milk production by producing prepartum milk, or colostrum. Stage II of lactogenesis begins with birth as progesterone levels drop sharply when the placenta is removed. For the first 2 to 3 days after birth, the baby receives colostrum, a clear, yellowish fluid that is rich in antibodies and higher in protein but lower in fat than mature milk. The high protein level of colostrum facilitates binding of bilirubin, and the laxative action of colostrum promotes the early passage of meconium. Colostrum is important in establishing normal *Lactobacillus bifidus* flora in the infant's digestive tract. It gradually changes to transitional milk. By 3 to 5 days after birth, the woman experiences a noticeable increase in milk production. While this is often referred to as *the milk coming in*, it is a misnomer. It is more appropriate to use the phrase *transitioning from colostrum to mature milk*. To some women, the phrase *milk coming in* implies that the milk is not present. Breast milk continues to change in composition for approximately 10 days, when the mature milk is established. This is stage III of lactogenesis (Lawrence & Lawrence, 2016).

The composition of human milk changes over time as the infant grows and develops. Fat is the most variable component of human milk with changes in concentration over a feeding, over a 24-hour period, and across time. Variations in fat content exist between breasts and among individuals. During each feeding, the concentration of fat gradually increases from the lower fat foremilk to the richer hindmilk. The hindmilk contains the denser calories from fat necessary for ensuring optimal growth and contentment between feedings. Because of this changing composition of human milk during each feeding, breastfeeding the infant long enough to supply a balanced feeding is important.

Milk production gradually increases as the baby grows. Infants have fairly predictable growth spurts (at approximately 10 days, 3 weeks, 6 weeks, 3 months, and 6 months), when more frequent feedings stimulate increased milk production. These growth spurts usually last 24 to 48 hours, after which the infants resume their usual feeding pattern as the mother's milk supply increases.

CARE MANAGEMENT

Supporting Breastfeeding Mothers and Infants

Nurses interact with women in a variety of preconception, prenatal, intrapartum, and postpartum settings. These interactions are strategic opportunities to provide breastfeeding education and support to women and their families (AWHONN, 2015).

The key to encouraging mothers to breastfeed is education and anticipatory guidance, beginning as early as possible during and even before pregnancy. Each encounter with an expectant mother is an opportunity to educate, dispel myths, clarify misinformation, identify risk factors, and address concerns. Prenatal education and preparation for breastfeeding influence feeding decisions, breastfeeding success, and the amount of time that women breastfeed. Prenatal preparation ideally includes the father of the baby, partner, or another significant support person and provides information about benefits of breastfeeding and how he or she can participate in infant care and nurturing. Nurses begin by assessing knowledge of the woman and her family about breastfeeding, providing information, and helping them develop breastfeeding goals and a breastfeeding plan (AWHONN, 2015). Education about breastfeeding is provided through a variety of methods, including one-on-one or group sessions, printed materials, videos, and electronic media such as websites and phone apps.

As part of the admission assessment to the birthing unit, the nurse asks the woman if she is planning to breastfeed and if she and her partner or family members are knowledgeable about the benefits of breastfeeding and the risks of infants not receiving human milk. The nurse assesses the breasts and nipples and examines the obstetric and medical history for factors that may influence lactation. The events during labor and birth, including medications and any complications that occur such as emergent cesarean or neonatal resuscitation, can influence breastfeeding and should be communicated to the postpartum nurse who can share this information with the lactation consultant (AWHONN, 2015). The labor and birth nurse assists the mother with initial breastfeeding after birth while the infant is skin-to-skin, providing encouragement and support.

For women with limited access to health care, the postpartum period may provide the first opportunity for education about breastfeeding. Even women who have indicated the desire to formula-feed can benefit from information about the benefits of breastfeeding. Offering these women the chance to try breastfeeding with the assistance of a nurse or lactation consultant can influence a change in infant feeding practices.

Promoting feelings of competence and confidence in the breastfeeding mother and reinforcing the unequaled contribution she is making toward the health and well-being of her infant are the responsibility of the nurse and other health care professionals. The first 2 weeks of breastfeeding can be the most challenging as mothers are adjusting to life with a newborn, the baby is learning to latch on and feed effectively, and the mother may be experiencing nipple or breast discomfort. This is a time when support is critical. Anticipatory guidance during the prenatal period and especially during the hospital stay after birth can provide the mother with information and increase her confidence in her ability to successfully breastfeed her infant. New mothers need access to lactation support following discharge through primary care offices or outpatient lactation services.

Connecting expectant mothers with women from similar backgrounds who are breastfeeding or have successfully breastfed is often helpful. Nursing mothers' support groups, such as La Leche League, provide information about breastfeeding, along with opportunities for breastfeeding mothers to interact with one another and share concerns (Fig. 25.4). Community-based peer counseling programs such as those instituted by the WIC program are beneficial.

The most common reasons for breastfeeding cessation are insufficient milk supply, painful nipples, and problems getting the infant to feed (Lawrence & Lawrence, 2016). Early and ongoing assistance and support from health care professionals to prevent and address problems with breastfeeding can help promote a successful and satisfying breastfeeding experience for mothers and infants. Many health care agencies have certified lactation consultants on staff. These health care professionals, many who are nurses, have specialized training and experience in helping breastfeeding mothers and infants.

The U.S. Breastfeeding Committee (USBC, 2010a) has identified key competencies for health care professionals related to breastfeeding care and services. The competencies include knowledge, skills, and attitudes to promote and support breastfeeding. The USBC identifies specific competencies for those who provide more "hands-on" care (e.g., nurses and lactation consultants). The competencies are to "assist

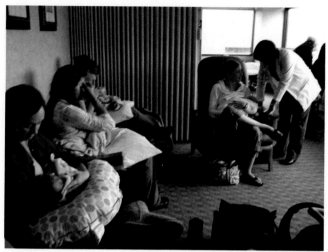

Fig. 25.4 Breastfeeding Mothers Support Group With Lactation Consultant. (Courtesy Shannon Perry, Phoenix, AZ.)

in early initiation of breastfeeding, assess the lactating breast, perform an infant feeding observation, recognize normal and abnormal infant feeding patterns, and develop and appropriately communicate a breastfeeding care plan" (USBC, 2010a, p. 5).

All parents are entitled to a birthing environment that promotes and supports breastfeeding. The Baby-Friendly Hospital Initiative (BFHI), sponsored by the WHO and UNICEF, was founded in 1991 to encourage institutions to offer optimal levels of care for lactating mothers. When a hospital or birthing facility achieves the "Ten Steps to Successful Breastfeeding for Hospitals," it is recognized as "Baby-Friendly" (Box 25.1). In 2018, more than 500 hospitals and birthing centers in the United States were designated as Baby-Friendly, and many others are working toward the designation. Approximately 25% of live births, or more than 1 million babies each year, are born in Baby-Friendly designated facilities in the United States (Baby-Friendly USA, 2019). Globally, only 10% of births occur in facilities with designation or re-assessment as Baby-Friendly in the previous 5 years (WHO, 2017). Women are more likely to achieve their goals for exclusive breastfeeding if they give birth in facilities where all or most of the 10 steps are in place.

The Joint Commission (TJC) issued a set of Perinatal Core Measures that includes exclusive breast milk feeding. In implementing the core measures, hospitals strive to improve their adherence to evidence-based best practices that can result in increased rates of exclusive breastfeeding (TJC, 2012; USBC, 2010b). Care management of the breastfeeding mother and infant requires that nurses and other health care professionals are knowledgeable about the benefits and basic anatomic and physiologic aspects of breastfeeding. They also need to know how to help the mother with feedings and discuss interventions for common problems. Ongoing support of the mother enhances her self-confidence and promotes a satisfying and successful breastfeeding experience. Mothers should be encouraged to ask for help with breastfeeding, especially while they are in the hospital. Women most likely to need assistance are primiparas as well as multiparas who formula-fed their other children or had difficulty breastfeeding previously. In many facilities, these women are routinely seen by lactation consultants.

Breastfeeding Initiation

The mother needs to understand infant behaviors in relation to breastfeeding and recognize signs that the baby is ready to feed. Infants exhibit **feeding-readiness cues** or early signs of hunger. Instead of waiting to feed until the infant is crying in a distraught manner or withdrawing into sleep, the mother should attempt to breastfeed when the baby exhibits feeding cues:

BOX 25.1 Ten Steps to Successful Breastfeeding (revised 2018)

Critical Management Procedures

1. a. Comply fully with the International Code of Marketing of Breast-milk Substitutes and relevant World Health Assembly resolutions.
   b. Have a written infant feeding policy that is routinely communicated to staff and parents.
   c. Establish ongoing monitoring and data-management systems.
2. Ensure that staff have sufficient knowledge, competence and skills to support breastfeeding.

Key Clinical Practices

3. Discuss the importance and management of breastfeeding with pregnant women and their families.
4. Facilitate immediate and uninterrupted skin-to-skin contact and support mothers to initiate breastfeeding as soon as possible after birth.
5. Support mothers to initiate and maintain breastfeeding and manage common difficulties.
6. Do not provide breastfed newborns any food or fluids other than breast milk, unless medically indicated.
7. Enable mothers and their infants to remain together and to practice rooming-in 24 hours a day.
8. Support mothers to recognize and respond to their infants' cues for feeding.
9. Counsel mothers on the use and risks of feeding bottles, teats and pacifiers.
10. Coordinate discharge so that parents and their infants have timely access to ongoing support and care.

From World Health Organization. (2018). *Protecting, promoting and supporting breastfeeding in facilities providing maternity and newborn services: The revised Baby-Friendly Hospital Initiative.* Geneva, Switzerland: Author.

- Sucking or mouthing motions
- Hand-to-mouth or hand-to-hand movements
- Rooting reflex—infant moves toward whatever touches the area around the mouth and attempts to suck

Babies normally consume small amounts of milk with feedings during the first 3 days of life. As the baby adjusts to extrauterine life and the digestive tract is cleared of meconium, milk intake increases from 5 to 15 mL per feeding in the first 24 hours to 60 to 90 mL by the end of the first week (Kellams, Harrel, Omage, et al., 2017).

In the postpartum period, interventions focus on helping the mother and the newborn initiate successful breastfeeding. An important goal is to build maternal confidence in breastfeeding. Interventions to promote successful breastfeeding include educating and assisting mothers and their partners with basics such as latch and positioning, signs of adequate feeding, and self-care measures such as prevention of engorgement. It is important to provide the parents with a list of resources that they can contact after discharge from the birthing facility.

The ideal time to begin breastfeeding is within the first hour after birth. Newborns without complications should be allowed to remain in direct skin-to-skin contact with the mother until the baby is able to breastfeed for the first time. This is true both for mothers who gave birth by cesarean and for those who gave birth vaginally. Routine procedures such as vitamin K injection, eye prophylaxis, weighing, and bathing should be delayed until the neonate has completed the first feeding (AAP Section on Breastfeeding, 2012).

Positioning

Each mother will determine which breastfeeding position or positions work best for her and her infant. Sometimes this takes experimenting with a variety of positions. The nurse can assist the mother and infant to try different positions prior to discharge from the birthing facility.

For the initial feedings, it can be advantageous to encourage and assist the mother to breastfeed in a semi-reclining position with the newborn lying prone, skin-to-skin on the mother's bare chest. Her body supports the baby. The mother is more relaxed, nipple pain is reduced or eliminated, and she has more freedom of movement to use her hands. The baby is able to use inborn reflexes to latch onto the breast and feed effectively. This approach to breastfeeding is based on the concept of "biological nurturing" (Colson, 2012) (www.biological-nurturing.com) and is often referred to as "laid-back nursing." Some mothers prefer this position even after the early days of breastfeeding

The four traditional positions for breastfeeding are the football or clutch hold (under the arm), across the lap (cross-cradle or modified cradle), cradle, and side-lying (Fig. 25.5). The mother should be encouraged to use the position that most easily facilitates latch while allowing maximal comfort. The football or clutch hold is often recommended for early feedings because the mother can see the baby's mouth easily as she guides the infant onto the nipple. Mothers who gave birth by cesarean often prefer the football or clutch hold. The modified cradle or across-the-lap hold works well for early feedings, especially with smaller babies. The side-lying position allows the mother to rest while breastfeeding. Women with perineal pain and swelling often prefer this position. Cradling is the most common breastfeeding position for infants who have learned to latch easily and feed effectively. Before discharge from the birth institution, the nurse can help the mother try all of the positions so she will be confident in trying these positions at home.

During breastfeeding, the mother should be as comfortable as possible. After arranging for privacy, the nurse might suggest that she empty her bladder and attend to other needs before starting a feeding session. The nurse or lactation consultant who is assisting with breastfeeding should be at the mother's eye level. The mother holds the infant securely at the level of the breast, supported by firm pillows or folded blankets, facing toward her. The baby's mouth is directly in front of the nipple. The mother should support the baby's neck and shoulders with her hand and not push on the occiput. The baby's body is held in alignment (ears, shoulders, and hips are in a straight line) during latch and feeding.

The nurse can teach and encourage the woman's partner to be involved with feedings; for example, the partner can assist the mother to find a comfortable position and help her with placement of pillows or other supportive surfaces (e.g., folded blankets) (Fig. 25.6). The degree of involvement by the partner often depends on the mother's desire for assistance from that person and on the partner's willingness and comfort level in providing assistance; the astute nurse is careful to assess their interactions prior to seeking partner involvement in breastfeeding.

Latch

Latch, or latch-on, is defined as placement of the infant's mouth over the nipple, areola, and breast, making a seal between the mouth and breast to create adequate suction for milk removal. In preparation for latch during early feedings, the mother should manually express a few drops of colostrum or milk and spread it over the nipple. This action lubricates the nipple and entices the baby to open the mouth as the milk is tasted.

To facilitate latch, the mother supports her breast in one hand with the thumb on top and four fingers underneath at the back edge of the areola. The breast is compressed slightly with the fingers parallel to the infant's lips, as one might compress a large sandwich in preparing to take a bite, so an adequate amount of breast tissue is taken into the mouth with latch. Most mothers need to support the breast during feeding until the infant is adept at feeding.

The mother holds the baby close to the breast with the infant's mouth directly in front of the nipple. The infant who is displaying the rooting reflex with the mouth opening widely may easily latch on. If the infant is not readily opening the mouth, the mother tickles the

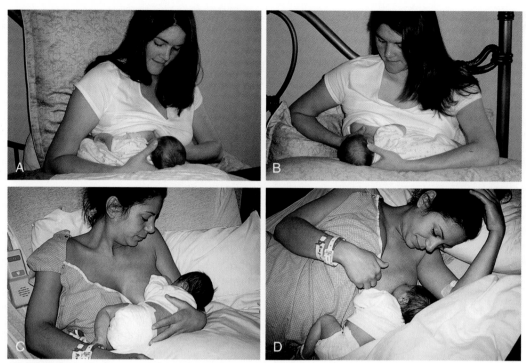

Fig. 25.5 Breastfeeding Positions. (A) Football or clutch (under the arm) hold. (B) Across the lap (modified cradle or cross-cradle). (C) Cradling. (D) Side-lying. ([A and B] Courtesy Allison and Matthew Wyatt, Eagle, CO; [C and D] Courtesy Marjorie Pyle, RNC, Lifecircle, Costa Mesa, CA.)

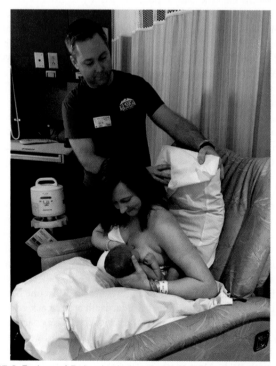

Fig. 25.6 Father of Baby Assisting the Breastfeeding Mother; Note Placement of Pillows for Support. Baby is in football (clutch) hold; mother is supporting her breast with "C-hold." Hospital grade breast pump is at right of the mother's chair. (Courtesy Erin and Josh Evans, Richmond, VA.)

baby's lips with her nipple, stimulating the mouth to open. When the mouth is open wide and the tongue is down, the mother quickly "hugs" the baby to the breast, bringing him or her onto the nipple. The amount of areola in the baby's mouth with correct latch depends on the size of the baby's mouth and the size of the areola and nipple. If breastfeeding is painful, the baby likely has not taken enough of the breast into the mouth, and the tongue is pinching the nipple.

Mothers may use the *asymmetric latch technique.* When the baby's mouth opens widely, the mother moves the baby in toward her body so the chin and lower mandible make contact with the breast first, followed by the top lip. When the baby is latched on, the nose is tilted slightly away from the mother's breast, and the chin is pressed into the underside of the breast. The infant's mouth placement is asymmetric on the areola; the lower part is covered by the baby's mouth, but the top is clearly visible above the top lip.

Once the infant is latched on and sucking (Fig. 25.7), there are signs that the feeding is going well. These include (1) the mother reports a firm tugging sensation on her nipple but feels no pinching or pain; (2) the baby sucks with cheeks rounded, not dimpled; (3) the baby's jaw glides smoothly with sucking; and (4) swallowing is usually audible. Sucking creates a vacuum in the intraoral cavity as the breast is compressed between the tongue and the palate. When the infant is latched on and sucking correctly, breastfeeding is not painful. If the mother feels pinching or pain after the initial sucks or does not feel a strong tugging sensation on the nipple, the latch and positioning are evaluated. Any time the signs of adequate latch and sucking are not present, the baby should be taken off the breast and latch should be attempted again. To prevent nipple trauma as the baby is taken off the breast, the mother is instructed to break the suction by inserting a finger in the side of the baby's mouth between the gums and leaving it there until the nipple is completely out of the mouth (Fig. 25.8; see Nursing Care Plan).

◉ NURSING CARE PLAN

Breastfeeding and Infant Nutrition

Client Problem or Need	Expected Outcome	Nursing Interventions	Rationale
Lack of knowledge about breastfeeding as evidenced by primiparity and no prenatal education related to breastfeeding	Mother will verbalize understanding and demonstrate correct positioning and latch technique. Mother will report no nipple pain with infant suckling.	Assess knowledge about breastfeeding. Observe feeding session at least once every shift and assist as needed with positioning and latch. Instruct mother about signs of effective feeding and other aspects of breastfeeding; give her a list of available resources (local and web-based).	To provide starting point for teaching. To provide baseline assessment and monitoring of progress. To prepare her for what to expect in the days ahead and to be able to seek help as needed.
Difficulty with latch and milk transfer related to sleepy infant as evidenced by infant's lack of output	Infant will latch and suck effectively with evidence of milk transfer. Infant will awaken and breastfeed every 2-3 h for least 15-20 min. Infant will void at least 2-3 times in the next 24 h and will have at least one bowel movement	Teach mother to observe for feeding-readiness cues. Assist mother with techniques to awaken infant, including skin-to-skin contact, massage, changing diaper; and assist her with latch and keeping the infant awake during feeding. Closely monitor and document infant's output; assess daily weight	To identify signs that the infant may be ready to feed. To gently awaken infant in readiness for feeding and to keep the infant awake and sucking to allow milk transfer. To assess for signs of dehydration
Anxiety about ability to produce adequate milk supply as evidenced by stated concerns	Mother will state signs that infant is receiving adequate breast milk. Mother will verbalize understanding of factors influencing milk production. Mother will identify resources for help with concerns related to milk supply postdischarge.	Teach mother signs of effective breastfeeding (e.g., infant urine and stool output, weight gain, behavior; breasts softening with feeding) Assess for factors that may impact milk production. Teach mother about supply meets demand principle of milk production and importance of regular feeding and/or pumping; teach her how to hand express her milk. Refer her to a lactation consultant and provide list of available resources in the community and through the internet.	To enable mother to recognize if milk supply may be in sufficient. To address any risk factors and to reduce her anxiety by empowering her with knowledge. To decrease her anxiety and provide needed information and support

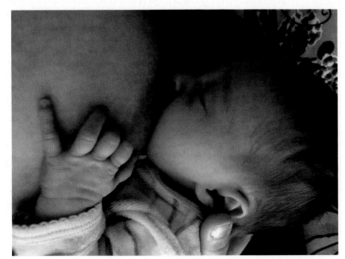

Fig. 25.7 Newborn Latched On and Feeding. (Courtesy Kathryn Alden, Apex, NC.)

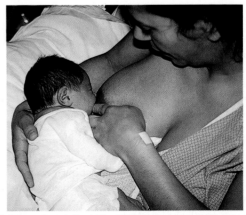

Fig. 25.8 Removing Infant From Breast by Inserting a Finger to Break Suction. (Courtesy Marjorie Pyle, RNC, Lifecircle, Costa Mesa, CA.)

Milk Ejection or Let-Down

As the baby begins sucking on the nipple, the milk ejection, or let-down, reflex is stimulated (see Fig. 25.3B). The following signs indicate that milk ejection has occurred:

- The mother may feel a tingling sensation in the nipples and breasts, although many women never feel when milk ejection occurs.
- The baby's suck changes from quick, shallow sucks to a slower, more drawing sucking pattern.
- Audible swallowing is heard as the baby sucks.
- In the early days, the mother feels uterine cramping and can have increased lochia during and after feedings.
- The mother feels relaxed or drowsy during feedings.
- The opposite breast may leak.

Frequency of Feedings

Feeding patterns vary because every mother-infant dyad is unique. Breastfeeding frequency is influenced by a variety of factors, including the infant's age, weight, maturity level, stomach capacity and gastric emptying time, and the storage capacity of the breast (i.e., the milk available when the breast is full).

Newborns need to breastfeed at least 8 to 12 times in a 24-hour period (AAP Section on Breastfeeding, 2012). Some infants breastfeed every 2 to 3 hours throughout a 24-hour period. Others cluster-feed, breastfeeding every hour or so for three to five feedings and then sleeping for 3 to 4 hours between clusters. During the first 24 to 48 hours after birth, most babies do not awaken often enough to feed. Parents need to understand that they need to awaken the baby to feed at least every 3 hours during the day and at least every 4 hours at night. (Feeding frequency is determined by counting from the beginning of one feeding to the beginning of the next.) Once the infant is feeding well and gaining weight adequately, going to demand feeding is appropriate, in which case the infant determines the frequency of feedings. (With demand feeding, the infant should still receive at least eight feedings in 24 hours.)

⚡ SAFETY ALERT

Nurses should caution parents against attempting to place newborn infants on strict feeding schedules. Strict scheduling of feedings (forcing the baby to wait for a set amount of time before feeding) can result in failure to meet the nutritional needs of infants.

Infants should be fed whenever they exhibit feeding cues. This is known as "cue-based feeding." Keeping the baby close is the best way to observe and respond to these cues. Newborns should remain with mothers during the recovery period after birth and room-in during the hospital stay. At home, babies should be kept nearby so parents can observe signs that the baby is ready to feed. The mother and breastfeeding infant should sleep in proximity (in the same room but not in the same bed) to promote breastfeeding (AAP Section on Breastfeeding, 2012).

Duration of Feedings

The duration of breastfeeding sessions varies greatly because the timing of milk transfer differs for each mother-baby pair. The average time for early feedings is 30 to 40 minutes or approximately 15 to 20 minutes per breast. As infants grow, they become more efficient at breastfeeding, and consequently the length of feedings decreases. The amount of time an infant spends breastfeeding is not a reliable indicator of the amount of milk the infant consumes because some of the time at the breast is spent in nonnutritive sucking.

In the early days after birth, the mother may be instructed to feed on the first breast until the neonate falls asleep and try to wake the baby and offer the second breast. Some mothers prefer one-sided nursing, which means that the baby nurses only one breast at each feeding. The first breast offered should be alternated at each feeding to ensure that each breast receives equal stimulation and emptying.

Instead of instructing mothers to feed for a set number of minutes, nurses should teach them to look for signs that the baby has finished feeding (e.g., the baby's sucking and swallowing pattern has slowed, the breast is softened, the baby appears content and may fall asleep or release the nipple).

If a baby seems to be feeding effectively and urine output and bowel movements are adequate but the weight gain is not satisfactory, the mother may be switching to the second breast too soon. Feeding on the first breast until it softens ensures that the baby receives the higher-fat hindmilk, which usually results in increased weight gain.

Indicators of Effective Breastfeeding

One of the most common concerns of breastfeeding mothers is how to determine if the baby is getting enough milk. In the newborn period, when breastfeeding is becoming established, parents should be taught about the signs that breastfeeding is going well. Awareness of these signs helps them recognize when problems arise so they can seek appropriate assistance (Box 25.2).

During the early days of breastfeeding, keeping a feeding diary can be helpful. This involves recording the time and length of feedings and infant urine output and bowel movements. The data from the diary provide evidence of the effectiveness of breastfeeding and are useful to health care providers in assessing adequacy of feeding. Parents are instructed to take this feeding diary to the follow-up visit with the infant's health care provider. There are smartphone apps that parents can use to track infant feedings and urine/stool output.

The infant's output is highly indicative of feeding adequacy. It is important that parents are aware of the expected changes in the characteristics of urine output and bowel movements during the early newborn period. As the volume of breast milk increases, urine becomes more dilute and should be light yellow; dark, concentrated urine can be associated with inadequate intake and possible dehydration. (Note: Infants with jaundice often have darker urine as bilirubin is excreted.)

BOX 25.2   Signs of Effective Breastfeeding

Mother

- Onset of copious milk production (milk is "in") by day 3 or 4
- Firm tugging sensation on nipple as infant sucks but no pain
- Uterine contractions and increased vaginal bleeding while feeding (first week or less)
- Feels relaxed and drowsy while feeding
- Increased thirst
- Breasts soften or feel lighter while feeding
- With milk ejection (let-down), can feel warm rush or tingling in breasts, leaking of milk from opposite breast

Infant

- Latches without difficulty
- Has bursts of 15 to 20 sucks/swallows at a time
- Audible swallowing is present
- Easily releases breast at end of feeding
- Infant appears content after feeding
- Has at least three substantive bowel movements and six to eight wet diapers every 24 hrs after day 4.

Infants should have at least six to eight sufficiently wet diapers (light yellow urine) every 24 hours after day 4. The first 1 to 2 days after birth, newborns pass meconium stools, which are greenish black, thick, and sticky. By day 2 or 3, the stools become greener, thinner, and less sticky. If the mother's milk has transitioned by day 3 or 4, the stools start to appear greenish yellow and are looser. By the end of the first week, breast milk stools are yellow, soft, and seedy (they resemble a mixture of mustard and cottage cheese). If an infant is still passing meconium stool by day 3 or 4, breastfeeding effectiveness and milk transfer should be assessed.

Infants should have at least three stools (quarter-size or larger) per day for the first month. Some babies stool with every feeding. The stooling pattern gradually changes; breastfed infants can continue to stool more than once per day, or they may stool only every 2 or 3 days. As long as the baby continues to gain weight and appears healthy, this decrease in the number of bowel movements is normal.

Assessment of Effective Breastfeeding

The nurse should observe at least one breastfeeding session every 8 to 12 hours to assess feeding effectiveness while the mother and newborn are in the hospital; at least one assessment is needed during the 8 hours prior to discharge (Evans, Marinelli, Taylor, et al., 2014). The assessment should include positioning, latch, and milk transfer. Using a standard breastfeeding scoring tool such as the LATCH tool (Jenson, Wallace, & Kelsay, 1994) to document observations provides consistency in assessment criteria. With the LATCH assessment tool, each letter represents a scored item: *L*atch, *A*udible swallowing, *T*ype of nipple, *C*omfort level of the mother, and *H*old (positioning). During the feeding assessment, the nurse can provide education about breastfeeding, help with feeding techniques, and offer support. If the mother's partner or other family members are present, the nurse can include them in the teaching and demonstrate how they can help the mother and provide support.

Other parameters of the feeding effectiveness assessment relate to the well-being of the neonate. The nurse examines the infant for clinical jaundice and performs daily weights to assess for weight loss. The infant's output is closely monitored; assessment includes the number of voidings and stools, stool color and transition, and presence of uric acid crystals (Evans et al., 2014).

Supplements, Bottles, and Pacifiers

Unless a medical indication exists, no supplements should be given to breastfeeding infants (AAP Section on Breastfeeding, 2012; Kellams, et al., 2017). With sound breastfeeding knowledge and practice, supplements are rarely needed. Early supplementation by hospital staff undermines a new mother's confidence and models behavior that is counterproductive to establishing breastfeeding.

When supplementation is deemed necessary, giving the baby expressed breast milk is best. If the mother is not able to provide the milk, the recommended alternative is pasteurized donor milk from a milk bank. However, in many cases donor milk is not readily accessible and a commercial infant formula is used. The use of a protein-hydrolasate formula instead of standard infant formula avoids exposure to intact cow's milk proteins and may help lower bilirubin levels (Kellams et al., 2017). Before supplementation, it is important to perform a careful evaluation of the mother-infant dyad.

Possible indications for supplementary feeding include infant factors such as hypoglycemia, dehydration, weight loss of more than 8% by day 5 or weight loss exceeding 75th percentile for age associated with delayed lactogenesis, delayed passage of bowel movements or meconium stool continued to day 5, or hyperbilirubinemia (Kellams et al., 2017).

Maternal indications for possible supplementation include delayed lactogenesis, intolerable pain during feedings, or temporary cessation of breastfeeding because of maternal medications. Women with insufficient glandular tissue as those who have had previous breast surgery such as augmentation or reduction may need to provide supplementary feedings for their infants (Kellams et al., 2017).

Newborns can become confused going from breast to bottle or bottle to breast when breastfeeding is first being established. Breastfeeding and bottle-feeding require different oral motor skills. It is best to avoid bottles until breastfeeding is well established, usually after 3 or 4 weeks.

If supplemental feeding is needed, nurses or lactation consultants can help parents select and use an appropriate method. Supplemental nursing devices allow the baby to be supplemented with expressed breast milk or infant formula while still breastfeeding (Fig. 25.9). Infants can also be fed with a spoon, dropper, cup, or syringe. If parents choose to use bottles, a slow-flow nipple is recommended. Although some parents combine breastfeeding and bottle-feeding, some infants never take a bottle and go directly from the breast to a cup.

Because of the correlation between pacifier use and a decreased risk for SIDS, experts recommend pacifier use for healthy term infants at nap or sleep time, but only after breastfeeding is well established at about 3 or 4 weeks of age (AAP Section on Breastfeeding, 2012).

Special Considerations
Sleepy Baby

Some babies need to be awakened for feedings for the first few days after birth. If the infant is awakened from a sound sleep, attempts at feeding may be unsuccessful. Babies are more likely to feed if they are

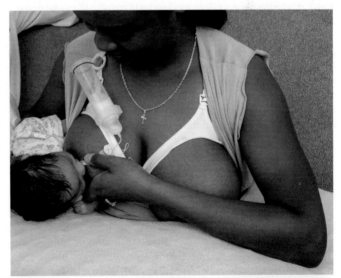
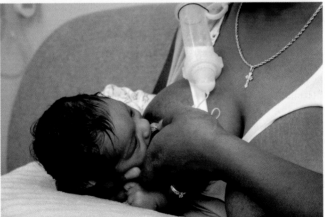

Fig. 25.9 Supplemental Nursing Device. (Copyright 2019 by Medela LLC.)

awakened from a light or active sleep state. Signs that the infant is in this sleep state are movements of the eyelids, body movements, and making sounds while sleeping. Unwrapping the baby, changing the diaper, sitting the baby upright, talking to him or her with variable pitch, gently massaging his or her chest or back, and stroking the palms or soles may bring the baby to an alert state. It is helpful to place the sleepy baby skin-to-skin with the mother; she can move the infant to the breast when feeding-readiness cues are apparent.

Fussy Baby

Babies sometimes awaken from sleep crying frantically. Although they are hungry, they cannot focus on feeding until they are calmed. Parents can swaddle the baby, hold him or her close, talk soothingly, and allow him or her to suck on a clean finger until calm enough to latch on to the breast. Placing the baby skin-to-skin with the mother can be very effective in calming a fussy infant. Fussiness during feeding can be the result of birth injury such as bruising of the head or fractured clavicle. Changing the feeding position can help alleviate this problem.

Infants who were suctioned extensively or intubated at birth can demonstrate an aversion to oral stimulation. The baby may scream and stiffen if anything approaches the mouth. Parents need to spend time holding and cuddling the baby before attempting to breastfeed.

An infant can become fussy and appear discontented when sucking if the nipple does not extend far enough into the mouth. The feeding can begin with well-organized sucks and swallows, but the infant soon begins to pull off the breast and cry. The mother should support her breast throughout the feeding so the nipple stays in the same position as the feeding proceeds and the breast softens.

Fussiness can be related to GI distress (e.g., cramping, gas pains, gastroesophageal reflux). It can occur in response to an occasional feeding of infant formula, or it can be related to something the mother has ingested, although most women are able to eat a normal diet without causing GI distress to the breastfeeding infant. Persistent crying or refusing to breastfeed can indicate illness. Parents are instructed to notify the health care provider if either circumstance occurs.

Some mothers find that their babies are less fussy when placed in a sling or carrier. Some slings make it easy to breastfeed without removing the baby from the sling (Fig. 25.10).

Slow Weight Gain

Newborn infants typically lose 5% to 10% of body weight after birth before they begin to gain weight. Weight loss of more than 7% in a breastfeeding infant during the first 3 days of life needs to be investigated (Lawrence & Lawrence, 2016). After the early milk has transitioned to mature milk, infants should gain approximately 110 to 200 g (3.9 to 7 oz) per week or 20 to 28 g (0.7 to 1 oz) per day for the first 3 months. Breast-fed infants usually do not gain weight as quickly as formula-fed infants.

Parents are taught the warning signs of ineffective breastfeeding, including inadequate weight gain, minimal output, and feeding constantly. If any of these warning signs is present, the parent should notify the pediatric health care provider.

At times, slow weight gain is related to inadequate breastfeeding. Feedings can be short or infrequent, or the infant can be latching incorrectly or sucking ineffectively or inefficiently. Other possibilities are illness or infection, malabsorption, or circumstances that increase the baby's energy needs such as congenital heart disease, cystic fibrosis, or being small for gestational age. Slow weight gain must be differentiated from failure to thrive; this can be a serious problem that warrants medical intervention.

Maternal factors can be the cause of slow weight gain. The mother can have a problem with inadequate emptying of the breasts, pain with feeding, or inappropriate timing of feedings. Inadequate glandular breast tissue or previous breast surgery can affect milk supply. Severe

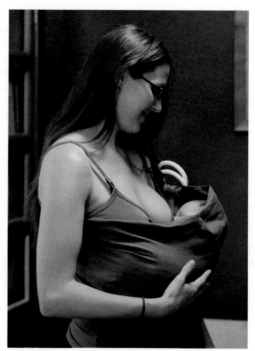

Fig. 25.10 Baby Breastfeeding While in Sling. (Courtesy Julie Perry Nelson, Loveland, CO.)

intrapartum or postpartum hemorrhage (Sheehan syndrome), illness, or medications can decrease milk supply. Stress and fatigue also negatively affect milk production (Lawrence & Lawrence, 2016).

In most instances, the solution to slow weight gain is to increase feeding frequency and to improve the feeding technique. Positioning and latch are evaluated, and adjustments are made. Adding a feeding or two in a 24-hour period can help. If the problem is a sleepy baby, parents are instructed in waking techniques.

Using alternate breast massage during feedings can help increase the amount of milk going to the infant. With this technique, the mother massages her breast from the chest wall to the nipple whenever the baby has sucking pauses. This technique also can increase the fat content of the milk, which aids in weight gain.

When babies are calorie deprived and need supplementation, they can receive expressed breast milk or formula with a supplemental nursing device (see Fig. 25.9), spoon, cup, syringe, or bottle. In most cases, supplementation is necessary only for a short time until the baby gains weight and is feeding adequately.

Jaundice

Chapters 23 and 24 discuss jaundice (hyperbilirubinemia) in the newborn in detail. Breastfeeding infants can develop early-onset jaundice or breastfeeding-associated jaundice, which is associated with insufficient feeding and infrequent stooling. Colostrum has a natural laxative effect and promotes early passage of meconium. Bilirubin is excreted from the body primarily through the intestines. Infrequent stooling allows bilirubin in the stool to be resorbed into the infant's system, thus increasing bilirubin levels (Blackburn, 2018).

To prevent early-onset, breastfeeding-associated jaundice, newborns should breastfeed frequently (at least 8 to 12 times in 24 hours) during the first several days of life. Increased frequency of feedings is associated with decreased bilirubin levels (Kamath-Rayne, Thilo, Deacon, et al., 2016).

To treat early-onset jaundice, breastfeeding is evaluated in terms of frequency and length of feedings, positioning, latch, and milk transfer. Factors such as a sleepy or lethargic infant or maternal breast engorgement can interfere with effective breastfeeding and should be corrected. If the infant is not breastfeeding effectively, the mother can use a mechanical breast pump to stimulate her milk supply and the expressed milk can be fed to the infant. In some cases, donor milk or formula supplementation is needed. Bilirubin levels are closely monitored (Kamath-Rayne et al., 2016).

Late-onset jaundice or breast milk jaundice affects a small number of breastfed infants and develops between 5 and 10 days of age. Affected infants typically thrive, gain weight, and stool normally; all pathologic causes of jaundice have been ruled out. In the presence of other risk factors, hyperbilirubinemia can be severe enough to require phototherapy. In most cases of breast milk jaundice, no intervention is necessary. Some health care providers recommend temporary interruption of breastfeeding for 12 to 24 hours to allow bilirubin levels to decrease (Newton, 2017).

Any breastfeeding infant who develops jaundice should be evaluated carefully for weight loss greater than 7%, decreased milk intake, infrequent stooling (fewer than three stools per day), and decreased urine output (fewer than four to six wet diapers per day). Bilirubin levels should be assessed by serum testing or transcutaneous monitoring (see Chapter 24).

Preterm Infants

Human milk is the ideal food for preterm infants, with benefits that are unique and in addition to those received by term healthy infants. Breast milk enhances retinal maturation in the preterm infant and improves neurocognitive outcomes; it also decreases the risk for sepsis and necrotizing enterocolitis. Greater physiologic stability occurs with breastfeeding compared to bottle-feeding (AAP Section on Breastfeeding, 2012; Lawrence & Lawrence, 2016).

Initially, breast milk from mothers of preterm infants contains higher concentrations of protein, sodium, chloride, potassium, iron, and magnesium than breast milk from mothers of term infants. Within 4 to 6 weeks after birth, milk from mothers of preterm infants becomes more similar to milk produced by mothers of term infants. Depending on gestational age and physical condition, many preterm infants are capable of breastfeeding for at least some feedings each day. Mothers of preterm infants who are not able to breastfeed their infants should begin pumping their breasts as soon as possible after birth with a hospital-grade electric pump. Pumping frequency depends on the mother's breastfeeding goals but may be recommended up to 8 to 10 times every 24 hours to establish the milk supply. These women are taught proper handling and storage of breast milk to minimize bacterial contamination and growth. Kangaroo care (skin-to-skin contact) is encouraged until the baby is able to breastfeed and while breastfeeding is established because it enhances milk production.

Mothers of preterm infants often receive specific emotional benefits in breastfeeding or providing breast milk for their babies. They find rewards in knowing that they can provide the healthiest nutrition for the infant and believe that breastfeeding enhances feelings of closeness to the infant.

Late Preterm and Early Term Infants

Neonates born at 34 0/7 to 36 6/7 weeks of gestation are categorized as *late preterm* infants. Those born at 37 0/7 to 38 6/7 weeks are considered *early term*. Both categories of newborns are at risk for breastfeeding difficulties because of their low energy stores and high energy demands. Compared to term infants, they are more prone to hypothermia, hypoglycemia, respiratory problems, and hyperbilirubinemia. They tend to be sleepy, with minimal and short wakeful periods. These

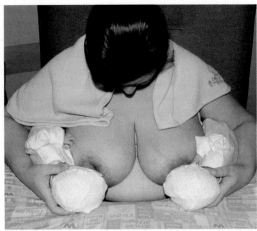

Fig. 25.11 Breastfeeding Twins. (Courtesy Cheryl Briggs, RNC, Annapolis, MD.)

infants may tire easily while feeding and have a weak suck and low tone; these factors can contribute to inadequate milk intake resulting in dehydration and poor weight gain. This predisposes mothers to delayed onset of lactogenesis II and inadequate milk supply (Boies, Vaucher, & ABM, 2016).

Goals of care are to nourish the infant and protect the mother's milk supply. A lactation consultant should be involved in planning and providing appropriate care that usually includes hand expression, use of a hospital-grade electric breast pump, and supplementation of the infant with expressed breast milk or infant formula.

Early and extended skin-to-skin contact promotes breastfeeding and helps prevent hypothermia. These infants need to have free access to the breast and should be fed ad libitum and on demand; if not waking within 4 hours of the previous feeding, the infant should be awakened to breastfeed (Boies et al., 2016). Because these infants are more prone to positional apnea than term infants, mothers may find it advantageous to use the clutch (under the arm or football) or cross-cradle hold for feeding, and avoid flexing the head, which can impede breathing. When supplementation is needed, expressed breast milk is the optimal supplement. Close follow-up care is needed to monitor weight gain.

Breastfeeding Multiple Infants

Breastfeeding is especially beneficial to twins, triplets, and other higher-order multiples because of the immunologic and nutritional advantages and the opportunity for the mother to interact with each baby frequently. Most mothers are capable of producing an adequate milk supply for multiple infants. Multiple gestation often results in the birth of late preterm or early term infants with inherent risks as discussed in the previous section. Supplemental feedings are often necessary. Parenting multiples can be overwhelming; mothers and their husbands or partners need extra support and help to learn how to manage infant care and feedings (Fig. 25.11). Parents of multiples can find breastfeeding information and support through groups such as La Leche League International (www.lalecheleague.org/nb/nbmultiples.html).

Expressing and Storing Breast Milk

Breast milk expression is a common practice, typically performed to obtain breast milk for someone other than the mother to feed to the baby. It is most often associated with maternal employment. In some situations, expression of breast milk is necessary or desirable such as when engorgement occurs, when the mother's nipples are sore or damaged, when the mother and baby are separated, as in the case of a preterm infant who remains in the hospital after the mother is discharged, or when the mother leaves the infant with a caregiver and will not be present for feeding. Some women express milk to have an emergency supply. Some women choose to pump exclusively, providing breast milk for their infants but never allowing the baby to suckle at the breast. Because pumping and hand expression are rarely as efficient as a baby in removing milk from the breast, the milk supply is never judged based solely on the volume expressed. Milk volume can be more accurately assessed using prefeeding and postfeeding infant weights, also known as *test weights*.

Hand Expression

All mothers should be instructed in hand expression. This simple technique can actually be more effective than an electric breast pump for expressing colostrum, which tends to be thicker than mature milk (Morton, Hall, & Pessl, 2013–2014). Hand expression during the first 3 days after birth can has a positive effect on milk production during the early weeks. A video of hand expression of breast milk is available at https://med.stanford.edu/newborns/professional-education/breast-feeding/hand-expressing-milk.html.

Mechanical Milk Expression (Pumping)

For most women, recommendations are to initiate pumping only after the milk supply is well established and the infant is latching and breastfeeding well. However, when breastfeeding is delayed after birth such as when babies are ill or preterm, mothers should begin pumping with an electric breast pump as soon as possible and continue to pump regularly until the infant is able to breastfeed effectively. Early pumping may be initiated if the baby is too sleepy to feed effectively or if there are issues with latching or milk transfer. Milk expression is essential to maintaining milk supply if breastfeeding is interrupted. Double pumping (pumping both breasts at the same time) saves time and can stimulate the milk supply more effectively than single pumping (Fig. 25.12).

The amount of milk obtained when pumping depends on the type of pump being used, the time of day, the time since the baby breastfed, the mother's milk supply, how practiced she is at pumping, and her comfort level (pumping is uncomfortable for some women). Breast milk can vary in color and consistency, depending on the time of day, the age of the baby, and foods the mother has eaten.

Types of pumps. Many types of breast pumps are available, varying in price and effectiveness. Before purchasing or renting a breast pump, the mother will benefit from professional advice from a nurse, lactation consultant, or health care provider to determine which pump best suits her needs (Meier, Patel, Hoban, et al., 2016).

The flange (funnel-shaped device that fits over the nipple or areola) should fit the nipple to prevent nipple pain, trauma, and possible reduction in milk supply (Fig. 25.13). Mothers are advised to use the lowest suction setting on electric pumps, increasing gradually if needed. Breast massage before and during pumping can increase the amount of milk obtained.

Manual, battery-operated, or mini-electric pumps are the least expensive and can be the most appropriate when portability and quietness of operation are important. These pumps are most often used by mothers who are pumping for an occasional bottle.

Full-service electric pumps, or hospital-grade pumps (see Figs. 25.6 and 25.12), most closely duplicate the sucking action and pressure of the breastfeeding infant. When breastfeeding is delayed after birth (e.g., preterm or ill newborn) or when the mother and baby are separated for lengthy periods, these pumps are most appropriate (Meier et al., 2016). Portable versions of these pumps are available to rent for home use.

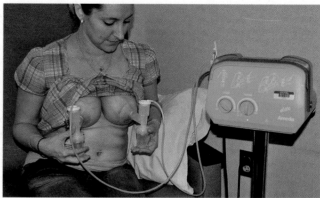

Fig. 25.12 Bilateral Breast Pumping. (Courtesy Cheryl Briggs, RNC, Annapolis, MD.)

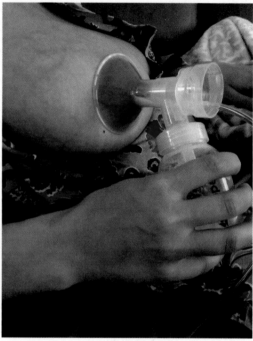

Fig. 25.13 Close-Up View of Milk Expression Using Electric Breast Pump. Note flange fits over nipple and areola. (Courtesy Kathryn Alden, Apex, NC)

Electric self-cycling double pumps are efficient and easy to use. They are designed for working mothers or for use during brief periods (1 to 2 days) of separation by women with established lactation (Meier et al., 2016). Some of these pumps come with carry bags containing coolers to store pumped milk.

Storage of Breast Milk

Mothers who express and feed breast milk to their infants need to be educated about safe practices for handling, storing, and feeding. Attention to hand hygiene and proper cleaning of equipment reduces the risk for bacterial contamination. This is especially important when mothers are providing milk for preterm or ill neonates. Guidelines for storing expressed breast milk for a healthy term infant are listed in Teaching for Self-Management: Breast Milk Storage Guidelines for Home Use for Term Infants.

TEACHING FOR SELF-MANAGEMENT

Breast Milk Storage Guidelines for Home Use for Term Infants

- Before expressing or pumping breast milk, wash your hands; if soap and water are not available, use an alcohol-based hand sanitizer (≥60% alcohol).
- Containers for storing milk should be washed in hot, soapy water and rinsed thoroughly; they can also be washed in a dishwasher. If the water supply may not be clean, boil containers after washing. Plastic bags designed specifically for breast milk storage can be used for short-term storage (<72 hours).
- Write the date of expression on the container before storing milk. A waterproof label is best.
- Store milk in serving sizes of 2 to 4 ounces to prevent waste.
- Freshly expressed or pumped breast milk can be stored safely at room temperature (≤77° F [25°C]) for up to 4 hours and in the refrigerator for up to 4 days. The optimal storage time in the freezer is 6 months, but it is acceptable up to 1 year.
- Storing breast milk in the refrigerator or freezer with other food items is acceptable.
- You can combine milk from pumping sessions in the same day; cool freshly expressed milk before adding it to the refrigerated container. Do not add warm milk to a container of refrigerated milk.
- When storing milk in a refrigerator or freezer, place containers in the back of the freezer, not on the door.
- When filling a storage container that will be frozen, fill only three quarters full, allowing space at the top of the container for expansion.
- To thaw frozen breast milk, place container in the refrigerator for gradual thawing or under warm, running water for quicker thawing. A waterless warmer can also be used. Never boil or microwave.
- Milk thawed in the refrigerator can be stored for 24 hours.
- Thawed breast milk should never be refrozen.
- Gently shake milk container before feeding baby, and test the temperature of the milk on the inner aspect of your wrist.
- Any unused milk left in the bottle after feeding is discarded within 1 to 2 hours.

Data from Centers for Disease Control and Prevention. (2018). Proper storage and preparation of breast milk. Retrieved from https://www.cdc.gov/breastfeeding/recommendations/handling_breastmilk.htm; Eglash, A., Simon, L., & the Academy of Breastfeeding Medicine. (2017). ABM clinical protocol no. 8: Human milk storage information for home use for full-term infants, revised 2017. *Breastfeeding Medicine, 12*(7), 390-395.

⚡ SAFETY ALERT

Breast milk is never thawed or heated in a microwave oven. Microwaving does not heat evenly and can cause encapsulated boiling bubbles to form in the center of the liquid, which may not be detected when drops of milk are checked for temperature. Babies have sustained severe burns to the mouth, throat, and upper gastrointestinal tract as a result of microwaved milk. In addition, microwaving significantly decreases the antiinfective properties and vitamin C content. The safety of low-temperature microwaving is questionable (Lawrence & Lawrence, 2016).

Maternal Employment

Returning to work after birth is associated with a decrease in the duration of breastfeeding. Women who return to work often face workplace challenges in breastfeeding, such as lack of flexibility in work schedules, inadequate breaks to allow time for pumping, lack of privacy,

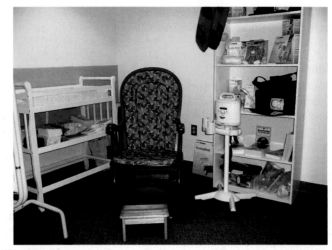

Fig. 25.14 Lactation Room. Note breast pump, rocking chair, nursing foot stool, changing table, books, and supplies. (Courtesy Cheryl Briggs, RNC, Annapolis, MD.)

lack of space for pumping, and lack of support from supervisors or coworkers. Mothers who are students in educational settings face similar challenges. Issues that can affect continued breastfeeding include fatigue, child care concerns, competing demands, and household responsibilities.

Employed mothers can continue breastfeeding with appropriate guidance and support (Robertson, 2014). They are encouraged to set realistic goals for employment and breastfeeding, with accurate information regarding the costs, risks, and benefits of available feeding options. Women need information about planning for their return to work; nurses and lactation consultants can provide guidance. Websites such as www.workandpump.com include information about choosing pumps and other supplies, making a plan for breastfeeding and expressing milk, and preparing for their return to work.

Women who are able to breastfeed their infants during the workday tend to breastfeed longer. With increasing numbers of women having the option of working from home, this situation is becoming more common. In some settings, mothers are able to breastfeed during the workday, either by going to an on-site daycare center or by having a friend or relative bring the baby to her for some feedings. Many working mothers pump their milk while they are at work and save the milk for later feedings. Working mothers who are unable to pump or breastfeed their infants during the workday have the shortest duration of breastfeeding.

Because women are a significant proportion of the workforce, many companies make provisions for breastfeeding women returning to work. Ideally, employers should provide accommodations for breastfeeding mothers, specifically reasonable breaks during the workday and a nonbathroom space for milk expression until the child's first birthday. Breastfeeding programs typically include on-site lactation rooms (Fig. 25.14) and education and consulting services. Some employers provide on-site child care and high-quality breast pumps for their employees (Marinelli, Moren, Taylor, et al., 2013). Workplace support for breastfeeding mothers has improved significantly in recent years. However, further efforts are needed to educate employers about the importance of supporting their breastfeeding employees. Employers need to realize that breastfeeding programs can provide short- and long-term cost savings with significant health benefits for mothers, infants, and families. The Health Resources and Services Administration offers a free toolkit for employers: the "Business Case for Breastfeeding" outlines steps that employers can take to support breastfeeding employees (https://www.womenshealth.gov/breastfeeding/breastfeeding-home-work-and-public/breastfeeding-and-going-back-work/business-case).

Weaning

Weaning may be defined as the process of transferring the infant's dependence on the mother's milk for nutrition to other sources of nutrition (Lawrence & Lawrence, 2016). For infants who are exclusively breastfed, the process of weaning is initiated when babies are introduced to foods other than breast milk and concludes with the last breastfeeding, which ideally continues until the infant is 1 year of age and beyond as desired. Gradual weaning over weeks or months is easier for mothers and infants than abrupt weaning. Abrupt weaning is likely to be distressing for mother and baby and physically uncomfortable for the mother because it can cause engorgement and mastitis.

Weaning is initiated by either the infant or the mother. With infant-led weaning, the infant moves at his or her own pace in omitting feedings, which usually facilitates a gradual decrease in the mother's milk supply. In most cases, the mother determines when weaning will occur. Mother-led weaning means that the mother decides which feedings to drop. This approach is most easily undertaken by omitting the feeding of least interest to the baby or the one through which the infant is most likely to sleep. Every few days thereafter, the mother drops another feeding until the infant is gradually weaned from the breast.

Infants can be weaned directly from the breast to a cup. Bottles are usually offered to infants younger than 6 months of age. If the infant is weaned before 1 year of age, he or she should receive iron-fortified formula instead of cow's milk (AAP Section on Breastfeeding, 2012).

If abrupt weaning is necessary, breast engorgement can occur. To relieve the discomfort, the mother can take mild analgesics such as ibuprofen, wear a supportive bra, apply ice packs or cabbage leaves to the breasts, and pump small amounts if needed. When possible, it is best to avoid pumping because the breasts should remain full enough to promote a decrease in the milk supply.

Weaning is often a very emotional time for mothers; many believe that it is the end to a special, satisfying relationship with the infant and experience feelings of sadness or depression. Some women go through a grieving period after weaning. Sudden weaning can evoke feelings of guilt and disappointment. Nurses and others can help the mother by discussing other ways to continue this nurturing relationship with the infant such as skin-to-skin contact while bottle-feeding or holding and cuddling the baby. Support from the father or partner and other family members is essential at this time.

Milk Banking

The AAP recommends pasteurized donor milk for preterm infants if the mother's own milk is not available despite substantial lactation support (AAP Section on Breastfeeding, 2012). For infants who cannot be breastfed but who also cannot survive except on human milk, banked donor milk is critically important. Because of the antiinfective and growth-promoting properties of human milk and its superior nutrition, processed donor milk is used in some neonatal intensive care units, primarily for very-low-birth-weight infants as well as for other preterm or sick infants when the mother's own milk is not available. Donor milk may be used therapeutically in other situations, such as for infants with abdominal wall defects (omphalocele, gastroschisis), necrotizing enterocolitis, or congenital heart disease (AAP Committee on Nutrition, Section on Breastfeeding, & Committee on Fetus and Newborn, 2017). It is also used for infants with IgA deficiency who are not breastfed, and older children or adults with IgA deficiency (Lawrence & Lawrence, 2016).

The Human Milk Banking Association of North America (HMBANA) (www.hmbana.org) has established annually reviewed guidelines for the operation of not-for-profit donor human milk banks (HMBANA, 2018). There is no federal oversight or regulation of milk banking in the United States. However, some states have laws and regulations that specify how donor milk is to be procured, processed, and distributed. Currently there are 27 HMBANA milk banks in the United States and Canada, with more in various stages of planning and development (HMBANA, 2019). The milk banks collect, screen, process, and distribute the milk donated by lactating mothers. All donors are screened both by interview and serologically for communicable diseases. Donor milk is stored frozen until it is pasteurized (heat processed) to kill potential pathogens; it is then refrozen for storage until it is dispensed for use. The heat processing adds a level of protection for the recipient that is not possible with any other donor tissue or organ. Banked milk is dispensed only by prescription. A per-ounce fee is charged by the bank to pay for the processing costs, but the HMBANA guidelines prohibit payment to donors.

The demand for human milk far exceeds the supply that is available through the non-profit HMBANA facilities. There are for-profit companies who offer payment to women who donate their breast milk. This raises bioethical issues surrounding the sale of human milk, the compensation to donors, and diverting the supply of donor milk from non-profit milk banks. There is also concern about the quality and safety of the milk (Thibeau & Ginsberg, 2018). Another concern about for-profit milk banking is the potential for predatory recruitment of low-income women as donors (See Community Focus box.)

🏠 COMMUNITY FOCUS

Milk Donation

The Human Milk Banking Association of North America is a nonprofit organization that provides donor milk that has been safely pasteurized and tested. It is dispensed only by hospital purchase order or health care provider prescription. Visit the website www.hmbana.org, and read about how milk is processed. Also explore how a woman can become a milk donor.

Milk Sharing

In some situations when a mother is unable to provide breast milk in sufficient quantity for her infant, or is unable to breastfeed because of a contraindication such as HIV, or in the case of maternal death when the family wants human milk for the surviving infant, women and families may turn to alternative sources for human milk. In such cases, the family is unlikely to be considered a priority for milk from a human milk bank, or they may not have the financial resources to purchase the milk. They may resort to cross-nursing or wet-nursing, where the infant is breastfed by a woman other than the birth mother. Some families acquire donor milk for their babies through internet-based milk sharing or community sharing of donor human milk (see Community Focus box). In these cases, there is a lack of screening of milk donors in terms of diseases, medications, or illicit substances (Martino & Spatz, 2014). The U.S. Food and Drug Administration (FDA, 2015) warns against milk sharing, recommending that potential users should consult a health care provider before obtaining milk from a source other than the baby's own mother. They warn individuals against feeding donor milk procured directly from individuals or through the internet, citing safety risks including exposing the infant to infectious diseases or chemical contaminants in donor milk. Samples of milk purchased through the internet have been shown to have high overall bacterial growth and contamination with pathogenic bacteria; this is likely related to improper techniques for collecting, storing, and shipping the milk. As informal milk sharing is becoming increasingly more common, it is the role of health care professionals to help mothers and families make informed choices, providing information about risks and benefits, stressing the importance of medical screening of donors and safe milk handling practices, and strongly discouraging internet-based milk sharing, especially purchasing milk over the internet (Sriraman, Evans, Lawrence, et al. 2018).

> ### ⚡ SAFETY ALERT
>
> Nurses and lactation consultants should be aware of the safety concerns associated with milk sharing. Parents who indicate an interest in obtaining donor human milk for their infant should be directed to one of the HMBANA milk banks and should be cautioned about the safety risks associated with feeding donor milk from an alternative source.

Care of the Mother

Nutrition

In general, the breastfeeding mother should eat a healthy, well-balanced diet. Caloric intake during lactation should be sufficient to achieve the goal of balancing energy intake and expenditure. Most women are able to achieve that balance by adding 450 to 500 calories per day (AAP Section on Breastfeeding, 2012). Even with the increased caloric intake, women who are breastfeeding tend to lose weight more quickly than those who are formula-feeding (Lawrence & Lawrence, 2016).

Medications or diets that promote weight loss are not recommended for breastfeeding mothers. Rapid loss of large amounts of weight can be detrimental, given that fat-soluble contaminants to which the mother has been exposed are stored in body fat reserves, and these can be released into the breast milk. Another potential consequence of weight loss is reduced milk production (Newton, 2017). For most women, a weight loss of 1 to 2 kg (2.2 to 4.4 lb) per month is safe; however, if weight loss exceeds this amount, careful evaluation of infant weight and feeding pattern is recommended. The mother's diet is also evaluated.

No specific foods that the breastfeeding mother should avoid have been identified. In most cases, the woman can consume a normal diet, according to her personal preferences and cultural practices. However, there is clinical evidence that some breastfeeding infants are sensitive to specific foods in the mother's diet; for example, garlic, onions, cabbage, broccoli, turnips, or beans have been known to cause temporary GI distress (colic). Breastfed infants can have food-induced allergic disorders; cow's milk protein in the mother's diet is a common cause of allergic response in the infant. Symptoms of food allergy are eczema, GI discomfort, bloody stools, and slow weight gain. If a mother thinks that her infant is reacting to something she has eaten, she can avoid the food completely, or try eating it again and closely observe the infant for distress during the next 24 hours (Lawrence & Lawrence, 2016; Matson, Marinelli, & ABM, 2011).

Women may be told to continue taking their prenatal vitamins as long as they are breastfeeding. Vitamin D supplements are recommended, especially for women with limited sun exposure or darker skin (Newton, 2017).

It is recommended that breastfeeding mothers consume 200 to 300 mg of the omega-3 long-chain polyunsaturated fatty acids (DHA) daily. A DHA supplement and a multivitamin may be needed for women who are undernourished and those on vegan diets (AAP Section on Breastfeeding, 2012).

Women on vegetarian diets are at risk for dietary deficiencies including B vitamins (especially B_{12}), total protein, and some amino acids. Recommendations for lactating women on vegetarian diets include (1) supplementing protein intake with soy flour, nuts, and molasses; and using complementary protein combinations; (2) avoiding excessive intake of phylates and bran; and (3) taking vitamin supplements of B_{12}, B_2, and D (Lawrence & Lawrence, 2016; Newton, 2017).

Mothers are encouraged to drink fluids in response to thirst (women often report feeling thirsty when they are breastfeeding). It can be helpful for the mother to know that if her urine appears light yellow (like lemonade), she is probably consuming adequate fluids. Excessive consumption of water or other fluids by the mother does not increase milk supply, and overhydration can actually decrease milk production.

Rest

The breastfeeding mother should rest as much as possible, especially in the first 1 or 2 weeks after birth. Fatigue, stress, and worry can negatively affect milk production and ejection (let-down). The nurse can encourage the mother to sleep when the baby sleeps. Breastfeeding in a side-lying position promotes rest for the mother. The father or partner, grandparents, other relatives, and friends can help with household chores and caring for other children.

Breast Care

The breastfeeding mother's normal routine bathing is all that is necessary to keep her breasts clean. Soap can have a drying effect on nipples; therefore, the mother should avoid washing the nipples with soap. Breast creams should not be used routinely because they can block the natural oil secreted by the Montgomery glands on the areola.

If a mother needs breast support, she will likely be uncomfortable unless she wears a bra because otherwise the ligament that supports the breast (Cooper ligament) will stretch and be painful. Bras should fit well and provide nonbinding support. Underwire or improperly fitting bras can cause clogged milk ducts.

If milk leakage between feedings is a problem, mothers can wear breast pads (disposable or washable) inside the bra. Plastic-lined breast pads are not recommended because they trap moisture and can contribute to sore nipples. Pads should be changed when they are damp.

Breastfeeding and Contraception

Although breastfeeding confers a period of infertility, it is not considered an effective method of contraception unless the mother is strictly following guidelines for the lactational amenorrhea method of contraception (see Chapter 8). Breastfeeding delays the return of ovulation and menstruation; however, ovulation can occur before the first menstrual period after birth.

The contraceptives least likely to affect breastfeeding and milk production are the nonhormonal methods such as the lactational amenorrhea method, natural family planning, barrier methods (diaphragm/cap, spermicides, condoms), and intrauterine devices (Berens, Labbok, & ABM, 2015).

Hormonal contraceptives containing estrogen, including combined estrogen-progesterone pills or injectables, are not recommended for breastfeeding mothers because of the potential for reducing milk supply. Progestin-only contraceptives (pill, injection, or implant) are better options for breastfeeding mothers, although their use is not recommended during the first 6 weeks after birth (Berens et al., 2015) (see Chapter 8).

Breastfeeding During Pregnancy

Breastfeeding women who become pregnant can continue to breast-feed if there are no medical contraindications (e.g., risk for preterm labor). For pregnant women who are breastfeeding, adequate nutrition is especially important to promote normal fetal growth.

Nipple tenderness associated with early pregnancy can cause discomfort when breastfeeding the older child. The taste and composition of breast milk are altered during pregnancy, which can prompt some children to self-wean (Lawrence & Lawrence, 2016).

The practice of breastfeeding a newborn and an older child is called **tandem nursing**. When the baby is born, colostrum is produced. The nurse should remind the mother always to feed the newborn first to ensure that he or she is receiving the colostrum, which is high in immune properties and prepares the infant's gut for future feedings. The supply-meets-demand principle works in this situation, just as with breastfeeding multiples.

Breastfeeding After Breast Surgery

Any type of previous breast or chest surgery (biopsy, augmentation, reduction, reconstructive surgery) can affect the ability to produce breast milk and transfer it to the infant. Surgical procedures can damage nerves and interrupt milk ducts (Newton, 2017). Before undergoing breast surgery, all women should discuss their lactation potential with their surgeon. During preconception or prenatal care, obstetric health care providers should identify women who have had breast surgery, discuss potential concerns related to breastfeeding, and refer women to lactation professionals for further counseling and assistance.

Women who have had augmentation mammoplasty (breast implants) may be able to breastfeed successfully. Many women have breast augmentation surgery purely for cosmetic reasons. However, if the procedure was done because of hypoplastic or asymmetric breasts or for breast reconstruction following cancer surgery, there can be concerns about adequate milk production. Submuscular implants are less likely to cause these problems; implants placed through periareolar incisions are more likely to result in breastfeeding problems. Large implants can impede milk flow by compressing milk ducts. Women with silicone implants can safely breastfeed without adverse effects on the infant (Newton, 2017).

Reduction mammoplasty causes problems with milk production and transfer because of interference with milk ducts, removal of glandular tissue, and nerve damage (Newton, 2017). Even so, many women are still able to breastfeed while also supplementing with infant formula or banked donor milk.

! NURSING ALERT

Women may not self-report previous breast or chest surgery such as breast biopsy, augmentation, or reduction mammoplasty. If surgical scars are present on the breast, the nurse should inquire about the type of surgery and the reason it was performed. Mothers with a history of breast surgery should be informed about the risk for interference with milk production and transfer. They are instructed to monitor their infants carefully for signs of adequate feeding.

It is possible for some women with a history of breast cancer to breastfeed. However, treatment for breast cancer (surgery, radiation, chemotherapy) can result in reduced milk supply or absence of lactation in the affected breast.

Breastfeeding and Nipple Piercing

Women who have nipple piercings can safely breastfeed. It can take as long as a year after piercing for the nipples to completely heal, placing the woman at risk for infection such as mastitis. Therefore, it is best if the piercing is done 18 to 24 months prior to pregnancy or at least 3 months after weaning. Piercings can damage milk ducts, obstructing the flow of milk. There can be leakage of milk from the piercing sites or fast flow of milk through the holes. Pierced nipples may have increased sensitivity. To prevent infant choking, breastfeeding mothers who have nipple piercings must remove the jewelry from the nipples before breastfeeding.

Breastfeeding and Obesity

Women who are overweight or obese are less likely to breastfeed, and the duration of breastfeeding tends to be shortened. These women are more likely to experience delayed onset of lactogenesis stage II and to experience problems with insufficient milk production compared with women of average weight (Turcksin et al., 2014).

For women who have had bariatric surgery and plan to breast-feed, nutritional deficiencies are a primary concern. Monitoring of the breastfeeding mother's micronutrient levels is recommended as frequently as every 3 months (Kominiarek & Rajan, 2016). Breastfeeding mothers who have had a malabsorptive procedure such as a Roux-en-Y gastric bypass should take daily dietary supplements, including a prenatal vitamin, vitamin B_{12}, iron with vitamin C (to maximize absorption), and calcium. It is important to monitor infant weight gain. Vitamin B_{12} deficiency or decreased milk production can cause failure to thrive. In addition, vitamin B_{12} deficiency can result in infant anemia, developmental delays, and neurologic problems. Women with a history of bariatric surgery can benefit from referrals to registered dieticians and lactation consultants during pregnancy and in the postpartum period to discuss optimizing their nutritional status in preparation for and while breastfeeding (Caplinger, Cooney, Bledsoe et al., 2015).

Medications, Alcohol, Smoking, and Caffeine

Although much concern exists about the compatibility of drugs and breastfeeding, few drugs are absolutely contraindicated during lactation. Considerations in evaluating the safety of a specific medication during breastfeeding include the pharmacokinetics of the drug in the maternal system and the absorption, metabolism, distribution, storage, and excretion in the infant. The gestational and chronologic age of the infant, body weight, and breastfeeding pattern are also considered. In general, any medication that is given to an infant routinely is safe for a mother who is breastfeeding. The benefits of breastfeeding should be weighed against any risks of the medication to the infant (Hale & Rowe, 2017; Sachs & Committee on Drugs, 2013).

⊘ MEDICATION ALERT

Breastfeeding mothers should be cautioned about taking any medications, except those that are deemed essential. They are advised to check with their health care provider before taking any medication, even over-the-counter drugs.

Information about the safety of medications and breastfeeding can be accessed through the Drugs and Lactation Database (LactMed), a website provided by National Library of Medicine: http://toxnet.nlm.nih.gov/c-gi-bin/sis/htmlgen?LACT (Anderson, 2016). The AAP recommends that providers consult this resource for the most current evidence-based information about specific medications for breastfeeding mothers (Sachs & Committee on Drugs, 2013).

Breastfeeding should be discontinued temporarily when the mother undergoes imaging procedures that use radiopharmaceuticals. Mothers are advised to pump and discard milk for a period of time based on the properties of the specific radioactive agent (Sachs & Committee on Drugs, 2013).

Drugs that are associated with adverse effects on the breastfeeding infant include antimetabolite and cytotoxic medications and drugs of abuse such as cocaine, heroin, amphetamines, and phencyclidine. These substances are not compatible with breastfeeding (Hale & Rowe, 2017).

Women with a history of opioid use (prescription medications or heroin) who are on a medication-assisted treatment program may be encouraged to breastfeed as long as they are not using other illicit substances. Methadone and buprenorphine are considered safe during breastfeeding. Infants may have decreased severity of neonatal abstinence symptoms when they are receiving breast milk from mothers taking these medications (Hale & Rowe, 2017; Reece-Stremtan, Marinelli, & ABM, 2015).

Pain in postpartum breastfeeding mothers is most safely managed with nonopioid analgesics such as ibuprofen. When opioid analgesia is used, breastfeeding infants are at risk for sedation and sucking difficulties. Parenteral doses of morphine or butorphanol are preferred over meperidine. Oral hydrocodone is often used and is considered safe in standard doses; maternal doses should be limited to no more than 30 mg/day (Hale & Rowe, 2017). Oxycodone is considered less desirable because relatively high amounts are transferred to the nursing infant and can lead to central nervous system depression (Sachs & Committee on Drugs, 2013).

As the use of antidepressant, antianxiety, mood stabilizing, and antipsychotic medications rises among childbearing women, there are increasing concerns about the effects of these medications on breastfeeding infants (see Chapter 31). There is a lack of evidence about the long-term effects on infants and children. Psychotropic medications are prescribed for breastfeeding mothers based on risk/benefit considerations. Commonly used antidepressant medications that are considered safe during lactation include nortriptyline, sertraline, and paroxetine (Sriraman, Melvin, Meltzer-Brody, et al., 2015).

Although there is no standard recommendation about avoiding alcohol use when breastfeeding, it is important for mothers to be aware of potential risks. Alcohol intake by breastfeeding women should be minimal. Alcohol passes freely from the blood into breast milk, with peak levels occurring in 30 to 90 minutes. Potential effects on the infant include sedation and poor feeding. The MER and milk production can be adversely affected by maternal alcohol intake. Breastfeeding mothers should limit their alcohol intake to the equivalent of 2 beers or 8 ounces of wine, and should not breastfeed for at least 2 hours (Reece-Stremtan et al., 2015). Contrary to popular belief, pumping and discarding milk do not accelerate removal of alcohol from the milk (Lawrence & Lawrence, 2016). Some mothers use test strips for alcohol content of breast milk; however, there is a lack of evidence to support the accuracy or reliability of these strips.

Smoking by breastfeeding mothers should be strongly discouraged (AAP Section on Breastfeeding, 2012). Smoking can impair milk production; it also exposes the infant to the risks of secondhand smoke, including the risk of SIDS and respiratory allergies. Nicotine and other chemicals are transferred to the infant in breast milk, whether through smoking or use of nicotine replacement products (e.g., patches, gum) (U.S. National Library of Medicine, 2018). Lactating mothers who continue to smoke should be advised not to smoke within 2 hours before breastfeeding and never to smoke in the same room with the infant (AAP Section on Breastfeeding, 2012).

Moderate intake of caffeine by breastfeeding mothers appears to pose no risk to normal full-term infants. Minimal amounts of caffeine pass through to the infant in the breast milk. However, caffeine accumulates in infants, especially if they are preterm, and can cause irritability and insomnia. There is some evidence that chronic coffee-drinking may reduce iron content in breast milk (Hale & Rowe, 2016; Lawrence & Lawrence, 2016).

Herbs and Herbal Preparations

Herbs and herbal preparations such as teas are often recommended for breastfeeding women, especially when there is a need to increase milk supply. Herbs that are commonly used as galactagogues include fenugreek, milk thistle, goat's rue, fennel seeds, moringa leaf, charavari, and torbangun (Brodribb & ABM, 2018). Although these herbal preparations may seem to be effective for some women, the recommendations are based on anecdotal information. There is a lack of evidence related to the prevalence, effectiveness, and safety of herbs during breastfeeding. Herbals are not regulated by the FDA because they are considered dietary supplements. Consequently, there is a lack of quality control; unknown additives in and unknown side effects from herbal preparations can be harmful to the infant. Although some herbs may be considered safe, others contain pharmacologically active compounds that can have unfavorable effects. A thorough maternal history should include the use of any herbal remedies. Each remedy should then be evaluated for its compatibility with breastfeeding. LactMed provides information about the safety of herbal preparations and breastfeeding. In addition, regional poison control centers can provide information on the active properties of herbs (Brodribb & ABM; Lawrence & Lawrence, 2016).

Common Concerns of the Breastfeeding Mother

The breastfeeding mother can experience some common problems. In most cases, these complications are preventable if the mother receives appropriate education about breastfeeding and assistance as needed. Early recognition and prompt resolution of these problems are important to prevent interruption of breastfeeding and to promote the mother's comfort and sense of well-being. Emotional support provided by nurses or lactation consultants is essential to help allay maternal frustration and anxiety and prevent early cessation of breastfeeding.

Engorgement. Engorgement is a common response of the breasts to the sudden change in hormones and the onset of significantly increased milk volume in lactogenesis stage II. It usually occurs 3 to 5 days after birth as the milk transitions from colostrum to mature milk. At this time, there is increased blood flow to the breasts, and increased uptake of glucose and oxygen by the breasts. Milk production is copious (Newton, 2017). As milk production rapidly increases, the volume can exceed the storage capacity of the alveoli in the breasts. If milk is not removed, the alveoli become distended, causing impairment of capillary blood flow surrounding the alveolar cells. As the blood vessels become more congested, fluid leaks into the surrounding tissue, resulting in edema. The milk ducts can be compressed by the tissue edema so milk cannot flow easily from the breasts. The breasts can become firm, tender, and hot, and can appear shiny and taut. The areolae are firm, and the nipples can flatten, making it difficult for the infant to latch on to the breast (see Clinical Reasoning Case Study: Breastfeeding: Engorgement). Because back pressure on full milk glands inhibits milk production, if milk is not removed from the breasts, the milk supply can diminish.

❓ CLINICAL REASONING CASE STUDY

Breastfeeding: Engorgement

The nurse on the mother-baby unit is caring for Johanna, a 37-year-old primipara who gave birth to a baby girl by emergency cesarean 3 days ago. She has been breastfeeding but has needed much support with positioning due to the pain in her incision. She has had frequent visitors throughout the day. During the evening assessment, the nurse observes that Johanna's breasts are engorged, her areolae are edematous, and her nipples appear flatter. Johanna requested bottles of infant formula for the night feedings because she was exhausted. Johanna is scheduled for discharge this morning.

1. What is the priority concern or client need in this situation? Support your answer with data as stated in the case.
2. List other client needs/problems in this case.
3. Identify any additional information or assessment data that are needed by the nurse in planning care for this client.
4. What nursing actions are appropriate in this situation?
   a. What is the priority nursing action?
   b. Describe other nursing interventions that are important to providing optimal client care.
5. Describe the roles/responsibilities of the interprofessional health care team members (other than nurses) who may be involved in providing care for this client.

Engorgement does not occur in all breastfeeding mothers. The frequency and effectiveness of feedings during the first 2 to 3 days after birth seem to affect the development of engorgement. Early and frequent feedings may help prevent engorgement. Keeping the mother and infant together is an important strategy to help with recognizing and responding to feeding cues. Emptying one breast at each feeding and alternating which breast is offered first at each feeding may also help prevent engorgement. The risk for engorgement appears to be increased among primiparas, women who received large amounts of IV fluids during labor and birth, and women who had previous breast surgery (Berens, Brodribb, & ABM, 2016).

When engorgement occurs it is a temporary condition that is usually resolved within 24 hours. The mother is instructed to feed 8 to 12 times in 24 hours, softening at least one breast and pumping or hand expressing the other breast as needed to soften it. Pumping during engorgement does not cause a problematic increase in milk supply. Sometimes during feeding, the opposite breast will leak milk, and the mother may use a milk collection device; such a device uses gentle suction to attach to the breast and provides a clean receptacle for milk that can be fed to the infant or stored for later use (Fig. 25.15).

A variety of interventions are used to treat engorgement, although there is a lack of research evidence confirming the effectiveness of any specific treatment regimen (Berens, Brodribb, & ABM, 2016; Mangesi & Zakarija-Grkovic, 2016). Frequently used interventions for engorgement include the use of cold (ice packs, gel packs, cold compresses), warmth (warm compresses, warm showers), cabbage leaves, anti-inflammatory medications, breast massage, and hand expression or pumping. Other treatment techniques for engorgement include the use of ultrasound, acupressure, acupuncture, and Gua sha (usually part of acupuncture therapy).

To reduce swelling of breast tissue surrounding the milk ducts, ice packs are often recommended in a 10- to 15-minutes-on, 45-minutes-off rotation between feedings. The ice packs should cover both breasts. Large bags of frozen peas make easy packs and can be refrozen between uses.

Fresh, raw cabbage leaves placed over the breasts between feedings can help relieve engorgement. It is thought that the effect of the cabbage leaves is related to the coolness of the leaves and phytoestrogens within them. They are washed, dried, chilled in the refrigerator or freezer, and then placed over the breasts for 15 to 20 minutes (Fig. 25.16). Some clinicians recommend crushing the leaves slightly to break up the veins in the leaves prior to placing them over the breasts. This treatment can be repeated for two or three sessions. Frequent application of cabbage leaves can decrease milk supply. Cabbage leaves should not be used if the mother is allergic to cabbage or develops a skin rash.

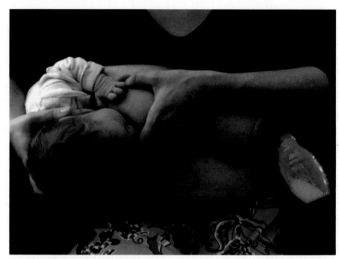

Fig. 25.15 Breastfeeding Newborn on One Breast While Collecting Milk From the Other Breast. Note fullness of breasts. (Courtesy Kathryn Alden, Apex, NC)

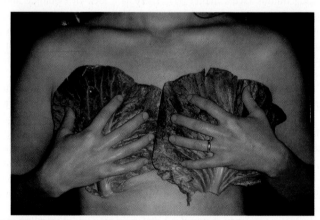

Fig. 25.16 Cabbage Leaves to Treat Engorgement. (Courtesy Kathryn Alden, Apex, NC.)

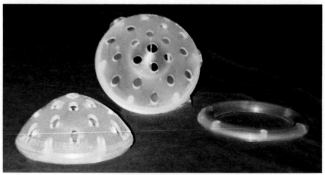

Fig. 25.17 Breast Shells.

Antiinflammatory medications such as ibuprofen can help reduce the pain and swelling associated with engorgement. Ibuprofen also helps reduce fever and aching in the breasts that are often associated with engorgement.

Because heat increases blood flow, its application to an already congested breast is usually counterproductive. However, occasionally standing in a warm shower starts the milk leaking, or the mother may be able to manually express enough milk to soften the areola sufficiently to allow the baby to latch and breastfeed.

As a result of engorgement, excessive intravenous fluids during labor, or oxytocin for labor induction or augmentation, the nipple and areola can become distended, making it difficult for the newborn to latch successfully. A technique called *reverse pressure softening* manually displaces the areolar interstitial fluid inward, softening the areola and making it easier for the infant's mouth to grasp the nipple and areola with latch (Berens, Brodribb, & ABM, 2016).

Sore nipples. Mild nipple tenderness during the first few days of breastfeeding is common. Severe soreness or painful, abraded, cracked, or bleeding nipples are not normal and most often result from poor positioning, incorrect latch, improper suck, or infection. Suboptimal positioning can result in a shallow latch and abnormal nipple compression with sucking. Latch and sucking difficulties can be related to infant issues such as prematurity, oral and mandibular anatomy, muscle tone, congenital anomalies, ankyloglossia, biting, or jaw-clenching. Latch problems can also be due to maternal issues such as nipple size or anatomy (e.g., flat or inverted nipples), breast size, engorgement, or milk flow. Painful nipples can be due to eczematous conditions such as atopic dermatitis, contact dermatitis, psoriasis, or in rare cases, Paget disease. Severe nipple pain can be related to vasospasm or Raynaud phenomenon. Bacterial, viral, or candida infections of the nipple and/or breast can cause pain (Berens, Eglash, Malloy, et al., 2016).

The key to preventing sore nipples is correct breastfeeding technique. Limiting the time at the breast does not prevent sore nipples. Soreness is often the result of the mother allowing the baby to latch on to the breast before the mouth is open wide.

For the first few days after birth, the mother can experience some mild discomfort with the infant's initial sucks. This should quickly dissipate as the milk begins to flow and acts as a lubricant. To make the initial sucks less painful, the mother can express a few drops of colostrum or milk to moisten the nipple and areola before latch. If the mother continues to experience nipple pain or discomfort after the first few sucks, the nurse or lactation consultant helps her evaluate the latch and baby's position at the breast. If the nipple pain continues, the mother needs to remove the baby from the breast, breaking suction with her finger in the baby's mouth (see Fig. 25.8). Repositioning the mother or infant can be helpful in resolving the nipple discomfort. The mother then proceeds to attempt latch again, making sure that the baby's mouth is open wide before latching him or her on to the breast.

The nurse, health care provider, or lactation consultant can assess the infant's suck by inserting a clean, gloved finger into the mouth and stimulating the infant to suck. If the tongue is not extruding over the lower gum and the mother reports pain or pinching with sucking, the baby may have ankyloglossia, which is a short or tight frenulum (commonly known as *tongue-tie*). In some instances, this condition is corrected surgically to free the tongue for less painful, more effective breastfeeding (Lawrence & Lawrence, 2016).

The treatment for sore nipples is first to identify the cause and then attempt to correct the problem. Early assessment and intervention are essential to increase the likelihood that the mother will continue to breastfeed. Once the problem is identified and corrected, sore nipples should heal within a few days, even though the baby continues to breastfeed regularly. When sore nipples occur, the woman is advised to start the feeding on the least sore nipple. It is important to assess the nipples for cracking or other damage to the skin integrity, which increases the risk for infection. If there is any break in the skin, the mother is advised to wipe the nipples with water after feeding to remove the baby's saliva. Expressing a few drops of colostrum or breast milk and rubbing it into the nipples may be recommended. A thin coating of a topical antibiotic on damaged nipples may help reduce the risk for infection and promote healing; if not absorbed prior to the next feeding, the antibiotic cream or ointment should be gently removed before breastfeeding. Sore nipples should be open to air as much as possible. To promote comfort, breast shells can be worn inside the bra; these devices allow air to circulate while keeping clothing off sore nipples (see Fig. 25.17).

Rapid healing of sore nipples is critical to relieve the mother's discomfort, maintain breastfeeding, and prevent mastitis. Although numerous creams, ointments, gels, and gel pads have been used to treat sore nipples, there is a lack of conclusive evidence related to the effectiveness of any particular method (Dennis, Jackson, & Watson, 2014). However, because they have not been shown to cause harm, many health care professionals recommend their use. Some women report increased comfort for sore nipples with the application of purified lanolin, petroleum jelly, edible oils, or hydrogel pads. If nipples are extremely sore or damaged and if the mother cannot tolerate breastfeeding, she may need to use an electric breast pump for 24 to 48 hours to allow the nipples to begin healing before resuming breastfeeding. She should use a pump that effectively empties the breasts (see Figs. 25.6 and 25.12).

Insufficient milk supply. A common reason that women stop breastfeeding is perceived or actual insufficient milk supply (Odom, Li, Scanlon, et al., 2013; Stuebe, 2014). This often leads to formula supplementation and early weaning. Careful evaluation of the mother-infant dyad is needed, including assessment of infant weight gain or loss, feeding technique, milk transfer, and consideration of possible medical causes for low supply (e.g., medications, glandular insufficiency, previous breast surgery). Stress and fatigue can cause decreased milk production.

The key to establishing and maintaining milk supply is frequent emptying of the breasts. Interventions for increasing milk supply are based on causative factors. In many cases, the mother is told to spend time with the baby skin-to-skin, increase feeding frequency, express milk using an electric pump, rest as much as possible, consume a healthy diet, and reduce stress. If nonpharmacologic measures to increase milk supply are not effective, galactagogues or lactagogues (medications or other substances that are believed to increase milk supply) may be recommended. Mothers often use herbal galactagogues such as fenugreek, blessed thistle, goat's rue, and shatavari to increase milk production. However, there is a lack of evidence to support the use of these substances (ABM, 2018; Sachs & Committee on Drugs, 2013).

Pharmaceutical galactagogues must be prescribed by the health care provider. Metoclopramide and domperidone are the most commonly prescribed medications; both are dopamine antagonists typically used to treat gastroesophageal reflux. It is thought that they increase prolactin levels, which enhances milk production. There is a lack of evidence to support the use of these medications in breastfeeding women (Sachs & Committee on Drugs, 2013).

Domperidone is often prescribed for lactating women in Canada and other countries, although it is not available in the United States, except in special circumstances for clients with severe GI motility disorders. Domperidone has been associated with increased risk for cardiac arrhythmias, cardiac arrest, and sudden cardiac death. The USFDA has issued warnings against its use by lactating women to increase milk production (USFDA, 2004).

Plugged milk ducts. A milk duct can become plugged or clogged, causing an area of the breast to become swollen and tender. This area typically does not empty or soften with feeding or pumping. A small white pearl may be visible on the tip of the nipple; this pearl is the curd of milk blocking the flow. The mother is afebrile and has no generalized symptoms.

Plugged milk ducts are most often the result of inadequate removal of milk from the breast, which can be caused by clothing that is too tight, a poorly fitting or underwire bra, or always using the same position for feeding. Application of warm compresses to the affected area and to the nipple before feeding helps promote emptying of the breast and release of the plug.

Frequent feeding is recommended, with the baby beginning the feeding on the affected side to foster more complete emptying. The mother is advised to massage the affected area while the infant nurses or while she is pumping. Varying feeding positions and feeding without wearing a bra may be useful in resolving a plugged duct. Plugged milk ducts can increase susceptibility to breast infection. For recurrent plugged ducts, taking lecithin, a fat emulsifier, may be useful (Lawrence & Lawrence, 2016).

Mastitis. Although the term mastitis means inflammation of the breast, it is most often used to refer to infection of the breast. It is characterized by the sudden onset of influenza-like symptoms, including fever, chills, malaise, body aches, headache, nausea, and vomiting. The woman usually has localized breast pain and tenderness and a hot, reddened area on the breast. Mastitis most commonly occurs in the upper outer quadrant of the breast; one or both breasts can be affected. Most cases occur during the first 2 to 4 weeks postpartum, although mastitis can occur at any time (Newton, 2017).

Certain factors can predispose a woman to mastitis. Inadequate emptying of the breasts is common; this can be related to engorgement, plugged ducts, a sudden decrease in the number of feedings, abrupt weaning, or wearing underwire bras. Sore, cracked nipples can lead to mastitis by providing a portal of entry for causative organisms (*Staphylococcus*, *Streptococcus*, and *Escherichia coli* are most common). Stress, fatigue, maternal illness, ill family members, breast trauma, and poor maternal nutrition also are predisposing factors for mastitis (Amir & the Academy of Breastfeeding Medicine, 2014). Breastfeeding mothers should be taught the signs of mastitis before they are discharged from the hospital after birth, and they need to know to call the health care provider promptly if the symptoms occur.

Treatment includes antibiotics such as cephalexin or dicloxacillin for 10 to 14 days and analgesic and antipyretic medications such as ibuprofen. In most cases, mothers with mastitis can continue to breastfeed. Health care providers usually prescribe antibiotics that will not cause harm to the breastfeeding infant. The infection cannot be transmitted to the infant. The mother is advised to rest as much as possible and breastfeed or pump frequently, striving to empty the affected side

adequately. Warm compresses to the breast before feeding or pumping can be useful. Adequate fluid intake and a balanced diet are important for the mother with mastitis (Newton, 2017).

Complications of mastitis include breast abscess, chronic mastitis, and fungal infections of the breast. Most complications can be prevented by early recognition and treatment.

Follow-Up After Discharge

Problems with sore nipples, engorgement, and jaundice are likely to occur after discharge from the birthing facility. Nurses and lactation consultants educate the mother about potential problems she may encounter once she is home. She should be given a list of resources for help with breastfeeding concerns. Community resources for breastfeeding mothers include lactation consultants in hospitals, primary care offices, or private practice; nurses in pediatric or obstetric offices; support groups such as La Leche League; and peer counseling programs (e.g., those offered through WIC). Many websites contain current and correct information about breastfeeding (e.g., www.womenshealth.gov/breastfeeding). The National Breastfeeding Helpline (1-800-994-9662) through the Office of Women's Health provides breastfeeding information and counseling by English- and Spanish-speaking counselors.

Telephone follow-up by nurses or lactation consultants in hospitals, birth centers, clinics, or offices within the first day or two after discharge can help identify problems and offer needed advice and support. It often takes at least 2 weeks for breastfeeding to become established, so ongoing contact with the mother is important in providing her with needed support.

Follow-up care of the breastfeeding mother and infant is interprofessional. Breastfeeding infants should be seen by a pediatric health care provider at 3 to 5 days of age and again at 2 to 3 weeks of age to assess weight gain and offer encouragement and support to the mother (AAP Section on Breastfeeding, 2012). A lactation consultant or a nurse in the pediatric office or clinic will assess breastfeeding and provide education and counseling. Referral may be made to a home health agency or peer counselor for further lactation assistance and support. If the mother encounters problems such as mastitis, she will need to be evaluated by her obstetric or primary health care provider. If the mother is taking any medications, a pharmacist can help evaluate safety of use in lactation.

FORMULA-FEEDING

Parent Education

Many infants receive at least some amount of commercial infant formula during their first year of life. Some parents choose formula-feeding instead of breastfeeding; others combine the two methods. If the infant is weaned from breastfeeding before the first birthday, iron-fortified infant formula should be given (AAP Section on Breastfeeding, 2012).

It is important for nurses and other health care professionals to be intentional about providing education for parents related to formula preparation, feeding, and common problems they can encounter. Because of the lack of clear information about the practical aspects of formula-feeding, parents often rely on advice from friends and family. If that advice is incorrect and the parents use unsafe practices for formula preparation and feeding, the infant is at risk for foodborne illness and burns (see Teaching for Self-Management: Formula Preparation and Feeding).

Readiness for Feeding

Ideally the first feeding of formula is given after the neonate's initial transition to extrauterine life. Feeding-readiness cues include stability of vital signs, effective breathing pattern, presence of bowel sounds, an active sucking reflex, and signs described earlier for breastfed infants.

Feeding Patterns

In the first 24 to 48 hours of life, a newborn typically consumes 15 to 30 mL of formula at a feeding. Intake gradually increases during the first week of life. Most newborns drink 90 to 150 mL at a feeding by the end of the second week or sooner. Many parents do not understand about the capacity of the newborn stomach and will tend to overfeed the newborn infant. In explaining to parents about how the stomach capacity gradually increases, it can be helpful to use analogies. This is also helpful in teaching parents of breastfeeding infants. On day 1, the newborn stomach is about the size of a cherry or a shooter marble and can hold about 5 to 7 mL (approximately 1 to 1½ teaspoons). By the third day, the stomach is about the size of a walnut or ping-pong ball, and the capacity increases to 22 to 27 mL (approximately 1 oz). By 1 week, the stomach is about the size of an apricot with a capacity of 45 to 60 mL (1.5 to 2 oz). By 2 weeks, the stomach is about the size of a large egg with a capacity of 80 to 150 mL (2.5 to 5 oz).

The newborn infant should be fed on demand, not going longer than 4 hours between feeds, even if it is necessary to wake him or her for the feedings; however, rigid feeding schedules are not recommended. The infant showing an adequate weight gain may be allowed to sleep at night and be fed only on awakening. Most newborns need six to eight feedings in 24 hours; the number of feedings decreases as the infant matures and consumes more at each feeding. By 3 to 4 weeks after birth, a fairly predictable feeding pattern has usually developed. Scheduling feedings arbitrarily at predetermined intervals may not meet a newborn's needs, but initiating feedings at convenient times often moves the feedings to times that work for the family.

Mothers usually notice increases in the infant's appetite at the age of approximately 10 days, 3 weeks, 6 weeks, 3 months, and 6 months. These appetite spurts correspond to growth spurts. Mothers should increase the amount of formula per feeding by approximately 30 mL to meet the baby's needs at these times.

Feeding Technique

Infants should be held for all feedings. During feedings parents are encouraged to sit comfortably, holding the infant close in a semi-upright position with good head support. Feedings provide opportunities to bond with the baby through touching, talking, singing, or reading to the infant. Parents should consider feedings a time of peaceful relaxation with the infant. Mothers who bottle-feed should be encouraged to spend some time with their newborns in skin-to-skin contact.

> ### ⚡ SAFETY ALERT
>
> A bottle should never be propped with a pillow or other inanimate object and left with the infant. This practice can result in choking, and it deprives the infant of important interaction during feeding. Moreover, propping the bottle has been implicated in causing nursing-bottle caries or decay of the first teeth resulting from continuous bathing of the teeth with carbohydrate-containing fluid as the infant sporadically sucks the nipple.

Newborns must learn to coordinate sucking, swallowing, and breathing as they feed. The typical fast flow of milk from bottles can create difficulty for an infant trying to learn to feed. A slow-flow nipple is often used for the first few weeks.

Traditionally parents are told to position the infant in a semi-reclining position and to hold the bottle so that fluid fills the nipple and none of the air in the bottle is allowed to enter it (Fig. 25.18A).

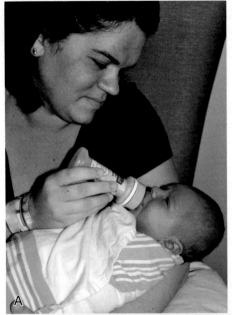

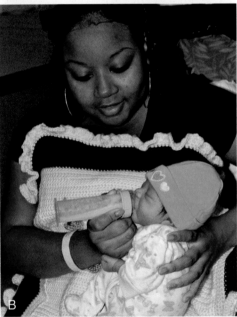

Fig. 25.18 Bottle-feeding. (A) Traditional technique with infant semi-reclining. (B) Paced bottle-feeding: infant is more upright. (Courtesy Cheryl Briggs, RNC, Annapolis, MD.)

A more physiologic approach to bottle-feeding is called paced bottle-feeding. With this method of feeding, the bottle is held at more of a horizontal angle (approximately 45 degrees); when the baby pauses between bursts of sucking, the parent withdraws the nipple, allowing it to rest on the baby's lip until he or she is ready to resume sucking (Lauwers & Swisher, 2016). This position slows the flow of milk from the bottle so the infant is more in control. Paced bottle-feeding works well for infants who are primarily breastfeeding but are occasionally fed from a bottle.

If the infant falls asleep, spits out the nipple, seals the lips, turns the head away, or ceases to suck, it usually indicates that he or she has consumed enough formula to feel satiated. Teach parents to look for these cues and avoid overfeeding, which can contribute to obesity (see Evidence-Based Practice box).

EVIDENCE-BASED PRACTICE
Caregiver Feeding Styles and Childhood Obesity

Ask the Question
Does caregiver responsiveness to infant feeding cues have an effect on obesity in early childhood and beyond?

Search for the Evidence
Search Strategies: English language research-based publications on infant, feeding, satiety, breastfeeding, overweight, obesity were included.
Databases Used: Cochrane Collaborative Database, National Guideline Clearinghouse (AHRQ), CINAHL, PubMed, and UpToDate

Critical Appraisal of the Evidence
Childhood obesity can have its roots in the feeding patterns established in infancy (Gross, Mendelsohn, Fierman, et al., 2014). Overfeeding can impair the infant's ability to self-regulate. Infants whose caregivers are responsive to an infant's hunger and satiety (full) cues are significantly less likely to be overweight (Bahorski, Childs, Loan, et al., 2019).

Discordant responsiveness occurs when the caregiver perceives that the infant cannot recognize hunger or satiety. Restrictive feeding style is associated with maternal fear of causing obesity. Pressuring feeding style is associated with caregiver concern that the infant has poor appetite and will be underweight (Bahorski et al., 2019).

Low-income, food-insecure mothers are more likely to be discordant, either restrictive or pressuring, than food-secure mothers (Gross et al., 2014). Authoritative parenting style is associated with pressuring to eat (Collins, Duncanson, & Burrows, 2014).

Apply the Evidence: Nursing Implications
(Evidence derived from Arikpo, Edet, Chibuzor, et al., 2018; Bahorski, et al., 2019; Feldman-Winters, Burnham, Grossman, et al., 2018; Hodges, Wasser, & Colgan, 2017; McNally, Hugh-Jones, Caton, et al., 2016.)

- Parents can be taught typical feeding cues that let them know their baby's readiness to eat, as well as cues that the baby is satisfied. The nurse should point out the infant cues, and praise the parents for appropriate responsiveness.
- Videos and printed material, as well as warm lines, should be made available to new parents. Specific suggestions as to how much formula to feed initially and as the infant grows, and how voiding and stool patterns and weight gain reflect adequate nutrition can provide education guidelines.
- Clients need to be aware that infant feeding cues are diverse and vary across factors such as age, sex, genotype, developmental level, and method of feeding. Both infant and maternal characteristics affect how feeding cues are perceived. Hunger cues are easier to perceive than cues that the baby is satisfied.
- Education regarding the various newborn cries and their possible reasons can reassure parents and their extended families that feeding should not be the first and only option.
- Overfeeding during the first week of life increases the risk of becoming overweight by age 2. Babies who are exclusively breastfed are least likely to gain extra weight during the first week of life. Parents can be taught about how overfeeding affects the infant's health.
- Parents need information about the risks of overfeeding and the health implications of childhood obesity.
- Education of parents should include that complementary foods are introduced no earlier than 6 months of age.

References
Arikpo, D., Edet, E. S., Chibuzor, M. T., et al. (2018). Educational interventions for improving primary caregiver complementary feeding practices for children aged 24 months and under. *Cochrane Database of Systematic Reviews*, 5, CD011768.
Bahorski, J. S., Childs, G. D., Loan, L. A., et al. (2019). Self-efficacy, infant feeding practices, and infant weight gain: An integrative review. *Journal of Child Health Care*. 23(2), 286–310.
Collins, C., Duncanson, K., & Burrows, T. (2014). A systematic review investigating associations between parenting style and child feeding behaviours. *Journal of Human Nutrition and Dietetics*, 27(6), 557–568.
Feldman-Winter, L., Burnham, L., Grossman, X., et al. (2018). Weight gain in the first week of life predicts overweight at 2 years: A prospective cohort study. *Maternal Child Nutrition*, 14(1), 1–8.
Gross, R. S., Mendelsohn, A. L., Fierman, A. H., et al. (2014). Maternal infant feeding behaviors and disparities in early child obesity. *Childhood Obesity*, 10(2), 145–152.
Hodges, E. A., Wasser, H. M., & Colgan, B. K. (2016). Development of feeding cues during infancy and toddlerhood. *American Journal of Maternal Child Nursing*, 41(4), 244–251.
McNally, J., Hugh-Jones, S., Caton, S., et al. (2016). Communicating hunger and satiation in the first 2 years of life: A systematic review. *Maternal and Child Nutrition*, 12(2), 205–228.

Jennifer Taylor Alderman

Instruct parents to observe the infant for signs of stress during feeding, including turning the head, arching the back, choking, sputtering, changing color, moving the arms, and tensing fists. When these signs occur, the parent should stop feeding and attempt to calm the infant before resuming. The signs can indicate that the infant is finished with the feeding and does not want to drink any more.

Most infants swallow air when fed from a bottle and need a chance to burp several times during a feeding. Parents are taught various positions that can be used for burping (Fig. 25.19).

Common Concerns

Parents need to know what to do if the infant spits up. They may need to decrease the amount of feeding or feed smaller amounts more frequently. Burping the infant several times during a feeding such as when the infant's sucking slows down or stops can decrease spitting. Holding the baby upright for 30 minutes after feeding and avoiding bouncing or placing him or her on the abdomen soon after the feeding is finished also can help. Spitting can be a result of overfeeding, or it can be symptomatic of gastroesophageal reflux. Parents should report vomiting one third or more of the feeding at most feeding sessions or projectile vomiting to the health care provider and should be cautioned to refrain from changing the infant's formula without consulting the health care provider.

Bottles and Nipples

Various brands and styles of bottles and nipples are available. Most infants feed well with any bottle and nipple. Bottles may be standard, angled, wide neck, vented, disposable, or with disposable liners. They may be made of plastic, glass, or stainless steel. Nipples range in shape, size, and flow; they are made of latex or silicon. Preterm and term infants often begin with smaller nipples that have a slow flow rate, moving to larger size nipples with faster flow as age and feeding skills increase.

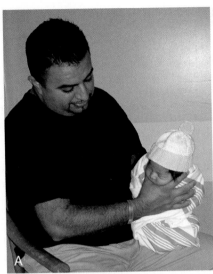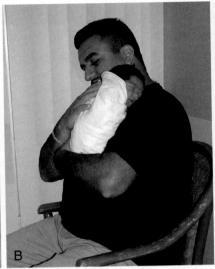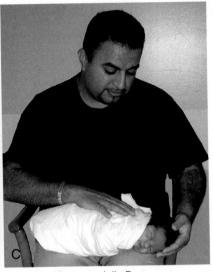

Fig. 25.19 Positions for Burping an Infant. (A) Sitting. (B) On shoulder. (C) Across lap. (Courtesy Julie Perry Nelson, Loveland, CO.)

⚡ **SAFETY ALERT**

Because of concerns about potential harmful effects of bisphenol A (BPA), parents should be cautioned about using hard plastic polycarbonate baby bottles or containers. BPA is a chemical that is used to harden plastics, prevent bacterial contamination of foods, and prevent can rusting. It is in many food and liquid containers, including baby bottles. The AAP (2012) recommends avoiding clear plastic bottles or containers imprinted with the recycling number 7 and the letters PC and purchasing bottles that are certified or identified as BPA-free. Glass bottles are an alternative, but parents must be aware of the risk for injury if the bottle is dropped or broken. Because heat can cause the release of BPA from plastic, polycarbonate bottles should never be boiled, heated in the microwave, or washed in a dishwasher.

Parents should be instructed in proper cleaning of all equipment used in formula preparation and feeding. See Teaching for Self-Management: Formula Preparation and Feeding.

Infant Formulas

Commercial Formulas

Commercial infant formulas are designed to resemble human milk as closely as possible, although none has ever duplicated it. The exact composition of infant formula varies with the manufacturer, but all must meet specific standards. The FDA regulates the manufacture of infant formula in the United States to ensure product safety.

Infants who are not breastfed should be given commercial iron-fortified formulas. The AAP recommends iron-fortified formulas from birth to 1 year of age for infants who are not breastfed and for those who are partially breastfed (Baker et al., 2010).

⚡ **SAFETY ALERT**

The type of commercial infant formula that parents choose should be based on the recommendation of the pediatric health care provider. Specialty formulas are designed for infants with specific needs and should be used only if recommended or prescribed by the health care provider.

The most widely used commercially prepared formulas are cow's milk–based formulas that have been modified to closely resemble the nutritional content of human milk. The caloric content of standard infant formula is 19 to 20 kcal/oz. These formulas are altered from cow's milk by removing butterfat, decreasing the protein content, and adding vegetable oil and carbohydrate. The major carbohydrate is lactose. Regardless of the commercial brand, the standard cow's milk–based formulas have essentially the same compositions of vitamins, minerals, protein, carbohydrates, and essential amino acids, with minor variations such as the source of carbohydrate; nucleotides to enhance immune function; and long-chain polyunsaturated fatty acids (DHA and ARA), which are thought to improve visual and cognitive function. Some formulas contain added probiotic and others are fortified with prebiotics in the form of oligosaccharides to mimic natural oligosaccharides in human milk. Some parents choose to feed only organic infant formulas. Many desire a natural formula without preservatives; without artificial flavors, colors, or sweeteners; made from milk produced by cows fed only organic foods, without pesticides or herbicides, growth hormones, antibiotics, steroids, or other harmful additives.

Protein hydrolysate formulas, also known as predigested formulas, contain proteins that are broken down into smaller particles for easier digestion; they are lactose free. These formulas are either partially hydrolyzed or extensively hydrolyzed. Infants at risk for atopic disease (e.g., eczema) and those with documented IgE allergies caused by cow's milk should be fed an extensively hydrolyzed protein formula. Extensively hydrolyzed formulas are recommended for infants with intolerance to cow milk or soy proteins. Amino acid formulas are used for infants who have dairy protein allergy and are unable to tolerate hydrolyzed formulas (Parks, Shaikhkhalil, Groleau, et al., 2016).

Soy protein–based formulas are free of cow milk–based protein and lactose; sucrose, corn syrup solids, and/or maltodextrin are added to meet the caloric content; fat content is similar to cow milk–based formulas. Uses of this type of infant formula are limited; soy protein–based formulas are recommended for infants with galactosemia and congenital lactase deficiency; infants with secondary lactase deficiency may benefit as well. Soy protein–based formulas have not been proven

TEACHING FOR SELF-MANAGEMENT
Formula Preparation and Feeding

Formula Preparation

- Using warm soapy water, wash your hands, and arms, and clean under your nails; rinse well. Clean and sanitize the surface where you will be preparing the bottles.
- In a basin that is only used for cleaning equipment used in formula preparation and feeding, thoroughly wash bottles, nipples, rings, caps, can opener, and other preparation utensils in hot soapy water and rinse thoroughly. Squeeze water through nipples to make sure that the holes are open.
- Place bottles, nipples, rings, and caps in a pot, and cover with water; boil for 5 minutes; remove items from pot with sanitized tongs, and allow them to air dry. (Do this before using items the first time; thereafter you can continue to do this or place items in the dishwasher.)
- Note the expiration date on the formula container. It should be used before the expiration date. Any unopened expired formula should be returned to the place of purchase.
- Read the label on the container of formula, and mix it exactly according to the directions.
- Mix formula with tap water deemed safe by the local health department. Allow cold water to run for 1 minute before collecting it. If water is unsafe or the safety is uncertain, it should be boiled for 1 minute and allowed to cool, but not for longer than 30 minutes, before mixing with formula. If using bottled water, make sure that it is labeled as "sterile"; unsterile bottled water must be boiled.
- If using a can of ready-to-feed or concentrated formula, wash the top of the can with hot soapy water and rinse well. Shake the can before opening.
- Mixing formula
  - Ready-to-feed: No mixing is needed; do not add water. Pour desired amount of formula into clean bottle; add nipple and ring.
  - Concentrate: Pour desired amount of formula into clean bottle and add equal amount of cooled boiled water. Add nipple and ring and shake well.
  - Powder: When first opening the container of powder, write the date on the lid. Using the scoop from the container, add 1 scoop of powdered formula for each 2 oz of boiled, cooled water in a clean bottle. For example, if 6 oz of water is in the bottle, add three scoops of powder. Add nipple and ring, and shake well.
- If preparing multiple bottles at the same time, place nipple right side up on each bottle and cover with a clean nipple cap. Use bottles within 48 hours.
- Opened cans of ready-to-feed or concentrated formula should be covered and refrigerated. Any unused portions must be discarded after 48 hours.
- Bottles or cans of unopened formula can be stored at room temperature.
- If the formula is refrigerated, warm it by placing the bottle in a pan of hot water. Never use a microwave to warm any food to be given to a baby. Test the temperature of the formula by letting a few drops fall on the inside of your wrist. If the formula feels comfortably warm to you, the temperature is correct. Milk at room temperature can be fed to the infant.
- A bottle of formula should be discarded within 1 hour after being fed to an infant; do not save the "leftovers" for another feeding.

Feeding Techniques and Tips

- Wash your hands with soap and water before feeding.

- Newborns should be fed at least every 3 to 4 hours and should never go longer than 4 hours without feeding until a satisfactory pattern of weight gain is established. This period can be as long as 2 weeks. If a baby cries or fusses between feedings, check to see if the diaper should be changed and if the baby needs to be picked up and cuddled. If the baby continues to cry and acts hungry, feed him or her. Babies do not get hungry on a regular schedule.
- Infants gradually increase the amount of milk they drink with each feeding. The first day or so, most newborns consume 15 to 30 mL (0.5 to 1 oz) with each feeding. This amount increases as the infant grows. If any formula remains in the bottle as the feeding ends, it must be thrown away because saliva from the baby's mouth can cause the formula to spoil.
- Keep a feeding diary, writing down the amount of formula the infant drinks with each feeding for the first week or so. Also record the number of the baby's wet diapers and bowel movements. Take this diary with you to the baby's first follow-up visit with the primary health care provider.
- For feeding, hold the infant close in a semi-reclining position. Talk to him or her during the feeding. This time is ideal for social interaction and cuddling.
- Place the nipple in the infant's mouth on the tongue. It should touch the roof of the mouth to stimulate the baby's sucking reflex. Hold the bottle like a pencil. Keep it tipped so the nipple stays filled with milk and the baby does not suck in air.
- Taking a few sucks and then pausing briefly before continuing to suck again is normal for infants. Some infants take longer to feed than others. Be patient. Keep the baby awake; encouraging sucking may be necessary. Moving the nipple gently in the infant's mouth may stimulate sucking.
- Another technique that can be used for bottle-feeding is *paced bottle-feeding*. The infant is placed in a more upright position, and the bottle is held at a more horizontal angle. When the baby pauses between bursts of sucking, withdraw the nipple and allow it to rest on the baby's lip until he or she is ready to resume sucking. This slows the flow of milk from the bottle so the infant is more in control. Paced bottle-feeding works well for infants who are primarily breastfeeding but are occasionally fed from a bottle.
- Newborns are apt to swallow air when sucking. Give the infant opportunities to burp several times during a feeding. As he or she gets older, you will know better when to stop for burping.
- Watch for signs that the infant is getting full: spitting out the nipple, sealing the lips together, slower sucking, or turning away from the nipple.
- After the first 2 or 3 days, the stools of a formula-fed infant are yellow and soft but formed. The infant may have a stool with each feeding in the first 2 weeks, although this amount can decrease to one or two stools each day. It is not abnormal for formula-fed infants to have a stool every other day.

Safety Tips

- Infants should be held and never left alone while feeding. Never prop the bottle. The infant might inhale formula or choke on any that was spit up. Infants who fall asleep with a propped bottle of milk can be prone to cavities when the first teeth come in.
- Know how to use the bulb syringe and help an infant who is choking.

Data from American Academy of Pediatrics. (2018). Ages and stages: Formula feeding: How to sterilize and warm baby bottles safely. Retrieved from https://www.healthychildren.org/English/ages-stages/baby/formula-feeding/Pages/How-to-Sterilize-and-Warm-Baby-Bottles-Safely.aspx; American Academy of Pediatrics Committee on Nutrition. (2014). Feeding the infant. In R. E. Kleinman & F. R. Greer (Eds.), *Pediatric nutrition* (7th ed.). Elk Grove Village, IL: American Academy of Pediatrics; Centers for Disease Control and Prevention. (2018). Infant formula preparation and storage. Retrieved from https://www.cdc.gov/nutrition/infantandtoddlernutrition/formula-feeding/infant-formula-preparation-and-storage.html.

to be effective against colic or in the prevention of allergy in healthy or high-risk infants (Bhatia, Greer, & AAP Committee on Nutrition, 2008; Parks, et al., 2016).

> ## ⚡ SAFETY ALERT
>
> Alternate milk sources such as goat's milk; skim or low-fat milk; condensed milk; or raw, unpasteurized milk from any animal source should not be fed to infants because they are inadequate to support growth and can contain excess protein or an inadequate calcium-to-phosphorus ratio, which can cause seizures.

Formula Preparation

Commercial formulas are available in three forms: powder, concentrate, and ready to feed. All forms are equivalent in terms of nutritional content, but they vary considerably in cost.

Ready-to-feed formula is the most expensive but the easiest to use. The desired amount is poured into the bottle. The opened can is refrigerated safely for 48 h. This type of formula can be purchased in individual disposable bottles for the most convenient feeding.

Concentrated formula is less expensive than ready to feed. It is diluted with equal parts of water and can be stored in the refrigerator for 48 h after opening.

Powdered formula is the least expensive. For most brands, it is easily mixed by using 1 scoop for every 60 mL of water.

The commercial infant formula must include label directions for preparation and use of the formula with pictures and symbols for the benefit of individuals who cannot read. Some manufacturers translate the directions into languages such as Spanish, French, Vietnamese, Chinese, and Arabic to prevent misunderstanding and errors in formula preparation.

> ## ⚡ SAFETY ALERT
>
> An important aspect to impress on families is that the proportions must not be altered (i.e., neither diluted to extend the amount of formula nor concentrated to provide more calories) unless advised by a medical professional. The newborn's kidneys are immature; giving the infant overly concentrated formula can provide protein and minerals in amounts that exceed the excretory ability of the kidneys. In contrast, if the formula is diluted too much (sometimes done to save money), the infant does not consume sufficient calories to grow appropriately and may become hyponatremic.

Sterilization of formula rarely is recommended when families have access to a safe public water supply. Instead formula is prepared with attention to cleanliness. When water from a private well is used, parents should be advised to contact the health department to have a chemical and bacteriologic analysis of the water performed before using the water in formula preparation. The presence of nitrates, excess fluoride, or bacteria can be harmful to the infant. If parents are concerned or uncertain about the safety of their water supply, they can prepare formula with bottled water or cold tap water that has been boiled for 1 minute and allowed to cool for no longer than 30 minutes. Otherwise, it is safe to mix formula with tap water (AAP, 2018).

If the conditions in the home appear unsanitary, the nurse should recommend the use of ready-to-feed formula or teach the mother to sterilize the formula. The two traditional methods for sterilization are terminal heating and the aseptic method. In the terminal heating method, the prepared formula is placed in the bottles, which are topped with the nipples placed upside down and covered with the caps and sealed loosely with the rings. The bottles are then boiled together in a water bath for 25 minutes. This would likely result in vitamin loss. A better method is the aseptic method in which the bottles, rings, caps, nipples, and any other necessary equipment such as a funnel are boiled separately, after which the formula is poured into the bottles. Instructions for formula preparation and feeding are provided in Teaching for Self-Management: Formula Preparation and Feeding.

Vitamin and Mineral Supplementation

Commercial iron-fortified formula has all of the nutrients that infants need for the first 6 months of life. After 6 months of age, fluoride supplementation is recommended based on levels in the water supply.

Weaning

The bottle-fed infant gradually learns to use a cup, and the parents find that they are preparing fewer bottles. The bottle-feeding before bedtime is often the last one to remain. Babies have a strong need to suck, and the baby who has the bottle taken away too early or abruptly compensates with nonnutritive sucking on his or her fingers, thumb, a pacifier, or even the tongue. Therefore, weaning from a bottle should be attempted gradually because the baby has learned to rely on the comfort that sucking provides.

Complementary Feeding: Introducing Solid Foods

Complementary feedings are defined as foods or liquids given to the infant in addition to breast milk or formula. The AAP recommends introducing solid foods after 6 months of age (AAP Committee on Nutrition, 2014; AAP Section on Breastfeeding, 2012). First foods should include iron- and zinc-fortified cereals and meats. New foods should be introduced slowly to assess for any allergic reaction or intolerance. It is best to wait 3 to 5 days before introducing a new food. Infants should be consuming foods from all food groups by 7 to 8 months of age. Fruit juices are not recommended before 6 months of age, and juice consumption should be limited because it is possible that the infant who drinks juice will consume less breast milk or formula. Consumption of low-nutrient foods such as fatty or sugary foods or restaurant foods should be limited (AAP Committee on Nutrition).

In spite of the recommendations from the AAP, many parents begin complementary feedings earlier than 4 months of age. They need to be informed that the infant receives the right balance of nutrients from breast milk or formula during the first 4 to 6 months. The notion that the feeding of solids helps the infant sleep through the night is not true. Parents should not put cereal into the infant's bottle. Introduction of solid foods before the infant is 4 to 6 months of age can result in overfeeding and decreased intake of breast milk or formula.

Cultural beliefs and traditions affect complementary feeding practices. First foods given to infants vary widely. For example, first foods for Egyptian infants include bread soaked in milk and tea or yogurt sweetened with honey. Chinese and Vietnamese infants are sometimes fed prechewed rice paste, rice, or sweetened porridge.

Nurses and other health care professionals educate parents regarding complementary feedings. This most often occurs during well-baby supervision visits with the pediatric health care provider. Early feeding practices have implications for long-term dietary patterns; therefore, it is essential to teach parents about proper nutrition.

KEY POINTS

- Breast milk is recommended for infants for the first year of life.
- Exclusive breastfeeding is recommended for the first six months.
- Breast milk is species specific and provides immunologic protection against many infections and diseases.
- Breast milk changes in composition with each stage of lactogenesis, during each feeding, and as the infant grows.
- During the prenatal period, expectant parents should be informed of the benefits of breastfeeding for infants, mothers, families, and society.
- Infants should be breastfed as soon as possible after birth, preferably during the first hour and at least 8 to 12 times every 24 hours thereafter.
- Parents should be taught the signs of effective feeding.
- Breast milk production is based on a supply-meets-demand principle: the more the infant nurses, the greater the milk supply.

- Infants go through predictable growth spurts.
- All women should be instructed in hand expression and if desired, assisted as needed in selecting the appropriate devices for mechanical milk expression.
- Sore nipples are most often caused by incorrect latch.
- Engorgement occurs around 3 days after birth and with appropriate treatment resolves within 24 hours.
- Iron-fortified commercial infant formula is recommended for the first year of life for infants who are not breastfed or are partially breastfed.
- Parents need instruction about formula preparation and feeding.
- Complementary feeding should begin at 6 months of age.
- Nurses must be knowledgeable about feeding methods and provide education and support for families.

REFERENCES

American Academy of Family Physicians. (2012). *Breastfeeding policy statement*. Retrieved from: www.aafp.org/online/en/home/policy/policies/b/breastfeedingpolicy.html.

American Academy of Pediatrics. (2012). *Ages and stages: Baby bottles and bisphenol A (BPA)*. Retrieved from: https://www.healthychildren.org/English/ages-stages/baby/feeding-nutrition/Pages/Baby-Bottles-And-Bisphenol-A-BPA.aspx.

American Academy of Pediatrics. (2018). *Ages and stages: Formula feeding: How to sterilize and warm baby bottles safely*. Retrieved from: https://www.healthychildren.org/English/ages-stages/baby/formula-feeding/Pages/How-to-Sterilize-and-Warm-Baby-Bottles-Safely.aspx.

American Academy of Pediatrics Committee on Nutrition. (2014). Feeding the infant. In R. E. Kleinman, & F. R. Greer (Eds.), *Pediatric nutrition* (7th ed.). Elk Grove Village, IL: American Academy of Pediatrics.

American Academy of Pediatrics Committee on Nutrition, Section on Breastfeeding, & Committee on Fetus and Newborn. (2017). Donor human milk for the high-risk infant: Preparation, safety, and usage options in the United States. *Pediatrics, 139*(1), e20163440.

American Academy of Pediatrics Section on Breastfeeding. (2012). Breastfeeding and the use of human milk—Policy statement. *Pediatrics, 129*(3), e827–e841.

American College of Nurse-Midwives. (2016). *Position statement: Breastfeeding*. Retrieved from: http://www.midwife.org/ACNM/files/ACNMLibraryData/UPLOADFILENAME/000000000248/Breastfeeding-statement-Feb-2016.pdf.

American College of Obstetricians and Gynecologists. (2018). Committee opinion no. 756: Optimizing support for breastfeeding as part of obstetric practice. *Obstetrics & Gynecology, 132*(4), e187–e196.

American Dietetic Association. (2009). Position of the American Dietetic Association: Promoting and supporting breastfeeding. *Journal of the American Dietetic Association, 109*(11), 1926–1942.

Amir, L. H., & & the Academy of Breastfeeding Medicine Protocol Committee. (2014). ABM clinical protocol no. 4: Mastitis, revised March 2014. *Breastfeeding Medicine, 9*(5), 239–243.

Anderson, P. O. (2016). LactMed update: An introduction. *Breastfeeding Medicine, 11*(2), 54–55.

Association of Women's Health, Obstetric and Neonatal Nurses. (2014). AWHONN position statement: Breastfeeding. *Journal of Obstetric, Gynecologic and Neonatal Nursing, 44*(1), 145–150.

Association of Women's Health, Obstetric and Neonatal Nurses. (2015). *Breastfeeding support: Preconception care through the first year* (3rd ed.). Washington, DC: Author.

Friendly, U. S. A. (2019). *The Baby-Friendly Hospital Initiative*. Retrieved from: https://www.babyfriendlyusa.org/about/.

Baker, R. D., Greer, F. R., & American Academy of Pediatrics Committee on Nutrition. (2010). Clinical report: Diagnosis and prevention of iron-deficiency and iron-deficiency anemia in infants and young children (0–3 years of age). *Pediatrics, 126*(5), 1–11.

Berens, P., Brodribb, W., & & the Academy of Breastfeeding Medicine. (2016). ABM clinical protocol no. 20: Engorgement, revised 2016. *Breastfeeding Medicine, 11*(4), 159–163.

Berens, P., Eglash, A., & Malloy, M. (2016). ABM clinical protocol no. 26: Persistent pain with breastfeeding. *Breastfeeding Medicine, 11*(2), 46–53.

Berens, P., Labbok, M., & & the Academy of Breastfeeding Medicine. (2015). ABM protocol no. 13: Contraception during breastfeeding, revised 2015. *Breastfeeding Medicine, 10*(1), 3–12.

Bhatia, J., Greer, F., & & American Academy of Pediatrics Committee on Nutrition.. (2008). Use of soy protein-based formulas in infant feeding. *Pediatrics, 121*(5), 1062–1068.

Blackburn, S. T. (2018). *Maternal, fetal, and neonatal physiology* (5th ed.). St. Louis: Elsevier.

Boies, E. G., Vaucher, Y. E., & & the Academy of Breastfeeding Medicine. (2016). ABM clinical protocol no. 10: Breastfeeding the late preterm (34-36 6/7 weeks of gestation) and early term infants (37-38 6/7 weeks of gestation), 2nd revision. *Breastfeeding Medicine, 11*(10), 494–500.

Brodribb, W., & & the Academy of Breastfeeding Medicine. (2018). ABM clinical protocol no. 9: Use of galactogogues in initiating or augmenting maternal milk production, second revision 2018. *Breastfeeding Medicine, 13*(5), 307–314.

Caplinger, P., Cooney, A. T., Bledsoe, C., et al. (2015). Breastfeeding outcomes following bariatric surgery. *Clinical Lactation, 6*(4), 144–152.

Centers for Disease Control and Prevention. (2018a). *Breastfeeding facts*. Retrieved from: http://www.cdc.gov/breastfeeding/data/facts.html.

Centers for Disease Control and Prevention. (2018b). *Breastfeeding report card*. Retrieved from: http://www.cdc.gov/breastfeeding/data/reportcard.htm.

Chantry, C. J., Eglash, A., & Labbok, M. (2015). Position on breastfeeding—Revised 2015. *Breastfeeding Medicine, 10*(9), 407–411.

Chowdhury, R., Sinha, B., Sankar, M. J., et al. (2015). Breastfeeding and maternal health outcomes: A systematic review and meta-analysis. *Acta Paediatrica, 104*(467), 96–113.

Colson, S. (2012). The laid-back breastfeeding revolution. *Midwifery Today With International Midwife,* (101), 9–11, 66.

Dell, K. M. (2015). Fluid, electrolytes, and acid-base homeostasis. In R. J. Martin, A. A. Fanaroff, & M. C. Walsh (Eds.), *Fanaroff and Martin's neonatal-perinatal medicine: Diseases of the fetus and infant* (10th ed.). St. Louis: Mosby.

Dennis, C., Jackson, K., & Watson, J. (2014). Interventions for treating painful nipples among breastfeeding women. *Cochrane Database of Systematic Reviews, 12*, CD007366.

Evans, A., Marinelli, K. A., Taylor, J. S., et al. (2014). ABM clinical protocol no. 2: Guidelines for hospital discharge of the breastfeeding term newborn and mother: "The going home protocol", revised 2014. *Breastfeeding Medicine*, *9*(1), 3–8.

Farrow, A. (2015). Lactation support and the LGBTQI community. *Journal of Human Lactation*, *31*(1), 26–28.

Grummer-Strawn, L. A., & Rollins, N. (2015). Summarising the health benefits of breastfeeding. *Acta Paediatrica*, *104*(467), 1–2.

Hale, T. W., & Rowe, H. E. (2017). *Medications and mothers' milk* (17th ed.). New York, N.Y.: Springer.

Human Milk Banking Association of North America. (2018). *Guidelines for the establishment and operation of a donor human milk bank*. Ft. Worth, TX: Author. Retrieved from: https://www.hmbana.org/publications.

Human Milk Banking Association of North America. (2019). *Find a milk bank*. Retrieved from: https://hmbana.org/find-a-milk-bank/.

Institute of Medicine. (2005). *Dietary reference intakes for energy, carbohydrate, fiber, fatty acids, cholesterol, protein, and amino acids*. Washington, DC: National Academies Press.

Jenson, D., Wallace, S., & Kelsay, P. (1994). LATCH: A breastfeeding charting system and documentation tool. *Journal of Obstetric, Gynecologic and Neonatal Nursing*, *23*(1), 27–32.

Kamath-Rayne, B. D., Thilo, E. H., Deacon, J., et al. (2016). Neonatal hyperbilirubinemia. In S. L. Gardner, B. S. Carter, M. Enzman Hines, et al. (Eds.), *Merenstein & Gardner's handbook of neonatal intensive care* (8th ed.). St. Louis: Elsevier.

Kanhadilok, S., & McGrath, J. M. (2015). An integrative review of factors influencing breastfeeding in adolescent mothers. *Journal of Perinatal Education*, *24*(2), 119–127.

Kellams, A., Harrel, C., Omage, S., et al. (2017). Supplementary feedings in the healthy term breastfed neonate, revised 2017. *Breastfeeding Medicine*, *12*(3), 188–198.

Kominiarek, M. A., & Rajan, P. (2016). Nutrition recommendations in pregnancy and lactation. *Medical Clinics of North America*, *100*(6), 1199–1215.

Lauwers, J., & Swisher, A. (2016). Breastfeeding techniques and devices. *Counseling the nursing mother* (6th ed.). Burlington MA: Jones & Bartlett.

Lawrence, R. M., & Lawrence, R. A. (2016). *Breastfeeding: A guide for the medical profession* (8th ed.). St. Louis: Elsevier.

Mangesi, L., & Zakarija-Grkovic, I. (2016). Treatments for breast engorgement during lactation. *Cochrane Database of Systematic Reviews*, 6, CD006946.

Marinelli, K. A., Moren, K., Taylor, J. S., et al. (2013). Breastfeeding support for mothers in workplace employment or educational settings: Summary statement. *Breastfeeding Medicine*, *8*(1), 137–142.

Martino, K., & Spatz, D. (2014). Informal milk sharing: What nurses need to know. *Maternal-Child Nursing Journal*, *39*(6), 369–374.

Matson, A. P., Marinelli, K. A., & & the Academy of Breastfeeding Medicine. (2011). ABM clinical protocol no. 24: Allergic proctocolitis in the exclusively breastfed infant. *Breastfeeding Medicine*, *6*(6), 435–440.

McMillan, D. (1997, reaffirmed 2016). *& Canadian Paediatric Society Fetus and Newborn Committee*. Position statement: Routine administration of vitamin K to newborns. Retrieved from: www.cps.ca/documents/position/administration-vitamin-K-newborns.

Meier, P. P., Patel, A. L., Hoban, R., et al. (2016). Which breast pump for which mother: An evidence-based approach to individualizing breast pump technology. *Journal of Perinatology*, *36*(7), 493–499.

Morton, J., Hall, J. Y., & Pessl, M. (2013–2014). Five steps to improve bedside breastfeeding care. *Nursing for Women's Health*, *17*(6), 478–488.

Mueffelmann, R. E., Racine, E. F., Warren-Findlow, J., et al. (2015). Perceived infant feeding preferences of significant family members and mothers' intentions to exclusively breastfeed. *Journal of Human Lactation*, *31*(3), 479–489.

Mueller, N. T., Bakacs, E., Combellick, J., et al. (2015). The infant microbiome development: Mom matters. *Trends in Molecular Medicine*, *21*(2), 109–117.

Newton, E. R. (2017). Lactation and breastfeeding. In S. G. Gabbe, J. R. Niebyl, J. L. Simpson, et al. (Eds.), *Obstetrics: Normal and problem pregnancies* (7th ed.). Philadelphia: Elsevier.

Odom, E. C., Li, R., Scanlon, K. S., et al. (2013). Reasons for earlier than desired cessation of breastfeeding. *Pediatrics*, *131*(3), e726–e732.

Odom, E. C., Li, R., Scanlon, K. S., et al. (2014). Association of family and health care provider opinion on infant feeding with mother's breastfeeding decision. *Journal of the Academy of Nutrition and Dietetics*, *114*(8), 1203–1207.

Office of Disease Prevention and Health Promotion. (2018). *Healthy People 2020: Maternal, infant, and child health*. Retrieved from: https://www.healthypeople.gov/2020/topics-objectives/topic/maternal-infant-and-child-health/objectives.

Parks, E. P., Shaikhkhalil, A., Groleau, V., et al. (2016). Feeding healthy infants, children, and adolescents. In R. M. Kliegman, B. F. Stanton, J. W. St Geme, III, et al. (Eds.), *Nelson textbook of pediatrics* (20th ed.). Philadelphia: Elsevier.

Reece-Stremtan, S., Marinelli, K. A., & & the Academy of Breastfeeding Medicine. (2015). ABM clinical protocol no. 21: Guidelines for breastfeeding and substance use or substance use disorder. *Breastfeeding Medicine*, *10*(3), 135–141.

Robertson, B. D. (2014). Working and breastfeeding: Practical ways you can support employed and breastfeeding mothers. *Clinical Lactation*, *5*(4), 137–140.

Roll, C. L., & Cheater, F. (2016). Expectant parents' views of factors influencing infant feeding decisions in the antenatal period: A systematic review. *International Journal of Nursing Studies*, *60*, 145–155.

Rosen-Carole, C., Hartman, S., & the Academy of Breastfeeding Medicine. (2015). ABM clinical protocol no. 19: Breastfeeding promotion in the prenatal setting. *Breastfeeding Medicine*, *10*(10), 451–457.

Sachs, H. C., & & Committee on Drugs.. (2013). The transfer of drugs and therapeutics into human breast milk: An update on selected topics. *Pediatrics*, *132*(3), e796–e809.

Sankar, M. J., Sinha, B., Chowdhury, R., et al. (2015). Optimal breastfeeding practices and infant and child mortality: A systematic review and meta-analysis. *Acta Paediatrica*, *104*(467), 3–13.

Sriraman, N. K., Evans, A. E., Lawrence, R., et al. (2018). Academy of Breastfeeding Medicine's 2017 position statement on informal breast milk sharing for the term healthy infant. *Breastfeeding Medicine*, *13*(1), 2–4.

Sriraman, N. K., Melvin, K., Meltzer-Brody, S., & the Academy of Breastfeeding Medicine. (2015). ABM clinical protocol no. 18: Use of antidepressants in breastfeeding mothers. *Breastfeeding Medicine*, *10*(6), 290–299.

Stuebe, A. M. (2014). Enabling women to achieve their breastfeeding goals. *Obstetrics & Gynecology*, *123*(3), 643–652.

Taylor, S. N., & & the Academy of Breastfeeding Medicine. (2018). ABM clinical protocol no. 29: Iron, zinc, and vitamin D supplementation during breastfeeding. *Breastfeeding Medicine*, *13*(6), 398–404.

The Joint Commission. (2012). *Specifications manual for Joint Commission national quality core measures (version 2013A1)*. Washington, DC: Author. Retrieved from: https://manual.jointcommission.org/releases/TJC2013A/MIF0170.html.

Thibeau, S., & Ginsberg, H. G. (2018). Bioethics in practice: The ethics surrounding the use of donor milk. *The Ochsner Journal*, *18*(1), 17–19.

Turcksin, R., Bel, S., Galjaard, S., et al. (2014). Maternal obesity and breastfeeding intention, initiation, intensity and duration: A systematic review. *Maternal and Child Nutrition*, *10*(2), 166–183.

U.S. Breastfeeding Committee. (2010a). *Core competencies in breastfeeding care and services for all health care professionals*. Washington, DC: Author.

U.S. Breastfeeding Committee. (2010b). *Implementing the Joint Commission perinatal care core measure on exclusive breast milk feeding*. Washington, DC: Author. rev. ed.

U.S. Food and Drug Administration. (2004). *FDA talk paper: FDA warns against women using unapproved drug, domperidone, to increase milk production*. Retrieved from: https://www.fda.gov/Drugs/DrugSafety/InformationbyDrugClass/ucm173886.htm.

U.S. Food and Drug Administration. (2015). *Use of donor milk*. Retrieved from: http://www.fda.gov/ScienceResearch/SpecialTopics/PediatricTherapeuticsResearch/ucm235203.htm.

U.S. National Library of Medicine. (2018). Nicotine. *LactMed*. Retrieved from: https://toxnet.nlm.nih.gov/.

Victora, C. G., Bahl, R., Barros, A. J., et al. (2016). Breastfeeding in the 21st century: Epidemiology, mechanisms, and lifelong effect. *Lancet*, *387*(10017), 475–490.

Wagner, C., Grier, F., & & American Academy of Pediatrics Section on Breastfeeding, and Committee on Nutrition. (2008). Prevention of rickets and vitamin D deficiency in infants, children and adolescents. *Pediatrics, 122*(5), 1142–1152.

Wilson, E., Perrin, M. T., Fogleman, A., et al. (2015). The intricacies of induced lactation for same-sex mothers of an adopted child. *Journal of Human Lactation, 31*(1), 64–67.

Wolfe-Roubatis, E., & Spatz, D. L. (2015). Transgender men and lactation. *Maternal-Child Nursing Journal, 40*(1), 32–38.

World Health Organization. (2013). *Essential nutrition actions: Improving maternal, newborn, infant, and young child health and nutrition.* Geneva, Switzerland: Author. Retrieved from: http://www.who.int/nutrition/publications/infantfeeding/essential_nutrition_actions/en/.

World Health Organization. (2016). *Exclusive breastfeeding. E-library of evidence for nutrition actions.* Geneva, Switzerland: Author. Retrieved from: http://www.who.int/elena/titles/exclusive_breastfeeding/en/.

World Health Organization. (2017). *National implementation of the Baby-Friendly hospital initiative.* Geneva, Switzerland: Author. Retrieved from: http://www.who.int/nutrition/publications/guidelines/breastfeeding-facilities-maternity-newborn/en/.

26

Assessment of High-Risk Pregnancy

Janet A. Tucker

http://evolve.elsevier.com/Lowdermilk/MWHC/

LEARNING OBJECTIVES

- Explore biophysical, psychosocial, sociodemographic, and environmental influences on high-risk pregnancy.
- Examine risk factors identified through history, physical examination, and diagnostic techniques.
- Differentiate among screening and diagnostic techniques, including when they are used in pregnancy and for what purposes.

- Discuss psychologic considerations for the woman and her family experiencing a high-risk pregnancy.
- Develop a teaching plan to explain screening and diagnostic techniques and implications of findings to women and their families.

In the most recent year for which figures are available, nearly 4 million births occurred in the United States (Martin, Hamilton, Osterman, et al., 2018). Many of these were the result of pregnancies considered to be *high risk* because the life or health of the mother, fetus, or newborn was jeopardized by circumstances coincidental with or unique to the pregnancy. Care of these high-risk clients requires the combined efforts of an interprofessional health care team. The team may be composed of obstetric clinicians, maternal/fetal medicine specialists, pediatric specialists, nurses, pharmacists, social workers, and dietitians. Factors associated with a diagnosis of a high-risk pregnancy are identified in this chapter. Diagnostic techniques often used to monitor the maternal-fetal unit at risk also are described.

ASSESSMENT OF RISK FACTORS

Pregnancies can be designated as high risk for any of several threats of undesirable outcomes. In the past, risk factors were evaluated only from a medical standpoint. Therefore, only adverse medical, obstetric, or physiologic conditions were considered to place the woman at risk. Today a more comprehensive approach to high-risk pregnancy is used, and the factors associated with high-risk childbearing are grouped into broad categories based on threats to health and pregnancy outcome. Categories of risk include biophysical, psychosocial, sociodemographic, and environmental (Box 26.1). Risk factors are interrelated and cumulative in their effects.

Biophysical risks include factors that originate within the mother or fetus and affect the development or functioning of either one or both. Examples include genetic disorders, nutritional and general health status, and medical or obstetric-related illnesses. Box 26.2 lists common risk factors for several pregnancy-related problems.

Psychosocial risks consist of maternal behaviors and adverse life events that have a negative effect on the health of the mother or fetus.

These risks may include emotional distress, history of depression or other mental health problems, disturbed interpersonal relationships such as intimate partner violence, substance use or abuse, inadequate social support, and unsafe cultural practices.

Sociodemographic risks arise from the context in which the mother and family live. These risks may place the mother and fetus at risk. Examples include lack of prenatal care, low income, single marital status, and being a member of an ethnic minority group (see Box 26.1).

Environmental factors include hazards in the workplace and the woman's general environment and may include environmental chemicals (e.g., lead, mercury), anesthetic gases, and radiation (Chambers & Friedman, 2019; Cunningham, Leveno, Bloom, et al., 2018).

ANTEPARTUM TESTING

Standard prenatal tests that are done for all pregnant women are discussed in Chapter 14 and listed in Table 14.1. This chapter concentrates on the testing that is done for high-risk pregnancies rather than for those considered routine. Antepartum testing has two major goals. The first is to identify fetuses at risk for injury caused by acute or chronic interruption of oxygenation so that permanent injury or death might be prevented. The second goal is to identify appropriately oxygenated fetuses so that unnecessary intervention can be avoided (Miller, Miller, & Cypher, 2017). In most cases monitoring begins by 32 to 34 weeks of gestation and continues regularly until birth. Assessment tests should be selected on the basis of their effectiveness, and the results must be interpreted in light of the complete clinical picture. Box 26.3 lists common maternal and fetal indications for antepartum testing that are supported by available evidence (Miller et al.).

The remainder of this chapter describes maternal and fetal assessment tests that are often used to monitor high-risk pregnancies.

BOX 26.1   Categories of High-Risk Factors

Biophysical Factors

Genetic Considerations: Genetic factors may interfere with normal fetal or neonatal development, result in congenital anomalies, or create difficulties for the mother. These factors include defective genes, transmissible inherited disorders and chromosomal anomalies, multiple pregnancy, large fetal size, and ABO incompatibility.

Nutritional Status: Adequate nutrition, without which fetal growth and development cannot proceed normally, is one of the most important determinants of pregnancy outcome. Conditions that influence nutritional status include the following: young age; three pregnancies in the previous 2 years; tobacco, alcohol, or drug use; inadequate dietary intake because of chronic illness or food fads; inadequate or excessive weight gain; and hematocrit value <33%.

Medical and Obstetric Disorders: Complications of current and past pregnancies, obstetric-related illnesses, and pregnancy losses put the woman at risk (see Box 26.2).

Psychosocial Factors

Smoking: Risks include low-birth-weight infants, higher neonatal mortality rates, increased rates of miscarriage, and increased incidence of prelabor rupture of membranes. These risks are aggravated by low socioeconomic status, poor nutritional status, and concurrent use of alcohol.

Caffeine: Birth defects in humans have not been related to caffeine consumption. However, pregnant women who consume more than 200 mg of caffeine daily (equivalent to about 12 ounces of coffee per day) may be at increased risk for giving birth to infants with intrauterine growth restriction (IUGR).

Alcohol: Although the exact effects of alcohol in pregnancy have not been quantified and its mode of action is largely unexplained, it exerts adverse effects on the fetus, resulting in fetal alcohol syndrome, fetal alcohol effects, learning disabilities, and hyperactivity.

Drugs: The developing fetus may be affected adversely by drugs through several mechanisms. They can be teratogenic, cause metabolic disturbances, produce chemical effects, or cause depression or alteration of central nervous system (CNS) function. This category includes medications prescribed by a health care provider or bought over the counter, and commonly abused drugs such as heroin, cocaine, and marijuana. (See Chapter 31 for more information about drug and alcohol abuse.)

Psychologic Status: Childbearing triggers profound and complex physiologic, psychologic, and social changes, with evidence to suggest a relationship between emotional distress and birth complications. This risk factor includes conditions such as specific intrapsychic disturbances and addictive lifestyles; a history of child abuse or intimate partner violence; inadequate support systems; family disruption or dissolution; maternal role changes or conflicts; noncompliance with cultural norms; unsafe cultural, ethnic, or religious practices; and situational crises.

Sociodemographic Factors

Low Income: Poverty underlies many other risk factors and leads to inadequate financial resources for food and prenatal care, poor general health, increased risk for medical complications of pregnancy, and greater prevalence of adverse environmental influences.

Lack of Prenatal Care: Failure to diagnose and treat complications early is a major risk factor arising from financial barriers or lack of access to care;

depersonalization of the system resulting in long waits, routine visits, variability in health care personnel, and unpleasant physical surroundings; lack of understanding of the need for early and continued care or cultural beliefs that do not support the need; and fear of the health care system and its providers.

Age: Women at both ends of the childbearing age spectrum have an increased incidence of poor outcomes; however, age may not be a risk factor in all cases. Physiologic and psychologic risks should be evaluated.

Adolescents: Possible pregnancy and birth complications include anemia, preeclampsia, prolonged labor, and contracted pelvis and cephalopelvic disproportion. Long-term social implications of early motherhood are lower educational attainment, lower income, increased dependence on government support programs, higher divorce rates, and higher parity.

Mature Mothers: The risks to older mothers (over 35 years of age) are not from age alone but from other considerations such as number and spacing of previous pregnancies, genetic disposition of the parents, medical history, lifestyle, nutrition, and prenatal care. The increased likelihood of chronic diseases and complications that arise from more invasive medical management of a pregnancy and labor combined with demographic characteristics put an older woman at risk. Conditions more likely to be experienced by mature women include chronic hypertension and preeclampsia, diabetes, prolonged labor, cesarean birth, placenta previa, placental abruption, and death. Her fetus is at greater risk for low birth weight and macrosomia, chromosomal abnormalities, congenital malformations, and neonatal death.

Parity: The number of previous pregnancies is a risk factor associated with age and includes all first pregnancies, especially a first pregnancy at either end of the childbearing age continuum. The incidence of preeclampsia and dystocia is increased with a first birth.

Marital Status: The increased mortality and morbidity rates for unmarried women, including an increased risk for preeclampsia, are often related to inadequate prenatal care and a young childbearing age.

Social Determinants of Health: The availability and quality of prenatal care vary widely with geographic residence. Women in metropolitan areas have more prenatal visits than those in rural areas who have fewer opportunities for specialized care and consequently a higher incidence of maternal mortality. Health care in the inner city, where residents are usually poorer and begin childbearing earlier and continue longer, may be of lower quality than in a more affluent neighborhood.

Ethnicity: Although ethnicity by itself is not a major risk, race is associated with some poor pregnancy outcomes. In the United States, for example, African American women have the highest rates of preterm birth, almost twice as high as those of other racial and ethnic groups.

Environmental Factors

Various environmental substances can affect fertility and fetal development, the chance of a live birth, and the child's subsequent mental and physical development. Environmental influences include infections, radiation, chemicals such as mercury and lead, therapeutic drugs, illicit drugs, industrial pollutants, cigarette smoke, stress, and diet. Paternal exposure to mutagenic agents in the workplace has been associated with an increased risk for miscarriage.

Data from Simhan, H. N., Iams, J. D., & Romero, R. (2017). Preterm labor and birth. In S. G. Gabbe, J. R. Niebyl, J. L. Simpson, et al. (Eds.), *Obstetrics: Normal and problem pregnancies* (7th ed.). Philadelphia: Elsevier.

BIOPHYSICAL ASSESSMENT

Daily Fetal Movement Count

Assessment of fetal activity by the mother is a simple yet valuable method for monitoring the condition of the fetus. The daily fetal movement count (DFMC) (also called *kick count*) can be assessed at home and is noninvasive, inexpensive, and simple to understand and usually does not interfere with a daily routine. It is frequently used to monitor the fetus in pregnancies complicated by conditions that may affect fetal oxygenation (see Box 26.2). The presence of movements is generally a reassuring sign of fetal health. During the third trimester, the fetus makes about 30 gross body movements each hour. The mother is able to recognize 70% to 80% of these movements (Greenberg & Druzin, 2017).

BOX 26.2 Specific Pregnancy Problems and Related Risk Factors

Polyhydramnios
Poorly controlled diabetes mellitus
Fetomaternal hemorrhage
Fetal congenital anomalies (e.g., gastrointestinal obstruction, central nervous system abnormalities)
Genetic disorders
Twin-to-twin transfusion syndrome

Intrauterine Growth Restriction
Maternal Causes
Hypertensive disorders
Pregestational diabetes
Cyanotic heart disease
Autoimmune disease
Restrictive pulmonary disease
Multifetal gestation
Malabsorptive disease/malnutrition
Living at a high altitude
Tobacco/substance abuse
Fetal Causes
Genetic disorders
Teratogenic exposure
Fetal infection

Oligohydramnios
Renal agenesis (Potter syndrome)
Prelabor rupture of membranes
Prolonged pregnancy
Uteroplacental insufficiency
Severe intrauterine growth restriction (IUGR)
Maternal hypertensive disorders
Maternal dehydration/hypovolemia

Chromosomal Abnormalities
Advanced maternal age
Parental chromosomal rearrangements
Previous pregnancy with autosomal trisomy
Abnormal ultrasound findings during the current pregnancy (e.g., fetal structural anomalies, IUGR, amniotic fluid volume abnormalities)
Increased risk, as calculated from noninvasive screening results (e.g., nuchal translucency and maternal serum analytes)

Data from Baschat, A. A., & Galan, H. L. (2017). Intrauterine growth restriction. In S. G. Gabbe, J. R. Niebyl, J. L. Simpson, et al. (Eds.), *Obstetrics: Normal and problem pregnancies* (7th ed.). Philadelphia: Elsevier; Driscoll, D. A., Simpson, J. L., Holzgreve, W., et al. (2017). Genetic screening and prenatal genetic diagnosis. In S. G. Gabbe, J. R. Niebyl, J. L. Simpson, et al. (Eds.), *Obstetrics: Normal and problem pregnancies* (7th ed.). Philadelphia: Elsevier; Gilbert, W. M. (2017). Amniotic fluid disorders. In S. G. Gabbe, J. R. Niebyl, J. L. Simpson, et al. (Eds.), *Obstetrics: Normal and problem pregnancies* (7th ed.). Philadelphia: Elsevier.

BOX 26.3 Common Maternal and Fetal Indications for Antepartum Testing

Chronic hypertension
Preeclampsia (with or without severe features)
Suspected or confirmed fetal growth restriction
Multiple gestation
Oligohydramnios
Preterm prelabor rupture of membranes
Late term or postterm gestation
Previous stillbirth
Decreased fetal movement
Systemic lupus erythematosus
Renal disease
Cholestasis of pregnancy

From Miller, L., Miller, D., & Cypher, R. (2017). *Mosby's pocket guide to fetal monitoring: A multidisciplinary approach* (8th ed.). St. Louis: Elsevier.

Several different protocols are used for counting. One recommendation is to count once a day for 60 minutes (Fig. 26.1 is an example of a form used to record fetal kick counts). Other common recommendations are that mothers count fetal activity two or three times daily (e.g., after meals or before bedtime) for 2 hours or until 10 movements are counted, or all fetal movements in a 12-hour period each day until a minimum of 10 movements are counted. Smart phone apps (e.g., Baby Kicks Monitor and Count the Kicks) are also available for recording fetal movements. Except for establishing a very low number of daily fetal movements or a trend toward decreased motion, the clinical value of the absolute number of fetal movements has not been established, other than in the situation in which fetal movements cease entirely for 12 hours (the so-called *fetal alarm signal*). A count of fewer than 3 fetal movements within 1 hour warrants further evaluation by a nonstress test (NST) or a contraction stress test (CST) and a complete or modified biophysical profile (BPP). See later discussion about these tests. Women should be taught the significance of the presence or absence of fetal movements, the procedure for counting, how to record findings on a daily fetal movement record, and when to notify the health care provider.

SAFETY ALERT

When assessing fetal movements it is important to remember that they are usually not present during the fetal sleep cycle; they may be reduced temporarily if the woman is taking depressant medication, drinking alcohol, or smoking a cigarette. They do not decrease as the woman nears term. Obesity decreases perception of fetal movements and consequently the ability of the mother to count them.

Ultrasonography

Diagnostic ultrasonography is an important, safe technique in antepartum fetal surveillance. It is considered by many to be the most valuable diagnostic tool used in obstetrics (Richards, 2017). It provides critical information to health care providers regarding fetal activity and gestational age, normal versus abnormal fetal growth curves, fetal and placental anatomy, fetal well-being, and visual assistance with which invasive tests can be performed more safely (Driscoll, Simpson, Holzgreve, et al., 2017; Richards).

Sound is a form of wave energy that causes small particles in a medium to oscillate. The frequency of sound, which refers to the number of peaks or waves that move over a given point per unit of time, is expressed in hertz (Hz). Sound with a frequency of one cycle, or one peak per second, has a frequency of 1 Hz. When directional beams of sound strike an object, an echo is returned. The time delay between the emission of the sound and the return and direction of the echo is noted. From these data, the distance and location of an object can be calculated. Ultrasound is sound frequency higher than that detectable by humans (>20,000 Hz). Ultrasound images are a reflection of the strength of the sending beam, the strength of the returning echo, and the density of the medium (e.g., muscle [uterus], bone, tissue [placenta], fluid, or blood) through which the beam is sent and returned.

An ultrasound examination can be performed either transvaginally or abdominally during pregnancy. Ultrasound scans produce a two- or three-dimensional view of the area being examined and can be used to create pictorial images (Fig. 26.2A and B). Box 26.4 explains the differences in these scans and the views they produce.

Transvaginal ultrasonography, in which the probe is inserted into the vagina, allows pelvic anatomic features to be evaluated in greater detail and intrauterine pregnancy to be diagnosed earlier. A transvaginal ultrasound examination does not require that the woman have a full bladder. It is especially useful in obese women whose thick abdominal layers cannot be penetrated adequately with an abdominal approach. A transvaginal ultrasound may be performed with the woman in a lithotomy position or with her pelvis elevated by towels, cushions, or a folded pillow. This pelvic tilt is optimal to image the pelvic structures. A protective cover such as a condom, the finger of a clean surgical glove, or a special probe cover provided by the manufacturer is used to cover the transducer probe. The probe is lubricated with a water-soluble gel and placed in the vagina either by the examiner or by the woman herself. During the examination, the position of the probe or the tilt of the examining table may be changed so the complete pelvis is in view. The procedure is not physically painful, although the woman feels pressure as the probe is moved. Transvaginal ultrasonography is optimally used in the first trimester to detect ectopic pregnancies, monitor the developing embryo, help identify abnormalities, and help establish gestational age. In some instances it may be used along with abdominal scanning to evaluate preterm labor in second- and third-trimester pregnancies.

Abdominal ultrasonography is more useful after the first trimester when the pregnant uterus becomes an abdominal organ. During the procedure the woman should have a full bladder to displace the uterus upward to provide a better image of the fetus. Transmission gel or paste is applied to the woman's abdomen to enhance the transmission and reception of the sound waves before a transducer is moved over the skin. She is positioned with small pillows under her head and knees. The display panel is positioned so the woman or her partner (or both) can observe the images on the screen if they desire.

Levels of Ultrasonography

The American College of Obstetricians and Gynecologists (ACOG) and several other organizations, including the American College of Radiology, the American Institute for Ultrasound in Medicine (AIUM), and the Society for Maternal Fetal Medicine (SMFM), describe three levels of ultrasonography (ACOG & AIUM, 2016c/2018):

Fetal Movement Chart

This chart will help to keep track of your baby's well-being. Carefully count the number of movements your baby makes during the same hour every evening, when babies are typically most active. For example, between 9 and 10 p.m.

If your baby has not moved for 12 hours, please contact 602.406.3521. Be sure to bring this chart with you when visiting your doctor.

Daily Chart of Baby Kicks							
DAYS OF WEEK	MONDAY	TUESDAY	WEDNESDAY	THURSDAY	FRIDAY	SATURDAY	SUNDAY
DATE							
KICKS							
DATE							
KICKS							
DATE							
KICKS							
DATE							
KICKS							
DATE							
KICKS							
DATE							
KICKS							
DATE							
KICKS							
DATE							
KICKS							
DATE							
KICKS							
DATE							
KICKS							

Fetal movement (kick count) chart. Courtesy of St. Joseph's Hospital and Medical Center, Phoenix, AZ.

Fig. 26.1 Fetal Movement (Kick Count) Chart. (Courtesy St. Joseph Hospital and Medical Center, Phoenix, AZ.)

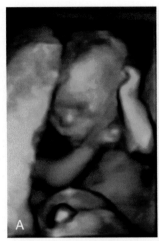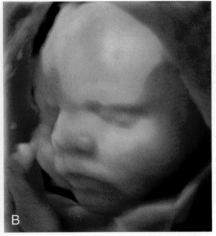

Fig. 26.2 Fetus Seen on Three-Dimensional Ultrasound. (A) View of fetus at 15 weeks and 3 days of gestation. (B) Close-up view of fetal face later in pregnancy. ([A] Courtesy Christina and Eva Gardner, Memphis, TN; [B] Courtesy Mandi and Chase Steele, Millington, TN.)

BOX 26.4 Types of Ultrasound Scans

Two-Dimensional (2D)
- Sound waves are sent straight down from the ultrasound transducer.
- The image produced includes only two dimensions (length and width), so it appears flat.
- The image is viewed in black, white, or shades of gray.
- This is the standard medical scan used in pregnancy.

Three-Dimensional (3D)
- Sound waves are sent out at different angles. The returning echoes are processed by a computer program, which adds a third dimension (depth) to the 2D scan, producing a 3D image.
- The image is usually displayed in sepia tones rather than in black and white.
- This scan can be used for diagnostic or management purposes. Viewing certain anomalies using a 3D scan provides further information that assists in planning for care at birth and for the neonate. These images are also often requested by pregnant women and families simply for their own enjoyment.

Four-Dimensional (4D)
- This scan adds a fourth dimension (time) to the 3D scan.
- The images produced are recorded and played back in succession. As the image is continuously updated, the fetus is viewed in real time.

TABLE 26.1 Major Uses of Ultrasonography During Pregnancy

First Trimester	Second Trimester	Third Trimester
Confirm pregnancy	Establish or confirm dates	Confirm gestational age
Confirm viability	Confirm viability	Confirm viability
Determine gestational age	Detect polyhydramnios, oligohydramnios	Detect macrosomia
Rule out ectopic pregnancy	Detect congenital anomalies	Detect congenital anomalies
Detect multiple gestation	Detect intrauterine growth restriction (IUGR)	Detect IUGR
Determine cause of vaginal bleeding	Assess placental location	Determine fetal position
Visualization during chorionic villus sampling	Visualization during amniocentesis	Detect placenta previa or placental abruption
Detect maternal abnormalities such as bicornuate uterus, ovarian cysts, fibroids	Evaluate for preterm labor	Visualization during amniocentesis, external version
		Biophysical profile
		Amniotic fluid volume assessment
		Doppler flow studies
		Detect placental maturity
		Evaluate for preterm labor

- *Standard* (also called *basic*) examinations are done most frequently and can be performed by ultrasonographers or other health care professionals, including nurses, who have had special training. Indications for standard ultrasonography are described in detail in the next section. In the second and third trimesters a standard ultrasound examination is used to evaluate fetal presentation, amniotic fluid volume (AFV), cardiac activity, placental position, fetal growth parameters, and number of fetuses. It is also used to perform an anatomic survey of the fetus.
- *Limited* examinations are performed to determine a specific piece of information about the pregnancy such as identifying fetal presentation during labor or estimating AFV. These examinations are usually performed by the woman's obstetric health care provider in the office or clinic, or the labor and birth unit.
- *Specialized* (also called *detailed*) or *targeted* examinations are performed when a woman is suspected of carrying an anatomically or physiologically abnormal fetus. Indications for this comprehensive examination

include abnormal history or laboratory findings, or the results of a previous standard or limited ultrasound examination. Specialized ultrasonography is performed by highly trained and experienced personnel.

Indications for Use

Major indications for obstetric sonography are listed by trimester in Table 26.1. During the first trimester, ultrasound examination is performed to obtain information regarding the number, size, and location of gestational sacs; the presence or absence of fetal cardiac activity and body movements; the presence or absence of uterine abnormalities (e.g., bicornuate uterus or fibroids) or adnexal masses (e.g., ovarian cysts or an ectopic pregnancy); and pregnancy dating.

During the second and third trimesters, ultrasonography is used to assess fetal viability, number, position, gestational age, growth pattern, and anomalies; AFV; placental location and condition; presence of uterine fibroids or anomalies; presence of adnexal masses; and cervical length.

Ultrasonography provides early diagnoses, allowing therapy to be instituted early in the pregnancy, thereby decreasing the severity and

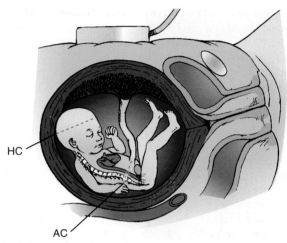

Fig. 26.3 Appropriate planes of sections *(dotted lines)* for head circumference *(HC)* and abdominal circumference *(AC)*.

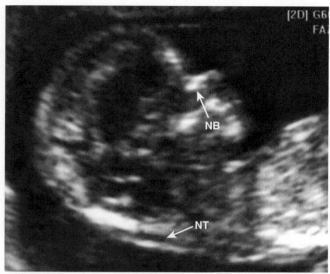

Fig. 26.4 Midsagittal view of a 12-week fetus showing the nuchal translucency *(NT)* and nasal bone *(NB)*. (From Gabbe, S. G., Niebyl, J. R., Simpson, J. L., et al. [Eds.]. [2017]. *Obstetrics: Normal and problem pregnancies* [7th ed.]. Philadelphia: Elsevier.)

duration of morbidity, both physical and emotional, for the family. For instance, early diagnosis provides time for the family to make informed decisions regarding possible intrauterine interventions, termination of the pregnancy, or preparing to care for an infant with special health care needs.

Fetal heart activity. Fetal cardiac activity can be demonstrated by about 6 weeks of gestation using transvaginal ultrasound. When the fetus is in a favorable position, good views of the fetal cardiac anatomy are possible in most women at 13 weeks of gestation (Richards, 2017). Fetal death can be confirmed by lack of heart motion along with the presence of fetal scalp edema, and maceration and overlap of the cranial bones.

Gestational age. Gestational dating by ultrasonography is indicated for conditions such as uncertainty regarding the date of the last normal menstrual period, recent discontinuation of oral contraceptives, a bleeding episode during the first trimester, uterine size that does not correlate with dates, and other high-risk conditions. Gestational dating may best be done using ultrasound measurements and ignoring menstrual dates. However, all recent guidelines on establishing gestational age include references to menstrual dates. A standard set of measurements has been accepted as being the most useful for determining gestational age. These measurements include the crown-rump length in the first trimester and the biparietal diameter (BPD), head circumference, abdominal circumference, and femur length after the first trimester (Fig. 26.3). Gestational age calculation using a combination of these measurements is the most accepted method of ultrasound dating after the first trimester. An ultrasound examination performed for pregnancy dating before 22 weeks of gestation is comparable to one performed during the first trimester in terms of accuracy. However, after that time ultrasound dating is less reliable because of variability in fetal size (Richards, 2017).

Fetal growth. Fetal growth is determined by both intrinsic growth potential and environmental factors. Conditions that require ultrasound assessment of fetal growth include poor maternal weight gain or pattern of weight gain, previous pregnancy with intrauterine growth restriction (IUGR), chronic infections, substance use (e.g., tobacco, alcohol), maternal diabetes, hypertension, multifetal pregnancy, and other medical or surgical complications.

Serial evaluations of BPD, limb length, and abdominal circumference can allow differentiation among size discrepancies resulting from inaccurate dates, true IUGR, and macrosomia (estimated weight of 4000 g or more). IUGR may be symmetric (the fetus is small in all parameters) or asymmetric (head and body growth do not match). Symmetric IUGR reflects a chronic or long-standing insult and may be caused by low genetic

growth potential, intrauterine infection, chromosomal anomaly, maternal undernutrition, or heavy smoking. Asymmetric growth suggests an acute or late-occurring deprivation such as placental insufficiency resulting from hypertension, renal disease, or cardiovascular disease. Reduced fetal growth is still one of the most frequent conditions associated with stillbirth. Macrosomic infants are at increased risk for traumatic injury and asphyxia during birth. Macrosomia also may be characterized as symmetric or asymmetric.

Fetal anatomy. Anatomic structures that can be identified by ultrasonography (depending on the gestational age) include the following: head (including ventricles and blood vessels), neck, spine, heart, stomach, small bowel, liver, kidneys, bladder, and limbs. Ultrasonography permits the confirmation of normal anatomy and detection of major fetal malformations. The presence of an anomaly may influence the location of birth (e.g., a subspecialty center versus a basic care center) and the method of birth (vaginal versus cesarean) to optimize neonatal outcomes. For example, plans are often made for a fetus with a condition that will require immediate surgery to be born in or near a hospital that is able to provide that care rather than in a small community hospital that is totally unequipped to meet the newborn's needs.

Fetal genetic disorders and physical anomalies. A prenatal screening technique called *nuchal translucency* (NT) screening uses ultrasound measurement of fluid in the nape of the fetal neck between 10 and 14 weeks of gestation to identify possible fetal abnormalities (Fig. 26.4). Mandatory training and quality assurance for professionals who perform NT measurement are critical to ensure accurate results. A fluid collection greater than 3 mm is considered abnormal (ACOG & SMFM, 2016b/2018). When combined with abnormal maternal serum marker levels, elevated NT indicates a possible increased risk of certain chromosomal abnormalities in the fetus, including trisomies 13, 18, and 21. An elevated NT alone indicates an increased risk for congenital heart defects. If the NT is abnormal, diagnostic genetic testing is recommended (ACOG & AIUM, 2016c/2018; Driscoll et al., 2017). Other ultrasound findings that predict trisomy 21 include an absent nasal bone, shortened femur or humerus, echogenic intracardiac focus, echogenic bowel, pyelectasis (enlargement of the renal pelvis, the part of the kidney that collects urine), and an abnormally fast or slow fetal heart rate (FHR) (Driscoll et al.; Richards, 2017). These findings are considered soft markers only; they are not diagnostic for the anomaly. Women with positive screening results for a chromosomal abnormality should be referred for genetic counseling and offered an invasive diagnostic test (Driscoll et al.).

Placental position and function. Ultrasonography is also valuable in diagnosing problems related to placental location or appearance. The pattern of uterine and placental growth and the fullness of the maternal bladder influence the apparent location of the placenta by ultrasonography. During the first trimester differentiation between the endometrium and small placenta is difficult. By 14 to 16 weeks the placenta is clearly defined, but if it is seen to be low lying, its relationship to the internal cervical os can sometimes be altered dramatically by varying the fullness of the maternal bladder. When ultrasound scanning is performed between 18 and 23 weeks of gestation, the edge of the placenta extends to or covers the internal os of the cervix in about 2% of pregnancies. However, at least 90% of placentas identified earlier in pregnancy as previa or low-lying ultimately resolve by the third trimester. This occurs because the placenta grows toward the uterine fundus, where the blood supply is better than in the lower uterine segment and because of the elongation of the lower uterine segment as pregnancy advances. Therefore, if placenta previa is diagnosed during the second trimester, repeated ultrasounds should be performed as pregnancy progresses until the placenta moves well away from the cervical os or it becomes clear that the previa will persist (Hull, Resnik, & Silver, 2019; Richards, 2017).

Many changes observed in the appearance of the placenta are related to calcification, fibrosis, and infarction. These changes tend to become more apparent as pregnancy progresses, but their clinical significance is not clear. It has recently been recognized that a "globular" placenta, with a narrow base in comparison to height, is associated with an increased rate of IUGR, fetal death, and other complications (Richards, 2017).

Adjunct to other invasive tests. The safety of amniocentesis is increased when the positions of the fetus, placenta, umbilical cord, and pockets of amniotic fluid can be identified accurately. Ultrasound scanning has reduced risks previously associated with amniocentesis, such as fetomaternal hemorrhage from a pierced placenta. Percutaneous umbilical blood sampling (PUBS) and chorionic villus sampling (CVS) also are guided by ultrasonography to accurately identify the cord and chorion frondosum.

Fetal well-being. Physiologic parameters of the fetus that can be assessed with ultrasound scanning include AFV, vascular waveforms from the fetal circulation, heart motion, fetal breathing movements (FBMs), fetal urine production, and fetal limb and head movements. Assessment of these parameters, alone or in combination, yields a fairly reliable picture of fetal well-being. The significance of these findings is discussed in the following sections.

Doppler blood flow analysis. One of the major advances in perinatal medicine is the ability to study blood flow in the woman, fetus, and placenta noninvasively using ultrasound. Doppler blood flow analysis uses systolic/diastolic flow ratios and resistance indices to estimate blood flow in various arteries. Thus, it provides an indication of fetal adaptation and reserve. The vessels most often studied are the fetal umbilical and middle cerebral arteries and the maternal uterine arteries. Severe restriction of umbilical artery blood flow as indicated by absent or reversed flow during diastole has been associated with IUGR (Fig. 26.5) (Miller et al., 2017). Doppler ultrasound has been demonstrated to be of value in reducing perinatal mortality and unnecessary obstetric interventions in fetuses with IUGR (Greenberg & Druzin, 2017). Significantly increased peak systolic velocity in the middle cerebral artery has been found to predict moderate to severe fetal anemia. Abnormal maternal uterine artery Doppler waveforms have been used to predict fetal growth restriction (Miller et al.).

Amniotic fluid volume. Accurate measurement of AFV using ultrasound is difficult, and evidence indicates that the estimates produced poorly predict abnormal values. However, the measurement is still frequently performed in clinical practice. Differences in the amount of pressure placed on the ultrasound transducer by the sonographer can affect the accuracy of measurement. Use of greater pressure when placing the ultrasound transducer on the maternal abdomen can yield a lower measurement, while less pressure can result in a higher measurement (Gilbert, 2017).

Abnormalities in AFV are frequently associated with fetal disorders. Subjective determinants of oligohydramnios (decreased fluid) include a fundal height that is small for gestational age and a fetus that is easily palpated. An objective criterion of decreased AFV is met if the maximum vertical pocket of amniotic fluid is less than 1 to 2 cm (Gilbert, 2017). Increased amniotic fluid is called polyhydramnios or sometimes just *hydramnios*. Subjective criteria for polyhydramnios include a fundal height that is large for gestational age and a fetus that cannot easily be palpated or that is ballotable. Polyhydramnios is usually objectively defined as pockets of amniotic fluid measuring more than 8 cm (Gilbert).

The total AFV can be evaluated by a method in which the vertical depths (in centimeters) of the largest pocket of amniotic fluid in all four quadrants surrounding the maternal umbilicus are totaled, providing an amniotic fluid index (AFI). An AFI of less than 5 cm indicates oligohydramnios. With polyhydramnios, the AFI is 25 cm or more (Gilbert, 2017). Oligohydramnios is associated with congenital anomalies (e.g., renal agenesis [Potter syndrome]), and prelabor rupture of membranes. Polyhydramnios is associated with gastrointestinal and central nervous system (CNS) abnormalities, multiple fetuses, and fetal hydrops (Gilbert).

Biophysical profile. Real-time ultrasound permits detailed assessment of the physical and physiologic characteristics of the developing fetus and cataloging of normal and abnormal biophysical responses to stimuli. The biophysical profile is a noninvasive dynamic assessment of a fetus that is based on acute and chronic markers of fetal disease. The BPP includes AFV, FBMs, fetal movements, and fetal tone determined by ultrasound and FHR reactivity determined by means of the NST. Therefore, the BPP can be considered a physical examination of the fetus, including determination of vital signs. FHR reactivity, FBMs, fetal movement, and fetal tone reflect current CNS status, whereas the AFV demonstrates the adequacy of placental function over a longer period of time (Miller et al., 2017). BPP scoring and management are detailed in Tables 26.2 and 26.3.

The BPP is used frequently in the late second and the third trimester for antepartum fetal testing because it is a reliable predictor of fetal well-being. A BPP of 8 or 10 with a normal AFV is considered normal. Advantages of the test include excellent sensitivity and a low false-negative rate (Miller et al., 2017). One limitation of the test is that if the fetus is in a quiet sleep state, the BPP can require a long period of observation. Also, unless the ultrasound examination is videotaped, it cannot be reviewed (Greenberg & Druzin, 2017).

Modified biophysical profile. The modified BPP (mBPP) is being used increasingly as a way to shorten the testing time required for the complete BPP by assessing the components that are most predictive of perinatal outcome. The mBPP combines the NST, which assesses the current fetal condition, with measurement of the quantity of amniotic fluid, an indicator of placental function over a longer period of time. It is recommended that the AFV be determined by measuring a single deepest pocket of fluid instead of using the AFI. Desired test results are a reactive NST and a single deepest vertical pocket of amniotic fluid that is more than 2 cm (Greenberg & Druzin, 2017; Miller et al., 2017).

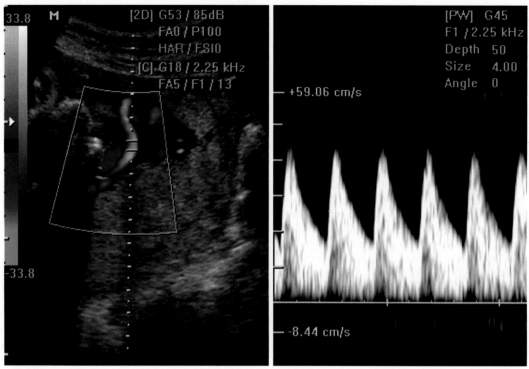

Fig. 26.5 Color and Spectral Doppler Evaluation of the Umbilical Artery. In the left panel the coiling arteries and vein are shown. Red indicates flow toward the transducer, and blue is flow away. The sample gate for the pulse Doppler is superimposed. On the right is the result of the pulse Doppler, depicting a normal flow velocity waveform. (From Gabbe, S. G., Niebyl, J. R., Simpson, J. L., et al. [Eds.]. [2017]. *Obstetrics: Normal and problem pregnancies* [7th ed.]. Philadelphia: Elsevier.)

TABLE 26.2   Scoring the Biophysical Profile

Biophysical Variable	Score 2	Score 0
Fetal breathing movements (FBM)	At least one episode of FBM of at least 30 seconds duration in a 30-min observation	Absent FBM or <30 seconds of sustained FBM in 30 min
Fetal movements	At least three trunk/limb movements in 30 min	Fewer than three episodes of trunk/limb movements in 30 min
Fetal tone	At least one episode of active extension with return to flexion of fetal limb or trunk; opening and closing of hand considered normal tone	Absence of movement or slow extension/flexion
Amniotic fluid index (AFI)	Deepest vertical pocket >2 cm	Deepest vertical pocket ≤2 cm
Nonstress test	Reactive	Nonreactive

From Miller, L., Miller, D., & Cypher, R. (2017). *Mosby's pocket guide to fetal monitoring: A multidisciplinary approach* (8th ed.). St. Louis: Elsevier.

TABLE 26.3   Biophysical Profile Management

Score	Interpretation	Management
10	Normal; low risk for chronic asphyxia	Repeat testing at weekly to twice-weekly intervals.
8	Normal; low risk for chronic asphyxia	Repeat testing at weekly to twice-weekly intervals.
6	Suspect chronic asphyxia	If ≥36-37 weeks of gestation or <36 weeks with positive testing for fetal pulmonary maturity, consider delivery; if <36 weeks and/or fetal pulmonary maturity testing negative, repeat biophysical profile in 4-6 h; deliver if oligohydramnios is present.
4	Suspect chronic asphyxia	If ≥36 weeks of gestation, deliver; if <32 weeks of gestation, repeat score.
0-2	Strongly suspect chronic asphyxia	Extend testing time to 120 min; if persistent score ≤4, deliver, regardless of gestational age.

Modified from Manning, F. A., Harman, C. R., Morrison, I., et al. (1990). Fetal assessment based on fetal biophysical profile scoring. *American Journal of Obstetrics and Gynecology, 162*(3), 703–700; and Manning, F. A. (1992). Biophysical profile scoring. In J. Nijhuis (Ed.), *Fetal behavior.* New York: Oxford University Press.

Nursing Role

Although a growing number of nurses with additional training/education perform ultrasound scans and BPPs in certain centers, the main role of nurses is counseling and educating women about the procedure. Ultrasound is widely used and in fact is considered a standard part of current prenatal care. Unlike many diagnostic tests, most women look forward to and enjoy their prenatal ultrasound. Exposure to diagnostic ultrasonography during pregnancy appears to be safe for the fetus. Nevertheless, because there is the possibility that unrecognized harm exists, ultrasound should be used only by qualified health professionals to provide medical benefit to clients (Richards, 2017).

Nonmedical Ultrasounds

Three- and four-dimensional ultrasonography for nonmedical purposes has become increasingly popular with pregnant women and their families. Although insurance does not cover the cost, women can have ultrasound images made of the fetus, just as professional photographs are often taken of infants and children. Both AIUM and ACOG have published statements that strongly discourage this practice. Although ultrasonography is considered safe, exposure of the fetus to high-frequency soundwaves without a clear medical indication for doing so should be avoided. In addition, casual ultrasonography performed by people who are not qualified health care professionals could give false reassurance to women or result in the discovery of abnormalities in settings that are not conducive to discussion and follow-up of findings (ACOG & AIUM, 2016c/2018; AIUM, 2012; Richards, 2017). Helping the expectant family to understand the role of ultrasound beyond providing a picture of the fetus is a component of prenatal education.

Magnetic Resonance Imaging

Magnetic resonance imaging (MRI) is a noninvasive radiologic technique used for obstetric and gynecologic diagnosis. Similar to computed tomography (CT), MRI provides excellent pictures of soft tissue. Unlike CT, ionizing radiation is not used. Therefore, vascular structures within the body can be visualized and evaluated without injecting an iodinated contrast medium, thus eliminating any known biologic risk. Similar to sonography, MRI is noninvasive and can provide images in multiple planes, but no interference occurs from skeletal, fatty, or gas-filled structures, and imaging of deep pelvic structures does not require a full bladder.

With MRI the examiner can evaluate fetal structure (CNS, thorax, abdomen, genitourinary tract, musculoskeletal system) and overall growth, the placenta (position, density, and presence of gestational trophoblastic disease), and the quantity of amniotic fluid. Maternal structures (uterus, cervix, adnexa, and pelvis), the biochemical status (pH, adenosine triphosphate content) of tissues and organs, and soft-tissue, metabolic, or functional anomalies can also be evaluated.

The woman is placed on a table in the supine position with one hip elevated if possible and moved into the bore of the main magnet, which is similar in appearance to a CT scanner. Depending on the reason for the study, the procedure may take from 20 to 60 min, during which time the woman must be perfectly still except for short breaks. Because of the long time needed to produce MRIs, the fetus will probably move, which will obscure anatomic details. The only way to ensure that this problem does not occur is to administer a sedative to the mother, but this approach should be reserved for selected cases in which visualization of fetal detail is critical.

MRI has little effect on the fetus. Concerns that the FHR or fetal movement would decrease have not been supported.

BIOCHEMICAL ASSESSMENT

Biochemical assessment involves biologic examination (e.g., of chromosomes in exfoliated cells) and chemical determinations (e.g., lecithin/sphingomyelin [L/S] ratio, phosphatidylglycerol [PG], or lamellar body count [LBC] (Table 26.4). Procedures used to obtain the needed specimens include amniocentesis, PUBS, CVS, and maternal blood sampling (Box 26.5).

Amniocentesis

Amniocentesis is performed to obtain amniotic fluid, which contains fetal cells. Under direct ultrasonographic visualization, a needle is inserted transabdominally into the uterus and amniotic fluid is withdrawn into a syringe. Then the various assessments are

TABLE 26.4 Summary of Biochemical Monitoring Techniques

Test	Possible Findings	Clinical Significance
Maternal Blood		
Coombs test	Titer of 1:8 and increasing	Significant Rh incompatibility
Cell-free DNA screening	Normal amount of DNA from specific chromosomes	Fetus with trisomy 13, 18, or 21
AFP	See AFP later in table	
Amniotic Fluid Analysis		
Lung profile:		Fetal lung maturity
L/S ratio	2:1	
Phosphatidylglycerol	Present	
LBC	≥50,000/μL	
Creatinine	>2 mg/dL	Gestational age >36 weeks
Lipid cells	>10%	Gestational age >35 weeks
AFP	High levels after 15 weeks of gestation	Open neural tube or other defect
Osmolality	Declines after 20 weeks of gestation	Advancing gestational age
Genetic disorders: Sex-linked Chromosomal Metabolic	Dependent on cultured cells for karyotype and enzymatic activity	Counseling possibly required

AFP, α-fetoprotein; *L/S*, lecithin/sphingomyelin; *LBC*, lamellar body count.

BOX 26.5 Fetal Rights

Amniocentesis, percutaneous umbilical blood sampling (PUBS), and chorionic villus sampling (CVS) are prenatal tests used for diagnosing fetal defects in pregnancy. They are invasive and carry risks to the mother and fetus. A consideration of induced abortion is linked to the performance of these tests because no treatment for genetically affected fetuses has been developed; therefore, the issue of fetal rights is a key ethical concern in prenatal testing for fetal defects.

performed on the fluid sample (Fig. 26.6). Amniocentesis is possible after week 14 of pregnancy, when the uterus becomes an abdominal organ and sufficient amniotic fluid is available for testing. Indications for the procedure include prenatal diagnosis of genetic disorders or congenital anomalies (neural tube defects [NTDs] in particular), assessment of pulmonary maturity, and (rarely) diagnosis of fetal hemolytic disease.

Complications in the mother and fetus occur only rarely and include the following:

Maternal: leakage of amniotic fluid, hemorrhage, fetomaternal hemorrhage with possible maternal Rh isoimmunization, infection, labor, placental abruption, inadvertent damage to the intestines or bladder, and amniotic fluid embolism (anaphylactoid syndrome of pregnancy)

Fetal: death, hemorrhage, infection (amnionitis), and direct injury from the needle

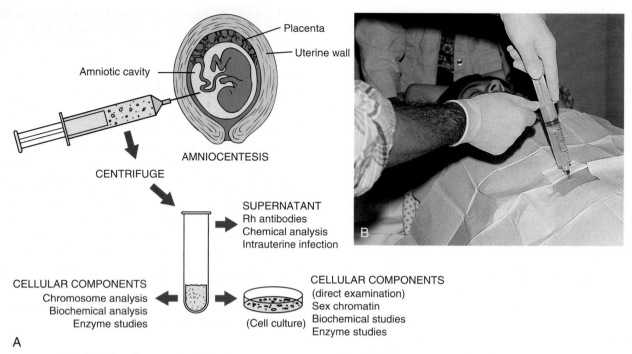

Fig. 26.6 Amniocentesis. (A) Amniocentesis and laboratory use of amniotic fluid aspirant. (B) Transabdominal amniocentesis. (B, Courtesy Marjorie Pyle, RNC, Lifecircle, Costa Mesa, CA.)

Many of the complications have been minimized or eliminated by using ultrasonography to direct the procedure.

> ⚡ **SAFETY ALERT**
>
> Because of the possibility of fetomaternal hemorrhage, administering Rh_0D immune globulin to the woman who is Rh negative is standard practice after an amniocentesis.

Indications for Use

Genetic concerns. Families in several different categories are considered to be at increased risk for having a child with a genetic disorder. These include the following (ACOG & SMFM, 2016a/2018):

- Older maternal age (35 years of age or older)
- Older paternal age (there is no consensus, but usually considered to be 40 to 50 years of age)
- Parents who are affected by or are carriers of genetic disorders, including sickle cell anemia, Tay-Sachs disease, and cystic fibrosis
- Women with a prior child with a structural birth defect or with a structural fetal defect identified by ultrasound during their current pregnancy
- Women with a prior child with a chromosomal abnormality

In the past, prenatal assessment of genetic disorders focused on women and their partners who were included in one of these categories. Now, however, ACOG and SMFM (2016a/2018) recommend that all pregnant women, regardless of age or other risk factors, be offered genetic screening or diagnostic testing (Box 26.6).

Biochemical analysis of enzymes in amniotic fluid can detect inborn errors of metabolism or fetal structural anomalies. For example, α-fetoprotein (AFP) levels in amniotic fluid are assessed as a follow-up for elevated levels in maternal serum. High AFP levels in amniotic fluid help confirm the diagnosis of a NTD such as spina bifida or anencephaly, or an abdominal wall defect such as omphalocele. The elevation results from the increased leakage of cerebrospinal or abdominal fluid into the amniotic fluid through the closure defect.

> ## BOX 26.6 Prenatal Screening and Testing for Fetal Genetic Disorders
>
> All pregnant women should be offered the option of screening or diagnostic testing for fetal genetic disorders, regardless of age or other risk factors. Genetic testing should be discussed as early as possible in pregnancy, ideally at the first prenatal visit. Health care providers must carefully explain the difference in screening tests, which assess whether a woman is at increased risk for having a fetus affected by a genetic disorder, and diagnostic tests, which determine with as much certainty as possible whether a specific genetic disorder or condition is present in the fetus. It is also important that women understand the benefits and limitations of all prenatal screening and diagnostic testing, including the conditions for which tests are available and the conditions that will not be detected by testing (ACOG & SMFM, 2016a/2018).

Data from American College of Obstetricians and Gynecologists, & Society for Maternal Fetal Medicine. (2016a, reaffirmed 2018). Practice bulletin no. 162: Prenatal diagnostic testing for genetic disorders. *Obstetrics & Gynecology*, 127(5), e108–e122.

Fetal lung maturity. Late in pregnancy, accurate assessment of fetal lung maturity is possible by examining amniotic fluid to determine the L/S ratio or for the presence of PG. However, because both of these tests require considerable time, technical expertise, and cost to perform, they are generally used as secondary tests if simpler and less expensive automated tests indicate lung immaturity (Mercer, 2019).

The LBC is a test commonly performed to determine fetal pulmonary maturity. Lamellar bodies are surfactant-containing particles secreted by type II pneumocytes. The number of lamellar bodies found in the amniotic fluid increases with the onset of functional fetal pulmonary maturity. The LBC compares favorably with the L/S ratio and the PG test in predicting fetal lung maturity. The automated test is simple to perform, and almost all hospital laboratories have the equipment used to perform it (Mercer, 2019) (see Table 26.4).

Fetal hemolytic disease. In the past amniocentesis was used for identification and follow-up of fetal hemolytic disease in cases of isoimmunization. Doppler velocimetry of the fetal middle cerebral artery has now replaced serial amniocentesis as the method of choice to accurately and noninvasively monitor for fetal anemia in isoimmunized pregnancies (Moise, 2017).

Chorionic Villus Sampling

The combined advantages of earlier diagnosis and rapid results made chorionic villus sampling a popular technique for genetic studies in the first trimester. Indications for CVS are similar to those for amniocentesis, although CVS cannot be used for maternal serum marker screening because no fluid is obtained. CVS performed in the second trimester carries no greater risk of pregnancy loss than amniocentesis and is considered equal to amniocentesis in diagnostic accuracy. When performed after the first trimester, the procedure is better known as *late CVS* or *placental biopsy* (Driscoll et al., 2017).

CVS can be performed in the first or second trimester, ideally between 10 and 13 weeks of gestation, and involves the removal of a small tissue specimen from the fetal portion of the placenta (Driscoll et al., 2017). Because chorionic villi originate in the zygote, this tissue reflects the genetic makeup of the fetus.

CVS procedures can be accomplished either transcervically or transabdominally. In transcervical sampling, a sterile catheter is introduced through the cervical canal toward the placenta under continuous ultrasonographic guidance, and a small portion of the chorionic villi is aspirated with a syringe. If the abdominal approach is used, an 18- or 20-gauge spinal needle with stylet is inserted under sterile conditions through the abdominal wall into the placenta under ultrasound guidance. The stylet is then withdrawn and the chorionic tissue is aspirated into a syringe. The transabdominal approach is preferred if genital herpes, cervicitis, or a bicornuate uterus is present (Driscoll et al., 2017).

CVS is a relatively safe procedure. Pregnancy loss with CVS is similar to that of second-trimester amniocentesis. The incidence of IUGR, placental abruption, and preterm birth is no higher in women undergoing CVS than would be expected in the general population. In the early 1990s there was controversy concerning an increased risk for fetal limb reduction defects associated with CVS. However, the consensus of further studies is that, when CVS is performed by experienced individuals after 9 completed weeks of gestation, the risk for limb reduction defects is no higher than it is in the general population (Driscoll et al., 2017)

⚡ SAFETY ALERT

Because of the possibility of fetomaternal hemorrhage, women who are Rh negative should receive Rh₀D immune globulin after CVS to prevent isoimmunization, regardless of whether the procedure is performed transcervically or transabdominally, unless the fetus is known to be Rh negative (Driscoll et al., 2017).

Because amniocentesis and CVS are invasive tests, their use is associated with a small but concerning risk for pregnancy loss and infection. Noninvasive diagnostic tests, which will someday replace them, are currently in development. These tests will be able to isolate and analyze fetal deoxyribonucleic acid (DNA) in maternal serum to diagnose multiple disorders such as single gene disorders and chromosomal aberrations, in addition to trisomies (Latendresse & Deneris, 2015) (see later discussion and the Evidence-Based Practice box).

Percutaneous Umbilical Blood Sampling

Direct access to the fetal circulation during the second and third trimesters is possible through percutaneous umbilical blood sampling (also called *cordocentesis* or *funipuncture*). PUBS can be used for fetal

blood sampling and transfusion. However, PUBS has been replaced in many centers by placental biopsy because it is a safer, easier, and faster alternative. Improvements in cytogenetic and molecular diagnostic testing have decreased the need for fetal blood samples. Many tests that were once performed using fetal blood can now be done using DNA-based analysis of chorionic villi (Driscoll et al., 2017).

PUBS involves the insertion of a needle directly into a fetal umbilical vessel, preferably the vein, under ultrasound guidance (Figs. 26.7 and 26.8). Puncture of the umbilical cord near its insertion into the placenta is technically easier, but is associated with a higher risk for contamination with maternal blood. Alternatively, free loops of umbilical cord or the intrahepatic vein may be used as puncture sites instead. Generally, a small amount of blood is removed and tested immediately to ensure that it is fetal in origin (Driscoll et al., 2017). The most common genetic indication for the use of PUBS is evaluation of mosaic results found on amniocentesis or CVS, when a sample of fetal blood is required to determine the specific mutation. PUBS is also used to assess for fetal anemia, infection, and thrombocytopenia (Wapner & Dugoff, 2019). Bleeding from the cord puncture site is the most common complication of the procedure. Transient fetal bradycardia can also occur. Maternal complications are rare but include amnionitis and transplacental hemorrhage (Driscoll et al.).

Maternal Assays

α-Fetoprotein

Maternal serum α-fetoprotein levels are used as a screening tool for NTDs in pregnancy. Through this technique approximately 85% to 92% of open NTDs and almost all cases of anencephaly can be detected early (Wapner & Dugoff, 2019). Screening is recommended for all pregnant women.

The cause of NTDs is not well understood, but 95% of all affected infants are born to women with no family history of similar anomalies (Wapner & Dugoff, 2019). The defect occurs in approximately 1 in 1000 live births. Risk factors for NTDs include a history of this disorder in a prior pregnancy, folic acid deficiency, pregestational diabetes, and teratogen exposure (e.g., valproic acid [Depakote], carbamazepine [Tegretol]) (Wolf, 2019).

AFP is produced in the fetal gastrointestinal tract and liver, and increasing levels are detectable in the serum of pregnant women beginning at 7 weeks of gestation. Although amniotic fluid AFP measurement is diagnostic for NTD, maternal serum AFP (MSAFP) is a screening tool only. MSAFP screening can be performed between 15 and 20 weeks of gestation, with 16 to 18 weeks being ideal (Wapner & Dugoff, 2019).

Once the maternal level of AFP is determined, it is compared with normal values for each week of gestation. Values also should be correlated with maternal age, weight, race, presence of a multifetal pregnancy, and whether the woman has insulin-dependent diabetes. If the MSAFP level is elevated, the next step is ultrasound evaluation to confirm gestational age and the presence of a singleton pregnancy, and search for other causes for the elevation. In up to half of all women, incorrect dating is identified as the cause of the elevated MSAFP level. If ultrasound evaluation does not reveal the cause, further testing using amniocentesis or a targeted ultrasound is necessary (Wapner & Dugoff, 2019).

Multiple Marker Screens

Screening to detect fetal chromosomal abnormalities, particularly trisomy 21 (Down syndrome), is available beginning in the first trimester of pregnancy at 11 to 14 weeks of gestation (Cunningham et al., 2018). This first-trimester screen includes measurement of two maternal biochemical markers, pregnancy-associated plasma protein A (PAPP-A) and human chorionic gonadotropin (hCG) or the free β-human chorionic gonadotropin (β-hCG) subunit, and evaluation of fetal NT. In the

EVIDENCE-BASED PRACTICE

Cell-Free Fetal DNA Testing for Trisomies

Ask the Question

For women at risk for trisomies or sex chromosome aneuploidies, is there a non-invasive screening test?

Search for the Evidence

Search Strategies English language research-based publications since 2014 on noninvasive prenatal screening, cell-free fetal DNA, trisomy, and aneuploidy were included.

Databases Used Cochrane Collaborative Database, National Guideline Clearinghouse (AHRQ), CINAHL, PubMed, UpToDate, and the professional websites for ACOG and AWHONN

Critical Appraisal of the Evidence

In the past, women at risk for genetic abnormality had the option of screening maternal blood for serum analytes ("triple screen"), with or without ultrasound for nuchal translucency, an early visible marker for trisomy 21. These combinations had a detection rate ranging from 50% to 95% (Gregg, Skotko, Benkendorf, et al., 2016). Other diagnostic tests, such as chorionic villus sampling and amniocentesis, are definitive but invasive.

- Introduced in 2011 as a noninvasive pregnancy screening test, cell-free DNA (cfDNA) testing isolates fetal DNA fragments from maternal blood to determine sex and to screen for trisomies 13, 18, and 21 with an excellent negative predictive value, high detection rate, and a lower false-positive rate. Screening has now expanded to include sex and other chromosome aneuploidies, microdeletion screening, and whole-exome sequencing (WES) (Gregg et al., 2016; Post, Mottola, & Kuller, 2017).
- Offered at 10 to 20 weeks of gestation, cfDNA has limited sensitivity in the presence of a high body mass index. In addition, it may reflect placental DNA, which may have mosaicism and differ from the true fetal karyotype. A "vanishing twin" or later fetal loss may confound the results. For these reasons professional recommendations advocate that in the event of abnormal cfDNA results, direct fetal DNA sampling using invasive techniques be used for confirmation (Gregg et al., 2016; Post et al., 2017).

- First-trimester ultrasound is still the gold standard for confirming dating and identifying some structural abnormalities, as well as multiple fetuses and large cystic hygromas. Maternal blood test for α-fetoprotein, although variable in sensitivity, is still recommended at 15 to 18 weeks of gestation as a screening test for open neural tube defects (American College of Obstetricians and Gynecologists, 2017).

Apply the Evidence: Nursing Implications

- Earlier screening for trisomies provides pregnant women with either earlier reassurance of a normal fetus or more time to adjust to abnormality. The timing allows for the option for a less risky first trimester termination.
- Pretest counseling recommendations include the benefits and limitations of cfDNA testing. This includes the recommendation for further diagnostic testing using invasive techniques prior to any irrevocable obstetric decisions (Post et al., 2017).
- Women and families may need help sorting out the bewildering array of tests available during pregnancy. Tests are only useful if they provide usable information, so health care providers should have knowledge and information ready to assist clients for all possible test result outcomes.
- This test may help women avoid routine invasive procedures, a cost savings. However, cfDNA is expensive, costing up to $2,000 or more. As with all new tests, much research and discussion are needed regarding cost analysis, appropriate population, and economic justice.
- Ethical debates will undoubtedly multiply with the eventual availability of more prenatal genetic testing, including whole-genome sequencing.

References

American College of Obstetricians and Gynecologists. (2017). Practice bulletin no. 187: Neural tube defects. *Obstetrics and Gynecology, 130*(6), e279–e290.
Gregg, A. R., Skotko, B. G., Benkendorf, J. L., et al. (2016). Noninvasive prenatal screening for fetal aneuploidy. *Genetics in Medicine, 18*(10), 1056–1065.
Post, A. L., Mottola, A. T., & Kuller, J. A. (2017). What's new in prenatal genetics? A review of current recommendations and guidelines. *Obstetrical and Gynecological Survey, 72*(10), 610–617.

Jennifer Taylor Alderman

DNA, Deoxyribonucleic acid.

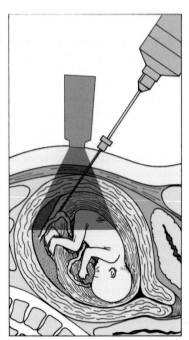

Fig. 26.7 Technique for Percutaneous Umbilical Blood Sampling Guided by Ultrasound.

presence of a fetus with trisomy 21, hCG levels and the NT measurement are higher than normal in the first trimester, whereas PAPP-A levels are lower than normal. In contrast, levels of both hCG and PAPP-A are lower in fetuses with trisomy 18 and trisomy 13. First-trimester screening using PAPP-A and hCG or β-hCG levels has been shown to be as accurate for detecting fetuses with trisomy 21 as quadruple screening in the second trimester (Cunningham et al; Driscoll et al., 2017; Wapner & Dugoff, 2019).

Another biochemical marker that can be measured during the first trimester, ideally at 8 to 10 weeks of gestation, is a disintegrin and metalloproteinase 12 (ADAM 12), a glycoprotein that is synthesized by the placenta and secreted throughout pregnancy. Decreased levels of ADAM 12 are found in women carrying a fetus with trisomy 21 (Wapner & Dugoff, 2019).

When used as a single marker, NT detects about two-thirds of fetuses with trisomy 21. However, NT alone is generally used for this purpose only in multifetal gestations, when serum screening is less accurate or may not be available. Combining the serum marker and NT values results in the detection of Down syndrome in 84% of cases. These results are comparable to those obtained with quad screening (see discussion following) in the second trimester (Cunningham et al., 2018).

Assessment of the fetal nasal bone by ultrasound during the first trimester provides another method to predict trisomy 21. The nasal bone cannot be identified on ultrasound in about one-third to one-quarter of fetuses who have trisomy 21 (Wapner & Dugoff, 2019).

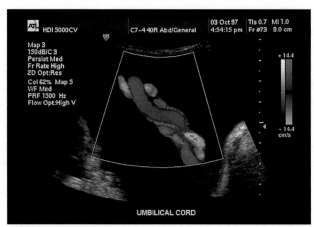

Fig. 26.8 Umbilical Cord as Seen on Ultrasound at 26 Weeks of Gestation. (Courtesy Advanced Technology Laboratories, Bothell, WA.)

In the second trimester the only widely used multiple marker test in the United States is the quadruple marker or "quad" test, used to screen for fetuses with trisomy 21 and trisomy 18. The quad screen, performed at 15 to 21 weeks of gestation, measures the levels of four maternal serum markers: MSAFP, unconjugated estriol, hCG, and inhibin (Cunningham et al., 2018). The addition of inhibin to the other three markers increases the detection rate for Down syndrome to about 75% in women who are less than 35 years old and to more than 80% in women 35 years of age or older (Driscoll et al. 2017). In the presence of a fetus with trisomy 21 the MSAFP and unconjugated estriol levels are lower, whereas the hCG and inhibin levels are elevated. Low MSAFP, unconjugated estriol, and hCG values are associated with trisomy 18. Inhibin is not included in determining the trisomy 18 screen result (Cunningham et al.).

The ability of multiple marker tests to detect chromosomal abnormalities depends on the accuracy of gestational age assessment. These tests are screening procedures only and are not diagnostic. A positive screening test result indicates an increased risk but is not diagnostic of trisomy 21 or another chromosome abnormality. Women with positive screening results should be offered genetic counseling and diagnostic testing by amniocentesis or CVS for fetal karyotyping (see Box 26.6) (Cunningham et al., 2018). In the future, noninvasive prenatal diagnosis will likely replace amniocentesis and CVS as diagnostic, or confirmatory, testing (Latendresse & Deneris, 2015).

Coombs Test

The indirect Coombs test is a screening tool for Rh incompatibility. If the maternal titer for Rh antibodies is greater than 1:8, amniocentesis for determination of bilirubin in amniotic fluid is indicated to establish the severity of fetal hemolytic anemia. However, middle cerebral artery Doppler studies to determine the degree of fetal hemolysis have almost entirely replaced serial amniocentesis (see earlier discussion) (Moise, 2017). The Coombs test can also detect other antibodies that may place the fetus at risk for incompatibility with maternal antigens.

Cell-Free Deoxyribonucleic Acid Screening in Maternal Blood

The newest screening test for aneuploidy, cell-free DNA (cfDNA), is performed using a sample of maternal blood (see the Evidence-Based Practice box). The cfDNA screening test is an example of *noninvasive prenatal testing (NIPT)*. *Aneuploidy* is defined as having one or more extra or missing chromosomes in the 23 pairs each individual normally possesses (ACOG & SMFM, 2016b/2018). Common aneuploidies are trisomies 13, 18, and 21, each of which results from an extra chromosome. cfDNA also provides a definitive diagnosis noninvasively for fetal Rh status, fetal gender, and certain paternally transmitted single gene disorders (ACOG & SMFM, 2016b/2018; Cunningham et al., 2018; Driscoll et al., 2017; Latendresse & Deneris, 2015).

Maternal plasma contains small fragments of cfDNA, resulting from the breakdown of both maternal and fetal cells (Driscoll et al., 2017; Latendresse & Deneris, 2015). Normal amounts of cfDNA, which vary throughout pregnancy, are known and compared with those obtained from the maternal sample. The test cannot actually distinguish fetal from maternal DNA, but it can accurately predict the fetal status by measuring the amount of cfDNA circulating in maternal blood and comparing it with known standards. If the fetus has a normal karyotype, the amount of DNA is consistent with the known standard for the normal amount. However, if more than the expected amount of chromosome 21 DNA, for example, is detected, it can then be assumed that the fetus is contributing the extra amount and therefore has trisomy 21. The same is true for trisomies 13 and 18. The test has a detection rate of more than 99% for trisomies 21 and 18, but a lower rate (approximately 80%) for trisomy 13 (Latendresse & Deneris, 2016b/2018). Women should understand that although the cfDNA screen results nearly match those of diagnostic tests, cfDNA is still a screening test. Therefore, women with positive cfDNA results are referred for amniocentesis or CVS to confirm the findings (ACOG & SMFM, 2016b/2018; Latendresse & Deneris) (see Box 26.6).

The accuracy of the test depends on the proportion of fetal to maternal DNA in the maternal plasma, which must be at least 4%. As pregnancy progresses, the fetal contribution to the amount of cfDNA in maternal circulation increases. cfDNA screening for the detection of fetal chromosomal abnormalities is optimally performed at 10 to 12 weeks of gestation, by which time the average fetal DNA fraction should have reached approximately 10% of the maternal DNA (Driscoll et al., 2017; Latendresse & Deneris, 2015). The test is offered to women considered to be at greater risk for chromosomal abnormalities (i.e., aneuploidies), including those with advanced maternal age, screen-positive maternal serum screens, or ultrasound abnormalities. Women who have previously given birth to a child with a chromosomal abnormality are also candidates for the screen (Cunningham et al., 2018; Latendresse & Deneris). The cfDNA test is simple to perform; a sample of maternal blood is obtained by venipuncture and sent to a commercial laboratory. The test is less sensitive in women who are obese. Currently cfDNA testing is not recommended for use in multifetal pregnancies (Latendresse & Deneris).

FETAL CARE CENTERS

With developing technology, diagnosis and subsequent treatment options exist for some fetal anomalies. Fetal care centers have evolved in response to the need to provide diagnostic and therapeutic options as well as support services for families with a fetal anomaly diagnosis (ACOG, 2011/2017). These families need access to an interprofessional team that is able to provide multiple services such as genetic counseling, support from social workers and chaplains, a palliative care team skilled in perinatal issues, and ethics consultation because of the complex emotional stressors they face. Care coordination is critical for the successful management of high-risk pregnancies. Many fetal care centers have a staff member, often a nurse, who coordinates care and assists the family in navigating multiple appointments with members of the interprofessional team.

ANTEPARTUM ASSESSMENT USING ELECTRONIC FETAL MONITORING

Indications

First- and second-trimester antepartum assessment is directed primarily at the diagnosis of fetal anomalies. The goal of third-trimester testing is to determine whether the intrauterine environment continues to support the fetus. The testing is often used to determine the timing of birth for women at risk for interrupted oxygenation to the fetus by any of several mechanisms (see Box 26.2). Evidence-based recommendations for condition-specific testing schemes in cases of identified risk factors have been difficult to develop and often do not exist. Condition-specific testing used as a strategy to prevent fetal death is unlikely to be effective, given the many fetal deaths that occur in pregnancies considered to be low risk or with no identifiable risk factors. There is no ideal single test or testing strategy for all high-risk pregnancies (Greenberg & Druzin, 2017).

The ability to detect and prevent impending fetal death depends on the group of pregnant women selected for testing, the predictive value of the tests used, and the clinician's ability to respond to abnormal test results. Maternal assessment of fetal movement is suggested as a first-line screening test for fetal well-being (see earlier discussion of daily fetal movement count). When electronic fetal monitoring and ultrasound are used for antepartum fetal evaluation, the NST and the mBPP are the primary tests performed. The complete BPP and the CST are used for follow-up evaluation in women who have a persistently nonreactive NST or abnormal mBPP. Traditionally, testing has begun at 32 to 34 weeks of gestation, with earlier initiation of testing recommended for women with multiple high-risk conditions. Testing is usually performed once or twice weekly (Greenberg & Druzin, 2017).

Nonstress Test

The nonstress test (NST) is the most widely applied technique for antepartum evaluation of the fetus. The basis for the NST is that the normal fetus produces characteristic heart rate patterns in response to fetal movement, uterine contractions, or stimulation. In the term fetus, accelerations are associated with movement more than 85% of the time. The most common reason for the absence of FHR accelerations is the quiet fetal sleep state. However, CNS depressant medications, chronic smoking, and the presence of fetal malformations can also adversely affect the test results (Greenberg & Druzin, 2017). The NST can be performed easily and quickly in an outpatient setting because it is noninvasive, easy to perform and interpret, relatively inexpensive, and has no known contraindications. Disadvantages include the requirement for twice-weekly testing, a high false-positive rate, and a higher false-negative rate than is achieved with most other methods. The test also is slightly less sensitive in detecting fetal compromise than the CST or the BPP (Greenberg & Druzin; Miller et al., 2017).

Procedure

The woman is seated in a reclining chair (or in the semi-Fowler position) with a slight lateral tilt to optimize uterine perfusion and prevent supine hypotension. The FHR is recorded with a Doppler transducer, and a tocodynamometer is applied to detect uterine contractions or fetal movements. The tracing is observed for signs of fetal activity and a concurrent acceleration of FHR. If evidence of fetal movement is not apparent on the tracing, the woman may be asked to depress a button on a handheld event marker connected to the monitor when she feels fetal movement. The movement is then noted on the tracing. Because almost all accelerations are accompanied by fetal movement, the movements need not be recorded for the test to be considered reactive. The test is usually completed within 20 to 30 minutes, but more time may be required if the fetus must be awakened from a sleep state.

Health care professionals sometimes attempt to increase fetal activity by manually stimulating the fetus or having the woman drink orange juice to increase her blood sugar level. Although these practices are common, there is no evidence that they increase fetal activity (Greenberg & Druzin, 2017).

Vibroacoustic stimulation (VAS; see later discussion) is often used to change the fetal state from quiet to active sleep if the initial NST result is nonreactive. After 26 weeks of gestation, VAS may significantly increase the number of reactive NSTs obtained, thus shortening the time required to complete the test (Greenberg & Druzin, 2017).

Interpretation

NST results are either reactive (Fig. 26.9) or nonreactive (Fig. 26.10). Box 26.7 lists criteria for both results. A reactive NST is considered normal, while a nonreactive test requires further evaluation. The testing period is often extended, usually for an additional 20 minutes, with the expectation that the fetal sleep state will change and the test will become reactive. During this time, VAS (see later discussion) may be used to stimulate fetal activity. If the test does not meet the criteria after 40 minutes, a CST or BPP should be performed. Once the NST testing is initiated, it is usually repeated once or twice weekly for the remainder of the pregnancy (Greenberg & Druzin, 2017; Miller et al., 2017) (see Clinical Reasoning Case Study).

 CLINICAL REASONING CASE STUDY

Fetal Assessment Using the Nonstress Test

Emily is a 30-yr-old G5 T3 P0 A1 L3 who is now at 32 weeks of gestation. Emily was diagnosed with diabetes 4 years ago and also has chronic hypertension. Her physician has scheduled her for twice-weekly nonstress testing, and this appointment is her first. You are the nurse assigned to perform Emily's nonstress test (NST) today. As you help her get comfortable and attach the fetal heart rate and contraction monitors, Emily grumbles, "I don't see why I had to come get this test done. It was really hard to find a babysitter for my kids, and it is hard to have gas money to come so often!"

1. What is the priority concern or client need in this situation? Support your answer with data as stated in the case.
2. List other client needs/problems in this case.
3. Identify any additional information or assessment data that is needed by the nurse in planning care for this client.
4. What nursing actions are appropriate in this situation?
   a. What is the priority nursing action? (What should the nurse do first?)
   b. Describe other nursing interventions that are important to providing optimal client care.
5. Describe the roles/responsibilities of the interprofessional health care team members (other than nurses) who may be involved in providing care for this client.

Vibroacoustic Stimulation

Vibroacoustic stimulation (also called the *fetal acoustic stimulation test [FAST]*) is another method of testing antepartum FHR response. This test is generally performed in conjunction with the NST and uses a combination of sound and vibration to stimulate the fetus. Whether the acoustic or the vibratory component alters the fetal state is unclear. The fetus is monitored for 5 minutes before stimulation to obtain a baseline FHR. If the fetal baseline pattern is nonreactive, the sound source (usually a laryngeal stimulator) is then activated for 3 seconds on the maternal abdomen over the fetal head. The desired result is a reactive NST, which usually occurs within 3 minutes of stimulation. The accelerations produced may have a significant increase in duration (Fig. 26.11). The stimulus may be repeated at 1-minute intervals up to three times when no response is noted. Further evaluation is needed with BPP or a CST if the pattern is still nonreactive. VAS is safe for use during pregnancy. No long-term evidence of hearing loss has been found in children followed up to 4 years of age who were exposed to VAS during pregnancy (Greenberg & Druzin, 2017).

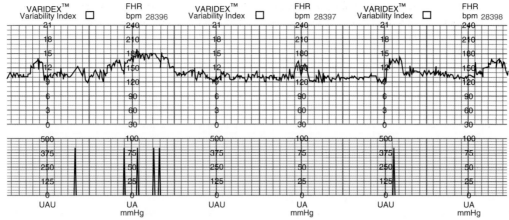

Fig. 26.9 Reactive Nonstress Test. (From Gabbe, S. G., Niebyl, J. R., Simpson, J. L., et al. [Eds.]. [2017]. *Obstetrics: Normal and problem pregnancies* [7th ed.]. Philadelphia: Elsevier.)

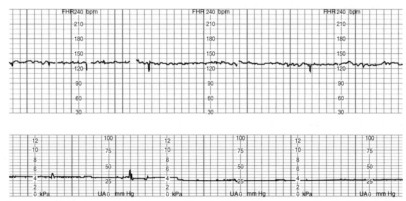

Fig. 26.10 Segment of Nonreactive Nonstress Test in Term Pregnancy. The lack of accelerations meeting minimum criteria continued for 40 minutes. (From Miller, L., Miller, D., & Cypher, R. [2017]. *Mosby's pocket guide to fetal monitoring: A multidisciplinary approach* [8th ed.]. St. Louis: Elsevier.)

BOX 26.7 Interpretation of the Nonstress Test

Reactive test: Two accelerations in a 20-min period, each lasting at least 15 seconds and peaking at least 15 beats/min above the baseline. (Before 32 weeks of gestation, an acceleration is defined as a rise of at least 10 beats/min lasting at least 10 seconds from onset to offset; see Fig. 26.9.)

Nonreactive test: A test that does not demonstrate at least two qualifying accelerations within a 20-min window (see Fig. 26.10).

From Miller, L., Miller, D., & Cypher, R. (2017). *Mosby's pocket guide to fetal monitoring: A multidisciplinary approach* (8th ed.). St. Louis: Elsevier.

Contraction Stress Test

The contraction stress test or *oxytocin challenge test (OCT)* was the first widely used electronic fetal assessment test. It was devised as a graded stress test of the fetus, and its purpose was to identify the jeopardized fetus that was stable at rest but showed evidence of compromise after stress. Uterine contractions decrease uterine blood flow and placental perfusion. If this decrease is sufficient to produce hypoxia in the fetus, a deceleration in FHR results.

❗ NURSING ALERT

In a healthy fetoplacental unit, uterine contractions do not usually produce late decelerations, whereas if interrupted oxygenation is present, contractions produce late decelerations.

The CST provides an earlier warning of fetal compromise than the NST and produces fewer false-positive results. Like most methods of antepartum fetal surveillance, however, it cannot predict acute fetal compromise (e.g., umbilical cord accidents, placental abruption, or rapid deterioration of glucose control in a woman with diabetes). The CST is more time consuming and expensive than the NST. It is also an invasive procedure if oxytocin stimulation is required. In general, the CST cannot be performed on women who should not give birth vaginally at the time the test is done. Absolute contraindications for the CST are the following: preterm labor, placenta previa, vasa previa, cervical insufficiency, multiple gestation, and previous classical incision for cesarean birth (Greenberg & Druzin, 2017; Miller et al., 2017). Because of these disadvantages, the CST is generally used as a backup, rather than a primary method of antepartum testing.

Procedure

The woman is placed in the semi-Fowler position or sits in a reclining chair with a slight lateral tilt to optimize uterine perfusion and avoid supine hypotension. She is monitored electronically with a fetal ultrasound transducer and a uterine tocodynamometer. The tracing is observed for 10 to 20 minutes for baseline rate and variability and the possible occurrence of spontaneous contractions. The two methods of CST are the nipple-stimulated contraction test and the more commonly used oxytocin-stimulated contraction test.

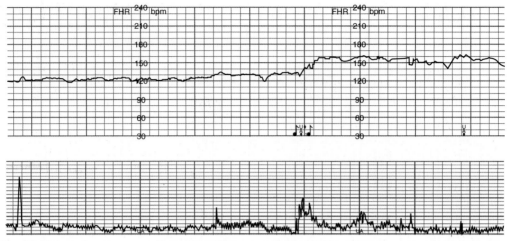

Fig. 26.11 Reactive Nonstress Test After Vibroacoustic Stimulation. The stimulus was applied at the point marked by the musical notes. A sustained fetal heart rate acceleration was produced. *FHR*, Fetal heart rate. (From Gabbe, S. G., Niebyl, J. R., Simpson, J. L., et al. [Eds.]. [2017]. *Obstetrics: Normal and problem pregnancies* [7th ed.]. Philadelphia: Elsevier.)

Nipple-stimulated contraction test. Several methods of nipple stimulation have been described. In one approach, the woman applies warm, moist washcloths to both breasts for several minutes. She is then asked to massage one nipple for 10 minutes. Massaging the nipple causes a release of oxytocin from the posterior pituitary gland. An alternative approach is for her to massage one nipple through her clothes for 2 minutes, rest for 5 minutes, and repeat the cycles of massage and rest as necessary to achieve adequate uterine activity. When adequate contractions or hyperstimulation (defined as uterine contractions lasting more than 90 seconds, or five or more contractions in 10 minutes) occur, stimulation should be stopped.

Oxytocin-stimulated contraction test. Exogenous oxytocin also can be used to stimulate uterine contractions. An intravenous (IV) infusion is begun, and a dilute solution of oxytocin (e.g., 30 units in 500 mL of fluid) is infused into the tubing of the main IV line through a piggyback port and delivered by an infusion pump to ensure an accurate dose. One method of oxytocin infusion is to begin at 0.5 milliunits/min and double the dose every 20 minutes until three uterine contractions of moderate intensity, each lasting 40 to 60 seconds, are observed within a 10-minute period. These criteria for contractions were selected to approximate the stress experienced by the fetus during the first stage of labor (Greenberg & Druzin, 2017).

Interpretation

CST results are negative, positive, equivocal, suspicious, or unsatisfactory. If no late decelerations are observed with the contractions, the findings are considered negative (Fig. 26.12A). Repetitive late decelerations render the test results positive (see Fig. 26.12B). Table 26.5 lists criteria for each possible test result and the clinical significance of each.

The desired CST result is negative because it has consistently been associated with good fetal outcomes. The likelihood of fetal death occurring within 1 week of a negative CST is less than 1 in 1000. Positive CST results have been associated with intrauterine fetal death, late FHR decelerations in labor, IUGR, and meconium-stained amniotic fluid (Greenberg & Druzin, 2017). A positive CST result usually leads to hospitalization for further close observation or birth. Unsatisfactory, suspicious, and equivocal tests require further evaluation, either by prolonged monitoring or repeat testing, often the following day (Miller et al., 2017).

PSYCHOLOGIC CONSIDERATIONS RELATED TO HIGH-RISK PREGNANCY

Once a pregnancy has been identified as high risk, the pregnant woman and her fetus are monitored carefully throughout the remainder of the pregnancy. All women who undergo antepartum assessments are at risk for real and potential problems and may feel anxious. In most instances the tests are ordered because of suspected fetal compromise, deterioration of a maternal condition, or both. In the third trimester, pregnant women are most concerned about protecting themselves and their fetuses and consider themselves most vulnerable to outside influences. The label of *high risk* often increases this sense of vulnerability.

When a woman is diagnosed with a high-risk pregnancy, she and her family will likely experience stress related to the diagnosis. The woman may exhibit various psychologic responses, including anxiety, low self-esteem, guilt, frustration, and inability to function. A high-risk pregnancy can also affect parental attachment, accomplishment of the tasks of pregnancy, and family adaptation to the pregnancy. If the woman is fearful for her well-being, she may continue to feel ambivalent about the pregnancy or may not accept its reality. She may not be able to complete preparations for the baby or go to childbirth classes if she is placed on restricted activity at home or hospitalized. The family may become frustrated because they cannot engage in activities that prepare them for parenthood. The nurse can help the woman and her family regain control and balance in their lives by providing support and encouragement, information about the pregnancy problem and its management, and opportunities to make as many choices as possible about the woman's care.

THE NURSE'S ROLE IN ASSESSMENT AND MANAGEMENT OF THE HIGH-RISK PREGNANCY

Nursing interventions for all pregnant women include education, anticipatory guidance, counseling for family adaptation, assessment, and planning of appropriate interventions. Providing care to women facing a high-risk pregnancy draws on the nurse's unique knowledge in understanding the physiologic and psychosocial needs when a pregnancy is complicated by a maternal or fetal issue. Along with receiving a diagnosis of a maternal or fetal health concern, women

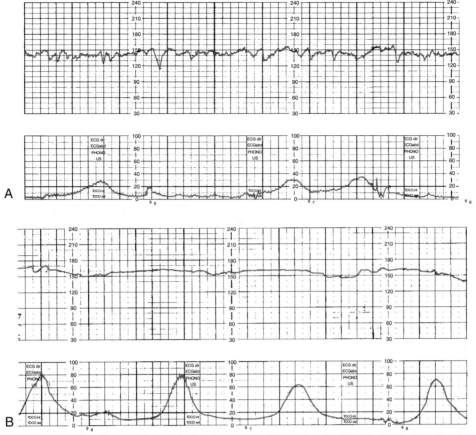

Fig. 26.12 Contraction Stress Test. (A) Negative contraction stress test (CST). (B) Positive CST. (From Tucker, S. [2004]. *Pocket guide to fetal monitoring and assessment* [5th ed.]. St. Louis: Mosby.)

TABLE 26.5 Interpretation of the Contraction Stress Test

Interpretation	Clinical Significance
Negative	
At least three uterine contractions in a 10-min period, with no late or significant variable decelerations	Usually resume routine weekly testing schedule
Positive	
Late decelerations occur with 50% or more of contractions, even if there are fewer than three contractions in 10 min	Usually warrants hospital admission for further evaluation and/or birth
Suspicious or Equivocal	
Prolonged, variable, or late decelerations occurring with less than 50% of the contractions	Further evaluation needed, either by prolonged monitoring or by repeat testing the next day
Equivocal-Hyperstimulatory	
Decelerations that occur in the presence of contractions more frequent than every 2 min or lasting longer than 90 seconds	Further evaluation needed, either by prolonged monitoring or repeat testing the next day
Unsatisfactory	
Failure to produce three contractions within a 10-min window or inability to trace the fetal heart rate	Further evaluation needed, either by prolonged monitoring or repeat testing the next day

From Miller, L., Miller, D., & Cypher, R. (2017). *Mosby's pocket guide to fetal monitoring: A multidisciplinary approach* (8th ed.). St. Louis: Elsevier.

may experience loss and grief, increased stress, uncertainty, information needs, and decision-making dilemmas (Lalor, Begley, & Galavan, 2009).

High-risk pregnancies are often accompanied by additional testing and procedures. In these situations, the nurse's role is to provide education and support as women undergo procedures such as ultrasonography, MRI, CVS, PUBS, and amniocentesis. In some instances, the nurse may assist the health care provider with the test or procedure. When educating the woman and her family, the nurse must explain the purpose of each test, how it is performed, and the difference between screening and diagnostic tests. The nurse must also be aware of potential moral and ethical implications associated with certain tests. For example, women and their families may need to make a decision about pregnancy termination based on test results.

In many settings nurses actually perform tests such as NSTs, CSTs, and BPPs; conduct an initial assessment; and begin necessary interventions for nonreassuring results. Nurses who perform these tests have had additional education and training and function under guidance of established protocols and in collaboration with obstetric care providers. Client teaching, which is an integral component of this role, involves preparing the woman for the test, interpreting the findings, and providing psychosocial support when needed.

Women with high-risk pregnancies will likely receive many different services from multiple care providers. For all childbearing families effective care management requires that members of the interprofessional health care team cooperate, communicate, and collaborate to provide care that promotes the best possible outcomes for mothers and babies. This coordination of care is even more essential in meeting the needs of families who are dealing with the additional stressors associated with a high-risk pregnancy (Barron, 2014).

▌KEY POINTS

- A high-risk pregnancy is one in which the life or well-being of the mother or infant is jeopardized by a biophysical or psychosocial disorder coincident with or unique to pregnancy.
- Biophysical, sociodemographic, psychosocial, and environmental factors place the pregnancy and fetus or neonate at risk.
- Biophysical assessment techniques include DFMCs, ultrasonography, and MRI.
- Biochemical monitoring techniques include amniocentesis, PUBS, CVS, MSAFP, multiple marker screens, and cell-free DNA screening in maternal blood.

- Fetal care centers have evolved in response to the need to provide diagnostic and therapeutic options as well as care coordination and other support services for families with a fetal anomaly diagnosis.
- Reactive NSTs and negative CSTs suggest fetal well-being.
- Most assessment tests have some degree of risk for the mother and fetus and usually cause some anxiety for the woman and her family.
- The nurse's roles in assessment and management of the high-risk pregnancy are primarily those of educator and support person.

REFERENCES

American College of Obstetricians and Gynecologists. (2011, reaffirmed 2017). Committee opinion no. 501: Maternal-fetal intervention and fetal care centers. *Obstetrics and Gynecology, 118*(2 Pt 1), 405–410.

American College of Obstetricians and Gynecologists, & American Institute of Ultrasound in Medicine. (2016c, reaffirmed 2018). Practice bulletin no. 175: Ultrasound in Pregnancy. *Obstetrics & Gynecology, 128*(6), e241–e256.

American College of Obstetricians and Gynecologists, & Society for Maternal Fetal Medicine. (2016a, reaffirmed 2018). Practice bulletin no. 162: Prenatal diagnostic testing for genetic disorders. *Obstetrics & Gynecology, 127*(5), e108–e122.

American College of Obstetricians and Gynecologists, & Society for Maternal Fetal Medicine. (2016b, reaffirmed 2018). Practice bulletin no. 163: Screening for fetal aneuploidy. *Obstetrics & Gynecology, 127*(5), e123–e137.

American Institute of Ultrasound in Medicine. (2012). *Official statement: Prudent use in pregnancy.* Laurel, MD: American Institute of Ultrasound in Medicine.

Barron, M. L. (2014). Antenatal care. In K. R. Simpson, & P. Creehan (Eds.), *Awhonn's perinatal nursing* (4th ed.). Philadelphia: Lippincott Willliams & Wilkins.

Chambers, C., & Friedman, J. M. (2019). Teratogenesis and environmental exposure. In R. Resnik, C. J. Lockwood, T. R. Moore, et al. (Eds.), *Creasy and Resnik's maternal-fetal medicine: Principles and practice* (8th ed.). Philadelphia: Elsevier.

Cunningham, F., Leveno, K., Bloom, S., et al. (2018). *Williams obstetrics* (25th ed.). New York: McGraw-Hill Education.

Driscoll, D. A., Simpson, J. L., Holzgreve, W., et al. (2017). Genetic screening and prenatal genetic diagnosis. In S. G. Gabbe, J. R. Niebyl, J. L. Simpson, et al. (Eds.), *Obstetrics: Normal and problem pregnancies* (7th ed.). Philadelphia: Elsevier.

Gilbert, W. M. (2017). Amniotic fluid disorders. In S. G. Gabbe, J. R. Niebyl, J. L. Simpson, et al. (Eds.), *Obstetrics: Normal and problem pregnancies* (7th ed.). Philadelphia: Elsevier.

Greenberg, M. B., & Druzin, M. L. (2017). Antepartum fetal evaluation. In S. G. Gabbe, J. R. Niebyl, J. L. Simpson, et al. (Eds.), *Obstetrics: Normal and problem pregnancies* (7th ed.). Philadelphia: Elsevier.

Hull, A. D., Resnik, R., & Silver, R. M. (2019). Placenta previa and accreta, vasa previa, subchorionic hemorrhage, and abruptio placentae. In R. Resnik, C. J. Lockwood, T. R. Moore, et al. (Eds.), *Creasy and Resnik's maternal-fetal medicine: Principles and practice* (8th ed.). Philadelphia: Elsevier.

Lalor, J., Begley, C., & Galavan, E. (2009). Recasting hope: A process of adaptation following fetal anomaly diagnosis. *Social Science & Medicine, 68*(3), 462–472.

Latendresse, G., & Deneris, A. (2015). An update on current prenatal testing options: First trimester and noninvasive prenatal testing. *Journal of Midwifery & Women's Health, 60*(1), 24–36.

Martin, J. A., Hamilton, B. E., Osterman, M. J. K., et al. (2018). Births: Final data for 2017. *National Vital Statistics Reports, 67*(8), 1–49.

Mercer, B. M. (2019). Assessment and induction of fetal pulmonary maturity. In R. Resnik, C. J. Lockwood, T. R. Moore, et al. (Eds.), *Creasy and Resnik's maternal-fetal medicine: Principles and practice* (8th ed.). Philadelphia: Elsevier.

Miller, L., Miller, D., & Cypher, R. (2017). *Mosby's pocket guide to fetal monitoring: A multidisciplinary approach* (8th ed.). St. Louis: Elsevier.

Moise, K. (2017). Red cell alloimmunization. In S. G. Gabbe, J. R. Niebyl, J. L. Simpson, et al. (Eds.), *Obstetrics: Normal and problem pregnancies* (7th ed.). Philadelphia: Elsevier.

Richards, D. S. (2017). Obstetrical ultrasound: Imaging, dating, growth, and anomaly. In S. G. Gabbe, J. R. Niebyl, J. L. Simpson, et al. (Eds.), *Obstetrics: Normal and problem pregnancies* (7th ed.). Philadelphia: Elsevier.

Wapner, R.J., & Dugoff, L. (2019). Prenatal diagnosis of congenital disorders. In R. Resnik, C. J. Lockwood, T. R. Moore, et al. (Eds.), *Creasy and Resnik's maternal-fetal medicine: Principles and practice* (8th ed.). Philadelphia: Elsevier.

Wolf, R. B. (2019). Skeletal imaging. In R. Resnik, C. J. Lockwood, T. R. Moore, et al. (Eds.), *Creasy and Resnik's maternal-fetal medicine: Principles and practice* (8th ed.). Philadelphia: Elsevier.

27

Hypertensive Disorders

Dusty Dix

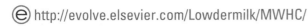
http://evolve.elsevier.com/Lowdermilk/MWHC/

LEARNING OBJECTIVES

- Differentiate among gestational hypertension, preeclampsia, and chronic hypertension.
- Describe etiologic theories and the pathophysiology of preeclampsia.
- Compare the care management of women with gestational hypertension and preeclampsia with or without severe features.

- Describe appropriate nursing actions during and after an eclamptic seizure.
- Discuss the preconception, antepartum, intrapartum, and postpartum management of the woman with chronic hypertension.

Pregnancy-associated hypertensive disorders develop during pregnancy, labor, or after birth. These disorders include gestational hypertension and preeclampsia–eclampsia. Chronic hypertensive disorders precede pregnancy. Women with chronic hypertension can also develop superimposed preeclampsia. The classification, pathophysiologic changes, assessment, and management of pregnancy-associated hypertensive disorders are discussed in this chapter, with a primary focus on preeclampsia. The care of women with hypertensive disorders during the perinatal period requires a collaborative effort by members of an interprofessional health care team. Care management is directed toward early detection, thorough assessment, and timely intervention.

SIGNIFICANCE AND INCIDENCE

Hypertensive disorders are common medical complications of pregnancy, occurring in approximately 5% to 10% of all pregnancies. The incidence varies among hospitals, regions, and countries. Hypertensive disorders are a major cause of perinatal morbidity and mortality worldwide. The three most common types of hypertensive disorders occurring in pregnancy are gestational hypertension, preeclampsia, and chronic essential hypertension (Sibai, 2017).

CLASSIFICATION

The classification of hypertensive disorders in pregnancy is confusing because standard definitions are not used consistently by all health care providers. The classification system most commonly used in the United States since 2000 was based on recommendations from the American College of Obstetricians and Gynecologists (ACOG) and the National High Blood Pressure Education Program Working Group on High Blood Pressure in Pregnancy. In 2013, ACOG convened a task force of experts in the management of hypertension in pregnancy. The Task Force on Hypertension in Pregnancy chose to continue use of this classification system, although it modified some of the system components (ACOG, 2013). The current classification system is summarized in Table 27.1.

Gestational Hypertension

Gestational hypertension is the onset of hypertension without proteinuria or other systemic findings diagnostic for preeclampsia after week 20 of pregnancy (ACOG, 2013). *Hypertension* is defined as a systolic blood pressure (BP) greater than 140 mm Hg or a diastolic BP greater than 90 mm Hg. The hypertension should be recorded on two

TABLE 27.1 Classification of Hypertensive States of Pregnancy

Type	Description
Gestational Hypertensive Disorders	
Gestational hypertension	Development of hypertension after week 20 of pregnancy in a previously normotensive woman without proteinuria or other systemic findings (see description of preeclampsia in the text)
Preeclampsia	Development of hypertension and proteinuria in a previously normotensive woman after 20 weeks of gestation or in the early postpartum period. In the absence of proteinuria, the development of new-onset hypertension with the new onset of any of the following: thrombocytopenia, renal insufficiency, impaired liver function, pulmonary edema, or cerebral or visual symptoms
Eclampsia	Development of seizures or coma not attributable to other causes in a preeclamptic woman
Chronic Hypertensive Disorders	
Chronic hypertension	Hypertension in a pregnant woman present before pregnancy
Superimposed preeclampsia	Chronic hypertension in association with preeclampsia

Data from American College of Obstetricians and Gynecologists. (2013). Executive summary: Hypertension in pregnancy. *Obstetrics & Gynecology, 122*(5), 1122–1131.

occasions at least 4 hours apart after 20 weeks of gestation in a woman with a previously normal BP (ACOG). Only one pressure (either systolic or diastolic) must be elevated to meet the definition of hypertension (Witcher & Shah, 2019).

The definitions of gestational hypertension are the same as the definitions for BP readings for preeclampsia (Table 27.2). Gestational hypertension resolves after giving birth, although it may require 6 to 12 months to do so (Witcher & Shah, 2019). Some women who are initially thought to have gestational hypertension are eventually diagnosed with chronic hypertension instead. About 25% to 50% of women with gestational hypertension go on to develop preeclampsia (Snydal, 2014).

EVIDENCE-BASED PRACTICE

What's Up With Preeclampsia?

Ask the Question

For pregnant women, what are the new best practices for identifying and treating preeclampsia?

Search for the Evidence

Search Strategies English language research-based publications since 2014 on preeclampsia and gestational hypertension were included.

Databases Used Cochrane Collaborative Database, National Guideline Clearinghouse (AHRQ), CINAHL, PubMed, UpToDate, and the professional websites for ACOG and AWHONN

Critical Appraisal of the Evidence

Risk factors for preeclampsia include advanced maternal age, nulliparity, unmarried status, African American race, multiple fetuses, chronic hypertension, diabetes, and history of preeclampsia.

Recent research has also found the following to be risk factors for preeclampsia:

- For women with normal prepregnancy weight, excessive (>10) increase in body mass index (BMI) during pregnancy is associated with increased risk for preeclampsia. For overweight and obese women, even moderate BMI increase (5-10) can increase risk (Swank, Caughey, Farinelli, et al., 2014; Wang, Hao, Sampson, & Xia, 2017). Being overweight or obese is a prevalent risk factor (Pare, Parry, McElrath et al., 2014).
- Levels of C-reactive protein, blood urea nitrogen, serum uric acid, and alanine transaminase, as well as platelet count are associated with the presence and severity of preeclampsia (Maged, Aid, Bassiouny et al., 2017).
- Low levels of placental growth factor, an angiogenic factor, combined with increased levels of anti-angiogenic factors are predictive of preeclampsia (Ngene & Moodley, 2018).

The ACOG Task Force on Hypertension in Pregnancy (2013) has issued the following guideline changes for diagnosis and treatment of preeclampsia:

- Although proteinuria may still be used for diagnosis, a massive amount (>5 g in a 24-h urine collection) is no longer considered to be a severe feature of preeclampsia. Routine screening, beyond an appropriate medical history, is not recommended.
- Vitamins C and E are not recommended to prevent preeclampsia.
- Daily low-dose aspirin can help high-risk women.
- Antihypertensives (labetalol or hydralazine) are useful for severe hypertension.

- Magnesium sulfate is used for seizure prevention but not as an antihypertensive agent.

Apply the Evidence: Nursing Implications

- Preconception counseling for modifiable risk factors, such as smoking and weight gain, can decrease preeclampsia risk.
- Physical activity has a protective effect against preeclampsia (Magro-Malosso, Saccone, Tommaso et al., 2017).
- Teaching stress management techniques for lifelong stress and pregnancy stress is important, especially in the presence of chronic hypertension.
- In addition to assessing BP, alert nurses are often the first to note subtle clinical changes indicating preeclampsia, such as sudden weight gain, edema, headache, oliguria, right-sided pain, and fetal distress.
- In the event of emergent hypertensive crisis, nurses must be familiar and proficient with assessments, including reflexes and fetal monitoring; must understand medications; and must be proactive in environmental alteration, such as limiting visitors and lowering lights and sound in the room.

References

ACOG Task Force on Hypertension in Pregnancy. (2013). *Hypertension in pregnancy.* Washington, DC: ACOG. Retrieved from: https://www.acog.org/~/media/Task%20Force%20 and%20Work%20Group%20Reports/public/HypertensioninPregnancy.pdf.

Maged, A. M., Aid, G., Bassiouny, N., et al. (2017). Association of biochemical markers with the severity of preeclampsia. *International Journal of Gynecology & Obstetrics, 136* (2), 138–144.

Magro-Malosso, E. R., Saccone, G., Tommaso, M., et al. (2017). Exercise during pregnancy and risk of gestational hypertensive disorders: A systematic review and meta-analysis. *Acta Obstetricia et Gynecologica Scandinavica, 96*(8), 921–931.

Ngene, N. C., & Moodley, J. (2018). Role of angiogenic factors in the pathogenesis and management of pre-eclampsia. *International Journal of Gynecology & Obstetrics, 141*(1), 5–13.

Pare, E., Parry, S., McElrath, T. F., et al. (2014). Clinical risk factors for preeclampsia in the 21st century. *Obstetrics & Gynecology, 124*(4), 763–770.

Swank, M. L., Caughey, A. B., Farinelli, C. K., et al. (2014). The impact of change in pregnancy body mass index on the development of gestational hypertensive disorders. *Journal of Perinatology, 34*(3), 181–185.

Wang, Y., Hao, M., Sampson, S., & Xia, J. (2017). Elective delivery versus expectant management for pre-eclampsia: A meta-analysis of RCTs. *Archives of Gynecology and Obstetrics, 295*(3), 607–622.

Jennifer Taylor Alderman

Preeclampsia

Preeclampsia is a pregnancy-specific condition in which hypertension and proteinuria develop after 20 weeks of gestation in a woman who previously had neither condition. The signs and symptoms of preeclampsia also can develop for the first time during the postpartum period. Preeclampsia is a leading cause of maternal and perinatal morbidity and mortality in the United States and Canada (Huwe, Puck, Vasher et al., 2019). The 2013 ACOG Task Force on Hypertension in Pregnancy eliminated several criteria that had traditionally been used to diagnose severe features of preeclampsia. These include proteinuria, oliguria, presence of intrauterine growth restriction (IUGR), or fetal growth restriction as a requirement for the diagnosis of preeclampsia (Sibai, 2017). In the absence of proteinuria, preeclampsia may be defined as hypertension along with either thrombocytopenia, impaired liver function, new-onset renal insufficiency, pulmonary edema, or new-onset cerebral or visual disturbances (see Table 27.2) (ACOG,

TABLE 27.2	Diagnostic Criteria for Preeclampsia and Preeclampsia With Severe Features	
	Preeclampsia	**Preeclampsia With Severe Features**
Component		
Hypertension	Blood pressure (BP) reading ≥140/90 mm Hg × 2, at least 4 hrs apart after 20 weeks of gestation in a previously normotensive woman	BP reading ≥160/110 mm Hg × 2, at least 4 hrs apart while the woman is on bed rest (unless antihypertensive therapy has already been initiated)
Proteinuria	Proteinuria of ≥300 mg in a 24-hr specimen Protein/creatinine ratio ≥0.3 (with each measured as mg/dL) ≥1+ on dipstick (used only if quantitative measurement is not available)	Massive proteinuria (>5 g in a 24-hr specimen) is no longer used as a diagnostic criterion
Thrombocytopenia	Platelet count <100,000/μL	Platelet count <100,000/μL
Impaired liver function	Elevated blood levels of liver enzymes to twice the upper level of normal concentration or higher	Abnormally elevated blood concentrations of liver enzymes to twice the normal concentration; severe persistent epigastric or right upper quadrant abdominal pain unresponsive to medication and not accounted for by alternative diagnoses, or both
Renal insufficiency	New development of serum creatinine >1.1 mg/dL or a doubling of the serum creatinine concentration in the absence of other renal disease	Progressive renal insufficiency (serum creatinine concentration >1.1 mg/dL or a doubling of the serum creatinine concentration) in the absence of other renal disease
Pulmonary edema	Absent	Present
Cerebral or visual disturbances	Absent	New onset

Modified from American College of Obstetricians and Gynecologists. (2013). Executive summary: Hypertension in pregnancy. *Obstetrics & Gynecology, 122*(5), 1122–1131; Witcher, P. M., & Shah, S. S. (2019). Hypertension in pregnancy. In N. H. Troiano, P. M. Witcher, & S. M. Baird (Eds.), *AWHONN's high risk and critical care obstetrics* (4th ed.). Philadelphia: Wolters Kluwer.

2013). Table 27.3 lists common laboratory changes that occur in preeclampsia. (See Community Activity box: Learning About Preeclampsia box.)

 COMMUNITY ACTIVITY

Learning About Preeclampsia

Visit the Preeclampsia Foundation website, https://www.preeclampsia.org/, which provides education and support for women with preeclampsia and other hypertensive disorders of pregnancy. Review the information under the Health Information tab: about signs and symptoms, about preeclampsia, cause of preeclampsia, HELLP syndrome, heart disease and stroke, FAQs, and preeclampsia tests.

Eclampsia

Eclampsia is the onset of seizure activity or coma in a woman with preeclampsia who has no history of preexisting pathology that can result in seizure activity (Harper, Tita, & Karumanchi, 2019; Witcher & Shah, 2019). In developed countries, eclampsia occurs in approximately 1 in 2000 to 1 in 3448 births. The incidence is usually higher in tertiary referral centers, with multifetal gestation, and in women who did not receive prenatal care (Sibai, 2017). Although eclamptic seizures can occur before, during, or after birth, approximately 50% of cases occur during the antepartum period (Poole, 2014).

CHRONIC HYPERTENSIVE DISORDERS

Chronic Hypertension

Chronic hypertension is defined as hypertension that is present before the pregnancy (ACOG, 2013). Women may be diagnosed with chronic hypertension once it is evident that hypertension persists after the postpartum period (Witcher & Shah, 2019).

Chronic Hypertension With Superimposed Preeclampsia

Women with chronic hypertension may develop superimposed preeclampsia. This condition, which is associated with adverse maternal or fetal outcomes, can be difficult to diagnose (ACOG, 2013).

PREECLAMPSIA

Etiology

Preeclampsia is a condition unique to human pregnancy. It occurs in approximately 2% to 7% of healthy nulliparous pregnant women. The incidence and severity of preeclampsia is substantially higher in women with multifetal gestation, a history of preeclampsia, chronic hypertension, preexisting diabetes, and preexisting thrombophilias. Women with limited sperm exposure with the same partner before conception also have a greater risk for developing preeclampsia. Paternal factors also contribute to the risk for preeclampsia. Men who have fathered a preeclamptic pregnancy are nearly twice as likely to father another preeclamptic pregnancy with a different woman, regardless of whether the new partner has a history of a preeclamptic pregnancy (Sibai, 2017). Common risk factors associated with the development of preeclampsia are listed in Box 27.1.

The precise etiology of preeclampsia is unknown. Current thought is that preeclampsia is caused by a complex interaction of maladaptive cardiovascular and uteroplacental responses to pregnancy (Witcher & Shah, 2019).

Pathophysiology

Preeclampsia is a progressive disorder, with the placenta as the root cause. Therefore the disease begins to resolve after the placenta has

TABLE 27.3   Common Laboratory Changes in Preeclampsia

	Normal Nonpregnant	Preeclampsia	HELLP
Hemoglobin, hematocrit	12-16 g/dL, 37%-47%	May ↑	↓
Platelets (cells/mm³)	150,000-400,000/mm³	<100,000/mm³	<100,000/mm³
Prothrombin time (PT), partial thromboplastin time (PTT)	12-14 secs, 60-70 secs	Unchanged	Unchanged
Fibrinogen	200-400 mg/dL	300-600 mg/dL	↓
Fibrin split products (FSPs)	Absent	Absent or present	Present
Blood urea nitrogen (BUN)	10-20 mg/dL	↑	↑
Creatinine	0.5-1.1 mg/dL	>1.1 mg/dL	↑
Lactate dehydrogenase (LDH)[a]	45-90 units/L	↑	↑ (>600 units/L)
Aspartate aminotransferase (AST)	4-20 units/L	↑	↑ (>70 units/L)
Alanine aminotransferase (ALT)	3-21 units/L	↑	↑
Creatinine clearance	80-125 mL/min	130-180 mL/min	↓
Burr cells or schistocytes	Absent	Absent	Present
Uric acid	2-6.6 mg/dL	>5.9 mg/dL	>10 mg/dL
Bilirubin (total)	0.1-1 mg/dL	Unchanged or ↑	↑ (>1.2 mg/dL)

[a]LDH values differ according to the test or assays being performed.
Data from American College of Obstetricians and Gynecologists (ACOG). (2002). *Practice bulletin no. 33: Diagnosis and management of pre-eclampsia and eclampsia.* Washington, DC: ACOG; American College of Obstetricians and Gynecologists. (2013). Executive summary: Hypertension in pregnancy. *Obstetrics & Gynecology, 122*(5), 1122–1131; Dildy, G. (2004). Complications of preeclampsia. In G. Dildy, M. Belfort, G. Saade, et al. (Eds.), *Critical care obstetrics* (4th ed.). Malden, MA: Blackwell Science; Witcher, P. M., & Shah, S. S. (2019). Hypertension in pregnancy. In N. H. Troiano, P. M. Witcher, & S. M. Baird (Eds.), *AWHONN's high risk and critical care obstetrics* (4th ed.). Philadelphia: Wolters Kluwer.

BOX 27.1   Risk Factors for Preeclampsia

- Nulliparity
- Age >40 years
- Pregnancy with assisted reproductive technology
- Interpregnancy interval >7 years
- Family history of preeclampsia
- Woman born small for gestational age
- Obesity/gestational diabetes mellitus
- Multifetal gestation
- Preeclampsia in previous pregnancy
- Poor outcome in previous pregnancy
- Preexisting medical/genetic conditions
- Chronic hypertension
- Renal disease
- Type 1 (insulin-dependent) diabetes mellitus
- Antiphospholipid antibody syndrome
- Factor V Leiden mutation

From Sibai, B. (2017). Preeclampsia and hypertensive disorders. In S. G. Gabbe, J. R. Niebyl, J. L. Simpson, et al. (Eds.), *Obstetrics: Normal and problem pregnancies* (7th ed.). Philadelphia: Elsevier.

been expelled. Current thought is that the pathologic changes that occur in the woman with preeclampsia are caused by disruptions in placental perfusion and endothelial cell dysfunction (ACOG, 2013; Sibai, 2017; Snydal, 2014; Witcher & Shah, 2019). These changes develop early in pregnancy, long before the signs and symptoms of pre-eclampsia become evident (Harper et al., 2019; Sibai Snydal). Normally in pregnancy, the spiral arteries in the uterus widen from thick-walled muscular vessels to thinner, saclike vessels with much larger diame-ters. This change increases the capacity of the vessels, allowing them to handle the increased blood volume of pregnancy. Because this vascular

remodeling does not occur or only partially develops in women with preeclampsia, decreased placental perfusion and endothelial dysfunc-tion result (Witcher & Shah).

Placental ischemia is thought to cause endothelial cell injury and subsequent dysfunction by stimulating the release of sub-stances that are toxic to endothelial cells. This causes generalized vasospasm, which results in poor tissue perfusion in all organ sys-tems, increased peripheral resistance and BP, and increased endo-thelial cell permeability, leading to intravascular protein and fluid loss and ultimately to less plasma volume. The main pathogenic factor is not an increase in BP but poor perfusion as a result of vasospasm and reduced plasma volume. There is increasing evi-dence that endothelial injury can play an important role in the pathophysiology of preeclampsia (Fig. 27.1) (Harper et al., 2019; Poole, 2014). Fig. 27.2 demonstrates how endothelial cell dys-function causes many of the common signs and symptoms of preeclampsia.

Reduced kidney perfusion decreases the glomerular filtration rate and can lead to degenerative glomerular changes and oliguria. Patho-logic changes in the endothelial cells of the glomeruli (glomerular endotheliosis) are uniquely characteristic of preeclampsia. Protein, pri-marily albumin, is lost in the urine. Uric acid clearance is decreased, but serum uric acid levels increase. Sodium and water are retained. Acute tubular necrosis and renal failure may occur (Poole, 2014; Sny-dal, 2014; Witcher & Shah, 2019).

Plasma colloid osmotic pressure decreases as serum albumin lev-els decrease. Intravascular volume is reduced as fluid moves out of the intravascular compartment, resulting in hemoconcentration, increased blood viscosity, and tissue edema. The hematocrit value increases as fluid leaves the intravascular space. Arteriolar vasospasm can lead to endothelial damage and increased capillary permeability, predisposing the woman to pulmonary edema (see Fig. 27.2) (Poole, 2014; Snydal, 2014).

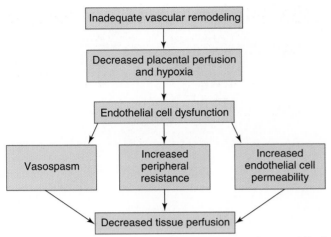

Fig. 27.1 Etiology of Preeclampsia: Disruptions in Placental Perfusion and Endothelial Cell Dysfunction. (Data from Witcher, P. M., & Shah, S. S. [2019]. Hypertension in pregnancy. In N. H. Troiano, P. M. Witcher, & S. M. Baird [Eds.], *AWHONN's high risk and critical care obstetrics* [4th ed.]. Philadelphia: Wolters Kluwer; Harper, L. M., Tita, A., & Karumanchi, S.A. [2019]. Pregnancy-related hypertension. In R. Resnik, C. J. Lockwood, T. R. Moore, et al. (Eds), *Creasy & Resnik's maternal-fetal medicine: Principles and practice* [8th ed.]. Philadelphia: Elsevier; Poole, J. H. [2014]. Hypertensive disorders of pregnancy. In K. R. Simpson, & P. Creehan [Eds.], *AWHONN's perinatal nursing* [4th ed.]. Philadelphia: Lippincott Williams & Wilkins.)

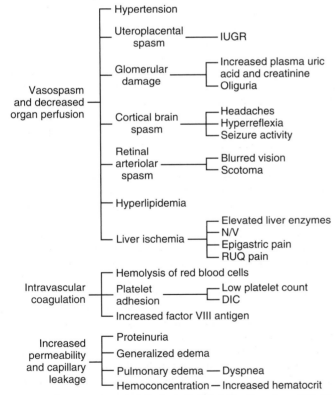

Fig. 27.2 Consequences of Endothelial Cell Dysfunction. *DIC*, Disseminated vascular coagulation; *IUGR*, intrauterine growth restriction; *N/V*, nausea/vomiting; *RUQ*, right upper quadrant. (From Gilbert, E. [2011]. *Manual of high risk pregnancy & delivery* [5th ed.]. St. Louis: Mosby.)

Decreased liver perfusion can lead to impaired liver function and elevated liver enzyme levels. If hepatic edema and subcapsular hemorrhage develop, the woman may complain of epigastric or right upper quadrant abdominal pain. Hemorrhagic necrosis in the liver can result in a subcapsular hematoma, which is a rare occurrence. Rupture of a subcapsular hematoma is a life-threatening complication and a surgical emergency (Snydal, 2014; Witcher & Shah, 2019) (see Fig. 27.2).

Neurologic complications associated with preeclampsia include cerebral edema and hemorrhage and increased central nervous system (CNS) irritability. CNS irritability manifests as headaches, hyperreflexia, positive ankle clonus, and seizures. Arteriolar vasospasms and decreased blood flow to the retina can lead to visual disturbances such as scotoma (dim vision or blind or dark spots in the visual field) and blurred or double vision (Poole, 2014; Snydal, 2014; Witcher & Shah, 2019).

HELLP Syndrome

HELLP syndrome is a laboratory diagnosis for a variant of preeclampsia that involves hepatic dysfunction, characterized by hemolysis *(H)*, elevated liver enzymes *(EL)*, and low platelet *(LP)* count. HELLP syndrome can develop in women who do not have hypertension or proteinuria. Specific laboratory findings are needed to diagnose HELLP syndrome and distinguish it from other serious diseases that share the same signs and symptoms (Witcher & Shah, 2019). Table 27.3 lists laboratory changes that occur in HELLP syndrome.

> **! NURSING ALERT**
>
> An extremely important point to understand is that many women with HELLP syndrome may not have signs or symptoms of preeclampsia with severe features. For example, although most women have hypertension, BP may be only mildly elevated in 15% to 50% of cases. Proteinuria may be absent. As a result, women with HELLP syndrome are often misdiagnosed with a variety of other medical or surgical disorders (Sibai, 2017).

HELLP syndrome appears to occur more frequently in Caucasian women versus women of other races. A diagnosis of HELLP syndrome is associated with an increased risk for maternal death and adverse perinatal outcomes, including pulmonary edema, acute renal failure, disseminated intravascular coagulation (DIC), placental abruption, liver hemorrhage or failure, acute respiratory distress syndrome (ARDS), sepsis, and stroke (Sibai, 2017). The reported perinatal mortality rate ranges from 7.4% to 34%, with a maternal mortality rate of approximately 1% (Sibai). The rate of preterm birth in women with HELLP syndrome is approximately 70%, with 15% of these births occurring before 28 weeks of gestation. Most of the perinatal deaths occur before 28 weeks of gestation in association with placental abruption or severe fetal growth restriction (Sibai).

CARE MANAGEMENT

Identifying and Preventing Preeclampsia

Numerous clinical trials have examined various interventions to prevent preeclampsia, including protein or salt restriction; zinc, magnesium, fish oil, or vitamin C and E supplementation; use of diuretics or other antihypertensive medications; and use of heparin. All of these interventions demonstrated minimal to no benefit in preventing or reducing the incidence of preeclampsia (Sibai, 2017). However, low-dose aspirin has been found to reduce preeclampsia and adverse outcomes in selected high-risk women. ACOG and the Society for Maternal-Fetal Medicine (SMFM) recommend that women at high risk for developing preeclampsia begin daily low-dose (81 mg/day) aspirin therapy between 12 and 28 weeks of gestation for the prevention of preeclampsia. This includes women with one or more of the following high-risk factors: history of preeclampsia, especially if accompanied by an adverse outcome; multifetal gestation; chronic hypertension; preexisting diabetes (type 1 or type 2); renal disease; and autoimmune disease (e.g., systemic lupus erythematosus, antiphospholipid syndrome). In addition, low-dose aspirin prophylaxis should be considered in women who have one or more of the following moderate risk factors for preeclampsia: first pregnancy, maternal age of 35 years or older, BMI greater than 30, family history of preeclampsia, sociodemographic characteristics, and personal history factors (ACOG & SMFM, 2018).

No reliable test that can be used as a routine screening tool for predicting preeclampsia has yet been developed. However, the search for biomarkers that can identify individual women who will develop hypertension during pregnancy is ongoing. For example, decreased circulating levels of the angiogenic proteins vascular endothelial growth factor (VEGF) and placental-like growth factor (PlGF) and increased levels of the antiangiogenic proteins soluble fms-like tyrosine kinase-I (sFlt-I) and soluble endoglin (sEng) have been found to precede the development of preeclampsia by weeks or months (Harper et al., 2019; Witcher & Shah, 2019). Adding biomarkers such as these proteins to a risk assessment for preeclampsia remains investigational, however. Further research is needed before their use is implemented clinically (Witcher & Shah).

Evaluation of maternal clinical factors and biophysical or biochemical markers measured during the first trimester is useful only for predicting women who will go on to develop preeclampsia and will need to give birth before 34 weeks of gestation. At this time, the use of first-trimester screening tests for predicting preeclampsia in clinical practice is not recommended (Sibai, 2017). Abnormal uterine artery Doppler findings in the second trimester of pregnancy have also been noted in women who go on to develop preeclampsia. At this time, however, data do not support the use of Doppler studies for routine screening of pregnant women for preeclampsia (Sibai).

Although research offers future promise, much work remains before a screening test for preeclampsia is available for widespread clinical use. Nurses should be aware of strategies that are being studied and use the most valid results so they can counsel pregnant women about interventions that are evidence-based. Meanwhile, the best preeclampsia prevention methods include early prenatal care for the identification of women at risk and early detection of the disease.

Assessment

Accurate measurement of BP is essential in the early detection of hypertensive disorders. Many factors influence BP measurement, including accuracy of the equipment used, size of the sphygmomanometer cuff, duration of the rest period before recording the BP, posture of the client, and the Korotkoff phase used (phase IV or phase V) for diastolic BP measurement (see Box 14.4) (Sibai, 2017).

Electronic BP devices, often used in inpatient settings, produce different BP measurements from those obtained using a manual cuff and stethoscope. Electronic devices consistently underestimate diastolic BPs by approximately 10 mm Hg and overestimate systolic BP values by 4 to 6 mm Hg. Therefore BP readings taken using different measurement devices are not interchangeable. BP assessment should focus on trends over time, rather than on a single measurement (Poole, 2014).

Assessment for edema is another component of the physical examination, although the presence of edema is no longer included in the definition of preeclampsia. Edema is assessed for distribution, degree, and pitting. Dependent edema is edema of the lowest or most dependent parts of the body, where hydrostatic pressure is greatest. If a pregnant woman is ambulatory, the edema may first be evident in the feet and ankles. If she is confined to bed, it is more likely to occur in the

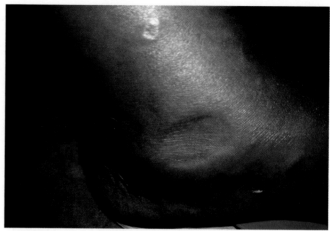

Fig. 27.3 Pitting Edema. (Courtesy Shannon Perry, Phoenix, AZ.)

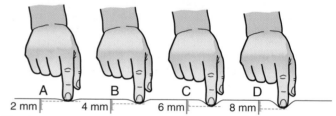

Fig. 27.4 Assessment of Pitting Edema of Lower Extremities. (A) +1; (B) +2; (C) +3; (D) +4.

sacral region. Pitting edema leaves a small depression or pit after finger pressure is applied to the swollen area (Fig. 27.3). The pit, which is caused by movement of fluid to adjacent tissue away from the point of pressure, normally disappears within 10 to 30 seconds. Although the amount of edema is difficult to quantify, the method shown in Fig. 27.4 may be used to record relative degrees of edema formation.

Deep tendon reflexes (DTRs) reflect the balance between the cerebral cortex and spinal cord. They are evaluated as a baseline and to detect any changes. The biceps and patellar reflexes are assessed and the findings recorded (Fig. 27.5 and Table 27.4). To elicit the biceps reflex, the examiner strikes a downward blow over the thumb, which is situated over the biceps tendon (see Fig. 27.5A). Normal response is flexion of the arm at the elbow, described as a 2+ response. The patellar reflex is elicited with the woman's legs hanging freely over the end of the examining table or with the woman lying on her side with the knee slightly flexed (see Fig. 27.5D). The patellar tendon (inferior to the patella) is tapped with a percussion hammer. Normal response is the extension or kicking out of the leg.

To assess for hyperactive reflexes (clonus) at the ankle joint, the examiner supports the leg with the knee flexed (see Fig. 27.5F). With one hand, the examiner sharply dorsiflexes the foot, maintains the position for a moment, and then releases it. Normal (negative clonus) response is elicited when no rhythmic oscillations (jerks) are felt while the foot is held in dorsiflexion. When the foot is released, no oscillations are seen as the foot drops to the plantar-flexed position. Abnormal (positive clonus) response is recognized by rhythmic oscillations of one or more "beats" felt when the foot is in dorsiflexion and seen as the foot drops to the plantar-flexed position.

The presence of proteinuria is ideally determined by evaluation of a 24-hour urine collection. In a 24-hour specimen, proteinuria is defined as a concentration at or greater than 300 mg or a protein/creatinine ratio greater than 0.3. If it is not possible to obtain either of these measurements, proteinuria can be diagnosed by a dipstick measurement of at least 1+ on two occasions. Proteinuria is influenced by

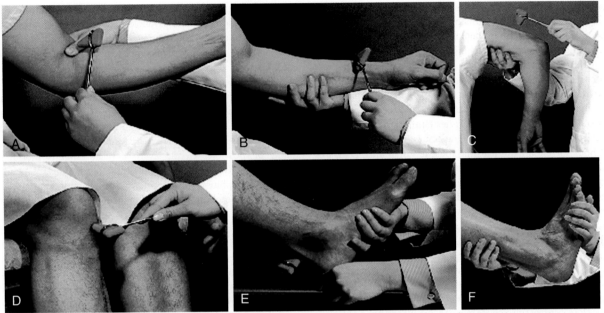

Fig 27.5 Location of Tendons for Evaluation of Deep Tendon Reflexes. (A) Biceps. (B) Brachioradial. (C) Triceps. (D) Patellar. (E) Achilles. (F) Evaluation of ankle clonus. (From Ball, J. W., Dains, J. E., Flynn, J. A., et al. [2019]. *Seidel's guide to physical examination: An interprofessional approach* [9th ed.]. St. Louis: Elsevier.)

TABLE 27.4	**Scoring Deep Tendon Reflexes**
Grade	**Deep Tendon Reflex Response**
0	No response
1+	Sluggish or diminished
2+	Active or expected response
3+	More brisk than expected, slightly hyperactive
4+	Brisk, hyperactive, with intermittent or transient clonus

From Ball, J. W., Dains, J. E., Flynn, J. A., et al. (2019). *Seidel's guide to physical examination: An interprofessional approach* (9th ed.). St. Louis: Elsevier.

contamination with vaginal secretions, blood, bacteria, or amniotic fluid. It also varies with urine specific gravity and pH, exercise, and posture (Sibai, 2017).

Although proteinuria may still be used to define preeclampsia, studies have shown little relationship between the degree of proteinuria in women with preeclampsia and pregnancy outcome. Therefore massive proteinuria (>5 g) is not considered to be a severe feature of preeclampsia. Because a 24-hour collection to measure the quantity of protein and creatinine clearance is more reflective of true renal status, it is preferred over dipstick testing, which should not be used for diagnosis of preeclampsia if at all possible (ACOG, 2013).

During the examination, the woman is evaluated for signs and symptoms considered to be severe features of preeclampsia such as severe headaches (usually frontal), epigastric pain (heartburn), right upper quadrant abdominal pain, or visual disturbances such as scotoma, photophobia, or double vision.

Client Problems

Problems often experienced by the woman with preeclampsia include the following:

- *Anxiety* related to
  - Preeclampsia and its effects on the woman and infant
- *Need for Health Teaching* related to
  - Management of preeclampsia (maternal and fetal assessment, medications, activity restriction, plans for labor and birth)

- *Disabled Family Coping* related to
  - Restricted activity and concern over a high-risk pregnancy
  - Financial concerns
- *Potential for Injury* to the woman related to
  - Hypertension
  - Central nervous system (CNS) irritability secondary to cerebral edema
  - Vasospasm
  - Decreased renal perfusion
- *Potential for Injury* to the fetus related to
  - Disruption of oxygen transfer from environment to fetus
  - Intrauterine growth restriction (IUGR)
  - Placental abruption
  - Preterm birth

Interventions

Gestational Hypertension and Preeclampsia Without Severe Features

In the past, both gestational hypertension and preeclampsia were usually described as either "mild" or "severe." Because preeclampsia is a dynamic disease process, this terminology is no longer recommended. A diagnosis of "mild preeclampsia" applies only at the time it is made. Women must be evaluated frequently to determine if the disease has progressed to the point that severe features are present (see Table 27.2) (ACOG, 2013).

The goals of therapy for women with gestational hypertension and preeclampsia without severe features are to ensure maternal safety and to deliver a healthy newborn as close to term as possible. Prior to 37 gestational weeks, care management is expectant with close monitoring of the maternal and fetal status. Most women with gestational hypertension or preeclampsia without severe features can be safely managed at home, provided they have frequent maternal and fetal evaluation (Sibai, 2017). Vaginal birth by induction of labor, preceded by cervical ripening (if necessary), is recommended beginning at 37 gestational weeks. At this gestational age, the risks to the fetus outweigh any potential benefits of continuing the pregnancy (ACOG, 2013; Sibai).

Outpatient management can be considered for reliable women who have a systolic BP of 155 mm Hg or less or a diastolic BP of 105 mm

Hg or less and no accompanying symptoms (Sibai, 2017). A regular diet without salt restriction is recommended. Women should be taught to go to the hospital or outpatient facility immediately if they develop abdominal pain, significant headache, uterine contractions, vaginal spotting, or decreased fetal movement (Sibai). Successful home care requires the woman to be well educated about preeclampsia and highly motivated to follow the plan of care (see Teaching for Self-Management box: Assessing and Reporting Clinical Signs of Preeclampsia). All teaching should include the woman and her family, and time must be allowed for them to absorb information, ask questions, and voice concerns. Methods for enhancing learning include visual aids, DVDs or internet videos, handouts, and demonstrations with return demonstrations. Furthermore, the effects of illness, language, age, cultural beliefs, and support systems must be considered.

TEACHING FOR SELF-MANAGEMENT

Assessing and Reporting Clinical Signs of Preeclampsia

- Take your BP as directed. Always sit to take your BP, and use your right arm each time for consistent and accurate readings. Support your arm on a table in a horizontal position at heart level.
- Report any increase in your BP to your health care provider immediately.
- Dipstick test your clean-catch urine sample as directed to assess proteinuria.
- Report to your health care provider if proteinuria is 1+ or more or if you have a decrease in urine output.
- Assess your baby's activity daily. Decreased activity (four or fewer movements per hour) may indicate fetal compromise and should be reported.
- Be sure to keep your scheduled prenatal appointments so that any changes in your or your baby's condition can be detected.
- Keep a daily log or diary of your assessments for your home health care nurse, or take it with you to your next prenatal visit.
- Report any headache, dizziness, blurred vision or "seeing spots" to your health care provider immediately.

Maternal and fetal assessment. Initial laboratory evaluation for women with gestational hypertension or preeclampsia without severe features includes measurement of serum creatinine, platelet count, and liver enzymes. Thereafter, hematocrit, platelet count, serum creatinine, and liver function tests should be performed weekly. Women are also evaluated for signs or symptoms of severe features, such as severe headaches, blurred or double vision, mental confusion, right upper quadrant abdominal or epigastric pain, nausea or vomiting, shortness of breath, and decreased urinary output (ACOG, 2013; Sibai, 2017). BP should be monitored twice weekly and proteinuria assessed weekly (ACOG).

Fetal evaluation generally includes daily fetal movement counts and nonstress testing or a biophysical profile once or twice weekly until birth (see Chapter 26 for more information on fetal assessment tests). Ultrasound evaluation of amniotic fluid status and determination of estimated fetal weight are performed at the time preeclampsia is diagnosed and serially thereafter, depending on findings. Doppler blood flow studies are recommended if IUGR is suspected (Sibai, 2017).

Activity restriction. Complete or partial bed rest for the duration of the pregnancy is still recommended frequently by health care providers. However, no evidence has been found that this practice improves pregnancy outcomes. Moreover, prolonged bed rest is known to increase the risk for venous thromboembolism (VTE) (Sibai, 2017). Other adverse physiologic outcomes related to complete bed rest include cardiovascular

deconditioning; diuresis with accompanying fluid, electrolyte, and weight loss; muscle atrophy; and psychologic stress. These changes begin on the first day of bed rest and continue for the duration of therapy. Therefore restricted activity rather than complete bed rest is recommended (ACOG, 2013; Sibai).

Women with preeclampsia generally feel reasonably well; therefore, boredom from activity restriction is common. Diversionary activities, including television and computer or smartphone use, visits from friends, and a comfortable and convenient environment are ways to cope with the boredom. Participation in online prenatal classes also may be possible. Gentle exercise (e.g., range-of-motion exercises, stretching, Kegel exercises, pelvic tilts) is important in maintaining muscle tone, blood flow, regular bowel function, and a sense of well-being (see Teaching for Self-Management box: Coping With Activity Restriction).

A high-risk pregnancy can be very stressful for a woman and her family. Family stressors include separation from family members when hospitalized; need for activity restriction; financial concerns; and inability to manage the household, family activities, and child care. The family needs to use coping mechanisms and support systems to help them through this crisis. Relaxation techniques also may help reduce stress and prepare the woman for labor and birth. An excellent web-based support group for pregnant women on restricted activity is Sidelines (www.sidelines.org).

Gestational Hypertension and Preeclampsia With Severe Features

Women with severe levels of gestational hypertension are at greater risk for pregnancy complications than women who have preeclampsia without severe features. Therefore these women should be managed as if they have preeclampsia with severe features. Women diagnosed with severe levels of gestational hypertension or preeclampsia with severe features should be hospitalized immediately for a thorough evaluation of maternal-fetal status (Sibai, 2017). These women are placed on magnesium sulfate to prevent eclamptic seizures and antihypertensive medication if necessary to lower severe levels of hypertension. Maternal assessments include BP, urine output, cerebral status, presence of epigastric pain and/or tenderness, labor, and vaginal bleeding (Sibai). Laboratory evaluation includes a platelet count, liver enzymes, and serum creatinine (see Table 27.3). Fetal assessment includes continuous electronic fetal heart rate (FHR) monitoring, a biophysical profile, and ultrasound evaluation of fetal growth and amniotic fluid volume (Sibai). If evidence of fetal growth restriction is found, umbilical artery Doppler velocimetry is recommended (ACOG, 2013; Sibai).

After this initial assessment period, an interprofessional plan of care is developed with the woman and her family. The goals of care management are to promote maternal safety, assess the degree of maternal and fetal risk, formulate a plan for giving birth, and prevent eclampsia and other serious complications such as placental abruption, HELLP syndrome, fetal growth restriction, and fetal demise. If the disease develops after 34 weeks of gestation, it is recommended that the woman give birth promptly because preeclampsia with severe features has been associated with increased rates of maternal morbidity and mortality and with significant fetal risks (Sibai, 2017).

Expectant management. Women who are less than 34 0/7 weeks of gestation and have no indication for giving birth immediately may be candidates for expectant management. These women should be hospitalized at a tertiary care facility that is able to provide both maternal and neonatal intensive care. Care management decisions should be made by an interprofessional health care team that includes a **perinatologist** (a maternal fetal medicine specialist), a neonatologist, an obstetrician, a nurse, and a social worker. Client and family

TEACHING FOR SELF-MANAGEMENT

Coping With Activity Restriction

At Home

- Clarify with your health care provider: What is "limited" or "restricted" activity? Question your activity level, positioning, bathroom privileges, children's visits, activities, personal hygiene, mobility, diet, and visitors.
- Have your computer, tablet, or smartphone available at your bedside. These devices can be used to communicate with friends, conduct business, and shop as necessary. Also use your computer or smartphone to communicate with internet support groups and obtain information.
- Have a television and DVD player to watch television programs or movies (can also watch on a computer, tablet, or smartphone) and a radio, CD player, or MP3 player to listen to music.
- Delegate responsibilities to family members or friends as much as possible (e.g., attend to the laundry, pick up groceries, drop off and pick up dry cleaning, meet repair people, attend to child care, organize meals).
- Have these available for use on your bed or couch:
  - Eggcrate mattress
  - Pillows and more pillows (body pillow)
- Keep a big trash basket near your bed and daytime resting place.
- Place a box or crate near the bed/sofa to store items such as:
  - Post-it Notes
  - Cups with lids and flexible straws
  - Paper plates
  - Plastic forks, spoons, and knives
  - Baby monitor or walkie-talkie
  - Wet wipes
  - Notebook to record questions for providers, telephone numbers, and to-do lists
  - Envelopes and stationery
  - Take-out menus
  - Reading materials
  - Books
  - Audiobooks
  - Magazines

- Stock a mini-refrigerator or cooler with water or other beverages or healthy snacks.
- Plan for family time—visits and interaction, particularly with small children (see Teaching for Self-Management box: Activities for Children of Women on Activity Restriction in Chapter 32).
- Explore your interest in a new hobby.
- Work crossword or jigsaw puzzles.
- Learn to embroider, smock, crochet, or knit.
- Do mending or sewing.
- Do craft projects; make something for the baby.
- Identify relaxation exercises and activities (music) and implement.
- Arrange to have a facial, manicure/pedicure, neck massage, or other special treat when you need a lift.

In the Hospital

- Clarify with your health care provider: What is "limited" or "restricted" activity? Question your activity level, positioning, bathroom privileges, children's visits, activities, personal hygiene, mobility, diet, and visitors.
- In addition to survival tips for the home, the following may be useful in the hospital setting:
  - Bring your own pillow, shampoo, and conditioner.
  - Have a wheelchair for outside visits or visiting other antepartal women if allowed.
  - If possible, bring a laptop computer or a tablet so you can watch movies or television programs if internet access is available.
  - Ask friends to bring healthy food and snacks rather than flowers when visiting.
  - Explore your interest in handheld games.
  - Work with staff regarding scheduling (e.g., obstetric provider examinations, vital signs, nursing assessments).
  - Bring earplugs to block the hospital noise.
  - Ask for a room with a view.
  - Have a large calendar and clock for easy viewing. Record significant events on the calendar.

counseling by a neonatologist should be provided (ACOG, 2013; Sibai, 2017).

Expectant management includes the use of oral antihypertensive medications to maintain a systolic BP between 140 and 155 mm Hg and a diastolic BP between 90 and 105 mm Hg. Management also includes ongoing maternal and fetal assessment for indicators of worsening condition (see the previous discussion) (Sibai, 2017). Corticosteroids (betamethasone or dexamethasone) are ordered to enhance fetal lung maturation for gestations less than 34 weeks. The dose of betamethasone is 12 mg intramuscularly, repeated in 24 hours, while dexamethasone is given intramuscularly as four doses of 6 mg each, 12 hours apart. Neonatal benefit is maximized when the interval between the first dose and birth is longer than 48 hours. The duration of benefit after a single course of betamethasone or dexamethasone is unclear (see Medication Guide: Antenatal Glucocorticoid Therapy With Betamethasone or Dexamethasone in Chapter 32) (Sibai; Simhan, Iams, & Romero, 2017).

Most women managed expectantly develop a maternal or fetal indication for giving birth within 2 weeks, although some are able to continue their pregnancies safely for several more weeks. Immediate birth is indicated if any of the following complications are present: imminent or actual eclampsia, uncontrollable severe hypertension, pulmonary edema, placental abruption, DIC, evidence of nonreassuring fetal status, fetal gestational age less than 24 weeks, or fetal demise (ACOG, 2013; Sibai, 2017).

Intrapartum care. Intrapartum nursing care is directed toward the early identification of FHR abnormalities and the prevention of maternal complications. Continuous FHR and uterine contraction monitoring are initiated, and the woman is assessed for signs of placental abruption such as a tense, tender uterus. Maternal evaluation also includes assessment of the central nervous, cardiovascular, pulmonary, hepatic, and renal systems (Poole, 2014). Vital signs and assessments are performed as ordered and per hospital policy. Client and family education and supportive measures are also initiated (see Nursing Care Plan: Preeclampsia With Severe Features).

The woman with preeclampsia with severe features is maintained on bed rest with the side rails up in a quiet, darkened environment. Emergency drugs, oxygen, and suction equipment should be checked and readily available (Box 27.2). To reduce the risk of pulmonary edema, total intravenous (IV), and oral fluids should not exceed 125 mL/hr. Intensive hemodynamic monitoring with a pulmonary artery (Swan-Ganz) catheter to evaluate central venous and pulmonary artery pressures is not a routine standard of care for preeclampsia with severe features. It is indicated only in selected women, such as those with oliguria unresponsive to a fluid challenge (Harper et al., 2019; Poole, 2014).

⚙ CLINICAL REASONING CASE STUDY

Preeclampsia With Severe Features

Karen is a 30-year-old G1 P0 who is currently 32 weeks of gestation. At 28 weeks of gestation, Karen developed preeclampsia. Since then she has been home on modified bed rest. A home health nurse visits her twice a week and calls her daily.

Today when the home health nurse visits, Karen tells her, "I have a terrible headache and hardly slept at all last night." When asked about other symptoms Karen replies, "My vision is blurry, I'm seeing spots, and my stomach hurts." Karen's BP is 154/100, she has pitting edema in her legs, and her first voided urine this morning tested 3+ for protein. The nurse calls Karen's physician, who decides to admit her to the labor and birth unit immediately. At the hospital Karen continues to complain of a severe headache and seeing spots. Physical assessment reveals a BP of 160/110 and 4+ DTRs with 3 beats of ankle clonus. The electronic monitor reveals minimal FHR variability and periodic late decelerations.

1. What is the priority concern or client need in this situation? Support your answer with data as stated in the case.
2. List other client needs/problems in this case.
3. Identify any additional information or assessment data that is needed by the nurse in planning care for this client.
4. What nursing actions are appropriate in this situation?
   a. What is the priority nursing action? (What should the nurse do first?)
   b. Describe other nursing interventions that are important to providing optimal client care.
5. Describe the roles/responsibilities of the interprofessional health care team members (other than nurses) who may be involved in providing care for this client.

BOX 27.2   Hospital Precautionary Measures for Women With Preeclampsia

- Environment
  - Quiet
  - Nonstimulating
  - Lighting subdued
- Seizure precautions
  - Suction equipment tested and ready to use
  - Oxygen administration equipment tested and ready to use
  - Call button within easy reach
- Emergency medications available on the unit
  - Hydralazine
  - Labetalol
  - Nifedipine
  - Magnesium sulfate
  - Calcium gluconate
- Emergency birth pack easily accessible

Magnesium sulfate. Magnesium sulfate is the medication of choice for preventing and treating seizure activity (eclampsia). It is almost always administered intravenously as a secondary infusion (piggyback) by a volumetric infusion pump. Per protocol or health care provider's order, an initial loading dose of 4 to 6 g of magnesium sulfate is infused over 15 to 30 minutes. This dose is followed by a maintenance dose of magnesium sulfate that is diluted in an IV solution (e.g., 40 g of magnesium sulfate in 1000 mL of lactated Ringer's solution [1 g = 25 mL]) and administered

---

◎ NURSING CARE PLAN

Preeclampsia With Severe Features

Client Problem	Expected Outcome	Interventions	Rationales
Potential for Injury related to CNS irritability (seizures)	Woman will show diminished signs of CNS irritability (e.g., DTRs ≤2+, absence of clonus) and have no seizure activity.	Assess vital signs, LOC, DTRs, IV rate, I&O, proteinuria as ordered.	To determine need for and effectiveness of treatment measures
		Initiate seizure precautions and administer IV magnesium sulfate as ordered. Make certain that oxygen and suction equipment are readily available.	To minimize risk of seizure activity and associated complications
		Teach woman to report signs and symptoms of worsening condition: headache, visual changes, RUQ pain.	So complications can immediately be reported to the obstetric health care provider
Decreased Tissue Perfusion secondary to preeclampsia related to vasospasm	Woman will exhibit signs of adequate tissue perfusion (i.e., adequate urine output and normal FHR tracing).	Assess BP, IV fluid intake, output via indwelling urinary catheter, breath sounds, edema, FHR and pattern.	To determine need for and effectiveness of treatment measures
		Administer antihypertensive medications as ordered.	To reduce vasoconstriction by relaxing vasospasms, thereby decreasing BP and increasing uteroplacental oxygenation
		Teach woman to remain on bed rest in side-lying position.	To maximize uteroplacental blood flow and reduce blood pressure
Potential for Decreased Gas Exchange related to pulmonary edema secondary to increased vascular resistance	Woman will exhibit signs of normal gas exchange (i.e., normal breath sounds, respiratory rate, and full orientation to person, time, and place).	Assess color, capillary refill, LOC, breath sounds (crackles). Monitor woman for signs of impaired gas exchange (increased respiratory rate, dyspnea, oxygen saturation <95%).	To detect potential complications
		Notify obstetric health care provider immediately if signs of impaired gas exchange are detected. Administer oxygen and medications (likely a diuretic) as ordered.	To improve woman's oxygenation status and increase oxygen levels in vital organs
		Teach woman to turn, cough, and take deep breaths regularly and to immediately report any perceived difficulty with breathing.	To enable timely interventions

BP, Blood pressure; *CNS,* central nervous system; *DTR,* deep tendon reflex; *FHR,* fetal heart rate; *I&O,* Intake and output; *IV,* intravenous. *LOC,* level of consciousness; *RUQ,* right upper quadrant (of the abdomen).

by an infusion pump at 2 to 3 g/h. This dose should maintain a therapeutic serum magnesium level of 4 to 7 mEq/L. Contrary to popular belief, magnesium sulfate has little effect on maternal BP when administered in this fashion (Harper et al., 2019; Poole, 2014).

Magnesium sulfate is rarely given intramuscularly because the absorption rate cannot be controlled, injections are painful, and tissue necrosis may occur. However, the intramuscular (IM) route may be used in low-resource settings or with some women who are being transported to a tertiary care center. Use of the ventral gluteal site for injection is recommended. The IM dose is a 10-g loading dose (administered as two separate injections of 5 g in each buttock). The maintenance dosage is 5 g administered every 4 hours in alternating buttocks. Local anesthetic can be added to the solution to reduce injection pain (Cunningham, Leveno, Bloom et al., 2018). The Z-track technique should be used for the deep IM injection, followed by gentle massage at the site.

It is unclear how magnesium sulfate works to prevent and treat eclamptic seizures. It may cause vasodilation in the peripheral and cerebral circulation, prevent or decrease cerebral edema, or function as a central anticonvulsant (Witcher & Shah, 2019). Common side effects of magnesium sulfate are a feeling of warmth, flushing, diaphoresis, and burning at the IV site. Because magnesium is excreted in the urine, accurate measurements of maternal urine output must be obtained. If renal function declines, excretion of magnesium sulfate is inadequate, resulting in magnesium toxicity. Symptoms of magnesium toxicity include absent DTRs, decreased respiratory rate, and decreased level of consciousness (Huwe et al., 2019). Blood can be drawn to determine the serum magnesium level if toxicity is suspected (Box 27.3; see Medication Guide: Tocolytic Therapy for Preterm Labor in Chapter 32).

> ### ⚕ MEDICATION ALERT
>
> High serum levels of magnesium can cause relaxation of smooth muscle, such as the uterus. However, when administered as a 4- to 6-g loading dose followed by a 1- to 2-g/hr maintenance dose, magnesium sulfate has not been shown to significantly affect uterine contractility, other than a brief period of uterine muscle relaxation during and immediately after administration of the loading dose (Cunningham et al., 2018).

> ### ⚕ MEDICATION ALERT
>
> If magnesium toxicity is suspected, prompt actions are needed to prevent respiratory or cardiac arrest. The magnesium infusion should be discontinued immediately. Calcium gluconate (antidote for magnesium sulfate) can be given intravenously (Huwe et al., 2019).

> ### ❗ NURSING ALERT
>
> The effect of magnesium sulfate on FHR baseline variability is controversial. Because fetal levels of magnesium approximate those of the mother, fetal sedation is possible. However, absent or minimal baseline variability should not be assumed to be the result of magnesium sulfate therapy until other causes of fetal hypoxemia have been ruled out (Poole, 2014). Neonatal serum magnesium levels are almost identical to those of the mother (Harper et al., 2019).

> ### ⚡ SAFETY ALERT
>
> Magnesium sulfate is considered a high-alert medication because it has a heightened risk for causing significant client harm when used in error. Measures to improve the safe use of this medication include developing detailed policies, procedures, protocols, and standing orders and thorough assessment and documentation. *Never* abbreviate magnesium sulfate as $MgSO_4$ anywhere in the medical record (Huwe et al., 2019; Institute for Safe Medication Practices, 2014).

Control of blood pressure. Antihypertensive medications are indicated when the systolic BP exceeds 160 mm Hg or the diastolic BP exceeds 110 mm Hg. Maternal risks associated with severe hypertension include left ventricular failure, cerebral hemorrhage, and placental abruption. To maintain uteroplacental perfusion, antihypertensive therapy must not decrease the arterial pressure too much or too rapidly. The goal of antihypertensive therapy is to achieve a systolic pressure of 140 to 150 mm Hg and a diastolic pressure of 90 to 100 mm Hg. Hydralazine (Apresoline), labetalol (Trandate), and nifedipine (Procardia) are effective drugs for treating hypertension intrapartum. They may also be used during pregnancy or in the postpartum period for BP control (ACOG, 2013; Witcher & Shah, 2019). Table 27.5 compares antihypertensive agents commonly used to treat hypertension in pregnancy.

Postpartum care. Throughout the postpartum period, the woman needs careful assessment of her vital signs, intake and output, DTRs, and level of consciousness. The magnesium sulfate infusion is continued after birth for seizure prophylaxis as ordered, usually for 24 hours. Assessments for effects and side effects continue until the medication is discontinued. Given that magnesium sulfate potentiates the action of opioids, CNS depressants, and calcium channel blockers, these medications must be administered with caution (Poole, 2014). The signs and symptoms of preeclampsia usually resolve within 48 hours after birth. Clinical signs that demonstrate resolution of preeclampsia include diuresis and decreased edema.

The nurse should assess the postpartum woman regularly for any symptoms of preeclampsia such as headaches, visual disturbances, or epigastric pain. Some women develop signs and symptoms of preeclampsia for the first time after giving birth. Women who develop hypertension and severe features of preeclampsia such as headaches or blurred vision or severe hypertension should be placed on IV magnesium sulfate for seizure prophylaxis. Nonsteroidal anti-inflammatory pain medications should be used with caution when hypertension persists for more than 1 day after birth because these agents can contribute to an increase in BP. Women should be taught to contact their obstetric health care provider or return to the hospital immediately if they develop headaches, visual disturbances, or epigastric pain after discharge (ACOG, 2013; Sibai, 2017).

Because preeclampsia is a major cause of IUGR and preterm birth, the baby may be cared for in a neonatal intensive care unit (NICU). Nursing care that facilitates bonding and attachment while the infant is in the NICU includes providing the family with photographs of the infant, keeping the family informed of the infant's status, encouraging the partner to visit the NICU, and taking the woman to the NICU by wheelchair after her condition has stabilized (Poole, 2014). Postpartum and neonatal nurses can collaborate to provide family-centered care in this situation.

Most women with gestational hypertension become normotensive during the first week after giving birth. On the other hand, hypertension may take longer to resolve in women with preeclampsia. For women with gestational hypertension, preeclampsia, or superimposed preeclampsia, it is recommended that BP be monitored in the hospital or that equivalent outpatient surveillance be performed for at least 72

BOX 27.3   Care of the Woman With Preeclampsia Receiving Magnesium Sulfate

Client and Family Teaching

- Explain technique, rationale, and reactions to expect (route and rate).
  - Purpose of "piggyback" infusion
- Reasons for use
  - Tailor information to woman's readiness to learn.
  - Explain that magnesium sulfate is used to prevent disease progression.
  - Explain that magnesium sulfate is used to prevent seizures, *not* to decrease blood pressure.
- Reactions to expect from medication
  - Initially the woman appears flushed and feels hot, sedated, and nauseated. She may experience diaphoresis and burning at the IV site, especially during the bolus.
  - Sedation continues.
- Monitoring to anticipate
  - *Maternal:* Blood pressure, pulse, respiratory rate, DTRs, level of consciousness, urine output (indwelling catheter), headache, visual disturbances, epigastric pain
  - *Fetal:* FHR and activity

Administration

- Verify health care provider's order.
- Position woman in side-lying position.
- Prepare solution and administer with an infusion control device (pump).
- Piggyback solution of 40 g of magnesium sulfate in 1000 mL lactated Ringer's solution with infusion-control device at the ordered rate: loading dose—initial bolus of 4-6 g over 15-30 min; maintenance dose—2 g/hr, according to unit protocol or health care provider's specific order.

Maternal and Fetal Assessments

- Vital signs and assessments are performed as ordered by the health care provider and per hospital protocol.
- Monitor blood pressure, pulse, respiratory rate every 15-30 min, depending on woman's condition.
- Monitor FHR and contractions continuously.
- Monitor level of consciousness, intake and output, proteinuria, DTRs, headache, visual disturbances, and epigastric pain at least hourly.
- Restrict hourly fluid intake to a total of no more than 125 mL/hr; urinary output should be at least 25-30 mL/hr.

Reportable Conditions

- Blood pressure: systolic ≥160 mm Hg or diastolic ≥110 mm Hg
- Respiratory rate: <12 breaths/min
- Urinary output: <25-30 mL/hr
- Presence of headache, visual disturbances, decrease in level of consciousness, or epigastric pain
- Increasing severity or loss of DTRs, increasing edema, proteinuria
- Any abnormal laboratory values (magnesium level, platelet count, creatinine clearance, protein/creatinine ratio, levels of uric acid, AST, ALT, prothrombin time, partial thromboplastin time, fibrinogen, fibrin split products)
- Any other significant change in maternal or fetal status

Emergency Measures

- Keep emergency drugs and intubation equipment immediately available.
- Keep side rails up.
- Keep lights dimmed, and maintain a quiet environment.

ALT, Alanine aminotransferase; *AST,* aspartate aminotransferase; *DTR,* deep tendon reflex; *FHR,* fetal heart rate; *IV,* intravenous.

hours after birth. The BP should then be rechecked at 7 to 10 days postpartum, or earlier in women who are symptomatic. Women with a BP of 150/100 mm Hg or higher (on two occasions that are 4 to 6 hours apart) should be placed on an antihypertensive medication, often labetalol or nifedipine (ACOG, 2013). If this is the case, the BP needs to be checked frequently either at home or at the health care provider's office. Within a few weeks after birth, antihypertensive medications often can be discontinued.

Future Health Care

Women with preeclampsia with severe features have a significantly increased risk for developing preeclampsia in a future pregnancy, especially those who had early-onset (diagnosed during the second trimester) preeclampsia. Even if these women remain normotensive in a subsequent pregnancy, they may have a greater likelihood of an adverse pregnancy outcome such as preterm birth, small-for-gestational-age infant, and perinatal death (Sibai, 2017).

Ideally, women who have had preeclampsia in a previous pregnancy should receive counseling during a preconception visit before the next planned pregnancy. At this visit, the previous pregnancy history should be reviewed and the prognosis for the upcoming pregnancy discussed. Potential lifestyle modifications such as weight loss and increased physical activity should be encouraged. The current status of any chronic medical conditions, such as diabetes or chronic hypertension, should be assessed, so that they are brought into the best control possible before the upcoming pregnancy. Current medications should be reviewed and their administration modified if necessary for the upcoming pregnancy (ACOG, 2013). The use of low-dose aspirin during the upcoming pregnancy will likely be recommended, especially if an adverse outcome accompanied the previous pregnancy complicated by preeclampsia (ACOG & SMFM, 2018).

Women with preeclampsia (especially early-onset and preeclampsia with severe features) also have an increased risk for developing chronic hypertension and cardiovascular disease later in life. It is believed that preeclampsia does not cause cardiovascular disease but rather that preeclampsia and cardiovascular disease share common risk factors. Further research is needed to determine how to take advantage of this information relating preeclampsia to cardiovascular disease later in life. For now, women should be educated about lifestyle changes (maintaining a healthy weight, increasing physical activity, and avoiding smoking) that may decrease the risk for developing future health problems (ACOG, 2013; Sibai, 2017).

Eclampsia

Eclampsia is usually preceded by premonitory signs and symptoms, including persistent headache, blurred vision, photophobia, severe epigastric or right upper quadrant abdominal pain, and altered mental status. However, seizures can appear suddenly and without warning in a seemingly stable woman with only minimal BP elevations (Sibai, 2017). Eclamptic seizures are frightening to observe. Tonic contraction of all body muscles (seen as arms flexed, hands clenched, legs inverted) precedes the tonic-clonic convulsion. During this stage muscles alternately relax and contract. Respirations are halted and then begin again with long, deep, stertorous inhalations. Hypotension follows; and muscular twitching, disorientation, and amnesia persist for a while after the seizure. The woman may also vomit or be incontinent of urine or stool.

Immediate Care

Nursing actions during a seizure are directed toward ensuring a patent airway and client safety (see Emergency box: Eclampsia). It is important to note the time of onset and duration of the seizure. The nurse should call for help but remain at the bedside. The side rails on the bed

TABLE 27.5	**Pharmacologic Control of Hypertension in Pregnancy**			
Action	**Target Tissue**	**Maternal Effects**	**Fetal Effects**	**Nursing Actions**
Hydralazine (Apresoline, Neopresol)				
Arteriolar vasodilator	Peripheral arterioles: to decrease muscle tone, decrease peripheral resistance; hypothalamus and medullary vasomotor center for minor decrease in sympathetic tone	Headache, flushing, palpitations, tachycardia, some decrease in uteroplacental blood flow, increase in heart rate and cardiac output, increase in oxygen consumption, nausea and vomiting	Tachycardia; late decelerations and bradycardia if maternal diastolic pressure <90 mm Hg	Assess for effects of medication; alert woman (family) to expected effects of medication; assess blood pressure frequently because precipitous drop can lead to shock and perhaps placental abruption; if giving multiple doses, wait at least 20 min after the first dose is given to administer an additional dose to allow time to assess the effects of the initial dose; assess urinary output; maintain bed rest in lateral position with side rails up; use with caution in presence of maternal tachycardia.
Labetalol Hydrochloride (Normodyne, Trandate)				
Combined alpha- and beta-blocking agent causing vasodilation without significant change in cardiac output	Peripheral arterioles (see Hydralazine)	Lethargy, fatigue, sleep disturbances; Minimal: flushing, tremulousness, orthostatic hypotension; minimal change in pulse rate	Minimal, if any. May be associated with small-for-gestational-age infant	See hydralazine; less likely to cause excessive hypotension and tachycardia; less rebound hypertension than hydralazine. Do not use in women with asthma, heart disease, or congestive heart failure. Do not exceed 80 mg in a single dose. Do not give more than 300 mg total in a 24-hr period.
Methyldopa (Aldomet)				
Maintenance therapy if needed: 250-500 mg orally every 8 hr (α_2-receptor agonist)	Postganglionic nerve endings: interferes with chemical neurotransmission to reduce peripheral vascular resistance; causes CNS sedation	Sleepiness, postural hypotension, constipation, hepatic dysfunction and necrosis, hemolytic anemia; rare: drug-induced fever in 1% of women and positive Coombs test result in 20% of women	After 4 months of maternal therapy, positive Coombs test result in infant	See Hydralazine.
Nifedipine (Adalat, Procardia)				
Calcium channel blocker	Arterioles: to reduce systemic vascular resistance by relaxation of arterial smooth muscle	Headache, flushing, tachycardia; may interfere with labor	Minimal	See Hydralazine. Avoid concurrent use with magnesium sulfate because skeletal muscle blockade can result. Avoid immediate release or sublingual form due to increased risk for profound maternal hypotension

CNS, Central nervous system.
Data from Harvey, C., & Sibai, B. (2013). Hypertension in pregnancy. In N. Troiano, C. Harvey, & B. Chez (Eds.), *AWHONN's high risk and critical care obstetrics* (3rd ed.). Philadelphia: Wolters Kluwer/Lippincott Williams & Wilkins; Poole, J. H. (2014). Hypertensive disorders of pregnancy. In K. R. Simpson, & P. Creehan (Eds.), *AWHONN's perinatal nursing* (4th ed.). Philadelphia: Lippincott Williams & Wilkins; Sibai, B. (2017). Preeclampsia and hypertensive disorders. In S. G. Gabbe, J. R. Niebyl, J. L. Simpson, et al. (Eds.), *Obstetrics: Normal and problem pregnancies* (7th ed.). Philadelphia: Elsevier; Witcher, P. M. (2017). Caring for the laboring woman with hypertensive disorders complicating pregnancy. In B. B. Kennedy, & S. M. Baird (Eds.), *Intrapartum management modules: A perinatal education program* (5th ed.). Philadelphia: Wolters Kluwer.

must be raised and should be padded with a folded blanket or pillow if possible. Women with eclampsia have been known to sustain fractures from falling out of bed during the seizure. Immediately after the seizure, the nurse should lower the head of the bed and turn the woman onto her side. This helps prevent aspiration of vomitus.

✚ EMERGENCY

Eclampsia

Tonic-Clonic Convulsion Signs
- Stage of invasion: 2-3 secs, eyes fixed, twitching of facial muscles
- Stage of contraction: 15-20 secs, eyes protrude and are bloodshot, all body muscles in tonic contraction
- Stage of convulsion: Muscles relax and contract alternately (clonic), respirations halted and then begin again with long, deep, stertorous inhalation; coma ensues

Intervention
- Keep airway patent: turn head to one side, place pillow under one shoulder or back if possible.
- Call for assistance. Do not leave bedside.
- Raise side rails, and pad them with a folded blanket or pillow, if possible.
- Observe and record convulsion activity.

After Convulsion
- Do not leave unattended until fully alert.
- Observe for postconvulsion confusion, coma, incontinence.
- Use suction as needed.
- Administer oxygen via nonrebreather face mask at 10 L/min.
- Start IV fluids, and monitor for potential fluid overload.
- Give magnesium sulfate or other anticonvulsant drug as ordered.
- Insert indwelling urinary catheter.
- Monitor BP, pulse, and respirations frequently until stabilized.
- Monitor fetal and uterine status.
- Expedite laboratory work as ordered to monitor kidney function, liver function, coagulation system, and drug levels.
- Provide hygiene and a quiet environment.
- Support the woman and her family, and keep them informed.
- Be prepared to assist with birth when woman is in stable condition.

Nursing actions after a seizure are directed toward maternal stabilization. First, the status of the woman's airway, breathing, and pulse should be assessed. If apnea is present, the nurse should immediately open the airway, begin bag/mask ventilation, and activate the hospital's code for respiratory or cardiac arrest. If respirations are present, secretions should be suctioned from the woman's glottis to clear the airway and oxygen administered at 10 L/min by face mask. If an IV infusion is not in place, one should be started with an 18-gauge needle. If an IV line was in place before the seizure, it may have infiltrated and will need to be restarted immediately. As soon as IV access is obtained, magnesium sulfate should be administered as ordered.

If eclampsia develops after initiating magnesium sulfate therapy, additional magnesium sulfate should be administered. Magnesium sulfate is the drug of choice for treating eclamptic seizures and preventing repeated seizures. One of its advantages over other antiseizure medications such as diazepam (Valium) is that it reduces the risk for aspiration because it does not depress the gag reflex (Witcher & Shah, 2019). Occasionally a woman will experience recurrent eclamptic seizures while receiving adequate and therapeutic doses of magnesium

sulfate. If this occurs, lorazepam (Ativan) 2 mg, given intravenously over 3 to 5 minutes, may be administered (Sibai, 2017).

After the woman is stabilized, uterine activity, cervical status, and fetal status must be assessed. During a seizure, the uterus becomes hypercontractile and hypertonic. As a result, the membranes may have ruptured or the cervix may have dilated rapidly, and birth may be imminent (Poole, 2014). The FHR tracing may demonstrate bradycardia, late decelerations, absent or minimal baseline variability, or compensatory tachycardia. These findings usually resolve soon after the seizure ends and the woman's hypoxia is corrected (Sibai, 2017).

⚡ SAFETY ALERT

Immediately after a seizure, a woman may be very confused and combative. Restraints may be necessary temporarily. Several hours may be needed for the woman to regain her usual level of mental functioning.

After stabilizing the woman and fetus, a decision is made regarding the timing and method of birth. Eclampsia alone is not an indication for immediate cesarean birth. The route of birth (induction of labor versus cesarean birth) is determined based on the maternal and fetal condition, fetal gestational age, presence of labor, and cervical Bishop score (ACOG, 2013; Sibai, 2017).

Regional anesthesia is not recommended for eclamptic women with coagulopathy or a platelet count less than 50,000/mm^3 (Sibai, 2017). If cesarean birth is necessary for these women, it is performed using general anesthesia.

Chronic Hypertension

An increasing number of women who give birth have chronic hypertension, which affects approximately 1% to 5% of all pregnancies. African American women are much more likely to have a pregnancy complicated by chronic hypertension than women of other races or ethnicities. In addition to race, other risk factors for chronic hypertension in pregnancy are older age and obesity. As more women delay childbearing and are obese, the number of pregnancies complicated by chronic hypertension is expected to increase (Sibai, 2017).

More than 90% of women with chronic hypertension have primary or essential hypertension. In the remaining 10%, the hypertension is secondary to a medical condition such as renal or collagen vascular disease, an endocrine disorder, or arteriosclerosis (Witcher & Shah, 2019). Chronic hypertension in pregnancy is associated with maternal complications such as superimposed preeclampsia, stroke, acute kidney injury, heart failure, placental abruption, and death. Fetal risks include IUGR, death, and preterm birth (Cunningham et al., 2018; Sibai, 2017).

Ideally the management of chronic hypertension in pregnancy begins before conception. An evaluation is performed to assess the cause and severity of the hypertension and the presence of any target organ damage (e.g., heart, eye, and kidney) (Sibai, 2017). Moreover, the woman should be encouraged to make lifestyle changes before conception, such as smoking and alcohol cessation, participating in aerobic exercise, and losing weight if indicated. A diet that includes a maximum of 2.4 g sodium per day is recommended (Sibai). These lifestyle modifications should continue throughout the pregnancy.

Based on the BP and presence of target organ damage, women with chronic hypertension are classified as either high or low risk for pregnancy complications. Antihypertensive medications are frequently discontinued before pregnancy in women with low-risk chronic hypertension. This decreases the risk of fetal exposure to some medications (e.g., angiotensin-converting enzyme [ACE] inhibitors) that can be teratogenic. Women who are high risk are managed with anti-hypertensive medication and frequent assessments of maternal and fetal well-being. Methyldopa (Aldomet) is most often recommended for treating chronic hypertension in pregnancy. However, because it is rarely used for treating chronic hypertension in nonpregnant women, it may not be practical to switch medications because of pregnancy. Labetalol, nifedipine, and a thiazide diuretic are other antihypertensive medications used during pregnancy (see Table 27.5). Women who are high risk are monitored closely, and the route and timing of the birth depend on the maternal and fetal status.

After giving birth, the woman should be monitored closely for complications such as pulmonary edema, hypertensive encephalopathy, and renal failure. Women with chronic hypertension can breastfeed if they desire. All antihypertensive medications are present to some degree in breast milk.

Levels of methyldopa in breast milk appear to be low and are considered safe. Labetalol also has a low concentration in breast milk. Little is known about the transfer of calcium channel blockers such as nifedipine in breast milk, but no apparent side effects have been noted in infants. Concentrations of diuretic agents in breast milk are low, but their use may cause a decrease in milk production (Sibai, 2017). Any medications given to a breastfeeding mother should be checked for safety. LactMed (https://toxnet.nlm.nih.gov/newtoxnet/lactmed.htm) is an excellent online resource.

▮ KEY POINTS

- Hypertensive disorders during pregnancy are a leading cause of maternal and perinatal morbidity and mortality worldwide.
- The cause of preeclampsia is unknown, and no reliable test that can be used as a routine screening tool for predicting preeclampsia has yet been developed.
- Preeclampsia is a multisystem disease, and the pathologic changes are present long before clinical manifestations such as hypertension become evident.
- HELLP syndrome, which is usually diagnosed during the third trimester, is a variant of preeclampsia, not a separate illness.

- Magnesium sulfate, the anticonvulsant of choice for preventing or controlling eclamptic seizures, requires careful monitoring of reflexes, respirations, and renal function.
- Women with preeclampsia (especially early-onset and preeclampsia with severe features) also have an increased risk for developing chronic hypertension and cardiovascular disease later in life.
- The intent of emergency interventions for eclampsia is to prevent injury, enhance oxygenation, reduce aspiration risk, and establish control with magnesium sulfate.

REFERENCES

American College of Obstetricians and Gynecologists. (2013). Executive summary: Hypertension in pregnancy. *Obstetrics & Gynecology, 122*(5), 1122–1131.

American College of Obstetricians and Gynecologists, & Society for Maternal Fetal Medicine. (2018). Committee opinion no. 743: Low-dose aspirin use during pregnancy. *Obstetrics & Gynecology, 132*(1), e44–e52.

Cunningham, F., Leveno, K., Bloom, S., et al. (2018). *Williams obstetrics* (25th ed.). New York: McGraw-Hill Education.

Harper, L.M., Tita, A., & Karumanchi, S.A. (2019). Pregnancy-related hypertension. In R. Resnik, C.J. Lockwood, T.R. Moore, et al. (Eds), *Creasy & Resnik's maternal-fetal medicine: Principles and practice* (8th ed.). Philadelphia: Elsevier.

Huwe, V. Y., Puck, A. L., Vasher, J., et al. (2019). Guidelines for the care of the patient with hypertension during pregnancy. In N. H. Troiano, P. M. Witcher, & S. M. Baird (Eds.), *AWHONN's high risk and critical care obstetrics* (4th ed.). Philadelphia: Wolters Kluwer.

Institute for Safe Medication Practices. (2014). *ISMP's list of high-alert medications*. Retrieved from: www.ismp.org.

Poole, J. H. (2014). Hypertensive disorders of pregnancy. In K. R. Simpson, & P. Creehan (Eds.), *AWHONN's perinatal nursing* (4th ed.). Philadelphia: Lippincott Willliams & Wilkins.

Sibai, B. (2017). Preeclampsia and hypertensive disorders. In S. G. Gabbe, J. R. Niebyl, J. L. Simpson, et al. (Eds.), *Obstetrics: Normal and problem pregnancies* (7th ed.). Philadelphia: Elsevier.

Simhan, H. N., Iams, J. D., & Romero, R. (2017). Preterm labor and birth. In S. G. Gabbe, J. R. Niebyl, J. L. Simpson, et al. (Eds.), *Obstetrics: Normal and problem pregnancies* (7th ed.). Philadelphia: Elsevier.

Snydal, S. (2014). Major changes in diagnosis and management of preeclampsia. *Journal of Midwifery & Women's Health, 59*(6), 596–605.

Witcher, P. M., & Shah, S. S. (2019). Hypertension in pregnancy. In N. H. Troiano, P. M. Witcher, & S. M. Baird (Eds.), *AWHONN's high risk and critical care obstetrics* (4th ed.). Philadelphia: Wolters Kluwer.

28

Hemorrhagic Disorders

Kristen S. Montgomery

 http://evolve.elsevier.com/Lowdermilk/MWHC/

Bleeding in pregnancy can jeopardize maternal and fetal well-being. Maternal blood loss decreases oxygen-carrying capacity, which places the woman at increased risk for hypovolemia, anemia, infection, and preterm labor and adversely affects oxygen delivery to the fetus. Fetal risks from maternal hemorrhage include blood loss or anemia, hypoxemia, hypoxia, anoxia, and preterm birth. Hemorrhagic disorders in pregnancy are medical emergencies. The incidence and type of bleeding vary by trimester. Ruptured ectopic pregnancy and abruptio placentae (placental abruption) have the highest incidence of maternal mortality. Prompt assessment and intervention by the interprofessional health care team are essential to save the lives of both the woman and her fetus.

EARLY PREGNANCY BLEEDING

Bleeding during early pregnancy is alarming to the woman and of concern to health care providers. The common bleeding disorders of early pregnancy include miscarriage (spontaneous abortion), cervical insufficiency, ectopic pregnancy, and hydatidiform mole (molar pregnancy).

Miscarriage (Spontaneous Abortion)

A pregnancy that ends as a result of natural causes before fetal viability is defined as a **miscarriage** (**spontaneous abortion**). The National Center for Health Statistics, the Centers for Disease Control and Prevention, and the World Health Organization define spontaneous abortion as a loss that occurs before 20 weeks of gestation. A fetal weight less than 500 g also may be used to define an abortion. However, state laws may define abortion more widely (Cunningham, Leveno, Bloom, et al., 2018). The term *miscarriage* rather than *abortion* is used throughout this discussion because it is more appropriate to use with clients. Abortion may be perceived as an insensitive term by families who are grieving a pregnancy loss. Therapeutic or elective induced abortion is discussed in Chapter 8.

Incidence and Etiology

Approximately 10% to 15% of all clinically recognized pregnancies end in miscarriage (Simpson & Jauniaux, 2017). The majority—greater than 80% of miscarriages—are early pregnancy losses, occurring before 12 weeks of gestation and are not clinically recognized. In many cases the woman does not realize that she is pregnant (Cunningham et al., 2018).

Approximately half of all miscarriages are chromosomally normal, while the other half have a chromosomal abnormality. Other possible causes of miscarriage include various medical disorders (e.g., poorly controlled diabetes mellitus, obesity, thyroid disease, and systemic lupus erythematosus). Regular and heavy alcohol consumption, excessive (>500 mg/day) caffeine intake, environmental toxins, and increasing paternal age are other possible causes of miscarriage. Infections, however, are not a common cause of miscarriage (Cunningham et al., 2018.).

Types

The types of miscarriages include threatened, inevitable, incomplete, complete, and missed. All types of miscarriage can recur in subsequent pregnancies. All types except the threatened miscarriage can lead to infection (Fig. 28.1).

Clinical Manifestations

Signs and symptoms of miscarriage depend on the duration of pregnancy. The presence of uterine bleeding, uterine contractions, or abdominal pain is an ominous sign during early pregnancy and must be considered a threatened miscarriage until proven otherwise.

If miscarriage occurs before the sixth week of pregnancy, the woman may report what she believes is a heavy menstrual flow. Miscarriage that occurs between weeks 6 and 12 of pregnancy causes moderate discomfort and blood loss. After week 12, miscarriage is typified by severe pain, similar to that of labor, because the fetus must be expelled. Diagnosis and management of miscarriage is based on the signs and symptoms present (Table 28.1).

Recurrent (habitual) miscarriage is classically defined as three or more spontaneous pregnancy losses before 20 weeks of gestation or with a fetal weight of less than 500 g. Some authorities now recommend that the definition of recurrent miscarriage be two or more prior pregnancy losses. The most widely accepted causes of recurrent miscarriage are parental chromosomal abnormalities, antiphospholipid

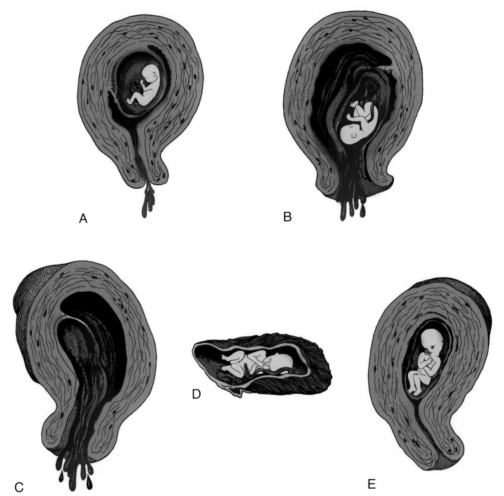

Fig. 28.1 Miscarriage. (A) Threatened. (B) Inevitable. (C) Incomplete. (D) Complete. (E) Missed.

TABLE 28.1 Assessing Miscarriage and the Usual Management

Type of Miscarriage	Amount of Bleeding	Uterine Cramping	Passage of Tissue	Cervical Dilation	Management
Threatened	Slight, spotting	Mild	No	No	Bed rest is often ordered but has not proven to be effective in preventing progression to actual miscarriage. Repetitive transvaginal ultrasounds and assessment of human chorionic gonadotropin (β-hCG) and progesterone levels may be done to determine if the fetus is still alive and in the uterus. Further treatment depends on whether progression to actual miscarriage occurs.
Inevitable	Moderate	Mild to severe	No	Yes	Expectant management may be instituted if no pain, bleeding, or infection is present. If pain, bleeding, or infection is present, then prompt termination of pregnancy is accomplished, usually surgically by dilation and suction curettage.
Incomplete	Heavy, profuse	Severe	Yes	Yes, with tissue in cervix	May or may not require additional cervical dilation before curettage Suction curettage is often performed but medical management with misoprostol (Cytotec) is also a treatment option.
Complete	Slight	Mild	Yes	No (cervix has already closed after tissue passed)	No further intervention may be needed if uterine contractions are adequate to prevent hemorrhage and no infection is present. If an expelled complete gestational sac is not identified, transvaginal ultrasound is performed to differentiate a complete miscarriage from a threatened miscarriage or an ectopic pregnancy.
Missed	None, spotting	None	No	No	If expectant management is not desired, pregnancy is terminated either medically using misoprostol (Cytotec) given orally or vaginally or surgically by dilation and suction curettage.
Septic	Varies, usually malodorous	Varies	Varies	Yes, usually	Immediate termination of pregnancy, usually by suction curettage, followed by broad-spectrum antibiotic therapy. Treatment for septic shock is initiated if necessary.

Data from Cunningham, F., Leveno, K., Bloom, S., et al. (2018). *William's obstetrics* (25th ed.). New York: McGraw-Hill Education.

antibody syndrome, and certain uterine abnormalities (Cunningham et al., 2018).

The evaluation of couples experiencing recurrent pregnancy loss usually includes karyotyping of both partners and miscarriage specimens and assessment of the placenta; evaluating the woman's uterine cavity; and screening for abnormalities of prolactin and thyroid disease. Evaluation should also address the psychological response to this diagnosis because women and their partners often report feelings of guilt, anxiety, and depression. Thus couples experiencing recurrent pregnancy loss should be screened for depression and post-traumatic stress disorder (Williams & Scott, 2019).

Miscarriages can become septic, although this is uncommon. Symptoms of a septic miscarriage include fever and abdominal tenderness. Vaginal bleeding, which may be slight to heavy, is usually malodorous.

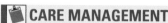 CARE MANAGEMENT

Assessment

Whenever a woman has vaginal bleeding early in pregnancy, a thorough assessment should be performed. The data to be collected include pregnancy history, vital signs, type and location of pain, quantity and nature of bleeding, and emotional status. Laboratory tests may include evaluation of human chorionic gonadotropin (β-hCG) (pregnancy), hemoglobin level (anemia), and white blood cell count (infection).

Client Problems

Problems often identified in women experiencing a miscarriage include:

- *Anxiety* related to unknown outcome and unfamiliarity with medical procedures
- *Disrupted fluid balance (intravascular dehydration)* related to
  - excessive bleeding secondary to miscarriage
- *Acute pain* related to
  - uterine contractions
- *Decreased self-esteem* related to
  - inability to carry a pregnancy successfully to term gestation
- *Potential for infection* related to
  - surgical treatment
  - dilated cervix

Initial Care

Management depends on the classification of the miscarriage and on signs and symptoms (see Table 28.1). Traditionally, threatened miscarriages have been managed expectantly with supportive care. However, there are no proven effective therapies for this condition. Bed rest, although often prescribed, does not prevent progression to actual miscarriage. Repetitive transvaginal ultrasounds and measurement of β-hCG and progesterone levels may be performed to determine if the fetus is alive and within the uterus (Cunningham et al., 2018).

Follow-up treatment depends on whether the threatened miscarriage progresses to actual miscarriage or symptoms subside and the pregnancy remains intact. If bleeding and infection do not occur, observation is implemented. Acetaminophen-based analgesia may be given to relieve pain from cramping (Cunningham et al., 2018).

Once the cervix begins to dilate, the pregnancy cannot continue and miscarriage becomes inevitable. If all the products of conception are passed, no surgical intervention is necessary. If heavy bleeding, excessive cramping, or infection is present, however, the remaining embryonic, fetal, or placental tissue must be removed from the uterus, usually by suction curettage (surgical management). In women who are clinically stable, expectant management of an incomplete miscarriage to allow spontaneous resolution or medical management using the prostaglandin misoprostol (Cytotec) administered orally or vaginally are other treatment options (Cunningham et al., 2018).

Most missed miscarriages eventually end spontaneously, although weeks may pass between the diagnosis of a failed pregnancy and spontaneous miscarriage. Miscarriage completion rates with expectant management range from 50% to 85%. After pregnancy loss has been confirmed, women may be offered medical or surgical management. While medical management is less invasive, more bleeding, longer completion times, and lower success rates are associated with this option, compared with surgical management (Cunningham et al., 2018).

If medical management is chosen, nursing care is similar to the care for any woman whose labor is induced (see Chapter 32). Special care may be needed for management of side effects of prostaglandin, such as nausea, vomiting, and diarrhea. If the products of conception are not passed completely, the woman may be prepared for manual or surgical evacuation of the uterus.

The surgical management option, one that is often chosen, is **dilation and curettage (D&C)**, a procedure in which the cervix is dilated if necessary and uterine contents are removed by suction curettage using a catheter attached to an electric-powered vacuum source. Pain relief during a D&C is usually achieved by administering analgesics or sedatives intravenously or orally (conscious sedation). A paracervical block using a local anesthetic may also be administered. Alternatively, the procedure may be performed under regional or general anesthesia (Cunningham et al., 2018). Before a surgical procedure is performed, a full history should be obtained and general and pelvic examinations conducted. General preoperative and postoperative care is appropriate for the woman requiring surgical intervention for miscarriage. The nurse reinforces explanations, answers any questions or concerns, and prepares the woman for surgery. Postoperative care includes recovery from anesthesia, pain management, and discharge instructions.

After evacuation of the uterus, oxytocin is often given to prevent hemorrhage. For excessive bleeding after the miscarriage, ergot products such as ergonovine (Methergine) or a prostaglandin derivative such as methylcarboprost tromethamine (Hemabate) may be given to contract the uterus. (See Medication Guide: Drugs Used to Manage Postpartum Hemorrhage in Chapter 33.) Antibiotics are given as necessary. Analgesics, such as antiprostaglandin agents (e.g., nonsteroidal antiinflammatory drugs [NSAIDs]), may decrease discomfort from cramping. Transfusion therapy may be required for shock or anemia. The woman who is Rh negative and is not isoimmunized is given $Rh_o(D)$ immune globulin (see Medication Guide: Rh Immune Globulin in Chapter 21) (Cunningham et al., 2018).

Psychosocial aspects of care focus on what the pregnancy loss means to the woman and her family. Grief from perinatal loss is complex and unique to each individual (see Chapter 37). Explanations are provided regarding the nature of the miscarriage, expected procedures, and possible future implications for childbearing.

As with other fetal or neonatal losses, the woman should be offered the option of seeing the products of conception. She may also want to know what the hospital does with the products of conception or whether she needs to make a decision about final disposition of fetal remains.

! NURSING ALERT

Procedures for disposition of the fetal remains vary from hospital to hospital and state to state. The nurse should know what the usual procedures are in his or her setting.

Follow-up Care

The woman will likely be discharged home within a few hours after a D&C or as soon as her vital signs are stable, vaginal bleeding remains minimal, and she has recovered from anesthesia. Discharge teaching emphasizes the need for rest. If significant blood loss has occurred, iron supplementation may be ordered. Teaching includes information

TEACHING FOR SELF-MANAGEMENT

Care After Miscarriage

- Clean the perineum after each voiding or bowel movement and change perineal pads often.
- Shower (avoid tub baths) for 2 weeks.
- Avoid tampon use, douching, and vaginal intercourse for 2 weeks.
- Notify your health care provider if an elevated temperature or a foul-smelling vaginal discharge develops.
- Eat foods high in iron and protein to promote tissue repair and red blood cell replacement.
- Seek assistance from support groups, clergy, or professional counseling as needed.
- Allow yourself (and your partner) to grieve the loss before becoming pregnant again.

about normal physical findings, such as cramping, type and amount of bleeding, resumption of sexual activity, and family planning (see Teaching for Self-Management box: Care After Miscarriage).

Frequently the woman and her partner want to know when she should attempt to become pregnant again. Emphasis is placed on the importance of completely resolving the loss before attempting another pregnancy. Follow-up care should assess the woman's emotional as well as physical recovery. Referrals to local support groups are provided as needed. Share: Pregnancy and Infant Loss Support, Inc. (www.nationalshare.org) is an excellent online resource for families who have experienced an early pregnancy loss.

Follow-up telephone calls after a loss are important. The woman may appreciate a telephone call on what would have been her due date. These calls provide opportunities for the woman to ask questions, seek advice, and receive information to help process her grief.

EVIDENCE-BASED PRACTICE

Interventions for Short Cervix

Ask the Question
For pregnant women in the second trimester with short cervix and previous preterm birth, what interventions can protect against preterm birth?

Search for the Evidence
Search Strategies English language research-based publications since 2014 on antenatal, short cervix, preterm, cerclage, pessary, and progesterone were included.
Databases Used Cochrane Collaborative Database, National Guideline Clearinghouse (AHRQ), CINAHL, PubMed, UpToDate, and the professional websites for ACOG and AWHONN

Critical Appraisal of the Evidence
Normally the cervix remains thick until the end of pregnancy. If the cervix is short (<25 mm), there is a risk for premature cervical opening. Sometimes called "cervical insufficiency," often the first symptom is pregnancy loss in the second trimester. Women with a history of second-trimester loss and preterm birth should have their cervix measured via ultrasound. To prevent preterm birth, three options provide additional mechanical support.

- **Cerclage:** First used in 1902, a cervical suture is placed surgically to tie the cervix closed and clipped at term. Meta-analysis of 15 trials found that compared with no treatment, cerclage decreased preterm births. However, there were no differences in perinatal morbidity or mortality (Alfirevic, Stampalija, & Medley, 2017).
- **Pessaries:** Used for centuries to support a prolapsed uterus, pessaries are rings inserted into the vagina that distribute the weight of the uterus away from the cervix and obstruct the internal cervical os. The insertion of a pessary is non-invasive. When women with short cervices began using pessaries mid-pregnancy, they experienced significantly less preterm birth, less use of tocolytic medications, and fewer neonatal intensive care admissions (Saccone, Maruotti, Giudicepietro, & Martinelli, 2017).
- **Progesterone:** This essential hormone of pregnancy maintenance can be given by oral, vaginal, or intramuscular route. Meta-analysis of trials for women with a short cervix showed that those who received progesterone vaginally had significantly less incidence of preterm birth. Their babies had less morbidity and mortality, respiratory distress syndrome, neonatal intensive care admissions, and need for mechanical ventilation compared with women who were treated with a placebo (Romero, Conde-Agudelo, Da Fonseca, et al., 2018).
Comparisons: A systematic review found no difference between cerclage and progesterone in preventing preterm birth in women with short cervix, previous

preterm birth, and singleton pregnancy (Alfirevic et al., 2017). The evidence supports the use of vaginal progesterone in singleton pregnancies with a short cervix. Cerclage works best in women with prior preterm birth and cervix less than or equal to 25 mm (Saccone et al., 2017). Ha and McDonald (2017) found that women preferred close-monitoring to any interventions (cerclage, progesterone, or pessary) aimed at preventing preterm birth.

Apply the Evidence: Nursing Implications
Cerclage is a surgical procedure, requiring skill, sterile technique, and fetal monitoring. Anesthesia is usually spinal, epidural, or general. For this reason, it is usually an outpatient procedure done in proximity to a hospital setting. Clients may be NPO prior to surgery and need rest afterward. Surgery can be stressful, invasive, and expensive.

Vaginal progesterone may cause minor irritation and must be administered every day. Oral progesterone may have side effects of sleepiness, headache, and fatigue. Intramuscular progesterone is given weekly.

The risk of very preterm birth and perinatal loss is frightening, and much clinical decision making is based on client history of prior pregnancy loss. Clients frequently carry guilt or anxiety about something they did or did not do into the current pregnancy. The nurse can explore their understanding and feelings about prior losses and their current pregnancy.

Because the cervix provides protection against pathogens, couples may be instructed to avoid intercourse until 1 week after a cerclage placement and to use condoms thereafter. Clients and partners need pictures, literature, websites, and warm lines to call with questions.

References
Alfirevic, Z., Stampalija, T., & Medley, N. (2017). Cervical stitch (cerclage) for preventing preterm birth in singleton pregnancy. *Cochrane Database of Systematic Reviews* (6), CD008991.
Ha, V., & McDonald, S. D. (2017). Pregnant women's preferences for and concerns about preterm birth prevention: A cross-sectional survey. *BMC Pregnancy and Childbirth, 17* (1), 49–59.
Romero, R., Conde-Agudelo, A., Da Fonseca, E., et al. (2018). Vaginal progesterone for preventing preterm birth and adverse perinatal outcomes in singleton gestations with a short cervix: A meta-analysis of individual patient data. *American Journal of Obstetrics and Gynecology, 218* (12), 161–180.
Saccone, G., Maruotti, G., Giudicepietro, A., & Martinelli, P. (2017). Effect of cervical pessary on spontaneous preterm birth in women with singleton pregnancies and short cervical length: A randomized controlled trial. *Journal of the American Medical Association, 318* (23), 2317–2324.

Jennifer Taylor Alderman

Cervical Insufficiency

One cause of late miscarriage is cervical insufficiency, which has traditionally been defined as passive and painless dilation of the cervix leading to recurrent preterm births during the second trimester in the absence of other causes. It was believed that these criteria defined women whose early births were caused solely by structural weakness of cervical tissue that could be corrected surgically by cerclage placement. Measurement of cervical length has been used as a way to diagnose cervical insufficiency. However, it is now known that an abnormally short cervix identified during the second trimester can also represent an early step in the process of preterm labor. Therefore, the challenge is to identify women who have cervical changes because of impaired cervical strength before conception or in early pregnancy rather than when preterm labor begins. However, assessment of cervical function to diagnose or rule out cervical insufficiency can be done only during pregnancy (Simhan, Berghella, & Iams, 2019).

Etiology

Cervical insufficiency may be either acquired or congenital. Congenital risk factors for cervical insufficiency include collagen disorders, uterine anomalies, and ingestion of diethylstilbestrol (DES) by the woman's mother while pregnant with the woman. Because DES has not been used since the early 1970s, however, it is now rare to encounter women who have this risk factor (Simhan et al., 2019). A risk factor for acquired cervical insufficiency is a history of previous cervical trauma resulting from lacerations during birth or mechanical dilation of the cervix during gynecologic procedures. Women who have had prior cervical surgery such as a biopsy in which a large cone specimen was removed or destroyed are also at risk for cervical insufficiency (Ludmir, Owen, & Berghella, 2017; Simhan et al., 2019).

Diagnosis

Cervical insufficiency is a clinical diagnosis, made by a thorough obstetric history along with speculum and digital pelvic examinations and a transvaginal ultrasound examination. Speculum and digital examinations allow identification of an opening at the internal cervical os, prolapsed fetal membranes, or both. A vaginal ultrasound examination will reveal an abnormally short (<25 mm) cervix. Often the short cervix is accompanied by *cervical funneling* (beaking), effacement of the internal cervical os, although the external cervical os remains closed (Cunningham et al., 2018; Ludmir et al., 2017; Simhan et al., 2019).

📋 CARE MANAGEMENT

Cervical cerclage placement has been the treatment of choice for women with cervical insufficiency due to cervical weakness. Indications for cerclage placement are a poor obstetric history, which should include at least 1 previous early preterm birth, a short (<25 mm) cervical length identified on transvaginal ultrasound, and an open cervix found on digital or speculum examination (Simhan et al., 2019). The McDonald technique is often the procedure of choice because of its proven effectiveness and ease of placement and removal. In this procedure, a suture is placed around the cervix beneath the mucosa to constrict the internal os of the cervix (Fig. 28.2) (Cunningham et al., 2018).

A cerclage may be placed either prophylactically or as a therapeutic or rescue procedure after cervical change has been identified (Cunningham et al., 2018; Simhan et al., 2019). (See the Evidence-Based Practice box: Interventions for Short Cervix for additional management options.) A history-indicated cerclage is usually placed at 12 to 14 weeks of gestation. An ultrasound-indicated cerclage may be placed therapeutically at 14 to 23 weeks of gestation in women with a singleton pregnancy and a history of a prior preterm birth if a short (<25 mm) cervix is identified on vaginal ultrasound. Finally, a rescue cerclage may be placed between 16 and 23 weeks of gestation in women who are found to have cervical

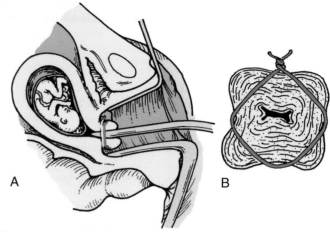

Fig. 28.2 Vaginal Cerclage. (A) Cerclage correction of premature dilation of the cervical os. (B) Cross-sectional view of closed internal os.

change (>1 cm dilated or prolapsed membranes) on physical examination. The cerclage is removed if preterm prelabor rupture of membranes or advanced preterm labor that puts pressure on the stitch occurs. If the pregnancy progresses without further complications, the cerclage is removed when the woman reaches 36 weeks of gestation (Simhan et al.).

The only indication for an abdominal cerclage that has been proven to be of benefit is failure of a prior history-indicated transvaginal cerclage, where spontaneous preterm birth occurred before 33 weeks of gestation. This procedure is usually done at 11 to 12 weeks of gestation or before conception by means of a laparotomy. Suture (Mersilene tape) is placed at the junction of the lower uterine segment and the cervix (Fig. 28.3). Cesarean birth is necessary following an abdominal cerclage, and the suture is left in place if future pregnancies are desired (Ludmir et al., 2017).

The nurse assesses the woman's feelings about her pregnancy and her understanding of cervical insufficiency. Evaluating the woman's support systems is also important. Because the diagnosis of cervical insufficiency is usually not made until the woman has lost one or more pregnancies, she may feel guilty or to blame for this impending loss. Assessing for previous reactions to stresses and appropriateness of coping responses is therefore important. The woman needs the support of health care professionals and her family.

Follow-up Care

Bed rest following cerclage was recommended in the past as a theoretical way to place less pressure on the cervix while in the recumbent position. However, the validity of bed rest has not been scientifically proven. In fact, some data suggest poorer outcomes in women on bed rest. Progesterone therapy, given either intramuscularly or vaginally, may be recommended for some women. Decisions about physical activity and intercourse are individualized, based on the status of the woman's cervix, as determined by digital and ultrasound examination (Ludmir et al., 2017).

The woman must understand the need for close observation and supervision for the remainder of the pregnancy. Additional instruction includes the need to watch for and report signs of preterm labor, rupture of membranes, and infection. Finally, the woman should know the signs that would warrant an immediate return to the hospital, including strong contractions less than 5 minutes apart, preterm prelabor rupture of membranes, severe perineal pressure, and an urge to push. If management is unsuccessful and the fetus is born before viability, appropriate grief support should be provided. If the fetus is born prematurely, appropriate anticipatory guidance and support will be necessary. (See Chapter 34 for information on high-risk newborns and Chapter 37 for information on perinatal loss and grief.)

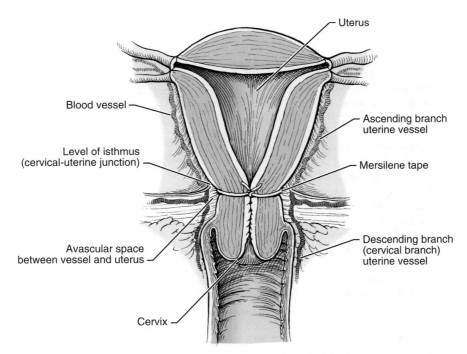

Fig. 28.3 Abdominal Cerclage. Surgical placement of circumferential Mersilene tape around uterine isthmus and median to uterine vessel. Knot is tied anteriorly. (From Gabbe, S. G., Niebyl, J. R., Simpson, J. L., et al. [Eds.]. [2017]. *Obstetrics: Normal and problem pregnancies* [7th ed.]. Philadelphia: Elsevier.)

Ectopic Pregnancy

Incidence and Etiology

An ectopic pregnancy is one in which the fertilized ovum is implanted outside the uterine cavity (Fig. 28.4). Of all first-trimester pregnancies in the United States, 0.5% to 1.5% are ectopic, and these account for 3% of all pregnancy-related maternal deaths. Women are less likely to have a successful subsequent pregnancy after an ectopic pregnancy (Cunningham et al., 2018). Ectopic pregnancy is also a leading cause of infertility.

Ectopic pregnancies are often called *tubal pregnancies* because at least 90% are located in the uterine tube (Weant, Bailey, Baum, et al., 2017). Of all tubal ectopic pregnancies, approximately 70% are located in the ampulla, or largest portion of the tube (Cunningham et al., 2018). Although they are much less common, ectopic pregnancies can also occur in the abdominal cavity, on an ovary, on the cervix, or on a previous cesarean scar.

Ectopic pregnancies probably account for about 2% of all pregnancies in the United States. The actual number is difficult to determine, however, because many women are treated in outpatient settings where events are not tracked. Moreover, national surveillance data on ectopic pregnancies have not been updated in over 25 years (American College of Obstetricians and Gynecologists [ACOG], 2018). Some of the increased incidence is likely because of improved diagnostic techniques, such as more sensitive β-hCG measurement and transvaginal ultrasound, resulting in the identification of more cases. Other causes for the rise include a history of past surgeries for a prior tubal pregnancy, for fertility restoration, or for sterilization and prior sexually transmitted infection or another tubal infection. Smoking is associated with ectopic pregnancy, although the reason for this association is unclear. Finally, the use of assisted reproductive technologies or certain contraceptive methods such as copper or progestin-releasing intrauterine devices (IUDs) increases a woman's risk for an ectopic pregnancy (Cunningham et al., 2018). Ectopic pregnancy is classified according to site of implantation (e.g., tubal, ovarian, or abdominal). The uterus is

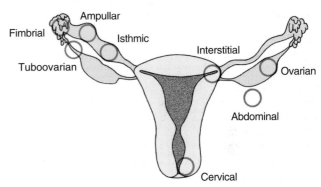

Fig. 28.4 Sites of Implantation of Ectopic Pregnancies. Order of frequency of occurrence is ampulla, isthmus, interstitium, fimbria, tuboovarian ligament, ovary, abdominal cavity, and cervix (external os).

the only organ capable of containing and sustaining a term pregnancy. Most abdominal pregnancies are thought to be the result of early tubal rupture, followed by reimplantation. Surgery to remove the embryo or fetus is usually performed as soon as an abdominal pregnancy is identified because of the high risk for hemorrhage at any time during the pregnancy (Fig. 28.5). There is a risk for fetal malformations and deformations in an abdominal pregnancy as a result of pressure deformities caused by oligohydramnios.

Clinical Manifestations

Most cases of ectopic (tubal) pregnancy are diagnosed before rupture based on the three most classic symptoms: (1) abdominal pain, (2) delayed menses, and (3) abnormal vaginal bleeding (spotting). Abdominal pain occurs in almost every case. It usually begins as a dull, lower quadrant pain on one side. The discomfort can progress from a dull pain to a colicky pain when the tube stretches, to sharp, stabbing pain. It progresses to a diffuse, constant, severe pain that is generalized

Uterus

Gestational sac

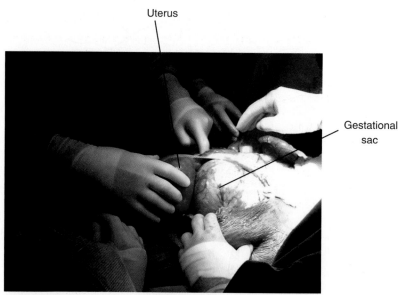

Fig. 28.5 Ectopic Pregnancy, Abdominal, Diagnosed on a Routine Ultrasound at 25 Weeks of Gestation. Note that the gestational sac is clearly outside the uterus. The placenta was attached to the right uterine tube and right ovary. (Courtesy Danielle L. Tate, MD, Memphis, TN.)

throughout the lower abdomen. The majority of women with an ectopic pregnancy report a period that is delayed 1 to 2 weeks or lighter than usual, or an irregular period. Mild to moderate dark red or brown intermittent vaginal bleeding occurs in many of these women.

If the ectopic pregnancy is not diagnosed until after rupture has occurred, referred shoulder pain may be present in addition to generalized, one-sided, or deep lower quadrant acute abdominal pain. Referred shoulder pain results from diaphragmatic irritation caused by blood in the peritoneal cavity. The woman may need medication to manage severe, excruciating pain while she is being prepared for surgery. She may exhibit signs of shock, such as faintness and dizziness, related to the amount of bleeding in the abdominal cavity and not necessarily related to obvious vaginal bleeding. An ecchymotic blueness around the umbilicus (Cullen sign), indicating hematoperitoneum (blood in the peritoneal cavity), may also develop in an undiagnosed ruptured intraabdominal ectopic pregnancy.

Diagnosis

The differential diagnosis of ectopic pregnancy involves consideration of numerous disorders that share many signs and symptoms. Many of these women go to the emergency department because of first-trimester bleeding or pain. Miscarriage, ruptured corpus luteum cyst, appendicitis, salpingitis, ovarian cysts, torsion of the ovary, and urinary tract infection are possible diagnoses. The key to early detection of ectopic pregnancy is having a high index of suspicion for this condition. *Every woman with abdominal pain, vaginal spotting or bleeding, and a positive pregnancy test should undergo screening for ectopic pregnancy.*

The most important screening tools for ectopic pregnancy are quantitative β-hCG levels and transvaginal ultrasound examinations. The term discriminatory zone addresses the concept that there is a β-hCG level above which a normal intrauterine pregnancy should be visible on ultrasound. Discriminatory levels can be set at different thresholds. When β-hCG levels are greater than 1500 to 2000 milli-International Units/mL, for example, a normal intrauterine pregnancy should be visible on transvaginal ultrasound. Therefore, if β-hCG levels are greater than 1500 milli-International Units/mL but no intrauterine pregnancy is seen on transvaginal ultrasound, an ectopic pregnancy is very likely. Other institutions set their discriminatory threshold at an even higher

level. β-hCG levels will probably be redrawn every 48 hours to determine if the pregnancy is viable. A transvaginal ultrasound may also be repeated to determine if the pregnancy is inside the uterus. Sometimes the location of an ectopic pregnancy will be visible on transvaginal ultrasound (Cunningham et al., 2018).

Another laboratory test that can be ordered to determine if the pregnancy is developing normally is a progesterone level. A progesterone level greater than 25 ng/mL almost always rules out the presence of an ectopic pregnancy. However, a progesterone level less than 5 ng/mL suggests either an ectopic pregnancy or an abnormal intrauterine pregnancy (Cunningham et al., 2018).

The woman should also be assessed for the presence of active bleeding, which is associated with tubal rupture. If internal bleeding is present, assessment may reveal vertigo, shoulder pain, hypotension, and tachycardia. A vaginal examination should be performed only once, and then with great caution. Approximately 20% of women with a tubal pregnancy have a palpable mass on examination. Rupturing the mass is possible during a bimanual examination; thus, a gentle touch is critical.

CARE MANAGEMENT

Medical Management

Many women with an early diagnosis of ectopic pregnancy can be managed medically with methotrexate (ACOG, 2018). Methotrexate is an antimetabolite and folic acid antagonist that destroys rapidly dividing cells. It is classified as a hazardous drug and can cause serious toxic side effects even when given in low doses. These side effects can cause safety risks for health care providers if the drug is not handled appropriately. Additionally, the Institute for Safe Medication Practices considers methotrexate to be a high-alert drug (Box 28.1) (ACOG, 2018; National Institute for Occupational Safety and Health, 2016).

Methotrexate therapy avoids surgery and is a safe, effective, and cost-effective way of managing many cases of tubal pregnancy. The woman must be hemodynamically stable and have normal liver and kidney function to be eligible for methotrexate therapy. The best results following methotrexate therapy are usually obtained if the mass is unruptured and measures less than 3.5 cm in diameter by ultrasound, if

BOX 28.1 Methotrexate Administration

- Obtain the woman's height and weight. These measurements are used to calculate her body surface area in order to determine the correct dose of methotrexate, so they must be accurate.
- The standard dose of methotrexate used to treat ectopic pregnancy is 50 mg/m² given intramuscularly, although it may also be ordered as 1 mg/kg.
- The dose of methotrexate should be prepared in the hospital pharmacy under a biologic safety cabinet. Syringe(s) containing the methotrexate should be dispensed from the pharmacy no more than three-quarters full in a sealed plastic bag without a needle attached.
- Don two pairs of gloves before removing the syringe(s) from the sealed plastic bag.
- Remove the syringe cap and replace with an appropriate needle for intramuscular injection.
- Do not expel air from the syringe or prime the needle because these actions could aerosolize the methotrexate.
- Check the client's identity and the medication and dosage before injecting the methotrexate. Another nurse should also perform an independent check before the injection is given.
- Dispose of any items worn or used to prepare, dispense, or administer the methotrexate injection in a waste container designated specifically for hazardous drugs.
- Wash hands thoroughly after removing gloves.

Data from Shastay, A., & Paparella, S. (2010). Ectopic pregnancies and methotrexate: Are you prepared to manage this hazardous drug? *Journal of Emergency Nursing, 36*(1), 57–59.

no fetal cardiac activity is noted on ultrasound, and if the initial serum β-hCG level is less than 1000 milli-International Units/L (Cunningham et al., 2018). The woman must also be willing to comply with post-treatment lifestyle restrictions and monitoring. She is informed of how the medication works, possible side effects, general self-care guidelines, and the importance of follow-up care (see Box 28.2).

BOX 28.2 Instructions for Women Receiving Methotrexate Therapy for Ectopic Pregnancy

- Explain that methotrexate dissolves ectopic (tubal) pregnancies by destroying rapidly dividing cells.
- Explain that urine contains levels of drug metabolite that could be considered toxic for approximately 72 hrs after receiving methotrexate. The levels are highest during the first 8 hrs after treatment. Teach the woman to avoid getting urine on the toilet seat and to double flush the toilet (with the lid down) after urinating. Also explain that her stools may contain residual drug for up to 7 days.
- Inform the woman of possible side effects. Gastric distress, nausea and vomiting, stomatitis, and dizziness are common. Rare side effects include severe neutropenia, reversible hair loss, and pneumonitis.
- Advise the woman to do the following:
  - Avoid foods and vitamins containing folic acid.
  - Avoid "gas-forming" foods.
  - Avoid sun exposure.
  - Avoid sexual intercourse until the β-hCG level is undetectable.
  - Keep all scheduled follow-up appointments.
  - Take no analgesic stronger than acetaminophen and contact her health care provider immediately if she has severe abdominal pain, which may be a sign of impending or actual tubal rupture.

Data from Weant, K. A., Bailey, A. M., Baum, R. A., et al. (2017). Chemotherapy in the emergency department? There is a role for that: Methotrexate for ectopic pregnancy. *Advanced Emergency Nursing Journal, 39*(1), 18–25.

SAFETY ALERT

Women receiving methotrexate to treat an ectopic pregnancy should not take any analgesic stronger than acetaminophen. Stronger analgesics can mask symptoms of tubal rupture.

Surgical Management

Surgical management depends on the location and cause of the ectopic pregnancy, the extent of tissue involvement, and the woman's desires regarding future fertility. One option is removal of the entire tube (salpingectomy). If the tube has not ruptured and the woman desires future fertility, salpingostomy may be performed instead. In this procedure an incision is made over the pregnancy site in the tube and the products of conception are gently and very carefully removed. The incision is not sutured but left to close by secondary intention instead, given that this method results in less scarring.

If surgery is planned, general preoperative and postoperative care is appropriate for the woman with an ectopic pregnancy. Before surgery, vital signs (pulse, respirations, and blood pressure [BP]) are assessed every 15 minutes or as needed, according to the severity of the bleeding and the woman's condition. Preoperative laboratory tests include determination of blood type and Rh status, complete blood cell count, and serum quantitative β-hCG level. Ultrasonography is used to confirm an extrauterine pregnancy. Blood component replacement may be necessary. The nurse verifies the woman's Rh and antibody status and administers Rh₀(D) immune globulin postoperatively if appropriate (see Medication Guide: Rh Immune Globulin in Chapter 21).

Follow-up Care

Women who have received methotrexate therapy have their β-hCG level measured weekly to make certain that it continues to drop steadily until it becomes undetectable. Complete resolution of an ectopic pregnancy usually occurs in 2 to 3 weeks but can require as long as 6 to 8 weeks (Fields & Hathaway, 2017).

Whether treated medically or surgically, the woman and her family should be encouraged to share their feelings and concerns related to the loss. Future fertility should be discussed. A contraceptive method should be used for at least three menstrual cycles to allow time for the woman's body to heal. *Every* woman who has been diagnosed with an ectopic pregnancy should be instructed to contact her health care provider as soon as she suspects that she might be pregnant because of the increased risk for recurrent ectopic pregnancy. These women may need referral to grief or infertility support groups. In addition to the loss of the current pregnancy, they are faced with the possibility of future pregnancy losses or infertility. (See Chapter 37 for information on perinatal loss and grief.)

Molar Pregnancy (Hydatidiform Mole)

Molar pregnancy (also called *hydatidiform mole*) is a benign proliferative growth of the placental trophoblast in which the chorionic villi develop into edematous, cystic, avascular transparent vesicles that hang in a grapelike cluster. Molar pregnancy is one of a group of pregnancy-related cancers without a viable fetus known as gestational trophoblastic neoplasia (GTN) that are caused by abnormal fertilization. GTN have the potential for local invasion, distant metastasis, and death from disease. In addition to partial and complete molar pregnancies, gestational choriocarcinoma and placental site trophoblastic tumors are also GTNs (Cohn, Ramaswamy, Christian, & Bixel, 2019).

Incidence and Etiology

Molar pregnancy occurs in 1 in 1000 pregnancies in the United States (Cohn et al., 2019). The cause is unknown, although it may be related to an ovular defect or a nutritional deficiency. Women at increased risk for hydatidiform mole formation are those who have had a prior molar pregnancy and those who are at the extremes of age for reproduction (Salani & Copeland, 2017). Asian, Hispanic, and Native American women are more likely than women of other races/ethnicities to develop hydatidiform mole (Cunningham et al., 2018).

Types

Molar pregnancies typically result from chromosomally abnormal fertilization. They are further categorized as a complete or partial mole. The complete mole results from fertilization of an egg in which the nucleus has been lost or inactivated. The nucleus of a sperm (23,X or 23,Y) duplicates itself (resulting in the diploid number 46,XX [most common] or 46,XY) because the ovum has no genetic material or the material is inactive. It is also possible for an "empty" egg to be fertilized by two normal sperm, thereby producing either a 46,XX or 46,XY genotype (Moore, 2019). The mole resembles a bunch of white grapes. The hydropic (fluid-filled) vesicles grow rapidly, causing the uterus to be larger than expected for the duration of the pregnancy. The complete mole contains no fetus, placenta, amniotic membranes, or fluid (Fig. 28.6). Maternal blood has no placenta to receive it; therefore hemorrhage into the uterine cavity and vaginal bleeding occur.

In a partial mole one apparently normal ovum is fertilized by two or more sperm. Triploidy (69XXY) or quadraploidy (92XXXY) genotypes then result (Moore, 2019). Partial moles often have embryonic or fetal parts and an amniotic sac (Fig. 28.7). Congenital anomalies, severe growth restriction, or both are usually present. The risk of persistent GTN is less than with a complete mole (Cunningham et al., 2018).

Clinical Manifestations

In the early stages the clinical manifestations of a complete hydatidiform mole cannot be distinguished from those of normal pregnancy. Later, vaginal bleeding occurs in almost all cases. The vaginal discharge may be dark brown (resembling prune juice) or bright red and either scant or profuse. It may continue for only a few days or intermittently for weeks. Usually the uterus is larger than indicated from menstrual dates, although some women will have a uterus that is smaller than would be expected. Anemia from blood loss, excessive nausea and vomiting (hyperemesis gravidarum), and abdominal cramps caused by uterine distention are relatively common findings. Women may also pass vesicles, which are frequently avascular edematous villi, from the uterus. Preeclampsia occurs in approximately 70% of women with large, rapidly growing hydatidiform moles and occurs earlier than usual in the pregnancy. If preeclampsia is diagnosed before 24 weeks of gestation, hydatidiform mole should be suspected and ruled out. Hyperthyroidism is another serious complication of hydatidiform mole. Treatment of the hydatidiform mole restores thyroid function to normal. Partial moles cause few of these symptoms and may be mistaken for an incomplete or missed miscarriage (Harper, Tita, & Karumanchi, 2019; Moore, 2019; Nader, 2019).

Diagnosis

Transvaginal ultrasound and serum hCG levels are used for diagnosis. Transvaginal ultrasound is the most accurate tool for diagnosing a hydatidiform mole. In the past, about half of all molar pregnancies were not diagnosed until molar tissue was passed from the vagina. Currently, however, many women are diagnosed by ultrasound while asymptomatic or by ultrasound done to evaluate vaginal bleeding or cramping symptoms. A characteristic pattern of multiple diffuse intrauterine masses, often called a *snowstorm pattern*, is seen in place of or along with an embryo or a fetus. The trophoblastic tissue secretes the hCG hormone. In a molar pregnancy, hCG levels are persistently high or rising beyond the time they would begin to decline in a normal pregnancy (Cohn et al, 2019; Moore, 2019; Salani & Copeland, 2017).

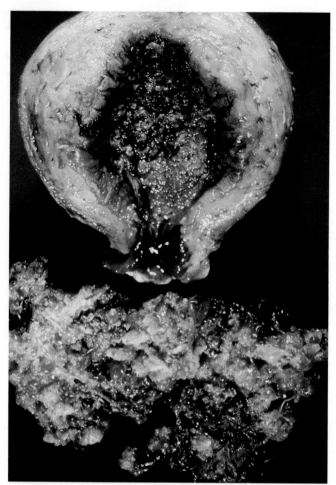

Fig. 28.6 Gross Specimen in a Woman Treated for Complete Hydatidiform Mole with Primary Hysterectomy. (Courtesy John Soper, MD.) (From DiSaia, P., & Creasman, W. [2007]. *Clinical gynecologic oncology* [7th ed.]. Philadelphia: Mosby.)

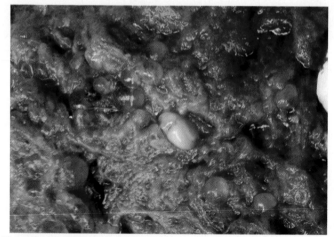

Fig. 28.7 Partial Hydatidiform Mole. (Courtesy Norman L. Meyer, MD, PhD, Memphis, TN.)

CARE MANAGEMENT

Although most moles abort spontaneously, suction curettage offers a safe, rapid, and effective method of evacuating a hydatidiform mole if necessary. Older women who desire sterilization may undergo hysterectomy instead of suction curettage (Cunningham et al., 2018; Salani & Copeland, 2017. Induction of labor with oxytocic agents or prostaglandin is not recommended because of the increased risk for embolization of trophoblastic tissue (Salani & Copeland).

The nurse provides the woman and her family with information about the disease process, the necessity for a long course of follow-up, and the possible consequences of the disease. The nurse also helps the woman and her family cope with the pregnancy loss and recognize that the pregnancy was not normal. In addition, the woman and her family are encouraged to express their feelings, and information is provided about local support groups or counseling and spiritual resources as needed. Internet resources such as Share: Pregnancy and Infant Loss Support, Inc., and the International Society for the Study of Trophoblastic Diseases at www. isstd.org may also be useful. Explanations about the importance of postponing a subsequent pregnancy and contraceptive counseling are provided to emphasize the need for consistent and reliable use of the method chosen.

To avoid confusion in regard to rising levels of hCG that are normal in pregnancy but could indicate GTN, pregnancy should be avoided during the follow-up assessment period. IUDs should not be used until β-hCG levels are undetectable. Combination oral contraceptives are preferred because they are highly effective. Injectable medroxyprogesterone acetate or a progestin implant are also effective contraceptive methods and are practical options for women who have difficulty complying with the daily dosing required for oral contraceptive use (Cunningham et al., 2018).

Follow-up Care

After the molar pregnancy has been evacuated, the woman is still at risk for recurrence or the development of invasive mole or choriocarcinoma (Moore, 2019). Therefore, close follow-up is essential. Follow-up care includes frequent physical and pelvic examinations along with weekly measurements of the β-hCG level until the level decreases to normal and remains normal for 3 consecutive weeks. Monthly measurements are then taken for 6 to 12 months. The follow-up assessment period usually continues for 1 year. During that time rising β-hCG levels and an enlarging uterus may indicate GTN (see Chapter 11 for further discussion) (Salani & Copeland, 2017).

🏠 COMMUNITY ACTIVITY

Loss of Pregnancy

Talk with someone who has experienced an early pregnancy loss, either a miscarriage, an ectopic pregnancy, or a hydatidiform mole. What helpful things did her health care providers say or do at the time of the loss? What things did they say or do that were not helpful? Are there things that she wishes had been done or said differently? Which of her suggestions do you think would be helpful to people experiencing a different kind of loss?

LATE PREGNANCY BLEEDING

The major causes of bleeding in late pregnancy are placenta previa and premature separation of the placenta (abruptio placentae, or placental abruption). Rapid assessment and diagnosis of the cause of bleeding are essential to reduce maternal and perinatal morbidity and mortality (Table 28.2).

Placenta Previa

Because of advances in ultrasonography, especially transvaginal ultrasound, and an increased understanding of the changing relationship between the placenta and the internal cervical os as pregnancy progresses, definitions and classifications of placenta previa have changed. In **placenta previa** the placenta is implanted in the lower uterine segment such that it completely or partially covers the cervix or is close enough to the cervix to cause bleeding when the cervix dilates or the lower uterine segment effaces (Fig. 28.8) (Hull, Resnik, & Silver, 2019). When transvaginal ultrasound is used, the placenta is classified as a *complete placenta previa* if it totally covers the internal cervical os. In a *marginal placenta previa* the edge of the placenta is seen on transvaginal ultrasound to be 2.5 cm or closer to the internal cervical os. When the exact relationship of the placenta to the internal cervical os has not been determined or in the case of apparent placenta previa in the second trimester, the term *low-lying placenta* is used (Hull et al.).

Incidence and Etiology

Placenta previa affects approximately 1 in 200 pregnancies at term. Some evidence suggests that the incidence of placenta previa is increasing, perhaps as a result of more cesarean births. In addition to a history of previous cesarean birth, other risk factors for placenta previa include advanced maternal age (more than 35 to 40 years of age), multiparity, history of prior suction curettage, and smoking (Hull et al., 2019). Living at a higher altitude is also a risk factor for placenta previa. Like cigarette smoking, a higher altitude causes a decrease in uteroplacental oxygenation and thus a need for increased placental surface area. Maternal race is another factor associated with placenta previa. It appears that Asian women have the highest risk for placenta previa. Placenta previa occurs more frequently in women carrying male fetuses. A possible explanation for this is that placental sizes are larger in pregnancies involving male fetuses (Francois & Foley, 2017). Multiple gestation is also a risk factor for placenta previa (Cunningham et al., 2018), possibly because of the larger placental area in these pregnancies. Women who had placenta previa in a previous pregnancy are more likely than others to develop the problem in a subsequent pregnancy, perhaps as a result of a genetic predisposition. Previous cesarean birth and curettage in the past for miscarriage or induced abortion are risk factors for placenta previa because both result in endometrial damage and uterine scarring (Francois & Foley; Hull et al.). (See Clinical Reasoning Case Study: Third Trimester Vaginal Bleeding.)

❓ CLINICAL REASONING CASE STUDY

Third-Trimester Vaginal Bleeding

Crystal is a 41-year-old G5 P2 1 1 4 (one set of twins) who presents to the emergency department with heavy vaginal bleeding. She has had no prenatal care but is approximately 33 weeks of gestation by her LMP. Crystal said, "I was fine when I went to bed last night. In the middle of the night I woke up and found a huge puddle of blood in my bed. I called the ambulance right away and they brought me here." During her medical screening exam you learn that Crystal has had one cesarean birth (with her twins) and a D&C after a miscarriage 5 years ago. She also smokes 1 pack of cigarettes per day.

1. What is the priority concern or client need in this situation? Support your answer with data as stated in the case.
2. List other client needs/problems in this case.
3. Identify any additional information or assessment data that is needed by the nurse in planning care for this client.
4. What nursing actions are appropriate in this situation?
   a. What is the priority nursing action?
   b. Describe other nursing interventions that are important to providing optimal client care.
5. Describe the roles/responsibilities of the interprofessional health care team members (other than nurses) who may be involved in providing care for this client.

TABLE 28.2   Summary of Findings: Placental Abruption and Placenta Previa

Findings	PLACENTAL ABRUPTION			PLACENTA PREVIA
	Grade 1 Mild Separation (10%-20%)	Grade 2 Moderate Separation (20%-50%)	Grade 3 Severe Separation (>50%)	
Physical and Laboratory Findings				
Bleeding, external, vaginal	Minimal	Absent to moderate	Absent to moderate	Minimal to severe and life threatening
Total amount of blood loss	<500 mL	1000-1500 mL	>1500 mL	Varies
Color of blood	Dark red	Dark red	Dark red	Bright red
Shock	Rare; none	Mild shock	Common, often sudden, profound	Uncommon
Coagulopathy	Rare, none	Occasional DIC	Frequent DIC	None
Uterine tonicity	Normal	Increased, may be localized to one region or diffuse over uterus, uterus fails to relax between contractions	Tetanic, persistent uterine contractions, boardlike uterus	Normal
Tenderness (pain)	Usually absent	Present	Agonizing, unremitting uterine pain	Absent
Ultrasonographic Findings				
Location of placenta	Normal, upper uterine segment	Normal, upper uterine segment	Normal, upper uterine segment	Abnormal, lower uterine segment
Station of presenting part	Variable to engaged	Variable to engaged	Variable to engaged	High, not engaged
Fetal position	Usual distribution[a]	Usual distribution[a]	Usual distribution[a]	Commonly transverse, breech, or oblique
Gestational or chronic hypertension	Usual distribution[a]	Commonly present	Commonly present	Usual distribution[a]
Fetal effects	Normal fetal heart rate and pattern	Abnormal fetal heart rate and pattern	Abnormal fetal heart rate and pattern; fetal death can occur	Normal fetal heart rate and pattern

[a]Usual distribution refers to the expected variations of incidence seen when there is no concurrent problem.
DIC, Disseminated intravascular coagulation.

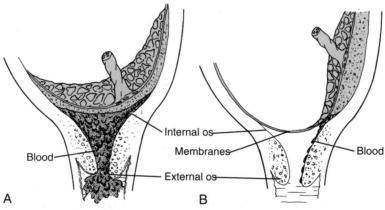

Fig. 28.8 Types of Placenta Previa. (A) Complete. (B) Marginal.

Clinical Manifestations

Placenta previa is typically characterized by painless bright red vaginal bleeding during the second or third trimester. In the past, placenta previa was usually diagnosed after an episode of bleeding. Currently, however, most cases are diagnosed by ultrasound before significant vaginal bleeding occurs. This bleeding is associated with the disruption of placental blood vessels that occurs with stretching and thinning of the lower uterine segment. Between 70% and 80% of women with placenta previa will have at least one episode of vaginal bleeding. Of women with vaginal bleeding, one-third will present before 30 weeks of gestation, one-third between 30 and 36 weeks of gestation, and one-third after 36 weeks of gestation (Francois & Foley, 2017).

Vital signs may be normal, even with heavy blood loss, because a pregnant woman can lose up to 40% of her blood volume without showing signs of shock. Clinical presentation and decreasing urinary output may be better indicators of acute blood loss than vital signs alone. The fetal heart rate (FHR) is normal unless a major detachment of the placenta occurs.

Abdominal examination usually reveals a soft, relaxed, nontender uterus with normal tone. The presenting part of the fetus usually remains high because the placenta occupies the lower uterine segment. Thus, the fundal height is often greater than expected for gestational age. Because of the abnormally located placenta, fetal malpresentation (breech and transverse or oblique lie) is common.

Maternal and Fetal Outcomes

The major maternal complication associated with placenta previa is hemorrhage. Another serious complication is development of a *morbidly adherent placenta*, an abnormally firm placental attachment (e.g., *placenta accreta, increta,* or *percreta*) (see Chapter 33). If excessive bleeding cannot be controlled, hysterectomy may be necessary (Cunningham et al., 2018; Hull et al., 2019). Because most women with placenta previa give birth by cesarean, surgery-related trauma to structures adjacent to the uterus and anesthesia complications are also possible. In addition, blood transfusion reactions, anemia, venous thromboembolism (VTE), and infection may occur.

Preterm birth is a major cause of perinatal morbidity and mortality for infants born to women with placenta previa. Intrauterine growth restriction (IUGR) has also been associated with placenta previa, although the risk for developing this condition is low. The incidence of fetal anomalies is increased in pregnancies complicated by placenta previa (Cunningham et al., 2018).

Diagnosis

All women with painless vaginal bleeding after 20 weeks of gestation should be assumed to have a placenta previa until proven otherwise. A transabdominal ultrasound examination should be performed initially followed by a transvaginal scan, unless the transabdominal ultrasound clearly shows that the placenta is not located in the lower uterine segment. A transvaginal ultrasound is better than a transabdominal scan for accurately determining placental location (Hull et al., 2019). If ultrasonographic scanning reveals a normally implanted placenta, a speculum examination may be performed to rule out local causes of bleeding (e.g., cervicitis, polyps, carcinoma of the cervix), and a coagulation profile is obtained to rule out other causes of bleeding.

📋 CARE MANAGEMENT

Once placenta previa has been diagnosed, a management plan is developed. The woman will be managed either expectantly or actively, depending on the gestational age, amount of bleeding, and fetal condition.

Problems often experienced by women with placenta previa include the following:

- *Inadequate tissue perfusion* related to excessive blood loss secondary to placenta previa
- *Dehydration* related to excessive blood loss secondary to placenta previa
- *Decreased placental perfusion* related to hypovolemia and shunting of blood to central circulation
- *Anxiety* related to maternal condition and pregnancy outcome
- *Grieving* related to actual or perceived threat to self, pregnancy, or infant

Expectant Management

Expectant management (observation and bed rest) is implemented if the fetus is at less than 36 to 37 weeks of gestation with normal fetal growth and if no other pregnancy-associated complications exist (Francois & Foley, 2017). The woman initially is hospitalized in a labor and birth unit for continuous FHR and contraction monitoring. Large-bore IV access should be initiated immediately. Initial laboratory tests include hemoglobin, hematocrit, platelet count, and coagulation studies. A "type and screen" blood sample should be maintained at all times in the transfusion services department of the hospital to allow for immediate crossmatch of blood component therapy if necessary. If the woman is at less than 34 weeks of gestation, antenatal corticosteroids

should be administered. Tocolytic medications may be given if the vaginal bleeding is preceded by or associated with uterine contractions (Francois & Foley, 2017).

If the bleeding stops, the woman will most likely be placed on bed rest with bathroom privileges and limited activity (e.g., able to use the bathroom, shower, and move around her hospital room for 15 to 30 minutes at a time, four times a day). No vaginal or rectal examinations are performed, and the woman is told to avoid intercourse. Ultrasound examinations are performed serially to assess placental location and fetal growth. The woman will also receive nutritional counseling and iron supplementation to avoid anemia (Francois & Foley, 2017).

Placenta previa should always be considered a potential emergency because massive blood loss with resulting hypovolemic shock can occur quickly if bleeding resumes. The possibility always exists that the woman will require an emergency cesarean birth. Placenta previa in a preterm gestation may be an indication for transfer to a tertiary- or quaternary-care perinatal center, given that a neonatal intensive care unit may be necessary for care of the preterm infant. Because many community hospitals are not prepared to perform emergency surgery 24 hours per day, 7 days per week, transfer of the woman to a tertiary- or quaternary-care center may be necessary to ensure constant access to cesarean birth. Also, the transfusion services departments in many community hospitals do not have immediate access to large amounts of blood products, which will be necessary if massive hemorrhage occurs.

Home Care

Sometimes women with placenta previa are discharged from the hospital before giving birth to be managed at home. The woman's condition should be stable, and she should have experienced no vaginal bleeding for at least 48 hours before discharge (Hull et al., 2019). A candidate for home care must meet other strict criteria as well. She should be willing and able to comply with activity restrictions (bed rest with bathroom privileges and pelvic rest); live within a short distance of the hospital; have constant access to transportation; and verbalize a thorough understanding of the risks associated with placenta previa (Francois & Foley, 2017). If bleeding resumes, she needs to return to the hospital immediately. She must also be able to keep all appointments for fetal testing, laboratory assessments, and prenatal care. Visits by a perinatal home care nurse may be arranged.

If hospitalization or home care with activity restriction is prolonged, the woman can have concerns about her work- or family-related responsibilities or become bored with inactivity. She should be encouraged to participate in her own care and decisions about care as much as possible. Providing diversionary activities or encouraging her to participate in activities she enjoys and can perform while sedentary are necessary. Participating in a support group made up of other women on activity restriction while hospitalized or online if at home may be a helpful coping mechanism (see Teaching for Self-Management box: Coping with Activity Restriction in Chapter 27).

Active Management

If the woman definitely has placenta previa and she is at or beyond 36 weeks of gestation, birth is appropriate. If bleeding is excessive or continues or there are concerns about the condition of the fetus, immediate birth is indicated, regardless of gestational age (Hull et al., 2019). Almost all women with placenta previa will give birth by cesarean. If the placenta is located between 1 mm and 20 mm from the internal cervical os, however, as many as 60% of women may choose to attempt vaginal birth. If vaginal birth is attempted, health care providers must be prepared for the possibility of an emergent cesarean birth and the need for blood transfusion (Francois & Foley, 2017).

If cesarean birth is planned, the nurse continually assesses maternal and fetal status while preparing the woman for surgery. Maternal vital signs are assessed frequently for decreasing BP, increasing pulse rate, changes in level of consciousness, and oliguria. Fetal assessment is maintained by continuous electronic fetal monitoring (EFM) to assess for signs of hypoxia.

Blood loss may not stop with the birth of the infant. The large vascular channels in the lower uterine segment may continue to bleed because of the diminished muscle content of that segment. The natural mechanism to control bleeding so characteristic of the upper part of the uterus (i.e., the interlacing muscle bundles, the "living ligature" contracting around open vessels) is absent in the lower part of the uterus. Therefore postpartum hemorrhage may occur even if the fundus is contracted firmly (see Chapter 33).

Emotional support for the woman and her family is extremely important. The actively bleeding woman is concerned not only for her own well-being but also for that of her fetus. All procedures should be explained, and a support person should be present. The woman should be encouraged to express her concerns and feelings. If the woman and her support person or family desire pastoral support, the nurse can notify the hospital chaplain service or provide information about other supportive resources.

Premature Separation of the Placenta (Abruptio Placentae [Placental Abruption])

Premature separation of the placenta, or abruptio placentae, is the detachment of part or all of a normally implanted placenta from the uterus (Fig. 28.9). Separation occurs in the area of the decidua basalis after 20 weeks of gestation and before the birth of the infant.

Incidence and Etiology

Premature separation of the placenta is a serious complication that accounts for significant maternal and fetal morbidity and mortality. The overall incidence of placental abruption is 1 in 100 births, but a range of 1 in 80 to 1 in 250 pregnancies has been reported. The range in incidence likely reflects both variable criteria for diagnosis and an increased recognition of milder forms of abruption. Approximately one-third of all antepartum bleeding is caused by placental abruption (Francois & Foley, 2017). Maternal hypertension, whether chronic or pregnancy related, is the most consistently identified risk factor for abruption. Cocaine use is also a risk factor because it causes vascular disruption in the placental bed. Blunt external abdominal trauma, most often the result of motor vehicle accidents (MVAs) or maternal battering, is another frequent cause of placental abruption (Cunningham et al., 2018; Francois & Foley). Other risk factors include cigarette smoking, a history of abruption in a previous pregnancy, and preterm prelabor rupture of membranes. There has been great interest in a possible association between thrombophilic disorders and abruption. However, both retrospective and prospective studies of women with the factor V Leiden mutation have shown no increase in risk for abruption (Hull et al., 2019). Abruption is more likely to occur in twin gestations than in singletons (Francois & Foley). Women who have had two previous abruptions have a recurrence risk of 25% in the next pregnancy (Hull & Resnik).

Classification

The most common classification of placental abruption is according to type and severity. This classification system is summarized in Table 28.2.

Clinical Manifestations

Clinical symptoms vary with degree of separation (see Table 28.2). Classic symptoms of placental abruption include vaginal bleeding,

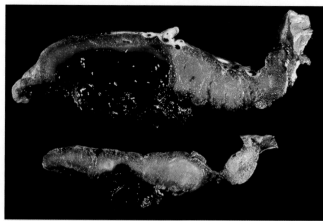

Fig. 28.9 Abruptio Placentae. A large retroplacental abruption at 30 weeks' gestation. (From Resnik, R., Lockwood, C. J., Moore, T. R., et al. [Eds.]. [2019]. *Creasy & Resnik's maternal-fetal medicine: principles and practice* [8th ed.]. Philadelphia: Elsevier.)

abdominal pain, uterine tenderness, and contractions (Cunningham et al., 2018; Hull et al., 2019). Bleeding may result in maternal hypovolemia (i.e., shock, oliguria, anuria) and coagulopathy. Mild-to-severe uterine hypertonicity is present. Pain is mild to severe and localized over one region of the uterus or diffusely over the uterus with a board-like abdomen.

Extensive myometrial bleeding damages the uterine muscle. If blood accumulates between the separated placenta and the uterine wall, it may produce a Couvelaire uterus. The uterus appears purple or blue, rather than its usual "bubble-gum pink" color, and contractility is lost. Shock may occur and is out of proportion to blood loss. Laboratory findings include a positive Apt test result (blood in the amniotic fluid); a decrease in hemoglobin and hematocrit levels, which may appear later; and a decrease in coagulation factor levels. Clotting defects (e.g., disseminated intravascular coagulation) may be present, but most abruptions are not accompanied by maternal coagulopathy (Francois & Foley, 2017). A Kleihauer-Betke (KB) test may be ordered to determine the presence of fetal-to-maternal bleeding (transplacental hemorrhage), although it is of no diagnostic value. The KB test may be useful, however, to guide $Rh_o(D)$ immune globulin therapy in Rh-negative women who have had an abruption (Hull et al., 2019).

Maternal and Fetal Outcomes

The mother's prognosis depends on the extent of placental detachment, overall blood loss, degree of coagulopathy present, and the time that passes between placental detachment and birth. Maternal complications are associated with the abruption or its treatment. Hemorrhage, hypovolemic shock, hypofibrinogenemia, and thrombocytopenia are associated with severe abruption. Renal failure and pituitary necrosis may result from ischemia. In rare cases, women who are Rh negative can become sensitized if fetal-to-maternal hemorrhage occurs and the fetal blood type is Rh positive.

Fetal complications, which include IUGR, oligohydramnios, preterm birth, hypoxemia, and stillbirth, are related to the severity and timing of the hemorrhage. Fetal survival is related to the size of the hemorrhage. Large (>60 mL) retroplacental hemorrhages have been associated with a fetal mortality rate of 50% or greater (Francois & Foley, 2017). Neonatal deaths are also common following placental abruption. Morbidity, including cerebral palsy, is common in surviving infants. Some authorities believe that adverse neurodevelopmental outcomes are more related to preterm birth than to placental abruption (Cunningham et al., 2018).

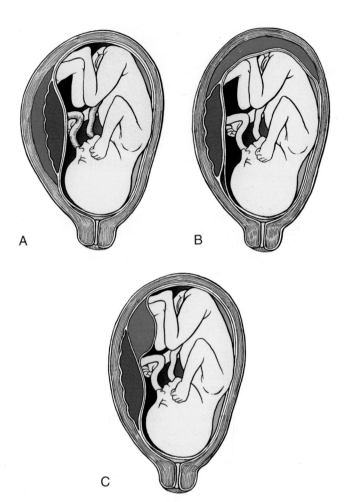

Fig. 28.10 The Classification System of Placental Abruption. (A) Retroplacental abruption. The bright red area represents a blood collection behind the placenta *(dark red)*. (B) Subchorionic abruption. The bright red area represents subchorionic bleeding, which is observed to dissect along the chorion. (C) Preplacental abruption. The bright red area represents a blood collection anterior to the placenta within the amnion and chorion (subamniotic). (From Gabbe, S. G., Niebyl, J. R., Simpson, J. L., et al. [Eds.]. [2017]. *Obstetrics: Normal and problem pregnancies* [7th ed.]. Philadelphia: Elsevier.)

Diagnosis

Placental abruption is primarily a clinical diagnosis. Although ultrasound can be used to rule out placenta previa, it cannot detect all cases of abruption. A retroplacental mass may be detected with ultrasonographic examination, but negative findings do not rule out a life-threatening abruption. In fact, at least 50% of abruptions cannot be identified on ultrasound (Hull et al., 2019). Recent advances in imaging and interpretation have improved detection of placental abruption using ultrasound. Ultrasound can identify three main sources of abruption: *subchorionic* (between the placenta and the membranes), *retroplacental* (between the placenta and the uterine wall), and *preplacental* (between the placenta and the amniotic fluid) (see Figs. 28.9 and 28.10). The location of the placental abruption is clinically significant. Retroplacental hematomas are associated with a worse fetal prognosis than is subchorionic hemorrhage (Francois & Foley, 2017). The diagnosis of abruption is confirmed after birth by visual inspection of the placenta. Adherent clot on the maternal surface of the placenta and depression of the underlying placental surface are usually present (see Fig. 28.9) (Francois & Foley).

Placental abruption should be highly suspected in the woman who experiences a sudden onset of intense, usually localized, uterine pain, with or without vaginal bleeding. Initial assessment is much the same as for placenta previa. Physical examination usually reveals abdominal pain, uterine tenderness, and contractions. The fundal height may be measured over time because an increasing fundal height indicates concealed bleeding. Approximately 60% of live fetuses exhibit abnormal FHR patterns, and elevated uterine resting tone may also be noted on the monitor tracing (Francois & Foley, 2017). Coagulopathy, as evidenced by abnormal clotting studies, may be present if a large or complete abruption has occurred.

CARE MANAGEMENT

Expectant Management

Management depends on the severity of blood loss and fetal maturity and status. If the fetus is between 20 and 34 weeks of gestation and both the woman and fetus are stable, expectant management can be implemented. The woman is monitored closely because the abruption may extend at any time. The fetus is assessed regularly for evidence of appropriate growth because there is risk for IUGR. In addition, assessments of fetal well-being (e.g., nonstress testing, biophysical profile) are performed regularly. See Chapter 26 for further discussion of these tests. Corticosteroids are given to accelerate fetal lung maturity (Hull et al., 2019).

Active Management

Immediate birth is the management of choice if the fetus is at term gestation or the bleeding is moderate to severe and the mother or fetus is in jeopardy. At least one large-bore (16- to 18-gauge) IV line should be inserted. Maternal vital signs are monitored frequently to observe for signs of declining hemodynamic status, such as increasing pulse rate and decreasing blood pressure. Serial laboratory studies include hematocrit or hemoglobin determinations and clotting studies. Continuous EFM is mandatory. An indwelling catheter is inserted for continuous assessment of urine output, an excellent indirect measure of maternal organ perfusion. Fluid volume replacement may be necessary, along with administration of blood products to correct any coagulation defects.

Although vaginal birth is usually preferable, cesarean birth may become necessary. Cesarean birth should not be attempted when the woman has severe and uncorrected coagulopathy because it can result in uncontrollable bleeding (Francois & Foley, 2017).

Nursing care of women experiencing moderate to severe abruption is demanding because it requires constant close monitoring of the maternal and fetal condition. Information about placental abruption, including the cause, treatment, and expected outcome, is given to the woman and her family. Emotional support is also extremely important because the woman and her family may be experiencing fetal loss and grief in addition to the woman's critical illness.

Cord Insertion and Placental Variations

When fetal vessels lie over the cervical os, the condition is termed vasa previa. In vasa previa the vessels are implanted into the fetal membranes rather than into the placenta. Usually these vessels are protected only by the membranes (not by Wharton jelly); thus they are at risk for rupture or compression (Hull et al., 2019). In the past, vasa previa was usually diagnosed after rupture of membranes occurred, followed by acute-onset vaginal bleeding caused by a lacerated fetal vessel. Currently, however, vasa previa is often diagnosed during pregnancy by ultrasound using color and pulsed Doppler imaging (Francois & Foley, 2017).

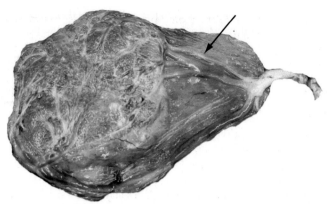

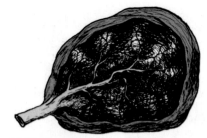

Fig. 28.13 Battledore (Marginal) Cord Insertion.

Fig. 28.11 Vasa Previa (Velamentous Insertion of Cord). Arrow shows velamentous cord insertion in the placenta. (From Resnik, R., Lockwood, C. J., Moore, T. R., et al. [Eds.]. [2019]. *Creasy & Resnik's maternal-fetal medicine: principles and practice* [8th ed.]. Philadelphia: Elsevier.)

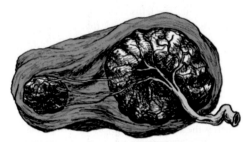

Fig. 28.12 Vasa Previa (Succenturiate Placenta).

Vasa previa is rare, affecting between 1 in 1275 and 1 in 8333 pregnancies (Hull et al., 2019). Risk factors for vasa previa include a history of second-trimester placenta previa or low-lying placenta, pregnancies resulting from assisted reproductive technology, and multiple gestations (Francois & Foley, 2017).

There are two variations of vasa previa. In both situations artificial or spontaneous rupture of the membranes or traction on the cord may rupture one or more of the fetal vessels. As a result, the fetus may rapidly bleed to death (Francois & Foley, 2017; Sosa, 2014).

One variation of vasa previa, *velamentous insertion of the cord*, occurs when the cord vessels begin to branch at the membranes and then course onto the placenta (Fig. 28.11). The other variant of vasa previa occurs when the placenta has divided into two or more lobes rather than remaining as a single mass. This is known as a *succenturiate* placenta (Fig. 28.12). Fetal vessels then run between the lobes of the placenta. The vessels collect at the periphery, and the main trunks eventually unite to form the vessels of the cord. During the third stage of labor one or more of the separate lobes may remain attached to the decidua basalis, preventing uterine contraction and increasing the risk for postpartum hemorrhage.

Another placental variation is *Battledore* (marginal) insertion of the cord (Fig. 28.13). This variation also increases the risk of fetal hemorrhage, especially after marginal separation of the placenta.

Clotting Disorders in Pregnancy
Normal Clotting
Normally a delicate balance (homeostasis) exists between the opposing hemostatic and fibrinolytic systems. The hemostatic system stops the flow of blood from injured vessels, first by a platelet plug, then by the formation of a fibrin clot. The coagulation process involves an interaction of the coagulation factors that constantly circulate in the

> **BOX 28.3**   **Common Causes of Disseminated Intravascular Coagulation in Pregnancy**
>
> - Placental abruption
> - Preeclampsia or eclampsia/HELLP syndrome
> - Amniotic fluid embolism
> - Postpartum hemorrhage
> - Sepsis
> - Acute fatty liver of pregnancy
> - Retained IUFD (delayed birth of a dead fetus)

HELLP syndrome, Hemolysis of red blood cells, elevated liver enzymes, low platelet count; *IUFD*, intrauterine fetal demise.
Data from Sisson, M. C., & Hamner, L. (2019). Disseminated intravascular coagulation in pregnancy. In N. H. Troiano, P. M. Witcher, & S. M. Baird (Eds.), *AWHONN's high risk and critical care obstetrics* (4th ed.). Philadelphia: Wolters Kluwer.

bloodstream, in which each factor sequentially activates the factor next in line (the "cascade effect" sequence). The fibrinolytic system is the process through which the fibrin clot is split into fibrinolytic degradation products and circulation is restored.

Clotting Problems
Disseminated intravascular coagulation. Disseminated intravascular coagulation (DIC), sometimes called *consumptive coagulopathy* or *defibrination syndrome*, is an acquired syndrome characterized by intravascular activation of coagulation which is widespread, rather than localized, and results in excessive clot formation and hemorrhage (Sisson & Hamner, 2019). DIC is never a primary diagnosis. Instead it results from some event that triggered coagulation. Current thought is that tissue factor, a glycoprotein found in body organs containing many blood vessels, such as the brain, lungs, and placenta, and in amniotic fluid, activates circulating clotting factors when it is released from damaged tissues. This eventually results in the widespread formation of fibrin clots within blood vessels (Cunningham et al., 2018; Sisson & Hamner).

In the obstetric population, DIC is most often triggered by the release of large amounts of tissue factor as a result of placental abruption (the most common cause of severe consumptive coagulopathy in obstetrics). Box 28.3 lists common causes of DIC in pregnancy. Clinical manifestations of and laboratory test results found in DIC are summarized in Box 28.4. Although bleeding is often the presenting sign of DIC, it is always preceded by clot formation (Sisson & Hamner, 2019).

🛈 CARE MANAGEMENT

Medical management in all cases of DIC involves correction of the underlying cause (e.g., removal of an abrupted placenta or the dead

BOX 28.4 Clinical Manifestations and Laboratory Results for Women With Disseminated Intravascular Coagulation

Common Physical Examination Findings

- Signs of thrombosis (e.g., peripheral cyanosis, renal impairment, drowsiness, confusion, coma, cardiorespiratory failure)
- Bleeding from at least 3 unrelated sites
- Spontaneous epistaxis (nosebleed)
- Oozing from venipuncture sites or other sites of trauma
- Petechiae (e.g., on the arm where blood pressure cuff was placed)
- Ecchymosis (bruising)
- Large subcutaneous hematomas
- Hypotension
- Tachycardia

Common Laboratory Coagulation Test Results

- Platelet count—decreased
- Fibrinogen—decreased
- Prothrombin time—prolonged
- Activated partial thromboplastin time—prolonged
- Fibrin degradation products (fibrin split products)—increased
- D-dimer test (specific fibrin degradation fragment)—increased

Data from Sisson, M. C., & Hamner, L. (2019). Disseminated intravascular coagulation in pregnancy. In N. H. Troiano, P. M. Witcher, & S. M. Baird (Eds.), *AWHONN's high risk and critical care obstetrics* (4th ed.). Philadelphia: Wolters Kluwer.

fetus or treatment of existing infection or preeclampsia/eclampsia). Volume expansion, rapid replacement of blood products and clotting factors, optimization of oxygenation, achievement of normal body temperature, and continued reassessment of laboratory parameters are the usual forms of treatment. Vitamin K administration, recombinant activated factor VIIa, fibrinogen concentrate, and hemostatic agents should be considered as additional therapies (Francois & Foley, 2017).

Nursing interventions include assessment for signs of bleeding (see Box 28.4) and complications from the administration of blood products, administering fluid or blood products as ordered, and protecting the woman from injury. Because renal failure is one consequence of DIC, urinary output is closely monitored by using an indwelling catheter. Urinary output must be maintained at more than 30 mL/h. Vital signs are assessed frequently. If DIC develops before birth, continuous EFM is necessary. The woman should be maintained in a side-lying tilt to maximize blood flow to the uterus. Oxygen may be administered through a nonrebreather face mask at 10 L/min or per hospital protocol or health care provider order. DIC usually is "cured" with the birth and as coagulation abnormalities resolve.

The woman and her family will be anxious and concerned about her condition and prognosis. The nurse offers explanations about care and provides emotional support to the woman and her family through this critical time.

KEY POINTS

- Vaginal bleeding during pregnancy should always be regarded as a warning sign and determining the cause is a priority.
- The cause of a miscarriage is often unknown; some of the known causes relate to maternal or fetal problems.
- The type of miscarriage and signs and symptoms direct care management.
- Cervical insufficiency may be treated with a cerclage placed cervically or sometimes abdominally; the woman is instructed to recognize the warning signs of preterm labor, preterm prelabor rupture of membranes, and infection.
- Ectopic pregnancy is a significant cause of maternal morbidity and mortality.

- Molar pregnancy (hydatidiform mole) is a gestational trophoblastic neoplasia (GTN). GTN is a group of pregnancy-related cancers without a viable fetus that are caused by abnormal fertilization.
- Placenta previa and placental abruption are differentiated by type of bleeding, uterine tonicity, and presence or absence of pain.
- Management of late-pregnancy bleeding requires immediate evaluation; care is based on diagnosed cause of the bleeding, gestational age, amount of bleeding, and fetal condition.
- DIC is characterized by widespread intravascular activation of coagulation which results in excessive clot formation and hemorrhage. It is never a primary diagnosis but always results from some event that triggered intravascular clotting.

REFERENCES

American College of Obstetricians and Gynecologists. (2018). Practice bulletin no. 193: Tubal ectopic pregnancy. *Obstetrics & Gynecology, 131*(3), e91–e103.

Cohn, D., Ramaswamy, B., Christian, B., & Bixel, K. (2019). Malignancy and pregnancy. In R. Resnik, C. J. Lockwood, T. R. Moore, et al. (Eds.), *Creasy & Resnik's maternal-fetal medicine: Principles and practice* (8th ed.). Philadelphia: Elsevier.

Cunningham, F., Leveno, K., Bloom, S., et al. (2018). *Williams obstetrics* (25th ed.). New York: McGraw-Hill Education.

Fields, L., & Hathaway, A. (2017). Key concepts in pregnancy of unknown location: Identifying ectopic pregnancy and providing patient-centered care. *Journal of Midwifery and Women's Health, 62*(2), 172–179.

Francois, K., & Foley, M. (2017). Antepartum and postpartum hemorrhage. In S. G. Gabbe, J. R. Niebyl, J. L. Simpson, et al. (Eds.), *Obstetrics: Normal and problem pregnancies* (7th ed.). Philadelphia: Elsevier.

Harper, L.M., Tita, A., & Karumanchi, S.A. (2019). Pregnancy-related hypertension. In R. Resnik, C.J. Lockwood, T.R. Moore, et al. (Eds), *Creasy & Resnik's maternal-fetal medicine: Principles and practice* (8th ed.). Philadelphia: Elsevier.

Hull, A. D., Resnik, R. & Silver, R. M. (2019). Placenta previa and accreta, vasa previa, subchorionic hemorrhage, and abruptio placentae. In R. Resnik, C. J. Lockwood, T. R. Moore, et al. (Eds.), *Creasy & Resnik's maternal-fetal medicine: Principles and practice* (8th ed.). Philadelphia: Elsevier.

Ludmir, J., Owen, J., & Berghella, V. (2017). Cervical insufficiency. In S. G. Gabbe, J. R. Niebyl, J. L. Simpson, et al. (Eds.), *Obstetrics: Normal and problem pregnancies* (7th ed.). Philadelphia: Elsevier.

Moore, T. R. (2019). Placenta and umbilical cord imaging. In R. Resnik, C. J. Lockwood, T. R. Moore, et al. (Eds.), *Creasy & Resnik's maternal-fetal medicine: Principles and practice* (8th ed.). Philadelphia: Elsevier.

Nader, S. (2019). Thyroid disease and pregnancy. In R. Resnik, C. J. Lockwood, T. R. Moore, et al. (Eds.), *Creasy & Resnik's maternal-fetal medicine: Principles and practice* (8th ed.). Philadelphia: Elsevier.

National Institute for Occupational Safety and Health. (2016). NIOSH list of antineoplastic and other hazardous drugs in healthcare settings. Retrieved from: www.ced.gov/niosh/topics/hazdrug.

Salani, R., & Copeland, L. J. (2017). Malignant diseases and pregnancy. In S. G. Gabbe, J. R. Niebyl, J. L. Simpson, et al. (Eds.), *Obstetrics: Normal and problem pregnancies* (7th ed.). Philadelphia: Elsevier.

Simhan, H. N., Berghella, V., & Iams, J. D. (2019) Prevention and management of preterm parturition. In R. Resnik, C. J. Lockwood, T. R. Moore, et al. (Eds.), *Creasy & Resnik's maternal-fetal medicine: Principles and practice* (8th ed.). Philadelphia: Elsevier.

Simpson, J. L., & Jauniaux, E. R. M. (2017). Early pregnancy loss and stillbirth. In S. G. Gabbe, J. R. Niebyl, J. L. Simpson, et al. (Eds.), *Obstetrics: Normal and problem pregnancies* (7th ed.). Philadelphia: Elsevier.

Sisson, M. C., & Hamner, L. (2019). Disseminated intravascular coagulation in pregnancy. In N. H. Troiano, P. M. Witcher, & S. M. Baird (Eds.), *AWHONN's high risk and critical care obstetrics* (4th ed.). Philadelphia: Wolters Kluwer.

Sosa, M. E. B. (2014). Bleeding in pregnancy. In K. R. Simpson, & P. Creehan (Eds.), *AWHONN's perinatal nursing* (4th ed.). Philadelphia: Lippincott Williams & Wilkins.

Weant, K. A., Bailey, A. M., Baum, R. A., et al. (2017). Chemotherapy in the emergency department? There is a role for that: Methotrexate for ectopic pregnancy. *Advanced Emergency Nursing Journal, 39*(1), 18–25.

Williams, Z., & Scott, J. R. (2019). Recurrent pregnancy loss. In R. Resnik, C.J. Lockwood, T. R. Moore, et al. (Eds.), *Creasy & Resnik's maternal-fetal medicine: Principles and practice* (8th ed.). Philadelphia: Elsevier.

29

Endocrine and Metabolic Disorders

Deborah R. Bambini

http://evolve.elsevier.com/Lowdermilk/MWHC/

LEARNING OBJECTIVES

- Describe normal changes in metabolic pathways during pregnancy.
- Differentiate the types of diabetes mellitus and their respective risk factors in pregnancy.
- Compare insulin requirements during pregnancy, postpartum, and with lactation.
- Identify maternal and fetal risks or complications associated with diabetes in pregnancy.
- Develop a plan of care for the pregnant woman with pregestational or gestational diabetes.

- Explain the effects of hyperemesis gravidarum on maternal and fetal well-being.
- Discuss management of the woman with hyperemesis gravidarum.
- Explain the effects of thyroid disorders on pregnancy.
- Compare the management of a pregnant woman with hyperthyroidism with one who has hypothyroidism.
- Discuss care management for the woman with phenylketonuria during the perinatal period.
- Examine the effects of maternal phenylketonuria on pregnancy outcome.

Pregnancy is naturally a state of endocrine upheaval. The normal changes that occur in the endocrine and metabolic systems during pregnancy present a challenge for healthy women. For women with an endocrine or metabolic disorder, the ability to adapt to the normal changes is compromised. This chapter reviews normal endocrine changes, as well as what happens when adaptation is compromised by specific endocrine or metabolic disorders, including diabetes mellitus, hyperemesis gravidarum, hyperthyroidism, hypothyroidism, and phenylketonuria (PKU). The primary care objective is to promote optimal outcomes for both the pregnant woman and the fetus. This requires the active participation of well-motivated women in the treatment plan and careful management by an interprofessional health care team.

METABOLIC CHANGES ASSOCIATED WITH PREGNANCY

Normal pregnancy is characterized by complex alterations in maternal glucose metabolism, insulin production, and metabolic homeostasis. During normal pregnancy, adjustments in maternal metabolism allow for adequate nutrition for the mother and the developing fetus. Glucose, the primary fuel used by the fetus, is transported across the placenta through the process of carrier-mediated facilitated diffusion, meaning that the glucose levels in the fetus are directly proportional to maternal levels. Although glucose crosses the placenta, insulin does not. During the first trimester of pregnancy the pregnant woman's metabolic status is significantly influenced by the rising levels of estrogen and progesterone. These hormones stimulate the β cells in the pancreas to increase insulin production, which promotes increased peripheral use of glucose and decreased blood glucose, with fasting levels being reduced by approximately 10% (Fig. 29.1A). At the same time, an increase in tissue glycogen stores and a decrease in hepatic glucose production occur, which further encourage lower fasting glucose levels. As a result of these

normal metabolic changes of pregnancy, women with insulin-dependent diabetes are prone to hypoglycemia during the first trimester.

During the second and third trimesters, pregnancy exerts a "diabetogenic" effect on the maternal metabolic status. Because of the major hormonal changes, decreased tolerance to glucose, increased insulin resistance, decreased hepatic glycogen stores, and increased hepatic production of glucose occur. Rising levels of human chorionic somatomammotropin, estrogen, progesterone, prolactin, cortisol, and insulinase increase insulin resistance through their actions as insulin antagonists. Insulin resistance is a glucose-sparing mechanism that ensures an abundant supply of glucose for the fetus. Maternal insulin requirements gradually increase from approximately 18 to 24 weeks of gestation to approximately 36 weeks of gestation. Maternal insulin requirements may double or quadruple by the end of the pregnancy (see Fig. 29.1B and C).

At birth, expulsion of the placenta prompts an abrupt drop in levels of circulating placental hormones, cortisol, and insulinase (see Fig. 29.1D). Maternal tissues quickly regain their prepregnancy sensitivity to insulin. For the nonbreastfeeding mother, the prepregnancy insulin-carbohydrate balance usually returns in approximately 7 to 10 days (see Fig. 29.1E). Lactation uses maternal glucose; therefore the breastfeeding mother's insulin requirements remain lower during lactation. On completion of weaning, the mother's prepregnancy insulin requirement is reestablished (see Fig. 29.1F).

DIABETES MELLITUS

The worldwide incidence of diabetes mellitus is growing at a rapid rate, mostly because of increases in overweight, obesity, and physical inactivity. An estimated 422 million people are currently diabetic (World Health Organization [WHO], 2017). In 2017 an estimated 30.3 million people in the United States (9.4% of the total population) had diabetes.

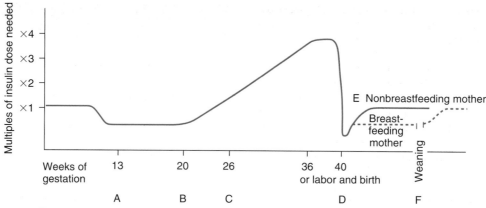

Fig. 29.1 Changing Insulin Needs During Pregnancy. *A,* First trimester: Insulin need is reduced because of increased insulin production by pancreas and increased peripheral sensitivity to insulin; nausea, vomiting, and decreased food intake by mother and glucose transfer to embryo or fetus contribute to hypoglycemia. *B,* Second trimester: Insulin needs begin to increase as placental hormones, cortisol, and insulinase act as insulin antagonists, decreasing insulin's effectiveness. *C,* Third trimester: Insulin needs may double or even quadruple but usually level off after 36 weeks of gestation. *D,* Day of birth: Maternal insulin requirements decrease dramatically to approach prepregnancy levels. *E,* Breastfeeding mother maintains lower insulin requirements, as much as 25% less than those of prepregnancy; insulin needs of nonbreastfeeding mother return to prepregnancy levels in 7 to 10 days. *F,* Weaning of breastfeeding infant causes mother's insulin needs to return to prepregnancy levels.

Of these, 7.2 million were undiagnosed (Centers for Disease Control and Prevention [CDC], 2017). If this trend continues, it is predicted that by 2050 as many as one in three adults in the United States will have diabetes. The prevalence of diabetes among women of childbearing age is increasing in the United States, which will greatly affect the care of mothers and children for years to come (Moore, Hauguel-DeMouzon, & Catalano, 2019).

It is estimated that diabetes complicates as many as 6% to 7% of pregnancies. Although 90% of women with diabetes during pregnancy have gestational diabetes, the number of pregnant women who have type 1 or type 2 diabetes is growing (American Diabetes Association [ADA], 2018; Landon, Catalano, & Gabbe, 2017; Moore et al., 2019). The perinatal mortality rate for well-managed pregnancies complicated by diabetes, excluding major congenital malformations, is approximately the same as for any other pregnancy. The key to an optimal pregnancy outcome is strict maternal glucose control before conception and throughout the gestational period (Landon et al., 2017). Consequently, for women with diabetes, much emphasis is placed on preconception counseling.

Pregnancy complicated by diabetes is considered high risk. It is most successfully managed by an interprofessional team approach involving the obstetrician, perinatologist, internist or endocrinologist, ophthalmologist, nephrologist, neonatologist, nurse, nutritionist or dietitian, and social worker. A favorable outcome also requires commitment and active participation by the pregnant woman and her family.

Pathogenesis

Diabetes mellitus refers to a group of metabolic diseases characterized by hyperglycemia resulting from defects in insulin secretion, insulin action, or both (ADA, 2017). Insulin, produced by the β cells in the islets of Langerhans in the pancreas, regulates blood glucose levels by enabling glucose to enter adipose and muscle cells, where it is used for energy. When insulin is insufficient or ineffective in promoting glucose uptake by the muscle and adipose cells, glucose accumulates in the bloodstream, and hyperglycemia results. Hyperglycemia causes hyperosmolarity of the blood, which attracts intracellular fluid into the vascular system, resulting in cellular dehydration and expanded blood volume. Consequently, the kidneys function to excrete large volumes

of urine (polyuria) in an attempt to regulate excess vascular volume and to excrete the unusable glucose (glycosuria). Polyuria, along with cellular dehydration, causes excessive thirst (polydipsia).

The body compensates for its inability to convert carbohydrate (glucose) into energy by burning proteins (muscle) and fats. However, the end products of this metabolism are ketones and fatty acids, which, in excess quantities, produce ketoacidosis and acetonuria. Weight loss occurs as a result of the breakdown of fat and muscle tissue. This tissue breakdown causes a state of starvation that compels the individual to eat excessive amounts of food (polyphagia).

Over time, diabetes causes significant changes in the microvascular and macrovascular circulations. These structural changes affect a variety of organ systems, particularly the heart, eyes, kidneys, and nerves. Complications resulting from diabetes include premature atherosclerosis, retinopathy, nephropathy, and neuropathy.

Diabetes may be caused either by impaired insulin secretion, when the β cells of the pancreas are destroyed by an autoimmune process, or by inadequate insulin action in target tissues at one or more points along the metabolic pathway. Both of these conditions are commonly present in the same person, and determining which, if either, abnormality is the primary cause of the disease is difficult (ADA, 2017). For additional information on diabetes, visit the ADA's website at www.diabetes.org.

Classification of Diabetes Mellitus

The current classification system includes four groups: type 1 diabetes, type 2 diabetes, other specific types (e.g., diabetes caused by genetic defects in β cell function or insulin action, disease or injury of the pancreas, or drug-induced diabetes), and gestational diabetes mellitus (GDM) (ADA, 2018; Moore et al., 2019). *Pregestational diabetes mellitus* is the label sometimes given to type 1 or type 2 diabetes that existed before pregnancy.

Type 1 accounts for 5% to 10% of all diabetes and includes cases that are caused primarily by pancreatic islet β-cell destruction and that are prone to ketoacidosis. People with type 1 diabetes usually have an abrupt onset of illness at a young age and an absolute insulin deficiency. Type 1 diabetes includes cases thought to be caused by an autoimmune process and those for which the cause is unknown (ADA, 2017; Landon et al., 2017).

Type 2 is the most prevalent form of the disease, accounting for 90% to 95% of all diabetes, and includes individuals who have insulin resistance and usually relative (rather than absolute) insulin deficiency (ADA, 2017). Although type 2 diabetes was once believed to affect mostly older individuals, increasing numbers of children and adolescents have been diagnosed with the disorder since the early 1990s (Moore et al., 2019). Specific causes of type 2 diabetes are unknown at this time. It often goes undiagnosed for years because hyperglycemia develops gradually and is often not severe enough for the person to recognize the classic signs of polyuria, polydipsia, and polyphagia. Most people who develop type 2 diabetes are obese or have an increased amount of body fat distributed primarily in the abdominal area. Other risk factors for the development of type 2 diabetes include aging, a sedentary lifestyle, family history and genetics, puberty, hypertension, and prior gestational diabetes. Type 2 diabetes often has a strong genetic predisposition (ADA, 2017; Moore et al.).

Gestational diabetes mellitus is defined as carbohydrate intolerance with the onset or first recognition occurring during pregnancy (American College of Obstetricians and Gynecologists [ACOG], 2018a). This definition is appropriate whether or not management includes medication in addition to dietary changes or the diabetes persists after pregnancy. It does not exclude the possibility that the glucose intolerance preceded the pregnancy or that medication might be required for optimal glucose control (Landon et al., 2017). The ADA has adopted a new definition for gestational diabetes that excludes women with preexisting diabetes (type 1 or type 2) that is diagnosed during pregnancy. This definition for GDM is simply diabetes diagnosed during pregnancy that is clearly not overt (preexisting) diabetes (ADA, 2017).

Classification of Diabetes in Pregnancy

Dr. Priscilla White, a physician who worked with pregnant women with diabetes during the 1940s, developed a system specifically to further classify diabetes in pregnant women (Table 29.1). White's system was based on age at diagnosis, duration of illness, and presence of end-organ, especially eye and kidney, involvement (Landon et al., 2017; Moore et al., 2019). Her classification system has been modified through the years, changing her original definitions and adding increasing complexity (Bennett, Tita, Owen, et al., 2015). However, it is still frequently used to assess maternal and fetal risk.

A new system has since been developed by the ADA that further classifies type 1 and type 2 diabetes as (a) without vascular complications and (b) with vascular complications that are specified. This distinction is important because perinatal risk increases with vascular complications regardless of the duration of illness. Only women whose glucose intolerance was diagnosed during pregnancy but who do not meet the criteria defining type 1 or type 2 diabetes are included in the gestational diabetes category. It has been suggested that White's modified classification system be replaced by the new ADA system in clinical practice (ADA, 2018).

PREGESTATIONAL DIABETES MELLITUS AND PREGNANCY

Only approximately 10% of pregnancies complicated by diabetes occur in women who have preexisting disease (Landon et al., 2017). Women who have pregestational diabetes mellitus can have either type 1 or 2 diabetes, which may be complicated by vascular disease, retinopathy, nephropathy, or other diabetic complications. Type 2 is a more common diagnosis than type 1. Almost all women with pregestational diabetes are insulin dependent during pregnancy. According to White's classification system, these women fall into classes B through T (see Table 29.1).

The diabetogenic state of pregnancy imposed on the compromised metabolic system of the woman with pregestational diabetes has

TABLE 29.1	White's Classification of Diabetes in Pregnancy
Gestational Diabetes	
Class A₁	Woman has two or more abnormal values on OGTT but her fasting and postprandial glucose values are diet controlled.
Class A₂	Woman was not known to have diabetes before pregnancy but requires either insulin or oral hypoglycemic medication for blood glucose control.
Pregestational Diabetes	
Class B	Onset of disease occurs after 20 years of age, and duration of illness is <10 years.
Class C	Onset of disease occurs between 10 and 19 years of age, duration of illness is 10-19 years, or both.
Class D	Onset of disease occurs before 10 years of age, duration of illness is >20 years, or both.
Class F	Woman has developed diabetic nephropathy.
Class R	Woman has developed retinitis proliferans.
Class T	Woman has had a renal transplant.

OGTT, Oral glucose tolerance test.
Data from Landon, M. B., Catalano, P. M., & Gabbe, S. G. (2017). Diabetes mellitus complicating pregnancy. In S. G. Gabbe, J. R. Niebyl, J. L. Simpson, et al. (Eds.), *Obstetrics: Normal and problem pregnancies* (7th ed.). Philadelphia: Elsevier; and Moore, T. R., Hauguel-deMouzon, S., & Catalano, P. (2019). Diabetes in pregnancy. In R. Resnik, C. J. Lockwood, T. R. Moore, et al. (Eds.), *Creasy & Resnik's maternal-fetal medicine: Principles and practice* (8th ed.). Philadelphia: Elsevier.

significant implications. The normal hormonal adaptations of pregnancy affect glycemic control, and pregnancy may accelerate the progress of vascular complications.

During the first trimester, when maternal blood glucose levels are normally reduced and the insulin response to glucose is enhanced, glycemic control may be improved. The insulin dose for the woman with well-controlled diabetes may have to be reduced to prevent hypoglycemia. Nausea, vomiting, and cravings typical of early pregnancy result in dietary fluctuations that influence maternal glucose levels and may necessitate a reduction in the insulin dose.

Because insulin requirements steadily increase after the first trimester, the insulin dose must be adjusted accordingly to prevent hyperglycemia. Insulin resistance begins as early as 14 to 16 weeks of gestation and continues to rise until it stabilizes during the last few weeks of pregnancy.

Preconception Counseling

Preconception counseling is recommended for all women of reproductive age who have diabetes, because it is associated with less perinatal morbidity and mortality and fewer congenital anomalies (Landon et al., 2017; Moore et al., 2019). Under ideal circumstances, women with pregestational diabetes are counseled before the time of conception to plan the optimal time for pregnancy, establish glycemic control before conception, and diagnose any vascular complications of diabetes. However, estimates indicate that in the United States fewer than 20% of women with diabetes participate in preconception counseling (Landon et al.).

The woman's partner should be included in the counseling to assess the couple's level of understanding related to the effects of pregnancy on the diabetic condition and the potential complications of pregnancy as a result of diabetes. The couple should also be informed of the anticipated alterations in management of diabetes during pregnancy and the need for an interprofessional team approach to health care. Financial implications of diabetic pregnancy and other demands related to frequent maternal and fetal surveillance should be discussed. In addition, medications the woman is currently taking must be assessed for safety during pregnancy. Medications that carry risk for adverse maternal or fetal outcomes should be changed to ones that are safer but equally effective. Preconception counseling should also include discussion of microvascular and macrovascular complications that carry significant risk for maternal morbidity and mortality during pregnancy such as coronary artery disease and renal insufficiency. Rarely, renal transplantation may be necessary prior to conception. Contraception is another important aspect of preconception counseling to assist the couple in planning effectively for pregnancy. They should be encouraged to use reliable contraception until glycemic control is optimal.

Maternal Risks and Complications

Although maternal morbidity and mortality rates have improved significantly, the pregnant woman with diabetes remains at risk for the development of complications during pregnancy. Poor glycemic control around the time of conception and in the early weeks of pregnancy is associated with an increased incidence of miscarriage. However, women with excellent glycemic control before conception and in the first trimester are no more likely to miscarry than women who do not have diabetes (Moore et al., 2019).

Poor glycemic control later in pregnancy, particularly in women without vascular disease, increases the rate of fetal macrosomia. Macrosomia has been defined as a birthweight more than 4000 to 4500 g or greater than the 90th percentile. It occurs in approximately 40% of pregestational diabetic pregnancies and up to 50% of pregnancies complicated by GDM (Landon et al., 2017). Infants born to women with diabetes tend to have a disproportionate increase in shoulder, trunk, and chest size. Because of this tendency the risk for shoulder dystocia is greater in these babies than in other macrosomic infants. Therefore women with diabetes face an increased likelihood of cesarean birth because of failure of fetal descent or labor progress or of operative vaginal birth (birth involving the use of episiotomy, forceps, or vacuum extractor) (Moore et al., 2019).

Women with preexisting diabetes are at risk for several obstetric and medical complications, including hypertension, preeclampsia, cesarean birth, preterm birth, and maternal mortality. In general, the risk of developing these complications increases with the duration and severity of the woman's diabetes. For example, more than one-third of women who have had diabetes for more than 20 years develop preeclampsia. Women with nephropathy and hypertension in addition to diabetes are also increasingly likely to develop preeclampsia. Poor glycemic control at the beginning of pregnancy is also related to the development of preeclampsia. The rate of hypertensive disorders in all types of pregnancies complicated by diabetes is 15% to 30%. Chronic hypertension occurs in 10% to 20% of all pregnant women with diabetes and in up to 40% of women who have preexisting renal or retinal vascular disease (Moore et al., 2019).

Hydramnios (polyhydramnios) frequently develops during the third trimester of pregnancy in women with diabetes. Its cause is unknown. One theory is that hydramnios in women with diabetes is caused by an increased glucose concentration in amniotic fluid resulting from maternal and fetal hyperglycemia, which induces fetal polyuria. The complications most frequently associated with hydramnios (defined as an amniotic fluid index [AFI] > 24 cm) are placental abruption, uterine dysfunction, and postpartum hemorrhage (Cunningham, Leveno, Bloom, et al., 2018).

Infections are more common and more serious in pregnant women with diabetes than in those without the disease. Disorders of carbohydrate metabolism alter the normal resistance of the body to infection. The inflammatory response, leukocyte function, and vaginal pH are all affected. Vaginal infections, particularly monilial vaginitis, are more common. Urinary tract infections (UTIs) are also more prevalent. Infection is serious because it causes increased insulin resistance and may result in ketoacidosis.

Ketoacidosis (accumulation of ketones in the blood resulting from hyperglycemia and leading to metabolic acidosis) occurs most often during the second and third trimesters, when the diabetogenic effect of pregnancy is greatest. When the maternal metabolism is stressed by illness or infection, the woman is at increased risk for diabetic ketoacidosis (DKA). DKA can also be caused by poor compliance with treatment or the onset of previously undiagnosed diabetes (Moore et al., 2019). The use of β-mimetic drugs such as terbutaline (Brethine) for tocolysis to treat preterm labor or corticosteroids given to enhance fetal lung maturation may also contribute to the risk for hyperglycemia and subsequent DKA (Mercer, 2019; Simhan, Berghella, & Iams, 2019).

DKA may occur with blood glucose levels barely exceeding 200 mg/dL, compared with 300 to 350 mg/dL in the nonpregnant state. During times of stress, such as infection or illness, stress hormones cause an increase in hepatic glucose production and decreased peripheral uptake of glucose, leading to hyperglycemia (a greater than normal amount of glucose in the blood). Fatty acids are mobilized into the circulation from fat stores in an attempt to meet the needs for energy for the cells. As the fatty acids are oxidized, ketone bodies are released into the peripheral circulation. The woman's buffering system is unable to compensate, and metabolic acidosis develops. The excessive blood glucose and ketone bodies result in osmotic diuresis with subsequent loss of fluid and electrolytes, volume depletion, and cellular dehydration. DKA is a medical emergency. Prompt treatment is necessary to prevent maternal coma or death. Ketoacidosis occurring at any time during pregnancy can lead to intrauterine fetal death. The incidence of DKA has decreased in recent years because of advances in clinical management and blood glucose monitoring. Currently it affects only approximately 1% to 2% of pregnant women with diabetes. The rate of intrauterine fetal demise (IUFD) with DKA, formerly approximately 35%, is 10% or less (Moore et al., 2019) (Table 29.2).

The risk for hypoglycemia (a less than normal amount of glucose in the blood) is also increased during pregnancy. Early in pregnancy, when hepatic production of glucose is diminished and peripheral use of glucose is enhanced, hypoglycemia occurs frequently, often during sleep. Later in pregnancy it may also result as insulin doses are adjusted to maintain euglycemia (a normal blood glucose level). Women with a prepregnancy history of severe hypoglycemia are at increased risk for severe hypoglycemia during gestation. Mild-to-moderate hypoglycemic episodes do not appear to have significant damaging effects on fetal well-being (see Table 29.2).

Fetal and Neonatal Risks and Complications

From the moment of conception, the infant of a woman with diabetes faces an increased risk of complications that may occur during the antepartum, intrapartum, or neonatal periods. Infant morbidity and mortality rates associated with diabetic pregnancy are significantly reduced with strict control of maternal glucose levels before and during pregnancy.

Despite improvements in the care of pregnant women with diabetes, the perinatal mortality rate is three times higher for women with diabetes than for women who do not have this disease. Miscarriage rates for women with preexisting diabetes are as high as 30%. Major causes of perinatal mortality are congenital malformations, respiratory distress syndrome, and extreme prematurity. IUFD (sometimes called *stillbirth*) remains a major concern. Approximately 4% of all stillbirths occur in women whose pregnancies are complicated by preexisting diabetes. Poor glycemic control is the most consistent finding in women who had a stillbirth. In addition to hyperglycemia, other causes of stillbirth include

TABLE 29.2 Differentiation of Hypoglycemia (Insulin Shock) and Hyperglycemia (Diabetic Ketoacidosis)

Causes	Onset	Symptoms	Interventions
Hypoglycemia (Insulin Shock)			
Excess insulin	Rapid (regular insulin)	Irritability	Check blood glucose level when symptoms first appear.
Insufficient food (delayed or missed meals)	Gradual (modified insulin or oral hypoglycemic agents)	Hunger	If blood glucose is <70 mg/dL, eat 2-4 glucose tablets or gel (8-16 g carbohydrate) immediately.
Excessive exercise or work		Sweating	Recheck blood glucose level in 15 min. If glucose level is still <70 mg/dL, eat 2-4 additional glucose tablets.
Indigestion, diarrhea, vomiting		Nervousness	Recheck blood glucose level in 15 min. If glucose level is still <70 mg/dL, notify health care provider immediately.
		Personality change	
		Weakness	
		Fatigue	If woman is unconscious, administer 50% dextrose IV push, 5%–10% dextrose in water IV drip, or 1 mg glucagon intramuscularly.
		Blurred or double vision	
		Dizziness	Obtain blood and urine specimens for laboratory testing.
		Headache	
		Pallor; clammy skin	
		Shallow respirations	
		Rapid pulse	
		Laboratory values	
		Urine: negative for sugar and acetone	
		Blood glucose: <70 mg/dL	
Hyperglycemia (DKA)			
Insufficient insulin	Slow (hours to days)	Thirst	Notify primary health care provider.
Excess or wrong kind of food		Nausea or vomiting	Administer insulin in accordance with blood glucose levels.
Infection, injuries, illness		Abdominal pain	Give IV fluids such as normal saline solution or one-half normal saline solution; potassium when urinary output is adequate; bicarbonate for pH < 7.
Emotional stress		Constipation	
Insufficient exercise		Drowsiness	Monitor laboratory testing of blood and urine.
		Dim vision	
		Increased urination	
		Headache	
		Flushed, dry skin	
		Rapid breathing	
		Weak, rapid pulse	
		Acetone (fruity) breath odor	
		Laboratory values	
		Urine: positive for sugar and acetone	
		Blood glucose: >200 mg/dL	

DKA, Diabetic ketoacidosis; *IV,* intravenous.

congenital abnormalities, placental insufficiency or fetal growth restriction, macrosomia or polyhydramnios, or obstructed labor (intrapartum stillbirth) (Inturrisi, 2017; Reddy & Silver, 2019).

Hyperglycemia during the first trimester of pregnancy, when organs and organ systems are forming, is the main cause of diabetes-associated birth defects. Anomalies commonly seen in infants born to women with diabetes affect primarily the cardiovascular system and the central nervous system (CNS) (Inturrisi, 2017; Moore et al., 2019).

The fetal pancreas begins to secrete insulin at 10 to 14 weeks of gestation. The fetus responds to maternal hyperglycemia by secreting large amounts of insulin (hyperinsulinism). Insulin acts as a growth hormone, causing the fetus to produce excess stores of glycogen, protein, and adipose tissue and leading to increased fetal size, or macrosomia. Birth injuries are more common in infants born to mothers with diabetes compared with mothers who do not have diabetes, and macrosomic fetuses have the highest risk for this complication (Inturrisi, 2017; Moore et al., 2019). Common birth injuries associated with diabetic pregnancies include brachial plexus palsy, facial nerve injury, humerus or clavicle fracture, and cephalhematoma. Most of these injuries are associated with difficult vaginal birth and shoulder dystocia (Moore et al.).

Hypoglycemia at birth is also a risk for infants born to mothers with diabetes (for further discussion of neonatal complications related to maternal diabetes, see Chapter 35).

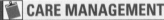 **CARE MANAGEMENT**

Assessment

When a pregnant woman with diabetes initiates prenatal care, a thorough evaluation of her health status is completed. At the initial visit a complete physical examination is performed. In addition to the routine prenatal examination, specific efforts are made to assess for acute and chronic complications of diabetes (Daley, 2014), especially retinopathy, nephropathy, peripheral and autonomic neuropathy, and peripheral vascular and cardiac involvement.

Routine prenatal laboratory tests are performed, and baseline renal function may be assessed with a 24-hour urine collection for total protein excretion and creatinine clearance. Urinalysis and culture are performed to assess for the presence of a UTI, which is common in diabetic pregnancy. Because of the risk for coexisting thyroid disease, thyroid function tests may also be performed (see later discussion of thyroid disorders). The **glycosylated hemoglobin A1c** level may be measured to assess recent glycemic control.

With prolonged hyperglycemia, some of the hemoglobin remains saturated with glucose for the life of the red blood cell (RBC). Therefore a test for glycosylated hemoglobin provides a "diabetic report card," an evaluation of past glycemic control. Because RBCs turn over more rapidly during pregnancy, A1c levels are normally lower in pregnant women than in nonpregnant individuals. Therefore the estimation of glycemic control provided by the test applies to a shorter period of time, only the previous 2 to 6 weeks. Hemoglobin A1c levels less than 6 to 6.5 in early pregnancy have been associated with the lowest rates of adverse fetal outcomes (ADA, 2017; Inturrisi, 2017). Fasting blood glucose or random (1 to 2 hours after eating) glucose levels may be assessed during antepartum visits (Fig. 29.2).

> **! NURSING ALERT**
>
> Iron deficiency anemia falsely increases the A1c level (Inturrisi, 2017).

Client Problems

Problems often experienced by the woman with pregestational diabetes include the following:

- *Need for health teaching* related to
  - diabetic pregnancy, management, and potential effects on pregnant woman and fetus
  - insulin administration and its effects
  - hypoglycemia and hyperglycemia
  - diabetic diet
- *Anxiety, grieving, decreased ability to cope, decreased adherence, decreased self-esteem* related to
  - stigma of being labeled "diabetic"
  - effects of diabetes and its potential sequelae on the pregnant woman and the fetus
- *Potential for injury to fetus* related to
  - disruption of oxygen transfer from environment to fetus
  - birth trauma
- *Potential for injury to mother* related to
  - improper insulin administration
  - hypoglycemia and hyperglycemia
  - cesarean or operative vaginal birth
  - postpartum infection

Antepartum Care

Because of her high-risk status, a woman with pregestational diabetes is monitored much more frequently and thoroughly than other pregnant women. During the first and second trimesters of pregnancy, her routine prenatal care visits are scheduled every 1 to 2 weeks. In the last trimester she will likely be seen 1 or 2 times each week. In the past, routine hospitalization for management of the diabetes, such as for insulin dose changes, was common. With the availability of improved home glucose monitoring and the growing reluctance of third-party payers to reimburse for hospitalization, pregnant women with diabetes generally currently are managed as outpatients. Some client and family education and maternal and fetal assessment may be performed in the home, depending on the woman's insurance coverage and care provider preference.

Achieving and maintaining constant euglycemia is the primary goal of medical therapy. Blood glucose levels should be in the range of 60 to 105 mg/dL before meals and 140 mg/dL or less when measured 1 hour after a meal. Postmeal glucose levels at 2 hours should be no higher than 120 mg/dL (Landon et al., 2017) (Table 29.3). Euglycemia is achieved through a combination of diet, insulin, and exercise. Providing the woman with the knowledge, skill, and motivation she needs to achieve and maintain excellent blood glucose control is the primary nursing goal.

Achieving euglycemia requires commitment on the part of the woman and her family to make the necessary lifestyle changes, which can sometimes seem overwhelming. Maintaining tight blood glucose control necessitates that the woman follows a consistent daily schedule. She must get up, go to bed, eat, exercise, and take insulin at the same time each day. Blood glucose measurements are done frequently (6 to 8 times each day) to determine how well the major components of therapy (diet, insulin, and exercise) are working together to control blood glucose levels. The pregnant woman with diabetes should wear a medical identification bracelet at all times and carry insulin, syringes or pens, a blood glucose meter, and glucose tablets with her whenever she is away from home (see Community Focus: Accessibility of Diabetes Supplies).

TABLE 29.3 Target Blood Glucose Levels During Pregnancy	
Time of Day	**Target Plasma Glucose Level (mg/dL)**
Premeal or fasting	60-105
Postmeal (1 h)	<140
Postmeal (2 h)	≤120
2 a.m. to 6 a.m.	>60

Data from Landon, M. B., Catalano, P. M., & Gabbe, S. G. (2017). Diabetes mellitus complicating pregnancy. In S. G. Gabbe, J. R. Niebyl, J. L. Simpson, et al. (Eds.), *Obstetrics: Normal and problem pregnancies* (7th ed.). Philadelphia: Elsevier.

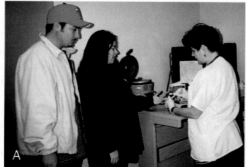 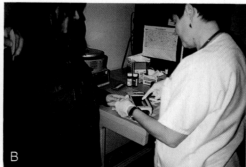

Fig. 29.2 Blood Glucose Monitoring. (A) Clinic nurse collects blood to determine glucose level. (B) Nurse interprets glucose value displayed by monitor. (Courtesy Dee Lowdermilk, UNC Ambulatory Care Clinics, Chapel Hill, NC.)

Accessibility of Diabetes Supplies

Visit your local pharmacy, and examine the diabetes equipment and supplies that are available. Locate glucose meters, urine test strips, insulin syringes, and insulin pens. How much does each of these items cost? Check to see which items are covered by most types of insurance and Medicaid. Read the instructions for use of each item. How easily could you follow the instructions? Could a woman with low literacy skills read and understand them? Do the instructions contain illustrations? Are the instructions written in more than one language (e.g., in Spanish or French) in addition to English? Does the pharmacy have someone who can teach women? How can you use the information you have obtained in this exercise in your client teaching?

Because the woman with pregestational diabetes is at increased risk for infections, eye problems, and neurologic changes, foot and general skin care are important. A daily bath that includes thorough perineal and foot care is important. For dry skin, lotions, creams, or oils can be applied. Tight clothing should be avoided. Shoes or slippers that fit properly should be worn at all times and are best worn with socks or stockings. Feet should be inspected regularly; toenails should be cut straight across, and professional help should be sought for any foot problems. Extremes of temperature should be avoided.

Diet

The woman with pregestational diabetes has usually had nutrition counseling regarding managing her diabetes. However, because pregnancy produces special nutritional concerns and needs, the woman must be educated to incorporate these changes into dietary planning. The woman who has "controlled" her diabetes for several years may find it difficult to adjust to the changes in her insulin and dietary needs mandated by pregnancy. Nutritional counseling is usually provided by a registered dietitian. Counseling should address general nutrition principles appropriate for all pregnant women as well as diabetes-specific nutritional needs.

Dietary management during diabetic pregnancy must be based on blood (not urine) glucose levels. The diet is individualized to allow for increased fetal and metabolic requirements, with consideration of such factors as prepregnancy weight and dietary habits, overall health, ethnic background, lifestyle, stage of pregnancy, knowledge of nutrition, and insulin therapy. The dietary goals are to provide weight gain consistent with a normal pregnancy, prevent ketoacidosis, and minimize wide fluctuation of blood glucose levels.

For women with a body mass index (BMI) of 22 to 27, dietary counseling includes advice to consume approximately 35 kcal/kg of ideal body weight per day. In contrast, obese women with a BMI of 30 or greater may be managed with a caloric intake as low as 15 kcal/kg of actual weight per day (Landon et al., 2017). The average diet includes 2200 calories (first trimester) to 2500 calories (second and third trimesters). Total calories are best distributed among three meals and three snacks. Meals should be eaten on time and never skipped. Going more than 4 hours without food intake increases the risk for episodes of hypoglycemia. Snacks must be planned carefully in accordance with insulin therapy to prevent fluctuations in blood glucose levels. A large bedtime snack of at least 25 g of complex carbohydrate with some protein or fat is recommended to help prevent hypoglycemia and starvation ketosis during the night (Moore et al., 2019).

The ideal diet is composed of 40% to 60% complex high-fiber carbohydrates, 20% protein, and 30% to 40% fat, with less than 10% as saturated fat (Landon et al., 2017) (see Teaching for Self-Management box: Dietary Management for Pregnant Women With Diabetes).

Simple carbohydrates are limited. Complex carbohydrates that are high in fiber content are recommended because the starch and protein in such foods help to regulate the blood glucose level by producing a more gradual release of glucose into the bloodstream (Moore et al., 2019).

TEACHING FOR SELF-MANAGEMENT

Dietary Management for Pregnant Women With Diabetes

- Follow the prescribed diet plan.
- Eat a well-balanced diet, including daily food requirements for a normal pregnancy.
- Divide daily food intake among three meals and two or three snacks, depending on individual needs.
- Eat a substantial bedtime snack to prevent a severe drop in blood glucose level during the night.
- Take daily vitamins and iron as prescribed by your health care provider.
- Avoid foods high in refined sugar.
- Eat consistently each day; never skip meals or snacks.
- Eat foods high in dietary fiber.
- Avoid alcohol and nicotine; limit caffeine.
- Avoid excessive use of nonnutritive sweeteners.

Exercise

Being active for 30 to 60 min/day is encouraged. Daily activity has been shown to: increase insulin sensitivity, thus lowering blood glucose levels; increase utilization of glucose, especially after a meal; improve glucose control, perhaps eliminating the need for insulin therapy; reduce the risk for excessive weight gain; and reduce the weight of the newborn by approximately 150 g. Physical activity can be divided into 10- to 20-minute periods after each meal (Daley, 2014; Inturrisi, 2017).

Women with pregestational diabetes who are poorly controlled or have vascular disease should avoid vigorous exercise during pregnancy. Walking and swimming are two forms of exercise with minimal risk and may be the exercises of choice for previously sedentary women (Daley, 2014). Women should check their blood glucose levels before, during, and after exercising. If the blood glucose is less than 100 mg/dL, they should consume 15 to 30 g of carbohydrate to prevent hypoglycemia. Women should avoid exercise if they have positive urine ketones or a blood glucose greater than 200 mg/dL, because hyperglycemia and ketosis can worsen with physical activity (Inturrisi, 2017). Exercising with another person is prudent for safety reasons.

❗ NURSING ALERT

Uterine contractions may occur during exercise. The woman should be advised to stop exercising immediately if they are detected.

Insulin Therapy

Adequate insulin is the primary factor in the maintenance of euglycemia during pregnancy, thus ensuring proper glucose metabolism of the woman and fetus. Insulin requirements during pregnancy change dramatically as the pregnancy progresses, necessitating frequent adjustments in the dose. In the first trimester, from weeks 6 to 10 of gestation, the insulin dose should be reduced by 10% to 25% to avoid hypoglycemia. The commonly prescribed insulin dose is 0.6 units/kg in the first trimester for women with type 1 diabetes. During the second and third trimesters, because of insulin resistance, the dose must be increased significantly to maintain target glucose levels. Insulin requirements normally peak at 36 weeks of gestation and drop significantly after that (Moore et al., 2019).

For the woman with type 1 pregestational diabetes who has typically been accustomed to one injection per day of intermediate-acting insulin, multiple daily injections of mixed insulin are a new experience. The woman with type 2 diabetes previously treated with oral hypoglycemics is faced with the task of learning to self-administer injections of insulin. The nurse is instrumental in educating and supporting women with pregestational diabetes in regard to insulin administration and adjustment of the insulin dose to maintain euglycemia (see Teaching for Self-Managment box: Self-Administration of Insulin and Box 29.1).

TEACHING FOR SELF-MANAGEMENT

Self-Administration of Insulin

Procedure for Mixing NPH (Intermediate-Acting) and Rapid-Acting Insulin

- Wash hands thoroughly, and gather supplies. Be sure that insulin syringe corresponds to concentration of insulin you are using.
- Check insulin bottle to be certain that it is the appropriate type, and check expiration date.
- Gently rotate (do not shake) the insulin vial to mix the insulin.
- Wipe off the rubber stopper of each vial with alcohol.
- Draw into syringe the amount of air equal to the total dose.
- Inject air equal to NPH dose into NPH vial. Remove syringe from vial.
- Inject air equal to rapid-acting insulin dose into vial, and leave syringe in vial.
- Invert rapid-acting vial, and withdraw insulin dose.
- Without adding more air to NPH vial, carefully withdraw NPH dose.

Procedure for Self-Injection of Insulin

- Select proper injection site.
- Injection site should be clean. There is no need to use alcohol. If alcohol is used, let it dry before injecting.
- Puncture the skin at a 90-degree angle.
- Slowly inject the insulin.
- As you withdraw the needle, cover the injection site with sterile gauze and apply gentle pressure to prevent bleeding.
- Record insulin dose and time of injection.

Since 1982 most insulin preparations have been produced by inserting portions of deoxyribonucleic acid (DNA) ("recombinant DNA") into special laboratory-cultivated bacteria or yeast cells. The cells then produce synthetic human insulin (Humulin), which is less likely to cause antibody formation than animal-derived (beef or pork) insulin. More recently, insulin products called insulin analogs, in which the structure differs slightly from human insulin, have been produced. This small alteration in insulin structure results in changes in the onset and peak of action of the medication. The most commonly used insulin preparations include rapid acting, short acting, intermediate acting, and long acting (Landon et al., 2017) (Table 29.4). Mixtures of short- and intermediate-acting insulins in several proportions are also available but usually are not in the correct percentages to be effective in pregnancy. Therefore they are rarely used.

Lispro (Humalog) and aspart (NovoLog) are commonly prescribed rapid-acting insulin analogs that have replaced regular insulin (Landon et al., 2017). Rapid-acting insulins have a faster onset of action and peak effect than regular insulin, so their use may help to prevent hypoglycemia between meals (Daley, 2014). Rapid-acting insulins are convenient to use because they are injected immediately before mealtime. Because their effects last only 3 to 5 hours, most clients require a longer-acting insulin in addition to the rapid-acting insulin to maintain optimal blood glucose levels (see Table 29.4).

BOX 29.1 **Helpful Hints for Using Insulin**

- Unopened vials of insulin should be stored in the refrigerator until reaching their expiration date. Insulin should not be frozen. Vials currently in use can be stored at room temperature for up to 1 month. They should not be left in a car or exposed to extreme heat as in the sun.
- Regular insulin can be mixed with NPH insulin in the same syringe. Lispro insulin can also be mixed in a syringe with NPH insulin. Once mixed, the syringe can be used immediately or stored for future use. If it is used later, the syringe should be rotated 20 times before injection.
- Glargine insulin is usually administered at bedtime. It cannot be mixed with any other insulin in the same syringe. Prepared syringes are stable for 2 weeks in the refrigerator.
- Insulin may be administered by pen injector, jet injector, or insulin pump, in addition to syringe.
- The abdomen is the preferred injection site because insulin is best absorbed there. Other possible injection sites are the upper outer arm (not the deltoid area), thighs, and buttocks.
- Each injection should be given 2 inches from the previous injection in one quadrant before moving to another quadrant.

Glargine (Lantus) and detemir (Levemir) are long-acting insulin analogs that have been designed to more accurately mimic basal insulin secretion. Small amounts of these insulins are released slowly, with no pronounced peak. Glargine insulin may be combined with rapid-acting insulin to prevent hypoglycemia. When it is administered with rapid-acting insulin, unpredictable spikes in insulin levels and resulting hypoglycemia appear to occur less often. Both glargine and detemir appear to be safe for use during pregnancy (Landon et al., 2017) (see Table 29.4).

Insulin is usually administered in three to five injections per day. Many women with insulin-dependent diabetes take a combination of intermediate-acting and rapid-acting insulin before breakfast and dinner. Usually two-thirds of the daily insulin dose, with intermediate-acting and rapid-acting insulin combined in a 2:1 ratio, is given before breakfast. The remaining one-third is administered in the evening. It may be given as a combination of rapid- and intermediate-acting insulin before dinner or split, with rapid-acting insulin at dinner and intermediate-acting insulin at bedtime (Landon et al., 2017).

Insulin is still usually administered by drawing up the correct dose from a vial into a syringe and injecting it subcutaneously. However, some women may have difficulty drawing up the dose correctly, especially if mixing insulins in a syringe is required. Using prefilled syringes that have been stored in a refrigerator is one solution to this problem. Prefilled insulin pens are also available for use (Fig. 29.3). In addition to ensuring that the correct dose of insulin is administered, the pen is convenient for use away from home because there is no need to carry vials and syringes. The woman simply turns a dial on the pen to select her correct dose and then injects it. Some individuals believe that pen injections, because of the needle's small length and gauge, are less painful than those administered using a traditional syringe and needle. However, a disadvantage of insulin pens is that they are more expensive than syringes and needles.

The continuous subcutaneous insulin infusion (CSII) system, commonly referred to as the *insulin pump*, is used increasingly during pregnancy. The CSII system is designed to mimic more closely the function of the pancreas in secreting insulin (Fig. 29.4). This portable battery-powered device is worn similar to a pager during most daily activities. The pump infuses rapid-acting insulin (usually lispro) (Landon et al., 2017) at a set basal rate. It has the capacity to deliver up to 24 different basal rates in 24 hours, although only three or four rates are necessary to provide individualized glycemic control. The pump also delivers bolus

TABLE 29.4 Common Insulin Preparations

Type of Insulin	Examples Generic (Trade) Name	Onset of Action	Peak of Action	Duration of Action
Rapid acting	Lispro (Humalog)	15 min	30-90 min	4-5 hr
	Aspart (NovoLog)	15 min	1-3 hr	3-5 hr
Short acting	Humulin R	30 min	2-4 hr	5-7 hr
	Novolin R	30 min	2.5-5 hr	6-8 hr
Intermediate acting	Humulin NPH	1-2 hr	6-12 hr	18-24 hr
	Novolin N	1.5 hr	4-20 hr	24 hr
	Humulin L	1-3 hr	6-12 hr	18-24 h
	Novolin L	2.5 hr	7-15 hr	22 hr
Long acting	Glargine (Lantus)	1 hr	None	24 hr
	Detemir (Levemir)	1-2 hr	None	24 hr

h, Hour; *L,* lente; *min,* minutes; *NPH* (or *N*), neutral protamine Hagedorn; *R,* regular.
Data from Landon, M. B., Catalano, P. M., & Gabbe, S. G. (2017). Diabetes mellitus complicating pregnancy. In S. G. Gabbe, J. R. Niebyl, J. L. Simpson, et al. (Eds.), *Obstetrics: Normal and problem pregnancies* (7th ed.). Philadelphia: Elsevier.

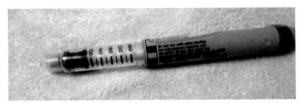

Fig. 29.3 An Insulin Pen Provides an Accurate and Convenient Way to Administer Insulin. (Courtesy of Barbra Manning, RN, MSN, Senatobia, MS.)

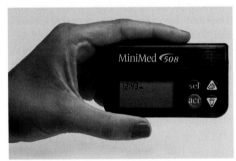

Fig. 29.4 Insulin Pump Shows Basal Rate for Pregnant Women With Diabetes. (Courtesy MiniMed, Inc., Sylmar, CA.)

doses of insulin before meals to control postprandial blood glucose levels or to correct elevations in blood glucose. A fine-gauge plastic catheter is inserted into subcutaneous tissue, usually in the abdomen, and attached to the pump syringe by connecting tubing. The subcutaneous catheter and connecting tubing are changed every 2 to 3 days. Although the insulin pump is convenient and generally provides good glycemic control, complications such as pump failure, precipitation of insulin inside the pump mechanism, abscess formation, and poor uptake from the infusion site still can occur. To safely use the pump during pregnancy, the woman must monitor her blood glucose levels frequently. Therefore use of the insulin pump requires a knowledgeable, motivated woman and skilled health care providers (Daley, 2014).

Self-Monitoring of Blood Glucose

Blood glucose testing at home using a glucose meter is considered the standard of care for monitoring blood glucose levels during pregnancy. It provides the most important tool available to the woman to assess her degree of glycemic control. The newer meters are calibrated to provide plasma (rather than whole blood) glucose values. The nurse must be knowledgeable about the specific glucose meter that the woman uses in order to troubleshoot problems, assess accuracy of technique, and determine accuracy of reported results. To perform blood glucose monitoring a drop of blood is obtained and placed on a test strip. Most glucose meters allow the user to obtain the blood sample from the forearm or palm rather than a finger. However, fingersticks are recommended during pregnancy because use of other sites can affect the accuracy of results. After a specified amount of time the glucose level is displayed by the meter (see Teaching for Self-Management box: Self-Monitoring of Blood Glucose). Blood glucose levels are routinely measured at various times throughout the day such as before breakfast, lunch, and dinner; 1 to 2 hours after each meal; at bedtime; and in the middle of the night if nighttime insulin is being adjusted. When any adjustment in the insulin dose or diet is made, more frequent measurement of blood glucose is warranted. If nausea, vomiting, or diarrhea occurs or if infection is present, the woman is asked to monitor her blood glucose levels more closely than usual.

TEACHING FOR SELF-MANAGEMENT
Self-Monitoring of Blood Glucose

- Gather supplies, check expiration date, and read instructions on testing materials. Prepare glucose meter for use according to manufacturer's instructions.
- Wash hands in warm water (warmth increases circulation).
- Select site on side of any finger (all fingers should be used in rotation).
- Pierce site with lancet (may use automatic spring-loaded, puncturing device). Cleaning the site with alcohol is not necessary.
- Drop hand down to side; with other hand, gently squeeze finger from hand to fingertip.
- Allow blood to be drawn into glucose test strip.
- Determine blood glucose value using glucose reflectance meter following manufacturer's instructions.
- Record results displayed.
- Repeat as instructed by health care provider and as needed for signs of hypoglycemia or hyperglycemia.

! NURSING ALERT

Hyperglycemia is most likely to be identified in 2-h postmeal values because blood glucose levels peak approximately 2 h after a meal.

Target levels of blood glucose during pregnancy are lower than non-pregnant values (see Table 29.3). Acceptable fasting levels are generally between 60 and 90 mg/dL, and 1-hour postmeal levels should be 140 mg/dL or less. Two-hour postmeal levels should be 120 mg/dL or less (Landon et al., 2017). The woman should be told to report recurrent episodes of hypoglycemia (<70 mg/dL) and hyperglycemia (>200 mg/dL) to her health care provider so adjustments in diet or insulin therapy can be made.

Pregnant women with diabetes are much more likely to develop hypoglycemia than hyperglycemia. Most episodes of mild or moderate hypoglycemia can be treated with oral intake of 15 g of carbohydrate, preferably in the form of commercial glucose tablets (see Teaching for Self-Management box: Treatment for Hypoglycemia). If severe hypoglycemia occurs and the woman experiences a decrease in or loss of consciousness or an inability to swallow, she will require a parenteral injection of glucagon or intravenous (IV) glucose. Because hypoglycemia can develop rapidly and impaired judgment can be associated with even moderate episodes, family members, friends, and work colleagues must be able to recognize signs and symptoms quickly and initiate proper treatment if necessary.

TEACHING FOR SELF-MANAGEMENT
Treatment for Hypoglycemia

- Be familiar with signs and symptoms of hypoglycemia (nervousness, headache, fatigue, shaking, irritability, tachycardia, hunger, blurred vision, sweaty skin, tingling of mouth or extremities).
- Check blood glucose level immediately when hypoglycemic symptoms occur.
- If blood glucose is less than 70 mg/dL, immediately eat 2 to 4 glucose tablets or gel (8 to 16 g carbohydrate). If glucose tablets or gel are not available, then other simple carbohydrates (15 g) can be eaten or drunk instead. Examples are as follows:
  - ½ cup (4 oz) unsweetened orange juice
  - ½ cup (4 oz) regular (not diet) soda
  - 5 or 6 hard candies
  - 1 cup (8 oz) skim milk
- Rest for 15 minutes, and then recheck blood glucose.
- If glucose level is greater than 70 mg/dL, eat a meal to stabilize the sugar level.
- If glucose level is still less than 70 mg/dL, eat 2 to 4 additional glucose tablets.
- Wait 15 minutes, and then recheck blood glucose. If level is still less than 70 mg/dL, notify your health care provider immediately.
- If nausea related to hypoglycemia prevents ingestion of carbohydrates, inject 0.15 mg glucagon intramuscularly. This will elevate the blood glucose enough to allow eating.

Some women with long-term pregestational diabetes develop hypoglycemia unawareness, a condition in which early symptoms of hypoglycemia are not recognized. Women with hypoglycemia unawareness should test their blood glucose levels more frequently, especially during the night, to detect hypoglycemia earlier. Glycemic thresholds in women with hypoglycemia unawareness should be higher than for other women with diabetes, to avoid dangerous hypoglycemia. The threshold for recognition of hypoglycemia should be determined at the first prenatal visit so that individual guidelines for hypoglycemia can be determined and the woman and her family educated.

Hyperglycemia is less likely to occur than hypoglycemia, although it can rapidly progress to DKA, which is associated with an increased risk for fetal death (Inturrisi, 2017; Landon et al., 2017). Women and family members should be particularly alert for signs and symptoms of hyperglycemia when infections or other illnesses occur (see Teaching for Self-Management box: What to Do When Illness Occurs).

TEACHING FOR SELF-MANAGEMENT
What to Do When Illness Occurs

- Be sure to take insulin even if unable to eat or appetite is less than normal. (Insulin needs are increased with illness or infection.)
- Call your health care provider, and relay the following information:
  - Symptoms of illness (e.g., nausea, vomiting, diarrhea)
  - Elevated temperature
  - Most recent blood glucose level
  - Urine ketones
  - Time and amount of last insulin dose
- Increase oral intake of fluids to prevent dehydration.
- Rest as much as possible.
- If you are unable to reach your health care provider and blood glucose exceeds 200 mg/dL with moderate urine ketones present, seek emergency treatment at the nearest health care facility. Do not attempt to self-treat for this condition.

Urine Testing

Urine testing for glucose is not beneficial during pregnancy. Because of the lowered renal threshold for glucose, the degree of glycosuria does not accurately reflect the blood glucose level. However, urine testing for ketones continues to have a place in diabetic management. Monitoring for urine ketones may detect inadequate caloric or carbohydrate intake or skipped meals or snacks. Testing may also be performed when illness occurs or when the blood glucose level is 250 mg/dL or greater, because of the increased risk for ketoacidosis. The woman should be told to report moderate levels of urine ketones to her health care provider (Daley, 2014).

Complications Requiring Hospitalization

Occasionally, hospitalization is necessary to regulate insulin therapy and stabilize glucose levels. Infection, which can lead to hyperglycemia and DKA, may be an indication for hospitalization, regardless of gestational age. Hospitalization during the third trimester for close maternal and fetal observation may be indicated for women whose diabetes is poorly controlled. In addition, women with diabetes are more likely than women who do not have diabetes to also have preexisting hypertension or develop preeclampsia, which may necessitate hospitalization.

Fetal Surveillance

Diagnostic techniques for fetal surveillance are often performed to assess fetal growth and well-being. The goals of fetal surveillance are to detect fetal compromise as early as possible and prevent IUFD or unnecessary preterm birth.

Early in pregnancy the estimated date of birth is determined. A baseline ultrasound is obtained during the first trimester to assess gestational age. Follow-up ultrasound examinations are usually performed during the pregnancy (as often as every 3 to 4 weeks) to monitor fetal growth; estimate fetal weight; and detect hydramnios, macrosomia, and congenital anomalies.

Because the fetus of a woman with diabetes is at increased risk for neural tube defects such as spina bifida, anencephaly, or microcephaly, measurement of maternal serum α-fetoprotein is performed between

15 and 20 weeks of gestation (ideally between 16 and 18 weeks of gestation) (Wapner & Dugoff, 2019). In addition, a detailed ultrasound study to examine the fetus for neural tube defects and other anomalies should be performed between 18 and 20 weeks of gestation (Moore et al., 2019).

Women with pregestational diabetes are also more likely to give birth to infants with congenital cardiac anomalies. Fetal echocardiography may be performed between 20 and 22 weeks of gestation to detect cardiac anomalies, especially when cardiac imaging during a second trimester anatomy scan was suboptimal and in women who had less than desirable glucose control early in pregnancy, as demonstrated by a hemoglobin A1c level greater than 10% (Moore et al., 2019). Most fetal surveillance measures are concentrated in the third trimester, when the risk of fetal compromise is greatest. The goals of antepartum testing during the third trimester are to monitor fetal growth and ensure fetal well-being. Pregnant women should be taught how to make daily fetal movement counts, beginning at 28 weeks of gestation (see Chapter 26) (Moore et al., 2019).

The nonstress test (NST) is the preferred primary method to evaluate fetal well-being. It is usually begun by 32 weeks of gestation and performed at least twice weekly. If the NST is nonreactive, a biophysical profile or contraction stress test will be performed. Testing often begins earlier, between 28 and 32 weeks of gestation, in women who have vascular disease, poor glucose control, or suspected fetal growth restriction (Landon et al., 2017) (see Chapter 26).

Determination of Birth Date and Mode of Birth

The optimal time for birth is between 39 and 40 weeks of gestation, as long as good metabolic control is maintained and parameters of antepartum fetal surveillance remain within normal limits. Induction of labor at 39 weeks of gestation is often planned for women with well-controlled diabetes who do not have vascular disease (Landon et al., 2017). Reasons to proceed with birth before term include poor metabolic control, coexisting hypertension, and nonreassuring responses to fetal testing (Moore et al., 2019).

To confirm fetal lung maturity, an amniocentesis should be performed when birth will occur before 38 weeks of gestation. For the pregnancy complicated by diabetes, fetal lung maturation is best predicted by the amniotic fluid phosphatidylglycerol (>3%) or the equivalent. If the fetal lungs are still immature, birth should be postponed until 40 weeks of gestation as long as fetal assessment test results remain reassuring. However, after that time, the benefits of conservative management are outweighed by the increasing risk of fetal compromise if the pregnancy is allowed to continue. Birth, despite poor fetal lung maturity, may be necessary before 39 weeks of gestation because of compelling maternal or fetal reasons such as preeclampsia with severe features or nonreassuring fetal status (Moore et al., 2019).

Although vaginal birth is expected for most women with pregestational diabetes, the cesarean rate for these women is as high as 80% (Cunningham et al., 2018). ACOG (2016) states that, although the diagnosis of fetal macrosomia is imprecise, prophylactic cesarean birth may be considered when the estimated fetal weight is at least 4500 g in women with diabetes. This recommendation may reduce the risk for shoulder dystocia to some degree for an individual woman, but the benefit to a larger group of women is less clear (Moore et al., 2019.).

Intrapartum Care

During the intrapartum period the woman with pregestational diabetes must be monitored closely to prevent complications related to dehydration, hypoglycemia, and hyperglycemia. An IV line is inserted for infusion of a maintenance fluid. Initially this infusion will be either normal saline or lactated Ringer's solution. Once active labor begins or glucose levels fall to less than 70 mg/dL, a piggybacked pump-controlled infusion of a solution containing 5% dextrose should be added (Landon et al., 2017). The dextrose provides the energy (calories) necessary for the woman to accomplish the work and manage the stress of labor and birth. Most commonly, insulin is administered by continuous infusion, piggybacked into the main IV line. Only rapid- or short-acting insulin can be administered intravenously. Insulin may also be given intermittently by subcutaneous injection as needed to maintain glucose levels within the target range. Determinations of blood glucose levels are made every hour, and fluids and insulin are adjusted to maintain the blood glucose level between 90 and 110 mg/dL (Moore et al., 2019). Maintaining this target glucose level is essential because hyperglycemia during labor can cause metabolic problems in the neonate, particularly hypoglycemia (Daley, 2014).

During labor, continuous fetal heart monitoring is necessary. The woman should assume an upright or side-lying position during labor to prevent supine hypotension caused by a large fetus or polyhydramnios. Labor, whether spontaneous or induced, is allowed to progress as long as expected rates of cervical dilation and fetal descent are maintained and fetal well-being is evident. Failure to progress in labor may indicate a macrosomic infant and cephalopelvic disproportion, necessitating a cesarean birth. The woman is observed and treated during labor for complications of diabetes such as hyperglycemia, ketosis, and ketoacidosis. During second-stage labor, shoulder dystocia may occur with the birth of a macrosomic infant (see Chapter 32). A neonatologist, pediatrician, or neonatal nurse practitioner will likely be present at the birth to initiate assessment and neonatal care.

If a cesarean birth is planned, it should be scheduled in the early morning to facilitate glycemic control. Women should take their full dose of insulin the night before surgery. No morning insulin is given on the day of surgery, and the woman is given nothing by mouth (Daley, 2014; Landon et al., 2017). Regional (spinal or epidural) anesthesia is recommended because hypoglycemia can be detected earlier if the woman is awake. After surgery, glucose levels should be monitored carefully.

Postpartum Care

During the first 24 hours postpartum, insulin requirements decrease substantially because the major source of insulin resistance, the placenta, has been removed. Women with preexisting diabetes usually require only 50% to 60% of their most recent pregnancy insulin dose on the first postpartum day, provided they are eating a full diet (Daley, 2014). Women who give birth by cesarean may need an IV infusion of glucose and insulin until they resume a regular diet (Moore et al., 2019). A subcutaneous dose of insulin should be given at least 1 hour before discontinuing IV insulin.

After birth, several days may be required to reestablish carbohydrate homeostasis (see Fig. 29.1D and E). Blood glucose levels are carefully monitored in the postpartum period, and the insulin dose is adjusted appropriately. The woman who has insulin-dependent diabetes must realize the importance of eating on time even if the baby needs feeding or other pressing demands exist. Women with type 2 diabetes may resume taking their prepregnancy oral hypoglycemics if these medications are compatible with breastfeeding and provide adequate glycemic control.

Possible postpartum complications include preeclampsia or eclampsia, hemorrhage, and infection. Hemorrhage is a possibility if the mother's uterus was overdistended (hydramnios, macrosomic fetus) or overstimulated (oxytocin induction). Postpartum infections such as endometritis are more likely to occur in women with diabetes than in women who do not have diabetes.

Women with diabetes are encouraged to breastfeed. In addition to the benefits of breastfeeding for all mothers and infants, breastfeeding may offer longer-term benefits for both women with diabetes and their children. Weight control and glucose levels may both be improved in breastfeeding women in the first 3 months postpartum. Infants of women with diabetes have a decreased risk for childhood obesity, if they are breastfed for at least 6 months (ADA, 2018; Inturrisi, 2017). Children who were exclusively breastfed also have a significantly lower risk for developing non–insulin-dependent diabetes (Moore et al., 2019).

Insulin requirements in breastfeeding women decrease because of the carbohydrate used in human milk production. Because glucose levels are lower than normal, breastfeeding women are at increased risk for hypoglycemia after breastfeeding, particularly after late-night nursing sessions (Moore et al., 2019). Women should check their blood glucose level just before breastfeeding. If it is less than 100 mg/dL, they should consume 15 g carbohydrate (see Teaching for Self-Management box: Treatment for Hypoglycemia) without taking insulin. Women should also be aware that frequent hypoglycemia can reduce breast milk production. Breastfeeding mothers with diabetes are at increased risk for mastitis (see Chapter 25) (Inturrisi, 2017). The insulin dose, which is decreased during lactation, must be recalculated at weaning (see Fig. 29.1F).

The mother may have early breastfeeding difficulties. Poor metabolic control may delay lactogenesis and contribute to decreased milk production (Moore et al., 2019). Initial contact with an opportunity to breastfeed the infant may be delayed for mothers who gave birth by cesarean or if infants are placed in neonatal intensive care units or special care nurseries for observation during the first few hours after birth. Support and assistance from nursing staff and lactation specialists can facilitate the mother's early experience with breastfeeding and encourage her to continue.

The new mother needs information about family planning and contraception. Although family planning is important for all women, it is essential for the woman with diabetes to safeguard her own health and promote optimal outcomes in future pregnancies. The risks and benefits of contraceptive methods should be discussed with the mother and her partner before discharge from the hospital. Barrier methods have become the preferred interim method of contraception for women with diabetes because they are safe, inexpensive options that do not affect carbohydrate metabolism or have no inherent risks. An intrauterine device (IUD) may also be used without concerns about an increased risk for infection (Landon et al., 2017).

Use of oral contraceptives by women with diabetes is controversial because of the possible increased risk of thromboembolic and vascular complications and the effect on carbohydrate metabolism (Landon et al., 2017). In nonsmoking women who are less than 35 years old and do not have vascular disease, combination low-dose oral contraceptives may be prescribed if they are not breastfeeding. Progestin-only oral contraceptives also may be used because they do not significantly affect glucose levels (Cunningham et al., 2018). Close monitoring of blood pressure and lipid levels is necessary to detect complications (Landon et al., 2017).

Opinion is divided about the use of long-acting parenteral progestins, such as medroxyprogesterone (Depo-Provera). Some health care providers recommend their use, particularly in women who are noncompliant with daily dosing oral contraceptives. In contrast, other health care providers believe this method may adversely affect glycemic control. In addition, although Depo-Provera may lower serum triglyceride and high-density lipoprotein (HDL) cholesterol levels, it does not lower total cholesterol or low-density lipoprotein (LDL) levels. For this reason it is not recommended as a first-choice method for contraception for women with diabetes (Landon et al., 2017). Implants that contain only progesterone (e.g., Nexplanon) can be used by many women with diabetes because they do not significantly affect glucose levels (Cunningham et al., 2018).

Transdermal (patch) and transvaginal (vaginal ring) are also contraceptive options, particularly effective in women who prefer weekly or every-third-week dosing, respectively. For women weighing more than 90 kg (198 lb), the contraceptive failure rate with transdermal administration is higher than in normal-weight women. Therefore this method is contraindicated in obese women. In addition, women who use the patch may be at increased risk for developing thromboembolic disease, compared with women who use other contraceptives that contain both estrogen and progesterone (Cunningham et al., 2018). The risks associated with pregnancy increase with the duration and severity of diabetes. In addition, pregnancy may contribute to the vascular changes associated with diabetes. This information needs to be thoroughly discussed with the woman and her partner. Sterilization is often recommended for the woman who has completed her family, who has poor metabolic control, or who has significant vascular problems. Vasectomy for the partner is very effective and is safer than surgical sterilization in the woman with diabetes.

GESTATIONAL DIABETES MELLITUS

Gestational diabetes mellitus (GDM) complicates approximately 9.2% of all pregnancies in the United States (a range of 2% to 18%, depending on the population and the method of diagnosis) (Inturrisi, 2017). It currently occurs more often worldwide than in the past, probably because of increasing rates of overweight and obesity and the stricter criteria for diagnosis currently being used by some health care practitioners (Landon et al., 2017). According to White's classification system, women with GDM fall into classes A_1 and A_2 (see Table 29.1). It is more likely to occur among Hispanic, African-American, Native-American, Asian, and Pacific Islander women than in Caucasians and is likely to recur in future pregnancies; the risk for development of overt diabetes later in life is also increased (Inturrisi; Landon et al.). This tendency is especially true of women whose GDM is diagnosed early in pregnancy and who have elevated fasting glucose levels (Landon et al.). Classic risk factors for GDM include a family history of diabetes and a previous pregnancy that resulted in an unexplained stillbirth or the birth of a malformed or macrosomic fetus. Other risk factors for GDM include obesity, hypertension, glycosuria, and maternal age older than 25 years. However, more than half of all women diagnosed with GDM do not have these risk factors (Landon et al.).

GDM is diagnosed during the second half of pregnancy. As fetal nutrient demands rise during the late second and the third trimesters, maternal nutrient ingestion induces greater and more sustained levels of blood glucose. At the same time, maternal insulin resistance is also increasing because of the insulin-antagonistic effects of the placental hormones, cortisol, and insulinase. Consequently, maternal insulin demands rise as much as threefold. Most pregnant women are capable of increasing insulin production to compensate for insulin resistance and maintain euglycemia. However, when the pancreas is unable to produce sufficient insulin or the insulin is not used effectively, GDM can result.

Screening for Gestational Diabetes Mellitus
Early Pregnancy Screening
All pregnant women not known to have pregestational diabetes should be screened for GDM by history, clinical risk factors, and laboratory screening of blood glucose levels (ACOG, 2018a). Although most women are screened for GDM between 24 and 28 weeks of gestation, those with strong risk factors should be screened earlier in pregnancy. Increasing rates of obesity and diabetes have resulted in more women of childbearing age with type 2 diabetes, many of

EVIDENCE-BASED PRACTICE

Debating Gestational Diabetes Diagnosis

Ask the Question

For pregnant women with hyperglycemia, at what level do diagnosis and treatment for gestational diabetes become most beneficial for the baby?

Search for the Evidence

Search Strategies: English language research-based publications since 2014 on gestational diabetes screening or diagnosis, hyperglycemia, American Diabetes Association (ADA), American College of Obstetricians and Gynecologists (ACOG), and National Institutes of Health (NIH) were included.

Databases Used: Cochrane Collaborative Database, National Guideline Clearinghouse (AHRQ), CINAHL, PubMed, UpToDate, and the professional websites for ACOG, ADA, and AWHONN

Toward a Diagnosis of Gestational Diabetes Mellitus
Background

- High serum glucose in pregnancy is associated with complications such as preeclampsia, macrosomia, operative vaginal birth, shoulder dystocia, birth injury, cesarean birth, neonatal hypoglycemia, need for neonatal intensive care, respiratory distress, and neonatal hyperbilirubinemia. A commonly accepted method of diagnosing gestational diabetes mellitus (GDM) has been a nonfasting glucose challenge test at 24-28 weeks of gestation (Moyer, 2014). For a 50-g glucose challenge test, the most common cutoff was 140 mg/dL. An elevated result triggered a fasting 2- or 3-hour oral glucose tolerance test (OGTT). A second abnormal result yielded a diagnosis of GDM (Ogunleye, Davidson, Gregg, & Egerman, 2017).

Conflicting Guidelines

- **ACOG:** In 2006, at least nine different criteria were used to identify gestational diabetes, using 50-100 g of glucose as the challenge. The ACOG's approach used two-step screening, clinical criteria, and history. Critics of this approach questioned its reliance on maternal, rather than newborn, outcomes; its acceptance of clinical criteria or history alone for diagnosis; and its ambiguous screening cutoffs (Benhalima, Devlieger, & Van Assche, 2015; Ogunleye et al., 2017).
- **ADA:** In 2008 the International Association of Diabetes in Pregnancy Study Group set out to identify levels at which treatment would benefit the baby. They proposed a one-step approach, consisting of a 75-g OGTT. A single abnormal value confirmed the diagnosis (Ogunleye et al., 2017). The ADA endorsed this approach (ADA, 2018).

Perinatal Outcomes Using Both Approaches

- Ogunleye et al. (2017) conducted a retrospective study in which they examined the outcomes of two cohorts. The first cohort was screened and diagnosed with GDM using the two-step ACOG approach. The second cohort was evaluated using the one-step approach supported by the ADA. Twenty-six women were diagnosed with GDM from the first cohort, and 53 women from the second cohort were diagnosed with GDM. There were no statistically significant maternal or neonatal outcomes between groups.

Other Perinatal Outcomes

- In a Cochrane systematic review, it was determined that the ideal screening method for GDM that results in the best outcomes for moms and their babies is not clear (Tieu, McPhee, Crowther, et al., 2017). Strong evidence supports treatment of GDM, but determining if screening every pregnant woman for GDM improves outcomes has yet to be firmly supported by evidence (Tieu et al.).
- Feghali, Abebe, Comer, et al. (2018) looked retrospectively at whether early diagnosis of GDM had affected outcomes. Women diagnosed with GDM before 24 weeks of gestation were more likely to be obese and less likely to have excess weight gain in their overall pregnancy. The only potentially adverse outcome women with an early diagnosis (before 24 weeks) of GDM experienced was an increased risk for macrosomia.

References

American Diabetes Association. (2018). Management of diabetes in pregnancy: Standards of medical care in diabetes—2018. *Diabetes Care, 41*(Suppl. 1), s137–s143.

Benhalima, K., Devlieger, R., & Van Assche, A. (2015). Screening and management of gestational diabetes. *Best Practice & Research Clinical Obstetrics and Gynaecology, 29*(3), 339–349.

Feghali, M. N., Abebe, K. Z., Comer, D. M., et al. (2018). Pregnancy outcomes in women with an early diagnosis of gestational diabetes mellitus. *Diabetes Research and Clinical Practice, 138*, 177–186.

Moyer, V. A. (2014). Screening for gestational diabetes mellitus: U.S. Preventive Services Task Force recommendation statement. *Annals of Internal Medicine, 160*(6), 414–420.

Ogunleye, O. K., Davidson, K. D., Gregg, A. R., & Egerman, R. S. (2017). Perinatal outcomes after adopting 1-versus 2-step approach to diagnosing gestational diabetes. *Journal of Maternal-Fetal and Neonatal Medicine, 30*(2), 186–190.

Tieu, J., McPhee, A. J., Crowther, C. A., et al. (2017). Screening for gestational diabetes mellitus based on different risk profiles and settings for improving maternal and infant health. *Cochrane Database of Systematic* Reviews, 8, CD007222.

Jennifer Taylor Alderman

---

whom are undiagnosed when they become pregnant. Both the ADA and ACOG recommend that women with high-risk factors for type 2 diabetes (i.e., severe obesity, a strong family history of type 2 diabetes, and a history of GDM in a previous pregnancy) be tested for preexisting diabetes at their initial prenatal visit by one of the methods used to diagnose diabetes in the nonpregnant population (ADA, 2017; Inturrisi, 2017; Landon et al., 2017). Screening early in pregnancy diagnoses women with preexisting diabetes so that appropriate treatment and postpartum follow-up are possible. If early screening indicates that these women do not have preexisting diabetes, they should be rescreened at 24 to 28 weeks of gestation for GDM (ADA; Inturrisi; Landon et al.).

Screening at 24 to 28 Weeks of Gestation

Two different blood glucose screening methods for GDM are used in the United States. ACOG recommends the two-step screening method that has been used for many years. The first step is a screen consisting of a 50-g oral glucose load followed by a plasma glucose measurement 1 hour later. The woman need not be fasting when the screen is done. A glucose value of 130 to 140 mg/dL, or higher, is considered a positive screen. An initial positive screening result is followed by step 2, a 3-hour (100-g) oral glucose tolerance test (OGTT) on another day. ACOG recommends use of the two-step screening procedure because there is no evidence that the one-step method leads to clinically significant improvement in maternal or newborn outcomes. However, use of the one-step method does significantly increase health care costs because more women will be diagnosed with GDM and thus will require more visits, tests, and procedures than pregnant women who do not have this disease (ACOG, 2018a).

The OGTT is administered after an overnight fast and at least 3 days of unrestricted diet (at least 150 g of carbohydrate) and physical activity. The woman is instructed to avoid caffeine because it increases glucose levels

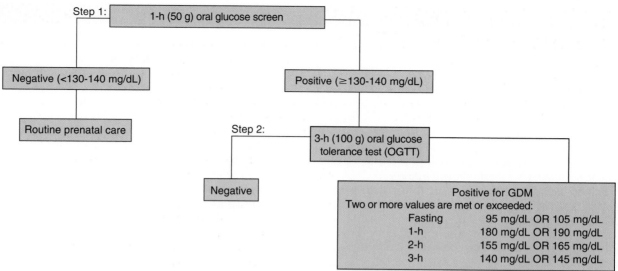

Fig. 29.5 Two-Step Method for Diagnosing Gestational Diabetes Mellitus (GDM), Recommended by the American College of Obstetricians and Gynecologists (ACOG). (Data from American College of Obstetricians and Gynecologists. (2018). Gestational diabetes mellitus. Practice bulletin no: 190. *Obstetrics & Gynecology, 131*(2), e49–e64.)

and to abstain from smoking for 12 hours before the test. The 3-hour OGTT requires a fasting blood glucose level, which is drawn before giving a 100-g glucose load. Blood glucose levels are then drawn 1, 2, and 3 hours later. The woman is diagnosed with GDM if two or more values are met or exceeded (ACOG, 2018a). Two different sets of glucose values are commonly used to diagnose GDM following the 100-g OGTT (Fig. 29.5). Currently, use of one set of glucose values cannot be clearly recommended over the other. Therefore providers are urged to select one set of blood glucose values and use it consistently in their practice (ACOG).

An international consensus group, the International Association of Diabetes and Pregnancy Study Groups (IADPSG), consisting of representatives from multiple obstetric and diabetic organizations including the ADA, recommends a different (one-step) method of screening and diagnosis. If the tests done early in pregnancy for overt diabetes are normal, a 75-g OGTT diagnostic test is administered between 24 and 28 weeks of gestation. The 75-g OGTT requires a fasting blood glucose level, which is drawn before giving the glucose load. Blood glucose levels are then drawn 1 and 2 hours later. A diagnosis of GDM is made if only one glucose value is exceeded (Fig. 29.6). This one-step method of screening and diagnosis significantly increases the incidence of GDM, likely double that found using the two-step method, because the upper limit of normal for the blood glucose value at each sampling time is lower than in the two-step method. Therefore more cases of GDM are diagnosed. Approximately 95% of all obstetricians in the United States continue to use the two-step approach to screening for GDM (ACOG, 2018a). However, many countries in Europe and Asia, as well as some health care providers in the United States, have adopted the IADPSG recommendations for screening and diagnosing GDM (ADA, 2017; Inturrisi, 2017; Landon et al., 2017). (See the Evidence-Based Practice box: Debating Gestational Diabetes Diagnosis.)

Maternal Risks

Women with gestational diabetes have fewer risks than women with pregestational diabetes; however, they are significant. These risks include preeclampsia (9.8% if well controlled, 18% if not well controlled), cesarean birth (17% to 25%), and the development of type 2 diabetes later in life (up to 70%) (ACOG, 2018a).

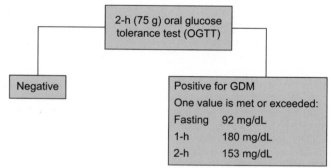

Fig. 29.6 One-Step Method for Diagnosing Gestational Diabetes Mellitus *(GDM)*, Recommended by the International Association of Diabetes in Pregnancy Study Groups (IADPSG). (Data from American College of Obstetricians and Gynecologists. (2018). Practice bulletin no: 190: Gestational diabetes mellitus. *Obstetrics & Gynecology, 131*(2), e49–e64.)

Fetal Risks

No increase in the incidence of birth defects has been found among infants of women who develop GDM after the first trimester because the critical period of organ formation has already passed by the time that blood glucose levels increase (Moore et al., 2019). However, it is important to note that obesity (BMI >30) also contributes to congenital defects even in the absence of GDM. As with pregestational diabetes, infants born to women with GDM are at risk for macrosomia and associated risks for birth trauma and electrolyte imbalances including neonatal hypoglycemia and hyperinsulinemia (ACOG, 2018a).

📋 CARE MANAGEMENT

Client problems and expected outcomes of care for women with GDM are basically the same as those for women with pregestational diabetes. However, the time frame for planning may be shortened with GDM because the diagnosis is made later in pregnancy (see Nursing Care Plan).

NURSING CARE PLAN

The Pregnant Woman With Gestational Diabetes

Client Problem	Expected Outcome	Interventions	Rationales
Reduced glucose regulation related to physiologic stress and processes of pregnancy	The woman will maintain a euglycemic state throughout pregnancy.	Assess woman's current knowledge base of the disease process, management, effects on mother and fetus, and potential complications	To provide foundation for teaching
		Teach woman the principles of a diabetic diet and the procedure for self-monitoring of blood glucose	To promote self-management and competence with following her plan of care
		Review signs and symptoms of hypoglycemia and hyperglycemia and appropriate interventions for both	To promote prompt recognition of complications and self-management
Potential for fetal injury related to elevated maternal glucose levels	The fetus will remain free of injury and be born at term in a healthy state.	Assess woman's current diabetic control by reviewing the blood glucose values she obtains and reports using self-monitoring of blood glucose	To identify risk for fetal macrosomia
		Assess fetal movement and heart rate during each prenatal visit and schedule and/or perform other fetal assessment tests that may be ordered during the third trimester	To monitor fetal well-being
		Teach woman to perform daily fetal movement counts. Explain the results that indicate she needs to immediately contact her health care provider	To monitor fetal well-being
Anxiety related to threat to maternal and fetal well-being as evidenced by the woman's verbal expressions of concern	The mother will report a lower level of perceived anxiety	Use therapeutic communication and private, unhurried environment to encourage verbalization of concerns	To promote trust
		Identify misinformation or missing information in woman's stated understanding	To correct any misconception or misinformation that may be contributing to anxiety
		Teach woman about her treatment plan, including scheduled visits, fetal assessment tests, and anticipated management of labor and birth	To promote compliance with the plan

Antepartum Care

When the diagnosis of GDM is made, treatment begins immediately, allowing little or no time for the woman and her family to adjust to the diagnosis before they are expected to participate in the treatment plan. With each step of the treatment plan, the nurse and other health care providers educate the woman and her family, providing detailed and comprehensive explanations to ensure understanding, participation, and adherence to the necessary interventions. Potential complications are discussed and the need for maintaining euglycemia throughout the remainder of the pregnancy reinforced. Knowing that GDM typically disappears when the pregnancy is over may be reassuring for the woman and her family (see Clinical Reasoning Case Study: The Pregnant Woman with Gestational Diabetes).

As with pregestational diabetes, the aim of therapy in women with GDM is strict blood glucose control. Fasting blood glucose levels less than 95 mg/dL, 1-hour postmeal blood glucose levels less than 140 mg/dL, and 2-hour postmeal glucose levels less than 120 mg/dL are recommended (Landon et al., 2017; ACOG, 2018a). These levels are very similar to but not exactly the same as those recommended for women with preexisting diabetes (see Table 29.3).

Diet

Dietary modification is the mainstay of treatment for GDM. The woman with GDM is placed on a standard diabetic diet. The usual prescription is 2000 to 2500 kcal/day, which represents approximately 35 kcal/kg/day of present pregnancy weight. For overweight or obese women, a

CLINICAL REASONING CASE STUDY

The Pregnant Woman With Gestational Diabetes

Anijah is a 30-year-old African-American woman, gravida 2, para 1, in the 26th week of her second pregnancy. During her first pregnancy, 2 years ago, she had elevated blood glucose levels that she was able to control with diet. She did not lose the weight she gained during her first pregnancy and now is approximately 30 pounds over her ideal weight. She had a two-step screening for gestational diabetes last week. Her initial 1-h glucola result was 150 mg/dL, which is a positive screen. This was followed 4 days later by a 3-h (100 g) oral glucose tolerance test. Those results were: fasting blood sugar 114, 1-h 192, 2-h 160, and 3-h 150. Her urine was positive for ketones. Anijah is upset: "I am worried that I will have to take shots this time! I don't think I can do this!"

1. What is the priority concern or client need in this situation? Support your answer with data as stated in the case.
2. List other client needs/problems in this case.
3. Identify any additional information or assessment data that are needed by the nurse in planning care for this client.
4. What nursing actions are appropriate in this situation?
    a. What is the priority nursing action? (What should the nurse do first?)
    b. Describe other nursing interventions that are important to providing optimal client care.
5. Describe the roles/responsibilities of the interprofessional health care team members (other than nurses) who may be involved in providing care for this client.

reduction to 25 kcal/kg/day and 15 kcal/kg/day (present pregnancy weight), respectively, may be advised. The usual carbohydrate intake is restricted to approximately 50% to 60% of caloric intake. However, some authorities believe that a diet containing this much carbohydrate will cause excessive weight gain and postmeal hyperglycemia, resulting in a need for insulin therapy in 50% of women with GDM. Therefore they recommend limiting carbohydrate intake to 33% to 40% of calories (Landon et al., 2017; ACOG, 2018a), 20% protein, and 40% fat, across three meals and two snacks (ACOG, 2018a). Dietary counseling by a registered dietitian is recommended.

Exercise

There are few published studies on the benefits of exercise in women with GDM. In adults who are not pregnant, exercise increases lean muscle mass and improves sensitivity to insulin. Therefore a moderate exercise program is recommended for overweight or obese women with GDM to improve blood sugar control and facilitate weight loss (ACOG, 2018a).

Self-Monitoring of Blood Glucose

Blood glucose monitoring is necessary to determine whether euglycemia can be maintained by diet and exercise. The frequency and timing of blood glucose monitoring should be individualized for each woman. A typical schedule for monitoring blood glucose is on rising in the morning, 1 or 2 hours after breakfast, before and after lunch, before dinner, and at bedtime (Moore et al., 2019). Alternatively, women may be instructed to check a fasting blood glucose level and then continue to monitor their values 2 hours after each meal (Inturrisi, 2017; Landon et al., 2017). Women with GDM usually perform self-monitoring at home with a review of their results at prenatal visits to determine the effectiveness of diet and exercise. If glycemic thresholds are not met with diet and exercise management, then pharmacologic intervention is indicated.

Pharmacologic Therapy

If fasting plasma glucose levels are persistently greater than 95 mg/dL, 1-hour postmeal levels are persistently greater than 140 mg/dL, or 2-hour postmeal levels are persistently greater than 120 mg/dL, pharmacologic therapy is begun (ACOG, 2018a). Approximately 25% to 50% of women with GDM require insulin or oral medication during the pregnancy to maintain satisfactory blood glucose levels, despite compliance with the prescribed diet (Landon et al., 2017).

Women who are unable or unwilling to take insulin by injection or are cognitively impaired may be candidates for oral hypoglycemic medication. Oral hypoglycemic therapy has become increasingly used as an alternative to insulin, despite lack of approval by the U.S. Food and Drug Administration (FDA) for such use. Metformin and glyburide are both used for blood glucose control in women with GDM.

Metformin works by decreasing hepatic glucose production and increasing peripheral sensitivity to insulin (Landon et al., 2017). It readily crosses the placenta in levels as high as maternal levels but does not appear to be teratogenic. Glyburide works by causing the maternal pancreas to produce more insulin. It also crosses the placenta, in smaller amounts, but has not proven to be more effective than metformin. There is ongoing debate whether one of these oral medications is better than the other for treating GDM. Current recommendations suggest the use of metformin over glyburide (ACOG, 2018a). Although both medications appear to be safe for use during pregnancy, long-term studies on the effects of metformin and glyburide over time on women with GDM and their children are lacking (ADA, 2017; Daley, 2014). Hence insulin remains the preferred treatment (ACOG, 2018a).

Fetal Surveillance

Women with GDM whose blood glucose levels are well controlled by diet are at low risk for IUFD. Therefore antepartum fetal testing is not performed routinely in these women unless they also have hypertension, a history of a prior stillbirth, or suspected macrosomia. Women with these complications or those who require insulin or oral hypoglycemic agents for blood glucose control may have twice-weekly NSTs beginning at 32 weeks of gestation (ACOG, 2018a; Landon et al., 2017). They should also be monitored for polyhydramnios, a consequence of fetal hyperglycemia (ACOG, 2018a). In women with excellent diet-controlled glucose levels and normal fetal growth, pregnancy may continue until 41 weeks of gestation. If the pregnancy extends beyond 40 weeks of gestation, twice-weekly fetal testing (NST and assessment of amniotic fluid volume) should be performed (Inturrisi, 2017). However, monitoring of fetal growth should be considered because of an apparent increasing risk for macrosomia as gestational age advances. In women whose glucose control is suboptimal, decisions regarding birth before 39 weeks of gestation should be individualized (Landon et al.).

Intrapartum Care

During the labor and birth process, blood glucose levels are monitored hourly to maintain levels at 80 to 110 mg/dL. Levels within this range decrease the incidence of neonatal hypoglycemia. Infusing rapid-acting insulin intravenously may be necessary during labor to maintain the desired blood glucose levels. However, it is usually possible to maintain excellent glucose control in women with GDM during labor by avoiding the use of IV fluids containing dextrose (Moore et al., 2019). If glucose-containing solutions are given, they should be administered by an infusion device so that inadvertent boluses are avoided. Although GDM is not an indication for cesarean birth, this procedure may be necessary in the presence of preeclampsia or macrosomia.

Postpartum Care

Although most women with GDM return to normal glucose levels after birth, up to one-third will be found to have diabetes or impaired glucose metabolism when they are screened postpartum. These women are also at high risk for recurrent GDM in future pregnancies (Landon et al., 2017). In addition, women who had GDM have as high as a 70% chance of developing type 2 diabetes within 10 to 20 years. Children born to women with GDM are at risk for future health-related complications because they may develop obesity and type 2 diabetes later in life (ACOG, 2018a; ADA, 2018; Inturrisi, 2017).

ACOG recommends assessing all women who had GDM for carbohydrate intolerance with a 75-g, 2-hr OGTT or a fasting plasma glucose level at 6 to 12 weeks postpartum (Landon et al., 2017). The optimal frequency of subsequent testing has not been established. However, the ADA recommends lifelong repeat screening at least every 3 years for women with a history of GDM and normal postpartum glucose testing results. The exact frequency of screening depends on the presence of other risk factors, including family history, prepregnancy BMI, and need for insulin or oral hypoglycemic medication during pregnancy. This ongoing screening may be done using hemoglobin A1c, fasting plasma glucose, or 75-g 2-hour OGTT, using nonpregnant values (ADA, 2018).

However, it is important to remember that progression to type 2 diabetes is not inevitable. Women with a history of GDM who exercise, become less sedentary, and eat a healthy diet decrease their likelihood for developing type 2 diabetes in the future (Ortiz, Jimenez, Boursaw, et al., 2016).

Low-dose combined oral contraceptives may be safely used by women with a history of GDM. The rate of subsequent diabetes in these women is no different from that in women without a history of GDM who use low-dose oral contraceptives. At present, little information is available concerning the use of long-acting progestins by women with a history of GDM, although a deterioration in carbohydrate tolerance has been reported in depot medroxyprogesterone acetate (DMPA) users (Landon et al., 2017).

HYPEREMESIS GRAVIDARUM

Etiology

Nausea and vomiting complicate 50% to 80% of all pregnancies, typically beginning at 4 to 10 weeks of gestation. These symptoms are usually confined to the first 20 weeks of gestation (ACOG, 2018b). The cause of nausea and vomiting in pregnancy (NVP) is not well understood. Many theories have been proposed. The most common include increasing levels of estrogen, progesterone, and human chorionic gonadotropin (hCG), gastric changes, and thyroid changes. Some authorities have suggested that nausea and vomiting are evolutionary adaptations that occur during pregnancy to protect the woman and fetus from potentially harmful foods (ACOG, 2018b; Antony, Racusin, Aagaard, et al., 2017; Kelly & Savides, 2019). Whether a psychological component contributes to NVP has been disputed. Pregnancies complicated by nausea and vomiting generally have a more favorable outcome than those without these symptoms (Antony et al.).

Although NVP is typically benign, with no significant metabolic alterations or risks to the mother or fetus, it may affect quality of life. See Chapter 13 for additional discussion of NVP.

When vomiting during pregnancy becomes excessive enough to cause weight loss, electrolyte imbalance, nutritional deficiencies, and ketonuria, the disorder is termed hyperemesis gravidarum. This disorder occurs in approximately 0.3% to 3% of pregnancies (ACOG, 2018b). Hyperemesis gravidarum usually begins during the first trimester, but approximately 10% of women with the disorder continue to have symptoms throughout the pregnancy (Kelly & Savides, 2019). Hyperemesis gravidarum is the second most common reason for hospitalization during pregnancy in the United States (ACOG, 2018b).

There are a number of maternal characteristics associated with an increased risk for the development of hyperemesis gravidarum, including younger maternal age, nulliparity, a BMI less than 18.5 or greater than 25, and low socioeconomic status. Women with asthma, migraines, preexisting diabetes, psychiatric illness, hyperthyroid disorders, gastrointestinal disorders, or a previous pregnancy complicated by hyperemesis gravidarum are also more likely to develop hyperemesis. Factors related to the current pregnancy that make a woman more likely to develop hyperemesis gravidarum are carrying a female fetus, multifetal gestation, and gestational trophoblastic disease. In addition, a maternal family history of hyperemesis is associated with the disorder (Bustos, Venkataramanan, & Caritis, 2017; Castillo & Phillippi, 2015).

Hyperemesis gravidarum can cause complications for both women and infants. Severe but rare maternal complications of hyperemesis gravidarum include esophageal rupture, pneumomediastinum, and deficiencies of vitamin K and thiamine with resulting Wernicke encephalopathy (CNS involvement) (ACOG 2018b; Kelly & Savides, 2019). Infants born to women who had poor pregnancy weight gain because of hyperemesis may be small for gestational age, have a low birthweight, or be born prematurely (Castillo & Phillippi, 2015; Kelly & Savides).

Clinical Manifestations

The woman with hyperemesis gravidarum usually has significant weight loss and dehydration. She may have dry mucous membranes, decreased BP, increased pulse rate, and poor skin turgor. Frequently she is unable to keep down even clear liquids taken by mouth. Laboratory tests may reveal electrolyte imbalances.

CARE MANAGEMENT

Assessment

Whenever a pregnant woman has nausea and vomiting, the first priority is a thorough assessment to determine the severity of the problem. The physical assessment should include:

- Frequency, severity, and duration of episodes of nausea and vomiting, including approximate amount and color of the vomitus
- Presence of diarrhea, indigestion, and abdominal pain or distention
- Precipitating and alleviating factors
- Any pharmacologic or nonpharmacologic treatment measures used
- Complete physical examination with special attention to measures of fluid and electrolyte balance, nutritional status, and gastric, liver, thyroid, heart, and lung function
- Prepregnancy weight and gain or loss during pregnancy

The most important initial laboratory test to be obtained is a determination of ketonuria. Other laboratory tests that may be ordered are a urinalysis, a complete blood cell count, electrolytes, liver enzymes, and bilirubin levels. These tests help to rule out underlying diseases such as gastroenteritis, pyelonephritis, pancreatitis, cholecystitis, peptic ulcer, and hepatitis (Cunningham et al., 2018). Because of the recognized association between hyperemesis gravidarum and hyperthyroidism, thyroid levels may also be measured (Nader, 2019).

Psychosocial assessment includes asking the woman about anxiety, fears, and concerns related to her own health and the effects on pregnancy outcome. Family members should be assessed both for anxiety and their role in providing support for the woman.

Client Problems

Common problems identified in women experiencing hyperemesis gravidarum include:

- *Dehydration* related to excessive vomiting as evidenced by fluid and electrolyte imbalance
- *Inadequate weight gain*, related to nausea and persistent vomiting as evidenced by weight decrease as compared with prepregnant weight
- *Anxiety* related to effects of hyperemesis on fetal well-being as evidenced by woman's statements of concern

Interventions

Initial Care

Initially the woman who is unable to retain clear liquids by mouth requires IV therapy for correction of fluid and electrolyte imbalances. In the past, women requiring IV therapy were admitted to the hospital. More recently, they are successfully managed as outpatients or at home, even if on enteral therapy.

Medications may be used if nausea and vomiting are uncontrolled. The current ACOG guidelines for treatment of NVP recommend the use of pyridoxine (vitamin B_6), either alone or in combination with doxylamine (Unisom) as initial medical management. Since 2013 a single drug combination of pyridoxine and doxylamine (Diclegis) has been available for use in the United States. Advantages to the use of Diclegis are that it is a single tablet and provides delayed-release effects (ACOG, 2018b; Castillo & Phillippi, 2015). Cost is a disadvantage to the use of Diclegis, because no generic form of the medication is currently available.

Other frequently prescribed drugs include dopamine antagonists such as promethazine (Phenergan), chlorpromazine (Thorazine), and prochlorperazine (Compazine). These medications have been found to be effective, but their safety in pregnancy has not been proven. Moreover, they have side effects such as dry mouth, dystonia, and sedation (ACOG, 2018b; Kelly & Savides, 2019). Antihistamines such as diphenhydramine (Benadryl) act on the vestibular system, decreasing stimulation of the vomiting center (Bustos et al., 2017). They have efficacy and side effects similar to the dopamine antagonists listed previously, with the addition of lightheadedness and constipation as side effects.

Metoclopramide (Reglan) accelerates gastric emptying and corrects gastric dysrhythmias. It has been demonstrated in some small studies to be both safe and effective. Ondansetron (Zofran) and droperidol (Inapsine) have been used to treat postoperative nausea and vomiting, but their use in pregnancy has not been well studied (Kelly & Savides, 2019).

Corticosteroids (methylprednisolone [Medrol] or hydrocortisone) may be prescribed for women who do not respond well to the medications previously discussed, but their use is controversial. These medications affect the chemoreceptor trigger zone in the brain (Bustos et al., 2017), but they have not been proven to treat hyperemesis effectively in all women. Because exposure to corticosteroids may increase the risk for facial clefting, they should be used with caution and avoided if possible during the first trimester, when organs and organ systems are developing (Kelly & Savides, 2019).

In addition to antiemetic drugs, medications to control heartburn or reflux may also be prescribed. Use of antacids, histamine blockers, and proton pump inhibitors has been associated with improved symptom management and quality of life (Castillo & Phillippi, 2015).

Finally, enteral or parenteral nutrition may be used as a last resort in women who are nonresponsive to other medical therapies (Kelly & Savides, 2019). Because of potential risks, parenteral therapy should be used only after multiple medical management and enteral tube feeding attempts have been unsuccessful.

Nursing care of the woman with hyperemesis gravidarum involves implementing the medical plan of care, whether in the hospital or home setting. Interventions may include initiating and monitoring IV therapy, administering drugs and nutritional supplements, and monitoring the woman's response to interventions. The nurse observes the woman for any signs of complications such as metabolic acidosis (secondary to starvation), jaundice, or hemorrhage and alerts the health care provider should these occur. Monitoring includes assessing the woman's nausea, retching without vomiting (sometimes called *dry heaves*), and vomiting, given that these symptoms, although related, are separate. Intake and output, including the amount of emesis, should be measured accurately and recorded. Oral hygiene while the woman is receiving nothing by mouth and after episodes of vomiting helps to lessen associated discomforts. Assistance with positioning and providing a quiet, restful environment that is free from odors may increase the woman's comfort.

Once the vomiting has stopped, feedings are started in small amounts at frequent intervals. In the beginning, limited amounts of oral fluids and bland foods such as crackers, toast, or baked chicken are offered. The diet progresses slowly as tolerated by the woman until she is able to consume a nutritionally sound diet. Because sleep disturbances may accompany hyperemesis gravidarum, promoting adequate rest is important. The nurse can help to coordinate treatment measures and periods of visitation to provide opportunity for rest periods.

Follow-Up Care

Most women are able to take nourishment by mouth after several days of treatment. They should be encouraged to eat small, frequent meals and foods that sound appealing (e.g., nongreasy, dry, sweet, and salty foods). In many instances, women discover that foods they normally like have no appeal at all during this time. (See Teaching for Self-Management: Diet for Hyperemesis for more suggestions.) Many pregnant women find exposure to cooking odors nauseating. Having other family members cook may lessen the woman's nausea and vomiting, even if only temporarily. The woman is counseled to contact her health care provider immediately if the nausea and vomiting recur.

The woman with hyperemesis gravidarum needs calm, compassionate, and sympathetic care, with recognition that the manifestations of hyperemesis can be physically and emotionally debilitating to her and stressful for her family. Irritability, tearfulness, and mood changes are often consistent with this disorder. Fetal well-being is a primary concern of the woman. The nurse can provide an environment conducive to discussion of concerns and help the woman to identify and mobilize sources of support. The family should be included in the plan of care whenever possible. Their participation may help alleviate some of the emotional stress associated with this disorder.

THYROID DISORDERS

The thyroid undergoes physiologic changes during pregnancy, including an increase in size and a 50% increase in production levels of thyroxine (T_4) and triiodothyronine (T_3), while hCG stimulates thyroid-stimulating hormone (TSH) receptors, resulting in a decrease in TSH reference ranges (Alexander, Pearce, Brent, et al., 2017). These changes are also different for each stage of pregnancy, which further makes the interpretation of laboratory results for diagnosis of dysfunction difficult. In addition, many of the signs and symptoms of thyroid disorders (e.g., nausea, anxiety, fatigue, and increased heart rate) are also common complaints during pregnancy. Thus careful assessment and analysis of any symptoms is critical to early diagnosis and intervention to prevent fetal and maternal harm.

Hyperthyroidism

Hyperthyroidism in pregnancy is rare. The incidence varies, occurring in approximately 2 to 17 of every 1000 births (Cunningham et al., 2018). In 90% to 95% of pregnant women, it is caused by Graves disease (Nader). Clinical manifestations of hyperthyroidism include heat intolerance, diaphoresis, fatigue, anxiety, emotional lability, and tachycardia. Signs that may help to differentiate hyperthyroidism from normal pregnancy changes include weight loss, goiter, and a pulse rate greater than 100 beats/min. Laboratory findings typically include elevated T_3 and T_4 levels and greatly suppressed TSH levels (Nader).

Moderate and severe hyperthyroidism must be treated during pregnancy. Untreated or inadequately treated women have an increased risk of miscarriage, preterm birth, and giving birth to infants with goiter, hyperthyroidism, or hypothyroidism. However, most neonates born to women with hyperthyroidism have normal thyroid function. Women with hyperthyroidism are at increased risk for developing severe preeclampsia and heart failure (Cunningham et al., 2018; Nader, 2019).

The primary treatment of hyperthyroidism during pregnancy is drug therapy. The medications most often prescribed in the United States are propylthiouracil (PTU) or methimazole (MMI). Both drugs are effective at controlling symptoms, but both have potentially dangerous maternal and fetal side effects. PTU can cause hepatic toxicity serious enough to require liver transplantation. When taken during the first trimester of pregnancy, MMI can cause choanal atresia or esophageal atresia, facial anomalies, hearing loss, developmental delay, and congenital cardiac malformations in exposed fetuses. Although the likelihood of maternal and fetal side effects from both drugs is low, a panel convened by the FDA and the American Thyroid Association recommended that PTU be used only in the first trimester of pregnancy. After the first trimester, women requiring drug therapy for hyperthyroidism should be switched to MMI for the remainder of pregnancy (Mestman, 2017).

The usual starting dose of PTU is 100 to 150 mg three times a day. For MMI the initial dose is generally 20 mg/day. Women usually show clinical improvement (weight gain and less tachycardia) within 2 to 6 weeks after beginning therapy. Once clinical improvement occurs, the dose of PTU or MMI may be cut in half. If symptoms worsen, the medication dosage is doubled (Mestman, 2017). During therapy thyroid test results are used to taper the drug to the smallest effective dose to prevent development of unnecessary fetal or neonatal hypothyroidism. In many women the medication can be discontinued by 32 to 36 weeks of gestation. PTU readily crosses the placenta and may cause fetal hypothyroidism, which is characterized by goiter, bradycardia, and intrauterine growth restriction (IUGR) (Nader, 2019).

Both medications work well in and are well tolerated by most women. The most common maternal side effects of both PTU and MMI are pruritus and skin rash. Other possible side effects include drug-related fever, bronchospasm, migratory polyarthritis, a lupus-like syndrome, and cholestatic jaundice (Mestman, 2017; Nader, 2019). The most severe side effect is agranulocytosis, which occurs rarely and usually develops only in older women and in those taking high doses of the drug. Symptoms of agranulocytosis are fever and unexpected sore throat, which should be reported to the health care provider; in addition, the woman should immediately stop taking the medication (Mestman; Nader). β-Adrenergic blockers such as propranolol (Inderal) or atenolol (Tenormin) may be used in severe hyperthyroidism to control maternal symptoms, especially elevated heart rate. However, long-term use of these medications is not recommended because of the potential for IUGR, bradycardia, and hypoglycemia (Nader).

! NURSING ALERT

A serious but uncommon complication of undiagnosed or partially treated hyperthyroidism is thyroid storm, which can occur in response to stress such as labor and vaginal birth, infection, preeclampsia, or surgery. A woman with this emergency disorder may have fever, restlessness, tachycardia, vomiting, or stupor. Prompt treatment is essential. IV fluids and oxygen are administered, along with high doses of PTU. After administration of PTU, iodide is given. Other medications include antipyretics, dexamethasone, and β-blockers (Cunningham et al., 2018; Nader, 2019).

After birth, women taking either PTU or MMI who choose to breastfeed may do so, if their daily dose of PTU or MMI is less than 300 mg/day or 20 mg/day, respectively. Women should be informed that the medications do not appear to adversely affect the neonate's thyroid

function. Antithyroid medication should be given in divided doses and taken just after breastfeeding, thus allowing a 3- to 4-hour period before nursing again (Mestman, 2017; Nader, 2019; Spencer, 2015).

Radioactive iodine must not be used in diagnosis or treatment of hyperthyroidism in pregnancy because therapeutic doses given to treat maternal thyroid disease may also destroy the fetal thyroid. There is no evidence that radioactive iodine given before pregnancy causes fetal anomalies if enough time has passed to allow the radiation effects to disappear and if the woman has normal thyroid function (Cunningham et al., 2018).

In severe cases, surgical treatment of hyperthyroidism, subtotal thyroidectomy, can be performed during pregnancy. Surgery is best performed during the early second trimester of pregnancy when the risk for teratogenesis and preterm labor is lower, although it can be done during the first or third trimester if necessary. Surgery is usually reserved for women with severe disease, those for whom drug therapy proves toxic, and those who are unable to follow the prescribed medical regimen. Risks associated with the surgery are hypoparathyroidism, recurrent laryngeal nerve paralysis, and anesthesia-related complications (Nader, 2019).

Hypothyroidism

Hypothyroidism occurs in 2 to 12 pregnancies per 1000. Because severe hypothyroidism is often associated with infertility and an increased risk of miscarriage, it is not often seen during pregnancy (Cunningham et al., 2018). Although iodine deficiency is rare in the United States, it is a common cause of maternal, fetal, and neonatal hypothyroidism in the rest of the world (Nader, 2019). Adult hypothyroidism is usually caused by glandular destruction by autoantibodies, most commonly because of Hashimoto thyroiditis. Characteristic symptoms of hypothyroidism include weight gain, lethargy, decrease in exercise capacity, and cold intolerance. Women who are moderately symptomatic can also develop constipation, hoarseness, hair loss, brittle nails, and dry skin. Laboratory values in pregnancy include elevated levels of TSH, with or without low T_4 levels (Nader).

Pregnant women with untreated hypothyroidism are at increased risk for miscarriage, preeclampsia, placental abruption, preterm birth, and stillbirth. Infants born to mothers with hypothyroidism may also be of low birthweight (Alexander et al., 2017; Cunningham et al., 2018; Nader, 2019). These outcomes can be improved with early treatment (Nader).

Thyroid hormone supplements are used to treat hypothyroidism. Levothyroxine (e.g., T_4 [Synthroid]) is most often prescribed during pregnancy. The usual beginning dosage is 0.1 to 0.15 mg/day, with adjustment by 25 to 50 μg every 4 to 6 weeks as necessary based on the maternal TSH level (Cunningham et al., 2018; Nader, 2019). The aim of drug therapy is to maintain the TSH level at the lower end of the normal range for pregnant women. Women with little or no functioning thyroid tissue require higher doses of levothyroxine. In addition, as pregnancy progresses, increased doses of thyroid hormone are usually required. This increased demand during pregnancy is probably related to increased estrogen levels (Cunningham et al.; Nader). Women with hypothyroidism will likely continue treatment with levothyroxine postpartum. This medication is considered safe for use while breastfeeding (Spencer, 2015).

⬦ MEDICATION ALERT

If taking iron supplementation, pregnant women should be told to take levothyroxine at a different time of day, at least 4 h apart, from their iron tablets, because ferrous sulfate decreases absorption of T_4 (Nader, 2019).

The fetus depends on maternal thyroid hormones until approximately 18 weeks of gestation, when fetal production begins. Normal maternal T_4 levels early in pregnancy are important for proper fetal brain development. Results of two studies suggested that normalizing thyroid function by midpregnancy in women with hypothyroidism avoids neurodevelopmental deficits in their children (Mestman, 2017).

Nursing Interventions

Education of the pregnant woman with thyroid dysfunction is essential to promote compliance with the plan of treatment. Important points to discuss with the woman and her family include the disorder and its potential effect on her, her family, and her fetus; the medication regimen and possible side effects; the need for continuing medical supervision; and the importance of adherence. In addition, teaching about how to manage the discomforts and frustrations associated with symptoms of the disorder should be provided. For example, a woman with hyperthyroidism who has nervousness and hyperactivity along with weakness and fatigue can benefit from suggestions to channel excess energies into quiet diversional activities such as reading or crafts. Discomfort associated with hypersensitivity to heat (hyperthyroidism) or cold intolerance (hypothyroidism) can be minimized by appropriate clothing and regulation of environmental temperatures and by avoiding temperature extremes.

Nutrition counseling with a registered dietitian may provide guidance in selecting a well-balanced diet. The woman with hyperthyroidism who has increased appetite and poor weight gain and the hypothyroid woman who has anorexia and lethargy need counseling to ensure adequate intake of nutritionally sound foods to meet both maternal and fetal needs.

MATERNAL PHENYLKETONURIA

Phenylketonuria (PKU), a recognized cause of cognitive impairment, is an inborn error of metabolism caused by an autosomal recessive trait that creates a deficiency in the enzyme phenylalanine hydrolase. Absence of this enzyme impairs the body's ability to metabolize the amino acid phenylalanine found in all protein foods. Consequently, toxic accumulation of phenylalanine in the blood occurs, which interferes with brain development and function. Individuals with this disorder also have hypopigmentation of hair, eyes, and skin because phenylalanine inhibits melanin production (Cunningham et al., 2018). The prevalence of PKU varies worldwide, but it is present in every racial and ethnic group. In the United States, PKU affects approximately 1 in 20,000 live births (Banta-Wright, Kodadek, Houck, et al., 2015).

PKU was the first inborn error of metabolism to be universally screened for in the United States. Since 1961, all newborns have been tested soon after birth for this disorder. Prompt diagnosis and therapy with a phenylalanine-restricted diet significantly decrease the incidence of cognitive impairment (Douglas & Aminoff, 2019). Currently, lifelong dietary restriction and therapy are recommended because they improve the quality of life for individuals with PKU (ACOG, 2015/2017). The keys to the prevention of fetal anomalies caused by maternal PKU are the identification of women in their reproductive years with the disorder and dietary compliance for women who are diagnosed. Screening for undiagnosed homozygous maternal PKU at the first prenatal visit may be warranted, especially in individuals with a family history of the disorder, with low intelligence of uncertain origin, or who have given birth to microcephalic infants. Ideally women with PKU begin dietary phenylalanine restriction before conception and continue it throughout early pregnancy (Douglas & Aminoff). (See Chapter 36 for more information regarding the diet recommended for individuals with PKU.) Experts recommend that maternal phenylalanine levels be less than 6 mg/dL for at least 3 months before conception and range between 2 and 6 mg/dL throughout pregnancy. These levels are associated with a decrease in fetal sequelae (ACOG, 2015/2017; Cunningham et al., 2018). High maternal phenylalanine levels are associated with intellectual disability, microcephaly, seizures, growth impairment, and cardiac anomalies in their children (Douglas & Aminoff; Cunningham et al.).

Breastfeeding is safe for women with PKU, so long as the baby does not also have PKU (ACOG, 2015/2017). If infants with PKU are breastfed, their blood phenylalanine levels are measured once or twice weekly and the dietary feeding plan is adjusted, based on the results. Infants are fed both breast milk and phenylalanine-free medical formula. If the infant's phenylalanine level is diminished, breastfeeding is increased. On the other hand, if the phenylalanine level is elevated, breastfeeding is decreased (Banta-Wright et al., 2015).

▮ KEY POINTS

- In pregnant women with pregestational diabetes, lack of glycemic control before conception and in the first trimester of pregnancy may be responsible for fetal congenital malformations.
- For pregnant women who have diabetes and are insulin dependent, insulin requirements increase as the pregnancy progresses and may quadruple by term as a result of insulin resistance created by placental hormones, insulinase, and cortisol. After birth, levels decrease dramatically; breastfeeding affects insulin needs.
- Poor glycemic control before and during pregnancy in women who have diabetes can lead to maternal complications such as miscarriage, infection, and dystocia (difficult labor) caused by fetal macrosomia.
- Careful glucose monitoring, insulin administration when necessary, and dietary counseling are used to create a normal intrauterine environment for fetal growth and development in the pregnancy complicated by diabetes mellitus.

- Because gestational diabetes mellitus (GDM) is asymptomatic in most cases, all women who are not known to have pregestational diabetes undergo routine screening by history, clinical risk factors, and laboratory assessment of blood glucose levels during pregnancy. Two different methods for diagnosing GDM are currently used.
- The woman with hyperemesis gravidarum may have significant weight loss and dehydration. Management focuses on restoring fluid and electrolyte balance and preventing recurrence of nausea and vomiting.
- Thyroid dysfunction, hyperthyroidism or hypothyroidism, during pregnancy requires close monitoring of thyroid hormone levels to regulate therapy and prevent fetal insult.
- High levels of phenylalanine in the maternal bloodstream cross the placenta and are teratogenic to the developing fetus. Damage can be prevented or minimized by dietary restriction of phenylalanine before and during pregnancy.

REFERENCES

Alexander, E. K., Pearce, E. N., Brent, G. A., et al. (2017). Guidelines for the diagnosis and management of thyroid disease during pregnancy and the postpartum. *Thyroid, 27*(3), 316–389.

American College of Obstetricians and Gynecologists. (2015, reaffirmed 2017). Committee opinion no. 636: Management of women with phenylketonuria. *Obstetrics & Gynecology, 125*(6) 1548-50.

American College of Obstetricians and Gynecologists. (2016, reaffirmed 2018). Practice bulletin no. 173: Fetal macrosomia. *Obstetrics & Gynecology, 128*(5), e195–e209.

American College of Obstetricians and Gynecologists. (2018a). Practice bulletin no. 190: Gestational diabetes mellitus. *Obstetrics & Gynecology, 131*(2), e49–e64.

American College of Obstetricians and Gynecologists. (2018b). Practice bulletin no. 189: Nausea and vomiting of pregnancy. *Obstetrics & Gynecology, 131*(1), e15–e30.

American Diabetes Association. (2017). Classification and diagnosis of diabetes. *Diabetes Care, 40*(Suppl. 1), S11–S24.

American Diabetes Association. (2018). Management of diabetes in pregnancy: Standards of medical care in diabetes – 2018. *Diabetes Care, 41*(Suppl. 1), S137–143.

Antony, K. M., Racusin, D. A., Aagaard, K., et al. (2017). Maternal physiology. In S. G. Gabbe, J. R. Niebyl, J. L. Simpson, et al. (Eds.), *Obstetrics: Normal and problem pregnancies* (7th ed.). Philadelphia: Elsevier.

Banta-Wright, S. A., Kodadek, S. M., Houck, G. M., et al. (2015). Commitment to breastfeeding in the context of phenylketonuria. *Journal of Obstetric, Gynecologic and Neonatal Nursing, 44*(6), 726–736.

Bennett, S., Tita, A., Owen, J., et al. (2015). Assessing White's classification of pregestational diabetes in a contemporary diabetic population. *Obstetrics & Gynecology, 125*(5), 1217–1223.

Bustos, M., Venkataramanan, R., & Caritas, S. (2017). Nausea and vomiting of pregnancy: What's new? *Autonomic Neuroscience: Basic and Clinical, 202*, 62–72.

Castillo, M. J., & Phillippi, J. C. (2015). Hyperemesis gravidarum: A holistic overview and approach to clinical assessment and management. *Journal of Perinatal & Neonatal Nursing, 29*(1), 12–22.

Centers for Disease Control and Prevention (CDC). (2017). *National diabetes statistics report*, 2017. Retrieved from: https://www.cdc.gov/diabetes/data/statistics/statistics-report.html.

Cunningham, F., Leveno, K., Bloom, S., et al. (2018). *Williams Obstetrics* (25th ed.). New York: McGraw-Hill Education.

Daley, J. M. (2014). Diabetes in pregnancy. In K. R. Simpson, & P. Creehan (Eds.), *AWHONN's perinatal nursing* (4th ed.). Philadelphia: Lippincott Willliams & Wilkins.

Douglas, V. C., & Aminoff, M. J. (2019). Neurologic disorders. In R. Resnik, C. J. Lockwood, T. R. Moore, et al. (Eds.), *Creasy & Resnik's maternal-fetal medicine: Principles and practice* (8th ed.). Philadelphia: Elsevier.

Inturrisi, M. (2017). Care of the laboring woman with diabetes. In B. B. Kennedy, & S. M. Baird (Eds.), *Intrapartum management modules: A perinatal education program* (5th ed.). Philadelphia: Wolters Kluwer.

Kelly, T. F., & Savides, T. J. (2019). Gastrointestinal disease in pregnancy. In R. Resnik, C. J. Lockwood, T. R. Moore, et al. (Eds.), *Creasy & Resnik's maternal-fetal medicine: Principles and practice* (8th ed.). Philadelphia: Elsevier.

Landon, M. B., Catalano, P. M., & Gabbe, S. G. (2017). Diabetes mellitus complicating pregnancy. In S. G. Gabbe, J. R. Niebyl, J. L. Simpson, et al. (Eds.), *Obstetrics: Normal and problem pregnancies* (7th ed.). Philadelphia: Elsevier.

Mercer, B. M. (2019). Assessment and Induction of fetal pulmonary maturity. In R. Resnik, C. J. Lockwood, T. R. Moore, et al. (Eds.), *Creasy & Resnik's maternal-fetal medicine: Principles and practice* (8th ed.). Philadelphia: Elsevier.

Mestman, J. H. (2017). Thyroid and parathyroid diseases in pregnancy. In S. G. Gabbe, J. R. Niebyl, J. L. Simpson, et al. (Eds.), *Obstetrics: Normal and problem pregnancies* (7th ed.). Philadelphia: Elsevier.

Moore, T. R., Hauguel-deMouzon, S., & Catalano, P. (2019). Diabetes in pregnancy. In R. Resnik, C. J. Lockwood, T. R. Moore, et al. (Eds.), *Creasy & Resnik's maternal-fetal medicine: Principles and practice* (8th ed.). Philadelphia: Elsevier.

Nader, S. (2019). Thyroid disease and pregnancy. In R. Resnik, C. J. Lockwood, T. R. Moore, et al. (Eds.), *Creasy & Resnik's maternal-fetal medicine: Principles and practice* (8th ed.). Philadelphia: Elsevier.

Ortiz, F. M., Jimenez, E. Y., Boursaw, B., et al. (2016). Postpartum care for women with gestational diabetes. *American Journal of Maternal Child Nursing, 41*(2), 116–122.

Reddy, U. M., & Silver, R. M. (2019). Stillbirth. In R. Resnik, C. J. Lockwood, T. R. Moore, et al. (Eds.), *Creasy & Resnik's maternal-fetal medicine: Principles and practice* (8th ed.). Philadelphia: Elsevier.

Simhan, H. N., Berghella, V., & Iams, J. D. (2019). Prevention and management of preterm parturition. In R. Resnik, C. J. Lockwood, T. R. Moore, et al. (Eds.), *Creasy & Resnik's maternal-fetal medicine: Principles and practice* (8th ed.). Philadelphia: Elsevier.

Spencer, B. (2015). Medications and breastfeeding for mothers with chronic illness. *Journal of Obstetric, Gynecologic and Neonatal Nursing, 44*(4), 543–552.

Wapner, R. J., & Dugoff, L. (2019). Prenatal diagnosis of congenital disorders. In R. Resnik, C. J. Lockwood, T. R. Moore, et al. (Eds.), *Creasy & Resnik's maternal-fetal medicine: Principles and Practice* (8th ed.). Philadelphia: Elsevier.

World Health Organization. (2017). *Diabetes: Fact sheet*. Retrieved from: http://www.who.int/mediacentre/factsheets/fs312/en/.

30

Medical-Surgical Disorders

Kristen S. Montgomery

http://evolve.elsevier.com/Lowdermilk/MWHC/

LEARNING OBJECTIVES

- Describe the management of selected cardiovascular disorders in pregnant women.
- Identify nursing interventions for a pregnant woman with a cardiovascular disorder.
- Discuss anemia during pregnancy.
- Explain the care of pregnant women with pulmonary disorders.
- Examine the effect of a gastrointestinal disorder on gastrointestinal function during pregnancy
- Identify the effects of neurologic disorders on pregnancy.

- Describe the care of women whose pregnancies are complicated by autoimmune disorders.
- Differentiate signs and symptoms and management of urinary tract infections during pregnancy.
- Explain the basic principles of care for a pregnant woman who is having surgery.
- Discuss the implications of trauma in regard to mother and fetus.
- Identify priorities in assessment and stabilization measures for the pregnant trauma survivor.

For most women, pregnancy represents a normal part of life. This chapter discusses the care of women for whom pregnancy represents a significant risk because it is superimposed on a preexisting medical condition. Care of women with uncomplicated pregnancies who develop medical or surgical problems that could happen to anyone at any time of life but occur during pregnancy is also discussed. With the active participation of well-motivated women in the treatment plan and careful management from an interprofessional health care team, positive pregnancy outcomes are often possible in both of these situations.

This chapter focuses on the care of pregnant women with disorders of the cardiovascular, hematologic, respiratory, integumentary, neurologic, gastrointestinal, and urinary systems, as well as those with autoimmune disorders. Care of the pregnant woman undergoing surgery or experiencing trauma is also discussed.

CARDIOVASCULAR DISORDERS

During a normal pregnancy, the maternal cardiovascular system undergoes many changes that place a physiologic strain on the heart (see Chapter 13). The major cardiovascular changes that occur during a normal pregnancy and affect the woman with cardiac disease are increased intravascular volume, decreased systemic vascular resistance, cardiac output changes occurring during labor and birth, and the intravascular volume changes that occur just after birth. These physiologic changes are present during pregnancy and continue for a few weeks after birth. The normal heart can compensate for the increased workload, so pregnancy, labor, and birth are generally well tolerated, but the diseased heart is hemodynamically challenged.

If the cardiovascular changes are not well tolerated, cardiac failure can develop during pregnancy, labor, or the postpartum period. In addition, if myocardial disease develops, valvular disease exists, or a congenital heart defect is present, *cardiac decompensation* (inability of the heart to maintain a sufficient cardiac output) may occur. Fever is

the major cause of cardiac decompensation during pregnancy (Deen, Chandrasekaran, Stout, et al., 2017).

About 1% of pregnancies are complicated by serious heart disease. The risk of maternal morbidity and mortality ranges from low to high, depending on the cardiac defect (Elkayam, Goland, Pieper, & Silversides, 2016). A perinatal mortality of up to 50% is anticipated with persistent cardiac decompensation. The rates of congenital heart disease and mitral valve disease are increasing in women of childbearing age, whereas the incidence of rheumatic fever has diminished. The presence of a maternal congenital cardiac defect increases the risk to the fetus for a congenital heart defect from 1% to about 4% to 6% (Elkayam et al.). Box 30.1 lists maternal cardiac disease risk groups.

The degree of disability experienced by the woman with cardiac disease is often more important in the treatment and prognosis of cardiac disease complicating pregnancy than is the diagnosis of cardiovascular disease. The New York Heart Association's (NYHA) functional classification of organic heart disease has been a widely accepted standard for many years:

- Class I: asymptomatic without limitation of physical activity
- Class II: symptomatic with slight limitation of activity
- Class III: symptomatic with marked limitation of activity
- Class IV: symptomatic with inability to carry on any physical activity without discomfort

No classification of heart disease can be considered rigid or absolute, but the NYHA classification offers a basic practical guide for treatment, assuming that frequent prenatal visits, good client cooperation, and appropriate obstetric care occur. The functional classification may change for the pregnant woman because of the hemodynamic changes that occur in the cardiovascular system during pregnancy. A 30% to 45% increase in cardiac output occurs compared with nonpregnancy resting values, with most of the increase in the first trimester and the peak at 20 to 26 weeks of gestation (Blanchard & Daniels, 2019; Elkayam et al., 2016). The functional classification of the disease is determined at 3 months and again at 7 or 8 months

BOX 30.1 Maternal Cardiac Disease Risk Groups

Group I (Mortality Rate <1%)
Atrial septal defect
Ventricular septal defect (uncomplicated)
Patent ductus arteriosus
Pulmonic and tricuspid disease
Biosynthetic valve prosthesis (porcine and human allograft)
Tetralogy of Fallot (corrected)
Mitral stenosis (New York Heart Association [NYHA] classes I and II)

Group II (Mortality Rate 5%-15%)
Mitral stenosis (NYHA classes III and IV or with atrial fibrillation)
Aortic stenosis
Coarctation of the aorta (uncomplicated)
Uncorrected tetralogy of Fallot
Previous myocardial infarction
Marfan syndrome with normal aorta
Mechanical valve prosthesis

Group III (Mortality Rate 25%-50%)
Pulmonary hypertension
Coarctation of the aorta (complicated)
Endocarditis
Marfan syndrome with aortic involvement

Data from Krening, C., Troiano, N. H., & Shah, S. S. (2019). Maternal cardiac disorders. In N. H. Troiano, P. M. Witcher, & S. M. Baird (Eds.), *AWHONN's high risk and critical care obstetrics* (4th ed.). Philadelphia: Wolters Kluwer.

of gestation. Pregnant women may progress from class I or II to III or IV during the pregnancy as cardiac output increases and more stress is placed on the heart. Women with cyanotic congenital heart disease do not fit into the NYHA classification because their exercise-induced symptoms have causes unrelated to heart failure.

A diagnosis of cardiac disease depends on the history, physical examination, radiographic and electrocardiographic findings, Holter monitoring, and, if indicated, ultrasonographic results. Most diagnostic studies are noninvasive and can be safely performed during pregnancy. The differential diagnosis of heart disease also involves ruling out respiratory problems and other potential causes of chest pain.

Pregnancy in a woman with heart disease is associated with increased risks for decompensation of maternal cardiac status and pregnancy complications, including maternal arrhythmias, heart failure, preterm birth, fetal growth restriction, and a small but significant risk for maternal and fetal death (Deen et al., 2017). The highest risk of complications or death occurs in women with pulmonary hypertension, complicated coarctation of the aorta, and Marfan syndrome with aortic involvement (Elkayam et al., 2016).

Cardiac diseases vary in their effect on pregnancy depending on whether they are acute or chronic conditions. The following discussion focuses on selected congenital and acquired cardiac conditions and other cardiac disorders. A review of the care of the pregnant woman who has had a heart transplant concludes this section.

Congenital Cardiac Disease

Septal Defects

Atrial septal defect. Atrial septal defect (ASD) (an abnormal opening between the atria), one of the causes of a left-to-right shunt, is one of the most common congenital defects seen during pregnancy. This defect may go undetected because the woman is usually asymptomatic. The pregnant woman with an ASD will most likely have an uncomplicated pregnancy.

Some women may have right-sided heart failure or arrhythmias as the pregnancy progresses as a result of increased plasma volume. Another possible complication is the development of emboli (blood clots) (Krening, Troiano, & Shah, 2019) The risk for congenital heart disease in the fetus of a woman with ASD is 4% to 10% (Elkayam et al., 2016).

Ventricular septal defect. Ventricular septal defect (VSD) (an abnormal opening between the right and left ventricles), another cause of a left-to-right shunt, is usually diagnosed and corrected early in life. As a result, a VSD is not very common in pregnancy. A VSD may occur as a single lesion or in combination with other cardiac anomalies such as tetralogy of Fallot. Women with small, uncomplicated VSDs usually do not have pregnancy complications. For women with a large VSD, there is a higher risk for arrhythmias, heart failure, and pulmonary hypertension. As with ASD, consequences from blood clots can be serious, so thromboembolic prophylaxis is a priority (Krening et al., 2019). The risk for a congenital heart defect to the fetus of a woman with VSD is 6% to 10% (Elkayam et al., 2016).

Patent ductus arteriosus. Patent ductus arteriosus (PDA) is another cause of a left-to-right shunt that is usually diagnosed and corrected during infancy. Possible complications of a PDA include those of VSD as well as endocarditis and pulmonary emboli. Medical management is the same as for VSD (Blanchard & Daniels, 2019).

Acyanotic Lesions

Coarctation of the aorta. Coarctation of the aorta (localized narrowing of the aorta near the insertion of the ductus) is an example of an acyanotic congenital heart lesion. Women with this lesion have hypertension in the upper extremities but hypotension in the lower extremities. If at all possible the lesion should be corrected surgically before pregnancy (Blanchard & Daniels, 2019). However, pregnancy is usually relatively safe for the woman with uncomplicated, uncorrected coarctation. The maternal mortality rate is about 3% for uncorrected defects (Blanchard & Daniels). Complications include hypertension, heart failure, aortic dissection, rupture of associated cranial berry aneurysms and hemorrhagic stroke, ischemic heart disease associated with cephalic hypertension, and infective endocarditis (Blanchard & Daniels; Deen et al., 2017). Preeclampsia also occurs more frequently in women with coarctation (Blanchard & Daniels). The mainstays of treatment for uncorrected coarctation of the aorta during pregnancy are rest and antihypertensive medications, preferably β-adrenergic blocking agents. Vaginal birth is preferable, with epidural anesthesia and shortening of the second stage with vacuum extraction or use of forceps, if necessary. β-Blockers should be continued throughout labor.

Cyanotic Lesions

Tetralogy of fallot. Tetralogy of Fallot is by far the most common cyanotic heart disease during pregnancy (Elkayam et al., 2016). Components of tetralogy of Fallot include a VSD, pulmonary stenosis, overriding aorta, and right ventricular hypertrophy, leading to a right-to-left shunt. Women with tetralogy of Fallot are encouraged to have surgical repair before conception. Pregnancy usually does not pose a significant risk once the VSD and pulmonary stenosis have been repaired but complications such as arrhythmias and heart failure can still develop. Women with uncorrected tetralogy of Fallot, however, experience more right-to-left shunting during pregnancy, resulting in reduced blood flow through the pulmonary circulation and increasing hypoxemia. Women with uncorrected tetralogy of Fallot who have a prepregnancy hematocrit greater than 65%, a history of syncopal episodes, congestive heart failure, oxygen saturation of less than 90%, high right ventricular pressures, or cardiomegaly have a poor prognosis (Krening et al., 2019). Maintenance of venous return in women with uncorrected tetralogy of Fallot is critical. Therefore the most dangerous time for these women is the late third trimester of pregnancy and the early postpartum period, when venous return is reduced by the large pregnant uterus and by peripheral venous pooling after birth.

Use of pressure-graded support hose is recommended. Blood loss during birth may also adversely affect venous return; thus blood volume must be adequately maintained. Prophylactic antibiotics should be given during the intrapartum period (Blanchard & Daniels, 2019).

Acquired Cardiac Disease
Mitral Valve Prolapse
Mitral valve prolapse (MVP) is a fairly common, usually benign, condition. More specific echocardiographic diagnostic criteria have resulted in significantly reduced prevalence estimates for MVP (perhaps 1% of the female population) than previously thought (Blanchard & Daniels, 2019). In MVP, the mitral valve leaflets prolapse into the left atrium during ventricular systole, allowing some backflow of blood. Midsystolic click and late systolic murmur are hallmarks of this syndrome. Most cases are asymptomatic. A few women have atypical chest pain (sharp and located in the left side of the chest) that occurs at rest and does not respond to nitrates. They may also have anxiety, palpitations, dyspnea on exertion, and syncope. If women are symptomatic, β-blocking medications are given to relieve chest pain and palpitations and reduce the risk of life-threatening arrhythmias (Cunningham, Leveno, Bloom, et al., 2018). If symptoms are unusually severe, thyroid function should also be checked (Blanchard & Daniels). Pregnancy and its associated hemodynamic changes may alter or alleviate the murmur and click of MVP, as well as symptoms (Deen et al., 2017). Antibiotic prophylaxis for bacterial endocarditis is no longer recommended for women with uncomplicated MVP. Pregnancy, labor, and birth are usually safe and well tolerated (Blanchard & Daniels; Cunningham et al.).

Mitral Stenosis
Mitral stenosis is almost always caused by rheumatic heart disease (RHD), a consequence of rheumatic fever (Deen et al., 2017). Rheumatic fever develops suddenly, often several symptom-free weeks after an inadequately treated group A β-hemolytic streptococcal throat infection. Episodes of rheumatic fever create an autoimmune reaction in the heart tissue, leading to permanent damage of heart valves (usually the mitral valve) and the chordae tendineae cordis. This damage is classified as RHD. RHD may be evident during acute rheumatic fever or discovered years later. Recurrences of rheumatic fever are common, each with the potential to increase the severity of heart damage.

Mitral stenosis (narrowing of the opening of the mitral valve caused by stiffening of valve leaflets) obstructs blood flow from the left atrium to the left ventricle. As the mitral valve narrows, dyspnea worsens, occurring first on exertion and eventually at rest. A tight stenosis plus the increase in blood volume and cardiac output of normal pregnancy may cause pulmonary edema, atrial fibrillation, right-sided heart failure, infective endocarditis, pulmonary embolism, and massive hemoptysis (Blanchard & Daniels, 2019; Cunningham et al., 2018). Maternal mortality is related to functional capacity. Almost all maternal deaths related to mitral stenosis occur in women who are classified as NYHA class III or class IV (Cunningham et al.).

Women with a history of RHD who are at risk for exposure to streptococcal infection should receive prophylaxis with daily oral penicillin G or monthly benzathine penicillin (Bicillin) injections. Pregnant women are usually considered at high risk for exposure because they generally live around groups of children (Deen et al., 2017). In addition, women with mitral stenosis may receive diuretics such as furosemide (Lasix) to prevent pulmonary edema and a β-blocker to reduce heart rate, improve diastolic blood flow across the valve, and relieve pulmonary congestion (Deen et al.). A combination of drugs will most likely be needed. Women who have chronic atrial fibrillation may require digoxin and β-blockers or calcium channel blockers to control the heart rate. In addition, anticoagulant therapy may be needed to prevent embolism (Blanchard & Daniels, 2019). About 25% of women with mitral valve stenosis experience cardiac failure for the first time during pregnancy (Cunningham et al., 2018).

Care of the woman with mitral stenosis is typically managed by reducing her activity, restricting dietary sodium, and administering diuretics. The pregnant woman with mitral stenosis should be assessed clinically for symptoms and with echocardiograms to monitor the atrial and ventricular size and heart valve function (Blanchard & Daniels, 2019; Deen et al., 2017).

During labor, adequate pain control is required to prevent tachycardia. Epidural analgesia for labor is preferred (Deen et al., 2017; Elkayam et al., 2016). Laboring and birthing in the side-lying position are desirable. The lithotomy position, with the woman supine and her feet in stirrups, will likely cause pulmonary edema (Blanchard & Daniels, 2019). Shortening the second stage of labor by vacuum- or forceps-assisted birth is recommended to decrease the cardiac workload. Even with close monitoring, the woman with moderate to severe mitral stenosis is at risk for pulmonary edema and arrhythmias, the most commonly seen complications. Central hemodynamic monitoring may be necessary for some women during the intrapartum period (Deen et al.).

Medical management alone may not be adequate to control symptoms. For women with NYHA class III or IV cardiac disease, percutaneous balloon mitral valvuloplasty is the treatment of choice for most women with symptomatic mitral stenosis. The procedure appears to be safer for the fetus than open mitral commissurotomy. Mitral balloon valvuloplasty is optimally performed after the first trimester to decrease radiation risks to the fetus (Blanchard & Daniels, 2019).

Aortic Stenosis
Aortic stenosis (narrowing of the opening of the aortic valve leading to an obstruction of left ventricular ejection) is rarely encountered as a complication of pregnancy because most women who develop this condition do so after their reproductive years are over. In the past, the maternal mortality rate was reported to be as high as 17%, but it has decreased over the past several decades (Deen et al., 2017). Medical management is similar to that for mitral stenosis.

Ischemic Heart Disease
Myocardial Infarction
Myocardial infarction (MI) (an acute ischemic event) is rare in reproductive-aged women. It usually occurs during the third trimester of pregnancy (Elkayam et al., 2016).

It is estimated to occur in only 1 of 16,000 pregnancies. However, experts anticipate that the incidence will rise, considering the number of women who delay childbearing until later in life (Krening et al., 2019). Women with coronary artery disease frequently have classic risk factors such as diabetes, hypertension, tobacco use, hyperlipidemia, and family history. The cardiac changes that normally occur in a pregnant woman may provoke symptoms for the first time. It is also possible for women with a history of MI to become pregnant (Krening et al.).

MI occurs most frequently in multigravid women older than 33 years of age. The maternal mortality rate from an MI during pregnancy is approximately 21%. Women are most likely to die at the time of the infarction or within 2 weeks of giving birth (Krening et al., 2019).

Medical management for pregnant women with MI is the same as that for nonpregnant women and includes the administration of morphine, nitrates, lidocaine, β-blockers, aspirin, magnesium sulfate, and calcium antagonists. Coronary angioplasty and stenting procedures have been performed during pregnancy. These procedures should not be avoided if they are considered to be appropriate for treating the woman (Deen et al., 2017). Thrombolytic agents such as urokinase, streptokinase, and tissue plasminogen activator (tPA) do not appear to cross the placenta. However, their use is considered to be relatively contraindicated in pregnancy because of the risk for subsequent maternal and fetal hemorrhage, particularly if they are given at the time of birth (Krening et al., 2019).

Because pain can lead to tachycardia and increased cardiac demands, pain control during labor, usually accomplished with regional anesthesia, is crucial. The side-lying position is preferred to prevent pressure on the vena cava. Vaginal birth is preferred although maternal pushing should be avoided. Vacuum- or forceps-assisted birth may be used to shorten the second stage of labor (Deen et al.).

Other Cardiac Diseases and Conditions

Primary Pulmonary Hypertension

Women with primary pulmonary hypertension (PPH) have constriction of the arteriolar vessels in the lungs, leading to an increase in the pulmonary artery pressure. As a result of this pathology, there is right ventricular hypertension, right ventricular hypertrophy and dilation, and right ventricular failure with tricuspid regurgitation and systemic congestion. The major physiologic difficulty in PPH is maintaining blood flow to the lungs. Any event that significantly decreases venous return to the heart, such as hypotension, impairs the ability of the right ventricle to pump blood through the pulmonary vessels with their high, fixed vascular resistance. Because hypotension can occur quickly and is often unresponsive to medical therapy, it must be avoided (Blanchard & Daniels, 2019).

Symptoms may be vague. Dyspnea on exertion is the most common symptom. Orthopnea and nocturnal dyspnea are also usually present (Cunningham et al., 2018).

PPH is diagnosed by electrocardiography (ECG). Although cardiac catheterization remains the standard procedure for measuring pulmonary artery pressures, noninvasive echocardiography is often used to provide an estimate of these pressures (Cunningham et al., 2018). Mortality rates reported during pregnancy approach 50%, so pregnancy is not advised in women with this condition (Blanchard & Daniels, 2019).

Medical management of women with PPH during pregnancy includes limiting activity and avoiding supine positioning. Diuretics, supplemental oxygen, and vasodilator medications will also be ordered. During labor and birth, hypotension must be avoided by carefully establishing epidural analgesia and preventing blood loss (Cunningham et al., 2018).

Marfan Syndrome

Marfan syndrome is an autosomal dominant disorder characterized by generalized weakness of the connective tissue, resulting in the characteristic feature of the disease, aortic root dilation. Associated cardiovascular changes include MVP, mitral regurgitation, aortic regurgitation, and possible dissection or rupture of the aortic root. Other signs and symptoms associated with Marfan syndrome include dislocation of the optic lens, deformity of the anterior thorax, scoliosis, long limbs, joint laxity, and arachnodactyly. Diagnosis is usually based on family history and physical examination, including ocular, cardiovascular, and skeletal features (Deen et al., 2017; Smith & Gros, 2017).

The majority of deaths from Marfan syndrome are caused by aortic dissection and rupture. Overall, the maternal mortality rate associated with Marfan syndrome is greater than 50%. However, it is significantly increased if the aortic root diameter measures more than 4 cm (Deen et al., 2017; Smith & Gros, 2017).

Preconception counseling for women with Marfan syndrome is essential to make them aware of the risks of pregnancy with this condition. Because the condition is inherited, each child born to a woman with Marfan syndrome has a 50% chance of having the disorder (Krening et al., 2019). An accurate assessment of the aortic root must be obtained to assess the woman's specific risk and make management recommendations. Elective repair of the aorta prior to pregnancy is recommended when the aortic root diameter measures 4 cm or more. On the other hand, women with an aortic root diameter less than 4 cm can attempt pregnancy with only modest risk (Deen et al., 2017).

Management during pregnancy includes restricted activity and use of β-blockers to maintain a resting heart rate of approximately 70 beats/min. Tachycardia should also be prevented during labor. Women with aortic root diameters less than 4 cm may give birth vaginally, reserving cesarean birth for obstetric indications. Some authorities believe that women with larger aortic root diameters should give birth by elective cesarean because of concerns about increased pressure in the aorta during labor. However, data do not exist to make this a firm recommendation (Deen et al., 2017).

Infective Endocarditis

Infective endocarditis is inflammation of the innermost lining—the endocardium—of the heart, caused by invasion of microorganisms. In the United States, women at greatest risk to develop infective endocarditis are those who have congenital heart lesions, degenerative valve disease, or intracardiac devices or who use drugs intravenously (Cunningham et al., 2018). Bacterial endocarditis, leading to incompetence of heart valves and thus congestive heart failure and cerebral emboli, can result in death. Treatment is with antibiotics. Prophylactic treatment with antibiotics is used only for women at highest risk for this condition.

Eisenmenger Syndrome

Eisenmenger syndrome is caused by a congenital communication between the systemic and pulmonary circulations and elevated pulmonary vascular resistance which can result in right-to-left shunting. It is associated with an underlying structural cardiac defect, either a VSD (most common) or a PDA (Blanchard & Daniels, 2019). Eisenmenger syndrome is associated with high maternal mortality (between 30% and 50%). Because of the poor pregnancy outcomes, pregnancy should be avoided by women with the syndrome. Termination (therapeutic abortion) (see Chapter 8 for more information) may be recommended if pregnancy occurs (Krening et al., 2019). Although sudden death can occur at any time, the intrapartum and especially the early postpartum periods seem to be the most dangerous (Blanchard & Daniels). Maternal morbidity is associated with right ventricular failure and associated cardiogenic shock (Cunningham et al., 2018).

In women who continue pregnancy despite the risks, management includes measures to maintain pulmonary blood flow. Physical activity is strictly limited. Other interventions include the use of pressure-graded elastic support hose and oxygen therapy. Antepartal hospitalization may be necessary to provide optimal care (Blanchard & Daniels, 2019; Deen et al., 2017). During labor and birth, regional anesthesia using an opioid analgesic provides pain relief without causing excessive hemodynamic instability. Hypotension must be prevented because it results in more right-to-left shunting. A pulmonary artery catheter and a peripheral arterial catheter may be used to guide hemodynamic management. Cesarean birth should be performed only for obstetric indications and avoided whenever possible (Deen et al.).

Peripartum Cardiomyopathy

Peripartum cardiomyopathy (PCM) is congestive heart failure with cardiomyopathy. The classic criteria for the diagnosis of PCM include development of congestive heart failure in the last month of pregnancy or within the first 5 postpartum months, absence of heart disease before the last month of pregnancy, a left ventricular ejection fraction (EF) of less than 45%, and, most important, lack of another cause for heart failure. The cause of the disease is unknown. The U.S. incidence is 1 in 3000 to 4000 live births (Blanchard & Daniels, 2019).

Associated risk factors include maternal age older than 30 years, multiparity, black race, obesity, multifetal gestation, tocolytic use, preeclampsia, and chronic hypertension. Clinical findings are those of congestive heart failure (left ventricular failure). Clinical manifestations include dyspnea, fatigue, and peripheral or pulmonary edema. Cardiomegaly, pulmonary edema, and occasionally pleural effusions are noted on chest x-ray. The diagnosis is confirmed by echocardiography that demonstrates left ventricular systolic dysfunction with a dilated or normal left ventricular size (Krening et al., 2019).

Medical management of PCM includes a regimen used for congestive heart failure: diuretics, sodium and fluid restriction, afterload-reducing agents, and digoxin. β-blockers have been shown to improve cardiac function and increase the chance of survival. Anticoagulation may be necessary if the cardiac chambers are significantly dilated and contract poorly because of the increased risk for clot formation. Angiotensin-converting enzyme inhibitors, often prescribed to achieve afterload reduction, can be used only in the postpartum period because they are associated with fetal renal dysfunction. During labor, epidural anesthesia is often used for pain control to decrease the cardiac workload and reduce tachycardia. Cesarean birth should be performed only for obstetric indications (Deen et al., 2017).

In one-half of all women with PCM, left ventricular dysfunction resolves within 6 months. These women generally do well. If left ventricular dysfunction does not resolve within 6 months, however, approximately 85% of women with PCM will die in the next 4 to 5 years. Death is usually the result of progressive congestive heart failure, arrhythmia, or thromboembolism (Deen et al., 2017). The recurrence rate for cardiomyopathy in a subsequent pregnancy is high—anywhere from 20% to 50%. The risk of recurrence is increased in women who did not have complete recovery of left ventricular function after the initial episode of PCM (Blanchard & Daniels, 2019).

Valve Replacement

Pregnant women with bioprosthetic or mechanical heart valves require specialized care for this high-risk situation. The primary medical management, anticoagulation, is both controversial and complicated. A high risk for thromboembolism exists because of the hypercoagulability of pregnancy. At the same time, the use of anticoagulants during pregnancy presents the possibility of maternal and fetal hemorrhage. Some oral anticoagulants pose a significant risk to the fetus for abnormalities and intracranial hemorrhage. However, prosthetic heart valve thrombosis is a life-threatening emergency during pregnancy and requires clot removal surgery, which carries a high mortality rate (Elkayam et al., 2016).

Women with bioprosthetic heart valves usually do not require anticoagulation during pregnancy. This type of valve may be used in reproductive-aged women because it has a relatively low rate of complications during pregnancy. However, bioprosthetic valves are not as durable as mechanical valves. In addition, pregnancy accelerates the deterioration of bioprosthetic valves (Deen et al., 2017).

Anticoagulation is required with a mechanical valve. Management of anticoagulation during pregnancy is quite controversial because commonly used medications have significant maternal and fetal adverse effects, and no single agent is safe for use throughout the entire prenatal period. Often low-molecular-weight heparin (Lovenox) is used during the first trimester. In the second and third trimesters, warfarin (Coumadin) may be used instead. If Lovenox is used during the second and third trimesters, it should be discontinued several weeks before the anticipated date of birth and the woman started on heparin. Anticoagulation therapy should be discontinued during labor and resumed in the postpartum period. Warfarin is generally used for long-term postpartum anticoagulation and is safe for use in breastfeeding women (Deen, et al., 2017).

Heart Transplantation

Increasing numbers of heart recipients are successfully completing pregnancies. It is recommended that pregnancy be avoided for at least 1 year after the transplant, because by that time, the risk for rejection and the intensity of immunosuppression are considerably less (Blanchard & Daniels, 2019). Before conception, the woman should be assessed for quality of ventricular function and potential rejection of the transplant. Additionally, she should be stabilized on her immunosuppressant regimen. Women who have no evidence of rejection and have normal cardiac function at the beginning of the pregnancy appear to do well during pregnancy,

labor, and birth. Research has shown that the transplanted heart responds normally to pregnancy-related changes. Complications that are common in women who have had a heart transplant include hypertension and at least one episode of rejection (Cunningham et al., 2018).

CARE MANAGEMENT

The presence of cardiac disease is a significant influencing factor in the decision-making process for or against becoming pregnant. Couples planning a pregnancy must understand the risks involved in their situation. If the pregnancy is unplanned, the nurse should explore the couple's desire to continue the pregnancy in light of the risks involved. Pregnancy termination is one option, depending on the severity of the cardiac defect. The family may need further information to make an informed decision regarding the future of the pregnancy.

Assessment

The pregnant woman with a cardiac disorder is in a high-risk situation. She requires detailed assessment throughout the peripartum period to determine the potential for optimal maternal health and a viable fetus. Her care will be provided by an interprofessional team, including a cardiologist, obstetrician, perinatologist, and registered nurse experienced in the care of women with high-risk pregnancies (see Community Activity box). If she chooses to continue the pregnancy, the woman's condition may be assessed as often as weekly. For additional information on cardiac disease, visit the American Heart Association's website at www.americanheart.org.

COMMUNITY ACTIVITY
Care for Women With High-Risk Pregnancies

- Identify a major medical center near where you live. Check to see if they offer maternity services. If they do, see if they have information related to high-risk pregnancies and the staff available to care for them. Maternal-fetal medicine physicians (perinatologists) are physicians who specialize in high-risk maternal care. Determine how many providers are at the facility and what types of resources they offer online for women with a high-risk pregnancy. Also find out if the hospital offers high-risk neonatal care. Many infants born to women with medical complications need to be cared for in a neonatal intensive care unit (NICU). Review the website for information on what the NICU is like and resources to support the family with an infant in the NICU.
- Review the local newspaper or community websites to determine if there are support groups in your area for women with high-risk pregnancies. Also check online sites because many women connect with online communities when they are pregnant.

Client Problems

Problems often experienced by a woman with a cardiac disorder include:
- *Fear* related to increased peripartum risk
- *Potential for decreased ability to cope* related to
  - the woman's cardiac condition
  - changes in role performance
- *Decreased tissue perfusion* related to hypotensive syndrome
- *Reduced stamina* related to cardiac condition
- *Need for health teaching* related to
  - cardiac condition
  - pregnancy and how it affects cardiac condition
  - medication: dosages and possible side effects
  - requirements to alter self-care activities
- *Reduced functional ability (bathing, dressing, toileting)* related to
  - fatigue or activity intolerance
  - need for bed rest and/or limited activity level

Interventions

Antepartum

Therapy for the pregnant woman with heart disease is focused on minimizing stress on the heart, which intensifies as cardiac output increases. Cardiac output begins to rise significantly early in pregnancy and probably peaks somewhere between 25 and 30 weeks of gestation (Antony, Racusin, Aagaard, et al., 2017). Factors that increase the risk of cardiac decompensation are avoided. The workload of the cardiovascular system is reduced by appropriate treatment of any coexisting emotional stress, hypertension, anemia, hyperthyroidism, or obesity.

Signs and symptoms of cardiac decompensation are taught at the first prenatal visit and reviewed at each subsequent visit (see boxes Signs of Potential Complications: Cardiac Decompensation and Teaching for Self-Management: The Pregnant Woman at Risk for Cardiac Decompensation).

SIGNS OF POTENTIAL COMPLICATIONS

Cardiac Decompensation

Pregnant Woman: Subjective Symptoms

- Increasing fatigue or difficulty breathing, or both, with her usual activities
- Feeling of smothering
- Frequent cough
- Palpitations; feeling that her heart is "racing"
- Generalized edema: swelling of face, feet, legs, fingers (e.g., rings no longer fit)

Nurse: Objective Signs

- Irregular, weak, rapid pulse (≥100 beats/min)
- Progressive, generalized edema
- Crackles at base of lungs after two inspirations and exhalations that do not clear after coughing
- Orthopnea; increasing dyspnea
- Rapid respirations (≥25 breaths/min)
- Moist, frequent cough
- Cyanosis of lips and nailbeds

TEACHING FOR SELF-MANAGEMENT

The Pregnant Woman at Risk for Cardiac Decompensation

- Watch for and immediately report signs of cardiac decompensation or congestive heart failure: generalized edema; distention of neck veins; dyspnea; frequent, moist cough; or palpitations.
- Watch for and immediately report signs of thromboembolism: pain, redness, tenderness, or swelling in extremities or chest pain.
- Avoid constipation and thus straining with bowel movements (Valsalva maneuver) by taking in adequate fluids and fiber. A stool softener may also be helpful.
- Weigh yourself daily, at the same time each day.
- Keep all prenatal appointments.
- Limit activity as instructed by your health care provider.

Modified from Gilbert, E. S. (2011). *Manual of high risk pregnancy and delivery* (5th ed.). St. Louis: Mosby.

Infections are treated promptly because they can complicate the condition by accelerating the heart rate and by direct spread of organisms (e.g., streptococci) to the heart structures. Infections are a major cause of cardiac decompensation during pregnancy. Bacteriuria screens should be performed. The woman should be instructed to notify her health care provider at the first sign of an upper respiratory infection, especially if fever is present. Vaccination against influenza and pneumococci is appropriate (Deen et al., 2017).

Many women with heart disease, especially adolescents, recent immigrants, and those living in poverty, are at risk for iron deficiency anemia. Iron and folate supplementation may help to prevent anemia, and thus decrease cardiac workload (Deen et al., 2017).

Nutrition counseling is necessary, optimally with the woman's family present. The pregnant woman needs a well-balanced diet with iron and folic acid supplementation, high protein levels, and adequate calories to gain weight. Iron supplements tend to cause constipation, so the woman should increase her intake of fluids and fiber. A stool softener may also be prescribed. It is important that the woman with a cardiac disorder avoid straining during defecation, thus causing the Valsalva maneuver (forced expiration against a closed airway, which when released, causes blood to rush to the heart and overload the cardiac system). Sodium restriction may be necessary. The woman's intake of potassium may be monitored to prevent hypokalemia, especially if she is taking diuretics. Depending on the specific cardiac condition, some women may be limited in their total daily fluid intake. A referral to a registered dietitian may be necessary for a nutritional plan of care.

Cardiac medications are prescribed as needed, with attention to fetal well-being. The hemodynamic changes that occur during pregnancy, such as increased plasma volume and increased renal clearance of drugs, can alter the amount of medication needed to establish and maintain a therapeutic drug level. Therefore monitoring drug levels during pregnancy is crucial to maintain effective therapy for the woman while minimizing risk to the fetus. Table 30.1 lists information on medications that are often used to treat cardiac disorders during pregnancy.

Anticoagulant therapy may be prescribed during pregnancy for several conditions such as recurrent venous thrombosis, pulmonary embolus, RHD, prosthetic valves, or cyanotic congenital heart defects. If anticoagulant therapy is required during pregnancy, a number of various regimens may be recommended (see the section on valve disorders for more discussion of anticoagulant therapy). The woman may need to learn to self-administer injectable agents such as heparin or Lovenox. A woman taking warfarin (Coumadin) requires specific nutritional teaching to avoid foods high in vitamin K, such as raw, dark green leafy vegetables, which counteract the effects of warfarin. In addition, she will require a folic acid supplement.

Tests for fetal maturity and well-being and placental sufficiency may be necessary. Other therapy is directly related to the functional classification of heart disease. The nurse must reinforce the need for close medical supervision (see the Nursing Care Plan).

Heart surgery during pregnancy. Ideally, surgery to correct a cardiac lesion should be performed prior to pregnancy. In some women, however, cardiac disease is diagnosed for the first time during pregnancy. The maternal mortality risk does not increase, but there is a fetal mortality risk of 10% to 15% if heart surgery is performed, especially if cardiopulmonary bypass is used. Hypothermia should also be avoided because it appears to be especially dangerous for the fetus. If possible, surgery should be postponed until the third trimester of pregnancy, when the risk to the fetus is considerably decreased (Blanchard & Daniels, 2019).

Intrapartum

For all pregnant women, the intrapartum period is the one that causes the most apprehension in clients and caregivers. The woman with impaired cardiac function has more reasons to be anxious because

TABLE 30.1 Selected Drugs Used in Treatment of Cardiac Disorders in the Pregnant Woman

Generic (Trade) Name	Use in Pregnancy	Potential Side Effects
Digoxin (Lanoxin)	Maternal and fetal arrhythmias, heart failure	No evidence for unfavorable side effects on the fetus
Procainamide (Procanbid, Pronestyl)	Maternal and fetal arrhythmias	Limited data; no fetal side effects reported
Verapamil (Calan, Isoptin)	Maternal and fetal arrhythmias	Limited data; other than one case of fetal death of uncertain cause, no adverse fetal or newborn effects reported
β-Blockers (a class of drugs)	Hypertension, maternal arrhythmias, myocardial ischemia, mitral stenosis, hypertrophic cardiomyopathy, hyperthyroidism, Marfan syndrome	Fetal bradycardia, low placental weight, possible IUGR, hypoglycemia; no information on carvedilol
Heparin	Anticoagulation	None reported
Warfarin (Coumadin)	Anticoagulation	Crosses placenta; fetal hemorrhage, embryopathy, CNS abnormalities
Diuretics (a class of drugs)	Hypertension, congestive heart failure	Hypovolemia leads to reduced uteroplacental perfusion, fetal hypoglycemia, thrombocytopenia, hyponatremia, hypokalemia; thiazide diuretics can inhibit labor and suppress lactation.
Lidocaine (Xylocaine)	Local anesthesia, maternal arrhythmias	No evidence for unfavorable fetal effects; high serum levels may cause CNS depression at birth.
Quinidine (Quinidex)	Maternal and fetal arrhythmias	Minimal oxytocic effect; high dosages may cause premature labor or miscarriage; transient neonatal thrombocytopenia and damage to eighth cranial nerve reported
Nifedipine (Procardia, Adalat)	Hypertension, tocolysis	Fetal distress related to maternal hypotension reported.
ACE inhibitors (a class of drugs)	Hypertension	Oligohydramnios, IUGR, prematurity, neonatal hypotension, renal failure, anemia, death, skull ossification defect, limb contractures, patent ductus arteriosus
Sodium nitroprusside	Hypertension, aortic dissection	Limited data; potential thiocyanate fetal toxicity, fetal mortality reported in animals

ACE, Angiotensin-converting enzyme; *CNS,* central nervous system; *IUGR,* intrauterine growth restriction.
Data from Blanchard, D. G., & Daniels, L. B. (2014). Cardiac diseases. In R. K. Creasy, R. Resnik, J. D. Iams, et al. (Eds.), *Creasy and Resnik's maternal-fetal medicine: Principles and practice* (7th ed.). Philadelphia: Saunders.

labor and giving birth place an additional burden on her already compromised cardiovascular system.

Assessments include the routine assessments for all laboring women and those for cardiac decompensation. In addition, arterial blood gases (ABGs) may be needed to assess for adequate oxygenation. A pulmonary artery catheter may be inserted to monitor hemodynamic status accurately during labor and birth. ECG monitoring and continuous monitoring of blood pressure (BP) and oxygen saturation (pulse oximetry) are usually instituted for the woman, and continuous electronic fetal heart rate (FHR) monitoring is used to monitor the fetus.

❗ NURSING ALERT

A pulse rate of 100 beats/min or greater or a respiratory rate of 25 breaths/min or greater is a concern. The nurse checks the respiratory status frequently for developing dyspnea, coughing, or crackles at the base of the lungs. The color and temperature of the skin are noted, as well. Pale, cool, clammy skin may indicate cardiac shock.

LEGAL TIP

Cardiac and Metabolic Emergencies

The management of emergencies such as maternal cardiopulmonary distress or arrest or maternal metabolic crisis should be documented in policies, procedures, and protocols. Any independent nursing actions that are appropriate to the emergency should be clearly identified.

Nursing care during labor and birth focuses on promoting cardiac function. A calm atmosphere in the labor and birth rooms helps to minimize anxiety. The nurse provides anticipatory guidance by keeping the woman and her family informed of labor progress and events that can occur, as well as answering any questions. It is important to support the woman's labor and birth preparation method and birth plan to the degree it is feasible for her cardiac condition. Nursing interventions that promote comfort, such as back massage, also are used.

Cardiac function is supported by keeping the woman's head and shoulders elevated and body parts resting on pillows. The side-lying position usually facilitates positive hemodynamics during labor. Discomfort is relieved with medication and supportive care. Physiologically, the ideal labor for a woman with heart disease is one that is short and pain free. Therefore use of epidural anesthesia is encouraged, although care must be taken to avoid hypotension, a common side effect of regional anesthesia (Deen et al., 2017; Krening et al., 2019).

β-Adrenergic agents such as terbutaline (Brethine) are associated with various side effects, including tachycardia, irregular pulse, myocardial ischemia, and pulmonary edema. Therefore these medications should not be used in women with known or suspected heart disease (Simhan, Berghella, & Iams, 2019; Simhan, Iams, & Romero, 2017). Spontaneous or induced (with a favorable cervix) labor followed by vaginal birth is preferred for women with cardiac disease. If no obstetric problems exist, vaginal birth may be accomplished with the woman in the side-lying position to facilitate uterine perfusion. The supine position should be avoided. If it is used, a pad or small wedge is placed under one hip to displace the uterus laterally and minimize the danger of supine hypotension. The woman can flex her knees and place her feet flat on the bed. The use of stirrups is contraindicated because stirrups can compress the popliteal veins, thereby increasing the blood volume in the chest and trunk as a result of the effects of gravity. Open-glottis pushing is recommended. The woman should avoid the Valsalva maneuver when pushing in the second stage of labor because it reduces diastolic ventricular filling and obstructs left ventricular outflow. Mask oxygen is important. Episiotomy and vacuum extraction or outlet forceps are often used to decrease the length of the second stage of labor and the heart's workload at that time. Cesarean birth is not routinely recommended for women who have cardiovascular disease because of the risks of dramatic fluid shifts, sustained hemodynamic changes, and increased blood loss.

Routine intrapartum antibiotic prophylaxis for the prevention of bacterial endocarditis is not recommended by the American Heart Association or the American College of Cardiology, but it is optional in women at the highest risk for adverse outcomes from endocarditis who give birth vaginally. This includes women with cyanotic cardiac disease or prosthetic valves, or both. Because bacteremia is common during both vaginal and cesarean birth, many practitioners routinely give antibiotic prophylaxis to all high-risk women. Ampicillin, cefazolin (Ancef), ceftriaxone (Rocephin), and clindamycin (Cleocin) are the antibiotics recommended for prophylaxis. One of these antibiotics is administered as a one-time dose as close as feasible to within 30 to 60 minutes of giving birth (American College of Obstetricians and Gynecologists [ACOG], 2018; Deen et al., 2017; Krening et al., 2019). Oxytocin is usually given immediately after birth to prevent hemorrhage. Ergot products (e.g., methylergonovine [Methergine]) should not be used because they increase BP. Fluid balance should be maintained, and blood loss replaced. If tubal sterilization is desired, it is best to delay surgery until

the woman is hemodynamically near normal, afebrile, nonanemic, and able to ambulate normally (Cunningham et al., 2018).

Postpartum

Monitoring for cardiac decompensation in the postpartum period is essential. The first 24 to 48 hours after birth are the most hemodynamically difficult for the woman. Hemorrhage or infection, or both, may worsen the cardiac condition. The woman with a cardiac disorder may continue to require a pulmonary artery catheter and ABG monitoring after giving birth.

> ### ⚡ SAFETY ALERT
>
> The immediate postbirth period is hazardous for a woman whose heart function is compromised. Cardiac output increases rapidly as extravascular fluid is remobilized into the vascular compartment. At the moment of birth, intraabdominal pressure is reduced dramatically; pressure on veins is removed, the splanchnic vessels engorge, and blood flow to the heart is increased.

Care in the postpartum period is tailored to the woman's functional capacity. Postpartum assessment of the woman with cardiac disease includes vital signs, oxygen saturation levels, lung and heart auscultation, presence and degree of edema, amount and character of bleeding, uterine tone and fundal height, urinary output, pain (especially chest pain), the activity-rest pattern, dietary intake, mother-infant interactions, and emotional state. The head of the bed is elevated, and the woman is encouraged to lie on her side. Bed rest may be ordered, with or without bathroom

◎ NURSING CARE PLAN

The Pregnant Woman With Heart Disease

Client Problem	Expected Outcome	Nursing Interventions	Rationales
Fatigue related to effects of pregnancy on the woman with cardiac disease	Woman will verbalize a plan to modify lifestyle throughout pregnancy so as to reduce the risk of cardiac decompensation	Assist the woman in identifying factors that decrease activity tolerance and explore extent of limitations	To establish a baseline for evaluation
		Teach the woman to monitor physiologic responses to activity (e.g., pulse rate, respiratory rate) and reduce activity that causes fatigue	To maintain sufficient cardiac output and prevent potential injury to the fetus
		Suggest that the woman maintain an activity log that records activities, time, duration, intensity, and physiologic response	To evaluate effectiveness of and adherence to the activity program
Need for health teaching related to the woman's cardiac condition and her perceived sense of wellness	Woman will participate in an effective therapeutic regimen for pregnancy complicated by cardiac disease	Identify factors such as insufficient knowledge about the effect of cardiac disease on pregnancy that might inhibit the woman from participating in a therapeutic regimen	To promote early interventions, such as teaching about the importance of rest
		Teach the woman and her family about factors such as lack of rest or not taking prescribed medications that might adversely affect the pregnancy	To provide information and promote empowerment over the situation
		Encourage expression of feelings about the disease and its potential effect on the pregnancy	To promote a sense of trust
Potential for fluid overload related to increased circulatory volume secondary to pregnancy and cardiac disease	Woman will exhibit signs of adequate cardiac output (i.e., normal pulse and blood pressure; normal heart and breath sounds; normal skin color, tone, and turgor; normal capillary refill; normal urine output; no evidence of edema)	Teach the woman and her family members the signs of cardiac decompensation	To provide information about when to contact the health care provider
		Monitor intake and output and check for edema	To assess for renal complications or venous return problems

privileges. Progressive ambulation may be permitted as tolerated. The nurse or family members may need to help the woman meet her grooming and hygiene needs and other activities. Bowel movements without stress or strain are promoted with stool softeners, diet, and fluids.

The woman may need a family member to help care for the infant. Breastfeeding is not contraindicated, but some women with heart disease (particularly those with life-threatening disease) may be unable to breastfeed. The woman who chooses to breastfeed will need the support of her family and the nursing staff to be successful. For example, she may need assistance in positioning herself or the infant for feeding. Lactation consultants can assist women with breastfeeding positions and other strategies to minimize stress on the cardiovascular system. To further conserve the woman's energy, the infant can be brought to her and taken from her after the feeding. Most medications used to manage cardiac disorders are compatible with breastfeeding. However, diuretics such as furosemide (Lasix) and hydrochlorothiazide (HCTZ) may decrease the milk supply (Blanchard & Daniels, 2019; Spencer, 2015). Because diuretics can cause neonatal diuresis that can lead to dehydration, lactating women must be monitored closely to determine if medication doses can be reduced and still be effective. Neonatal nurses should be alerted to watch for voiding patterns and amounts and to monitor the infant closely for signs of dehydration.

If the woman is unable to breastfeed and her energies do not allow her to bottle feed the infant, the baby can be kept at the bedside so she can look at and touch her baby to establish an emotional bond with a low expenditure of energy. The infant should be held at the mother's eye level and near her lips and brought to her fingers. Assisting the mother to hold her baby skin-to-skin can promote maternal-infant bonding. At the same time, involving the mother passively in her infant's care helps the mother feel vitally important—as she is—to the infant's well-being (e.g., "You can offer something no one else can; you can provide your baby with your sounds, touch, and rhythms that are so comforting"). Perhaps the woman can be encouraged to make a recording of her talking, singing, or whispering, which can be played for the baby in the nursery to help the infant feel her presence and be in contact with her voice. This also enhances maternal-infant bonding.

Preparation for discharge is carefully planned with the woman and family. Provision of help for the woman in the home by relatives, friends, and others must be addressed. If necessary, the nurse or social worker refers the family to community resources (e.g., for assistance with household activities). Rest and sleep periods, activity, and diet must be planned.

Monitoring for cardiac decompensation continues after birth. During the first 2 postpartum weeks, extravascular fluid is mobilized, diuresis begins, and vascular resistance increases, as the woman returns to a nonpregnant state (Deen et al., 2017). Women who have demonstrated little or no evidence of cardiac compromise during the antepartum or intrapartum period may do so postpartum when intravascular fluid mobilization and reduction of peripheral vascular resistance place higher demands on the heart (Cunningham et al., 2018). Maternal cardiac output usually returns to normal by 2 weeks postpartum (Deen et al.).

The couple may need information about reestablishing sexual relations and contraception or sterilization. Women with congenital heart disease should be offered contraceptive counseling. In general, the complications associated with pregnancy are usually greater than the risks associated with any form of contraception (Deen et al., 2017). Women at particular risk for thromboembolism should avoid combined estrogen-progestin oral contraceptives, but progestin-only pills may be used. Parenteral progestins (e.g., medroxyprogesterone [Depo-Provera]) are safe for use by women with cardiac disease and are extremely effective. However, they cause irregular bleeding, which may be problematic for women on anticoagulant therapy. An intrauterine device (IUD) may be used by some women with congenital heart lesions (Deen et al.).

Women, as well as men with congenital heart disease are at increased risk for having children who also have congenital heart disease. The risk for affected mothers is greater, approximately two to more than three times that of affected fathers. Children born with congenital heart disease to parents with congenital heart defects appear to inherit the risk for a defect in general rather than for a specific defect (Deen et al., 2017). Therefore preconception counseling and genetic counseling before a subsequent pregnancy are essential.

OTHER MEDICAL DISORDERS IN PREGNANCY

Anemia

Anemia is a common medical disorder of pregnancy, affecting from 20% to 52% of pregnant women (Kilpatrick & Kitahara, 2019). It results in a reduction of the oxygen-carrying capacity of the blood; the heart tries to compensate by increasing the cardiac output. This effort increases the workload of the heart and stresses ventricular function. Therefore anemia that occurs with any other complication (e.g., preeclampsia) may result in congestive heart failure.

An indirect index of the oxygen-carrying capacity is the packed red blood cell (RBC) volume, or hematocrit level. The normal hematocrit range in nonpregnant women is 37% to 47%. However, the mean hematocrit for pregnant women at term is 33.8% (Blackburn, 2018). According to the Centers for Disease Control and Prevention (CDC), anemia in pregnancy is defined as hemoglobin less than 11 g/dL in the first and third trimesters and less than 10.5 g/dL in the second trimester (Kilpatrick & Kitahara, 2019). A hemoglobin level less than 6 to 8 mg/dL is considered severe anemia (Blackburn).

When a woman has anemia during pregnancy, the loss of blood at birth, even if minimal, is not well tolerated. She has an increased risk for requiring blood transfusions. Women with anemia have a higher incidence of puerperal complications, such as infection, than postpartum women with normal hematologic values.

Care of the anemic pregnant woman requires that the health care provider distinguish between the normal physiologic anemia of pregnancy and disease states. The majority of cases of anemia in pregnancy are caused by iron deficiency. The other types include a considerable variety of acquired and hereditary anemias, such as folic acid deficiency, sickle cell anemia, and thalassemia.

Iron Deficiency Anemia

Iron deficiency anemia is by far the most common anemia of pregnancy, accounting for approximately 75% of cases. In developing countries, it is alarmingly common and is a major cause of maternal morbidity and mortality. It is diagnosed by checking the woman's serum ferritin level in addition to her hemoglobin and hematocrit levels. The serum ferritin level reflects iron reserves (Samuels, 2017). A serum ferritin value less than 12 mcg/L along with a low hemoglobin value indicates iron deficiency anemia (Blackburn, 2018). An association appears to exist between maternal iron deficiency anemia, especially severe anemia, and preterm birth and low-birth-weight infants, although it is uncertain whether these poor pregnancy outcomes are caused by iron deficiency anemia (Samuels). Usually, even the fetus of an anemic woman will receive adequate iron stores from the mother, at the cost of further depleting the mother's iron level (Blackburn).

Generally, iron deficiency anemia is preventable or easily treated with iron supplements. Because of the increased amounts of iron needed for fetal development and maternal stores, pregnant women are often encouraged to take prophylactic iron supplementation (Blackburn, 2018). Most women with iron deficiency anemia can absorb as much iron as they need by taking one 325-mg tablet of ferrous sulfate twice each day (Samuels, 2017). Women who cannot or will not take oral iron therapy but are not anemic enough to require blood transfusion may receive parenteral iron therapy (e.g., iron dextran, iron sucrose [Venofer], or sodium ferric gluconate complex). These medications can be given either intravenously or intramuscularly, although the intramuscular injection is very painful. Women who are severely anemic may require blood transfusions (Samuels).

The nurse teaches the importance of iron supplements for preventing or treating iron deficiency anemia. In addition, the nurse teaches about increasing dietary intake of iron-rich foods and how to decrease the gastrointestinal side effects of iron therapy (see Teaching for Self-Management box: Iron Supplementation in Chapter 15).

Folic Acid Deficiency Anemia

Folate is a water-soluble vitamin found naturally in dark green leafy vegetables, citrus fruits, eggs, legumes, and whole grains. Even in well-nourished women, folate deficiency is common. Poor diet, cooking with large volumes of water, and increased alcohol use may contribute to folate deficiency. During pregnancy, the need for folate increases, both because of fetal demands and because it is less well absorbed from the gastrointestinal (GI) tract during gestation.

Folic acid is the form of the vitamin used in vitamin supplements. The recommended daily intake of folic acid for women planning a pregnancy or capable of becoming pregnant is 400 mcg (ACOG, 2017). Pregnant women need 50% more, or 600 mcg/day (March of Dimes, 2017). Since 1998, the U.S. Food and Drug Administration (FDA) has required the addition of folic acid to cereals, pasta, breads, and other foods that are labeled "enriched." However, the amount added is small, and most pregnant women need a supplement. Both prescription and nonprescription prenatal vitamins contain more than the recommended amount of folic acid and should be sufficient to prevent and treat folate deficiency. Women at particular risk for folate deficiency include those who have significant hemoglobinopathies, take an anticonvulsant medication, are pregnant with a multifetal gestation, or have frequent pregnancies. These women require larger doses of folic acid (Samuels, 2017).

Folate deficiency is the most common cause of megaloblastic anemia during pregnancy, but a vitamin B_{12} deficiency must also be considered. Vitamin B_{12} deficiency in pregnant women is seen much more often now than in the past because of the increasing numbers of women who become pregnant after undergoing bariatric surgery (Kilpatrick & Kitahara, 2019). Other women at risk for developing vitamin B_{12} deficiency are those with gastrointestinal disease such as Crohn disease or who take the medication metformin (Samuels, 2017).

Megaloblastic anemia rarely occurs before the third trimester of pregnancy. Women with megaloblastic anemia caused by folic acid deficiency have the usual presenting symptoms and signs of anemia: pallor, fatigue, and lethargy, as well as glossitis and skin roughness, which are associated specifically with megaloblastic anemia (Kilpatrick & Kitahara, 2019). Folate deficiency usually improves rapidly with folic acid therapy. It rarely occurs in the fetus and is not a significant cause of perinatal morbidity. Iron deficiency often occurs along with folate deficiency (Samuels, 2017).

Sickle Cell Hemoglobinopathy

Sickle cell hemoglobinopathy is a disease caused by the presence of abnormal hemoglobin in the blood. Sickle cell trait (SA hemoglobin pattern) is sickling of the RBCs but with a normal RBC life span. Most people with sickle cell trait are asymptomatic. Approximately 1 in 12 African American adults in the United States has sickle cell trait (Samuels, 2017). Women with sickle cell trait require genetic counseling and

partner testing to determine the risk of their children having sickle cell trait or disease.

Women with sickle cell trait usually do well in pregnancy. However, they are at increased risk for preeclampsia, intrauterine fetal death, preterm birth, low-birth-weight infants, and postpartum endometritis. They are also at increased risk for urinary tract infections (UTIs) (Kilpatrick, 2019; Samuels, 2017).

Sickle cell anemia (sickle cell disease) is a recessive, hereditary, familial hemolytic anemia that affects people of African or Mediterranean ancestry. These individuals usually have abnormal hemoglobin types (SS or SC). The average life span of RBCs in a person with sickle cell anemia is only 5 to 10 days, compared to the 120-day life span of a normal RBC. Sickle cell anemia occurs in 1 in 708 African Americans in the United States (Samuels, 2017). People with sickle cell anemia have recurrent attacks (crises) of fever and pain, most often in the abdomen, joints, or extremities, although virtually all organ systems can be affected. These attacks are attributed to vascular occlusion when RBCs assume a characteristic sickled shape. Crises are usually triggered by dehydration, hypoxia, or acidosis (Samuels).

Women with sickle cell anemia require genetic counseling before pregnancy. All children born to a woman with sickle cell anemia will be affected in some way by the disease. The woman's partner must be tested to determine the couple's risk for having children with sickle cell disease rather than sickle cell trait. Women with sickle cell anemia are at risk for poor pregnancy outcomes, including miscarriage, preterm birth, intrauterine growth restriction (IUGR), and stillbirth. Although maternal mortality is rare, maternal morbidity is significant and includes an increased risk for preeclampsia and infection, particularly in the urinary tract and in the lungs. The frequency of painful crises also appears to be increased during pregnancy (Samuels, 2017).

Folic acid supplementation of at least 1 mg/day should begin as soon as pregnancy is diagnosed. The woman is monitored carefully during pregnancy for the development of UTI or preeclampsia. Fetal surveillance includes serial ultrasound examinations throughout pregnancy to monitor fetal growth and antepartum fetal testing (e.g., nonstress test) during the third trimester. Infections are treated aggressively with antibiotics. If crises occur, they are managed with analgesia, oxygen, and hydration. Prophylactic transfusions, which replace the woman's sickle cells with normal RBCs, have not been shown to improve perinatal outcome. However, although there is no difference in perinatal morbidity or mortality, prophylactic transfusions appear to significantly decrease the incidence of painful crises (Samuels, 2017).

If no complications occur, pregnancy can continue until term. Women with sickle cell disease should be encouraged to labor in a side-lying position. They may require supplemental oxygen. Adequate hydration should be maintained while preventing fluid overload. Regional anesthesia (e.g., epidural or combined spinal epidural anesthesia) is recommended because it provides excellent pain relief. Vaginal birth is preferred. Cesarean birth should be performed only for obstetric indications (Samuels, 2017).

> **⚡ SAFETY ALERT**
>
> Women with sickle cell anemia are not iron deficient. Therefore routine iron supplementation, even in prenatal vitamins, should be avoided because these women can develop iron overload (Samuels, 2017).

Thalassemia

Thalassemia is a relatively common anemia in which an insufficient amount of hemoglobin is produced to fill the RBCs. It is a hereditary disorder that involves the abnormal synthesis of the α or β chains of hemoglobin. β thalassemia is the more common variety in the

United States and usually occurs in people of Mediterranean, Middle Eastern, and Asian descent (Kilpatrick & Kitahara, 2019).

β thalassemia minor is the heterozygous form of thalassemia and has different forms of expression. Some women with this disorder are asymptomatic, while others have splenomegaly and significant anemia. They may require numerous transfusions during pregnancy (Samuels, 2017). Women with pregnancies complicated by β thalassemia minor generally do not experience associated maternal or infant complications if their condition is stable (Blackburn, 2018). These women are managed similarly to women with sickle cell anemia during pregnancy. Iron therapy should only be prescribed for women who are iron deficient, although folic acid supplementation is recommended for all women with β thalassemia minor (Samuels).

The homozygous form of β thalassemia is thalassemia major, formerly called *Cooley anemia*. People with this form of the disease usually have hepatosplenomegaly and bone deformities caused by massive marrow tissue expansion. These individuals usually die of infection or cardiovascular complications fairly early in life. If women live to reach childbearing age, infertility is common. If women with this disorder do become pregnant, they usually experience severe anemia and congestive heart failure, although successful full-term pregnancies have been reported. Women with β thalassemia major are managed much like those with sickle cell anemia during pregnancy (Samuels, 2017).

Pulmonary Disorders

As pregnancy advances and the enlarged uterus presses on the thoracic cavity, any pregnant woman may experience increased respiratory difficulty. This difficulty is compounded by pulmonary disease.

Asthma

Asthma is a chronic inflammatory disorder involving the tracheobronchial airways, with increased airway responsiveness to a variety of stimuli. It is characterized by periods of exacerbations and remissions. Exacerbations are usually triggered by stimuli such as allergens, medications (i.e., aspirin, β-blockers), marked change in ambient temperature, or emotional tension. In many cases, the actual cause may be unknown, although a family history of allergy is common in people with asthma. In response to stimuli, there is widespread but reversible narrowing of the hyperreactive airways, making it difficult to breathe. The clinical manifestations are expiratory wheezing, productive cough, thick sputum, dyspnea, or any combination.

Asthma may be the most common potentially serious medical condition to complicate pregnancy. It affects approximately 4% to 8% of all pregnancies. The prevalence and morbidity rates are increasing, although the asthma-related mortality rate has dropped in recent years (Whitty & Dombrowski, 2019). For clinical convenience, asthma has been divided into four classifications based on severity: mild intermittent, mild persistent, moderate persistent, and severe persistent. Management is determined based on the woman's clinical classification (Mason & Burke, 2019).

The effect of pregnancy on asthma is unpredictable. In one large study, 23% of women with asthma improved during pregnancy, whereas 30% became worse. Pregnant women with severe asthma were much more likely than those with mild or moderate asthma to have exacerbations and require hospitalization. Asthma appears to be associated with preterm birth, preeclampsia, small for gestational age fetuses, IUGR, and an increased rate of cesarean birth, in women with moderate or severe disease or who have daily symptoms. A significant increase in congenital malformations has been associated with asthma exacerbations during the first trimester of pregnancy (Whitty & Dombrowski, 2019). Although poorly controlled asthma greatly increases pregnancy risk, well-controlled asthma is associated with positive pregnancy outcomes (Mason & Burke, 2019).

The ultimate goal of asthma therapy in pregnancy is maintaining adequate oxygenation of the fetus by preventing hypoxic episodes in the mother. Achieving this goal requires monitoring lung function objectively (e.g., peak expiratory flow rate and forced expiratory volume in 1 second), avoiding or controlling asthma triggers (e.g., dust mites, animal dander, pollen, wood smoke), educating women about the importance of controlling asthma during pregnancy, and drug therapy (Whitty & Dombrowski, 2017). Current drug therapy for asthma emphasizes treatment of airway inflammation to decrease airway hyperresponsiveness and prevent asthma symptoms. Inhaled corticosteroids are widely used for managing persistent asthma during pregnancy (Mason & Burke, 2019; Whitty & Dombrowski, 2019).

During pregnancy, women with poorly controlled asthma may benefit from ultrasound examinations and antenatal testing. Because asthma has been associated with IUGR and preterm birth, accurate pregnancy dating should be established by a first-trimester ultrasound if possible. Evaluation of fetal growth by serial ultrasound examinations may be considered for women who have suboptimally controlled asthma or moderate persistent or severe persistent asthma (beginning at 32 weeks of gestation) and after recovery from a severe asthma exacerbation. All women with asthma should be encouraged to monitor fetal activity (see Chapter 26 for information on daily fetal movement counts) (Whitty & Dombrowski, 2019). Acute exacerbations are managed with albuterol, inhaled ipratropium bromide (Atrovent), systemic corticosteroids, β-adrenergic agents, and oxygen. Women with severe exacerbations unresponsive to treatment may require intubation and mechanical ventilation (Whitty & Dombrowski, 2017).

Although asthma exacerbations during labor are rare, medications for asthma are continued during labor and the postpartum period. Women who are currently taking or have received several short courses of systemic corticosteroids during pregnancy should be given stress doses of corticosteroids during labor and for the first 24 hours after birth to prevent adrenal crisis (Whitty & Dombrowski, 2017). Pulse oximetry should be instituted during labor. Epidural anesthesia reduces oxygen consumption and minute ventilation and is recommended for pain relief. Fentanyl (Sublimaze) or butorphanol (Stadol) are safer choices for systemic analgesia than morphine and meperidine (Demerol), which can cause histamine release. If tocolytic medications are necessary, indomethacin (Indocin) should be avoided because it may induce bronchospasm in aspirin-sensitive women (Whitty & Dombrowski, 2017).

During the postpartum period, women who have asthma are at increased risk for hemorrhage. If excessive bleeding occurs, prostaglandin (PG) E_1 or E_2 can be given, although the woman's respiratory status should be monitored. Because carboprost (15-methyl $PGF_{2\alpha}$ [Hemabate]) and ergonovine and methylergonovine (Methergine) can cause bronchospasm, their use should be avoided (Whitty & Dombrowski, 2017). In general, only small amounts of asthma medications enter breast milk; therefore their use is not considered a contraindication to breastfeeding. However, in sensitive neonates, theophylline in breast milk can cause vomiting, feeding difficulties, jitteriness, and cardiac arrhythmias (Whitty & Dombrowski, 2017). The woman usually returns to her prepregnancy asthma status within 3 months after giving birth.

Cystic Fibrosis

Cystic fibrosis (CF) is a common autosomal recessive genetic disorder in which the exocrine glands produce excessive viscous secretions, which causes problems with both respiratory and digestive functions. Most people with CF have chronic obstructive pulmonary disease, pancreatic exocrine insufficiency, and elevated levels of sweat electrolytes. Morbidity and mortality are usually caused by progressive chronic bronchial pulmonary disease (Whitty & Dombrowski, 2019).

Because the gene for CF was identified in 1989, data can be collected for the purpose of genetic counseling for couples regarding carrier status. In the United States, approximately 4% of the Caucasian population are carriers of the CF gene. CF occurs in 1 in 3200 Caucasian live births. People with CF live longer than in the past because of earlier diagnosis and intervention, along with advances in antibiotic therapy and nutritional support. More than 45% of all individuals in the United States with CF are more than 18 years old (Whitty & Dombrowski, 2019). Men tend to live a little longer (median age of survival is 29.6 years) compared with women, whose median age of survival is 27.3 years. Although most men with CF are infertile, women with the disease are often fertile. The number of women with CF who achieve pregnancy is steadily increasing (Whitty & Dombrowski, 2017).

Pregnancy is well tolerated in women with mild CF who have good prepregnancy nutritional status and less impairment of lung function (Whitty & Dombrowski, 2017). In women with severe disease, the pregnancy is often complicated by chronic hypoxemia and frequent pulmonary infections. Risk factors that may predict a poor pregnancy outcome are poor prepregnancy nutritional status, significant pulmonary disease with hypoxemia, pulmonary hypertension, liver disease, and diabetes mellitus. The incidence of IUGR and uteroplacental insufficiency is increased (Whitty & Dombrowski, 2019).

Care of the pregnant woman with CF requires an interprofessional health team effort. Ideally the woman should lose or gain (she usually needs to gain) weight to reach 90% of her ideal body weight before becoming pregnant. A weight gain of 11 to 12 kg (24 to 26 lb) is recommended during pregnancy. Women who are unable to achieve the recommended weight gain through oral supplements may require nasogastric tube feedings at night (Whitty & Dombrowski, 2017). Pancreatic insufficiency may put the woman at risk for malnutrition because she cannot meet the increased nutritional requirements of pregnancy. If malnutrition is severe, total parenteral hyperalimentation may be necessary. Fat-soluble vitamins may not be well absorbed, resulting in deficiency in those nutrients. Throughout pregnancy, frequent monitoring of the woman's weight, blood glucose, hemoglobin, total protein, serum albumin, prothrombin time, and fat-soluble vitamins A and E is suggested. Pancreatic enzymes should be adjusted as necessary (Whitty & Dombrowski, 2019).

Women with CF are followed closely with serial pulmonary function testing. Test results are used both to guide management and to predict pregnancy outcome. Inhaled recombinant human deoxyribonuclease I may be given to improve lung function by decreasing sputum viscosity. Inhaled 7% saline also produces both short- and long-term benefits (Cunningham et al., 2018). Early detection and treatment of infection are critical. Management of infection includes IV antibiotics along with chest physical therapy and bronchial drainage (Whitty & Dombrowski, 2017).

Fetal assessment is essential, given that the fetus is at risk for uteroplacental insufficiency and IUGR. Maternal nutritional status and weight gain during pregnancy significantly affect fetal growth. Fundal height should be measured routinely, and ultrasound examinations performed to evaluate fetal growth and amniotic fluid volume. Fetal movement counts are often recommended, starting at 28 weeks of gestation. Nonstress tests (NSTs) should be initiated at 32 weeks of gestation or sooner if evidence of fetal compromise exists (see Chapter 26 for more information on fetal assessment tests) (Whitty & Dombrowski, 2017).

During labor, increased cardiac output stresses the cardiovascular system and can lead to cardiopulmonary failure in the woman with pulmonary hypertension or cor pulmonale. These women are also more likely to develop right-sided heart failure. Epidural or local analgesia is the preferred analgesic for birth, with vaginal birth recommended. Cesarean birth should be reserved for obstetric indications. If general anesthesia is needed for cesarean birth, anticholinergic medications should not be given before surgery because they tend to promote airway drying (Whitty & Dombrowski, 2017).

Mothers with pulmonary and pancreatic disease can breastfeed, and their infants do well. It is appropriate, however to test milk samples occasionally for sodium, chloride, and total fat, and to monitor the infant's growth pattern carefully (Lawrence & Lawrence, 2016).

Integumentary Disorders

Dermatologic disorders induced by pregnancy include melasma (chloasma), vascular "spiders," palmar erythema, and striae gravidarum (see Chapter 13). A number of chronic skin disorders may complicate pregnancy. These disorders may be present prior to pregnancy or appear for the first time during pregnancy. The course of these disorders varies during pregnancy. Acne is unpredictably affected by pregnancy. Psoriasis is also unpredictable during pregnancy, but postpartum flares are common. Lesions from neurofibromatosis may increase in size and number during pregnancy (Cunningham et al., 2018). Explanation, reassurance, and common sense measures should suffice for normal skin changes. In contrast, disease processes during and soon after pregnancy may be extremely difficult to diagnose and treat.

> ### ⚡ SAFETY ALERT
>
> Isotretinoin (Accutane), commonly prescribed for cystic acne, is highly teratogenic. There is a risk for craniofacial, cardiac, and central nervous system (CNS) malformations in exposed fetuses. This drug should not be taken during pregnancy.

Pruritus Gravidarum

Pruritus (itching) is a major symptom in several pregnancy-related skin diseases. *Pruritus gravidarum,* generalized itching without the presence of a rash, develops in up to 14% of pregnant women. It is often limited to the abdomen and is usually caused by skin distention and development of striae. Pruritus gravidarum is associated with twin gestation, fertility treatment, diabetes, and nulliparity. It is not associated with poor perinatal outcomes. It is treated symptomatically with skin lubrication, topical antipruritics, and oral antihistamines. Ultraviolet light and careful exposure to sunlight decrease itching. Pruritus gravidarum usually disappears shortly after birth but can recur in approximately one-half of all subsequent pregnancies (Rapini, 2019).

Pruritic Urticarial Papules and Plaques of Pregnancy

Another common pregnancy-specific cause of pruritus is pruritic urticarial papules and plaques of pregnancy (PUPPP) (Fig. 30.1), a rash also known as *polymorphic eruption of pregnancy.* PUPPP classically appears in primigravidas during the mid to late third trimester and occurs slightly more often in women carrying male fetuses. The lesions usually appear first on the abdomen but can spread to the arms, thighs, back, and buttocks. PUPPP almost always causes pruritus, and the itching is severe in 80% of cases. It is associated with increased maternal weight gain, an increased rate of twin gestation, hypertension, and induction of labor. It is not, however, associated with poor maternal or fetal outcomes. Therefore the goal of therapy is simply to relieve maternal discomfort. Antipruritic topical medications, topical steroids, and oral antihistamines usually provide relief. Women with severe symptoms may require oral prednisone. PUPPP usually resolves before birth or within several weeks after birth. It rarely persists or begins after birth. PUPPP does not usually recur in subsequent pregnancies (Rapini, 2019; Wang & Kroumpouzos, 2017).

Intrahepatic Cholestasis of Pregnancy

Intrahepatic cholestasis of pregnancy (ICP) is the most common liver disease of pregnancy (Gabzdyl & Schlaeger, 2015). It is characterized by

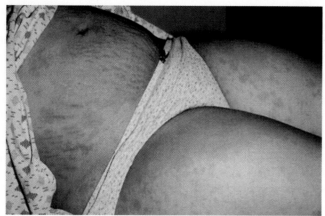

Fig. 30.1 Pruritic Urticarial Papules and Plaques of Pregnancy. Lesions commonly begin in the abdominal striae. Confluent, erythematous urticarial papules and plaques are seen on the thighs in this woman. (From Rapini, R. P. (2019). The skin and pregnancy. In R. Resnik, C. J. Lockwood, T. R. Moore, et al. (Eds.), *Creasy & Resnik's maternal-fetal medicine: Principles and practice* (8th ed.). Philadelphia: Elsevier.)

generalized pruritus that usually begins in the third trimester of pregnancy. The itching commonly affects the palms and soles but can occur on any part of the body and is usually worse at night. No skin lesions are present. Women with ICP have elevated serum bile acids and elevated liver function tests. Jaundice may be present. Up to one-half of women with ICP develop dark urine and light-colored stools. The cause of ICP is unknown, but approximately one-half of women have a family history of the disorder. ICP occurs more frequently during the winter months. It is also seen more commonly in women with multiple gestations and women who are older than 35 years of age. A geographic variance in the prevalence of the disease also exists. ICP occurs most often in Southeast Asia, Chile, Bolivia, and Scandinavia, although it is seen less frequently now in Chile and in Scandinavia than in the past (Cappell, 2017b; Lee, Chung, & Pringle, 2019).

Treatment consists of giving ursodeoxycholic acid, which effectively controls the pruritus and laboratory abnormalities associated with ICP, and continued monitoring of liver function tests and bile acid levels (Cappell, 2017b; Lee et al., 2019). Antihistamines such as diphenhydramine (Benadryl) or chlorpheniramine (Chlor-Trimeton) may be prescribed. Other comfort measures that may provide relief from itching include cool baths, oatmeal products added to a bath, oatmeal cream or lotion, baking soda baths, or an aqueous cream containing 2% menthol (Gabzdyl & Schlaeger, 2015).

The major fetal complications associated with ICP are asphyxial events, meconium staining, stillbirth, and preterm birth. The cause of these complications is likely related to increased levels of fetal serum bile acids (Cappell, 2017b; Lee et al., 2019). Antepartum fetal assessment with twice-weekly NSTs will probably be performed (Cappell).

As long as fetal assessment test results remain reassuring, birth at approximately 37 weeks of gestation should be considered. Symptoms usually disappear and laboratory abnormalities resolve soon after birth (Cappell, 2017b). ICP can recur in approximately two-thirds of subsequent pregnancies, however, or with oral contraceptive use (Cappell, 2017b; Gabzdyl & Schlaeger, 2015).

Neurologic Disorders

The pregnant woman with a neurologic disorder may have to deal with potential teratogenic effects of prescribed medications, changes of mobility during pregnancy, and impaired ability to care for the baby. The nurse should be aware of all medications the woman is taking and the associated potential for producing congenital anomalies. As the pregnancy progresses, the woman's center of gravity shifts and causes balance and gait changes. The nurse should advise the woman of these expected changes and suggest safety measures as appropriate. Family and community resources may be needed to assist in providing infant care for the neurologically impaired woman.

Epilepsy

Epilepsy (often called *seizure disorder*) is a disorder of the brain that causes recurrent seizures and is the most common major neurologic disorder accompanying pregnancy. Less than 1% of all pregnant women have a seizure disorder (Douglas & Aminoff, 2019). Seizure disorders are divided into *generalized* and *focal* epilepsies. Focal epilepsy is the most common type of epilepsy in adults. The cause of most focal epilepsies remains unknown. Women with epilepsy are much more likely to die during the perinatal period than are women who do not have epilepsy. However, through comprehensive care by an interprofessional health care team that includes an obstetrician, neurologist, pharmacist, nurse, and social worker, most women with a seizure disorder can have a successful pregnancy with minimal risk to mother and fetus (Gerard & Samuels, 2017).

Women with epilepsy should receive preconception counseling if at all possible. A detailed history of medication use and seizure frequency should be obtained. If the woman has frequent seizures before conception, she is likely to continue this pattern during pregnancy; therefore achieving effective seizure control before conception is extremely important. In most cases, she should be encouraged to delay pregnancy until better seizure control is established (Gerard & Samuels, 2017).

Infants born to women taking anticonvulsant medications have an increased incidence of congenital anomalies, including cleft lip and palate, congenital heart disease, neural tube defects (NTDs), and hypospadias. These anomalies are often related to the dose, type, and number of anticonvulsant medications taken, not to epilepsy itself (Gerard & Samuels, 2017). However, epilepsy itself can be associated with an increased risk for fetal malformations (Douglas & Aminoff, 2019).

> ⚡ **SAFETY ALERT**
>
> Valproate (Depakote) should be avoided if possible during pregnancy because its use is associated with major congenital malformations, as well as adverse cognitive outcomes, including lower IQ and an increased risk for autism (Gerard & Samuels, 2017).

Lamotrigine (Lamictal) and levetiracetam (Keppra) are now the most commonly prescribed antiepileptic medications for women of childbearing age. Both appear to have relatively low major malformation rates associated with their use. More information is needed regarding the fetal effects of these medications. Carbamazepine (Tegretol) is also a reasonable choice for use in women who plan to conceive, although its use is declining (Gerard & Samuels, 2017) (see the Evidence-Based Practice box: Using Newer Antiepileptic Medications to Treat Epilepsy During Pregnancy and Table 31.2 for more information on these medications).

All women of childbearing age who take an anticonvulsant medication are advised to take a folic acid supplement of 0.4 mg to 1 mg daily, which may decrease the incidence of NTDs in their children. More research is needed to determine the optimal dose of folic acid for women with epilepsy. Many practitioners recommend a dose of 4 mg/day for women with epilepsy who are trying to conceive or are already pregnant. Vitamin D deficiency is common in women with epilepsy, because anticonvulsant medications can interfere with production of the active form of this vitamin. Therefore pregnant women with epilepsy are

EVIDENCE-BASED PRACTICE BOX

Using Newer Antiepileptic Medications to Treat Epilepsy During Pregnancy

Ask the Question

For pregnant women, what effects do new medications used to treat epilepsy have on fetuses, as compared to older medications?

Search for the Evidence

Search Strategies: English research-based publications since 2014 on epilepsy in pregnancy, new epilepsy medications were included.

Databases Used: Cochrane Collaborative Database, National Guideline Clearinghouse (AHRQ), CINAHL, PubMed, UpToDate, and the professional websites for ACOG and AWHONN.

Critical Appraisal of the Evidence

- Epilepsy is the second most common neurologic disorder for pregnant women, after headache. Most pregnant women with epilepsy have successful, uneventful pregnancies. Pregnant women with epilepsy are often prescribed medications to manage their symptoms. A systematic review and metaanalysis showed that newer antiepileptic drugs such as lamotrigine and levetiracetam were not linked to increased risk of congenital malformations (Veroniki, Cogo, Rios, et al., 2017). Sodium valproate is an older drug typically prescribed for pregnant women with epilepsy. It is considered a pregnancy category D drug. The American Academy of Neurology recommends using the lowest dose possible when managing epilepsy in pregnant women (Doyle, Geraghty, & Folan, 2016).
- Some medications prescribed for epilepsy have been known to cause negative consequences to the fetus, such as fetal loss, growth restriction, congenital malformations, and compromised neurodevelopmental issues in newborns (Hugill & Meredith, 2017).
- In one systematic review (Bromley & Baker, 2017), many antiepileptic medications were examined for effects on the fetus. A review of carbamazepine was found to have mixed results. Generally, this drug does not cause adverse consequences in the neonate. However, some studies associated it with poorer neurodevelopmental outcomes. One of the newer antiepileptic drugs, lamotrigine, has not been shown to be detrimental to the fetus. Some studies have shown that children exposed to lamotrigine in utero have higher IQ scores and language function, while some have shown that these children have decreased motor and sensory integration (Bromley & Baker).
- Evidence for the other newer antiepileptic drug, levetiracetam, is very limited. The few studies that exist have not shown this drug to have detrimental effects on children exposed to it in utero (Bromley & Baker, 2017).

Apply the Evidence: Nursing Implications

- Pregnant women should be counselled about the risks of taking antiepileptic drugs during pregnancy. Seizure control is a consideration when making decisions about the benefits of taking antiepileptic drugs during pregnancy (Veroniki et al., 2017). Nurses should provide information to women as they weigh risks of taking medications during pregnancy with the need to control seizures.
- Nurses can teach women that antiepileptic drugs tend to be safe for breastfeeding (Hugill & Meredith, 2017).
- Nurses should also understand that normal physiological changes during pregnancy impact the effectiveness of antiepileptic drugs. Decreases in drug concentrations occur because of increased extracellular fluid, decreased intestinal absorption, and increased elimination and liver metabolism (Doyle et al., 2016).

References

Bromley, R. L., & Baker, G. A. (2017). Fetal antiepileptic drug exposure and cognitive outcomes. *Seizure, 44*, 225–231.

Doyle, L., Geraghty, S., & Folan, M. (2016). Epilepsy in pregnancy: Pharmacodynamics and pharmacokinetics. *British Journal of Midwifery, 24*(12), 830–835.

Hugill, K., & Meredith, D. (2017). Caring for pregnant women with long-term conditions: Maternal and neonatal effects of epilepsy. *British Journal of Midwifery, 25*(5), 301–307.

Veroniki, A. A., Cogo, E., Rios, P., et al. (2017). Comparative safety of anti-epileptic drugs during pregnancy: A systematic review and network meta-analysis of congenital malformations and prenatal outcomes. *BMC Medicine, 15*(95), 1–20.

Jennifer Taylor Alderman

---

encouraged to take a supplemental dose of 1000 to 2000 IU of vitamin D daily, in addition to a prenatal vitamin (Gerard & Samuels, 2017).

If possible, only one anticonvulsant medication—at the lowest dose that is effective at keeping the woman seizure-free—should be prescribed during pregnancy. The increase in plasma volume that is a normal pregnancy change can affect drug metabolism and distribution. Therefore, blood levels of anticonvulsant medications should be checked and drug dosages adjusted as necessary (Douglas & Aminoff, 2019; Gerard & Samuels, 2017). Often the dosage will need to be increased as pregnancy progresses. With client cooperation and close monitoring, most women with epilepsy should experience no change in seizure frequency from their baseline seizure frequency (Gerard & Samuels).

In addition to congenital anomalies, the fetus of a woman with epilepsy is also at risk for IUGR. Determining an accurate gestational age as early as possible is important. This information decreases any confusion later in pregnancy in regard to fetal growth issues. Maternal serum α-fetoprotein screening around 16 weeks of gestation should be performed to assess for the presence of an NTD or other fetal anomalies. A specialized, detailed anatomic ultrasound examination should be performed at 18 to 22 weeks of gestation to determine whether congenital malformations, including NTDs, are present. Nonstress testing later in pregnancy is not necessary for all women with epilepsy, but it should be considered for those who have seizures during the third trimester (Gerard & Samuels, 2017).

The risk for seizures during labor is small. Seizures are most likely to occur in women who have had seizures during pregnancy. They are usually treated with short-acting benzodiazepines (e.g., lorazepam [Ativan]). Most women with epilepsy successfully give birth vaginally (Gerard & Samuels, 2017).

After birth, the levels of anticonvulsant medications must be monitored frequently for the first few weeks because they can rise rapidly. If medication doses were increased during pregnancy, they need to be reduced within the first 3 weeks postpartum to slightly higher than or at prepregnancy levels (Gerard & Samuels, 2017). All of the major anticonvulsant medications are found in breast milk to varying degrees but few data suggest neonatal harm from exposure through breast milk (Gerard & Samuels). Safety measures related to the new baby should be discussed with the woman and her family members. In addition to the safety measures that apply to all newborns, specific precautions should be observed with babies whose mothers have epilepsy. The sleep deprivation that can be associated with breastfeeding a newborn may put the woman at risk for seizures. Partners or other members of the woman's support system should assist with night feedings so that the woman can have a prolonged period (typically 6 to 8 hours) of uninterrupted sleep. Other recommendations include bathing the baby only when another adult is present and changing diapers on a pad placed on the floor, instead of on a changing table. In addition, avoiding stairs whenever possible and using a stroller to transport the baby, rather than an infant carrier strapped to the mother, are safety measures that should be considered (Gerard & Samuels).

Contraceptive counseling is an important part of postpartum and preconception planning for women with epilepsy. Certain anticonvulsant medications may interfere with the effectiveness of oral contraceptives and implantable progestins, resulting in unplanned pregnancy (Douglas & Aminoff, 2019). The most reliable form of contraception is the IUD. The IUD, either the copper or the levonorgestrel type, is considered the contraceptive method of choice for most women with epilepsy (Gerard & Samuels, 2017). In terms of planning for future childbearing, couples should be informed that their risk for passing epilepsy along to their children is higher than that of the general population, but still relatively low. Interestingly, mothers with epilepsy have a much greater chance of having a child with epilepsy than do fathers with epilepsy (Gerard & Samuels).

Multiple Sclerosis

Multiple sclerosis (MS), a patchy demyelination of the spinal cord and CNS, may be a viral disorder. It affects women more often than men. Onset of symptoms, which include weakness, paresthesias, or numbness of one or both lower extremities, visual complaints, and loss of coordination, is subtle and usually occurs between 20 and 40 years of age. The disease is characterized by exacerbations and remissions. Pregnancy likely does not have an adverse long-term effect on the course of the disease (Gerard & Samuels, 2017).

Remissions during pregnancy are common. If an exacerbation occurs, it is more likely to do so during the postpartum period. The mainstay of treatment for acute MS relapses is corticosteroids and, rarely, other immunosuppressive agents. In 1993, the first disease-modifying agent (DMA), interferon-β, a new class of medications for treating MS, was introduced for use. Since then, there has been a steady increase in the number of available DMAs. Their use in pregnancy has been limited; thus few data and no controlled studies are available. Because MS exacerbations are rare during pregnancy and few data are available regarding the safety of DMA use during pregnancy, most experts recommend stopping DMA use prior to conception. A few studies have suggested that the use of DMAs prior to conception or during gestation decreases the risk for postpartum MS relapses. Postpartum relapses are also less likely to occur in women whose MS activity had been well controlled in the year prior to pregnancy (Gerard & Samuels, 2017).

No specific changes in routine obstetric care are recommended for the woman with MS, because MS in the mother does not pose significant risk to the fetus. The woman should take a prenatal vitamin daily. Vitamin D deficiency may affect her susceptibility to MS and MS relapses, as well as her child's subsequent risk for developing MS. Therefore experts recommend that the woman take 1000 to 2000 IU of vitamin D daily. Women with disturbances in bladder function are more likely to develop UTIs during pregnancy. Therefore they should be screened routinely. If an acute and severe MS relapse occurs during pregnancy, it can be treated with corticosteroids or intravenous immunoglobulin (IVIG) (Gerard & Samuels, 2017).

In the past, there were concerns that epidural use during labor and birth might somehow worsen MS or promote relapses. However, studies have shown that this does not seem to be the case. Cesarean birth is usually not indicated for women with MS. Only rare cases of severe or active disease that affect the spinal cord prevent a woman with MS from laboring safely (Gerard & Samuels, 2017).

Breastfeeding in women with MS is controversial. Some authorities believe that breastfeeding does not affect disease activity. Others believe that breastfeeding may reduce the likelihood of MS relapses during the postpartum period. Most experts recommend that DMAs not be used during breastfeeding because of a lack of evidence regarding their safety. Others believe that the DMA interferons β1a and β1b are safer for breastfeeding because of their large molecular weight and low oral bioavailability (Gerard & Samuels, 2017; Spencer, 2015). Depression is common among women with MS; thus they should be assessed frequently for evidence of postpartum depression. All hormonal contraceptives may be used by women with MS.

Bell Palsy

Bell palsy is an acute idiopathic facial paralysis. The cause is unknown, but it may be related to the reactivation of herpes simplex virus or herpes zoster virus. Bell palsy occurs fairly often, especially in women of reproductive age. Pregnant women are affected four times more often than nonpregnant women. Women who develop Bell palsy during pregnancy have an increased risk for gestational hypertension or preeclampsia (Cunningham et al., 2018).

The clinical manifestations of Bell palsy typically include the sudden development of a unilateral facial weakness, with maximal weakness within 48 hours after onset. There is often associated pain surrounding the ear, difficulty closing the eye on the affected side, hyperacusis (abnormal acuteness of the sense of hearing), and a loss of taste (Cunningham et al., 2018; Douglas & Aminoff, 2019).

Outcome is generally good unless a complete block in nerve conduction occurs. Most women recover without treatment. Steroid therapy is the only medical treatment that has been shown to influence the outcome of Bell palsy. To be effective, treatment should begin within the first 3 to 5 days after the paralysis develops (Douglas & Aminoff, 2019). Supportive care includes prevention of injury to the constantly exposed cornea, facial muscle massage, careful chewing and manual removal of food from inside the affected cheek, and reassurance. Although 80% of affected men and nonpregnant women recover to a satisfactory level within a year, only approximately half of women who develop the disorder during pregnancy do so (Cunningham et al., 2018).

Autoimmune Disorders

Autoimmune disorders, also called *collagen vascular diseases*, make up a large group of conditions that disrupt the function of the immune system of the body. In these types of disorders, the body's immune system is unable to distinguish "self" from "nonself." As a result, antibodies develop that attack its normally present antigens, causing tissue damage. More women than men are affected by autoimmune disorders. Autoimmune disorders can occur during pregnancy because a large percentage of women with an autoimmune disease manifest it at some time during their reproductive years (Carpenter & Branch, 2017). Common autoimmune diseases include systemic lupus erythematosus (SLE), myasthenia gravis (MG), antiphospholipid syndrome, rheumatoid arthritis, and systemic sclerosis.

Systemic Lupus Erythematosus

SLE is a chronic, multisystem inflammatory disease that affects the skin, joints, kidneys, lungs, nervous system, liver, and other body organs. The exact cause is unknown but probably involves the interaction of immunologic, environmental, hormonal, and genetic factors. SLE is one of the most common serious autoimmune diseases encountered during pregnancy. It occurs four times more often in African American women than in Caucasian women and is nine times more common in women than in men. Most cases of SLE are diagnosed in adolescence or young adulthood (Carpenter & Branch, 2017; Sammaritano, Salmon, & Branch, 2019).

Common symptoms, including myalgias, fatigue, weight change, and fevers, occur in nearly all women with SLE at some time during the course of the disease. Although a diagnosis of SLE is suspected based on clinical signs and symptoms, it is confirmed by laboratory testing that demonstrates the presence of circulating autoantibodies. As is the case with other autoimmune diseases, SLE is characterized by a series of exacerbations (flares) and remissions (Carpenter & Branch, 2017; Sammaritano et al., 2019).

Pregnancy probably does not increase the likelihood of serious SLE flares (Sammaritano et al., 2019). However, it appears that disease activity at the beginning of pregnancy is an important predictor of exacerbations during pregnancy. Therefore women are advised to wait until they have been in remission for at least 6 months before attempting conception. In addition to exacerbations, other maternal risks include an increased rate of miscarriage, a possible need to give birth at a preterm gestation, and preeclampsia. Fetal risks include stillbirth, IUGR, and preterm birth (Carpenter & Branch, 2017).

Medical therapy during pregnancy is kept to a minimum in women who are in remission or who have a mild form of SLE. Occasional doses of nonsteroidal antiinflammatory drugs (NSAIDs) can be given to treat arthralgia. These medications should not be used chronically, however, because of related oligohydramnios or ductus arteriosus closure. Low-dose aspirin can be used throughout pregnancy (Cunningham et al., 2018). Glucocorticoids such as prednisone are often used to treat SLE during pregnancy, either as maintenance therapy or as short-term treatment for flares. There is a small risk for fetal cleft lip and palate if glucocorticoids are used during the first trimester. Prolonged use of this group of medications also increases the risk for maternal bone loss, gestational diabetes, hypertension and preeclampsia, and adrenal suppression. Given the significant risks associated with long-term glucocorticoid use, hydroxychloroquine (Plaquenil), an antimalarial drug, may be the best medication for maintenance SLE therapy during pregnancy. It significantly reduces SLE disease activity but appears to cause no adverse effects on the fetus (Carpenter & Branch, 2017).

Prenatal care otherwise focuses on close monitoring to detect common pregnancy complications such as hypertension, proteinuria, and IUGR. Ultrasound examinations are performed monthly after 24 to 28 weeks of gestation to monitor fetal growth. Fetal assessment tests, including weekly or twice-weekly NSTs and amniotic fluid volume assessments or biophysical profiles, are performed beginning at 32 weeks of gestation unless indicated earlier in pregnancy due to IUGR (see Chapter 26) (Carpenter & Branch, 2017).

It is recommended that women with SLE give birth by 39 weeks of gestation. Birth may be necessary earlier in gestation if complications such as IUGR, preeclampsia, or worsening renal function develop.

Women who have received chronic glucocorticoid therapy (20 mg or more of prednisone daily for at least 3 weeks) need larger (stress) doses of steroids during labor (Carpenter & Branch, 2017). Vaginal birth is preferred, but cesarean birth is common because of maternal and fetal complications.

Close monitoring of all women with SLE should continue after birth because some of them will experience a disease flare during the postpartum period. It is usually recommended that the woman follow up with her rheumatologist within 1 to 3 months after giving birth (Carpenter & Branch, 2017).

Women with SLE and chronic vascular or renal disease should limit their number of pregnancies because of maternal complications associated with the illness and increased adverse perinatal outcomes. If desired, the safest time for tubal sterilization is during the postpartum period or when the disease is in remission. Combined oral contraceptive pills do not appear to increase the incidence of lupus flares. Progestin-only implants and injections provide effective contraception with no known effects on lupus flares. Evidence does not support concerns regarding an increased risk of infection when IUDs are prescribed for women receiving immunosuppressive therapy (Cunningham et al., 2018).

Myasthenia Gravis

MG, an autoimmune motor (muscle) end-plate disorder that involves acetylcholine use, affects the motor function at the myoneural junction. Muscle weakness results, particularly of the eyes, face, tongue, neck, limbs, and respiratory muscles. In addition, women may experience ptosis, diplopia, and dysphagia. Women are affected twice as often as men, and the incidence peaks between the ages of 20 and 30 years. Because the greatest period of risk is during the first year after diagnosis, pregnancy should probably be avoided until symptomatic improvement occurs (Cunningham et al., 2018). The response of women with MG to pregnancy is unpredictable; remission, exacerbation, or continued stability during pregnancy can occur (Douglas & Aminoff, 2019).

Pregnancy does not appear to affect the overall course of MG, but as the uterus enlarges, respirations may be compromised. Also, the normal fatigue experienced by many pregnant women may be tolerated poorly by those with MG (Cunningham et al., 2018). Treatment during pregnancy is the same as for nonpregnant women. Usual medications include glucocorticoids and acetylcholinesterase inhibitors. Thymectomy may result in remission of the disease. For severe weakness, plasmapheresis or IVIG therapy may be needed (Douglas & Aminoff, 2019).

Because MG does not affect smooth muscle, most women usually tolerate labor well. Vaginal birth is desired, but vacuum or forceps assistance may be required because of muscle weakness. Oxytocin may be given, but all medications that cause muscular relaxation should be avoided if at all possible. Opioids must be used cautiously because they may cause respiratory depression, and women with MG are already at risk for respiratory muscle weakness. Regional analgesia is preferred (Cunningham et al., 2018; Douglas & Aminoff, 2019). After birth, women must be carefully supervised because relapses often occur during the postpartum period.

> **⚡ SAFETY ALERT**
>
> Magnesium sulfate must not be administered to women with MG because it inhibits the release of acetylcholine and can trigger myasthenic crisis (Douglas & Aminoff, 2019).

Approximately 10% to 15% of neonates born to women with MG develop neonatal myasthenia. This transient disorder results from the transfer of the maternal antibody against acetylcholine receptors across the placenta. Symptoms, including a weak cry, respiratory difficulties, weakness in suckling, a weak Moro reflex, and feeble limb movements, usually appear within the first 72 hours after birth. Neonatal myasthenia can be treated with anticholinesterase medications and usually resolves by 6 weeks after birth (Douglas & Aminoff, 2019).

Gastrointestinal Disorders

Compromise of GI function during pregnancy is a concern. Obvious physiologic alterations, such as the greatly enlarged uterus, and less apparent changes, such as hormonal differences and hypochlorhydria (deficiency of hydrochloric acid in the stomach's gastric juice), require understanding for proper diagnosis and treatment. Gallbladder disease and inflammatory bowel disease are examples of GI disorders that may occur during pregnancy.

Cholelithiasis and Cholecystitis

Cholelithiasis (the presence of gallstones in the gallbladder) occurs more often in women than in men. Its incidence increases during pregnancy, probably because of increased hormone levels and pressure from the enlarged uterus that interferes with the normal circulation and drainage of the gallbladder. Most gallstones are asymptomatic during pregnancy. Usually the first symptom of cholelithiasis is biliary colic presenting as epigastric or right upper quadrant pain that can radiate to the back or shoulders. Pain may occur spontaneously or after eating a high-fat meal. Approximately two-thirds of clients with biliary colic have recurrent attacks (Cappell, 2017b). Cholecystitis (inflammation of the gallbladder) is usually caused when a gallstone obstructs a cystic duct. As in biliary colic that occurs with cholelithiasis, epigastric or right upper quadrant pain is present, but the pain is usually more severe and prolonged. Nausea, vomiting, and fever may also be present. Acute cholecystitis is the third most common indication for nonobstetric surgical intervention in pregnancy, occurring in about 4 cases per 10,000 pregnancies (Cappell, 2017b).

Often gallbladder surgery is postponed until the postpartum period. The woman can usually be managed conservatively for the remainder of the pregnancy (see Teaching for Self-Management box: Nutritional Counseling for the Pregnant Woman With Cholelithiasis or Cholecystitis). However, women with recurrent biliary colic or acute cholecystitis generally require immediate cholecystectomy. Although the second trimester has traditionally been considered the safest time for this surgery, it is increasingly performed at any time during pregnancy because of improved surgical techniques and outcomes. Both laparoscopic and open cholecystectomy procedures are acceptable during pregnancy (Cappell, 2017b; Cunningham et al., 2018).

TEACHING FOR SELF-MANAGEMENT

Nutritional Counseling for the Pregnant Woman With Cholelithiasis or Cholecystitis

- Assess your diet for foods that cause discomfort and gas, and omit foods that trigger episodes.
- Reduce dietary fat intake to 40 to 50 g/day.
- Limit protein to 10% to 12% of total calories.
- Choose foods so that most of the calories come from carbohydrates.
- Prepare food without adding fats or oils as much as possible.
- Avoid fried foods.

Inflammatory Bowel Disease

Inflammatory bowel disease refers to ulcerative colitis and Crohn disease. It is relatively common in young women, so these disorders are seen during pregnancy. The incidence of an inflammatory bowel disease flare is not increased in pregnancy and no evidence suggests that pregnancy significantly affects either ulcerative colitis or Crohn disease (Cunningham et al., 2018; Kelly & Savides, 2019). In general, infants born to mothers with inflammatory bowel disease have a higher risk for preterm birth, low birth weight, and being small for gestational age. However, these infants do not have an increased risk for congenital anomalies (Kelly & Savides). Active disease early in pregnancy increases the risk for a poor pregnancy outcome (Cunningham et al.).

Treatment of inflammatory bowel disease is usually the same for the pregnant woman as it is for the nonpregnant woman. Discontinuing her prepregnancy medications can cause the woman to have a relapse or disease flare. The medications 5-aminosalicylates, prednisone, and 6-mercaptopurine or azathioprine are often prescribed for treatment of inflammatory bowel disease. Occasionally biologic agents such as infliximab also are ordered. Antibiotics such as metronidazole and ciprofloxacin may also be necessary from time to time. These drugs appear to be safe for use during pregnancy (Kelly & Savides, 2019). Daily dosage of 4 mg of folic acid taken before conception and during the first trimester is recommended. The high dose of folic acid counteracts

the antifolate actions of some medications used to treat inflammatory bowel disease. Calcium supplementation is also necessary because osteoporosis is a significant complication in up to one-third of these women. Women with prolonged flares may require total parenteral nutrition (Cunningham et al., 2018). Surgery during pregnancy is done for emergencies such as intestinal obstruction, perforation, abscess, or fulminant colitis. In these situations, surgery is required for the mother's health (Kelly & Savides).

Urinary Tract Infections

UTIs are a common medical complication of pregnancy, occurring in up to 20% of all pregnancies. They are also responsible for 10% of all hospitalizations during pregnancy (Duff, 2019). UTIs include asymptomatic bacteriuria, cystitis, and pyelonephritis. They are usually caused by coliform organisms that are a normal part of the perineal flora. By far the most common cause is *Escherichia coli*, a gram-negative bacterium responsible for at least 80% of initial cases and about 70% of recurrent cases. *Klebsiella pneumoniae* and *Proteus* species are other common pathogens, particularly in women with a history of recurrent infections. Up to 10% of infections are caused by gram-positive organisms such as group B streptococci, enterococci, and staphylococci (Duff & Birsner, 2017).

Asymptomatic Bacteriuria

Asymptomatic bacteriuria refers to the persistent presence of bacteria within the urinary tract of women who have no symptoms. A clean-voided urine specimen containing more than 100,000 organisms per mL is diagnostic. If asymptomatic bacteriuria is not treated, about one-third of pregnant women will develop acute pyelonephritis. Therefore, all women should be screened for asymptomatic bacteriuria at their first prenatal visit (Duff & Birsner, 2017). Asymptomatic bacteriuria has been associated with preterm birth and low-birth-weight infants (Cunningham et al., 2018).

Asymptomatic bacteriuria should be treated with an antibiotic. Antibiotics that are often prescribed include amoxicillin, ampicillin, cephalosporins such as cephalexin (Keflex) or ciprofloxacin (Cipro), levofloxacin (Levaquin), nitrofurantoin (Macrodantin), and trimethoprim-sulfamethoxazole (Bactrim DS). Several different regimens, including single-dose or 3-, 7-, and 10-day treatment may be used (Cunningham et al., 2018). In women who experience a prompt response to treatment of an initial infection, a urine culture for test of cure may not be clinically necessary or cost effective. Conversely, urine cultures during or immediately after the completion of therapy are indicated for women who have a poor response to therapy or a history of recurrent infection (Duff & Birsner, 2017). Women who have persistent or frequent bacteriuria recurrences may be placed on suppressive therapy, often nitrofurantoin each night at bedtime, for the remainder of the pregnancy (Cunningham et al.).

Cystitis

Cystitis (bladder infection) is characterized by dysuria, urgency, and frequency, along with lower abdominal or suprapubic pain. Usually white blood cells (WBCs), as well as bacteria, are found in the urine. Microscopic or gross hematuria also may be present. Typically, symptoms are confined to the bladder rather than becoming systemic. Cystitis is usually uncomplicated, but it may lead to ascending UTI if untreated. Approximately 40% of pregnant women with pyelonephritis experience symptoms of bladder infection before developing pyelonephritis (Cunningham et al., 2018).

Cystitis is often treated with a 3-day course of antibiotic therapy, which is usually 90% effective in curing the infection (see Clinical Reasoning Case Study: Urinary Tract Infection). Antibiotics often prescribed include amoxicillin, ampicillin, a cephalosporin such as cephalexin

(Keflex), ciprofloxacin (Cipro), levofloxacin (Levaquin), nitrofurantoin (Macrodantin), and trimethoprim-sulfamethoxazole (Bactrim DS) (Cunningham et al., 2018). Phenazopyridine (Pyridium), a urinary analgesic, is often prescribed along with an antibiotic for relief of symptoms caused by irritation of the urinary tract. Although phenazopyridine is effective at relieving dysuria, urgency, and frequency, women should be taught that the medication colors urine and tears orange. Therefore, they should be instructed to avoid wearing contact lenses while taking this medication and warned that it will stain underwear.

🔎 CLINICAL REASONING CASE STUDY

Urinary Tract Infection

Emily is a 23-year-old G1 P0 who has her initial prenatal visit at 8 weeks of gestation. She is complaining of urinary frequency and burning with urination. During the visit a routine urine sample is collected and sent to the lab. Emily declines antibiotics because she wants to be sure she really has an infection, choosing to wait on the lab results. Two days later Emily receives a call at work from her health care provider, telling her that she needs to pick up a prescription for an antibiotic because her lab results indicated that she has a UTI. Emily asks, "Is the antibiotic okay for the baby? I thought medications should be avoided in the first trimester."

1. What is the priority concern or client need in this situation? Support your answer with data as stated in the case.
2. List other client needs/problems in this case.
3. Identify any additional information or assessment data that is needed by the nurse in planning care for this client.
4. What nursing actions are appropriate in this situation?
   a. What is the priority nursing action?
   b. Describe other nursing interventions that are important to providing optimal client care.
5. Describe the roles/responsibilities of the interprofessional health care team members (other than nurses) who may be involved in providing care for this client.

Pyelonephritis

Renal infection (pyelonephritis) is one of the most frequent serious medical complications of pregnancy and a leading cause of septic shock during pregnancy (Cunningham et al., 2018). The most common maternal complications associated with pyelonephritis include sepsis, acute respiratory distress syndrome (ARDS), and preterm labor (Duff & Birsner, 2017).

Pyelonephritis is most often caused by the *E. coli* organism. Infection develops only in the right kidney in more than half of all cases. The onset of pyelonephritis is often abrupt, with fever, chills, flank pain, dysuria, urgency, and frequency. Nausea and vomiting can also be present. Usually, one or both costovertebral angles are tender to palpation (Duff, 2019).

Until recently, most pregnant women diagnosed with pyelonephritis were usually admitted to the hospital immediately for treatment with parenteral antibiotics. Although more recent studies have shown that women with mild to moderate disease may be managed on an outpatient basis instead, most experts currently recommend that pregnant women with pyelonephritis be hospitalized for 12 to 24 hours for assessment before a decision about outpatient management is made (Duff, 2019).

Treatment with IV antibiotics is started as soon as urine (and possibly blood) samples for culture and sensitivity have been collected (Cunningham et al., 2018). Ceftriaxone (Rocephin) is often prescribed because it provides excellent coverage against many of the organisms that commonly cause pyelonephritis. Some authorities prefer initial treatment with ampicillin and gentamicin instead (Duff, 2019). The woman must be monitored closely for complications such as sepsis, ARDS, and preterm labor (Duff & Birsner, 2017). Administering intravenous fluids to maintain adequate urine output (50 mL or more per hour) is extremely important (Cunningham et al.).

Clinical symptoms generally resolve within a couple of days after antibiotic therapy is begun. Most women are afebrile after 72 hours. If no clinical improvement is seen within 48 to 72 hours, an ultrasound should be performed to assess for a urinary tract obstruction or some other complication (Cunningham et al., 2018). Once a woman has been afebrile and asymptomatic for 24 hours, she can be discharged to complete a 14-day course of antibiotics as an outpatient. She may be treated with oral antibiotics such as amoxicillin-clavulanic acid (Augmentin) or trimethoprim-sulfamethoxazole (Bactrim DS). Alternatively, arrangements may be made for a home care nurse to administer an antibiotic, such as ceftriaxone (Rocephin) either intravenously or intramuscularly (Duff, 2019; Duff & Birsner, 2017).

Recurrent bacteriuria develops in 30% to 40% of women after completion of treatment for pyelonephritis. If this infection is left untreated, 25% of these women will develop recurrent pyelonephritis. Many women are maintained on a prophylactic antibiotic (often nitrofurantoin [Macrodantin] taken daily at bedtime) for the remainder of the pregnancy. An acceptable alternative to daily prophylactic antibiotics is to obtain urine cultures every 2 weeks for the remainder of the pregnancy to detect and treat recurrent bacteriuria (Duff, 2019).

Client Education

Nurses are often responsible for teaching pregnant women about taking medications safely and effectively. This education is especially important in regard to antibiotics because this type of medication is so often misused by the general public. The woman should be instructed to finish the entire course of prescribed antibiotic therapy rather than stopping the medication as soon as she feels better. Failure to complete treatment can lead to the creation of additional drug-resistant organisms. Antibiotics should be taken on time and around the clock so that medication levels in the body remain constant. Finally, many women develop a yeast infection while taking antibiotics because the medication kills normal flora in the genitourinary tract as well as pathologic organisms. Therefore, they should be encouraged to take probiotics and include yogurt, cheese, or milk-containing active acidophilus cultures in their diet while on antibiotics.

The woman should also be taught simple ways to prevent future UTIs. See Teaching for Self-Management box: Prevention of Genital Tract Infections in Chapter 7 for several suggestions.

SURGERY DURING PREGNANCY

Approximately 1 in 500 women require nonobstetric surgery during pregnancy. However, pregnancy can make the diagnosis more difficult. An enlarged uterus and displaced internal organs can make abdominal palpation more difficult, alter the position of an affected organ, and/or change the usual signs and symptoms associated with a particular disorder. Two common nonobstetric abdominal conditions requiring surgery during pregnancy are appendicitis and symptomatic cholelithiasis (see earlier discussion of cholecystectomy) (Schwartz & Ludmir, 2017).

Appendicitis

The most common nonobstetric surgical emergency during pregnancy is appendicitis, occurring in about 1 in 1000 pregnancies (Cappell, 2017a). The diagnosis of appendicitis is often delayed because the usual signs and symptoms mimic some normal changes of pregnancy such as nausea and vomiting and increased WBC count. As pregnancy progresses, the appendix is pushed upward and to the right from its usual anatomic location (see Fig. 13.8) (Cunningham et al., 2018). Because of these changes, rupture of the appendix and the subsequent development of peritonitis occur in up to 25% of pregnant women with appendicitis (Cappell, 2017a).

The most common symptom of appendicitis in pregnant women is right lower quadrant abdominal pain, regardless of gestational age. Nausea and vomiting are often present, but loss of appetite is not a reliable indicator of appendicitis. Fever, tachycardia, a dry tongue, and localized abdominal tenderness are commonly found in nonpregnant people with appendicitis, but they are less likely indicators for the disorder in pregnant women. Because of the physiologic increase in WBCs that occurs in pregnancy, this test is not helpful in making the diagnosis. A urinalysis and a chest x-ray should be performed to rule out UTI and right lower lobe pneumonia, given that both of these conditions can cause lower abdominal pain (Kelly & Savides, 2019). Appendicitis can also be confused with other disorders such as cholecystitis, labor, pyelonephritis, renal colic, uterine leiomyoma degeneration, or placental abruption (Cunningham et al., 2018).

Radiologic imaging is necessary if appendicitis is suspected after history, physical examination, and laboratory studies have been completed. Although computed tomography (CT) is the imaging test of choice in nonpregnant clients because it is highly accurate, the use of ultrasound during pregnancy is preferred to avoid fetal exposure to radiation from CT (Cappell, 2017a). Magnetic resonance imaging (MRI) is the appropriate next step in a pregnant woman if appendicitis has not been confirmed by other imaging techniques (Cappell; Kelly & Savides, 2019).

Prompt surgical intervention to remove the appendix is still the standard treatment (Kelly & Savides, 2019). Laparoscopic surgery may be performed during the first and second trimesters of pregnancy if the appendix has not ruptured or the diagnosis is uncertain. Appendectomy is recommended, even if appendicitis is not evident at surgery. Antibiotics are often administered for uncomplicated appendicitis and are definitely necessary if rupture, abscess, or peritonitis has occurred. Clindamycin and gentamicin are often prescribed because they are considered both effective and safe. The maternal mortality rate from ruptured appendix is about 4%. The fetal mortality rate from ruptured appendix is much higher, more than 30% (Cappell, 2017a).

📋 CARE MANAGEMENT

Assessment

Initial assessment of the pregnant woman requiring surgery focuses on her presenting signs and symptoms. A thorough history and physical examination are performed. Laboratory testing includes, at a minimum, a complete blood cell count with differential and a urinalysis. Additional laboratory and other diagnostic tests may be necessary to reach a diagnosis. In addition, FHR and activity, along with uterine activity, should be monitored, and constant vigilance for symptoms of impending obstetric complications maintained. The extent of preoperative assessment is determined by the immediacy of surgical intervention and the specific disorder that requires surgery.

Hospital Care

When surgery becomes necessary during pregnancy, the woman and her family are concerned about the effects of the procedure and medication on fetal well-being and the course of pregnancy. An important aspect of preoperative nursing care is encouraging the woman to express her fears, concerns, and questions.

Preoperative procedures such as preparation of the operative site and time of insertion of IV lines and urinary retention catheters vary with the surgeon and the facility. However, in every instance there is a total restriction of solid foods and liquids or a clear specification of the type, amount, and time at which clear liquids may be taken before surgery. Some bowel preparation such as clear liquids and laxatives may be required before surgery. Food by mouth is restricted for several hours before a scheduled procedure. Even if she has had nothing by mouth but, more important, if surgery is unexpected, the woman is in danger of vomiting and aspirating; special precautions are taken before anesthetic is administered (e.g., administering an antacid).

Intraoperatively, perinatal nurses may collaborate with the surgical staff to increase their knowledge about the special needs of pregnant women undergoing surgery. One intervention to improve fetal oxygenation is positioning the woman on the operating table with a lateral tilt to avoid compression of the maternal vena cava. Continuous FHR and uterine contraction monitoring during surgery may be performed if the fetus is considered viable. Monitoring may be accomplished by using sterile Aquasonic gel and a sterile sleeve for the transducer. During abdominal surgery, uterine contractions may be palpated manually. However, many practitioners simply monitor the fetus before and after the procedure.

In the immediate recovery period general observations and care pertinent to postoperative recovery are initiated. Frequent assessments are carried out for several hours after surgery. Whether the woman is cared for in the surgical postanesthesia recovery area or in a labor and birth unit, continuous fetal and uterine monitoring are likely to be initiated or resumed because of the potential risk for preterm labor. Tocolysis may be necessary if preterm labor occurs (see Chapter 32).

Home Care

Plans for the woman's return home and for convalescent care should be completed as early as possible before discharge. Depending on her insurance coverage, nursing care may be provided through a home health agency. If not, the woman and other support people must be taught necessary skills and procedures, such as wound care. Ideally the woman and other caregivers should have opportunities for supervised practice before discharge so that they can feel comfortable with their knowledge and ability before being totally responsible for providing care. Box 30.2 lists information that should be included in discharge teaching for the postoperative client. The woman may also need referrals to various community agencies for evaluation of the home situation, child care, home health care, and financial or other assistance.

BOX 30.2   Discharge Teaching for Home Care After Surgery

- Care of incision site
- Diet and elimination related to gastrointestinal (GI) function
- Signs and symptoms of developing complications: wound infection, venous thromboembolism (VTE), pneumonia
- Equipment needed and technique for assessing temperature
- Recommended schedule for resumption of activities of daily living
- Treatments and medications ordered
- List of resource people and their telephone numbers
- Schedule of follow-up visits
  If birth has not occurred:
- Assessment of fetal activity (kick counts)
- Signs of preterm labor

TRAUMA DURING PREGNANCY

Trauma remains a common complication during pregnancy because most pregnant women in the United States continue their usual activities. Approximately 30,000 pregnant women in the United States experience treatable injuries each year because of trauma (Brown, 2017).

Significance

As pregnancy progresses, the risk of trauma increases because more cases of trauma are reported in the third trimester than earlier in gestation. Trauma, especially from motor vehicle accidents (MVAs), is a major cause of maternal injury and death (Hawkins, 2019; Ruth & Mighty, 2019). Serious injuries are more likely to occur in an MVA if the woman is not wearing a seat belt with a shoulder harness and is ejected from the vehicle. Therefore, to improve chances of survival for mother and fetus, pregnant women should wear properly positioned restraints at all times when in a motor vehicle (see Fig. 14.14). However, approximately one-third of pregnant women do not wear seat belts because of discomfort, inconvenience, or fear of hurting the baby. Other sources of trauma include intimate partner violence, falls, burns, homicide, suicide, and penetrating trauma (Ruth & Mighty).

Trauma is one of the leading causes of nonobstetric maternal death in the United States (Ruth & Mighty, 2019). The effect of trauma on pregnancy is influenced by the length of gestation, type and severity of the trauma, and degree of disruption of uterine and fetal physiologic features. Fortunately, most trauma injuries during pregnancy are relatively minor and have no adverse effect on pregnancy outcome (Ruth & Mighty). However, each case must be evaluated carefully because pregnancy can mask signs of severe injury.

Fetal morbidity and mortality are also significantly affected by maternal trauma. An increased risk for fetal death is associated with maternal trauma, as well as a greater chance of other adverse maternal, fetal, and neonatal outcomes, including miscarriage, preterm birth, preterm prelabor rupture of membranes, uterine rupture, cesarean birth, placental abruption, and stillbirth (Brown, 2017). Fetal death rates related to maternal trauma are reported to be as high as 41% if the maternal injuries are life threatening (Ruth & Mighty, 2019). This information is probably underestimated because reporting of fetal death or injury resulting from maternal trauma is not standardized (Brown). Special considerations for mother and fetus are necessary when trauma occurs during pregnancy because of the physiologic alterations that accompany pregnancy and because of the presence of the fetus.

Maternal Physiologic Characteristics

Optimal care for the pregnant woman after trauma depends on understanding the physiologic state of pregnancy and its effects on trauma. The pregnant woman's body exhibits responses that are different from those of a nonpregnant person to the same traumatic insults. Because of the different responses to injury during pregnancy, management strategies must be adapted for appropriate resuscitation, fluid therapy, positioning, assessments, and most other interventions. Significant maternal adaptations and the relation to trauma are summarized in Table 30.2.

The uterus and bladder are confined to the bony pelvis during the first trimester of pregnancy and are at reduced risk for injury in cases of abdominal trauma. After pregnancy progresses beyond the 14th week, the uterus becomes an abdominal organ, and the risk for injury in cases of abdominal trauma increases. During the second and third trimesters, the distended bladder becomes an abdominal organ and is at increased risk for injury and rupture. Bowel injuries occur less often during pregnancy because of the protection provided by the enlarged uterus.

> **! NURSING ALERT**
>
> The unconscious pregnant woman is at increased risk for regurgitation of gastric contents and aspiration whenever her head is positioned lower than her stomach or if abdominal pressure is applied.

The elevated levels of progesterone that accompany pregnancy relax smooth muscle and profoundly affect the GI tract. GI motility decreases, with a resultant increased time required for gastric emptying, whereas the production of hydrochloric acid increases in the last trimester, and the gastroesophageal sphincter relaxes (Ruth & Mighty, 2019). Because of these changes, airway management of the unconscious pregnant woman is critically important.

A pregnant woman has decreased tolerance for hypoxia and apnea because of her decreased functional residual capacity and increased renal loss of bicarbonate. Acidosis develops more quickly in the pregnant than in the nonpregnant state.

Cardiac output increases 30% to 50% over prepregnancy values and is position dependent in the third trimester. Because of compression of the inferior vena cava and descending aorta by the pregnant uterus, cardiac output decreases dramatically if the woman is placed in the supine position. Therefore the supine position must be avoided, even in women with cervical spine injuries. It is a primary priority that lateral uterine displacement be accomplished without any head movement. As soon as the neck is immobilized, the stretcher should be tilted laterally (Brown, 2017; Ruth & Mighty, 2019).

The increase in circulating blood volume during pregnancy allows the woman to tolerate significant intraabdominal or intrauterine blood loss with only minimal changes in vital signs. By the time maternal tachycardia and hypotension, which are considered hallmark symptoms of blood loss, are evident, massive hemorrhage has likely already occurred (Ruth & Mighty, 2019).

Fetal Physiologic Characteristics

Perfusion of the uterine arteries, which provide the primary blood supply to the uteroplacental unit, depends on adequate maternal arterial pressure because these vessels lack autoregulation. Therefore maternal hypotension decreases uterine and fetal perfusion. Maternal shock results in splanchnic and uterine artery vasoconstriction, which decreases blood flow and oxygen transport to the fetus. Electronic fetal monitoring (EFM) tracings can assist in evaluating maternal status after trauma. They reflect fetal cardiac responses to hypoxia and hypoperfusion, including tachycardia or bradycardia, minimal or absent baseline variability, and late decelerations.

Careful monitoring of fetal status assists greatly in maternal assessment because the fetal monitor tracing serves as an "oximeter" of internal maternal well-being. Hypoperfusion can be present in the pregnant woman before the onset of clinical signs of shock. The EFM tracings may show the first signs of maternal compromise (e.g., when maternal heart rate, BP, and color appear normal), yet the EFM tracing shows signs of fetal hypoxia (Brown, 2017; Miller, Miller, & Cypher, 2017).

Mechanisms of Trauma
Blunt Abdominal Trauma

Blunt abdominal trauma is most commonly the result of MVAs but also may be the result of intimate partner violence or falls. Maternal and fetal mortality and morbidity rates are directly correlated with whether the mother remains inside the vehicle or is ejected. Maternal death is usually the result of a head injury or exsanguination from a

TABLE 30.2 Maternal Adaptations During Pregnancy and Relation to Trauma

System	Alteration	Clinical Responses
Respiratory	↑ Oxygen consumption	↑ Risk for acidosis
	↑ Tidal volume	↑ Risk for respiratory mismanagement
	↓ Functional residual capacity	
	Chronic compensated alkalosis	↓ Blood-buffering capacity
	↓ PaCO₂	
	↓ Serum bicarbonate	
Cardiovascular	↑ Circulating volume, 1600 mL	Can lose 1000 mL blood
	↑ CO	No signs of shock until blood loss >30% of total blood volume
	↑ Heart rate	
	↓ SVR	↓ Placental perfusion in supine position
	↓ Arterial blood pressure	
	Heart displaced upward to left	Point of maximal impulse, fourth intercostal space
Renal	↑ Renal plasma flow	
	Dilation of ureters and urethra	↑ Risk for stasis, infection
	Bladder displaced forward	↑ Risk for bladder trauma
Gastrointestinal	↓ Gastric motility	↑ Risk for aspiration
	↑ Hydrochloric acid production	
	↓ Competency of gastroesophageal sphincter	Passive regurgitation of stomach acid if head lower than stomach
Reproductive	↑ Blood flow to organs	Source of ↑ blood loss
	Uterine enlargement	Vena caval compression in supine position
Musculoskeletal	Displacement of abdominal viscera	↑ Risk for injury, altered rebound response
	Pelvic venous congestion	Altered pain referral
	Cartilage softened	↑ Risk for pelvic fracture
		Center of gravity changed
	Fetal head in pelvis	↑ Risk for fetal injury
Hematologic	↑ Clotting factors	↑ Risk for thrombus formation
	↓ Fibrinolytic activity	

CO, Cardiac output; *PaCO₂,* arterial partial pressure of carbon dioxide; *SVR,* systemic vascular resistance.

major vessel rupture. Serious retroperitoneal hemorrhage after lower abdominal and pelvic trauma is reported more frequently during pregnancy. Serious maternal abdominal injuries are usually the result of splenic rupture or liver or renal injury.

Blunt trauma to the maternal abdomen is an important cause of placental abruption (Brown, 2017). Placental separation is thought to be a result of deformation of the elastic myometrium around the relatively inelastic placenta. Shearing of the placental edge from the underlying decidua basalis results and is worsened by the increased intrauterine pressure resulting from the impact. It is critical that all pregnant survivors be carefully evaluated for signs and symptoms of placental abruption after even minor blunt abdominal trauma.

> **! NURSING ALERT**
>
> Signs and symptoms of placental abruption include uterine tenderness or pain, uterine irritability, uterine contractions, vaginal bleeding, leaking of amniotic fluid, or a change in fetal heart rate characteristics.

Pelvic fracture may result from severe injury and may produce bladder trauma or retroperitoneal bleeding with the two-point displacement of pelvic bones that usually occurs. One point of displacement is commonly at the symphysis pubis, and the second point is posterior because of the structure of the pelvis. Careful evaluation for clinical signs of internal hemorrhage is indicated.

Direct fetal injury as a complication of trauma during pregnancy most often involves the fetal skull and brain. Most commonly this injury accompanies maternal pelvic fracture in late gestation, after the fetal head becomes engaged. When the force of the impact is great enough to fracture the maternal pelvis, the fetus often sustains a skull fracture. Evaluation for fetal skull fracture or intracranial hemorrhage is indicated.

Uterine rupture as a result of blunt trauma is rare, occurring in less than 1% of severe cases. Rupture is more likely to occur in a previously scarred uterus. When uterine rupture occurs, it is usually associated with a direct blow delivered with substantial force (Cunningham et al., 2018). Although maternal death can and does occur, traumatic uterine rupture almost always results in fetal death (Ruth & Mighty, 2019).

Penetrating Abdominal Trauma

Bullet and stab wounds are the most frequent causes of penetrating abdominal trauma in pregnant women. When the uterus sustains penetrating wounds, the fetus is more likely than the mother to be seriously injured. The enlarged uterus may protect other maternal organs, particularly the bowel, but the fetus is more vulnerable (Ruth & Mighty, 2019).

Numerous factors determine the extent and severity of maternal and fetal injury from a bullet wound, including the size and velocity of the bullet, anatomic region penetrated, angle of entry, path of the bullet, organs damaged, gestational age, and exit wound. Once the bullet enters the body, it may ricochet several times as it encounters organs or bone, or it may sever a large blood vessel. During the second half of pregnancy, the fetus usually sustains a direct injury from the bullet. Gunshot wounds require surgical exploration to determine the extent of injury and repair damage as needed.

Stab wounds are limited by the length and width of the penetrating object and are usually confined to the pathway of the weapon. Maternal and fetal injury is less if the stab wound is located in the upper abdomen and is from movement of the penetrating object from above the head downward toward the abdomen than from movement from the ground upward toward the lower abdomen. Stab wounds usually require surgical exploration to clean out debris, determine extent of injury, and repair damage.

Thoracic Trauma

Thoracic trauma is reported to produce 25% of all trauma deaths. Pulmonary contusion results from nearly 75% of blunt thoracic trauma and is a potentially life-threatening condition. Pulmonary contusion can be difficult to recognize, especially if flail chest is also present or if there is no evidence of thoracic injury. Pulmonary contusion should be suspected in cases of thoracic injury, especially after blunt acceleration or deceleration trauma, such as that occurring when a rapidly moving vehicle crashes into an immovable object.

Penetrating wounds into the chest can result in pneumothorax or hemothorax. This type of injury is usually caused by an MVA that results in impalement by the steering column or a loose article in the vehicle that became a projectile with the force of impact. Stab wounds into the chest also may occur as a result of violence.

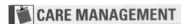 CARE MANAGEMENT

Immediate Stabilization

Immediate priorities for stabilization of the pregnant woman after trauma should be identical to those of the nonpregnant trauma client. Pregnancy should not result in any restriction of the usual diagnostic, pharmacologic, or resuscitative procedures or maneuvers (American Academy of Pediatrics [AAP] & ACOG, 2017). The initial response of many trauma team members when caring for the pregnant woman is to assess fetal status first because of the concern for a healthy neonate. Instead the trauma team should follow a methodic evaluation of maternal status to ensure complete assessment and stabilization of the mother. Fetal survival depends on maternal survival, and stabilizing the mother improves the chance of fetal survival.

> ### ⚡ SAFETY ALERT
>
> Priorities of care for the pregnant woman after trauma must be to resuscitate the woman and stabilize her condition first and then consider fetal needs.

Primary Survey

The systematic evaluation begins with a primary survey and the initial *CABDs* of resuscitation: *compressions, airway, breathing,* and *defibrillation.* Increased oxygen needs during gestation necessitate a rapid response. The presence of a cervical spine injury is always assumed.

> ### ⚡ SAFETY ALERT
>
> Hyperextension of the neck is avoided; instead, jaw thrust is used to establish an airway for the trauma survivor.

Once an airway is established, assessment should focus on adequacy of oxygenation. The chest wall is observed for movement. If breathing is absent, ventilations and endotracheal intubation are initiated. Supplemental oxygen should be administered with a tight-fitting, nonrebreathing face mask at 10 to 12 L/min to maintain adequate oxygen availability to the fetus. The chest wall is assessed for penetrating chest wound or flail chest. Breathing with a flail chest is rapid and labored; chest wall movements are uncoordinated and asymmetric; crepitus from bony fragments may be palpated.

Immediate placement of two large-bore (14- to 16-gauge) IV lines is recommended. This facilitates initial rapid fluid replacement and intravascular volume expansion and provides a route for possible blood and blood products, if necessary. Normal saline, a crystalloid solution, is the universal fluid of choice for quick volume expansion (Ruth & Mighty, 2019). Hypovolemia has traditionally been managed by administering large volumes of crystalloid fluids until bleeding is controlled. However, studies have shown that this practice can lead to fluid overload, with resulting complications of tissue edema, acute respiratory distress syndrome, dilutional coagulopathy, and disruptions in regulatory processes. Therefore, low-volume resuscitation, which includes limiting the volume of crystalloid fluids used in resuscitation, is now recommended. Currently there is no specific recommendation regarding the optimal volume of fluid to be infused (Ruth & Graves, 2019).

Another component of therapy during the primary survey is balanced ratio administration of blood products. Administering platelets, plasma, and packed RBCs in a 1:1:1 ratio is intended to mimic the composition of whole blood. Balanced ratio resuscitation has been shown to improve outcomes (Ruth & Graves, 2019). If blood loss continues and the woman is unstable, type O Rh-negative blood may be administered until type-specific or cross-matched donor blood is available (Ruth & Mighty, 2019).

Hypovolemia should be presumed to be the cause of hypotension until proven otherwise. Careful volume replacement (as described earlier) is the treatment of choice for maternal hypotension. Administering vasopressor drugs to treat maternal hypotension should be avoided if possible. These medications may significantly reduce uterine blood flow and thus decrease oxygen delivery to the fetus (Ruth & Mighty, 2019).

After 20 weeks of gestation, venous return to the heart is best accomplished by positioning the uterus to one side to eliminate the weight of the uterus compressing the inferior vena cava or the descending aorta. This facilitates efforts to establish the forward flow of blood through resuscitation and stabilization. If a lateral position is not possible because of resuscitative efforts or cervical spine immobilization, the uterus can be manually deflected, or a wedge should be inserted underneath one side of the backboard or stretcher.

Cardiopulmonary Resuscitation of the Pregnant Woman

The most common underlying causes of maternal cardiac arrest are hemorrhage, heart failure, amniotic fluid embolism, and sepsis (Hawkins, 2019). Special modifications are necessary when cardiopulmonary resuscitation (CPR) is performed during the second half of pregnancy. In nonpregnant women, chest compressions produce a cardiac output of only about 30% of normal. Cardiac output in pregnant women may be even less as a result of aortocaval compression caused by the gravid uterus. Therefore, uterine displacement during resuscitation efforts is critical (Cunningham et al., 2018). The uterus may be displaced laterally either manually or by placing a wedge, rolled blanket, or towel under one of the woman's hips. If defibrillation is needed, the paddles must be placed one rib interspace higher than usual because the heart is displaced slightly by the enlarged uterus (see Emergency: Cardiopulmonary Resuscitation for the Pregnant Woman).

Complications, including laceration of the liver, rupture of the spleen or uterus, hemothorax, hemopericardium, or fracture of ribs or sternum may be associated with CPR on a pregnant woman. Fetal complications, including cardiac arrhythmia or asystole related to maternal defibrillation and medications and CNS depression related to antiarrhythmic drugs and inadequate uteroplacental perfusion, with possible fetal hypoxemia and acidemia, may also occur.

If the resuscitation is successful, the woman must be monitored carefully afterward. She remains at increased risk for recurrent cardiac arrest and arrhythmias (e.g., ventricular tachycardia, supraventricular tachycardia, bradycardia). Therefore her cardiovascular, pulmonary, and neurologic status should be assessed continually. If the pregnancy remains intact, uterine activity and resting tone must be monitored. Fetal status and gestational age should also be determined and used in decision making regarding continuation of the pregnancy or the timing and route of birth.

Another common reason for performing CPR on a pregnant woman is airway obstruction caused by choking. Clearing an airway obstruction is usually accomplished by performing abdominal thrusts. However, during the second and third trimesters of pregnancy, chest thrusts rather than abdominal thrusts should be used (see Emergency: Relief of Foreign Body Airway Obstruction) (Fig. 30.2).

Secondary Survey

After immediate resuscitation and successful stabilization measures, a more detailed *secondary survey* of the mother and fetus should be accomplished. A complete physical assessment including all body systems is performed.

➕ EMERGENCY

Cardiopulmonary Resuscitation for the Pregnant Woman

Assessment
- Determine unresponsiveness and no breathing or no normal breathing.
- Activate emergency medical system and get AED if available.
- Return to woman and check for pulse.
- Begin chest compressions if no pulse is felt.

Compressions
- Position the woman on a flat, firm surface with her uterus displaced laterally with a wedge (e.g., a rolled towel placed under her hip) or manually or place her in a left lateral position.
- Begin chest compressions at a rate of 100/min to 120/min. Push hard and push fast! At the end of each compression, allow the chest to recoil (reexpand) completely.
- Chest compressions should be performed to a depth of at least 5 cm (2 inches) for an average adult, but no greater than 6 cm (2.4 inches).
- Chest compressions may be performed slightly higher on the sternum if the uterus is enlarged enough to displace the diaphragm into a higher position.
- After five cycles of 30 compressions and two breaths (or approximately 2 min), check for a pulse. If no pulse is present, continue CPR. Rotate the compressor role every 2 min if possible to prevent fatigue.

Airway
- Open airway using head tilt-chin lift maneuver.

Breathing
- Deliver breaths using a face mask or bag-mask device if possible.
- Deliver each breath over 1 sec, watching for chest rise.
- Deliver breaths using a ratio of 30 chest compressions to 2 breaths.

Defibrillation
- Use an AED according to standard protocol to analyze heart rhythm and deliver shock if indicated.

AED, Automated external defibrillator; *CPR,* cardiopulmonary resuscitation. Data from Kleinman, M. E., Brennan, E. E., Goldberger, Z. D., et al. (2015). Part 5: Adult basic life support and cardiopulmonary resuscitation quality: 2015 American Heart Association guidelines update for cardiopulmonary resuscitation and emergency cardiovascular care. *Circulation, 132*(2 suppl), S414–S435.

➕ EMERGENCY

Relief of Foreign Body Airway Obstruction

If the pregnant woman is unable to speak or cough, perform chest thrusts. Stand behind her and place your arms under her armpits to encircle her chest. Press backward with quick thrusts until the foreign body is expelled (see Fig. 30.2). If the woman becomes unconscious, carefully support her to the ground, immediately activate EMS, and begin CPR.

EMS, Emergency medical services; *CPR,* cardiopulmonary resuscitation. Data from Berg, R. A., Hemphill, R., Abella, B. S., et al. (2010). Part 5: Adult basic life support: 2010 American Heart Association guidelines for cardiopulmonary resuscitation and emergency cardiovascular care science. *Circulation, 122*(Suppl 3), S685–S705.

The maternal abdomen should be evaluated carefully because a large percentage of serious injuries involve the uterus, intraperitoneal structures, and the retroperitoneum. The greatest clinical concern after severe blunt abdominal trauma is placental abruption because as many as 40% to 50% of these women have a clinically evident abruption (Brown, 2017). Assessments should focus on recognition of this complication, with careful

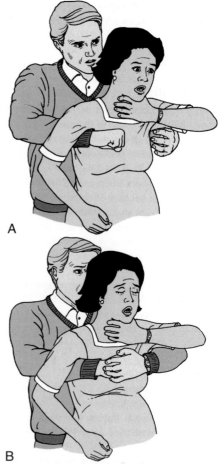

A

B

Fig. 30.2 Clearing Airway Obstruction in Woman in Late Stage of Pregnancy. (A) Standing behind woman, place your arms under woman's armpits and across chest. Place thumb side of your clenched fist against middle of sternum, and place other hand over fist. (B) Perform backward chest thrusts until foreign body is expelled or woman becomes unconscious (see Emergency: Relief of Foreign Body Airway Obstruction). (Data from Berg, R. A., Hemphill, R., Abella, B. S., et al. [2010]. Part 5: Adult basic life support: 2010 American Heart Association guidelines for cardiopulmonary resuscitation and emergency cardiovascular care science. *Circulation, 122*[Suppl 3], S685–S705.)

evaluation of fetal monitor tracings, uterine tenderness, labor, or vaginal bleeding. Ultrasound examination may be performed to determine gestational age, viability of the fetus, and placental location. However, ultrasound studies cannot exclude placental abruption (Ruth & Mighty, 2019).

If trauma is the result of a penetrating wound, the woman should be completely undressed and carefully examined for all entrance and exit wounds. Focused *a*ssessment *s*onographic *t*rauma (FAST) ultrasound and CT are commonly used to assess the likelihood of intraabdominal bleeding. The standard FAST examination is now used instead of peritoneal lavage to identify intraabdominal bleeding because of its ability to detect intraperitoneal fluid (Brown, 2017).

Exploratory laparotomy is necessary after a gunshot wound to assess the abdominal cavity for organ damage and to repair any damage, with careful examination of all organs, the entire bowel, and posterior vessels. If uterine injury is found, a careful evaluation of the risks and benefits of cesarean birth is quickly accomplished. A cesarean birth is desirable if the fetus is alive and near term and may be necessary for the preterm fetus because of the high incidence of direct fetal injury in these cases. The fetus usually tolerates surgery and anesthesia if adequate uterine perfusion and oxygenation are maintained. Tetanus prophylaxis guidelines are not changed by pregnancy so vaccine is given if needed.

Trauma may affect numerous systems in the maternal body and may affect more than the pregnancy. External signs of maternal trauma should suggest the possibility of internal trauma. Back and neck pain suggest spine injury, abrasions on the chest suggest chest injury, and limb pain and malposition suggest limb fractures. If head injury results in nonresponsiveness, spinal, thoracic, and abdominal injuries are suspected. Hypovolemic shock can occur with internal hemorrhage, fracture of long bones, ruptured liver or spleen, hemothorax, or arterial dissection.

All female trauma survivors of childbearing age should be considered pregnant until proven otherwise. Determination of the health history and a history of the events preceding the trauma are important components of care. If the pregnant woman was involved in an MVA, it should be determined whether she was the driver or a passenger, if air bags were deployed, and if she was ejected from the vehicle or used a restraining device and remained within the vehicle.

Electronic Fetal Monitoring

External FHR and contraction monitoring is recommended after blunt trauma in a viable gestation for a minimum of 4 hours, regardless of injury severity. Fetal monitoring should be initiated soon after the woman is stable (Cunningham et al., 2018). Continuous EFM may show early signs of placental abruption, including a change in baseline rate, loss of accelerations, or the presence of late decelerations, especially when accompanied by absent or minimal variability. The external device to monitor uterine activity, the tocodynamometer, is unable to measure pressures, so the pattern made with this device only shows the frequency and duration of contractions. Palpation is required to evaluate the intensity of contractions and the uterine resting tone. It is important to palpate between contractions to verify that the uterus is well relaxed. If the uterus does not relax between contractions, placental abruption could be present.

The exact duration of FHR and contraction monitoring required after blunt abdominal trauma is not known. Monitoring should be continued indefinitely if uterine contractions, abnormal FHR characteristics, vaginal bleeding, uterine tenderness or irritability, serious maternal injury, or ruptured membranes are present (Cunningham et al., 2018). Most serious complications develop within 4 to 6 hours following the traumatic event (Ruth & Mighty, 2019). Women without contractions or with less than one contraction in 10 minutes may be removed from the electronic fetal monitor and discharged, as long as there is evidence of fetal movement, normal FHR characteristics, and no vaginal bleeding or indication of ruptured membranes (Miller et al., 2017).

LEGAL TIP

Care of the Pregnant Woman Involved in a Minor Trauma Situation

After minor trauma, the pregnant woman may be discharged after an adequate period of electronic fetal monitoring that demonstrates a normal (category I) tracing (see Chapter 18) and absence of uterine contractions. However, clear instructions must be given for immediate return to the health care facility if vaginal bleeding, leaking of amniotic fluid, decreased fetal movement, or severe abdominal pain occurs.

Fetomaternal Hemorrhage

The potential for fetomaternal hemorrhage exists after trauma, particularly blunt trauma. Hemorrhage can lead to fetal anemia, distress, or even death. If the pregnant trauma survivor is Rh negative, fetomaternal hemorrhage can result in sensitization and hemolytic disease of the neonate. The Kleihauer-Betke assay may be performed in women following blunt abdominal trauma to estimate the amount of fetal blood within the maternal circulation. Because most cases of fetomaternal hemorrhage involve less than 30 mL of blood, the routine administration of 300 mcg of $Rh_o(D)$ immune globulin is sufficient to protect almost all Rh-negative pregnant trauma clients from isoimmunization (Brown, 2017).

Ultrasound

Ultrasound after trauma is not as sensitive as EFM for diagnosing placental abruption. It may be useful to help establish gestational age, locate the placenta, evaluate cardiac activity (to determine whether the fetus is alive), and determine amniotic fluid volume. It may also be used to evaluate the presence of intraabdominal fluid that would suggest the presence of intraabdominal hemorrhage.

Radiation Exposure

If the pregnant woman has sustained serious injuries, any necessary radiographic examination should be performed, regardless of fetal exposure. If radiographic examination would be performed for the nonpregnant trauma survivor, it also should be performed for the pregnant woman. Abdominal or pelvic CT scanning can be used to visualize extraperitoneal and retroperitoneal structures and the genitourinary tract. Radiation exposure of less than 5 rads has not been associated with fetal abnormalities or pregnancy loss, and the radiation level associated with abdominal or pelvic CT scans is far below this amount (Brown, 2017). MRI can also be safely used to assess injuries because it does not produce ionizing radiation (Brown).

Perimortem Cesarean Birth

In the presence of multisystem trauma, perimortem cesarean birth may be indicated. Emptying the uterus early in the process of resuscitation may increase the chance for a favorable outcome for the fetus and also improve maternal resuscitative efforts (Arafeh & Abir, 2019; Brown, 2017). Therefore if the pregnancy is at or beyond fetal viability (23 to 24 weeks of gestation) a cesarean birth should be performed after 4 minutes of resuscitative efforts if there is no spontaneous return of circulation (Brown, 2017; Lavonas et al., 2015) so that the fetus can be born within 5 minutes of pulselessness (Arafeh & Abir). It has been suggested that *perimortem cesarean birth* be replaced by the term *resuscitative hysterectomy*, because this term better describes a procedure that has the potential to benefit both mother and fetus (Ruth & Mighty, 2019).

KEY POINTS

- The normal hemodynamic values are significantly altered as a result of pregnancy.
- The stress of the normal maternal adaptations to pregnancy on a heart whose function is already taxed may cause cardiac decompensation.
- Maternal morbidity and mortality are significant risks in a pregnancy complicated by mitral stenosis.
- Anemia, a common medical disorder of pregnancy, affects at least 20% of pregnant women.
- Asthma is a common medical condition to complicate pregnancy, and the prevalence and morbidity from this disorder are increasing.
- Pruritus is a common symptom in pregnancy-specific inflammatory skin diseases.

- If possible, a pregnant woman with epilepsy should take only one anticonvulsant medication at the lowest dose that is effective at keeping her seizure-free.
- Autoimmune disorders can occur during pregnancy because a large percentage of people with an autoimmune disorder are women of childbearing age. Common autoimmune diseases include SLE and MG.
- Cholecystitis and cholelithiasis are common GI problems in pregnancy.
- UTIs are a common medical complication of pregnancy.
- Pyelonephritis is one of the most frequent serious medical complications of pregnancy and a leading cause of septic shock during pregnancy.
- In the pregnant woman, an enlarged uterus, displaced internal organs, and altered laboratory values may confuse the diagnosis when the need for immediate abdominal surgery occurs.

- Trauma is one of the leading causes of nonobstetric maternal death in the United States. Pregnancy does not limit or restrict resuscitative, diagnostic, or pharmacologic treatment after trauma.
- Fetal survival depends on maternal survival. After a trauma, the first priority, before consideration of fetal concerns, is to resuscitate and stabilize the mother.
- Optimal care for the pregnant survivor of trauma depends on knowledge of the physiologic state of pregnancy.
- In the case of a cardiac arrest in a pregnant woman, the standard advanced cardiac life support guidelines should be implemented with a few slight modifications: the uterus must be displaced to the left, and the defibrillation paddles should be placed one rib interspace higher.

REFERENCES

American Academy of Pediatrics & American College of Obstetricians and Gynecologists. (2017). *Guidelines for perinatal care* (8th ed.). Washington, DC: American College of Obstetricians and Gynecologists.

American College of Obstetricians and Gynecologists. (2017). Practice bulletin no. 187: Neural tube defects. *Obstetrics & Gynecology, 130*(6), e279–286.

American College of Obstetricians and Gynecologists. (2018). Practice bulletin no. 199: Use of prophylactic antibiotics in labor and delivery. *Obstetrics & Gynecology, 132*(3), e103–e119.

Antony, K. M., Racusin, D. A., Aagaard, K., et al. (2017). Maternal physiology. In S. G. Gabbe, J. R. Niebyl, J. L. Simpson, et al. (Eds.), *Obstetrics: Normal and problem pregnancies* (7th ed.). Philadelphia: Elsevier.

Arafeh, J. M. R., & Abir, G. (2019). Cardiopulmonary resuscitation in pregnancy. In N. H. Troiano, P. M. Witcher, & S. M. Baird (Eds.), *AWHONN's high risk and critical care obstetrics* (4th ed.). Philadelphia: Wolters Kluwer.

Blackburn, S. T. (2018). *Maternal, fetal, and neonatal physiology: A clinical perspective* (5th ed.). St. Louis: Elsevier.

Blanchard, D. G., & Daniels, L. B. (2019). Cardiac diseases. In R. Resnik, C. J. Lockwood, T. R. Moore, et al. (Eds.), *Creasy & Resnik's maternal-fetal medicine: Principles and practice* (8th ed.). Philadelphia: Elsevier.

Brown, H. L. (2017). Trauma and related surgery in pregnancy. In S. G. Gabbe, J. R. Niebyl, J. L. Simpson, et al. (Eds.), *Obstetrics: Normal and problem pregnancies* (7th ed.). Philadelphia: Elsevier.

Cappell, M. S. (2017a). Gastrointestinal disorders during pregnancy. In S. G. Gabbe, J. R. Niebyl, J. L. Simpson, et al. (Eds.), *Obstetrics: Normal and problem pregnancies* (7th ed.). Philadelphia: Elsevier.

Cappell, M. (2017b). Hepatic disorders during pregnancy. In S. G. Gabbe, J. R. Niebyl, J. L. Simpson, et al. (Eds.), *Obstetrics: Normal and problem pregnancies* (7th ed.). Philadelphia: Elsevier.

Carpenter, J. R., & Branch, D. W. (2017). Collagen vascular diseases. In S. G. Gabbe, J. R. Niebyl, J. L. Simpson, et al. (Eds.), *Obstetrics: Normal and problem pregnancies* (7th ed.). Philadelphia: Elsevier.

Cunningham, F., Leveno, K., Bloom, S., et al. (2018). *Williams obstetrics* (25th ed.). New York: McGraw-Hill Education.

Deen, J., Chandrasekaran, S., Stout, K., et al. (2017). Heart disease in pregnancy. In S. G. Gabbe, J. R. Niebyl, J. L. Simpson, et al. (Eds.), *Obstetrics: Normal and problem pregnancies* (7th ed.). Philadelphia: Elsevier.

Douglas, V. C., & Aminoff, M. J. (2019). Neurologic disorders. In R. Resnik, C. J. Lockwood, T. R. Moore, et al. (Eds.), *Creasy & Resnik's maternal-fetal medicine: Principles and practice* (8th ed.). Philadelphia: Elsevier.

Duff, P. (2019). Maternal and fetal infections. In R. Resnik, C. J. Lockwood, T. R. Moore, et al. (Eds.), *Creasy & Resnik's maternal-fetal medicine: Principles and practice* (8th ed.). Philadelphia: Elsevier.

Duff, P., & Birsner, M. (2017). Maternal and perinatal infection in pregnancy: Bacterial. In S. G. Gabbe, J. R. Niebyl, J. L. Simpson, et al. (Eds.), *Obstetrics: Normal and problem pregnancies* (7th ed.). Philadelphia: Elsevier.

Elkayam, U., Goland, S., Pieper, P. G., & Silversides, C. K. (2016). High risk cardiac disease in pregnancy. Part 1. *Journal of the American College of Cardiology, 68*(4), 396–410.

Gabzdyl, E. M., & Schlaeger, J. M. (2015). Intrahepatic cholestasis of pregnancy: A critical clinical review. *Journal of Perinatal & Neonatal Nursing, 29*(1), 41–50.

Gerard, E. E., & Samuels, P. (2017). Neurological disorders in pregnancy. In S. G. Gabbe, J. R. Niebyl, J. L. Simpson, et al. (Eds.), *Obstetrics: Normal and problem pregnancies* (7th ed.). Philadelphia: Elsevier.

Hawkins, J. L. (2019). Anesthesia considerations for complicated pregnancies. In R. Resnik, C. J. Lockwood, T. R. Moore, et al. (Eds.), *Creasy & Resnik's maternal-fetal medicine: Principles and practice* (8th ed.). Philadelphia: Elsevier.

Kelly, T. F., & Savides, T. J. (2019). Gastrointestinal disease in pregnancy. In R. Resnik, C. J. Lockwood, T. R. Moore, et al. (Eds.), *Creasy & Resnik's maternal-fetal medicine: Principles and practice* (8th ed.). Philadelphia: Elsevier.

Kilpatrick, S. J., & Kitahara, S. (2019). Anemia and pregnancy. In R. Resnik, C. J. Lockwood, T. R. Moore, et al. (Eds.), *Creasy & Resnik's maternal-fetal medicine: Principles and practice* (8th ed.). Philadelphia: Elsevier.

Krening, C., Troiano, N. H., & Shah, S. S. (2019). Maternal cardiac disorders. In N. H. Troiano, P. M. Witcher, & S. M. Baird (Eds.), *AWHONN's high risk and critical care obstetrics* (4th ed.). Philadelphia: Wolters Kluwer.

Lavonas, E. J., Drennan, I. R., Gabrielli, A., et al. (2015). Part 10: Special circumstances of resuscitation: 2015 American Heart Association guidelines update for cardiopulmonary resuscitation and emergency cardiovascular care. *Circulation, 132*(2 Suppl), S501–S518.

Lawrence, R. A., & Lawrence, R. M. (2016). *Breastfeeding: A guide for the medical profession* (8th ed.). Philadelphia: Elsevier.

Lee, R. H., Chung, R. T., & Pringle, P. (2019). Diseases of the liver, biliary system, and pancreas. In R. Resnik, C. J. Lockwood, T. R. Moore, et al. (Eds.), *Creasy & Resnik's maternal-fetal medicine: Principles and practice* (8th ed.). Philadelphia: Elsevier.

March of Dimes. (2017). *Folic acid.* Retrieved from: www.marchofdimes.org/pregnancy/folic-acid.aspx#.

Mason, B. A., & Burke, C. (2019). Pulmonary disorders in pregnancy. In N. H. Troiano, P. M. Witcher, & S. M. Baird (Eds.), *AWHONN's high risk and critical care obstetrics* (4th ed.). Philadelphia: Wolters Kluwer.

Miller, L., Miller, D., & Cypher, R. (2017). *Mosby's pocket guide to fetal monitoring: A multidisciplinary approach* (8th ed.). St. Louis: Elsevier.

Rapini, R. P. (2019). The skin and pregnancy. In R. Resnik, C. J. Lockwood, T. R. Moore, et al. (Eds.), *Creasy & Resnik's maternal-fetal medicine: Principles and practice* (8th ed.). Philadelphia: Elsevier.

Ruth, D., & Graves, C. R. (2019). Volume resuscitation and blood component therapy. In N. H. Troiano, P. M. Witcher, & S. M. Baird (Eds.), *AWHONN's high risk and critical care obstetrics* (4th ed.). Philadelphia: Wolters Kluwer.

Ruth, D., & Mighty, H. E. (2019). Trauma in pregnancy. In N. H. Troiano, P. M. Witcher, & S. M. Baird (Eds.), *AWHONN's high risk and critical care obstetrics* (4th ed.). Philadelphia: Wolters Kluwer.

Sammaritano, L. R., Salmon, J. E., & Branch, D. W. (2019). Pregnancy and rheumatic diseases. In R. Resnik, C. J. Lockwood, T. R. Moore, et al. (Eds.), *Creasy & Resnik's maternal-fetal medicine: Principles and practice* (8th ed.). Philadelphia: Elsevier.

Samuels, P. (2017). Hematologic complications of pregnancy. In S. G. Gabbe, J. R. Niebyl, J. L. Simpson, et al. (Eds.), *Obstetrics: Normal and problem pregnancies* (7th ed.). Philadelphia: Elsevier.

Schwartz, N., & Ludmir, J. (2017). Surgery during pregnancy. In S. G. Gabbe, J. R. Niebyl, J. L. Simpson, et al. (Eds.), *Obstetrics: Normal and problem pregnancies* (7th ed.). Philadelphia: Elsevier.

Simhan, H. N., Berghella, V., & Iams, J. D. (2019). Prevention and management of preterm parturition. In R. Resnik, C. J. Lockwood, T. R. Moore, et al. (Eds.), *Creasy & Resnik's maternal-fetal medicine: Principles and practice* (8th ed.). Philadelphia: Elsevier.

Simhan, H. N., Iams, J. D., & Romero, R. (2017). Preterm labor and birth. In S. G. Gabbe, J. R. Niebyl, J. L. Simpson, et al. (Eds.), *Obstetrics: Normal and problem pregnancies* (7th ed.). Philadelphia: Elsevier.

Smith, K., & Gros, B. (2017). Pregnancy-related acute aortic dissection in Marfan syndrome: A review of the literature. *Congenital Heart Disease, 12*(3), 251–260.

Spencer, B. (2015). Medications and breastfeeding for mothers with chronic illness. *Journal of Obstetric, Gynecologic and Neonatal Nursing, 44*(4), 543–552.

Wang, A. R., & Kroumpouzos, G. (2017). Skin disease and pregnancy. In S. G. Gabbe, J. R. Niebyl, J. L. Simpson, et al. (Eds.), *Obstetrics: Normal and problem pregnancies* (7th ed.). Philadelphia: Elsevier.

Whitty, J. E., & Dombrowski, M. P. (2017). Respiratory disease in pregnancy. In S. G. Gabbe, J. R. Niebyl, J. L. Simpson, et al. (Eds.), *Obstetrics: Normal and problem pregnancies* (7th ed.). Philadelphia: Elsevier.

Whitty, J. E., & Dombrowski, M. P. (2019). Respiratory diseases in pregnancy. In R. Resnik, C. J. Lockwood, T. R. Moore, et al. (Eds.), *Creasy & Resnik's maternal-fetal medicine: Principles and practice* (8th ed.). Philadelphia: Elsevier.

31

Mental Health Disorders and Substance Abuse

Genae Strong

(e) http://evolve.elsevier.com/Lowdermilk/MWHC/

LEARNING OBJECTIVES

- Describe mental health disorders occurring in the perinatal period, including mood disorders, anxiety disorders, posttraumatic stress disorder, and bipolar disorder.
- Compare postpartum blues, postpartum depression, and postpartum psychosis, including risk factors, assessment, and management.

- Evaluate the role of the nurse in caring for women with mental health disorders during pregnancy and the postpartum period.
- Examine substance abuse during pregnancy, including prevalence, barriers to treatment, legal considerations, and commonly abused drugs.
- Discuss the care of pregnant women who use, abuse, or are dependent on alcohol or illicit or prescription drugs.

This chapter covers the most common maternal mental health disorders: perinatal mood disorders, anxiety disorders, postpartum depression, and postpartum psychosis, which usually manifests as bipolar disorder. Issues related to substance abuse during pregnancy also are discussed.

PERINATAL MENTAL HEALTH DISORDERS

Management of mental health disorders takes place primarily in community settings. Compared with births in the general non–mentally ill population, women with mental illness who give birth have a higher risk for obstetric complications (Ogunyemi, Jovanovski, Liu, et al., 2017). However, mentally ill women who are treated are at lower risk than women who are not treated.

Perinatal mental health problems are common worldwide, though they are widely underrecognized and underreported. Many women experience these disorders but do not seek care. Perinatal depression is one of the most common medical complications during pregnancy and the postpartum period, affecting one in seven women (American Academy of Pediatrics [AAP] & American College of Obstetricians and Gynecologists [ACOG], 2017). In high-income countries, about 10% of pregnant women and 15% of women who have just given birth experience a mental disorder, primarily depression or anxiety. Depression accounts for $30 to $50 billion in lost productivity and direct medical costs in the United States each year. High rates of common perinatal mental disorders have also been seen among women from low- and lower-middle-income countries (AAP & ACOG; Dennis, Falah-Hassani, & Shiri, 2017).

Women are at greatest risk for developing a mental health disorder between the ages of 18 and 45 years—the childbearing years. Women who have serious mental disorders may be engaging in sexual activities that can result in pregnancy. The pregnant woman may have a history of disorder in mood, anxiety, substance use, schizophrenia, personality, or development. Assessment throughout pregnancy and the postpartum period is critical to the mother's and the infant's health. With a history or current symptoms of mental illness, referral to a mental health care provider for evaluation is recommended, with care managed by an interprofessional health care team. Mental health disorders have implications for the pregnant woman, the fetus, the infant and the entire family.

Perinatal Mood Disorders

Although the general public commonly uses the term *depression,* the term connotes a range of disorders that are collectively termed mood disorders. Perinatal mood disorders (PMDs) are a set of disorders, including depression, anxiety, bipolar disorder, and postpartum psychosis, that can occur any time during pregnancy as well as in the first year postpartum (Association of Women's Health, Obstetric and Neonatal Nurses [AWHONN], 2015; Kendig, Keats, Hoffman, et al., 2017).

A mood disorder that emerges during childbearing requires a thorough medical and family history, review of systems, and complete physical examination. The use of prescribed and over-the-counter medications as well as commonly abused substances must be assessed. Thyroid abnormalities and anemia, which are common in childbearing women, should be ruled out (Meltzer-Brody & Jones, 2015).

DIAGNOSIS

Depression

To be diagnosed with major depression, at least five of the following signs or symptoms must be present nearly every day: depressed mood, often with spontaneous crying; markedly diminished interest in all activities; insomnia or hypersomnia; weight changes (increases or decreases); psychomotor retardation or agitation; fatigue or loss of energy; feelings of worthlessness or inappropriate guilt; diminished ability to concentrate; and suicidal ideation with or without a suicidal plan (American Psychiatric Association [APA], 2013). The 10-item Edinburgh Postnatal Depression Scale (see later discussion) accurately identifies depression in pregnant and postpartum women (ACOG, 2018; Clark, Sit, Driscoll, et al., 2015).

Depression *during* pregnancy is a major risk factor for postpartum depression (PPD). PPD has been associated with negative effects on child development, including a difficult infant and childhood temperament, attachment insecurity, and increased risk of developmental delay and lower IQ scores. A substantial rate of suicide occurs postpartum, because maternal suicide accounts for up to 20% of postpartum deaths in depressed women (Grigoriadis, Wilton, Kurdyak, et al., 2017). In fact, more maternal deaths are caused by suicide than by hemorrhage and hypertensive disorders (American College of Obstetricians and Gynecologists [ACOG], 2018).

Untreated maternal depression can negatively affect an infant's psychologic, cognitive, neurologic, and motor skill development. A mother's untreated depression can also negatively affect older children's mental health and behavior (AAP & ACOG, 2017; Gentile, 2017).

CARE MANAGEMENT

Medical management of depression is usually a combination of antidepressants and cognitive-behavioral therapy (CBT) or interpersonal psychotherapy (IPT). For mild cases of depression in pregnant women, psychotherapy is the treatment of choice as the initial intervention. Both IPT and CBT are time-limited treatments (usually 10 to 12 sessions) that focus on present problems and encourage the woman to regain control over her mood and functioning. Short-term therapies, such as CBT, may be delivered by psychiatrists and non-physician professionals such as psychologists, psychiatric clinical nurse specialists or practitioners, or licensed clinical social workers (McKeever, Alderman, Luff, & DeJesus, 2015).

Self-help strategies can be helpful. Such strategies include exercise, respite from caregiving, and self-help groups.

Antidepressant Medications

Pharmacotherapy has become a common treatment for perinatal depression. In the United States, prenatal use of antidepressants has more than doubled in the last 15 years. Estimates vary, but approximately 6 to 13% of women are prescribed an antidepressant at some point during pregnancy (Berard, Zhao, & Sheehy, 2017; Meltzer-Brody & Jones, 2015). The commonly used antidepressant drugs are often divided into four groups: selective serotonin reuptake inhibitors (SSRIs), serotonin/norepinephrine reuptake inhibitors (SNRIs), tricyclic antidepressants (TCAs), and monoamine oxidase inhibitors (MAOIs). The most common antidepressants are listed in Table 31.1.

No consensus exists regarding safety in the use of antidepressant medications by pregnant women. To date, the U.S. Food and Drug Administration (FDA) has not approved any psychotropic medication for use during pregnancy. Information about the safety of these medications during pregnancy or while breastfeeding is available at https:// toxnet.nlm.nih.gov/.

Because the majority of women are not aware of their pregnancy until at least 6 weeks of gestation, psychotropic medications may not be discontinued until after the period of greatest potential risk to

the fetus has passed. Risk-benefit analyses of depression treatment options should consider the potential risks that can accrue if depressive episodes go untreated in the pregnant woman. Risks include severe psychologic distress, suicide, financial hardships, and inability to plan for transition to parenthood. Most women who discontinue antidepressant medications relapse during pregnancy. The majority of relapses occur in the first trimester, and relapse is more prevalent in women with histories of chronic depression. Because randomized clinical trial data regarding the relative safety of available psychotropic medications are unavailable, clinical decision making is complicated.

Concerns regarding the safety of antidepressant medications are common (Lupattelli, Spigset, Bjornsdottir, et al., 2015). However, untreated depression can also cause adverse effects, such as preterm birth, small head circumference, low Apgar scores, and neonatal hypoxia, on the developing fetus and neonate (Ogunyemi et al., 2017). For women with a diagnosis of major depression, treatment with antidepressants is appropriate.

Use of antidepressants, including SSRIs, is indicated for vegetative signs accompanying a major depressive episode (MDE) that do not resolve with supportive interventions. There is a lack of definitive evidence to demonstrate a statistically significant association between fetal exposure to antidepressant medications and congenital abnormalities, although isolated cases have been reported. Reports have linked third-trimester use of SSRIs by pregnant women to a constellation of neonatal signs that include continuous crying, irritability, jitteriness, and restlessness; shivering; fever; tremors; hypertonia or rigidity; tachypnea or respiratory distress; feeding difficulty; sleep disturbance; hypoglycemia; and seizures. The onset of these signs can range from several hours to several days after birth and usually resolve within 1 to 2 weeks (Chisolm & Payne, 2015). Paroxetine has been associated with anencephaly, atrial septal defect, right ventricular outflow tract obstruction, gastroschisis and omphalocele. Venlafaxine has been associated with an increased risk of respiratory defects and citalopram with an increased risk of musculoskeletal defects. Fluoxetine has been significantly associated with right ventricular outflow tract obstruction and early closure of cranial sutures (Berard et al., 2017; Reefhuis, Devine, Friedman, et al., 2015).

Although less information is known regarding the use of SSRIs during pregnancy compared with the use of TCAs, drugs in this classification are emerging as first-line agents in treatment (McKeever et al., 2016; Tran & Robb, 2015) (see Table 31.1). These medications are relatively safe and carry fewer side effects than the TCAs. However, if an SSRI is taken with dextromethorphan, an agent found in cough syrup, the combination could trigger the serotonin syndrome (e.g., mental status changes, agitation, hyperreflexia, shivering, and diarrhea). The most frequent side effects with the SSRIs are gastrointestinal (GI) disturbances (e.g., nausea and diarrhea), headache, and insomnia. SSRIs also can inhibit specific P-450 isoenzymes, resulting in a marked elevation in drug concentration and a reduction in drug clearance.

The TCAs cause many central nervous system (CNS) and peripheral nervous system (PNS) side effects. In overdose, these medications can cause death (see Table 31.1). A common CNS effect is sedation. Other side effects include weight gain, tremors, grand mal seizures, nightmares, agitation or mania, and extrapyramidal side effects. Anticholinergic side effects include dry mouth, blurred vision (usually temporary), difficulty voiding, constipation, sweating, and difficulty with orgasm.

Antidepressant medications known as MAOIs are contraindicated during pregnancy and breastfeeding. Their reproductive safety has not been established.

TABLE 31.1	**Antidepressant Medications**		
	Pregnancy Risk Category[a]	**Lactation Risk Category**[a]	**Pregnancy-Lactation-Reproduction**
Selective Serotonin Reuptake Inhibitors (SSRIs)			
Citalopram (Celexa)	C	L3	There are no adequate well-controlled studies in pregnant women. Use during pregnancy only if potential benefits justify potential risk to the fetus.
			Use in third trimester may be linked to neonatal complications at birth. Consider risk versus benefit of treatment during this time.
			Drug appears in breast milk. Woman should either discontinue breastfeeding or discontinue drug, taking into account importance of drug to the woman.
Fluoxetine (Prozac)	C	L2 in older infants; L3 in neonates	Use cautiously in pregnant women and only if benefits justify possible risk to the fetus.
			Drug appears in breast milk. Use in breastfeeding women is not recommended.
Fluvoxamine (Luvox)	C	L2	Neonates exposed to the drug late in the third trimester have developed complications requiring prolonged hospitalization, respiratory support, and tube feeding.
			Neonates exposed to SSRIs in late pregnancy may have an increased risk of persistent pulmonary hypertension of the newborn, which is associated with substantial neonatal morbidity and mortality. Risks and benefits of treatment should be carefully considered on a case-by-case basis.
			Drug appears in breast milk. Woman should either discontinue breastfeeding or discontinue drug.
Paroxetine (Paxil)	D	L2	Drug can cause fetal harm. Manufacturer suggests discontinuing drug or switching to another antidepressant unless benefits justify continuing treatment. Consider other options for those planning to become pregnant.
			Contraindicated for treatment of vasomotor symptoms in pregnant women.
			Drug appears in breast milk. Use in breastfeeding only if benefits of treating postpartum depression with the drug outweigh risk. Monitor infants for growth.
Sertraline (Zoloft)	C	L2	There are no adequate well-controlled studies in pregnant women. Use during pregnancy only if potential benefits justify potential risk to the fetus.
			Neonates exposed to the drug late in the third trimester have developed complications requiring prolonged hospitalization, respiratory support, and tube feeding.
			Neonates exposed to SSRIs in late pregnancy may have an increased risk of persistent pulmonary hypertension of the newborn.
			It is not known if the drug appears in breast milk. Use cautiously in breastfeeding women.
Serotonin/Norepinephrine Reuptake Inhibitors (SNRIs)			
Bupropion (Wellbutrin) IR & SR	C	L3	Use during pregnancy only when potential benefits justify potential risk to the fetus.
			Prescriber should be notified if woman plans to become or becomes pregnant.
			Drug and its metabolites appear in breast milk. Recommendations for breastfeeding vary by individual product; refer to manufacturer's labeling.
Mirtazapine (Remeron)	C	L3	There are no adequate well-controlled studies in pregnant women. Use during pregnancy only if clearly needed.
			Drug appears in breast milk. Use cautiously in breastfeeding women.
Venlafaxine (Effexor)	C	L3	There are no adequate well-controlled studies in pregnant women. Use only if clearly needed and potential benefits justify potential fetal risk.
			Neonates exposed to the drug late in the third trimester have developed complications (sometimes immediately after birth) requiring prolonged hospitalization, respiratory support, and tube feeding.
			Drug appears in breast milk. Woman should either discontinue breastfeeding or discontinue drug.
Tricyclic Antidepressants (TCAs)			
Amitriptyline (Elavil)	D	L2	There are no adequate well-controlled studies in pregnant women. Use only if clearly needed and potential benefits justify potential fetal risk.
			Drug appears in breast milk. Woman should either discontinue breastfeeding or discontinue drug.

TABLE 31.1 Antidepressant Medications—cont'd

	Pregnancy Risk Category[a]	Lactation Risk Category[a]	Pregnancy-Lactation-Reproduction
Clomipramine (Anafranil)	C	L2	There are no adequate and well-controlled studies in pregnant women. Use only during pregnancy if the benefit outweighs the risk to the fetus. Women should notify their healthcare provider/s if they are pregnant or planning to become pregnant. Neonates whose mothers had taken this drug up until delivery have developed dyspnea, lethargy, colic, irritability, hypotension or hypertension, tremor or spasms, during the first few hours or days of life. If possible, this drug should be gradually withdrawn at least 7 weeks before the estimated date of birth. Animal studies have revealed evidence of fetotoxicity and embryotoxicity. There are no controlled data in human pregnancy.
Desipramine (Norpramin)	C	L2	Safe use in pregnant women has not been established. Use during pregnancy only if clearly needed and potential benefits justify potential risk to the fetus. Drug appears in breast milk. Woman should either discontinue breastfeeding or discontinue drug.
Imipramine (Tofranil)	D	L2	There are no adequate well-controlled studies in pregnant women. Use only if clearly needed and potential benefits justify potential fetal risk. Drug appears in breast milk. Use in breastfeeding women is not recommended.
Nortriptyline (Pamelor)	D	L2	Safe use in pregnancy and breastfeeding has not been established. Weigh potential benefits against possible risks. Monitor pregnant women and breastfeeding infants for adverse reactions.
Monoamine Oxidase Inhibitors (MAOIs)			
Phenelzine (Nardil)	C	Unknown	MAOIs are contraindicated during pregnancy and breastfeeding as reproductive safety has not been established.
Tranylcypromine (Parnate)	C	Unknown	MAOIs are contraindicated during pregnancy and breastfeeding as reproductive safety has not been established.

B = Animal studies have not shown fetal risk, but no controlled studies in pregnant women *or* animal studies showed adverse effect that was not confirmed in controlled studies in women in first trimester—no risk in later trimesters.

C = Animal studies show adverse effects on fetus, but no controlled studies in pregnant women *or* no studies available.

D = Positive evidence of human fetal risk.

L2 = Drug studied in limited number of breastfeeding women without an increase in adverse effects in infant *or* risk is remote.

L3 = No controlled studies in breastfeeding women *or* studies show minimal nonthreatening adverse effects.

L5 = Contraindicated because studies have shown significant and documented risk to infant.

[a]From Hale, T., & Rowe, H. (2017). *Medications and mother's milk* (17th ed.). New York: Springer; and Schatzberg, A., Cole, J. O., & DeBattista, C., (Eds.). (2015). *Manual of clinical psychopharmacology* (8th ed.). Arlington, VA: American Psychiatric Publishing.

NOTE: As of June 30, 2015, new prescription drugs submitted for approval no longer use the U.S. Food and Drug Administration lettering system to categorize drugs based on their potential to cause birth defects. Instead, a new, more comprehensive text is required in the label to explain the risks. Prescription drugs currently using the lettering system to identify potential for a drug to cause birth defects will be gradually phased into the new labeling requirement.

IR, Intermediate release; *SR,* sustained release.

Special Considerations for Psychotropic Medications During Pregnancy

Even though the basic rule is to avoid administering any medication to a pregnant woman, particularly during the first trimester, decisions about the use of medications during pregnancy should be made jointly by the woman, her partner, and her health care providers. If the woman is stable and appears likely to remain well while not taking medication, then discontinuation before pregnancy is a viable option. For those women with a history of relapse after medication discontinuation, remaining on the drug during pregnancy is advised. There is a lack of conclusive evidence that antipsychotic medications (either typical or atypical) are teratogenic (McKeever et al., 2016).

Although a pregnant woman should be receiving the lowest therapeutic dose, psychotropic medications may have to be increased over the course of pregnancy to maintain adequate therapeutic serum concentrations and response (Wisner, Sit, Bogen, et al., 2017). Administering psychotherapeutic medications at or near birth can cause a baby to be overly sedated at birth and require ventilatory support or to be physically dependent on the drug and require detoxification and treatment of a withdrawal syndrome (see Chapter 35).

If a woman becomes psychotic during pregnancy, it is usually either because she has stopped taking mood stabilizers or antipsychotics or because she has a history of schizophrenia. Psychosis is a medical emergency. To treat a psychotic state, antipsychotic medication or electroconvulsive therapy (ECT) can be used (McKeever et al., 2016). Lithium is currently considered the first-line medication for the treatment of psychosis during pregnancy (Meltzer-Brody & Jones, 2015).

TABLE 31.2 Mood Stabilizers

Mood Stabilizers	Pregnancy Risk Category[a]	Lactation Risk Category[a]	Pregnancy-Lactation-Reproduction
Carbamazepine (Tegretol XR)	C	L2	Drug may cause fetal harm, including major congenital malformations, when administered during pregnancy. If used in pregnant women, monotherapy, rather than use in combination with other anticonvulsants, is recommended to possibly reduce risk of teratogenic effects. Consider tests to detect defects using currently accepted procedures as part of routine prenatal care in pregnant women receiving drug. Pregnant women taking carbamazepine should enroll themselves in the North American Antiepileptic Drug Pregnancy Registry by calling 1-888-233-2334 or visiting www.aedpregnancyregistry. Drug and its metabolite appear in breast milk. Woman should either discontinue breastfeeding or discontinue drug, taking into account importance of drug to the woman.
Lamotrigine (Lamictal)	C	L3	There are no adequate studies in pregnant women; in animal studies, lamotrigine was developmentally toxic. Use during pregnancy only if potential benefits justify potential risk to the fetus. Pregnant women are encouraged to register in the North American Antiepileptic Drug Pregnancy Registry by calling 1-888-233-2334 or visiting www.aedpregnancyregistry.org. Drug appears in breast milk. Closely monitor breastfeeding infants for adverse events resulting from drug use. Women should discontinue breastfeeding if infants develop drug toxicity. Use cautiously in breastfeeding women.
Valproic acid (Depakene, Depakote, Depakote ER)	D	L2	Drugs that act directly on the renin-angiotensin-aldosterone system can cause injury and even death to the developing fetus. When pregnancy is detected, stop drug as soon as possible. It is not known if drug appears in breast milk. Women should either discontinue breastfeeding or discontinue drug.

C = Animal studies show adverse effects on fetus, but no controlled studies in pregnant women *or* no studies available.
D = Positive evidence of human fetal risk.
L2 = Drug studied in limited number of breastfeeding women without an increase in adverse effects in infant *or* risk is remote.
L3 = No controlled studies in breastfeeding women *or* studies show minimal nonthreatening adverse effects.
[a]From Hale, T., & Rowe, H. (2017). *Medications and mother's milk* (17th ed.). New York: Springer; and Schatzberg, A., & DeBattista, C., (Eds.). (2015). *Manual of clinical psychopharmacology* (8th ed.). Arlington, VA: American Psychiatric Publishing.
NOTE: As of June 30, 2015, new prescription drugs submitted for approval no longer use the U.S. Food and Drug Administration lettering system to categorize drugs based on their potential to cause birth defects. Instead, a new, more comprehensive text is required in the label to explain the risks. Prescription drugs currently using the lettering system to identify potential for a drug to cause birth defects will be gradually phased into the new labeling requirement.

Most of the mood-stabilizing medications such as lithium carbonate, carbamazepine (Tegretol), gabapentin (Neurontin), lamotrigine (Lamictal), and valproic acid (Depakote) are Category D (Table 31.2 for FDA categories of mood stabilizers). In women with preexisting illness, there is a high recurrence of mania during pregnancy that can present as psychosis; thus maintenance on lithium is important to deter the development of adverse effects in the mother and infant. Maintenance includes checking lithium levels more frequently, stopping the medicine at the onset of labor, and reinstating the regimen following birth when plasma level and electrolyte balance can be confirmed. Monitoring lithium levels at the time of birth is essential as well because of the tremendous fluctuation of fluids between the onset of labor and the immediate postpartum period. Mood stabilizers are often taken over the life span by women with bipolar disorder. Women with this disorder should receive preconception counseling. Those who have experienced a single manic episode may elect to have the medication tapered gradually and make an attempt to have a lithium-free pregnancy or, if indicated, reinstitute the lithium after the first trimester (Meltzer-Brody & Jones, 2015).

If the pregnant woman is receiving pharmacologic treatment, the nurse must make sure that she is being treated by a mental health care provider (e.g., psychiatrist or nurse practitioner). No woman should abruptly discontinue taking any psychotropic medication because of the risk of withdrawal symptoms.

Nursing Interventions

Nursing strategies include educating the woman about depression as an illness and the plan of care, including medications. For the woman who refuses medications during pregnancy, the nurse should discuss alternative treatments and respect her choice. The nurse also can be effective by maintaining a caring relationship, which includes being hopeful. The nurse can ask about a time when the woman was coping well and how she was able to combat her depression then.

POSTPARTUM MOOD DISORDERS

The weeks after birth are a time of vulnerability to psychologic complications for many women, causing significant distress for the mother, disrupting family life, and, if prolonged, negatively affecting the child's emotional and social development. Preexisting mood and anxiety disorders are particularly likely to recur or worsen during these weeks. Such conditions can interfere with attachment to the newborn and family integration, and some may threaten the safety and well-being of the mother, the newborn, and other children. Because birth is usually thought to be a happy event, a new mother's emotional distress can puzzle and immobilize family and friends. When she most needs the caring attention of loved ones, they may either criticize or withdraw because of their anxiety. Nurses can offer anticipatory guidance, assess the mental health of new mothers, offer therapeutic interventions, and make referrals when necessary. Failure to do so can result in tragic consequences. In rare cases, a disturbed mother may kill her infant, other family members, or herself.

Mood disorders are the predominant mental health disorder in the postpartum period (APA, 2013). Up to 85% of women experience a mild depression or "baby blues" after the birth of a child; however, the woman's functioning is usually not impaired. Baby blues are characterized by mood swings, feelings of sadness and anxiety, crying, difficulty sleeping, and loss of appetite. The symptoms resolve within a few days, and treatment is not needed (Paschetta, Berrisford, Coccia, et al., 2014).

Postpartum Depression

Prevalence estimates of postpartum depression (PPD) vary based on the definition and the period of time included. PPD is experienced by approximately 8% to 20% of women during the postpartum period (Isley & Katz, 2017). It is likely that the actual occurrence of PPD exceeds the reported estimates because it is often unrecognized and undiagnosed (ACOG, 2018).

The cause of PPD can be biologic, psychologic, situational, or multifactorial. The change from the high levels of estrogen and progesterone at the end of pregnancy to the much lower levels of both hormones that are present after birth is an important etiologic factor in the development of PPD. While all women experience these hormonal changes, there are some who are more sensitive to the mood-destabilizing effects of withdrawal from the pregnancy hormones and are therefore at risk for PPD (O'Hara & Wisner, 2014). Poor nutrition may also be a contributing factor. Folate and vitamin B_{12} are needed for the synthesis of serotonin and other neurotransmitters. A marginal or low folate level also increases the likelihood of a poor response to antidepressant medication as well as the potential for relapse in people who initially responded well to pharmacologic therapy (Wisner et al., 2017).

PPD frequently recurs. Up to 70% of women with a history of PPD will have a subsequent episode. Postpartum women with a history of PPD who are currently experiencing the "baby blues" have a very high risk for developing major depression (Cunningham, Leveno, Bloom, et al., 2018). Other risk factors for PPD include younger age, unintended pregnancy, personal history of severe premenstrual dysphoria, family history of mood disorder, unmarried status, marital discord, lack of social support, socioeconomic deprivation, lower education, substance abuse, low self-esteem, and stressful life events (O'Hara & McCabe, 2013; Wisner et al., 2017). Women facing multiple or severe psychosocial problems or chronic interpersonal difficulties are at increased risk for PPD. Complications of pregnancy and birth increase the risk for PPD. Having a preterm, low-birth-weight, and ill neonate is associated with higher rates of PPD (Alkozei, McMahon, & Lahav, 2014). Women who are survivors of intimate partner violence are at increased risk for PPD (Kothari, Liepman, Tareen, et al., 2016). Cultural practices can positively or negatively affect the development of PPD.

Screening for Postpartum Depression

When PPD is identified early, it is highly treatable. Screening for depression during pregnancy and the postpartum period may reduce the prevalence and symptoms of depression (O'Connor, Rossom, Henninger, et al., 2016). Screening for anxiety and depression during pregnancy and in the postpartum period is recommended by the American College of Obstetricians and Gynecologists (ACOG, 2018), the US Preventive Services Task Force (Siu & USPSTF, 2016), and the Association of Women's Health, Obstetric and Neonatal Nurses (AWHONN, 2015).

Postpartum nurses can screen for PPD before women are discharged from the birth setting. Although this identifies some who are at risk, it is important that follow-up screening is also done. PPD is most likely to occur around 4 weeks after birth. Follow-up assessments for risks and signs of PPD can be done by primary care providers during pediatric care visits for the infant and during postpartum follow-up visits for the mother. The American Academy of Pediatrics (AAP) recommends maternal depression screening at the infant's 1-, 2-, and 4-month visits (Earls & AAP Committee on Psychosocial Aspects of Child and Family Health, 2010). Women with a positive screen should be referred appropriately for evaluation and treatment.

In perinatal populations the most widely used and validated tools are the Edinburgh Postnatal Depression Screen (EPDS) and the Postpartum Depression Screening Scale (PDSS). Both are brief, self-report questionnaires specifically developed for use with perinatal women, which take between 5 and 10 minutes to complete (Milgrom & Gemmill, 2014).

The EPDS tool asks the woman to respond to 10 statements about the common symptoms of depression. The woman is asked to choose the response that is closest to describing how she has felt for the past week. A maximum score on the EPDS is 30; women with scores of 12 or higher may possibly have depression and need further assessment. One item on the tool addresses suicidal thoughts; responses to this item should be carefully examined (Cox, Holden, & Henshaw, 2014).

The PDSS is a 35-item Likert response scale that assesses for seven dimensions of depression: sleeping or eating disturbances, anxiety or insecurity, emotional lability, mental confusion, loss of self, guilt or shame, and suicidal thoughts (Myers, Aubuchon-Endsley, & Bastian, 2013). Both tools are designed to be used by nurses and other health care professionals to elicit information from the woman during an interview to assess risk.

In addition, a simple two-item tool has been shown to be effective in identifying women at risk for PPD. If the woman answers yes to either of the two questions, the screen is considered to be positive. The questions are as follows: "Over the past 2 weeks have you ever felt down, depressed, or hopeless?" and "Over the past 2 weeks have you felt little interest or pleasure in doing things?" (Earls & AAP Committee on Psychosocial Aspects of Child and Family Health, 2010).

The effectiveness of screening for PPD is related to the follow-up for positive screening results (Agency for Healthcare Research and Quality [AHRQ], 2018). If PPD screening results are positive or if the woman's self-report shows signs that she might be depressed, a formal screening is needed to determine the urgency of the referral and the type of provider. Also important is the need to include the woman's family because they may be able to offer valuable information, as well as need to express how they have been affected by the woman's emotional disorder.

Paternal Postpartum Depression

It is estimated that paternal perinatal depression (PPND) occurs in approximately 8% to 10% of men during the period of time from the first trimester of pregnancy through the first year after birth. During the first 6 months after birth, the incidence increases to approximately 25% (Cameron, Sedov, & Tomfohr-Madsen, 2016; Paulson & Bazemore, 2010).

The best predictor of PPND is having a partner with PPD. Other risk factors are a history of depression, age younger than 25 years, low socioeconomic status, unmarried status, an inadequate support system, and family and social stressors. Men may not exhibit classic symptoms of PPD but are likely to display fatigue, frustration, anger, irritability, indecisiveness, withdrawal from social situations, alcohol/drug use, marital conflict, partner violence, and somatic symptoms (Musser, Ahmed, Foli, & Coddington, 2013).

Men are not routinely screened for perinatal depressive symptoms. There is no depression scale designed for this specific use. Some experts recommend using the EPDS in combination with the Gotland Male Depression Scale to identify men with signs of PPND (Habib, 2012).

When both the father and the mother are depressed, life can be very difficult. Routine tasks of caring for the newborn and maintaining a household can present significant challenges. Interaction with the infant can be affected, and there can be negative effects on parenting.

Nurses should include partners in discussions about PPD, raising awareness that fathers can also suffer from depression, describing symptoms, and providing information about resources for help if the symptoms occur. During interactions with fathers, nurses can assess for signs of PPND, provide support and encouragement, and offer information about resources for further assessment and treatment (Letourneau, Tryphonopoulos, Duffett-Leger, et al., 2012). The nurse can direct fathers to online resources such as www.postpartummen.com or http://postpartumhealthalliance.org (Stadtlander, 2015).

Postpartum Depression Without Psychotic Features

PPD without psychotic features is often referred to as simply PPD. It is an intense and pervasive sadness with severe and labile mood swings. PPD is more serious and persistent than postpartum blues, lasting more than 2 weeks. Intense fears, anger, anxiety, and despondency that persist past the baby's first few weeks are not a normal part of postpartum blues. These symptoms rarely disappear without outside help. Most of these mothers seek help only after reaching a "crisis point."

The symptoms of postpartum major depression are very similar to those of adult depression except that the mother's ruminations of guilt and inadequacy feed her worries about being an incompetent and inadequate parent. In PPD, there can be loss of appetite or odd food cravings (often sweet desserts) and binges with abnormal appetite and weight gain. Sleep disturbance is common. Sleep deprivation is a factor in the development of PPD, and it can worsen the symptoms (Park, Meltzer-Brody, & Stickgold, 2013). (See Clinical Reasoning Case Study.)

❓ CLINICAL REASONING CASE STUDY

Postpartum Depression

Jennifer is a 35-year-old G1, P1 who gave birth by emergency cesarean 2 weeks ago, to a 7-lb 6-oz baby boy. She has come to the OB clinic for her 2-week follow-up visit and is accompanied by her husband and her mother. Jennifer appears tired, her color is pale, and she has dark circles under both eyes. Her affect is flat. Jennifer's husband reports that she is not sleeping, she cries often, her appetite is poor, and she seems to be constantly worried about breastfeeding. Jennifer's mother states that the baby cries much of the time and never seems satisfied after breastfeeding. She says that there have been times in the past when Jennifer was depressed and she took antidepressant medication, although she did not want to take any medication during pregnancy.

1. What is the priority concern or client need in this situation? Support your answer with data as stated in the case.
2. List other client needs/problems in this case.
3. Identify any additional information or assessment data that is needed by the nurse in planning care for this client.
4. Describe other nursing interventions that are important to providing optimal client care.
   a. What is the priority nursing action? (What should the nurse do first?)
   b. Describe other nursing interventions that are important to providing optimal client care.
5. Describe the roles/responsibilities of the interprofessional health care team members (other than nurses) who may be involved in providing care for this client.

A distinguishing feature of PPD is irritability. These episodes of irritability can flare up with little provocation, and they sometimes escalate to violent outbursts or dissolve into uncontrollable sobbing. Many of these outbursts are directed against significant others. Women with postpartum MDEs often have severe anxiety, panic attacks, and spontaneous crying long after the usual duration of baby blues.

Feelings of detachment toward the newborn or not feeling love for the newborn are common symptoms of PPD. Women feel guilt and shame for having these feelings and are not likely to verbalize or discuss this with anyone. Many women feel especially guilty about having depressive feelings at a time when they believe they should be happy. They can be reluctant to discuss their symptoms or their negative feelings toward the infant. A woman with PPD may have obsessive thoughts about harming the infant, and this can be very frightening to her. Often she does not share these thoughts because of embarrassment; when she does, other family members become very frightened. On the other hand, some women feel very emotionally attached and connected to their infants; this can prevent them from experiencing total despair (Puryear, 2014).

Antidepressants are the most commonly used treatment for PPD; one explanation for this is that primary care providers can prescribe these medications and monitor the woman's progress. In some communities, access to mental health care providers is limited and primary care providers treat women with PPD (see Table 31.1).

In March, 2019, brexanolone (Zulressa) became the first drug to be approved by the FDA specifically for treatment of PPD. In clinical trials, women who received the medication demonstrated an improvement in depressive symptoms. Currently women must receive Brexanolone only in a certified health care facility, so that they can be carefully monitored during treatment. The medication is administered as a continuous intravenous infusion for a total of 60 hours (FDA, 2019).

Psychotherapy without the use of medication can be effective for mild cases of PPD. It is often used in combination with antidepressants for moderate to severe cases. Psychotherapy methods include general counseling (listening visits), IPT, CBT, and psychodynamic therapy (O'Hara & McCabe, 2013). Peer support may be helpful; some women find that postpartum support groups are very beneficial (www.postpartum.net). Internet-based and telephone-based psychotherapy are increasing in use; there is a need for more evidence to support their effectiveness (Stuart & Koleva, 2014).

For more severe PPD, antidepressant medication is combined with some form of psychotherapy. Often, an SSRI is prescribed initially and if symptoms improve during a 6-week trial period, the medication is continued for at least 6 months to prevent relapse. If response to the medication is less than optimal, another SSRI may be prescribed instead (see Table 31.1) (Cunningham et al., 2018).

Sleep deprivation must be resolved; 4 to 5 hours of uninterrupted sleep for several days may help the woman begin the road to recovery from PPD. Planning with the woman and her family to promote her sleep as much as possible is essential to the plan of care (Puryear, 2014).

Postpartum Depression With Psychotic Features (Postpartum Psychosis)

The most severe of the PMDs, **postpartum psychosis,** also known as *postpartum depression with psychotic features,* occurs in 1 to 2 per 1000 births during the first month, although it usually manifests within the first 2 weeks postpartum (Wisner et al., 2017).

Because the recurrence rate is 50%, women with a history of postpartum psychosis are at significant risk for repeat psychosis following the current pregnancy. Primiparous women are more likely to suffer from postpartum psychosis, especially if they experienced obstetric complications (Cunningham et al., 2018).

Postpartum psychosis can be due to major depression. However, it is most commonly associated with **bipolar disorder** (or manic-depressive disorder) and presents with symptoms of mania, depression, or both (Wisner et al., 2017). Postpartum psychosis is defined by the presence of abnormally elevated energy levels, cognition, and mood; and one or more depressive episodes. The elevated moods are generally referred to as *mania*. Clinical manifestations of a manic episode include at least three of the following: grandiosity, decreased need for sleep, pressured speech, flight of ideas, distractibility, psychomotor agitation, and excessive involvement in pleasurable activities without regard for negative consequences (APA, 2013). Individuals who experience manic episodes also commonly experience depressive episodes or symptoms of mixed episodes in which features of both mania and depression are present at the same time. These episodes are usually separated by periods of normal mood, but in some individuals, depression and mania rapidly alternate. These rapid changes in mood are known as *rapid cycling*.

In general, postpartum psychosis is characterized by rapid onset of bizarre behavior, auditory or visual hallucinations, paranoid or grandiose delusions, elements of delirium or disorientation, and extreme deficits in judgment accompanied by high levels of impulsivity that can contribute to increased risk for suicide or infanticide (O'Hara & Wisner, 2014). Initially the woman may complain of fatigue, insomnia, and restlessness and can have episodes of tearfulness and emotional lability. Later, suspiciousness, confusion, incoherence, irrational statements, and obsessive concerns about the baby's health and welfare can be present. Hallucinations and delusions are common. Auditory hallucinations that command the mother to kill the infant can occur in severe cases. When delusions are present, they are often related to the infant. The mother may think the infant is possessed by the devil, has special powers, or is destined for a terrible fate. Grossly disorganized behavior can be manifested as a disinterest in the infant or an inability to provide care. Some women will insist that something is wrong with the baby or accuse nurses or family members of hurting or poisoning their child.

> **! NURSING ALERT**
>
> Nurses are advised to be alert for mothers who are agitated, overactive, confused, complaining, or suspicious.

Women with postpartum psychosis usually need inpatient psychiatric care. Antipsychotics, mood stabilizers, and benzodiazepines are the treatments of choice for postpartum psychosis (see Tables 31.2 and 31.3). Other psychotropic medications such as antidepressants may be used based on the underlying diagnosis (e.g., bipolar mania, bipolar depression) (see Table 31.1). It is usually advantageous for the mother to have contact with her baby if she so desires, but visits must be closely supervised. Psychotherapy is indicated after the period of acute psychosis has passed.

CARE MANAGEMENT

An interprofessional team approach to care is needed for the woman who presents with signs and symptoms of PPD. A nurse in the role of case manager can coordinate care management. The obstetric health care provider assesses her physical condition in relation to postbirth recovery as well as her current symptoms. The provider may order pharmacologic treatment (e.g., antidepressant medications) or may refer the woman to a mental health care provider for treatment of the depression. A pharmacist may consult with the provider regarding the optimal medications and their safety during breastfeeding and may provide education to the woman and her family about the medications (dose, schedule, side effects, when to expect improvement in symptoms). If the woman is experiencing a loss of appetite, a nutritionist may be a part of care management. A lactation consultant and pediatric health care provider may need to be consulted if the woman is experiencing breastfeeding difficulties. The pediatric health care provider will monitor the infant's weight and health status. Close follow-up and ongoing monitoring of the woman's mental and physical status and the infant's health, growth, and development are vital to optimizing outcomes.

> **! NURSING ALERT**
>
> Because mothers who have postpartum depression with psychotic features can harm their infants, extra caution is needed in assessment and intervention. The nurse needs to ask specifically if the mother has had thoughts about harming her baby.

Nursing Considerations

Postpartum nurses carefully observe all new mothers for signs of depression and conduct further assessments as necessary. Before discharge from the birthing facility, nurses educate the woman and her partner/family about signs of postpartum blues, PPD, and postpartum psychosis, as well as when and where to seek help (see Teaching for Self-Management: Signs of Postpartum Blues, Depression, and Psychosis). Nurses also provide suggestions about how to prevent PPD (see Teaching for Self-Management: Preventing Postpartum Depression). Nurses should provide women and their families with a current list of available community resources for treating PPD (AWHONN, 2015).

Before the mother is discharged from the birthing facility and in follow-up visits to clinics or health care provider offices, nurses are key to identifying symptoms of PPD. The nurse should be an active listener and demonstrate a caring attitude. Nurses cannot depend on women to volunteer unsolicited information about their depression or ask for help. Examples of ways to initiate conversation include the following: "Now that you've had your baby, how are things going for you? Have you had to change many things in your life since having the baby?" If the nurse believes that the new mother is showing signs of depression, the next step is to ask if the mother has thought about hurting herself or the baby. The woman may be more willing to answer honestly if the nurse says, "Many women feel depressed after having a baby, and some feel so badly that they think about hurting themselves or the baby. Have you had these thoughts?" (see Nursing Care Plan: Postpartum Depression).

Whenever a woman exhibits signs of PPD, the nurse notifies the obstetric or primary health care provider. Women with moderate to severe cases of PPD should be referred to a mental health professional such as a psychiatric nurse practitioner or psychiatrist for evaluation and therapy. Inpatient psychiatric hospitalization may be necessary. This decision is made when the safety of the mother, her infant, or other children is threatened.

Women who are at risk for PPD and those showing early signs of depression may be followed after discharge from the birthing facility through home visits or telephone calls. Postpartum home visits can reduce the incidence of or complications from depression (Dennis & Dowswell, 2013).

TABLE 31.3 Atypical Antipsychotic Medications

Antipsychotic Medications	Pregnancy Risk Category[a]	Lactation Risk Category[a]	Pregnancy-Lactation-Reproduction
Aripiprazole (Abilify)	C	L3	Drug is associated with increased risk of oral clefts (cleft lip or palate) in infants born to women treated with aripiprazole during pregnancy. Use in pregnant women only if potential benefit outweighs risk to the fetus. Consider alternative medications with a lower risk of adverse outcomes for those women. Pregnant women exposed to this medication should register with the National Pregnancy Registry for Atypical Antipsychotics (1-866-961-2388). Neonates exposed to this medication during the third trimester are at risk for developing extrapyramidal signs and symptoms (repetitive muscle movements of the face and body) and withdrawal symptoms (agitation, abnormally increased or decreased muscle tone, tremors, sleepiness, severe difficulty breathing, and difficulty feeding) after birth. Drug appears in breast milk. Use in breastfeeding women is not recommended.
Olanzapine (Zyprexa)	C	L2	There are no adequate studies in pregnant women. Use during pregnancy if clearly needed and potential benefit justifies potential risk to the fetus. When used during the third trimester, there is an increased risk for developing extrapyramidal signs and symptoms (repetitive muscle movements of the face and body) and withdrawal symptoms (agitation, abnormally increased or decreased muscle tone, tremors, sleepiness, severe difficulty breathing, and difficulty feeding) in the newborn that can be severe and require hospitalization. Pregnant women exposed to this medication should register with the National Pregnancy Registry for Atypical Antipsychotics (1-866-961-2388). Drug appears in breast milk. Women receiving drug should not breastfeed.
Quetiapine (Seroquel)	C	L4	Risk of use during pregnancy is unknown. When used during the third trimester, there is an increased risk for developing extrapyramidal signs and symptoms (repetitive muscle movements of the face and body) and withdrawal symptoms (agitation, abnormally increased or decreased muscle tone, tremors, sleepiness, severe difficulty breathing, and difficulty feeding) in the newborn that can be severe and require hospitalization. Pregnant women exposed to this medication should register with the National Pregnancy Registry for Atypical Antipsychotics (1-866-961-2388). Drug appears in breast milk. Women receiving drug should not breastfeed.
Risperidone (Risperdal)	C	L3	Risk of use during pregnancy is unknown. When used during the third trimester, there is an increased risk for developing extrapyramidal signs and symptoms (repetitive muscle movements of the face and body) and withdrawal symptoms (agitation, abnormally increased or decreased muscle tone, tremors, sleepiness, severe difficulty breathing, and difficulty feeding) in the newborn that can be severe and require hospitalization. Pregnant women exposed to this medication should register with the National Pregnancy Registry for Atypical Antipsychotics (1-866-961-2388). Drug appears in breast milk. Women receiving drug should not breastfeed. Drug may cause hyperprolactinemia, which may decrease reproductive function in both men and women.
Ziprasidone (Geodon)	C	L4	There are no adequate studies in pregnant women. Use during pregnancy if clearly needed and potential benefit justifies potential risk to the fetus. When used during the third trimester, there is an increased risk for developing extrapyramidal signs and symptoms (repetitive muscle movements of the face and body) and withdrawal symptoms (agitation, abnormally increased or decreased muscle tone, tremors, sleepiness, severe difficulty breathing, and difficulty feeding) in the newborn that can be severe and require hospitalization. Pregnant women exposed to this medication should register with the National Pregnancy Registry for Atypical Antipsychotics (1-866-961-2388). It is not known if drug or its metabolites appear in breast milk. Breastfeeding is not recommended.

C = Animal studies show adverse effects on fetus, but no controlled studies in pregnant women *or* no studies available.
L2 = Drug studied in limited number of breastfeeding women without an increase in adverse effects in infant *or* risk is remote.
L3 = No controlled studies in breastfeeding women *or* studies show minimal nonthreatening adverse effects.
L4 = Possibly hazardous.

[a]From Hale, T., & Rowe, H. (2017). *Medications and mother's milk* (17th ed.). New York: Springer; and Schatzberg, A., & DeBattista, C., (Eds.). (2015). *Manual of clinical psychopharmacology* (8th ed.). Arlington, VA: American Psychiatric Publishing.

NOTE: As of June 30, 2015, new prescription drugs submitted for approval no longer use the U.S. Food and Drug Administration lettering system to categorize drugs based on their potential to cause birth defects. Instead, a new, more comprehensive text is required in the label to explain the risks. Prescription drugs currently using the lettering system to identify potential for a drug to cause birth defects will be gradually phased into the new labeling requirement.

◎ NURSING CARE PLAN

Postpartum Depression

Client Problem	Expected Outcome	Interventions	Rationales
Potential for injury to the woman and/or newborn related to woman's emotional state and/or treatment	The mother and newborn will remain free of injury.	Provide information about signs of postpartum depression (PPD) to woman and family.	To promote prompt recognition of problems
		Counsel woman and family to contact health care provider if behaviors indicating depression, such as crying, are identified.	To provide prompt care and referral if necessary and avoid injury to newborn and mother
		Assist family to develop a plan for maternal and infant supervision.	To provide for safety of woman and infant
Impaired family functioning related to postpartum maternal depression	Family will identify positive coping mechanisms and initiate a plan to cope with the woman's depression.	Provide opportunity for family and significant others to verbalize feelings and concerns.	To establish a trusting relationship
		Give information regarding postpartum depression to the family.	To clarify any misconceptions or misinformation
		Assist family to identify positive coping mechanisms that have been effective during past crises.	To promote active participation in care
Potential for inadequate parenting related to inability of mother to attach to infant	Woman demonstrates appropriate attachment behaviors in infant interactions. Woman expresses satisfaction with infant.	Observe maternal-infant interactions.	To assess quality of interactions and to determine need for interventions
		Encourage the woman to have as much contact with the infant as possible.	To minimize separation and to promote attachment
		Demonstrate infant care and explain infant behaviors.	To enhance mother's care abilities and understanding of infant's abilities

TEACHING FOR SELF-MANAGEMENT

Signs of Postpartum Blues, Depression, and Psychosis

- Signs of baby blues (these should go away in a few days or a week):
  - Sad, anxious, or overwhelmed feelings
  - Crying spells
  - Loss of appetite
  - Difficulty sleeping
- Signs of postpartum depression (can begin any time in the first year):
  - Same signs as baby blues, but they last longer and are more severe
  - Thoughts of harming yourself or your baby
  - Not having any interest in the baby
- Signs of postpartum psychosis:
  - Seeing or hearing things that are not there
  - Feelings of confusion
  - Rapid mood swings
  - Trying to hurt yourself or your baby
- When to call your health care provider:
  - The baby blues continue for more than 2 weeks
  - Symptoms of depression get worse
  - Difficulty performing tasks at home or at work
  - Inability to care for yourself or your baby
  - Thoughts of harming yourself or your baby

Data from US Department of Health and Human Services Office of Women's Health. (2018). *Depression during and after pregnancy fact sheet*. Retrieved from http://www.womenshealth.gov/publications/our-publications/fact-sheet/depression-pregnancy.html.

TEACHING FOR SELF-MANAGEMENT

Preventing Postpartum Depression

- Share knowledge about postpartum emotional problems with close family and friends.
- At least once each day or every other day, purposely relax for 15 min by deep breathing, meditating, or taking a hot bath.
- Take care of yourself: eat a balanced diet.
- Exercise on a regular basis, at least 30 min a day.
- Sleep as much as possible; make a promise to yourself to try to sleep when the baby sleeps.
- Get out of the house: try to leave home for 30 min a day; take a walk outdoors or walk at the mall.
- Share your feelings with someone close to you; don't isolate yourself at home with the television.
- Don't overcommit yourself or feel like you need to be a superwoman. Ask for help from family and friends.
- Don't place unrealistic expectations on yourself; no mother is perfect!
- Be flexible with your daily activities.
- Go to a new mothers' support group: for example, take a postpartum exercise class or attend a breastfeeding support group.

Supervision of the mother with emotional complications can become a prime concern. Depression can greatly interfere with a woman's ability to care for herself, her infant, and other children. This is a time for family and friends to provide assistance; the nurse can work with them to ensure adequate supervision and their understanding of the woman's mental illness.

When the woman has PPD, her partner often reacts with confusion, shock, denial, and anger and feels neglected and blamed. The nurse can provide nonjudgmental opportunities for the partner to verbalize feelings and concerns, help the partner identify positive coping strategies, and be a source of encouragement for the partner to continue supporting the woman. Suggestions for partners of women with PPD include helping around the house, setting limits with family and friends, going with her to appointments with the health care provider, educating himself or herself, writing down concerns and questions to take to the primary care provider or therapist, and just being with her—sitting quietly, hugging her, and demonstrating concern and compassion. Both the woman and her partner need an opportunity to express their needs, fears, thoughts, and feelings in a nonjudgmental environment.

Even if the woman is severely depressed, hospitalization may be avoided if adequate resources can be mobilized to ensure safety for mother and infant. The nurse in home health care needs to make frequent telephone calls or home visits for assessment and counseling. Community resources that may be helpful are temporary child care or foster care, homemaker services, parenting guidance centers, mother's-day-out programs, and support groups such as Postpartum Support International (http://postpartum.net) and Depression After Delivery (www.depressionafterdelivery.com).

Safety Concerns

When a woman is suffering from depression, there can be safety concerns related to risk for self-harm or harm to the infant. If delusional thinking about the baby is suspected, the nurse asks, "Have you thought about hurting your baby?" When depression is suspected, the nurse asks, "Have you thought about hurting yourself?" Four criteria can be used to measure the seriousness of a suicidal plan: method, availability, specificity, and lethality. Has the woman specified a method? Is the method of choice available? How specific is the plan? If the method is concrete and detailed, with access to carry it out at hand, the suicide risk increases. How lethal is the method? The most lethal method is shooting, with hanging a close second. The least lethal is slashing one's wrists.

❗ NURSING ALERT

Suicidal or homicidal ideations and/or attempt to cause harm to self or others (including the infant) are among the most serious symptoms of postpartum depression. This is considered a psychiatric emergency and warrants immediate assessment, evaluation, and intervention by a mental health care professional.

LEGAL TIP

Commitment for Psychiatric Care

If a woman with postpartum depression or postpartum psychosis is experiencing active suicidal ideation or harmful delusions about the baby and is unwilling to seek treatment, legal intervention may be necessary to commit the woman to an inpatient setting for treatment.

When a mother is hospitalized, she is separated from her infant. After her condition is stabilized, and if allowed within the inpatient psychiatric setting, the reintroduction of the baby to the mother can occur at the mother's own pace. A schedule is set for increasing the number of hours the mother cares for the baby over several days, culminating in the infant's staying overnight in the mother's room. This method allows the mother to experience meeting the infant's needs and giving up sleep for the baby, a situation difficult for new mothers even under ideal conditions. The mother's readiness for discharge

and caring for the baby is assessed. Her interactions with her baby are carefully supervised and guided. A postpartum nurse is often asked to assist the psychiatric nursing staff in assessment of the mother-infant interactions.

Nurses should observe the mother for signs of bonding with the baby. Attachment behaviors are defined as eye-to-eye contact; physical contact that involves holding, touching, cuddling, and talking to the baby and calling the baby by name; and the initiation of appropriate care. A staff member is assigned to observe the baby at all times. Praise and encouragement are used to bolster the mother's self-esteem and self-confidence.

Medical Management

The natural course is one of gradual improvement over the 6 months after birth. Treatment options for PPD include psychotherapy and antidepressant medication (see Table 31.1). Women with postpartum psychosis usually need inpatient psychiatric care. Antipsychotics, mood stabilizers, and benzodiazepines are the treatments of choice (see Tables 31.2 and 31.3).

Psychotropic Medications

Antidepressant medications are the most widely used treatment for PPD. Paroxetine, sertraline, fluoxetine, venlafaxine, nortriptyline, and nefazodone (see Table 31.1) have been evaluated and are associated with improvement in PPD symptoms over 2 to 3 months of treatment (O'Hara & Wisner, 2014). If the woman with PPD is not breastfeeding, in most cases antidepressants can be prescribed without special precautions. A variety of medications can be prescribed for these women, including TCAs, SSRIs, SNRIs, mood stabilizers, and antipsychotic medications.

Mood stabilizers are used in the treatment of severe psychiatric syndromes such as schizophrenia, bipolar disorder, or psychotic depression (see Table 31.2). Women taking mood stabilizers must be taught about the many side effects, and especially for those taking lithium, the need to have serum lithium levels determined every 6 months. Most of the mood stabilizing medications can cause sedation and orthostatic hypotension—both of which can interfere with the mother being able to care safely for her baby. They also can cause PNS effects such as constipation, dry mouth, blurred vision, tachycardia, urinary retention, weight gain, and agranulocytosis. CNS effects may include akathisia, dystonias, parkinsonian-like symptoms, tardive dyskinesia (irreversible), and neuroleptic malignant syndrome (potentially fatal). Medication education is especially important when caring for women who are taking antipsychotic medications. The nurse should use discretion in selecting the content to be shared because of the women's altered thought processes and the large number of side/toxic effects. The nurse may choose to do more extensive education with a close family member. The newer, atypical antipsychotic medications such as aripiprazole, olanzapine, quetiapine, risperidone, and ziprasidone are usually safer and have fewer side effects than the older, more traditional antipsychotics (see Table 31.3). Their safety in breastfeeding women, however, has not been established.

Psychotropic Medications and Lactation

Use of any psychotropic medication in a breastfeeding mother is done with consideration of risks and benefits. The risk of not treating the mother versus not breastfeeding the infant prompts providers to prescribe medications that reduce maternal symptoms without harming the infant. Concerns about many psychotropic drugs are related to the long-term use and potential effects on the infant (Lawrence & Lawrence, 2016; Sriraman, Melvin, Meltzer-Brody, & Academy of Breastfeeding Medicine, 2015) (see Tables 31.1–31.4).

Factors that affect the passage of a medication through breast milk include the size of the molecule, the solubility in lipids and water, the protein-binding capacity, the drug's pH, and the rate of diffusion. Infant factors to consider relate to the gestational and chronologic age of the infant, weight, health, and frequency and amount of feeding (Lawrence & Lawrence, 2016). To minimize the infant's exposure to maternal medication, the mother should avoid breastfeeding when the blood levels of the medication are peaking.

SSRIs are the most common pharmacologic treatment for PPD; they are also prescribed for anxiety disorders (see Table 31.1). Research has shown that themajority of the SSRIs taken by breastfeeding mothers pass through the milk to the infant in small amounts and have no untoward effects on the infant. Paroxetine (Paxil), sertraline (Zoloft), and nortriptyline (Pamelor) provide less infant exposure than fluoxetine (Prozac) and citalopram (Celexa). All breastfeeding mothers who take SSRIs should be taught to monitor their infants for signs of irritability, poor feeding, and alterations in sleep pattern (Hudak, Tan, & AAP Committee on Fetus and Newborn, 2012; Sriraman et al., 2015).

Benzodiazepines, mood stabilizers, and antipsychotic medications are used frequently in the treatment of postpartum psychiatric disorders despite the lack of research in this population (see Tables 31.2 and 31.3). No long-term effects have been reported in exclusively breastfed infants whose mothers were taking benzodiazepines on a regular basis. The shorter-acting agents (alprazolam [Xanax], lorazepam [Ativan]) are favored over those with longer half-lives (clonazepam [Klonopin], diazepam [Valium]) (Lawrence & Lawrence, 2016). Mood-stabilizing medications are present in the breast milk of women who take these drugs. Lithium has been the most extensively studied. Lithium can be used safely in breastfeeding mothers with dosing based on maternal serum drug levels (Sriraman et al., 2015). Infants should be monitored for signs of toxicity (hypotonia, lethargy, feeding problems) (Wisner et al., 2017). Valproic acid (Depakote) and carbamazepine (Tegretol) are considered reasonably safe while breastfeeding, although careful monitoring for infant hepatotoxicity is recommended. The benefits of breastfeeding and the potential risks must be carefully considered before using mood stabilizers.

In summary, all psychotropic medications studied to date are excreted in breast milk. The best psychotropic medications for breastfeeding women are those with the greatest documentation of prior use, few or no metabolites, and fewer side effects.

When breastfeeding women have emotional complications and need psychotropic medications, referral to a mental health care provider who specializes in postpartum disorders is preferred. The woman should be informed of the risks and benefits to her and her infant of the medications to be taken. Depressed women will need the nurse to reinforce the importance of taking antidepressants as ordered. Because antidepressants usually do not exert any significant effect for approximately 2 weeks and usually do not reach full effect for 4 to 6 weeks, many women discontinue taking the medication on their own. Client and family teaching should reinforce the need for taking medications until therapeutic effects are present and for as long as prescribed by the health care provider.

Current information about breastfeeding and drug compatibility can be found at the Drugs and Lactation Database (LactMed; http://toxnet.nlm.nih.gov/cgi-bin/sis/htmlgen?LACT). This is a peer-reviewed and fully referenced database of drugs to which breastfeeding mothers may be exposed. Among the data included are maternal and infant levels of drugs, possible effects on breastfed infants and on lactation, and alternate drugs to consider (Anderson, 2016).

Other Treatments for Postpartum Depression

Other treatments for PPD include hormone therapy, complementary or alternative therapies (herbs, dietary supplements, massage,

aromatherapy, acupuncture, exercise, bright light therapy), and ECT. ECT, especially when bilaterally administered, has been shown to be highly effective. The safety and efficacy of these other treatment modalities relative to standard treatments must still be systematically determined (Deligiannidis & Freeman, 2014).

ANXIETY DISORDERS

Anxiety disorders are the most common psychiatric disorders, and some (e.g., panic disorder, generalized anxiety disorder, posttraumatic stress disorder [PTSD], agoraphobia) are twice as likely to be diagnosed in women compared with men. The estimated prevalence of anxiety disorders during the perinatal period ranges from 4% to 39%. If left untreated, the cost of anxiety disorders in the United States reaches nearly $5.7 billion annually (Dennis et al., 2017). High prevalence rates suggest anxiety disorders range from excessive worrying to panic attacks throughout pregnancy and postpartum. Often comorbid with depression, anxiety disorders can be difficult to diagnose, missed, or go undiagnosed leading to suboptimal treatment. Anxiety and stress during pregnancy are associated with miscarriage, preterm birth, preeclampsia, and birth complications, although a direct causal relationship has not been established (Goodman, Watson, & Stubbs, 2016; Marchesi, Ossola, & Amerio, 2016).

Anxiety disorders are characterized by prominent symptoms of anxiety that impair functioning. Examples are obsessive-compulsive disorder (OCD), PTSD, generalized anxiety disorder, panic disorder, and social anxiety phobia (AWHONN, 2015).

Diagnosis

Although panic attacks are often associated with panic disorder, they occur in a variety of disorders including anxiety, mood, substance use, psychotic spectrum, and personality disorders. Panic attacks can occur within a chronic disorder or in an otherwise healthy individual exposed to acute stress. Panic attacks are characterized by the rapid onset of intense fear (typically peaking at 10 minutes) with at least four physiological symptoms (e.g., palpitations, sweating, shortness of breath, choking, nausea, abdominal discomfort, dizziness, unsteadiness, numbness or tingling, chills, hot flashes) or cognitive symptoms such as a fear of going crazy, fear of dying, or fear of losing control (Locke, Kirst, & Shultz, 2015). Notably, the existence of panic attacks indicates greater severity, higher rates of comorbidity and suicidality, and poorer treatment response resulting in negative outcomes (Brown, LeBeau, Liao, et al., 2016).

Panic disorder is diagnosed if panic attacks are recurrent or associated with a continuing fear of future attacks, which results in anxiety between attacks. The most disabling consequence of panic disorder, agoraphobia, occurs in 30% to 40% of women with untreated panic disorder. Individuals with agoraphobia (fear of certain places or situations from which escape may be difficult or embarrassing) restrict their activities outside the home or insist on being accompanied by another individual due to fear of having a panic attack where help is unavailable (Locke et al., 2015).

Generalized anxiety disorder is characterized by excessive worrying or the inability to let go of worrying, feeling keyed up, restlessness, inability to relax, difficulty concentrating, distress about making decisions, and obsession over things that are out of proportion to the impact of the event. The issues of concern to people with generalized anxiety disorder are realistic but the level of worry is much more intense than appropriate (McKeever et al., 2016). The pregnant woman also may have persistent thoughts that something is wrong with the fetus.

Individuals with generalized anxiety disorder often have physical symptoms associated with worrying, such as muscle tension, irritability, restlessness, insomnia, fatigue, headache, nausea, diarrhea, or irritable bowel syndrome. To meet criteria for the disorder, individuals must have significant impairment of functioning and intrusive anxiety for at least 6 months, affecting multiple domains such as finances, work, and health (Locke et al., 2015).

PTSD can occur as a result of serious injury, actual or threat of death, or sexual violence. (See Chapter 5.) PTSD has been found to be more prevalent in women who have experienced severe complications in pregnancy or during birth such as premature birth, emergency cesarean birth, or stillbirth, with rates of 15% to 18% (Yildiz, Ayers, & Phillips, 2017). Symptoms include reexperiencing the traumatic event, persistent avoidance of stimuli, and numbing, as well as difficulty sleeping, irritability or angry outbursts, difficulty concentrating, hypervigilance, and exaggerated startle response, lasting for at least a month and significantly impairing women's ability to function. Nurses can support the healing process of individuals with PTSD by being alert to what the woman is experiencing during pregnancy and labor.

If the current pregnancy is a result of rape, the woman may be extremely ambivalent about the baby. If the rape occurred some time ago, the whole experience of pregnancy with prenatal visits and physical examinations can trigger memories of the original trauma. She may avoid prenatal care because of the anxiety triggered by bodily touch and vaginal examinations. Some pregnant women with PTSD may feel more comfortable with a female nurse midwife or a female physician. Giving birth can trigger memories of being out of control, and she may lose contact with reality. The nurse can verbalize understanding of the anxiety and orient the woman to current reality by saying, "You're having an examination to make sure the baby is okay," or, "You're in labor preparing to give birth to your baby. I am your nurse. You're in the hospital. I will check on you frequently. You are safe here." Treatment usually includes psychotherapy and referral to support groups.

📋 CARE MANAGEMENT

When anxiety substantially impairs work, family, or social adjustment, mental health evaluation is indicated and treatment is appropriate. Both panic disorder and generalized anxiety disorder respond to a variety of antidepressant medications as well as psychotherapy (Locke et al., 2015). Psychotherapy includes many different approaches such as cognitive-behavioral therapy (CBT), interpersonal psychotherapy (IPT), and relaxation. CBT may use applied relaxation, exposure therapy, breathing, cognitive restructuring, or education. Psychotherapy is as effective as medication in both generalized anxiety disorder and panic disorder. Panic disorder responds to most antidepressant medications, which are first-line therapies for this disorder (Locke et al.) (see Table 31.1). Benzodiazepines are also effective but can be associated with abuse and physical dependence in some women. Prenatal benzodiazepine exposure remains controversial regarding the risk for oral cleft. Maternal benzodiazepine use shortly before birth has been associated with temperature dysregulation, apnea, reduced Apgar scores, hypotonia, and poor feeding in neonates (Chisolm & Payne, 2015; Marchesi, et al., 2016).

Note that most of the antianxiety medications such as alprazolam (Xanax) and lorazepam (Ativan) are FDA Category D (evidence of human fetal risk) or Category X (demonstrated fetal abnormalities and use is contraindicated). However, benzodiazepines should not be abruptly discontinued during pregnancy. Instead, they should be tapered sufficiently before the birth to limit neonatal withdrawal syndrome.

OCD is effectively treated with SSRIs. A behavioral therapy technique, exposure and response prevention, is also effective for OCD (Marchesi et al., 2016). PTSD is partially responsive to antidepressant medication, but high-intensity trauma-informed psychotherapy and psychoeducation are recommended for women who have PTSD resulting from traumatic birth, miscarriage, stillbirth, or neonatal death (National Institute for Clinical Excellence [NICE], 2015). The first-line medication treatment for social phobia is SSRIs; cognitive therapy also can be very helpful. Specific phobias are most effectively treated with focused desensitization psychotherapy rather than medication (McKeever et al., 2016).

A risk-to-benefit evaluation for treatments during pregnancy must be individualized for the pregnant woman with anxiety disorder, which, like an MDE, can have a negative effect on pregnancy outcome. If psychotherapy treatment is refused, not available, or ineffective, pharmacologic treatment should be considered (Chisolm & Payne, 2015).

Strategies to reduce anxiety include empowerment through education; sensory interventions such as music therapy and aromatherapy; medication; behavioral interventions such as breathing exercises, progressive muscle relaxation, and guided imagery; and cognitive strategies such as encouraging positive self-talk and questioning negative thinking.

Nurses and other members of the interprofessional health care team should educate women about the dangers of benzodiazepines during pregnancy, assess for use during pregnancy, and help pregnant women find other ways to handle their anxiety and insomnia, or refer them to a psychiatrist who specializes in psychiatric disorders in pregnancy.

PERINATAL SUBSTANCE ABUSE

Large numbers of women of childbearing age abuse potentially addictive and mood-altering drugs. Misuse of tobacco, alcohol, marijuana, opioids, cocaine, methamphetamines, prescription drugs, and many other substances can lead to chemical dependency. Chemical dependency is a chronic, relapsing, and progressive disease. Without treatment or participation in recovery activities, it can progress and result in disability or premature death.

This section discusses only substance abuse during pregnancy. Chapter 4 contains additional information related to substance abuse in the general population. See Chapter 35 for information regarding effects of maternal substance abuse on neonates.

Pregnant women who abuse drugs can display warning signs such as receiving no prenatal care, late entry into care, or sporadic care with multiple missed appointments. They may keep prenatal appointments but leave without being seen. Another warning sign in pregnant substance abusers is noncompliance with recommended treatment (Baird, Kennedy, & Dalton, 2017). They may also show evidence of poor nutrition, have frequent encounters with law enforcement officials, or engage in marital and family disputes.

Drugs that affect the mother can also affect the fetus in multiple ways either directly or indirectly. Early in gestation drugs can cause significant teratogenic effects. During the fetal period, after major structural development is complete, drugs exert more subtle effects, including abnormal growth and maturation, alterations in neurotransmitters and their receptors, and brain organization. These are considered to be the direct effects of drugs (Behnke, Smith, Committee on Substance Abuse, & Committee on Fetus and Newborn, 2013). Drugs that exert a pharmacologic effect on the mother can indirectly affect the fetus. Indirect effects include altered delivery of nutrition to the fetus, either because of placental insufficiency or altered maternal health behaviors attributable to the mother's addiction.

Maternal factors can indirectly place the fetus at risk. Examples include decreased access/compliance with health care, increased exposure to violence, and increased risk for mental illness and infection (Behnke et al., 2013).

Prevalence

Substance use in the United States is a problem that continues to grow. Women make up about 30% of the addicted population, and many of them are in their childbearing years (Baird et al., 2017). Illicit drug use also occurs among pregnant women. Rates of use are generally higher in the first and second trimesters of pregnancy than in the third (Wisner et al., 2017). Universal screening for drug use in pregnant women is recommended. Because substance use is prevalent in all populations, providers should never make assumptions based on age, race, or socioeconomic status. Universal screening is nonbiased and nonstigmatizing (Baird et al.; Wisner et al.).

Maternal and Fetal Effects of Selected Drugs of Abuse

Tobacco

Maternal effects related to cigarette smoking include thromboembolic disease and respiratory complications. Pregnancy-related complications include miscarriage, preterm birth, intrauterine growth restriction (IUGR), placenta previa, placental abruption, low-birth-weight, and preterm prelabor rupture of membranes (AAP & ACOG, 2017; Wisner et al., 2017).

Alcohol

Prenatal alcohol exposure increases the chance of birth defects significantly. No amount of alcohol use at any time during pregnancy is considered safe. Health care providers should advise women that low-level consumption of alcohol in early pregnancy is not an indication for pregnancy termination. However, women who have already consumed alcohol during a current pregnancy should be advised to stop to minimize further risk (AAP & ACOG, 2017). Although fetal alcohol syndrome (FAS) is a known consequence of prenatal alcohol intake, other consequences include an increased risk for miscarriage, stillbirth, and preterm birth. Fetal exposure to alcohol is the most common preventable cause of cognitive impairment (AAP & ACOG; Wisner et al., 2017).

Marijuana

Marijuana is the most commonly used illicit drug in pregnancy and many women continue to use it throughout their pregnancies. As more states legalize the use of marijuana for medical or recreational purposes, it will likely be used more often to treat such conditions as pregnancy-associated hyperemesis. No safe threshold limits for marijuana use have been determined. Its use during pregnancy has been associated with intrauterine growth restriction (Wisner et al., 2017).

Opioids

Opioid use among pregnant women has greatly increased in recent years, just as it has in the general population. This class of drugs includes, among others, morphine, heroin, codeine, meperidine, methadone, and buprenorphine. Opioid users can develop withdrawal symptoms once the drug has been metabolized. The box Signs of Potential Complications: Maternal Opioid Abstinence Syndrome (Opioid/Narcotic Withdrawal) in Chapter 17 lists common signs and symptoms of opioid withdrawal in women. During pregnancy, chronic untreated addiction to heroin is associated with IUGR, placental abruption, intrauterine passage of meconium, preterm labor, and fetal death (ACOG, 2017).

Cocaine

Cocaine is a powerful CNS stimulant that is addictive because of the tremendous sense of euphoria that it creates. When used during pregnancy, there is an increased incidence of miscarriage, preterm labor, small-for-gestational-age babies, placental abruption, and stillbirth. Fetal anomalies have been reported with its use.

Methamphetamines

Methamphetamines are CNS stimulants with vasoconstrictive characteristics similar to those of cocaine, and they are used similarly. Pregnancy-associated complications with amphetamine use include IUGR, preterm birth, and placental abruption.

Barriers to Treatment

Many pregnant women who are substance abusers do not receive treatment for their addictions. Social stigma, labeling, and guilt are significant barriers to receiving necessary care. Women often do not seek help because of the fear of losing custody of their child or children or criminal prosecution. Pregnant women who abuse substances commonly have little understanding of the ways in which these substances affect them, their pregnancies, and their babies. In many instances pregnant mothers who use psychoactive substances receive negative feedback from society and health care providers, who may not only condemn them for endangering the life of the fetus but may also even withhold support as a result. Barriers within the drug treatment system can also deter these women from receiving the help they need. Traditionally substance-abuse treatment programs have not addressed issues that affect pregnant women such as concurrent need for obstetric care and child care for other children. Long waiting lists and lack of health insurance present further barriers to treatment. Pregnant women with co-occurring substance abuse and psychiatric disorders face unique barriers because of the social stigma attached to both conditions and insufficient knowledge and training to manage coexisting disorders.

Legal Considerations

Pregnant women in some states have been prosecuted under existing criminal laws because of substance abuse during pregnancy. Pregnant substance abusers in Alabama and South Carolina, for example, have been convicted of criminal child abuse in those states (Guttmacher Institute, 2018). Substance abuse in pregnancy is defined as child abuse in 23 states and the District of Columbia, with 3 states defining it as reason for civil commitment. Suspected drug abuse in pregnant women is reason for required reporting by health care professionals in 24 states and the District of Columbia, and prenatal drug exposure testing is required in 8 states if health care providers suspect substance abuse (Guttmacher Institute). Because reporting requirements vary widely, health care professionals must be aware of current laws in the state(s) where they practice (AAP & ACOG, 2017).

CARE MANAGEMENT

Screening

All pregnant women should be screened at their first prenatal visit regarding their past and present use of tobacco, alcohol, and other drugs, including the recreational use of prescription and over-the-counter medications as well as herbal remedies. When inquiring about tobacco, it is important to ask about all forms of use, including smoking, chewing, vaping, or an electronic nicotine delivery system. Substance use information can be obtained by interview or use of a validated screening tool. The overall approach and emotional tone of the clinician is more important than the specific wording or content used. Women are more likely to report substance use when asked in a nonjudgmental manner by an empathic interviewer and within the context of general health questions. Screening when the woman is alone with the health care provider (i.e., no family members or friends present in the room) is another strategy to increase the likelihood of truthful responses (AAP & ACOG, 2017; ACOG, 2017; Wisner et al., 2017).

When questioning a woman about her drug use, it is usually best to begin by asking about her intake of over-the-counter and prescribed medications. Questions about these types of drugs are usually

BOX 31.1   Screening With the *4Ps Plus*

Parents: Did either of your parents ever have a problem with alcohol or drugs?

Partner: Does your partner have a problem with alcohol or drugs?

Past: Have you ever had any beer or wine or liquor?

Pregnancy: In the month before you knew you were pregnant, how many cigarettes did you smoke? In the month before you knew you were pregnant, how much beer, wine, or liquor did you drink?

From Chasnoff, I. J., & Hung, W. C. (1999). *The 4Ps plus.* Chicago: NTI Publishing.

perceived as nonthreatening. Next, her use of legal drugs such as caffeine, nicotine, and alcohol should be determined. Finally, she should be asked about her use of illicit drugs such as cocaine, heroin, and methamphetamines. The approximate frequency and amount should be documented for each drug used.

Use of validated screening questionnaires, along with the assurance of confidentiality, improves client-provider communication and can increase the truthfulness of client responses (AAP & ACOG, 2017). The *4Ps Plus* is a screening tool designed specifically to identify pregnant women who need in-depth assessment (Box 31.1). It consists of five questions and takes less than 1 minute to complete. Because women frequently deny or greatly underreport usage when asked about drug or alcohol consumption during pregnancy, asking about substance use before pregnancy is often an effective screening method (Wisner et al., 2017). CRAFFT is a substance abuse screening tool designed specifically for use with adolescents and young adults. It consists of six questions. A "yes" answer to two or more questions suggests a serious problem and indicates a need for further assessment (AAP & ACOG).

Toxicologic testing is often performed to screen for illicit drug use. Because positive test results have implications for women beyond their health, informed consent should be obtained before testing is done (AAP & ACOG, 2017). Information that should be communicated to the woman includes the test planned, purpose of the test, management based on test results, and benefits or consequences of testing (Baird et al., 2017).

Several biologic specimens can be used to screen for drug exposure. The three specimens most commonly used to establish drug exposure during the prenatal and perinatal periods are urine, meconium, and hair. There are practical limitations, however, with testing all three substances (Wisner et al., 2017).

LEGAL TIP

Toxicologic Testing

The legal implications of testing and the need for consent from the mother can vary among states. Therefore, health care providers should be aware of local laws and legislative changes that can influence regional practice (AAP & ACOG, 2017).

Assessment

Because substance-abusing pregnant women are at risk for a variety of infections and medical conditions, a comprehensive medical history should be obtained, and a complete physical examination performed. Laboratory assessments will likely include screening for syphilis, hepatitis B and C, and human immunodeficiency virus (HIV). A complete blood count and a skin test to screen for tuberculosis may also be ordered. In addition, the woman may be tested for other common sexually transmitted infections such as gonorrhea and chlamydia. Initial and serial ultrasound studies are usually performed to determine gestational age because the woman may have had amenorrhea as a result of her drug use or have no idea when her last menstrual period occurred.

Interventions

Intervention with substance-abusing pregnant women is best accomplished by an interprofessional health care team. Team members should

include, at a minimum, an obstetrician or nurse-midwife, mental health provider, substance abuse counselor, nurse, and social worker.

Medical Management

Intervention with the pregnant substance abuser begins with education about specific effects on pregnancy, the fetus, and the newborn for each drug used. Consequences of perinatal drug use should be clearly communicated, and abstinence recommended as the safest course of action unless the woman is abusing opioids. Women are often more receptive to making lifestyle changes during pregnancy than at any other time in their lives. The casual, experimental, or recreational drug user is frequently able to achieve and maintain sobriety when she receives education, support, and continued monitoring throughout the remainder of the pregnancy. Periodic screening throughout pregnancy of women who have admitted to drug use may help them to continue abstinence.

Treatment for substance abuse is individualized for each woman. Specific recommendations will vary depending on the type of drug used and the frequency and amount of use.

Women are more likely to attempt to stop smoking during pregnancy than at any other time in their lives. Women who quit smoking by the first trimester have infants whose growth is comparable to those born to nonsmokers. Smoking-cessation programs during pregnancy are effective and should be offered to all pregnant smokers. These programs should continue throughout the postpartum period as well, because women who quit smoking during pregnancy tend to relapse within 1 year of giving birth (Wisner et al., 2017). The U.S. Preventive Services Task Force (USPSTF) states that insufficient evidence is available to assess the risks and benefits of pharmacotherapy interventions for tobacco cessation during pregnancy. Therefore, the USPSTF recommends that pregnant women who use tobacco be advised to quit and provided only with behavioral interventions to assist with cessation (Siu & USPSTF, 2015). Many smoking-cessation resources are available, both in print and online, and smoking "quit lines" (for example, 1-800-QUIT-NOW) are effective in assisting pregnant women to quit smoking (Wisner et al.). For more information on smoking cessation, visit the American Lung Association website at www.lungusa.org or the CDC website at www.cdc.gov/tobacco/quit_smoking/index.htm.

Detoxification, short-term inpatient or outpatient treatment, long-term residential treatment, aftercare services, and self-help support groups are all possible options for alcohol and drug abuse. Women for Sobriety (https://womenforsobriety.org/) may be a more helpful organization for women than Alcoholics Anonymous or Narcotics Anonymous, which were originally developed for male substance abusers. In general, long-term treatment of any sort is becoming increasingly difficult to obtain, particularly for women who lack insurance coverage. Although some programs allow a woman to keep her children with her at the treatment facility, far too few of them are available to meet the demand (see Community Activity: Visiting a Twelve-Step Meeting).

🏠 **COMMUNITY ACTIVITY**

Visiting a Twelve-Step Meeting

Search online to find an "open" (one that welcomes visitors) twelve-step meeting in your community. Alcoholics Anonymous, Narcotics Anonymous, and Cocaine Anonymous are all examples of twelve-step recovery groups. Attend an open meeting held by one of these groups. Discuss your experience with your clinical group. Did pregnant women or new mothers attend the meeting? What was your impression of the meeting format and the discussion that occurred? Did you notice anything at the meeting that surprised you? Do you think that attending twelve-step meetings would be helpful for pregnant women or new mothers attempting to achieve and maintain sobriety? Give reasons to support your answer to the last question.

Pregnant women requiring withdrawal from alcohol should be admitted for inpatient management. In pregnant women, alcohol withdrawal tends to begin within 6 to 24 hours after the last drink. Alcohol withdrawal treatment during pregnancy consists of the administration of benzodiazepines. Chlordiazepoxide (Librium) and diazepam (Valium) are considered the benzodiazepine agents of choice for treatment of pregnant women (Wisner et al., 2017).

Since the 1970s, opioid agonist therapy (also referred to as *medication-assisted treatment*) has been considered the standard of care for pregnant women with an opioid use disorder. Opioid agonist therapy includes methadone and buprenorphine (Subutex or Suboxone) (AAP & ACOG, 2017). Neither buprenorphine nor methadone is associated with an increased risk for birth defects (Wisner et al., 2017). (See the Evidence-Based Practice box: Treating Opioid Dependence During Pregnancy.) Opioid agonist pharmacotherapy is preferred over supervised medical withdrawal, because withdrawal is associated with high relapse rates and poorer outcomes (AAP & ACOG).

Medical withdrawal from opioids during pregnancy is currently not recommended, in part, because of a potential risk for fetal distress or fetal demise. However, a study of more than 600 pregnant women who were medically withdrawn from opioids reported no fetal harm during the process. These data highly suggest that medical withdrawal in opioid-addicted pregnant women is not harmful (Bell, Towers, Hennessy, et al., 2016).

Anywhere from 30% to 80% of infants exposed to opioids, including methadone or buprenorphine, in utero require treatment for neonatal abstinence syndrome (NAS). Neither the incidence nor the severity of NAS correlates directly with the maternal methadone dose at birth. Therefore, limiting the methadone dose to minimize the risk for NAS is not warranted (Wisner et al., 2017). See Chapter 25 for additional information on NAS.

Pregnant women who use cocaine should be advised to stop using immediately and be referred for substance abuse treatment. Effective psychosocial and behavioral treatments have been developed for pregnant substance abusers. Communication between obstetric care providers and substance abuse treatment staff is necessary for treatment success (Wisner et al., 2017).

As is the case with cocaine users, methamphetamine users are urged to immediately stop all use during pregnancy. Because methamphetamine users are extremely psychologically addicted, the rate of relapse is very high.

The most effective treatments for methamphetamine addiction at this time are behavioral therapies, such as cognitive-behavioral and contingency-management interventions. There are currently no medications that counteract the specific effects of methamphetamine or that prolong abstinence from and reduce the abuse of methamphetamine (National Institute on Drug Abuse [NIDA], 2013).

Nursing Interventions

Although substance abusers can be difficult to care for at any time, they are often particularly challenging during the intrapartum and postpartum periods because of manipulative and demanding behavior. Typically these women display poor control over their behavior and a low threshold for pain. Increased dependency needs and lack of involvement with infant care may also be apparent.

Nurses must understand that substance abuse is an illness and that these women deserve to be treated with patience, kindness, consistency, and firmness when necessary (Box 31.2). Even women who

---

EVIDENCE-BASED PRACTICE

Treating Opioid Dependence During Pregnancy

Ask the Question

For pregnant women, what is the most effective treatment for opioid dependence?

Search for the Evidence

Search Strategies: English research-based publications since 2014 on suboxone, methadone, detox, and opioid dependence in pregnancy were included.

Databases Used: Cochrane Collaborative Database, National Guideline Clearinghouse (AHRQ), CINAHL, PubMed, UpToDate, and the professional websites for ACOG and AWHONN.

Critical Appraisal of the Evidence

- Opioid dependence during pregnancy increased 127% from 1998 to 2011. It is associated with significant obstetrical morbidity and mortality. Identifying therapeutic interventions for pregnant women is an important priority (Maeda, Bateman, Clancy, et al., 2014).
- Suboxone (buprenorphine plus naloxone) is used to treat opioid dependence outside of pregnancy. The use of buprenorphine alone in pregnancy is preferred to prevent prenatal naloxone exposure. Methadone is also used to treat opioid dependence during pregnancy. Buprenorphine is associated with decreased time in treatment, decreased medications needed to treat neonatal abstinence syndrome, and shorter hospital stays for newborns. Use of methadone or buprenorphine is considered standard of care for opioid dependent mothers during pregnancy, yet both are underutilized (Tran, Griffin, Stone, et al., 2017).
- Opioid agonist pharmacotherapy is the best treatment for women with opioid use disorder. It is more effective than medically supervised withdrawal, which is linked to high rates of relapse (American College of Obstetricians and Gynecologists [ACOG], 2017).

Apply the Evidence: Nursing Implications

- Nurses in the perinatal setting have been affected by the opioid crisis. Nurses must be mindful that providing care for opioid-dependent mothers can lead to burnout, moral distress, and frustration (Sander, Henderson, Metz, et al., 2018).
- Nurses need education about best practices in caring for women with opioid dependence. Standardizing care, including terminology, interventions, and education have been shown to improve outcomes for opioid-dependent pregnant women and their newborns. Interprofessional care for these women is critical to ensure that they are offered all available resources (Sander et al., 2018).
- Nurses should know that substance use disorders cross all lines of socioeconomic status, race and ethnicity, and rural, urban, or suburban settings. Nurses can encourage early screening of pregnant women for opioid use disorder (ACOG, 2017).

References

American College of Obstetricians and Gynecologists. (2017). Committee opinion no. 711: Opioid use and opioid use disorder in pregnancy. *Obstetrics & Gynecology, 130*(2), 488–489.

Maeda, A., Bateman, B. T., Clancy, C. R., et al. (2014). Opioid abuse and dependence during pregnancy: Temporal trends and obstetrical outcomes. *Anesthesiology, 121*(6), 1158–1165.

Sander, A., Henderson, C., Metz, G., et al. (2018). Specialized care of women and newborns affected by opioids with a CORE team of nurses. *Nursing for Women's Health, 22*(4), 327–331.

Tran, T. H., Griffin, B., Stone, R., et al. (2017). Methadone, buprenorphine, and naltrexone for the treatment of opioid use disorder in pregnant women. *Pharmacotherapy, 37*(7), 824–839.

Jennifer Taylor Alderman

BOX 31.2 Caring for Pregnant Substance Abusers

Realize that the decision to become and remain sober can *only* be made by the substance abuser.

Understand that nurses do not have the power to cure anyone. They only serve as educators, supporters, and advocates.

Educate yourself about the effects of drug use in general and effects on pregnancy and the newborn specifically.

Treat substance abusers with the same respect and consideration that you show other people.

Become familiar with your local treatment centers. Learn which of them accept pregnant women. Keep an up-to-date list of groups meeting in your community.

Remember that there are no "hopeless cases." It is *never* too late to quit!

Practice patience and persistence. It may take months or years to see the effects of your work.

are actively abusing drugs experience pain during labor and after giving birth and may need both pharmacologic and nonpharmacologic interventions. Developing a standardized plan of care so clients have limited opportunities to play staff members against one another is helpful. Mother-infant attachment should be promoted by identifying the woman's strengths and reinforcing positive maternal feelings and behaviors. Staffing should be sufficient to ensure strict surveillance of visitors and prevent unsupervised drug use.

Advice regarding breastfeeding must be individualized. Although all abused substances appear in breast milk, some in greater amounts than others, breastfeeding is definitely contraindicated in women who use amphetamines, alcohol, cocaine, heroin, or marijuana. However, methadone use is not a contraindication to breastfeeding. The baby's nutrition and safety needs are of primary importance in this consideration. For some women a desire to breastfeed can provide strong motivation to achieve and maintain sobriety.

Smoking can interfere with the milk ejection (let-down) reflex. Women who smoke and breastfeed should avoid smoking for 2 hours before a feeding to minimize the amount of nicotine in the milk and improve the milk ejection reflex. All smokers should be discouraged from smoking in the same room with the infant because exposure to secondhand smoke can increase the likelihood that the infant will experience behavioral and respiratory health problems.

Follow-up Care

Before a known substance abuser is discharged with her baby, the home situation must be assessed to determine that the environment is safe and that someone will be available to meet the infant's needs if the mother is unable to do so. The social services department of the birthing facility is usually involved in interviewing the mother before discharge to ensure that the infant's needs will be met. Family members or friends are sometimes asked to become actively involved with the mother and infant after discharge. A home care or public health nurse may be asked to make home visits to assess the mother's ability to care for the baby and provide guidance and support. If serious questions about the infant's well-being exist, the case is likely to be referred to the state child protective services agency for further action.

KEY POINTS

- Because pregnant women may have a history of mental disorder or substance abuse, careful assessment is extremely important at the first and each subsequent prenatal and postpartum visit.
- Mood disorders account for most mental health disorders in the postpartum period.
- Psychotherapy is the first-line treatment option for women with mild to moderate peripartum depression.
- Antidepressant medications are the usual treatment for postpartum depression; however, specific precautions are needed for breastfeeding women.
- Treatment of anxiety disorders requires a combination of medication, education, supportive measures, and psychotherapy.
- Treatment of both depression and anxiety is critical to improving mental health.

- Perinatal depression with suicidal or homicidal intent or plan as well as postpartum depression with psychotic features is a psychiatric emergency. Immediate evaluation by a mental health professional is warranted.
- Identification of women at greatest risk for substance abuse during pregnancy and depression in the postpartum period can be facilitated by use of validated screening tools.
- Alcohol abuse during pregnancy is the leading cause of cognitive disability in the United States, and it is entirely preventable.
- Treatment programs must start with an understanding that substance abuse in women is a complex problem surrounded by multiple individual, familial, and social issues that require many levels of intervention and treatment.

REFERENCES

Agency for Healthcare Research and Quality. (2018). Efficacy and safety of screening for postpartum depression. Retrieved from: http://www.ahrq.gov/research/findings/postpartumdep.html.

Alkozei, A., McMahon, E., & Lahav, A. (2014). Stress levels and depressive symptoms in NICU mothers in the early postpartum period. *Journal of Maternal, Fetal, and Neonatal Medicine, 27*(17), 1738–1743.

American Academy of Pediatrics & American College of Obstetricians and Gynecologists. (2017). *Guidelines for perinatal care* (8th ed.). Washington, DC: American College of Obstetricians and Gynecologists.

American College of Obstetricians and Gynecologists. (2017). Committee opinion no. 711: Opioid use and opioid use disorder in pregnancy. *Obstetrics & Gynecology, 130*(2), e81–94.

American College of Obstetricians and Gynecologists. (2018). Committee opinion no. 757: Screening for perinatal depression. *Obstetrics & Gynecology, 132*(5), e208–e212.

American Psychiatric Association. (2013). *Diagnostic and statistical manual of mental disorders* (5th ed.). Washington, DC: American Psychiatric Association.

Anderson, P. O. (2016). LactMed update: An introduction. *Breastfeeding Medicine, 11*(2), 54–55.

Association of Women's Health, Obstetric and Neonatal Nurses. (2015). AWHONN position statement: Mood and anxiety disorders in pregnant and postpartum women. *Journal of Obstetric, Gynecologic, and Neonatal Nursing, 44*(5), 561–563.

Baird, S. M., Kennedy, B. B., & Dalton, J. (2017). Special considerations for individualized care of the laboring woman. In B. B. Kennedy, & S. M. Baird (Eds.), *Intrapartum management modules: A perinatal education program* (5th ed.). Philadelphia: Wolters Kluwer.

Behnke, M., Smith, V. C., & Committee on Substance Abuse, & Committee on Fetus and Newborn. (2013). Prenatal substance abuse: Short- and long-term effects on the exposed fetus. *Pediatrics, 131*(3), e1009–e1024.

Bell, J., Towers, C. V., Hennessy, M. D., et al. (2016). Detoxification from opiate drugs during pregnancy. *American Journal of Obstetrics & Gynecology, 215*(3), 374.e1–374.e6.

Berard, A., Zhao, J., & Sheehy, O. (2017). Antidepressant use during pregnancy and the risk of major congenital malformations in a cohort of depressed pregnant women: An updated analysis of the Quebec pregnancy cohort. *British Medical Journal Open, 7*(1), 1–13.

Brown, L., LeBeau, R., Liao, B., et al. (2016). A comparison of the nature and correlates of panic attacks in the context of panic disorder and social anxiety disorder. *Psychiatry Research, 235*, 69–76.

Cameron, E. E., Sedov, I. D., & Tomfohr-Madsen, L. M. (2016). Prevalence of paternal depression in pregnancy and the postpartum: An updated meta-analysis. *Journal of Affective Disorders, 206*, 189–203.

Chisolm, M., & Payne, J. (2015). Management of psychotropic drugs during pregnancy. *British Medical Journal, 351*, 1–15.

Clark, C., Sit, D., Driscoll, K., et al. (2015). Does screening with the MDQ and EPDS improve identification of bipolar disorder in an obstetrical sample? *Depression and Anxiety, 32*(7), 518–526.

Cox, J., Holden, J., & Henshaw, C. (2014). *Perinatal mental health: The Edinburgh postnatal depression scale (EPDS) manual*. London, UK: RCPsych Publications.

Cunningham, F., Leveno, K., Bloom, S., et al. (2018). *Williams obstetrics* (25th ed.). New York: McGraw-Hill Education.

Deligiannidis, K. M., & Freeman, M. P. (2014). Complementary and alternative medicine therapies for perinatal depression. Best practice & research. *Clinical Obstetrics & Gynaecology, 28*(1), 85–95.

Dennis, C., Falah-Hassani, K., & Shiri, R. (2017). Prevalence of antenatal and postnatal anxiety: Systematic review and meta-analysis. *British Journal of Psychiatry, 210*, 315–323.

Dennis, C. L., & Dowswell, T. (2013). Psychosocial and psychological interventions for preventing postpartum depression (review). *Cochrane Database of Systematic Reviews, 2013*(2), CD001134.

Earls, M. F., & American Academy of Pediatrics Committee on Psychosocial Aspects of Child and Family Health. (2010). Incorporating recognition and management of perinatal and postpartum depression into pediatric practice. *Pediatrics, 126*(5), 1032–1039.

Gentile, S. (2017). Untreated depression during pregnancy: Short- and long-term effects in offspring. A systematic review. *Neuroscience, 342*, 154–166.

Goodman, J., Watson, G., & Stubbs, B. (2016). Anxiety disorders in postpartum women: A systematic review and meta-analysis. *Journal of Affective Disorders, 203*, 292–331.

Grigoriadis, S., Wilton, A., Kurdyak, P., et al. (2017). Perinatal suicide in Ontario, Canada: A 15-year population-based study. *Canadian Medical Association Journal, 189*(34), 1085–1092.

Guttmacher Institute. (2018). *Substance abuse during pregnancy*. Retrieved from: https://www.guttmacher.org/state-policy/explore/substance-use-during-pregnancy.

Habib, C. (2012). Paternal perinatal depression: An overview and suggestions towards an intervention model. *Journal of Family Studies, 18*(1), 4–16.

Hudak, M. L., Tan, R. C., & American Academy of Pediatrics Committee on Fetus and Newborn. (2012). Neonatal drug withdrawal. *Pediatrics, 129*(2), e540–e560.

Isley, M. M., & Katz, V. L. (2017). Postpartum care and long-term health considerations. In S. G. Gabbe, J. R. Niebyl, J. L. Simpson, et al. (Eds.), *Obstetrics: Normal and problem pregnancies* (7th ed.). Philadelphia: Elsevier.

Kendig, S., Keats, J., Hoffman, C., et al. (2017). Consensus bundle on maternal mental health: Perinatal depression and anxiety. *Journal of Obstetric, Gynecologic, & Neonatal Nursing, 46*(2), 272–281.

Kothari, C. L., Liepman, M. R., Tareen, R. S., et al. (2016). Intimate partner violence associated with postpartum depression, regardless of socioeconomic status. *Maternal and Child Health Journal, 20*(6), 1237–1246.

Lawrence, R. A., & Lawrence, R. M. (2016). *Breastfeeding: A guide for the medical profession* (8th ed.). Philadelphia: Elsevier.

Letourneau, N., Tryphonopoulos, P. D., Duffett-Leger, L., et al. (2012). Support intervention needs and preferences of fathers affected by postpartum depression. *Journal of Perinatal & Neonatal Nursing, 26*(1), 69–80.

Locke, A., Kirst, N., & Shultz, C. (2015). Diagnosis and management of generalized anxiety disorder and panic disorder in adults. *American Family Physician, 91*(9), 617–624.

Lupattelli, A., Spigset, O., Bjornsdottir, I., et al. (2015). Patterns and factors associated with low adherence to psychotropic medications during pregnancy – A cross-sectional, multinational web-based study. *Depression and Anxiety, 32*(6), 426–436.

Marchesi, C., Ossola, P., Amerio, A., et al. (2016). Clinical management of perinatal anxiety disorders: A systematic review. *Journal of Affective Disorders, 190*, 543–550.

McKeever, A., Alderman, S., Luff, S., & DeJesus, B. (2015). Assessment and care of childbearing women with severe and persistent mental illness. *Nursing for Women's Health, 20*(5), 485–499.

Meltzer-Brody, S., & Jones, I. (2015). Optimizing the treatment of mood disorders in the perinatal period. *Dialogues in Clinical Neuroscience, 17*(2), 207–218.

Milgrom, J., & Gemmill, A. W. (2014). Screening for perinatal depression. Best practice & research. *Clinical Obstetrics & Gynaecology, 28*(1), 13–23.

Musser, A. K., Ahmed, A. H., Foli, K. J., & Coddington, J. A. (2013). Paternal postpartum depression: What health care providers should know. *Journal of Pediatric Health Care, 27*(6), 479–485.

Myers, E. R., Aubuchon-Endsley, N., & Bastian, L. A. (2013). *Efficacy and safety of screening for postpartum depression*. Comparative effectiveness review 106. Rockville, MD: Agency for Healthcare Research and Quality.

National Institute for Clinical Excellence. (2015). *Antenatal and postnatal mental health: Clinical management and service guidance*. Available at: https://www.nice.org.uk/guidance/cg192#.

National Institute of Drug Abuse. (2013). *Methamphetamine*. Retrieved from: https://www.drugabuse.gov/publications/research-reports/methamphetamine.

O'Connor, E., Rossom, R. C., Henninger, M., et al. (2016). Primary care screening for and treatment of depression in pregnant and postpartum women: Evidence report and systematic review for the U.S. Preventive Services Task Force. *Journal of the American Medical Association, 315*(4), 388–406.

Ogunyemi, D., Jovanovski, A., Liu, J., et al. (2017). The contribution of untreated and treated anxiety and depression to prenatal, intrapartum, and neonatal outcomes. *American Journal of Perinatology Reports, 8*(3), 146–157.

O'Hara, M. W., & McCabe, J. E. (2013). Postpartum depression: Current status and future directions. *Annual Review of Clinical Psychology, 9*, 379–407.

O'Hara, M. W., & Wisner, K. L. (2014). Perinatal mental illness: Definition, description, aetiology. Best practice & research. *Clinical Obstetrics & Gynaecology, 28*(1), 3–12.

Park, E. M., Meltzer-Brody, S., & Stickgold, R. (2013). Poor sleep maintenance and subjective sleep quality are associated with postpartum maternal depression symptom severity. *Archives of Women's Mental Health, 16*(6), 539–547.

Paschetta, E., Berrisford, G., Coccia, F., et al. (2014). Perinatal psychiatric disorders: An overview. *American Journal of Obstetrics & Gynecology, 210*(6), 501–509 e6.

Paulson, J. F., & Bazemore, S. D. (2010). Prenatal and postpartum depression in fathers and its association with maternal depression: A meta-analysis. *Journal of the American Medical Association, 303*(19), 1961–1969.

Puryear, L. J. (2014). Postpartum adjustment: What is normal and what is not? In D. L. Barnes (Ed.), *Women's reproductive mental health across the lifespan*. Cham, Switzerland: Springer International.

Reefhuis, J., Devine, O., Friedman, J., et al. (2015). National birth defects prevention study. Specific SSRIs and birth defects: Bayesian analysis to interpret new data in the context of previous reports. *British Medical Journal, 351*, 48–50.

Siu, A. L., & U.S. Preventive Services Task Force. (2015). Behavioral and pharmacotherapy interventions for tobacco smoking cessation in adults, including pregnant women: U.S. Preventive Services Task Force recommendation. *Annals of Internal Medicine, 163*(8), 622–634.

Siu, A. L., & US Preventive Services Task Force (2016). Screening for depression in adults: US Preventive Services Task Force recommendation statement. *Journal of the American Medical Association, 315*(4), 380–387.

Sriraman, N. K., Melvin, K., Meltzer-Brody, S., & Academy of Breastfeeding Medicine (2015). ABM clinical protocol no. 18: Use of antidepressants in breastfeeding mothers. *Breastfeeding Medicine, 10*(6), 290–299.

Stadtlander, L. (2015). Paternal postpartum depression. *International Journal of Childbirth Education, 30*(2), 11–13.

Stuart, S., & Koleva, H. (2014). Psychological treatments for perinatal depression. Best practice and research. *Clinical Obstetrics and Gynaecology, 28*(1), 61–70.

Tran, H., & Robb, A. (2015). SSRI use during pregnancy. *Seminars in Perinatology, 28*(15), 101–109.

U.S. Food and Drug Administration. (2019). FDA approves first treatment for post-partum depression. Retrieved from: https://www.fda.gov/news-events/press-announcements/fda-approves-first-treatment-post-partum-depression.

Wisner, K. L., Sit, D. K. T., Bogen, D. L., et al. (2017). Mental health and behavioral disorders in pregnancy. In S. G. Gabbe, J. R. Niebyl, J. L. Simpson, et al. (Eds.), *Obstetrics: Normal and problem pregnancies* (7th ed.). Philadelphia: Elsevier.

Yildiz, P., Ayers, S., & Phillips, L. (2017). The prevalence of posttraumatic stress disorder in pregnancy and after birth: A systematic review and meta-analysis. *Journal of Affective Disorder, 208*, 634–645.

32

Labor and Birth Complications

Deborah R. Bambini

LEARNING OBJECTIVES

- Differentiate between preterm birth and low birth weight.
- Describe the criteria for very preterm, early preterm, and late preterm and the implications of each.
- Discuss major risk factors associated with preterm labor.
- Analyze current interventions to prevent spontaneous preterm birth.
- Discuss the use of tocolytics and antenatal glucocorticoids for management of preterm labor.
- Design a nursing care plan for women with preterm prelabor rupture of membranes (preterm PROM).

- Explain the care of a woman with postterm pregnancy.
- Explain the challenge of caring for obese women during labor and birth.
- Summarize the nursing care for a woman experiencing a trial of labor, the induction and augmentation of labor, forceps- and vacuum-assisted birth, cesarean birth, and vaginal birth after a cesarean birth.
- Discuss obstetric emergencies and their appropriate management.

When complications arise during labor and birth, the risk for perinatal morbidity and mortality increases. Some complications are anticipated, especially if the woman is identified to be at high risk during the antepartum period; other complications are unexpected or unforeseen. It is crucial for nurses to understand the normal birth process to prevent and detect deviations from normal labor and birth and to promptly implement nursing interventions when complications arise. Optimal care of the laboring woman, fetus, and family experiencing complications is possible only when members of the interprofessional health care team use their knowledge and skills in a collaborative effort to provide competent and compassionate care. This chapter focuses on the problems of preterm labor and birth, prelabor rupture of membranes, postterm pregnancy, dysfunctional labor/dystocia, obesity, and obstetric emergencies.

PRETERM LABOR AND BIRTH

Preterm labor is generally diagnosed clinically as regular contractions along with a change in cervical effacement or dilation or both, or presentation with regular uterine contractions and cervical dilation of at least 2 cm that occurs at a preterm gestation. **Preterm birth** is any birth that occurs between 20 0/7 and 36 6/7 weeks of gestation (American College of Obstetricians and Gynecologists [ACOG], 2016/2018). Since 2014, gestational age at birth has been reported in the United States as the *obstetric estimate*, rather than according to the date of the woman's last menstrual period. The obstetric estimate represents the birth attendant's best estimate of the newborn's gestational age, as determined by using a number of sources. Thus the gestational ages reported as national statistics now are more accurate than they have been in the past (Martin, Osterman, Kimeyer, et al., 2015). The preterm birth rate for all races in the United States, which had been decreasing for nearly a decade, increased slightly to 9.85% in 2016, the most recent year for which data are available (Martin, Hamilton, Osterman, et al.,

2018). Three major practice changes have impacted reported rates: (1) improved fertility practices that reduce the risk for higher-order multiple gestations; (2) quality improvement programs that limit scheduled late preterm and near-term births to only those with valid indications; and (3) increased use of strategies to prevent recurrent preterm birth (Simhan, Iams, & Romero, 2017). In addition, the number of births to teens and young mothers has declined from 2007 to 2014 (Martin et al., 2018).

Preterm birth is also a worldwide problem. Every year, an estimated 15 million babies are born preterm and the preterm birth rate is increasing in almost all countries with reliable data (World Health Organization [WHO], 2018). The rate of preterm birth is highest in Africa and South Asia and lowest in Europe (Simhan et al., 2017). The rate of preterm birth in the United States is disproportionately distributed by race. Of the 9.85% preterm births in 2016, rates ranged from a high of 13.77% to black mothers to a low of 8.63% to Asian mothers (Martin et al., 2018).

Preterm births are categorized as *very preterm* (<32 weeks of gestation), *moderately preterm* (32 to 34 weeks of gestation), and *late preterm* (34 0/7 to 36 6/7 weeks of gestation). The degree of risk for an infant born prematurely is directly related to the degree of prematurity. About 75% of all preterm births in the United States are categorized as late preterm. Late preterm infants are at increased risk for early death and long-term health problems when compared with infants who are born full term (see Chapter 34). Although late preterm babies do experience significant problems, the great majority of infant deaths and the most serious morbidity occur among the infants who are born before 32 weeks of gestation (very preterm birth) (Simhan et al., 2017).

Preterm Birth Versus Low Birth Weight

Although they have distinctly different meanings, the terms *preterm birth* or *prematurity* and *low birth weight* were often interchanged in the past. Preterm birth describes length of gestation (i.e., <37 0/7 weeks regardless of the weight of the infant), whereas low birth weight describes only weight at the time of birth (i.e., 2500 g or less). Because birth weight was far easier to determine than gestational age, in many settings and publications low birth weight was used as a substitute term for preterm birth. Preterm birth, however, is a more dangerous health condition for an infant because less time in the uterus correlates with immaturity of body systems. Low-birth-weight babies can be, but are not necessarily, preterm; low birth weight can be caused by conditions other than preterm birth, such as intrauterine growth restriction (IUGR), a condition of inadequate fetal growth not necessarily correlated with initiation of labor. Pregnant women who have various complications of pregnancy that interfere with uteroplacental perfusion, such as gestational hypertension or poor nutrition, may give birth to a baby at term who is low birth weight because of IUGR. However, infants born at a preterm gestation can weigh more than 2500 g at birth. Currently, thanks to advances in pregnancy dating, outcomes related to gestational age can increasingly be distinguished from outcomes related to birth weight. Therefore use of birth weight as a substitute for gestational age in developed countries is no longer considered acceptable (Simhan, Berghella, & Iams, 2019).

Spontaneous Versus Indicated Preterm Birth

Preterm births can be divided into two categories: spontaneous and indicated. Spontaneous preterm births occur following an early initiation of the labor process in the apparent absence of maternal or fetal illness and make up nearly 75% of all preterm births in developed countries. Conditions such as preterm labor with intact membranes and preterm PROM often result in preterm birth (Simhan et al., 2019). Box 32.1 lists risk factors for the development of spontaneous preterm labor.

Indicated preterm births are *iatrogenic* because they occur as a means to resolve maternal or fetal risk related to continuing the pregnancy. About 25% of all preterm births in the United States are indicated because of medical or obstetric conditions that affect the mother, the fetus, or both (Simhan et al., 2017). An increase in the number of indicated preterm births between 34 and 36 weeks of gestation accounts for much of the rise in late preterm births. Box 32.2 lists common causes of indicated preterm births. The remainder of this section deals with spontaneous preterm labor and birth.

BOX 32.1 Risk Factors for Spontaneous Preterm Labor

- History of genital tract colonization, infection, or instrumentation
- African-American race
- Bleeding of uncertain origin in pregnancy
- History of a previous spontaneous preterm birth between 16 and 36 weeks of gestation[a]
- Uterine anomaly
- Use of assisted reproductive technology
- Multifetal gestation
- Cigarette smoking, substance abuse
- Prepregnancy underweight (BMI < 19.6) and prepregnancy obesity (BMI > 30)
- Periodontal disease
- Limited education and low socioeconomic status
- Late entry into prenatal care
- High levels of personal stress in one or more domains of life

[a]Strongest historic risk factor for spontaneous preterm birth.
BMI, Body mass index.
Data from Simhan, H. N., Iams, J. D., & Romero, R. (2017). Preterm labor and birth. In S. G. Gabbe, J. R. Niebyl, J. L. Simpson, et al. (Eds.), *Obstetrics: Normal and problem pregnancies* (7th ed.). Philadelphia: Elsevier.

Causes of Spontaneous Preterm Labor and Birth

Causes of spontaneous preterm labor and birth are multifactorial. Infection is definitely associated with preterm labor. Prepregnancy colonization of the upper and lower genital tract and the maternal immune response to that colonization are increasingly recognized as important factors in the infection-related risk for preterm labor. Women in spontaneous preterm labor with intact membranes commonly have organisms that are normally found in the lower genital tract present in their amniotic fluid, placenta, and membranes (Simhan et al., 2019). Clinical and laboratory evidence of infection are more common when birth occurs earlier than 30 to 32 weeks of gestation rather than closer to term. Intraabdominal infections (e.g., appendicitis) also have been related to preterm birth (Simhan et al., 2017). Women with periodontal disease have been shown to have an increased risk for preterm birth. However, the risk is not reduced by periodontal care, suggesting that the link between periodontal disease and preterm birth is not a cause-and-effect relationship (Simhan et al., 2017).

Preterm labor may also be caused by congenital structural abnormalities of the uterus, which can affect the cervix, the body of the uterus, or both. Implantation of the placenta on a uterine septum may lead to preterm birth as a result of placental separation and hemorrhage. Women who experience unexplained vaginal bleeding after the first trimester of pregnancy also have an increased risk for preterm birth. The risk rises as the number of bleeding episodes increases (Simhan et al., 2017). Genetic predisposition, gene-environment interaction, maternal and fetal stress, uterine overdistention, fetal allergy, and a decrease in progesterone are other factors that can play a part in

---

BOX 32.2 Common Causes of Indicated Preterm Birth

- Preexisting or gestational diabetes
- Chronic hypertension
- Preeclampsia
- Obstetrical disorders or risk factors in the current or a previous pregnancy
  - Previous cesarean birth via a vertical or T-shaped uterine incision
  - Cholestasis
  - Placental disorders (abruption or previa)
- Medical disorders
  - Seizures
  - Thromboembolism
  - Connective tissue disorders
  - Asthma and chronic bronchitis
  - Maternal HIV or active herpes infection
  - Obesity
  - Smoking
- Advanced maternal age
- Fetal disorders
  - Fetal compromise
    - Chronic (poor fetal growth)
    - Acute (abnormal results on a NST or BPP)
  - Excessive (polyhydramnios) or inadequate (oligohydramnios) amount of amniotic fluid
  - Fetal hydrops, ascites, blood group alloimmunization
  - Birth defects
  - Fetal complications of multifetal gestation (e.g., growth deficiency, twin-to-twin transfusion syndrome)

BPP, Biophysical profile; *HIV,* human immunodeficiency virus; *IUGR,* intrauterine growth restriction; *NST,* nonstress test.
Data from Simhan, H., Iams, J., & Romero, R. (2017). Preterm labor and birth. In S. Gabbe, J. Niebyl, J. Simpson, et al. (Eds.), *Obstetrics: Normal and problem pregnancies* (7th ed.). Philadelphia: Elsevier.

initiating preterm labor. It is becoming increasingly clear that preterm labor is caused by multiple pathologic processes that eventually result in uterine contractions, cervical changes, and rupture of membranes (Simhan et al., 2019).

Predicting Spontaneous Preterm Labor and Birth

Risk Factors

Predicting those at risk for spontaneous preterm labor and birth includes identification of risk factors. In addition to the risk factors listed in Box 32.1, social determinants such as living in a disadvantaged neighborhood, state, or region and lack of access to prenatal care also have been identified as risk factors. The risk for preterm birth also appears to be genetically related. For example, women who were themselves born prematurely have an increased risk for giving birth prematurely. Women whose sisters gave birth prematurely are also more likely to do so, and the grandparents of women who give birth prematurely are more likely to have been born prematurely themselves than the grandparents of women who give birth at term (Simhan et al., 2017; Simhan et al., 2019). Researchers have developed many risk scoring systems based on history, demographic characteristics, and current pregnancy risk factors in an attempt to determine which women might go into labor prematurely. No risk scoring system has been very successful in lowering the preterm birth rate, however, because at least 50% of all women who ultimately give birth prematurely have no identifiable risk factors (Simhan et al., 2017).

Cervical Length

One possible predictor of preterm labor is endocervical length. Changes in cervical length occur before uterine activity, so cervical measurement can identify women in whom the labor process has begun. However, because preterm cervical shortening occurs over a period of weeks, neither digital nor ultrasound cervical examination is very sensitive for predicting imminent preterm birth. Women whose cervical length as measured by transvaginal ultrasound is greater than 30 mm in the second and third trimesters of pregnancy are unlikely to give birth prematurely even if they have symptoms of preterm labor (Simhan et al., 2017; Simhan et al., 2019).

Fetal Fibronectin Test

Fetal fibronectin (fFN) has been studied extensively and is marketed in the United States as a diagnostic test for preterm labor. fFN is a glycoprotein "glue" found in plasma and produced during fetal life. It normally appears in cervical and vaginal secretions early in pregnancy and then again in late pregnancy. The test is performed by collecting fluid from the woman's vagina using a swab during a speculum examination. The presence of fFN during the late second and early third trimesters of pregnancy may be related to placental inflammation, which is thought to be one cause of spontaneous preterm labor. The presence of fFN alone is not very sensitive as a predictor of preterm birth, however. Often the test is used to predict who will *not* go into preterm labor because its negative predictive value is high. Women with a negative test have less than a 1% chance of giving birth within 2 weeks (McCue & Torbenson, 2017).

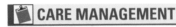

CARE MANAGEMENT

Assessment

Because all pregnant women must be considered at risk for preterm labor, assessment for factors that contribute to this risk begins early in pregnancy and continues throughout the prenatal period. The onset of preterm labor is often insidious and can be easily mistaken for normal discomforts of pregnancy, thus client education is crucial. Client problems, expected outcomes of care, and evidence-based interventions are established for each woman based on her assessment findings (see the Nursing Care Plan).

NURSING CARE PLAN

Preterm Labor

Client Problem	Expected Outcome	Nursing Interventions	Rationales
Need for health teaching related to recognition of preterm labor	Woman and partner accurately describe signs and symptoms of preterm labor.	Assess what woman and partner know about preterm labor and birth and how to recognize its presence.	To identify areas of deficit
		Discuss signs and symptoms that serve as warning signs of preterm labor so that woman or her partner has adequate information.	To identify problems early
		Provide written supplemental materials that include a list of warning signs and instructions regarding what to do if any of listed signs occur.	Couple can reinforce and review learning and act swiftly and appropriately should a sign occur
Potential injury (maternal/fetal) related to recurrence of preterm labor	Woman demonstrates ability to assess self for signs of recurring labor; maternal-fetal well-being is maintained.	Teach woman and partner how to monitor uterine contraction activity daily.	To provide immediate evidence of worsening condition
		Instruct woman and partner to report rupture of membranes, vaginal bleeding, cramping, pelvic pressure, or low backache to appropriate health care resource immediately.	Because such symptoms can be signs of labor
		Teach woman to take tocolytic or other medications per physician's orders.	To inhibit uterine contractions
		Teach woman and partner about and have them report any medication side effects immediately.	To prevent medication-induced complications
Anxiety related to preterm labor and potential birth of premature neonate	Symptoms of anxiety are reduced.	Provide calm, soothing atmosphere, and encourage family to provide emotional support.	To facilitate coping
		Encourage verbalization of fears.	To decrease intensity of emotional response
		Help woman identify and use appropriate coping strategies and support systems.	To reduce fear and anxiety

Interventions

Prevention

Primary prevention strategies that address risk factors associated with preterm labor and birth are less costly in human and financial terms than the high-tech and often long-term care required by preterm infants and their families. Programs aimed at health promotion and disease prevention that encourage healthy lifestyles for the population in general and women of childbearing age in particular should be developed. Preconception counseling and care for women, especially those with a history of preterm birth, can identify correctable risk factors and provide a means to encourage women to participate in health-promotion activities. Smoking cessation, for example, has been shown to prevent preterm labor and birth (Reedy, 2014; Simhan et al., 2017).

Preterm birth can be prevented in some women by administering prophylactic progesterone supplementation. Daily vaginal suppositories or creams or weekly intramuscular (IM) injections of 17-α hydroxyprogesterone caproate (17-P or 17-OHP [Makena]) have been shown to decrease the rate of preterm birth by about 40% in women with a history of prior preterm birth or with a short (<15-mm to 20-mm length) cervix before 24 weeks of gestation. Supplementation begins at 16 weeks and continues until 36 weeks of gestation. Progesterone supplementation does not affect the rate of preterm birth in women with multiple gestations. Exactly how progesterone works to prevent preterm birth is unclear (Simhan et al., 2017).

Early Recognition and Diagnosis

Although preterm birth is often not preventable, early recognition of preterm labor is essential to implement interventions that have been demonstrated to reduce neonatal and infant morbidity and mortality. These interventions include the following (Simhan et al., 2017):

- Transferring the mother before birth to a hospital equipped to care for her preterm infant
- Administering antibiotics during labor to prevent neonatal group B streptococci infection
- Administering antenatal glucocorticoids (e.g., betamethasone, dexamethasone) to women at risk for preterm birth to prevent or reduce neonatal and infant morbidity and mortality from health problems including respiratory distress syndrome, intraventricular hemorrhage, necrotizing enterocolitis, and other causes
- Administering magnesium sulfate to women giving birth before 32 weeks of gestation to reduce the incidence of cerebral palsy in their infants (see Evidence-Based Practice Box)

EVIDENCE-BASED PRACTICE

Magnesium Sulfate for Neuroprotection Against Cerebral Palsy

Ask the Question

For women anticipating preterm birth, can any prenatal treatment protect the premature newborn from cerebral palsy?

Search for the Evidence

Search Strategies: English research-based publications since 2014 on magnesium sulfate, neuroprotection, preterm, premature were included.

Databases Used: Cochrane Collaborative Database, National Guideline Clearinghouse (AHRQ), CINAHL, PubMed, UpToDate, and the professional websites for ACOG and AWHONN.

Critical Appraisal of the Evidence

Among the many challenges for a premature baby is the risk for cerebral palsy, the most common motor disability in children. Alert clinicians noticed that newborns whose mothers had been given magnesium sulfate for tocolysis or preeclampsia were less likely to have cerebral palsy. Further research confirmed its benefit and safety (Zeng, Xue, Tian, et al., 2016).

- Although magnesium sulfate is widely used in clinical settings, the exact mechanism by which neuroprotection occurs is not clear. It is thought that antioxidant and antiinflammatory properties of magnesium sulfate promote hemodynamic stability, thus preventing excitatory injury to neurons (Escalona-Vargas, Thagard, McGrail, et al., 2016).
- Although magnesium sulfate is no longer recommended for stopping preterm labor, the American College of Obstetricians and Gynecologists and the Society for Maternal-Fetal Medicine (2016/2018) still recommend magnesium sulfate for neuroprotection against cerebral palsy in women anticipating imminent preterm birth at less than 32 weeks of gestation. To optimize fetal neuroprotection and prevent cerebral palsy, a maternal serum magnesium level should be between 3.7 and 4.4 mg/dL at birth (Brookfield, Elkomy, Su, et al., 2017).
- Antenatal administration of magnesium sulfate prior to preterm birth prevents cerebral palsy and reduces the risk of infant death from cerebral palsy. Similar results have been seen across a range of preterm gestational ages and varied treatment protocols (Crowther, Middleton, Voysey, et al., 2017).
- Administering magnesium sulfate requires intravenous infusion and close monitoring. In a systematic review of the economic evaluation of cost of interventions for cerebral palsy, researchers found that magnesium sulfate improves newborn outcomes and results in cost savings (Shih, Tonmukayakul, Imms, et al., 2018).

Apply the Evidence: Nursing Implications

- Magnesium sulfate should be given in settings where staff are familiar with its use, monitoring is available, and emergency resuscitation and ventilation equipment are available.
- Typical use in women in active preterm labor or with preterm prelabor rupture of membranes is a 4-g loading dose given over 30-60 min, followed by the maintenance dose of 1 g/h, given until birth or for up to 24 h, whichever comes first. Other tocolytics are discontinued.
- To improve safety, the infusion should be given via infusion device in prepackaged concentrations clearly labeled as loading and maintenance doses, and double-checked by another nurse.
- Neonatal hypermagnesemia, although rare, can present as apnea, respiratory depression, lethargy, poor feeding, and hyporeflexia. An interprofessional team skilled in neonatal resuscitation should be available.

References

American College of Obstetricians and Gynecologists & Society for Maternal-Fetal Medicine. (2016, reaffirmed 2018). Committee opinion no. 652: Magnesium sulfate use in obstetrics. *Obstetrics & Gynecology, 127*(1), e52–e53.

Brookfield, K. F., Elkomy, M., Su, F., et al. (2017). Optimization of maternal magnesium sulfate administration for fetal neuroprotection: Application of a prospectively constructed pharmacokinetic model to the BEAM cohort. *The Journal of Clinical Pharmacology, 57*(11), 1419–1424.

Crowther, C. A., Middleton, P. F., Voysey, M., et al. (2017). Assessing the neuroprotective benefits for babies of antenatal magnesium sulfate: An individual participant data meta-analysis. *PLOS Medicine, 14*(10) e1002398.

Escalona-Vargas, D., Thagard, A. S., McGrail, K., et al. (2016). Observations of fetal brain activity via non-invasive magnetoencephalography following administration of magnesium sulfate for neuroprotection in preterm labor. *Prenatal Diagnosis, 36*(10), 982–984.

Shih, S. T., Tonmukayakul, U., Imms, C., et al. (2018). Economic evaluation and cost of interventions for cerebral palsy: A systematic review. *Developmental Medicine and Child Neurology, 60*(6), 543–558.

Zeng, X., Xue, Y., Tian, Q., et al. (2016). Effects and safety of magnesium sulfate on neuroprotection: A meta-analysis based on PRISMA guidelines. *Medicine, 95*(1) e2451.

Jennifer Taylor Alderman

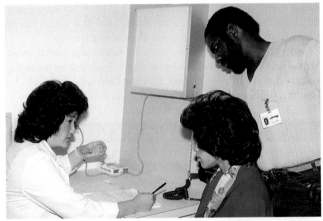

Fig. 32.1 A Nurse Teaching a Couple Signs and Symptoms of Preterm Labor. (Courtesy Marjorie Pyle, RNC, Lifecircle, Costa Mesa, CA.)

In some cases, it is both wise and possible to transport pregnant women in preterm labor to a tertiary or quaternary care center (e.g., if a woman lives in a small town where there is only a community hospital with no neonatal intensive care unit). Although maternal transport helps ensure a better health outcome for the mother and the baby, it also has a downside. Women may be transported to tertiary or quaternary centers far from home, making visits by family and friends difficult and increasing the anxiety levels of the woman and her family. Attention to the needs of the woman and her family before, during, and after the transport is essential to comprehensive nursing care (see Chapter 34).

Because more than half of preterm births occur in women without obvious risk factors, it is essential that all pregnant women are taught the symptoms of preterm labor (Box 32.3). The nurse caring for women in a prenatal setting should educate them about how to recognize symptoms of preterm labor and then assess for these symptoms at each prenatal visit. Women also must be taught the significance of these symptoms of preterm labor and what to do should they occur (see Teaching for Self-Management box: What to Do If Symptoms of Preterm Labor Occur).

In particular, client education regarding any symptoms of uterine contractions, pain, and vaginal discharge occurring between 20 0/7 and 36 6/7 weeks of gestation must emphasize that these symptoms are not just normal discomforts of pregnancy but indications of possible preterm labor (Fig. 32.1). Waiting too long to see a health care provider could result in inevitable preterm birth without sufficient time to implement the interventions that have been shown to improve infant outcomes (see preceding discussion).

As mentioned, the diagnosis of preterm labor is based on three major diagnostic criteria (ACOG, 2016/2018):

- Gestational age between 20 0/7 and 36 6/7 weeks
- Regular uterine activity, accompanied by a change in cervical effacement, dilation, or both
- Initial presentation with regular contractions and cervical dilation of at least 2 cm

If the presence of fFN is used as another diagnostic criterion, a sample of cervical fluid for testing should be obtained by sterile speculum exam. This should be obtained before any digital examination for cervical changes, because the lubricant used to examine the cervix can reduce the accuracy of the test for fFN. The presence of vaginal bleeding or ruptured membranes or a history of intercourse within the past 24 hours also can reduce the accuracy of the test results (Swanson & Baird, 2017).

The pregnant woman at 30 weeks of gestation with an irritable uterus but no documented cervical change is not in preterm labor, although she should be carefully evaluated during follow-up care to determine whether she has progressed to active preterm labor (e.g., effacement, dilation, or both). Women with preterm contractions without cervical change, especially those with a cervical dilation of less than 2 cm, should not be given tocolytic medications (ACOG, 2016/2018).

Lifestyle Modifications

Activity restriction. Bedrest, hydration, and limited work are often recommended to reduce the risk for preterm birth in women at risk for giving birth prematurely. There is no evidence, however, to support the effectiveness of these interventions, and they should not be routinely recommended. In fact, both bed rest and excessive hydration can cause potentially harmful maternal complications. Research indicates that bed rest causes adverse physical effects, including risk for thrombus formation, muscle atrophy, bone loss, cardiovascular deconditioning, and endocrine system changes (Simhan et al., 2017; Swanson & Baird, 2017). In addition, bed rest affects women and their families psychologically, emotionally, socially, and financially. Many health care providers now recommend only modified bed rest. With modified bed rest, women are usually allowed bathroom privileges for toileting and showering and can be up to the table for meals. (See the Community Activity box.)

TEACHING FOR SELF-MANAGEMENT

What to Do If Symptoms of Preterm Labor Occur

- Stop what you are doing.
- Lie down on your side.
- Drink two to three glasses of water or juice.
- Wait 1 hr.
- If symptoms get worse, call your health care provider or go to the birthing facility.
- If symptoms go away, tell your health care provider what happened at your next prenatal visit.
- If symptoms come back, call your health care provider.

Data from Reedy, N. J. (2014). Preterm labor and birth. In K. R. Simpson & P. Creehan (Eds.), *AWHONN's perinatal nursing* (4th ed.). Philadelphia: Lippincott Williams & Wilkins.

Restriction of sexual activity. Restriction of sexual activity, sometimes referred to as *pelvic rest*, is frequently recommended for women at risk for preterm birth. Evidence is lacking that this is an effective intervention for preventing preterm birth (Simhan et al., 2017).

🏠 **COMMUNITY ACTIVITY**

Activity Restriction for Preterm Labor

Identify a website intended for pregnant women who are on activity restriction for preterm labor. What criteria did you use to evaluate the website to determine the quality of the information provided? List at least three suggestions found on the website that would be helpful for women on activity restriction and their families.

Home Care

Home care of the woman at risk for preterm birth is a challenge for the nurse, who must assist the woman and her family in dealing with the many difficulties faced by families in which one member is unable to fulfill usual role responsibilities.

The woman's environment can be modified for convenience by using tables and storage units around her bed or daytime resting place to keep essential items within reach (e.g., cell or smart phone, television, radio, MP3 player, CD player, computer with Internet access, snacks, books, magazines, newspapers, and items for hobbies) (Fig. 32.2). Ensuring that the bed or couch is near a window and the bathroom is also helpful. Covering the bed with an eggcrate mattress can relieve discomfort. Women often find that a daily schedule of smaller, more frequent meals, activities (e.g., paying bills, planning and helping with meal preparation, hobbies), limited naps, and hygiene and grooming (e.g., shower, dressing in street clothes, applying makeup) reduces boredom and helps them maintain control and normalcy. (See Teaching for Self-Management box: Activities for Children of Women on Activity Restriction for additional ideas and suggestions. Also see Teaching for Self-Management: Coping with Activity Restriction in Chapter 27 for more information.) With modified bed rest, women are usually allowed bathroom privileges for toileting and showering and can be up to the table for meals.

Suppression of Uterine Activity

Tocolytics are medications given to arrest labor after uterine contractions and cervical change have occurred. No medications are currently approved for use as tocolytics by the U.S. Food and Drug Administration (FDA). Drugs marketed for other purposes, such as treatment of asthma or hypertension or as antiinflammatory or analgesic agents, are used on an "off-label" basis (i.e., drugs known to be effective for a specific purpose, although not specifically developed and tested for this purpose) to suppress preterm labor (Simhan et al., 2019). No tocolytic has been shown to reduce the rate of preterm birth. Rather, the rationale for giving these medications is to delay birth long enough to allow time for maternal transport to a Level III or Level IV neonatal care center and for corticosteroids to reach maximum benefit to reduce neonatal morbidity and mortality. Studies of individual drugs used for tocolysis rarely contain information about whether delaying birth improved infant outcomes (Simhan et al., 2017). Selecting the appropriate tocolytic medication requires consideration of each drug's effectiveness, risks, and side effects. Important contraindications exist to the use of all tocolytics. Maternal and fetal contraindications to tocolytic therapy are listed in Box 32.4. Box 32.5 describes nursing care for women receiving tocolytic therapy.

Magnesium sulfate is the most commonly used tocolytic agent, because maternal and fetal or neonatal adverse reactions are less severe and less common than with the β-adrenergic agonists. Clinicians are familiar with its use as a treatment for preeclampsia and believe it is safer to use when

---

TEACHING FOR SELF-MANAGEMENT

Activities for Children of Women on Activity Restriction

- Schedule brief play periods throughout the day.
- Keep a few favorite toys in a box or basket close to the bed or couch.
- Read to the children.
- Put puzzles together.
- Watch videos or play video games (remote control for television is ideal).
- Play card or board games.
- Color in coloring books.
- Cut out pictures from magazines and paste them on cardboard.
- Play bed basketball with a soft (sponge) ball or rolled up sock and a trash can or empty laundry basket.

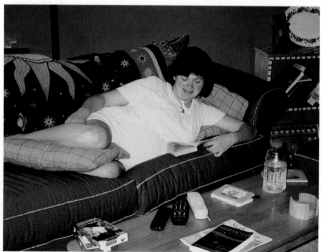

Fig. 32.2 Woman at Home on Restricted Activity for Preterm Labor Prevention. Note how she has arranged her daytime resting area so that needed items are close at hand. (Courtesy Amy Turner, Cary, NC.)

BOX 32.4   Contraindications to Tocolysis

Maternal
- Preeclampsia with severe features or eclampsia
- Bleeding with hemodynamic instability
- Contraindications to specific tocolytic medications

Fetal
- Intrauterine fetal demise
- Lethal fetal anomaly
- Nonreassuring fetal status
- Chorioamnionitis
- Preterm prelabor rupture of membranes (preterm PROM)

Data from American College of Obstetricians and Gynecologists. (2016, reaffirmed 2018). Practice bulletin no. 171: Management of preterm labor. *Obstetrics & Gynecology, 128*(4), e155–e164.

BOX 32.5   Nursing Care for the Woman Receiving Tocolytic Therapy

- Explain the purpose and side effects of the tocolytic medication(s) to the woman and her family.
- Position the woman on her side to enhance placental perfusion and reduce pressure on the cervix.
- Monitor maternal vital signs including lung sounds and respiratory effort, FHR and pattern, and labor status according to hospital protocol and professional standards.
- Assess the mother and fetus for signs of adverse reactions related to the tocolytic medication(s) being administered (see the Medication Guide: Tocolytic Therapy for Preterm Labor).
- Determine maternal fluid balance by measuring the daily weight and intake and output.
- Limit fluid intake to 2500-3000 mL/day, especially if a β-adrenergic agonist or magnesium sulfate is being administered.
- Provide psychosocial support and opportunities for the woman and family to express feelings and concerns.
- Offer comfort measures as needed.
- Encourage diversional activities and relaxation techniques.

compared with the β-adrenergic agonists. However, although magnesium sulfate is still frequently used, its effectiveness as a tocolytic is not supported by the literature (see the Medication Guide: Tocolytic Therapy for Preterm Labor) (Simhan et al., 2019; Swanson & Baird, 2017).

⚡ SAFETY ALERT

Because magnesium sulfate depresses the function of the central nervous system, it is essential that the nurse frequently assesses the woman's respiratory status, deep tendon reflexes, and level of consciousness to identify signs that the serum level of magnesium sulfate is reaching toxic levels.

β₂-adrenergic agonists (e.g., ritodrine and terbutaline [Brethine]) have been widely used as tocolytics. They have many maternal and fetal adverse reactions, however, including β_1-stimulated cardiopulmonary (e.g., tachycardia) effects and β_2-stimulated metabolic (e.g., hyperglycemia) effects. Therefore β_2-adrenergic agonists are increasingly being replaced by medications that are safer and have fewer adverse reactions. They should not be used in women with known or suspected heart disease, preeclampsia with severe features or eclampsia, pregestational or gestational diabetes, or hyperthyroidism (Simhan et al., 2017; Simhan et al., 2019). These drugs are

MEDICATION GUIDE

Tocolytic Therapy for Preterm Labor

Medication and Action	Dosage and Route	Adverse Effects	Nursing Considerations
Magnesium Sulfate CNS depressant; relaxes smooth muscle, including uterus	IV fluid should contain 40 g in 1000 mL, piggyback to primary infusion, and administer using controller pump: Loading dose: 4-6 g over 20-30 min Maintenance dose: 1-4 g/hr Use for stabilization only Discontinue within 24-48 hr at the maintenance dose or if intolerable adverse effects occur	**Maternal:** • Hot flushes, sweating, burning at the IV insertion site, nausea and vomiting, dry mouth, drowsiness, blurred vision, diplopia, headache, ileus, generalized muscle weakness, lethargy, dizziness • Hypocalcemia • Dyspnea • Transient hypotension • Some reactions may subside when loading dose is completed **Intolerable:** • Respiratory rate fewer than 12 breaths/min • Pulmonary edema • Absent DTRs • Chest pain • Severe hypotension • Altered level of consciousness • Extreme muscle weakness • Urine output <25-30 mL/hr or <100 mL/4 hr • Serum magnesium level of 10 mEq/L (9 mg/dL) or greater **Fetal (uncommon):** Decreased breathing movement Reduced FHR variability Nonreactive NST	Assess woman and fetus to obtain baseline before beginning therapy and then before and after each incremental change; follow frequency of agency protocol. Drug is almost always given IV but can also be administered IM. Monitor serum magnesium levels with higher doses; therapeutic range is 4-7.5 mEq/L or 5-8 mg/dL. Discontinue infusion and notify health care provider if intolerable adverse effects occur. Ensure that calcium gluconate is available for emergency administration to reverse magnesium sulfate toxicity. Do not give to women with myasthenia gravis. Total IV intake should be limited to 125 mL/hr.
β-Adrenergic Agonist (β-Mimetic) Terbutaline (Brethine) relaxes smooth muscle, inhibiting uterine activity and causing bronchodilation	Subcutaneous injection of 0.25 mg every 4 hr Treatment should last no longer than 24 hr Discontinue use if intolerable adverse effects occur	**Maternal (most are mild and of limited duration):** • Tachycardia, chest discomfort, palpitations, arrhythmias • Tremors, dizziness, nervousness • Headache • Nasal congestion • Nausea and vomiting • Hypokalemia • Hyperglycemia • Hypotension **Intolerable:** • Tachycardia > 130 beats/min • BP < 90/60 • Chest pain • Cardiac arrhythmias • Myocardial infarction • Pulmonary edema	Should not be used in women with known or suspected heart disease, pregestational or gestational diabetes, preeclampsia with severe features or eclampsia, hyperthyroidism, or with significant hemorrhage or possible chorioamnionitis. Myocardial infarction leading to death has been reported after use.

Continued

MEDICATION GUIDE—cont'd

Tocolytic Therapy for Preterm Labor

Medication and Action	Dosage and Route	Adverse Effects	Nursing Considerations

β-Adrenergic Agonist (β-Mimetic)—cont'd		**Fetal:**
		• Tachycardia
		• Hyperinsulinemia
		• Hyperglycemia
			Assess woman and fetus according to agency protocol, being alert for adverse effects.
			Assess maternal glucose and potassium levels before treatment is initiated and periodically during treatment. Significant hyperglycemia (>180 mg/dL) and hypokalemia (<2.5 mEq/L) may occur.
			Notify health care provider if the following are noted:
			  Maternal heart rate > 130 beats/min; arrhythmias, chest pain
			  BP < 90/60 mm Hg
			  Signs of pulmonary edema (e.g., dyspnea, crackles, decreased SaO$_2$).
			  Fetal heart rate > 180 beats/min.
			Hyperglycemia occurs more frequently in women who are being treated simultaneously with corticosteroids.
			Ensure that propranolol (Inderal) is available to reverse adverse effects related to cardiovascular function.

Prostaglandin Synthetase Inhibitors (NSAIDs)			
Indomethacin (Indocin) relaxes uterine smooth muscle by inhibiting prostaglandins	Loading dose: 50 mg orally, then 25-50 mg orally every 6 hr for 48 hr	**Maternal (common):** • Nausea and vomiting • Heartburn **(Less common but more serious):** • GI bleeding • Prolonged bleeding time • Thrombocytopenia • Asthma in aspirin-sensitive clients **Fetal:** • Constriction of ductus arteriosus • Oligohydramnios, caused by reduced fetal urine production • Neonatal pulmonary hypertension	The long-acting formulations decrease the incidence of adverse effects. Used only if gestational age is < 32 weeks. Administer for 48 hr or less. Do not use in women with renal or hepatic disease, active peptic ulcer disease, poorly controlled hypertension, asthma, or coagulation disorders. Can mask maternal fever. Assess woman and fetus according to agency policy, being alert for adverse effects. Determine amniotic fluid volume and function of fetal ductus arteriosus before initiating therapy and within 48 hr of discontinuing therapy; assessment is critical if therapy continues for more than 48 hr. Administer with food to decrease GI distress. Monitor for signs of postpartum hemorrhage.
Calcium Channel Blockers			
Nifedipine (Adalat, Procardia) relaxes smooth muscle including the uterus by blocking calcium entry	Initial dose: 10-20 mg, orally, every 3-6 hr until contractions are rare, followed by long-acting formulations of 30 or 60 mg every 8-12 hr for 48 hr while corticosteroids are being given (however, the ideal dose has not been established)	**Maternal (most effects are mild):** • Hypotension • Headache • Flushing • Dizziness • Nausea **Fetal:** • Hypotension (questionable)	Avoid concurrent use with magnesium sulfate because skeletal muscle blockade can result. Should not be given simultaneously with or immediately after terbutaline because of effects on heart rate and blood pressure. Assess woman and fetus according to agency protocol, being alert for adverse effects. Do not use sublingual route of administration.

NOTE: There are variations in recommended administration protocols; always consult agency protocol, which should be evidence based.
BP, Blood pressure; *CNS,* central nervous system; *DTRs,* deep tendon reflexes; *FHR,* fetal heart rate; *GI,* gastrointestinal; *IM,* intramuscular; *IV,* intravenous; *NSAIDs,* nonsteroidal antiinflammatory drugs; *NST,* nonstress test; *SaO$_2$,* arterial oxygen saturation; *SOB,* shortness of breath.
Data from Gilbert, E. (2011). *Manual of high risk pregnancy and delivery* (5th ed.). St. Louis: Mosby; Simhan, H. N., Berghella, V., & Iams, J. D. (2019). Prevention and management of preterm parturition. In R. Resnik, C. J. Lockwood, T. R. Moore, et al. (Eds.), *Creasy & Resnik's maternal-fetal medicine: Principles and practice* (8th ed.). Philadelphia: Elsevier; and Simhan, H. N., Iams, J. D., & Romero, R. (2017). Preterm labor and birth. In S. G. Gabbe, J. R. Niebyl, J. L. Simpson, et al. (Eds.), *Obstetrics: Normal and problem pregnancies* (7th ed.). Philadelphia: Elsevier.

also contraindicated when preterm labor is complicated by maternal fever, fetal tachycardia, or other signs of possible chorioamnionitis (Simhan et al., 2019).

Terbutaline, the most commonly administered β-adrenergic agonist used for tocolysis, relaxes uterine smooth muscle by stimulating β$_2$-receptors in the uterine smooth muscle. Terbutaline is often given subcutaneously to facilitate maternal transfer to a tertiary or quaternary center or to initiate tocolytic therapy while another agent with a slower onset of action is administered concurrently. Additionally, a subcutaneous injection of 0.25 mg may be given to suppress uterine tachysystole during labor induction or augmentation or to suppress contractions prior to cesarean birth. Long-term oral or subcutaneous administration (e.g., terbutaline pump) as maintenance therapy to suppress preterm labor has not been proven to be effective in reducing prematurity or neonatal morbidity, so terbutaline should not be used for this purpose. In addition, terbutaline has the potential to cause serious maternal cardiac problems and death (Simhan et al., 2017; Simhan et al., 2019) (see Medication Guide: Tocolytic Therapy for Preterm Labor).

Nifedipine (Adalat, Procardia), a calcium channel blocker, is a tocolytic agent that can suppress contractions. It works by preventing calcium from entering smooth muscle cells, thus reducing uterine contractions. Because of its ease of administration and low incidence of significant maternal and fetal side effects, nifedipine's use is increasing. However, the ideal dosage is not clear. It should not be administered to women with hypertension or cardiac disease (see Medication Guide: Tocolytic Therapy for Preterm Labor) (Simhan et al., 2017; Simhan et al., 2019).

⚡ **SAFETY ALERT**

Administering nifedipine and magnesium sulfate simultaneously can cause skeletal muscle blockade. In addition, nifedipine should not be given along with or immediately following a β_2-adrenergic agonist (e.g., terbutaline) because of effects on maternal heart rate and blood pressure (Simhan et al., 2017; Simhan et al., 2019).

⚡ **SAFETY ALERT**

Because using a calcium channel blocker can result in orthostatic hypotension and dizziness, it is essential to instruct women to slowly change position from supine to upright and then sit until any dizziness disappears before standing. In addition, it is important to maintain adequate fluid balance to reduce the drop in blood pressure that can occur with the drug-related vasodilation.

Indomethacin (Indocin), a nonsteroidal antiinflammatory drug (NSAID), has been shown in some trials to suppress preterm labor by blocking the production of prostaglandins. Serious maternal side effects are uncommon, and indomethacin is usually well tolerated. However, serious fetal or neonatal side effects have caused major concerns about its use as a tocolytic. Therefore limiting the use of indomethacin to a period no longer than 48 hours in women with preterm labor at less than 32 weeks of gestation is recommended (Simhan et al., 2017; Simhan et al., 2019). (see Medication Guide: Tocolytic Therapy for Preterm Labor).

Promotion of Fetal Lung Maturity

Antenatal glucocorticoids, given as IM injections to the mother to accelerate fetal lung maturity by stimulating fetal surfactant production, are now considered one of the most effective and cost-efficient interventions for preventing morbidity and mortality associated with preterm birth. Antenatal glucocorticoids have been shown to significantly reduce the incidence of respiratory distress syndrome, intraventricular hemorrhage, necrotizing enterocolitis, and death in neonates, without increasing the risk of infection in either mothers or newborns (Mercer, 2017, 2019). ACOG (2016/2018) recommends that all women between 24 and 34 weeks of gestation be given a single course of antenatal glucocorticoids when preterm birth is threatened. Because recent data indicate that betamethasone decreases neonatal respiratory morbidity when given to women between 34 0/7 and 36 6/7 weeks of gestation who are at risk for giving birth within the next 7 days and who have not previously received glucocorticoids during the current pregnancy, ACOG (2016/2018) also recommends that a course of betamethasone be given to these women. A single course of steroids may also be considered for women at 23 weeks of gestation if it seems likely that they will give birth within the next 7 days (ACOG, 2016/2018). A single repeat (rescue) course of antenatal steroids may be given to women who received their initial course more than 2 weeks previously if their gestational age remains less than 32 6/7 weeks and they are still considered likely to give birth within the next week. More than two courses of antenatal glucocorticoids, however, are not recommended (Simhan et al., 2017). The regimen for administration of antenatal glucocorticoids is given in the Medication Guide: Antenatal Glucocorticoid Therapy With Betamethasone or Dexamethasone.

💊 **MEDICATION ALERT**

All women between 24 and 34 weeks of gestation who are at risk for preterm birth should receive treatment with a single course of antenatal glucocorticoids (ACOG, 2016/2018). Because 48 hr from the time of the first injection are required for the fetus to receive optimal benefit, timely administration of the medication is essential.

MEDICATION GUIDE

Antenatal Glucocorticoid Therapy With Betamethasone or Dexamethasone

Action
Stimulates fetal lung maturation by promoting release of enzymes that induce production or release of lung surfactant. Glucocorticoids have similar maturational effects on other organs, including the brain, kidneys, and gut. **Note:** The U.S. Food and Drug Administration has not approved these medications for this use (i.e., this is an off-label use for obstetrics).

Indication
To prevent or reduce the severity of neonatal respiratory distress syndrome by accelerating lung maturity in fetuses between 24 and 34 weeks of gestation. Infants born to women who received antenatal glucocorticoids are also less likely to experience intraventricular hemorrhage, necrotizing enterocolitis, or neonatal death.

Dosage and Route
- *Betamethasone:* 12 mg intramuscular (IM) for two doses 24 hrs apart
- *Dexamethasone:* 6 mg IM for four doses 12 hrs apart

Maternal Effects
- Transient (lasting 72 hrs) increase in white blood cell and platelet counts
- Hyperglycemia

Fetal Effects
Transient (typically lasting 48-72 hrs after the last dose) decrease in fetal breathing and body movements

Nursing Considerations
- Give deep IM in ventral gluteal or vastus lateralis muscle.
- Medication *must* be given by IM injection; oral administration is *not* an acceptable alternative.
- Injection is painful.
- Medication should *not* affect maternal blood pressure.
- Assess blood glucose levels. Women with diabetes whose blood sugars have previously been well controlled may require increased insulin doses for several days.

Data from Simhan, H. N., Iams, J. D., & Romero, R. (2017). Preterm labor and birth. In S. G. Gabbe, J. R. Niebyl, J. L. Simpson, et al. (Eds.), *Obstetrics: Normal and problem pregnancies* (7th ed.). Philadelphia: Elsevier.

Management of Inevitable Preterm Birth

When preterm birth appears inevitable (i.e., is expected to occur within the next 24 hours), magnesium sulfate may be administered to reduce or prevent neonatal neurologic morbidity (e.g., cerebral palsy). The current recommendation is that magnesium sulfate for neuroprotection be given to women who are at least 24 but less than 32 weeks of gestation at the time birth is expected to occur. The magnesium sulfate infusion should not be continued longer than 24 hours if birth has not occurred. How magnesium sulfate works to provide neuroprotection is not well understood. Although it is likely that the neuroprotective effects are the result of residual concentrations of the medication in the neonate's system, data are insufficient to determine the precise maternal dose necessary to achieve the benefit (Simhan et al., 2017; Simhan et al., 2019). The recommended dose of magnesium sulfate for neuroprotection is a loading dose of 4 g given intravenously over 30 minutes, followed by a maintenance dose of 1 g/h (Simhan et al., 2017) (see Medication Guide: Tocolytic Therapy for Preterm Labor). Labor that has progressed to a cervical dilation of 4 cm or more is likely to lead to inevitable preterm birth. If birth appears imminent, members of the interprofessional health care team will make preparations to care for a small, immature neonate. Women in preterm labor can rapidly progress to birth, and a very small fetus can be born through a partially dilated cervix. Also malpresentation (e.g., breech presentation) occurs much more frequently in preterm than in term fetuses. Therefore nurses must be prepared to handle the emergency birth of a preterm infant, from either cephalic or breech presentation, without the woman's obstetric health care provider being present. Personnel skilled at neonatal resuscitation should be present at the time of birth. Equipment, supplies, and medications used for neonatal resuscitation should be gathered in advance and prepared for immediate use. If birth occurs in a hospital that is not prepared to provide continuing care for a preterm neonate, plans should be made for transfer of the baby as soon as possible to a facility with a higher level of care.

Fetal and Early Neonatal Loss

Preterm birth or the presence of congenital anomalies or genetic disorders incompatible with life are major reasons for intrauterine fetal demise (stillbirth) or early neonatal death. In many of these situations the parents will already have been told that the fetus has died or that the baby has a condition that is incompatible with life and will most likely die very soon after birth. Sometimes, however, the fetal death is unexpected, diagnosed only after the woman has been admitted to the labor and birth unit. Whatever the case, labor and birth nurses must be prepared to provide sensitive care to these women and their families (see Chapter 37).

If fetal or early neonatal death is expected, the parents and members of the interprofessional health care team need to discuss the situation before the birth and decide on a management plan that is acceptable to everyone. Despite counseling about the likelihood of a poor outcome, some parents want "everything possible" to be done for the baby including cesarean birth for an abnormal fetal heart rate (FHR) tracing. If such intervention is not desired, usually the FHR is not monitored during labor.

Another major decision is whether to attempt neonatal resuscitation. Sometimes the feasibility of neonatal resuscitation cannot be determined until the baby's size and physical appearance have been assessed. If the baby is too small, too immature, or too malformed for effective resuscitation, palliative care can be provided instead. The baby is kept warm and comfortable, at the mother's bedside, in the nursery, or at home, depending on the parents' desires, until death occurs. Parents can choose to view and hold the baby as they wish.

After the birth the woman should be given the opportunity to decide if she wants to stay on the maternity unit or be moved to another hospital unit. She may prefer to be away from the sound of crying babies and exposure to other families who have had healthy infants. However,

postpartum care and grief support may not be as sensitive or effective on another hospital unit, where the staff is not experienced in postpartum and bereavement care. Whether death occurs in utero or after birth, parents are faced with the same needs. See Chapter 37 for additional information on dealing with families experiencing a perinatal loss.

PRELABOR RUPTURE OF MEMBRANES

Prelabor rupture of membranes (PROM) (formerly termed *premature rupture of membranes*) is the spontaneous rupture of the amniotic sac and leakage of amniotic fluid beginning before the onset of labor at any gestational age. **Preterm prelabor rupture of membranes (preterm PROM or pPROM)** (i.e., membrane rupture before 37 0/7 weeks of gestation) complicates approximately 3% of all pregnancies in the United States (ACOG, 2018b). Preterm PROM occurs twice as often in African Americans as in other racial groups. The frequency of preterm PROM appears to have decreased since the 1990s (Mercer, 2017).

Preterm PROM most likely results from pathologic weakening of the amniotic membranes caused by inflammation, stress from uterine contractions, or other factors that cause increased intrauterine pressure (IUP). Infection of the urogenital tract is a major risk factor associated with preterm PROM (Mercer, 2017; Mercer & Chien, 2019). Box 32.6 lists other risk factors. PROM or preterm PROM is diagnosed after the woman reports either a sudden gush of fluid or a slow leak of fluid from the vagina.

Chorioamnionitis is the most common maternal complication of preterm PROM, making it a major complication of pregnancy (see later discussion). Other less common but serious maternal complications include placental abruption, retained placenta and hemorrhage, sepsis, and death (Mercer, 2017; Mercer & Chien, 2019). Fetal complications from preterm PROM are primarily related to intrauterine infection, cord prolapse, umbilical cord compression associated with oligohydramnios, and placental abruption. Pulmonary hypoplasia is a common complication of PROM that occurs before 20 weeks of gestation (Mercer; Mercer & Chien).

📋 CARE MANAGEMENT

Management of PROM, regardless of the gestational age at which it occurs, is determined for each woman based on an assessment of the estimated risk for maternal, fetal, and neonatal complications if pregnancy is allowed to continue or immediate labor and birth are attempted.

BOX 32.6 Risk Factors for Preterm Prelabor Rupture of Membranes

- History of prior preterm birth, especially if associated with preterm PROM
- History of cervical conization or cerclage
- Urinary or genital tract infection
- Short (<25 mm) cervical length identified by transvaginal ultrasound
- Preterm labor or symptomatic contractions in the current pregnancy
- Uterine overdistention
- Second- or third-trimester bleeding
- Pulmonary disease
- Connective tissue disorders
- Low socioeconomic status
- Low body mass index
- Nutritional deficiencies (copper and ascorbic acid)
- Cigarette smoking

Data from Mercer, B. (2017). Premature rupture of the membranes. In S. Gabbe, J. Niebyl, J. Simpson, et al. (Eds.), *Obstetrics: Normal and problem pregnancies* (7th ed.). Philadelphia: Elsevier.

At term (at or after 37 0/7 weeks of gestation), because infection is the greatest maternal, fetal, and neonatal risk, birth is the best option. Labor will most likely be induced if it does not begin spontaneously soon after PROM occurs (Mercer, 2017; Mercer & Chien, 2019).

Active pursuit of labor and birth, rather than expectant management, is usually recommended for women who experience preterm PROM between 34 and 36 weeks of gestation. Although infants born at this gestational age have a higher risk for complications than babies born at or after 37 0/7 weeks, serious morbidity and mortality is uncommon. Because conservative management at this gestational age prolongs pregnancy by only a few days, significantly increases the risk for chorioamnionitis, and has not been shown to improve neonatal outcomes, immediate birth is generally considered to be the best management option (Mercer & Chien, 2019). If pulmonary maturity can be documented, women with preterm PROM at 32 to 33 weeks gestation may also be offered immediate birth because with conservative management they have an increased risk for complications such as umbilical cord compression (Mercer, 2017; Mercer & Chien).

Preterm PROM before 32 weeks of gestation is usually managed expectantly or conservatively, because the risks to the fetus and newborn associated with preterm birth are considered to be greater than the risk for infection. Women will likely be hospitalized in an attempt to prolong the pregnancy and allow additional time for fetal maturation unless intrauterine infection, significant vaginal bleeding, placental abruption, or advanced labor is evident; or fetal assessment becomes nonreassuring. Conservative management may require transfer to a hospital that is prepared to provide 24-hour neonatal resuscitation and intensive care (Mercer & Chien, 2019). Ideally transfer should occur early in the course of care, before birth becomes imminent or complications arise (Mercer, 2017). Nursing support of the woman and her family is critical at this time. They are often anxious about the health of the baby and the woman may fear that she was responsible in some way for the membrane rupture. Other nursing interventions include encouraging expression of feelings and concerns, providing information, and making referrals as needed.

Conservative management of preterm PROM includes fetal assessment at least daily because of the risk for FHR abnormalities as a result of umbilical cord compression. Often this assessment will be performed using the nonstress test (NST) and biophysical profile (BPP) (Mercer & Chien, 2019). The woman should also be taught how to assess her fetus using daily fetal movement counts (DFMCs) because a slowing of fetal movement is a warning sign of severe fetal compromise. (See Chapter 26 for further discussion of these tests.) In addition, the woman will be monitored for signs of labor, placental abruption, and the development of intrauterine infection (Mercer & Chien).

ACOG (2018b) recommends that all women with preterm PROM between 24 0/7 and 34 0/7 weeks of gestation be given a single course of antenatal glucocorticoids. A single course of glucocorticoids may also be considered for women as early as 23 0/7 weeks of gestation if they are at risk for giving birth within the next 7 days. Current data suggest that antenatal glucocorticoid use is not associated with an increased risk for either maternal or neonatal infection. Whether to give a single rescue course of glucocorticoids to women with preterm PROM is controversial and there is insufficient evidence at this time to make a recommendation (ACOG, 2018b).

A 7-day course of broad-spectrum antibiotics (e.g., ampicillin/amoxicillin and erythromycin) is administered. Antibiotic treatment has been shown to significantly prolong the time between membrane rupture and birth, decrease the incidence of maternal chorioamnionitis, and reduce infections and gestational age-dependent complications in the neonate such as the need for oxygen or surfactant therapy and intraventricular hemorrhage (Mercer, 2017).

Administering magnesium sulfate for fetal neuroprotection to women with preterm PROM before 32 weeks of gestation who are thought to be at imminent risk for giving birth prematurely is recommended (ACOG, 2018; Simhan et al., 2017) (see the earlier discussion for more information on magnesium sulfate administration for this reason).

Vigilance for signs of infection is a major part of the client education and nursing care after preterm PROM. The woman must be taught how to keep her genital area clean and that nothing should be introduced into her vagina. Signs of infection (e.g., fever, foul-smelling vaginal discharge, maternal and fetal tachycardia) should be reported immediately. If chorioamnionitis develops, the woman is placed on broad-spectrum antibiotics and birth is accomplished (Mercer, 2017).

CHORIOAMNIONITIS

Chorioamnionitis, bacterial infection of the amniotic cavity, is a major cause of complications for both mothers and newborns at any gestational age. It occurs in approximately 1% to 5% of term births but in as many as 25% of preterm births (Duff & Birsner, 2017). Other terms for this condition include *amnionitis* and *intrapartum infection*. Chorioamnionitis is usually diagnosed by the clinical findings of maternal fever, maternal and fetal tachycardia, uterine tenderness, and purulent amniotic fluid in the absence of another evident source of infection (Duff & Birsner; Mercer, 2017).

Chorioamnionitis most often occurs after membranes rupture or labor begins, as organisms that are part of the normal vaginal flora ascend into the amniotic cavity. Many of the risk factors for chorioamnionitis are associated with a long labor, such as prolonged membrane rupture, multiple vaginal examinations, and use of internal FHR and contraction monitoring modes (Duff, 2019). Other risk factors include young maternal age, low socioeconomic status, nulliparity, and preexisting infections of the lower genital tract (Duff & Birsner, 2017).

Women with chorioamnionitis can develop bacteremia. They are also more likely to have dysfunctional labor, which can result in the need for cesarean birth (see later discussion). If cesarean birth is necessary, wound infection or pelvic abscess are complications that can occur (Duff & Birsner, 2017).

Neonatal risks include pneumonia, bacteremia, and meningitis. Death is more likely to occur in preterm than in term infants (Duff & Birsner, 2017). There is increasing evidence that intrauterine infection is associated with increased risks for respiratory distress syndrome, periventricular leukomalacia, and cerebral palsy. It is thought that intrauterine infection leads to fetal infection that eventually produces a fetal inflammatory response syndrome with resulting pulmonary and central nervous system (CNS) damage (Duff, 2019).

In order to prevent maternal and neonatal complications, prompt treatment with intravenous (IV) broad-spectrum antibiotics and birth of the fetus are necessary. Ampicillin or penicillin and gentamicin are the antibiotics most often used to treat chorioamnionitis during labor. After cesarean birth, an antibiotic that provides coverage for anaerobic organisms, such as clindamycin (Cleocin) or metronidazole (Flagyl), should be added (Duff & Birsner, 2017; Duff, 2019). One additional dose of a combination of broad-spectrum antibiotics (e.g., ampicillin and gentamicin) given postpartum is usually sufficient treatment for women with chorioamnionitis (Duff).

The increased use of intrapartum antibiotic prophylaxis during labor in women who are group B streptococci (GBS) positive to prevent neonatal GBS infection has decreased the incidence of chorioamnionitis. Other measures that have proven to be effective in decreasing the frequency of chorioamnionitis are active management of labor (see later discussion), induction of labor, rather than expectant management, following rupture of membranes at term, and use of prophylactic antibiotics in selected women with preterm PROM (Duff, 2019).

POSTTERM PREGNANCY, LABOR, AND BIRTH

A postterm pregnancy (also sometimes referred to as a *postdates* or *prolonged* pregnancy) is one that reaches 42 0/7 weeks of gestation or more (ACOG & Society for Maternal-Fetal Medicine [SMFM], 2013/2017). According to the Centers for Disease Control and Prevention, less than 0.5% of all births in the United States were postterm in 2016, a percentage that essentially has not changed for the past several years (Martin et al., 2018). Many pregnancies are misdiagnosed as postterm. The use of first-trimester ultrasound for pregnancy dating has confirmed that the first day of the last menstrual period (LMP), traditionally used for pregnancy dating, is much less reliable as a predictor of true gestational age. Therefore use of the LMP alone for pregnancy dating tends to greatly overestimate the number of postterm gestations (Rampersad & Macones, 2017).

The exact cause of true postterm pregnancy is still unknown. However, it is clear that the timing of labor is determined by complex interactions among the mother, fetus, and placenta. For example, placental sulfatase deficiency causes low estrogen production. Women with this disorder generally do not go into spontaneous labor. This is an example of a genetic cause for postterm pregnancy that supports the important role of the placenta in labor initiation. Risk factors for postterm pregnancy include a first pregnancy, prior postterm pregnancy, a male fetus, obesity, and a genetic predisposition (Rampersad & Macones, 2017).

Clinical manifestations of postterm pregnancy include maternal weight loss (more than 1.4 kg [approximately 3 lb]/week) and decreased uterine size (related to decreased amniotic fluid), meconium in the amniotic fluid, and advanced bone maturation of the fetal skeleton with an exceptionally hard fetal skull.

Maternal and Fetal Risks

A number of factors related to postterm pregnancy, including labor dystocia, severe perineal injuries, chorioamnionitis, endomyometritis, postpartum hemorrhage, and cesarean birth are associated with significant maternal risk for morbidity during the intrapartum period (Rampersad & Macones, 2017; Sheibani & Wing, 2017). Each intervention, such as induction of labor with prostaglandins or oxytocin, forceps- or vacuum-assisted birth, and cesarean birth carries its own set of risks. The woman also may experience fatigue, physical discomfort, and psychologic reactions such as anxiety, depression, frustration, and feelings of inadequacy as she passes her estimated date of birth. Relationships with close friends and family members may become strained, and the woman's negative feelings about herself may be projected as feelings of resentment toward the fetus.

Another complication associated with postterm pregnancy is abnormal fetal growth. Although the risk for having a small for gestational age infant is increased, only 10% to 20% of postterm fetuses are undernourished. The risk for macrosomia increases as gestational age advances. Macrosomia occurs when the placenta continues to provide adequate nutrients to support fetal growth after 40 weeks of gestation. Macrosomic infants have an increased risk for operative birth and shoulder dystocia, leading to fetal injury (Rampersad & Macones, 2017).

Other fetal risks associated with postterm gestation are related to the intrauterine environment. Decreased amniotic fluid, or *oligohydramnios*, is a common finding in postterm pregnancy. Because of the decreased amount of amniotic fluid, there is a potential for cord compression and resulting hypoxemia. Other potential complications include meconium-stained amniotic fluid and increased risk for meconium aspiration (Rampersad & Macones, 2017).

Postmaturity syndrome occurs in 10% to 20% of neonates born following postterm pregnancies. The postmature infant has decreased subcutaneous fat and lacks lanugo and vernix. Other characteristics of postmature infants include dry, cracked, peeling skin; long nails; and meconium staining of skin, nails, and umbilical cord (see Chapter 34) (Rampersad & Macones, 2017).

📋 CARE MANAGEMENT

The management of postterm pregnancy is somewhat controversial. Because of the increased risk for stillbirth, antepartum fetal assessment beginning at 41 0/7 weeks of gestation may be considered (ACOG, 2014/2019). There are several options for performing fetal surveillance, including the NST, contraction stress test (CST), BPP, or modified BPP. Once begun, fetal assessment is usually performed once or twice per week for the remainder of the pregnancy. Data are not sufficient to make a recommendation regarding the best assessment test or the optimal frequency of testing (ACOG, 2014/2019) (see Chapter 26 for a discussion of these tests). If the cervix is favorable, labor can be induced at 41 weeks of gestation. Studies have shown a significantly increased rate of perinatal mortality after 41 weeks of gestation (Sheibani & Wing, 2017). Currently it is recommended that birth occur after 42 0/7 weeks and by 42 6/7 weeks of gestation to decrease the risk for perinatal morbidity and mortality (ACOG, 2014/2019; Rampersad & Macones, 2017).

During the postterm period the woman is encouraged to assess fetal activity daily, assess for signs of labor, and keep appointments with her obstetric health care provider (see Teaching for Self-Management box: Postterm Pregnancy). The woman and her family should be encouraged to express their feelings (e.g., frustration, anger, impatience, fear) about the prolonged pregnancy and helped realize that these feelings are normal. At times the emotional and physical strain of a postterm pregnancy can seem overwhelming. Referral to a support group or another supportive resource may be needed.

TEACHING FOR SELF-MANAGEMENT

Postterm Pregnancy

- Perform daily fetal movement counts.
- Assess for signs of labor.
- Call your obstetric health care provider if your membranes rupture or if you notice a decrease in or no fetal movement.
- Keep appointments for fetal assessment tests and cervical checks.
- Go to the hospital soon after labor begins.

During labor the fetus of a woman with a postterm pregnancy should be continuously monitored electronically to accurately assess the FHR and pattern. The aging placenta in a woman with a postterm pregnancy can produce disruption in oxygen transfer to the fetus during contractions, resulting in late decelerations caused by transient fetal hypoxemia. Inadequate fluid volume, often noted in women with postterm pregnancy, can lead to compression of the umbilical cord, which results in fetal hypoxemia that is reflected in variable or prolonged deceleration patterns. If oligohydramnios is present, an amnioinfusion may be performed to restore amniotic fluid volume to maintain a cushioning of the cord. See Chapter 18 for additional information on causes and management of these FHR deceleration patterns and amnioinfusion.

CLINICAL REASONING CASE STUDY

Postterm Pregnancy

Angela is a 31-year-old primigravida, presenting to the office for a routine prenatal visit. She is 40 weeks and 2 days of gestation and expresses her concern, stating, "I am really tired and just want this baby out! But he just seems to have settled in; he's gotten really quiet lately. It's a good thing, though, because I'm not really ready, I still need to borrow a car seat."

Assessment reveals:

Weight—3 pound (1.4 kg) increase in past week

Blood pressure—124/68

Urine—trace protein, trace glucose

1. What is the priority concern or client need in this situation? Support your answer with data as stated in the case.
2. List other client needs/problems in this case.
3. Identify any additional information or assessment data that is needed by the nurse in planning care for this client.
4. What nursing actions are appropriate in this situation?
   a. What is the priority nursing action? (What should the nurse do first?)
   b. Describe other nursing interventions that are important to providing optimal client care.
5. Describe the roles/responsibilities of the interprofessional health care team members (other than nurses) who may be involved in providing care for this client.

DYSFUNCTIONAL LABOR (DYSTOCIA)

Dystocia refers to a lack of progress in labor for any reason (Kilpatrick & Garrison, 2017). **Dysfunctional labor** is defined as a long, difficult, or abnormal labor. Dystocia/dysfunctional labor is responsible for approximately 30% of all cesarean births (Berghella, Mackeen, & Jauniaux, 2017) and the most common indication for primary cesarean birth (ACOG & SMFM, 2014). It can be caused by any of the following factors (Cunningham, Leveno, Bloom, et al., 2018):

- Ineffective uterine contractions or maternal bearing-down efforts (the *powers*)
- Fetal causes, including abnormalities of presentation, position, or development (the *passenger*)
- Alterations in the pelvic structure, including abnormalities of the maternal bony pelvis or soft-tissue abnormalities of the reproductive tract (the *passage*)

These factors are interdependent. Each may exist alone or in combination with others. In assessing the woman for an abnormal labor pattern, the nurse must consider the ways in which these factors interact and influence labor progress. Dysfunctional labor is suspected when there is an alteration in the characteristics of uterine contractions, a lack of progress in the rate of cervical dilation, or a lack of progress in fetal descent and expulsion, resulting in an abnormal labor pattern.

Abnormal Uterine Activity

Abnormal uterine activity can occur throughout first-stage labor. Ineffective contractions that are either hypertonic or hypotonic can result from abnormal uterine activity. Common labor disorders caused by abnormal uterine activity are discussed next.

Latent Phase Disorders

A common labor disorder that occurs during the latent phase of first-stage labor is *hypertonic uterine dysfunction*. The woman experiencing hypertonic uterine dysfunction, or primary dysfunctional labor, often is an anxious first-time mother who is having painful and frequent contractions that are ineffective in causing cervical dilation or effacement to progress. These contractions usually occur in the latent phase of first-stage labor (cervical dilation of <6 cm) and are usually uncoordinated. The force of the contractions may be in the midsection of the uterus rather than in the fundus; therefore the uterus cannot apply downward pressure to push the presenting part against the cervix. The uterus may not relax completely between contractions. Some women can spend days in protracted latent labor.

Women with hypertonic uterine dysfunction may be exhausted and express concern about loss of control because of the intense pain they are experiencing and the lack of progress. They can be managed expectantly, because most women will eventually enter the active phase of labor. Another management approach is to provide therapeutic rest, which is achieved with a warm bath or shower and an analgesic, such as morphine, to inhibit uterine contractions, reduce pain, and encourage sleep (Sheibani & Wing, 2017). In the absence of pain, zolpidem (Ambien) may be used to facilitate rest and sleep. After several hours of rest, these women are likely to awaken in active labor with a normal uterine contraction pattern.

Active-Phase Disorders

Active-phase labor disorders can be divided into either *protraction disorders,* where progress in labor is slower than normal, or *arrest disorders,* where there is no progress in labor (ACOG & SMFM, 2014; Sheibani & Wing, 2017). The most common cause of an active-phase protraction disorder is inadequate uterine activity (*hypotonic uterine dysfunction*) (Sheibani & Wing, 2017). The woman initially makes normal progress into the active phase of first-stage labor, but then the contractions become weak and inefficient or stop altogether. The uterus is easily indented, even at the peak of contractions. Intrauterine pressure during the contraction (usually < 25 mm Hg) is insufficient for progress of cervical effacement and dilation. Cephalopelvic disproportion (CPD) (see later discussion) and fetal malposition are other common causes of active-phase labor protraction disorders. Examples of fetal malposition are an extended (rather than flexed) fetal head, brow or face presentation, and occiput posterior presentation (Sheibani & Wing, 2017).

Evaluation of arrest during the first stage of labor includes an assessment of uterine activity using an intrauterine pressure catheter (IUPC) (see Chapter 18 for more information on the IUPC). Fetal presentation, position, station, and estimated fetal weight must also be evaluated. If findings are normal, labor augmentation measures may be implemented (e.g., ambulation, hydrotherapy, rupture of membranes, nipple stimulation, or oxytocin infusion). Most women respond to these interventions by resuming progression of cervical dilation and are able to give birth vaginally (Sheibani & Wing, 2017).

Secondary Powers

Secondary powers, or bearing-down efforts, are compromised when large amounts of analgesic medications are given. Anesthesia may also block the bearing-down reflex and, as a result, alter the effectiveness of voluntary bearing-down efforts. Exhaustion resulting from lack of sleep or long labor and fatigue resulting from inadequate hydration and food intake reduce the effectiveness of the woman's voluntary bearing-down efforts. Maternal position can work against the forces of gravity and decrease the strength and efficiency of the contractions. Table 32.1 summarizes the characteristics of dysfunctional labor.

Abnormal Labor Patterns

Six abnormal labor patterns were identified and classified by Friedman (1989) decades ago according to the nature of the cervical dilation and fetal descent. These patterns are (1) prolonged latent phase, (2) protracted active-phase dilation, (3) secondary arrest: no change,

TABLE 32.1   Dysfunctional Labor: Primary and Secondary Powers

PRIMARY POWERS (ABNORMAL UTERINE ACTIVITY)		SECONDARY POWERS
Hypertonic Uterine Dysfunction	**Hypotonic Uterine Dysfunction**	**Inadequate Voluntary Expulsive Forces**
Description		
Usually occurs early in latent phase labor; cause unknown, may be related to fear and tension	Cause is usually cephalopelvic disproportion or fetal malposition	Involves abdominal and levator ani muscles Occurs in second stage of labor; cause may be related to nerve block anesthetic, analgesia, exhaustion
Change in Pattern of Progress		
Pain out of proportion to intensity of contractions and to effectiveness of contractions in effacing and dilating the cervix Contractions increase in frequency and are uncoordinated Uterus is contracted between contractions, cannot be indented	Contractions decrease in frequency and intensity Uterus easily indented even at peak of contractions Uterus relaxed between contractions (normal)	No voluntary urge to push or bear down or inadequate or ineffective pushing
Potential Maternal Effects		
Loss of control related to intensity of pain and lack of progress Exhaustion Fear regarding unexpected nature of labor	Infection Exhaustion Stress regarding change in progress	Spontaneous vaginal birth prevented; assisted birth likely
Potential Fetal Effects		
Fetal asphyxia with meconium aspiration	Fetal infection Fetal and neonatal death	Fetal asphyxia
Care Management		
Initiate therapeutic rest measures Administer analgesic (e.g., morphine) if membranes are intact and pelvic adequacy is confirmed Relieve pain to permit woman to rest Assist with measures to enhance rest and relaxation (e.g., hydrotherapy, massage, music, distracting activities)	Rule out cephalopelvic disproportion Augment labor with oxytocin (Pitocin) Perform amniotomy Assist with measures to enhance the progress of labor (e.g., position changes, ambulation, hydrotherapy)	Coach woman in bearing down with contractions; assist with relaxation between contractions Position woman in favorable position for pushing Reduce epidural infusion rate Assist with forceps- or vacuum-assisted birth Prepare for cesarean birth if abnormal fetal status occurs

(4) protracted descent, (5) arrest of descent, and (6) failure of descent. These patterns may result from a variety of causes, including ineffective uterine contractions, pelvic contractures, CPD, abnormal fetal presentation or position, early use of analgesics, nerve block analgesia or anesthesia, and anxiety and stress. Progress in either the first or the second stage of labor can be protracted (prolonged) or arrested (stopped). Abnormal progress can be identified by plotting cervical dilation and fetal descent on a labor graph (partogram) at various intervals after the onset of labor and comparing the resulting curve with the expected labor curve for a nulliparous or multiparous labor. If a woman exhibits an abnormal labor pattern, the obstetric health care provider should be notified.

Maternal morbidity and mortality from uterine rupture, infection, severe dehydration, and postpartum hemorrhage are higher for women experiencing dysfunctional labor. The fetus is at increased risk for hypoxia. A long and difficult labor also can have an adverse psychologic effect on the mother, father or partner, and family.

Studies done within the past 2 decades indicate that the contemporary pattern of labor progression is different from what Friedman observed in the 1950s. In general, modern labor progresses at a slower rate for both nulliparous and multiparous women. The active labor phase now begins at 6 cm cervical dilation and lasts twice as long as Friedman described. It is common for more than 2 hours to pass in the active phase of labor without cervical dilation. Maternal characteristics have changed considerably since Friedman's work was published.

In general, women giving birth now are older and heavier, and both of these factors are associated with longer labors. Clinical guidelines incorporating this new information are being developed by organizations such as ACOG and SMFM to assist health care providers in managing contemporary labor and birth (ACOG & SMFM, 2014).

Precipitous Labor

Precipitous labor is defined as labor that lasts less than 3 hours from the onset of contractions to the time of birth. This abnormal labor pattern occurs in approximately 3% of all births in the United States. Precipitous birth alone is not usually associated with significant maternal or infant morbidity or mortality (Cunningham et al., 2018).

Precipitous labor may result from hypertonic uterine contractions that are tetanic in intensity. Conditions often associated with this type of uterine contraction include placental abruption, uterine tachysystole, and recent cocaine use. Maternal complications can include uterine rupture, lacerations of the birth canal, amniotic fluid embolus (AFE) (anaphylactoid syndrome of pregnancy), and postpartum hemorrhage caused by uterine atony. Fetal complications include hypoxia caused by decreased periods of uterine relaxation between contractions, and, in rare instances, intracranial trauma related to rapid birth (Cunningham et al., 2018).

Women who have experienced precipitous labor often describe feelings of disbelief that their labor began so quickly, alarm that their labor progressed so rapidly, panic about the possibility they would not make it to the hospital in time to give birth, and finally, relief when they arrived at the hospital. In addition, women have expressed frustration when nurses did not believe them when they reported their readiness to push. Progress can be so rapid in some women that they may have difficulty remembering the details of their labor and birth. They should be provided with an opportunity to discuss their labor and birth experiences with caregivers who were present.

Alterations in Pelvic Structure

Pelvic Dystocia

Pelvic dystocia can occur whenever there are contractures of the pelvic diameters that reduce the capacity of the bony pelvis, including the inlet, the midpelvis, the outlet, or any combination of these planes. Pelvic contractures may be caused by congenital abnormalities, maternal malnutrition, neoplasms, or lower spinal disorders. An immature pelvic size predisposes some adolescent mothers to pelvic dystocia. Pelvic deformities also can be the result of vehicular or other accidents or trauma.

Soft-Tissue Dystocia

Soft-tissue dystocia results from obstruction of the birth passage by an anatomic abnormality other than that involving the bony pelvis. The obstruction can result from placenta previa (low-lying placenta) that partially or completely obstructs the internal cervical os. Other causes, such as leiomyomas (uterine fibroids) in the lower uterine segment, ovarian tumors, and a full bladder or rectum, may prevent the fetus from entering the pelvis. Occasionally cervical edema occurs during labor when the cervix is caught between the presenting part and the symphysis pubis or when the woman begins bearing-down efforts prematurely, thereby inhibiting complete dilation. Sexually transmitted infections (e.g., human papillomavirus) can alter cervical tissue integrity and thus interfere with adequate effacement and dilation.

Fetal Causes

Dystocia of fetal origin can be caused by anomalies, excessive fetal size (macrosomia), malpresentation, malposition, or multifetal pregnancy. Complications associated with dystocia of fetal origin include neonatal asphyxia, fetal injuries or fractures, and maternal vaginal lacerations. Although spontaneous vaginal birth is possible in these instances, a forceps-assisted, vacuum-assisted, or cesarean birth often is necessary.

Anomalies

Gross ascites, large tumors, open neural tube defects (e.g., myelomeningocele), and hydrocephalus are examples of fetal anomalies that can cause dystocia. The anomalies affect the relationship of the fetal anatomy to the maternal pelvic capacity, with the result that the fetus cannot descend through the pelvis and birth canal.

Cephalopelvic Disproportion

Cephalopelvic disproportion (CPD), also called *fetopelvic disproportion (FPD)*, is disproportion between the size of the fetus and the size of the mother's pelvis. With CPD the fetus cannot fit through the maternal pelvis to be born vaginally. Although CPD is often related to excessive fetal size, or macrosomia (i.e., 4000 g or more), the problem in many cases is malposition of the fetal presenting part rather than true CPD (Sheibani & Wing, 2017). Fetal macrosomia is associated with maternal diabetes mellitus, obesity, multiparity, or the large size of one or both parents. If the maternal pelvis is too small, abnormally shaped, or deformed, CPD may be of maternal origin. In this case, the fetus may be of average size or even smaller. CPD cannot be accurately predicted (Sheibani & Wing).

Malposition

The most common fetal malposition is persistent occipitoposterior position (i.e., right occipitoposterior [ROP] or left occipitoposterior [LOP]; see Chapter 16), which is present in 20% of early labors, though

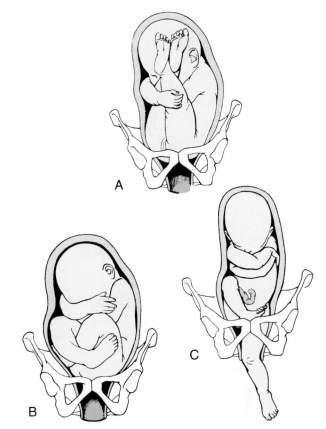

Fig. 32.3 Breech Presentation. (A) Frank breech. (B) Complete breech. (C) Single footling breech. (From Gilbert, E. [2011]. *Manual of high risk pregnancy & delivery* [5th ed.]. St. Louis: Mosby.)

only 5% of these are persistent through the end of labor (Verhaeghe, Parot-Schinkel, Bouet, et al., 2018). Labor, especially the second stage, is prolonged. The woman typically complains of severe back pain from the pressure of the fetal head (occiput) pressing against her sacrum. See Box 19.8 for suggested positions to relieve back pain and encourage rotation of the fetal occiput to an anterior position, which will facilitate birth.

Malpresentation

Malpresentation (the fetal presentation is something other than cephalic or head first) is another commonly reported complication of labor and birth. Breech presentation is the most common form of malpresentation, occurring in 3% to 4% of all labors (Thorp & Grantz, 2019). The three types of breech presentation are as follows (Lanni, Gherman, & Gonik, 2017) (Fig. 32.3):

- Frank breech (hips flexed, knees extended)
- Complete breech (hips and knees flexed)
- Footling breech (one or both hips are partially or fully extended). One foot (single footling) or both feet (double footling) present before the buttocks.

Breech presentations are associated with multifetal gestation, preterm birth, fetal and maternal anomalies, polyhydramnios, and oligohydramnios. High rates of breech presentation are also noted in fetuses with certain genetic disorders (e.g., trisomies 13, 18, and 21; Potter syndrome [renal agenesis]; and myotonic dystrophy). Fetuses with neuromuscular disorders have a high rate of breech presentation, perhaps because they are less capable of movement within the uterus. Abnormal amniotic fluid volume (both increased and decreased) also contributes to more breech presentations because it affects fetal mobility. Breech presentation is diagnosed by abdominal palpation (e.g., Leopold maneuvers) and vaginal examination and confirmed by ultrasound scan (Lanni et al., 2017; Thorp & Grantz, 2019).

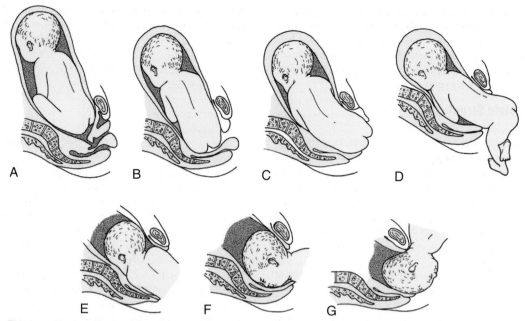

Fig. 32.4 Mechanism of Labor in Breech Presentation. (A) Breech before onset of labor. (B) Engagement and internal rotation. (C) Lateral flexion. (D) External rotation or restitution. (E) Internal rotation of shoulders and head. (F) Face rotates to sacrum when occiput is anterior. (G) Head is born by gradual flexion during elevation of fetal body.

During labor the descent of the fetus in a breech presentation may be slow because the breech is not as effective a dilating wedge as is the fetal head. There is risk for prolapse of the cord if the membranes rupture in early labor. The presence of meconium in amniotic fluid is not necessarily a sign of fetal distress because it results from pressure on the fetal abdominal wall as it travels through the birth canal. Assessment of FHR and pattern should be used to determine whether the passage of meconium is an expected finding associated with breech presentation or is an abnormal sign associated with fetal hypoxia. In a breech presentation, fetal heart tones (FHTs) are best heard at or above the umbilicus.

External cephalic version (ECV) (see later discussion) may be tried to turn the fetus from a breech to a vertex presentation. If the attempt at ECV is unsuccessful, the woman usually gives birth by cesarean (Lanni et al., 2017).

Vaginal birth is accomplished by mechanisms of labor that manipulate the buttocks and lower extremities as they emerge from the birth canal (Fig. 32.4). Risks associated with vaginal birth from a breech presentation include prolapse of the umbilical cord (especially in single or double footling breech presentations), trapping of the after-coming fetal head (especially with preterm infants), and trauma resulting from extension of the fetal head or nuchal position of the arms. Safe vaginal birth from a breech presentation is largely dependent on the experience, judgment, and skill of the health care provider who assists the birth. Criteria for attempting a vaginal birth from a breech presentation are as follows (Thorp & Grantz, 2019):
- Frank or complete breech presentation
- Estimated fetal weight between 2000 and 3800 g
- Normal (gynecoid) maternal pelvis with adequate measurements
- Flexed fetal head

Face and brow presentations are uncommon and are associated with increased parity, prematurity, prelabor rupture of membranes, and CPD. Face and brow presentations are not associated with fetal anomalies other than anencephaly, which almost always results in a face presentation. Spontaneous vaginal birth is possible if the fetus flexes to a vertex presentation. Cesarean birth is indicated if the presentation persists or if fetal distress occurs (Thorp & Grantz, 2019).

ECV may be attempted for a fetus in a transverse lie (i.e., shoulder) presentation at or after 36 to 37 weeks of gestation if membranes are intact and CPD and placenta previa are not present. Cesarean birth may be necessary, however, with a transverse lie presentation (Thorp & Grantz, 2019).

Multifetal Pregnancy

Multifetal pregnancy is the gestation of twins, triplets, quadruplets, or more infants. Twin gestations accounted for more than 3.3% of all live births in the United States in 2016. The rate of triplet or higher-order multiple births in 2016 was 101.4/100,000 births, the lowest rate in 18 years (Martin et al., 2018). The number of multiple-gestation pregnancies rose dramatically in the 1980s and 1990s, most likely due to fertility-enhancing medications and procedures as well as more women older than age 35 continuing childbearing. When compared with younger women, those 35 years and older are naturally more likely to have a multifetal pregnancy. The rate of triplet and higher-order multiple pregnancies peaked at an all-time high rate of 193.5/100,000 in 1998. Since then, the rate has either dropped slightly or remained unchanged. The decrease has been attributed to refinements in the treatments used for infertility, particularly limiting the number of embryos transferred during in vitro fertilization (IVF) procedures, and to the availability and acceptability of multifetal pregnancy reduction procedures (Malone & D'Alton, 2019; Newman & Unal, 2017).

Multiple births are associated with more complications (e.g., dysfunctional labor) than single births. The higher incidence of fetal and newborn complications and greater risk for perinatal mortality stem primarily from the birth of low-birth-weight infants resulting from preterm birth or IUGR (or both), in part related to placental dysfunction and twin-to-twin transfusion. Fetuses can experience distress and asphyxia during the birth process as a result of cord prolapse and the onset of placental separation with the birth of the first fetus. As a result, the risk for long-term problems such as cerebral palsy is higher among infants who were part of a multiple birth.

In addition, fetal complications such as congenital anomalies and abnormal presentations can result in dysfunctional labor and an increased incidence of cesarean birth. For example, in only 40% to 45%

of all twin pregnancies do both fetuses present in the vertex position, the most favorable for vaginal birth. In 35% to 40% of the pregnancies, one twin presents in the vertex position and the other in a breech or transverse lie presentation (Bowers, 2014; Malone & D'Alton, 2019).

The health status of the mother can be compromised by an increased risk for hypertension, anemia, and hemorrhage associated with uterine atony, placental abruption, and multiple or adherent placentas. Duration of the phases and stages of labor can vary from the duration experienced with singleton births.

Teamwork and planning are essential components of the management of labor and birth in multiple pregnancies, especially those of higher-order multiples. The nurse plays a key role in coordinating the activities of the interprofessional health care team. Early detection and management of the maternal, fetal, and newborn complications associated with multiple births are essential to achieve a positive outcome for mother and babies. Maternal positioning and active support are used to enhance labor progress and placental perfusion. Stimulation of labor with oxytocin, epidural anesthesia, internal or external version, and forceps or vacuum assistance may be used to accomplish the vaginal birth of twins. Cesarean birth is almost always performed with higher-order multiple births. Each infant will have its own interprofessional health care team present at the birth. Nurses provide important emotional support to women and their families to help reduce anxiety and stress. They explain events as they occur and offer updates on the status of the mother and infants.

Position of the Woman

The functional relationship among the uterine contractions, the fetus, and the mother's pelvis are altered by the maternal position. In addition, the position can provide a mechanical advantage or disadvantage to the mechanisms of labor by altering the effects of gravity and the body-part relationships that are important to the progress of labor. See Box 19.8 for suggested positions to enhance fetal descent.

Discouraging maternal movement or restricting labor to the recumbent or lithotomy position can compromise progress. The incidence of dysfunctional labor in women confined to these positions is increased, resulting in a greater need for augmentation of labor or forceps-assisted, vacuum-assisted, or cesarean birth.

Psychologic Responses

Hormones and neurotransmitters released in response to stress (e.g., catecholamines) can cause dysfunctional labor. Sources of stress vary for each woman, but pain and the absence of a support person are often related to dysfunctional labor. Confinement to bed and restriction of maternal movement can be a source of psychologic stress that compounds the physiologic stress caused by immobility in the unmedicated laboring woman. When anxiety is excessive it can inhibit cervical dilation and result in prolonged labor and increased pain perception. Anxiety also causes increased levels of stress-related hormones (e.g., β-endorphin, adrenocorticotropic hormone, cortisol, and epinephrine). These hormones act on the smooth muscles of the uterus. Increased levels can cause dysfunctional labor by reducing uterine contractility.

CARE MANAGEMENT

Risk assessment is a continual process in the laboring woman. By reviewing the woman's history of past labor or labors and observing her physical and psychologic responses to the current labor, any factors that might contribute to dysfunctional labor should be identified. The initial and ongoing physical assessments provide information about maternal well-being; status of labor in terms of the characteristics of uterine contractions and progress of cervical effacement and dilation; fetal well-being in terms of FHR and pattern, presentation, station, and position; and status of the amniotic membranes. Common problems that might be identified in women experiencing dysfunctional labor include the following:

- *Potential injury* to mother or fetus related to
  - interventions implemented for dystocia
- *Anxiety related to*
  - loss of control
- *Decreased ability to cope related to*
  - inadequate support system
  - exhaustion secondary to a prolonged labor process
  - pain
- *Potential for impaired self-concept as parent related to*
  - separation from infant associated with emergency cesarean birth
  - emotional responses to a traumatic childbirth experience

Client problems, expected outcomes of care, and interventions are established for each woman based on assessment findings. Many interventions for dysfunctional labor (e.g., ECV, cervical ripening, induction or augmentation of labor, and operative procedures [forceps- or vacuum-assisted birth, cesarean birth]) are implemented collaboratively with other members of the interprofessional health care team. Commonly performed interventions are discussed in detail in the Obstetric Procedures section later in this chapter. Nursing interventions are identified with each procedure.

When providing care for a woman who is experiencing labor or birth complications, all members of the health care team are responsible for complying with professional standards of care. This promotes client safety and helps improve outcomes.

OBESITY

Excessive weight is an increasingly serious problem for children, adolescents, and adults living in affluent nations, including the United States, and pregnant women are no exception. The body mass index (BMI) is used to define obesity. People with a BMI of 25 or greater are categorized as overweight, whereas those with a BMI of 30 or greater are considered obese. Individuals with a BMI of 40 or greater are classified as severely obese (Baird, Kennedy, & Dalton, 2017; Dalton & Strehlow, 2019; Gibbs Pickens, Kramer, Howards, et al., 2018).

Obese women are more likely to begin pregnancy with preexisting medical conditions such as chronic hypertension and type 2 diabetes. They are at higher risk for spontaneous abortion and stillbirth, and are more likely to develop pregnancy-associated hypertensive disorders, or gestational diabetes. They also have a higher risk for fetal congenital abnormalities, such as neural tube defects; hydrocephaly; and cardiovascular, orofacial, and limb reduction anomalies (ACOG, 2015/2018; Dalton & Strehlow, 2019). Additionally, obese women have an increased incidence of postterm pregnancy and longer labor (Dalton & Strehlow). All of these factors can increase the likelihood that labor will be induced. In addition to an increased risk for cesarean birth in general, obese women are also more likely to require emergency cesarean birth (ACOG, 2015/2018). During the postpartum period they are at risk for thromboembolism and wound disruption and infection after cesarean birth (Dalton & Strehlow, 2019; Gibbs Pickens et al., 2018). Obese women also have a higher risk for postpartum hemorrhage because of an increased likelihood of induction, resulting in prolonged labor, birth of a macrosomic infant, and caregiver difficulty with locating the uterine fundus to provide effective fundal massage (Baird et al., 2017).

CARE MANAGEMENT

Care of obese women during labor and birth is challenging for a number of reasons. Sometimes standard furniture such as beds, chairs, and operating tables is simply not large enough to accommodate the

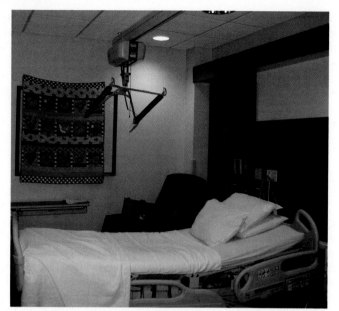

Fig. 32.5 Room Specifically Designed to Accommodate Obese Pregnant Clients. Note lift attached to ceiling for use in transferring women from the bed to chairs or stretchers. (Courtesy Dee Lowdermilk, Chapel Hill, NC.)

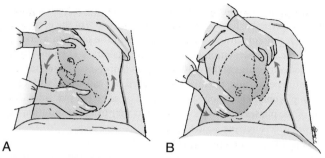

A   B

Fig. 32.6 External Version of Fetus From Breech to Vertex Presentation. This must be achieved without force. (A) Breech is pushed up out of pelvic inlet while head is pulled toward inlet. (B) Head is pushed toward inlet while breech is pulled upward.

of action is chosen, the woman and other family members are taught to perform dressing changes and wound care.

OBSTETRIC PROCEDURES

Version

Version is the turning of the fetus from one presentation to another. It may be performed externally or internally by the health care provider.

External Cephalic Version

External cephalic version (ECV) is used in an attempt to turn the fetus from a breech or shoulder presentation to a vertex presentation for birth. It may be attempted in a labor and birth setting at 36 to 37 weeks of gestation. ECV is accomplished using gentle, constant pressure on the abdomen (Fig. 32.6) (Lanni et al., 2017). At this gestational age, the success rate for ECV is approximately 65% and the risk for caesarean birth is reduced by 50% (Thorp & Grantz, 2019). Therefore ECV should be offered and performed whenever possible as one strategy to safely lower the primary cesarean birth rate (ACOG & SMFM, 2014).

Before ECV is attempted, ultrasound scanning is done for the following reasons (Thorp & Grantz, 2019):

* To confirm the breech presentation
* To detect multiple gestation, oligohydramnios, or fetal abnormalities
* To measure fetal dimensions

An NST is performed to confirm fetal well-being, or the FHR and pattern are monitored for a period of time (i.e., 10 to 20 minutes). Informed consent is obtained. A tocolytic agent such as terbutaline often is given to relax the uterus and facilitate the maneuver. ECV is sometimes performed under regional anesthesia (Lanni et al., 2017; Thorp & Grantz, 2019).

Contraindications to ECV include the following (Thorp & Grantz, 2019):

* Uterine anomalies
* Third-trimester bleeding
* Multiple gestation
* Oligohydramnios
* Evidence of uteroplacental insufficiency
* A nuchal cord (identified by ultrasound)
* Previous cesarean birth or other significant uterine surgery
* Obvious CPD

ECV is most successful in a nonobese multiparous woman with a nonanterior placenta who has an abundant amount of amniotic fluid and whose fetus is not yet engaged in the pelvis (Cunningham et al., 2018). The procedure should be performed in a hospital equipped to provide emergency surgery in case a non-reassuring FHR tracing unresponsive to resuscitative measures occurs (Thorp & Grantz, 2019).

woman's size. Extra-large furniture may not fit through a standard doorway, so room renovation may be necessary. Some hospitals have created rooms specifically designed to accommodate obese clients (Fig. 32.5). Continuous external FHR and contraction monitoring can be extremely difficult if not impossible to perform. Special equipment, such as extra-large blood pressure cuffs, is necessary to properly assess the woman's condition.

Even routine procedures require more time and effort to accomplish when a woman is obese. This can slow essential interventions and increase risks to the mother and fetus, such as when an emergency cesarean birth is needed. Establishing IV access, for example, may require multiple attempts, sometimes by multiple people. Mobility is often a problem. Moving the woman from a labor room to the operating room and transferring her from a bed to the operating table can require the assistance of additional personnel or special equipment, especially if regional anesthesia is already in effect. If it is not, surgery may be further delayed by anesthetic complications, such as difficulty establishing an epidural or spinal block or accomplishing endotracheal intubation.

In the immediate recovery period, use of thromboembolic deterrent anti-embolism stockings (TED hose) and sequential compression devices (SCDs) boots helps decrease the chance for venous thromboembolism (VTE) formation. Some women may also be given heparin prophylactically to prevent VTE (Simpson & O'Brien-Abel, 2014). In the postpartum period women should also be encouraged to get out of bed and begin ambulating as soon as possible.

Keeping the incision clean and dry to prevent wound infection and promote healing is another postoperative challenge. Many obese women have a *pannus* (large roll of abdominal fat) that overlies a lower abdominal transverse skin incision made just above the pubic area. The pannus causes the area to remain moist, which encourages the development of infection. Women should be taught to wash the incision with soap and water several times a day, thoroughly drying the area afterward. Using a handheld hair dryer on a low setting works well for this purpose. Sutures or staples used to close the skin incision are generally left in place longer than usual to avoid possible wound disruption when they are removed. Sometimes the skin and subcutaneous layers of the incision are left open to heal by secondary intention to avoid possible dehiscence. If this course

During an attempted ECV the nurse continuously monitors the FHR and pattern, especially for bradycardia and variable decelerations; checks the maternal vital signs; and assesses the woman's level of comfort because the procedure can be painful. After the procedure is completed, the nurse continues to monitor maternal vital signs and uterine activity and assess for vaginal bleeding until the woman's condition is determined to be stable. FHR and pattern monitoring should continue for at least 1 hour. Women who are Rh negative should receive Rh immune globulin because the manipulation can cause fetomaternal bleeding (Thorp & Grantz, 2019).

Internal Version

With internal version the fetus is turned by the obstetric health care provider, who inserts a hand into the uterus and changes the presentation to cephalic (head) or podalic (foot). Internal version is only rarely used, most often in twin gestations to assist with the birth of the second fetus. The safety of this procedure has not been documented; maternal and fetal injury is possible. Cesarean birth is the usual method for managing malpresentation in multifetal pregnancies. The nurse's role is to monitor the status of the fetus and to provide support to the woman.

Induction of Labor

Induction of labor is the chemical or mechanical initiation of uterine contractions before their spontaneous onset for the purpose of bringing about birth. Induction of labor is a significant intervention, accounting for up to 25% of term births around the world and up to 23% of all births in the United States (Bakker, Pierce, & Myers, 2017). Chemical, mechanical, physical, and alternative methods are used to induce labor. IV oxytocin (Pitocin) and amniotomy are the most common methods used in the United States.

Labor may be induced for *indicated* reasons when the risk of continuing the pregnancy becomes more dangerous for either the mother or the fetus and there are no contraindications for artificial rupture of the membranes (amniotomy) or augmenting uterine contractions with oxytocin. Prior to labor induction, gestational age should be determined and any potential risks to the maternal-fetal unit evaluated. Women must be fully counseled regarding risks, benefits, and alternatives of labor stimulation methods as part of the process for informed consent (ACOG, 2009/2019; Thorp & Grantz, 2019). Box 32.7 lists indications and contraindications for labor induction.

Elective Induction of Labor

An elective induction is one in which labor is initiated without a medical indication. Many elective inductions are purely for the convenience of the woman or her obstetric health care provider. At times, however, labor may be electively induced to allay maternal fears and anxieties associated with prior perinatal losses or to ensure that an experienced interprofessional health care team is available to handle anticipated maternal or neonatal complications immediately following birth (Sheibani & Wing, 2017). Elective induction of labor has also been used in cases of maternal obesity and maternal diabetes (Gibbs Pickens, et al., 2018), before complications arise.

To prevent iatrogenic prematurity, elective induction of labor should not be initiated until the woman reaches 39 completed weeks of gestation (ACOG, 2009/2019). The March of Dimes and the Association of Women's Health, Obstetric and Neonatal Nurses (AWHONN) have created informational campaigns to educate pregnant women and their families about the dangers of early-term births (visit their websites at www.health4mom.org/zones/go-the-full-40 and https://www.marchofdimes.org/pregnancy/why-at-least-39-weeks-is-best-for-your-baby.aspx).

Birth data from the United States for 2016 indicate that the percentage of infants born early term (37 to 38 weeks) rose 2% from

---

BOX 32.7 Indications and Contraindications for Labor Induction

Maternal Indications
- Hypertensive complications of pregnancy: gestational hypertension, preeclampsia, eclampsia
- Fetal death
- Chorioamnionitis

Fetal Indications

Any condition in which a variety of fetal tests demonstrate significant fetal jeopardy in any of the following situations:
- Diabetes
- Postterm pregnancy, especially when oligohydramnios is present
- Hypertensive complications of pregnancy
- Intrauterine growth restriction
- Isoimmunization
- Chorioamnionitis
- Premature rupture of membranes with established fetal maturity

Contraindications
- Acute, severe fetal distress
- Shoulder presentation (transverse lie)
- Floating fetal presenting part
- Uncontrolled hemorrhage
- Placenta previa
- Previous uterine incision that prohibits a trial of labor

Relative Contraindications
- Grand multiparity (five or more pregnancies that ended after 20 weeks of gestation)
- Multiple gestation
- Suspected cephalopelvic disproportion
- Breech presentations
- Inability to adequately monitor the fetal heart rate throughout labor

Data from Thorp, J. M., & Grantz, K. L. (2019). Clinical aspects of normal and abnormal labor. In R. Resnik, C. J. Lockwood, T. R. Moore, et al. (Eds.), *Creasy & Resnik's maternal-fetal medicine: Principles and practice* (8th ed.). Philadelphia: Elsevier.

2015 to 2016, from 24.99% to 25.47%, and the full-term birth rate declined slightly, from 58.47% to 57.94%. From 2007 to 2014, the early-term birth rate had generally been on the decline, and the full-term (39 weeks of gestation or more) rate had been on the rise, so these numbers represent a change in the opposite direction for both early- and full-term birth rates for the second consecutive year (Martin et al., 2018). These data may indicate a need for continued recommendations and efforts to reduce nonmedically indicated births prior to 39 weeks (see the Community Activity box).

COMMUNITY ACTIVITY

Elective Induction of Labor

Visit the March of Dimes website (www.marchofdimes.org) and download client teaching materials regarding the importance of avoiding an elective early-term birth by waiting until at least 39 weeks of gestation for labor induction. Then talk with a woman who is 36-38 weeks pregnant. Ask if she wants to have her labor induced immediately. If so, what are her reasons? Share the information you obtained from the March of Dimes website with her. Were you able to change her mind?

Success rates for induction of labor are higher when the condition of the cervix is favorable, or inducible. Cervical ripeness is the most important predictor of successful induction. A rating system such as the Bishop score (Table 32.2) can be used to evaluate inducibility. For example, a score of 8 or more on this 13-point scale indicates that the cervix is soft, anterior, 50% or more effaced, and dilated 2 cm or more and that the presenting part is engaged. When the Bishop score totals 8 or more, the likelihood of vaginal birth is similar whether labor is spontaneous or induced (Sheibani & Wing, 2017). The Bishop score should be documented prior to the use of methods to ripen the cervix or induce labor.

TABLE 32.2 Bishop Score

	SCORE			
	0	**1**	**2**	**3**
Dilation (cm)	0	1-2	3-4	≥5
Effacement (%)	0-30	40-50	60-70	≥80
Station (cm)	−3	−2	−1, 0	+1, +2
Cervical consistency	Firm	Medium	Soft	Soft
Cervical position	Posterior	Midposition	Anterior	Anterior

Modified from Bishop, E. H. (1964). Pelvic scoring for elective induction. *Obstetrics & Gynecology, 24*(2), 266–268.

Cervical Ripening Methods

Chemical agents. Preparations of prostaglandins E_1 (PGE_1) and E_2 (PGE_2) have been shown to be effective when used before induction to "ripen" (soften and thin) the cervix (see Medication Guides: Prostaglandin E_1 [PGE_1]: Misoprostol [Cytotec] and Prostaglandin E_2 [PGE_2]: Dinoprostone [Cervidil Insert; Prepidil Gel]) (ACOG, 2009/2019; Bakker et al., 2017). In some cases, women spontaneously begin laboring after the administration of prostaglandin, thereby eliminating the need to administer oxytocin to induce labor. Additional advantages of prostaglandin use for cervical ripening include decreased oxytocin induction time and a decrease in the amount of oxytocin required for successful induction (Sheibani & Wing, 2017). PGE_1, although much less expensive and more effective than PGE_2 for inducing labor and birth, is associated with a higher risk for uterine tachysystole with abnormal FHR and pattern changes and passage of meconium into the amniotic fluid. Most of these adverse outcomes are associated with higher-dose protocols (ACOG 2009/2019; Bakker et al.; Sheibani & Wing). Although the drug's manufacturer has acknowledged for several years that PGE_1 is effective for cervical ripening and labor induction, it has not yet been approved by the FDA for these uses (Thorp & Grantz, 2019). ACOG, however, considers the use of PGE_1 for preinduction cervical ripening to be a safe and effective off-label use of the medication (Sheibani & Wing). PGE_2 in the form of a vaginal insert (dinoprostone [Cervidil]), although more expensive than PGE_1, has the major advantage of easy removal should adverse reactions, including uterine tachysystole, occur (Bakker et al., 2017).

MEDICATION GUIDE

Prostaglandin E1 (PGE1): Misoprostol (Cytotec)

Action

PGE_1 ripens the cervix, making it softer and causing it to begin to dilate and efface; it stimulates uterine contractions.

Indications

- PGE_1 is used for preinduction cervical ripening (ripen the cervix before oxytocin induction of labor when the Bishop score is 4 or less) and to induce labor or abortion (abortifacient agent); it has not yet been approved by the FDA for cervical ripening or labor induction (i.e., this is an off-label use for obstetrics).
- It should not be used if the woman has a history of previous cesarean birth or other major uterine surgery.

Dosage and Administration

- Misoprostol is available either as a 100- or a 200-mcg tablet. Therefore tablets must be broken to prepare the correct dose. This preparation should take place in the pharmacy to ensure accurate doses.
- Recommended initial dose is 25 mcg. Insert intravaginally into the posterior vaginal fornix using the tips of index and middle fingers without the use of a lubricant. Repeat every 4 hrs or until an effective contraction pattern is established (three or more uterine contractions in 10 min), the cervix ripens (Bishop score of 8 or greater), or significant adverse effects occur.

Adverse Effects

Higher doses (e.g., 50 mcg every 6 hrs) are more likely to result in adverse reactions such as nausea and vomiting, diarrhea, fever, uterine tachysystole with or without an abnormal FHR and pattern, or fetal passage of meconium.

The risk for adverse reactions is reduced with lower dosages and longer intervals between doses.

Nursing Considerations

- Explain the procedure to the woman and her family; ensure that an informed consent has been obtained as per agency policy.
- Assess the woman and fetus before each insertion and during treatment following agency protocol for frequency. Assess maternal vital signs and health status, FHR and pattern, and status of pregnancy, including indications for cervical ripening or induction of labor, signs of labor or impending labor, and the Bishop score. Recognize that an abnormal FHR and pattern; maternal fever, infection, vaginal bleeding, or hypersensitivity; and regular, progressive uterine contractions contraindicate the use of misoprostol.
- Avoid giving aluminum hydroxide and magnesium-containing antacids along with misoprostol.
- Use with caution in women with renal failure because the medication is eliminated through the kidneys.
- Have the woman void before insertion.
- Assist the woman to maintain a supine position with a lateral tilt or a side-lying position for 30-40 min after insertion.
- Prepare to (1) swab the vagina to remove unabsorbed medication using a saline-soaked gauze wrapped around fingers or (2) administer terbutaline 0.25 mg subcutaneously if significant adverse effects occur.
- Initiate oxytocin for induction of labor no sooner than 4 hrs after the last dose of misoprostol was administered, following agency protocol, if ripening has occurred and labor has not begun.
- Document all assessment findings and administration procedures.

FDA, U.S. Food and Drug Administration; *FHR,* fetal heart rate.
Data from Hill, W., & Harvey, C. (2013). Induction of labor. In N. Troiàno, C. Harvey, & B. Chez (Eds.), *AWHONN's high risk and critical care obstetrics* (3rd ed.). Philadelphia: Wolters Kluwer/Lippincott Williams & Wilkins; Moleti, C. (2009). Trends and controversies in labor induction. *American Journal of Maternal/Child Nursing, 34*(1), 40–47; and Thorp, J. M., & Grantz, K. L. (2019). Clinical aspects of normal and abnormal labor. In R. Resnik, C. J. Lockwood, T. R. Moore, et al. (Eds.), *Creasy & Resnik's maternal-fetal medicine: Principles and practice* (8th ed.). Philadelphia: Elsevier.

MEDICATION GUIDE

Prostaglandin E2 (PGE2): Dinoprostone (Cervidil Insert; Prepidil Gel)

Action

PGE$_2$ ripens the cervix, making it softer and causing it to dilate and efface; it stimulates uterine contractions. Dinoprostone is the only FDA-approved medication for cervical ripening or labor induction.

Indications

- PGE$_2$ is used for preinduction cervical ripening (ripen the cervix before oxytocin induction of labor when the Bishop score is 4 or less) and for induction of labor or abortion (abortifacient agent).
- It is not recommended for use if the woman has a history of previous cesarean birth or other major uterine surgery.

Dosage and Route

Cervidil Insert

Dosage is 10 mg of dinoprostone designed to be gradually released (approximately 0.3 mg/hr) over 12 hrs. Insert is placed transvaginally into the posterior fornix of the vagina. The insert is removed after 12 hrs or at the onset of active labor or earlier if tachysystole or abnormal FHR and patterns occur.

Prepidil Gel

Dosage is 0.5 mg of dinoprostone in a 2.5-mL syringe. Gel is administered through a catheter attached to the syringe into the cervical canal just below the internal cervical os. Dose may be repeated every 6 hrs as needed for cervical ripening up to a maximum cumulative dose of 1.5 mg (3 doses) in a 24-hr period.

Adverse Effects

Potential adverse effects include headache, nausea and vomiting, diarrhea, fever, hypotension, uterine tachysystole with or without an abnormal FHR and pattern, or fetal passage of meconium.

Nursing Considerations

- Explain the procedure to the woman and her family. Ensure that an informed consent has been obtained as per agency policy.

- Assess the woman and fetus before each insertion and during treatment following agency protocol for frequency. Assess maternal vital signs and health status, FHR and pattern, and status of pregnancy, including indications for cervical ripening or induction of labor, signs of labor or impending labor, and the Bishop score. Recognize that an abnormal FHR and pattern; maternal fever, infection, vaginal bleeding, or hypersensitivity; and regular, progressive uterine contractions contraindicate the use of dinoprostone.
- Avoid use in women with asthma, glaucoma, and hypotension or hypertension.
- Use with caution if the woman has cardiac, renal, or hepatic disease; anemia; jaundice; diabetes; epilepsy; or genitourinary (GU) infections.
- Bring the gel to room temperature just before administration. Do not force the warming process by using a warm-water bath or other source of external heat such as microwave because heat may cause inactivation.
- Keep the insert frozen until just before insertion. No warming is needed.
- Have the woman void before insertion.
- Assist the woman to maintain a supine position with a lateral tilt or a side-lying position for at least 30 min after insertion of the gel or for 2 hrs after placement of the insert.
- Allow the woman to ambulate after the recommended period of bed rest and observation.
- Prepare to pull the string to remove the insert and to administer terbutaline 0.25 mg subcutaneously if significant adverse effects occur. There is no effective way to remove the gel from the vagina if uterine tachysystole or abnormal FHR and pattern occur.
- Delay the initiation of oxytocin for induction of labor for 6-12 hrs after the last instillation of the gel or for 30-60 min after removal of the insert, or follow agency protocol for induction if ripening has occurred but labor has not begun.
- Document all assessment findings and administration procedures.

FDA, U.S. Food and Drug Administration; *FHR*, fetal heart rate.
Data from Hill, W., & Harvey, C. (2013). Induction of labor. In N. Troiano, C. Harvey, & B. Chez (Eds.), *AWHONN's high risk and critical care obstetrics* (3rd ed.). Philadelphia: Wolters Kluwer/Lippincott Williams & Wilkins; Moleti, C. (2009). Trends and controversies in labor induction, *American Journal of Maternal/Child Nursing, 34*(1), 40–47.

Mechanical and physical methods. Mechanical dilators ripen the cervix by stimulating the release of endogenous prostaglandins. Balloon catheters (e.g., Foley catheter) can be inserted through the intracervical canal to ripen and dilate the cervix. The catheter balloon is inflated above the internal cervical os with 30 to 50 mL of sterile water. This process results in pressure and stretching of the lower uterine segment and the cervix, as well as the release of endogenous prostaglandins. It is especially helpful for women who cannot receive exogenous prostaglandins for cervical ripening. The balloon usually falls out within 8 to 12 hours, when cervical dilation reaches approximately 3 cm. Evidence supports the insertion of a balloon catheter as a cervical ripening method because of its low cost compared with prostaglandins, stability at room temperature, and reduced risk for uterine tachysystole with or without FHR changes (ACOG, 2009/2019).

Hydroscopic dilators (substances that absorb fluid from surrounding tissues and then enlarge) also can be used for cervical ripening. Laminaria tents (natural cervical dilators made from desiccated seaweed) and synthetic dilators containing magnesium sulfate (Lamicel) are inserted into the endocervix without rupturing the membranes. As they absorb fluid, they expand and cause cervical dilation and the release of endogenous prostaglandins. These dilators are left in place for 6 to 12 hours before being removed to assess cervical dilation. Fresh

dilators are inserted if further cervical dilation is necessary. Synthetic dilators swell faster than natural dilators and become larger with less discomfort. When compared with prostaglandins, these mechanical methods achieved a lower rate of birth within 24 hours, but caused no change in the cesarean birth rate. Additionally, they were less likely to cause uterine tachysystole with or without changes in the FHR (ACOG, 2009/2019; Thorp & Grantz, 2019).

Hydroscopic dilators compare favorably with prostaglandins in their effectiveness in ripening the cervix but are associated with increased discomfort at insertion and during expansion and a higher incidence of postpartum maternal and newborn infections. They are a reliable alternative when prostaglandins are contraindicated or are unavailable.

Nursing responsibilities for women who have dilators inserted include the following:

- Documenting the number of dilators and sponges inserted during the procedure, as well as the number removed
- Assessing for urinary retention, rupture of membranes, uterine tenderness or pain, contractions, vaginal bleeding, infection, and fetal distress

Amniotic membrane stripping or sweeping is a method of inducing labor through the release of prostaglandins and oxytocin. The procedure involves separation of the membrane from the wall of the cervix and lower uterine segment by inserting a finger into the internal cervical os and rotating it 360 degrees. Studies have suggested that membrane stripping increases the rate of spontaneous vaginal birth and shortens the induction to birth interval. Harmful side effects that could be attributed to the procedure have not been reported. Research has not demonstrated an increase in either maternal or fetal infection associated with membrane stripping. However, because there is limited data available on the risk for infection in women who are known to be GBS positive, potential risks and benefits of the procedure should be carefully considered before performing membrane stripping on this group of women (Sheibani & Wing, 2017).

Physical methods such as sexual intercourse (prostaglandins in the semen and stimulation of contractions with orgasm), nipple stimulation (release of endogenous oxytocin from the pituitary gland), and walking (gravity applies pressure to the cervix, which stimulates the secretion of endogenous oxytocin) may be used by women to "self-induce" labor. Breast (nipple) stimulation has been shown to increase the number of women who go into labor within 72 hours, but safety issues associated with this method have not been fully evaluated. Although orgasm does stimulate uterine contractions, there is inadequate evidence to support the belief that sexual intercourse enhances cervical ripening (Thorp & Grantz, 2019).

Alternative methods. Various alternative methods have been used by women to stimulate cervical ripening and the onset of labor. For example, blue cohosh and castor oil can be used for their labor stimulation effects, and black cohosh and evening primrose oil can ripen the cervix. Nurses must be knowledgeable about these preparations and ask about their use when assessing women during prenatal visits and on admission during labor. Women may accidentally take too much of the preparation or use it incorrectly. Also these preparations may potentiate the effect of pharmacologic methods to stimulate cervical ripening and uterine contractions, thereby increasing the potential for tachysystole and precipitous labor and birth.

Acupuncture has been used effectively to induce labor and has been found, in several studies, to reduce the duration of labor, the use of oxytocin, and the rate of cesarean birth. Specific points have been identified to stimulate uterine contractions or to facilitate cervical dilation. More than one treatment may be required to establish labor.

Amniotomy

Amniotomy (i.e., artificial rupture of membranes [AROM]) can be used to induce labor when the condition of the cervix is favorable (ripe) or to augment labor if progress begins to slow. Labor usually begins within 12 hours of AROM. Amniotomy can decrease the duration of labor by up to 2 hours, even without oxytocin administration. However, if amniotomy does not stimulate labor, the resulting prolonged rupture may lead to chorioamnionitis. Variable FHR deceleration patterns can occur as a result of cord compression associated with umbilical cord prolapse or a decreased amount of amniotic fluid. Once an amniotomy is performed, the woman is committed to labor with an unknown outcome for how and when she will give birth. For this reason amniotomy often is used in combination with oxytocin induction.

Before the procedure the woman should be told what to expect. She also should be assured that the actual rupture of the membranes is painless for her and the fetus, although she may experience some discomfort when the Amnihook or other sharp instrument is inserted through the vagina and cervix (Box 32.8). The presenting part of the fetus should be engaged and well applied to the cervix prior to the procedure to prevent cord prolapse. The woman should also be free of active infection of the genital tract (e.g., herpes) and should be human immunodeficiency virus (HIV) negative. After rupture the amniotic fluid is allowed to drain slowly. The color, odor, and consistency of the fluid are assessed (i.e., for the presence or absence of meconium or blood). The time of rupture is recorded (Simpson & O'Brien-Abel, 2014).

BOX 32.8 Procedure: Assisting With Amniotomy

Procedure
- Explain to the woman what will be done.
- Assess the fetal heart rate (FHR) and pattern before the procedure begins to obtain a baseline reading.
- Place several underpads under the woman's buttocks to absorb the fluid.
- Position the woman on a padded bedpan, fracture pan, or rolled-up towel to elevate her hips.
- Assist the obstetric care provider who is performing the procedure by providing sterile gloves and lubricant for the vaginal examination.
- Unwrap the sterile package containing an Amnihook or Allis clamp and pass the instrument to the obstetric health care provider, who inserts it alongside the fingers and then hooks and tears the membranes.
- Reassess the FHR and pattern.
- Assess the color, consistency, and odor of the fluid.
- Assess the woman's temperature every 2 hrs or per protocol.
- Evaluate the woman for signs and symptoms of infection.

Documentation
Record the following:
- FHR and pattern before and after the procedure
- Time of rupture
- Color, odor, and consistency of the fluid
- Maternal status (how well procedure was tolerated)

⚡ SAFETY ALERT

The fetal heart rate is assessed before and immediately after the amniotomy to detect any changes. Transient tachycardia is common. Bradycardia and variable decelerations can indicate cord compression or prolapse.

The woman's temperature should be checked at least every 2 hours after rupture of membranes, more frequently if signs or symptoms of infection are noted. If her temperature is 38°C (100.4°F) or higher, the nurse notifies the obstetric health care provider. The nurse assesses for other signs and symptoms of infection, such as maternal chills, uterine tenderness on palpation, foul-smelling vaginal drainage, and fetal tachycardia. Comfort measures, such as frequently changing the woman's underpads and perineal cleansing, are implemented.

LEGAL TIP

Performing Amniotomy

Performing amniotomy is outside the scope of practice of nurses. In some locations, however, nurses have been asked to perform this procedure. A policy that is consistent with professional standards of care and clearly explains the nurse's role in amniotomy should be in place in all labor and birth areas.

Oxytocin

Oxytocin is a hormone normally produced by the posterior pituitary gland. It stimulates uterine contractions and aids in milk ejection (letdown). Synthetic oxytocin (Pitocin) may be used either to induce labor or to augment a labor that is progressing slowly because of inadequate uterine contractions. Synthetic oxytocin is the most commonly used agent for labor induction in the United States (Huwe, 2017; Simpson & O'Brien-Abel, 2014). It is also the drug most commonly associated with adverse events during labor and birth. The most common errors involving oxytocin administration during labor are dose related (Simpson & O'Brien-Abel, 2014).

⚡ SAFETY ALERT

Oxytocin is included on the list of high-alert medications designated by the Institute for Safe Medication Practices because it has a heightened risk for causing significant client harm when used in error (Institute for Safe Medication Practices [ISMP], 2014).

Oxytocin use can present hazards to the mother and fetus. Maternal hazards include placental abruption, uterine rupture, unnecessary cesarean birth because of abnormal FHR and pattern, postpartum hemorrhage, and infection. When placental perfusion is diminished by contractions that are too frequent or prolonged, the fetus can experience hypoxemia and acidemia, which eventually result in late decelerations and minimal or absent baseline variability. The goal of oxytocin use is to produce contractions of normal intensity, duration, and frequency using the lowest dose of medication possible (Huwe, 2017).

The obstetric health care provider writes the order for the induction or augmentation of labor with oxytocin. The nurse implements the order by initiating the primary IV infusion and administering the oxytocin solution through a secondary line. The nurse's actions related to the assessment and care of a woman whose labor is being induced are guided by hospital protocol and professional standards (Fig. 32.7 and the Medication Guide: Oxytocin [Pitocin]).

MEDICATION GUIDE

Oxytocin (Pitocin)

Action

Oxytocin is a hormone produced in the posterior pituitary gland that stimulates uterine contractions and aids in milk ejection (let-down). Pitocin is a synthetic form of this hormone.

Indications

Oxytocin is used primarily for labor induction and augmentation; it is also used to control postpartum bleeding.

Dosage

- The IV solution containing oxytocin should be mixed in a standard concentration. Concentrations often used are 10 units in 1000 mL of fluid, 20 units in 1000 mL of fluid, or 30 units in 500 mL of fluid.
- Oxytocin is administered intravenously through a secondary line connected to the main line at the proximal port (connection closest to the IV insertion site). Oxytocin is always administered by infusion pump.
- Begin oxytocin administration at 1 milliunit/min. Increase the rate by 1-2 milliunits/min, no more frequently than every 30-60 min based on the response of the woman and fetus and the progress of labor.
- The goal of oxytocin administration is to produce acceptable uterine contractions as evidenced by:
  - Consistent achievement of 200-220 MVUs *or*
  - A consistent pattern of one contraction every 2-3 min, lasting 80-90 secs, and strong to palpation

Adverse Effects

- Possible maternal adverse effects include uterine tachysystole, placental abruption, uterine rupture, unplanned cesarean birth caused by abnormal FHR and pattern, postpartum hemorrhage, infection, and death from water intoxication (e.g., severe hyponatremia).
- Possible fetal adverse effects include hypoxemia and acidosis, eventually resulting in abnormal FHR and pattern.

Nursing Considerations

- Oxytocin is considered a high-alert medication because it has a heightened risk for causing significant client harm when used in error.
- Client and partner teaching and support:
  - Reasons for use of oxytocin (e.g., start or improve labor)

- Reactions to expect concerning the nature of contractions: the intensity of the contraction increases more rapidly, holds the peak longer, and ends more quickly; contractions come regularly and more often
- Monitoring to anticipate
- Continue to keep woman and her partner informed regarding progress.
- Remember that women vary greatly in their response to oxytocin; some require only very small amounts of medication to produce adequate contractions, whereas others need larger doses.
- Assessment:
  - Assess fetal status using electronic fetal monitoring; evaluate tracing every 15 min and with every change in dose during the first stage of labor and every 5 min during the active pushing phase of the second stage of labor.
  - Monitor the contraction pattern and uterine resting tone every 15 min and with every change in dose during the first stage of labor and every 5 min during the second stage of labor.
  - Monitor blood pressure, pulse, and respirations every 30-60 min and with every change in dose.
  - Assess intake and output; limit IV intake to 1000 mL in 8 hrs; urine output should be 120 mL or more every 4 hrs.
  - Perform a vaginal examination as indicated.
  - Monitor for side effects, including nausea, vomiting, headache, and hypotension.
  - Observe emotional responses of the woman and her partner.
- Use a standard definition for uterine tachysystole that does not include an abnormal FHR and pattern or the woman's perception of pain (see Emergency box: Uterine Tachysystole with Oxytocin [Pitocin] Infusion).
- The rate of oxytocin infusion should be continually titrated to the lowest dose that achieves acceptable labor progress. Usually the oxytocin dose can be decreased or discontinued after rupture of membranes and in the active phase of first-stage labor.
- Documentation:
  - The time the oxytocin infusion is begun, and each time the infusion is increased, decreased, or discontinued
  - Assessment data as described earlier
  - Interventions for uterine tachysystole and abnormal FHR and pattern and the response to the interventions
  - Notification of the obstetric health care provider and that person's response

FHR, Fetal heart rate; *IV,* intravenous; *MVUs,* Montevideo units.

Data from American College of Obstetricians and Gynecologists. (2009, reaffirmed 2019). Practice bulletin no. 107: Induction of labor. *Obstetrics & Gynecology, 114*(2, pt 1), 386–397; Clark, S., Simpson, K., Knox, G., & Garite, T. J. (2009). Oxytocin: New perspectives on an old drug. *American Journal of Obstetrics and Gynecology, 200*(1), 35.e1-35.e6; Hill, W., & Harvey, C. (2013). Induction of labor. In N. Troiano, C. Harvey, & B. Chez (Eds.), *AWHONN's high risk and critical care obstetrics* (3rd ed.). Philadelphia: Wolters Kluwer/Lippincott Williams & Wilkins; Mahlmeister, L. (2008). Best practices in perinatal care: Evidence-based management of oxytocin induction and augmentation of labor. *Journal of Perinatal and Neonatal Nursing, 22*(4), 259–263; Simpson, K. R., & O'Brien-Abel, N. (2014). Labor and birth. In K. R. Simpson & P. Creehan (Eds.), *AWHONN's perinatal nursing* (4th ed.). Philadelphia: Lippincott; and Simpson, K., & Knox, G. (2009). Oxytocin as a high-alert medication: Implications for perinatal patient safety. *American Journal of Maternal/Child Nursing, 34*(1), 8–15.

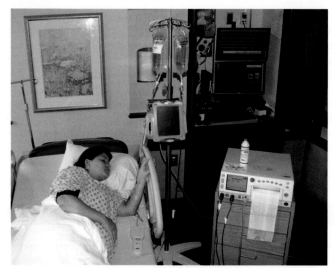

Fig. 32.7 Woman in Side-Lying Position Receiving Oxytocin. (Courtesy Cheryl Briggs, RNC, Annapolis, MD.)

The most commonly used regimen in the United States for administering oxytocin is to begin with a starting dose of 1 milliunit/min and to increase by 1 to 2 milliunits/min no more frequently than every 30 to 40 minutes (Simpson & O'Brien-Abel, 2014). This recommendation is based on research findings related to the pharmacokinetics of oxytocin. The uterus responds to oxytocin within 3 to 5 minutes of IV administration. The half-life of oxytocin (the time required to metabolize and eliminate half the dose) is approximately 10 to 12 minutes. Approximately 40 minutes is required to reach a steady state of oxytocin (the point in time when the rate of oxytocin administered intravenously equals the rate of oxytocin elimination) and for the full effect of a dosage increment to be reflected in more intense, frequent, and longer contractions (ACOG, 2009/2019; Simpson & O'Brien-Abel, 2014) (see Medication Guide: Oxytocin [Pitocin] and Fig. 32.7). Low-dose (physiologic) protocols such as the one described result in decreased risk for oxytocin-induced tachysystole. High-dose protocols, in which the initial dose of oxytocin is larger and the dosage is increased more rapidly, have been found to result in shorter labors, fewer failed inductions, less forceps-assisted births, and fewer cesarean births because of failure to progress in labor, less chorioamnionitis, and less neonatal sepsis. However, high-dose protocols have been associated with an increased incidence of uterine tachysystole and more cesarean births related to fetal stress (Sheibani & Wing, 2017).

Nursing considerations. An evidence-based protocol for preparing and administering oxytocin should be established and utilized by the obstetric department (health care providers and nurses) in each institution. Other safety measures recommended for use of this high-alert drug are using a standard concentration of oxytocin and a standard definition of uterine tachysystole that does not include an abnormal FHR or pattern or the woman's perception of pain. Additionally, standardized treatment of oxytocin-induced uterine tachysystole is recommended (Huwe, 2017; Simpson & O'Brien-Abel, 2014) (see Emergency box: Uterine Tachysystole With Oxytocin [Pitocin] Infusion).

The definition of excessive uterine contractions needs to be standardized. The Eunice Kennedy Shriver National Institute of Child Health and Human Development, along with ACOG and SMFM, sponsored a workshop in April 2008 to review definitions, interpretation, and research recommendations for intrapartum fetal monitoring.

✚ EMERGENCY

Uterine Tachysystole With Oxytocin (Pitocin) Infusion

Signs
- More than five contractions in 10 min *or*
- A series of single contractions lasting greater than 2 min *or*
- Contractions of normal duration occurring within 1 min of each other

Interventions (With Normal [Category I] FHR Tracing)
- Reposition or maintain woman in side-lying position (either side).
- Administer IV fluid bolus with 500 mL of lactated Ringers solution.
- If uterine activity has not returned to normal after 10 min, decrease the oxytocin dose by at least half.
- If uterine activity has not returned to normal after another 10 min, discontinue the oxytocin infusion until fewer than five contractions occur in 10 min.

Interventions (With Indeterminate [Category II] or Abnormal [Category III] FHR Tracing)
- Discontinue oxytocin infusion immediately.
- Reposition or maintain woman in side-lying position (either side).
- Administer IV fluid bolus with 500 mL of lactated Ringers solution.
- Consider giving oxygen at 10 L/min via nonrebreather face mask if the above interventions do not resolve the indeterminate or abnormal (category II or category III) FHR tracing.
- If still no response, consider giving 0.25 mg terbutaline subcutaneously according to unit protocol or standing orders.
- Notify obstetric health care provider of actions taken and maternal and fetal response.

Resumption of Oxytocin After Resolution of Tachysystole
- If the oxytocin infusion has been discontinued for less than 20-30 min, resume at no more than one half the rate that caused the tachysystole.
- If the oxytocin infusion has been discontinued for more than 30-40 min, resume at the initial starting dose.

FHR, Fetal heart rate; *IV,* intravenous.
Data from Huwe, V. Y. (2017). Induction and augmentation of labor. In B. B. Kennedy & S. M. Baird (Eds.), *Intrapartum management modules: A perinatal education program* (5th ed.). Philadelphia: Wolters Kluwer; and Simpson, K. (2011). Clinicians' guide to the use of oxytocin for labor induction and augmentation. *Journal of Midwifery & Women's Health, 56*(3), 214–221.

Workshop participants also recommended standardizing definitions regarding uterine contractions for use in clinical practice. This group defined uterine tachysystole as more than five contractions in 10 minutes, averaged over a 30-minute window. The term tachysystole applies to both spontaneous and stimulated labor. Participants also recommended that use of the terms *hyperstimulation* and *hyperactivity* be abandoned because they are not defined (Macones, Hankins, Spong, et al., 2008).

Augmentation of Labor

Augmentation of labor is the stimulation of uterine contractions after labor has started spontaneously and progress is unsatisfactory. Augmentation is usually implemented to manage hypotonic uterine dysfunction that resulted in a slowing of the labor process (protracted active phase). Common augmentation methods include oxytocin infusion and amniotomy. Noninvasive methods such as emptying the bladder, ambulation and position changes, relaxation measures, nourishment and hydration, and hydrotherapy should be attempted before initiating invasive interventions. The administration procedure and nursing assessment and care measures for augmenting labor with oxytocin are similar to those used for induction of labor with oxytocin (see Medication Guide: Oxytocin [Pitocin]).

Some physicians advocate active management of labor, that is, augmentation to establish efficient labor with the aggressive use of oxytocin so that the woman gives birth within 12 hours of admission to the labor unit. The physicians who developed the original protocol for active management of labor found that intervening early (as soon as a nulliparous woman was not dilating her cervix at least 1 cm/hr) with use of higher (pharmacologic) oxytocin doses administered at frequent increment intervals (e.g., a starting dose of 6 milliunits/min with increases of 6 milliunits/min every 15 minutes) shortened labor for most women and significantly decreased the cesarean birth rate at their institution (Simpson & O'Brien-Abel, 2014).

Additional components of the active management of labor include (1) strict criteria to diagnose that the woman is indeed in active labor with 100% cervical effacement, (2) amniotomy within 1 hour of admission of a woman in labor if spontaneous rupture of the membranes has not occurred, and (3) continuous presence of a personal nurse who provides one-on-one care for the woman while she is in labor. Many obstetricians in the United States emphasize using high-dose oxytocin protocols but do not implement all the other components of active management (Simpson & O'Brien-Abel, 2014). The presence of a personal nurse who provides constant emotional and physical support is the only component of active management of labor that is associated with shorter labors and lower rates of cesarean birth.

Operative Vaginal Birth

Operative vaginal birth is the term used for vaginal births that are assisted with either forceps or a vacuum extractor to apply direct traction on the fetal skull/scalp. The use of both devices has declined over the last two decades, as cesarean delivery has increased. In 2013, approximately 3.3% of all births in the United States were accomplished using forceps or vacuum assistance. Indications and prerequisites for the use of both instruments are identical (Nielsen, Deering, & Galan, 2017). The decision to use forceps or a vacuum extractor is based on the experience and personal preference of the physician performing the procedure. There are several types of operative vaginal births (American Academy of Pediatrics [AAP] & ACOG, 2017).

Forceps-Assisted Birth

A **forceps-assisted birth** is one in which an instrument with two curved blades is used to assist in the birth of the fetal head. The cephalic-like curve of the forceps commonly used is similar to the shape of the fetal head, with a pelvic curve to the blades conforming to the curve of the pelvic axis. The blades are joined by a pin, screw, or groove arrangement. These locks prevent the forceps from compressing the fetal skull (Fig. 32.8). There are several types of forceps-assisted births, classified by the station of the fetal head at application and the degree of rotation necessary for birth to occur (Table 32.3) (AAP & ACOG, 2017).

Maternal indications for forceps-assisted birth include a prolonged second stage of labor and the need to shorten the second stage of labor for maternal reasons (e.g., maternal exhaustion or maternal cardiopulmonary or cerebrovascular disease) (Nielsen et al., 2017).

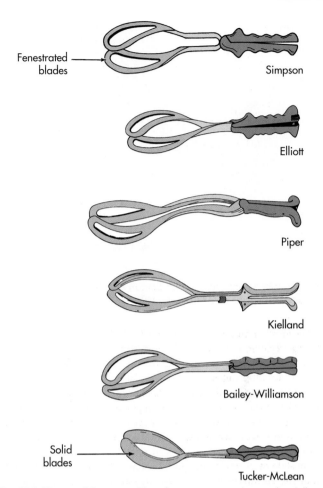

Fig. 32.8 Types of Forceps. Piper forceps are used to assist delivery of the head in a breech birth.

TABLE 32.3	Definitions for Forceps- and Vacuum-Assisted Births	
Outlet	Fetal scalp is visible on the perineum without manually separating the labia
Low	Fetal head is at least at the +2 station
Midpelvis	Fetal head is engaged (no higher than 0 station) but above +2 station

Data from American Academy of Pediatrics & American College of Obstetricians and Gynecologists. (2017). *Guidelines for perinatal care* (8th ed.). Washington, DC: American College of Obstetricians and Gynecologists.

The major fetal indication is suspicion of immediate or potential fetal compromise (i.e., a nonreassuring FHR tracing). The use of forceps during birth has been decreasing, replaced by vacuum extraction or cesarean birth (Nielsen et al.; Thorp & Grantz, 2019).

Certain conditions are required for a forceps-assisted birth to be successful. The woman's cervix must be fully dilated to prevent lacerations and hemorrhage. The bladder should be empty. The presenting part must be engaged—vertex presentation is desired. Membranes must be ruptured so that the position of the fetal head can be precisely determined and the forceps can firmly grasp the head during birth (Fig. 32.9). In addition, the size of the maternal pelvis must be assessed as adequate for the estimated fetal head circumference and weight (Nielsen et al., 2017).

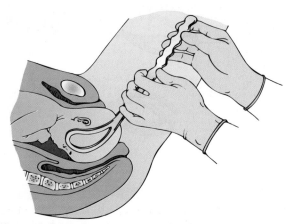

Fig. 32.9 Outlet Forceps-Assisted Extraction of the Head.

⚡ **SAFETY ALERT**

Because compression of the cord between the fetal head and the forceps will cause a decrease in fetal heart rate (FHR), the FHR is assessed, reported, and recorded before and after application of the forceps.

Medical management. Both blades are positioned by the physician, and the handles are locked. Traction is usually applied during contractions. The mother may or may not be instructed to push during contractions, depending on physician preference. If a decrease in the FHR occurs, the forceps are removed and reapplied.

Nursing interventions. When a forceps-assisted birth is deemed necessary, the nurse obtains the type of forceps requested by the physician. The nurse can explain to the mother that the forceps blades fit the same way two tablespoons fit around an egg, with the blades placed in front of the baby's ears.

After birth the mother should be assessed for vaginal or cervical lacerations, urinary retention, and hematoma formation in the pelvic soft tissues, which can result from blood vessel damage. The infant should be assessed for bruising or abrasions at the site of the blade applications, facial palsy resulting from pressure of the blades on the facial nerve, and subdural hematoma. Newborn and postpartum caregivers should be told that a forceps-assisted birth was performed.

Vacuum-Assisted Birth

Vacuum-assisted birth, or *vacuum extraction,* is a birth method involving the attachment of a vacuum cup to the fetal head, using negative pressure to assist in the birth of the head (Fig. 32.10). It is generally not used to assist birth before 34 weeks of gestation. Indications for its use are the same as those for outlet forceps. Prerequisites for use include informed consent, a completely dilated cervix, ruptured membranes, engaged head, vertex presentation, and no suspicion of CPD. Other prerequisites are an experienced operator and adequate anesthesia (Cunningham et al., 2018). The types of vacuum-assisted births are classified the same as for forceps-assisted births—by the station of the fetal head at application and the degree of rotation necessary for birth to occur (see Table 32.3) (AAP & ACOG, 2017). Advantages of vacuum-assisted birth compared with forceps-assisted birth are the ease with which the vacuum can be placed and the need for less anesthesia. Also it is far easier to teach and to learn the skills necessary to safely use the vacuum than to gain a similar level of skill with forceps (Thorp & Grantz, 2019).

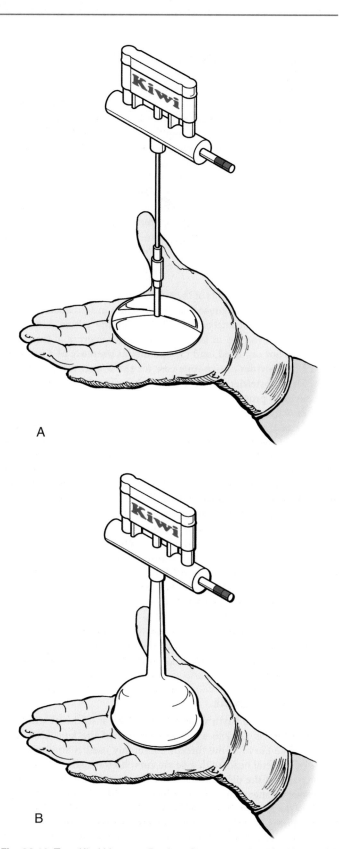

A

B

Fig. 32.10 Two Kiwi Vacuum Devices Demonstrating the Handheld Pump and Pressure Gauge Device. (From Gabbe, S. G., Niebyl, J. R., Simpson, J. L., et al. [Eds.]. (2017). *Obstetrics: Normal and problem pregnancies* [7th ed.]. Philadelphia: Elsevier.)

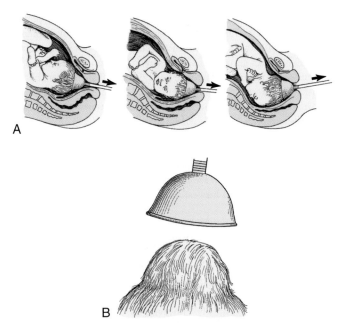

Fig. 32.11 Use of Vacuum Extraction to Rotate Fetal Head and Assist With Descent. (A) Arrow indicates direction of traction on the vacuum cup. (B) Caput succedaneum formed by the vacuum cup.

Medical management. The vacuum cup is applied to the fetal head by the physician. There are basically two types of vacuum devices. One is a self-contained unit, which allows the physician to both position the cup on the baby's head and generate the desired amount of negative pressure to create a vacuum. When the other type of vacuum device is used, the physician applies the cup to the baby's head, after which the nurse connects the suction tubing attached to the cup to wall suction or a separate hand pump and generates the amount of pressure requested by the physician. With both devices, a caput develops inside the cup as the pressure is initiated (Fig. 32.11). The woman is encouraged to push as traction is applied by the physician. The vacuum cup is released and removed after birth of the head. If vacuum extraction is not successful, a forceps-assisted or cesarean birth is usually performed.

Risks to the newborn include cephalohematoma, scalp lacerations, and subdural hematoma. These complications can be reduced by strict adherence to the manufacturer's recommendations for method of application, amount of pressure to be generated, and duration of application. Maternal risks include perineal, vaginal, or cervical lacerations and soft-tissue hematomas.

Nursing interventions. The nurse provides education and support for the woman who has a vacuum-assisted birth. The nurse can prepare the woman for birth and encourage her to remain active in the birth process by pushing during contractions. The FHR should be assessed frequently during the procedure. Documentation of the procedure in the medical record is important and is often the nurse's responsibility (Box 32.9). Neonatal caregivers should be told that the birth was vacuum assisted. After the birth, the newborn is observed for signs of trauma and infection at the application site and for cerebral irritation (e.g., seizures, lethargy, increased irritability or poor feeding) (Simpson & O'Brien-Abel, 2014). The newborn can be at risk for hyperbilirubinemia and neonatal jaundice as bruising resolves. The parents need to be reassured that the caput succedaneum usually disappears in 3 to 5 days (see Fig. 32.11B).

BOX 32.9 Assisting With Birth by Vacuum Extraction

- Assess the fetal heart rate frequently during the procedure.
- Encourage the woman to push during contractions.
- If responsible for generating pressure for the vacuum, do not exceed the "green zone" indicated on the pump. Verify with the physician the amount of pressure to be generated.
- Document the number of pulls attempted, the maximum pressure used, and any pop-offs that occur.

Cesarean Birth

Cesarean birth is the birth of a fetus through a transabdominal incision of the uterus. Whether cesarean birth is planned (scheduled) or unplanned, the loss of experiencing a vaginal birth can have a negative effect on a woman's self-concept. An effort is therefore made to maintain the focus on the birth of the baby rather than on the operative procedure.

The purpose of cesarean birth is to preserve the well-being of the mother and her fetus. It may be the best choice for birth when evidence exists of maternal or fetal complications. Since the advent of modern surgical methods and care and the use of antibiotics, maternal and fetal morbidity and mortality have decreased. In addition, incisions are usually made into the lower uterine segment rather than in the muscular body of the uterus, thus promoting more effective healing. However, despite these advances, cesarean birth still poses threats to the health of the mother and infant.

Birth data for 2016, the most recent available, indicate that the cesarean birth rate in the United States declined for the fourth consecutive year, to a rate of 31.9%. This is the lowest rate since 2007 (Martin et al., 2018). Despite recent small decreases, the cesarean birth rate in the United States remains very high. Part of the reason is that a number of common risk factors for cesarean birth are increasing in frequency, especially in developed countries. These factors include fetal macrosomia, advanced maternal age, increased maternal BMI, gestational diabetes, multifetal pregnancy, and dystocia in nulliparous women (Thorp & Grantz, 2019). Limited use of a trial of labor (TOL) after cesarean, due in part to concerns about safety and medicolegal considerations, is another reason for the high cesarean birth rate (Berghella et al., 2017).

ACOG and SMFM (2014) have recommended several measures to safely reduce the rate of primary cesarean births in the United States (Box 32.10). These measures involve the combined efforts of health care professionals and women and their families.

Indications

Few absolute indications exist for cesarean birth. Currently most are performed for conditions that might pose a threat to both the mother and the fetus if vaginal birth occurred, such as complete placenta previa or placental abruption (Berghella et al., 2017). Box 32.11 lists common indications for cesarean birth.

Elective Cesarean Birth

Elective cesarean birth, sometimes referred to as *cesarean on maternal request,* refers to a primary cesarean birth without medical or obstetric indication. Reasons given for elective cesarean birth include fear of pain during labor and birth and the mistaken belief that the surgery will prevent future problems with pelvic support, bladder and bowel incontinence, or sexual dysfunction. There is currently insufficient evidence to recommend elective caesarean delivery to prevent long-term urinary or anal incontinence (Thorp & Grantz, 2019). Although some nulliparous women may fear the pain of labor because of no firsthand experience, multiparous women may request a cesarean birth after a previous traumatic vaginal birth. Other women desire an elective cesarean birth because of the convenience of planning a date, or having control and choice about when to give birth. Less than 10% of women prefer a cesarean birth based solely on their own desires (Berghella et al., 2017).

Only limited data are available comparing cesarean births on request with planned vaginal births. ACOG, (2018a) states that planned cesarean birth requires a longer hospital stay than vaginal birth. Also,

postpartum hemorrhage occurs less frequently following planned cesarean birth than after planned vaginal birth followed by unplanned cesarean birth. Cesarean birth on request should not be performed before 39 weeks of gestation. Also, cesarean birth on request is not recommended for women who desire several additional children, because the risks for placenta previa, placenta accreta, and cesarean hysterectomy increase with each cesarean birth and are substantial with more than three surgeries (ACOG, 2018a; Berghella et al., 2017).

Scheduled Cesarean Birth

Cesarean birth is scheduled or planned if any of the following occur:
- Labor and vaginal birth are contraindicated (e.g., complete placenta previa, active genital herpes, positive HIV status with a high viral load)
- Birth is necessary but labor is not inducible (e.g., hypertensive states that cause a poor intrauterine environment that threatens the fetus)
- This course of action has been chosen by the obstetric health care provider and the woman (e.g., a repeat cesarean birth)

Women who are scheduled for a cesarean birth usually have time to prepare for it psychologically. However, the psychologic responses of these women may differ. Those having a repeat cesarean birth may have disturbing memories of the conditions preceding the initial (primary) cesarean birth and of their experiences in the postoperative recovery period. They may be concerned about the added burdens of caring for the infant and perhaps other children while recovering from surgery. Others may feel glad that they have been relieved of the uncertainty about the date and time of the birth and are free of the pain of labor.

Unplanned Cesarean Birth

The psychosocial outcomes of unplanned or emergency cesarean birth are usually more pronounced and negative when compared with the outcomes associated with a scheduled or planned cesarean birth. Women and their families experience abrupt changes in their expectations for birth, postpartum care, and care of the new baby at home. This can be an extremely traumatic experience for all.

The woman may approach the procedure tired and discouraged after an ineffective and difficult labor. Fear may predominate as she worries about her own safety and well-being and that of her fetus. She may be dehydrated, with low glycogen reserves. Because preoperative procedures must be done rapidly, there is often little time for explanation of the procedures and the operation itself. Because maternal and family anxiety levels are high at this time, much of what is said can be forgotten or misunderstood. The woman can experience feelings of anger or guilt in the postpartum period. Fatigue is often noticeable in these women, and they need much supportive care.

Forced Cesarean Birth

A woman's refusal to undergo cesarean birth when indicated for fetal reasons is often described as a *maternal-fetal conflict*. Health care providers are ethically obliged to protect the well-being of mother as well as fetus; a decision for one affects the other. If a woman refuses a cesarean birth that is recommended because of fetal jeopardy, health care providers must make every effort to find out why she is refusing and provide information that may persuade her to change her mind. If the woman continues to refuse surgery, then health care providers must decide if it is ethical to get a court order for the surgery. Every effort, however, should be made to avoid this legal step.

Surgical Techniques

The skin incision will either be vertical, extending from near the umbilicus to the mons pubis or transverse (Pfannenstiel) in the lower abdomen (Fig. 32.12). The transverse incision, sometimes referred to as the "bikini" incision, is performed more often in the United States. The type of skin incision is generally determined by the urgency of the surgery, prior incision type, the presence of known placental disorders (i.e., anterior complete placenta previa, placenta accreta), and the possible need to explore the upper abdomen for nonobstetric pathology (Berghella et al., 2017). The type of skin incision does *not* necessarily indicate the type of uterine incision.

The two main types of uterine incisions are the low transverse (Fig. 32.13A) or vertical incision, which may be either low or classical (see Fig. 32.13B and C). Occasionally an initial low transverse incision will be extended into a *J* shape (see Fig. 32.13D) or a *T* shape (see Fig. 32.13E). Ideally the vertical incision is contained entirely within the lower uterine segment, but extension into the contractile portion of the uterus (e.g., a classical incision) is common. The vertical uterine incision is only rarely performed, but occasionally it is necessary. Indications for a vertical incision include an underdeveloped lower uterine segment, a transverse lie presentation, an anterior placenta previa or

accreta, or if uterine leiomyomas (fibroids) obstruct the lower uterine segment (Berghella et al., 2017). Because it is associated with a higher incidence of uterine rupture in subsequent pregnancies than is lower-segment cesarean birth, vaginal birth after a classical uterine incision is contraindicated.

The low transverse uterine incision is performed in more than 90% of cesarean births (see Fig. 32.13A). Compared with the vertical incision, the transverse incision is preferred because it is easier to perform and repair and is associated with less blood loss. It also provides for the option of TOL and vaginal birth after cesarean (VBAC) in subsequent pregnancies (Berghella et al., 2017).

Complications and Risks

Possible maternal complications related to cesarean birth include anesthesia events (problems with intubation, drug reactions, aspiration pneumonia), hemorrhage, bowel or bladder injury, amniotic fluid embolism, and air embolism. Possible postpartum complications include atelectasis; endomyometritis; urinary tract infection; abdominal wound hematoma formation, dehiscence, infection, or necrotizing fasciitis; thromboembolic disease; and bowel dysfunction (Thorp & Grantz, 2019). In addition to these risks, the woman is also at economic risk because the cost of cesarean birth is higher than that of vaginal birth, and a longer recovery period may require additional expenditures.

Cesarean birth is associated with uncommon but significant dangers to the infant. The fetus may be born prematurely if the gestational age has not been accurately determined (iatrogenic prematurity). Fetal asphyxia can occur if the uterus and placenta are poorly perfused as a result of maternal hypotension caused by regional anesthesia (epidural or spinal) or maternal positioning. Fetal injuries (e.g., injuries caused by scalpel lacerations) can also occur during the surgery. The newborn is more likely to require resuscitation efforts and develop respiratory complications (Thorp & Grantz, 2019).

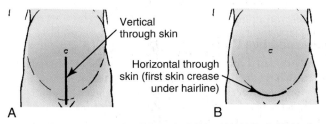

Fig. 32.12 Skin Incisions for Cesarean Birth. (A) Vertical. (B) Horizontal (Pfannenstiel).

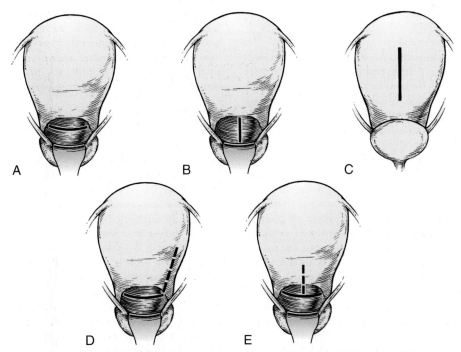

Fig. 32.13 Uterine Incisions for Cesarean Birth. (A) Low transverse. (B and C) Vertical. (D) Low transverse J-shaped. (E) Low transverse T-shaped. (From Gabbe, S. G., Niebyl, J. R., Simpson, J. L., et al. [Eds.]. [2017]. *Obstetrics: Normal and problem pregnancies* [7th ed.]. Philadelphia: Elsevier.)

Anesthesia

Spinal, epidural, and general anesthetics are used for cesarean births (see Chapter 17). Epidural blocks are popular because women want to be awake for and aware of the birth experience. However, the choice of anesthetic depends on several factors. The mother's medical history or present condition, such as a spinal injury, hemorrhage, or coagulopathy, may rule out the use of regional anesthesia. Time is another factor, especially if there is an emergency and the life of the mother or infant is at stake. In an emergency general anesthesia will most likely be used unless the woman already has an epidural block in effect. The woman herself is a factor. Either she may not know all the options or may have fears about having "a needle in her back" or about being awake and feeling pain. She needs to be fully informed about the risks and benefits of the different types of anesthesia so that she can participate in the decision whenever there is a choice.

 CARE MANAGEMENT

Prenatal Preparation

A discussion of cesarean birth should be included in all childbirth preparation classes. No woman can be guaranteed a vaginal birth, even if she is in good health and no indication of danger to the fetus exists before the onset of labor. Therefore every woman needs to be aware of and prepared for the possibility of having a cesarean birth.

Childbirth educators should emphasize the similarities and differences between a cesarean and a vaginal birth. In support of the philosophy of family-centered birth, many hospitals have instituted policies that permit fathers or partners and family members to share in these births as they do in vaginal births. Women who have undergone cesarean birth agree that the continued presence and support of their partners helped them respond more positively to the entire experience. In addition to preparing women for the possibility of cesarean birth, childbirth educators should empower them to believe in their ability to give birth vaginally and to seek care measures during labor that will enhance the progress of their labors and reduce their risk for cesarean birth.

Preoperative Care

Preparing a woman for cesarean birth is the same as that for other elective or emergency surgery. The obstetric health care provider discusses with the woman and her family the need for the cesarean birth and the prognosis for the mother and infant. A member of the anesthesia care team assesses the woman's cardiopulmonary status and describes the options for anesthesia. Women who are scheduled for an elective cesarean are often told to remain NPO (nothing by mouth) for at least 8 hours before the surgery. Informed consent is obtained for the procedure.

Blood tests are usually done 1 or 2 days before a planned cesarean birth or on admission to the labor and birth unit. Laboratory tests commonly ordered include a complete blood cell count and blood type and Rh status. Maternal vital signs and FHR and pattern are assessed according to hospital protocol until the operation begins. IV fluids are started to maintain hydration and to provide an open line for the administration of medications and blood products, if needed. Other preoperative preparations include ensuring that an informed consent form has been signed, inserting a retention (Foley) catheter to keep the bladder empty, and administering prescribed preoperative medications. In addition to medications given to prevent aspiration pneumonia, women may also receive prophylactic antibiotics to prevent postoperative infection. In the rare instance that an abdominal-mons shave or a clipping of pubic hair is ordered by the obstetric health care provider, it is performed in the operating room just before making the incision because shaving can result in injury of the integument, thereby increasing the risk for infection. Often, TED hose or SCD boots will be placed on the woman's legs to prevent blood clot formation. Removal of contact lenses, dentures, nail polish, and jewelry may be optional, depending on hospital policies and the type of anesthesia used. If the woman wears glasses and is going to be awake, the nurse should make sure her glasses accompany her to the operating room so she can see her infant.

During the preoperative preparation, the support person is encouraged to remain with the woman as much as possible to provide continuing emotional support (if this action is culturally acceptable to the woman and support person). The nurse provides essential information about the preoperative procedures during this time. Although the nursing actions may be carried out quickly if a cesarean birth is unplanned, verbal communication, particularly explanations, is important. Silence can be frightening to the woman and her support person. The nurse's use of touch (if culturally appropriate) can communicate feelings of care and concern for the woman. The nurse can assess the woman's and her partner's perceptions about cesarean birth. As the woman expresses her feelings, the nurse may identify the potential for a disturbance in self-concept during the postpartum period that would need to be addressed. If there is time before the birth, the nurse can teach the woman about postoperative expectations and about pain relief, position changes, leg exercises, coughing, and deep-breathing measures.

Intraoperative Care

Family-centered care is the goal for the woman who is undergoing cesarean birth and for her family. For the past several years, increasing efforts have been made to help women and their families optimize the cesarean birth experience while still maintaining safety. Options that can be offered to improve the cesarean birth experience include playing music chosen by the woman and her partner, softening the overhead lighting, using a surgical drape with a window if desired by the woman, and limiting extraneous conversation in the operating room. Implementing skin-to-skin care and breastfeeding in the operating room for infants who appear to be at term gestation and healthy are other interventions that are often desired by women and their families. Even seemingly "small" interventions, such as inserting the IV line into the woman's nondominant arm or hand, can enhance her birth experience (Schorn, Moore, Spetalnick, & Morad, 2015).

Cesarean births occur in operating rooms in the surgical suite or in the labor and birth unit. Staff members from the labor and birth unit may scrub and circulate during the surgery or these functions may be assumed by members of the hospital's surgery staff (Fig. 32.14). If possible, the partner or another person, dressed appropriately for the operating room, accompanies the mother to the operating room and remains close to her for continued comfort and support. In unplanned cesarean birth, the nurse who cared for the woman during labor should be part of the nursing care team in the operating room if possible.

The nurse who is circulating may assist with positioning the woman on the birth (operating) table. It is important to position her so that the uterus is displaced laterally to prevent compression of the inferior vena cava, which causes decreased placental perfusion. This is usually accomplished by placing a wedge under the hip or tilting the table to one side. The woman's legs should be strapped to the table to ensure proper positioning during surgery. A retention (Foley) catheter is inserted into the bladder at this time if one is not already in place.

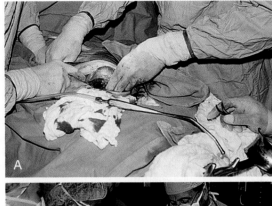

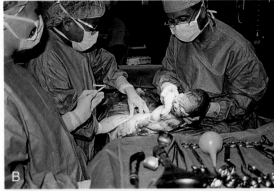

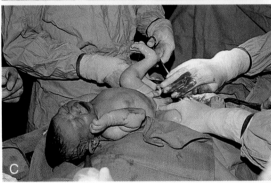

Fig. 32.14 Cesarean Birth. (A) "Bikini" incision has been made, the muscle layer is separated, the abdomen is entered, and the uterus has been exposed and incised; suctioning of amniotic fluid continues as head is brought up through the incision. Note small amount of bleeding. (B) The neonate's birth through the uterine incision is nearly complete. (C) A quick assessment is performed; note extreme molding of head resulting from cephalopelvic disproportion. (Courtesy Marjorie Pyle, RNC, Lifecircle, Costa Mesa, CA.)

As is done in other surgical procedures, a "time out" should be conducted just before the surgery begins. This is an opportunity for all members of the surgical team to participate in confirming the woman's identity and the planned procedure(s) to be performed. The circulating nurse is usually responsible for ensuring that the operative consent form has been signed and witnessed and is in the woman's chart. Members of the surgical team confirm that ordered preoperative medications have been given and that blood products, if ordered, are available. Information about drug or other allergies is also shared.

If the woman has general anesthesia, the partner likely will not be allowed in the operating room. If the partner or another person is not allowed or chooses not to be present, the nurse can stay in communication with him or her and give progress reports whenever possible. If the

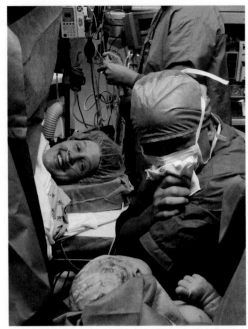

Fig. 32.15 New Parents' First View of Baby Born by Cesarean, While Surgery Is Still in Progress. (Courtesy Amber and Zack Gaynor, Apex, NC.)

woman is awake during the birth, the nurse, anesthesia care provider, or both can tell her what is happening and provide support. She may be anxious about the sensations she is experiencing, such as the coldness of solutions used to cleanse the abdomen and pressure or pulling during the actual birth of the infant. She also may be apprehensive because of the bright lights or the presence of unfamiliar equipment and masked and gowned personnel in the room. Explanations can help decrease her anxiety.

A nurse from the labor and birth unit is usually present to provide care for the infant. In addition, a neonatal or pediatric health care provider or an interprofessional team skilled in neonatal resuscitation may also be present for the surgery because these infants are considered to be at risk until evidence of physiologic stability after the birth is observed. A radiant warmer bed with resuscitation equipment is readied before surgery. Personnel who are responsible for care are expert not only in resuscitative techniques but also in detecting normal and abnormal infant responses (AAP & American Heart Association [AHA], 2016). After the birth, if the infant's condition permits and the mother is awake, the baby can be placed skin-to-skin on the mother or can be given to the woman's partner or another person to hold (Fig. 32.15). The infant whose condition is compromised is transported after initial stabilization to the nursery for observation and the implementation of appropriate interventions. In some institutions the partner or another person may accompany the infant; if not, personnel keep the family informed of the infant's progress and parent-infant contacts are initiated as soon as possible.

If family members cannot accompany the woman during surgery, they are directed to the surgical or obstetric waiting room. The physician then reports on the condition of the mother and infant to the family members after the birth is completed. Family members may be allowed to accompany the infant as she or he is transferred to the nursery, giving them an opportunity to see and admire the new baby.

Immediate Postoperative Care

Once surgery is completed, the mother is transferred to a postanesthesia recovery area. After a cesarean birth, women have postoperative and postpartum needs that must be addressed. They are surgical clients as well as new mothers. Assessments in this immediate postbirth period follow agency protocol and include degree of recovery from the effects of anesthesia, postoperative and postbirth status, and degree of pain. A patent airway is maintained, and the woman is positioned to prevent possible aspiration. Blood pressure and pulse are taken at least every 15 minutes for 2 hours but more frequently and for longer duration if there are complications. Temperature should be assessed every 4 hours for the first 8 hours after birth and then at least every 8 hours (AAP & ACOG, 2017). The condition of the incisional dressing and the fundus and the amount of lochia are assessed, as well as the IV intake and the urine output through the retention (Foley) catheter. Oxytocin usually is added to at least the first liter of the IV infusion to ensure that the fundus remains firmly contracted, thereby reducing blood loss. The woman is assisted to cough, deep-breathe, turn, and perform leg exercises. Medications for pain relief should be administered before postoperative pain becomes severe.

If the baby is present, the woman and her partner or another person are given some time alone with him or her to facilitate bonding and attachment, perhaps utilizing skin-to-skin contact. Breastfeeding may be initiated if the woman desires. The woman is ready for discharge from the postanesthesia recovery area once her condition is stable and the effects of anesthesia have worn off (i.e., she is alert and oriented and able to feel and move her extremities).

Postoperative Postpartum Care

The attitude of the nurse and other interprofessional health care team members can influence the woman's perception of herself after a cesarean birth. The caregivers should stress that the woman is a new mother first and a surgical client second. This attitude helps the woman perceive herself as having the same problems and needs as other new mothers, while requiring supportive postoperative care.

The woman's physiologic concerns may be dominated initially by pain at the incision site and later by pain resulting from intestinal gas. For the first 24 hours after surgery, pain relief is usually provided by epidural opioids, patient-controlled analgesia, or IV or IM injections. The most commonly used analgesics include opioids (e.g., hydromorphone [Dilaudid], morphine sulfate, nalbuphine [Nubain]) and NSAIDs (e.g., ketorolac [Toradol]). If opioids are used, an antiemetic (e.g., metoclopramide [Reglan]) is often administered either as needed by the woman or scheduled as long as the opioid is used. Palpation of the fundus with the possibility of massage should be performed after an analgesic is given to decrease pain. By 24 hours after surgery, pain management is generally changed to oral analgesics. Other comfort measures such as position changes, splinting of the incision with pillows, and relaxation and breathing techniques (e.g., those learned in childbirth classes) may be implemented (see Teaching for Self-Management box: Nonpharmacologic Postpartum Pain Relief After Cesarean Birth).

Women are often the best judges of what their bodies need and can tolerate, including the postoperative ingestion of foods and fluids.

Some health care providers keep women NPO or allow only "sips and chips" (sips of clear fluids and teaspoons of crushed ice) until bowel sounds return. The diet is then advanced to full liquids. After women are passing flatus they can resume a regular diet. Because most women have an epidural or spinal anesthetic for surgery, many health care providers allow the early introduction of solid food if desired and tolerated. IV fluids are usually continued until the woman is tolerating fluids orally. Ambulation and rocking in a rocking chair may relieve gas pains. Women should be taught to avoid gas-forming foods, ice chips, carbonated beverages, and using a straw to drink beverages to help limit gas formation, thereby minimizing the severity of gas pains (see Teaching for Self-Management box: Nonpharmacologic Postpartum Pain Relief After Cesarean Birth).

Nursing Interventions

Nurses must be alert to a woman's physiologic needs, managing care to ensure adequate rest and pain relief. Mother-baby care (couplet care) for a cesarean birth mother may have to be modified according to her physical limitations as a surgical client.

Daily care includes perineal care, breast care, and routine hygienic care. The woman may shower after the original incisional dressing is removed, usually on the first postoperative day (if showering is acceptable according to the woman's cultural beliefs and practices). The indwelling (Foley) catheter is usually also removed on the first postoperative day. The woman is encouraged to be out of bed and ambulating several times each day as soon as the urinary catheter is removed. Use of TED hose or SCD boots should continue as long as the woman remains in bed. They may be removed when she begins ambulating. The nurse assesses the woman's vital signs, incision, fundus, and lochia according to hospital policies, procedures, or protocols. Breath sounds, bowel sounds, circulatory status of lower extremities, and urinary and bowel elimination patterns also are assessed. It is important to observe maternal emotional status and progress of attachment to her baby.

During the postpartum period the nurse provides care that meets the psychologic and teaching needs of women who have had cesarean births. She or he can explain postpartum procedures to help the woman participate in her recovery from surgery. The nurse can help the woman plan care and visits from family and friends that will allow for adequate rest periods. Providing information on and assistance with infant care can facilitate adjustment to her role as a mother. With adequate support these women can benefit from providing baby care to facilitate attachment and enhance involvement in newborn care. The woman is supported as she breastfeeds her baby by receiving individualized assistance to comfortably hold and position the baby at her breast. Use of the side-lying or football-hold (under the arm or clutch hold) positions and supporting the newborn with pillows can enhance comfort and facilitate successful breastfeeding. The partner and other family members can be included in teaching sessions about infant care and the woman's recovery.

⚡ SAFETY ALERT

When holding her baby or breastfeeding, a woman may become drowsy and even fall asleep because of the sedation that occurs with the use of analgesics. It is important that someone be with her during these times to prevent newborn injury.

The couple also should be encouraged to express their feelings about the birth experience. Some parents are angry, frustrated, or disappointed that a vaginal birth was not possible. Some women express feelings of low self-esteem or a negative self-image. Others express relief and gratitude that the baby is healthy and safely born. It may be helpful for them to have the nurse who was present during the birth visit and help fill in "gaps" about the experience.

Discharge after cesarean birth is usually by the third postoperative day if not sooner. The nurse provides discharge teaching to prepare the woman for self-care and newborn care while trying to ensure that she is comfortable and able to rest. The nurse assesses the woman's information needs and coordinates the interprofessional health care team's efforts to meet them. Discharge teaching and planning should include information about nutrition; measures to relieve pain and discomfort; exercise and specific activity restrictions; time management that includes periods of uninterrupted rest and sleep; hygiene, breast, and incision care; timing for resumption of sexual activity and contraception; signs of complications (see Teaching for Self-Management box: Signs of Postoperative Complications After Discharge Following Cesarean Birth and Teaching for Self-Management box: Signs of Postpartum Blues, Depression, and Psychosis in Chapter 31); and infant care. The nurse assesses the woman's need for continued support or counseling to facilitate her emotional recovery from the birth. The woman's family and friends should be educated regarding her needs during the recovery process, and their assistance should be requested before discharge. Referral to support groups (e.g., www.birthrites.org) or to community agencies may be indicated to further promote the recovery process. A postdischarge program of telephone follow-up and home visits can facilitate the woman's full recovery after cesarean birth.

TEACHING FOR SELF-MANAGEMENT

Signs of Postoperative Complications After Discharge Following Cesarean Birth

Report the following signs to your health care provider:
- Temperature exceeding 38°C (100.4°F)
- Urination: painful urination, urgency, cloudy urine
- Lochia: heavier than a normal menstrual period, clots, odor
- Cesarean incision: redness, swelling, bruising, foul-smelling discharge or bleeding, wound separation
- Severe, increasing abdominal pain

Trial of Labor

A trial of labor (TOL) is the observance of a woman and her fetus for a reasonable period (e.g., 4 to 6 hours) of spontaneous active labor to assess the safety of vaginal birth for the mother and infant. It may be initiated if the mother's pelvis is of questionable size or shape or if the fetus is in an abnormal presentation or position. By far the most common reason for a TOL is if the woman wishes to have a vaginal birth after a previous cesarean birth. A woman who has had a previous cesarean birth with a low transverse uterine incision and who has no contraindications for vaginal birth should be counseled regarding TOL (ACOG, 2009/2019). Fetal sonography, maternal pelvimetry, or both may be done before a TOL to rule out CPD. During a TOL the woman is evaluated for active labor, including adequate contractions, engagement and descent of the presenting part, and effacement and dilation of the cervix.

The nurse assesses maternal vital signs and FHR and pattern and is alert for signs of potential complications. If complications develop, the nurse is responsible for initiating appropriate actions, including notifying the obstetric health care provider, and for evaluating and documenting the maternal and fetal responses to the interventions. Nurses must recognize that the woman and her partner are often anxious about maternal and fetal well-being. Supporting and encouraging the woman and her partner and providing information regarding progress can reduce stress and enhance the labor process and facilitate a successful outcome.

Vaginal Birth After Cesarean

Indications for primary cesarean birth, such as breech presentation or abnormal FHR or pattern, often are nonrecurring. Therefore a woman who has had a cesarean birth with a low transverse uterine incision may subsequently become pregnant, experience no contraindications to labor and vaginal birth during the pregnancy, and choose to attempt a vaginal birth after cesarean (VBAC).

A VBAC is contraindicated for women at high risk for uterine rupture. It should not be attempted by women with a previous classical or T-shaped uterine incision or extensive transfundal uterine surgery, a previous uterine rupture, or medical or obstetric complications that prevent vaginal birth (Landon & Grobman, 2017).

The overall success rate of VBAC is approximately 60% to 80% (Landon & Grobman, 2017). The strongest predictors for a successful VBAC are a prior vaginal birth and spontaneous (rather than induced or augmented) labor (AAP & ACOG, 2017). Women whose first cesarean birth was performed because of a nonrecurring indication (e.g., breech presentation) also are likely to have a successful VBAC (Landon & Grobman). Women with the following characteristics are less likely to have a successful VBAC (Landon & Grobman):
- Recurrent indication (e.g., labor dystocia) for initial cesarean birth
- Increased maternal age
- Non-Caucasian race or ethnicity
- Gestational age at or beyond 40 weeks
- Maternal obesity (BMI > 30)
- Estimated fetal weight greater than 4000 g
- Labor induction

ACOG (2019) also lists a short (<19 months) interbirth interval and preeclampsia at the time of birth as characteristics that are associated with a reduced chance for a successful VBAC.

Women who succeed in having a VBAC and thus avoid major abdominal surgery have lower rates of hemorrhage, thromboembolism, and infection, and a shorter recovery period than do women who give birth by repeat cesarean. Additionally, for women considering future pregnancies, VBAC may decrease the risk for maternal consequences related to multiple cesarean births, such as abnormal placentation (i.e., placenta previa or placenta accreta) (ACOG, 2019). The major risk associated with VBAC is uterine rupture (see later discussion) (Landon

& Grobman, 2017). Other maternal risks include infection, operative injury, blood transfusion, hysterectomy, and death (ACOG, 2019).

Women are most often the primary decision makers with regard to choice of birth method. During the prenatal period the woman should be given information about VBAC and encouraged to choose it as an alternative to repeat cesarean birth, as long as no contraindications exist. VBAC support groups (e.g., www.vbac.com) and prenatal classes can help prepare the woman psychologically for labor and vaginal birth. Women need to believe not only that their efforts during a TOL will be successful but also that they are fully capable of doing what is necessary to give birth vaginally. They must be given the opportunity to discuss their previous labor experience, including feelings of failure and loss of control, and to express concerns they may have about how they will manage during their upcoming labor and birth. Not everyone is enthusiastic about TOL and VBAC. After being fully informed about the benefits and risks, more than 25% of potential candidates choose to have a repeat cesarean birth instead (Thorp & Grantz, 2019). In 2016, for the first time, national data regarding VBAC was collected in the United States. In that year, 12.4% of women with a history of previous cesarean birth successfully gave birth vaginally (Martin et al., 2018).

If a woman chooses TOL, the nurse is attentive to her psychologic as well as physical needs during the TOL. Anxiety increases the release of catecholamines and can inhibit the release of oxytocin, thus delaying the progress of labor and possibly leading to a repeat cesarean birth. To reduce or alleviate such anxiety the nurse can encourage the woman to use breathing and relaxation techniques and to change positions to promote labor progress. The woman's partner can be encouraged to provide comfort measures and emotional support. Collaboration among the woman in labor, her partner, the nurse, and other health care providers often results in a successful VBAC. If a TOL does not result in vaginal birth, the woman will need support and encouragement to express her feelings about having another cesarean birth. It is very important that this outcome not be labeled a "failed" VBAC.

VBAC is a reasonable option for many women who have had a previous cesarean birth. However, many women who are appropriate candidates for TOL and VBAC lack access to providers and health care facilities that are able and willing to offer this option. ACOG (2019) continues to recommend that TOL and VBAC be offered only in facilities that have staff immediately available to provide emergency care. Because resources for immediate cesarean birth may not be available in all birthing facilities, the best alternative in some situations may be to refer interested women to other facilities that have the resources necessary to offer TOL and VBAC (Landon & Grobman, 2017).

OBSTETRIC EMERGENCIES

Meconium-Stained Amniotic Fluid

Meconium-stained amniotic fluid indicates that the fetus has passed meconium (first stool) before birth. Meconium-stained amniotic fluid is green. The consistency of the meconium fluid is often described as either thin (light) or thick (heavy), depending on the amount of meconium present. Three possible reasons for the passage of meconium are (1) it is a normal physiologic function that occurs with maturity (meconium passage being infrequent before weeks 23 or 24, with an increased incidence after 38 weeks) or with a breech presentation; (2) it is the result of hypoxia-induced peristalsis and sphincter relaxation; or (3) it can be a sequel to umbilical cord compression–induced vagal stimulation in mature fetuses.

The major risk associated with meconium-stained amniotic fluid is the development of meconium aspiration syndrome (MAS) in the newborn. MAS causes a severe form of aspiration pneumonia that occurs most often in term or postterm infants who have passed meconium in utero. MAS most likely results from a long-standing intrauterine process, rather than from aspiration immediately following birth as respirations are initiated (see Chapter 34) (Rozance & Rosenberg, 2017).

 CARE MANAGEMENT

The presence of an interprofessional team skilled in neonatal resuscitation is required at the birth of any infant with meconium-stained amniotic fluid. When meconium-stained amniotic fluid is present, the AAP and AHA's Neonatal Resuscitation Program no longer recommends routine suctioning of the newborn's mouth and nose on the perineum (after the head is out but before the rest of the baby is born) followed by endotracheal suctioning after birth. Instead, management of a newborn with meconium-stained amniotic fluid is based only on assessment of the baby's condition at birth. No clinical studies warrant basing tracheal suctioning guidelines simply on meconium consistency (AAP & AHA, 2016). See the Emergency box: Immediate Management of the Newborn with Meconium-Stained Amniotic Fluid for specific interventions.

 EMERGENCY

Immediate Management of the Newborn With Meconium-Stained Amniotic Fluid

Before Birth
- Assess the amniotic fluid for the presence of meconium after rupture of membranes.
- If the amniotic fluid is meconium stained, gather equipment and supplies that might be necessary for neonatal resuscitation.
- Have at least one person capable of performing endotracheal intubation on the newborn present at the birth.

Immediately After Birth
- Assess the newborn's respiratory efforts, heart rate, and muscle tone.
- Suction only the newborn's mouth and nose, using either a bulb syringe or a large-bore suction catheter if the baby has:
  - Strong respiratory efforts
  - Good muscle tone
  - Heart rate greater than 100 beats/min
- Suction the trachea using an endotracheal tube connected to a meconium aspiration device and suction source to remove any meconium present before many spontaneous respirations have occurred or assisted ventilation has been initiated if the newborn has:
  - Depressed respirations
  - Decreased muscle tone
  - Heart rate less than 100 beats/min

Data from American Academy of Pediatrics & American Heart Association. (2016). *Textbook of neonatal resuscitation* (7th ed.). Elk Grove Village, IL: American Academy of Pediatrics.

⚡ SAFETY ALERT

Every birth should be attended by at least one person whose only responsibility is the newborn and who is capable of initiating resuscitation. Either that person or someone else who is immediately available should have the skills required to perform a complete resuscitation, including endotracheal suctioning to remove meconium, if necessary.

Shoulder Dystocia

Shoulder dystocia is an uncommon obstetric emergency that increases the risk for fetal and maternal morbidity and mortality during the attempt to accomplish birth vaginally. Shoulder dystocia is a condition in which the head is born, but the anterior shoulder cannot pass under the pubic arch. It results from a size discrepancy between the fetal shoulders and the pelvic inlet, which may be absolute or may be relative, because of malposition. It is estimated that 0.2% to 3% of all vaginal births are complicated by shoulder dystocia (Lanni et al., 2017). The incidence of shoulder dystocia has increased in recent years, perhaps because of larger birth weights or simply because more attention is now paid to documenting the condition.

Fetopelvic disproportion related to excessive fetal size (more than 4000 g) or maternal pelvic abnormalities can cause shoulder dystocia, although 40% to 50% of all cases of shoulder dystocia occur with smaller fetuses (Simpson & O'Brien-Abel, 2014; Thorp & Grantz, 2019). Other risk factors for shoulder dystocia include maternal diabetes (risk for macrosomia), a history of shoulder dystocia with a previous birth, and a prolonged second stage of labor. In one-half of all cases of shoulder dystocia, however, no risk factors are identified (Thorp & Grantz). Shoulder dystocia cannot be accurately predicted or prevented (Simpson & O'Brien-Abel).

Signs that indicate the presence of shoulder dystocia include slowing of the progress of the second stage of labor and formation of a caput succedaneum that increases in size. The nurse should observe for retraction of the fetal head against the perineum immediately following its emergence (turtle sign), an early sign of shoulder dystocia. External rotation does not occur (Simpson & O'Brien-Abel, 2014; Thorp & Grantz, 2019).

Fetal injuries are usually caused either by asphyxia related to the delay in completing the birth or by trauma from the maneuvers used to accomplish the birth. The most common complications related to trauma include fracture of the humerus or clavicle and unilateral brachial plexus injuries. The right arm is typically the one affected. Evidence now exists that brachial plexus injuries can result from intrauterine forces during the second stage of labor rather than from the maneuvers used to accomplish birth (Lanni et al., 2017; Thorp & Grantz, 2019). If brachial plexus injuries are recognized early and treated properly, 80% to 90% heal completely. Therefore permanent neurologic injury is rare, occurring in only 1 or 2 of every 10,000 births. The major maternal complications associated with shoulder dystocia are postpartum hemorrhage and rectal injuries (Lanni et al.; Thorp & Grantz).

📋 CARE MANAGEMENT

Many maneuvers have been suggested and tried to free the anterior shoulder. The McRoberts maneuver and suprapubic pressure are usually the first-line interventions for shoulder dystocia because they are noninvasive, easily learned, and can be performed quickly. The specific interventions used are less important than is being prepared at every vaginal birth to deal with shoulder dystocia using a planned sequence of interventions if the need arises (Lanni et al., 2017).

In the McRoberts maneuver (Fig. 32.16), the woman's legs are hyperflexed on her abdomen (Lanni et al., 2017). This maneuver causes the sacrum to straighten, and the pelvis and symphysis pubis to rotate toward the mother's head. The angle of pelvic inclination is decreased, which frees the shoulder. Suprapubic pressure can then be applied over the anterior shoulder (Fig. 32.17) in an attempt to dislodge the shoulder (Lanni et al., 2017). Use of the McRoberts maneuver and suprapubic pressure may relieve more than one-half of all cases of shoulder dystocia. Fundal pressure as a method of relieving shoulder dystocia

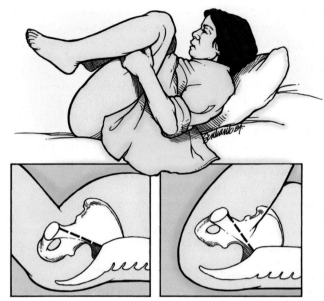

Fig. 32.16 McRoberts Maneuver. (From Gabbe, S. G., Niebyl, J. R., Simpson, J. L., et al. [Eds.]. [2017]. *Obstetrics: Normal and problem pregnancies* [7th ed.]. Philadelphia: Elsevier.)

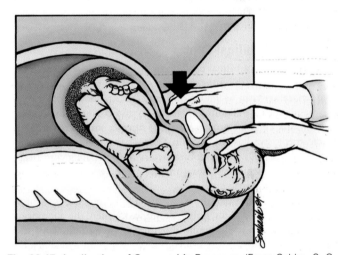

Fig. 32.17 Application of Suprapubic Pressure. (From Gabbe, S. G., Niebyl, J. R., Simpson, J. L., et al. [Eds.]. [2017]. *Obstetrics: Normal and problem pregnancies* [7th ed.]. Philadelphia: Elsevier.)

should be avoided because it will only further impact the anterior shoulder behind the symphysis pubis (Lanni et al., 2017). The Gaskin maneuver (having the woman move to a hands-and-knees position) has also been highly effective in resolving cases of shoulder dystocia. However, the Gaskin maneuver may be difficult to accomplish if the woman has significant loss of motor function caused by regional anesthesia (Baird & Kennedy, 2017).

When shoulder dystocia is diagnosed, the nurse should stay calm and immediately call for additional assistance (i.e., extra nurses, anesthesia care provider, and neonatal resuscitation team). The nurse then helps the woman assume the position or positions that may facilitate birth of the shoulders, assists the obstetric health care provider with these maneuvers and techniques during birth, and documents the maneuvers, including the total amount of time required to resolve the

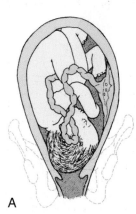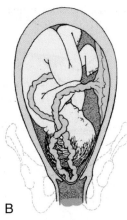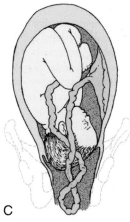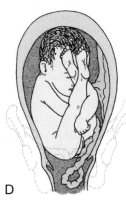

A B C D

Fig. 32.18 Prolapse of Umbilical Cord. Note pressure of presenting part on umbilical cord, which endangers fetal circulation. (A) Occult (hidden) prolapse of cord. (B) Complete prolapse of cord. Note that membranes are intact. (C) Cord presenting in front of the fetal head may be seen in the vagina. (D) Frank breech presentation with prolapsed cord.

shoulder dystocia. The nurse also provides encouragement and support to reduce the anxiety of the woman and her partner. Newborn assessment should include examination for fracture of the clavicle or humerus as well as brachial plexus injuries and asphyxia. Maternal assessment should focus on early detection of hemorrhage and trauma to the vagina, perineum, and rectum.

Prolapsed Umbilical Cord

Prolapse of the umbilical cord occurs when the cord lies below the presenting part of the fetus. Umbilical cord prolapse may be occult (hidden, rather than visible) at any time during labor whether or not the membranes are ruptured (Fig. 32.18A and B). It is most common to see frank (visible) prolapse directly after rupture of membranes, when gravity washes the cord in front of the presenting part (see Fig. 32.18C and D). Contributing factors include a long cord (longer than 100 cm), malpresentation (breech or transverse lie), or an unengaged presenting part.

If the presenting part does not fit snugly into the lower uterine segment (e.g., as in polyhydramnios), when the membranes rupture, a sudden gush of amniotic fluid may cause the cord to be displaced downward. Similarly, the cord may prolapse during amniotomy if the presenting part is high. A small fetus may not fit snugly into the lower uterine segment; as a result, cord prolapse is more likely to occur.

CARE MANAGEMENT

Prompt recognition of a prolapsed umbilical cord is important because fetal hypoxia resulting from prolonged cord compression (i.e., occlusion of blood flow to and from the fetus for more than 5 minutes) usually results in CNS damage or death of the fetus. Pressure on the cord may be relieved by the examiner putting a sterile gloved hand into the vagina and holding the presenting part off the umbilical cord (Fig. 32.19A and B). The woman may also be assisted into a position such as a modified Sims (see Fig. 32.19C), Trendelenburg, or knee-chest (see Fig. 32.19D) position, in which gravity keeps the pressure of the presenting part off the cord. If the cervix is fully dilated, a forceps- or vacuum-assisted birth can be performed for the fetus in a cephalic presentation; otherwise, a cesarean birth is likely to be performed. Abnormal FHR and pattern (e.g., bradycardia, absent or minimal variability, and variable or prolonged decelerations), inadequate uterine relaxation, and

bleeding also can occur as a result of a prolapsed umbilical cord. Indications for immediate interventions are presented in the Emergency box: Prolapsed Umbilical Cord. Ongoing assessment of the woman and her fetus is critical to determine the effectiveness of each action taken. The woman and her family are often aware of the seriousness of the situation; therefore the nurse must provide support by giving explanations for the interventions being implemented and their effect on the status of the fetus.

✚ EMERGENCY
Prolapsed Umbilical Cord

Signs
- Variable or prolonged deceleration during uterine contractions
- Woman reports feeling the cord after membranes rupture
- Cord is seen or felt in or protruding from the vagina

Interventions
- Call for assistance. Do not leave the woman alone.
- Have someone notify the obstetric health care provider immediately.
- Glove the examining hand quickly and insert two fingers into the vagina to the cervix. With one finger on either side of the cord or both fingers to one side, exert upward pressure against the presenting part to relieve compression of the cord (see Fig. 32.19A and B). Do not move your hand! Another person may place a rolled towel under the woman's right or left hip.
- Place woman into the extreme Trendelenburg or a modified Sims position (see Fig. 32.19C) or a knee-chest position (see Fig. 32.19D).
- If cord is protruding from vagina, wrap loosely in a sterile towel saturated with warm sterile normal saline solution. Do not attempt to replace cord into cervix.
- Administer oxygen to the woman by nonrebreather mask at 8-10 L/min until birth is accomplished.
- Start intravenous fluids or increase existing flow rate.
- Continue to monitor fetal heart rate continuously, by internal fetal scalp electrode, if possible.
- Explain to woman and support person what is happening and the way it is being managed.
- Prepare for immediate vaginal birth if cervix is fully dilated or cesarean birth if it is not.

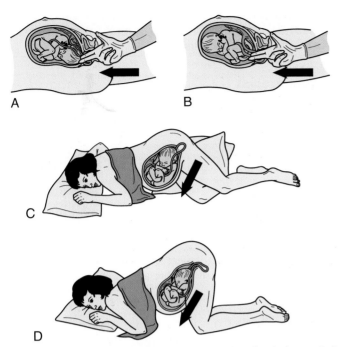

Fig. 32.19 Interventions for Prolapsed Umbilical Cord. Arrows indicate direction of pressure against presenting part to relieve compression of prolapsed umbilical cord. Pressure exerted by the examiner's fingers in (A) vertex presentation, and (B) breech presentation. (C) Gravity relieves pressure when woman is in modified Sims' position with hips elevated as high as possible with pillows. (D) Knee-chest position.

Rupture of the Uterus

Uterine rupture is defined as the symptomatic disruption and separation of the layers of the uterus or previous scar. Uterine rupture can result in the ejection of fetal parts or the entire fetus into the peritoneal cavity. The incidence of uterine rupture is approximately 1%. During labor and birth, the major risk factor for uterine rupture is a scarred uterus as a result of previous cesarean birth or other uterine surgery (Baird & Kennedy, 2017). Rupture most commonly occurs during a TOL for VBAC; symptomatic rupture is rarely observed in planned, repeat cesarean births. The likelihood of uterine rupture depends on the type and location of the previous uterine scar. Other factors that increase the risk for uterine rupture include prior uterine rupture, trauma, abortion, instrumentation injury or uterine perforation; grand multiparity; and uterine overdistension (i.e., macrosomic fetus, multiple gestation, polyhydramnios, and fetal malpresentation) (Baird & Kennedy).

Uterine dehiscence, sometimes called *incomplete uterine rupture*, is separation of a prior scar. It may go unnoticed unless the woman undergoes a subsequent cesarean birth or other uterine surgery. The potential for maternal or fetal complications as a result of uterine dehiscence is negligible because separation of a prior scar does not result in hemorrhage (Landon & Grobman, 2017).

Signs and symptoms vary with the extent of the uterine rupture. The most common finding is an abnormal (category II or category III) FHR tracing, as evidenced by an abrupt decrease in FHR, late or variable decelerations, absent baseline variability, or tachycardia or bradycardia. A loss of fetal station or no fetal descent also can occur. The woman can experience sudden sharp abdominal pain or a ripping or tearing sensation that is not associated with contractions. She may also exhibit bright red vaginal bleeding and signs of hypovolemic shock caused by hemorrhage (i.e., hypotension,

tachypnea). Fetal parts may be palpable through the abdomen (Baird & Kennedy, 2017).

📋 CARE MANAGEMENT

Prevention is the best treatment. Women who have had a cesarean birth with a classical uterine incision are advised not to labor or attempt vaginal birth in subsequent pregnancies. Those at risk for uterine rupture are assessed closely during labor. Women whose labor is induced with oxytocin or prostaglandin (especially if their previous birth was cesarean) are monitored for signs of uterine tachysystole because this can precipitate uterine rupture. If tachysystole occurs, the oxytocin infusion is decreased or discontinued, and a tocolytic medication may be given to decrease the intensity of the uterine contractions (see the Emergency box: Uterine Tachysystole with Oxytocin [Pitocin] Infusion). After giving birth, the woman is assessed for excessive bleeding, especially if the fundus is firm and signs of hemorrhagic shock are present.

If rupture occurs, management depends on the severity. A small rupture may be managed with a laparotomy and birth of the infant, repair of the laceration, and blood transfusions, if needed. Hysterectomy may be necessary if the rupture is large and difficult to repair or if the woman is hemodynamically unstable.

The nurse's role can include starting IV fluids, transfusing blood products, administering oxygen, and assisting with preparations for immediate surgery. Supporting the woman's family and providing information about the treatment are important during this emergency. Fetal prognosis is largely determined by whether significant placental abruption occurs and the degree of associated maternal hemorrhage and hypovolemia. Maternal morbidity and mortality also can be substantial. Rates of perinatal morbidity and mortality are also high (Cunningham et al., 2018). Providing information about spiritual support services or suggesting that the family contact their own support system may be warranted.

Amniotic Fluid Embolus

Amniotic fluid embolus (AFE), also known as *anaphylactoid syndrome of pregnancy*, is a rare but devastating complication of pregnancy characterized by the sudden, acute onset of hypotension, hypoxia, and hemorrhage caused by coagulopathy. AFE is considered to be unpreventable. AFE is neither an embolism or amniotic fluid-related, although it's timing suggests a breach of the normal physiologic barriers between woman and fetus (Hawkins, 2019). The true incidence of AFE is unknown because it is a diagnosis of exclusion with variations in diagnostic criteria. Because AFE is such a rare event, obtaining reliable information regarding risk factors, incidence, and outcomes is extremely challenging (Drummond & Yeomans, 2019). AFE is estimated to occur in 1 in 40,000 to1 in 50,000 births (Cunningham et al., 2018).

AFE occurs during labor, during birth, or within 30 minutes after birth. This combination of sudden respiratory and cardiovascular collapse, along with coagulopathy, is similar to that observed in clients with systemic inflammatory response syndrome or anaphylaxis (Hawkins, 2019).

The exact factor that initiates AFE has not been identified. In the past, particles of fetal debris (e.g., vernix, hair, skin cells, or meconium) found in amniotic fluid were thought to be responsible for initiating the syndrome; however, fetal debris can be found in the pulmonary circulation of most healthy laboring women. Also fetal debris is not identified in many women diagnosed with AFE. Therefore AFE is diagnosed clinically (Drummond & Yeomans, 2019; Hawkins, 2019; Simpson & O'Brien-Abel. 2014). Neonatal outcome in cases of AFE is poor. The neonatal mortality rate is estimated to be between 20% and 60%. Only half of the neonates who survive are neurologically intact (Drummond & Yeomans).

Predisposing conditions for AFE are rapid labor, meconium-stained amniotic fluid, and tears into uterine and other large pelvic veins that permit an exchange of fluids between the maternal and fetal compartments. Other commonly cited risk factors for AFE include older maternal age; postterm pregnancy; labor induction or augmentation; eclampsia; cesarean birth; forceps- or vacuum-assisted birth; placental abruption or placenta previa; and hydramnios (Cunningham et al., 2018). Previously it was thought that the hypertonic uterine contractions that often accompany AFE actually caused the event. Instead, it appears that the physiologic response to AFE produces the hypertonic contractions (Drummond & Yeomans, 2019).

CARE MANAGEMENT

The immediate interventions for AFE are summarized in the Emergency box: Amniotic Fluid Embolus. Care must be instituted immediately. If AFE occurs during labor, cesarean birth should be performed to aid in resuscitation of the woman and improve the chances of fetal survival (Hawkins, 2019). The nurse's immediate responsibility is to assist with the resuscitation efforts.

If the woman survives she is usually moved to a critical care unit. Additional interventions include replacing blood and clotting factors and maintaining adequate hydration and blood pressure. The woman is usually placed on ventilatory support (Hawkins, 2019).

Support of the woman's partner and family is needed; they will be anxious and distressed. Brief explanations of what is happening are important during the emergency and can be reinforced after the immediate crisis is over. If the woman dies, emotional support and involvement of the perinatal loss support team or other resources for grief counseling are needed. Referral to loss and grief support groups also is appropriate (see Chapter 37). The nursing staff also may need help in coping with feelings and emotions that result from a maternal death.

✚ EMERGENCY

Amniotic Fluid Embolus

Signs
- Respiratory distress
  - Restlessness
  - Dyspnea
  - Cyanosis
  - Pulmonary edema
  - Respiratory arrest
- Circulatory collapse
  - Hypotension
  - Tachycardia
  - Shock
  - Cardiac arrest
- Hemorrhage
  - Coagulation failure: bleeding from incisions, venipuncture sites, trauma (lacerations); petechiae, ecchymoses, purpura
  - Uterine atony

Interventions
- Oxygenate
  - Administer oxygen by nonrebreather face mask (8-10 L/min) or resuscitation bag delivering 100% oxygen.
  - Prepare for intubation and mechanical ventilation.
  - Initiate or assist with cardiopulmonary resuscitation. Tilt pregnant woman 30 degrees to her side to displace uterus.
- Maintain cardiac output, and replace fluid losses.
  - Position woman onto her side.
  - Administer intravenous fluids.
  - Administer blood products: packed cells, fresh-frozen plasma.
  - Insert indwelling catheter, and measure hourly urine output.
- Correct coagulation failure.
- Monitor fetal and maternal status.
- Prepare for emergency birth once woman's condition is stabilized.
- Provide emotional support to woman, her partner, and family.

▌ KEY POINTS

- Preterm birth is any birth that occurs between 20 0/7 and 36 6/7 weeks of gestation. Preterm birth is divided into two categories, *spontaneous* and *indicated*.
- Spontaneous preterm labor is generally diagnosed clinically as regular contractions along with a change in cervical effacement or dilation or both or presentation with regular uterine contractions and cervical dilation of at least 2 cm.
- The incidence of spontaneous preterm birth varies considerably by race. In the United States, non-Hispanic black women have the highest rate of preterm birth.
- The cause of spontaneous preterm labor is unknown and is assumed to be multifactorial; therefore it is not possible to predict with certainty which women will experience preterm labor and birth.
- Because the onset of spontaneous preterm labor is often insidious and can be mistaken for normal discomforts of pregnancy, nurses should teach all pregnant women how to detect the early symptoms of preterm labor and to call their obstetric health care provider when symptoms occur.

- The best reason to use tocolytic therapy is to achieve sufficient time to administer glucocorticoids in an effort to accelerate fetal lung maturity. Additionally, time is allowed for transport of the woman prior to birth to a center equipped to care for preterm infants.
- If fetal or early neonatal death is expected, the parents and members of the interprofessional health care team need to discuss the situation before the birth and decide on a management plan that is acceptable to everyone.
- Vigilance for signs of infection is an essential component of the care management for women with preterm prelabor rupture of membranes.
- Dysfunctional labor can be caused by ineffective uterine contractions or maternal bearing down efforts; fetal causes including abnormalities of presentation, position, or development; or alterations in the pelvic structure including abnormalities of the maternal bony pelvis or soft-tissue abnormalities of the reproductive tract.
- Obese women are at risk for several pregnancy complications, including cesarean birth. Even routine procedures require more time and effort to accomplish when the client is obese.

■ KEY POINTS—cont'd

- Uterine contractility is increased by the effects of oxytocin and prostaglandin and is decreased by tocolytic agents.
- Labor should not be induced electively until the woman has reached at least 39 weeks of gestation.
- Cervical ripening using chemical or mechanical measures can increase the success of labor induction.
- Expectant parents benefit from learning about operative obstetrics (e.g., forceps-assisted, vacuum-assisted, or cesarean birth) during the prenatal period.

- The basic purpose of cesarean birth is to preserve the well-being of the mother and her fetus.
- Unless contraindicated, vaginal birth is possible after a previous cesarean birth.
- Obstetric emergencies (e.g., meconium-stained amniotic fluid, shoulder dystocia, prolapsed cord, rupture of the uterus, and amniotic fluid embolism) occur rarely but require immediate intervention to preserve the health or life of the mother and fetus or newborn.

REFERENCES

American Academy of Pediatrics & American College of Obstetricians and Gynecologists. (2017). *Guidelines for perinatal care* (8th ed.). Washington, DC: American College of Obstetricians and Gynecologists.

American Academy of Pediatrics & American Heart Association. (2016). *Textbook of neonatal resuscitation* (7th ed.). Elk Grove Village, IL: American Academy of Pediatrics.

American College of Obstetricians and Gynecologists. (2009, reaffirmed 2019). Practice bulletin no. 107: Induction of labor. *Obstetrics & Gynecology, 114*(2 pt 1), 386–397.

American College of Obstetricians and Gynecologists. (2014, reaffirmed 2019). Practice bulletin no. 146: Management of late-term and postterm pregnancies. *Obstetrics & Gynecology, 124*(2 pt 1), 390–396.

American College of Obstetricians and Gynecologists. (2015, reaffirmed 2018). Practice bulletin no. 156: Obesity in pregnancy. *Obstetrics & Gynecology, 126*(6), e112–e126.

American College of Obstetricians and Gynecologists. (2016, reaffirmed 2018). Practice bulletin no. 171: Management of preterm labor. *Obstetrics & Gynecology, 128*(4), e155–e164.

American College of Obstetricians and Gynecologists. (2018a). Committee opinion no. 761: Cesarean delivery on maternal request. *Obstetrics & Gynecology, 133*(1), e73–e77.

American College of Obstetricians and Gynecologists. (2018b). Practice bulletin no. 188: Prelabor rupture of membranes. *Obstetrics & Gynecology, 131*(1), e1–14.

American College of Obstetricians and Gynecologists. (2019). Practice bulletin no. 205: Vaginal birth after cesarean delivery. *Obstetrics & Gynecology, 133*(2), e110–e127.

American College of Obstetricians and Gynecologists & Society for Maternal-Fetal Medicine. (2013, reaffirmed 2017). Committee opinion no. 579: Definition of term pregnancy. *Obstetrics & Gynecology, 122*(5), 1139–1140.

American College of Obstetricians and Gynecologists & Society for Maternal-Fetal Medicine. (2014). Safe prevention of the primary cesarean delivery. *Obstetrics & Gynecology, 123*(3), 693–711.

Baird, S. M., & Kennedy, B. B. (2017). Obstetric emergencies. In B. B. Kennedy, & S. M. Baird (Eds.), *Intrapartum management modules: A perinatal education program* (5th ed.). Philadelphia: Wolters Kluwer.

Baird, S. M., Kennedy, B. B., & Dalton, J. (2017). Special considerations for individualized care of the laboring woman. In B. B. Kennedy, & S. M. Baird (Eds.), *Intrapartum management modules: A perinatal education program* (5th ed.). Philadelphia: Wolters Kluwer.

Bakker, R., Pierce, S., & Myers, D. (2017). The role of prostaglandins E1 and E2, dinoprostone, and misoprostol in cervical ripening and the induction of labor: A mechanistic approach. *Archives of Gynecology and Obstetrics, 296*(2), 167–179.

Berghella, V., Mackeen, D., & Jauniaux, E. R. M. (2017). Cesarean delivery. In S. G. Gabbe, J. R. Niebyl, J. L. Simpson, et al. (Eds.), *Obstetrics: Normal and problem pregnancies* (7th ed.). Philadelphia: Elsevier.

Bowers, N. A. (2014). Multiple gestation. In K. R. Simpson, & P. Creehan (Eds.), *AWHONN's perinatal nursing* (4th ed.). Philadelphia: Lippincott, Williams & Wilkins.

Cunningham, F., Leveno, K., Bloom, S., et al. (2018). *Williams obstetrics* (25th ed.). New York: McGraw-Hill Education.

Dalton, J., & Strehlow, S. (2019). Maternal obesity. In N. H. Troiano, P. M. Witcher, & S. M. Baird (Eds.), *AWHONN's high risk and critical care obstetrics* (4th ed.). Philadelphia: Wolters Kluwer.

Drummond, S., & Yeomans, E. R. (2019). Amniotic fluid embolism. In N. H. Troiano, P. M. Witcher, & S. M. Baird (Eds.), *AWHONN's high risk and critical care obstetrics* (4th ed.). Philadelphia: Wolters Kluwer.

Duff, P. (2019). Maternal and fetal infections. In R. Resnik, C. J. Lockwood, T. R. Moore, et al. (Eds.), *Creasy & Resnik's maternal-fetal medicine: Principles and practice* (8th ed.). Philadelphia: Elsevier.

Duff, P., & Birsner, M. (2017). Maternal and perinatal infection in pregnancy: Bacterial. In S. G. Gabbe, J. R. Niebyl, J. L. Simpson, et al. (Eds.), *Obstetrics: Normal and problem pregnancies* (7th ed.). Philadelphia: Elsevier.

Friedman, E. (1989). Normal and dysfunctional labor. In W. Cohen, D. Ackers, & E. Friedman (Eds.), *Management of labor* (6th ed.). Rockville, MD: Aspen.

Gibbs Pickens, C. M., Kramer, M. R., Howards, P. P., et al. (2018). Term elective induction of labor and pregnancy outcomes among obese women and their offspring. *Obstetrics & Gynecology, 131*(1), 12–22.

Hawkins, J. L. (2019). Anesthesia considerations for complicated pregnancies. In R. Resnik, C. J. Lockwood, T. R. Moore, et al. (Eds.), *Creasy & Resnik's maternal-fetal medicine: Principles and practice* (8th ed.). Philadelphia: Elsevier.

Huwe, V. Y. (2017). Induction and augmentation of labor. In B. B. Kennedy, & S. M. Baird (Eds.), *Intrapartum management modules: A perinatal education program* (5th ed.). Philadelphia: Wolters Kluwer.

Institute for Safe Medication Practices. (2014). *ISMP's list of high-alert medications*. Retrieved from: http://www.ismp.org/Tools/highAlertMedication-Lists.asp.

Kilpatrick, S., & Garrison, E. (2017). Normal labor and delivery. In S. G. Gabbe, J. R. Niebyl, J. L. Simpson, et al. (Eds.), *Obstetrics: Normal and problem pregnancies* (7th ed.). Philadelphia: Elsevier.

Landon, M. B., & Grobman, W. A. (2017). Vaginal birth after cesarean delivery. In S. G. Gabbe, J. R. Niebyl, J. L. Simpson, et al. (Eds.), *Obstetrics: Normal and problem pregnancies* (7th ed.). Philadelphia: Elsevier.

Lanni, S. M., Gherman, R., & Gonik, B. (2017). Malpresentations. In S. G. Gabbe, J. R. Niebyl, J. L. Simpson, et al. (Eds.), *Obstetrics: Normal and problem pregnancies* (7th ed.). Philadelphia: Elsevier.

Macones, G., Hankins, G., Spong, C., et al. (2008). The 2008 National Institute of Child Health and Human Development workshop report on electronic fetal monitoring: Update on definitions, interpretation, and research guidelines. *Journal of Obstetric, Gynecologic & Neonatal Nursing, 37*(5), 510–515.

Malone, F. D., & D'Alton, M. E. (2019). Multiple gestation: Clinical characteristics and management. In R. Resnik, C. J. Lockwood, T. R. Moore, et al. (Eds.), *Creasy & Resnik's maternal-fetal medicine: Principles and practice* (8th ed.). Philadelphia: Elsevier.

Martin, J. A., Hamilton, B. E., Osterman, M. J. K., et al. (2018). Births: Final data for 2016. *National Vital Statistics Reports, 67*(1), 1–55.

Martin, J. A., Osterman, M. J. K., Kimeyer, S. E., & Gregory, E. C. W. (2015). Measuring gestational age in vital statistics data: Transitioning to the obstetric estimate. *National Vital Statistics Reports, 64*(5), 1–20.

McCue, B., & Torbenson, V. E. (2017). Fetal fibronectin: The benefits of a high negative predictive value in management of preterm labor. *Contemporary OB/GYN, 62*(9), 1–6.

Mercer, B. M. (2017). Premature rupture of the membranes. In S. G. Gabbe, J. R. Niebyl, J. L. Simpson, et al. (Eds.), *Obstetrics: Normal and problem pregnancies* (7th ed.). Philadelphia: Elsevier.

Mercer, B. M. (2019). Assessment and induction of fetal pulmonary maturity. In R. Resnik, C. J. Lockwood, T. R. Moore, et al. (Eds.), *Creasy & Resnik's maternal-fetal medicine: Principles and practice* (8th ed.). Philadelphia: Elsevier.

Mercer, B. M., & Chien, E. K. S. (2019). Premature rupture of the membranes. In R. Resnik, C. J. Lockwood, T. R. Moore, et al. (Eds.), *Creasy & Resnik's maternal-fetal medicine: Principles and practice* (8th ed.). Philadelphia: Elsevier.

Newman, R. B., & Unal, E. R. (2017). Multiple gestations. In S. G. Gabbe, J. R. Niebyl, J. L. Simpson, et al. (Eds.), *Obstetrics: Normal and problem pregnancies* (7th ed.). Philadelphia: Elsevier.

Nielsen, P. E., Deering, S. P., & Galan, H. L. (2017). Operative vaginal delivery. In S. G. Gabbe, J. R. Niebyl, J. L. Simpson, et al. (Eds.), *Obstetrics: Normal and problem pregnancies* (7th ed.). Philadelphia: Elsevier.

Rampersad, R., & Macones, G. A. (2017). Prolonged and postterm pregnancy. In S. G. Gabbe, J. R. Niebyl, J. L. Simpson, et al. (Eds.), *Obstetrics: Normal and problem pregnancies* (7th ed.). Philadelphia: Elsevier.

Reedy, N. J. (2014). Preterm labor and birth. In K. R. Simpson, & P. Creehan (Eds.), *AWHONN's perinatal nursing* (4th ed.). Philadelphia: Lippincott, Williams & Wilkins.

Rozance, P. J., & Rosenberg, A. A. (2017). The neonate. In S. G. Gabbe, J. R. Niebyl, J. L. Simpson, et al. (Eds.), *Obstetrics: Normal and problem pregnancies* (7th ed.). Philadelphia: Elsevier.

Schorn, M. N., Moore, E., Spetalnick, B. M., & Morad, A. (2015). Implementing family-centered cesarean birth. *Journal of Midwifery & Women's Health, 60*(6), 682–690.

Sheibani, L., & Wing, D. A. (2017). Abnormal labor and induction of labor. In S. G. Gabbe, J. R. Niebyl, J. L. Simpson, et al. (Eds.), *Obstetrics: Normal and problem pregnancies* (7th ed.). Philadelphia: Elsevier.

Simhan, H. N., Berghella, V., & Iams, J. D. (2019). Prevention and management of preterm parturition. In R. Resnik, C. J. Lockwood, T. R. Moore, et al. (Eds.), *Creasy & Resnik's maternal-fetal medicine: Principles and practice* (8th ed.). Philadelphia: Elsevier.

Simhan, H. N., Iams, J. D., & Romero, R. (2017). Preterm labor and birth. In S. G. Gabbe, J. R. Niebyl, J. L. Simpson, et al. (Eds.), *Obstetrics: Normal and problem pregnancies* (7th ed.). Philadelphia: Elsevier.

Simpson, K. R., & O'Brien-Abel, N. (2014). Labor and birth. In K. R. Simpson, & P. Creehan (Eds.), *AWHONN's perinatal nursing* (4th ed.). Philadelphia: Lippincott, Williams & Wilkins.

Swanson, D., & Baird, S. M. (2017). Preterm labor and preterm premature rupture of membranes. In B. B. Kennedy, & S. M. Baird (Eds.), *Intrapartum management modules: A perinatal education program* (5th ed.). Philadelphia: Wolters Kluwer.

Thorp, J. M., & Grantz, K. L. (2019). Clinical aspects of normal and abnormal labor. In R. Resnik, C. J. Lockwood, T. R. Moore, et al. (Eds.), *Creasy & Resnik's maternal-fetal medicine: Principles and practice* (8th ed.). Philadelphia: Elsevier.

Verhaeghe, C., Parot-Schinkel, E., Bouet, P. E., et al. (2018). *The impact of manual rotation of the occiput posterior position on spontaneous vaginal delivery rate: Study protocol for a randomized clinical trial (RMOS). Trials, 19:109.*

World Health Organization. Preterm birth. Retrieved from: http://www.who.int/en/news-room/fact-sheets/detail/preterm-birth.

Postpartum Complications

Rhonda K. Lanning

LEARNING OBJECTIVES

- Identify the causes, signs and symptoms, and interprofessional management of postpartum hemorrhage.
- Describe hemorrhagic shock as a complication of postpartum hemorrhage, including management and hazards of therapy.

- Describe thromboembolic disorders, including incidence, etiology, signs and symptoms, and interprofessional management.
- Differentiate the causes of postpartum infection.
- Summarize the assessment and care of women with postpartum infection.

The postpartum period is a time of change and transition for mothers and newborns. Mothers experience incredible physiologic shifts and emotional adjustments in the hours and days following birth. Perinatal nurses provide education, care, and support for mothers, newborns, and families during this critical time. In addition, nurses are responsible for identifying signs and symptoms of complications. The nurse collaborates with other members of the interprofessional health care team to provide safe and effective care to women experiencing postpartum physiologic complications. The nurse's rapid and skillful responses to complications such as hemorrhage, thromboembolic disorders, and infection are critical to the well-being of the new mother. This chapter focuses on these important postpartum complications. Postpartum mental health issues are addressed in Chapter 31.

POSTPARTUM HEMORRHAGE

Definition and Incidence

Postpartum hemorrhage (PPH) is an obstetric emergency and a leading cause of maternal morbidity and mortality in the United States and throughout the world (World Health Organization [WHO], 2015). It can occur with little warning and often is not recognized until the mother has profound symptoms. Early recognition, preparation, and appropriate management are critical to achieve a good outcome.

Definitions of PPH vary considerably in the literature. The American College of Obstetricians and Gynecologists (ACOG) revised their definition of PPH from the classic one (≥500 mL after vaginal birth or ≥1000 mL after cesarean) to (1) cumulative blood loss ≥1000 mL or (2) bleeding associated with signs/symptoms of hypovolemia within 24 hours of the birth process regardless of type of birth (ACOG, 2017). In practice settings, diagnosis is often based on subjective observations, with blood loss often being underestimated by as much as 50% (Cunningham, Leveno, Bloom, et al., 2018). (See Clinical Reasoning Case Study: Postpartum Hemorrhage.)

PPH is classified as early or late with respect to the time of birth. Early, acute, or primary PPH occurs within 24 hours of the birth. Late or secondary PPH occurs more than 24 hours but less than 6 weeks after the birth (Francois & Foley, 2017). Today's health care environment encourages shortened hospital stays after birth, which increases the potential for acute episodes of PPH to occur outside the traditional hospital or birth center setting.

❓ CLINICAL REASONING CASE STUDY

Postpartum Hemorrhage

Maria is a 30-year-old woman who had an uncomplicated 2-hr labor and a spontaneous vaginal birth of a 4-kg baby boy. You are the mother-baby nurse providing their care. When she calls you to her room, Maria is skin-to-skin and breastfeeding her 2-hr-old son. She notes that she has been "cramping" and is concerned that her peripad feels "wet." You check her pad and find that it is soaked through with blood. You help her lie back and then assess her fundus. It is soft and three fingerbreadths above the umbilicus and deviated to the right.

1. What is the priority concern or client need in this situation? Support your answer with data as stated in the case.
2. List other client needs/problems in this case.
3. Identify any additional information or assessment data that are needed by the nurse in planning care for this client.
4. Describe other nursing interventions that are important to providing optimal client care.
   a. What is the priority nursing action? (What should the nurse do first?)
   b. Describe other nursing interventions that are important to providing optimal client care.
5. Describe the roles/responsibilities of the interprofessional health care team members (other than nurses) who may be involved in providing care for this client.

Etiology and Risk Factors

From birth of the infant until separation of the placenta, the character and quantity of blood expelled from the vagina can suggest excessive bleeding. For example, dark red blood is likely of venous origin, perhaps from varices or superficial lacerations of the birth canal. Bright blood is arterial and can indicate deep lacerations of the cervix. Excessive bleeding that occurs during the period from the separation of the placenta to its expulsion or removal is commonly the result of incomplete placental separation, undue manipulation of the fundus, or excessive traction on the umbilical cord. Persistent or excessive blood loss occurring after the expulsion or removal of the placenta is usually the result of uterine atony or prolapse of the uterus into the vagina. Late PPH can be the result of subinvolution of the uterus, endometritis, or retained placental fragments (Francois & Foley, 2017). Predisposing factors for PPH are listed in Box 33.1.

Uterine Atony

The greatest risk for early PPH is during the first hour after birth. The body of the uterus is like a basket-weave of strong, interlacing smooth muscle bundles through which many large maternal blood vessels pass (see Fig. 4.3). After the expulsion or removal of the placenta, the uterus controls bleeding by contracting these smooth muscle fibers. If inadequate uterine contraction occurs, the uterus remains flaccid and rapid blood loss can follow. This hypotonia of the uterus is called **uterine atony**.

Uterine atony is the leading cause of early PPH. It is associated with high parity, polyhydramnios, fetal macrosomia, obesity, and multiple gestations. In such conditions the uterus is overdistended and may not contract as well after birth. See Box 33.1 for other risk factors and causes of uterine atony (Francois & Foley, 2017).

Placental Complications

When the placenta has not been expelled within 30 minutes after birth despite an upright posture of the woman, gentle traction on the umbilical cord, and uterine massage, it is described as a *retained placenta*. Initial management of a retained placenta consists of manual separation and removal by the nurse-midwife or physician. This involves the provider reaching into the uterus and gently separating the placenta from the uterine wall and removing it manually. When the woman has regional anesthesia for labor, supplementary anesthesia is usually not needed. For other women, administration of light nitrous oxide and oxygen inhalation anesthesia or intravenous (IV) pain medications should be considered. A tocolytic medication such as nitroglycerin IV may be given to promote uterine relaxation (Francois & Foley, 2017). After removal of a retained placenta, the woman has an increased risk for PPH and infection.

Fragments of the placenta can remain in the uterus after spontaneous separation of the placenta during the third stage of labor. In this case, the woman will have excessive bleeding and the uterus feels boggy (soft) due to uterine atony. Ultrasonography can be used to detect placental fragments. The nurse-midwife or physician may attempt manual exploration to remove the fragments; uterine curettage (removal of uterine contents using a curette or vacuum suction) may be necessary.

PPH can also be due to an abnormally implanted, invasive, or adhered placenta; this is known as *placenta accrete syndrome* or a *morbidly adherent placenta*. Abnormal placental adherence can be total, partial, or focal, depending on how much placental tissue is involved. The following degrees of abnormal placental attachment are recognized:

Placenta accreta—Slight penetration of myometrium

Placenta increta—Deep penetration of myometrium

Placenta percreta—Perforation of myometrium and uterine serosa, possibly involving adjacent organs

Placenta accrete syndrome has an increased incidence in association with the rise in cesarean birth rates (Cunningham et al., 2018). Other risk factors include placenta previa, prior uterine surgery, endometrial defects, submucosal fibroids, multiparity, and older maternal age (Francois & Foley, 2017). Placenta accrete syndrome can be diagnosed before birth using ultrasound and magnetic resonance imaging (MRI), but often it is not recognized until there is excessive bleeding after birth. Cesarean birth is recommended when the diagnosis is made prenatally. Bleeding may not occur unless manual removal of the placenta is attempted. With more extensive involvement, bleeding becomes profuse when removal of the placenta is attempted. Less blood is lost if the diagnosis is made antenatally and no attempt is made to manually remove the placenta. Treatment includes blood component replacement therapy. Hysterectomy can be indicated for all three types of placental adherence if bleeding is uncontrolled and is almost always required for a placenta percreta or placenta increta (Cunningham et al., 2018). Attempts to remove the placenta in the usual manner are unsuccessful, and laceration or perforation of the uterine wall can result, putting the woman at great risk for severe PPH and infection (Francois & Foley).

Lacerations of the Genital Tract

Lacerations of the cervix, vagina, and perineum also are causes of PPH. Hemorrhage related to lacerations should be suspected if bleeding continues despite a firm, contracted uterine fundus. This bleeding can be a slow trickle, an oozing, or frank hemorrhage. Factors that influence the causes and incidence of obstetric lacerations of the lower genital tract include operative birth, precipitous or rapid birth, congenital abnormalities of the maternal soft tissue, and contracted pelvis. Other possible causes of lacerations are increased size, abnormal presentation, and position of the fetus; relative size of the presenting part and the birth canal; previous scarring from infection, injury, or surgery; and vulvar, perineal, and vaginal varicosities.

Lacerations of the perineum are the most common of all injuries in the lower portion of the genital tract. These are classified as first, second, third, and fourth degree (see Chapter 19). An episiotomy can extend to become either a third- or fourth-degree laceration.

Prolonged pressure of the fetal head on the vaginal mucosa ultimately interferes with the circulation and may produce ischemic or pressure necrosis. The state of the tissues in combination with the type of birth can result in deep vaginal lacerations, with consequent predisposition to vaginal hematomas.

Cervical lacerations usually occur at the lateral angles of the external os. Most are shallow, and bleeding is minimal. More extensive lacerations may extend into the vaginal vault or into the lower uterine segment.

Lacerations are usually identified and sutured immediately after birth. After the bleeding has been controlled, the care of the woman with lacerations of the perineum includes position changes, analgesia as needed for pain, and warm or cold applications as necessary. The need for increased fiber in the diet and increased intake of fluids is emphasized to reduce the risk for constipation. Stool softeners may be used to assist the woman in reestablishing bowel habits without straining and putting stress on the sutures.

> ### ! NURSING ALERT
>
> To avoid injury to healing tissues, a woman with third- or fourth-degree lacerations is not given rectal suppositories or enemas.

Hematomas

Pelvic hematomas (i.e., a collection of blood in the connective tissue) can be vulvar, vaginal, or retroperitoneal in origin. Vulvar hematomas are the most common. Pain is the most common symptom, and most vulvar hematomas are visible. Vaginal hematomas occur more commonly in association with a forceps-assisted birth, an episiotomy, or primigravidity (Francois & Foley, 2017).

Retroperitoneal hematomas are the least common but are life threatening. They are caused by laceration of one of the vessels attached to the hypogastric artery, usually associated with rupture of a cesarean scar during labor. During the postpartum period, if the woman reports persistent perineal or rectal pain or a feeling of pressure in the vagina, a careful examination is made. However, a retroperitoneal hematoma can cause minimal pain and the initial symptoms may be signs of shock (Francois & Foley, 2017).

Hematomas are generally surgically evacuated. Once the bleeding has been controlled, usual postpartum care is provided with careful attention to pain relief, monitoring the amount of bleeding, replacing fluids, and reviewing laboratory results (hemoglobin and hematocrit).

Inversion of the Uterus

Inversion (turning inside out) of the uterus after birth is a rare but potentially life-threatening complication. The incidence of uterine inversion varies from 1 in 2000 to 1 in 20,000 births and differs, depending on which risk factors for the condition are present (Cunningham et al., 2018). Uterine inversion can be incomplete, complete, or prolapsed. Incomplete inversion cannot be seen; a smooth mass can be palpated through the dilated cervix. In complete inversion, the lining of the fundus crosses through the cervical os and forms a mass in the vagina. Prolapsed inversion of the uterus is obvious—a large, red, rounded mass (perhaps with the placenta attached) protrudes 20 to 30 cm (approximately 8 to 12 in) outside the introitus. The primary presenting signs of uterine inversion are sudden and include hemorrhage, shock, and pain. The uterus is not palpable abdominally.

The two most likely causes of uterine inversion are excessive umbilical cord traction with a fundally attached placenta and fundal pressure in the setting of a relaxed uterus. Although a causal relationship between active management of the third stage of labor and uterine inversion remains unproven (Francois & Foley, 2017), the umbilical cord should *not* be pulled forcefully unless there are clear signs of placental separation (see Chapter 19). Uterine inversion is an obstetric emergency requiring immediate interventions that include maternal fluid resuscitation, replacement of the uterus within the pelvic cavity, and correction of associated clinical conditions. Tocolytics or halogenated anesthetics may be given to relax the uterus before attempting replacement (Francois & Foley, 2017). Oxytocic agents are administered after the uterus is repositioned; broad-spectrum antibiotics are initiated. The woman's response to treatment is monitored closely to prevent shock or fluid overload. If the uterus has been repositioned manually, care must be taken to avoid aggressive fundal massage.

Subinvolution of the Uterus

Late postpartum bleeding can result from subinvolution of the uterus (delayed return of the enlarged uterus to nonpregnant size and function). Recognized causes of subinvolution include retained placental fragments and pelvic infection. Signs and symptoms include prolonged lochial discharge, irregular or excessive bleeding, and sometimes hemorrhage. A pelvic examination usually reveals a larger-than-normal uterus that can be boggy.

Treatment of subinvolution depends on the cause. Ergonovine (Ergotrate) or methylergonovine (Methergine), 0.2 mg every 3 to 4 hours for 24 to 48 hours, is often recommended. Dilation and curettage (D&C) may be performed to remove retained placental fragments or to débride the placental site. If the cause of subinvolution is infection, antibiotic therapy is needed (Cunningham et al., 2018).

CARE MANAGEMENT

Care of women experiencing PPH requires the collaboration of an interprofessional health care team. Nurses and obstetric care providers work closely with personnel from transfusion services (blood bank), pharmacy, and laboratory to manage this obstetric emergency. Each birthing facility should have an obstetric hemorrhage team that is called into action when hemorrhage occurs. The woman's obstetric health care provider is not considered a member of the obstetric hemorrhage team, although he or she may work with the other team members. The hemorrhage team should include health care providers who can perform surgical procedures (e.g., general obstetrics, maternal-fetal medicine, anesthesia), critical care nursing, blood bank, and laboratory (Fleischer & Meirowitz, 2016; Lyndon, Lagrew, Shields, et al., 2015).

In order for the health care team to be optimally prepared for obstetric hemorrhage, institutions must develop standardized management protocols and regularly conduct emergency drills. The California Maternal Quality Care Collaborative (www.cmqcc.org) has developed best-practice approaches that can be adopted by other institutions (Lyndon et al., 2015). The use of obstetric rapid-response teams and massive transfusion protocols is vital to promoting safe, effective care and improving outcomes.

The Council on Patient Safety in Women's Health Care, representing all major professional organizations dealing with women's health, developed a safety bundle for obstetric hemorrhage. This bundle consists of evidence-based recommendations for care management and is organized in four action domains: (1) *Readiness*—hemorrhage cart, immediate access to hemorrhage medications, a response team, massive and emergency-release transfusion protocols, and unit-based education with drills; (2) *Recognition and Prevention*—assessment of risk for hemorrhage, measurement of blood loss, and active management of third stage of labor; (3) *Response*—emergency management plan with checklists and support program for clients, families, and staff when significant hemorrhage occurs; and (4) *Reporting and Systems Learning*—huddling and post event debriefs, multidisciplinary review of serious hemorrhages, and monitoring outcomes and processes (http://www.safehealthcarefor-everywoman.org/) (Main, Goffman, Scavone, et al., 2015).

Assessment

Early recognition and treatment of PPH are critical to care management (Fig. 33.1). Risk assessment beginning during pregnancy and continuing during the intrapartum and postpartum periods is important in identifying women who are at risk for PPH. This increases the awareness of the health care team in planning and implementing care and in preventing hemorrhage and its sequelae. Team members should be made aware whenever a woman with identified risk factors is admitted to the birthing facility (Fleischer & Meirowitz, 2016).

Excessive blood loss is the clinical finding that warrants prompt action. In general, health care professionals are highly inaccurate in estimating blood loss in terms of volume (Hancock, Weeks, & Lavender, 2015). Most often blood loss is estimated by visual assessment and results in low estimates compared to actual blood loss. Accuracy of estimating blood loss can be improved by interventions that can quantify the amount of blood the woman loses during and after birth.

The Association of Women's Health, Obstetric and Neonatal Nurses (AWHONN, 2015) published a practice brief on quantification of blood loss (QBL), recommending that cumulative blood loss be measured with every birth, whether vaginal or cesarean. For vaginal birth, QBL should begin immediately after birth, prior to delivery of the placenta, using a calibrated under-buttocks drape and weighing all blood-soaked items. With cesarean birth, QBL begins when the membranes are ruptured or after birth of the neonate, measuring fluids in suction canisters (subtracting irrigation fluid) and weighing all blood-soaked materials and clots.

Whenever blood loss appears to be excessive, the first step is to evaluate the contractility of the uterus. If the uterus is hypotonic or boggy, management is directed toward increasing contractility and minimizing blood loss.

If the uterus is firmly contracted and bleeding continues, the source of bleeding still must be identified and treated. Assessment may include visual or manual inspection of the perineum, the vagina, the uterus, the

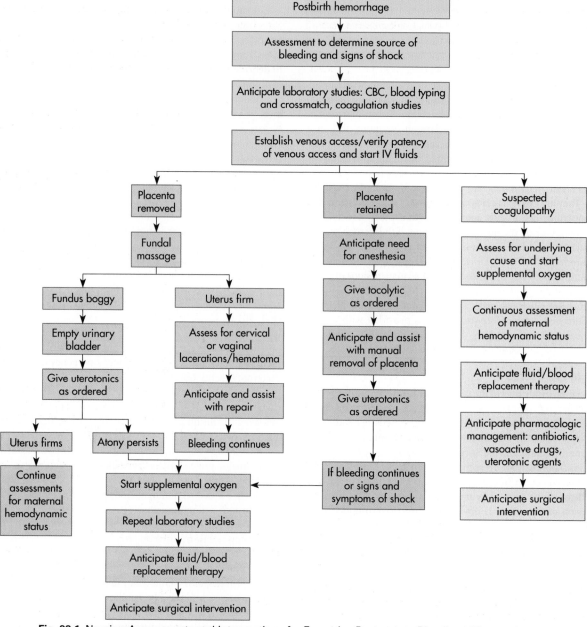

Fig. 33.1 Nursing Assessments and Interventions for Excessive Postpartum Bleeding. (Uterotonics are medications to contract the uterus; tocolytics are medications to relax the uterus.) *CBC,* Complete blood count; *IV,* intravenous.

cervix, or the rectum, as well as laboratory studies (e.g., hemoglobin, hematocrit, coagulation studies, platelet count). Treatment depends on the source of the bleeding.

Medical Management

The initial intervention in management of excessive postpartum bleeding due to uterine atony is firm massage of the uterine fundus (see Fig. 21.2). Expression of any clots in the uterus, elimination of bladder distention, and continuous IV infusion of 10 to 40 units of oxytocin added to 1000 mL of lactated Ringers or normal saline solution also are primary interventions. If the uterus does not contract in response to oxytocin, other uterotonic medications are administered. Misoprostol (Cytotec), a synthetic prostaglandin E_1 analog, is often used. An advantage of misoprostol is that it can be given rectally, sublingually, or orally. Methylergonovine may be given intramuscularly to produce sustained uterine contractions. A derivative of prostaglandin $F_{2\alpha}$ (carboprost tromethamine [Carboprost; Hemabate]) may be given intramuscularly. It can also be given intramyometrially at cesarean birth or intra-abdominally after vaginal birth. Prostaglandin E_2 (Dinoprostone) vaginal or rectal suppository can be used for PPH. (See Medication Guide: Uterotonic Drugs to Manage Postpartum Hemorrhage for a comparison of uterotonic drugs and common dosages used to manage PPH.) See the Evidence-Based Practice box: Tranexamic Acid Treatment for Postpartum Hemorrhage for information on another management option for postpartum hemorrhage. In addition to the medications used to contract the uterus, rapid administration of crystalloid solutions or blood products or both will be needed to restore the woman's intravascular volume (Francois & Foley, 2017).

MEDICATION ALERT

The use of ergonovine or methylergonovine is contraindicated in the presence of hypertension or cardiovascular disease. Prostaglandin $F_{2\alpha}$ should not be given to women with a history of asthma as it can cause bronchoconstriction (Francois & Foley, 2017).

Oxygen can be given by nonrebreather face mask to enhance oxygen delivery to the cells. An indwelling urinary catheter is usually inserted to monitor urine output as a measure of renal perfusion, which in turn reflects perfusion of other vital organs (Cunningham et al., 2018). Laboratory studies usually include a complete blood count with platelet count, fibrinogen, fibrin split products, prothrombin time, and partial thromboplastin time. Blood type and antibody screen are done if not previously performed.

If bleeding persists, bimanual compression may be performed by the obstetrician or nurse-midwife. This procedure involves inserting a fist into the vagina and pressing the knuckles against the anterior side of the uterus, and then placing the other hand on the abdomen and massaging the posterior uterus with it. If the uterus still does not become firm, the health care provider performs manual exploration of the uterine cavity for retained blood clots or placental fragments.

Surgical Management

If the preceding procedures are ineffective, surgical management is needed. Surgical management options include uterine tamponade

MEDICATION GUIDE

Uterotonic Drugs to Manage Postpartum Hemorrhage

Drug	Action	Side Effects	Contraindications	Dosage and Route	Nursing Considerations
Oxytocin (Pitocin)	Contraction of uterus; decreases bleeding	Infrequent: water intoxication, nausea and vomiting	None for PPH	10-20 units/L up to 80 units/L diluted in lactated Ringers solution or normal saline at 125-200 milliunits/min IV; or 10-20 units IM	Continue to monitor vaginal bleeding and uterine tone.
Misoprostol (Cytotec)	Contraction of uterus	Headache, nausea, vomiting, diarrhea, fever, chills	None	600-1000 mcg rectally once or 400 mcg sublingually or PO once	Continue to monitor vaginal bleeding and uterine tone.
Methylergonovine (Methergine)	Contraction of uterus	Hypertension, hypotension, nausea, vomiting, headache	Hypertension, preeclampsia, cardiac disease	0.2 mg IM q2-4hr up to five doses; may also be given intrauterine or orally	Check blood pressure before giving, and do not give if >140/90 mm Hg; continue monitoring vaginal bleeding and uterine tone.
15-Methylprostaglandin $F_{2\alpha}$ (Prostin/15 m; Carboprost, Hemabate)	Contraction of uterus	Headache, nausea and vomiting, fever, chills, tachycardia, hypertension, diarrhea	Avoid with asthma or hypertension	250 mcg IM or intrauterine injection q15-90 min up to eight doses	Continue to monitor vaginal bleeding and uterine tone.
Dinoprostone (Prostin E_2)	Contraction of uterus	Headache, nausea and vomiting, fever, chills, diarrhea	Use with caution with history of asthma, hypertension, or hypotension	20 mg vaginal or rectal suppository q2hr	Continue to monitor vaginal bleeding and uterine tone.

IM, Intramuscular; *IV,* intravenous; *PO,* by mouth; *PPH,* postpartum hemorrhage.
Data from Francois, K. E., & Foley, M. R. (2017). Antepartum and postpartum hemorrhage. In S. G. Gabbe, J. R. Niebyl, J. L. Simpson, et al. (Eds.), *Obstetrics: Normal and problem pregnancies* (7th ed.). Philadelphia: Elsevier; and Lyndon, A., Lagrew, D., Shields, L., et al. (Eds.). (2015). *California maternal quality care collaborative toolkit to transform maternity care: Improving health care response to obstetric hemorrhage version 2.0.* Stanford, CA: California Maternal Quality Care Collaborative (CMQCC). Retrieved from https://www.cmqcc.org/ob_hemorrhage.

EVIDENCE-BASED PRACTICE

Tranexamic Acid Treatment for Postpartum Hemorrhage

Ask the Question

For women experiencing postpartum hemorrhage, is tranexamic acid an effective treatment?

Search for the Evidence

Search Strategies: English research-based publications since 2014 were included.

Databases Used: Cochrane Collaborative Database, National Guideline Clearinghouse (AHRQ), CINAHL, PubMed, UpToDate, and the professional websites for ACOG and AWHONN.

Critical Appraisal of the Evidence

- In 2017, the World Health Organization (WHO) issued an update to 2012 guidelines about the management of postpartum hemorrhage (PPH). Intravenous (IV) tranexamic acid is recommended for administration to women experiencing postpartum hemorrhage within 3 hrs of birth in addition to the usual care for postpartum hemorrhage (WHO, 2017).
- Administration of tranexamic acid should be considered part of the standard postpartum hemorrhage treatment plan. It should be used in all cases of PPH (WHO, 2017).
- Tranexamic acid is contraindicated when a client has a history of a thromboembolic event during her pregnancy (WHO, 2017).
- Tranexamic acid should be deployed to all settings in which women give birth. If tranexamic acid is only used in hospitals, maternal mortality from PPH would be reduced by 2%. If it is also used in home and clinic settings, maternal mortality from PPH could be reduced by 30% (McClure, Jones, Rouse, et al., 2015).

Apply the Evidence: Nursing Implications

- Nurses can provide client education about tranexamic acid, explaining that it has been shown to decrease blood loss and prevent PPH in women undergoing vaginal or cesarean birth (Novikova, Hofmeyr, & Cluver, 2015).
- Nurses should know evidence-based dosing recommendations for tranexamic acid. The first dose should be 1 g (100 mg/mL) IV at 1 mL/min. A second dose of 1 g IV may follow if bleeding has not stopped in 30 min, or if bleeding resumes within 24 hrs after the first dose (WHO, 2017). In most cases, one dose is effective (Pacheco, Hankins, Saad, et al., 2017).
- Nurses can teach women that administration of tranexamic acid does not pose a barrier to breastfeeding (Pacheco et al., 2017).

References

McClure, E. M., Jones, B., Rouse, D. J., et al. (2015). Tranexamic acid to reduce postpartum hemorrhage: A MANDATE systematic review and analyses of impact on maternal mortality. *American Journal of Perinatology, 32*(5), 469–474.

Novikova, N., Hofmeyr, G. J., & Cluver, C. (2015). Tranexamic acid for preventing postpartum haemorrhage. *Cochrane Database of Systematic Reviews, 6,* Art. No. CD007872.

Pacheco, L. D., Hankins, G., Saad, A. F., et al. (2017). Tranexamic acid for the management of obstetric hemorrhage. *Obstetrics & Gynecology, 130*(4), 765–769.

World Health Organization. (2017). *WHO recommendation on tranexamic acid for the treatment of postpartum haemorrhage.* Retrieved from: http://apps.who.int/iris/bitstream/handle/10665/259379/WHO-RHR-17.21-eng.pdf?sequence=1.

Jennifer Taylor Alderman

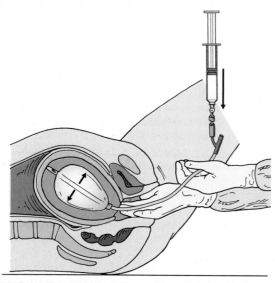

Fig. 33.2 Bakri Tamponade Balloon. (From Bakri, Y. N., & Arulkumaran, S. [2015]. *Intrauterine balloon tamponade for control of postpartum hemorrhage.* Retrieved from http://www.uptodate.com/contents/intrauterine-balloon-tamponade-for-control-of-postpartum-hemorrhage.)

(uterine packing or an intrauterine tamponade balloon) (Fig. 33.2), bilateral uterine artery ligation, ligation of utero-ovarian arteries and infundibulopelvic vessels, and selective arterial embolization. Uterine compression suturing (e.g., B-Lynch or Hayman vertical sutures) may be performed and is sometimes combined with a tamponade balloon (see Fig. 33.2). If these treatment measures are ineffective, hysterectomy will likely be needed (Cunningham et al., 2018; Francois & Foley, 2017).

Nursing Interventions

The nurse must be alert to the signs and symptoms of hemorrhage and be prepared to act quickly to minimize blood loss. Common problems, expected outcomes of care, and interventions are based on the cause of PPH as previously discussed (see Nursing Care Plan).

The woman and her family will be anxious about her condition. The nurse can intervene by calmly providing explanations about interventions being performed and the need to act quickly. Family members will likely be asked to leave the room while the hemorrhage team is intervening. After the event, it is important that the nurse help the woman and her family understand what occurred and the interventions that were needed.

Once the woman's condition is stabilized and she has begun the recovery process, preparations for discharge are made. Discharge instructions for the woman who experienced PPH are similar to those for any postpartum woman. In addition, the woman should be told that she will probably feel fatigue, even exhaustion, and will need to limit her physical activities to conserve her strength. She may need instructions about increasing her dietary iron and protein intake and iron supplementation to rebuild lost red blood cell (RBC) volume. She may need assistance with infant care and household activities until she has regained strength. The nurse should assess the woman's anticipated level of support from family and friends and help her plan how to ask for help when returning home. Some women experiencing a PPH have problems with delayed lactogenesis, insufficient milk production, or postpartum depression. Interprofessional care providers may include lactation consultants, obstetric and pediatric health care providers, mental health providers, social workers, and home care nurses. Referrals for home care follow-up or to community resources may be needed, including lactation support or a postpartum doula service.

NURSING CARE PLAN
Postpartum Hemorrhage

Client Problem	Expected Outcome	Nursing Interventions	Rationale
Disrupted fluid balance related to postpartum hemorrhage	Woman will demonstrate acceptable fluid balance as evidenced by stable vital signs, prompt capillary refill time, and balanced ___ output	Monitor vital signs, especially heart rate and blood pressure.	To assess effectiveness of treatment
		Measure and record amount and type of bleeding by weighing and counting saturated pads; save clots and tissue for further examination.	To estimate type and amount of blood loss for fluid replacement
		Administer medications as ordered, such as oxytocin, misoprostol, methylergonovine, or prostaglandin $F_2\alpha$.	To increase contractility of uterus
___ tissue perfusion related to hypovolemia	Woman will have stable vital ___ oxygen saturation, ___ arterial blood gases and adequate hematocrit and hemoglobin levels.	Monitor vital signs, oxygen saturation, arterial blood gases, and hematocrit and hemoglobin.	To assess for hypovolemic shock and decreased tissue perfusion
		Assess capillary refill, mucous membranes, and skin temperature.	To note indicators of vasoconstriction
		Give supplementary oxygen by nonrebreather mask as ordered.	To provide additional oxygenation to tissues
Potential for infection related to blood loss and invasive procedures	Woman will demonstrate no signs of infection.	Maintain Standard Precautions and use proper hand hygiene when providing care.	To prevent introduction of or spread of infection
		Teach woman to maintain proper hand hygiene (particularly before handling her newborn) and to maintain scrupulous perineal care with frequent change and careful disposal of perineal pads.	To avoid spread of microorganisms
		Monitor for signs of infection (fever, foul-smelling lochia, increased pain or tenderness of uterus, etc.).	To detect signs of infection

HEMORRHAGIC (HYPOVOLEMIC) SHOCK

Hemorrhage can result in hemorrhagic (hypovolemic) shock. Shock is an emergency situation in which the perfusion of body organs can become severely compromised and death can occur. Physiologic compensatory mechanisms are activated in response to hemorrhage. The adrenal glands release catecholamines, causing arterioles and venules in the skin, lungs, gastrointestinal tract, liver, and kidneys to constrict. The available blood flow is diverted to the brain and heart and away from other organs, including the uterus. If shock is prolonged, the continued reduction in cellular oxygenation results in an accumulation of lactic acid and acidosis (from anaerobic glucose metabolism). Acidosis (lowered serum pH) causes arteriolar vasodilation; venule vasoconstriction persists. A circular pattern is established (i.e., decreased perfusion, increased tissue anoxia and acidosis, edema formation, and pooling of blood further decrease the perfusion). Cellular death occurs. See Emergency box: Hemorrhagic Shock for assessments and interventions for hemorrhagic shock.

CARE MANAGEMENT

As noted previously, birthing institutions must develop standardized management protocols and regularly conduct emergency drills to be adequately prepared for PPH (Lyndon et al., 2015). Interprofessional teamwork and collaboration are key to managing care of postpartum women who experience hemorrhagic shock. The woman is likely to be transferred to a critical care unit for stabilization and ongoing care and monitoring.

EMERGENCY
Hemorrhagic Shock

Assessments	Characteristics
• Respirations	• Rapid and shallow
• Pulse	• Rapid, weak, irregular
• Blood pressure	• Decreasing (late sign)
• Skin	• Cool, pale, clammy
• Urinary output	• Decreasing
• Level of consciousness	• Lethargy → coma
• Mental status	• Anxiety → coma
• Central venous pressure	• Decreased

Interventions
• Summon assistance and equipment.
• Start intravenous infusion per standing orders.
• Ensure patent airway; administer oxygen.
• Continue to monitor status.

LEGAL TIP

Standard of Care for Bleeding Emergencies
The standard of care for obstetric emergency situations such as postpartum hemorrhage or hypovolemic shock is that provision should be made for the nurse to implement nursing actions independently. Policies, procedures, standing orders or protocols, and clinical guidelines should be established by each health care facility in which births occur and should be agreed to by health care providers involved in the care of obstetric clients.

Vigorous treatment is necessary to prevent adverse outcomes. Management of hypovolemic shock involves restoring circulating blood volume and eliminating the cause of the hemorrhage (e.g., lacerations, uterine atony, or inversion). Venous access with a large-bore IV catheter is critical to successful management of the woman with a hemorrhagic complication. Establishing two IV lines facilitates fluid resuscitation. Fluid resuscitation includes administering crystalloids (lactated Ringers, normal saline solution), colloids (albumin), and blood components. To restore circulating blood volume, a rapid IV infusion of crystalloid solution is given at a rate of 3 mL infused for every 1 mL of estimated blood loss (e.g., 3000 mL infused for 1000 mL of blood loss). Packed red blood cells (PRBCs) are usually infused if the woman is still actively bleeding and no improvement in her condition is noted after the initial crystalloid infusion. Infusion of fresh frozen plasma may be needed if clotting factors and platelet counts are below normal values (Cunningham et al., 2018; Francois & Foley, 2017).

Hemorrhagic shock can occur rapidly, but the classic signs of shock may not appear until the postpartum woman has lost 30% to 40% of blood volume. By the time vital signs are abnormal, the woman may be in an advanced stage of shock. The shock index has been proposed as a parameter to identify early stages of hypovolemic shock. Shock index is the ratio of heart rate to systolic blood pressure; with shock, as the heart rate increases, the blood pressure decreases. For example, with a heart rate of 120 and a systolic blood pressure of 90, the shock index is 1.3. A shock index greater than 1.1 suggests significant blood loss, even before there are notable changes in the vital signs (Fleischer & Meirowitz, 2016).

Major goals of care are to restore oxygen delivery to the tissues and to maintain cardiac output. Fluid resuscitation must be monitored carefully because fluid overload can occur. Intravascular fluid overload occurs most often with colloid therapy.

If transfusion of blood products is necessary, there should be protocols in place for emergency release of blood products. These products may be universally compatible (e.g., O-negative red blood cells or AB plasma) or type-specific if the woman's blood type is known and a supply is available. A massive transfusion protocol facilitates timely access to and administration of blood products (Fleischer & Meirowitz, 2016).

Transfusion reactions can follow administration of blood components, including cryoprecipitates. Even in an emergency, each unit of blood products should be carefully checked per hospital protocol. Complications of fluid or blood replacement therapy include hemolytic reactions, febrile reactions, allergic reactions, circulatory overload, and air embolism.

The nurse continues to monitor the woman's pulse and blood pressure. If invasive hemodynamic monitoring is ordered, the nurse may assist with placement of a central venous pressure (CVP) or pulmonary artery (Swan-Ganz) catheter. Subsequently, the nurse monitors CVP, pulmonary artery pressure, or pulmonary artery wedge pressure as ordered.

Additional assessments include evaluating skin temperature, color, and turgor and mucous membranes. Breath sounds should be auscultated before fluid volume replacement to provide a baseline for future assessment. The nurse inspects for signs of disseminated intravascular coagulation (DIC) such as oozing at the sites of incisions or injections. Assessment for the presence of petechiae or ecchymosis in areas not associated with surgery or trauma is also critical in evaluating for DIC (see Chapter 28).

Oxygen is administered, preferably by a nonrebreather face mask, at 10 to 12 L/min to maintain oxygen saturation. Oxygen saturation should be monitored with a pulse oximeter, although measurements are not always accurate in a client with hypovolemia or decreased perfusion. Level of consciousness is assessed frequently and provides additional indications of blood volume and oxygen saturation. In early stages of decreased blood flow, the woman may report "seeing stars" or feeling dizzy or nauseated. She can become restless and orthopneic. As cerebral hypoxia increases, she can become confused and react slowly or not at all to stimuli. Some women complain of headaches.

Continuous electrocardiographic monitoring may be indicated for the woman who is hypotensive or tachycardic, or continues to bleed profusely. An indwelling (Foley) catheter is inserted, and a urometer is attached to allow hourly assessment of urine output. The most objective and least invasive assessment of adequate organ perfusion and oxygenation is a urine output of at least 30 mL/hr and preferably ≥50 mL/hr (Cunningham et al., 2018). Hemoglobin and hematocrit levels, platelet count, and coagulation studies are closely monitored.

COAGULOPATHIES

When bleeding is continuous and there is no identifiable source, a coagulopathy can be the cause. The woman's coagulation status must be assessed quickly and continuously. Abnormal laboratory results depend on the cause and can include increased prothrombin time, increased partial thromboplastin time, decreased platelets, decreased fibrinogen level, increased fibrin degradation products, and prolonged bleeding time. Causes of coagulopathies can include pregnancy complications such as idiopathic or immune thrombocytopenic purpura, von Willebrand disease (vWD), or DIC.

Idiopathic Thrombocytopenic Purpura

Idiopathic or immune thrombocytopenic purpura (ITP) is an autoimmune disorder in which antiplatelet antibodies decrease the life span of the platelets. Thrombocytopenia, capillary fragility, and increased bleeding time are diagnostic findings. ITP can cause severe hemorrhage after cesarean birth or cervical or vaginal lacerations. The incidence of postpartum uterine bleeding and vaginal hematomas is also increased. Neonatal thrombocytopenia can result, but serious bleeding is unusual (Samuels, 2017).

Medical management focuses on control of platelet stability. If ITP was diagnosed during pregnancy, the woman likely was treated with corticosteroids or IV immunoglobulin. Platelet transfusions are usually given when there is significant bleeding. A splenectomy may be needed if the ITP does not respond to medical management (Cunningham et al., 2018).

von Willebrand Disease

von Willebrand disease (vWD), a type of hemophilia, is the most common congenital bleeding disorder. It results from a deficiency or defect in a blood clotting protein called *von Willebrand factor (vWF)*. There are as many as 20 variations of vWD, most of which are inherited as autosomal dominant traits; types I and II are the most common. Symptoms include recurrent bleeding episodes such as nosebleeds, bruising easily, and excessive bleeding with surgery or other trauma. Laboratory results include prolonged bleeding time, prolonged partial thromboplastin time, decreased vWF antigen levels, decreased factor VIII immunological and coagulation-promoting activity, and inability of platelets from a person with vWD to react to various stimuli. Although pregnancy outcomes are generally good, up to half of all women with vWD will experience PPH (Cunningham et al., 2018).

The treatment of choice is IV administration of desmopressin (DDAVP), which promotes the release of vWF and factor VIII. Cryoprecipitate may be administered if significant bleeding occurs. Concentrates of factor VIII (Humate-P or Alphanate) also can be administered (Cunningham et al., 2018).

VENOUS THROMBOEMBOLIC DISORDERS

Venous thromboembolism (VTE) results from the formation of a blood clot or clots inside a blood vessel and is caused by inflammation (**thrombophlebitis**) or partial obstruction of the vessel. Three thromboembolic conditions are of concern in the postpartum period:
Superficial venous thrombosis—Involvement of the superficial saphenous venous system

Deep venous thrombosis (DVT)—Occurs most often in the lower extremities; involvement varies but can extend from the foot to the iliofemoral region

Pulmonary embolism (PE)—Complication of DVT occurring when part of a blood clot dislodges and is carried to the pulmonary artery, where it occludes the vessel and obstructs blood flow to the lungs

Incidence and Etiology

The incidence of VTE is approximately 1 in 1500 pregnancies (Pettker & Lockwood, 2017). VTE can occur in any trimester of pregnancy and in the postpartum period. The highest incidence of postpartum VTE is during the first 3 weeks after birth (Tepper, Boulet, Whiteman, et al., 2014). DVT occurs most often during pregnancy, and PE is more common in the postpartum period. The incidence of VTE in the postpartum period has declined because early ambulation after childbirth has become standard practice. However, PE is a major cause of maternal death.

The primary causes of thromboembolic disease are venous stasis and hypercoagulation, both of which are present in pregnancy and continue into the postpartum period. Cesarean birth nearly doubles the risk for VTE; therefore routine preoperative placement of pneumatic compression devices is recommended. Women with risk factors such as obesity, immobility, malignancy, or other chronic medical conditions may be given prophylactic low-dose heparin prior to cesarean birth. Other risk factors include operative vaginal birth; history of venous thrombosis, PE, or varicosities; maternal age older than 35 years; multiparity; and smoking (Pettker & Lockwood, 2017). Women who experience complications such as preeclampsia, hemorrhage, or postpartum infection also have an increased risk for VTE (Tepper et al., 2014).

Clinical Manifestations

Superficial venous thrombosis is the most common form of postpartum thrombophlebitis. It is characterized by pain and tenderness in the lower extremity. Physical examination may reveal warmth, redness, and an enlarged, hardened vein over the site of the thrombosis.

The clinical signs and symptoms of DVT can be difficult to distinguish from normal pregnancy changes. In fact, a diagnosis of DVT is ultimately not confirmed in up to 90% of pregnant women in whom the disorder is suspected. On the other hand, many pregnant women who are diagnosed with the disorder do not exhibit the classic features of DVT: unilateral extremity edema, erythema, warmth, pain, tenderness, or a positive Homans sign (Fig. 33.3) (Leung, Sottile, & Lockwood, 2019).

Acute PE usually results from dislodged deep vein thrombi. The most common presenting symptoms are dyspnea and chest pain. Other signs of PE include tachypnea (more than 20 breaths/min), tachycardia (more than 100 beats/min), apprehension, cough, hemoptysis, elevated temperature, and sweating. Syncope is rare and usually indicates a massive embolism (Cunningham et al., 2018; Leung et al., 2019).

Physical examination is not a sensitive diagnostic indicator for thrombosis. Compression ultrasonography with or without color Doppler is the most commonly used diagnostic test for evaluating pregnant women at risk for DVT. Contrast-enhanced magnetic resonance venography is relatively contraindicated in pregnancy because of concerns regarding long-term effects on the fetus. While D-dimer assays may be used in the non-pregnant population to rule out a DVT diagnosis, the role of D-dimer testing during pregnancy is uncertain. There is no validated clinical prediction rule for DVT in pregnant women. Moreover, the safety of D-dimer testing during pregnancy has not been validated (Leung et al., 2019). With PE, echocardiographic abnormalities may be seen in right ventricular size or function. Pregnancy limits the usefulness of arterial blood gases and oxygen saturation for diagnosis. A ventilation-perfusion scan, spiral computed tomography scan, magnetic resonance angiography, and pulmonary arteriogram may be used for diagnosis (Leung et al., 2019).

CARE MANAGEMENT

Superficial venous thrombosis is treated with analgesia, support from elastic compression stockings, heat, and rest. If it does not quickly improve or if DVT is suspected, appropriate diagnostic testing is performed (Cunningham et al., 2018).

DVT is initially treated with IV anticoagulant therapy, bed rest with the affected leg elevated, and analgesia. After the symptoms have decreased, the woman may be fitted with elastic compression stockings to wear when ambulating. She is taught how to put on the stockings before getting out of bed. After several days, anticoagulant therapy will be changed to oral administration. If a breastfeeding mother is on long-term anticoagulant therapy, the infant's prothrombin time should be monitored at least monthly and vitamin K should be given to the infant if necessary (Lawrence & Lawrence, 2016).

Acute PE is an emergent situation that requires prompt treatment. Massive pulmonary emboli can lead to pulmonary hypertension and right ventricular dysfunction; if right ventricular dysfunction is present, mortality can be as high as 25% (Cunningham et al., 2018). Immediate treatment of PE is anticoagulant therapy. Continuous IV heparin therapy is used for PE until symptoms have resolved. Intermittent subcutaneous heparin or oral anticoagulant therapy (usually warfarin [Coumadin]) is often continued for up to 6 months (Pettker & Lockwood, 2017).

In the birthing facility, nursing care of the woman with a thrombosis consists of ongoing assessments: inspecting and palpating the affected area; palpating the peripheral pulses; checking the Homans sign; and measuring and comparing leg circumferences (see Fig. 33.3). Signs of PE, including chest pain, coughing, dyspnea, and tachypnea, and respiratory status for presence of crackles are also assessed. Laboratory reports are monitored for prothrombin or partial thromboplastin

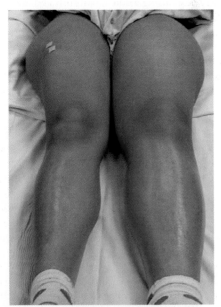

Fig. 33.3 Deep Vein Thrombosis. (From Murphy, E. H., Davis, C. M., Journeycake, J. M., et al. [2009]. Symptomatic ileofemoral DVT after onset of oral contraceptive use in women with previously undiagnosed May-Thurner Syndrome. *Journal of Vascular Surgery, 49*[3], 697–703.)

times. The nurse assesses for unusual bleeding. Increased lochia, generalized petechiae, hematuria, or oozing from venipuncture sites should be reported to the health care provider immediately (James, 2014). In addition, the woman and her family are assessed for their level of understanding about the diagnosis and their ability to cope during the unexpected extended period of recovery.

Interventions include explanations and education about diagnosis and treatment. The woman will need assistance with personal care while on bed rest; the family should be encouraged to participate in the care if that is what she and they wish. The woman should be encouraged to change positions frequently but to avoid placing her knees in a sharply flexed position that could cause pooling of blood in the lower extremities. She should avoid rubbing the affected area because this action could cause the clot to dislodge. Heparin and warfarin are administered as ordered, and the health care provider is notified if clotting times are outside the therapeutic level. If the woman is breastfeeding, she is informed that neither heparin nor warfarin is excreted in significant quantities in breast milk (Lawrence & Lawrence, 2016). If the infant has been discharged, the family is encouraged to bring the infant for feedings and the woman may express milk to be sent home. Pain can be managed with position changes, elevation of the affected leg, and application of moist heat. Analgesics and antiinflammatory medications may also be necessary.

The woman is usually discharged home on oral anticoagulants and will need an explanation of the treatment schedule and possible side effects. It is not known if any of the newer oral anticoagulants, such as rivaroxaban (Xarelto) and apixaban (Eliquis), are excreted in breast milk. Postpartum women who require anticoagulant therapy should either avoid breastfeeding or use an alternative anticoagulant, such as warfarin, because of the potential for infant harm (Cunningham et al., 2018).

If subcutaneous injections are to be given, the woman and family are taught how to administer the medication and about site rotation. They should also be given information about possible dietary restrictions (e.g., limited intake of green, leafy vegetables) and safe care practices to prevent bleeding and injury while she is on anticoagulant therapy (e.g., using a soft toothbrush and an electric razor). She will need information about follow-up with her health care provider to monitor clotting times and regulate the correct dosage of anticoagulant therapy. The woman should also use a reliable form of contraception if taking warfarin, because this medication is considered teratogenic. Combination oral contraceptives (containing both estrogen and progesterone) are contraindicated in women with acute or prior VTE (Cunningham et al., 2018).

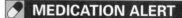

🗝 MEDICATION ALERT

Medications containing aspirin are not given to women on anticoagulant therapy because aspirin inhibits synthesis of clotting factors and can lead to prolonged clotting time and increased risk for bleeding.

POSTPARTUM INFECTION

Postpartum infection, or *puerperal infection*, is any clinical infection of the genital tract that occurs within 28 days after miscarriage, induced abortion, or birth. The definition used in the United States continues to be the presence of a fever of 38°C (100.4°F) or more on 2 successive days of the first 10 postpartum days (not including the first 24 hours after birth).

Endometritis is the most common puerperal infection (Isley & Katz, 2017). Other common postpartum infections include wound infections, urinary tract infections (UTIs), and respiratory tract infections. Mastitis, or breast infection, should also be considered as a possible diagnosis among breastfeeding mothers, with symptoms such as fever, malaise, flulike symptoms, and a sore area on a breast (Lawrence & Lawrence, 2016) (Fig. 33.4; see Chapter 25 for further discussion of mastitis).

The most common infecting organisms are the numerous streptococcal and anaerobic organisms. Postpartum infections are more common in women who have concurrent medical or immunosuppressive conditions or who had a cesarean or other operative birth. Intrapartal factors such as prolonged rupture of membranes, prolonged labor, and multiple vaginal examinations increase the risk for infection (Cunningham et al., 2018). Factors that predispose the woman to postpartum infection are listed in Box 33.2.

Endometritis

Endometritis is an infection of the lining of the uterus. It usually begins as a localized infection at the placental site but can spread to the entire endometrium. The highest incidence occurs in women who gave birth by cesarean after prolonged labor and rupture of membranes. Prophylactic antibiotics administered during labor and during cesarean surgery can help reduce the incidence and severity of endometritis.

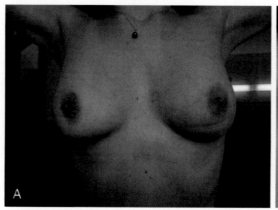
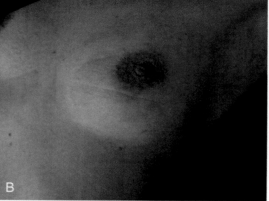

Fig. 33.4 Mastitis. (A) Comparison of left breast with mastitis to normal right breast. (B) Closer view of inflamed right lower quadrant of left breast. (From Boutet, G. [2012]. Breast inflammation: Clinical examination, aetiological pointers. *Diagnostic and Interventional Imaging, 93*[2], 78–84.)

Signs of endometritis include fever (usually greater than 38°C [100.4°F]), increased pulse, chills, anorexia, nausea, fatigue and lethargy, pelvic pain, uterine tenderness, and foul-smelling, profuse lochia. Leukocytosis and a markedly increased RBC sedimentation rate are typical laboratory findings of postpartum infections. Anemia can also be present. Blood cultures or intracervical or intrauterine bacterial cultures are not clinically useful and increase the cost of care (Cunningham et al., 2018).

Management

Management of endometritis consists of IV broad-spectrum antibiotic therapy (cephalosporins, penicillins, or clindamycin and gentamicin) and supportive care, including hydration, rest, and pain relief. Antibiotic therapy is usually discontinued 24 hours after the woman is asymptomatic. Assessments of lochia, vital signs, and changes in the woman's condition continue during treatment. Comfort measures depend on the symptoms and may include cool compresses, warm blankets, perineal care, and sitz baths. Teaching should include side effects of therapy, prevention of spread of infection, signs and symptoms of worsening condition, adherence to the treatment plan, and the need for follow-up care. Women may need additional support to maintain mother–infant interactions and breastfeeding.

Wound Infections

Wound infections are common postpartum infections that often develop after women are discharged home. Rates of wound infection after cesarean birth are 3% to 5% (Duff & Birsner, 2017). Women can also develop infection in the perineum in a repaired laceration or episiotomy site. Predisposing factors are similar to those for endometritis (see Box 33.2). Signs of wound infection include fever, erythema, edema, warmth, tenderness, pain, seropurulent drainage, and wound separation.

BOX 33.2 Predisposing Factors for Postpartum Infection

Preconception or Antepartal Factors
- History of previous venous thrombosis, urinary tract infection, mastitis, pneumonia
- Diabetes mellitus
- Alcoholism or substance use disorder
- Immunosuppression
- Anemia
- Malnutrition
- Obesity
- Preeclampsia

Intrapartal Factors
- Cesarean birth
- Operative vaginal birth
- Prolonged rupture of membranes
- Chorioamnionitis
- Prolonged labor
- Bladder catheterization
- Internal fetal heart rate or uterine contraction monitoring
- Multiple vaginal examinations after rupture of membranes
- Epidural analgesia/anesthesia
- Retained placental fragments
- Postpartum hemorrhage
- Episiotomy or lacerations
- Hematomas

Management

Wound exudate may be cultured to identify the causative organism. Wound infections are treated with IV antibiotic therapy. When pus is present in the incision, the wound is opened and drained. Wounds are irrigated with normal saline and redressed several times daily; healing occurs by secondary intention. In some cases, a wound vacuum device is used. Antibiotic treatment is continued until the base of the wound appears clear and there are no apparent signs of cellulitis (Duff & Birsner, 2017).

Nursing care includes frequent assessments of temperature and vital signs; wound assessment and care; and comfort measures such as analgesics, sitz baths, warm compresses, and perineal care. Teaching includes hygienic care techniques (e.g., changing perineal pads front to back, hand hygiene before and after perineal care), self-care measures, and signs of worsening conditions to report to the obstetric health care provider. Wound care and assessment will continue after discharge from the birthing facility. The woman and her family are instructed in how to perform wound care and dressing changes. Home visits by nurses may be provided to assess the wound, reinforce teaching, and offer support.

Urinary Tract Infections

UTIs occur in 2% to 4% of postpartum women. Risk factors include urinary catheterization, frequent pelvic examinations, regional (epidural or spinal) anesthesia, genital tract injury, history of UTI, and cesarean birth. Signs and symptoms include dysuria, frequency and urgency, low-grade fever, urinary retention, hematuria, and pyuria. Costovertebral angle tenderness or flank pain can indicate upper UTI. The most common infecting organism is *Escherichia coli,* although other gram-negative aerobic bacilli can cause UTIs.

Management

Medical management for UTIs consists of antibiotic therapy, analgesia, and hydration. Postpartum women are usually treated on an outpatient basis; therefore teaching should include instructions on how to monitor temperature, bladder function, and appearance of urine. The woman should also be taught about signs of potential complications and the importance of taking all antibiotics as prescribed. Other suggestions for prevention of UTIs include proper perineal care, wiping from front to back after urinating or having a bowel movement, and increasing fluid intake. Unsweetened cranberry juice or cranberry supplements may be beneficial in preventing UTI.

📋 CARE MANAGEMENT

Assessment

Women who are predisposed to postpartum infection (see Box 33.2) should be assessed carefully. Signs and symptoms associated with postpartum infection were discussed with each infection. Elevation of temperature, redness, and swelling are common signs. The woman may also complain of chills, fever, localized tenderness, or pain. Depending on the type of infection, laboratory tests usually include a complete blood count and urine culture. Assessment includes a review of the woman's history, and the laboratory results should be included in the assessment. Common client problems for women experiencing postpartum infection are listed in Box 33.3.

Interventions

The most effective treatment of postpartum infection is prevention. Preventive measures include good prenatal nutrition to reduce risk of anemia. Proper maternal perineal hygiene with thorough hand hygiene is emphasized. Strict adherence to aseptic techniques by all health care

BOX 33.3 Common Problems of Women Experiencing Postpartum Infection

- *Need for health teaching* related to:
  - Cause, management, course of infection
  - Transmission and prevention of infection
- *Delayed wound healing* related to:
  - Effects of infection process
- *Acute pain* related to:
  - Mastitis
  - Puerperal infection
  - Urinary tract infection
- *Decreased coping* related to:
  - Unexpected complication to expected postpartum recovery
  - Possible separation from newborn
- *Risk for inadequate parenting* related to:
  - Fear of spread of infection to newborn

personnel caring for women during labor, birth, and the postpartum period is very important. Specific medical, surgical, and nursing interventions were discussed with each infection.

Postpartum women are usually discharged to home by 48 hours after birth. This is often before signs of infection are evident. Nurses in birth centers and hospital settings must be able to identify women at risk for postpartum infection and provide anticipatory teaching and guidance before discharge (see Community Activity box: Fact Sheet About Postpartum Infection). Teaching should include the signs of infection and when to notify the health care provider. After discharge, telephone follow-up, hotlines, support groups, lactation counselors, home visits by nurses, and teaching materials can be used to decrease the risk for postpartum infections.

🏠 COMMUNITY ACTIVITY

Fact Sheet About Postpartum Infection

After giving birth, many women are discharged home before an infection can develop. Prepare a fact sheet regarding postpartum infections that could be distributed to postpartum women on discharge from the hospitals or birth centers in your community. The fact sheet should include a brief summary of the types of common infections, signs and symptoms, ways to help prevent infection, and when to call the health care provider. If your community has a large population of women who do not speak English, consider translating the fact sheet into Spanish or another language as appropriate.

▌ KEY POINTS

- Postpartum hemorrhage is a major cause of obstetric morbidity and mortality throughout the world and is the leading cause of obstetric intensive care unit admissions.
- Hemorrhagic (hypovolemic) shock is an emergency in which the perfusion of body organs can become severely compromised and death can result.
- The potential side effects of therapeutic interventions can further compromise the woman with a hemorrhagic disorder.

- Clotting disorders are associated with many obstetric complications.
- Postpartum infection is a major cause of maternal morbidity and mortality throughout the world.
- Postpartum urinary tract infections are common because of trauma experienced during labor.
- Prevention is the most effective treatment of postpartum infection.

REFERENCES

American College of Obstetricians and Gynecologists. (2017). Postpartum hemorrhage. Practice Bulletin No. 183. *Obstetrics & Gynecology, 130*(4), e168–e186.

Association of Women's Health, Obstetric and Neonatal Nurses. (2015). AWHONN practice brief no. 1: Quantification of blood loss. *Journal of Obstetric, Gynecologic and Neonatal Nursing, 44*(1), 158–160.

Cunningham, F., Leveno, K., Bloom, S., et al. (2018). *Williams obstetrics* (25th ed.). New York: McGraw-Hill.

Duff, P., & Birsner, M. (2017). Maternal and perinatal infection in pregnancy: Bacterial. In S. G. Gabbe, J. R. Niebyl, J. L. Simpson, et al. (Eds.), *Obstetrics: Normal and problem pregnancies* (7th ed.). Philadelphia: Elsevier.

Fleischer, A., & Meirowitz, N. (2016). Care bundles for management of postpartum hemorrhage. *Seminars in Perinatology, 40*(2), 99–108.

Francois, K. E., & Foley, M. R. (2017). Antepartum and postpartum hemorrhage. In S. G. Gabbe, J. R. Niebyl, J. L. Simpson, et al. (Eds.), *Obstetrics: Normal and problem pregnancies* (7th ed.). Philadelphia: Elsevier.

Hancock, A., Weeks, A. D., & Lavender, D. T. (2015). Is accurate and reliable blood loss estimation the "crucial step" in early detection of postpartum haemorrhage: An integrative review of the literature. *BMC Pregnancy and Childbirth, 15*, 1–9.

Isley, M. M., & Katz, V. L. (2017). Postpartum care and long-term health considerations. In S. G. Gabbe, J. R. Niebyl, J. L. Simpson, et al. (Eds.), *Obstetrics: Normal and problem pregnancies* (7th ed.). Philadelphia: Elsevier.

James, D. C. (2014). Postpartum care. In K. R. Simpson & P. A. Creehan (Eds.), *AWHONN's perinatal nursing* (4th ed.). Philadelphia: Lippincott Williams & Wilkins.

Lawrence, R. A., & Lawrence, R. M. (2016). *Breastfeeding: A guide for the medical profession* (8th ed.). St. Louis: Elsevier.

Leung, A., Sottile, P., & Lockwood, C. J. (2019). Thromboembolic disease in pregnancy. In R. Resnik, C. J. Lockwood, T. R. Moore, et al. (Eds.), *Creasy & Resnik's maternal-fetal medicine: Principles and practice* (8th ed.). Philadelphia: Elsevier.

Lyndon, A., Lagrew, D., Shields, L., et al. (2015). *A California toolkit to transform maternity care: Improving health care response to obstetric hemorrhage version 2.0.* Stanford, CA: California Maternal Quality Care Collaborative (CMQCC). Retrieved from: http://www.cmqcc.org/ob_hemorrhage.

Main, E. K., Goffman, D., & Scavone, B. M. (2015). National Partnership for Maternal Safety: Consensus bundle on obstetric hemorrhage. *Obstetrics & Gynecology, 126*(5), 155–162.

Pettker, C. M., & Lockwood, C. J. (2017). Thromboembolic disorders. In S. G. Gabbe, J. R. Niebyl, J. L. Simpson, et al. (Eds.), *Obstetrics: Normal and problem pregnancies* (7th ed.). Philadelphia: Elsevier.

Samuels, P. (2017). Hematologic complications of pregnancy. In S. G. Gabbe, J. R. Niebyl, J. L. Simpson, et al. (Eds.), *Obstetrics: Normal and problem pregnancies* (7th ed.). Philadelphia: Elsevier.

Tepper, N. K., Boulet, S. L., Whiteman, M. K., et al. (2014). Postpartum venous thrombosis: Incidence and risk factors. *Obstetrics & Gynecology, 123*(5), 987–996.

World Health Organization. (2015). *Maternal mortality fact sheet no. 348.* Retrieved from: http://www.who.int/mediacentre/factsheets/fs348/en.

Nursing Care of the High-Risk Newborn

Debbie Fraser

LEARNING OBJECTIVES

- Compare characteristics of preterm, late preterm, and postterm neonates.
- Discuss respiratory distress syndrome and the approach to treatment.
- Describe strategies for respiratory support of preterm infants.
- Analyze appropriate nursing interventions for nutritional care of the preterm infant.
- Discuss the care management of retinopathy of prematurity, bronchopulmonary dysplasia, patent ductus arteriosus, necrotizing enterocolitis, and intraventricular hemorrhage.
- Discuss pain assessment and management in the preterm infant.

- Describe the signs and symptoms of perinatal asphyxia.
- Explain the pathophysiology of meconium aspiration syndrome and its clinical signs.
- Plan developmentally appropriate care for high-risk infants.
- Discuss the needs of parents of high-risk infants.
- Describe nursing care for late preterm infants and list specific discharge teaching needs for parents of late preterm infants.
- Analyze common problems experienced by small and large for gestational age infants.
- Discuss nursing interventions for families of preterm and high-risk infants experiencing anticipatory loss and grief.

Modern technology and expert nursing care have made important contributions to improving the health and overall survival of high-risk infants. However, infants who are born considerably before term and survive are particularly susceptible to developing problems related to their preterm birth. These problems can also occur in term and late preterm infants (LPIs), although not as frequently, and include necrotizing enterocolitis (NEC), bronchopulmonary dysplasia (BPD), intraventricular and periventricular hemorrhage, and retinopathy of prematurity (ROP).

High-risk infants are most often classified according to birth weight, gestational age, and predominant pathophysiologic problems (Box 34.1). Intrauterine growth rates differ among infants; factors such as heredity, placental insufficiency, and maternal disease influence intrauterine growth and birth weight. For the high-risk infant, an accurate assessment of gestational age (see Chapter 24) is critical in helping the nurse anticipate problems. The response of the preterm, late preterm, or postterm infant to extrauterine life differs from that of the term infant. By understanding the physiologic basis of these differences, the nurse can assess these infants with a keen awareness of the potential problems they are most likely to encounter.

PRETERM INFANTS

The vast majority of high-risk infants are those born at less than 37 weeks of gestation: preterm and LPIs. The preterm birth rate in the United States showed a fairly steady increase from the early 1980s to 2006. Then, in 2006, the rate began to steadily decline to a low of 9.57 in 2014. Rates of preterm births increased in 2015 to 9.63% and in 2016 to 9.85%. Most of the recent increases were among LPIs (34 to 36 weeks). The rates of early term birth (37 to 38 weeks) rose in 2016 to a rate of 25.47% (Martin, Hamilton, Osterman, et al., 2018).

For some preterm or high-risk births it is possible to anticipate problems, such as when a woman is admitted in preterm labor. At other times the birth of a high-risk infant is unexpected. In either case the personnel and equipment necessary for immediate care of the infant must be available.

Preterm infants are at risk because their organ systems are immature and they lack adequate nutrient reserves. The potential problems and care needs of the preterm infant weighing 2000 g (4.4 lb) differ from those of the term or postterm infant of equal weight. If these infants have physiologic disorders and anomalies as well, they affect the infant's response to treatment. In general, the closer infants are to term in relation to gestational age and birth weight, the easier their adjustment to the external environment.

Preterm, low–birth-weight (LBW), and extremely low–birth-weight (ELBW) infants require hospitalization beyond the typical 48 hours after birth. Their physiologic immaturity and associated problems may require extensive use of technologic and pharmacologic interventions. The cost of the care of preterm and LBW infants is estimated to be billions of dollars each year and continues to rise as the use of technology increases.

Varying opinions exist about the practical and ethical dimensions of resuscitation of extremely low–birth-weight infants (those infants whose birth weight is 1000 g [2.2 lb] or less). Ethical issues associated with resuscitation of such infants include:

Classification According to Size

Low–birth-weight (LBW) infant: an infant whose birth weight is less than 2500 g (5.5 lb), regardless of gestational age

Very low–birth-weight (VLBW) infant: an infant whose birth weight is less than 1500 g (3.3 lb)

Extremely low–birth-weight (ELBW) infant: an infant whose birth weight is less than 1000 g (2.2 lb)

Appropriate for gestational age (AGA) infant: an infant whose birth weight falls between the 10th and 90th percentiles on intrauterine growth curves

Small for date (SFD) or small for gestational age (SGA) infant: an infant whose rate of intrauterine growth was slow and whose birth weight falls below the 10th percentile on intrauterine growth curves

Large for gestational age (LGA) infant: an infant whose birth weight falls above the 90th percentile on intrauterine growth curves

Intrauterine growth restriction (IUGR): found in infants whose intrauterine growth does not reach the expected potential

Symmetric IUGR: growth restriction in which the weight, length, and head circumference are all affected

Asymmetric IUGR: growth restriction in which the head circumference remains within normal parameters while the birth weight falls below the 10th percentile

Classification According to Gestational Age

- *Preterm (premature):* an infant born before completion of 37 weeks of gestation
- *Late preterm:* an infant born from 34 {0/7} through 36 {6/7} weeks of gestation
- *Early term:* an infant born from 37 {0/7} through 38 {6/7} weeks of gestation
- *Full term:* an infant born from 39 {0/7} weeks through 40 {6/7} weeks of gestation
- *Late term:* an infant born from 41 {0/7} through 41 {6/7} weeks of gestation
- *Postterm (postmature):* an infant born at 42 {0/7} or more weeks of gestation.

Data from American Academy of Pediatrics & American College of Obstetricians and Gynecologists. (2017). *Guidelines for perinatal care* (8th ed.). Elk Grove Village, IL: Author; and American College of Obstetricians and Gynecologists. (2013, reaffirmed 2017). Committee opinion no. 579: Definition of term pregnancy. *Obstetrics & Gynecology, 122*(5), 1139–1140.

- Should resuscitation be attempted and to what extent should it be continued?
- Who should decide?
- Is the cost of resuscitation justified?
- Do the benefits of technology outweigh the burdens in relation to the quality of life?

Interprofessional health care teams (health care providers, nurses, ethicists, clergy, attorneys, etc.) should participate with parents in discussions addressing these controversial questions. Although there are no clear answers, such discussions help clarify the issues and promote family-centered approaches to care. That care can involve sustaining life or providing care and support for a peaceful death. Nurses are key to the care of these infants and their families.

Physiologic Functions
Respiratory Function

The preterm infant is likely to have difficulty making the pulmonary transition from intrauterine to extrauterine life. Numerous problems can affect the respiratory systems of preterm infants:

- Decreased number of functional alveoli

- Deficient surfactant levels
- Smaller lumen in the airways
- Greater collapsibility or obstruction of respiratory passages
- Insufficient calcification of the bony thorax
- Weak or absent gag reflex
- Immature and friable capillaries in the lungs
- Greater distance between functional alveoli and the capillary bed

In combination, these deficits have the potential to severely hinder the preterm infant's respiratory efforts and can produce respiratory distress or apnea. Nurses must be alert to signs of respiratory distress or apnea and ready to intervene to promote adequate oxygenation.

Respiratory difficulty often follows a progressive pattern. Infants normally breathe between 30 and 60 times/min, relying significantly on their abdominal muscles to accomplish this. However, the respiratory rate can increase without a change in rhythm. Early signs of respiratory distress include flaring of the nares and an expiratory grunt. Depending on the cause, retractions can begin as subcostal, suprasternal, or intercostal. If the infant shows increasing respiratory effort (e.g., seesaw breathing patterns, retractions, flaring of the nares, expiratory grunting, and/or apneic spells), this indicates deepening distress. A compromised infant's color progresses from pink to circumoral cyanosis and then to generalized cyanosis.

> **! NURSING ALERT**
>
> Acrocyanosis is a normal finding in the neonate, but central cyanosis indicates an underlying problem that requires immediate evaluation.

Periodic breathing is a respiratory pattern commonly seen in preterm infants. Such infants exhibit 5- to 10-second respiratory pauses followed by 10 to 15 seconds of compensatory rapid respirations. Periodic breathing should not be confused with *apnea,* which is a cessation of breathing of 20 seconds or greater, or a shorter pause accompanied by bradycardia, cyanosis, or hypotonia (Patel, Mohr, Lake, et al., 2016).

Cardiovascular Function

Evaluation of heart rate and rhythm, skin color, blood pressure (BP), perfusion, pulses, oxygen saturation, and acid–base status provides information on cardiovascular status. The nurse must be prepared to intervene if symptoms of hypovolemia, shock, or both are found. These symptoms include hypotension, slow (>3 seconds) capillary refill, and continued respiratory distress despite the provision of oxygen and ventilation.

An accurate and timely BP reading can assist in making an early diagnosis of cardiorespiratory disease and in monitoring the effects of fluid therapy. BP is monitored routinely in the sick neonate by internal or external means. Direct recording with arterial catheters is often used but carries the risks inherent in any procedure in which a catheter is introduced into an artery. Oscillometric BP measurements are often done. This cuff BP is a noninvasive, effective means for detecting alterations in systemic BP (hypotension or hypertension) and for identifying the need to implement appropriate therapy to maintain cardiovascular function.

Thermoregulation

Preterm infants are susceptible to temperature instability. Because of their large body surface in relation to their weight, preterm infants are at high risk for heat loss. Other factors that place preterm infants at risk for temperature instability include:

- Minimal insulating subcutaneous fat
- Limited stores of brown fat (an internal source for the generation of heat present in normal term infants)

- Fragile capillaries
- Decreased or absent reflex control of skin capillaries
- Inadequate muscle mass activity (rendering the preterm infant unable to produce his or her own heat)
- Poor muscle tone, resulting in more body surface area being exposed to the cooling effects of the environment
- An immature temperature regulation center in the brain

The goal of thermoregulation is to create a *neutral thermal environment* (NTE), which is the environmental temperature at which oxygen consumption is minimal but adequate to maintain body temperature (Blackburn, 2018). With the knowledge of the four mechanisms of heat transfer (convection, conduction, radiation, and evaporation), the nurse can create an environment for the preterm infant that prevents temperature instability (see Chapter 23). The infant is kept in a radiant warmer bed or in an incubator with control settings to maintain an NTE. Because the preterm infant has few reserves in terms of calories and fat stores, this infant can easily lose heat and develop hypothermia. *Cold stress* results when the infant tries to conserve heat and burns more calories, causing the metabolism to increase, further stressing the already compromised neonate (see Chapter 23).

A critical nursing role is to prevent or minimize hypothermia and cold stress (see Fig. 23.3) by recognizing the risk factors and using intervention strategies to prevent and treat such stress. Signs of hypothermia and cold stress are listed in Box 34.2.

Hyperthermia is also detrimental as it results in an increase in oxygen and calorie consumption. The preterm infant is not able to sweat and thus dissipate heat. Overheating can lead to apnea, tachycardia, and eventually bradycardia, as well as consumption of calories that the preterm infant cannot afford to expend (see Box 34.2).

Central Nervous System Function

The preterm infant's central nervous system (CNS) is susceptible to injury as a result of:

- Birth trauma with damage to immature structures
- Bleeding from fragile capillaries
- An impaired coagulation process, including prolonged prothrombin time
- Recurrent hypoxic and hyperoxic episodes
- Predisposition to hypoglycemia
- Fluctuating systemic BP with concomitant variation in cerebral blood flow and pressure

In the preterm neonate, neurologic function is dependent on gestational age, associated illness factors, and predisposing factors such as intrauterine asphyxia that can cause neurologic damage. Clinical signs of neurologic dysfunction can be subtle, nonspecific, or specific. Five categories of clinical manifestations should be thoroughly evaluated in the preterm infant: seizure activity, hyperirritability, CNS depression, increased intracranial pressure (ICP), and abnormal movements such as decorticate posturing. Primary and tendon reflexes are generally present in preterm infants by 28 weeks of gestation; evaluation of these reflexes should be part of the neurologic examination (see Table 23.1).

The developing nervous system has the ability to reorganize neural connection after injury, meaning that some injuries that would be permanent in adults are not so in infants. Certain neurologic signs appear to be predictive of later abnormalities. These signs include hypotonia, decreased level of activity, weak cry for more than 24 hours, and inability to coordinate suck and swallow. Ongoing assessment and documentation of these neurologic signs are needed for the purpose of discharge teaching and making follow-up recommendations, as well as for their predictive value.

BOX 34.2 Signs of Hypothermia and Hyperthermia

Hypothermia (Cold Stress)

Apnea
Bradycardia
Central cyanosis
Coagulation defects (i.e., pulmonary hemorrhage)
Hypoglycemia
Hypotonia
Hypoxia
Feeding intolerance (abdominal distention, emesis, increased residuals)
Increased metabolic rate
Irritability
Lethargy
Metabolic acidosis
Peripheral vasoconstriction (persistent pulmonary hypertension of the newborn)
Poor weight gain (chronic hypothermia)
Shivering (mature infants in presence of severe hypothermia)
Weak cry or suck

Hyperthermia

Apnea
Central nervous system depression
Dehydration (increased insensible water loss)
Flushed/red skin
Hypernatremia
Irritability
Lethargy
Poor feeding
Seizures
Sweating
Tachycardia
Tachypnea
Warm to touch
Weak or absent cry

Data from Blackburn, S. (2018). *Maternal, fetal, and neonatal physiology: A clinical perspective* (4th ed.). St. Louis: Elsevier; and Gardner, S., & Hernández, J. (2016). Heat balance. In S. L. Gardner, B. S. Carter, M. Enzman-Hines, et al. (Eds.), *Merenstein & Gardner's handbook of neonatal intensive care* (8th ed.). St. Louis: Elsevier.

Nutrition

The goal of neonatal nutrition is to promote normal growth and development. However, maintaining adequate nutrition in the preterm infant is complicated by problems with intake and metabolism. Based on the gestational age, the preterm infant may have weak or absent suck, swallow, and gag reflexes; difficulty coordinating sucking, swallowing, and breathing; small stomach capacity; decreased gastric emptying time; and weak abdominal muscles. The preterm infant's metabolic functions are compromised by a limited store of nutrients, a decreased ability to digest proteins or absorb nutrients, and immature enzyme systems.

The nurse must continually assess the infant's feeding tolerance. Some preterm infants require gavage or intravenous (IV) feedings instead of oral feedings. In very low–birth-weight (VLBW) infants (<1500 g [3.3 lb]), minimal enteral nutrition (MEN) feedings are initiated as soon as the infant is medically stable (Kim, 2016). These feedings stimulate the gastrointestinal (GI) system with small amounts of breast milk or formula, usually given via gavage, so that when enteral feedings of greater volume can begin, the GI system is primed for nutrient absorption. They also may help protect LBW infants from sepsis (Brown, Hendrickson, Evans, et al., 2016).

Renal Function

The preterm infant's immature renal system is unable to adequately excrete metabolites and drugs, concentrate urine, or maintain acid–base, fluid, or electrolyte balance. Therefore intake and output must be assessed. Laboratory tests are done to determine acid–base and electrolyte balance. Medication levels are monitored in preterm infants because certain medications can overwhelm the immature system's ability to excrete them.

Hematologic Status

The preterm infant is predisposed to hematologic problems because of:
- Increased capillary fragility
- Increased tendency to bleed (prolonged prothrombin time and partial thromboplastin time)
- Slowed production of red blood cells (RBCs) resulting from rapid decrease in erythropoiesis after birth
- Loss of blood due to frequent blood sampling for laboratory tests
- Decreased RBC survival related to the relatively larger size of the RBC and its increased permeability to sodium and potassium

The nurse assesses preterm infants for any evidence of bleeding from puncture sites and the GI tract. Infants are examined for signs of anemia; these include decreased hemoglobin and hematocrit levels, pale skin, increased apnea, lethargy, tachycardia, and poor weight gain. The amount of blood drawn for laboratory testing is closely monitored and kept to a minimum.

Immunity

Preterm infants are at increased risk for infection because they have a shortage of stored maternal immunoglobulins, an impaired ability to make antibodies, and a compromised integumentary system (thin skin and fragile capillaries). Preterm infants exhibit various nonspecific signs and symptoms of infection (Box 34.3). Early identification and treatment of sepsis are essential (see Chapter 35). As with all aspects of care, strict attention to hand hygiene is the single most important measure to prevent health-care-associated infections.

Growth and Development

The age of a preterm newborn is corrected by adding the gestational age and the postnatal age. For example, an infant born 4 weeks ago at 32 weeks of gestation would now be considered 36 weeks of age. The infant's **corrected age** at 6 months after the birth date is then 4 months, and the infant's responses are accordingly evaluated against the norm expected for a 4-month-old. The growth and development milestones (e.g., motor milestones, vocalization, growth) are corrected for gestational age until the child is approximately 2½ years old.

Certain measurable factors predict normal growth and development. The preterm infant experiences catch-up body growth during the first 2 years of life. The head is the first to experience catch-up growth, followed by a gain in weight and height. At the infant's discharge from the hospital, which usually occurs between 36 and 40 weeks of postconception age, the infant should exhibit:
- An ability to cry vigorously when hungry
- An appropriate amount and pattern of weight gain according to growth curves
- Neurologic responses appropriate for corrected age

BOX 34.3   Signs and Symptoms of Infection

- Temperature instability
  - Hypothermia
  - Hyperthermia
- Central nervous system changes
  - Lethargy
  - Irritability
- Changes in color
  - Cyanosis, pallor
  - Jaundice
- Cardiovascular instability
  - Poor perfusion
  - Hypotension
  - Bradycardia/tachycardia
- Respiratory distress
  - Tachypnea
  - Apnea
  - Retractions, nasal flaring, grunting
- Gastrointestinal problems
  - Feeding intolerance
  - Vomiting
  - Diarrhea
  - Glucose instability
- Metabolic acidosis

Data from Bodin, M. B. (2014). Immune system. In C. Kenner, & J. W. Lott (Eds.), *Comprehensive neonatal care* (5th ed.). New York: Springer; and Leonard, E., & Dobbs, K. (2015). Postnatal bacterial infections. In R. J. Martin, A. A. Fanaroff, & M. C. Walsh (Eds.), *Fanaroff & Martin's neonatal-perinatal medicine: Diseases of the fetus and infant* (10th ed.). St. Louis: Saunders.

At 39 to 40 weeks of corrected age, the infant should be able to focus on the examiner's or parent's face and to follow with his or her eyes. The infant should also be able to raise the head when prone and be able to hold the head parallel with the body when tested for head lag.

VLBW survivors are at increased risk for neurologic and cognitive disabilities, particularly learning disabilities (Carter, Gratny, & Carter, 2016). Ongoing research focuses on examining other factors including environmental ones that can cause adverse cognitive and neurodevelopmental outcomes for VLBW and ELBW babies as they grow and develop.

Care Management

The goal of care for the preterm infant is to promote normal growth and development by providing an extrauterine environment that approximates that of the fetus. An interprofessional team of physicians, nurses, nurse practitioners, infant developmental specialists, pharmacists, dieticians, and respiratory therapists collaborates to provide the intensive care needed.

The admission of a preterm newborn to the intensive care nursery is usually an emergent situation. A rapid initial evaluation determines the infant's need for lifesaving treatment. Resuscitation is started in the birthing unit, and the newborn's needs for warmth and oxygen are provided for during transfer to the nursery.

Nursing care is focused on the continual assessment and analysis of the infant's physiologic status (see Nursing Care Plan and Clinical Reasoning Case Study). In addition to caring for the infant, nurses are the support persons and teachers during the first phase of the parents' adjustment to the birth of their preterm infant. Interventions for specific aspects of care including nursing actions are discussed in the following sections.

◎ NURSING CARE PLAN

The High-Risk Preterm Newborn

Client Problem	Expected Outcome	Nursing Interventions	Rationales
Acute respiratory distress and/or decreased gas exchange	Infant exhibits adequate gas exchange (i.e., blood gases and acid–base balance within normal limits [WNL]; oxygen saturation within the target range, respiratory rate and pattern WNL; breath sounds clear; absence of grunting and nasal flaring, minimal retractions, skin color WNL).	Position neonate prone or supine, avoiding neck hyperextension.	To promote optimum air exchange
		Administer oxygen and monitor neonatal response.	To maintain oxygen saturation
		Monitor blood gases, acid–base balance, oxygen saturation, respiratory rate and pattern, breath sounds, and airway patency; observe for grunting, nasal flaring, retractions, and cyanosis.	To conserve oxygen use
			To detect signs of respiratory distress
Temperature instability	Infant maintains stable body temperature within normal range for postconceptional age (36.5°C-37°C [97.7°F-99°F]).	Place neonate in a prewarmed radiant warmer or incubator.	To maintain stable temperature.
		Avoid infant exposure to cool air and drafts, cold scales, cold stethoscopes, cold examination tables, and prolonged bathing.	To prevent heat loss
		Transfer infant to a servo-controlled incubator.	Double-walled incubators reduce evaporative and convective heat losses and reduce environmental stimulation
Potential for sepsis	Infant exhibits no evidence of health-care-associated infection.	Institute scrupulous hand hygiene techniques before and after handling neonate, ensure all supplies and/or equipment are clean before use, and ensure strict aseptic technique with invasive procedures.	To minimize exposure to infective organisms
		Instruct parents in infection-control procedures.	To minimize infection risk
		Administer prescribed antibiotics.	To provide coverage for infection during sepsis workup

❓ CLINICAL REASONING CASE STUDY

The Preterm Infant

A 1400-g (3-lb) female infant is born at an estimated gestational age of 33 weeks. The parents are very excited about this birth because they have been trying for 6 years to become pregnant. They name the baby Anna. After skin-to-skin care with her mother, Anna is taken to the special care nursery for observation. She is placed on an open-bed warmer to maintain her temperature; pulse oximetry and cardiorespiratory monitoring are initiated. Anna's oxygen levels are within normal limits in room air and she does not require any respiratory support.

1. What is the priority concern for the infant in this situation? Support your answer with data from the case study.
2. List other needs or problems that Anna might experience.
3. Identify any additional information or assessment data that is needed by the nurse in planning care for this client.
4. What nursing actions are appropriate in this case?
   a. What is the priority nursing action? (What should the nurse do first?)
   b. Describe other nursing interventions that are important in providing optimal care for Anna.
5. Describe the roles/responsibilities of other members of the interprofessional health care team who may be involved in providing care for Anna.

The nurse uses many technologic support systems to monitor the body responses and maintain the body functions of the infant. Technical skill must be combined with a gentle touch and concern about the traumatic effects of harsh lighting and loud machinery noise. Provision of individualized behavioral and environmental care has been shown to reduce infant stress, conserve energy, and promote better neurobehavioral outcomes (Gardner, Goldson, & Hernández, 2016).

The environmental support measures for the preterm infant typically consist of the following equipment and procedures:
- An incubator or radiant warmer to control body temperature
- Oxygen administration or ventilatory support, depending on the infant's cardiopulmonary and circulatory status
- Electronic monitors as needed for the ongoing assessment of respiratory and cardiac functions
- Assistive devices for positioning the infant in neutral flexion and with boundaries
- Clustering of care and minimizing stimulation according to infant cues

Various metabolic support measures that can be instituted consist of the following:
- Parenteral fluids to help support nutrition and maintain normal blood gas levels and acid–base balance
- IV access to facilitate the administration of antibiotic therapy if sepsis is a concern
- Blood work to monitor oxygen and carbon dioxide levels, pH, blood glucose levels, electrolytes, and the status of blood cultures

Maintaining Body Temperature

The high-risk infant is susceptible to heat loss and its complications. In addition, LBW infants have a limited capacity to increase their metabolic rate because of impaired gas exchange, caloric intake restrictions, or poor thermoregulation. Transepidermal water loss is greater because of skin immaturity in very preterm infants (those at less than 28 weeks of gestation) and can contribute to temperature instability.

The preterm infant should be transferred from the birthing room in a prewarmed incubator; ELBW infants can be placed in a polyethylene bag to decrease heat and water loss (Fig. 34.1). Skin-to-skin contact (kangaroo care) between the stable preterm infant and parent is a viable option for interaction because of the maintenance of appropriate body temperature by the infant (see later in this chapter for further discussion of kangaroo care).

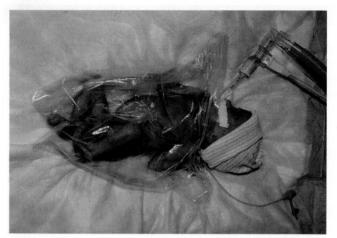

Fig. 34.1 Preterm Infant in Polyethylene Bag to Protect Against Heat Loss. (Courtesy Cheryl Briggs, RNC, Annapolis, MD.)

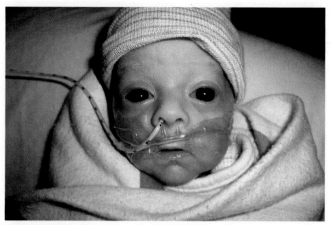

Fig. 34.2 Infant With Nasal Cannula. Note nasogastric tube in place. (Courtesy Cheryl Briggs, RNC, Annapolis, MD.)

High-risk infants are cared for in the thermoneutral environment created by use of an external heat source. A probe to an external heat source supplied by a radiant warmer or a servo-controlled incubator is attached to the infant. The infant acts as a thermostat to regulate the amount of heat supplied by the external source. This idealized environment maintains an infant's normal body temperature between 36.5°C and 37°C (97.9°F and 99°F). Maintaining a thermoneutral condition in the youngest, most immature infants decreases the need for them to generate additional heat, increasing physiologic stability and decreasing oxygen consumption (Blackburn, 2018; Gardner & Hernández, 2016a).

When hypothermia occurs, the infant can appear pale and mottled; the skin is cool to touch, especially the extremities. Acrocyanosis and respiratory distress can occur as oxygen consumption increases in an effort to generate heat. Glucose consumption may also be higher resulting in an increased risk of hypoglycemia. As hypothermia worsens, the infant can have apnea, bradycardia, and central cyanosis.

When an infant becomes hypothermic, rewarming should begin immediately by providing external heat. However, rapid changes in body temperature can cause apnea and acidosis. For the infant with mild hypothermia, slow rewarming is recommended. External heat sources should be slightly warmer than skin temperature and increased gradually until the infant's temperature is within the range of NTE. Use of radiant heaters or heated water mattresses helps prevent prolonged metabolic acidosis and hypoglycemia and reduces mortality (Gardner & Hernández, 2016a).

Respiratory Care

Neonatal resuscitation. In 2016, the American Heart Association (AHA) and American Academy of Pediatrics (AAP) updated their neonatal resuscitation guidelines (AHA & AAP, 2016). A rapid assessment of infants can identify those who do not require resuscitation: those born at term gestation, with no evidence of meconium or infection in the amniotic fluid; those who are breathing or crying; and those with good muscle tone. If any of these characteristics is absent, the infant should receive the following actions in sequence: (1) initial steps in stabilization: provide warmth by placing the baby under a radiant warmer, position the head to open the airway, clear the airway with a bulb syringe or suction catheter, dry the baby, stimulate breathing, and reposition the baby; (2) ventilation; (3) chest compressions; and (4) administration of epinephrine or volume expansion or both. The decision to move from one category of action to the next is based on the assessment of respirations, heart rate, and color. Rapid decision

making is imperative. The condition of the infant is reevaluated and the decision made whether to progress to the next step (see Fig. 24.1).

Resuscitation of asphyxiated newborns with 21% oxygen (room air) rather than 100% oxygen is recommended (AHA & AAP, 2016). Proponents for room air resuscitation suggest that fewer complications are associated with oxidative stress and hyperoxemia when room air is administered. Targeted oxygen saturation levels measured by pulse oximetry should be used to determine the need for, and amount of supplemental oxygen that should be provided. The goal is to minimize oxidative stress by preventing hyperoxia using supplemental oxygen at levels less than 100% (Niermeyer, Clarke, & Hernández, 2016). Neonatal mortality is reduced when room air instead of 100% oxygen is used for neonatal resuscitation (Katheria & Finer, 2018). Fluctuations in oxygen saturation are also deemed harmful especially in ELBW infants.

Oxygen therapy. Clinical criteria that indicate the need for oxygen administration include increased respiratory effort, respiratory distress with apnea, tachycardia, bradycardia, and central cyanosis with or without hypotonia. The need for oxygen should be substantiated by biochemical data (arterial oxygen pressure [PaO_2] of less than 60 mm Hg or an oxygen saturation of less than 92%).

Oxygen administered to an infant is warmed and humidified to prevent cold stress and drying of the respiratory mucosa. During the administration of oxygen, the concentration, volume, temperature, and humidity of the gas are carefully controlled. Delivery of oxygen for more than a few minutes requires the use of special equipment (nasal cannula, positive-pressure mask, or endotracheal tube) because the concentration of free-flow oxygen cannot be monitored accurately. Free-flow oxygen into an incubator should not be used because the concentration fluctuates dramatically each time the doors or portholes are opened. The indiscriminate use of oxygen can be hazardous. Possible complications of oxygen therapy include ROP and BPD.

Infants who need oxygen should have their respiratory status assessed at least hourly and should have continuous pulse oximetry monitoring. There should be hourly documentation of pulse oximetry readings as well as the amount of oxygen being administered and the mode of delivery (Gardner, Enzman-Hines, & Nyp, 2016). Necessary interventions are then determined on the basis of the clinical assessment findings. The interventions ordered are those that can directly manage the underlying disease process and range from nasal cannula oxygen administration to ventilator therapy.

Nasal cannula. Infants requiring low-flow amounts of oxygen can benefit from the use of a nasal cannula (Fig. 34.2). These work well for older infants who are recuperating but still require supplemental oxygen. They are the preferred method for home oxygen administration. Nasal

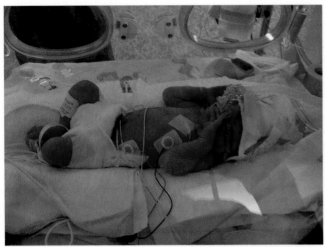

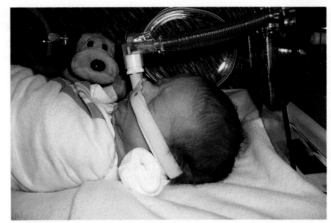

Fig. 34.4 Infant Intubated and on Ventilator. (Courtesy Cheryl Briggs, RNC, Annapolis, MD.)

Fig. 34.3 Infant Receiving Ventilatory Assistance With Nasal Continuous Positive Airway Pressure. (Courtesy Randi and Jacob Wills, Clayton, NC.)

cannulas permit the infant to receive an adequate, continuous flow of oxygen while allowing optimal vision, positioning, and parental holding. Infants can breastfeed or bottle feed while receiving oxygen by this method. Nasal cannulas come in various sizes; proper fit is important. The nasal prongs must be inspected and cleaned frequently to make sure they are not partially obstructed by milk or secretions.

Continuous positive airway pressure therapy. Infants who are unable to maintain an adequate Pao_2 despite the administration of oxygen by nasal cannula may require continuous positive airway pressure (CPAP). CPAP infuses oxygen or air under a preset pressure by means of nasal prongs or a face mask (Fig. 34.3). It may be achieved by sending the oxygen bubbling through water to the infant (bubble CPAP) or via a mechanical ventilator or a dedicated CPAP device. Researchers are investigating whether the failure rate is improved with bubble CPAP versus variable-flow devices (Bhatti, Khan, Murki, et al., 2015). In either case, an orogastric tube should be in place for decompression of the stomach during use of nasal prongs. CPAP increases the functional residual capacity, improves the diffusion time of pulmonary gases, including oxygen, and can decrease pulmonary shunting. CPAP can also preclude the need for mechanical ventilation (Gardner, Enzman-Hines, & Nyp, 2016). Complications of CPAP include mechanical injury to the nasal septum and feeding intolerance related to increased swallowing of air.

Mechanical ventilation. Mechanical ventilation must be implemented if other methods of therapy cannot correct abnormalities in oxygenation (Fig. 34.4). Its use is indicated whenever blood gas values demonstrate severe hypoxemia or severe hypercapnia. Intubation and ventilation can be needed for infants who have apnea with bradycardia, ineffective respiratory effort, shock, asphyxia, infection, meconium aspiration syndrome, respiratory distress syndrome (RDS), or congenital defects that affect ventilation (Gardner, Enzman-Hines, & Nyp, 2016). Ventilator settings are determined by the infant's individual needs. The ventilator is set to provide a predetermined amount of oxygen during spontaneous respirations and during mechanical ventilation in the absence of spontaneous respirations. Newer technologies in ventilation allow oxygen to be delivered at lower pressures and in assist modes, thereby preventing the overriding of the infant's spontaneous breathing and providing distending pressures within a physiologic range. Barotrauma and associated complications such as *pneumothorax* (accumulation of air in the pleural space) and *pulmonary interstitial emphysema* (free air

that accumulates in interstitial tissue) are decreased. See Table 34.1 for a description of the types of mechanical ventilation used in newborns.

High-frequency ventilation (HFV) is accomplished through the use of jet ventilators, oscillators, or high-frequency flow interrupters (Gardner, Enzman-Hines, & Nyp, 2016). These methods provide smaller volumes of oxygen at a significantly more rapid rate (more than 300 breaths/min) than traditional mechanical ventilators. As a result, the intrathoracic pressure is decreased and the risk of barotrauma is reduced. HFV is beneficial in treating infants with pulmonary hypoplasia, diaphragmatic hernia, and meconium aspiration (Bancalari, Claure & Jain, 2018).

> **⚡ SAFETY ALERT**
>
> Rates of retinopathy of prematurity and bronchopulmonary dysplasia are reduced when arterial oxygen saturation (Sao_2) is kept in the lower range of normal (88%-92%). Individualized target saturation ranges should be determined for each ELBW infant.

Surfactant administration. *Surfactant* is a surface-active phospholipid secreted by the alveolar epithelium. Acting much the same as a detergent, this substance reduces the surface tension of fluids that line the alveoli and respiratory passages, resulting in uniform expansion and maintenance of lung volumes at low intraalveolar pressure. Before 28 weeks of gestation, most infants do not produce adequate amounts of surfactant. As a result, lung compliance is decreased, and inadequate gas exchange occurs as the lungs become atelectatic and require greater pressures to expand.

Surfactant can be administered as an adjunct to oxygen and ventilation therapy. With administration of artificial surfactant, respiratory compliance is improved until the infant can generate sufficient surfactant. Exogenous surfactant is given in several doses through an endotracheal tube. The AAP recommends the use of surfactant in infants with RDS as soon as possible after birth, especially for ELBW infants and those not exposed to maternal antenatal steroids (Polin, Carlo, & Committee on Fetus and Newborn, 2014). The administration of antenatal steroids to the mother and surfactant replacement has decreased the incidence of RDS and concomitant morbidities. Use of exogenous surfactant has been associated with a significantly reduced length of time on ventilators and oxygen therapy, and an increased survival rate in preterm infants (Polin et al.). As with any drug therapy, the infant must be monitored for potential side effects such as a patent ductus arteriosus and pulmonary hemorrhage (see Medication Guide: Surfactant Replacement).

TABLE 34.1   Common Methods for Assisted Ventilation in Neonatal Respiratory Distress

Method	Description	How Provided
Continuous distending pressure—continuous positive airway pressure (CPAP)	Provides constant distending pressure to airway in spontaneously breathing infant	Nasal prongs or nasopharyngeal tubes Face mask Bubble CPAP uses water resistance
Intermittent mandatory ventilation (IMV)	Allows infant to breathe spontaneously at own rate but provides mechanical cycled respirations and pressure at regular preset intervals; infant can maintain asynchronous ventilation efforts, which diminishes effective gas exchange; uses positive end-expiratory pressure (PEEP)	Endotracheal intubation
Synchronized intermittent mandatory ventilation (SIMV)	Mechanically delivered breaths are synchronized to the onset of spontaneous infant breaths; assist or control (A/C) mode facilitates full inspiratory synchrony; involves signal detection of onset of spontaneous respiration from abdominal movement, thoracic impedance, and airway pressure or flow changes; pressure support ventilation provides an inspiratory pressure assist when spontaneous breathing is detected to decrease infant's work of breathing	Patient-triggered infant ventilator with signal detector and A/C mode; endotracheal tube; SIMV, A/C, and pressure support are also referred to as patient-triggered ventilation
Volume guarantee ventilation	Delivers a predetermined volume of gas using an inspiratory pressure that varies according to the infant's lung compliance (often used in conjunction with SIMV)	Volume guarantee ventilator with flow sensor; endotracheal tube
High-frequency oscillation (HFO)	Application of high-frequency, low-volume, sine-wave flow oscillations to airway at rates between 480 and 1200 breaths/min	Variable-speed piston pump (or loudspeaker, fluidic oscillator); endotracheal tube
High-frequency jet ventilation (HFJV)	Uses a separate, parallel, low-compliant circuit and injector port to deliver small pulses or jets of fresh gas deep into airway at rates between 250 and 900 breaths/min	May be used alone or with low-rate IMV; endotracheal tube

MEDICATION GUIDE

Surfactant Replacement

Drug/Source
- Beractant[a] (Survanta)—Exogenous surfactant from bovine lung extract
- Poractant alpha[a] (Curosurf)—Modified porcine-derived minced lung extract
- Calfactant[a] (Infasurf)—Natural surfactant extracted from calf lung lavage
- Lucinactant (Surfaxin): Synthetic surfactant

Action
These medications provide exogenous surfactant to promote lung maturity.

Indications
Surfactants are used to reduce the severity of respiratory distress syndrome (RDS) in preterm infants. The drug should be administered to infants with RDS as soon as possible after intubation and initial stabilization. It should be given prophylactically to extremely preterm infants at high risk for RDS, especially if there was no exposure to antenatal steroids. Early rescue surfactant treatment may be given to infants less than 2 hrs of age with signs of RDS. Late rescue surfactant treatment may be administered to infants at 4 to 6 hrs of age who require mechanical ventilation. Rescue surfactant may be given to infants with hypoxic respiratory failure that results from secondary surfactant deficiency; this includes meconium aspiration syndrome, sepsis or pneumonia, and pulmonary hemorrhage.

Dosage and Route
Dosage depends on the drug used. Administer via endotracheal tube as a bolus or in smaller amounts into the endotracheal tube through an adaptor port.
- Beractant[a] (Survanta)—4 mL/kg
- Poractant alpha[a] (Curosurf)—2.5 mL/kg
- Calfactant[a] (Infasurf)—3 mL/kg
- Lucinactant (Surfaxin)—5.8 mL/kg

Adverse Reactions
Adverse events are most often related to the administration procedure and include oxygen desaturation, transient bradycardia, alterations in blood pressure, and drug reflux.

Nursing Considerations
The nurse observes the infant for changes. Diuresis can occur with improvement. Ventilator settings may need changing as the infant's ability to oxygenate increases.

[a]Bovine and porcine products can be objectionable to parents because of religious or cultural beliefs (e.g., Jewish, Islam, Hindu); prior to administering surfactant to infant informed consent from parents is essential.

Data from Gardner, S., Enzman-Hines, M., & Nyp, N. (2016). Respiratory diseases. In S. L. Gardner, B. S. Carter, M. Enzman-Hines, et al. (Eds.), *Merenstein & Gardner's handbook of neonatal intensive care* (8th ed.). St. Louis: Mosby; and Polin, R. A., Carlo, W. A., & Committee on Fetus and Newborn. (2014). Surfactant replacement therapy for preterm and term neonates with respiratory distress. *Pediatrics, 133*(1), 156–163.

Additional therapies

Nitric oxide therapy. Inhaled nitric oxide (INO), delivered as a gas, causes potent and sustained pulmonary vasodilation in the pulmonary circulation. Nitric oxide is a colorless, highly diffusible gas that can be administered through the ventilator circuit or with nasal cannula blended with oxygen. It binds with hemoglobin in RBCs and is inactivated after metabolism. INO is used to decrease or reverse pulmonary hypertension, pulmonary vasoconstriction, acidosis, and hypoxemia in term and LPIs with conditions such as persistent pulmonary hypertension, meconium aspiration syndrome, pneumonia, sepsis, and congenital diaphragmatic hernia. INO therapy can be used in conjunction with surfactant replacement therapy, HFV, or extracorporeal membrane oxygenation (ECMO). In the few studies conducted with human infants, positive results were seen: oxygen saturation improved, and no toxic effects from methemoglobin or increased levels of nitrogen oxide were documented. INO shows much promise in reducing adverse respiratory sequelae of prematurity. Its use has reduced the need for invasive technologies such as ECMO (Gardner, Enzman-Hines, & Nyp, 2016).

Extracorporeal membrane oxygenation. ECMO is a very complex and costly treatment that is sometimes used to support life and allow treatment of intractable hypoxemia due to severe cardiac or respiratory failure. This therapy involves a modified heart-lung machine, although in ECMO the heart is not stopped, and blood does not entirely bypass the lungs. Blood is shunted from a catheter in the right atrium or right internal jugular vein by gravity to a servo-regulated roller pump, pumped through a membrane lung, where it is oxygenated, and through a small heat exchanger, where it is warmed, and then returned to the systemic circulation via a major artery such as the carotid artery to the aortic arch. ECMO provides oxygen to the circulation, allowing the lungs to "rest," and decreases pulmonary hypertension and hypoxemia in such conditions as persistent pulmonary hypertension of the newborn, congenital diaphragmatic hernia, sepsis, meconium aspiration, and severe pneumonia. ECMO is contraindicated for preterm infants younger than 34 weeks of gestation because of the anticoagulant therapy required in the pump and circuits, which can increase the potential for intraventricular hemorrhage (Gardner, Enzman-Hines, & Nyp, 2016).

Weaning from respiratory assistance.

The goal of weaning is the withdrawal of all respiratory support. Respiratory assistance is weaned slowly as the infant's status improves. The infant is ready to be weaned from respiratory assistance once the blood gas and oxygen saturation levels are maintained within normal limits. A spontaneous, adequate respiratory effort must be present, and the infant must show improved muscle tone during increased activity. Weaning is done in a stepwise and gradual manner. This can consist of the infant being extubated, placed on CPAP, and then weaned to oxygen by means of nasal cannula. Throughout the weaning process, the infant's oxygen levels are monitored by pulse oximetry and blood gas measurements. The infant is assessed for signs and symptoms indicating poor tolerance of the process. These include an increased pulse, increase in periods of apnea, respiratory distress or cyanosis, or a combination of these. If these occur, the amount of respiratory support being delivered is increased and weaning proceeds more slowly as assessments continue. Underlying causes of intolerance of weaning can be BPD, a PDA, or CNS damage.

Some infants do not tolerate weaning from oxygen therapy before discharge from the hospital. They can require supplementary oxygen at home for weeks or months.

Nutritional Care

It is not always possible to provide enteral (by the GI route) nourishment to a high-risk infant. Such infants are often too ill or weak to breastfeed or bottle feed because of respiratory distress or sepsis. Early enteral feeding of the asphyxiated neonate with a low Apgar score also is avoided to prevent bowel necrosis. In such cases, nutrition is provided parenterally. Infants who require parenteral nutrition are likely to have one or more of the following problems:

- Extreme prematurity where feedings must be introduced slowly
- Respiratory distress requiring aggressive ventilator support
- Asphyxiation with a potential for NEC

Type of nourishment.

The type, mode, volume, and schedule of feedings are based on:

- Initially, the birth weight, and then the current weight of the preterm infant
- Pattern of weight gain or loss (infants weighing less than 1500 g [3.3 lb] require more energy for growth and thermoregulation and can gain weight poorly with either breast- or bottle feedings)
- Presence or absence of suck-and-swallow reflex in all infants at less than 35 weeks of gestation
- Behavioral readiness to take oral feedings
- Physical condition, including presence or absence of bowel sounds, abdominal distention, or bloody stools, as well as presence and degree of respiratory distress or apneic episodes
- Residual from previous feeding, if being gavage fed
- Malformations (especially GI defects such as gastroschisis, omphalocele, or esophageal atresia), including the need for a gastrostomy feeding tube
- Renal function, including urinary output and laboratory values (nitrogen balance, electrolyte balance, glucose level); preterm infants are especially susceptible to altered renal function

Human milk. Human milk is the best source of nutrition for term and preterm infants. Even small preterm (32 to 36 weeks) infants are able to breastfeed if they have adequate sucking and swallowing reflexes and no other contraindications, such as respiratory complications or concurrent illness. Preterm infants who are breastfed rather than bottle fed demonstrate fewer oxygen desaturations, absence of bradycardia, warmer than normal skin temperature, and improved coordination of sucking, swallowing, and breathing (Gardner & Lawrence, 2016). Mothers who wish to breastfeed their preterm infants are encouraged to express their milk using a hospital-grade electric pump until their infants are sufficiently stable to tolerate feeding at the breast, and to continue pumping after feedings until the infant is able to exclusively breastfeed, usually after discharge from the hospital (Briere, Lucas, McGrath, et al., 2015). Appropriate guidelines for the storage of expressed mother's milk should be used to decrease the risk of milk contamination and destruction of its beneficial properties (Peters, McArthur, & Munn, 2016).

Infant formula. Commercially available preterm formulas are cow's milk based and whey predominant and have a higher concentration of protein, calcium, and phosphorus than term formulas to meet the unique needs of the preterm infant (Brown et al., 2016). Most preterm formulas are either 22 or 24 cal/oz. Human milk with commercial human milk fortifier is recommended for LBW preterm infants because it increases weight gain and improves bone mineralization better than nonfortified human milk (Gardner & Lawrence, 2016). Supplementation with iron, vitamin D, and multivitamins may be considered in exclusively breastfed LBW infants.

Weight and fluid balance.

The caloric, nutrient, and fluid requirements of high-risk infants are greater than those of the healthy term newborn. Premature or dysmature (malnourished) newborns have limited stores of nutrients and fluids. In addition, hypoglycemia, electrolyte imbalances, or other metabolic disturbances can develop in an infant whose nutritional intake is poor. Hypoglycemia can cause serious damage to carbohydrate-dependent brain cells.

The infant's weight is measured and recorded daily, and the rate of weight loss or gain is calculated. Further depletion of weight and

metabolic stores can occur as a result of one or a combination of the following factors:
- Birth asphyxia
- Increased respirations or respiratory effort
- Patent ductus arteriosus
- Hypothermia or hyperthermia
- Insensible fluid loss caused by evaporation (with radiant heat or phototherapy)
- Vomiting, diarrhea, and dysfunctional absorption from the GI tract
- Growth demands (a preterm infant's growth rate approximates that of fetal growth during the last trimester and is at least two times faster than a term infant's growth rate after birth)
- Inability of the renal system to concentrate urine and maintain an adequate rate of urea excretion, as well as infant's inadequate response to antidiuretic hormone

The high-risk newborn is predisposed to weight and fluid losses because of the greater amount of fluid and calories needed to meet the demands of the increased cellular metabolic processes (resulting from stress, repair, and growth). Preterm infants have higher water content than that of their full-term counterparts (Blackburn, 2018). Most of this water is in the extracellular fluid compartment. Even with the early institution of fluid and nutritional intake, the preterm infant's weight and fluid losses seem exaggerated. Inadequate fluid intake, resulting from either delayed administration or insufficient volume, can further cause weight and fluid losses in the preterm infant.

Insensible water loss (IWL) is an evaporative loss that occurs largely through the skin (70%) and through the respiratory tract (30%). The basal IWL in a term infant is approximately 20 mL/kg/day. It is significantly increased in preterm infants, and especially in ELBW infants with thin, gelatinous skin (Blackburn, 2018). The effects of radiant warmers, incubators, phototherapy, and other factors can increase the IWL. Humidifying the respiratory gases administered can prevent some of this loss.

During the first week of extrauterine life the preterm infant can lose up to 15% of his or her birth weight. In contrast, a weight loss up to 10% is acceptable in a term, appropriate for gestational age (AGA) infant. After the initial week, a preterm infant's loss or gain during each 24-hour period should not exceed 2% of the previous day's weight. (To calculate a weight loss or gain, see Box 34.4.)

Increased stooling or voiding, increased evaporative losses, inadequate volume or incorrect fluid administration, and problems with malabsorption can cause weight loss. Common interventions to correct weight loss include adjusting the incubator temperature; increasing the ambient humidity levels; monitoring and adjusting the volume and type of fluid being administered; assessing the urinary output; and assessing the blood glucose levels. Hyperglycemia results in urinary loss of glucose that can cause osmotic diuresis, which increases the risk of dehydration (Burris, 2017).

If the infant is gaining more than the expected amount of weight, this can be due to overfeeding or fluid retention. The nurse reports and records the findings and continues to assess the infant's fluid status, urinary output, and blood glucose levels. Interventions are determined by the infant's specific disorder and nutritional needs.

Elimination patterns. The infant's elimination patterns are assessed and documented. This includes the frequency of urination, as well as the amount and color of the urine. The assessment of the infant's bowel movements includes the frequency of stooling and the character of the stool, as well as whether there is constipation, diarrhea, or loss of fats (steatorrhea). Infants with unexplained abdominal distention are assessed carefully to rule out the presence of feeding intolerance or NEC.

Feeding methods

Oral feeding. Nourishment by the oral route is preferred for the infant who has adequate strength and GI function. The best milk for an infant is from the mother. Breast milk can be fed by breast, bottle, cup, or spoon. Throughout the feeding the nurse assesses the newborn's tolerance of the procedure. Preterm infants can be put to breast for nonnutritive suckling and practice feeds as soon as medically stable. The nurse or lactation consultant assists the mother by providing support and help as necessary when the infant breastfeeds.

Many high-risk infants cannot suck well enough to breastfeed or bottle feed until they have recovered from their initial illness or matured physically (corrected age more than 32 weeks of gestation). Mothers of high-risk infants are encouraged to continue expressing breast milk with a hospital-grade electric pump, especially if their infant is a very premature infant who will not breastfeed for many weeks. Because of the significant breastfeeding attrition rates among these mothers, they need ongoing support and encouragement to continue pumping while their infant is not yet able to nurse. If human milk is not available from the mother, donor breast milk from a milk bank or commercial formula is used. The calories, protein, and mineral content of commercial formulas vary. The type of bottle and nipple selected ("preemie," regular, orthodontic) depends on the infant's ability to suck from the specific type of nipple. The nurse also considers the energy the infant needs to expend in the process. However, the practice of delaying breastfeeding until the baby is able to effectively bottle feed is not evidence-based because studies continue to confirm that breastfeeding is less stressful than bottle feeding (Gardner & Lawrence, 2016).

Feedings are carefully monitored. Overfeeding of the preterm infant should be avoided because this can lead to abdominal distention, with apnea, vomiting, and possibly aspiration of the feeding.

Gavage feeding. Gavage feeding is a method of providing nourishment to the infant who is compromised by respiratory distress, the infant who is too immature to have a coordinated suck-and-swallow reflex, or the infant who is easily fatigued by sucking. In gavage feeding, human milk or commercial infant formula is given to the infant through a nasogastric or orogastric tube (Fig. 34.5). This spares the infant the work of sucking.

Gavage feeding can be done with an intermittently placed tube providing a bolus feeding or continuously through an indwelling catheter. Infants who cannot tolerate large bolus feedings are given continuous feedings. MEN, sometimes referred to as minimal enteral feeds; GI priming; or trophic feeding can be used to stimulate or prime the GI tract to achieve better absorption of nutrients when bolus or regular intermittent gavage feedings can be given (Blackburn, 2018).

BOX 34.4 Calculation of a Weight Loss or Gain

Example 1

Day 1	1750 g (birth weight)	$\dfrac{70}{1750} = \dfrac{X}{100}$
Day 3	1680 g 70-g loss	$1750X = 7000$
		$X = 4\%$ weight loss

Example 2

Day 3	1680 g	$\dfrac{40}{1680} = \dfrac{X}{100}$
Day 4	1720 g 40-g gain	$1680X = 4000$
		$X = 2.4\%$ weight gain

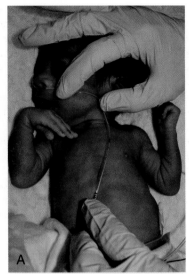

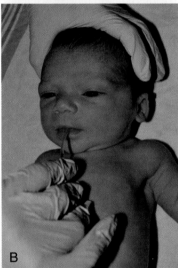

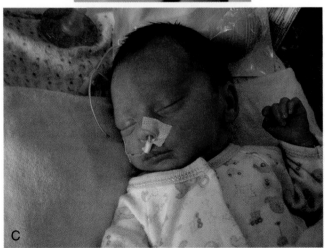

Fig. 34.5 Gavage Feeding. (A) Measurement of gavage feeding tube from tip of nose to earlobe and to midpoint between end of xiphoid process and umbilicus. Tape may be used to mark correct length on tube. For accurate measure the infant should be facing up. (B) Insertion of gavage tube using orogastric route. (C) Indwelling gavage tube, nasogastric route. After feeding by orogastric or nasogastric tube, infant is propped on right side or placed prone (preterm infant) for 1 hour to facilitate emptying of stomach into small intestine. (A and B, Courtesy Cheryl Briggs, RNC, Annapolis, MD; C, Courtesy Randi and Jacob Wills, Clayton, NC.)

BOX 34.5 Procedure for Inserting a Gavage Feeding Tube

Equipment

- Infant feeding tube
  - For infants less than 1 kg (2.2 lb), size 4 Fr
  - For infants more than 1 kg (2.2 lb), size 5 to 6 Fr
- Stethoscope
- Sterile water (lubricant)
- Syringe: 5-10 mL
- Tape, optional transparent dressing
- Gloves

Procedure

- Measure the length of the gavage tube from the tip of the nose to the earlobe to the midpoint between the xiphoid process and the umbilicus (see Fig. 34.5A). Mark the tube with indelible ink or a piece of tape.
- Lubricate the tip of the tube with sterile water and insert gently through the nose or mouth (see Fig. 34.5B) until the predetermined mark is reached. Placement of the tube in the trachea will cause the infant to gag, cough, or become cyanotic.
- Check correct placement of the tube by:
  a. Pulling back on the plunger to aspirate stomach contents. Lack of stomach aspirate or fluid is not necessarily evidence of improper placement. Aspiration of respiratory secretions can be mistaken for stomach contents; however, the pH of the stomach contents is much lower (more acidic) than the pH of respiratory secretions.
  b. Injecting a small amount of air (1-3 mL) into the tube while listening for gurgling by using a stethoscope placed over the stomach. Ensure that the tube is inserted to the mark; air entering the stomach can be heard even if the tube is positioned above the gastroesophageal (cardiac) sphincter.
  c. Abdominal or chest radiography. This is the only definitive way to verify tube placement.
- Using tape or a transparent dressing, secure the tube in place and tape it to the cheek to prevent accidental dislodgment and incorrect positioning (see Fig. 34.5C).
  a. Assess the infant's skin integrity before taping the tube.
  b. Edematous or very preterm infants should have a pectin barrier placed under the tape to prevent abrasions, or a hydrocolloid adhesive should be used to prevent epidermal stripping.
- Tube placement *must* be assessed before each feeding.

Breast milk or formula can be supplied intermittently via gavage by using a syringe with gravity-controlled flow, or it can be given continuously by using an infusion pump. The type of fluid instilled is recorded with every syringe change. The volume of the continuous feedings is recorded hourly, and the residual gastric aspirate is measured every 2 to 4 hours. Aspirates of less than a 1-hour volume can be re-fed to the infant. For intermittent feedings, residuals of less than 50% of the previous feeding can be re-fed to the infant to prevent the loss of gastric electrolytes. Feeding is usually stopped if the residual is greater than 50% of the feeding or if residuals are increasing and is not resumed until the infant can be assessed for a possible feeding intolerance (Brown et al., 2016).

The orogastric route for gavage feedings is preferred because most infants are preferential nose breathers. In addition, when indwelling nasogastric tubes are used, there is a risk for necrosis of the nares. However, some infants do not tolerate oral tube placement. A small nasogastric feeding tube can be placed in older infants who would otherwise gag or vomit or in ones who are learning to suck. To insert the tube and give the feeding, the nurse should follow the sequence given in Box 34.5.

Gastrostomy feedings. Gastrostomy feedings are used for infants with neurologic problems or certain congenital malformations that require long-term tube feedings. This involves the surgical placement of a tube through the skin of the abdomen into the stomach. The tube is then taped in an upright position to prevent trauma to the incision site. After the procedure the nurse initiates small bolus feedings per the health care provider's orders. Feedings by gravity are done slowly over 20- to 30-minute periods. Special care must be taken to prevent rapid bolusing of the fluid because this can lead to abdominal distention, GI reflux into the esophagus, or respiratory compromise. Meticulous skin care at the tube insertion site is necessary to prevent skin breakdown or infection. In addition, intake and output are closely monitored because these infants are prone to diarrhea until regular feedings are established.

Parenteral nutrition. Supplemental parenteral fluids are indicated for infants who are unable to obtain sufficient fluids or calories by enteral feeding. Some of these infants are dependent on total parenteral nutrition (TPN) for extensive periods. The nurse assesses and documents the following in infants receiving parenteral fluids or TPN:
- Type and infusion rate of the solution
- Functional status of the infusion equipment, including the tubing and infusion pump
- Infusion site for possible complications (phlebitis, infiltration, dislodgment)
- Caloric intake
- Infant's responses to therapy

The health care provider orders TPN per the hospital protocol. These orders must specify the electrolytes and nutrients desired, as well as the volume and rate of infusion. The composition of calories, protein, and fats is calculated on an individual basis.

While caring for the infant receiving parenteral fluids or TPN, the nurse secures and protects the insertion site. Scrupulous hand hygiene is used before handling the TPN tubing or IV sites. Strict sterile technique is implemented for dressing changes especially when the TPN is infusing through a central line (Olsen, Leick-Rude, Dustin, et al., 2016). The nurse must observe the principles of neonatal skin care. The nurse carefully inspects the infusion site for signs of infiltration and repositions the infant frequently to maintain body alignment and protect the site. Parents need explanations about TPN and the ways in which the IV equipment and solutions affect their infant.

Advancing infant feedings. Feedings are advanced as assessment data and the infant's ability to tolerate the feedings warrant. Documentation of a preterm infant's sucking patterns also can be used to determine readiness to nipple feed. Feedings are advanced from passive (parenteral and gavage) to active (breastfeeding or bottle feeding). At each step the nurse must carefully assess the infant's response to prevent stress to the infant.

The infant receiving nutrition parenterally is gradually weaned off this type of nutrition. To do this the nourishment given by continuous or intermittent gavage feedings is increased and the parenteral fluids are decreased. Even the smallest infants are given MEN to stimulate the GI system to mature and to enhance caloric intake (Blackburn, 2018).

Feedings are advanced slowly and cautiously because if advanced too rapidly, the infant can develop vomiting (with an attendant risk of aspiration), abdominal distention, and apneic episodes.

If the infant needs additional calories, a commercial human milk fortifier can be added to the breast milk, or the number of calories per 30 mL of commercial formula can be increased. Elemental formulas are used only for infants with very special dietary needs, such as allergies to cow's milk or chronic malabsorption. Calories in breast milk can be lost if the cream separates and adheres to the tubing during

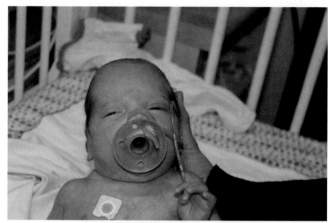

Fig. 34.6 Nonnutritive Sucking. (Courtesy Debbie Fraser, Winnipeg, Manitoba.)

continuous infusion. This problem is decreased if microbore tubing is used for both continuous and intermittent gavage feedings and if the infusion pump is positioned so that the tip of the syringe faces upward instead of horizontal.

The infant receiving gavage feedings progresses to breastfeeding or bottle feedings. To do this the gavage feedings are decreased as the infant's ability to suckle breast milk or formula improves. Often during this transition the infant is fed by both bottle or breast and gavage feeding to ensure the intake of both the prescribed volume of food and nutrients. However, when there is an indwelling tube, during breastfeeding or bottle feeding some infants experience increased respiratory effort, so nurses must watch for this. The parents need support during this transition because many families measure their parenting competence by how well they can feed their infant. For breastfed infants, it is important to weigh the infant before and after breastfeeding to determine the infant's intake (Gardner & Lawrence, 2016).

As the time of discharge nears, the appropriate method of feeding and the assessments pertaining to the method (e.g., tolerance of feedings, status of gavage tube placement) are reviewed with the parents. The parents should be encouraged to interact with the infant by talking and making eye contact with the infant during the feeding. This stimulates the psychosocial development of the infant and facilitates bonding and attachment.

Nonnutritive sucking. If the infant is receiving only TPN or gavage feeds, *nonnutritive sucking* should be encouraged for several reasons (Fig. 34.6). Allowing the infant to suck on a pacifier during gavage or between oral feedings can improve oxygenation. In addition, such nonnutritive sucking can lead to decreased energy expenditure with less restlessness. It also promotes positive weight gain and better sucking skills (Gardner & Lawrence, 2016).

Mothers of preterm infants should be encouraged to allow their infants to start sucking at the breast during kangaroo care (skin-to-skin). In some infants, the suck-and-swallow reflexes are coordinated as early as 32 weeks of gestation. If the neonate is unable to suck, the mother can place the infant near the nipple to encourage nuzzling or licking.

Skin Care

The skin of preterm infants is characteristically immature compared with that of full-term infants. Because of its increased sensitivity and fragility, the use of alkaline-based soap that might destroy the acid mantle of the skin is avoided. *Vernix caseosa* has benefits for the preterm infant's skin. Vernix acts as an epidermal barrier, decreases bacterial contamination of the skin through its antimicrobial peptides and proteins, and decreases transepidermal water loss (Blackburn, 2018).

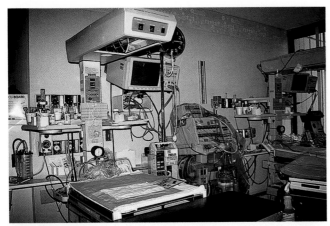

Fig. 34.7 Neonatal Intensive Care Unit Environment. Note bed, wall oxygen attachments, monitor, ventilator, incubator, and pumps, all of which have alarm systems. (Courtesy Marjorie Pyle, RNC, Lifecircle, Costa Mesa, CA.)

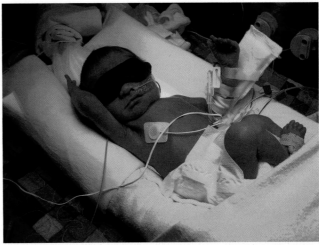

Fig. 34.8 Developmental Care: Positioning of Preterm Infant Using Containment While Undergoing Phototherapy. (Courtesy Randi and Jacob Wills, Clayton, NC.)

Experts recommend that a validated skin assessment tool such as the Neonatal Skin Condition Score (NSCS) be used once daily to evaluate the high-risk infant's skin condition so as to implement interventions aimed at minimizing skin breakdown (Lund & Durand, 2016).

Environmental Concerns

Infants in neonatal intensive care units (NICUs) are exposed to high levels of auditory input from the various machine alarms, and this can have adverse effects (Fig. 34.7). In addition, continual noise levels of 38 to 90 decibels (db) are common in NICUs. An incubator alone produces a constant noise level of 50 to 75 db, and each new piece of life-support equipment used adds more background noise. Hearing can be damaged if the infant is exposed to a constant decibel level of 85 db. Cochlear damage has been recognized as a side effect of the NICU environment. Hearing losses have been identified in NICU graduates; these losses lead to long-term speech and language deficits. Over time more emphasis has been placed on noise in the NICU and the adverse or long-term effects on neonates (Gardner, Goldson, & Hernández, 2016).

Respiratory equipment or a phototherapy mask can alter the infant's vision, making it difficult to interact with parents and caregivers. The infant may be unable to establish diurnal and nocturnal rhythms because of the continuous exposure to overhead lighting. In addition, sedation or pain medications affect the way in which the infant perceives the environment.

An additional concern in the care of infants is that some medications can potentiate environmental hazards. Drugs such as aminoglycosides can potentiate noise-induced hearing loss (Garinis, Kemph, Tharpe, et al., 2017). Routine hearing screening should be performed in all infants before discharge, with follow-up audiologic evaluation completed by no later than the third month of life (Sahai & Levy, 2018).

Research is ongoing to determine the long-term effects of light and noise on the preterm infant (Philpott-Robinson, Lane, Korostenski, et al., 2017). Cycling of light and covering of incubators to reduce direct light hitting the retina are two areas of research. The retina of the immature infant has little protection from the nearly translucent eyelid, thus allowing light to almost constantly penetrate the retina unless it is artificially protected by dimming the lights or using incubator covers. Cycled lighting has been shown to have a positive effect on growth (Vasquez-Ruiz, Maya-Barrios, Torres-Narváez, & Vega-Martinez, 2014). Light and sound can be adverse stimuli for the preterm infant

who is already stressed. Signs of stress include increased metabolic rate, increased oxygen and caloric use, and depression of the immune system. The nurse must monitor the macroenvironment and the microenvironment (unit and immediate environments) for sources of overstimulation. Providing a developmentally supportive environment can lead to decreased complications and length of stay. There are national recommendations for sound and light levels in the NICU.

Nurses can modify the environment to provide a developmentally supportive milieu. In that way the infant's neurobehavioral and physiologic needs can be better met, the infant's developing organization can be supported, and growth and development can be fostered (Gardner, Goldson, & Hernández, 2016).

Developmental Care

The goal of developmental care is to support each infant's efforts to become as well organized, competent, and stable as possible. The caregiver uses the infant's own behavior and physiologic functioning as the basis for planning care and providing interventions. Through caregiver observation, the infant's strengths, thresholds for disorganization, and vulnerable areas can be identified. The family is included in developmental care. Working together, the family and other caregivers provide opportunities to enhance the strengths of the family and the infant and to reduce the stress that is associated with the birth and care of high-risk infants.

Reducing light and noise levels by instituting "quiet hours" at regularly scheduled times and positioning are just two ways in which nurses can support infants in their development. Sleep interruptions are minimized, and positioning and bundling the infant help promote self-regulation and prevent disorganization (Altimier & Phillips, 2016; Gardner, Goldson, & Hernández, 2016).

Positioning. The motor development of preterm infants permits less flexion than in term infants. Caregivers can provide a variety of positions for infants. While the infant remains on cardiorespiratory monitors, side-lying and prone positions are preferred to supine. Body containment with use of blanket rolls, swaddling, holding the infant's arms in a crossed position, and secure holding provide boundaries (Fig. 34.8). Use of facilitated tucking promotes self-regulation during feeding, procedures, and other stressful interventions. The prone position encourages flexion of the extremities; a sling or hip roll assists in maintaining flexion. Keeping the extremities close to the body helps calm the infant and decreases stimulation (Altimier & Phillips, 2016).

Proper body alignment is necessary to prevent developmental problems that can affect the ability to walk as the child matures (Madlinger-Lewis, Reynolds, Zarem, et al., 2014).

Reducing stimulation. NICU staff can reduce unnecessary noise by closing doors or portholes on incubators quietly, placing only necessary objects gently on top of incubators, keeping radios at low volume, speaking quietly, and handling equipment noiselessly. Another source is internal noise created by mechanical sources such as CPAP. These noise sources must be considered in terms of their long-term effects on hearing. Earmuffs can be used to reduce stress from noise (Gardner, Goldson, & Hernández, 2016).

Infants can be protected from light by dimming the lights during the night, placing a blanket over the incubator, or covering the infant's eyes with a mask. Sleep-wake cycles can be induced with such measures. Infants need periods in which there are no disruptions and sleep can occur.

Infant communication. Infants communicate their needs and ability to tolerate sensory stimulation through physiologic responses. The nurses and parents of high-risk infants must therefore be alert to such cues. Although term infants can thrive on stimulation, the same level of stimulation in high-risk infants can provoke physical symptoms of stress and anxiety (Gardner, Goldson, & Hernández, 2016).

Problems with noxious stimuli and barriers to normal contact can cause anxiety and tension. Clues to overstimulation include averting the gaze, hiccupping, finger splaying, gagging, or regurgitating food. Term infants exhibit a startle reflex, and preterm infants move all of their limbs in an uncoordinated fashion in response to noxious stimuli. An irregular respiratory rate or an increased heart rate can develop in severely distressed infants, and they can be unable to regain a calm state. Apnea and bradycardia may also occur.

A relaxed infant state is indicated by stabilization of vital signs, closed eyes, and a relaxed posture. Nonintubated infants may make soothing verbal sounds when they are relaxed. Infants requiring artificial ventilation cannot cry audibly and often show their distress through posturing; they relax once their needs are met. As high-risk infants heal and mature, they increasingly respond to stimuli in a self-regulated manner rather than with a dissociated response. Infants who do not show increased self-regulation should be evaluated for a neurologic problem.

Infant stimulation. The Newborn Individualized Developmental Care and Assessment Program (NIDCAP, 2019) (www.nidcap.org) routinely integrates aspects of neurodevelopmental theory with caregivers' observations, environmental interventions, and parental support. Routine reassessment is built into the program's design. Developmental stimuli may consist of such simple measures as kangaroo care or parental touch. The simplest calming technique is for the caregiver to use both hands to contain the infant's extremities close to the body. The care of the infant is organized to allow extended periods of undisturbed rest and sleep. Pain assessments should be done consistently per the unit's protocol.

Infants acquire a sense of trust as they learn the feel, sound, and smell of their parents. High-risk infants also must learn to trust their caregivers to obtain comfort. However, caregivers in the nursery also can inflict pain as part of the care they must give. For this reason it is important for parents and caregivers to use comforting interventions such as removing painful stimuli, relieving hunger, and changing wet or soiled clothing to foster trust. They can offer nonnutritive sucking or use oral sucrose for pain relief before painful procedures.

As the infant matures, additional sensory input can be provided. These measures can include cuddling, rocking, singing, talking to the infant, and using music therapy. These activities are beneficial and promote growth and weight gain as well as shorten the length of hospital

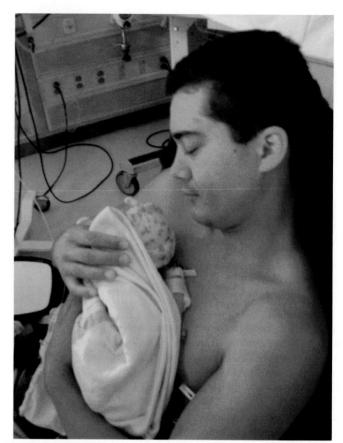

Fig. 34.9 Father Holding Infant in Kangaroo Care. (Courtesy Randi and Jacob Wills, Clayton, NC.)

stay. Stroking the infant's skin during medical therapy can provide tactile stimulation. The caregiver responds to the infant's cues by offering reassurance, providing nonnutritive sucking, stroking the infant's back, and talking to the infant. Infant massage is gaining evidence as a way to promote weight gain (Gardner, Goldson, & Hernández, 2016).

Mobiles and decals that can be changed frequently may be placed within the infant's visual range to stimulate the infant visually. Wind-up musical toys provide rhythmic distractions as long as they are not too loud. If the infant is receiving phototherapy, the protective eye patches are removed periodically (e.g., during feeding) to allow parent–infant or caregiver–infant interaction.

Kangaroo care. Kangaroo care and short periods of gentle massage can help reduce stress in preterm infants (Fig. 34.9). The parent is bare-chested or may wear a loose-fitting, open-front top that has a modified marsupial-like pocket carrier for the infant. The undressed (except for diaper) infant is placed in a vertical position on the parent's bare chest, which permits direct eye contact, skin-to-skin contact, and close proximity. Skin-to-skin contact can have a positive healing effect for the mother who had a high-risk pregnancy. Additional benefits include early contact with mechanically ventilated infants, maintenance of neonatal thermal stability and oxygen saturation, increased feeding vigor and enhanced breastfeeding, maintenance of organized state, decreased pain perception during painful heelsticks, and minimal untoward effects of being held (Conde-Agudelo & Díaz-Rossello, 2016; Lorenz, Dawson, Jones, et al., 2017).

Parental Adaptation to a Preterm Infant

Parents of premature infants often have difficulty in bonding and relating to their babies. The need to be empowered to recognize their competence and achieve competence is the basis of the Creating

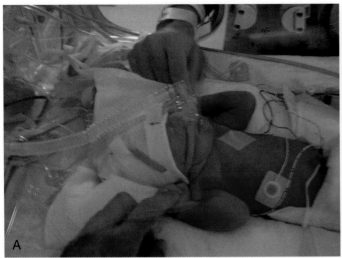
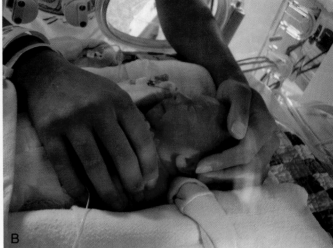

Fig. 34.10 Parent Interaction With Preterm Infant. (A) Mother and father touch preterm infant. (B) Mother caresses preterm infant. (Courtesy Randi and Jacob Wills, Clayton, NC.)

Opportunities for Parent Empowerment (COPE) program (www. copeforhope.com/nicu.php). This early educational-behavioral intervention model promotes more positive parent–infant interactions and enhanced ability to read and respond to infant cues (Gardner, Voos, & Hills, 2016; Kenner & Boykova, 2015).

Parental tasks. Parents of preterm infants must accomplish numerous psychologic tasks before effective relationships and parenting patterns can evolve. These tasks include the following:

- Experiencing anticipatory grief over the potential loss of an infant. The parent grieves in preparation for the infant's possible death, although the parent clings to the hope that the infant will survive. This process begins during labor (although it can begin during high-risk pregnancy) and lasts until the infant dies or shows evidence of surviving. Anticipatory grief occurs when families have knowledge of an impending loss, such as when a baby is admitted to a NICU with problems or when a diagnosis of an anencephalic fetus is made with ultrasonography. Being able to anticipate the loss gives families an opportunity to plan, feel more in control of their situation, and say goodbye in a special way. However, some individuals or family members distance or detach themselves from the experience or from their loved ones as a way of protecting themselves from the pain of loss and grief. How a parent responds to this situation depends on many factors including religious, spiritual, and cultural beliefs. These must be considered when planning care. The nurse's role is to advocate for the family so that other health care professionals realize that the family is grieving. Being fully present for these families and practicing active listening are important (see Chapter 37).
- The mother's acceptance of her failure to give birth to a healthy full-term infant. Grief and depression typify this phase, which persists until the infant is out of danger and is expected to survive.
- Resuming the process of relating to the infant. As the baby's condition begins to improve and the baby gains weight, is able to breast-feed or bottle feed, and is weaned from the incubator or radiant warmer, the parent can begin the process of developing an attachment to the infant that was interrupted by the infant's critical condition at birth.
- Learning about the ways in which this baby is unique in terms of his or her special needs and growth patterns, caregiving needs, and growth and development expectations
- Adjusting the home environment to accommodate the needs of the new infant. Parents are encouraged to limit the number of visitors

to minimize exposure of the infant to pathogens. The environmental temperature may have to be altered to optimize conditions for the infant.

Parental responses. Physical contact with the infant is important to establish early bonding and attachment. If it is not possible for parents to hold the infant, they can touch and stroke the baby as they speak softly (Fig. 34.10). As the infant's condition improves, parents can hold the neonate and provide kangaroo care (see Fig. 34.9). They gradually begin to participate in infant activities, such as feeding, bathing, and changing. Parents go through numerous phases of adjustment as they learn to parent their infant. Nurses facilitate the transition to parenthood through their teaching and support of parental efforts.

Parental support. The nurse as caregiver, support person, and educator is responsible for shaping the environment and responding with sensitivity to the needs of the parents and infant. Nurses are instrumental in helping parents learn who their infant is and to recognize behavioral cues in his or her development and to use these cues in the care they provide (Gardner, Goldson & Hernández, 2016).

When a high-risk birth is anticipated, the family can be given a tour of the NICU or shown a video to prepare them for the sights and activities of the unit. After an unexpected preterm birth, the parents can be given a booklet, view a video, or have someone describe what they will see when they go to the unit to see their infant.

As soon as possible, the parents should see and touch their infant so that they can begin to acknowledge the reality of the birth and the infant's true appearance and condition. The premature or sick baby's appearance can be stressful to the parents. They will need encouragement as they begin to accomplish the psychologic tasks imposed by the high-risk birth. For the following reasons, a nurse or health care provider should be present during the parents' first visit:

- To help them "see" the infant rather than focus on the equipment. The importance and purpose of the equipment that surrounds their infant should be explained to them.
- To explain the characteristics normal for an infant of their baby's gestational age; in this way parents do not compare their child with a term, healthy infant
- To encourage the parents to express their feelings about the pregnancy, labor, and birth, and the experience of having a high-risk infant
- To assess the parents' perceptions of the infant to determine the appropriate time for them to become actively involved in care

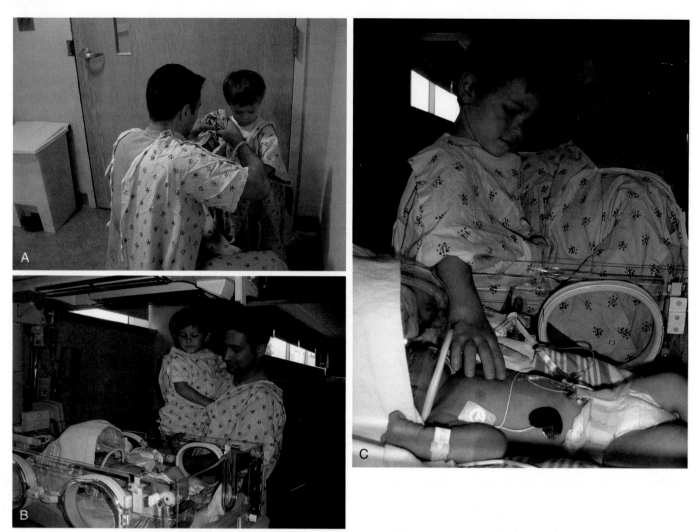

Fig. 34.11 Sibling Visits Newborn in the Neonatal Intensive Care Unit. (A) Father prepares older child for visit. (B) Sibling observes neonate at a safe distance. (C) He reaches out to touch the infant. (Courtesy Brian LiVecchi, Willow Spring, NC.)

When the parents cannot be present physically to visit with the infant, staff members devise appropriate methods to keep them informed and to help them feel connected to the newborn. Examples are daily phone calls, notes written as if by the infant, and photographs of the infant. Some NICUs have camera systems that allow parents to view their infant remotely.

The birth of a preterm or high-risk infant affects the entire family. Nurses need to consider responses and reactions of grandparents and siblings as they provide family-centered care for the infant and family. Grandparents may experience grief and sadness as they watch their own children experiencing the difficulties and challenges of having a preterm or high-risk infant. They worry about the well-being of their grandchild. Siblings also react to the birth of the preterm or high-risk infant. If they are old enough to realize that the mother was supposed to be bringing home a new baby, they can be very confused when the baby must remain in the hospital. When possible, it can be helpful to allow siblings to visit the new baby in the NICU environment so that they can see the infant (Fig. 34.11). Once the infant is brought home, some children are bewildered and angry at the seemingly disproportionate amount of parental time spent on the newborn. Nurses can facilitate visits by grandparents and siblings while the infant is hospitalized and can help parents anticipate possible reactions of siblings once the baby is discharged.

Some hospitals have support groups for the parents of infants in NICUs. These groups help parents experiencing anxiety and grief by encouraging them to share their feelings. Hospitals may arrange to have an experienced NICU parent make contact with a new group member to provide additional support. The volunteer parents provide support by making hospital visits, phone calls, and home visits. Mothers in particular are prone to posttraumatic stress that can hinder their ability to interact with or care for their infant (Borghini, Habersaat, Forcada-Guex, et al., 2014). They need help in expressing their feelings and, when appropriate, be referred for psychologic or family counseling.

Many NICUs use volunteers in varying capacities. After they have gone through the orientation program, volunteers can perform tasks such as holding the infants, stocking bedside cabinets, assembling parent packets, and, in some nurseries, feeding the infants.

Parental maladaptation. The incidence of physical and emotional abuse is increased in infants who, because of preterm birth or high-risk condition, are separated from their parents for a time after birth. Physical abuse includes varying degrees of poor nutrition, poor hygiene, and bodily harm. Emotional abuse ranges from subtle disinterest to outright dislike of the infant. Appropriate resources should be made available to assess the parents' feelings regarding the preterm infant's birth. In addition, proper guidance and counseling are made available, including post hospital discharge, to help families adjust to and care for the preterm infant. The ultimate goal is for the family to accept

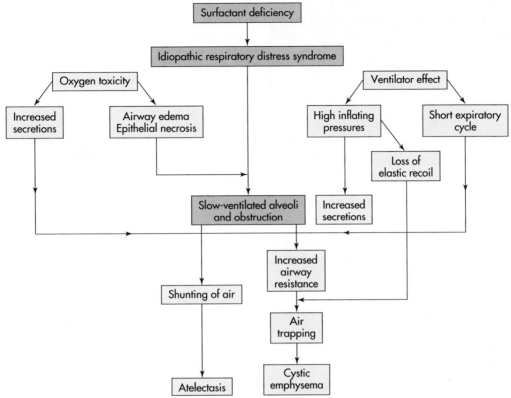

Fig. 34.12 Pathogenesis of Respiratory Distress Syndrome. (From Gardner, S. L., Enzman-Hines, M., & Nyp, M. [2016]. Respiratory diseases. In S. L. Gardner, B. S. Carter, M. Enzman-Hines, et al. [Eds.], *Merenstein & Gardner's handbook of neonatal intensive care* [8th ed.]. St. Louis: Elsevier.)

the infant and incorporate this new member into the existing family structure.

Parent education. The criteria indicating an infant's readiness for discharge are that the infant's physiologic condition is stable, the infant is consuming adequate nutrition, and the infant's body temperature is stable. The parents or other caregivers should demonstrate physical, emotional, and educational readiness to assume responsibility for the total care of the infant. Ideally, the home environment is adequate for meeting the needs of the infant. Resources for parents and health care professionals include http://premature-infant.com and www.neonatology.org.

Complications in High-Risk Infants

Respiratory Distress Syndrome

Respiratory distress syndrome (RDS) refers to a lung disorder usually affecting preterm infants. Maternal and fetal conditions associated with a decreased incidence and severity of RDS include African-American race, maternal gestational hypertension, illicit drug exposure, maternal steroid therapy (betamethasone), chronic retroplacental abruption, prolonged rupture of membranes, and intrauterine growth restriction (IUGR). The incidence and severity of RDS increase as gestational age decreases. Perinatal asphyxia, male sex, Caucasian race, maternal diabetes (types 1 and 2), second-born twin, familial predisposition, and cesarean birth without labor place an infant at increased risk for RDS. The incidence of RDS in infants weighing less than 1500 g (3.3 lb) is about 2% (Wambach & Hamvas, 2015).

RDS is caused by a lack of pulmonary surfactant, which leads to progressive atelectasis, loss of functional residual capacity, and ventilation-perfusion imbalance with an uneven distribution of ventilation. This surfactant deficiency can be caused by insufficient surfactant production, abnormal composition and function of surfactant, disruption of surfactant production, or a combination of these factors.

The weak respiratory muscles and an overly compliant chest wall, common among preterm infants, contribute to the sequence of events that occurs. Lung capacity is further compromised by the presence of fluid, proteinaceous material, and epithelial debris in the airways. The resulting decreased oxygenation, cyanosis, and metabolic or respiratory acidosis can cause the pulmonary vascular resistance (PVR) to be increased. This increased PVR can lead to right-to-left shunting and a reopening of the ductus arteriosus and foramen ovale (Fig. 34.12).

Clinical symptoms of RDS usually appear immediately after or within 6 hours of birth. Physical examination reveals crackles, poor air exchange, pallor, the use of accessory muscles (retractions), and, occasionally, apnea. Radiographic findings include a uniform reticulogranular appearance and air bronchograms (Gardner, Enzman-Hines, & Nyp, 2016; Jackson, 2018). The infant's clinical course is variable, usually with an increased oxygen requirement and increased respiratory effort, atelectasis, loss of functional residual capacity, and worsening of ventilation-perfusion imbalance.

RDS is a self-limiting disease that usually abates after 72 hours. This disappearance of respiratory signs coincides with the production of surfactant in the type 2 cells of the alveoli.

The treatment for RDS is supportive. Adequate ventilation and oxygenation must be established and maintained in an attempt to prevent ventilation-perfusion mismatch and atelectasis. Exogenous surfactant may be administered at birth or shortly after; this has the effect of shortening the typical course of RDS. Positive-pressure ventilation, nasal CPAP, and oxygen therapy may be necessary during the respiratory illness. The maintenance of an NTE reduces oxygen consumption (Hermansen & Mahajan, 2015).

The mortality and morbidity rates associated with RDS are attributed to the infant's immature organ systems and the complications associated with the treatment of the disease (Wambach &

TABLE 34.2 Normal Arterial Blood Gas Values for Neonates

Value	Range
pH	7.35-7.45
Arterial oxygen pressure (Pa_{O_2})	60-80 mm Hg
Carbon dioxide pressure (Pa_{CO_2})	35-45 mm Hg
Bicarbonate (HCO_3^-)	18-26 mEq/L
Base excess	−5 to +5
Oxygen saturation	92%-94%

From Barry, J. S., Deacon, J., Hernández, C., et al. (2016). Acid-base homeostasis and oxygenation. In S. L. Gardner, B. S. Carter, M. Enzman-Hines, et al. (Eds.), *Merenstein & Gardner's handbook of neonatal intensive care* (8th ed.). St. Louis: Mosby.

Hamvas, 2015). Preventing complications associated with mechanical ventilation is critical. These complications include PIE, pneumothorax, and chronic lung disease. Pulse oximetry documents trends in oxygenation. Arterial blood gases provide more detailed information on the infant's oxygenation status (Table 34.2).

The clinical and radiographic presentation (radiodense lung fields and air bronchograms) of neonatal pneumonia can be similar to that of RDS. Fluid in the minor fissure also can be noted in infants with neonatal pneumonia. Therefore sepsis evaluation, including blood culture and complete blood count (CBC) with differential, may be done in infants with RDS and risk factors to rule out neonatal pneumonia. Broad-spectrum antibiotics are begun until the results of cultures are available.

Fluid and nutrition must be maintained in the critically ill infant with RDS. TPN can be implemented to provide protein and fats to promote a positive nitrogen balance. Daily monitoring of the electrolyte values, urinary output, and weight help evaluate the infant's hydration status.

Frequent blood sampling can make blood transfusions necessary. The critically ill infant is usually maintained at a venous hematocrit level of more than 40% to maintain adequate oxygen-carrying capacity (Bagwell, 2014).

> **! NURSING ALERT**
>
> When transfusion is needed, the family may request directed donor blood. This donor blood usually is obtained from a family member or close friend of the family who has the same blood type as the infant or a compatible blood type. It may be necessary to notify the infant's family of the potential need for blood transfusion on admission to allow for the processing of directed-donor blood.

It is important to ask all parents to share any concerns and ask questions about blood transfusions. Reassuring the family about stringent testing of all blood products can help alleviate some of their anxiety about the transmission of blood-borne pathogens such as human immunodeficiency virus (HIV) and hepatitis B. Because some religions prohibit the use of blood transfusions, it is critical to obtain a complete history from the family, including their religious preference. Alternative strategies for maintaining the infant's hematocrit may be used in these instances.

Retinopathy of Prematurity

Retinopathy of prematurity (ROP) is a complex multifactorial disorder that affects the developing retinal vessels of preterm infants. The normal retinal vessels begin to form in utero at approximately 16 weeks in response to the release of growth factors. These vessels continue to develop until they reach maturity at approximately 42 to 43

weeks after conception. Once the retina is completely vascularized, the retinal vessels are not susceptible to ROP. The mechanism of injury in ROP is unclear. Oxygen tensions that are too high for the level of retinal maturity initially result in vasoconstriction. As the retinal tissue becomes hypoxic, neovascularization occurs in the retina and vitreous, with capillary hemorrhages, fibrotic resolution, and possible retinal detachment. Scar tissue formation and consequent visual impairment can be mild or severe. The entire disease process in severe cases can take as long as several months to evolve. The infant is examined by an ophthalmologist before discharge, and follow-up examinations are recommended as needed (Rubarth & Parker, 2014).

The key to the management of ROP is prevention of preterm birth and early detection. Blood oxygen levels in the preterm infant should be closely monitored and significant fluctuations avoided. Oxygen and ventilator settings should be adjusted to keep oxygen saturations within acceptable levels. Laser photocoagulation or intra-ocular injections of anti-bevacizumab, which inhibits vascular endothelial growth factor, are common treatments for ROP (Rubarth & Parker, 2014).

Bronchopulmonary Dysplasia

Bronchopulmonary dysplasia (BPD) is a chronic pulmonary condition occurring most commonly in preterm infants requiring mechanical ventilation. The etiology of BPD is multifactorial and includes pulmonary immaturity, surfactant deficiency, lung injury and stretch, barotrauma, inflammation caused by oxygen exposure, inadequate nutrition, fluid overload, ligation of a PDA, and a familial predisposition. With the advent of prenatal use of maternal steroids when preterm birth is expected, the risk of BPD or CLD has been reduced (Keller & Ballard, 2018).

Clinical signs of BPD include tachypnea, retractions, nasal flaring, increased work of breathing, and activity intolerance to handling and feeding. Infants with BPD can have an increase in ventilatory requirements or are unable to be weaned from the ventilator. The treatment for BPD includes oxygen therapy, nutrition, fluid restriction, and medications (diuretics, corticosteroids, and bronchodilators). However, the key to the management of BPD is prevention of prematurity and RDS. Other therapies that can aid in prevention of BPD include antenatal steroids, prophylactic surfactant, avoidance of mechanical ventilation when possible, use of CPAP, gentle ventilation in the birth setting, and administration of vitamin A (Gardner, Enzman-Hines, & Nyp, 2016).

The prognosis for infants with BPD depends on the degree of pulmonary dysfunction and on the infant's overall health status. Oxygen therapy may be continued in the home setting. There is usually progressive normalization of pulmonary function, although abnormalities of small airways can persist. Mortality after hospital discharge is usually due to complications such as respiratory infection (Gardner, Enzman-Hines & Nyp, 2016).

Patent Ductus Arteriosus

The ductus arteriosus is a normal muscular contractile structure in the fetus connecting the left pulmonary artery and the dorsal aorta, diverting blood to the placenta for gas exchange (see Fig. 12.13). The duct constricts after birth as oxygenation, the levels of circulating prostaglandins, and the muscle mass increase. Other factors that promote ductal closure include catecholamines, low pH, bradykinin, and acetylcholine. When the fetal ductus arteriosus fails to close after birth, patent ductus arteriosus (PDA) occurs. During the first few days of life when a preterm or sick infant is under stress, the ductus arteriosus can reopen, leading to mottling and cyanosis. The incidence of PDA in infants born at less than 1500 g is 30% (Sadowski, 2015).

Although a small PDA can be asymptomatic, the clinical presentation in an infant with a significant PDA includes systolic murmur, active precordium, bounding peripheral pulses, tachycardia, tachypnea, crackles, and hepatomegaly. Systemic hypotension and decreased urine output may be present. The systolic murmur is heard best at the second or third intercostal space at the upper left sternal border. An increased left ventricular stroke volume causes an active precordium.

Radiographic studies in infants with PDA typically show cardiac enlargement. Blood gases may indicate metabolic acidosis. Definitive diagnosis is through echocardiography, which can visualize a PDA and measure the amount of blood shunting across the PDA (Swanson & Erickson, 2016).

Medical management consists of respiratory support, fluid restriction, and the administration of indomethacin or ibuprofen (Clyman, 2018). Ibuprofen and indomethacin inhibit prostaglandin synthesis and cause the PDA to constrict. However, there is some concern that indomethacin reduces blood flow to the kidneys and inhibits platelet aggregation (Sadowski, 2015).

Respiratory support is adjusted based on assessment of the infant's respiratory status and blood gas values. Fluid restriction is implemented to decrease cardiovascular volume overload. Surgical ligation is done when a PDA is clinically significant and medical management is ineffective.

Nursing management of the infant with PDA focuses on supportive care. The infant needs an NTE, adequate oxygenation, meticulous fluid balance, and parental support.

Germinal Matrix Hemorrhage–Intraventricular Hemorrhage

Germinal matrix hemorrhage–intraventricular hemorrhage (GMH-IVH) is one of the most common types of brain injuries in neonates and is associated with some of the most severe long-term outcomes. It is the most common type of intracranial hemorrhage, occurring almost exclusively in preterm infants. The risk of GMH-IVH increases with decreasing gestational age. The incidence of GMH-IVH is estimated to be 5% to 11% and has shown a decline in recent years (de Vries, 2015). The decline is attributed to the prenatal use of corticosteroids and postnatal use of surfactant.

The germinal matrix is a loose network of cells abundantly supplied with tiny, fragile, thin-walled vessels. It lies beneath the lining of the lateral ventricles. This area is present and active until 34 to 35 weeks of gestation as a site for production of neurons and glial cells that gradually migrate to the cerebral cortex. The germinal matrix is especially vulnerable to alterations in cerebral blood flow related to BP changes. Hemorrhage occurs when the tiny blood vessels rupture; the hemorrhage can extend into the lateral ventricles, then to the third and fourth ventricles, the subarachnoid space, and even into the white matter of the brain. Large clots can develop and create outflow obstruction from the ventricles (de Vries, 2015).

Infants who experience GMH-IVH are usually less than 34 weeks of gestation with a history of hypoxia, birth asphyxia, RDS, or other events causing impaired venous return or increased venous pressure. In the majority of cases GMH-IVH is diagnosed within the first 2 weeks of life. Infants with GMH-IVH can be asymptomatic, develop symptoms gradually, or have an acute catastrophic presentation. Clinical signs suggestive of hemorrhage include decreasing hematocrit, full anterior fontanel, changes in activity level, and decreased muscle tone. With a catastrophic incident, the infant can develop stupor, coma, respiratory distress that progresses to apnea, decerebrate posturing, and seizures; there is a high mortality rate in these cases (Ditzenberger & Blackburn, 2014).

Morbidity and mortality related to GMH-IVH are based on the severity of the hemorrhage and the associated problems. Small hemorrhages are usually associated with good outcomes and high survival rates. Infants with more severe hemorrhages, posthemorrhagic

ventricular dilation, or periventricular leukomalacia have higher mortality rates and greater long-term morbidity. Neurodevelopmental outcomes of GMH-IVH include hydrocephalus, cerebral palsy, developmental delays, learning disorders, and sensory and attention problems (Ditzenberger & Blackburn, 2014).

Care management begins with prevention of preterm birth, birth trauma, and hypoxic-ischemic injury. Antenatal steroids help reduce the risk of GMH-IVH. Prompt and skilled resuscitation at birth minimizes hypoxia and ischemia. Nursing care focuses on recognition of factors that increase the risk of GMH-IVH, interventions to decrease the risk of bleeding, and supportive care to infants who have bleeding episodes. Ongoing assessment of vulnerable infants involves monitoring oxygenation and perfusion and avoiding or minimizing activities that increase cerebral blood flow. If GMH-IVH occurs, care is focused on maintaining oxygenation and perfusion, an NTE, and normoglycemia. The infant is positioned with the head in midline and the head of the bed elevated slightly to prevent or minimize fluctuations in intracranial BP. Rapid infusions of fluids should be avoided. BP is monitored closely for fluctuations. The use of developmental interventions such as swaddling or containment during painful procedures can help promote greater physiologic stability (Ditzenberger & Blackburn, 2014).

Nursing support for parents includes assessment of their understanding and concerns related to the infant's condition. They need opportunities to discuss their feelings and ask questions about the infant's condition and care as well as the long-term prognosis. Nurses can demonstrate to parents how they can interact with the infant in a developmentally appropriate manner. Nurses can provide anticipatory guidance regarding ways the infant's needs and care will change as he or she matures. For many of these infants an interprofessional approach to care is needed to address the neurodevelopmental sequelae of GMH-IVH and to plan for care after hospital discharge (Ditzenberger & Blackburn, 2014).

Necrotizing Enterocolitis

Necrotizing enterocolitis (NEC) is an acute inflammatory disease of the GI mucosa, commonly complicated by bowel necrosis and perforation. NEC occurs in up to 10% of all LBW infants. More than 90% of cases are preterm infants. Reported mortality rates due to NEC are as high as 40% (Caplan, 2015).

The exact etiology and pathophysiology of NEC are unclear, although many factors seem to contribute to its development (risk factors are listed in Box 34.6). Three primary conditions appear to be involved in the etiology of NEC. The first is intestinal ischemia that occurs as a result of asphyxia/hypoxia or events that cause a redistribution of blood flow away from the GI tract (e.g., hypotension, hypovolemia, severe stress). A second condition involved in the development of NEC seems to be bacterial colonization of the initially sterile GI tract with harmful organisms prior to the establishment of normal intestinal flora. *Klebsiella, Escherichia coli,* and *Clostridium* are common organisms involved in NEC. A third condition associated with the development of NEC is enteral feeding. The majority of infants with NEC had received some type of enteral feeding. It is thought that the feedings can provide a substrate for bacterial proliferation or that feedings can increase intestinal oxygen demand during absorption, resulting in tissue hypoxia. Breast milk seems to have a protective effect against the development of NEC—it is rare among infants who are exclusively fed breast milk. The use of probiotics such as *Bifidobacterium infantis* and *Streptococcus thermophilus* assist in the establishment of normal bowel flora and appear to decrease the incidence of NEC (AlFaleh & Anabrees, 2014). In addition, MEN can help reduce the risk of NEC.

BOX 34.6 Risk Factors for Necrotizing Enterocolitis

- Asphyxia
- Respiratory distress syndrome
- Umbilical artery catheter
- Exchange transfusion
- Early enteral feedings/hyperosmolar feedings
- Patent ductus arteriosus
- Congenital heart disease
- Myelomeningocele
- Intrauterine growth restriction
- Polycythemia
- Anemia
- Shock
- Gastrointestinal infection

Data from Caplan, M. S. (2015). Neonatal necrotizing enterocolitis. In R. J. Martin, A. A. Fanaroff, & M. C. Walsh (Eds.), *Fanaroff & Martin's neonatal-perinatal medicine: Diseases of the fetus and infant* (10th ed.). St. Louis: Saunders; and Bucher, B., Pacetti, A., Lovvorn, H., et al. (2016). Neonatal surgery. In S. L. Gardner, B. S. Carter, M. Enzman-Hines, et al. (Eds.), *Merenstein & Gardner's handbook of neonatal intensive care* (8th ed.). St. Louis: Mosby.

The onset of NEC in the term infant usually occurs between 1 and 3 days after birth, but can occur as late as 1 month. In the preterm infant NEC usually occurs within the first 7 days but can be delayed for up to 30 days. The signs of NEC are nonspecific, which is characteristic of many neonatal diseases. Some generalized signs include decreased activity, hypotonia, pallor, recurrent apnea and bradycardia, decreased oxygen saturation, respiratory distress, metabolic acidosis, oliguria, hypotension, decreased perfusion, temperature instability, and cyanosis. GI symptoms include abdominal distention, increasing or bile-stained residual gastric aspirates, grossly bloody stools, abdominal tenderness, and erythema of the abdominal wall (Bucher, Pacetti, Lovvorn, et al., 2016; Caplan, 2015).

A diagnosis is confirmed by a radiographic examination that reveals bowel loop distention, pneumatosis intestinalis (air in the wall of the bowel), pneumoperitoneum, portal air, or a combination of these findings. The abnormal radiographic findings are caused by the bacterial colonization of the GI tract associated with NEC, resulting in ileus. Pneumatosis intestinalis, pneumoperitoneum, and portal air are caused by gas produced by the bacteria that invade the wall of the intestines and escape into the peritoneum and portal system when perforation occurs. The laboratory evaluation in such infants consists of a CBC with differential, coagulation studies, blood gas analysis, measurement of serum electrolyte levels, C-reactive protein, and blood culture. The white blood cell count can be either increased or decreased. The platelet count and coagulation study findings can be abnormal, showing thrombocytopenia and disseminated intravascular coagulation (DIC). Electrolyte levels can be abnormal related to leaking capillary beds and fluid shifts with the infection (Bucher et al., 2016; Caplan, 2015). In some NICUs, bedside ultrasound is used to evaluate blood flow to the intestines and to identify inflammation associated with NEC.

Management strategies are based on the degree of bowel involvement and the severity of the disease. The goal of treatment is to prevent progression of the NEC, intestinal perforation, and shock.

For the infant with suspected or confirmed NEC, oral or tube feedings are discontinued to rest the GI tract. An orogastric tube is placed and attached to low suction to provide gastric decompression. TPN is begun.

Antibiotic therapy is instituted, and surgical resection is performed if perforation or clinical deterioration occurs. Therapy is usually prolonged, and recovery can be delayed by the formation of adhesions, the development of the complications associated with bowel resection, the occurrence of short-bowel syndrome (especially if the ileocecal valve is removed), or the development of intolerance to oral feedings (Bucher et al., 2016; Caplan, 2015).

Families need education and support when faced with the crisis of having an infant with NEC. As part of the interprofessional health care team, nurses can help parents understand the severity of the disease, treatment options, and care needed by the infant. When the disease is severe and the prognosis is poor, nurses are instrumental in supporting families with decision making and anticipatory grieving (Gardner & Carter, 2016; Gardner, Voos, & Hills, 2016).

Infant Pain Responses

The physiology of pain and pain assessment in the newborn are discussed in Chapter 24. This discussion focuses on pain assessment and management in the preterm infant.

Pain Assessment

Assessment of pain in the neonate is difficult because evaluation must be based on physiologic changes and behavioral observations. The Joint Commission (TJC, 2017) requires the assessment of pain using a valid and reliable tool. A scale that examines multiple dimensions facilitates accurate assessment of neonatal pain (Gardner, Enzman-Hines, & Agarwal, 2016). Although behaviors such as vocalizations, facial expressions, body movements, and general state are common to all infants, they vary with different situations. Crying associated with pain is more intense and sustained. Facial expression is the most consistent and specific characteristic; scales are available for systematic evaluation of facial features, such as eye squeeze or brow bulge (Gardner, Enzman-Hines, & Agarwal, 2016) (see Fig. 24.19). Most infants respond with increased body movements but can be experiencing pain even when lying quietly with eyes closed. The preterm infant's response to pain can be behaviorally blunted or absent. An infant who receives a muscle-paralyzing agent such as vecuronium is incapable of mounting a behavioral or visible pain response (Box 34.7) yet still feels pain.

! NURSING ALERT

When in doubt about the presence of pain in infants, the nurse should base the need for interventions on the following rule: whatever is painful to an adult or child is painful to an infant unless proved otherwise. The nurse should anticipate pain and intervene promptly, without waiting for physiologic or behavioral signs of pain to appear.

Several tools have been developed for the assessment of pain in the neonate. A commonly used tool is CRIES that assesses crying, oxygenation, vital signs, facial expression, and sleeplessness (Krechel & Bildner, 1995). Other instruments are the Pain Assessment Tool (PAT) (Hodgkinson, Bear, Thorn, & Van Blaricum, 1994); Scale for Use in Newborns (SUN) (Blauer & Gerstmann, 1998); Behavioral Pain Score (BPS) (Pokela, 1994); Distress Scale for Ventilated Newborn Infants (DSVNI) (Sparshott, 1995); Neonatal Infant Pain Scale (NIPS) (Lawrence, Alcock, McGrath, et al., 1993); and Premature Infant Pain Profile (PIPP) (Stevens, Johnston, Petryshen, & Taddio, 1996). The PIPP is one of the most widely used scales for preterm infants because it considers behavioral, physiologic, and contextual indicators (Gardner, Enzman-Hines, & Agarwal, 2016).

Memory of Pain

Preterm infants are subjected to a variety of repeated noxious stimuli including multiple heelsticks, venipuncture, endotracheal intubation

BOX 34.7 Manifestations of Acute Pain in the Neonate

Physiologic Responses

Vital Signs
- Increased heart rate
- Increased blood pressure
- Rapid, shallow respirations

Oxygenation
- Decreased transcutaneous O_2 saturation (TcPo$_2$)
- Decreased arterial O_2 saturation (Sao$_2$)
- Integumentary Changes
  - Pallor or flushing
  - Diaphoresis
  - Palmar sweating

Other Observations
- Increased muscle tone
- Dilated pupils
- Decreased vagal nerve tone
- Increased intracranial pressure
- Laboratory evidence of metabolic or endocrine changes
  - Hyperglycemia
  - Lowered pH
  - Elevated corticosteroids

Behavioral Responses

Vocalizations
- Crying
- Whimpering
- Groaning

Facial Expression
- Grimacing
- Brow furrowed
- Chin quivering
- Eyes tightly closed
- Mouth open and squarish

Body Movements and Posture
- Limb withdrawal
- Thrashing
- Rigidity
- Flaccidity
- Fist clenching

Change in State
- Changes in sleep-wake cycles
- Changes in feeding behavior
- Changes in activity level
- Fussiness, irritability
- Listlessness

Adapted from Blackburn, S. (2018). *Maternal, fetal, and neonatal physiology: A clinical perspective* (5th ed.). St. Louis: Elsevier; and Gardner, S. L., Enzman-Hines, M., & Agarwal, A. (2016). Pain and pain relief. In S. L. Gardner, B. S. Carter, M. Enzman-Hines, et al. (Eds.), *Merenstein & Gardner's handbook of neonatal intensive care* (8th ed.). St. Louis: Elsevier.

and suctioning, arterial sticks, chest tube placement, and lumbar puncture. The effects of pain caused by such procedures are not fully known, but researchers have begun to investigate potential consequences. From preliminary reports, it appears that a rewiring of the pain responses occurs in preterm infants who have been subjected to multiple painful treatments early in their lives. The nervous system networks of the preterm infant appear denser and have more branches than those in the average infant, leading to the conclusion that the pain threshold and sensitivity in once preterm infants is heightened for life. There are also changes when the infant has undergone anesthesia (Gardner, Enzman-Hines, & Agarwal, 2016).

Consequences of Untreated Pain in Infants

Despite research on the neonate's experience of pain, infant pain remains inadequately managed. This mismanagement is partially due to misconceptions regarding the effects of pain on the neonate, as well as a lack of knowledge of immediate and long-term consequences of untreated pain and the side effects associated with medications used to treat neonatal pain. Infants respond to noxious stimuli through physiologic indicators (increased heart rate and BP, variability in heart rate and ICP, and decreases in arterial oxygen saturations and skin blood flow) and behavioral indicators (muscle rigidity, facial expression, crying, withdrawal, and sleeplessness). The neurophysiologic responses to noxious stimulation are responsible for short- and long-term consequences of pain.

Pain Management

In 2001, the International Evidence-Based Group for Neonatal Pain developed a Consensus Statement for the Prevention and Management of Pain in the Newborn that stated that pain must be anticipated and prevented to avoid long-term consequences (Anand & International Evidence-Based Group for Neonatal Pain, 2001). This sentinel document continues to form the basis for work done to reduce the neonate's exposure to pain. In 2016, the AAP issued a follow-up document addressing procedural pain in the neonate (AAP, 2016).

Nonpharmacologic measures to alleviate pain include repositioning, swaddling, containment, cuddling, rocking, playing music, reducing environmental stimulation, providing tactile comfort measures and nonnutritive sucking, and using oral sucrose. However, nonpharmacologic measures may not be sufficient to decrease physiologic distress, even if behavioral responses such as crying are lessened. In preterm infants additional stimulation such as stroking or environmental light or noise can increase physiologic distress. The effect of the NICU environment must be considered along with other forms of stimuli that can produce stress and pain.

Morphine is the most widely used opioid analgesic for pharmacologic management of neonatal pain, with fentanyl as an effective alternative. Continuous or bolus epidural or IV infusion of opioids provides effective pain control. Other methods are epidural/intrathecal infusion, local and regional nerve blocks, and topical anesthetics, as well as general anesthesia for surgery (Walden, 2014).

Parents are universally concerned that their infants are feeling pain during procedures. Nurses need to address these concerns and encourage the parents to speak with the health care providers involved. Parents have the right to withhold consent for invasive procedures and are entitled to honest answers from those responsible for the infant's care. When appropriate, they also can help provide comfort measures for the infant. Kangaroo care and breastfeeding are parental interventions that comfort and calm the infant (Gardner, Goldson & Hernández, 2016). Oral sucrose has been studied for the relief of short-term procedural pain and is widely used for that purpose. The research supporting the use of oral sucrose suggests the need for more study in this area (Gao, Gao, Xu, et al., 2016).

Parents want to know that nurses recognize pain in their infants and that the infants will be comfortable when they (the parents) are not present. They want to know that the nurse will advocate for comfort care for their baby. Although pain is considered a fifth vital sign, it cannot be assessed only at the time of vital signs. There must be ongoing

TABLE 34.3   Late Preterm Infant Assessment and Interventions

Risk Factors	Assessment	Interventions[a]
Respiratory distress (RD)	Assess for cardinal signs of RD (nasal flaring, grunting, tachypnea, central cyanosis, retractions), for presence of apnea especially during feedings, and for hypothermia and hypoglycemia.	Perform gestational age assessment; observe for signs of RD; monitor oxygenation by pulse oximetry; provide supplemental oxygen judiciously.
Thermal instability	Monitor axillary temperature every 30 min immediately after birth until stable, thereafter every 1-4 h, depending on gestational age and ability to maintain thermal stability.	Provide skin-to-skin care immediately after birth for stable infant; implement measures to prevent excess heat loss (adjust environmental temperature, avoid drafts); bathe only after thermal stability has been maintained for 1 hr.
Hypoglycemia	Monitor for signs and symptoms of hypoglycemia; assess feeding ability (latch, nipple feeding); assess thermal stability, signs and symptoms of RD; monitor bedside glucose in infants with additional risk factors (mother with diabetes, prolonged labor, RD, poor feeding).	Initiate early feedings of human milk or formula; avoid dextrose water or water feedings; provide intravenous dextrose as necessary for hypoglycemia.
Jaundice	Observe for jaundice in first 24 hrs; evaluate maternal-fetal history for additional risk factors that may cause increased hemolysis and circulating levels of unconjugated bilirubin (Rh, ABO, spherocytosis, bruising); assess feeding method, voiding, stooling patterns.	Monitor transcutaneous bilirubin, and note risk zone on hour-specific nomogram.
Feeding problems	Assess suck-swallow and breathing; assess for respiratory distress, hypoglycemia, thermal stability; assess latch-on, maternal comfort with feeding method; weight loss no more than 10% of birth weight.	Initiate early feedings—human milk or formula; ensure maternal knowledge of feeding method and signs of inadequate feeding (sleepiness, lethargy, color changes during feeding, apnea during feeding, decreased or absent urinary output).

[a]This list is not exhaustive of nursing interventions; additional interventions include those discussed under the care of the high-risk infant in this chapter.

Portions adapted from Pappas, B. E., & Robey, D. L. (2015). Care of the late preterm infant. In M. T. Verklan & M. Walden (Eds.), *Core curriculum for neonatal intensive care nursing* (5th ed.). St. Louis: Elsevier; Association of Women's Health, Obstetric and Neonatal Nurses. (2017). *Assessment and care of the late preterm infant* (2nd ed.). Washington, DC: Author.

evaluation of the infant's pain level and the effectiveness of comfort measures used. This assessment is not lengthy but can be as simple as walking to the bedside and closely observing the infant's color, posture, movements, and breathing. Pain is a real phenomenon that is preventable in many instances. Pain management is a standard of care, and it is considered unethical not to prevent and effectively treat pain. Another growing area of neonatal nursing is end-of-life and palliative care. Most of this care centers on pain management. Palliative care is really comfort care that supports the needs of the preterm, sick neonate (Walden, 2014).

LATE PRETERM INFANTS

LPIs are those born between 34 {0/7} and 36 {6/7} weeks of gestation (Gardner & Hernández, 2016b). Because birth weights of LPIs often range from 2000 g (4.4 lb) to 2500 g (5.5 lb) and they appear relatively mature in comparison to the smaller, less mature infant, they are often cared for as if they are normal term infants. Risk factors for LPIs can easily be overlooked. Compared with term infants, LPIs are at increased risk for problems with thermoregulation, hypoglycemia, hyperbilirubinemia, feeding problems, sepsis, and respiratory function (Association of Women's Health, Obstetric and Neonatal Nurses [AWHONN], 2017; Mohan & Jain, 2018). Many of these healthy-appearing infants are admitted directly to postpartum units with their mothers or stay in the NICU only briefly (i.e., less than 24 hours). They are commonly discharged home at 2 to 3 days of age with their mothers. Discharge before 48 hours after birth is not recommended (Mohan & Jain, 2018).

Recognition of LPIs is essential to providing effective care. Initial physical assessment and assessment of gestational age are crucial to identifying these infants. Although the mother's estimated date of birth (EDB) can indicate a longer gestation, infant appearance, behaviors,

and/or weight can indicate otherwise. The obstetric estimate of gestational age is usually reliable if it is based on a first-trimester ultrasound. However, if there is a discrepancy between the gestational age based on the obstetric estimate and newborn examination, it is better to rely on the estimate based on the newborn examination. AWHONN (2017) published evidence-based clinical practice guidelines, the *Assessment and Care of the Late Preterm Infant*, for the education of perinatal nurses regarding the late preterm infant's risk factors and appropriate care and follow-up (Table 34.3).

Nursing care for LPIs and their parents is discussed in the following paragraphs. Frequent assessment is essential for detecting problems early so that appropriate interventions can be initiated.

Respiratory Distress

LPIs are at increased risk for respiratory problems, including apnea. Close monitoring of respiratory status is essential and any changes are reported promptly to the primary health care provider. Infants may go home on an apnea monitor. If possible, parents should attend an infant cardiopulmonary resuscitation (CPR) class or view a video about infant CPR. To help prevent respiratory infections, the nurse should instruct the parents to limit the infant's contact with others outside the home. The nurse should review signs and symptoms of respiratory problems with the parents.

Thermoregulation

LPIs have more difficulty with thermoregulation than term infants, and cold stress is a greater concern. They have less body fat than term infants, a higher ratio of surface area to body weight, decreased glycogen stores, and less mature mechanisms for increasing metabolism for heat. Stores of brown fat are smaller and quickly depleted. Cold stress can quickly lead to hypoglycemia. Nurses must closely monitor body temperature and teach parents to measure the infant's temperature.

Parents are encouraged to keep a record of this at home and to report high or low temperatures. Hypothermia can be an early sign of neonatal sepsis (Mohan & Jain, 2018).

Nutrition

LPIs are at greater risk of having breastfeeding difficulties and may have breastfeeding-associated rehospitalizations (Cartwright, Atz, Newman, et al., 2017). Feedings should occur at least every 2½ to 3 hours and according to infant feeding cues. They can have difficulty coordinating sucking, swallowing, and breathing. Breastfeeding can be more problematic if the infant is sleepy and difficult to arouse for feedings. LPIs are prone to early fatigue during feedings and often fall asleep before consuming adequate volumes of milk. Nurses should observe at least one breastfeeding session every 8 hours. Early and extended skin-to-skin contact promotes breastfeeding. If supplementation is needed, expressed breast milk is the best option. To maximize the milk supply and milk transfer to the infant, mothers should use the electric breast pump after feedings while in the hospital and continue this process at home until the infant is able to successfully remove milk from the breasts and until the milk supply is well established. The mother-baby nurse or lactation consultant can provide instruction and assist breastfeeding mothers with using a breast pump. Mothers also need information regarding safe milk handling and storage guidelines (Canadian Agency for Drugs in Technologies and Health, 2016). The Academy of Breastfeeding Medicine has developed an evidence-based protocol for breastfeeding the LPI (Boies & Vaucher, 2016).

Hypoglycemia

LPIs are more likely to develop hypoglycemia than are term infants (Mohan & Jain, 2018). Hospital protocols may require routine monitoring of blood glucose until levels are stabilized and the infant is feeding adequately. Although the cut-off value for treatment remains uncertain, blood glucose values of less than 40 or 45 mg/dL, or symptoms of hypoglycemia, should be treated (Blackburn, 2018).

Hyperbilirubinemia

Hyperbilirubinemia is more common in LPIs because of immaturity of the liver, decreased gastric motility, and increased breakdown of RBCs (Pappas & Robey, 2015). They are less able to conjugate and excrete bilirubin. Serum bilirubin levels tend to peak at 5 to 7 days and persist longer than in term infants. Hyperbilirubinemia is the most frequent reason for hospital readmission during the first week of life. Bilirubin levels are closely monitored before discharge, and parents are instructed regarding signs of jaundice and when to notify the health care provider. Follow-up visits soon after hospital discharge are important for monitoring rising bilirubin levels (Mohan & Jain, 2018).

Infection

The immune systems of LPIs are immature; thus they are more likely to experience infections. Nurses should assess the LPI for signs and symptoms of infection, including temperature instability, lethargy, irritability, poor feeding, or vomiting. Before discharge, nurses educate the parents about the common signs and symptoms of infection and when to notify the health care provider.

POSTMATURE INFANTS

A pregnancy that is prolonged beyond 42 {0/7} weeks is a *postterm* pregnancy, and the infant who is born is called postterm or *postmature*. Postmaturity can be associated with placental insufficiency, resulting in a fetus that has a wasted appearance (dysmaturity) at birth because of loss of subcutaneous fat and muscle mass. However, not all postterm infants show signs of dysmaturity; some continue to grow in utero and

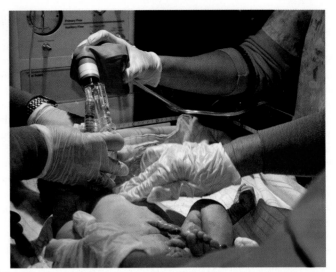

Fig. 34.13 Infant Being Resuscitated at Birth. Meconium was present on the abdomen and umbilical cord. Infant was not breathing, and heart rate was 65 beats/min at birth. Respirations and heart rate were normal at 2 minutes. (Courtesy Shannon Perry, Phoenix, AZ.)

are large at birth. Most postmature infants are oversized but otherwise normal, with advanced development and bone age. A postmature infant has some, but not necessarily all, of the following physical characteristics (Blickstein & Rimon, 2015):

- Dry, cracked (desquamating), parchment-like skin at birth
- Firm nails extending beyond the fingertips
- Depleted subcutaneous fat layers, leaving the skin loose and giving the infant an "old person" appearance
- Long and thin body
- Absent vernix
- Can have meconium staining (golden yellow to green) of skin, nails, and cord

The perinatal mortality rate is significantly higher in the postmature fetus and neonate. One reason for this is that during labor and birth the increased oxygen demands of the postmature fetus are not fully met. Insufficient gas exchange in the postmature placenta also increases the likelihood of intrauterine hypoxia, which can result in the passage of meconium in utero, thereby increasing the risk for meconium aspiration syndrome (MAS).

Parents may be concerned about the appearance of the postmature infant. Nurses can help them understand reasons for the dry, peeling, skin and other characteristics of postmaturity. Initial bathing should be done with a mild soap. It can be helpful to moisturize the skin with a petrolatum-based ointment. Nurses need to be alert to common problems associated with postmaturity, such as meconium aspiration, fetal distress, macrosomia, and birth injury (Blickstein & Rimon, 2015; Lund & Kuller 2014).

Meconium Aspiration Syndrome

Meconium staining of the amniotic fluid can be indicative of fetal distress, especially in a vertex presentation. It appears in 8% to 19% of all births. Many infants with meconium staining exhibit no signs of depression at birth; approximately 8% of newborns who are exposed to meconium develop **meconium aspiration syndrome (MAS)** (Gardner, Enzman-Hines & Nyp, 2016).

The presence of meconium in the amniotic fluid necessitates careful supervision of labor and close monitoring of fetal well-being. The presence of a team skilled in neonatal resuscitation is required at the birth of any infant with meconium-stained amniotic fluid (Fig. 34.13). The mouth and nares of the infant are not routinely suctioned on the perineum before the infant's first breath. Intubation for removal of meconium from the trachea is no longer routine practice. Intubation is reserved for those infants who do not respond to the initial steps of the Neonatal Resuscitation Program (NRP) (AHA & AAP, 2016; Gardner, Enzman-Hines & Nyp, 2016). See Chapter 32 for more information on immediate resuscitation of infants born with meconium-stained amniotic fluid.

Meconium can be aspirated into the airways either as the result of gasping respirations in utero or with the initial breaths following birth. This can lead to mechanical obstruction of the airways and MAS. Meconium aspiration can cause a chemical pneumonitis resulting in tachypnea and deactivation of surfactant. These infants can develop persistent pulmonary hypertension of the newborn, further complicating their management. Infants with MAS who receive surfactant experience improved oxygenation, decreased severity of respiratory failure, and reduced need for ECMO (Polin et al., 2014). Researchers are examining the use of surfactant lavage in treating meconium aspiration (Gardner, Enzman-Hines & Nyp, 2016).

Persistent Pulmonary Hypertension of the Newborn

The term persistent pulmonary hypertension of the newborn (PPHN) is applied to the combined findings of pulmonary hypertension, right-to-left shunting, and a structurally normal heart. PPHN can occur either as a primary problem or secondary to MAS, congenital diaphragmatic hernia, RDS, hyperviscosity syndrome, or neonatal pneumonia or sepsis. PPHN was formerly called persistent fetal circulation because the syndrome includes a reversion to fetal pathways for blood flow (Soltau & Carlo, 2014).

A brief review of the fetal blood flow can help in understanding the problems with PPHN. In utero, oxygen-rich blood leaves the placenta via the umbilical vein, goes through the ductus venosus, and enters the inferior vena cava. From there it empties into the right atrium where it is preferentially shunted across the foramen ovale to the left atrium, effectively bypassing the lungs. This blood enters the left ventricle, leaves via the aorta, and perfuses the carotid and coronary arteries. Thus the heart and brain receive the most oxygenated blood. Blood drains from the brain into the superior vena cava, reenters the right atrium, proceeds to the right ventricle, and exits via the main pulmonary artery. The fetus is relatively hypoxic in utero and, with the placenta supplying the oxygen, the fetal lungs need only enough perfusion for growth and nutrition. The ductus arteriosus (connecting the main pulmonary artery and the aorta) is the path of least resistance for the blood leaving the right side of the fetal heart, shunting most of the cardiac output away from the lungs and toward the systemic system. This right-to-left shunting is the key to fetal circulation (see Fig. 12.13).

After birth, both the foramen ovale and the ductus arteriosus close in response to various biochemical processes, pressure changes within the heart, and dilation of the pulmonary vessels. As air enters the lungs the fetal Po_2 rises and in response to increased oxygen levels, PVR drops. These changes allow virtually all of the cardiac output to enter and oxygenate the lungs and provide oxygen-rich blood to the tissues for normal metabolism.

The infant with PPHN is typically born at term or postterm and has tachycardia and cyanosis. Management depends on the underlying cause of the persistent pulmonary hypertension. The use of ECMO has improved the chances of survival in these infants (see earlier discussion); however, it is considered a very invasive procedure. In infants with PPHN, INO is used as a vasodilator to decrease the pulmonary hypertension while increasing oxygenation (Steinhorn & Abman, 2018). This therapy is proving to work well alone or with HFV. Another pharmacologic treatment is exogenous surfactant because some of these infants appear to be surfactant deficient. Use of environmental strategies such as decreasing adverse stimuli (excessive light and noise)

to reduce stress is an area of ongoing research. This intervention is used in conjunction with other therapies.

Another mode of treatment for PPHN and other respiratory disorders of the newborn is HFV, a group of assisted ventilation methods that deliver small volumes of gas at high frequencies and limit the development of high airway pressure, thus reducing barotrauma. HFV decreases carbon dioxide while increasing oxygenation. It can be effectively used in conjunction with INO (Soltau & Carlo, 2014).

It is important to understand that PPHN is considered a cardiovascular and a respiratory problem. The lungs of these infants are healthy, but the hypertension of the cardiovascular system leads to their oxygenation problems.

GROWTH-RESTRICTED INFANTS

Infants who are small for gestational age (SGA) (weight is less than the 10th percentile expected at term) and infants who have IUGR (rate of growth does not meet expected growth pattern) are considered high risk. The terms SGA and IUGR are sometimes used interchangeably but have different meanings. SGA infants are healthy but growing at a slower rate than expected and are less than the 10th percentile at birth. SGA may be related to factors such as small parental size or genetic predisposition. IUGR refers to a fetus who did not reach its growth potential usually because of environmental or genetic factors. Various conditions can affect and impede growth in the developing fetus. Conditions occurring in the first trimester that affect all aspects of fetal growth (e.g., infections, teratogens, chromosomal abnormalities) or extrinsic conditions early in pregnancy result in symmetric growth restriction (i.e., head circumference, length, and weight, are all less than the 10th percentile). Growth restriction in later stages of pregnancy, as a result of maternal or placental factors, results in asymmetric growth restriction (with respect to gestational age, weight will be less than the 10th percentile, whereas length and head circumference will be greater than the 10th percentile). Infants with asymmetric IUGR have the potential for normal growth and development. There is relative sparing of head and brain growth while weight and somatic organ growth are more seriously altered (Carlo, 2016).

Several physical findings are characteristic of the growth-restricted neonate (Gowen, 2015):

- Reduced subcutaneous fat stores
- Loose and dry skin
- Diminished muscle mass, especially over buttocks and cheeks
- Sunken abdomen (scaphoid) as opposed to the well-rounded abdomen seen in normal infants
- Thin, yellowish, dry umbilical cord (normal cord is gray, glistening, round, and moist)
- Wide skull sutures (inadequate bone growth)

Care of the growth-restricted infant is based on the presence of clinical problems and is the same for preterm infants with similar problems. Gas exchange is supported by maintaining a clear airway and preventing cold stress. Hypoglycemia is treated with oral feedings (e.g., breast, formula) or IV dextrose as the infant's condition warrants. An external heat source (radiant warmer or incubator) is used until the infant is able to maintain an adequate body temperature. Nursing support of parents is the same as that given to parents of preterm infants.

Common problems that affect growth-restricted infants are perinatal asphyxia, meconium aspiration, hypoglycemia, polycythemia, and temperature instability.

Perinatal Asphyxia

Commonly IUGR infants have been exposed to chronic hypoxia for varying periods before labor and birth. Labor is a stressor to the normal fetus, but it is an even greater stressor for the growth-restricted fetus. The chronically hypoxic infant is severely compromised even by a normal labor and has difficulty compensating after birth. Appropriate management and resuscitation are essential for these depressed infants.

The birth of growth-restricted infants with perinatal asphyxia can be associated with a maternal history of heavy cigarette smoking; preeclampsia; low socioeconomic status; multifetal gestation; gestational infections such as rubella, cytomegalovirus, and toxoplasmosis; advanced diabetes mellitus; and cardiac problems. The nursing staff must be alert to and prepared for possible perinatal asphyxia during the birth of an infant to a woman with such a history. Sequelae to perinatal asphyxia include MAS (see previous discussion), hypoxic-ischemia encephalopathy, and hypoglycemia.

Hypoglycemia

All high-risk infants have an increased likelihood of developing hypoglycemia (plasma glucose < 40 mg/dL) (Armentrout, 2015). Infants who experience physiologic stress can experience hypoglycemia as a result of a decreased glycogen supply, inadequate gluconeogenesis, or overuse of glycogen stored during fetal and postnatal life. Preterm infants can also become hypoglycemic because of inadequate intake and increased metabolic demands as a result of illness. There is insufficient evidence to support the concept that the preterm or high-risk infant can tolerate lower levels of serum glucose any better than healthy term infants (Blackburn, 2018) (see Chapter 24 for discussion of hypoglycemia). The IUGR infant, like the preterm infant, is at increased risk for hypoglycemia as a result of decreased fetal stores and decreased rate of gluconeogenesis (Rozance, McGowan, Price-Douglas, et al., 2016).

Symptoms of hypoglycemia include poor feeding, hypothermia, and diaphoresis. CNS symptoms can include tremors and jitteriness, weak cry, lethargy, floppy posture, and, with profound hypoglycemia, seizures or coma. Diagnosis is confirmed by point-of-care testing with products such as Accuchek or One-Touch or by laboratory confirmation. Blood glucose screening should be done on all high-risk infants soon after birth and frequently during the first few hours until glucose levels stabilize.

Polycythemia

Polycythemia or hyperviscosity of the blood is another common problem of the growth-restricted infant. With polycythemia there is an excess in circulating RBC mass. This condition is a result of fetal hypoxia and intrauterine stress that stimulates the fetus to produce more RBCs in an attempt to provide oxygen to body organs. Polycythemia is associated with maternal preeclampsia, maternal smoking, maternal diabetes, and delayed cord clamping (Diehl-Jones & Fraser, 2014). With hematocrit greater than 65% or venous hemoglobin greater than 22 g/dL, blood viscosity is increased. This can lead to compromised blood flow and reduced oxygenation of the body organs and increases the risk of neonatal stroke. Many infants with polycythemia are asymptomatic. Others present with plethora, cyanosis, CNS abnormalities (lethargy, jitteriness, seizures), respiratory distress, tachycardia, congestive heart failure, or hypoglycemia. Infants with polycythemia are at increased risk for hyperbilirubinemia. In some cases a partial exchange transfusion to reduce the viscosity of the blood is necessary.

Heat Loss

Growth-restricted infants are particularly susceptible to temperature instability as a result of decreased brown fat deposits, decreased adipose tissue, large body surface exposure, and, in many instances, poor flexion, as well as decreased glycogen storage in major organs such as the liver and heart. Therefore close attention must be given to maintaining an NTE. Nursing considerations focus on maintenance of thermoneutrality to promote recovery from perinatal asphyxia because cold stress jeopardizes such recovery.

LARGE FOR GESTATIONAL AGE INFANTS

The large for gestational age (LGA) infant is defined as weighing 4000 g (8.8 lb) or more at birth. An infant is considered LGA despite gestation when the weight is more than the 90th percentile on growth charts or two standard deviations greater than the mean weight for gestational age. The LGA infant is at greater risk for birth injuries, asphyxia, and congenital anomalies such as heart defects (Carlo, 2016).

All pregnancies of 42 {0/7} weeks gestation or longer must be thoroughly evaluated. All large fetuses are monitored during a trial of labor, and preparation is made for a cesarean birth if abnormal fetal heart rate patterns or poor progress of labor occurs. LGA newborns can be preterm, term, or postterm; they can be infants of mothers with diabetes; or they can be postmature. Each of these problems carries special concerns. Regardless of coexisting potential problems, the LGA infant is at risk by virtue of size alone.

The nurse assesses the LGA infant for hypoglycemia and trauma resulting from vaginal or cesarean birth. Any specific birth injuries are identified and treated appropriately (see Chapter 35).

DISCHARGE PLANNING

Discharge planning for the high-risk newborn begins early in the hospitalization. Throughout the infant's hospitalization the nurse gathers information from the interprofessional health care team members and the family. This information is used to determine the infant's and family's readiness for discharge. Discharge teaching for the family of a high-risk newborn is extensive, requires time and planning, and cannot be adequately accomplished on the day of discharge.

Information is provided about infant care, especially as it pertains to the particular infant's home care needs (e.g., supplemental oxygen, gastrostomy feedings, follow-up medical visits). Parents should be allowed to spend a night or two in a pre-discharge room providing care for the infant away from the NICU to become better acquainted with the necessary care and to have a time of transition in which questions can be answered regarding home care. Additional parent teaching should include bathing and skin care; requirements for meeting nutritional needs following discharge; safety in the home, including supine sleep position, avoiding exposure to cigarette smoke, prevention of infection (e.g., respiratory syncytial virus [RSV]); and medication administration.

🏠 COMMUNITY ACTIVITY

- Visit the March of Dimes website (www.marchofdimes.org/complications/touching-and-holding-your-baby-in-the-nicu.aspx) and explore the resources available for parents of preterm infants. Note the list of benefits of skin-to-skin holding. Think about some of the barriers that might prevent parents from holding their preterm infant skin-to-skin. What might help parents overcome some of these barriers?

- Visit https://www.healthychildren.org/English/ages-stages/baby/preemie/pages/Bringing-Baby-Home-Preparing-Yourself-Your-Home-and-Your-Family.aspx, sponsored by the American Academy of Pediatrics. Review the information for parents about caring for and bringing home a preterm infant. Explore the availability of support groups for parents of preterm infants in your community.

Durable medical equipment and supplies required for the care of the infant in the home should be delivered to the home before the infant is discharged; parents and other care providers should have education in the use of the equipment and ample opportunity to practice. Parents of infants being discharged with special needs such as gavage or gastrostomy feedings, nasal cannula oxygen, tracheostomy, or colostomy should receive several days of thorough education in the procedure before discharge. Preterm infants have a high rate of emergency department visits and readmission to acute care centers; the family absolutely must have a health care provider they can contact for questions regarding infant care and behavior once they are home. Parents should obtain an age-appropriate car seat before the discharge of their infant and demonstrate its correct use. Car seat safety is an essential aspect of discharge planning.

Before discharge, all high-risk or preterm infants should receive the appropriate immunizations, metabolic screening, hematologic assessment (bilirubin risk as appropriate), and hearing evaluation. Successful discharge of high-risk infants to their homes requires an interprofessional approach. Medical, nursing, social services, and other professionals (physical therapy, occupational therapy, developmental follow-up specialist) are crucial to the smooth transition of these infants and their families to the home and community. If the infant is transported back to the community hospital that referred either the mother before birth or the infant after birth, interfacility communication is essential to continuity of care.

Instruction in CPR is essential for parents of all infants but especially for those of infants at risk for life-threatening events. Infants considered at risk include those who are preterm, have apnea or bradycardia, or have a tendency to choke. Before taking their infant home, parents must be able to administer CPR. All parents should be encouraged to obtain instruction in CPR at their local Red Cross or other community agency, if it is not provided by the NICU.

TRANSPORT OF INFANTS

If a hospital is not equipped to care for a high-risk mother and fetus or a high-risk infant, transfer to a specialized perinatal, tertiary, or quaternary care center is arranged. Maternal transport ideally occurs with the fetus in utero because this has two distinct advantages: (1) the associated neonatal morbidity and mortality are decreased; and (2) infant–parent attachment is supported, thereby avoiding separation of the parents and infant. For a variety of reasons, however, it is not always possible to transport the mother before the birth. These reasons include imminent birth and unanticipated problems; therefore health care providers and nurses in level 1 and 2 facilities must have the skills and equipment necessary for making an accurate diagnosis and implementing emergency interventions to stabilize the infant's condition until transport can occur (Rojas, Craven, & Rush, 2016). The goal of these interventions is to maintain the infant's condition within the normal physiologic range. Specific attention is given to the following areas:

- Vital signs
- Oxygen and ventilation
- Thermoregulation
- Acid–base balance
- Fluid and electrolyte levels
- Glucose level
- Developmental interventions

Transport teams can include physicians, nurse practitioners, nurses with expertise in neonatal intensive care, and respiratory therapists. The team must have expertise in resuscitation, stabilization, and provision of critical care during the transport, which can occur on the ground or in the air. In a neonatal transport the team should provide information for the parents about the receiving center. Transport teams can integrate an individual developmental plan of care into their caregiving efforts, thereby initiating multidisciplinary interventions early in the infant's life.

Health care professionals who are responsible for the early stabilization of newborns need specialized training to provide timely, efficient, and effective care. The S.T.A.B.L.E. training program is an evidence-based continuing education program that focuses on the

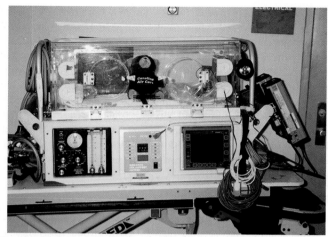

Fig. 34.14 Total Life Support System for Transport of High-risk Newborns. (Courtesy UNC Hospitals, Carolina Air Care, Chapel Hill, NC.)

postresuscitation and pretransport stabilization of sick neonates (S.T.A.B.L.E. Program, 2019). It has been endorsed by the March of Dimes and the AAP and is used internationally. The program consists of 7 modules: S= sugar and safe care, T= temperature, A= airway, B= blood pressure, L= lab work, E= emotional support, and the seventh module is on quality improvement. Training includes an interactive didactic presentation and a posttest (www.stableprogram.org).

The birth of any high-risk infant can cause profound parental stress. Parents may grieve the loss of the ideal infant. They are fearful of the possible eventual outcomes for the infant. They must deal with the technologic world surrounding their infant, and amid all the equipment, it is sometimes difficult for them to perceive the infant and respond to his or her needs. Parents of high-risk infants who have been transported to regional centers therefore need special support. As one way to deal with this problem, many intensive care units provide the family with a handbook or pictures of the tertiary or quarternary care unit to help them understand what is going on around them. Parents should have the name and telephone number of a contact person at the regional center.

Infants are sometimes transferred back to the referring facility; however, in most cases the infant is discharged home from the tertiary care center. Preterm infants who require thermoregulation and gavage feedings may be cared for in community hospitals closer to home, which allows parents to visit their infant more easily and to work with their personal health care provider on the long-range outcomes for the infant. Specialized incubators make these trips possible (Fig. 34.14). However, parents may express mixed feelings about such return transports and may be reluctant to adapt to a different facility and group of caregivers. To minimize some of these concerns, giving the parents clear information about return transports during the initial discharge planning is important.

ANTICIPATORY GRIEF

Families experience anticipatory grief when they are told of the impending death of their infant. Anticipatory grief prepares and protects parents who are facing a loss. Parents who have an infant with a debilitating disease (with or without a congenital deformity), but one that may not necessarily threaten the life of the child, also can experience anticipatory grief. An alteration in relationships, a change in lifestyle, and a very real threat to their hopes and dreams for the future can affect the day-to-day interaction of the family with their infant and the staff. Nurses can help facilitate the family's grieving process. If the nurse observes that a family member's daily interactions with the infant change, the nurse should assess the situation and request psychosocial support or intervention by a chaplain or social worker, if necessary.

Parents who know their infant is going to die have a very difficult time. The parents need to direct their attention, energy, and caregiving activities toward the dying infant. However, some parents find it difficult to visit their infant even for short periods once a terminal diagnosis has been made. Grandparents also grieve but often are unsure how to comfort their own child (the infant's parent) during the period of impending death. Health care professionals can help by involving the family in the infant's care, providing privacy, answering questions, and preparing them for the inevitability of the death (see Chapter 37). There is a growing emphasis on hospice and palliative care for infants and their families.

Nurses also experience grief. Many primary staff nurses find themselves grieving as if the infant were their own because they often have worked closely with the infant and family for weeks or even months. Managers and other staff members must acknowledge this grief. Talking about the infant or attending the funeral can help the staff members resolve their feelings about the infant's death.

KEY POINTS

- Preterm infants are at risk for problems stemming from the immaturity of their organ systems.
- Nurses who work with preterm, late preterm, and other high-risk infants observe them for respiratory distress and other early symptoms of physiologic disorders.
- The adaptation of parents to preterm, late preterm, or high-risk infants differs from that of parents to normal term infants.
- Nurses can facilitate the development of a positive parent–child relationship.
- Nurses' skills in interpreting data, making decisions, and initiating therapy in newborn intensive care units are crucial to ensuring infants' survival.
- Complications of prematurity include respiratory distress syndrome, necrotizing enterocolitis, and germinal matrix hemorrhage–intraventricular hemorrhage.
- Close monitoring of oxygen levels as well as oxygen and ventilator settings can reduce the risk of retinopathy of prematurity.
- Bronchopulmonary dysplasia is a chronic pulmonary condition that may require oxygen therapy in the home setting.

- Pain management requires vigilant ongoing assessment, anticipation of painful events, and early interventions to prevent and diminish such a response.
- Nurses need to assess the macroenvironments and microenvironments of the infant and family to create a developmentally positive atmosphere.
- Developmental care is a philosophy that embraces family-centered care and awareness of the effect of environmental stimuli on the physical and psychologic well-being of the infant and family.
- Parents need special instruction (e.g., CPR, oxygen therapy, suctioning, developmental care) before they take home a high-risk infant.
- SGA infants are considered at risk because of fetal growth restriction.
- The high incidence of fetal distress among postmature infants is related to the progressive placental insufficiency that can occur in a postterm pregnancy.
- Interprofessional health care teams including specially trained nurses transport high-risk infants to and from special care units.
- Parents need assistance as they cope with anticipatory grief or loss and grief.

REFERENCES

AlFaleh, K., & Anabrees, J. (2014). Probiotics for prevention of necrotizing enterocolitis in preterm infants. *Cochrane Database of Systematic Reviews, 4*, CD005496.

Altimier, L., & Phillips, R. M. (2016). The neonatal integrative developmental care model: Advanced clinical applications of the seven core measures for neuroprotective family-centered developmental care. *Newborn and Infant Nursing Reviews, 16*(4), 230–244.

American Academy of Pediatrics. (2016). Prevention and management of procedural pain in the neonate: An update. *Pediatrics, 137*(2), e20154271.

American Heart Association & American Academy of Pediatrics. (2016). *Textbook of neonatal resuscitation* (7th ed.). Elk Grove Village, IL: American Heart Association.

Anand, K. J., & International Evidence-Based Group for Neonatal Pain. (2001). Consensus statement for the prevention and management of pain in the newborn. *Archives of Pediatric and Adolescent Medicine, 155*(2), 173–180.

Armentrout, D. (2015). Glucose management. In M. T. Verklan & M. Walden (Eds.), *Core curriculum for neonatal intensive care nursing* (5th ed.). St. Louis, MO: Elsevier.

Association of Women's Health, Obstetric and Neonatal Nurses. (2017). *Assessment and care of the late preterm infant: Evidence-based clinical practice guidelines* (2nd ed.). Washington, DC: Author.

Bagwell, G. (2014). Hematologic system. In C. Kenner & J. W. Lott (Eds.), *Comprehensive neonatal care* (5th ed.). New York, NY: Springer.

Bancalari, E., Claure, N., & Jain, D. (2018). Neonatal respiratory therapy. In C. A. Gleason & S. E. Juul (Eds.), *Avery's diseases of the newborn* (10th ed.). Philadelphia: Elsevier.

Bhatti, A., Khan, J., Murki, S., et al. (2015). Nasal jet-CPAP (variable flow) versus bubble-CPAP in preterm infants with respiratory distress: An open-label, randomized control trial. *Journal of Perinatology, 35*(11), 935–940.

Blackburn, S. (2018). *Maternal, fetal, and neonatal physiology: A clinical perspective* (5th ed.). St. Louis: Elsevier.

Blauer, T., & Gerstmann, D. (1998). A simultaneous comparison of three neonatal pain scales during common NICU procedures. *Clinical Journal of Pain, 14*(1), 39–47.

Blickstein, I., & Rimon, O. (2015). Post-term pregnancy. In R. J. Martin, A. A. Fanaroff, & M. C. Walsh (Eds.), *Fanaroff & Martin's neonatal-perinatal medicine* (10th ed.). St. Louis, MO: Saunders.

Borghini, A., Habersaat, S., Forcada-Guex, M., et al. (2014). Effects of an early intervention on maternal post-traumatic stress symptoms and the quality of mother-infant interaction: The case of preterm birth. *Infant Behavior and Development, 37*(4), 624–631.

Boies, E. G., & Vaucher, Y. E. (2016). ABM clinical protocol #10: Breastfeeding the late preterm (34–36 6/7 weeks of gestation) and early term infants (37–38 6/7 weeks of gestation), second revision. *Breastfeeding Medicine, 11*(10), 494–500.

Briere, C. E., Lucas, R., McGrath, J. M., et al. (2015). Establishing breastfeeding with the late preterm infant in the NICU. *Journal of Obstetric, Gynecologic, and Neonatal Nursing, 44*(1), 102–113.

Brown, L., Hendrickson, K., Evans, R., et al. (2016). Enteral nutrition. In S. L. Gardner, B. S. Carter, M. Enzman-Hines, et al. (Eds.), *Merenstein & Gardner's handbook of neonatal intensive care* (8th ed.). St. Louis: Elsevier.

Bucher, B., Pacetti, A., Lovvorn, H., et al. (2016). Neonatal surgery. In S. L. Gardner, B. S. Carter, M. Enzman-Hines, et al. (Eds.), *Merenstein & Gardner's handbook of neonatal intensive care* (8th ed.). St. Louis: Elsevier.

Burris, H. (2017). Hypoglycemia and hyperglycemia. In E. Eichenwald, A. Hansen, C. Martin, et al. (Eds.), *Cloherty and Stark's manual of neonatal care* (8th ed). Philadelphia: Wolters Kluwer.

Canadian Agency for Drugs and Technologies in Health. (2016). *Storage, handling, and administration of expressed human breast milk: A review of guidelines.* Retrieved from https://www.ncbi.nlm.nih.gov/books/NBK368235/.

Caplan, M. (2015). Neonatal necrotizing enterocolitis: Clinical observations, pathophysiology, and prevention. In R. J. Martin, A. A. Fanaroff, & M. C. Walsh (Eds.), *Fanaroff & Martin's neonatal-perinatal medicine* (10th ed.). St. Louis: Saunders.

Carlo, W. A. (2016). The high-risk infant. In R. M. Kliegman, B. F. Stanton, J. W. St. Geme, III, et al. (Eds.), *Nelson textbook of pediatrics* (20th ed.). Philadelphia: Elsevier.

Carter, A., Gratny, L., & Carter, B. (2016). Discharge planning and follow-up of the neonatal intensive care unit infant. In S. L. Gardner, B. S. Carter, M. Enzman-Hines, et al. (Eds.), *Merenstein & Gardner's handbook of neonatal intensive care* (8th ed.). St. Louis: Elsevier.

Cartwright, J., Atz, T., Newman, S., et al. (2017). Integrative review of interventions to promote breastfeeding in the late preterm infant. *Journal of Obstetric, Gynecologic and Neonatal Nursing, 46*(3), 347–356.

Clyman, R. (2018). Patent ductus arteriosus in the preterm infant. In C. A. Gleason & S. E. Juul (Eds.), *Avery's diseases of the newborn* (10th ed.). St Louis: Elsevier.

Conde-Agudelo, A., & Díaz-Rossello, J. L. (2016). Kangaroo mother care to reduce morbidity and mortality in low birthweight infants. *Cochrane Database of Systematic Reviews, 8,* CD002771.

de Vries, L. (2015). Intracranial hemorrhage and vascular lesions in the neonate. In R. J. Martin, A. A. Fanaroff, & M. C. Walsh (Eds.), *Fanaroff & Martin's neonatal-perinatal medicine* (10th ed.). St. Louis: Saunders.

Diehl-Jones, W., & Fraser, D. (2014). Hematologic disorders. In M. Verklan & M. Walden (Eds.), *Core curriculum for neonatal intensive care nursing* (5th ed.). St. Louis: Elsevier.

Ditzenberger, G. R., & Blackburn, S. T. (2014). Neurologic system. In C. Kenner & J. W. Lott (Eds.), *Comprehensive neonatal care* (5th ed.). New York: Springer.

Gao, H., Gao, H., Xu, G., et al. (2016). Efficacy and safety of repeated oral sucrose for repeated procedural pain in neonates: A systematic review. *International Journal of Nursing Studies, 62,* 118–125.

Gardner, S. L., & Carter, B. S. (2016). Grief and perinatal loss. In S. L. Gardner, B. S. Carter, M. Enzman-Hines, et al. (Eds.), *Merenstein & Gardner's handbook of neonatal intensive care* (8th ed.). St. Louis: Elsevier.

Gardner, S. L., Enzman-Hines, M., & Agarwal, R. (2016). Pain and pain relief. In S. L. Gardner, B. S. Carter, M. Enzman-Hines, et al. (Eds.), *Merenstein & Gardner's handbook of neonatal intensive care* (8th ed.). St. Louis: Elsevier.

Gardner, S. L., Enzman-Hines, M., & Nyp, M. (2016). Respiratory diseases. In S. L. Gardner, B. S. Carter, M. Enzman-Hines, et al. (Eds.), *Merenstein & Gardner's handbook of neonatal intensive care* (8th ed.). St. Louis: Elsevier.

Gardner, S. L., Goldson, E., & Hernández, J. A. (2016). The neonate and the environment: Impact on development. In S. L. Gardner, B. S. Carter, M. Enzman-Hines, et al. (Eds.), *Merenstein & Gardner's handbook of neonatal intensive care* (8th ed.). St. Louis: Elsevier.

Gardner, S. L., & Hernández, J. A. (2016a). Heat balance. In S. L. Gardner, B. S. Carter, M. Enzman-Hines, et al. (Eds.), *Merenstein & Gardner's handbook of neonatal intensive care* (8th ed.). St. Louis: Elsevier.

Gardner, S. L., & Hernández, J. A. (2016b). Initial nursery care. In S. L. Gardner, B. S. Carter, M. Enzman-Hines, et al. (Eds.), *Merenstein & Gardner's handbook of neonatal intensive care* (8th ed.). St. Louis: Elsevier.

Gardner, S. L., & Lawrence, R. A. (2016). Breastfeeding the neonate with special needs. In S. L. Gardner, B. S. Carter, M. Enzman-Hines, et al. (Eds.), *Merenstein & Gardner's handbook of neonatal intensive care* (8th ed.). St. Louis: Elsevier.

Gardner, S. L., Voos, K., & Hills, P. (2016). Families in crisis: Theoretical and practical considerations. In S. L. Gardner, B. S. Carter, M. Enzman-Hines, et al. (Eds.), *Merenstein & Gardner's handbook of neonatal intensive care* (8th ed.). St. Louis: Elsevier.

Garinis, A. C., Kemph, A., Tharpe, A. M., et al. (2017). Monitoring neonates for ototoxicity. *International Journal of Audiology, 57*(Suppl. 4), S54–S61.

Gowen, C. (2015). Diseases of the fetus. In K. Marcdante & R. M. Kliegman (Eds.), *Nelson's essentials of pediatrics* (7th ed). Philadelphia: Elsevier.

Hermansen, C. L., & Mahajan, A. (2015). Newborn respiratory distress. *American Family Physician, 92*(11), 994–1002.

Hodgkinson, K., Bear, M., Thorn, J., & VanBlaricum, S. (1994). Measuring pain in neonates: Evaluating an instrument and developing a common language. *Australian Journal of Advanced Nursing, 12*(1), 17–22.

Jackson, J. C. (2018). Respiratory disorders in the preterm infant. In C. A. Gleason & S. E. Juul (Eds.), *Avery's diseases of the newborn* (10th ed.). St Louis: Elsevier.

Katheria, A., & Finer, N. (2018). Newborn resuscitation. In C. A. Gleason & S. E. Juul (Eds.), *Avery's diseases of the newborn* (10th ed.). St Louis: Elsevier.

Keller, R., & Ballard, R. (2018). Bronchopulmonary dysplasia. In C. A. Gleason & S. E. Juul (Eds.), *Avery's diseases of the newborn* (10th ed.). St Louis: Elsevier.

Kenner, C., & Boykova, M. (2015). Families in crisis. In M. T. Verklan & M. Walden (Eds.), *Core curriculum for neonatal intensive care nursing* (5th ed.). St. Louis: Elsevier.

Kim, M. J. (2016). Enteral nutrition for optimal growth in preterm infants. *Korean Journal of Pediatrics, 59*(12), 466–470.

Krechel, S. W., & Bildner, J. (1995). CRIES: A new neonatal postoperative pain measurement score. Initial testing of validity and reliability. *Paediatric Anaesthesia, 5*(1), 53–61.

Lawrence, J., Alcock, D., McGrath, P., et al. (1993). The development of a tool to assess neonatal pain. *Neonatal Network, 12*(6), 59–66.

Lorenz, L., Dawson, J. A., Jones, H., et al. (2017). Skin-to-skin care in preterm infants receiving respiratory support does not lead to physiological instability. *Archives of Disease in Childhood—Fetal and Neonatal Edition, 102*(4), F339–F344.

Lund, C. H., & Durand, D. J. (2016). Skin and skin care. In S. L. Gardner, B. S. Carter, M. Enzman-Hines, et al. (Eds.), *Merenstein & Gardner's handbook of neonatal intensive care* (8th ed.). St. Louis: Elsevier.

Lund, C. H., & Kuller, J. (2014). Integumentary system. In C. Kenner & J. W. Lott (Eds.), *Comprehensive neonatal care* (5th ed.). New York: Springer.

Madlinger-Lewis, L., Reynolds, L., Zarem, C., et al. (2014). The effects of alternative positioning on preterm infants in the neonatal intensive care unit: A randomized clinical trial. *Research in Developmental Disabilities, 35*(2), 490–497.

Martin, J. A., Hamilton, B. E., Osterman, M. J. K., et al. (2018). Births: Final data for 2016. *National Vital Statistics Reports, 67*(1), 1–54.

Mohan, S., & Jain, D. (2018). Late preterm infants. In C. A. Gleason & S. E. Juul (Eds.), *Avery's diseases of the newborn* (10th ed). St. Louis: Elsevier.

NIDCAP Federation International. (2019). *Overview: The Newborn Individualized Developmental Care And Assessment Program.* Retrieved from http://nidcap.org/en/programs-and-certifications/nidcap-training/overview-2/.

Niermeyer, S., Clarke, S. B., & Hernández, J. (2016). Delivery room care. In S. L. Gardner, B. S. Carter, M. Enzman-Hines, et al. (Eds.), *Merenstein & Gardner's handbook of neonatal intensive care* (8th ed.). St. Louis: Elsevier.

Olsen, S. L., Leick-Rude, M. K., Dustin, J., et al. (2016). Total parenteral nutrition. In S. L. Gardner, B. S. Carter, M. Enzman-Hines, et al. (Eds.), *Merenstein & Gardner's handbook of neonatal intensive care* (8th ed.). St. Louis: Elsevier.

Pappas, B., & Robey, D. (2015). Care of the late preterm infant. In M. T. Verklan & M. Walden (Eds.), *Core curriculum for neonatal intensive care nursing* (5th ed.). St. Louis: Elsevier.

Patel, M., Mohr, M., Lake, D., et al. (2016). Clinical associations with immature breathing in preterm infants: Part 2—periodic breathing. *Pediatric Research, 80*(1), 28–34.

Peters, M. D., McArthur, A., & Munn, Z. (2016). Safe management of expressed breast milk: A systematic review. *Women and Birth, 29*(6), 473–481.

Philpott-Robinson, K., Lane, S. J., Korostenski, L., et al. (2017). The impact of the neonatal intensive care unit on sensory and developmental outcomes in infants born preterm: A scoping review. *British Journal of Occupational Therapy, 80*(8), 459–469.

Pokela, M. (1994). Pain relief can reduce hypoxemia in distressed neonates during routine treatment procedures. *Pediatrics, 93*(3), 379–383.

Polin, R. A., Carlo, W. A., & Committee on Fetus and Newborn. (2014). Surfactant replacement therapy for preterm and term neonates with respiratory distress. *Pediatrics, 133*(1), 156–163.

Rojas, M. A., Craven, H., & Rush, M. G. (2016). Perinatal transport and levels of care. In S. L. Gardner, B. S. Carter, M. Enzman-Hines, et al. (Eds.), *Merenstein & Gardner's handbook of neonatal intensive care* (8th ed.). St. Louis: Elsevier.

Rozance, P. J., McGowan, J. E., Price-Douglas, W., et al. (2016). Glucose homeostasis. In S. L. Gardner, B. S. Carter, M. Enzman-Hines, et al. (Eds.), *Merenstein & Gardner's handbook of neonatal intensive care* (8th ed.). St. Louis: Elsevier.

Rubarth, L., & Parker, D. (2014). Ophthalmic system. In C. Kenner & J. W. Lott (Eds.), *Comprehensive neonatal care* (5th ed.). New York: Springer.

Sadowski, S. (2015). Cardiovascular disorders. In M. T. Verklan & M. Walden (Eds.), *Core curriculum for neonatal intensive care nursing* (5th ed.). St. Louis: Elsevier.

Sahai, I., & Levy, H. (2018). Newborn screening. In C. A. Gleason & S. E. Juul (Eds.), *Avery's diseases of the newborn* (10th ed.). St Louis: Elsevier.

Soltau, T. D., & Carlo, W. A. (2014). Respiratory system. In C. Kenner & J. W. Lott (Eds.), *Comprehensive neonatal nursing care* (5th ed.). New York: Springer.

Sparshott, M. (1995). Assessing the behaviour of the newborn infant. *Paediatric Nursing, 7*(7), 14–16.

S.T.A.B.L.E Program. (2019). *The S.T.A.B.L.E. Program.* Retrieved from https://stableprogram.org/.

Steinhorn, R., & Abman, S. (2018). Persistent pulmonary hypertension. In C. A. Gleason & S. E. Juul (Eds.), *Avery's diseases of the newborn* (10th ed). St. Louis: Elsevier.

Stevens, B., Johnston, C., Petryshen, P., & Taddio, A. (1996). Premature infant pain profile: Development and initial validation. *Clinical Journal of Pain, 12*(1), 13–22.

Swanson, T., & Erickson, L. (2016). Cardiovascular diseases and surgical interventions. In S. L. Gardner, B. S. Carter, M. Enzman-Hines, et al. (Eds.), *Merenstein & Gardner's handbook of neonatal intensive care* (8th ed.). St. Louis: Elsevier.

The Joint Commission. (2017). *Pain assessment and management standards for hospitals.* R3R Report Issue 11. Retrieved from https://jntcm.ae-admin.com/assets/1/6/R3_Report_Issue_11_Pain_Assessment_2_11_19_REV.pdf.

Vasquez-Ruiz, S., Maya-Barrios, J., Torres-Narváez, P., & Vega-Martinez, B.R. (2014). A light-dark cycle in the NICU accelerates body weight gain and shortens time to discharge in preterm infants. *Early Human Development, 90*(9), 535–540.

Walden, M. (2014). Pain in the newborn and infant. In C. Kenner & J. W. Lott (Eds.), *Comprehensive neonatal nursing care* (5th ed.). New York: Springer.

Wambach, J., & Hamvas, A. (2015). Respiratory distress syndrome in the neonate. In R. J. Martin, A. A. Fanaroff, & M. C. Walsh (Eds.), *Fanaroff & Martin's neonatal-perinatal medicine* (10th ed.). St. Louis: Saunders.

35

Acquired Problems of the Newborn

Patricia A. Scott

e http://evolve.elsevier.com/Lowdermilk/MWHC/

LEARNING OBJECTIVES

- Describe assessment and care of infants with soft-tissue, skeletal, and nervous system injuries resulting from birth trauma.
- Develop a plan of care for the neonate of a mother with diabetes.
- Describe the assessment and care of a newborn with a suspected infection or sepsis.
- Discuss common infections transmitted to the fetus during pregnancy, and to the neonate intrapartally and postnatally.
- Interpret the evidence available to guide the care of the infant at risk for group B streptococcal sepsis.

- Analyze fetal and neonatal effects of maternal substance abuse during pregnancy.
- Describe concerns for fetal and neonatal well-being related to maternal use of benzodiazepines, barbiturates, and selective serotonin reuptake inhibitors.
- Describe the assessment and care of a newborn experiencing drug withdrawal (neonatal abstinence syndrome); include the infant's family.

This chapter deals with acquired problems of the newborn. Acquired problems refer to those conditions resulting from environmental rather than genetic factors. The focus is on birth trauma, the infant of a mother with diabetes, neonatal infections, effects of maternal substance abuse on the fetus and neonate, and effects of maternal use of benzodiazepines, barbiturates, and antidepressant medications during pregnancy.

BIRTH TRAUMA

Birth trauma or birth injury refers to physical injury sustained by a newborn during labor and birth. According to the Agency for Healthcare Research and Quality (AHRQ, 2014), the incidence of birth injuries in the United States is 1.86/1000 live births. Despite improvements in obstetric techniques, increased use of cesarean surgery for births that would be difficult vaginally, and decreased use of forceps, vacuum extraction, and version; birth injuries still are an important source of neonatal morbidity. Therefore the clinician should consider the broad range of birth injuries in the differential diagnosis of neonatal clinical disorders (Mangurten, Puppala, & Prazad, 2015). The nurse's contribution to the welfare of the newborn begins with early observation and accurate documentation. The prompt reporting of signs that indicate deviations from normal permits early initiation of appropriate therapy. In addition, nurses provide essential support and education to parents whose newborn experiences a birth injury.

In theory, some birth injuries are avoidable, especially with careful assessment of risk factors and appropriate planning for birth. The use of ultrasonography allows antepartum diagnosis of macrosomia, hydrocephalus, and unusual presentations. Elective cesarean birth may be chosen for selected pregnancies to prevent significant birth injury. A small percentage of significant birth injuries are unavoidable despite skilled and competent obstetric care, as in especially difficult or prolonged labor or when the infant is in an abnormal presentation

(Mangurten et al., 2015). Some injuries cannot be anticipated until the specific circumstances occur during birth. Emergency cesarean birth can provide last-minute salvage, but in these circumstances the injury may be truly unavoidable.

Many injuries are minor and resolve readily in the neonatal period without treatment. Other injuries require intervention. A few injuries are considered major trauma and serious enough to be fatal. Major trauma can occur concomitantly with minor injuries. For example, a neonate who suffers a skull fracture is also likely to have a cephalhematoma (Mangurten et al., 2015).

Several factors predispose an infant to birth injuries. Maternal risk factors include age younger than 16 or older than 35, primigravida, uterine dysfunction that leads to prolonged or precipitous labor, preterm or postterm labor, and cephalopelvic disproportion. Oligohydramnios can increase the likelihood of birth trauma. Injury can result from dystocia caused by fetal macrosomia, multifetal gestation, abnormal or difficult presentation (not caused by maternal uterine or pelvic conditions), and congenital anomalies. Intrapartum events that can result in scalp injury include the use of internal monitoring of fetal heart rate (FHR) and collection of fetal scalp blood for acid–base assessment. Obstetric birth techniques can cause injury. Forceps- or vacuum-assisted birth and cesarean birth are potential contributory factors. Neonatal risk factors for birth injury include macrosomia, preterm or postterm birth, and congenital anomalies. Often more than one factor is present, and multiple predisposing factors can be related to a single maternal condition (Mangurten et al., 2015; Parsons, Seay, & Jacobson, 2018).

Birth injuries are usually classified according to their etiology (predisposing factors or mechanisms of injury) or anatomically. Table 35.1 shows an example of anatomic classification of birth injuries.

Soft-Tissue Injuries

Erythema; ecchymoses; petechiae (pinpoint hemorrhagic areas), abrasions; lacerations; and edema of the face, head, buttocks, and

TABLE 35.1 Anatomic Classification of Birth Injuries

Site of Injury	Type of Injury
Scalp	Caput succedaneum
	Cephalhematoma
	Subgaleal hemorrhage
Skull	Linear fracture
	Depressed fracture
	Occipital osteodiastasis
Intracranial	Epidural hematoma
	Subdural hematoma (laceration of falx, tentorium, or superficial veins)
	Subarachnoid hemorrhage
	Cerebral contusion
	Cerebellar contusion
	Intracerebellar hematoma
Spinal cord (cervical)	Vertebral artery injury
	Intraspinal hemorrhage
	Spinal cord transection or injury
Plexus injuries	Erb-Duchenne palsy
	Klumpke paralysis
	Total (mixed) brachial plexus injury
	Horner syndrome
	Diaphragmatic paralysis
	Lumbosacral plexus injury
Cranial and peripheral nerve injuries	Radial nerve palsy/nerve injuries
	Medial nerve palsy
	Sciatic nerve palsy
	Laryngeal nerve palsy
	Diaphragmatic paralysis
	Facial nerve palsy

From Parsons J., Seay A., & Jacobson, M. (2016). Neurologic disorders. In S. L. Gardner, B. S. Carter, M. Enzman-Hines, & J. A. Hernandez (Eds.), *Merenstein & Gardner's handbook of neonatal intensive care* (8th ed.). St.Louis: Mosby.

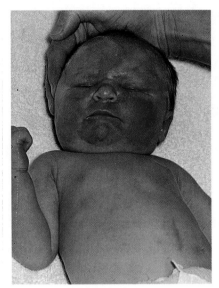

Fig. 35.1 Marked Bruising on the Entire Face of an Infant Born Vaginally After Face Presentation. Less severe ecchymoses were present on the extremities. Phototherapy was required for treatment of jaundice resulting from the breakdown of accumulated blood. (From O'Doherty, N. [1986]. *Neonatology: Microatlas of the newborn.* Nutley, NJ: Hoffmann-La Roche.)

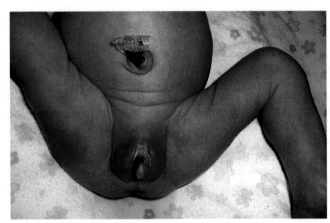

Fig. 35.2 Swelling of the Genitals and Bruising of the Buttocks of a Preterm Infant After a Breech Birth. Note the position of the infant's legs. (Courtesy Cheryl Briggs, RNC, Annapolis, MD.)

extremities can be present in a newborn. Localized discoloration can appear over presenting or dependent parts. Ecchymoses and edema can appear anywhere on the body and especially on the presenting body part from the application of forceps or vacuum cup. They also can result from the position of the infant within the bony pelvis or manipulation of the infant's body during birth.

Bruises over the face can be the result of face presentation (Fig. 35.1). In a breech presentation, bruising and swelling can occur over the buttocks or genitalia (Fig. 35.2). The skin over the entire head can be ecchymotic and covered with petechiae caused by a tight nuchal cord. Petechiae acquired during birth can extend over the upper portion of the trunk and face. These lesions are benign if they disappear within 2 days of birth and no new lesions appear. Ecchymoses and petechiae can also be signs of a more serious disorder, such as thrombocytopenic purpura, if the hemorrhagic areas do not disappear spontaneously in 2 days.

! NURSING ALERT

To differentiate hemorrhagic areas from skin rashes and discolorations such as mongolian spots, the nurse gently presses on the skin with two fingers. Because extravasated blood remains within the tissues, petechiae and ecchymoses do not blanch.

Forceps injury occurs at the site of application of the instrument. Forceps injury typically has a linear configuration across both sides of the face, outlining the placement of the forceps. The affected areas are kept clean to minimize the risk of secondary infection. These injuries usually resolve spontaneously within several days with no specific therapy.

Accidental lacerations can be inflicted with a scalpel during cesarean birth or with scissors during an episiotomy. These cuts can occur on any part of the body but most often are found on the scalp, buttocks, and thighs. Usually they are superficial, needing only to be kept clean. Adhesive wound closure strips or topical skin adhesive will usually hold together the edges of more serious lacerations. Rarely are sutures needed.

Two of the most commonly occurring birth injuries are subconjunctival (scleral) and retinal hemorrhages. These injuries result from rupture of capillaries caused by increased intracranial pressure (ICP) during birth. They usually clear within 7 to 10 days after birth and present no problems; however, parents need reassurance about their presence.

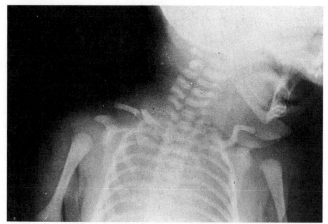

Fig. 35.3 Fractured Clavicle After Shoulder Dystocia. (From O'Doherty, N. [1986]. *Neonatology: Micro atlas of the newborn.* Nutley, NJ: Hoffmann-La Roche.)

Caput succedaneum and cephalhematoma are commonly seen in neonates, often as the result of pressure on the fetal head pushing through a dilated cervix (see Fig. 23.15A and B). A more serious injury is subgaleal hemorrhage, which is bleeding into the subgaleal compartment (see Fig. 23.15C). These are discussed in Chapter 23.

Skeletal Injuries

The newborn's immature flexible skull can withstand considerable deformation (molding) before fracture results (see Fig. 23.14). Substantial force is required to fracture the newborn's skull. Two types of skull fractures typically are identified in the newborn: linear fractures and depressed fractures. The location of the fracture and involvement of underlying structures determine its significance. Linear fractures are most common in the parietal bones, require no treatment, and are usually of no clinical significance. Skull fractures are common in infants with a cephalhematoma (Mangurten et al., 2015).

The soft skull can become indented without laceration of either the skin or the dural membrane. These depressed fractures, or "ping-pong ball" indentations, can occur during difficult births from pressure of the fetal head on the bony pelvis. They also can occur as a result of injudicious application of forceps. A computed tomography (CT) scan is done to rule out bone fragments or underlying injury of the brain tissue. Management of depressed skull fractures is controversial; many resolve without intervention. There are nonsurgical interventions that have been used if the fracture does not spontaneously resolve (Mangurten et al., 2015; Parsons et al., 2016).

The clavicle is the bone most often fractured during birth. Generally the break is in the middle third of the bone (Fig. 35.3). Difficult delivery of the shoulders with a vaginal birth or extension of the arms in a breech birth often results in clavicular fracture (Mangurten et al., 2015). Other risk factors include vacuum-assisted birth and birth weight greater than 4000 g (8 lbs, 13 oz). Limited movement of the arm, crepitus over the bone, and the absence of the Moro reflex on the affected side are diagnostic. Except for use of gentle rather than vigorous handling, no accepted treatment for fractured clavicle exists, and the prognosis is good. A sign posted on the bassinet will alert care providers to the need for careful handling. The figure-eight bandage appropriate for an older child should not be used for a newborn.

The humerus and femur can also be fractured during a difficult birth. Fractures in newborns generally heal rapidly. Immobilization is accomplished with slings, splints, swaddling, and other devices. Assessment and management of pain related to these injuries are important nursing responsibilities.

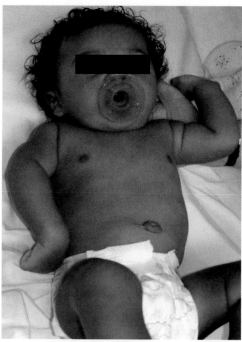

Fig. 35.4 Brachial Plexus Injury (Erb-Duchenne Palsy) in Newborn Infant. The Moro reflex was absent in right upper extremity. Recovery was complete. (From Chung, K. C., Yan, L., & McGillicuddy, J. E. [2012]. *Practical management of pediatric and adult brachial plexus palsies.* Philadelphia: Saunders.)

The parents need support in handling these infants because they often are fearful of hurting them. Parents are encouraged to practice handling, changing, and feeding the affected neonate under the guidance of nursing staff prior to discharge from the birth facility. This increases their confidence and knowledge and facilitates attachment. A plan for follow-up therapy is developed with the parents so that the times and arrangements for therapy are acceptable to them.

Peripheral Nervous System Injuries

Brachial plexus injury (Fig. 35.4) is the most common type of paralysis associated with a difficult birth and is defined as paralysis involving muscles of the upper extremity that follows mechanical trauma to spinal roots C5 through T1 (Mangurten et al., 2015). An increased risk of brachial plexus injury occurs with birth weight greater than 4000 g (8 lbs, 13 oz), vaginal breech birth, forceps- or vacuum-assisted birth, and a prolonged second stage of labor.

Erb-Duchenne paralysis or palsy is the result of injury to the upper plexus involving nerves C5 and C6 caused by stretching or pulling the head away from the shoulder during a difficult birth. The arm hangs limply alongside the body. The shoulder and arm are adducted and internally rotated. The elbow is extended, and the forearm is pronated, with the wrist and fingers flexed; a grasp reflex can be present because finger and wrist movement remains normal (Mangurten et al., 2015).

Damage to the lower plexus, also known as *Klumpke paralysis or palsy,* is less common. With lower arm paralysis the wrist and hand are flaccid, the grasp reflex is absent, and deep tendon reflexes are present; dependent edema and cyanosis can occur in the affected hand. This injury is a result of damage to the nerves between C8 and T1. There can also be a combination of Erb-Duchenne and Klumpke paralysis and the entire arm can be paralyzed (Verklan, 2015).

Treatment of brachial plexus injury involves intermittent immobilization across the upper abdomen, proper positioning, and range-of-motion (ROM) exercises. Gentle manipulation and ROM exercises are

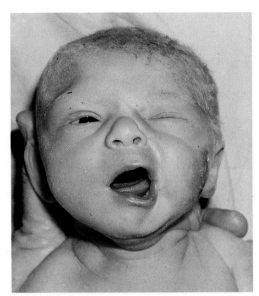

Fig. 35.5 Facial Paralysis 15 Minutes After Forceps Birth. Absence of movement on affected side is especially noticeable when infant cries. (From O'Doherty, N. [1986]. *Neonatology: Micro atlas of the newborn*. Nutley, NJ: Hoffmann-La Roche.)

delayed for 1 week to prevent additional injury to the brachial plexus. Immobilization can be accomplished with a brace or splint or by pinning the infant's sleeve to his or her shirt. Treatment for Klumpke palsy consists of placing the hand in a neutral position, padding the fist, and gently exercising the wrist and fingers (Mangurten et al., 2015).

If edema or hemorrhage is responsible for the paralysis, the prognosis is good and recovery can be expected in a few weeks. If laceration of the nerves has occurred and healing does not result in return of function within a few months, surgery may be indicated; however, return of function is variable. Full recovery is expected in the majority of infants (Mangurten et al., 2015).

Phrenic nerve injury (diaphragmatic paralyis) almost always occurs as a component of brachial plexus injury rather than as an isolated problem. Injury is usually the result of traction on the neck and arm during birth. Injury to the phrenic nerve is usually unilateral, but can be bilateral. Cyanosis and irregular thoracic respirations, with no abdominal movement on inspiration, are characteristic of paralysis of the diaphragm. Neonates with diaphragmatic paralysis usually require mechanical ventilatory support, at least for the first few days after birth, and are at risk of developing pneumonia. In the presence of persistent respiratory distress, diaphragmatic pacing or surgical correction may be necessary (Mangurten et al., 2015).

Facial paralysis (palsy) (Fig. 35.5) generally is caused by pressure on the facial nerve during birth. Risk factors include a prolonged second stage of labor and forceps-assisted birth. The face on the affected side is flattened and unresponsive to the grimace that accompanies crying or stimulation and the eye remains open on the affected side. Moreover, the forehead does not wrinkle. Usually the infant's face appears distorted, especially when crying. Often the condition is transitory, resolving within hours or days of birth, although total recovery can take weeks or months. Permanent paralysis is rare (Mangurten et al., 2015).

Treatment involves assistance with feeding, prevention of damage to the cornea of the open eye with the application of artificial tears or taping the eye closed, and supportive care of the parents. Feeding can be prolonged, with the milk flowing out the newborn's mouth around the nipple on the affected side. The parents will need understanding and sympathetic encouragement while learning how to feed and care for the infant (Verklan, 2015).

Central Nervous System Injuries

All types of intracranial hemorrhages (ICHs) occur in newborns. ICH as a result of birth trauma is more likely to occur in a large term newborn. Risk factors for ICH include vacuum- or forceps-assisted birth, presence of a coagulopathy, prematurity, chorioamnionitis, acidosis, hypotension, respiratory distress, and bicarbonate therapy (Shah & Wusthoff, 2016). More than one type of hemorrhage frequently occurs.

Subdural hemorrhage (hematoma), a collection of blood in the subdural space, most often is produced by the stretching and tearing of the large veins in the tentorium of the cerebellum, the dural membrane that separates the cerebrum from the cerebellum. When this type of bleeding occurs, the typical history includes a nulliparous mother, with the total labor and birth occurring in less than 2 or 3 hours; a difficult forceps-assisted birth; or a large for gestational age (LGA) infant. Subdural hematoma occurs less frequently today because of improvements in obstetric care. For most newborns, this injury is asymptomatic. If symptoms do present, this usually occurs at 24 to 48 hours of life with nonspecific signs such as apnea, respiratory distress, an altered neurologic exam, or seizures (deVries, 2015; Shah & Wusthoff, 2016).

Subarachnoid hemorrhage, a common type of ICH, occurs in term newborns as a result of trauma and in preterm infants as a result of hypoxia. Small hemorrhages are the most common. Bleeding is of venous origin, and underlying contusion also can occur. The clinical presentation of hemorrhage in the term newborn can vary considerably. In many newborns, the signs are absent and hemorrhaging is diagnosed only because of abnormal findings on lumbar puncture (e.g., red blood cells in the cerebrospinal fluid [CSF]). The initial clinical manifestations of neonatal subarachnoid hemorrhage can be the early onset of alternating depression and irritability, with refractory seizures or apnea. Occasionally the infant appears normal initially, then has seizures on the second or third day of life, followed by no apparent after effects (Verklan, 2015).

In general, nursing care of an infant with ICH is supportive and includes monitoring ventilatory and intravenous (IV) therapy, observing and managing seizures, and preventing increased ICP. Minimal handling to promote rest and reduce stress should guide nursing care (Shah & Wusthoff, 2016). Providing education and support to the family is also an important component of nursing care.

The most common cause of spinal cord injury in the neonate is a difficult breech birth. Stretching of the spinal cord, usually by forceful longitudinal traction on the trunk while the head is still firmly engaged in the pelvis, is the most common mechanism of injury. Fortunately, this injury is rarely seen today because cesarean birth is typically used for breech presentation. However, it can also occur with shoulder dystocia when traction is applied to the head. Brow and face presentations, dystocia, preterm birth, maternal nulliparity, and precipitous birth also have been identified as predisposing factors in spinal cord injury (Mangurten et al., 2015).

Clinical manifestations, treatment, and prognosis depend on the severity and location of the injury. Brainstem and high cervical cord injuries are likely to cause stillbirth or rapid death. Upper or midcervical lesions may not be recognized at birth but cause death after a few days. Infants can appear normal at birth but show progressive respiratory deterioration and signs of spinal shock, including flaccid extremities, diaphragmatic breathing, paralyzed abdominal movements, atonic anal sphincter, and distended bladder. Lower lesions can result in paraplegia and associated complications. Signs of partial spinal cord injuries such as spasticity can be less apparent (Mangurten et al., 2015).

Therapy is supportive and usually unsatisfactory. Infants who survive present a therapeutic challenge that requires combined treatment by an interprofessional health care team that includes a pediatrician, neurologist, neurosurgeon, urologist, orthopedist, nurse, physical therapist, and occupational therapist. Parents need to understand fully the implications of severe injury to the spinal cord and the overwhelming implications it presents for the newborn and family.

CARE MANAGEMENT

Nurses who perform initial and ongoing assessments of newborns should be alert for clinical signs of birth trauma such as bruising; edema; abrasions; or absence, limitation, or asymmetry of movement. There can be immediate evidence of injury following birth, or the signs of birth trauma may not appear until later. The neonate can experience impaired mobility, respiratory distress, or acute pain as a result of birth trauma. In some cases, more serious consequences of birth trauma can occur such as seizures or coma.

Care of the infant with a birth injury is individualized based on the type of injury. Through prompt identification of birth injury and notification of the health care provider, the nurse can proceed as directed with appropriate care measures. Based on the severity of the injury, the newborn may be transferred to the newborn intensive care unit (NICU).

Parents are likely to react to neonatal birth trauma with concern and anxiety. The nurse provides explanations about the type of injury and the treatment plan. Parents may need assistance and support from the nurse as they provide care for the newborn. For example, the nurse can demonstrate how to hold the infant to prevent discomfort from the injury. If the newborn is in the NICU, parents need even greater support from the nursing staff.

INFANTS OF MOTHERS WITH DIABETES

No single physiologic or biochemical event can explain the diverse clinical manifestations seen in the infants of mothers with diabetes. A better understanding of maternal and fetal metabolism, resulting in stricter control of maternal glucose levels and improved obstetric and neonatal intensive care, has led to a decrease in the perinatal mortality rate associated with diabetic pregnancy. However, maternal diabetes continues to play a significant role in neonatal morbidity and mortality. Compared with nondiabetic pregnancies, infants born to mothers with diabetes are at an increased risk for complications such as congenital anomalies, large fetal size, birth trauma, perinatal asphyxia, stillbirth, preterm birth, respiratory distress syndrome (RDS), hypoglycemia, hypocalcemia, hypomagnesemia, cardiomyopathy, hyperbilirubinemia, and polycythemia. The degree of risk depends on the severity and duration of maternal disease. For example, women with vascular complications are more likely to have infants who are small for gestational age (SGA). All infants born to mothers with diabetes are at some risk for complications. The likelihood of these complications is reduced when maternal glucose levels are maintained within normal limits during the periconception period and during pregnancy (Blickstein, Perlman, Hazan, et al., 2015).

Pathophysiology

The mechanisms responsible for the problems seen in infants of mothers with diabetes are not fully understood. In early pregnancy, fluctuations in blood glucose levels and episodes of ketoacidosis are believed to cause congenital anomalies. Later in pregnancy, when the mother's pancreas cannot release sufficient insulin to meet increased demands, maternal hyperglycemia results. Increased amounts of glucose cross the placenta and stimulate the fetal pancreas to release insulin. The combination of the increased supply of maternal glucose and other nutrients and increased fetal insulin results in excessive fetal growth. This excessive fetal growth is defined as *macrosomia* or LGA. Macrosomia is an absolute value defined as a birthweight greater than 4000 g (8 lbs, 13 oz). LGA is a relative term defined as a birth weight greater than the 90th percentile for gestational age.

Hyperinsulinemia accounts for many of the problems experienced by the fetus or newborn. In addition to fluctuating glucose levels, maternal vascular involvement or superimposed maternal infection adversely affects the fetus. Normally, maternal blood has a more alkaline pH than the carbon dioxide–rich fetal blood. This phenomenon encourages the exchange of oxygen and carbon dioxide across the placental membrane. When the maternal blood is more acidotic than the fetal blood, such as during ketoacidosis, little carbon dioxide or oxygen exchange occurs at the level of the placenta; this can lead to fetal death. In a recent study, the mortality rate for unborn babies resulting from an episode of maternal ketoacidosis was 15.6% (Morrison, Movassaghian, Seely, et al., 2017).

Congenital Anomalies

The incidence of congenital anomalies among mothers with pregestational diabetes is three to five times that of pregnant women who do not have diabetes. This increased risk of congenital malformations is related to the elevated glucose levels during the period of organogenesis that occurs between 5 and 8 weeks of gestation (Blickstein et al., 2015). Gestational diabetes that is diagnosed in mid- to late pregnancy is usually not associated with an increased incidence of congenital anomalies. This reinforces the importance of controlling blood glucose levels before conception and in the early stages of pregnancy. However, the risk of anomalies is increased in women who are diagnosed with gestational diabetes before 20 weeks' gestation, who had a previous pregnancy complicated by gestational diabetes, or who are obese (Blickstein et al., 2015).

The most frequently occurring anomalies involve the cardiac, renal, musculoskeletal, gastrointestinal (GI), and central nervous systems (CNS) (see Chapter 36). Infants of mothers with pregestational diabetes have a four times higher risk of having a congenital heart defect than the general population (Oyen, Diaz, Leirgul, et al., 2016). Coarctation of the aorta, transposition of the great vessels, and atrial or ventricular septal defects are the most common cardiac anomalies occurring in infants of mothers with diabetes. In the genitourinary system, renal agenesis (failure of the kidney to develop) and obstruction of the urinary tract have been associated with maternal diabetes. Central nervous system (CNS) anomalies include anencephaly, encephalocele, myelomeningocele, and hydrocephalus. The musculoskeletal system can be affected by *caudal regression syndrome* (*sacral agenesis*, with weakness or deformities of the lower extremities; malformation and fixation of the hip joints; and shortening or deformity of the femurs). Neonatal small left colon syndrome is a functional intestinal disorder often noted in these infants. This disorder is a transient dysmotility of the descending colon that usually is not associated with any long-term complications (Wood, Jinadatha, Agrawal, et al., 2018). It is suspected when the infant fails to pass meconium and has abdominal distention and bile-stained vomitus. Contrast enemas show a greatly diminished caliber of the left colon from the splenic flexure to the anus.

Macrosomia

Despite improvements in the control of maternal blood glucose levels, enlarged fetal size is common (Mitanchez, Yzydorczyk, & Simeoni, 2015). At birth the typical LGA infant has a round face, a chubby body, and a plethoric or flushed complexion. The infant has enlarged internal

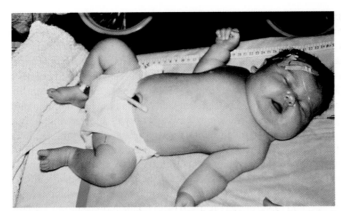

Fig. 35.6 Large for Gestational Age Infant. This infant of a diabetic mother weighed 5 kg (11 lb) at birth and exhibits the typical round face. (From Zitelli, B. J., & Davis, H. W. [2007]. *Atlas of pediatric physical diagnosis* [5th ed.]. Philadelphia: Mosby.)

organs (hepatosplenomegaly, splanchnomegaly, cardiomegaly) and increased body fat, especially around the shoulders. The placenta and umbilical cord are larger than average. These infants have normal head size; the brain is the only organ that is not enlarged. Infants of mothers with diabetes can be LGA but physiologically immature (Fig. 35.6).

Insulin is considered the primary growth hormone for intrauterine development. Maternal diabetes results in elevated maternal levels of amino acids and free fatty acids, along with hyperglycemia. As the nutrients cross the placenta, the fetal pancreas responds by producing insulin. The resulting accelerated protein synthesis, together with a deposition of excessive glycogen and fat stores, is responsible for the infant's enlarged size. The infant is at risk for hypoglycemia, hypocalcemia, hyperviscosity, and hyperbilirubinemia. The excessive amounts of metabolic fuels transported to the fetus from the mother and the consequent fetal hyperinsulinism represent the basic pathologic mechanism in diabetic pregnancy (Mangurten et al., 2015).

The excessive shoulder size in these infants often leads to dystocia. Macrosomic or LGA infants, born vaginally or by cesarean birth after a trial of labor, can incur birth trauma such as clavicle fracture or brachial plexus injury. Despite increased vigilance in screening and improvements in ultrasound techniques, the prenatal determination of fetal size can be difficult.

Birth Trauma and Perinatal Hypoxia

Birth injury (resulting from enlarged fetal size or method of birth) and perinatal hypoxia occur more often in infants of mothers with diabetes. Examples of birth trauma include cephalhematoma; paralysis of the facial nerve (cranial nerve VII) (see Fig. 35.5); fracture of the clavicle or humerus; brachial plexus paralysis, usually Erb-Duchenne palsy (see Fig. 35.4); and phrenic nerve paralysis, invariably associated with diaphragmatic paralysis.

Respiratory Distress Syndrome

RDS in infants of mothers with diabetes is much less common than in the past because of improved protocols to manage maternal glucose levels and enhanced antepartum fetal surveillance techniques to assess lung maturity (RDS is discussed in Chapter 34). Among infants born to women with well-controlled diabetes who give birth at term, the risk of RDS is similar to that of the general population. However, until the infant reaches 38 weeks' gestation, there is a significant increase in the risk of RDS (Blickstein et al., 2015). Maternal hyperglycemia can affect fetal lung maturity. In the fetus exposed to high levels of maternal glucose, synthesis of surfactant can be delayed because of the high

fetal serum levels of insulin and/or glucose. Late preterm birth may be indicated in cases where maternal glycemic control cannot be achieved as an inpatient or for those mothers who have abnormal antepartum fetal testing (American College of Obstetricians and Gynecologists [ACOG], 2018).

Hypoglycemia

Hypoglycemia affects many infants of diabetic mothers and is defined as a blood glucose concentration inadequate to support neurologic, organ, and tissue function; however, there is a lack of consensus among experts regarding the precise glucose level at which harm can occur. The lower limit for normal plasma glucose levels during the first 72 hours after birth is often cited as 40 to 45 mg/dL. There is concern about neurologic injury as a result of severe or prolonged hypoglycemia, especially in combination with ischemia (American Academy of Pediatrics [AAP] & ACOG, 2017; Rozance, McGowan, Price-Douglas, et al., 2016). Macrosomic, LGA, and preterm infants have the highest risk of hypoglycemia. After constant exposure to high circulating levels of glucose, hyperplasia of the fetal pancreas occurs, resulting in hyperinsulinemia. Disruption of the maternal glucose supply occurs with the clamping of the umbilical cord, and the neonate's blood glucose level decreases rapidly in the presence of fetal hyperinsulinism. It can take several days for the newborn to regulate the secretion of insulin in response to a lower postnatal supply of glucose. Hypoglycemia is most common in the macrosomic or LGA infant, but the nurse should monitor blood glucose levels in all infants of mothers with known or suspected diabetes.

Hypoglycemia most frequently occurs within the first 1 to 6 hours after birth. Signs of hypoglycemia include jitteriness, apnea, tachypnea, hypotonia, decreased activity, and cyanosis. Many infants with hypoglycemia remain asymptomatic. Asymptomatic hypoglycemia can be just as concerning as symptomatic hypoglycemia and has been associated with a dose-dependent increased risk of poor executive function and visual motor function (McKinlay, Alsweiler, Anstice, et al., 2017). Significant hypoglycemia can result in seizures. Physiologically, there is a direct correlation between temperature regulation, glucose homeostasis, and respiratory distress. Commonly a problem with one of these systems will result in challenges with one or both of the other systems. Regardless of the presence of clinical manifestations, severe or persistent hypoglycemia may require continuous IV glucose. Infants who require continuous IV fluids are typically cared for in the NICU.

Hypocalcemia and Hypomagnesemia

Hypocalcemia and hypomagnesemia can occur in infants of mothers with insulin-dependent diabetes although they are not usually present until 48 to 72 hours after birth. The likelihood of hypocalcemia is related to the severity and duration of maternal diabetes. It is often associated with preterm birth, birth trauma, and perinatal asphyxia. Hypomagnesemia is believed to develop because of maternal renal losses that occur in diabetes. Jitteriness is a sign of both hypocalcemia and hypomagnesemia, as well as hypoglycemia. Supplemental calcium therapy may be required. Magnesium levels usually return to normal without treatment (Blickstein et al., 2015).

Cardiomyopathy

All infants of mothers with diabetes need careful observation for cardiomyopathy (disease affecting the structure and function of the heart) because an increased heart size is often found in these infants. Cardiomyopathy is more likely to occur in cases of poorly controlled maternal diabetes. Two types of cardiomyopathies can occur: hypertrophic and nonhypertrophic. Clinicians must be able to identify the type of lesion correctly so that appropriate therapy is instituted. Both types of lesions are associated with respiratory symptoms and congestive heart failure.

Hypertrophic cardiomyopathy is characterized by a hypercontractile and thickened myocardium. The ventricular walls are thickened, as is the septum, which in severe cases results in outflow tract obstructions. Additionally, the mitral valve is poorly functioning. In nonhypertrophic cardiomyopathy, the myocardium is poorly contractile and overstretched. The ventricles are larger, and no outflow obstruction is found. Most infants are asymptomatic, but severe outflow obstruction can cause left ventricular heart failure (Blickstein et al., 2015).

Hyperbilirubinemia and Polycythemia

Infants of diabetic mothers are at increased risk of developing polycythemia and hyperbilirubinemia. Hyperinsulinism increases the newborn's metabolic rate which increases oxygen demand leading to mild chronic hypoxemia. This state of hypoxemia stimulates the production of red blood cells, also known as polycythemia (Blickstein et al., 2015). Polycythemia increases blood viscosity, thereby impairing circulation. In addition, this greater number of red blood cells to be hemolyzed increases the potential bilirubin load that the neonate must clear, thus increasing the likelihood of hyperbilirubinemia. Bruising associated with birth of a macrosomic or LGA infant further increases the overall bilirubin load that the neonate will need to clear.

Nursing Interventions

Nursing care depends on the neonate's particular problems. General care of the compromised infant is addressed in Chapter 34. If the maternal blood glucose level was well controlled throughout the pregnancy, the infant may require only monitoring. Because euglycemia (normal blood glucose levels) is not always possible, the nurse must promptly recognize and treat any consequences of maternal diabetes that arise. The most common problems experienced by infants of diabetic mothers that require intervention include birth trauma and perinatal asphyxia; RDS; difficult metabolic transition, including hypoglycemia and hypocalcemia; and congenital anomalies (see previous sections and the Clinical Reasoning Case Study)

❓ CLINICAL REASONING CASE STUDY

Infant of Diabetic Mother

Melissa is a female neonate born at 37 weeks of gestation to a G 2 P 1 mother, who was diagnosed with gestational diabetes. Following a spontaneous vaginal birth, Melissa received Apgar scores of 7 at 1 min and 8 at 5 min. Melissa weighs 3900 g (8 lbs 9 oz) and appears plethoric pink with a moderate amount of subcutaneous fat. She is noted to be slightly jittery at 30 min of age. In planning care for Melissa, the nurse needs to take into consideration the effects of maternal diabetes on the newborn.

1. What is the priority concern or client need in this situation? Support your answer with data as stated in the case.
2. List other client needs/problems in this case.
3. Identify any additional information or assessment data that is needed by the nurse in planning care for this client.
4. What nursing actions are appropriate in this situation?
    a. What is the priority nursing action? (What should the nurse do first?)
    b. Describe other nursing interventions that are important to providing optimal client care.
5. Describe the roles/responsibilities of the interprofessional health care team members (other than nurses) who may be involved in providing care for this client.

NEONATAL INFECTIONS

The newborn infant is susceptible to infection because of the immature immune system. Immunoglobulin G (IgG) crosses the placenta to provide protection to the newborn. IgG values typically reach a nadir at 3 to 4 months of age for term newborns and at 3 months for preterm infants. By 10 to 12 months of age, virtually all of the infant's IgG is endogenous (Weitkamp, Lewis, & Levy, 2018). IgA and IgM do not cross the placenta and both require time to reach optimal levels after birth. Phagocytosis is less efficient. Serum complement levels are inadequate; serum complement (C1 through C6) is involved in immunologic reactions, some of which kill or lyse bacteria and enhance phagocytosis. Dysmaturity seen with intrauterine growth restriction (IUGR) and preterm and postterm birth further compromises the neonate's immune system.

Neonatal infections can be acquired in utero (congenital infection), during the intrapartum period, and postnatally. Prenatal acquisition of infection occurs by organisms placentally transferred directly into the fetal circulatory system or transmitted from infected amniotic fluid, such as with herpes simplex virus (HSV), cytomegalovirus (CMV), or rubella. Microorganisms can ascend from the vagina and pass through the cervix into the uterus. Intrauterine infection can result in miscarriage, preterm birth, stillbirth, and neonatal infection at birth or in the postnatal period.

During birth, contact with an infected birth canal can result in generalized or local infection. The upper airway and the GI tract are the principal pathways for generalized infections. The conjunctiva and the oral cavity are the usual sites of local infection.

Postnatal infection is sometimes acquired during resuscitation or through the introduction of foreign objects such as indwelling catheters or endotracheal tubes, or through breastfeeding. Health care–associated infections can be transferred to the infant by the hands of the parents or health care personnel, or spread from contaminated equipment. The umbilicus is a receptive site for cutaneous infection leading to sepsis.

Sepsis

Neonatal sepsis is one of the most significant causes of neonatal morbidity and mortality. It can be defined as a systemic inflammatory response syndrome (SIRS) that occurs secondary to infection. SIRS is recognized by the presence of two or more of these signs/symptoms: hypothermia or fever, tachypnea or hyperventilation, tachycardia, and high or low white blood cell count (Leonard & Dobbs, 2015).

Neonatal sepsis is classified into two patterns according to the time of presentation. Early-onset sepsis is defined as invasive bacterial infection of the blood and/or CSF that occurs within the first 7 days of life (Kuzniewicz, Puopolo, Fischer, et al. 2017). The two most common microorganisms involved in early-onset infection are group B streptococci (GBS) and *Escherichia coli*; together they account for approximately 70% of early-onset infections. Other culprits include *Streptococci viridans*, *Streptococci pneumoniae*, *Enterococcus*, *Haemophilus influenzae*, and *Listeria monocytogenes*. Risk factors include prematurity, prolonged rupture of membranes, procedures during pregnancy or labor/birth, resuscitation after birth, maternal fever, and GBS colonization or bacteriuria (Table 35.2) (Leonard & Dobbs, 2015; Simonsen, Anderson-Berry, Delair, et al., 2014).

Late-onset sepsis, occurring at approximately 7 to 30 days of age, can include maternally derived infection or health care–acquired infection. The offending organisms are usually staphylococci, *Klebsiella* organisms, enterococci, *E. coli*, and *Pseudomonas*, or *Candida* species. Coagulase-negative staphylococci, considered to be primarily a contaminant in older children and adults, is the most common cause of

TABLE 35.2 Risk Factors for Neonatal Sepsis

Source	Risk Factors
Maternal	Low socioeconomic status
	Late or no prenatal care
	Poor nutrition
	Substance abuse
	Recently acquired sexually transmitted infection
	Untreated focal infection (urinary tract, vaginal, or cervical)
	Systemic infection
	Fever
Intrapartum	Premature rupture of membranes
	Maternal fever
	Chorioamnionitis
	Prolonged labor
	Preterm labor
	Use of fetal scalp electrode
Neonatal	Multiple gestation
	Male
	Birth asphyxia
	Meconium aspiration
	Congenital anomalies of skin or mucous membranes
	Metabolic disorders (e.g., galactosemia)
	Low birth weight
	Preterm birth
	Malnourishment
	Formula feeding
	Prolonged hospitalization
	Mechanical ventilation
	Umbilical artery catheterization or use of other vascular catheters

Data from Anderson-Berry, A. L., Bellig, L. L., & Ohning, B. L. (2015). Neonatal sepsis. *Medscape*. Retrieved from https://emedicine .medscape.com/article/978352-overview; and Ferrieri, P., & Wallen, L. D. (2018). Newborn sepsis and meningitis. In C. A. Gleason & S. E. Juul (Eds.), *Avery's diseases of the newborn* (10th ed.). Philadelphia: Elsevier.

BOX 35.1 Common Clinical Signs of Neonatal Sepsis

- Abnormal neurologic status: irritability, lethargy, poor feeding
- Abnormal temperature: hyperthermia or hypothermia
- Apnea
- Bleeding problems: petechiae, purpura, oozing
- Cardiovascular compromise: tachycardia, hypotension, poor perfusion
- Cyanosis
- Gastrointestinal symptoms: abdominal distention, emesis, diarrhea
- Jaundice
- Respiratory distress: tachypnea, increased work of breathing, hypoxemia
- Seizures

Data from Ferrieri, P., & Wallen, L. D. (2018). Newborn sepsis and meningitis. In C. A. Gleason, S. E. Juul, (Eds.), *Avery's diseases of the newborn* (10th ed.). Philadelphia: Elsevier.

with a high morbidity rate (Ku, Boggess, & Cohen-Wolkowiez, 2015). Gastroenteritis is sporadic, depending on epidemic outbreaks. Local infections such as conjunctivitis and omphalitis occur frequently, but incidence rates are unavailable. Sequelae to septicemia include meningitis, disseminated intravascular coagulation (DIC), and septic shock.

 ## CARE MANAGEMENT

The development of systemic infection in the newborn can be influenced by maternal, peripartum, and neonatal risk factors. Onset within the first 48 hours of life is more often associated with prenatal or perinatal predisposing factors. Onset after 2 or 3 days more frequently reflects disease acquired at or subsequent to birth.

Assessment

The earliest clinical signs of neonatal sepsis are nonspecific and include lethargy; poor feeding; and temperature instability, particularly hypothermia. The nurse or parent may simply note that the infant is just not doing as well as before. Differential diagnosis can be difficult because signs of sepsis are similar to signs of noninfectious neonatal problems such as anemia or hypoglycemia. Additional clinical and laboratory information and appropriate cultures supplement the findings described. Box 35.1 lists common signs and symptoms of sepsis.

Laboratory studies are key to diagnosis of neonatal infection. Specimens for cultures include blood, CSF, and urine. Fluids such as urine and CSF can be evaluated by counterimmunoelectrophoresis or latex agglutination to help identify the bacteria. A complete blood count (CBC) with differential is performed. The leukocyte count is not a reliable indicator of sepsis; however, the total neutrophil count, immature to total neutrophil ratio (I/T), absolute neutrophil count, platelet count, procalcitonin, and C-reactive protein can be used to diagnose sepsis. It is important to note that these tests are likely adjuncts for the confirmation of neonatal sepsis; a combination of these tests and clinical signs often alert the practitioner to the need for treatment. Additional diagnostic tests that may be used include sedimentation rate, cytokine assays, and nucleic acid amplification testing (Leonard & Dobbs, 2015; Simonsen et al., 2014).

Interventions

Standard treatment for early-onset sepsis includes ampicillin and an aminoglycoside. Late-onset sepsis is treated with vancomycin and an aminoglycoside. Results of blood cultures determine the need for

late-onset infection in the extremely low-birth-weight (ELBW) infant (Kuzniewicz et al., 2017; Simonsen et al., 2014). Bacterial invasion can occur through sites such as the umbilical stump; the skin; mucous membranes of the eye, nose, pharynx, and ear; and internal systems such as the respiratory, nervous, urinary, and GI systems.

Viral infections that are acquired perinatally can cause stillbirth, intrauterine infection, congenital malformations, and acute disease. These pathogens also can cause chronic infection, with subtle manifestations that can be recognized only after a prolonged period. It is important to recognize the manifestations of infections in the neonatal period to treat the acute infection, to prevent health care–associated infections in other infants, and to anticipate effects on the infant's subsequent growth and development.

Fungal infections are of great concern in the immunocompromised or premature infant. Occasionally fungal infections such as thrush are found in otherwise healthy term infants.

Infection continues to be a significant factor in fetal and neonatal morbidity and mortality. Pneumonia, the most common form of neonatal infection, is one of the leading causes of perinatal death and is caused by many of the same organisms that cause sepsis. Fortunately, the incidence of bacterial meningitis is low; it is a serious disease specific antimicrobial therapy. Duration of treatment depends on the site of infection and the neonate's clinical response (Leonard & Dobbs, 2015).

Antepartum viral infection can be treated with antiviral medications to decrease viral replication and fetal transmission of disease; neonates can also be treated with antiviral medications such as acyclovir and ganciclovir.

Breastfeeding or feeding the newborn expressed breast milk from the mother is encouraged. Breast milk provides protective mechanisms (see Chapter 25). Colostrum contains IgA, which offers protection against infection in the GI tract. Human milk contains iron-binding protein that exerts a bacteriostatic effect on *E. coli*. Human milk also contains macrophages and lymphocytes. The vulnerability of infants to common mucosal pathogens such as respiratory syncytial virus can be reduced by passive transfer of maternal immunity in the colostrum and breast milk.

Nursing considerations. Vigilant assessment continues during and after treatment. The nurse must be alert for signs of septicemia, meningitis, DIC, necrotizing enterocolitis, pneumonia, and septic shock.

Administering medications, monitoring IV infusions, taking precautions when performing treatments, and following isolation procedures are among nursing interventions for neonates with confirmed or suspected sepsis.

💊 MEDICATION ALERT

It is important to administer the prescribed dose of antimicrobial medication as soon as possible after it is prepared to avoid loss of drug stability. If the IV fluid the infant is receiving contains electrolytes, vitamins, or other medications, the nurse should check with the hospital pharmacy before adding antibiotics. The antibiotic (or any medication) can be deactivated or can form a precipitate when combined with other substances. To prevent this, a secondary line of the prescribed solution may be attached with a needleless connector at the infusion site.

Care must be taken in suctioning secretions from any newborn's oropharynx or trachea; the secretions may be infected. Routine suctioning is not recommended and can further compromise the infant's immune status, as well as cause hypoxia and increase ICP. Isolation procedures are implemented as indicated according to hospital policy. Isolation protocols change rapidly, and the nurse is urged to participate in continuing education and in-service programs to remain up-to-date.

Preventive measures. Hand hygiene is the single most important measure in preventing the spread of infection. Appropriate hand hygiene protocols should be in place and frequent education provided to ensure that good hand hygiene practices are followed by staff and families. Other measures include implementing Standard Precautions, carefully and thoroughly cleaning the environment and equipment, frequently replacing used equipment (e.g., changing IV tubing per hospital protocol, cleaning resuscitation and ventilation equipment), and appropriately disposing of excrement and linens. Overcrowding must be avoided in nurseries. Guidelines for space, visitation, and general infection control in areas where newborns receive care have been established and published (AAP & ACOG, 2017).

Specific newborn care procedures are intended to prevent infection. These include instilling antibiotic ointment in newborns' eyes 1 to 2 hours after birth, bathing, and cord care (see Chapter 24).

While the fetus and newborn may be affected by a plethora of infections, some of the more common ones are discussed in the following

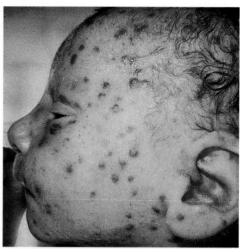

Fig. 35.7 Neonatal Cytomegalovirus Infection. Typical rash seen in a severely affected infant. (Courtesy David A. Clarke, Philadelphia, PA.)

sections. The infections are categorized according to the causative organism as viral, bacterial, protozoal, or fungal.

Viral Infections

Cytomegalovirus

CMV is the most common congenital viral infection in the U.S., occurring in approximately 0.5% to 1% of live births. Maternal-fetal transmission of CMV occurs in 40% of mothers with a primary CMV infection during pregnancy and approximately 1% to 2% of mothers who are already seropositive. CMV can be transmitted during birth or through breast milk while the mother has acute CMV infection; however, it is unlikely to result in clinical illness in the infant. It can also be transmitted by blood transfusion (AAP, 2018; Bialas, Swamy, & Permar, 2015).

Most newborns with congenital CMV infection are asymptomatic at birth. Death occurs in 3% to 10% of infants with symptomatic CMV disease. Clinical manifestations at birth can include rash, petechiae, jaundice, hepatosplenomegaly, IUGR, microcephaly, chorioretinitis, and intracerebral calcifications (Fig. 35.7). Approximately 10% to 15% of these newborns will show signs of CMV-associated sequelae which include thrombocytopenia, hepatitis, chorioretinitis, sensorineural hearing loss, cognitive impairment, and IUGR. In the United States, CMV is the primary nongenetic cause of sensorineural hearing loss in children (AAP, 2018; Bialas et al., 2015).

Improved neurodevelopmental and audiologic outcomes have been noted when symptomatic newborns are treated with oral valganciclovir for 6 months. Treatment is only recommended for infants who are symptomatic. Neutropenia is a serious side effect of valganciclovir therapy, necessitating frequent lab testing. Infants who are not able to tolerate the oral medication will be treated with IV ganciclovir. Because treatment can reduce these long-term sequelae, large-scale infant CMV testing is being investigated (AAP, 2018; Bialas et al., 2015).

Varicella

Varicella (chickenpox) is an acute infectious disease caused by the varicella-zoster virus (VZV), a highly contagious human herpesvirus (AAP & ACOG, 2017). After the primary infection, VZV remains in the body as a latent infection, usually in the sensory ganglia. If the latent infection reactivates, this causes herpes zoster (shingles).

Approximately 95% of women in the childbearing years are immune to varicella; therefore the risk of infection in pregnancy is low. For pregnant women with a primary varicella infection, the rate of transmission to the fetus is estimated to be approximately 25% (Schleiss & Marsh, 2018). When transmission to the fetus occurs during the first or early second trimester, congenital varicella can result in fetal death, limb hypoplasia, damage to the CNS, and eye abnormalities. When maternal varicella infection occurs between 8 and 20 weeks of gestation, the congenital varicella rate is 2%. Congenital varicella syndrome is rare after 20 weeks gestation (AAP, 2018). Maternal infection that occurs in the third trimester is not associated with congenital varicella infection, but it does increase the risk of the newborn having neonatal varicella (Schleiss & Marsh). Varicella infection is more serious for the newborn if the mother develops varicella between 5 days prior to and 2 days after birth because the infant's immune system is immature and there has been insufficient time for transplacental transfer of maternal antibodies. The death rate is high among these infants. Infants born to mothers with this time frame of exposure should receive varicella zoster immune globulin (VariZIG) or immune globulin intravenous (IGIV) as soon as possible after birth (AAP, 2018; Schleiss & Marsh, 2018).

Perinatal varicella may cause a generalized, pruritic, vesicular rash or only a few lesions. Complications can include pneumonia, CNS involvement, thrombocytopenia, and hepatitis (AAP, 2018). Neonatal varicella is treated with IV acyclovir.

Seroimmune pregnant women exposed to active chickenpox can be given VariZIG, which does not reduce the incidence of infection but should decrease the effects of the virus on the fetus. The immune globulin must be given within 96 hours of exposure to be effective (AAP, 2018).

Rubella

While congenital rubella syndrome (CRS) in the United States is rare, there are an estimated 100,000 cases worldwide each year (Centers for Disease Control and Prevention [CDC], 2017). The risk of a congenitally infected infant varies with the gestational age of the fetus when maternal infection occurs; the earlier in pregnancy that the infection occurs, the more severe the effects (Schleiss & Marsh, 2018). Rubella can cause miscarriage or fetal death. If the rubella infection is mild, there may be minimal or no effects on the fetus. Rubella infection in pregnancy is one of the few known causes of autism (AAP, 2018).

Congenital rubella syndrome includes cataracts or glaucoma, hearing loss (the most common sign), and cardiac defects (pulmonary artery stenosis, patent ductus arteriosus, or coarctation of the aorta). Multiple other abnormalities may also be present, including low birth weight, microphthalmia, hypotonia, hepatosplenomegaly, thrombocytopenic purpura, dermatoglyphic abnormalities, bony radiolucencies, microcephaly, and brain wave abnormalities. Severe infection can result in fetal death. Communication disorders, hearing deficits, microcephaly by 1 to 3 years of age, and cognitive or motor impairments have been reported after the newborn period (Schleiss & Marsh, 2018).

⚡ **SAFETY ALERT**

Contact isolation is recommended for 1 year for infants born with signs of CRS and for those whose mothers have a history of rubella during pregnancy. The contact isolation may be discontinued prior to 1 year if the infant has two cultures (e.g., urine, throat) that are negative for rubella, done 1 month apart after the age of 3 months (AAP, 2018).

Hepatitis B

The perinatal transmission of hepatitis B virus (HBV) from an infected mother to her fetus usually occurs during the blood exposure that occurs during labor and birth. The risk of transmission of HBV to the newborn ranges from 70% to 90% when the mother is seropositive for both hepatitis B surface antigen (HBsAg) and hepatitis B e antigen (HBeAg). If the mother is HBsAg positive but HBeAg negative, the risk of transmission is much lower (AAP, 2018).

Transmission can occur through breast milk, but antigens also develop in formula-fed infants at the same or a higher rate; thus breastfeeding is not contraindicated. Diagnosis is made by viral culture of amniotic fluid, as well as by the presence of HBsAg and IgM in the cord blood or infant serum.

The majority of infants who become HBsAg positive are asymptomatic at birth, although some show evidence of acute viral hepatitis. There is no specific treatment for acute HBV infection. Follow-up is essential to monitor for chronic liver disease (AAP, 2018).

The CDC recommends universal HBV immunization of all neonates prior to hospital discharge and subsequent completion of the recommended vaccine series (see Medication Guide: Chapter 24). Any infant born to a mother who is seropositive for HBV should receive HBV vaccine and hepatitis B immune globulin (HBIg) within 12 hours after birth and should complete the recommended vaccine series, followed by postvaccination serologic testing. If the mother's HBV status is unknown when she is admitted to the birthing facility, she should have serologic testing; her infant should receive the HBV vaccine within 12 hours after birth and if she is seropositive, HBIg should be administered to the newborn as soon as possible (Schille, Vellozzi, Reingold, et al., 2018).

Human Immunodeficiency Virus

HIV among newborns has declined significantly since the 1990s. If a pregnant woman with HIV takes her daily antiviral medication during pregnancy and in the perinatal period, and gives antiviral medication to her newborn for the recommended 4 to 6 weeks, the likelihood of neonatal infection is approximately 1% (CDC, 2019).

Preventive strategies have helped reduce the incidence of perinatal transmission of HIV. Universal HIV testing for all pregnant women allows for early identification and treatment of HIV-positive women during pregnancy, which decreases the risk of transmission to the fetus. Other strategies to prevent neonatal HIV infection include administration of antiviral medications to women with HIV viral loads greater than 1000 copies/mL, complete avoidance of breastfeeding, complete avoidance of premastication, and elective cesarean birth before labor and rupture of membranes after reaching 38 completed weeks of gestation (AAP, 2018; CDC, 2019).

Transmission of HIV from the mother to the fetus can occur transplacentally at various gestational ages. The risk of infection in an infant born to an untreated HIV-positive nonbreastfeeding mother is approximately 25%. Transmission most often occurs during birth. Globally, breastfeeding accounts for one third to one half of perinatal transmission; this is more likely in mothers who acquire HIV late in their pregnancy (AAP, 2018).

The preferred test for diagnosis of HIV infection in infants is the human immunodeficiency virus (HIV) deoxyribonucleic acid (DNA) nested polymerase chain reaction (PCR) assay, which is performed on neonatal blood, not cord blood. It may require 28 days for definitive results to become available (AAP, 2018). Follow-up testing for infants born to HIV-positive mothers is recommended at several intervals within the first year of life.

Typically the HIV-infected neonate is asymptomatic at birth. Early-onset illness (i.e., virus detected within 48 hours of birth) is attributed to prenatal infection. These infants develop opportunistic infections (*Candida* and *Pneumocystis jiroveci* pneumonia) and experience rapid progression of immunodeficiency that often results in death during the first 1 to 2 years of life.

The remainder of infants seroconvert over a period of months to years. By 1 year of age, the vast majority of perinatally infected infants show signs of infection. Some children infected at birth show no signs of disease 8 to 10 years later. The age of onset of symptoms predicts the length of survival.

The presenting signs and symptoms of HIV infection vary from severe immunodeficiency to nonspecific findings such as growth failure, parotitis, and recurrent or persistent upper respiratory tract infections. In the first year of life, lymphadenopathy and hepatosplenomegaly are common. The infant can have fever, chronic diarrhea, chronic dermatitis, interstitial pneumonitis, persistent thrush, and AIDS-defining opportunistic infections. Common secondary opportunistic infections include pneumonia, candidiasis, CMV, cryptosporidiosis, herpes simplex or herpes zoster, and disseminated varicella (AAP, 2018).

Although it is rare for an infant to be born with symptoms of HIV infection, all infants born to seropositive mothers should be presumed to be HIV positive until proven otherwise. Management begins by implementing Standard Universal Precautions. The infant should be bathed and cleansed of maternal secretions as soon as possible after birth. These newborns should also begin their antiretroviral (ARV) prophylaxis as soon as possible, preferably within 12 hours of life. When the mother has been adequately treated during pregnancy and labor and birth, the newborn is usually treated for 6 weeks. When the mother is not adequately treated, the newborn may be treated with a two- or three-drug ARV regimen (AAP, 2018).

Counseling regarding self-care of the mother, care of the infant, and future pregnancies should be provided for the mother and her partner. The risk for transmission among members of the same household is minimal. These families may benefit from social service involvement in their care. They must understand the importance of follow-up medical care for the mother and her newborn.

Herpes Simplex

HSV infections can cause significant morbidity and mortality in the newborn. Neonatal HSV infection occurs in 1 in 3000 to 1 in 20,000 live births in the U.S. (AAP, 2018).

Congenital infection is rare and is characterized by in utero destruction of normally formed organs, resulting in IUGR, microcephaly, hydranencephaly, chorioretinitis, or fetal death. In the majority of cases, HSV is transmitted from mother to neonate through viral shedding during labor and birth. This can occur whether or not the mother has active lesions. Primary maternal infections after 32 weeks of gestation present a higher risk for the fetus and newborn than recurrent infections or those occurring in early pregnancy. Less commonly, HSV is transmitted to the neonate after birth by the mother, family member, or hospital personnel (AAP, 2018; James & Kimberlin, 2015).

> ### ⚡ SAFETY ALERT
>
> Health care professionals (HCPs) with herpetic mouth lesions (cold sores) who provide care to newborns should practice strict hand hygiene and wear a mask to cover the lesions. Strict hand hygiene should prevent transmission of herpes simplex virus (HSV) infection to clients from HCPs with genital lesions. Any HCP with a herpetic whitlow (primary HSV infection of the terminal segment of a finger) should not provide care to immunocompromised clients or to newborns. Parents should be taught that household members with herpetic lesions of the mouth or skin should follow similar precautions plus avoid kissing or nuzzling the infant (AAP, 2018).

Clinically, neonatal HSV infections are classified as disseminated infection (25%); CNS disease (30%); or localized infection of the skin, eye, or mouth (SEM) (45%); there can be overlap of symptoms from these categories (AAP, 2018). Although the incubation period for HSV is

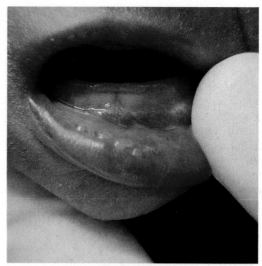

Fig. 35.8 Neonatal Herpes Simplex Virus Oral Lesions. (Courtesy David A. Clarke, Philadelphia, PA.)

1 to 7 days, the onset of symptoms varies with the type of infection. Disseminated infections are sepsis-like and can involve virtually every organ system but are most likely to involve the liver, adrenal glands, GI system, and lungs. In CNS disease, blood-borne seeding of the brain results in multiple lesions of cortical hemorrhagic necrosis. It also can occur alone or in association with SEM lesions. Brain involvement usually manifests in the second to fourth weeks of life. The presenting manifestations include lethargy, poor feeding, irritability, and local or generalized seizures. If untreated, the mortality rate in CNS disease approaches 50%; the vast majority of survivors experience severe sequelae such as microcephaly and blindness (AAP, 2018; James & Kimberlin, 2015).

The majority of newborns infected with HSV have a localized infection affecting their skin, eyes, and/or mouth (Fig. 35.8). Skin vesicles are often present at birth and tend to recur. Without treatment, CNS or disseminated disease develop in 70% of the infants with skin vesicles. Ocular involvement, which can occur alone, can be secondary to either HSV-1 or HSV-2. Ocular disease may not be discovered for months. Microphthalmos, cataracts, and corneal scarring can result from chorioretinitis, keratitis, and retinal hemorrhage (Baley & Gonzalez, 2015; James & Kimberlin, 2015).

Care.management depends on maternal history. Cesarean birth is recommended for women with active genital lesions. All infants born by cesarean or vaginal birth to women with active lesions should be placed on contact precautions and are closely monitored for signs of infection. Because neonatal risk of HSV is greatest if this is the mother's primary infection, surface cultures and blood and surface polymerase chain reaction (PCR) for HSV, serum alanine transaminase (ALT) and CSF cell count, chemistries, and PCR for HSV are done 24 hours after birth, or sooner if the infant is preterm, ill, or there was prolonged rupture of membranes. Treatment with acyclovir is started after the evaluation. If the maternal infection is deemed to be recurrent and neonatal testing is negative, the acyclovir may be discontinued. If the neonate is born to a mother with history of recurrent lesions, HSV cultures and PCR are done after 24 hours and the infant is observed carefully (AAP, 2018; Baley & Gonzalez, 2015).

The infant can be discharged with the mother if the infant's cultures are negative for the virus. Parents are instructed to observe the newborn for signs of HSV infection. As long as no suspicious lesions are present on the mother's breasts, breastfeeding is allowed.

For neonatal HSV, therapy includes general supportive measures, as well as treatment with acyclovir. Duration of treatment is 21 days for infants with disseminated or CNS disease and 14 days for the SEM form of the disease. For infants with ocular involvement, a topical ophthalmic medication (trifluridine or ganciclovir) is used (AAP, 2018).

All infants with HSV disease should have an ophthalmologic examination and neuroimaging to establish a baseline assessment of these areas. Those with CNS involvement should have a lumbar puncture near the end of treatment to ensure that the CSF has been cleared. The neurodevelopmental outcomes for these children can be improved by continuing oral acyclovir for 6 months following the treatment of acute HSV infection (AAP, 2018; James & Kimberlin, 2015).

Enteroviruses

Enteroviruses include coxsackieviruses, echoviruses, and numbered enteroviruses. Nonpolio enteroviruses are among the most common viruses that infect humans. Enteroviruses are spread primarily through fecal-oral and respiratory routes. Enteroviruses can survive on environmental surfaces for long periods of time, and may cause hospital nursery or other institutional outbreaks (AAP, 2018).

In utero transmission of enteroviruses can occur, but the most frequent mode of transmission to the neonate occurs during and after birth through contact with maternal blood, cervical or vaginal secretions, or fecal material (Schleiss & Marsh, 2018).

The usual incubation period is 3 to 6 days. Presenting symptoms can include fever, irritability, lethargy, poor feeding, rash, respiratory symptoms, and GI symptoms. Infection can be severe and include myocarditis, meningitis, respiratory distress, and hepatitis. Deaths are usually due to multiorgan involvement (AAP, 2018).

No specific therapy is available for the treatment of enterovirus infections. Intravenous immunoglobulin may be used in life-threatening situations or for the treatment of infections in immunocompromised clients. There are reports of treatment with the antiviral medication pleconaril, although it is not currently commercially available (AAP, 2018; Schleiss & Marsh, 2018).

Parvovirus B19

Parvovirus B19 infection is well known in older children as erythema infectiosum (EI) or fifth disease. It is often called the "slapped cheek illness" because of the characteristic facial appearance of the affected child. Other clinical manifestations include fever, malaise, myalgia, and a rash.

This infection is transmitted by vertical transmission from mother to fetus, contact with respiratory tract secretions, and exposure to blood or blood products. During pregnancy, infection can result in miscarriage, fetal anemia, hydrops fetalis, IUGR, or stillbirth. Parvovirus B19 does not appear to be a teratogen (AAP, 2018).

In most cases, only supportive care is needed. Intrauterine blood transfusions may be indicated for cases of hydrops fetalis (AAP, 2018).

Influenza

Pregnant women who contract influenza are at risk for complications, especially pulmonary problems. Complications appear to correlate with the severity of maternal infection and may include first trimester miscarriage, preterm birth, or stillbirth. Influenza vaccination is recommended for all pregnant women as maternal immunity is the only protection for the newborn against the influenza virus (AAP & ACOG, 2017).

Newborns who become ill with influenza are at high risk for severe complications. To help protect newborns, if the mother has influenza infection during the intrapartum or immediate postpartum period, she should be separated from her newborn. Separation should continue until the mother has received antiviral medication for 48 hours, she is afebrile without antipyretics for longer than 24 hours, and she is

capable of controlling her respiratory secretions and cough. If separation is not possible, the newborn should be kept at least 6 feet away from the mother and should be cared for by an adult who is well. If the mother is the only available caregiver, she should wear a face mask when feeding or in close contact with her infant. These practices should continue for at least 7 days after the onset of maternal symptoms (AAP & ACOG, 2017; CDC, 2018).

Zika

Zika virus is recognized as a mosquito-borne teratogen that can cause fetal loss, microcephaly, and other serious neurologic defects. The most severely affected fetuses with congenital Zika syndrome have microcephaly; brain, ocular, and optic nerve anomalies; congenital contractures; and other neurologic problems such as hearing loss, swallowing dysfunction, hypertonia, hypotonia, irritability, and tremors (AAP, 2018).

Bacterial Infections

Group B Streptococcus

GBS is a leading cause of perinatal infections, including bacteremia, endometritis, chorioamnionitis, and urinary tract infections (UTIs). In the newborn, it can cause focal or systemic disease. GBS commonly lives in the human GI and genitourinary tracts. Colonization during pregnancy can be continuous or intermittent (AAP, 2018). The practice of giving prophylactic antibiotics to women in labor who are GBS positive has significantly reduced the incidence and severity of early-onset GBS infection in the newborn. The incidence of early-onset neonatal GBS infection is 0.25/1000 live births (AAP, 2018).

Risk factors for the development of early-onset GBS infection include preterm birth, rupture of membranes of more than 18 hours before birth, intrapartum maternal fever (>38°C [100.4°F]), previous infant with invasive GBS disease, maternal GBS bacteriuria during the current pregnancy, intraamniotic infection (chorioamnionitis), maternal age less than 20 years old, intrauterine fetal monitoring, and African-American ethnicity (AAP, 2018; Ferrieri & Wallen, 2018).

Early-onset disease develops during the first 7 days, most often within 24 hours after birth, and usually results from vertical transmission from the birth canal. It manifests as systemic infection or respiratory illness that mimics the symptoms of severe respiratory distress. The infant can rapidly develop pneumonia, shock, or meningitis. The mortality rate for early-onset infection ranges from 1% to 3%, with higher rates among preterm infants. Late-onset GBS infections typically occur from 7 days to 3 months of age. Infection can result from vertical transmission or from health care–acquired infection or community exposure. Late-onset infection is associated with meningitis, osteomyelitis, and septic arthritis. Mortality rates are lower than for early-onset infection (AAP, 2018; Ferrieri & Wallen, 2018).

For newborns with suspected GBS infection, the usual treatment is ampicillin in combination with an aminoglycoside. If GBS is identified as the cause of infection, penicillin G alone may be given. The dosage of ampicillin and/or penicillin G and length of treatment are dependent on whether bacteremia or meningitis is being treated (AAP, 2018). Fig. 35.9 provides a sample algorithm for managing a neonate whose mother received intrapartum antibiotics for prevention (IAP) of GBS disease in the newborn or suspected chorioamnionitis.

Escherichia coli

E. coli is the second most common pathogen causing sepsis and meningitis in newborns (Ferrieri & Wallen, 2018). It is found in the GI tract soon after birth and makes up the bulk of human fecal flora. *E. coli* can cause a variety of neonatal infections, including omphalitis, diarrheal illness, pneumonia, peritonitis, UTI, and meningitis. Risk factors for the development of *E. coli* infections in the newborn include preterm birth, low birth weight, maternal infection, and prolonged rupture of membranes.

Neonates most often acquire *E. coli* from the maternal vagina or rectum during birth, although it also can be hospital acquired through person-to-person transmission or from the hospital environment. Exposure to *E. coli* can result in no infection, infection without illness, gastroenteritis, or rarely, septicemia. Symptoms can appear within the first 24 hours after birth or several weeks later. Clinical signs of *E. coli*

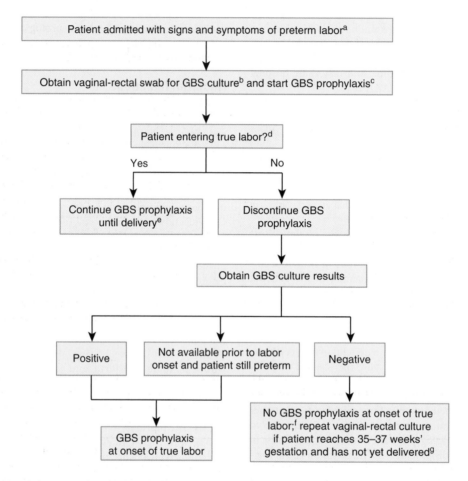

^a At <37 weeks and 0 days' gestation.

^b If patient has undergone vaginal-rectal GBS culture within the preceding 5 weeks, the results of that culture should guide management. GBS-colonized women should receive intrapartum antibiotic prophylaxis. No antibiotics are indicated for GBS prophylaxis if a vaginal-rectal screen within 5 weeks was negative.

^c See Figure 8 for recommended antibiotic regimens.

^d Patient should be regularly assessed for progression to true labor; if the patient is considered not to be in true labor, discontinue GBS prophylaxis.

^e If GBS culture results become available prior to delivery and are negative, then discontinue GBS prophylaxis.

^f Unless subsequent GBS culture prior to delivery is positive.

^g A negative GBS screen is considered valid for 5 weeks. If a patient with a history of PTL is re-admitted with signs and symptoms of PTL and had a negative GBS screen >5 weeks prior, she should be rescreened and managed according to this algorithm at that time.

Fig. 35.9 Sample algorithm for management of neonates for prevention of early-onset group B streptococcal *(GBS)* infection. *PTL,* Preterm labor. (From Verani, J. R., McGee, L., & Schrag, S. J. [2010]. Prevention of perinatal group B streptococcal disease. Revised guidelines from CDC. *Morbidity and Mortality Weekly Report, 59*(RR10), 1–32.)

sepsis are relatively nonspecific and include fever, temperature insta-bility, apnea, cyanosis, jaundice, hepatomegaly, lethargy or irritability, vomiting, abdominal distention, and diarrhea.

The usual treatment for *E. coli* infection in the newborn is ampi-cillin or an extended-spectrum cephalosporin and an aminoglycoside. Treatment is continued for 7 to 10 days for bacteremia and at least 14 days for meningitis (Ferrieri & Wallen, 2018).

Staphylococcus aureus

Most staphylococcal infections in the newborn develop after the first 72 hours of life and involve the skin and soft tissue. Conjunctivitis, presenting with purulent eye discharge, is also a common manifes-tation of *S. aureus* infection. Skin lesions are typically small vesicles or pustules that are easily treated with topical antimicrobial agents. The skin lesions can appear as large fragile bullae containing clear or purulent fluid. These bullae rupture easily and leave moist, red, denuded areas of skin. A more severe bullous eruption due to staph-ylococcal infection is *scalded skin syndrome* characterized by wide-spread bullous lesions that easily rupture; fever and irritability are also present (Boos & Sidbury, 2018).

S. aureus can cause serious problems such as abscesses, osteomyeli-tis, endocarditis, and septic arthritis. Breaks in the skin from IV cathe-ters or scalp electrodes present an opportunity for the development of *S. aureus* abscesses. Umbilical catheters and central lines may be col-onized with *S. aureus*, resulting in septicemia. The major sources of *S. aureus* are the hands of medical and nursing personnel. *S. aureus* is a common cause of health care-associated infections among neonates in NICU and nursery settings; such outbreaks are often caused by methi-cillin-resistant strains of *S. aureus* (Leonard & Dobbs, 2015).

Initial treatment includes nafcillin and vancomycin until definitive culture results are available. Although most strains of *S. aureus* are sen-sitive to semisynthetic penicillins, there are increasing concerns about methicillin-resistant strains (Leonard & Dobbs, 2015; Srinivasan & Evans, 2018).

Chlamydia

Neonatal infection caused by *Chlamydia trachomatis* is acquired by new-borns in approximately 50% of all vaginal births by infected mothers and is known to occur in some infants born by cesarean with intact membranes. *C. trachomatis* causes neonatal conjunctivitis (25% to 50% of exposed infants) and pneumonia (5% to 30% of exposed infants) (AAP, 2018).

Neonatal chlamydial conjunctivitis, with redness of the eyes, edema of the eyelids, and minimal discharge, develops within a few days to several weeks after birth and usually lasts 1 to 2 weeks. If untreated, it can progress to chronic follicular conjunctivitis with conjunctival scar-ring and corneal microgranulations.

Chlamydial pneumonia usually has a gradual onset, between 2 and 19 weeks of age. Manifestations can include tachypnea, otitis media, nasal stuffiness, and coughing (AAP, 2018). Signs can be subtle and often go unrecognized.

Chlamydial conjunctivitis is treated with oral erythromycin or azi-thromycin. The recommended treatment for chlamydial pneumonia is oral azithromycin for 3 days or a 14-day regimen of erythromycin. Erythromycin administration in infants younger than 6 weeks has been associated with an increased risk of infantile hypertrophic pyloric ste-nosis; therefore parents should be educated regarding the symptoms of the condition (feeding intolerance, projectile vomiting, and abdominal distention) (AAP, 2018).

Gonorrhea

In the United States, *Neisseria gonorrhoeae* infection is the second most commonly reported STI. Fortunately, screening during pregnancy and

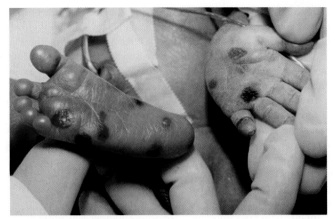

Fig. 35.10 Neonatal Syphilis Lesions on Hands and Feet. (Courtesy Mahesh Kotwal, MD, Phoenix, AZ.)

universal administration of neonatal eye prophylaxis (0.5% erythromy-cin ophthalmic ointment) during the first hour after birth have helped reduce the rates of neonatal infection, which occurs during birth when the infant is exposed to the mother's infected cervix (CDC, 2015). Infection in the neonate presents 2 to 5 days after birth and most often involves the eyes, causing *ophthalmia neonatorum*. Scalp abscesses, disseminated disease with bacteremia, arthritis, vaginitis, urethritis, or meningitis may also be seen. Eye prophylaxis alone does not prevent systemic infection; therefore infants with a gonococcal eye infection should receive one dose of ceftriaxone. These infants are hospitalized and evaluated for disseminated infection (e.g., sepsis, meningitis). Newborns with eye infections should have saline eye irrigations fre-quently until the discharge stops (AAP, 2018).

Infants with systemic gonococcal infection require hospitalization and 7 days of IV antibiotic therapy. If the newborn has gonococcal meningitis, 10 to 14 days of treatment is required (AAP, 2018).

Syphilis

Syphilis is caused by infection with the spirochete *Treponema pallidum*. Congenital syphilis can cause severe illness, miscarriage, stillbirth, and early infant death. The overall rate of reported cases of congenital syph-ilis decreased from 10.5 to 8.4 cases per 100,000 live births between 2008 to 2012, and then increased to 11.6 cases per 100,000 live births in 2014, the highest rate reported since 2001 (Bowen, Su, Torrone, et al. 2015). Risk factors for congenital syphilis include late or no prenatal care, failure of health care providers to follow maternal syphilis screen-ing recommendations, and infection with HIV (AAP, 2018).

This infection is contracted from an infected mother via transpla-cental transmission at any time during the pregnancy; however, the risk of infection increases as the pregnancy progresses. The infant can also become infected after birth if there is contact with maternal lesions. If the maternal syphilis is untreated, the rate of miscarriage, stillbirth, or perinatal death is approximately 40% (AAP, 2018). Prompt maternal treatment eliminates most fetal infections; however, delayed treatment or a failure to obtain treatment can result in fetal effects that range from minor anomalies to preterm birth or fetal death.

Clinical manifestations of congenital syphilis (Fig. 35.10) can include hepatosplenomegaly, snuffles, lymphadenopathy, mucocutaneous lesions, pneumonia, osteochondritis and pseudoparalysis, edema, rash, hemo-lytic anemia, or thrombocytopenia and may be present at birth or within the first 2 months of life. Newborns who were not treated at birth can also develop late manifestations that involve the CNS, bones and joints, teeth, eyes, and skin. There are also consequences that may not become appar-ent until the child is several years of age (AAP, 2018).

Importantly, newborns should not be discharged from the hospital without review of the mother's rapid plasma reagin (RPR) or Venereal Disease Research Laboratory (VDRL) test results. Usually mothers are tested early in their prenatal care and then again closer to birth. Mothers who have not had prenatal care will be tested for syphilis during their birth hospitalization.

Treatment of the newborn should be initiated when the diagnosis of congenital syphilis is confirmed or suspected or when maternal treatment status is unknown or not well documented. The neonate should be treated when the mother was treated within 1 month of giving birth or does not respond to treatment, when medications other than penicillin were used for the mother, or when the mother was treated appropriately but did not have sufficient serologic follow-up to assess response to treatment (AAP, 2018).

Infants who are symptomatic or whose mother was untreated or unsatisfactorily treated, should have a lumbar puncture (to evaluate for neurologic involvement), CBC, RPR or VDRL, and long-bone radiography prior to treatment. If the results of these tests are normal and follow-up is certain, a single intramuscular (IM) dose of penicillin G benzathine is recommended. If results are abnormal or there is concern about appropriate follow-up, a 10-day course of IV aqueous penicillin G or IM penicillin G procaine should be given. If the mother was adequately treated before giving birth and serologic testing of the infant does not show syphilis, the infant is usually not treated with antibiotics (AAP, 2018).

Listeriosis

Listeriosis, caused by *L. monocytogenes,* is primarily a foodborne infection that can cause maternal and neonatal illness. Mother-to-infant transmission occurs transplacentally through ascending infection or during birth. Prenatal infection causes chorioamnionitis or endometritis and should be suspected in cases of brown-stained amniotic fluid. It can also cause miscarriage, preterm birth, and stillbirth. Signs of early-onset infection are present at birth or in the first 1 to 2 days of life. Manifestations of infection are sepsis-like symptoms, acute respiratory distress, pneumonia, and more rarely, meningitis or myocarditis. With severe infection the infant can have granulomatosis infantisepticum causing an erythematous rash with small, pale papules. The mortality rate with early-onset infection ranges from 14% to 56%. Late-onset listeriosis is more insidious and usually manifests as meningitis. The mortality rates associated with late-onset infection are approximately 25%. Listeriosis in the newborn is usually treated with ampicillin and an aminoglycoside (AAP, 2018).

Protozoal Infection

Toxoplasmosis

Toxoplasmosis is a multisystem disease caused by the protozoan *Toxoplasma gondii* parasite, commonly found in cats, dogs, pigs, sheep, and cattle, with cats being the definitive host. Common ways that humans contract toxoplasmosis include eating raw or undercooked meats or seafoods, working with meat, drinking unpasteurized milk, handling cat litter that contains feces in which the *Toxoplasma* parasite was shed, or exposure to contaminated soil (CDC, 2018). The risk of maternal-fetal transmission of acute infection is approximately 40% with the risk of transmission increasing as the pregnancy progresses. When the maternal infection occurs earlier in the pregnancy, the clinical manifestations are more severe (Michaels, Sanchez, & Lin, 2018). Because many women are already seropositive for toxoplasmosis, the overall risk of a primary infection in pregnancy is quite low. The diagnosis of toxoplasmosis in the neonate is supported by elevated levels of cord blood serum IgM.

Most neonates infected with *T. gondii* in utero are asymptomatic at birth. The clinical manifestations of toxoplasmosis are often difficult to distinguish from other congenital infections. Approximately one-third of newborns have a generalized form of the disease that involves the reticuloendothelial system. The other two-thirds of infected newborns have neurologic signs (Michaels et al., 2018). The clinical features most commonly associated with a *T. gondii* infection include three key findings (classic triad): hydrocephalus, chorioretinitis, and cerebral calcifications. The majority of cases do not have all three symptoms (AAP, 2018). Severe toxoplasmosis is associated with preterm birth, IUGR, microcephaly or hydrocephaly, microphthalmos, chorioretinitis, CNS calcification, thrombocytopenia, jaundice, and fever. Petechiae or a maculopapular rash also can be evident.

Infants with congenital toxoplasmosis are treated with pyrimethamine, combined with oral sulfadiazine; folinic acid supplement is used to prevent anemia. Other medications may be added dependent on specific organ involvement; for example, corticosteroids may be helpful in the management of ocular complications (AAP, 2018).

Fungal Infection

Candidiasis

Candida infection, formerly known as moniliasis, can occur in the newborn. *Candida albicans,* the organism usually responsible, can cause disease in any organ system. It is a yeastlike fungus (producing yeast cells and spores) that is most often acquired during birth from a maternal vaginal infection; by person-to-person transmission; or from contaminated hands, bottles, nipples, or other articles. It usually is a benign disorder in the neonate, often confined to the oral and diaper regions (Boos & Sidbury, 2018).

Congenital candidiasis can occur as a result of ascending intrauterine infection. The newborn with congenital cutaneous candidiasis (CCC) presents with skin lesions most commonly on the back, extensor extremities, and in skin creases and folds. The lesions appear as erythematous macules, papules, and vesicopustules with background erythema. Most cases of CCC in healthy term newborns resolve without treatment in 1 to 2 weeks (Boos & Sidbury, 2018).

Diaper dermatitis is a common finding of candidiasis; it appears on the perianal area, inguinal folds, and lower portion of the abdomen. The affected area is intensely erythematous, with a sharply demarcated, scalloped edge, frequently with numerous satellite lesions that extend beyond the larger lesion. The source of the infection is through the GI tract, often the mouth. Treatment is an antifungal ointment, such as nystatin (Mycostatin), applied three times a day for 7 to 10 days. The infant also can be given an oral antifungal preparation to eliminate any GI source of infection (Boos & Sidbury, 2018).

Oral candidiasis (**thrush,** or mycotic stomatitis) is characterized by the appearance of white plaques on the oral mucosa, gums, and tongue. The white patches are easily differentiated from milk curds; the patches cannot be removed and tend to bleed when touched. In most cases the infant does not seem to be in discomfort from the infection. A few infants seem to have some difficulty swallowing. Topical application of 100,000 to 200,000 units of nystatin to the mouth 4 times daily for 14 to 21 days is usually sufficient to treat oral thrush (Boos & Sidbury, 2018). Gentian violet solution can be used in addition to one of the antifungal drugs in chronic cases of thrush; however, it does not treat GI candida and can irritate the oral mucosa.

The objectives of management are to eradicate the causative organism, to control exposure to *C. albicans,* and to improve the infant's resistance. Interventions include maintaining scrupulous cleanliness to prevent reinfection. Careful hand hygiene and proper cleanliness of the equipment and environment are essential.

Systemic candida infection is usually limited to critically ill neonates receiving antibiotic therapy for bacterial infections or who have indwelling catheters. For these infants, antifungal agents such as amphotericin B (Fungizone) or fluconazole (Diflucan) are given intravenously. Many NICUs administer prophylactic fluconazole to their premature infants who weigh less than 1000 g, the infants most at risk for systemic candida infections (Boos & Sidbury, 2018).

Infants who are breastfed can acquire candida infection from the mother. If the mother is colonized, treatment for mother and infant is recommended. Breastfeeding can continue even if the mother is receiving systemic antifungal medications (Boos & Sidbury, 2018).

SUBSTANCE ABUSE

Substance abuse during pregnancy is associated with significant fetal and neonatal risks. Other than alcohol and tobacco, cocaine and marijuana are the most commonly used substances by pregnant women. Maternal substance abuse is discussed in Chapter 31.

The adverse effects of exposure of the fetus to drugs are varied. They include transient behavioral changes such as alterations in fetal breathing movements or irreversible effects such as fetal death, IUGR, congenital anomalies, or cognitive impairment. Critical determinants of the effect of the drug on the fetus include the specific drug, the dosage, the route of administration, the genotype of the mother or fetus, and the timing of the drug exposure. Determining the specific effects of individual drugs on the fetus is made difficult by the common practice of polydrug use; errors or omissions in reporting drug use; and variations in the strength, purity, and types of additives found in illicit drugs. Maternal conditions such as poverty and malnutrition and comorbid conditions such as STIs further compound the difficulty in identifying the presence and consequences of intrauterine drug exposure.

Tobacco

Whether in the form of traditional cigarettes, electronic cigarettes, smokeless tobacco, or nicotine replacement patches, tobacco remains the most used substance during pregnancy. Low birth weight is the most widely recognized effect of maternal tobacco use. This may be related to the vasoconstrictive effects of nicotine and its metabolites. It is also known that carbon monoxide crosses the placenta, which can cause fetal hypoxemia. There may be a link between tobacco use and the risk of certain congenital anomalies. There is substantial evidence regarding the link between tobacco use and other adverse perinatal outcomes, including miscarriage, placental abruption, preterm birth, and placenta previa (Cunningham, Levino, Bloom et al., 2018; Wallen & Gleason, 2018).

Exposure to secondhand smoke increases the risk of ear infections, respiratory illnesses such as asthma and bronchitis, and sudden infant death syndrome (SIDS) (Wallen & Gleason, 2018). It is not clear whether the association between smoking and SIDS reflects in utero exposure or passive exposure postnatally, or both. Mothers and all others should refrain from smoking near the infant.

Alcohol

There is no quantity, frequency, or timing of alcohol intake during pregnancy that is considered safe (Williams, Smith, & Committee on Substance Abuse, 2015). Prenatal alcohol exposure (PAE) is associated with short- and long-term effects on the fetus and newborn, which are included under the term *fetal alcohol spectrum disorder (FASD)*. FASD includes five conditions: fetal alcohol syndrome (FAS), partial FAS, alcohol-related neurodevelopmental disorder, alcohol-related birth defects, and neurobehavioral disorder associated with PAE.

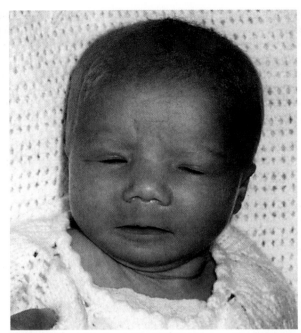

Fig. 35.11 Infant With Fetal Alcohol Syndrome. (From Markiewicz, M., & Abrahamson, E. [1999]. *Diagnosis in color: Neonatology*. St. Louis: Mosby.)

Ethanol easily crosses the placenta. The quantity of alcohol required to produce fetal effects is unclear, but it is known that the adverse effects of alcohol on the fetus are related to the gestational age at exposure, maternal age, the amount of alcohol consumed, the pattern of consumption, and maternal alcohol metabolism (Wallen & Gleason, 2018).

Fetal alcohol syndrome is the most severe FASD and can result in fetal death. The incidence of FAS in the United States has been estimated to vary from 0.5 to 9 cases per 1000 live births (Williams, et al., 2015). The criteria for FAS (Fig. 35.11) include specific dysmorphic facial features (short palpebral fissures, thin upper lip, smooth philtrum), growth deficiency, and CNS abnormalities (structural, neurologic, developmental, functional, or a combination of these). Less frequently, skeletal, renal, cardiac, and ophthalmologic abnormalities have been seen with FAS (Wallen & Gleason, 2018).

The term alcohol-related neurodevelopmental disorders (ARND) applies to children with confirmed PAE who lack facial features or growth deficits associated with FAS, yet they have structural CNS and cognitive abnormalities. Alcohol-related birth defects (ARBD) is the term used when there is confirmed PAE and congenital abnormalities that most often include cardiac and renal anomalies, orthopedic defects, and anomalies of the eyes and ears. These disorders run the gamut from learning disabilities and behavioral problems to speech or language problems and hyperactivity. Often these problems are not detected until the child goes to school and learning problems become evident (Wallen & Gleason, 2018; Williams et al., 2015).

Neurobehavioral disorder associated with PAE is a relatively new term that reflects the teratogenic effects of alcohol on the developing fetus. Children affected by this disorder lack the distinguishing physical features of FAS, but have CNS damage that is manifested in functional impairments of neurocognition, self-regulation, and adaptive functioning (Hagan, Balachova, Bertrand, et al., 2016).

Opioids

This class of drugs has been used as analgesics for centuries and continues to be the most widely used for pain control. The most popular opioids are morphine, heroin, methadone, meperidine, oxycodone,

BOX 35.2 Signs of Neonatal Abstinence Syndrome

Acute Signs and Symptoms That May Persist for Several Weeks

- Restlessness
- Tremors (disturbed at first to undisturbed)
- High-pitched cry
- Increased muscle tone
- Irritability and inconsolability
- Increased deep tendon reflexes
- Exaggerated Moro reflex
- Seizures in approximately 1%-2% of heroin-exposed neonates and approximately 7% of methadone-exposed neonates

Subacute Signs and Symptoms That May Persist for 4-6 months

- Irritability
- Sleep pattern disturbance
- Hyperactivity
- Feeding problems
- Hypertonia

Data from Weiner, S. M., & Finnegan, L. P. (2016). Drug withdrawal in the neonate. In S. L. Gardner, B. S. Carter, M. Enzman-Hines, & J. A. Hernandez (Eds.), *Merenstein & Gardner's handbook of neonatal intensive care* (8th ed.). St. Louis: Mosby.

codeine, and fentanyl. Over the last several years, there has been a significant increase in the use and misuse of opioids in the United States resulting in opioid dependence and addiction. This increase in use has also occurred in women of childbearing age.

Opioids readily cross the placenta and affect the fetus. Miscarriage, preterm labor, preterm birth, placental abruption, chorioamnionitis, IUGR, and fetal distress are obstetric complications associated with opioid dependence during pregnancy (Wallen & Gleason, 2018).

Neonates exposed to opioids while in utero experience drug withdrawal in the days and weeks after birth. Neonatal abstinence syndrome (NAS) describes the clinical signs that can be associated with withdrawal from opioids (Box 35.2). Signs of withdrawal develop in 55% to 94% of neonates exposed in utero to opioids (Wallen & Gleason, 2018).

Opioid receptors are located in the CNS and GI tract. This explains why the most common signs of NAS reflect CNS irritability, increased autonomic activity, and GI abnormalities. Withdrawal symptoms are more severe in newborns exposed to larger amounts of drugs for longer periods of time. The severity of withdrawal is also related to the timing of maternal drug use in relation to birth.

Scoring tools such as the Neonatal Abstinence Scoring System (Finnegan, 1990) (Fig. 35.12) are used to objectively review the infant's signs of withdrawal. Depending on the score, pharmacologic treatment may be necessary. The length of hospital stay varies for infants with NAS and is often several weeks. Those babies requiring medication have longer stays (Patrick, Dudley, Martin et al., 2015). All infants showing signs of withdrawal should receive nonpharmacologic care. Many mothers are in supervised opioid treatment programs. These programs typically use methadone or buprenorphine as the pharmacologic treatment for these mothers.

The Academy of Breastfeeding Medicine recommends that health care providers encourage stable methadone-or buprenorphine-maintained women to breastfeed. Breastfeeding is not recommended for women who are not in treatment or who are using opioids without physician supervision (Reece-Stremtan & Marinelli, 2015).

Marijuana

Marijuana is the most commonly used illicit drug in the United States (Azofeifa, Mattson, Schauer, et al., 2016). While it is illegal in the majority of U.S. states, it is increasingly becoming legalized by individual states. The primary chemical compound in marijuana—9-tetrahydro-cannabinol (THC)—easily crosses the placenta and can remain in the body for as long as 30 days, increasing fetal exposure and potential risk.

There is currently a lack of definitive evidence about the effects of marijuana on the developing fetus, primarily because pregnant women who use marijuana are likely to use other drugs (e.g., alcohol, tobacco, cocaine) and there may be other confounding exposures. Marijuana does not appear to have significant teratogenic effects. There may be some association with fetal growth restriction or preterm birth, but further study is needed. Long-term follow-up studies on exposed infants are needed to identify cognitive and behavioral effects of marijuana use during pregnancy (ACOG, 2017; Wallen & Gleason, 2018).

Until further evidence is available regarding perinatal effects of marijuana during pregnancy, pregnant women and those contemplating pregnancy should be encouraged to stop using marijuana. Likewise, women who are breastfeeding should be discouraged from using marijuana (ACOG, 2017).

Cocaine

Cocaine readily crosses the placenta and is found in breast milk. Amniotic fluid acts as a reservoir for cocaine and its metabolites, which prolongs fetal exposure. Confounding effects of other substances such as alcohol, tobacco, and marijuana, make it difficult to identify specific consequences of cocaine use (Wallen & Gleason, 2018).

Vasoconstrictive effects of cocaine in the maternal system decrease blood flow to the uterus and cause hypoxemia in the fetus. Cocaine is a recognized cause of placental abruption. Infants born to cocaine-abusing mothers have a high rate of IUGR, low birth weight, and preterm birth. There is a lack of evidence to support an association between cocaine use and congenital defects (Wallen & Gleason, 2018)

Cocaine-dependent neonates do not experience a process of withdrawal as do opioid-exposed infants, but rather they show signs of acute intoxication. Until the cocaine is cleared from their systems they are likely to be irritable; hypertonic; tremulous; and have abnormal feeding, sleeping, and crying patterns (Wallen & Gleason, 2018).

Prenatal cocaine exposure has been associated with longer-term effects. Children and adolescents may experience problems with attention, language development, and information processing (Wallen & Gleason, 2018).

Amphetamines

Methamphetamine is the primary form of amphetamine used by pregnant women. The fetal and neonatal effects associated with maternal use of methamphetamines in pregnancy are not well known. The limited data regarding the risk of congenital anomalies suggest little or no effect on organogenesis. Due to the vasoconstrictive effects of methamphetamine, women who use this drug during pregnancy are at increased risk for placental abruption, preterm birth, and an infant who is SGA (Wallen & Gleason, 2018).

Neonatal manifestations of methamphetamine withdrawal have not been clearly identified because of frequent maternal polydrug use. After birth, infants can experience bradycardia or tachycardia that resolves as the drug is cleared from the infant's system. Lethargy can continue for several months, along with frequent infections and poor weight gain. Emotional disturbances and delays in gross and fine motor coordination can be seen during early childhood. There is limited to no data available regarding the long-term effects of methamphetamine exposure (Wallen & Gleason, 2018).

NEONATAL ABSTINENCE SCORING SYSTEM

System	Signs and Symptoms	Score	AM						PM					Comments
Central Nervous System Disturbances	Excessive high-pitched (or other) cry	2												Daily weight:
	Continuous high-pitched (or other) cry	3												
	Sleeps <1 h after feeding	3												
	Sleeps <2 h after feeding	2												
	Sleeps <3 h after feeding	1												
	Hyperactive Moro reflex	2												
	Markedly hyperactive Moro reflex	3												
	Mild tremors disturbed	1												
	Moderate-severe tremors disturbed	2												
	Mild tremors undisturbed	3												
	Moderate-severe tremors undisturbed	4												
	Increased muscle tone	2												
	Excoriation (specific area)	1												
	Myoclonic jerks	3												
	Generalized convulsions	5												
Metabolic/Vasomotor/Respiratory Disturbances	Sweating	1												
	Fever <101° (99°F–100.8°F/37.2°C–38.2°C)	1												
	Fever >101° (38.4°C and higher)	2												
	Frequent yawning (>3 or 4 times/interval)	1												
	Mottling	1												
	Nasal stuffiness	1												
	Sneezing (>3 or 4 times/interval)	1												
	Nasal flaring	2												
	Respiratory rate >60/min	1												
	Respiratory rate >60/min with retractions	2												
Gastrointestinal Disturbances	Excessive sucking	1												
	Poor feeding	2												
	Regurgitation	2												
	Projectile vomiting	3												
	Loose stools	2												
	Watery stools	3												
	Total Score													
	Initials of Scorer													

Fig. 35.12 Neonatal Abstinence Scoring System. (From Finnegan, L. P. [1990]. Neonatal abstinence syndrome: Assessment and pharmacotherapy. In N. Nelson [Ed.], *Current therapy in neonatal-perinatal medicine* [2nd ed.]. St. Louis: Mosby.)

Other Drugs of Concern

Benzodiazepines and Barbiturates

Another class of drugs that infants may be exposed to in utero are benzodiazepines and barbiturates. Often signs of withdrawal from these substances are not seen until 7 to 21 days of age. Benzodiazepines (e.g. Ativan, diazepam) are associated with more severe signs and duration of withdrawal because they have longer half-lives. Common signs of withdrawal in these neonates include hypotonia, hypertonia, excessive or poor suck, and emesis. Depending on the severity of drug withdrawal, these infants may be managed with phenobarbital (Hudak, 2015).

Selective Serotonin Reuptake Inhibitors

Depression is one of the most common health disorders in the United States. Treatment of depression during pregnancy and lactation may be required to minimize negative outcomes to the mother, fetus, and newborn. Selective serotonin reuptake inhibitors (SSRIs) are the mainstay of treatment for depression and anxiety and are often prescribed during pregnancy. Commonly prescribed SSRIs include citalopram, escitalopram, fluoxetine, fluvoxamine, and sertraline (Tran & Robb, 2015) (see Table 31.1). All medications that have been studied are known to cross the placenta and are transferred in breast milk. Their use should be determined by a risk-benefit analysis of the risks to the fetus or neonate weighed against risks of not treating the mother's psychiatric condition.

Maternal use of SSRIs late in the pregnancy has been associated with preterm birth, low birth weight, and NICU admission (Tran & Robb, 2015). Fetal exposure to SSRIs during the third trimester predisposes the neonate to a behavioral syndrome resembling NAS. Symptoms during the first week of life include irritability, agitation, jitteriness, hypoglycemia, tachypnea, hypotonia, weak or absent cry, and lethargy (Tran & Robb). This syndrome is usually mild and lasts for no longer than 2 days. Persistent pulmonary hypertension in the newborn (PPHN) has been associated with maternal use of SSRIs late in pregnancy (Huybrechts, Bateman, Palmsten, et al., 2015). It is recommended that paroxetine be avoided during pregnancy as this SSRI has been shown to increase the risk of cardiovascular defects, specifically ventricular septal defects (ACOG, 2008/2018; Huybrechts, Palmsten, Avorn, et al., 2014).

For parents who are concerned about maternal use of psychiatric medications and the fetal or neonatal effects, they can talk with the nurse. The nurse can direct them to the following websites: REPROTOX (www.reprotox.org) and TERIS (http://depts.washington.edu/terisweb).

CARE MANAGEMENT

The maternal history is the key to identification of newborns who are at risk because of maternal substance abuse or use of other drugs during pregnancy and lactation. Review of the prenatal record can reveal a medical and social history of drug use or abuse and any detoxification treatment used. There can be other factors that contribute to neonatal outcomes and complications. For example, the woman who is addicted to opioids or cocaine can have infections that compound the risk to the infant, including hepatitis, septicemia, and STIs, including AIDS (Wallen & Gleason, 2018). In many cases there is no information in the prenatal record to suggest maternal substance abuse when the woman has, in fact, been using one or more substances during pregnancy.

A thorough assessment of the newborn is performed as described in Chapter 24. The infant's gestational age and maturity are noted. The infant can have IUGR or be preterm with low birth weight. In utero exposure to some drugs results in observable malformations or dysmorphism (abnormality of shape). Neonatal behavior can arouse suspicion. A standardized scoring system is used for assessing withdrawal

symptoms (NAS) (see Fig. 35.12). Because many women are multidrug users, the newborn initially can exhibit a confusing complex of signs. The nurse often is the first to observe the signs of drug withdrawal. The nurse's observations help the health care provider differentiate between signs of NAS and other conditions, such as CNS disorders, sepsis, hypoglycemia, and electrolyte imbalance (see Evidence-Based Practice box).

Urine or meconium screening can be used to identify substances abused by the mother. Urine screening is most commonly used, but its sensitivity is limited. It can also be challenging to obtain a urine specimen. To improve accuracy, it is important to collect the first urine specimen. Initially costly and of limited availability, tests of meconium collected before transitional stooling begins have been shown to be sensitive and reliable. Unfortunately, this test may take several days to collect. The accuracy is dependent on collecting as much meconium as possible. Meconium testing results also take as long as 1 to 2 weeks to receive. Recently, umbilical cord testing has been used. This method is able to test for more exposures, and because the tissue is immediately available, it can be sent, and results received, in a more time efficient manner (Wallen & Gleason, 2018).

Nursing Considerations

Planning for care of the infant born to a substance-abusing mother presents a challenge to the health care team. Parents are included in the planning for the newborn's care and for the care and support of the mother and her newborn at home. An interprofessional approach includes home health or community resource personnel (e.g., regulatory agencies such as child protective services).

Education and social support to prevent drug abuse provide the ideal approach. However, given the scope of the drug abuse problem, total prevention is an unrealistic goal.

Nursing care of the drug-dependent neonate involves supportive therapy for fluid and electrolyte balance, nutrition, infection control, and respiratory care. Swaddling, holding, and reducing stimuli, can be helpful in easing withdrawal (see the Nursing Care Plan: The Infant Experiencing Drug Withdrawal [Neonatal Abstinence Syndrome]). Specific suggestions for providing care to infants experiencing withdrawal are listed in Box 35.3.

Pharmacologic treatment is usually based on the severity of withdrawal symptoms, as determined by an assessment tool (see Fig. 35.12). When indicated, medications are given as ordered. The most commonly used medications to treat opioid withdrawal are methadone and morphine. In some cases, phenobarbital and clonidine may also be used. The dosage of medication is adjusted based on the newborn's specific withdrawal scores. (Wallen & Gleason, 2018). Treatment may be needed for 2 weeks or more.

> ### ⚠ MEDICATION ALERT
>
> The use of naloxone (Narcan) is contraindicated in infants born to opioid addicts because it can cause severe signs and symptoms of neonatal abstinence syndrome and even seizures.

The issue of breastfeeding in this population is a difficult one. Although breast milk remains the optimal source of nutrition for these infants, care must be taken to avoid exposing the infant to additional drugs through the breast milk. According to the Academy of Breastfeeding Medicine, mothers who use street drugs should not breastfeed. They also recommend that women enrolled in and committed to a methadone and/or buprenorphine treatment program should be encouraged to breastfeed (Reece-Stremtan & Marinelli, 2015).

The mother requires considerable support. Her ability to cope can be impaired due to her history of substance abuse and her life circumstances. She may blame herself for the infant's problems. The infant's withdrawal signs and decreased consolability stress her coping abilities even further. Family members also need support as they assist in caring for the infant. Home health care, treatment for addiction, and education are important. Sensitive exploration of the woman's options for the care of her infant and herself and for future fertility management may help her see that she has choices. This approach helps communicate respect for the new mother as a person who can make responsible decisions.

EVIDENCE-BASED PRACTICE

Nonpharmacologic Interventions for Neonatal Abstinence Syndrome

Ask the Question

For newborns withdrawing from maternal substances, what nonpharmacologic and relational interventions can improve outcomes?

Search for the Evidence

Search Strategies: English-language research-based publications since 2013 on neonatal abstinence, neonatal abstinence syndrome, Finnegan, substance abuse in pregnancy were included

Databases Used: Cochrane Collaborative Database, National Guideline Clearinghouse (AHRQ), CINAHL, PubMed, and the professional websites for ACOG and AWHONN.

Critical Appraisal of the Evidence

Newborns exposed to maternal substances in utero can develop neonatal abstinence syndrome (NAS) as they go through withdrawal, sometimes requiring medication, prolonged length of stay, and newborn intensive care unit (NICU) admission. Long accepted interventions have included swaddling, low light, quiet environment, minimal handling, and pacifier use, but not all are evidence-based.

- An integrative review of 14 articles on nonpharmacologic interventions revealed that breastfeeding, rooming-in, prone position, acupressure, and use of a nonoscillating newborn bed resulted in improved outcomes that included shorter length of stay, decrease in NAS scores, better sleep, and less pharmacologic treatment (Edwards & Brown, 2016).

- A systematic review of six studies found that providing multidisciplinary, integrated, and comprehensive perinatal services for substance-addicted women and caring relationships with their providers resulted in better neonatal outcomes of greater gestational age at birth, higher birth weight, shorter length of stay, lower NAS score, and discharge to home with mother (Kramlich & Kronk, 2015).

- A multidisciplinary quality improvement team implemented a protocol for standardized care that included training the nurses for interrater reliability when using the NAS scoring tool, scoring only after on-demand breastfeeding and skin-to-skin contact, rooming-in, standardizing the physician interpretation of NAS scores and medical decision-making, increasing prenatal teaching and family involvement in monitoring symptoms, and providing comfort care. Improved outcomes included shorter stays, fewer NICU admissions, less medication, and lower costs (Holmes, Atwood, Whalen, et al., 2016).

Apply the Evidence: Nursing Implications

- The nurse can utilize standardized NAS scoring by watching training videos and practicing scoring with coworkers and managers. Assessing the baby after breastfeeding and skin-to-skin contact ensures accurate equivalency.

- Family-centered care begins prenatally and includes education about the newborn's symptoms, coping strategies, and nonpharmacologic interventions. Institutional interdisciplinary commitment to rooming-in and breastfeeding is even more important for NAS babies.

- Prone position, if used, is contrary to what is taught for sudden infant death syndrome prevention, and should be explained to the family as a temporary measure to be used only until symptoms improve. Pulse and oxygen levels should be monitored.

- Relationships matter, both between the family and caregivers and within the health care team. A qualitative study of 16 NICU RNs identified six themes about caring for NAS newborns: "Learning the baby" via trial and error; core team support; role satisfaction; grief for the baby's present and future; making a difference; and caring for the mother (Nelson, 2016). Judgment and stigma were identified as toxic and barriers to family-centered care.

- The nurse needs to know the state laws regarding maternal substance abuse. The Association of Women's Health, Obstetric and Neonatal Nurses (AWHONN) has taken a position opposed to criminalization of substance abuse during pregnancy because the threat of incarceration is ineffective and counterproductive to getting women the interventions they need (AWHONN, 2015).

References

Association of Women's Health, Obstetric and Neonatal Nurses. (2015). Criminalization of pregnant women with substance use disorders. *Journal of Obstetric, Gynecologic and Neonatal Nursing, 44*(1), 155–157.

Edwards, L., & Brown, L. F. (2016). Nonpharmacologic management of neonatal abstinence syndrome: An integrative review. *Neonatal Network, 35*(5), 305–313.

Holmes, A. V., Atwood, E. C., Whalen, B., et al. (2016). Rooming-in to treat neonatal abstinence syndrome: Improved family-centered care at lower cost. *Pediatrics, 137*(6), e20152929.

Kramlich, D., & Kronk, R. (2015). Relational care for perinatal substance use: A systematic review. *American Journal of Maternal Child Nursing, 40*(5), 320–326.

Nelson, M. M. (2016). NICU culture of care for infants with neonatal abstinence syndrome: A focused ethnography. *Neonatal Network, 35*(5), 287–296.

Jennifer Taylor Alderman

⊚ NURSING CARE PLAN

The Infant Experiencing Drug Withdrawal (Neonatal Abstinence Syndrome)

Client Problem	Expected Outcome	Nursing Interventions	Rationales
Irritability and high-pitched crying	Infant will be less irritable, calmer, and have fewer episodes of high-pitched cry.	Administer prescribed medications per health care provider order.	To decrease central nervous system (CNS) irritability and prevent seizure activity
		Decrease environmental stimuli.	To minimize stimulation
		Plan care activities carefully. Wrap infant snugly and hold tightly.	To minimize stimulation
		If infant was cocaine exposed, position to avoid eye contact; swaddle infant, use vertical rocking techniques, and use a pacifier.	To reduce self-stimulation behaviors and protect skin from abrasions
Potential for inadequate weight gain or weight loss related to increased basal metabolic requirements, CNS irritability, poor suck reflex, vomiting, and diarrhea	Infant exhibits ingestion and retention of adequate nutrients and appropriate weight gain.	Feed in frequent, small amounts; elevate head during and after feeding, and burp well.	To diminish vomiting and aspiration
		Monitor weight daily and maintain strict intake and output.	To evaluate success of feeding
		If intake is insufficient, feed by oral gavage per provider order.	To ensure ingestion of needed nutrients
Potential for dehydration related to diarrhea and vomiting	Infant exhibits evidence of fluid homeostasis.	Administer oral and parenteral fluids per provider order.	To maintain fluid balance
		Monitor hydration status (skin turgor, weight, mucous membranes, fontanels, urine specific gravity, electrolytes) and intake and output.	To evaluate for evidence of dehydration

BOX 35.3   Nursing Care of the Infant Experiencing Withdrawal (Neonatal Abstinence Syndrome)

- Swaddle the infant with the legs flexed.
- Position the infant's hands in midline with the arms at the side.
- Carry the infant in a flexed position, holding firmly and close to your body. Use a soft-pack baby carrier.
- When interacting with the infant, introduce one stimulus at a time when the infant is in a quiet, alert state.
- Watch for signs of over-stimulation or distress signals (gaze aversion, yawning, sneezing, hiccups, arching, mottled color).
- When the infant is distressed, rock in a slow, rhythmic fashion.
- Offer pacifier for nonnutritive sucking.
- Place the infant in a sitting position with the chin tucked for feeding.
- Try feeding small amounts at frequent intervals or use a demand-feeding schedule.
- During feedings, avoid eye contact or talking.
- Reduce environmental stimuli (lights, noise).
- Organize care to minimize handling.

Data from Weiner, S. M., & L. P. Finnegan. (2016). Drug withdrawal in the neonate. In S. L. Gardner, B. S. Carter, M. Enzman-Hines, & J. A. Hernandez (Eds.), *Merenstein & Gardner's handbook of neonatal intensive care* (8th ed.). St. Louis: Mosby.

▮ KEY POINTS

- A small percentage of significant birth injuries occur despite skilled and competent obstetric care.
- The nurse's primary contribution to the welfare of the neonate begins with early observation, accurate recording, and prompt reporting of abnormal signs.
- Prepregnancy planning, along with strict glycemic control before and during pregnancy, can significantly reduce the embryonic, fetal, and neonatal conditions associated with pregnancies complicated by diabetes mellitus.
- Infants of diabetic mothers are at risk for complications, including congenital anomalies, stillbirth, macrosomia, birth injury, hypoglycemia, hyperbilirubinemia, and respiratory distress syndrome.
- Infection in the neonate can be acquired in utero, during labor and birth, or during the postnatal period.

- The most common maternal infections during early pregnancy that are associated with various congenital malformations are caused by viruses.
- HIV transmission from mother to infant occurs transplacentally at various gestational ages, perinatally by maternal blood and secretions, and by breast milk.
- Substance abuse by pregnant women has fetal and neonatal effects.
- Neonatal abstinence syndrome occurs in newborns experiencing drug withdrawal from maternal use of opioids.
- Newborns can experience withdrawal symptoms from maternal use of benzodiazepines, barbiturates, and selective serotonin reuptake inhibitors.
- Providing high-quality perinatal care to a varied population with multiple conditions is complicated by the special needs of high-risk drug-dependent mothers and families.

REFERENCES

Agency for Healthcare Research and Quality. (2014). *Data tables appendix: 2014 national healthcare quality and disparities reports*. Rockville, MD: Author.

American Academy of Pediatrics. (2018). Section 3: Summaries of infectious diseases. In D. W. Kimberlin, M. T. Brady, M. A. Jackson, et al. (Eds.), *Red book: 2018-2021 report of the Committee on Infectious Diseases* (31st ed.). Itasca, IL: Author.

American Academy of Pediatrics & American College of Obstetricians and Gynecologists. (2017). *Guidelines for perinatal care* (8th ed.). Elk Grove Village, IL: Author.

American College of Obstetricians and Gynecologists. (2017). Committee opinion no. 722: Marijuana use during pregnancy and lactation. *Obstetrics & Gynecology, 130*(4), e205–e209.

American College of Obstetricians and Gynecologists. (2018). Practice bulletin no. 190: Gestational diabetes mellitus. *Obstetrics & Gynecology, 131*(2), e49–e64.

American College of Obstetricians and Gynecologists. (2008, reaffirmed 2018). Practice bulletin no. 92: Use of psychiatric medication during pregnancy and lactation. *Obstetrics & Gynecology, 111*(4), 1001–1020.

Anderson-Berry, A. L., & Rosenkrantz, T. (2015). *Neonatal sepsis. Medscape.* Retrieved from https://emedicine.medscape.com/article/978352-overview.

Azofeifa, A., Mattson, M. E., Schauer, G., et al. (2016). National estimates of marijuana use and related indicators: National survey on drug use and health, United States, 2002-2014. *Morbidity and Mortality Weekly Report–Surveillance Summaries, 65*(11), 1–25.

Baley, J. E., & Gonzalez, B. E. (2015). Perinatal viral infections. In R. J. Martin, A. A. Fanaroff, & M. C. Walsh (Eds.), *Fanaroff & Martin's neonatal-perinatal medicine* (10th ed.). St. Louis: Saunders.

Bialas, K. M., Swamy, G. K., & Permar, S. R. (2015). Perinatal cytomegalovirus and varicella zoster virus infections: Epidemiology, prevention, and treatment. *Clinics in Perinatology, 42*(1), 61–75.

Blickstein, I., Perlman, S., Hazan, Y., et al. (2015). Diabetes mellitus during pregnancy. In R. J. Martin, A. A. Fanaroff, & M. C. Walsh (Eds.), *Fanaroff & Martin's neonatal-perinatal medicine* (10th ed.). St. Louis: Saunders.

Boos, M. D., & Sidbury, R. (2018). Infections of the skin. In C. A. Gleason & S. E. Juul (Eds.), *Avery's diseases of the newborn* (10th ed.). Philadelphia: Elsevier.

Bowen, V., Su, J., Torrone, E., et al. (2015). Increase in incidence of congenital syphilis – US, 2012-2014. *Morbidity and Mortality Weekly Report, 64*(44), 1241–1245.

Centers for Disease Control and Prevention. (2015). *Gonococcal treatment guidelines.* Retrieved from https://www.cdc.gov/std/tg2015/gonorrhea.htm.

Centers for Disease Control and Prevention. (2017). *Measles and rubella.* Retrieved from https://www.cdc.gov/globalhealth/measles/.

Centers for Disease Control and Prevention. (2018). *Parasites: Toxoplasmosis (toxoplasma infection).* Retrieved from https://www.cdc.gov/parasites/toxoplasmosis/.

Centers for Disease Control and Prevention. (2018). *Guidance for the prevention and control of influenza in the peri- and postpartum settings.* Retrieved from https://www.cdc.gov/flu/professionals/infectioncontrol/peri-post-settings.htm.

Centers for Disease Control and Prevention. (2019). *HIV among pregnant women, infants, and children.* Retrieved from https://www.cdc.gov/hiv/group/gender/pregnantwomen/index.html.

Cunningham, F. G., Leveno, K. J., & Bloom, S. L. (2018). *Williams obstetrics* (25th ed.). New York: McGraw-Hill.

deVries, L. (2015). Intracranial hemorrhage and vascular lesions in the neonate. In R. J. Martin, A. A. Fanaroff, & M. C. Walsh (Eds.), *Fanaroff & Martin's neonatal-perinatal medicine* (10th ed.). St. Louis: Saunders.

Ferrieri, P., & Wallen, L. D. (2018). Newborn sepsis and meningitis. In C. A. Gleason & S. E. Juul (Eds.), *Avery's diseases of the newborn* (10th ed.). Philadelphia: Elsevier.

Finnegan, L. P. (1990). Neonatal abstinence syndrome: Assessment and pharmacotherapy. In N. Nelson (Ed.), *Current therapy in neonatal-perinatal medicine* (2nd ed.). St. Louis: Mosby.

Hagan, J. F., Balachova, T., Bertrand, J., et al. (2016). Neurobehavioral disorder associated with prenatal alcohol exposure. *Pediatrics, 138*(4), e20151553.

Hudak, M. L. (2015). Infants with antenatal exposure to drugs. In R. J. Martin, A. A. Fanaroff, & M. C. Walsh (Eds.), *Fanaroff & Martin's neonatal-perinatal medicine* (10th ed.). St. Louis: Saunders.

Huybrechts, K. F., Bateman, B. T., Palmsten, K., et al. (2015). Antidepressant use late in pregnancy and risk of persistent pulmonary hypertension of the newborn. *Journal of the American Medical Association, 313*(21), 2142–2151.

Huybrechts, K. F., Palmsten, K., Avorn, J., et al. (2014). Antidepressant use in pregnancy and risk of cardiac defects. *New England Journal of Medicine, 370*(25), 2397–2407.

James, S. H., & Kimberlin, D. J. (2015). Neonatal herpes simplex virus infection: Epidemiology and treatment. *Clinics in Perinatology, 42*(1), 47–59.

Ku, L. C., Boggess, K. A., & Cohen-Wolkowiez, M. (2015). Bacterial meningitis in the infant. *Clinics in Perinatology, 42*(1), 29–45.

Kuzniewicz, M. W., Puopolo, K. M., Fischer, A., et al. (2017). A quantitative, risk-based approach to the management of neonatal early-onset sepsis. *Journal of the American Medical Association Pediatrics, 171*(4), 365–371.

Leonard, E. G., & Dobbs, K. (2015). Postnatal bacterial infections. In R. J. Martin, A. A. Fanaroff, & M. C. Walsh (Eds.), *Fanaroff & Martin's neonatal-perinatal medicine* (10th ed.). St. Louis: Saunders.

Mangurten, H., Puppala, B., & Prazad, P. (2015). Birth injuries. In R. J. Martin, A. A. Fanaroff, & M. C. Walsh (Eds.), *Fanaroff & Martin's neonatal-perinatal medicine* (10th ed.). St. Louis: Saunders.

McKinlay, C. J., Alsweiler, J. M., Anstice, N. S., et al. (2017). Association of neonatal glycemia with neurodevelopmental outcomes at 4.5 years. *JAMA Pediatrics, 171*(10), 972–983.

Michaels, M. G., Sanchez, P., & Lin, P. L. (2018). Congenital toxoplasmosis, syphilis, malaria, and tuberculosis. In C. A. Gleason & S. E. Juul (Eds.), *Avery's diseases of the newborn* (10th ed.). Philadelphia: Elsevier.

Mitanchez, D., Yzydorczyk, C., & Simeoni, U. (2015). What neonatal complications should the pediatrician be aware of in case of maternal gestational diabetes? *World Journal of Diabetes, 6*(5), 734–743.

Morrison, F. J., Movassaghian, M., Seely, E. W., et al. (2017). Fetal outcomes after diabetic ketoacidosis during pregnancy. *Diabetes Care, 40*(7), e77–e79.

Oyen, N., Diaz, L. J., Leirgul, E., et al. (2016). Prepregnancy diabetes and offspring risk of congenital heart disease: A nationwide cohort study. *Circulation, 133*(23), 2243–2253.

Parsons, J. A., Seay, A. R., & Jacobson, M. (2016). Neurologic disorders. In S. L. Gardner, B. S. Carter, M. Enzman Hines, et al. (Eds.), *Merenstein & Gardner's handbook of neonatal intensive care* (8th ed.). St. Louis: Elsevier.

Patrick, S. W., Dudley, J., Martin, P. R., et al. (2015). Prescription opioid epidemic and infant outcomes. *Pediatrics, 135*(5), 842–850.

Reece-Stremtan, S., & Marinelli, K. A. (2015). ABM clinical protocol no. 21: Guidelines for breastfeeding and substance use or substance use disorder, revised 2015. *Breastfeeding Medicine, 10*(3), 135–141.

Rozance, P. J., McGowan, J. E., Price-Douglas, W., et al. (2016). Glucose homeostasis. In S. L. Gardner, B. S. Carter, M. Enzman-Hines, et al. (Eds.), *Merenstein & Gardner's handbook of neonatal intensive care* (8th ed.). St. Louis: Elsevier.

Schleiss, M. R., & Marsh, K. J. (2018). Viral infections of the fetus and newborn. In C. A. Gleason & S. E. Juul (Eds.), *Avery's diseases of the newborn* (10th ed.). Philadelphia: Elsevier.

Schillie, S., Vellozzi, C., Reingold, A., et al. (2018). Prevention of hepatitis B virus infection in the United States: Recommendations of the Advisory Committee on Immunization Practices. *Morbidity and Mortality Weekly Report, 67*(1), 1–31.

Shah, N. A., & Wusthoff, C. J. (2016). Intracranial hemorrhage in the neonate. *Neonatal Network, 35*(2), 67–72.

Simonsen, K. A., Anderson-Berry, A. L., Delair, S. F., et al. (2014). Early-onset neonatal sepsis. *Clinical Microbiology Reviews, 27*(1), 21–47.

Srinivasan, L., & Evans, J. R. (2018). Health care-associated infections. In C. A. Gleason & S. E. Juul (Eds.), *Avery's diseases of the newborn* (10th ed.). Philadelphia: Elsevier.

Tran, H., & Robb, A. S. (2015). SSRI use during pregnancy. *Seminars in Perinatology, 39*(7), 545–547.

Verklan, M. T. (2015). Neurologic disorders. In M. T. Verklan & M. Walden (Eds.), *Core curriculum for neonatal intensive care nursing* (5th ed.). St. Louis: Elsevier.

Wallen, L. D., & Gleason, C. A. (2018). Prenatal drug exposure. In C. A. Gleason & S. E. Juul (Eds.), *Avery's diseases of the newborn* (10th ed.). Philadelphia: Elsevier.

Weitkamp, J. H., Lewis, D. B., & Levy, O. (2018). Immunology of the fetus and newborn. In C. A. Gleason & S. E. Juul (Eds.), *Avery's diseases of the newborn* (10th ed.). Philadelphia: Elsevier.

Williams, J. F., Smith, V. C., & Committee on Substance Abuse. (2015). Fetal alcohol spectrum disorders. *Pediatrics, 136*(5), e1395–e1406.

Wood, K., Jinadatha, A., Agrawal, K., et al. (2018). Rare but important left colon syndrome (NCLCS): Rare but important complication in an infant of diabetic mother. *BMJ Case Reports.*

36

Hemolytic Disorders and Congenital Anomalies

Christie W. Sawyer

http://evolve.elsevier.com/Lowdermilk/MWHC/

LEARNING OBJECTIVES

- Compare incompatibility of Rh and ABO blood types as causes of hemolytic disease of the newborn and the implications for neonatal outcomes.
- Present assessment strategies during the postnatal period to aid in diagnosing congenital disorders.
- Describe common congenital disorders that are apparent in the newborn period and care management for each.

- Develop a nursing care plan for parents of a newborn with a congenital abnormality.
- Discuss common inborn errors of metabolism that can be identified through newborn screening.
- Analyze the role of the interprofessional team in the management of infants with hemolytic disorders, congenital anomalies, and inborn errors of metabolism.

Many physiologic alterations occur in infants during the newborn period. In some cases, problems are anticipated when prenatal testing has identified specific actual or potential concerns related to the newborn's physiologic status. For example, if the mother's blood type is incompatible with that of her fetus, the newborn may be at risk of hemolysis and subsequent hyperbilirubinemia or anemia.

Prenatal testing may reveal an obvious congenital anomaly, such as myelomeningocele, whereas a less obvious abnormality, such as a congenital heart defect, may be asymptomatic at birth. Some anomalies are not identified before birth and present during the early postnatal period, whereas others may not be evident until much later. Inborn errors of metabolism (IEMs) are identified through newborn screening.

Using astute assessment skills and knowledge of normal adaptation to extrauterine life, the nurse is alert to deviations from normal physiologic adaptation and prepared to take appropriate actions for management in collaboration with the interprofessional health care team. The nurse must also be cognizant of the special needs of the family when a child is born with or acquires an abnormal condition.

HEMOLYTIC DISEASE OF THE NEWBORN

Hemolytic disorders occur when maternal antibodies are present naturally or form in response to an antigen from the fetal blood crossing the placenta and entering the maternal circulation. The maternal antibodies of the immunoglobulin G (IgG) class, in turn, cross the placenta, causing hemolysis of the fetal red blood cells (RBCs), resulting in possible hyperbilirubinemia, jaundice, and anemia.

Hemolytic disease of the newborn occurs most often when the blood groups of the mother and baby are different. The most common cause of hemolytic disease of the fetus and newborn is ABO incompatibility, followed by Rh(D) incompatibility. The incidence of Rh(D) incompatibility has been significantly reduced by immunoprophylaxis against Rh(D) sensitization (Rh immune globulin) (see Chapter 21); however, it is still a problem in underresourced countries (Christensen, 2018).

The four major blood groups in the ABO system are A, B, AB, and O. People with type A blood have A antigen; those with type B have B antigen; those with type AB have both A and B antigens; and those with type O have no antigens. In turn, people with type A blood have plasma antibodies to type B blood; those with type B blood have antibodies to type A blood; those with type AB blood have no antibodies; and those with type O blood have antibodies to types A and B blood. If a person receives or is exposed to an incompatible blood type, he or she will form antibodies against the antigen in that blood, with agglutination, or clumping, occurring as the antibodies in the plasma mix with the antigens of the different blood group.

The Rh factor, a genetically determined factor present on RBCs, can be a major source of incompatibility. Of the 48 forms of the Rh antigen, the D antigen is the most significant because it causes the most antibody production in a person who is Rh-negative. In general, referring to a person as Rh-negative means that she or he does not have the Rh(D) antigen, and Rh-positive means the presence of the Rh(D) antigen. A person who has the Rh factor is considered Rh-positive; a person without it is Rh-negative. For example, a mother who has A-negative blood has the A antigen, plasma antibodies to the B antigen, and no Rh(D) factor on her RBCs. The Rh(D)-negative blood type occurs in approximately 15% of Caucasians, 8% of African Americans, 1% to 2% of Native Americans and Intuit Eskimos, and less than 1% of Asians (Moise, 2018).

Rh Incompatibility

Rh incompatibility, or isoimmunization (also known as alloimmunization) occurs when an Rh-negative mother has an Rh-positive fetus who inherits the dominant Rh-positive gene from the father. If the mother is Rh-negative and the father is Rh-positive and homozygous for the Rh factor, all the offspring will be Rh-positive. If the father is heterozygous for the factor, there is a 50% chance that each infant born of the union will be Rh-positive and a 50% chance that each will be Rh-negative. An Rh-negative fetus is in no danger because it has the same Rh factor as the mother. An Rh-negative fetus with an Rh-positive mother is also in no danger. Only the Rh-positive fetus of an Rh-negative mother is at risk.

The pathogenesis of Rh incompatibility is as follows. Hematopoiesis (the formation, production, and maintenance of blood cells) in the fetus is well established by the ninth week of gestation. When fetal RBCs that contain the Rh antigen pass through the placenta into the maternal circulation of an Rh-negative woman, the maternal immune system produces antibodies against the foreign fetal antigens. The process of antibody formation is called *maternal sensitization.* Sensitization can occur during pregnancy, birth, miscarriage or induced abortion, amniocentesis, external cephalic version, or trauma. Usually Rh-negative women become sensitized in their first pregnancy with an Rh-positive fetus but do not produce enough antibodies to cause lysis (destruction) of fetal blood cells. During subsequent pregnancies, antibodies form in response to repeated contact with the antigen from the fetal blood, and lysis of fetal RBCs results. Multiple gestation, placental abruption, placenta previa, manual removal of the placenta, and cesarean birth increase the incidence of transplacental hemorrhage and the risk of isoimmunization (Blackburn, 2018; Moise, 2018).

In most cases of Rh incompatibility, hemolytic disease is mild; there is little or no anemia and mild hyperbilirubinemia. Treatment is not usually needed, although early phototherapy may be used if hyperbilirubinemia is present (Christensen, 2018).

Severe Rh incompatibility results in marked fetal hemolytic anemia because the fetal erythrocytes are destroyed by maternal Rh-positive antibodies. Although the placenta usually clears the bilirubin resulting from the RBC breakdown, in extreme cases fetal bilirubin levels increase. This results in fetal jaundice, also known as *icterus gravis.* The fetus compensates for the anemia by producing large numbers of immature erythrocytes to replace those hemolyzed; thus the name for this condition: erythroblastosis fetalis. In hydrops fetalis, the most severe complication of this disease, the fetus has marked anemia, cardiac decompensation, cardiomegaly, and hepatosplenomegaly. Hypoxia results from the severe anemia. In addition, because of decreased intravascular oncotic pressure, fluid leaks out of the intravascular space. This results in generalized edema as well as effusions into the peritoneal (ascites), pericardial, and pleural (hydrothorax) spaces (Speer, 2018). The placenta is often edematous, which, along with the edematous fetus, can cause uterine rupture.

Intrauterine or early neonatal death can occur as a result of hydrops fetalis, although intrauterine transfusions and early birth of the fetus can help to avert this. Intrauterine transfusion involves the infusion of Rh-negative type O blood into the umbilical vein. The frequency of intrauterine transfusions varies according to institutional protocol and fetal hydropic status, but it can be as often as every 2 weeks until the fetus reaches pulmonary maturity at approximately 37 to 38 weeks of gestation. Intrauterine transfusion is associated with high survival rates and a low risk of disabilities in surviving infants (Speer, 2018).

ABO Incompatibility

ABO incompatibility is the most common cause of hemolytic disease in the newborn. Of the 20% of newborns who have ABO incompatibility, only 5% have clinical effects (Cunningham, Leveno, Bloom, et al., 2018). The resulting anemia is usually mild. Hyperbilirubinemia is the most common result of ABO incompatibility (Christensen, 2018).

ABO incompatibility occurs if the fetal blood type is A, B, or AB and the maternal type is O. It occurs rarely in infants with type B blood born to mothers with type A blood. The incompatibility arises because naturally occurring anti-A and anti-B antibodies are transferred across the placenta to the fetus. Unlike the situation that pertains to Rh incompatibility, first-born infants can be affected because mothers with type O blood already have anti-A and anti-B antibodies in their blood. Such a newborn can have a weakly positive direct Coombs test (also referred to as a direct antiglobulin test [DAT]). The cord bilirubin level usually is less than 4 mg/dL, and any resulting hyperbilirubinemia can usually be treated with phototherapy. Exchange transfusions are required only occasionally.

Other Causes of Hemolysis

It is not within the scope of this text to discuss the many potential causes of hemolytic jaundice in childhood. However, a frequently encountered disorder is glucose-6-phosphate dehydrogenase (G6PD) deficiency. It is most common among neonates whose genetic heritage comes from Africa, Asia, the Mediterranean, and the Middle East. It is a known cause of bilirubin encephalopathy throughout the world (Watchko, 2018).

G6PD deficiency is a lack of the G6PD enzyme, which protects RBCs from reactive oxidative species and destruction. Because it is a sex-linked disease, male offspring are affected more often than females. A deficiency of the RBC enzyme in combination with exposure to an oxidant stressor (such as sepsis) results in hemolysis and a decreased RBC life. The increase in the destruction of RBCs overwhelms the immature neonatal liver's ability to conjugate the indirect bilirubin. Hyperbilirubinemia can be severe. Treatment is the same as for any newborn with rapidly rising serum bilirubin levels (see Chapter 24) (Glader, 2018; Watchko, 2018).

Other metabolic and inherited conditions cause hemolysis and hyperbilirubinemia in the newborn. These include galactosemia, Crigler-Najjar disease, hypothyroidism, Gilbert syndrome, pyruvate kinase deficiency, and spherocytosis (Calhoun, 2018).

📋 CARE MANAGEMENT

It is important to determine the blood type and Rh factor of the pregnant woman prenatally. Early identification of the Rh-negative woman is critical, and care must be taken to prevent sensitization. A thorough history is needed to identify events that could have caused the woman to develop antibodies to the Rh factor. Such events include (1) previous pregnancy with an Rh-positive fetus; (2) transfusion with Rh-positive blood, which causes immediate sensitization; (3) ectopic pregnancy, miscarriage, or induced abortion after 8 or more weeks of gestation or fetal death at any time; (4) chorionic villus sampling or amniocentesis; (5) placental abruption; (6) external cephalic version; and (7) trauma (Cunningham et al., 2018).

If any of these events has occurred, the nurse checks the woman's medical record to determine whether she has received Rh immune globulin, such as RhoGAM (WinGAM), which is a commercial preparation of passive antibodies against the Rh factor (see the Medication Guide in Chapter 21). This injection of anti-Rh antibodies destroys any fetal RBCs in the maternal circulation and blocks maternal antibody production. Rh immune globulin is 90% effective in preventing sensitization. It is recommended that it be given to an Rh-negative mother at 28 weeks of gestation, within 72 hours of delivery, after an invasive procedure, and any time there is a risk of fetal-maternal hemorrhage. It is also recommended after induced abortion, miscarriage, and ectopic pregnancy (American College of Obstetricians and Gynecologists [ACOG], 2017b).

At the first prenatal visit, the maternal blood type and antibody screen are routinely assessed, and an indirect Coombs test is done to detect unbound antibodies in maternal serum. If the test is positive, further testing is done to identify the specific antibodies and quantify titer levels. This titer indicates the degree of maternal sensitization. A level of 1:8 rarely results in fetal jeopardy. An anti-D titer between 1:16 and 1:32 is considered a critical titer, meaning that the fetus is at risk for hemolytic disease and follow-up is needed (Cunningham et al., 2018).

For the Rh-negative pregnant woman, the risk of the fetus being Rh positive must be determined. The first assessment is paternal zygosity testing to determine his Rh factor; an Rh-positive father increases the risk to the infant. If paternal testing is unavailable, cell-free DNA testing on the mother may be done to determine the fetal Rh factor. Owing to the associated risk, an amniocentesis is not usually done unless other methods are unavailable.

The indirect Coombs test is repeated at 28 weeks. If the result remains negative, indicating that sensitization has not occurred, the woman is given an intramuscular injection of $Rh_o(D)$ immune globulin (ACOG, 2017b). If the test result is positive, showing that sensitization has occurred, it is then repeated every 2 to 4 weeks to monitor the maternal antibody titer until a critical value is reached.

Once a critical value is noted, an assessment of fetal hemolytic process is needed. Serial measurement of the fetal middle cerebral artery peak systolic velocity (MCA-PSV) using Doppler ultrasound is the recommended method to detect fetal anemia (Society for Maternal-Fetal Medicine, Mari, Norton, et al., 2015). If the MCA-PSV shows fetal anemia or if there are signs of fetal hydrops, cordocentesis is performed to assess the fetal hematocrit. If the hematocrit is less than 30%, intrauterine transfusion is indicated (SMFM et al., 2015). Repeat intrauterine transfusion is performed based on decline in hematocrit, usually at 3- to 4-week intervals until 35 weeks. After that point, birth is planned at 38 weeks (Moise, 2018).

Postpartum interventions focus on preventing sensitization in the mother if it has not occurred already and treating any complications in the neonate resulting from the hemolysis of RBCs. The unsensitized Rh-negative mother whose baby is Rh positive should receive $Rh_o(D)$ immune globulin within 72 hours of birth to prevent her from producing antibodies to the fetal blood cells that entered her bloodstream during the birth. One dose accommodates approximately 15 mL of fetal RBCs (ACOG, 2017b).

At birth, the neonate's cord blood is sent to the laboratory to determine the infant's blood type and Rh status. A Coombs test is performed on this blood to determine whether it contains maternal antibodies. The antibody titer indicates the degree of maternal sensitization. In addition, the prevention of or prompt therapy for perinatal asphyxia, acidosis, cold stress, sepsis, and hypoglycemia will decrease the newborn's risk for severe hemolytic disease and susceptibility to acute bilirubin encephalopathy and kernicterus. Early feeding is initiated to stimulate stooling and thus facilitate the removal of bilirubin (see Chapter 24).

Severe hyperbilirubinemia can be caused by blood group incompatibility. Close monitoring of bilirubin levels and prompt treatment with phototherapy is needed to prevent acute bilirubin encephalopathy and kernicterus (see Chapter 24).

In some cases of severe hyperbilirubinemia, **exchange transfusion** may be needed. Partial exchange may be used in treatment of severe anemia due to hydrops. Exchange transfusion is accomplished by alternately removing a small amount of the infant's blood and replacing it with an equal amount of donor blood. Exchange transfusion replaces the RBCs that would otherwise be hemolyzed by circulating maternal antibodies, removes the antibodies responsible for hemolysis, and corrects the anemia caused by hemolysis of the infant's sensitized RBCs. It also reduces the serum bilirubin level in infants who have severe hyperbilirubinemia from any cause. If the infant has Rh incompatibility, type O Rh-negative blood is used for transfusion, so that the maternal antibodies still present in the infant do not hemolyze the transfused blood. Depending on the infant's size, maturity, and condition, amounts of 5 to 20 mL of the infant's blood are removed at one time and replaced with donor blood. The double-volume or two-volume exchange replaces approximately 170 mL/kg of body weight, or 86% of the infant's total blood volume. The procedure requires approximately 1 hour. After the procedure, phototherapy is continued and serial bilirubin levels are monitored (Bradshaw, 2015).

The infant is monitored closely during and after the procedure, including assessment of heart rate and rhythm, respirations, blood pressure, temperature, and perfusion. Preservatives in donor blood lower the infant's serum calcium and magnesium levels. It is not uncommon for calcium gluconate to be given during the exchange transfusion if symptoms of hypocalcemia become evident. Such symptoms include jitteriness, irritability, convulsions, tachycardia, and electrocardiographic changes. The nurse monitors the neonate for hypoglycemia during the several hours after the exchange because the high glucose content of the preservatives can stimulate insulin secretion. These high-risk neonates typically have dextrose support through an intravenous route.

If kernicterus occurs, planning for rehabilitative measures is necessary. The family will need the services of many community resources to care for the affected child. An interprofessional health care team approach that includes social services can help the parents identify early intervention services.

CONGENITAL ANOMALIES

A **congenital anomaly** is a structural or functional abnormality that occurs during intrauterine life and is identified prenatally, at birth, postnatally, during infancy, or thereafter. It is also known as a birth defect, congenital disorder, or congenital malformation. Although numerous genetic and environmental factors are known to cause congenital anomalies, up to 50% do not have an identifiable cause (World Health Organization [WHO], 2016). The WHO reported that during 2015, some 7.9 million infants worldwide were born with congenital anomalies; of those, 303,000 died during the first month (WHO). In the United States, congenital malformations and chromosomal abnormalities are the leading causes of death in infants less than 1 year of age, accounting for 20.8% of all infant deaths (Heron, 2018).

A variety of factors are related to the incidence of congenital anomalies. These include genetic, socioeconomic, demographic, and environmental factors. Maternal health factors that contribute to congenital anomalies include nutritional status (e.g., folic acid deficiency) and conditions such as diabetes and infections (e.g., cytomegalovirus, Zika, rubella) (WHO, 2016).

Advances in technology such as three- and four-dimensional sonography and fetal magnetic resonance imaging (MRI) allow for the early detection of many congenital abnormalities. Prenatal diagnosis allows for close monitoring, counseling for the woman and her partner, planning for the mode and timing of birth, fetal intervention, and planning for postnatal care (Sewell & Keene, 2018). In cases where an anomaly is severe and/or incompatible with life, women and their partners may opt to terminate the pregnancy (see Chapter 3). Whether a couple decides to continue or terminate, there are significant psychologic implications related to feelings of disappointment, disillusionment, loss, and grief (see Chapter 37).

An interprofessional health care team is vital for providing holistic, comprehensive care to infants and families affected by congenital anomalies. In addition to nurses, health care professionals who are likely to be involved in care management include the obstetrician, maternal-fetal medicine specialist, neonatologist, pediatric subspecialist, genetic counselor, social worker, and palliative care services. Anticipatory guidance and counseling are needed as families seek understanding and assistance in preparing for the birth of an infant with one or more abnormalities. Referral to a fetal care center may be needed if intervention is required before or immediately after birth. Most infants with congenital anomalies can be cared for in tertiary care centers (Sewell & Keene, 2018).

The most common anomalies that cause serious problems in the neonate are congenital heart disease, neural tube defects, cleft lip or palate, clubfoot, and developmental dysplasia of the hip. These are thought to result from the interaction of multiple genetic and environmental factors. Minor anomalies are less apparent but more common. It is important to identify them because they can be a part of a characteristic pattern of malformations. That is, they can point to the presence of a more serious major anomaly and aid in its diagnosis. The presence of a minor anomaly indicates the need for further evaluation of the neonate for other anomalies (Bacino, 2018).

This chapter describes some of the most common congenital anomalies. For some topics, statistics on prevalence and incidence are not included because the most current data available were published more than a decade ago. Refer to the Centers for Disease Control and Prevention (www.cdc.gov) or the March of Dimes (www.marchofdimes.org) for information.

Congenital Cardiac Defects

Congenital cardiac defects (CHDs) are structural abnormalities of the heart or intrathoracic vessels that are present at birth and affect cardiac function. They are the most common type of congenital abnormality and the leading cause of death from congenital anomalies. CHDs are often associated with other extracardiac defects such as renal agenesis, omphalocele, tracheoesophageal fistula, and diaphragmatic hernia.

In the United States, 25% of infants with congenital heart anomalies have a critical congenital heart defect (CCHD) that will likely require surgical intervention within the first year. In an effort to identify those infants with CCHDs who do not manifest symptoms prior to hospital discharge, current recommendations for newborn screening include routine pulse oximetry assessment prior to discharge from the birth facility (see Chapter 24). There is clear evidence that screening programs are effective in detecting CCHD and in reducing early infant deaths due to CCHD (Plana, Zamora, Suresh, et al., 2018; Rahi, Grosse, Ailes, et al., 2017).

The exact etiology of most CHDs is unknown. The majority of defects are thought to be multifactorial, resulting from a complex interaction of genetic and environmental factors. Certain maternal factors are known to be associated with a higher incidence of CHDs (Box 36.1). Family history of a CHD in a parent or sibling is a known risk factor. If one child is affected by a CHD, there is a high likelihood that others will also have a CHD.

Genetic factors are implicated in the pathogenesis of CHDs, with an increased percentage of CHDs attributed to single-gene mutations. An example of this is DiGeorge or 22q11.2 syndrome, which occurs when a small part of chromosome 22 is missing. This syndrome is associated with CHDs, cleft palate, poor immune function, hypocalcemia, and cognitive and emotional problems (Evans, Hing, & Cunningham, 2018). There is a well-known association of CHDs with other chromosomal abnormalities, including trisomies 13, 18, and 21 (Down syndrome) (Scholz & Reinking, 2018).

Although traditionally a CHD was classified as either cyanotic or acyanotic, a classification that categorizes cardiac defects physiologically by physiologic consequence is now considered more descriptive. This system is based on hemodynamic characteristics or blood flow patterns within the heart: (1) increased pulmonary blood flow, (2) decreased pulmonary blood flow, (3) obstruction to blood flow out of the heart, and (4) mixed blood flow (Fig. 36.1).

🏠 COMMUNITY ACTIVITY

Visit the National Heart, Lung, and Blood Institute website (www.nhlbi.nih.gov/health/health-topics/topics/chd). Under the types of defects, review the information on septal defects. In particular, familiarize yourself with the features of ventricular septal defects, the most common type of congenital heart defect. How could you explain this defect in simple terms to parents? Determine where infants from your community go to receive treatment for congenital heart defects.

BOX 36.1   Maternal Risk Factors for Congenital Heart Defects

- Infections: Rubella and cytomegalovirus
- Febrile illness in first trimester
- Medications: Anticonvulsants (phenytoin), lithium, opioids (early pregnancy)
- Alcohol intake
- Obesity
- Poor nutrition, folic acid deficiency
- Radiation or air pollution exposure
- Metabolic disorders such as diabetes mellitus
- Systemic lupus erythematosus
- Maternal age ≥40 years
- Maternal smoking >25 cigarettes per day

Data from Oster, M. (2018). Newborn screening for critical congenital heart disease using pulse oximetry. In D. R. Fulton & L. E. Weisman (Eds.), *UpToDate.* Retrieved from www.uptodate.com; Oyen, N., Diaz, L. J., Leirgul, E., et.al. (2016). Prepregnancy diabetes and offspring risk of congenital heart disease: A nationwide cohort study. *Circulation, 133*(23), 2243–2253; and Sadowski, S. (2015). Cardiovascular disorders. In M. T. Verklan & M. Walden (Eds.). *Core curriculum for neonatal intensive care nursing* (5th ed.). St. Louis: Elsevier.

CCHDs are often evident immediately after birth, especially those defects that cause cyanosis. Infants with these anomalies are transferred directly to neonatal intensive care units (NICUs), preferably those that are equipped to diagnose and medically or surgically treat these types of cardiac emergencies. Even though the structural or functional anomalies are always present at birth, the affected newborns can be asymptomatic because the defect is too small to interfere with sufficient blood flow to the lungs for oxygenation, or there is persistence of fetal circulation (i.e., patent ductus arteriosus) allowing alternate blood flow, or the defect does not interfere with delivery of oxygenated blood to the tissues. With growth and maturation, the defect can become apparent as the infant or child is exposed to stressors such as growth demands or infection.

If symptoms of a congenital heart defect are present at birth, they can be obvious with the first cry, which can be weak and muffled or loud and breathless. Newborns can exhibit cyanosis that is not relieved when the child is given supplemental oxygen. Other infants can be acyanotic but pale, with or without mottling on exertion and on crying, feeding, or stooling. The subjective assessment of an infant's color can be affected by several things, including skin pigmentation and hemoglobin level; therefore pulse oximetry is needed to assess oxygen saturation in an infant with abnormal coloration (Wycoff, Aziz, Escobedo, et al., 2015). The affected newborn may present with a variety of physical manifestations of the cardiac lesion. The activity level varies from restlessness to lethargy and possibly unresponsiveness. Irregular heart rhythm may be present as well as bradycardia (a resting heart rate of less than 80 beats/min) or tachycardia (a rate exceeding 160 beats/min). There may or may not be a murmur (turbulent blood flow).

Other findings include decreased peripheral pulses or bounding pulses, active precordium, decreased perfusion, and a blood pressure difference of more than 20 mm Hg between the upper and lower extremities (Sadowski, 2015).

❗ NURSING ALERT

The presence of a murmur does not indicate a congenital cardiac defect and the absence of a murmur does not rule out a congenital heart defect.

Congenital Cardiac Defects

Defects with Increased Pulmonary Blood Flow

Atrial septal defect (ASD)

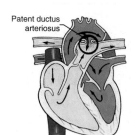

An ASD is an abnormal opening between the right and left atria. Basically, three types of abnormalities result from incorrect development of the atrial septum. An incompetent foramen ovale is the most common defect. The high ostium secundum defect results from abnormal development of the septum secundum. Improper development of the septum primum produces a basal opening known as an *ostium primum defect*, frequently involving the atrio-ventricular valves. In general, left-to-right shunting of the blood occurs in all atrial septal defects.

Ventricular septal defect (VSD)

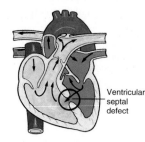

A VSD is an abnormal opening between the right and left ventricles. VSDs vary in size and may occur in either the membranous or muscular portion of the ventricular septum. Because of higher pressure in the left ventricle, a shunting of blood from the left to the right ventricle occurs during systole. If pulmonary vascular resistance produces pulmonary hypertension, the shunt of blood is then reversed from the right to the left ventricle, with cyanosis resulting.

Patent ductus arteriosus (PDA)

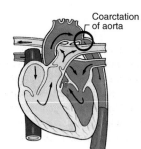

PDA is a vascular connection that, during fetal life, bypasses the pulmonary vascular bed and directs blood from the pulmonary artery to the aorta. Functional closure of the ductus normally occurs soon after birth. If the ductus remains patent after birth, the direction of blood flow in the ductus is reversed by the higher pressure in the aorta.

Atrioventricular canal (AVC) defect

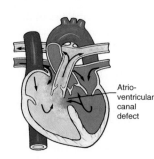

An AVC defect is an incomplete fusion of the endocardial cushions. It consists of a low atrial septal defect that is continuous, with a high ventricular septal defect and clefts of the mitral and tricuspid valves, creating a large central atrioventricular valve that allows blood to flow between all four chambers of the heart. Flow is generally from left to right. It is the most common cardiac defect in children with Down syndrome.

Obstructive Defects

Coarctation of the aorta (COA)

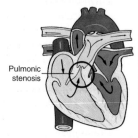

COA is characterized by localized narrowing of the aorta near the insertion of the ductus arteriosus, resulting in increased pressure proximal to the defect (head and upper extremities) and decreased pressure distal to the defect (body and lower extremities).

Aortic stenosis (AS)

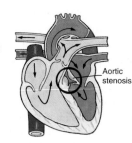

AS is a narrowing or stricture of the aortic valve, causing resistance to blood flow in the left ventricle, decreased cardiac output, left ventricular hypertrophy, and pulmonary vascular congestion. AS can be valvular, subvalvular, or supravalvular (rare). The most serious sequelae relate to the left ventricular hypertrophy (increased end-diastolic pressure, pulmonary hypertension, decreased coronary artery perfusion).

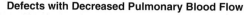

Pulmonic stenosis (PS)

PS is a narrowing at the entrance to the pulmonary artery. Resistance to blood flow causes right ventricular hypertrophy and decreased pulmonary blood flow. Pulmonary atresia is the extreme form of PS; no blood flows to the lungs.

Defects with Decreased Pulmonary Blood Flow

Tetralogy of Fallot (TOF)

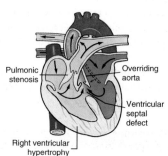

TOF is characterized by the combination of four defects: (1) pulmonary stenosis, (2) ventricular septal defect, (3) overriding aorta, and (4) hypertrophy of the right ventricle. It is the most common defect, causing cyanosis in children surviving beyond 2 years of age. The severity of symptoms depends on the degree of pulmonary stenosis, the size of the ventricular septal defect, and the degree to which the aorta overrides the septal defect.

Tricuspid atresia

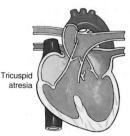

Tricuspid valvular atresia is characterized by a small right ventricle, a large left ventricle, and usually a diminished pulmonary circulation. Blood from the right atrium passes through an atrial septal defect into the left atrium, mixes with oxygenated blood returning from the lungs, flows into the left ventricle, and is propelled into the systemic circulation. The lungs may receive blood through one of three routes: (1) a small ventricular septal defect, (2) a patent ductus arteriosus, or (3) bronchial vessels.

Fig. 36.1 Congenital Heart Abnormalities. (Modified from Hockenberry, M.J., Wilson, D., & Rodgers, C. C. (2019). *Wong's nursing care of infants and children* (11th ed.). St. Louis: Elsevier.)

Mixed Defects

Transposition of the great vessels (TGV)

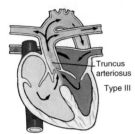

TGV is an embryologic defect caused by a straight division of the bulbar trunk without normal spiraling. As a result, the aorta originates from the right ventricle and the pulmonary artery from the left ventricle. An abnormal communication between the two circulations must be present to sustain life.

Total anomalous pulmonary venous connection (TAPVC)

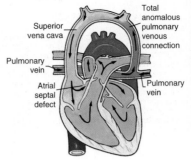

TAPVC is a rare defect characterized by a failure of the pulmonary veins to join the left atrium. Instead, the pulmonary veins are abnormally connected to the systemic venous circuit via the right atrium or various veins draining toward the right atrium (e.g., superior vena cava). The abnormal attachment results in mixed blood being returned to the right atrium and shunted from the right to the left through an atrial septal defect.

Connection

Truncus arteriosus (TA)

TA is a retention of the embryologic bulbar trunk. It results from the failure of normal septation and division of this trunk into an aorta and pulmonary artery. This single arterial trunk overrides the ventricles and receives blood from them through a ventricular septal defect. The entire pulmonary and systemic circulation is supplied from this common arterial trunk.

Hypoplastic left heart syndrome (HLHS)

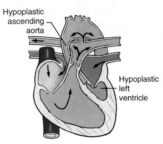

HLHS is characterized by underdevelopment of the left side of the heart, resulting in a hypoplastic left ventricle and aortic atresia. Most blood from the left atrium flows across the patent foramen ovale to the right atrium, to the right ventricle, and out the pulmonary artery. The descending aorta receives blood from the patent ductus arteriosus supplying systemic blood flow.

Fig. 36.1, cont'd.

Cardiac disease can be manifested by respiratory signs and symptoms. Tachypnea, a respiratory rate greater than 60 breaths/min without dyspnea, is typically a subtle clue that the infant possibly has a cardiac malformation. Increased respiratory depth or hyperpnea is often noted when the neonate has a cardiac lesion that is obstructing blood flow to the lungs. Signs that can indicate the development of congestive heart failure are feeding difficulties (e.g., tachypnea such that the infant has to stop feeding to breathe), increased work of breathing, crackles, and fatigue.

A major role of the nurse is to assess infants for abnormal findings, which must be reported immediately to the health care provider. Newborns exhibiting these symptoms require prompt diagnosis and appropriate therapy in a neonatal or pediatric intensive care unit. Immediate interventions include administering oxygen as ordered and placement of a pulse oximeter. Management may also include administering cardiotonic and other medications such as diuretics that rid the body of accumulated fluid, maintenance of a thermoneutral environment, feeding with the gavage method if necessary, and preventing crying (if this precipitates cyanosis). Various diagnostic tests such as echocardiography and cardiac catheterization are performed to obtain specific information about the defect and the need for surgical intervention. Significant improvements in diagnosis, medical management, and surgical treatment of CHDs have caused the death rate to decrease significantly, with the result that more of these children are reaching adulthood (Sadowski, 2015).

Central Nervous System Anomalies

Most congenital anomalies of the CNS result from defects in closure of the neural tube during fetal development. Although the cause of **neural tube defects (NTDs)** is unknown, they are thought to stem from the interaction of many genes that can be influenced by factors in the fetal environment. Environmental influences such as maternal treatment with anticonvulsants (e.g., valproic acid or carbamazepine), treatment

with methotrexate (a chemotherapeutic medication), use of opioids during the first trimester, maternal obesity, and maternal diabetes have been implicated. Excessive maternal body heat exposure during the early first trimester, significant febrile illness, and lower socioeconomic status can also increase the risk of an NTD (Dukhovny & Wilkins-Haug, 2018; March of Dimes, 2018). Maternal folic acid deficiency has a direct bearing on failure of the neural tube to close. Therefore, as a preventive measure, folic acid supplementation (0.4 mg/day) is recommended for women of childbearing age; those with history of NTDs should take 400 mg daily. Folic acid supplementation should continue for at least the first trimester of pregnancy (American Academy of Pediatrics [AAP] & American College of Obstetricians and Gynecologists [ACOG], 2017).

Globally, NTDs are among the most common congenital abnormalities, although prevalence is widely varied. The estimated worldwide prevalence is 18.6/10,000 births (including stillbirths and elective terminations of pregnancy) (Blencowe, Kancherla, Moorthie, et al., 2018). In the Americas, NTDs are estimated to occur in 5.3/10,000 live births (Zaganjor, Ahlia, Tsang, et al., 2016). The incidence of NTDs has decreased over the past 20 years because of the increased intake of folic acid before and during pregnancy.

There is genetic predisposition for NTDs. The risk for recurrence after one child has been found to be affected is 3% to 4%. The risk of recurrence is 10% after two previously affected children (Kinsman & Johnston, 2016).

Although an NTD is usually an isolated defect, it can occur with some chromosomal abnormalities and syndromes and with other defects such as cleft palate, ventricular septal defect, tracheoesophageal fistula, diaphragmatic hernia, imperforate anus, and renal anomalies. Some NTDs are diagnosed prenatally with fetal ultrasonography and the finding of elevated levels of alpha-fetoprotein in the amniotic fluid and maternal serum at 16 to 18 weeks. Increased use of prenatal diagnostic techniques such as chorionic villus sampling at 11 weeks allows earlier diagnosis and potential termination of pregnancies, having an

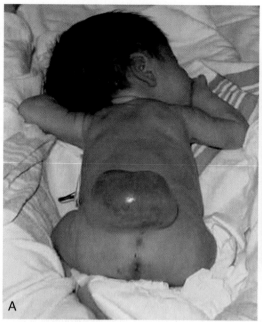

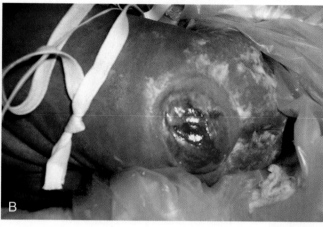

Fig. 36.2 Views of Meningomyelocele. (A) Myelomeningocele with an intact sac. (B) Myelomeningocele with a ruptured sac. (A, Courtesy Dr. Robert C. Dauser, Neurosurgery, Baylor College of Medicine, Houston, TX; B, Courtesy Cheryl Briggs, RNC, Annapolis, MD.)

effect on the overall birth rate of infants with NTDs (Greene & Copp, 2014).

Encephalocele and Anencephaly

Encephalocele and anencephaly are abnormalities resulting from failure of the anterior end of the neural tube to close. An encephalocele is a herniation of the brain and meninges through a skull defect, usually in the occipital area. Treatment consists of surgical repair and shunting to relieve hydrocephalus unless a major brain malformation is present. It is common for infants with encephalocele to have other major anomalies, such as congenital heart defects, cleft lip or palate, microcephaly, or craniosynostosis (Huang & Doherty, 2018).

Anencephaly, the most serious NTD, is the absence of both cerebral hemispheres and of the overlying skull. This condition is incompatible with life; the majority of affected infants are stillborn and the others die during the first few months due to respiratory failure. Palliative care and family support are provided (Verklan, 2015).

Spina Bifida

Spina bifida, the most common defect of the CNS, results from failure of the neural tube (the sheath that closes to form the brain and spinal cord) to close in early gestation. The two categories of spina bifida are spina bifida occulta and spina bifida manifesta, also known as open spina bifida.

Spina bifida occulta, the milder form, is a malformation in which the posterior portion of the laminae fails to close, but the spinal cord or meninges do not herniate or protrude through the defect and there is no abnormality of the spinal cord, nerve roots, or meninges; however, there can be tethering of the spinal cord. This occurs most frequently in the lumbosacral region (L5 and S1). Skin typically covers the opening in the spinal cord. There can also be a bulge under the skin where the ends of the spinal cord terminate in fatty tissue. There can be a hematoma, cutaneous dimple or abnormality, mass, or hair tuft in the lumbosacral region. Neurologic deficits in the newborn are typically absent, although sensory abnormalities in the lower extremities or sphincter abnormalities may occur (Robinson & Cohen, 2015).

Spina bifida manifesta occurs predominantly in the lumbar or lumbosacral region and includes meningocele and myelomeningocele. A meningocele occurs when meninges and spinal fluid extend through an irregular vertebral opening; the neural elements are usually not present. The lesion is usually covered with a layer of skin. Symptoms are rare, but they can include paralysis as well as bladder and bowel dysfunction. The infant's neurologic function tends to be normal unless other abnormalities are present.

A myelomeningocele is more severe and occurs when there is a herniation of the spinal cord and neural elements through an opening in the spine with or without skin or vertebral covering (Fig. 36.2). It results in partial or complete motor or sensory dysfunction of the body parts below the spinal opening. The impairment can cause bladder and bowel dysfunction and, in severe cases, paralysis. If covered, the sac can tear easily, allowing cerebrospinal fluid (CSF) to leak out and increasing the risk of CNS infection. A lesion in the thoracolumbar, lumbar, or lumbosacral region has the highest association with hydrocephalus. A lumbar lesion is often associated with an Arnold-Chiari malformation, resulting from the improper development and downward displacement of the hindbrain into the cervical spinal canal. This blocks the flow of CSF from communicating with the spinal column and results in the development of hydrocephalus. Other findings associated with myelomeningocele include kyphosis, club foot, hip dislocation, tethered cord, and seizure activity (Huang & Doherty, 2018).

Prenatal diagnosis allows for parental education and determination of their preference for prenatal or postnatal management. Intrauterine fetal surgery may be performed prior to 26 weeks of gestation to repair a myelomeningocele. ACOG (2017a) recommends that fetal surgery should be offered only at locations where there are extensive resources to care for these women and their families. Parents should be educated on the limited long-term information on fetal surgery and their wishes for management should be supported.

If parents do not choose prenatal surgery, birth should be scheduled at a facility with a level III NICU and with neurosurgery subspecialties. Birth at term is preferred, but if macrocephaly or ventriculomegaly is noted, earlier birth may be required.

Postnatal surgery for myelomeningocele is usually performed within the first 48 to 72 hours to close the defect. Based on the type and position of the lesion and the neonate's clinical condition, early surgical repair is advocated to preserve cognitive function, decrease the risk of sepsis, prevent further deterioration of the exposed spinal cord, and improve the prognosis for ambulation. Surgical shunt procedures such as a ventriculoperitoneal shunt to prevent increasing hydrocephalus may be needed (Dias, Parrington, & Section on Neurologic Surgery, 2015).

A major preoperative nursing intervention for a neonate with a myelomeningocele is to protect the protruding sac from injury, rupture, and resultant risk of CNS infection. Such infants should be positioned in a prone-kneeling position and the knees protected from skin breakdown. The sac should be covered with a sterile, moist, nonadherent dressing and cared for using sterile technique. A drape should be placed over the buttocks below the lesion and secured using the drape's adhesive to keep the lesion free of meconium or stool. If rupture of the lesion is noted, a culture of the specimen may be needed. Neurosurgery and urology consultations should occur as soon as possible after birth (Verklan, 2015).

A thorough physical examination is done to evaluate the level of the injury, sensory involvement, sphincter control (anal wink), and measurement of the fronto-occipital circumference to assess for hydrocephalus. Intake and output are recorded to document the number and character of the voids and stools as well as the leakage of urine and stool. Nursing assessment includes observations of movement or absence of movement as well as the quality of movements of the lower extremities.

Nurses provide support and information to parents as they begin to learn to cope with an infant who has immediate needs for intensive care and who will probably have long-term needs. Care should be provided by an interprofessional team of specialists representing nursing, pediatrics, neurosurgery, urology, physical therapy, endocrinology, orthopedics, and both rehabilitative and neuropsychiatric care (Huang & Doherty, 2018).

⚡ SAFETY ALERT

Infants with myelomeningocele are at increased risk for developing latex sensitivity, so they must not come into direct or secondary contact with any products or equipment containing latex.

Hydrocephalus

Hydrocephalus is a condition in which there is excess CSF in the ventricles of the brain due to overproduction (rare) or a decrease in reabsorption. The most common etiology for the neonate is excess ventricular CSF due to aqueductal flow obstruction. The obstruction prevents the CSF from leaving the head and flowing into the spinal column. It can be congenital or acquired. Congenital hydrocephalus can be due to a Dandy-Walker malformation, congenital viral infections (toxoplasmosis, cytomegalovirus), myelomeningocele with Arnold-Chiari malformation, and congenital masses or tumors. Hydrocephalus is also associated with spina bifida, holoprosencephaly, and encephalocele. Acquired hydrocephalus can result from neoplasm, intracranial hemorrhage, or meningitis. Preterm and low-birth-weight infants are at increased risk (Haridas & Tomita, 2018b; Robinson & Cohen, 2015).

In most cases hydrocephalus is a progressive condition. The neonate with congenital hydrocephalus presents with a large head and an increasing occipitofrontal circumference (OFC) (Fig. 36.3). The

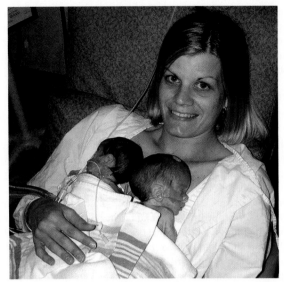

Fig. 36.3 A Mother Providing Kangaroo Care to Preterm Twins; the One on the Right has Hydrocephalus. The characteristic appearance is an enlarged head, thinning of the scalp, distended scalp veins, and a full fontanel. (Courtesy Cheryl Briggs, RNC, Annapolis, MD.)

sutures are widened and the fontanels are full or bulging and tense. Signs of increasing intracranial pressure include vomiting, lethargy, and irritability. The infant may have "setting sun eyes" (eyes that are rotated downward). Serial OFC measurements, serial head ultrasounds, and supplemental computed tomography (CT) and MRI scans are used to evaluate the evolving condition. The need for surgical intervention to drain the excess CSF is determined by the severity of symptoms and the results of diagnostic studies. Neurosurgery and genetics services are consulted to evaluate for the placement of a ventriculoperitoneal shunt versus placement of a reservoir and to assess for the presence of congenital anomalies (Haridas & Tomita, 2018a; Verklan, 2015).

The nurse provides support to the family by teaching and involving them in their infant's care as much as possible. Minimal stimulation protocols that promote the use of limited handling, dim lighting, and attention to the baby's cues will help keep the infant calm. The head must be positioned carefully and repositioned at least once every 4 hours; it is also important that the head not be positioned on the shunt side postoperatively. Gel-filled pillows can provide some comfort for the neonate. The OFC is measured serially; depending on the rate of increase, this is done every 4 to 24 hours. Neurologic assessments and observation for signs of increasing intracranial pressure should be done every 4 to 8 hours depending on the baby's clinical condition (Verklan, 2015).

The baby should be fed in a semi-reclining position with the head well supported. The method, amount, and frequency of feeding depend on the infant's tolerance and energy level. The nurse should be alert to the possibility of emesis, a frequent occurrence in the presence of increased intracranial pressure, and should maintain aspiration precautions. Nonnutritive sucking, touching, and cuddling needs should be met (Verklan, 2015).

The surgical correction of hydrocephalus involves the placement of a shunt that goes from the ventricles of the brain usually to the peritoneum to allow the drainage of excess CSF. Damaged or destroyed brain tissue cannot be restored. The long-term prognosis in affected infants depends on the presence and extent of such tissue damage along with the cause of the hydrocephalus, the presence of concurrent neurologic problems, and the long-term success of the shunt procedure.

Parent teaching regarding the shunt should be done both pre- and postoperatively. Parents must be taught about the signs of a blocked shunt (i.e., signs of increasing intracranial pressure), signs of infection, and changes in the baby's feeding patterns and to notify the health care provider if these symptoms occur (Portillo Medina, Franco, Ciapponi, et al., 2017).

Microcephaly

Microcephaly refers to an occipitofrontal head circumference that is more than two standard deviations smaller than the mean for gestational age, weight, and sex. It occurs because the brain did not develop properly or stopped growing. Microcephaly can be genetic or acquired (Huang & Doherty, 2018). Maternal risk factors include congenital viral infections (e.g., cytomegalovirus, rubella, varicella, Zika), chromosomal disorders, radiation exposure, maternal phenylketonuria, diabetes, and malnutrition. Fetal and neonatal factors include inflammation, birth trauma, and sequelae of hypoxic-ischemic encephalopathy. If the result of an in utero insult, the baby is typically born with a small head and brain, which gives the forehead a backward-sloping appearance. Diagnostic evaluations include a complete maternal history, evaluation of the events surrounding the birth, CT or MRI to evaluate brain volume, and a neurologic assessment. Genetics, neurology, and infectious disease consults are usually obtained. Although neurologic deficits are not present at birth, developmental delays will gradually become evident.

The baby's outcome and prognosis depend on the severity of the microcephaly. Nursing care is supportive and includes accurate OFC measurements and helping parents coordinate follow-up care. The parents will need support, resources, and education to help them learn to care for a child with cognitive impairment and developmental delays. Physical, occupational, and speech therapies are part of interprofessional management as the child grows (Verklan, 2015).

Respiratory System Anomalies

Screening for congenital anomalies of the respiratory system is necessary even in infants who are apparently normal at birth. Respiratory distress at birth or shortly thereafter can be the result of lung immaturity or anomalous development. This section focuses on the congenital anomalies of bilateral choanal atresia, diaphragmatic hernia, and tracheoesophageal fistula.

Choanal Atresia

Choanal atresia (Fig. 36.4) is the most common congenital anomaly of the nose. It is the congenital blockage of the posterior nares by a bony or soft-tissue obstruction. The obstruction can be unilateral or bilateral. Associated anomalies are common; for example, tracheoesophageal fistula, palatal abnormalities, CHARGE association (coloboma, heart defect, atresia choanae, restricted growth and development, genital hypoplasia, and ear anomalies/deafness). Since infants are obligate nose breathers for the first 4 to 6 weeks, symptoms of respiratory distress, low oxygen saturations, and cyanosis will be noted with rest, feeding, or pacifier use. However, when the infant cries, the saturations increase, the infant's color improves, and respiratory distress is alleviated. If choanal atresia is suspected, a small feeding tube or suction catheter may be passed through the nose into the pharynx. If it cannot be advanced, it is highly suggestive of the diagnosis. Caution must be taken when anything is inserted into the nares as it can cause edema or trauma. Securing an oral airway into the posterior pharynx and maintaining the baby in the prone position will provide a patent airway and time to evaluate for the presence of other abnormalities. Definitive diagnosis is usually by CT scan; treatment involves creating a patency through the bony or soft tissue obstruction and use of serial obturators to dilate the new airway passages (Evans et al., 2018; Otteson & Arnold, 2015).

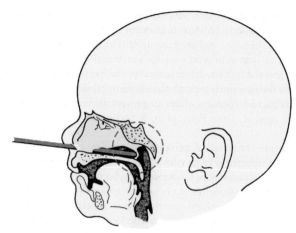

Fig. 36.4 Choanal Atresia. The posterior nares are obstructed by membrane or bone either bilaterally or unilaterally. The infant becomes cyanotic at rest. With crying, the newborn's color improves. Nasal discharge is present. Snorting respirations are often observed with increased respiratory effort. The newborn may be unable to breathe and eat at the same time. The diagnosis is made by noting an inability to pass small feeding tube through one or both nares. (Used with permission of Ross Products Division, Abbott Laboratories, Inc., Columbus, OH 43216. From Clinical Education Aid #6, Copyright 1963, Ross Products Division, Abbott Laboratories, Inc.)

Congenital Diaphragmatic Hernia

Congenital diaphragmatic hernia (CDH) results from a defect in the formation of the diaphragm, allowing the abdominal organs to be displaced into the thoracic cavity and interfering with the development of the lungs. Alveolar and capillary surface areas are decreased. Despite improvements in management, the mortality rate is high.

The etiology of CDH is unknown; however, it is not uncommon to find concomitant chromosomal anomalies, especially trisomies 12, 18, 21, or Turner syndrome. CDH is often associated with abnormalities of the cardiovascular and musculoskeletal systems and occurs more frequently in male infants. The vast majority of hernias occur posteriorly on the left side (Keller, Hirose, & Farmer, 2018).

Prenatal ultrasound will detect most cases of CDH. Fetuses with CDH tend to have polyhydramnios, which typically prompts the obstetrician to obtain an ultrasound. Fetal MRI aids in diagnosis and provides prognostic information. Prenatal diagnosis of CDH warrants referral to a tertiary or quarternary care center where the diagnosis can be confirmed and plans for birth can be made. Prenatal identification of CDH allows for assessment of associated physical and genetic abnormalities, consultation and counseling by an interprofessional health care team, and plans for management (Hedrick, 2017). There is currently insufficient evidence to recommend in utero intervention for fetuses with CDH as a part of routine clinical practice (Grivell, Andersen, & Dodd, 2015).

The spectrum of respiratory and hemodynamic problems associated with CDH varies and depends on the size of the defect, the degree of lung hypoplasia, and the development of persistent pulmonary hypertension. A small defect may not be symptomatic at birth; distress occurs when the infant is challenged with feedings. Newborns with large defects will have significant distress at birth due to lung hypoplasia and bowel in the chest; symptoms include respiratory distress, cyanosis, mottling, tachypnea, and pulmonary hypertension. Heart sounds are shifted to the right and blood pressure is low. Distress increases as the bowels fill with air. The abdomen may appear scaphoid and the chest barrel-shaped due to abdominal contents in the chest. Diagnosis can be made on the basis of the x-ray finding of loops of intestine in the thoracic cavity and the absence of intestine in the abdominal cavity (Hedrick & Adzick, 2018; Keller et al., 2018) (Fig. 36.5).

Surgical repair is timed on the basis of the infant's clinical status and comorbidities; immediate surgery is no longer the standard of care. Preoperative nursing interventions include participating in stabilizing the infant's cardiopulmonary condition until surgical repair can be done.

Persistent pulmonary hypertension is treated with oxygen and, in severe cases, inhaled nitric oxide (see Chapter 34). Gastric contents are aspirated and suction is applied to decompress the gastrointestinal (GI) tract and prevent further cardiothoracic compromise. Oxygen therapy, mechanical ventilation, and the correction of acidosis are necessary in infants with large defects. Extracorporeal membrane oxygenation (ECMO) or high-frequency oscillatory ventilation can be used in infants with severe circulatory and respiratory complications (see Chapter 34) (Hedrick & Adzick, 2018).

The prognosis depends largely on the degree of fetal pulmonary development and the success of surgical diaphragmatic closure, but the prognosis in severe cases is often poor. As a rule, liver herniation into the thorax is associated with the worst prognosis. Some infants with CDH die before they can have surgical repair. Of those who survive, lasting health issues include chronic lung disease, feeding difficulties, and gastroesophageal reflux (GER).

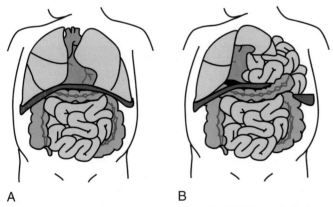

Fig. 36.5 Congenital Diaphragmatic Hernia. (A) Normal diaphragm separating the abdominal and thoracic cavities. (B) Diaphragmatic hernia with a small lung and abdominal contents in the thoracic cavity. (From Maheshwari, A., & Carlo, W. A. [2018]. Diaphragmatic hernia. In R. M. Kliegman, B. F. Stanton, J. W. St Geme III, et al. [Eds.], *Nelson textbook of pediatrics* [20th ed.]. Philadelphia: Elsevier.)

Gastrointestinal System Anomalies

Anomalies of the GI system can occur anywhere along the GI tract, from the mouth to the anus. Some anomalies—such as cleft lip, omphalocele, and gastroschisis—are apparent at birth. Others—including cleft palate, esophageal atresia, pyloric stenosis, intestinal obstructions, and imperforate anus—become apparent as the infant is further assessed or becomes symptomatic.

Cleft Lip and Palate

Cleft lip and cleft palate, also known as orofacial clefts, are among the most common congenital anomalies (Fig. 36.6). One or both deformities can occur, and nasal deformity can be present. Cleft lip is most often unilateral, although it can occur bilaterally. Cleft lip can range from a simple notch in the lip to complete separation of the lip extending to the floor of the nose. Cleft palate occurs midline in the secondary palate; it can range from a bifid uvula to a complete cleft extending from the soft to the hard palate. Orofacial clefting can occur as part of a syndrome (e.g., Pierre-Robin) or as an isolated defect.

Most cases of orofacial clefts are due to multifactorial inheritance, caused by a combination of genetic and environmental factors. Environmental influences include maternal infection, folic acid deficiency, maternal diabetes, maternal smoking, radiation exposure, obesity, alcohol ingestion, and treatment with medications such as corticosteroids, lithium, valproic acid, retinoids, and phenytoin (Wilkins-Haug, 2018).

Orofacial clefts occur in approximately 14.5/10,000 live births in the United States. Two-thirds of affected infants have cleft lip with cleft palate. Orofacial clefts are more common in male infants and among Native Americans and Alaska Natives. African Americans are the least likely affected (Mai, Cassell, Meyer, et al., 2014).

Surgical repair of cleft lip and nasal deformity is done by 6 months. Repair of a cleft palate is usually performed between 9 and 12 months of age to promote speech development. Advances in surgical techniques have made it possible for some infants, particularly those with unilateral cleft lip, to have a near normal appearance. The results of the repair depend on the severity of the defect, with more severe bilateral cleft lip requiring surgical repair in stages.

Airway management can be a concern for infants with orofacial clefts. Feeding can be difficult because the cleft lip renders the newborn unable to maintain a seal around a nipple; the cleft palate renders the infant unable to form a vacuum to maintain suction when feeding. In addition, the inability to suck and swallow normally allows milk to pool in the nasopharynx, which increases the likelihood of aspiration. Furthermore, as the infant attempts to suck, milk often comes out through the cleft and the nares. Although the degree of difficulty depends on the size of the cleft, feeding problems are greater in infants with a cleft palate than in those with a cleft lip. Breastfeeding is often

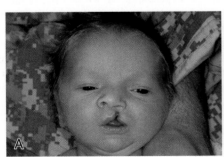
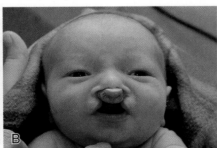
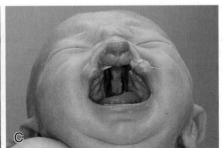

Fig. 36.6 Orofacial Clefts (A) An infant with unilateral incomplete cleft lip. (B and C) An infant with bilateral complete cleft lip and palate. (From Evans, K. N., Hing, A. V., & Cunningham, M. L. [2018]. Craniofacial malformations. In C. A. Gleason & S. E. Juul [Eds.], *Avery's diseases of the newborn* [10th ed.]. Philadelphia: Elsevier.)

possible if the infant has a cleft lip alone. Special nipples, bottles, and appliances (e.g., Haberman or pigeon feeder) are used for bottle feeding. In general, parents need education, support, and encouragement as they learn to feed their baby. This can help minimize anxiety and frustration while promoting competence and confidence in providing infant care.

Initial and ongoing care for children with orofacial defects involves the combined efforts of an interprofessional health care team that includes pediatrics, plastic surgery, otolaryngology, speech/language pathology, nursing, social work, dentistry, oral surgery, orthodontics, and psychology. Repair of the defects can involve a series of surgical procedures to allow the child to have a near normal appearance and adequate function (Evans et al., 2018).

Parents of infants with a cleft lip or palate need much support, particularly in the case of a cleft lip, because this is both a cosmetic and functional defect. Recognizing that this can interfere with normal parent-infant bonding in the neonatal period, the nurse must assess for this and intervene appropriately. Some communities have support groups for parents of children with orofacial clefts. Parents may also be referred to the following organizations for information and services: the American Cleft Lip Association (www.acpa-cpf.org), the Cleft Palate Foundation (www.cleftline.org), and the March of Dimes (www.marchforbabies.org).

❓ CLINICAL REASONING CASE STUDY

Cleft Lip and Cleft Palate

Michael, a 3.7-kg (8.2-lb) Caucasian neonate, was admitted to the newborn nursery after an uncomplicated vaginal birth at 40 weeks of gestation. He is his parents' first child. At birth Michael was noted to have a unilateral cleft lip and a cleft palate. Physical examination revealed no other congenital abnormalities, and Michael was otherwise vigorous and healthy.

1. What is the priority concern or client need in this situation? Support your answer with data as stated in the case.
2. List other client needs/problems in this case.
3. Identify any additional information or assessment data needed by the nurse in planning care for this client.
4. What nursing actions are appropriate in this situation?
   a. What is the priority nursing action?
   b. Describe other nursing interventions that are important to providing optimal client care.
5. Describe the roles/responsibilities of the interprofessional health care team (other than nurses) who may be involved in providing care for this client.

Esophageal Atresia and Tracheoesophageal Fistula

Esophageal atresia (EA) and tracheoesophageal fistula (TEF), the most life-threatening anomalies of the esophagus, typically occur together, although they can occur singly. EA/TEF occurs in 1 in 3000 to 1 in 5000 newborns (National Institutes of Health, 2018); it is more common in male infants and in Caucasians (Parry, 2015).

EA/TEF is rarely an isolated defect. Most often there is at least one other anomaly. Approximately 50% of EA/TEF cases are a component of VATER (*v*ertebral defects, imperforate *a*nus, *t*racheoesophageal fistula, and *r*adial and *r*enal dysplasia) or VACTERL (*v*ertebral, *a*nal, *c*ardiac, *t*racheal, *e*sophageal, *r*enal and *l*imb) association (Khan & Orenstein, 2016). Anomalies most often associated with EA/TEF (in order of frequency) are cardiovascular, GI, genitourinary (GU), skeletal, and neurologic (Parry, 2015).

With EA the esophagus ends in a blind pouch, thus failing to form a continuous passageway to the stomach. TEF is an abnormal connection between the esophagus and the trachea. There are four types of EA/TEF (A, B, C, and D), classified based on the presence or absence of a TEF, the site of the fistula, and the location and degree of the esophageal obstruction. The most common variant, type C, accounts for 85% of all cases. Type C is a combination of a proximal EA, in which the esophagus ends in a blind pouch, with a distal TEF, in which the lower esophagus exits the stomach and is connected to the trachea by a fistula rather than forming a continuous tube to the upper esophagus (Parry, 2015) (Fig. 36.7).

The cause of EA and TEF is not always identified, but known risk factors include older paternal age and assisted reproductive technology (CDC, 2017b). There does not appear to be a genetic link, although approximately 7% of infants with EA/TEF have an associated chromosomal abnormality (e.g., trisomy 13, 18, or 21) (Parry, 2015).

The defect can be diagnosed prenatally, but is usually diagnosed postnatally. A prenatal ultrasound finding of a small or absent stomach or polyhydramnios may indicate that the infant is unable to swallow the amniotic fluid, thus raising suspicion of an atresia.

At birth the clinical presentation depends on the type of anomaly present. Infants with EA and TEF show significant respiratory difficulty immediately after birth. EA, with or without TEF, results in excessive oral secretions, drooling, feeding intolerance, and the inability to pass a feeding tube. When fed, the infant may swallow but then cough and gag and return the fluid through the nose and mouth. Respiratory distress can result from aspiration or acute gastric distention. Choking, coughing, and cyanosis occur after even a small amount of fluid is taken by mouth.

⚡ SAFETY ALERT

Any infant with excessive oral secretions and respiratory distress should not be fed orally until a health care provider has been consulted.

Nursing interventions are supportive until surgery has been performed. The infant with EA and TEF should be kept in a supine position with the head of the bed elevated about 30 degrees to facilitate respiratory efforts and prevent reflux and aspiration of gastric contents. Antireflux and antacid medication may be given to minimize gastroesophageal reflux and prevent acid-induced pneumonitis. An orogastric tube (Replogle tube) is placed in the proximal esophageal pouch and attached to low continuous suction to remove secretions and decrease the possibility of aspiration. The infant requires close observation and intervention to maintain a patent airway. Other supportive measures include thermoregulation, maintaining fluid and electrolyte balance intravenously as well as acid-base balance, and preventing any further complications as a result of an associated defect (Bradshaw, 2015).

The timing and type of surgical intervention depend on the specific type of defect. Surgical correction is usually done within 1 week of birth. It consists of ligating the fistula and anastomosing the two segments of the esophagus. A staged repair may be necessary if there is too large a gap between the distal and proximal segments of the esophagus. In this situation, there is ligation of the TEF, placement of a gastrostomy tube for decompression and feeding, and drainage of the upper esophageal pouch.

Survival rates for otherwise healthy infants approach 100%. Outcomes for infants with EA/TEF depend on associated defects and the infant's birth weight. Preterm infants with cardiac or chromosomal anomalies have the highest mortality rate. GER and tracheomalacia are common postoperative complications among infants who have EA/TEF. Esophageal strictures can cause feeding difficulties and may

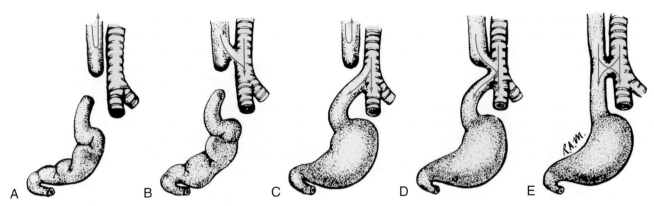

Fig. 36.7 Congenital Atresia of the Esophagus and Tracheoesophageal Fistula. (A) Upper and lower segments of the esophagus end in blind sac. (B) The upper segment of the esophagus ends in atresia and connects to the trachea by a fistulous tract. (C) The upper segment of the esophagus ends in a blind pouch; the lower segment connects with the trachea by small fistulous tract. (D) Both segments of the esophagus connect by fistulous tracts to the trachea. (E) The esophagus is continuous but connects by a fistulous tract to the trachea; this is known as the H type. (From Hockenberry, M. J., Wilson, D., & Rodgers, C. C. [2017]. *Wong's essentials of pediatric nursing* [10th ed.]. St. Louis: Elsevier.)

require serial dilation (Flynn-O'Brien, Rice-Townsend, & Ledbetter, 2018).

Omphalocele and Gastroschisis

Omphalocele and gastroschisis are the two most common congenital defects of the abdominal wall. Although both require surgical intervention to place herniated contents into the abdominal cavity, they represent distinctly different conditions (Ledbetter, Chabra, & Javid, 2018).

An omphalocele is a covered herniation of abdominal contents into the base of the umbilical cord (Fig. 36.8A). Omphalocele occurs in approximately 1.5 to 3/10,000 live births (Marshall, Salemi, Tanner, et al., 2015). Defects can be small, with only intestines present, or large, with liver and spleen herniation. The peritoneal sac covering the defect can rupture during or after birth. Chromosomal abnormalities (trisomy 12, 18, or 21) and other congenital anomalies (especially cardiac defects) are common. Omphalocele is a component of many syndromes of congenital abnormalities. Outcomes are poorer in infants with associated anomalies. Risk factors include younger or older maternal age; maternal obesity; and maternal use of selective serotonin reuptake inhibitors (SSRIs), alcohol, or tobacco (CDC, 2017b; Stephenson, Lockwood, & Mackenzie, 2018).

Gastroschisis is the herniation of the bowel through a defect in the abdominal wall lateral to umbilical ring (see Fig. 36.8B). No membrane covers the contents, as it does with an omphalocele. The exposure of bowel to amniotic fluid in utero leaves the intestines at risk for poor function after birth. Gastroschisis is not usually associated with other major congenital anomalies or syndromes, but intestinal atresia can occur. It is often associated with intrauterine growth restriction (Stephenson et al., 2018). Approximately 90% of cases are identified through routine prenatal care using ultrasonography (Ledbetter et al., 2018).

The prevalence of gastroschisis is increasing worldwide, especially among younger mothers. In recent years the prevalence of gastroschisis in the United States has risen significantly across all age groups and ethnicities to 4.9/10,000 live births. The highest prevalence is among mothers less than 20 years of age and among Hispanic and non-Hispanic white families (Jones, Isenburg, Salemi, et al., 2016). Risk factors include maternal age less than 20 years, maternal use of tobacco, recreational drugs, and antidepressants; low body mass index; unmarried

status; and genitourinary infections during pregnancy. Exposure to the agricultural chemical atrazine increases the risk of gastroschisis (Ledbetter et al., 2018; Stephenson et al., 2018).

Preoperative nursing care is similar for infants with either defect. Exposure of the viscera causes problems with thermoregulation and fluid and electrolyte balance. Immediately after birth, the neonate's torso should be placed in an impermeable, clear plastic bowel bag to decrease insensible water losses, maintain thermoregulation, and prevent contamination of the exposed viscera. It is essential for the nurse to assess the exposed viscera frequently to detect any changes in perfusion to the exposed abdominal contents. The infant should be placed in a side-lying position and the viscera supported with a blanket roll to prevent vascular compromise to a torqued intestine. Prior to surgery the exposed viscera should be kept covered with sterile moistened saline gauze and plastic wrap. Gastric decompression with a Replogle tube (a special type of gastric tube) connected to low intermittent wall suction is also necessary to prevent aspiration pneumonia and allow as much bowel as possible to be placed into the abdomen during surgery. Antibiotics, fluid and electrolyte replacement, and thermoregulation are needed for physiologic support (Bradshaw, 2015).

Surgery is usually performed soon after birth. If complete closure is impossible because of the small size of the defect and the large amount of viscera to be replaced, a prosthetic silo or patch is placed. This protects the contents as they are gradually placed back into the abdominal cavity and minimizes symptoms of respiratory distress as the increasing intra-abdominal pressure pushes against the diaphragm. The defect is closed surgically after the exposed visceral contents have been reduced; this reduction process usually takes 7 to 10 days. The prognosis depends on the size of the defect and the presence of associated anomalies. It is generally expected that there will be complications related to intestinal dysfunction—such as feeding difficulties, dysmotility, or short-gut syndrome—if a substantial portion of the intestine was removed (Stephenson et al., 2018).

Nursing care includes pain management, strict aseptic technique with dressing changes, monitoring of vital signs, and strict supervision of intake and output. Parental support is essential because the infant has an obvious disfiguring anomaly that can be shocking in appearance. Depending on the size of the defect, the infant can also be critically ill before surgery. The nurse must be aware of the effect this can

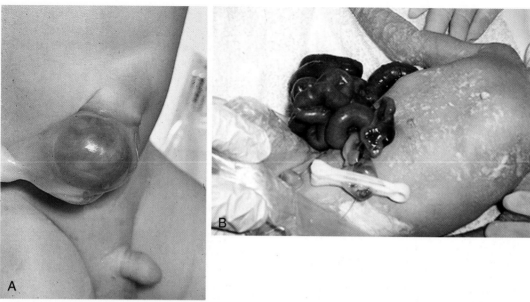

Fig. 36.8 Congenital Gastrointestinal Anomalies. (A) Omphalocele. (B) Gastroschisis of bowel and stomach. (A, From O'Doherty, N. [1986]. *Neonatology: Micro atlas of the newborn.* Nutley, NJ: Hoffmann-La Roche; B, Courtesy Cheryl Briggs, RNC, Annapolis, MD.)

have on parental bonding and intervene appropriately as the parents cope with this crisis.

Gastrointestinal Obstruction

Congenital intestinal obstruction can occur anywhere in the GI tract and takes one of the following forms: atresia, which is a complete obliteration of the passage; partial obstruction, in which the symptoms can vary in severity and sometimes are not detected in the neonatal period; or malrotation of the intestine, which leads to twisting of the intestine (volvulus) and obstruction. Common causes of neonatal GI obstruction include EA, duodenal atresia, midgut malrotation with or without volvulus, jejunoileal atresia, meconium ileus, meconium plug, and imperforate anus.

Meconium ileus is an obstruction caused by impacted, inspissated meconium in the distal ileum. These infants need follow-up with cystic fibrosis screening because more than 90% of infants with meconium ileus have cystic fibrosis (Flynn-O'Brien et al., 2018).

> **! NURSING ALERT**
>
> Any newborn who does not pass meconium during the first 24 hours after birth should be closely monitored for signs of distal intestinal obstruction (Flynn-O'Brien et al., 2018).

GI obstruction may be suspected prenatally when polyhydramnios is present. Postnatally, the common symptoms of neonatal intestinal obstruction include bilious (green-colored) emesis, abdominal distention, and failure to pass normal amounts of meconium in the first 48 hours. High intestinal obstruction is characterized by vomiting, even if the infant is not being fed orally. Distention usually indicates a low obstruction, with vomiting occurring later. Abdominal distention can elevate the diaphragm, causing respiratory difficulties (Flynn-O'Brien et al., 2018).

If an obstruction is suspected, oral feedings are withheld, an orogastric tube is placed to low intermittent wall suction, and intravenous therapy is initiated to provide needed fluid and electrolytes. In infants with an intestinal obstruction, surgery consists of resecting the obstructed area of bowel and anastomosing the unaffected bowel or creating an ostomy and allowing the bowel to rest.

> **! NURSING ALERT**
>
> Bilious emesis should always be considered abnormal and should be brought to the attention of the attending health care provider.

Anorectal Malformations

Anorectal malformations include a range of congenital defects involving the anus, rectum, and GU system (Fig. 36.9). These anomalies are relatively common, with an incidence of approximately 1 in 4000 to 5000 live births; they occur more often in male than in female infants (Parry, 2015). There is an association with trisomy 21 and other chromosomal abnormalities. Anorectal anomalies occur in isolation or as part of the VACTERL association (*v*ertebral, *a*nal atresia, *c*ardiac, *tr*acheoesophageal fistula, *r*enal agenesis and dysplasia, and *l*imb defects) (Flynn-O'Brien et al., 2018).

An imperforate anus exists when an infant's anus is absent or abnormally located. The defect may be high or low depending on the location above or below the levator muscle component of the anal sphincter muscles. With high defects, there is often a fistula (abnormal communication) from the distal rectum to the perineum or GU system. A fistula is evident when there is meconium coming through the vaginal opening, the perineum below the vagina, the male urethra, or the perineum beneath the scrotum. In some cases of imperforate anus there is obviously no anal opening, whereas in others there is a normal-appearing rectum and the abnormality is detected only when the infant does not pass meconium (Bradshaw, 2015; Parry, 2015).

Surgical repair is dependent on the anatomic characteristics and the extent of associated anomalies. If the anomaly involves only stenotic areas or a thin translucent membrane over the anal opening, treatment is anoplasty followed by daily dilation. The preoperative nursing care is similar to that described for other GI obstructions. Postoperative nursing interventions include pain management and assessment for wound healing, passage of stool, stricture, and rectal prolapse. Complications include chronic problems of bowel, bladder, and reproductive organs as well as psychosocial disturbances (Cairo, Gasior, Rollins, et al., 2018; Flynn-O'Brien et al., 2018).

Musculoskeletal System Anomalies

The two most common musculoskeletal system anomalies in neonates are developmental dysplasia of the hip and congenital clubfoot. Both of these conditions must be detected and treated early for successful correction.

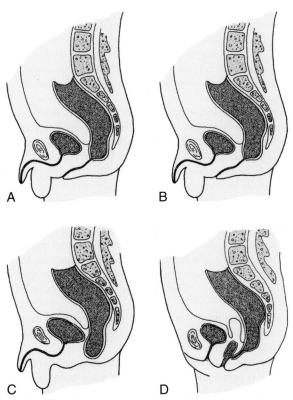

Fig. 36.9 Types of Anorectal Malformations (Imperforate Anus). The anal sphincter muscle may be present and intact. (A) A high lesion opening onto perineum through a narrow fistulous tract. (B) A high lesion ending in fistulous tract to the urinary tract. (C) A low lesion in the bowel passing through the puborectal muscle. (D) A high lesion ending in a fistulous tract to the vagina.

Developmental Dysplasia of the Hip

The broad term developmental dysplasia of the hip (DDH) describes a spectrum of disorders related to abnormal development of one or all of the components of the hip joint, which can develop at any time during fetal life, infancy, or childhood. DDH includes a variety of hip abnormalities in which there is an abnormal acetabulum and femoral head with mechanical instability of the hip (Rosenfield, 2017).

DDH occurs in approximately 1 in 1000 live births (Shaw, Segal, & Section on Orthopaedics, 2016). The etiology is unclear but it is likely multifactorial. The primary risk factors are female sex, breech presentation, and family history of DDH. Other factors that contribute to DDH are incorrect swaddling of the lower extremities and intrauterine factors that lead to tighter space and limitation of fetal movement (large fetal size, oligohydramnios, and multiple gestation) (Rosenfield, 2017; Shaw et al., 2016).

There are three degrees of DDH (Fig. 36.10):

Acetabular dysplasia (or preluxation)—the mildest form of DDH in which there is neither subluxation nor dislocation. There is a delay in acetabular development evidenced by osseous hypoplasia of the acetabular roof, which is oblique and shallow, although the cartilaginous roof is comparatively intact. The femoral head remains in the acetabulum; 80% of mild cases of DDH resolve spontaneously.

Subluxation—this accounts for the largest percentage of DDH. Subluxation implies incomplete dislocation of the hip and is sometimes regarded as an intermediate state in the development from primary dysplasia to complete dislocation. The femoral head remains in contact with the acetabulum, but a stretched capsule and ligamentum teres cause the head of the femur to be partially displaced. Pressure on the cartilaginous roof inhibits ossification and produces a flattened socket.

Dislocation—the femoral head loses contact with the acetabulum and is displaced posteriorly and superiorly over the fibrocartilaginous rim. The ligamentum teres is elongated and taut.

In the newborn period, dysplasia usually appears as hip joint laxity rather than as outright dislocation. Subluxation and the tendency to dislocate can be demonstrated by the Ortolani or Barlow test. These tests are most reliable from birth to 2 or 3 months of age (see Fig. 23.17). Other signs of DDH are shortening of the limb on the affected side, asymmetric thigh and gluteal folds (present only in unilateral DDH), decreased hip abduction on the affected side, and broadening of the perineum (in bilateral dislocation).

DDH is often not detected at the initial examination after birth; thus all infants should be carefully monitored for hip dysplasia at follow-up

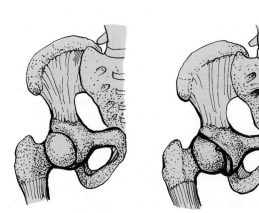
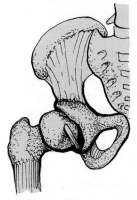
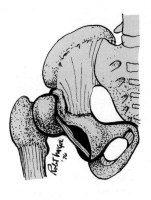

| Normal | Dysplasia | Subluxation | Dislocation |

Fig. 36.10 Configuration and Relationship of Structures in Developmental Dysplasia of the Hip.

visits throughout the first year of life or until the infant is walking (Choudry & Paton, 2018; Rosenfeld, 2017). If the physical exam was normal but risk factors are present, the American Academy of Pediatrics recommends imaging prior to 6 months of age (Shaw et al., 2016).

> ⚡ **SAFETY ALERT**
>
> To prevent fracture or other damage to the hip, the Ortolani and Barlow tests must be performed by an experienced clinician.

Treatment begins as soon as the condition is recognized. Early intervention is more favorable to the restoration of normal bony architecture and function. The longer treatment is delayed, the more severe the deformity, the more difficult the treatment, and the less favorable the prognosis. Treatment varies with the age of the infant and the extent of the dysplasia. The goal of treatment is to obtain and maintain a safe, congruent position of the hip joint and thus to promote normal hip joint development and ambulation.

The hip joint is maintained by dynamic splinting in a safe position with the proximal femur centered in the acetabulum in an attitude of flexion and abduction. The Pavlik harness (Fig. 36.11) is the most widely used, and with time, motion, and gravity, the hip works into a more abducted, reduced position. The harness is worn continually until the hip is proved stable on clinical and radiographic examination, typically around 6 to 12 weeks. This approach has an 80% success rate for the treatment of classic DDH. If not effective, traction, casting, and even open or closed reduction may be necessary to stabilize the hip (Judd & Clarke, 2014).

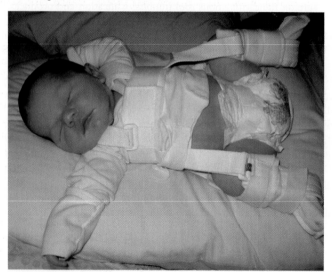

Fig. 36.11 An Infant in a Pavlik Harness. (Courtesy Amanda Politte, St. Louis, MO.)

> ⚡ **SAFETY ALERT**
>
> The former practice of double- or triple-diapering for developmental dysplasia of the hip is not recommended because it promotes hip extension, thus interfering with proper hip development.

As part of routine newborn assessment and care, the nurse may be the first person to detect DDH. If treatment for DDH is with a Pavlik harness, the nurse teaches the parents how to apply and maintain the device and how to care for the infant. The health care provider will determine if and when the harness can be removed (e.g., for bathing) and how long it

is needed; the nurse reinforces the instructions and reminds the parents not to make any adjustments in the harness. To prevent skin breakdown, parents are instructed to check the skin under the straps three or four times a day and to gently massage healthy skin under the straps at least once daily; the diaper is worn under the straps. Thorough and ongoing follow-up care is necessary, as is support for the family.

Foot Deformities

Congenital **clubfoot,** or talipes equinovarus, is a complex deformity involving the foot and ankle. The etiology is unknown, but a major factor is thought to be a single autosomal dominant gene. It occurs more often in males (2:1), and half of all cases are bilateral. It can occur as an insolated defect or in association with other disorders or syndromes such as chromosomal disorders, arthrogryposis (a generalized immobility of the joints), cerebral palsy, or spina bifida (Son-Hing & Thompson, 2015).

With congenital clubfoot the foot is rigid with excessive plantarflexion; there is adduction of the forefoot, varus of the heel, downward pointing of the foot and toes, and the sole facing inward. The foot appears stiff, small, and wide; the lower leg appears small because of hypoplasia of the calf muscles. If congenital clubfoot is untreated, further stiffening, bone changes and further deformities, infection, pain, and social stigma can result (Son-Hing & Thompson, 2015).

Positional clubfoot is not true clubfoot. The foot appears abnormal but it can easily be manipulated into normal position. This occurs due to intrauterine crowding or breech position. No treatment is needed (McKee-Garrett, 2016).

Treatment for congenital clubfoot is initiated soon after birth, most often using the Ponseti method, which involves serial manipulation, casting, and possible percutaneous tenoachilles tenotomy. Manipulation of the foot with passive stretching and replacement of the long-leg cast are done weekly to accommodate the rapid growth of early infancy. The extremity or extremities are often casted or splinted for 8 to 12 weeks, but bracing may be needed for up to 4 years. If surgical correction is required, it is done before the infant begins to walk (White, Bouchard, & Goldberg, 2018).

Metatarsus adductus is another common congenital foot defect. Although it is present at birth, it is often not diagnosed until later. It is more common in firstborn and twin gestations, 50% occur bilaterally, and it runs in families. The characteristic appearance includes medial deviation (adduction) of the forefoot while the hindfoot is in a normal position; this results in a "C" shape or concavity of the medial portion of the foot. Positional metatarsus adductus is flexible, does not have bone involvement, and usually resolves on its own. The structural type is fixed; the arch appears increased, and there is a deep medial crease. Regardless of the type, up to 90% will resolve spontaneously. If needed, initial treatment is stretching done by the parents; casting may be required in rare cases (McKee-Garrett, 2016).

Nursing interventions for infants with foot deformities include parent education on stretching, how to care for casting and to assess the toes for neurovascular compromise, and how to prevent skin breakdown. The nurse should be supportive of the parents as they learn how to meet the infant's normal needs as well as those brought about by his or her physical problem.

Genitourinary System Anomalies

Anomalies involving the GU system can be distressing to parents because they can be readily apparent and, in the case of some conditions, there may be the concern about sexuality and reproductive functioning. These anomalies range from obvious anomalies of the external genitalia, such as hypospadias, to those involving internal organs that are not obvious but can cause damage to the urinary tract.

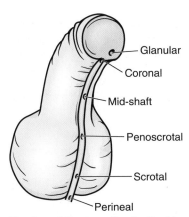

Fig. 36.12 Classification of Hypospadias by Position of the Urethral Meatus.

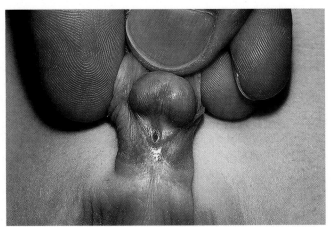

Fig. 36.13 Hypospadias. (Courtesy H. Gil Rushton, MD, Children's National Medical Center, Washington, DC.)

Hypospadias

The term *hypospadias* encompasses a range of penile anomalies associated with an abnormally located urinary meatus. The meatus can open below the glans penis or anywhere along the ventral surface of the penis, the scrotum, or the perineum. It is one of the most common congenital anomalies. Hypospadias is classified according to the location of the meatus and the presence or absence of chordee, which is a ventral curvature of the penis (Figs. 36.12 and 36.13). The cause is unknown, although it is thought to be of multifactorial inheritance. Hypospadias usually occurs as an isolated defect, but it can also occur as part of a syndrome with multiple anomalies (Merguerian & Rowe, 2018).

Mild cases of hypospadias are often repaired for cosmetic reasons and involve a single surgical procedure. In more severe cases, multiple surgeries are required to reconstruct the urethral opening and correct the chordee, thereby straightening the penis. The goals are to improve the appearance of the genitalia, make it possible for the child to urinate in a standing position, and have a sexually adequate organ. These infants are not circumcised because the foreskin may be needed during surgical repair. Repair is done early, between 1 and 2 years of age, so that the child's body image will not be impaired. There is a correlation between hypospadias and testicular cancer and also with cryptorchidism; therefore children with a history of hypospadias require long-term follow-up (Sherman, 2015).

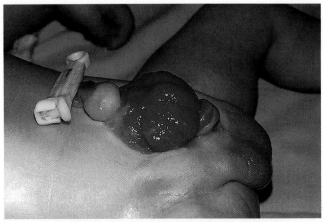

Fig. 36.14 Exstrophy of Bladder. (Courtesy H. Gil Rushton, MD, Children's National Medical Center, Washington, DC.)

Bladder Exstrophy

The most common bladder anomaly is exstrophy (Fig. 36.14). The bladder is visible in the suprapubic area as a red mass with numerous folds; the bladder plate is evaginated, and urine drips from the ureteric openings on the bladder surface. Bilateral inguinal hernias are commonly present. In males, the penis is shortened; the urethra is open and located on the top of the penis (epispadias). There is an upward curvature of the penis and the dorsal foreskin is absent; testes are typically descended. Females have a bifid clitoris, and the labia minora appear small and displaced laterally (Borer, 2018a).

Immediately after birth the exposed bladder should be covered with a sterile nonadherent dressing to protect its delicate surface until closure can be performed. Once the bladder has been stabilized, a transparent dressing that adheres to the surrounding skin is preferred. The timing of surgery is dependent on the clinical status of the infant. Immediate closure of the bladder is usually performed in the first 72 hours, but delayed closure can be as late as 6 to 12 weeks. A series of reconstructive surgeries may be needed. Parents need detailed instructions for care and dressing changes, along with support and encouragement as they cope with providing care for an infant with such an obvious defect. Repair is completed before school age, if possible, although some children never attain normal voiding patterns and may later be considered for urinary diversion surgery (Borer, 2018b).

Ambiguous Genitalia

Ambiguous genitalia refers to a disorder of sex development (DSD). In infants with a DSD there is a discrepancy between the external genitalia and the gonadal/chromosomal sex (Houk & Levitsky, 2017). The nurse is often the one to discover ambiguous genitalia in the newborn (Fig. 36.15) during a physical assessment. Erroneous or abnormal sexual differentiation can be due to virilization in the 46XX infant, undervirilization in the 46XY infant, disorders of gonadal differentiation, or a transient issue. Congenital adrenal hyperplasia (CAH) should be the primary consideration in any virilized infant with nonpalpable gonads. CAH is an inherited disorder that causes abnormally low levels of cortisol production. Diagnosis should be based on data gathered from the following sources: maternal and family history (including steroid use during pregnancy, relatives with ambiguous genitalia, neonatal deaths), physical examination, chromosomal analysis, endoscopy, ultrasonography, and radiographic contrast studies as well as biochemical tests (analysis of urinary steroid excretion to detect adrenocortical syndromes) and, in some instances, laparotomy or gonad biopsy (Houk & Levitsky; Indyk, 2017).

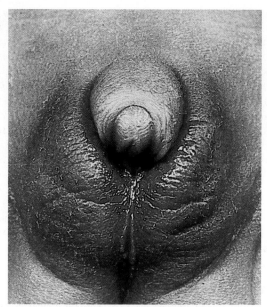

Fig. 36.15 Ambiguous External Genitalia. Structure may be an enlarged clitoral hood and clitoris or a malformed penis. (Courtesy Edward S. Tank, MD, Division of Urology, Oregon Health Science University, Portland.)

Assessment and management of a newborn with ambiguous genitalia require urgency and sensitivity. Therapeutic intervention, including any counseling and surgery, should be started as soon as possible. Care is best managed by an interprofessional health care team including the primary physician, pediatric endocrinologist, geneticist, surgeon, social worker, psychologist, and nurses. An infant born with ambiguous genitalia should not receive a sex assignment until diagnostic testing provides enough information for a well-informed decision (Indyk, 2017).

An appropriate gender assignment should be based on the following: diagnosis, karyotype, genital development and surgical options, cultural pressures, most likely adult gender identity, potential for mature sexual function, potential fertility, and the long-term psychologic and intellectual effect on the child and family (Indyk, 2017). Parents need much support as they learn to cope with this very challenging situation.

INBORN ERRORS OF METABOLISM

Inborn errors of metabolism (IEMs) are biochemical genetic disorders that result from defects in single genes; the majority are inherited as autosomal recessive conditions (Sutton, 2017). The genetic defect causes a blockage in a critical metabolic pathway. There can be absence of an essential enzyme, resulting in accumulation of precursors preceding a blocked step in a metabolic pathway. The defect can also result in a deficiency of a critical metabolic product. IEMs encompass a wide variety of disorders including defects of amino acid, carbohydrate, and organic acid metabolism; lysosomal storage disorders; energy metabolism disorders; and disorders of purine metabolism. This discussion focuses on selected IEMS that can be identified through newborn screening.

IEMs are individually rare, but collectively they are a common cause of disease in neonates. During the newborn period, IEMs may present with nonspecific signs in an otherwise healthy infant, making thorough evaluation critical. Some IEMs may not be evident until symptoms appear later in life. Others may show signs from birth or soon thereafter. Symptoms of an IEM are most often GI and neurologic. They can include poor feeding, respiratory distress, hypoglycemia, lethargy, seizures, metabolic acidosis or respiratory alkalosis, or cardiac arrhythmias. The presence of other congenital anomalies should not rule out the possibility of an IEM (Sutton, 2017; Zinn, 2015).

Diagnostic testing for IEMs is often ordered when other explanations for an infant's symptoms are not satisfactory. For example, if a neonate demonstrates signs of sepsis but testing fails to confirm the diagnosis, the provider may proceed with diagnostic measures for a metabolic disorder. Initial testing includes a broad range of blood and urine tests that are not diagnostic for IEMs but instead serve as screening measures. Further testing is required to confirm the diagnosis of an IEM, and a metabolic specialist is often involved. Biochemical studies for specific IEMs should be performed only by specialized laboratories that require compliance with very specific guidelines for collecting, storing, and shipping tissue samples.

It is critical that IEMs be identified as early as possible because undiagnosed and untreated IEMs can lead to severe consequences, such as cognitive impairment or even death. Presymptomatic identification of many IEMs is possible through routine newborn screening (see Chapter 24).

Care of an infant who has an IEM is managed by an interprofessional health care team including neonatal and pediatric providers, metabolic and genetic specialists, nutritionists, and nurses. If the infant is hospitalized when the diagnosis is made, all protein sources are eliminated, including feedings and amino acid solutions. Intravenous solutions of 10% glucose and electrolytes are administered until a specific diagnosis is made. Supportive care includes correction of volume and electrolyte imbalances, hypoglycemia, and metabolic acidosis. Neonates may be transferred to regional referral centers for further treatment. In severe cases, hemodialysis, ECMO, or even liver transplant may be needed.

Phenylketonuria

Phenylketonuria (PKU) is an autosomal recessive amino acid disorder that results from a deficiency of the enzyme phenylalanine dehydrogenase (see Chapter 3), which is needed to metabolize the essential amino acid phenylalanine. Classic PKU is one of a spectrum of disorders known as hyperphenylalaninemia; severity varies according to the degree of enzyme deficiency. This deficiency can cause elevated levels of phenylalanine that result in CNS damage. Severe effects of PKU are rare because of early recognition through newborn screening. The test for PKU is not reliable, however, until the newborn has ingested adequate amounts of breast milk or formula.

Treatment for PKU includes a diet low in protein plus the addition of a special amino acid–containing formula that does not contain phenylalanine. Breastfeeding may be allowed in conjunction with phenylalanine-free formula. Lack of treatment for PKU results in profound intellectual disability. Despite compliance with treatment, many affected children have some degree of cognitive impairment. Successful management and outcomes are largely dependent on early identification of the condition, modifying the diet, and compliance with the treatment regimen throughout life (Rezvani & Ficicioglu, 2016).

Galactosemia

Galactosemia is an autosomal recessive disorder caused by a deficiency of the enzyme galactose 1-phosphate uridyl transferase (GALT), resulting in the inability to convert galactose to glucose. Galactosemia is usually first suspected when absence of the GALT enzyme is found on newborn screening. Further testing includes blood and urine evaluation. There are no outward symptoms at birth, but once a newborn has ingested formula containing galactose, the symptoms will become evident. Early symptoms are vomiting, diarrhea, hypoglycemia, weight loss, persistent jaundice, and CNS symptoms (poor feeding, drowsiness, and seizures). If the disorder goes untreated, galactose levels continue to increase, and the affected infant shows failure to thrive, developmental delay, cataracts, jaundice, hepatomegaly, and cirrhosis of the liver, with death possibly occurring in the first month of life. Affected infants are at increased risk for *Escherichia coli* sepsis. Therapy consists of a galactose-free diet and supplementation with calcium. Breastfeeding is contraindicated because breast milk contains lactose (Kishnani & Chen, 2016; Merritt & Gallagher, 2018).

Congenital Hypothyroidism

Congenital hypothyroidism (CH) results from a deficiency of thyroid hormones; it can be permanent (requiring treatment for life) or transient (resolving spontaneously). The vast majority of cases are due to abnormal development of the thyroid gland; the remainder are the result of defects in thyroid hormone synthesis. This is the most common endocrine disorder found in neonates, affecting 1 in 2000 to 4000. CH affects female infants twice as often as males. It is a major cause of intellectual disability if not treated properly.

CH can be due to a single-gene defect or familial autoimmune factors; however, in the majority of cases it is caused by a nonfamilial embryogenic defect. Infants with Down syndrome are often affected with CH (Kim, Nandi-Munshi, & Diblasi, 2018; Wassner & Brown, 2015).

The majority of neonates with CH appear normal at birth, although some may exhibit signs of the disorder—such as hypotonia, large fontanel, poor feeding, or macroglossia. If the infant is untreated, symptoms usually appear after 6 weeks and include lethargy, bradycardia, hypothermia, hypotension, hyporeflexia, abdominal distention, umbilical hernia, hoarse cry, constipation, coarse dry hair, thick dry skin that feels cold, anemia, widely patent cranial sutures, and delayed bone age beginning at birth. The most disabling problem, however, is delayed development of the nervous system, leading to severe developmental delay. Once identified, treatment is started immediately using oral levothyroxine (L-T_4) as a thyroid replacement with close follow-up to monitor serum TSH and T4 levels (Kim et al., 2018). Approximately 30% of children with CH will regain normal thyroid function during early childhood; thyroid function is reevaluated around age 3 (LaFranchi, 2018).

Early diagnosis and treatment of congenital hypothyroidism is associated with a greater likelihood of normal mental development. Early recognition of the disorder is possible through routine newborn screening. All US states and Canadian provinces routinely screen for hypothyroidism by measuring T_4 or thyroid-stimulating hormone (TSH) levels. Screening is most accurate between 2 and 4 days of life. Screening done before 48 hours of age should be repeated by the primary care physician when the infant is 2 weeks old. Early screening can have false-positive results; preterm infants are more likely to have false-positive results. Any infant whose screening test is positive should be further evaluated for congenital hypothyroidism (Kim et al., 2018).

 CARE MANAGEMENT

Assessment

Congenital anomalies and disorders may be identified prenatally, at the time of birth, or in the days or weeks following birth. Although some prenatal and postnatal screening tests are routinely performed, diagnostic testing for specific congenital defects is performed on the basis of a variety of factors such as the results of screening tests, maternal and family history, prenatal course, and neonatal symptoms.

Prenatal

Refined prenatal testing procedures are available to monitor fetal development. Diagnostic techniques—such as amniocentesis, ultrasonography, alpha-fetoprotein measurements, chorionic villus sampling, percutaneous

umbilical cord blood sampling, fetal nuchal translucency screening, cell-free fetal DNA testing, and gene probes—contribute information to the database (see Chapter 26). Although they are a valuable adjunct to prenatal care, these tests cannot identify all congenital disorders. Furthermore, ethical issues surround such testing, and the nurse must be prepared to support the family's decision regarding it. If a disorder has been detected and the family decides to proceed with the pregnancy, the advantage is that appropriate care can be made available for the infant immediately at birth.

The nurse reviews the maternal history and medical information in the prenatal record for risk factors associated with congenital disorders. These factors include various medical, surgical, and social conditions and their treatment (see Chapter 30). Also see maternal infection (Chapter 7); maternal endocrine and metabolic disorders (Chapter 29); and infection and drug dependence in the newborn (Chapter 35). Family history is integral to diagnosing a congenital disorder. Data collection should include a three-generation pedigree (parents, siblings, grandparents, aunts, uncles, cousins) with information such as miscarriages, stillbirths, congenital anomalies, or childhood deaths.

Postnatal

If assessment or review of prenatal records raises the suspicion of a congenital disorder, further diagnostic evaluation is needed. A comprehensive physical exam of all neonates should be completed after birth and minor and major malformations noted. There can be mild malformations that in isolation are not clinically significant, but a pattern or combination of minor malformations can suggest a specific disorder or syndrome.

Diagnostic procedures for the detection of genetic disorders are performed after birth or at any time from the postnatal period through adulthood. Many tests exist for various disorders. The US National Library of Medicine, Genetics Home Reference, provides a guide to the different types of genetic tests (https://ghr.nlm.nih.gov/primer/testing/uses).

Cytogenic studies are done to rule out or confirm a suspected genetic diagnosis. Chromosome analysis and molecular deoxyribonucleic acid (DNA) analysis are often ordered. Results may take many weeks; however, in urgent situations, chromosome analysis from bone marrow samples can be available within hours. A variety of biochemical studies may be done, especially in seeking to diagnose an IEM. X-ray examination and organ imaging with MRI or CT scan may be used to identify skeletal abnormalities and structural anomalies of major organs.

The most widespread use of postnatal testing for congenital disorders is the routine screening of newborns in the United States and Canada for IEMs such as PKU, galactosemia, hemoglobinopathies (sickle cell disease and thalassemias), and hypothyroidism (see Chapter 24).

Interventions
Newborn Care

Many congenital anomalies require intervention soon after birth. A collaborative interprofessional team approach is needed, including medical specialists from maternal-fetal medicine, neonatology, pediatric subspecialties (e.g., surgery), nursing, social work, and others as needed according to the individual needs of each infant and family. Surgical intervention in the neonatal period may be necessary for the infant requiring either immediate correction or a palliative procedure to relieve the symptoms of the anomaly until definitive correction can be done.

The health care team must be highly skilled to meet the needs of these high-risk infants. Nurses are instrumental in stabilizing the infant (oxygenation and perfusion of tissues), performing preoperative interventions such as placing an orogastric tube for abdominal decompression, attending to thermoregulation and pain management, maintaining fluid and electrolyte balance, and providing support and education for the family.

Parents and Family Support

While the infant is receiving optimal care, the parents have needs that must be met as they deal with the crisis of having an infant with an abnormal condition. The nurse carefully assesses their reactions and facilitates their understanding of the information given them about their infant's condition. A newly diagnosed disorder often implies the need for implementing a therapeutic regimen. For example, the disorder can be an IEM, such as PKU, which requires rigid adherence to a special diet. The family may need help with securing the required commercial infant formula and receiving counseling from the clinical dietitian. The nurse stresses the importance of maintaining the diet, keeping an adequate supply of the prescribed infant formula, and not using unauthorized substitutions (see the Nursing Care Plan).

Referral to appropriate agencies is another essential component of follow-up management, and the nurse should make the parents aware of all possible sources of assistance, including pertinent literature, websites, parent groups, and national organizations. Many organizations and foundations provide services and counseling for families of affected children. There are also numerous parent groups that the family can join. There they can share experiences and receive mutual support in coping with problems similar to those of other group members. Nurses should be familiar with the services available in the parents' community that provide assistance and education to families with these special problems.

A major nursing function is providing emotional support to the family during all aspects of the care of the infant born with a defect or disorder. The feelings stemming from the real or imagined threat posed by a congenital anomaly are as varied as the people being counseled. Responses can include apathy, denial, anger, hostility, fear, embarrassment, grief, and loss of self-esteem (see Chapter 37).

Some parents benefit from seeing "before and after" pictures of other babies born with the same defect. Coupled with other verbal and nonverbal supportive care, this visual reassurance may be effective in allaying their concerns. Families need much information, guidance, and support as they make decisions regarding the care of their infants. Having heard risks and benefits of treatment and having received support and assistance in problem solving, the final decision regarding a course of action must be their own. It is then incumbent on the health care team to support the family's decision.

Genetic Evaluation and Counseling

Genetic counseling can help families assess the occurrence, or risk of occurrence, of a genetic disorder in a family. It involves relaying information about the diagnosis, treatment options, recurrence risk, and availability of prenatal diagnosis. It is essential that nurses understand the basic principles of genetics and the types of genetic testing available (see Chapter 3).

Nurses frequently encounter infants with genetic disorders and families for whom there is a risk that a disorder can be transmitted to or occur in an offspring. Nurses are responsible for identifying situations in which individuals can benefit from genetic evaluation and counseling. They should be aware of the local genetic resources and be prepared to help families find the needed services; they should also offer support and care for children and families affected by genetic conditions. Nurses can direct families to the appropriate resources. The Genetic Alliance (www.geneticalliance.org) is a nonprofit organization that has a database of support groups for genetic conditions. The National Society of Genetic Counselors (www.nsgc.org) lists genetic counselors by state. GeneTests (www.ncbi.nlm.nih.gov/sites/GeneTests) is a publicly funded medical genetics information resource developed for health care professionals; it is available at no cost to everyone.

◎ NURSING CARE PLAN

Parents and Family of Infant With Congenital Anomaly

Client Problem	Expected Outcome	Interventions	Rationales
Disappointment and grief related to birth of child with congenital abnormality	Parents will express their feelings and concerns.	Establish trusting relationship with family.	To facilitate their willingness to share their feelings
		Explain defect in simple terms before showing them the infant.	To prepare them for the appearance of their newborn
		Remain with the parents as they view and hold their newborn.	To provide support and assistance
		Present the infant as something precious and emphasize the normal, well-formed aspects of the infant's body.	To help the parents bond with the infant and not focus only on the anomaly
Lack of understanding about infant's condition	Parents will ask appropriate questions and state their understanding of the infant's condition.	Assess parents' knowledge about the infant's anomaly.	To identify learning needs before providing information
		Using simple language, explain the defect and the implications for care.	To aid in the parents' understanding during this emotional time
		Encourage parents to ask questions and provide honest, straightforward answers without undue optimism or pessimism.	To identify gaps in their understanding and to provide objective information
Anxiety about providing care for their infant's special needs after hospital discharge	Parents will acknowledge their anxiety and identify resources.	Encourage parents to express their specific concerns about infant care.	To identify and address areas of concern
		During hospital stay, provide teaching and support, involving parents in daily care of newborn as much as possible.	To provide information and allow parents to practice aspects of infant care under supervision and support of nursing staff and to assess their ability to provide care
		Consult with interprofessional care team to identify resources needed by the family.	To provide comprehensive care and help families find the resources they need

KEY POINTS

- Hemolytic disease of the newborn is most often due to Rh and ABO incompatibility. Erythroblastosis fetalis leads to anemia, edema, and the cytotoxic effects of unconjugated bilirubin.
- The administration of $Rh_o(D)$ immune globulin to Rh-negative and Coombs test–negative women provides passive immunity and minimizes the possibility of isoimmunization.
- Neonatal exchange transfusion with type O, Rh-negative red blood cells (RBCs) serves to treat anemia and acidosis and remove bilirubin, maternal antibodies, and fetal RBCs that are beginning to hemolyze.
- Major congenital defects are the leading cause of death in term neonates.
- The most common major congenital anomalies that cause serious problems in the neonate are congenital heart disease, neural tube defects, cleft lip or palate, and developmental dysplasia of the hip.
- Minor anomalies can be part of a characteristic pattern of malformations.

- Current technology permits the prenatal diagnosis of many congenital anomalies and disorders.
- The most widespread use of postnatal testing for genetic disease is the routine screening of newborns for inborn errors of metabolism.
- The curative and rehabilitative problems of an infant with a congenital disorder are often complex and require an interprofessional health team approach to management.
- Parents of newborns with congenital anomalies often need special instructions and support related to infant care (e.g., meeting nutrition requirements, cast care).
- Infants with inborn errors of metabolism are likely to need long-term treatment.
- The supportive care given to the parents of infants with an abnormal condition must begin at birth or at the time of diagnosis and continue for years.

REFERENCES

American Academy of Pediatrics & American College of Obstetricians and Gynecologists. (2017). *Guidelines for perinatal care* (8th ed.). Elk Grove Village, IL: Author.

American College of Obstetricians and Gynecologists. (2017a). Committee opinion no. 720: Maternal-fetal surgery for myelomeningocele. *Obstetrics & Gynecology, 130*(3), e164–e167.

American College of Obstetricians and Gynecologists. (2017b). Practice bulletin no. 191: Prevention of RhD alloimmunization. *Obstetrics & Gynecology, 130*(2), 57–70.

Bacino, C. A. (2018). Birth defects: Causes. In H. V. Firth & L. Wilkins-Haug (Eds.), *UptoDate*. Retrieved from: https://www.uptodate.com.

Blackburn, S. T. (2018). *Maternal, fetal, and neonatal physiology: A clinical perspective* (5th ed.). St. Louis: Elsevier.

Blencowe, H., Kancherla, V., Moorthie, S., et al. (2018). *Estimates of global and regional prevalence of neural tube defects for 2015: A systematic analysis* (pp. 31–46). Annals of the New York Academy of Sciences, 1414(1).

Borer, J. G. (2018a). Clinical manifestations and initial management of infants with bladder exstrophy. In L. S. Baskin (Ed.), *UpToDate*. Retrieved from: https://www.uptodate.com.

Borer, J. G. (2018b). Surgical management and postoperative outcome of children with bladder exstrophy. In L. S. Baskin (Ed.), *UpToDate*. Retrieved from: https://www.uptodate.com.

Bradshaw, W. T. (2015). Gastrointestinal disorders. In M. T. Verklan & M. Walden (Eds.), *Core curriculum for neonatal intensive care nursing* (5th ed.). St. Louis: Elsevier.

Cairo, S. B., Gasior, A., Rollins, M. D., et al. (2018). Challenges in transition of care for patients with anorectal malformations: A systematic review and recommendations for comprehensive care. *Diseases of the Colon and Rectum, 61*(3), 390–399.

Calhoun, D. A. (2018). *Postnatal diagnosis and management of hemolytic disease of the fetus and newborn*. UptoDate. Retrieved from: https://www.uptodate.com.

Centers for Disease Control and Prevention. (2018). *Data and statistics on birth defects*. Retrieved from: https://www.cdc.gov/ncbddd/birthdefects/data.html.

Centers for Disease Control and Prevention. (2017a). *Facts about esophageal atresia*. Retrieved from: *https://www.cdc.gov/ncbddd/birthdefects/esophagealatresia.html*.

Centers for Disease Control and Prevention. (2017b). *Facts about omphalocele*. Retrieved from: https://cdc.gov/ncbddd/birthdefects/omphalocele.html.

Choudry, Q. A., & Paton, R. W. (2018). Neonatal screening and selective sonographic imaging in the diagnosis of developmental dysplasia of the hip. *Bone and Joint Journal, 100-B*(6), 806–810.

Christensen, R. D. (2018). Neonatal erythrocyte disorders. In C. A. Gleason & S. E. Juul (Eds.), *Avery's diseases of the newborn* (10th ed.). Philadelphia: Elsevier.

Cunningham, F. G., Leveno, K. J., Bloom, S. L., et al. (2018). *Williams obstetrics* (25th ed.). New York: McGraw-Hill.

Dias, M., Parrington, M., & Section on Neurologic Surgery. (2015). Congenital brain and spinal cord malformations and their associated cutaneous markers. *Pediatrics, 136*(4), e1105–e1119.

Dukhovny, S., & Wilkins-Haug, L. (2018). Open neural tube defects: Risk factors, prenatal screening and diagnosis, and pregnancy management. In D. Levine, & L. L. Simpson (Eds.), *UpToDate*. Retrieved from: https://www.uptodate.com.

Evans, K. N., Hing, A. V., & Cunningham, M. L. (2018). Craniofacial malformations. In C. A. Gleason & S. E. Juul (Eds.), *Avery's diseases of the newborn* (10th ed.). Philadelphia: Elsevier.

Flynn-O'Brien, K. T., Rice-Townsend, S., & Ledbetter, D. J. (2018). Structural anomalies of the gastrointestinal tract. In C. A. Gleason & S. E. Juul (Eds.), *Avery's diseases of the newborn* (10th ed.). Philadelphia: Elsevier.

Glader, B. (2018). Genetics and pathophysiology of glucose-6-phosphate dehydrogenase (G6PD) deficiency. In S. L. Schrier & B. A. Raby (Eds.), *UpToDate*. Retrieved from: https://www.uptodate.com.

Greene, N. D., & Copp, A. J. (2014). Neural tube defects. *Annual Review of Neuroscience, 37*, 221–242.

Grivell, R. M., Andersen, C., & Dodd, J. M. (2015). Prenatal interventions for congenital diaphragmatic hernia for improving outcomes. *Cochrane Database of Systematic Reviews*, CD008925.

Haridas, A., & Tomita, T. (2018a). Hydrocephalus in children: Management and prognosis. In M. C. Patterson (Ed.), *UpToDate*. Retrieved from: https://www.uptodate.com.

Haridas, A., & Tomita, T. (2018b). Hydrocephalus in children: Physiology, pathogenesis, and etiology. In M. C. Patterson (Ed.), *UpToDate*. Retrieved from: https://www.uptodate.com.

Hedrick, H. L. (2017). Congenital diaphragmatic hernia: Prenatal diagnosis and management. In L. Wilkins-Haug (Ed.), *UpToDate*. Retrieved from: https://www.uptodate.com.

Hedrick, H. L., & Adzick, N. S. (2018). Congenital diaphragmatic hernia in the neonate. In L. E. Weisman (Ed.), *UpToDate*. Retrieved from: www.uptodate.com.

Heron, M. (2018). Deaths: Leading causes for 2016. *National Vital Statistics Reports, 67*(6), 1–76.

Houk, C. P., & Levitsky, L. L. (2017). Evaluation of the infant with atypical genitalia (disorder of sex development). In L. S. Baskin & M. E. Geffner (Eds.), *UpToDate*. Retrieved from: www.uptodate.com.

Huang, S. B., & Doherty, D. (2018). Congenital malformations of the central nervous system. In C. A. Gleason & S. E. Juul (Eds.), *Avery's diseases of the newborn* (10th ed.). Philadelphia: Elsevier.

Indyk, J. (2017). Disorders/differences of sex development for primary care: The approach to the infant with ambiguous genitalia. *Translational Pediatrics, 6*(4), 323–334.

Jones, A. M., Isenburg, J., Salemi, J. L., et al. (2016). Increasing prevalence of gastroschisis – 14 states, 1995-2012. *Morbidity and Mortality Weekly Report, 65*(2), 23–26.

Judd, J., & Clarke, N. M. (2014). Treatment and prevention of hip dysplasia in infants and young children. *Early Human Development, 90*(11), 731–734.

Keller, B. A., Hirose, S., & Farmer, D. L. (2018). Surgical disorders of the chest and airways. In C. A. Gleason & S. E. Juul (Eds.), *Avery's diseases of the newborn* (10th ed.). Philadelphia: Elsevier.

Khan, S., & Orenstein, S. R. (2016). Esophageal atresia and tracheoesophageal fistula. In R. M. Kliegman, B. F. Stanton, J. W. St Geme, et al. (Eds.), *Nelson textbook of pediatrics* (20th ed.). Philadelphia: Elsevier.

Kim, G., Nandi-Munshi, D., & Diblasi, C.C. (2018). Disorders of the thyroid gland. In C.A. Gleason & S.E. Juul (Eds.), *Avery's diseases of the newborn* (10th ed.). Philadelphia: Elsevier.

Kinsman, S. L., & Johnston, M. V. (2016). Myelomeningocele. In R. M. Kliegman, B. F. Stanton, J. W. St. Geme, et al. (Eds.), *Nelson textbook of pediatrics* (20th ed). Philadelphia: Elsevier.

Kishnani, P. S., & Chen, Y. (2016). Defects in galatose metabolism. In R. M. Kliegman, B. F. Stanton, J. W. St. Geme, et al. (Eds.), *Nelson textbook of pediatrics* (20th ed). Philadelphia: Elsevier.

LaFranchi, S. (2018). Treatment and prognosis of congenital hypothyroidism. In D. S. Ross & M. E. Geffner (Eds.), *UpToDate.* Retrieved from: https://www.uptodate.com.

Ledbetter, D. J., Chabra, S., & Javid, P. J. (2018). Abdominal wall defects. In C. A. Gleason & S. E. Juul (Eds.), *Avery's diseases of the newborn* (10th ed.). Philadelphia: Elsevier.

Mai, C. T., Cassell, C. H., Meyer, R. E., et al. (2014). Birth defects from populations-based birth defects surveillance programs in the United States, 2007 to 2011: Highlighting orofacial clefts. *Birth Defects Research Part A: Clinical and Molecular Teratology, 100*(11), 895–904.

March of Dimes. (2018). *Neural tube defects.* Retrieved from: http://www.marchofdimes.org/complications/neural-tube-defects.aspx.

Marshall, J., Salemi, J. L., Tanner, J. P., et al. (2015). Prevalence, correlates, and outcomes of omphalocele in the United States, 1995-2005. *Obstetrics & Gynecology, 126*(2), 284–293.

McKee-Garrett, T. M. (2016). Lower extremity positional deformations. In L. E. Weisman & W. Phillips (Eds.), *UpToDate.* Retrieved from: https://www.uptodate.com.

Merguerian, P. A., & Rowe, C. K. (2018). Developmental abnormalities of the genitourinary system. In C. A. Gleason & S. E. Juul (Eds.), *Avery's diseases of the newborn* (10th ed.). Philadelphia: Elsevier.

Merritt, J. L., & Gallagher, R. C. (2018). Inborn errors of carbohydrate, ammonia, amino acid, and organic acid metabolism. In C. A. Gleason & S. E. Juul (Eds.), *Avery's diseases of the newborn* (10th ed.). Philadelphia: Elsevier.

Moise, K. J. (2018). Overview of Rhesus D alloimmunization in pregnancy. In C. J. Lockwood (Ed.), *UpToDate.* Retrieved from: https://www.uptodate.com.

National Institutes of Health. (2019). *Esophageal atresia/tracheoesophageal fistula.* Retrieved from: https://ghr.nlm.nih.gov/condition/esophageal-atresia-tracheoesophageal-fistula#statistics.

Otteson, T. D., & Arnold, J. E. (2015). Upper airway lesions in the neonate. In R. J. Martin, A. A. Fanaroff, & M. C. Walsh (Eds.), *Fanaroff & Martin's neonatal-perinatal medicine: Diseases of the fetus and infant* (10th ed.). Philadelphia: Elsevier.

Parry, R. L. (2015). Selected gastrointestinal anomalies in the neonate. In R. J. Martin, A. A. Fanaroff, & M. C. Walsh (Eds.), *Fanaroff & Martin's neonatal-perinatal medicine: Diseases of the fetus and infant* (10th ed.). Philadelphia: Elsevier.

Plana, M. N., Zamora, J., Suresh, G., et al. (2018). Pulse oximetry screening for critical congenital heart defects. *Cochrane Database of Systematic Reviews, 3,* CD011912.

Portillo Medina, S. A., Franco, J., Ciapponi, A., et al. (2017). Ventriculo-peritoneal shunting devices for hydrocephalus (protocol). *Cochrane Database of Systematic Reviews, 7,* CD012726.

Rahi, A., Grosse, S. D., Ailes, E. C., et al. (2017). Association of U.S. state implementation of newborns screening policies for critical congenital heart disease with early infant deaths. *Journal of the American Medical Association, 318*(21), 1–8.

Rezvani, I., & Ficicioglu, C. H. (2016). Defects in metabolism of amino acids: Phenylalanine. In R. M. Kliegman, B. F. Stanton, J. W. St. Geme, et al. (Eds.), *Nelson textbook of pediatrics* (20th ed). Philadelphia: Elsevier.

Robinson, S., & Cohen, A. R. (2015). Myelomeningocele and related neural tube defects. In R. J. Martin, A. A. Fanaroff, & M. C. Walsh (Eds.), *Fanaroff & Martin's neonatal-perinatal medicine: Diseases of the fetus and infant* (10th ed.). Philadelphia: Elsevier.

Rosenfield, S. B. (2017). Developmental dysplasia of the hip: Clinical features and diagnosis. In W. Phillips (Ed.), *UpToDate.* Retrieved from: https://www.uptodate.com.

Sadowski, S. (2015). Cardiovascular disorders. In M. T. Verklan & M. Walden (Eds.), *Core curriculum for neonatal intensive care nursing* (5th ed.). St. Louis: Elsevier.

Scholz, T., & Reinking, B. E. (2018). Congenital heart disease. In C. A. Gleason & S. E. Juul (Eds.), *Avery's diseases of the newborn* (10th ed.). Philadelphia: Elsevier.

Sewell, E. K., & Keene, S. (2018). Perinatal care of infants with congenital birth defects. *Clinics in Perinatology, 45*(2), 213–230.

Shaw, B. A., Segal, L. S., & Section on Orthopaedics. (2016). Evaluation and referral for developmental dysplasia of the hip in infants. *Pediatrics, 138*(6), e20163107.

Sherman, J. (2015). Renal and genitourinary disorders. In M. T. Verklan & M. Walden (Eds.), *Core curriculum for neonatal intensive care nursing* (5th ed.). St. Louis: Elsevier.

Society for Maternal-Fetal Medicine, Mari, G., Norton, M. E., et al. (2015). Society for Maternal-Fetal Medicine clinical guideline no. 8: The fetus at risk for anemia – diagnosis and management. *American Journal of Obstetrics and Gynecology, 212*(6), 697–710.

Son-Hing, J. P., & Thompson, G. H. (2015). Congenital abnormalities of the upper and lower extremities and spine. In R. J. Martin, A. A. Fanaroff, & M. C. Walsh (Eds.), *Fanaroff & Martin's neonatal-perinatal medicine: Diseases of the fetus and infant* (10th ed.). Philadelphia: Elsevier.

Speer, M. E. (2018). Postnatal care of hydrops fetalis. In L. E. Weisman (Ed.), *UpToDate.* Retrieved from: https://www.uptodate.com.

Stephenson, C. D., Lockwood, C. J., & Mackenzie, A. P. (2018). Omphalocele. In L. Wilkins-Haug, & D. Levine (Eds.), *UpToDate.* Retrieved from: https://www.uptoddate.com.

Sutton, V. R. (2017). Inborn errors of metabolism: Epidemiology, pathogenesis, and clinical features. In S. Hahn (Ed.), *UpToDate.* Retrieved from: https://www.uptodate.com.

Verklan, M. T. (2015). Neurologic disorders. In M. T. Verklan & M. Walden (Eds.), *Core curriculum for neonatal intensive care nursing* (5th ed.). St. Louis: Elsevier.

Wassner, A. J., & Brown, R. S. (2015). Congenital hypothyroidism: Recent advances. *Current Opinion in Endocrinology, Diabetes, and Obesity, 22*(5), 407–412.

Watchko, J. F. (2018). Neonatal indirect hyperbilirubinemia and kernicterus. In C. A. Gleason & S. E. Juul (Eds.), *Avery's diseases of the newborn* (10th ed.). Philadelphia: Elsevier.

White, K. K., Bouchard, M., & Goldberg, M. J. (2018). Common neonatal orthopedic conditions. In C. A. Gleason & S. E. Juul (Eds.), *Avery's diseases of the newborn* (10th ed.). Philadelphia: Elsevier.

Wilkins-Haug, L. (2018). Etiology, prenatal diagnosis, obstetrical management, and recurrence of cleft lip and/or palate. *UpToDate.* Retrieved from: https://www.uptodate.com.

World Health Organization. (2016). *Congenital anomalies.* Retrieved from: http://www.who.int/news-room/fact-sheets/detail/congenital-anomalies.

Wycoff, M. H., Aziz, K., Escobedo, M. B., et al. (2015). Part 13: Neonatal resuscitation: 2015 American Heart Association guidelines update for cardiopulmonary resuscitation and emergency cardiovascular care. *Circulation, 132*(18 Suppl. 2), s543–s560.

Zaganjor, I., Ahlia, S., Tsang, B. L., et al. (2016). Describing the prevalence of neural tube defects worldwide: A systematic literature review. *PLoS One, 11*(4). https://doi.org.libproxy.lib.unc.edu/10.1371/journal.pone.0151586.

Zinn, A. B. (2015). Inborn errors of metabolism. In R. J. Martin, A. A. Fanaroff, & M. C. Walsh (Eds.), *Fanaroff & Martin's neonatal-perinatal medicine: Diseases of the fetus and infant* (10th ed.). Philadelphia: Elsevier.

37

Perinatal Loss, Bereavement, and Grief

Beth Perry Black

http://evolve.elsevier.com/Lowdermilk/MWHC/

LEARNING OBJECTIVES

- Define perinatal loss, bereavement, and grief.
- Describe the causes of perinatal loss.
- Describe the various responses parents and families may have to loss.
- Analyze the personal and societal issues complicating responses to loss.
- Identify actual and potential problems for persons experiencing loss.

- Discuss individualized nursing interventions to meet the special needs of bereaved women, their partners, and families with a perinatal loss and the ensuing grief.
- Differentiate between helpful and hurtful responses in caring for women, their partners, and families who experience a perinatal loss.
- Define complicated grief related to loss and how nurses can assess risk for complicated grief.

Most expectant parents anticipate the birth of their baby with joy and hope. However, for some women, their partners, and their families, pregnancy becomes a time of loss, resulting in profound grief and a period of bereavement in which they mourn the loss of their expected child. Loss associated with reproduction covers a wide range of conditions and events. Grief and loss in birth settings can pose a challenge for nurses, who should recognize the importance of self-care in confronting their own stress and grief (Carter, 2016); caring for healthy pregnant women who give birth to healthy infants is the more typical expectation for nurses in these settings. However, understanding grief and bereavement as a human response to loss is important because nurses in a variety of settings associated with women's health will encounter clients for whom the childbearing process results in loss.

The study of loss surrounding childbearing and the subsequent grief and bereavement is of great interest. For purposes of this chapter, **perinatal bereavement** is defined as the complex emotional responses experienced by women and their partners beginning immediately after the death of an expected child through miscarriage, stillbirth, neonatal death, or termination of pregnancy for fetal anomalies (TOPFA). Perinatal bereavement is often characterized by grief varying in intensity and duration across genders and is influenced by many situational, internal, and external factors (Fenstermacher & Hupcey, 2013). The purpose of this chapter is to prepare nurses to provide sensitive and supportive care to women, their partners, and families experiencing losses related to childbearing. An overview of loss, grief, and bereavement is presented as a guide for nurses to understand the responses of persons experiencing perinatal loss, to assess and then intervene appropriately in these distressing circumstances.

LOSS, BEREAVEMENT, AND GRIEF: BASIC CONCEPTS AND THEORIES

Much of the current understanding of loss, bereavement, and grief is based on the early work of Elisabeth Kübler-Ross, a Swiss-American psychiatrist who in 1969 published *On Death and Dying* (Kübler-Ross, 1969). In this important book, Kübler-Ross described five stages of grief—denial, anger, bargaining, depression, and acceptance—that she understood as being central to a person's movement through the emotional aftermath of loss. Her work was groundbreaking in that she began the conversation about how people experience loss, particularly death. Most researchers and clinicians who now study or work with dying clients and their families understand grief as a nonlinear process (i.e., people do not move uniformly through stages in a particular order at a specific time). Rather, the grief experience is individual and is influenced by many factors, including the meaning of the loss. Kübler-Ross identified elements of grief that many persons experience; the problem occurs when grieving individuals' responses are considered out-of-sequence or, worse, "abnormal" when they do not fit these stages as she described them. Despite the limits of Kübler-Ross's model, the value of understanding responses to grief is significant in assisting grieving individuals as they work through their sense of loss and sadness.

Nurses in perinatal settings may face challenges in addressing both the grief of their clients and their own distress. Nurses may not feel comfortable discussing grief and loss with women and families facing a pregnancy loss, stillbirth, or death of their newborn. Grief responses such as crying or questioning by the woman can be upsetting to nurses who feel inadequate in helping women and their families in these circumstances. Nurses may have their own grief responses that can be distressing, making it difficult to attend to the emotional care of the client. As a result, nurses and other providers may turn their attention to the mother's physical needs, which is very distressing when she and her partner may be focusing on the loss of their baby (Siassakos, Jackson, Gleeson, et al., 2018). Furthermore, nurses in maternity settings may witness many types of distressing events, including unexpected stillbirth, sudden life-threatening obstetric complications, and even maternal deaths; because these events are rare and unexpected, maternity nurses may be especially susceptible to distress and grief subsequent to their occurrence (Elmir, Pangas, Dahlen, et al., 2017).

The following two sections contain definitions of terms commonly used in end-of-life (EOL) care settings—loss, bereavement, grief, and mourning—and theoretical orientations to loss that may be useful for nurses in perinatal settings in understanding responses of their clients and their own reactions to loss. This in turn can increase nurses' expertise and comfort in providing care when a pregnancy ends in loss.

Defining Loss, Bereavement, Grief, and Mourning

Losses are any experiences in which a valued person or object can no longer be seen, touched, heard, known, or otherwise experienced. In childbearing settings, losses can be complicated in that the extent of the fetus being "known" is typically limited to the pregnant woman through fetal movements, ultrasound images, and pregnancy signs and symptoms. Her partner may have felt fetal movement through the woman's abdomen if the pregnancy is advanced; many partners are present for ultrasound exams. Early in pregnancy, women may not yet have even told their close family and friends of the pregnancy prior to a miscarriage.

The meaning of a loss will have a significant effect on how the loss is experienced. For many women, their partners, and families, a perinatal loss at any stage can mean the loss of hope for a planned-for child, plans for the future, an heir or legacy, or a "perfect" or healthy baby. Meanings of pregnancy are highly variable—a loss can hold great meaning for one woman and her family, whereas a woman in a different circumstance may feel relief that the pregnancy is over. However, thoughtful nurses are cautious in making assumptions about the meaning of a pregnancy loss for any one woman and family.

Bereavement is the state of being without a valued other, especially by death. Sometimes bereaved individuals are described as "bereft" or "the bereaved." Bereavement is characterized by the emotional state of grief, the profound feelings of sadness and despair accompanying loss. Grief is recognized as a *process* through which bereaved persons work to make meaning of and come to terms with their loss. Four attributes foundational to contemporary understanding of this complex issue are: (1) grief is *dynamic* and involves complex emotions, thoughts, and behaviors that shift and change; (2) grief is *a process* that is enduring and has no time limit; (3) grief is *highly individualized* and manifests differently from person to person; and (4) grief is *pervasive* involving psychological, social, physical, cognitive, behavioral, and affective responses and can affect every aspect of a person's life (Cowles & Rodgers, 2000). Although grief is a process, it is iterative. This means that people may return to earlier states of grief over time and somewhat unpredictably as they move forward from their loss.

Mourning, another word often associated with loss, involves culturally mandated traditions and rituals in the period after a death occurs. Bereaved persons are sometimes described as being "in mourning" for some time after the death of a loved one. Funerals, memorial services, wearing black, or otherwise acknowledging the death are common mourning rituals in the United States. Mourning rituals are intertwined with cultural norms and expectations and can vary greatly across families, religions, ethnicities, regions, and nationalities.

Useful Grief Theories in Perinatal Settings

EOL care theories provide an important basis for the care of women and their families with a perinatal loss. Although it is beyond the scope of this chapter to explain fully the theoretical foundations of EOL care, familiarity with these concepts assists perinatal nurses in understanding individual and family experiences of loss in a deeper way.

Ambiguous loss characterizes some types of perinatal loss such as a fetus that has never been physically seen or held by his or her parents and is unknown to others. Boss (2006) described ambiguous loss as occurring when the object of grief is missing. For women experiencing a miscarriage and their partners, for instance, a tangible loss may be never knowing the sex of their expected baby. Some intangible losses associated with miscarriage are the experience of being pregnant, a hoped-for baby, and a future with this child. Furthermore, the reason the miscarriage occurred is often unknown, adding to the ambiguity of the loss. Women and families might not, after certain perinatal losses, including stillbirth, observe or participate in conventional customs of mourning and thus may miss the solace and comfort often found in these rituals. Women have described their stillbirth experiences as "infused with ambiguity, uncertainty, and doubt" (Golan & Leichtentritt, 2016, p.147).

Disenfranchised grief occurs when a person's responses to loss are not openly acknowledged and mourned publicly, thereby limiting social support, which can lead to a sense of isolation in bereaved persons (Doka, 1989). Perinatal losses may be ambiguous because the loss is undefined or unseen, and thus the ensuing grief is disenfranchised because the sadness of bereaved women, partners, and families is unacknowledged. This can result in complicated grief, a complex situation in which grief may not resolve over time and the bereaved person grieves chronically. Wright (2016) noted that complicated grief responses may be characterized by numerous distressful chronic signs and symptoms, including strong preoccupation, yearning and longing for the deceased, intrusive thoughts, and sleep disturbances, among others. Murphy and Cacciatore (2017) noted that failure by others to recognize the significance of a pregnancy loss—specifically stillbirth—creates vulnerability in women, predisposing them to psychological, emotional, and other health risks.

Two established theories of grief and bereavement—continuing bonds theory and dual process model—expand understanding of the complexities of grief and are helpful to perinatal nurses. Developed by Klass, Silverman, and Nickman (1996), *continuing bonds theory* maintains that bonds of attachment forged in life continue into the survivors' future. Because these bonds continue, the full resolution of grief is not detachment but the incorporation of the loved one who has died into the bereaved person's own life. Perinatal losses pose a challenge because the bonds of attachment are newly formed, and time is often short to create meaningful memories to sustain parents and families in the future. Much of current nursing care of women and families who experience stillbirth or neonatal death is oriented around the creation of meaningful rituals that are often created jointly with families and become part of both their grief and their memories (Limbo & Kobler, 2016).

The *dual process model* first described by Stroebe and Schut (1999) emphasizes the processes and strategies individuals use to manage grief and bereavement, as opposed to stages of grief. Individuals move between behaviors oriented toward their losses (focusing on grief, their loss, and the past) and those oriented toward the restoration of their lives without their loved ones (focusing on the future, avoiding grief). Individuals can oscillate rapidly between these two orientations. Nurses who do not understand this phenomenon may be confused by what they construe as "denial" of a loss by their clients. For instance, a mother whose baby died at birth may stop crying soon thereafter, ask for food, take a shower, and talk on the phone.

This is *not* a sign that she is not grieving or that she is "in denial." She may be alleviating her profound grief by focusing for a while on less dramatic day-to-day activities. On the other hand, denial is a psychologic defense mechanism by which a person protects oneself from a distressful reality by removing that reality from conscious awareness. This defense mechanism is different from the restorative behaviors explained by the dual process model, in which the person is conscious of the loss but is seeking temporary relief from the expression of profound grief.

Caring Theory to Guide Nursing Practice When Pregnancy Ends in Loss

Women, their partners, and extended families look to the nursing staff for understanding and support during the time of loss. Caring theory provides a model for practice by which nurses can be particularly helpful to grieving individuals. Swanson developed her caring theory from her research with women and their partners experiencing miscarriage and first published her theory in 2009 (Swanson, Chen, Graham, et al., 2009). Swanson's caring theory has five concepts describing key elements in the nurse–client relationship:

1. Knowing
2. Being with
3. Doing for
4. Enabling
5. Maintaining belief

Knowing means that the nurse must assess the woman, partner, and family (as applicable and appropriate) to understand how they perceive the loss and what the loss means to them. *Being with* denotes the caring presence of the nurse, who as a function of professional caring conveys acceptance of the various feelings and perceptions of each family member. *Doing for* refers to those activities and interventions that the nurse performs on behalf of the woman and her family that provide physical care, comfort, and safety. *Enabling* occurs when the nurse offers the woman and her family options for care. Providing information, giving guidance, articulating choices for decision making, and giving support help the family to feel more in control of a situation in which they can feel out of control. Enabling allows families to feel more comfortable in asking for what they need, such as creating memories, spending time with their infant or with the infant's body, or garnering support from other sources such as friends and clergy. Women and their families then have more autonomy in working through their grief in a way consistent with their own traditions and needs. *Maintaining belief* involves encouraging the woman and her family to believe in their ability to survive their loss. By being with the family, the nurse becomes familiar with their strengths and coping abilities and helps them draw on these resources to grow from the loss (Swanson et al., 2009).

TYPES OF LOSSES ASSOCIATED WITH PREGNANCY

EOL care in perinatal settings brings together death—one of the most difficult of human experiences—and birth, one of life's most joyous occasions. When death and birth coexist, nurses face great challenges. Intervening effectively for women and families in this situation takes significant skill and sensitivity, which can be cultivated by a thorough understanding of the implications of types of pregnancy losses.

Defining Perinatal Losses

Perinatal refers to the period surrounding pregnancy and birth; however, women can have losses associated with reproduction such as infertility, miscarriage, intrauterine fetal death, stillbirth, and deaths of live-born infants soon after birth. In 2011, the American Academy of Pediatrics (AAP) recommended standard terminology for deaths associated with pregnancy (Barfield & Committee on Fetus and Newborn, 2011). Miscarriage is any in utero death prior to 20 weeks of gestation. Fetal death refers to any death prior to birth after 20 weeks of gestation. Fetal deaths are subdivided as early (20 to 27 weeks of gestation) or late (≥28 weeks of gestation). A stillbirth is a fetal death occurring at 20 weeks or later. Death of a live-born infant fewer than 7 days old is an early neonatal death; those occurring between 7 and 28 days are late neonatal deaths. Any live birth of a child who dies within the first year is defined as an infant death (Barfield & Committee on Fetus and Newborn, 2011). Nurses need to understand that these events not only mean distress for women and families but also are indicators of the health of women and infants. Health care practitioners are required to report fetal deaths, live births, and infant deaths, which are used collectively as data to determine perinatal and neonatal mortality rates at state and national levels. Policy makers, in turn, use these rates to influence policy decisions related to allocation of resources to improve care and outcomes.

Types of Perinatal Losses

Perinatal loss is a general term commonly used to describe losses associated with childbearing, particularly those losses occurring after conception and after the woman has recognized that she is pregnant. The complex emotional issues of infertility, including loss and grief for women and men, are discussed in Chapter 9. For the remainder of this chapter, the focus is on losses specific to pregnancy and the early neonatal period.

Miscarriage

Losses associated with childbearing are common. Early spontaneous losses are typically referred to as miscarriages. Specific information about the causes, symptoms, and signs of miscarriages are presented in Chapter 28. Although providers sometimes refer to these losses as "spontaneous abortions," miscarriage is the accepted term among providers to differentiate this form of loss from elective abortions. Grief from miscarriage is often suffered in isolation because other people in a woman's family and social network may not even know about the pregnancy and subsequent loss. Furthermore, grief after a miscarriage is sometimes disenfranchised because even if family and friends know about the pregnancy, their understanding of the meaning of the pregnancy or its importance to the woman may be underestimated or unappreciated.

Serious Fetal Diagnosis

Diagnosis of a serious fetal defect is a more recently described form of perinatal loss. Current standards of maternity care include at least one ultrasound examination, typically performed between 18 and 20 weeks of gestation, at which point the fetal anatomy can be assessed for growth and the presence of congenital defects. The increased use of ultrasonography in prenatal care has resulted in increased diagnosis of fetal defects; note that this is an increase in the *diagnosis* of defects, not in the actual *incidence* of defects. Because these diagnoses are made midpregnancy—later than the time most women would otherwise choose an abortion—most pregnancies with diagnosis of a severe fetal defect are pregnancies that are wanted. When a fetus is diagnosed with a severe defect, women then are confronted with the very difficult choice between continuing or terminating midpregnancy. The severity of the fetal defect, the certainty of both the diagnosis and prognosis, and the prospect of their expected child's suffering are typically taken into account as women make this difficult decision. Importantly, however, prenatal diagnostic technologies and interpretation of findings pose challenges to providers, for whom the abundance of information about the developing fetus may lead to more—not less—uncertainty about long-term outcomes (Kidszun, Linebarger, Walter, et al., 2016).

❓ CLINICAL REASONING CASE STUDY

Care of a Couple With a New Diagnosis of a Severe Fetal Defect

Diana is a 36-year-old multipara who is pregnant with her third child. She and her husband, James, are excited about today's 18-week ultrasound exam because they are hoping to find out the sex of the baby. They already have two sons and are hoping for a daughter. The pregnancy has been advancing without difficulty. Diana has felt fetal movement for approximately 2 weeks, and her early pregnancy symptoms have resolved. However, the ultrasound reveals that their expected baby has hypoplastic left heart syndrome and a severe diaphragmatic hernia. Diana and James learn that either one of these defects is life threatening; however, when they occur together, neonatal death is almost certain. They are devastated. Several consulting physicians come in to talk to them about the problems and what, if anything, can be done. Diana and James ask if they can go home and come back in 2 days once they have the chance to process the news. Diana is crying and tells the nurse that she "can't take in any more information today." When the nurse tells James that she is sorry about what they have found out, he snaps at her, "Mistakes happen all the time. This is one of those times. Our baby is fine." He appears angry and tells Diana to "pull herself together."

1. What is the priority concern or client need in this situation? Support your answer with data as stated in the case.
2. List other client needs/problems in this case.
3. Identify any additional information or assessment data that are needed by the nurse in planning care for this couple.
4. What nursing actions are appropriate in this situation?
   a. What is the priority nursing action?
   b. Describe other nursing interventions that are important to providing optimal client care.
5. Describe the roles/responsibilities of the interprofessional health care team members (other than nurses) who may be involved in providing care for this couple.

The diagnosis of a severe fetal defect causes several losses for pregnant women and their partners and families. Sandelowski and Barroso (2005), in a landmark article on the aftermath of a life-threatening fetal diagnosis, described the "loss of the joy of pregnancy, possibilities inherent in pregnancy, the dream child, innocence, and the world as they knew it" (p. 311). Many fetuses with particularly severe defects die in utero. Some live-born infants survive only a few minutes or hours after birth, and others stay days, weeks, or months in neonatal intensive care units (NICUs), where complex technologies and invasive treatments may be used to try to save their lives. Once these fragile infants are admitted to the NICU, parents are still confronted with making difficult EOL decisions about their baby.

Pregnancy Termination

Few topics in women's health are more controversial than elective abortion; however, nurses in perinatal settings sometimes encounter women who have chosen pregnancy termination or who have had an abortion in the past. These decisions are shaped by numerous,

varied, and often complex circumstances, and women choosing pregnancy termination or seeking care afterward require sensitive attention.

Women confronted with the diagnosis of a severe congenital fetal defect often choose pregnancy termination, sometimes referred to as TOPFA, especially if the prognosis for the fetus or newborn is dire or clearly fatal. In some states TOPFA is considered illegal. Sandelowski and Barroso (2005) described a severe fetal diagnosis as posing an "existential crisis" requiring women and their partners to "choose the fate of their unborn child and, in the process, confront, reconcile, and subsequently act on their beliefs about human imperfection and disability, the obligations of parenthood, and the acceptability of abortion" (p. 311). Couples who learn that their expected baby has a severe, life-threatening problem might, in a very short time, face a decision whether to terminate the pregnancy. The gestational age limit for legal abortion shortens the time women have to decide because the diagnosis is often made in midpregnancy. The gestational age limit for abortion varies across states.

A difficult situation of loss occurs when a woman is found to have a multifetal pregnancy and multifetal pregnancy reduction (MFPR) is recommended by her provider to reduce the number of developing embryos to a number that can be safely carried to near term. A multifetal pregnancy is one with three or more developing fetuses. Morbidity and mortality related to multifetal pregnancies are significant and are often related to complications from preeclampsia, preterm labor, and other conditions requiring significantly early birth. Although the procedure may be indicated medically or obstetrically, and despite the continuation of the development of one or two fetuses after an MFPR, expectant parents may feel deep grief and sadness. The American College of Obstetricians and Gynecologists (2017) published a Committee on Ethics opinion paper recommending that women may be referred for counseling by mental health professionals and support groups, among others. Key to their recommendations related to MFPR is a nondirective, nonjudgmental approach when working with women facing this difficult situation.

Women who choose abortion as a result of social and financial obstacles that preclude continuing the pregnancy can have coexisting, seemingly opposite feelings. Among women who have an abortion, sadness is not uncommon despite experiencing relief afterward. Women can mourn the end of the pregnancy despite determining that ending the pregnancy was the best option available at the time. Nurses who provide care for women in settings where pregnancy terminations are performed must be nonjudgmental and recognize that women can experience sadness even when the abortion was elective.

Other Losses

Other losses associated with childbearing can result in distress or even grief, even if the loss does not involve death. Preterm birth disrupts the pregnancy trajectory and can result in a transition to parenthood for women and their partners that is unexpected and for which they are unprepared. The full-term healthy baby for which they had hoped may be replaced by the reality of a small baby who is sick or requires lengthy hospitalization before going home. Breastfeeding can be delayed or foregone, resulting in another loss.

Other women grieve the loss of the birth experience they have dreamed of and planned for, specifically an uncomplicated vaginal birth. Despite being happy for the birth of their newborn that may have otherwise not survived a serious obstetric complication, some women feel sadness and even grieve the fact they required a cesarean birth. Sadness can be compounded when the cesarean surgery is done as an emergency procedure under general anesthesia, meaning that the woman and her partner are separated during the birth and the new mother does not hear her baby's first cries. The reality of the birth experience is inconsistent with the parents' hopes and expectations.

Perinatal Care Settings Where Nurses Encounter Loss

Nurses have a significant influence on how women, their partners, and families experience and cope with perinatal loss. Nurses encounter situations of loss in a variety of settings, including antepartum, labor and birth, neonatal, postpartum, and gynecologic inpatient units and prenatal, gynecologic, and infertility outpatient clinics, family planning settings, and general medical offices. In each of these settings, nurses can provide sensitive care to persons experiencing loss. Nurses in many inpatient settings have developed protocols that provide clear direction to all staff about how to help women and families through this difficult event. In some units, experienced nurses or social workers who are particularly comfortable in helping bereaved families are designated as perinatal grief consultants. They are available to help parents and assist, educate, and support staff in caring for grieving parents and families. In addition, many institutions have follow-up programs involving phone calls, home visits, and support groups that are effective in helping parents after discharge.

Perinatal palliative care (PPC) is a formalized interprofessional care model specifically aimed at intervening when pregnancy is expected to end in stillbirth or neonatal death. Perinatal care providers, including nurses, view perinatal palliative care as a positive way for families to have a voice in the planning and preparation for the birth and death of their expected baby (Wool, 2013). In 2016, the American Academy of Nursing published a policy statement in which it endorsed perinatal palliative care as an "essential element of childbearing choices" (Limbo, Brandon, Côté-Arsenault, et al., 2016, p. 123). Noting that perinatal palliative care is an interprofessional model of care for expectant parents who choose to continue pregnancy following a diagnosis of a life-limiting fetal condition, the Academy supported the development of perinatal palliative care models, workforce development of PPC team members, increasing awareness of PPC for women and families after diagnosis of a life-limiting fetal condition, and endorsed the role of nurses as key members of the PPC team (Limbo et al., 2016, p. 123).

Most palliative and hospice care for older clients with terminal illness is delivered by community-based palliative care and hospice agencies whose main purpose is to provide symptom management and grief and bereavement care. Perinatal palliative care occurs in three settings: large referral centers such as academic medical centers with maternal-fetal medicine specialists and NICUs; community hospital settings where staff members occasionally provide care for women and families experiencing stillbirth, preterm birth, or other types of perinatal losses; and traditional palliative care or hospice agencies that have expanded care options to families experiencing a perinatal loss (see Evidence-Based Practice box).

EVIDENCE-BASED PRACTICE

Perinatal Palliative Care

Ask the Question

Does perinatal palliative care make a difference in caring for women experiencing perinatal loss?

Search for the Evidence

Search Strategies: English-language research-based publications since 2014 on palliative care, perinatal palliative care, and perinatal loss were included.

Databases Used: Cochrane Collaborative Database, National Guideline Clearinghouse (AHRQ), CINAHL, PubMed, UpToDate, and the professional websites for ACOG and AWHONN.

Critical Appraisal of the Evidence

- Perinatal loss is defined as the death of a fetus at or after 20 weeks' gestation. The death of a newborn up to 4 weeks is also considered to be a perinatal loss (Wool, Black, & Woods, 2016).
- The primary goal of perinatal palliative care (PPC) is to alleviate suffering and promote healing for families experiencing perinatal loss. PPC is provided in a coordinated manner and includes health care disciplines such as nursing, maternal-fetal medicine, social work, chaplains or other clergy, surgery, neonatology, and genetics (Wool et al., 2016).
- A survey of palliative care programs across the United States revealed that most of the programs have a care coordinator position, but the duties of the role vary. The most important aspects of care included support and respect for the choices and preferences of families. The program outcomes included satisfaction of parents with both physical and psychosocial support from health care professionals, assistance with making decisions, and the chance to provide care and comfort for their infant (Denney-Koelsch, Black, Côté-Arsenault, et al., 2016).

- Health care organizations are increasingly measuring parent satisfaction with PPC programs as a measure of quality for the organization. A validated tool has been used to measure satisfaction. Results from use of the tool offer organizations valuable information about what parents want and need during their difficult circumstances of experiencing perinatal loss (Wool, Repke, & Woods, 2017).

Apply the Evidence: Nursing Implications

- Nurses are often front-line caregivers for women experiencing perinatal loss. Nurses should know if PPC resources are available in their workplace. The role of the nurse is to offer compassionate care and provide resources for families (Wool, et al., 2017).
- Nurses should provide consistent care for families experiencing perinatal loss. This continuity of care improves communication and satisfaction of families (Wool et al., 2017).
- Nurses are in the position to provide effective care for bereaved families by assessing patient knowledge and creating a family-centered plan of care that spans the course of the pregnancy, birth, and death of the baby (Wool et al., 2017).

References

Denney-Koelsch, E., Black, B. P., Côté-Arsenault, D., et al. (2016). A survey of perinatal palliative care programs in the United States: Structure, process, and outcomes. *Journal of Palliative Medicine, 19*(10), 1080–1086.

Wool, C., Black, B. P., & Woods, A. (2016). Quality indicators and parental satisfaction with perinatal palliative care in the intrapartum setting after diagnosis of a life-limiting fetal condition. *Advances in Nursing Science, 39*(4), 346–357.

Wool, C., Repke, J. T., & Woods, A. B. (2017). Parent reported outcomes of quality care and satisfaction in the context of a life-limiting fetal diagnosis. *Journal of Maternal-Fetal, and Neonatal Medicine, 30*(8), 894–899.

Jennifer Taylor Alderman

Each of these models has strengths and weaknesses. Large referral centers encounter perinatal losses frequently as a function of the number of high-risk pregnancies followed in these settings. Providers in these settings have experience with perinatal loss, and some medical centers have perinatal palliative care teams and well-developed protocols. However, follow-up grief and bereavement care can be difficult because the bereaved families often live in communities far from the medical center. Increasingly, community hospitals are developing interprofessional perinatal palliative care programs in response to the needs of bereaved families in the local community. Importantly, the programs may serve families for whom their expected baby has a congenital defect that usually results in stillbirth or neonatal death soon after birth (e.g., anencephaly, bilateral renal agenesis) and for whom high-tech interventions of a medical center would be futile. EOL care agencies have extensive experience in symptom management and grief and bereavement care; however, the specific needs of families with losses related to childbearing may be outside their usual expertise. Many of these agencies are developing programs to assist with perinatal losses with specific staff identified to provide care under these circumstances. A comprehensive list of agencies providing perinatal palliative care or hospice across the United States and in other parts of the world can be found at www.perinatalhospice.org. This website is updated frequently and contains other information about perinatal loss and EOL care that is helpful to both nurses and families.

MILES'S MODEL OF PARENTAL GRIEF RESPONSES

The previous section contained definitions of grief and several related concepts, and different types of perinatal loss were explained. However, putting concepts into practice involves using care models. For instance, perinatal palliative care involves using concepts germane to care of childbearing families and EOL care. A key goal of all care for women and families with a perinatal loss is supporting them in and through their grief. Understanding key elements of grief can help nurses be prepared to encounter the poignant, painful loss for families when their expected baby dies.

The model of grief presented here is based on years of clinical work by Margaret Miles, a nurse scientist who worked with bereaved parents in several settings and in community support groups throughout her career (Miles, 1984). Miles usually referred to pregnant women and their male partners as parents and often referred to them as mothers and fathers. However, it is important to recognize that not all pregnant women see themselves as mothers yet; neither are all of their partners necessarily male, nor do they always see themselves as fathers. Miles's work remains relevant with regard to grief responses of women and their partners; however, to be consistent with Miles's model, the terms *parents* and *parental* are used in the broadest manner possible across pregnancy and the early postpartum period.

Miles hypothesized that parental grief responses occur in three overlapping phases. Her work was instrumental in identifying parental responses in a broad manner and is useful for nurses to help grieving persons understand their responses and how they may change over time. Miles described an early period of *acute distress* and shock, followed by a period of *intense grief* that includes emotional, cognitive, behavioral, and physical responses. *Reorganization* occurs when they return to their usual level of functioning, although the distress associated with the death remains. Grief is a long-term process that can extend for months and years; some aspects of grief endure through life. This is consistent with continuing bonds theory discussed previously, in which the goal of the grief process is not resolution but rather the incorporation of the person who has died into one's own life moving forward.

Acute Distress

Pregnancy loss or the death of an infant can be an acute and distressing experience for women and their partners. The loss encompasses a loss of their identity or anticipated identity as a parent to this particular child and their dreams related to parenthood. A period of acute distress characterized by shock and numbness follows the diagnosis of an intrauterine death, impending stillbirth, or experiencing the death of an infant. Miles described parents' experiences as a sense of unreality, loss of innocence, and powerlessness; being devastated or feeling like they are in a bad dream, a fog, or trance; and having a sense of disbelief. Profound sadness accompanied by intense outbursts of emotion and crying is common. Occasionally a lack of affect, calmness, or even euphoria can reflect their numbness. (This phenomenon might be explained by the dual process model described earlier.) For some, their way of coping with a profound loss is to avoid emotional displays. Expressions of grief may be guided by deep sociocultural and religious/spiritual influences that are unfamiliar to the nurse who is expected to provide nonjudgmental support.

Women can develop mental health problems such as depression and anxiety from overwhelming grief and sense of loss. Depression is a medical condition that differs from grief. Recognizing symptoms of depression, especially in the presence of grief, can be very difficult. Nurses must be aware of the difference between grief and depression. Screening tools for depression are easily administered in clinical settings and can be very useful in helping determine if an individual has symptoms of depression. Nurses must seek referrals to mental health providers for those women and partners who show symptoms of depression. (See Chapter 31 for more information on perinatal and postpartum depression.) The coexistence of depression and grief can have serious implications for a person's health and daily functioning. Much of the literature and research on grief after perinatal loss or infant death have focused on the woman or mother. Similarly, much of the attention at the time of a loss is on the woman, and her partner is usually expected to be her main support. The partner's grief is sometimes not recognized or acknowledged.

The response of partners to reproductive losses tends to vary more than those of pregnant women and can depend on the level of identification with the pregnancy. Partners may hide their feelings from each other to protect the other during times of loss (Stroebe, Finkenhauer, Wijngaards-de Meij, et al., 2013). With early miscarriage or ectopic pregnancy, for instance, some partners may not yet have developed a strong investment in the expected child. However, many partners are profoundly affected and grieve deeply after perinatal loss. The nonbiological mother in a lesbian couple may be profoundly affected by the biological mother's loss; contextual issues related to the challenges of childbearing in a heteronormative society intensify the loss for lesbian couples (Wojnar, 2016).

Men are distressed by the grief of their partner and often see themselves as the partner's main support. Men's emotional responses may not be as intense or as long-lasting as their female partners' responses; however, they may be more likely to engage in behaviors such as alcohol consumption in response to the loss. Men's responses to a loss may be easily overlooked in comparison to what may be more outward expressions of grief by their partners (Due, Chiarolli, & Riggs, 2017). Because many men do not easily share feelings or ask for help, nurses may need to be intentional in addressing their grief and in helping them realize that they too need to receive support from others as they grieve. Experiences of grief are complex, and each partner within a couple (heterosexual or same sex) must come to terms with both the loss themselves, the effects of the loss on their partner, and the possible effect of the loss on their relationship with each other (Avelin, Rådestad, Säflund, et al., 2013).

During the acute distress period, parents face the first task of grief, accepting the reality of the loss. The pregnancy has ended or the baby has died, thereby changing their lives. They are often required to make many decisions during this period when normal functioning is impeded and decisions are difficult to make. This can be especially painful and difficult for young couples who have limited or no previous experience with death. These couples may turn to their own parents to help make difficult decisions regarding funeral arrangements or disposition of the body because they have more life experience. However, some well-meaning grandparents and other family members may try to make all the decisions to spare the bereaved parents additional grief associated with disposal of the baby's body or making funeral arrangements. The nurse as advocate can be very important in making sure that the bereaved parents are comfortable with the extent to which well-meaning family members are involved. An important goal of perinatal palliative care services is to help families make as many decisions as possible in advance of the birth, freeing them from having to make choices in the early acute phase of grief when decision making is very difficult.

Intense Grief

The phase of intense grief encompasses many difficult emotions as the parents work through their pain and adjust to life without the child they were expecting. This phase displaces the acute grief and will likely take longer to move through. In the early months after the loss, parents often experience feelings of loneliness, emptiness, and yearning. Women may report that their arms literally ache to hold the baby or they may think they hear a baby crying. Breast milk production still occurs for most women as part of the normal postpartum physiologic changes, even though there is no infant to feed. Lactation is a poignant reminder of the loss and requires careful planning by the nurse to assist the woman in managing the breast discomfort that can occur.

Preoccupation with the deceased expected baby is not uncommon. Women who have recently given birth often want to talk about details of the experience; women who had a stillbirth or whose baby died may have a particularly strong need to share details about the birth. Nurses can actively listen, taking time to allow women to work through their birth and loss stories as they try to make sense and meaning of the experience.

Going home without the baby is particularly difficult, and bereaved parents may face a decision about what to do with the nursery and baby items that they have collected or been given. Some women may want the nursery disassembled before they go home, whereas others want the room left intact until they have had time to grieve their loss. Well-meaning grandparents, relatives, or friends may rush to put away nursery furniture and baby items with the thought that they would be sparing the bereaved parents additional pain. In fact, these actions might serve to compound their grief if parents were not involved in the decision. The bereaved parents should have the opportunity to make the decision about when, and by whom, the nursery and baby items are stored or given away.

Guilt can accompany intense grief. During this phase, women may wonder what they did to cause the loss or if there was anything that they could have to done to prevent it. Women are particularly vulnerable to feelings of guilt because of their sense of responsibility for the well-being of the fetus and baby. Often, losses occur with no clear cause, leaving the woman to speculate about the cause of the loss and her role in it. Sometimes the guilt can be intense if the woman believes she is being punished for some unrelated event. Pressure to be "perfect" in one's lifestyle such as nutrition, exercise, and rest can encumber women with guilt if a pregnancy loss ensues. Women sometimes analyze their behaviors in detail in an effort to explain the loss; they may focus on occasions when they may have had a glass of wine or a cigarette or stayed out late, blaming themselves for an event that was inevitable or unavoidable. Women engaging in self-blame need emotional reassurance that they were not at fault. As their sadness begins to resolve, couples may experience guilt when they begin to socialize, enjoy their family and friends, and experience pleasure again despite the loss of their baby.

Anger, resentment, bitterness, or irritability are common during this phase of grief. Anger can be focused on the health care team who, in the opinion or belief of the bereaved parents, failed to save the pregnancy, fetus, or infant. Some parents direct their anger toward God, blaming God for allowing the loss to occur. Sometimes people experience a spiritual crisis as a result of the loss. Anger may be focused toward family, friends, and peers when they do not provide the support that bereaved parents need and want. Feeling anger at mothers and fathers who appear not to "deserve" or appreciate their children is common; bereaved parents may find that news of neglected or abused children is more intolerable than it was before their loss. Being around pregnant women can be very upsetting. Prolonged anger and generalized irritability may be signs of depression that needs treatment by a mental health care provider.

Deep sadness occurs when the parent faces the full awareness of the reality of the loss; this time can be characterized by *disorganization*, a time when individuals can experience a variety of changes. Cognitive changes can occur, such as an inability to concentrate, confused thought processes, difficulty in problem solving, and poor decision making. Disorganization may cause difficulty in keeping up with work and family expectations. Returning to work can be painful as bereaved parents face their colleagues and coworkers. However, some people find a great deal of comfort in returning to work; it gives them a sense of normalcy and routine in their grief. Families of children who have died have reported finding support from their friends as particularly useful, as is informal support from health care providers acting outside of their formal role as nurse, social worker, or physician (Gear, 2014). When couples begin to consider the next pregnancy, they are likely to experience fear and anxiety due to concerns about the potential for another loss (Côté-Arsenault & O'Leary, 2016). Some women want to become pregnant again right away; tension can arise between partners when one is ready to pursue pregnancy again and the other is not.

Physical symptoms of grief include fatigue, headaches, dizziness, or musculoskeletal aches and pains. Bereaved individuals can be immunosuppressed, leading them to contract respiratory and gastrointestinal infections more easily than before their loss. Lack of sleep, a common complaint among grieving individuals, contributes to their risk for health problems. Weight changes are common: appetites can be poor or individuals can turn to food as a coping response. Changes in health behaviors are common in grieving people.

Grief is very personal, ongoing, and difficult to endure. It is important for nurses to help grieving parents understand their responses and make sense of their feelings. Giving them a safe place to express their feelings is a key nursing intervention. The path to healing can be difficult but is eased to a degree when bereaved clients feel supported and their profound loss is affirmed.

Reorganization

From the time of the pregnancy loss or infant death, parents attempt to understand "why?" This leads to a long and intense search for meaning. At first the question of "why" is focused on the cause of death. Finding few good answers, parents focus next on "why me, why mine?" These questions lead some parents into an existential search about the meaning of life and death. The search for meaning involves questions such as, "What does this loss mean to my life?" "What is life all about?" "What do I do now?" This search continues into the phase of reorganization and can lead to profound changes in the bereaved parents' views and philosophies about life.

Time helps ease the painful feelings of grief. Although some grief models focus on "letting go" as an important step in the grief process, bereaved parents often want to hold on to their relationship with their child, a view that is consistent with continuing bonds theory. However, with perinatal loss, parents have few, if any, memories of their infant to provide a balance to their sense of loss. They usually cherish relics and mementos of birth and evidence of the life of their baby, even if by ultrasound photos. Some perinatal settings provide mementos to memorialize the baby, such as hand molds, footprints, locks of hair, clothing, and blankets. (Details of memorializations are included later in this chapter.)

Overwhelming feelings become less painful over time. Reorganization occurs when the parent is better able to function at home and work, experiences a return of self-esteem and confidence, can cope with new challenges, and has placed the loss in perspective. Reorganization often—but not always—occurs after several months or a year as parents begin to move forward with their lives. Enjoying pleasures without guilt, nurturing self and others, developing new interests, and reestablishing relationships are signs of moving on. For some women and families, another pregnancy and the birth of a subsequent child are important steps, although families report that their grief for their baby who died remains (Côté-Arsenault & O'Leary, 2016). However, the term *recovery* is not appropriate because the grief related to perinatal loss, as with any loss, can continue for life. Parents have reported that they will never forget the baby who died and that they are changed from the loss. They note certain anniversary dates related to the pregnancy and birth, such as the day they found out the woman was pregnant, the date they learned the baby had a congenital defect, the date of a miscarriage, the date of birth, and the date of death.

Resuming sexual activity can very complicated for grieving couples. Often, women are physically ready to resume sexual activity before they are emotionally ready. Some women and their partners find that sexual activity is important for emotional closeness and healing, whereas others have a decreased desire for sex. Partners may have divergent views about when and how to resume sex; nurses can help couples understand that this is common. Continuing conflicts around sex can be detrimental to a couple's relationship and may require professional counseling to help resolve this issue. Through careful assessment nurses can help women and their partners determine if they can benefit from professional counseling as they work through the many complicated issues, including sexuality, that are involved in living through grief.

Deciding to become pregnant again can involve intense and conflicting emotions. Fear of another loss can impede the decision. Couples may believe that their risk for another loss is higher than it actually is, so it is important that they understand why the previous loss occurred if possible. Often this is not possible; they need to understand that most losses are very unlikely to repeat, especially the first one. If a couple has had more than one pregnancy loss, genetic counselors may help determine if there is an explanation for the losses. Ambivalence is common. Expectant parents may feel anxiety during a subsequent pregnancy that tempers their excitement (Côté-Arsenault & O'Leary, 2016). This distress can continue even after the birth of a healthy infant and affect maternal attachment to the new baby. Expectant parents may delay emotional investment in a subsequent pregnancy and the developing fetus until after the midpregnancy ultrasound exam; some who had a loss late in the prior pregnancy will feel anxiety and distress throughout the subsequent pregnancy. At an extreme, mothers may withhold attachment to their new infant as a means of protecting themselves against the painful prospect of another loss.

FAMILY ASPECTS OF GRIEF

Nurses who care for grieving parents also often care for the extended family, including siblings of the expected baby and the parents of the bereaved woman and her partner (grandparents of the expected baby). The grief of grandparents is often complex because they are experiencing intense emotional pain related to the loss while witnessing and feeling the immense grief of their own child. It is extremely difficult to watch their son or daughter experience profound sadness with very few ways to comfort and ease their pain. As a result, the grief response can be complicated or delayed for grandparents. Some experience immense "survivor guilt" because they feel the death is out of order because they are alive and their grandchild has died.

Current understanding of care of families experiencing a perinatal loss is that effective care is relationship based (Limbo & Kobler, 2016). An important relationship that may be underestimated is that of children waiting for the birth of their expected sibling. When a pregnancy ends in fetal or neonatal death, the siblings of the expected infant also experience loss. Most parents begin to prepare their children for the arrival of a new baby at some point during the pregnancy. In assisting families in dealing with pregnancy loss, the children's age, development, and level of understanding must be considered. Understanding death requires some ability to think abstractly, and children do not fully understand the concept often until their early school years. Parents may create their own explanation to their children based on religious beliefs and their knowledge of their own child's development and abilities. Children can have a great deal of difficulty understanding why there suddenly is no baby or the baby has not come home. A young child will respond to the reactions of his or her parents, picking up on cues related to parents' sadness and behaviors. Young children may respond with clinging, changes in eating and sleeping patterns, or uncharacteristic behavior at the time when parents have limited patience for responding to and meeting the child's needs. Older children have a more complete understanding of the loss. School-aged children can be frightened by their parents' sadness, whereas teens can understand more fully but feel awkward in responding. Teenagers may feel more comfortable in talking with their friends than with adults in dealing with their loss and grief.

Nurses can help include siblings in grieving rituals to the extent the parents and their children feel comfortable, including seeing the baby's body. Nurses should follow the parents' lead but can suggest rituals and activities at the time of the loss that may be helpful for the children. The extent of the involvement of children is likely to be determined by the length of the pregnancy. An early miscarriage will be managed differently from an unexpected stillbirth at term. Nurses who are specifically interested in perinatal loss may want to consider additional training such as that offered by *Resolve Through Sharing* (http://www.bereavementservices.org/resolve-through-sharing) to increase their skills in working with families experiencing these distressful losses.

 CARE MANAGEMENT

Nursing care of women and their partners experiencing a perinatal loss begins the first time they are faced with the potential loss of the pregnancy or death of the fetus or infant. Supportive interventions are important when parents are anticipating loss, at the time of the loss, and after the family has returned home. To provide competent, compassionate, individualized care to grieving families, the nurse first does a thorough assessment. Several key areas to address include the following:

- The nature of the parental attachment to the pregnancy and developing fetus or infant, the meaning of the pregnancy and infant to the parent, and the related losses they are experiencing. Whether a woman has experienced a miscarriage or ectopic pregnancy, stillbirth, or death of an infant, it is important to understand parents' perceptions of their unique loss.

- Complex family and sociocultural influences on the meaning of the loss. Feelings about perinatal loss can range from feeling devastated to feeling relieved. Listening to parents tell their story and being sensitive to the language used to describe their experience can help nurses gain an understanding of the meaning of the loss. For example, if a woman refers to a miscarriage as "losing a pregnancy," nurses should be careful to edit their language not to refer to "your baby" but to use the cues the woman has given with regard to her view of the loss. Similarly, if a woman refers to the fetus by name or as her daughter or son, nurses should do the same. For instance, a woman who elects to terminate the pregnancy when the fetus is found to have a fatal defect might not even mention the fetus at all or may refer to the fetus as "it" or "the pregnancy." This is a distancing behavior that is protective and normal. Nurses' language surrounding grief and loss should follow the cues given by the bereaved woman and partner, who are likely to model the terms they prefer in referring to the loss.

- The circumstances surrounding the loss, including the time to prepare for the loss and the parents' level of understanding about the cause of the loss or death, and any related unresolved issues. Over the course of caring for women with a perinatal loss, nurses may discover that the women may have had experiences that make their losses even more poignant. A history of infertility, repeated pregnancy losses, a previous stillbirth, or infant death can make this loss even more painful. In addition, other life circumstances such as illness of another family member, loss of a job, or other family stresses can increase distress. The nonbiological mother in a lesbian relationship may have a history of losses of her own that are revisited when her partner experiences a loss. In addition, losses for which the expectant parents are unprepared, such as an obstetric accident late in pregnancy, can constitute a traumatic event that requires a great deal of sensitive and intense intervention.

- The immediate responses of the woman and partner to the loss, whether their responses are similar or different, and if their responses are consistent with their past experiences and sociocultural contexts. An understanding of common responses to grief described earlier can be helpful in attempting to understand the unique grief responses of the mother, partner, and other family members. As nurses work with families, they can find out how the individual or family responded to a previous loss or a personality or behavioral trait that may be involved in their responses to this grief. For instance, if a woman who has usually been outgoing and talkative is now withdrawn and silent, the nurse can ask her if in the past this is how she has grieved other losses. People tend to grieve various losses in their lives similarly, even though the meaning of each loss is unique. In helping women and their partners through a perinatal loss, it is important to know if there is a history of infertility, previous pregnancy losses, or infant deaths. The accumulation of losses can negatively affect grief responses. It also is important to be sensitive to varied expectations during grief for men and women from different cultural groups (see section on cultural and spiritual needs of parents later in this chapter).

- The social support network of the woman and her partner (e.g., extended family, friends, coworkers, church) and the extent to which it has been engaged. Social support in response to a perinatal loss can be very important; however, nurses should assess the amount and type of support that the bereaved family desires. Some prefer a few days alone to recover physically, whereas others find comfort in being surrounded immediately with supportive family and friends. In inpatient settings the nurse may need to be an advocate for a woman desiring solitude by limiting visitors. Other women want or need assistance in communicating with family members about the loss, in making necessary decisions, and in contacting clergy. The nurse should not assume that all women who have had a perinatal loss will want to be visited by clergy but should ask if the woman would like a visit by the hospital chaplain or her own clergyperson and, if so, to identify the specific religious tradition.

- Nursing care for women, partners, and families grieving the end of a pregnancy and death of their expected child or newborn is complex and should be comprehensive. The initial shock and numbness that accompany early grief can be misread if the nurse is not aware of the ebb and flow of sadness related to grief and misinterprets important cues (see Nursing Care Plan).

WHEN A LOSS IS DIAGNOSED: HELPING THE WOMAN AND HER FAMILY IN THE AFTERMATH

Learning of a loss or a potential loss is very distressing to most individuals. Under a great deal of stress, people are likely to have limited ability to take in anything but the most basic information and sometimes appear to "shut down." Simple, unambiguous, and consistent language is crucial. For example, a pregnant woman for whom English was her second language was visiting the United States. She began bleeding heavily at 32 weeks' gestation and noticed that her uterus was very hard. Her partner immediately transported her to a local medical center, where she was admitted directly to the high-risk maternal-fetal care unit. Her bleeding had subsided, but there were no fetal heart tones, and fetal death was confirmed by ultrasound. The resident physician told her that her "baby had passed," which she understood to mean that her pain was related to labor and that she had given birth. She asked where the baby was and began to look under the sheets. The nurse realized her misunderstanding of the word "passed" (as in "passed away" or "had died") and explained to the woman that the physician meant that the baby had died. Although the use of words like "death," "died," and "dying" are difficult in any setting, euphemisms or other veiled language can be misunderstood by women and their families under stress. The nurse's presence is crucial in hearing what other providers have told the woman and family and in clarifying any misunderstandings.

◎ NURSING CARE PLAN

Fetal Death and Stillbirth at 35 Weeks of Gestation

Client Problem	Expected Outcome	Interventions	Rationale
Grief related to unexpected fetal death	Parents will express feelings and demonstrate normal grieving behaviors.	Prepare family for viewing and holding infant. Allow family private, unhurried time with infant. Provide family with memorabilia (e.g., footprints, photos, lock of hair) as desired.	To initiate and support them in their grief. To provide evidence of the reality of the death while honoring the existence of their baby. To provide tangible evidence and memories of their baby's life as a means of creating bonds.
Potential for woman's decreased self-esteem and sense of failure to become a mother	Woman will exhibit positive self-comments as evidence of her decreasing sense of failure.	Provide private time for expression of feelings through therapeutic communication and active listening. Identify woman's perception and feelings about fetal death. Assist woman to identify positive coping mechanisms and support systems. Refer to appropriate health care professionals for counseling and care as needed.	To encourage her to openly express her feelings. To correct any misconceptions and alleviate guilt. To promote feelings of self-worth. To provide ongoing assistance.
Potential for disruption in the couple's relationship related to inadequate communication during period of grief.	Partners will discuss feelings involving their relationship with each other.	Provide information about how grief affects the family. Encourage partners to share feelings about the loss and how it affects the family. Refer to perinatal or family support group if appropriate.	To facilitate expression of grief and sadness. To clarify the possible effects on the family. To minimize the sense of isolation and facilitate communication and sharing of the experience of loss with others who have had similar experiences.

With early pregnancy loss, the word "miscarriage" should be used consistently. With fetal or neonatal death, providers should use the words "has died" or "there is no heartbeat," rather than "lost," "gone," or "passed" to eliminate ambiguity. Providing the opportunity for women and partners to ask questions, ask for more evidence of the loss, and get a referral for a second opinion gives them some element of control at a time when they have little if any control. Furthermore, in the case of a severe fetal defect, the couple may face a decision about whether to terminate the pregnancy and will want to make the decision with as little ambiguity or unanswered questions as possible.

Helping Parents Hold Their Fetus or Infant

Many women and partners find the experience of holding their stillborn or dying infant meaningful. Seeing and holding the fetus or baby may be important to them because it can help them face the reality of the loss, reduce painful fantasies, and facilitate their grief; however, they should be allowed to choose whether or not they want to see or hold their stillborn or dying baby. Encouraging reluctant individuals to hold or see the body by telling them that not seeing the body could make grieving more difficult is inappropriate. The nurse might ask questions such as, "Some parents have found it helpful to see or hold their baby. Would you like time to consider this?" is helpful. Because the need or willingness to see also can vary among family members, it is important to determine what each person desires and needs. Occasionally only one partner will desire to see or hold the baby's body, or a couple may want to limit holding the baby to themselves without involving other family members. These are difficult situations that have

to be handled with extreme tact and sensitivity by the nurse, always with the expectation that the nurse is advocating for what the client wants.

In preparation for holding the baby, parents appreciate explanations about what to expect. In preparing the baby's body for the parents to see, nurses generally cover the head with a small cap and clothe the baby. Many hospitals have volunteer groups that provide handcrafted hats and infant gowns for such use, items that may then be taken home by the family. The bodies of fetuses that died in utero must be handled extremely gently because of a process called *maceration* in which the upper layer of the skin begins to peel away from the deeper layers. Maceration often begins at the baby's lips, which then appear redder than usual. Bereaved parents often notice this redness, which actually enhances the baby's appearance. The nurse should remember that parents see their baby from a perspective quite different from that of health care professionals. Bathing the baby, applying lotion to the baby's skin, combing hair, placing identification bracelets on the arm and leg, dressing the baby in a diaper and special outfit, sprinkling powder in the baby's blanket, and wrapping the baby in a soft blanket convey to the parents that their baby has been cared for in a special way. Sometimes families will want to see the baby's body for a last time after the body has been taken to the morgue. There is no contraindication to this practice related to infection control. If the baby has been in the morgue, the nurse can place the body underneath a warmer for 20 to 30 minutes then wrap the body in a warm blanket.

When bringing the baby's body to the parents, it is important to treat the baby's body as one would a live baby. Holding the baby

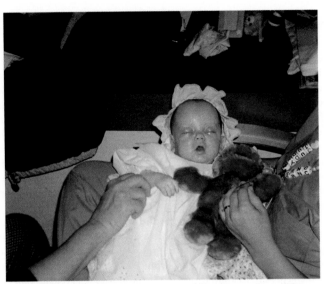

Fig. 37.1 Laura. (Courtesy Amy and Ken Turner, Cary, NC.)

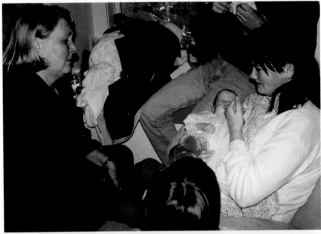

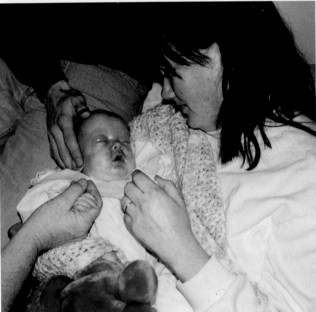

Fig. 37.2 Laura's Family Members Say a Special Goodbye. (Courtesy Amy and Ken Turner, Cary, NC.)

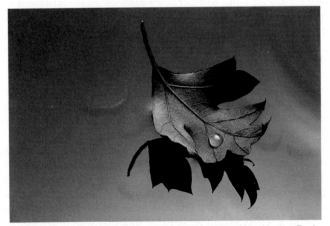

Fig. 37.3 Door Card for Room of Mother Who Has Had a Perinatal Loss. (Used with permission of Bereavement Services. Copyright Lutheran Hospital—La Crosse, Inc., A Gundersen Lutheran Affiliate, La Crosse, WI.)

close, touching a hand or cheek, using the baby's name, and talking with the parents about the special features of their child conveys that it is all right for them to do likewise. If a baby has a congenital anomaly that the family wants to see, the nurse can help explain what they are seeing. It is not unusual for parents to compare what they are seeing in "real life" with what they had seen on the ultrasound screen. Nurses can help parents explore the baby's body as they desire. Parents often seek to identify family resemblance and will point out characteristics of the baby that are similar to themselves or their previous children. Some families like to have the opportunity to bathe and dress their baby. Although the skin is fragile, parents can still apply lotion with cotton balls, sprinkle powder, tie ribbons, fasten the diaper, and place amulets, medallions, rosaries, or special toys or mementos in their baby's hands or alongside their baby. Parents may want to perform other parenting activities, such as combing the hair, dressing the baby in a special outfit, or wrapping the baby in a blanket (Fig. 37.1).

Parents need to be given time alone with their baby. They also need to know when the nurse will return and how to call if they should need anything. When possible, the family is placed in a private room with a rocking chair. This offers the parents time together with their baby and with other family members (Fig. 37.2). Marking the door to the room with a special card helps remind the staff that this family has experienced a loss (Fig. 37.3).

Parents and families vary in the amount of time they wish to have the baby's body with them. These moments are the only ones they will have to parent their child while their child's physical presence is still with them. Some parents need only a few minutes; others need hours; regardless of length of time they need, it is extremely painful for some parents to say goodbye to their baby. They will tell the nurse when they are ready verbally, or the nurse will observe nonverbal cues such as when parents and other family members are no longer holding their child close to them or have placed the baby back in the crib. There should be no institutional restrictions on how long a baby's body can remain in the room with the parents. Most parents become ready to hand the baby over to the nurses or to a funeral home at the time the baby's body shows obvious signs of deterioration, which for a baby who dies at birth will occur in approximately 24 to 36 hours. Stillborn babies, depending on how long they have been dead in utero prior to birth, will show signs of deterioration sooner. A position paper developed by the Perinatal Loss and Infant Death Alliance (PLIDA, 2005) notes that infection risks "are insignificant" in having the body of a deceased baby in the mother's room. Bereaved mothers and families should have unrestricted access to the baby's body, which allows them to "process the traumatic events surrounding their baby's death" in addition to allowing for a "more gradual goodbye, both of which are productive components of healthy grieving" (PLIDA, 2005, p. 1).

Helping Parents With Decisions Regarding Autopsies, Organ Donation, and Disposition of the Body

At a time when they are experiencing the great distress of a perinatal loss, parents have many decisions to make. Women, partners, and extended families often consult nurses for guidance in discerning what must be done immediately and what can wait and in understanding their options relative to each decision. The nurse's primary responsibility is to help them and to advocate for them, because choices made during the time of their loss will influence their memories for a lifetime.

Deciding on whether to agree to an autopsy can be challenging. An autopsy can be very important in answering the question "why" if there is a chance that the cause of death can be determined, and parents have reported that the need for knowledge eclipsed any barriers to agreeing to an autopsy (Breeze, Statham, Hackett, et al., 2012). This information can be helpful in decision making about future pregnancies and in working through grief. However, asking parents about an autopsy takes great sensitivity to personal, cultural, and religious views about an autopsy. Some religions prohibit autopsy or limit the choice to times when it may help prevent another loss. Options for the type of autopsy, such as excluding the head, are available to parents. Note that the cost of an autopsy must be considered because it is not covered by insurance and is expensive. The question of autopsy is often brought up in the prenatal period when the fetus has a life-limiting diagnosis for which the cause is unknown or the anatomic details of which are unclear.

If an infant is live-born but is expected to die soon after birth, organ donation may be a possibility. Organ donation can be an aid to grieving and an opportunity for the family to see something positive associated with their experience. The responsibility for determining organ donation potential rests with the state's organ procurement organization (OPO). States and hospitals have clear procedures for how and when to call the OPO. In general, if a death certificate is issued, a call must be made to the OPO. Once contacted, they will decide whether to talk to the family, and either an OPO representative or a designated requester will contact them. This allows requests to be made by trained personnel in a consistent and compassionate manner. The most common donation is corneas; donation of corneas from a baby can occur if the baby was born alive at 36 weeks of gestation or later. In some hospitals these situations are handled by descendent services, which manage a number of legal and practical issues related to a death that occurs in the hospital.

Another important decision relates to spiritual rituals that can be helpful and important to parents and families. The opportunity for support from the clergy should be offered to all bereaved individuals unless prior to the death they have made it clear that they do not want a clergy visit. Families may wish to have their own pastor, priest, rabbi, or spiritual leader contacted, or they may wish to see the hospital chaplain. Clergy or spiritual care providers can offer parents the opportunity for a blessing, naming ceremony, anointing, ritual of the sick, memorial service, baptism, or prayer as is appropriate to a family's beliefs and wishes.

One of the major decisions parents must make has to do with disposition of the body. Parents should be given information about the choices for the final disposition of their baby's body, regardless of gestational age. However, nurses must be aware of cultural and spiritual beliefs that can dictate the choices of parents, issues related to the cost of burial, alternatives to burial, and state laws related to burial. Depending on state regulations, a fetus of less than 20 weeks of gestation may be considered a product of conception, whereas embryos, uterine tubes removed with an ectopic pregnancy, and tissue from a pregnancy obtained during a dilation and curettage are considered tissue. Many hospitals will make arrangements for the cremation. The nurse should know the hospital's policies and procedures and answer the parents' questions honestly.

Respectful disposition refers to the safe handling and disposition of fetal tissue or remains by burial in a designated area. An increasing number of institutions are offering respectful disposition, and nurses can be at the forefront of establishing these procedures that honor women's preferences and wishes for disposition of fetal remains after an early pregnancy loss (Limbo, Kobler, & Levang, 2010). In most states if a fetus is at least 20 weeks and 1 day of gestational age or is born alive, it is the parents' responsibility to make the final arrangements for their baby's body, although some hospitals offer free cremation. In this case the family does not receive the ashes.

Final disposition of bodies, regardless of gestational age, can include burial or cremation. Depending on the cemetery's policies, caskets or ashes can be buried in a special place designated for babies, at the foot of a deceased relative, in a separate plot, or in a mausoleum. Ashes also may be scattered in a designated area; certain states may have regulations regarding where ashes may be scattered. A local funeral director or a state's vital statistics bureau should have information about the state's rules, codes, and regulations regarding live births, burial requirements, transportation of the body, and cremation.

Some parents want a special memorial or funeral service. They can choose to have a funeral service in the hospital chapel or in their own church, visitation at a funeral home or their own home, or a graveside service. Parents can make any of these services as special, personal, and memorable as they like, choosing special music, poetry, or prose written themselves or by others.

If the family has decided on a funeral and burial, they still have decisions about which funeral home to call and where to have the baby interred. Many couples live in an area distant from their family homes, and they may want to have a burial in their hometown or family cemetery. If the family desires cremation, they may want to have the option of obtaining the ashes. It is important to determine whether this will be done by the facility that does the cremation. Some families will keep the ashes ("cremains") in a small urn or other container in their home, and others will eventually take the ashes to a special place for release, such as the beach, the mountains, or a place with special sentimental meaning.

Families become unaware of time and are unaware of change of shifts or any needs the hospital system might have in the operations of the patient unit. When families are urged or rushed into making decisions, they may make a decision in response to the health care institution's needs, not their own. Actions such as naming the baby, seeing and holding the body, disposition of the body, and funeral arrangements should never be rushed. In some cases the mother is discharged home before these decisions are made. Then the family can think about them in the comfort of their home and contact the hospital in the following days to give their answers.

Helping the Bereaved Parents Acknowledge and Express Their Feelings

One of the most important goals of the nurse is to validate the experience and feelings of the parents by encouraging them to tell their stories and listening with care. Helping the parents talk about their loss and the meaning it has for their lives and to share their emotional pain is the next step. Because nurses tend to be very focused on the physical and emotional needs of the mother, it is especially important to ask the father or partner directly about his or her views of what happened and the associated feelings of loss. At the very least, the nurse should acknowledge the loss with a simple but sincere, "I am sorry."

Although listening can be difficult and sometimes painful, the nurse should listen patiently during the story of loss or grief. The emotions of expressed grief can overwhelm health care professionals. Being with someone who is sad and crying can be extremely difficult. The initial impulse to reduce one's sense of helplessness is to say or do something to reduce his or her pain. Although such a response seems supportive at the time, it can stifle the further expression of emotion. Bereaved parents have identified many unhelpful responses made to them by well-meaning health care professionals, family, and friends. The nurse should resist the temptation to give advice or use clichés in offering support to the bereaved (Box 37.1). Nurses need to be comfortable with their own feelings of loss and grief to support and care for bereaved individuals effectively. The nurse should have a presence of self and the willingness to be alongside, quietly supporting the bereaved in whatever expressions of feelings or emotions are appropriate for them. This presence is comforting for parents. Leaning forward, nodding the head, and words such as "Tell me more" is often encouragement enough for the bereaved person to tell his or her story. Sitting through the silence can be therapeutic; silence gives the bereaved person an opportunity to collect thoughts and to process what he or she is sharing. Furthermore, careful assessment is important before using touch as a therapeutic technique.

BOX 37.1   What to Say and What Not to Say to Bereaved Parents

What to Say
- "I'm sad for you."
- "How are you doing with all of this?"
- "This must be hard for you."
- "What can I do for you?"
- "I'm sorry."
- "I'm here, and I want to listen."

What Not to Say
- "God had a purpose for her."
- "Be thankful you have another child."
- "The living must go on."
- "I know how you feel."
- "It's God's will."
- "You have to keep on going for her sake."
- "You're young; you can have others."
- "We'll see you back here next year, and you'll be happier."
- "Now you have an angel in heaven."
- "This happened for the best."
- "Better for this to happen now, before you knew the baby."
- "There was something wrong with the baby anyway."

Used with permission of Bereavement Services. Copyright Lutheran Hospital-La Crosse, Inc., a Gundersen Lutheran Affiliate, La Crosse, WI.

For some, touch is a meaningful expression of concern, but for others it is an invasion of privacy or contrary to their cultural or religious beliefs.

As noted previously, a sense of guilt can pervade the experience of bereaved parents, who may raise many questions surrounding their loss that can leave them feeling guilty. This is particularly true for mothers. Such questions include, "What did I do?" "What caused this to happen?" "What do you think I should have, could have done?" Part of the grief process for bereaved parents is trying to make sense of what happened, why it happened to them, and why it happened to their baby. The nurse should recognize that the answers to these questions must be answered by the bereaved themselves; it is part of their healing. For example, a bereaved mother might ask, "Do you think that this was caused by painting the baby's room?" An appropriate response is, "Let's talk about what you are thinking." Trying to give bereaved parents answers when there are no clear answers or trying to assuage their feelings by telling them they should not feel guilty does not help them process their grief. Trying to figure out why something bad happened is a common human response, but often there are no answers. Sometimes simple factual information, such as the frequency of miscarriages in pregnant women or the fact that there usually is no clear cause of a stillbirth, can be helpful; however, for many people, understanding that something happens frequently is no consolation when it happens to them.

Feelings of anger, guilt, and sadness can occur immediately but often become more problematic in the early days and months after a loss. When a bereaved person expresses feelings of anger, it can be helpful to identify the feeling by simply saying, "You sound angry," or "You look angry." The nurse's willingness to sit down and listen to these feelings of anger can help the bereaved explore underlying feelings of powerlessness and helplessness in not being able to control the many aspects of the situation, which for many people will result in anger.

The attention needed to provide adequate care for grieving families can be time consuming, which can be difficult on a busy nursing unit; however, the nurse must create enough time to engage with them without being rushed. Nurses in inpatient settings who are caring for women and families whose baby has died may need assignments for their shift that allow time to give adequate attention to newly bereaved individuals in helping address their profound grief.

Helping the Bereaved Family Understand Differing Responses to Loss

Bereaved parents may need help in understanding their responses to their loss and in realizing that they are not alone in these painful responses. Most parents are not prepared for the raw feelings that they experience or the fact that these painful, complex feelings and related behavioral reactions continue for many weeks or months. Thus reassuring them that their responses are normal and preparing them for grief's potentially lengthy process can be useful.

The nurse can help parents prepare for the emptiness, loneliness, and yearning; for the feelings of helplessness that can lead to anger, guilt, and fear; for the cognitive processing problems, disorganization, difficulty making decisions; and for the sadness and depression that are part of the grief process. It is essential, then, for the nurse to reassure and educate bereaved parents about the grief process, including the physical, social, and emotional responses of individuals and families. Written materials about parental grief that are sensitive and brief can be very helpful. However, offering health teaching on the bereavement process alone is not enough. In the initial days after a loss, other strategies might include follow-up phone calls, referral to a perinatal grief support group, or providing a list of publications or websites intended for helping parents who have experienced a perinatal loss. Some important websites include www.compassionatefriends.org (death of a child), www.resolve.org (infertility), www.plida.org (perinatal loss and infant death), www.sidscenter.org (sudden infant death), http://www.gundersenhealth.org/resolve-through-sharing/ (bereavement education), and www.marchofdimes.com (information on prematurity and congenital defects, in addition to information about healthy pregnancy). However, as with any referral, the nurse should first review the materials or the websites for accuracy and appropriateness.

🏠 **COMMUNITY ACTIVITY**

- Visit the Healing Hearts Baby Loss Comfort website at www.babylosscomfort.com. Review the client information about the appropriate words to say, full-term baby loss, and stillbirth and grief resources. Also visit the website of the International Stillbirth Alliance (www.stillbirthalliance.org).
- Research the availability of a perinatal loss support group in your community or find online perinatal support groups. Visit the websites of the Compassionate Friends (www.compassionatefriends.org), Perinatal Loss and Infant Death Alliance (PLIDA) (www.plida.org), and Resolve Through Sharing (www.bereavementservices.org) for up-do-date information about organizations that provide support for bereaved parents.

People cope with grief in positive and negative ways. Nurses can reinforce positive coping efforts and attempt to prevent negative coping. Many women use the internet to locate other women who have experienced a pregnancy loss. Blogging and online support groups are increasingly used as means of sharing the experience, especially among well-educated white women. Many women have found decreased isolation in the convenience, access, privacy, and anonymity of message boards dedicated to perinatal loss and find social recognition for their loss in online communities (Davidson & Letherby, 2014). These sources of support should not be used to the exclusion of close friends and family. Many women have had children previously and find that care of their children day to day is healing.

Meeting the Physical Needs of the Bereaved Mother in the Postpartum Period

Coping with loss and grief after birth can be overwhelming for the woman and her family. While in the hospital or birthing center, it is especially difficult for them to hear the sound of crying babies and to witness the happiness of other families on the unit who have given birth to healthy infants. The mother should have the opportunity to decide if she wants to remain on the maternity unit or to move to another unit. Many institutions have cross-trained nurses to provide postpartum care on gynecology units for women whose babies have died; some nurses on these units have experience in dealing with death and bereavement as a function of working with gynecologic cancer clients and may provide highly sensitive and expert physical and emotional care.

The physical needs of a bereaved mother are the same as those of any woman who has given birth. Bereaved mothers still lactate, they have afterbirth pains, and they sometimes feel as though a baby is still moving inside. The issue of lactation is important. Many but not all women will want to suppress lactation (see Chapter 21). Careful attention to suppressing lactation should be a priority nursing intervention for those women who desire not to lactate. Engorgement associated with milk production is physically painful and can be emotionally distressing. Women experiencing a perinatal loss may benefit from a visit by a lactation consultant before being discharged home.

Women need the usual postpartum care instructions on discharge. They also need ideas about how to cope with problems with sleep, such as decreasing food or fluids that contain caffeine, limiting alcohol intake and nicotine use, exercising regularly, and using strategies to promote rest such as taking a warm bath or drinking caffeine-free or herbal tea before bedtime, doing relaxation exercises, listening to restful music, or having a massage.

Assisting the Bereaved Parents in Communicating and Establishing Support From Family Members

Sensitive care of bereaved parents may involve their own parents. A couple's parents and other children are particularly important when a perinatal loss has occurred. However, it is up to the parents to decide to what extent they want family involved in the acute phases of their grief. If it is the parents' desire, nursing staff should allow a couple's children, parents, extended family members, and friends to be involved in the rituals surrounding the death, such as seeing and holding the baby. Such visits afford others the opportunity to become acquainted with the baby, to understand the parents' loss, to offer their support, and to say goodbye (see Fig. 37.2). This experience helps parents explain to their children about their brother or sister and what death means, offers the children answers to their questions in a concrete manner, and helps the children in expressing their grief. Involving extended family and friends enables the parents to mobilize their social support system of people who will support the family not only at the time of loss but also in the future. Parents also need information about how grief affects a family. They may need help in understanding and coping with the potential differing responses of various family members. Frustrations can arise because of the insensitive or inadequate responses of other family members. Parents may need help in determining ways to let family members know how they feel and what they need.

Creating Memorabilia for Parents to Take Home

Parents may want tangible mementos of their baby. Some will bring in a previously purchased baby book. Special memory books, cards, and information on grief and mourning are available for purchase by parents or hospitals or clinics through national perinatal bereavement organizations (Fig. 37.4).

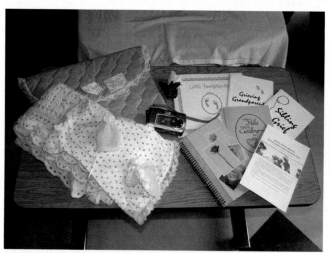

Fig. 37.4 A Memory Kit Assembled at John C. Lincoln Hospital, Phoenix, Arizona. Memory kits may include pictures of the infant, clothing, death certificate, footprints, identification bands, fetal monitor printout, and ultrasound picture. (Courtesy Julie Perry Nelson, Loveland, CO.)

The nurse can provide information about the baby's weight, length, and head circumference to the family. Footprints and handprints can be taken and placed with the other information on a special card or in a memory or baby book. Sometimes it is difficult to obtain clearly defined handprints or footprints. Alcohol or acetone applied to the palms or soles can help the ink adhere and improve the quality of the prints, especially for small babies. When making prints, it is helpful to have a hard surface underneath the paper to be printed. The baby's heel or palm is placed down first, and the foot or hand is rolled forward, keeping the toes or fingers extended. If the print is not clear or well defined, tracing around the baby's hands and feet can be done, although this distorts the actual size. A form of plaster of Paris can also be used to make an imprint of the baby's hand or foot.

Parents often appreciate articles that were in contact with or used in caring for the baby. This might include the tape measure used to measure the baby, baby lotions, combs or hairbrushes, clothing, hats, blankets, crib cards, and identification bands. The identification band helps the parents remember the size of the baby and personalizes the mementos. The nurse should ask parents if they wish to have these articles before giving them to the parents. A lock of hair can be another important keepsake. The nurse must ask the parents for permission before cutting a lock of hair, which can be removed from the nape of the neck, where it is not noticeable.

For some parents, pictures are the most important memento. Photographs are generally taken when it has been determined to be culturally acceptable to the family—the decision for photography is up to the parents. Photos should include close-ups of the baby's face, hands, and feet, with the baby both clothed and unclothed. Flowers, blocks, stuffed animals, or toys can be placed in the background, which serve to contextualize the photo and give an idea of the baby's approximate size. Parents may want their pictures taken holding the baby. Keeping a camera nearby and taking pictures when parents are spending time with their baby can provide special memories. The widespread use of smartphones means that most families have one or more people taking photos and videos of the occasion. Some parents may ask the nurse to record them as they bathe, dress, hold, or diaper their baby.

In some communities a volunteer organization of professional photographers (e.g., Now I Lay Me Down to Sleep [www.nowilaymedowntosleep.org]) has a photographer on-call around the clock to take photographs of families and their deceased baby free of charge. Some institutions will take photos with a digital camera and give families the camera's memory card containing their baby's photos for downloading when the parents are ready.

Nurses should be aware of the risk of family members and friends using social media such as Instagram, Twitter, and Facebook to post photos and videos of this intimate family event. A frank talk with the family about ownership of this occasion may help forestall this behavior.

Addressing Cultural and Spiritual Needs of Parents

Parents who experience perinatal loss can be from widely diverse cultural, ethnic, and spiritual groups. Many of the emotional responses and suggested interventions in this chapter are based on middle-class Euro-American views. Although there are likely no particular differences in the individual, intrapersonal experiences of grief based on culture, ethnicity, or religion, there are complex differences in the meaning of children and parenthood, the role of women and men, the beliefs and knowledge about modern medicine, views about death, mourning rituals and traditions, and behavioral expressions of grief. Thus the nurse must be sensitive to the responses and needs of parents from various cultural backgrounds and religious groups. To do this the nurse needs to be aware of his or her own values and beliefs and acknowledge the importance of understanding and accepting the values and beliefs of others who are different or even in conflict. Furthermore, it is critical to understand that the individual and unique responses of a parent to a perinatal loss cannot be entirely predicted by his or her cultural or spiritual backgrounds. The nurse approaches each partner as an individual needing support during a profoundly difficult and distressing life experience.

It would be impossible to address all of the specific differences and needs of parents from diverse cultural and religious groups because of the complexity of this task and the lack of adequate research in this area of practice. Instead, some key concepts are presented and a few examples of areas of particular concern are given. The cultural meaning of children has a strong effect on the response of parents, extended family, and the community when an infant dies or is stillborn. Cultural and religious beliefs often affect decision making surrounding stillbirth or death of an infant. For example, death of an infant or having a stillborn infant profoundly affects the foundations of a Jewish family and involves many specific cultural and religious traditions, such as naming of the baby, burial, and mourning rituals. Muslim women may turn to their husbands or family members as the main decision-makers and appreciate being reminded by their husbands, family, or close friends that their loss was a test from God (Sutan & Miskam, 2012). Some religious groups do not allow autopsies and cremation except under unusual circumstances, whereas making a decision to end life-sustaining measures is less acceptable for some cultural and ethnic groups. Photographs can conflict with beliefs of some cultures, such as among some Native Americans, Inuit, Amish, Hindus, and Muslims. Families from these cultures should be offered this opportunity sensitively, but there should be no insistence on photography. In many cultures, decisions do not reside solely with the individual woman or couple but with the extended family. In Hispanic families, the concept of *la familia* is critical. Family decisions are often made together and communicated through someone appointed by the family rather than the parents.

Culture and religious beliefs also influence the customs following death. Many religious groups have rituals that are performed at the time of death. They include prayers, ritualistic washing and shrouding, or anointing with oil. Nurses should ask parents about their needs as they relate to rituals at the time of and following death. For example, baptism is extremely important for Roman Catholics and some, but not all, Protestant groups. Baptism can be performed by a layperson such as a nurse in an emergency situation when a priest or other ordained clergy cannot arrive before the death of a live born infant. The nurse should inquire about parental beliefs and preferences related to infant baptism. The nurse can offer to contact the hospital chaplain or the family's own clergy who can help sort out theological questions related to rituals of faith.

Providing Sensitive Discharge and Follow-Up Care

When leaving the hospital, women are often transported from the nursing unit to their vehicle in a wheelchair. This can be very upsetting for the woman who has experienced a pregnancy loss. It is especially difficult if other women are seen leaving with babies; thus the timing of discharge of women who have experienced a perinatal loss should be done with great sensitivity. They should not be discharged at a time when other mothers with live babies are leaving. Some institutions give the bereaved mother some token of remembrance such as a teddy bear or a flower to carry as they leave.

The grief of the mother and her family does not end with discharge; rather it begins anew once they return home, attend the funeral, and continue their lives without a new baby. There are numerous models for providing follow-up care to parents after discharge, and, although there is no solid evidence from sound clinical trials regarding the benefit of these programs, nonexperimental studies and clinical evaluations suggest these programs are helpful. Programs include hospital-based bereavement teams who provide support during hospitalization and follow-up contacts. Follow-up phone calls after a loss are helpful to some but not all parents. The calls are made at times that are known to be difficult for bereaved persons such as the first week at home, 1 month to 6 weeks later, 4 to 6 months after the loss, and at the anniversary of the death. Families who experienced a miscarriage, ectopic pregnancy, or death of a preterm baby may appreciate a phone call on the estimated date of birth. The calls provide an opportunity for parents to ask questions, share their feelings, seek advice, and receive information to help them in processing their grief.

A grief conference can be planned when parents return for an appointment with their physician or midwife, nurses, and other members of the health care team. At the conference, the loss or death of the infant is discussed in detail, parents are given information about the baby's autopsy report and genetic studies, and they have opportunities to ask the questions that have arisen since their baby's death. Parents appreciate the opportunity to review the events of hospitalization, go over the baby's and mother's chart with their primary health care provider, and talk with those who cared for them and their baby while they were in the hospital or birthing facility. This is an important time to help parents understand the cause of the loss or to accept the fact that the cause will forever be unknown. This gives health care professionals the opportunity to assess how the family is coping with their loss and provide additional information and education on grief.

Some persons are very interested in finding a perinatal or parent grief support group. Talking with others who have been through similar experiences, sharing memories of the pregnancy and the baby, and gaining an understanding of the normality of the grief process can be very helpful. Over time it is possibly the only place where bereaved parents can talk about the wished-for child and their grief. However, not all parents find such groups helpful.

When referring to a group, it is important to know something about the group and how it operates. For example, if a group has a religious base for their interventions, a nonreligious parent would not likely find the group to be helpful. If parents experiencing a perinatal loss are referred to a general parental grief group, they might feel overwhelmed with the grief of parents whose older children have died of cancer, suicide, or homicide. In addition, other parents whose older children have died may inadvertently minimize the grief of parents following a perinatal loss. Thus the focus of the group needs to match the parents' needs.

Providing Postmortem Care

Preparing the baby's body and transporting it to the morgue depend on the procedures and protocols developed by individual hospitals. The Joint Commission (www.jointcommission.org) requires that appropriate care be offered to the body after death. A sensitive and respectful approach for taking the fetus or infant to the morgue is the use of a burial cradle, which makes the process more dignified for parents and the nursing staff. A burial cradle is a miniature casket usually made of Styrofoam or wood (Fig. 37.5).

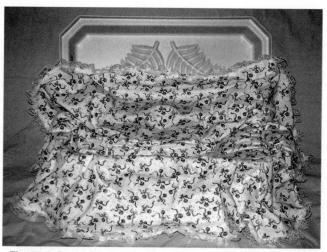

Fig. 37.5 Burial Cradle. (Courtesy Shannon Perry, Phoenix, AZ.)

Postmortem care can be an emotional and sometimes difficult task for the nurse. However, nurses can find that providing postmortem care helps them in their own grief related to a perinatal loss. This is particularly true for NICU nurses who have cared for an infant for several hours, days, or weeks.

> **! NURSING ALERT**
>
> An important caveat is needed for nurses providing care for newborns who are thought to be deceased: dying neonates may respond reflexively to the stimulation of cleaning and preparing for the morgue and sometimes will do this for several hours after being pronounced dead. This is extremely startling and upsetting when a baby who has been pronounced dead takes an agonal respiration or an extremity twitches. If this happens, the nurse should notify a physician for confirmation of death.

SPECIAL CIRCUMSTANCES

Prenatal Diagnoses With Poor Prognoses

Early prenatal diagnostic tests such as ultrasonography, chorionic villus sampling, and amniocentesis can determine the well-being of the embryo or fetus (see Chapter 26). Reasons for prenatal testing include history of chromosomal abnormality in the family; three or more miscarriages; maternal age over 35 years; lack of fetal growth, movement, or heartbeat; and diabetes, hypertension, lupus, sickle cell disease, or other chronic illnesses. If the health care provider is certain that the baby has a serious genetic defect that will lead to death in utero or after birth (congenital anomalies incompatible with life or genetic disorders with severe intellectual disability), the choice of interruption of a pregnancy via dilation and evacuation or induction of labor can be offered.

Foreknowledge of a congenital diagnosis in conjunction with the possibility of suffering by the baby can intensify parental grief. The decision to terminate a pregnancy is difficult and can lead to feelings such as guilt, despair, sadness, depression, and anger. The woman who decides to continue the pregnancy needs intensive support from the nursing staff. The time of labor and birth can be particularly difficult. The nurse should remember that expectant parents may be grieving for not only the loss of the "perfect child" but also loss of expectations for their child's future. Thus a nurse should assess how these parents feel about the experience, offer options for their memories as appropriate, and be a support person and good listener. Healing can be facilitated when words can be given to feelings. Perinatal palliative care or hospice care for parents experiencing prenatal diagnoses of lethal birth defects can be effective in helping families both before and after their loss (Carter, 2016; Limbo, et al., 2017). Perinatal palliative care, described in detail earlier, does not have to be a formal program, although many do exist. It is the provision of care for families as they plan for the birth and probable death of their baby and involves support, information, and resources. If the newborn infant lives to go home with his or her mother, pediatric palliative or hospice care may be needed from community EOL care agencies.

Death of a Fetus in a Multiple Gestation

The death of a fetus in a multifetal gestation during pregnancy, labor, birth, or after birth requires the mother and partner to both parent their live-born infant and grieve their dead or dying one at the same time. Such a death imposes a confusing and ambivalent transition into parenthood. They can experience difficulty parenting their surviving child with all the joy and enthusiasm of new parents because their surviving child reminds them of what they have lost. Yet they can also have difficulty fully grieving their loss because their surviving child demands their attention. These parents can be at risk for altered parenting and complicated bereavement.

It is important to help the parents acknowledge the birth of all their babies, although one or more may be stillborn. The nurse should plan the care of these families as they do all bereaved families, offering all the options previously noted. With the parents' consent, photographs should be taken of the babies and parents should be offered the opportunity to hold their babies and have time to say goodbye to the baby who has died.

It is helpful to alert bereaved parents that well-meaning family members or friends may say, "At least you have the other baby," implying that there should be no grief because they are lucky to have one living baby. Parents can anticipate insensitivity to their loss and may find it helpful to respond, "That is not how I feel." By simply setting a boundary on what their feelings are, they are able to acknowledge the baby who died and then have an opportunity to share more about their feelings if they so choose. When there is a loss of one or more babies in a multiple gestation, bereaved parents face specific issues in telling their surviving child about his or her twin, dealing with the possibility of that child's feelings of survivor guilt, and deciding on how to celebrate birthdays, special holidays, or anniversaries of the baby's death.

Adolescent Grief

Adolescents grieve the loss that occurs with miscarriage, stillbirth, or newborn death and have significant emotional, social, and cognitive responses that can differ from those of older women. Teens need a great deal of emotional support from the nurses who care for them. Adolescent pregnancy is often unplanned and in itself poses a developmental and situational crisis; despite the challenges pregnancy poses, the loss of a pregnancy for adolescents puts them at risk for both mental health problems, including depression, and becoming pregnant again quickly (Wheeler & Sefton, 2016).

Nurses and other health care professionals, as well as family members, may believe that the adolescent's loss of her baby, although sad, may open the opportunity for the young woman to complete her education and experience life without the demands of motherhood. Adolescent girls, then, may not receive the support they need from staff and family. In addition, adolescent girls sometimes do not have the support from the father of the baby that older women may have; thus there is a great need to provide sensitive care to all adolescents who experience any type of perinatal loss.

The first step for the nurse in caring for a bereaved adolescent is to develop a trusting relationship with her. Second, the nurse should acknowledge the significance of the loss, regardless of the mother's age. Third, as in the care of older women experiencing a perinatal loss, the nurse should provide anticipatory guidance, nonjudgmental support and information to meet the adolescent at the point of her need. Adolescents will process their grief differently from mature adults because of their lack of cognitive and emotional maturity, although this varies. Moreover, adolescents are often highly involved with their friends, who may lack maturity and perspective on the loss but at the same time are good sources of social support by simply being present. Encouraging the bereaved teen to seek out support from her friends can be very helpful. Being patient, saving mementos, and giving the adolescent information on how to contact the nurse are interventions that can help the adolescent accept the loss and work through her grief and sadness.

Complicated Grief

Although most parents cope adequately with the pain of their grief and return to some level of their usual functioning, some have extremely intense grief reactions that are prolonged and are characterized by sustained intense longing and persistent sadness that interferes with daily life; this response is complicated grief (Wright, 2016). Complicated grief can result when there is sudden or traumatic loss, as occurs with stillbirth or termination of pregnancy due to lethal fetal anomalies. Complicated grief differs from what is considered normal grief in its duration and the degree to which behavior and emotional state are affected. Risk factors for complicated grief include poor social support and history of mental health problems. In addition to prolonged and sustained longing and sadness, evidence of complicated grief may include inability to trust others, anger, difficulty moving on with one's life, feeling that life is empty or meaningless, hopelessness, loneliness, intense and continued guilt, and depression or anxiety interfering with daily functioning. Complicated grief can lead to abuse of drugs (including prescription medications) or alcohol, severe relationship difficulties, high levels of depressive symptoms, low self-esteem, feelings of inadequacy, and suicidal thoughts or threats years after the loss. Some persons grieving a perinatal loss may develop posttraumatic stress disorder, the symptoms of which include reliving the trauma, avoiding things and places that are reminders, intrusive thoughts about their baby who has died, disturbed sleep, and even hallucinations (Wright).

Persons showing signs of complicated grief or posttraumatic stress should be referred for counseling. Mental health professionals are qualified to determine whether individuals are experiencing a normal, albeit intense grief response, or whether they are also having a serious mental health problem such as depression. When referring a person struggling with the emotional aftermath of a loss, the referral should be made to a mental health professional with experience in grief responses and counseling. Making an appointment for counseling or therapy can be a difficult but important first step for persons struggling with emotional issues. Because cancellations and missed visits often occur on the first visit, anything the nurse can do for a family or individual to help them take this step is important. However, it also is important to remember that people can have symptoms but may not, for whatever reason, be ready to deal directly with these symptoms or may not have the energy to make the call. Enlisting a family member to encourage parents to seek such assistance can be helpful.

Posttraumatic Growth

Nurse researchers have noted that women and their partners can experience personal growth in the aftermath of a perinatal loss (Black & Sandelowski, 2010). Known as *posttraumatic growth* (PTG), this phenomenon is characterized by development along one or more of five dimensions: personal strength, appreciation for life, spirituality, relating to others, and new possibilities (Tedeschi & Calhoun, 1996, 2004, 2008). Growth can coexist with grief. In witnessing the grief of women, their partners, and families in the aftermath of a perinatal loss,

nurses should acknowledge that persons in fact can and do grow after highly traumatic events. Nurses should be alert for signs of growth in bereaved individuals; for instance, when a woman comes in for a 6-week postpartum check, she may indicate that she and her partner are closer because of this loss or note that she is beginning to look at opportunities to go back to school or change jobs. These are not indications that the woman's grief has gone away but that she has experienced growth from the trauma of her loss. The nurse should affirm these developments with simple comments such as, "I'm glad for you."

■ KEY POINTS

- Attachment to the idea of a baby can begin before pregnancy with many hopes and dreams for the future and can become more pronounced over the course of pregnancy.
- Women can feel profound grief regardless of the length of gestation; however, women tend to have higher levels of grief with longer gestations.
- When a fetus or a newborn dies, all members of a family are affected, but no two family members grieve in the same way.
- When birth and death coexist, sensitive care by a nurse is critical in assisting the woman and her family in their grief, regardless of the woman's age or stage of gestation.
- An understanding of the grief process is fundamental to care management of families experiencing perinatal loss.

- Assessment of each family member's perception and experience of the loss is important.
- Cultural and religious beliefs affect a family's response to and coping with perinatal death.
- Therapeutic communication and active listening can help women and their partners and families identify their feelings, feel comfortable in expressing their grief, and understand their bereavement process.
- Follow-up after discharge is important in providing care to families who have experienced a loss because of the evolving nature of grief.
- Nurses need to be aware of their own feelings of grief and loss to provide a nonjudgmental environment of care and support for bereaved families.

REFERENCES

American College of Obstetricians and Gynecologists. (2017). Committee opinion no. 719: Multifetal pregnancy reduction. *Obstetrics & Gynecology*, *130*(3), e158–e163.

Avelin, P., Rådestad, I., Säflund, K., et al. (2013). Parental grief and relationships after the loss of a stillborn baby. *Midwifery*, *29*(9), 668–673.

Barfield, W. D., & Committee on Fetus and Newborn. (2011). Standard terminology for fetal, infant, and perinatal deaths. *Pediatrics*, *128*(1), 177–181.

Black, B. P., & Sandelowski, M. (2010). Personal growth after severe fetal diagnosis. *Western Journal of Nursing Research*, *38*(2), 1011–1030.

Boss, P. (2006). *Loss, trauma and resilience: Therapeutic work with ambiguous loss*. New York: W.W. Norton.

Breeze, A. C., Statham, H., Hackett, G. A., et al. (2012). Perinatal postmortems: What is important to parents and how do they decide. *Birth*, *39*(1), 57–64.

Carter, L. (2016). Understanding our role in bereavement. *International Journal of Childbirth Education*, *31*(4), 28–30.

Côté-Arsenault, D., & O'Leary, J. (2016). Understanding the experience of pregnancy subsequent to a perinatal loss. In B. P. Black, P. M. Wright, & R. Limbo (Eds.), *Perinatal and pediatric bereavement for nursing and other health professions*. New York: Springer.

Cowles, K., & Rodgers, B. (2000). The concept of grief: An evolutionary perspective. In B. Rodgers & K. Knafl (Eds.), *Concept development in nursing: Foundations, techniques, and applications* (2nd ed.). Philadelphia: Saunders.

Davidson, D., & Letherby, G. (2014). Griefwork online: Perinatal loss, life-course disruption and online support. *Human Fertility*, *17*(3), 214–217.

Doka, K. J. (1989). Disenfranchised loss. In K. J. Doka (Ed.), *Disenfranchised grief: Recognizing hidden sorrow*. Lanham, MD: Lexington Books.

Due, C., Chiarolli, S., & Riggs, D. W. (2017). The impact of pregnancy loss on men's health and wellbeing: A systematic review. *BMC Pregnancy Childbirth*, *17*(1), 1–13.

Elmir, R., Pangas, J., Dahlen, H. S., et al. (2017). A meta-ethnographic synthesis of midwives' and nurses' experiences of adverse labour and birth events. *Journal of Clinical Nursing*, *26*(23-24), 4182–4200.

Fenstermacher, K., & Hupcey, J. E. (2013). Perinatal bereavement: A principle-based concept analysis. *Journal of Advanced Nursing*, *69*(11), 2389–2400.

Gear, R. (2014). Bereaved parents' perspectives on informal social support: "What worked for you?" *Journal of Loss and Trauma*, *19*(2), 173–188.

Golan, A., & Leichtentritt, R. D. (2016). Meaning reconstruction among women following stillbirth: A loss fraught with ambiguity and doubt. *Health & Social Work*, *41*(3), 147–154.

Kidszun, A., Linebarger, J., Walter, J. K., et al. (2016). What if the perinatal diagnosis of a lethal anomaly turns out to be wrong? *Pediatrics*, *137*(5), e20154514.

Klass, D., Silverman, P. R., & Nickman, S. L. (1996). *Continuing bonds: New understandings of grief*. Philadelphia: Taylor & Francis.

Kübler-Ross, E. (1969). *On death and dying*. New York: Scribner.

Limbo, R., Brandon, D., Côté-Arsenault, D., et al. (2017). Perinatal palliative care as an essential element of childbearing choices. *Nursing Outlook*, *65*(1), 123–125.

Limbo, R., & Kobler, K. (2016). Moments matter: Exploring the evidence of caring for grieving families and self. In B. P. Black, P. M. Wright, & R. Limbo (Eds.), *Perinatal and pediatric bereavement for nursing and other health professions*. New York: Springer.

Limbo, R., Kobler, K., & Levang, E. (2010). Respectful disposition in early pregnancy loss. *American Journal of Maternal/Child Nursing*, *35*(5), 271–277.

Miles, M. (1984). Helping adults mourn the death of a child. In H. Wass & C. Corr (Eds.), *Childhood and death*. New York: Hemisphere.

Murphy, S., & Cacciatore, J. (2017). The psychological, social, and economic impact of stillbirth on families. *Seminars in Fetal and Neonatal Medicine*, *22*(3), 129–134.

Perinatal Loss and Infant Death Alliance. (2005). *Position statement: Infection risks are insignificant*. Retrieved from PLIDA org/pdf/infectionRisks.pdf.

Sandelowski, M., & Barroso, J. (2005). The travesty of choosing after positive prenatal diagnosis. *Journal of Obstetric, Gynecologic and Neonatal Nursing*, *34*(3), 307–318.

Siassakos, D., Jackson, S., Gleeson, K., et al. (2018). All bereaved parents are entitled to good care after stillbirth: A mixed-methods multicenter study (INSIGHT). *BJOG: An International Journal of Obstetrics and Gynaecology, 125*(2), 160–170.

Stroebe, M., Finkenhauer, C., Wijngaards-de Meij, L., et al. (2013). Partner-oriented self-regulation among bereaved parents: The costs of holding in grief for the partner's sake. *Psychological Science, 24*(4), 395–402.

Stroebe, M., & Schut, H. (1999). The dual process model of coping with bereavement: Rationale and description. *Death Studies, 23*(3), 197–224.

Swanson, K., Chen, H., Graham, J., et al. (2009). Resolution of depression and grief during the first year after miscarriage: A randomized controlled clinical trial of couples-focused interventions. *Journal of Women's Health, 18*(8), 1245–1257.

Tedeschi, R. G., & Calhoun, L. G. (1996). The posttraumatic growth inventory: Measuring the positive legacy of trauma. *Journal of Traumatic Stress, 9*(3), 455–471.

Tedeschi, R. G., & Calhoun, L. G. (2004). Posttraumatic growth: Conceptual foundations and empirical evidence. *Psychological Inquiry, 15*(1), 1–18.

Tedeschi, R. G., & Calhoun, L. G. (2008). Beyond the concept of recovery: Growth and the experience of loss. *Death Studies, 32*(1), 27–39.

Wheeler, S. R., & Sefton, M. G. (2016). Early pregnancy loss during adolescence. In B. P. Black, P. M. Wright, & R. Limbo (Eds.), *Perinatal and pediatric bereavement for nursing and other health professions*. New York: Springer.

Wojnar, D. (2016). Lesbians, parenthood and reproductive loss. In B. P. Black, P. M. Wright, & R. Limbo (Eds.), *Perinatal and pediatric bereavement for nursing and other health professions*. New York: Springer.

Wool, C. (2013). Clinician confidence and comfort in providing perinatal palliative care. *Journal of Obstetric, Gynecologic and Neonatal Nursing, 42*(1), 48–58.

Wright, P. M. (2016). Complicated grief and perinatal loss. In B. P. Black, P. M. Wright, & R. Limbo (Eds.), *Perinatal and pediatric bereavement for nursing and other health professions*. New York: Springer.

GLOSSARY

abdominal Belonging or relating to the abdomen and its functions and disorders.

ABO incompatibility Hemolytic disease that occurs when the mother's blood type is O and the newborn's is A, B, or AB.

abortion Termination of pregnancy before the fetus is viable and capable of extrauterine existence, usually less than 20 weeks of gestation (or when the fetus weighs less than 500 g).

abruptio placentae (placental abruption) Premature separation of the placenta; the detachment of part or all of a normally implanted placenta from the uterus before the birth of the infant.

acceleration Visually apparent abrupt (onset to peak less than 30 seconds) increase in fetal heart rate to greater than the baseline rate. The peak is at least 15 beats/minute greater than the baseline, and the acceleration lasts 15 seconds or more, with a return to baseline less than 2 minutes from the beginning of the acceleration.

acculturation Changes that occur within one group or among several groups when people from different cultures come into contact with each other.

acquaintance Process used by parents to get to know or become familiar with their new infant; an important step in attachment.

acrocyanosis Peripheral cyanosis; bluish discoloration of hands and feet in most newborns at birth that is a normal finding for the first 24 hours.

active phase of labor Phase in first stage of labor which begins at 6 cm and ends with complete cervical dilation at 10 cm.

active pushing (descent) phase of labor Period during second stage of labor when the woman has strong urges to bear down as the fetal presenting part presses on the pelvic floor.

acute bilirubin encephalopathy Acute manifestations of bilirubin toxicity that occur during the first weeks after birth; symptoms can include lethargy, hypotonia, irritability, seizures, coma, and death.

adjuvant chemotherapy Chemotherapy administered soon after surgical removal of a tumor.

afterbirth pains See afterpains.

afterpains Uncomfortable uterine cramping that occurs intermittently for approximately 3 to 7 days after birth and that result from contractile efforts of the uterus to return to its normal involuted condition. Also called afterbirth pains.

agonist An agent that activates or stimulates a receptor to act.

alcohol-related birth defects (ARBDs) Congenital abnormalities that occur in infants with known prenatal alcohol exposure; most often ARBDs include cardiac, renal, and orthopedic abnormalities and anomalies of the eyes and ears but can also include cognitive and behavioral problems.

alcohol-related neurodevelopmental disorders (ARNDs) Refers to infants or children with confirmed prenatal alcohol exposure who lack facial features or growth deficits associated with fetal alcohol syndrome, yet they have structural central nervous system and cognitive abnormalities.

α-fetoprotein (AFP) Fetal antigen; elevated levels in amniotic fluid are associated with neural tube and open abdominal wall defects.

ambiguous loss Occurs when the object of grief is missing and includes intangible losses; for example, miscarriage and the associated losses of being pregnant, a hoped-for baby, and a future with the child.

amenorrhea Absence or suppression of menstruation or menstrual flow.

amniocentesis Procedure in which a needle is inserted through the abdominal and uterine walls under ultrasound guidance into the amniotic fluid; some fluid is withdrawn; used for assessment of fetal health and maturity.

amnioinfusion Infusion of room-temperature isotonic fluid (usually normal saline or lactated Ringer solution) into the uterine cavity if the volume of amniotic fluid is low, in an attempt to increase the fluid around the umbilical cord and prevent compression during uterine contractions.

amnion Inner membrane of two fetal membranes; accommodates the embryo/fetus and the surrounding amniotic fluid.

amniotic Pertaining or relating to the amnion.

amniotic fluid Fluid surrounding the fetus derived primarily from maternal serum and fetal urine.

amniotic fluid embolus (AFE) Rare but devastating complication of pregnancy characterized by the sudden, acute onset of hypoxia, hypotension, cardiovascular collapse, and coagulopathy. AFE usually occurs during labor, during birth, or within 30 minutes after birth. Also known as anaphylactoid syndrome of pregnancy.

amniotic fluid index (AFI) Evaluation of the total amount of amniotic fluid by measuring the vertical depths (in centimeters) of the largest pocket of amniotic fluid in all four quadrants surrounding the maternal umbilicus. A normal AFI is greater than 5 but less than 25 cm.

amniotomy Artificial rupture of the membranes, using a plastic amnihook or a surgical clamp.

analgesia Alleviating the sensation of pain or raising the threshold for pain perception without loss of consciousness.

anaphylactoid syndrome of pregnancy See amniotic fluid embolus (AFE).

anencephaly Congenital deformity characterized by the absence of both cerebral hemispheres (cerebrum and cerebellum) and the flat bones of the overlying skull.

anesthesia Encompasses analgesia, amnesia, relaxation, and reflex activity. Anesthesia abolishes pain perception by interrupting the nerve impulses to the brain. The loss of sensation may be partial or complete, sometimes with the loss of consciousness.

aneuploidy One of the two types of deviations from the correct number of chromosomes per cell, in which the numeric deviation is not an exact multiple of the haploid set. Having an abnormal number of chromosomes.

antagonist An agent that blocks a receptor or a medication designed to activate a receptor.

antenatal glucocorticoids Medications administered to the pregnant woman for the purpose of accelerating fetal lung maturity when an increased risk exists for preterm birth between 24 and 34 weeks of gestation.

anthropometric measurements Body measurements, such as height and weight.

anxiety disorders Mood disorders characterized by prominent symptoms that impair functioning. Examples are obsessive-compulsive disorder, posttraumatic stress disorder, generalized anxiety disorder, panic disorder, agoraphobia, and other phobias.

ARNDs See alcohol-related neurodevelopmental disorders (ARNDs).

appropriate for gestational age An infant whose birth weight falls between the 10th and 90th percentile on intrauterine growth curves.

APGAR score Numeric expression of the condition of a newborn obtained by rapid assessment at 1 and 5 minutes of age; developed by Dr. Virginia Apgar.

ARTs See assisted reproductive therapies (ARTs).

asphyxia Term used when fetal hypoxia results in metabolic acidosis.

assimilation Occurs when a cultural group loses its identity and becomes part of the dominant culture.

assisted reproductive technologies (ARTs) Treatments for infertility, including but not limited to in vitro fertilization procedures, embryo adoption, embryo hosting, and therapeutic insemination.

asymptomatic bacteriuria Persistent presence of bacteria within the urinary tract of women who have no symptom of infection. A clean-voided urine specimen containing more than 100,000 organisms per milliliter is diagnostic.

atony Absence of muscle tone. See also uterine atony.

attachment (1) The process by which a parent comes to love and accept a child and a child comes to love and accept a parent. (2) A specific and enduring affective tie to another person.

attitude The relation of the fetal body parts to one another. Normally the back of the fetus is rounded so that the chin is flexed on the chest, the thighs are flexed on the abdomen, the legs are flexed at the knees, and the arms are crossed over the thorax. This attitude is called general flexion.

augmentation of labor Stimulation of ineffective uterine contractions after labor has started spontaneously but is not progressing satisfactorily.

autolysis "Self-digestive" process by which the uterus returns to a nonpregnant state after birth. The decrease in estrogen and progesterone levels after birth results in this destruction of excess hypertrophied uterine tissue.

autosomal dominant inheritance disorder Condition in which only one copy of a variant allele is needed for phenotypic expression.

autosomal recessive inheritance disorder Condition in which both genes of a pair are forms associated with the disorder to be expressed.

autosomes Any of the paired chromosomes other than the sex (X and Y) chromosomes.

B

baby blues See postpartum blues.

balanced translocation Translocation in which parts of the two chromosomes are exchanged equally. The individual is phenotypically normal because there is no extra chromosome material; it is just rearranged.

ballottement (1) Movability of a floating object, such as a fetus. (2) Diagnostic technique using palpation: floating object, when tapped or pushed, moves away and then returns to touch the examiner's hand. (3) Passive movement of the unengaged fetus.

Bartholin cyst Most common benign lesion of the vulva; arises from obstruction of the Bartholin duct, which causes it to enlarge.

basalis, decidua See decidua basalis.

baseline fetal heart rate See fetal heart rate (FHR), baseline.

Bell palsy Acute idiopathic facial paralysis. The cause is unknown, but it may be related to the reactivation of herpes virus infection or acute human immunodeficiency virus type 1 retroviral infection. Bell palsy occurs fairly often, especially in women of reproductive age. Pregnant women are affected four times more often than nonpregnant women.

bereavement The state of being without a valued other, especially by death; characterized by the emotional state of grief.

biophysical profile (BPP) Noninvasive assessment of a fetus using ultrasound and the nonstress test. It includes the following components: fetal breathing movements, gross body movements, fetal tone, reactive fetal heart rate, and qualitative amniotic fluid volume.

biopsy Removal of a small piece of tissue for microscopic examination and diagnosis.

biorhythmicity Cyclic changes that occur with established regularity, such as sleeping and eating patterns.

biparietal diameter Largest transverse diameter of the fetal head; extends from one parietal bone to the other.

bipolar disorder Mood disorder defined by the presence of one or more episodes of abnormally elevated energy levels, cognition, and mood and one or more depressive episodes. Also called manic-depressive disorder. Postpartum psychosis is most commonly associated with a diagnosis of bipolar disorder. (See postpartum psychosis.)

birth control The device and/or practice used to decrease the risk of conceiving or bearing offspring. Also known as contraception.

birth injury See birth trauma.

birth plan A tool by which parents can explore their birth options and choose those that are most important to them.

birth rate Number of live births per 1000 population per year.

birth trauma Physical injury sustained by a neonate during labor and birth. Also called birth injury.

Bishop score Rating system to evaluate inducibility of the cervix; a higher score increases the rate of successful induction of labor.

blastocyst Stage in the development of a mammalian embryo, occurring after the morula stage, that consists of an outer layer, or trophoblast, and a hollow sphere of cells enclosing a cavity.

bloody show Vaginal discharge that originates in the cervix and consists of blood and mucus; increases as cervix dilates during labor.

BMI See body mass index (BMI).

body mass index (BMI) Method of calculating appropriateness of weight for height (BMI = weight [kilograms]/height^2 [meters]).

BPD See bronchopulmonary dysplasia (BPD).

brachial plexus injury Paralysis caused by physical injury to the upper brachial plexus of the newborn, resulting from difficult birth (e.g., shoulder dystocia).

bradycardia Baseline fetal heart rate of fewer than 110 beats/min for 10 minutes or longer. True bradycardia occurs rarely and is not specifically related to fetal oxygenation.

Braxton Hicks contractions Mild, intermittent, painless uterine contractions that occur during pregnancy. These contractions occur more frequently as pregnancy advances but do not represent true labor.

breast milk jaundice Also called late-onset jaundice; hyperbilirubinemia that occurs between days 5 and 10 of life, usually in a healthy, breastfed infant; may be related to factors in breastmilk that inhibit or decrease bilirubin excretion.

breast self-examination (BSE) Self-palpation of breasts to detect for changes in breast tissue.

breastfeeding-associated jaundice Also called early-onset jaundice; hyperbilirubinemia that begins at 2 to 5 days of life; associated with insufficient breastfeeding and infrequent stooling.

bronchopulmonary dysplasia (BPD) Chronic pulmonary condition most often affecting preterm infants requiring mechanical ventilation; usually requires oxygen therapy at home.

brown fat Source of heat unique to neonates that is capable of greater thermogenic activity than ordinary fat. Deposits are found around the adrenals, kidneys, and neck; between the scapulas; and behind the sternum for several weeks after birth.

C

café-au-lait Patches of skin pigmentation present in neurofibromatosis.

cancer of the cervix See cervical cancer.

caput Occiput of fetal head appearing at the vaginal introitus preceding birth of the head.

caput succedaneum Swelling of the tissue over the presenting part of the fetal head caused by pressure during labor.

carcinoma in situ (CIS) Diagnosed when the full thickness of epithelium is replaced with abnormal cells.

carpal tunnel syndrome Pressure on the median nerve at the point at which it goes through the carpal tunnel of the wrist. It causes soreness, tenderness, and weakness of the muscles of the thumb. Edema involving the peripheral nerves may result in carpal tunnel syndrome during the last trimester of pregnancy.

carrier Individual who carries a gene that does not exhibit itself in physical or chemical characteristics but that can be transmitted to offspring (e.g., a female carrying the trait for hemophilia, which is expressed in male offspring). Heterozygous individuals have only one variant allele and are unaffected clinically because their normal gene (wild-type allele) overshadows the variant allele. They are known as carriers of the recessive trait.

cell-free deoxyribonucleic acid (DNA) screening Screening method to detect the chromosomal abnormalities trisomy 21, 13, and 18. It also provides noninvasive prenatal genetic diagnosis of fetal Rh status, fetal gender, and certain paternally transmitted single gene disorders.

cephalhematoma NOTE: This is spelled cephalohematoma in some sources. Extravasation of blood from ruptured vessels between a skull bone and its external covering, the periosteum. Swelling is limited by the margins of the cranial bone affected (usually parietals).

cephalocaudal Head to rump.

cephalopelvic disproportion (CPD) Condition in which the fetal head is of such a shape, size, or position that it cannot pass through the mother's pelvis; can also be caused by maternal pelvic problems. Also called fetopelvic disproportion.

cerclage Use of nonabsorbable suture to constrict the internal os of a cervix that is dilating prematurely because of cervical weakness. The suture can be placed vaginally or abdominally. A cerclage can be placed either prophylactically or as a rescue procedure.

cervical cancer The third most common reproductive cancer; begins as neoplastic changes in the cervical epithelium. Also called cancer of the cervix.

cervical conization Excision of a cone-shaped section of tissue from the endocervix.

cervical insufficiency Passive and painless dilation of the cervix leading to recurrent preterm births during the second trimester in the absence of other causes. Measurement of cervical length has been used as a way to diagnose cervical insufficiency.

cervical intraepithelial neoplasia (CIN) Uncontrolled and progressive abnormal growth of cervical epithelial cells; preinvasive lesions.

cesarean birth Birth of a fetus by an incision through the abdominal wall and uterus. See also elective cesarean birth.

Chadwick sign Violet-blue color of the vaginal mucosa and cervix that is visible at approximately 6 to 8 weeks of pregnancy; caused by increased vascularity.

choanal atresia Complete obstruction of the posterior nares, which open into the nasopharynx, with membranous or bony tissue.

chorioamnionitis Bacterial infection of the amniotic cavity; usually diagnosed by the clinical findings of maternal fever, maternal and fetal tachycardia, uterine tenderness, and foul odor of amniotic fluid. Other terms for this condition include clinical chorioamnionitis, amnionitis, intrapartum infection, amniotic fluid infection, and intraamniotic infection.

chorion Fetal membrane closest to the intrauterine wall that gives rise to the placenta and continues as the outer membrane surrounding the amnion.

chorionic villi Tiny vascular protrusions on the chorionic surface that project into the maternal blood sinuses of the uterus and that help form the placenta and secrete human chorionic gonadotropin.

chorionic villus sampling (CVS) Removal of fetal tissue from the placenta for genetic diagnostic studies, which can be performed during either the first or second trimester. When performed after the first trimester, the procedure is better known as late CVS or placental biopsy.

chronic hypertension Hypertension that is present before pregnancy or that is initially diagnosed during pregnancy and persists longer than 12 weeks postpartum.

chronic hypertension with superimposed preeclampsia Condition that usually presents as elevated blood pressures in a woman whose blood pressure previously has been well controlled. Superimposed preeclampsia also may be diagnosed by the development of severe features of preeclampsia such as thrombocytopenia, impaired liver function, the new development of renal insufficiency, pulmonary edema, or new-onset cerebral or visual disturbances.

CIN See cervical intraepithelial neoplasia (CIN).

circumcision Removal of all or part of the foreskin (prepuce) of the penis.

CIS See carcinoma in situ (CIS).

claiming process Process by which the parents identify their new baby in terms of likeness to other family members, differences, and uniqueness; the unique newcomer is thus incorporated into the family.

cleft lip Orofacial cleft; most often it is unilateral but can be bilateral; ranges from a simple notch in the lip to complete separation of the lip extending to the floor of the nose.

cleft palate Orofacial cleft; incomplete closure of the palate or roof of mouth; a congenital fissure ranging from a bifid uvula to complete cleft extending from the soft to hard palate.

climacteric The period of a woman's life when she is passing from a reproductive to a nonreproductive state, with regression of ovarian function. The cycle of endocrine, physical, and psychosocial changes that occurs during the termination of the reproductive years. Also called climacterium.

clonus Hyperactive reflexes.

clubfoot Congenital deformity of the foot and ankle, also known as talipes equinovarus.

Cochrane Pregnancy and Childbirth Database Database of up-to-date systematic reviews and dissemination of views of randomized controlled trials of health care.

cohabiting-parent family Family form in which children live with two unmarried biologic parents or two adoptive parents.

cold stress Excessive loss of heat that results in increased respirations and nonshivering thermogenesis to maintain core body temperature; if not corrected, can lead to anaerobic glycolysis and metabolic acidosis.

colostrum The yellowish premilk fluid secreted by the breasts during the second trimester of pregnancy; the fluid in the breast from pregnancy into the early postpartal period. It is more concentrated than mature milk and is extremely rich in immunoglobulins; it has higher concentrations of protein and minerals but less fat than mature milk; it is also rich in antibodies, which provide protection from many diseases; high in protein, which binds bilirubin; and laxative acting, which speeds the elimination of meconium and helps loosen mucus.

colposcopy Examination of vagina and cervix with a colposcope (a stereoscopic binocular microscope that magnifies the view of the cervix) to identify neoplastic or other changes.

combined spinal-epidural (CSE) analgesia An epidural needle is inserted into the epidural space. Before the epidural catheter is threaded, a smaller-gauge spinal needle is inserted through the bore of the epidural needle into the subarachnoid space and a small amount of an opioid or a combination of an opioid and a local anesthetic is injected to rapidly provide analgesia. Afterward, the epidural catheter is inserted as usual. If pain relief is still needed after the effect of the medication injected into the subarachnoid space wears off, additional medication can be injected through the epidural catheter.

complicated bereavement See complicated grief.

complicated grief A complex situation in which grief may not resolve over time and the bereaved person grieves chronically; may be characterized by numerous distressful chronic signs and symptoms, including strong preoccupation, yearning and longing for the deceased, intrusive thoughts, sleep disturbances, etc.

conception Union of the sperm and a single egg (ovum) resulting in fertilization; formation of the one-celled zygote marks the beginning of a pregnancy.

congenital anomaly A defect that is present at birth and can be caused by genetic or environmental factors, or both; defined as a physical, metabolic, anatomic, or behavioral deviation from the normal pattern of development.

congenital diaphragmatic hernia Diaphragm malformation that allows displacement of the abdominal organs into the thoracic cavity.

congenital hypothyroidism Condition that affects infants from birth; partial or complete loss of thyroid gland function causing deficiency of thyroid hormones; can be permanent (requires treatment for life) or transient (spontaneously resolves).

congenital rubella syndrome Complex of problems, including hearing defects, cardiovascular abnormalities, and cataracts, caused by maternal rubella in the first trimester of pregnancy.

conization See cervical conization.

conjoined twins Twins who are physically united; Siamese twins.

continuing bonds theory An established theory of grief and bereavement; bonds of attachment forged in life continue into the survivors' future.

continuous positive airway pressure (CPAP) Method of infusing oxygen or air under a preset pressure by means of nasal prongs, a face mask, or an endotracheal tube.

contraception Intentional prevention of pregnancy (impregnation or conception) during sexual intercourse.

contraction stress test (CST) Test to stimulate uterine contractions for the purpose of assessing fetal response to stress; it identifies a fetus that is stable at rest but shows evidence of compromise after stress. This test is also known as the oxytocin challenge test.

Coombs test Indirect: determination of Rh-positive antibodies in maternal blood. Direct: determination of maternal Rh-positive antibodies in fetal cord blood. A positive test result indicates the presence of antibodies or titer.

cordocentesis See percutaneous umbilical blood sampling (PUBS).

corpus luteum cysts Occur after ovulation and are possibly caused by an increased secretion of progesterone that results in an increase of fluid in the corpus luteum.

corrected age Determined by adding the gestational age and the postnatal age of the preterm infant. Used when determining expectations for development.

counterpressure Pressure to the sacral area of the back during uterine contractions.

couplet care Care provided by one nurse, educated in both mother and infant care, who functions as the primary nurse for mother and infant. Also called mother-baby care or single-room maternity care.

couvade syndrome The phenomenon of expectant fathers' experiencing pregnancy-like symptoms.

couvelaire uterus Associated with placental abruption; occurs when blood accumulates between the separated placenta and the uterine wall. The uterus appears purple or blue rather than its usual "bubblegum pink" color, and contractility is lost.

CPAP See continuous positive airway pressure (CPAP).

crowning Occurs during the second stage of labor, when the top of the fetal head can be seen at the vaginal orifice as the widest part of the head distends the vulva.

cultural competence Awareness, acceptance, and knowledge of cultural differences and adaptation of services to acknowledge and support the client's culture.

cultural prescriptions Practices that are expected or acceptable.

cultural proscriptions Practices that are forbidden or taboo.

cultural relativism Learning about and applying the standards of another's culture to activities within that culture.

cystocele Bladder hernia; injury to the vesicovaginal fascia during labor and birth may allow herniation of the bladder into the vagina. Protrusion of the bladder downward into the vagina; develops when supporting structures in the vesicovaginal septum are injured.

D

daily fetal movement count (DFMC) Maternal assessment of fetal activity; the number of fetal movements within a specific time are counted. Also called kick count.

DDH See developmental dysplasia of the hip (DDH).

decidua Mucous membrane, lining of uterus, or endometrium of pregnancy that is shed after birth.

decidua basalis The portion of the endometrium directly under the blastocyst, where the chorionic villi tap into the maternal blood vessels. Maternal aspect of the placenta made up of uterine blood vessels, endometrial stroma, and glands. It is shed in lochial discharge after birth.

deletion Loss of chromosomal material and partial monosomy for the chromosome involved. The resulting clinical phenotype of either a terminal or an interstitial deletion depends on how much of the chromosome has been lost and the number and function of the genes contained in the missing segment.

demand feeding Feeding a neonate or infant when the baby exhibits signs of hunger, also known as feeding readiness cues.

deoxyribonucleic acid (DNA) Intracellular complex protein that carries genetic information, consisting of two purines (adenine and guanine) and two pyrimidines (thymine and cytosine).

dermoid cysts Germ cell tumors, usually occurring in childhood. These cysts contain substances such as hair, teeth, sebaceous secretions, and bones.

desquamation Shedding of epithelial cells of the skin and mucous membranes.

developmental dysplasia of the hip (DDH) Spectrum of disorders related to abnormal development of one or all components of the hip joint; includes a variety of hip abnormalities involving a shallow acetabulum, subluxation, or dislocation.

diabetes mellitus A group of metabolic diseases characterized by hyperglycemia resulting from defects in insulin secretion, insulin action, or both. The current classification system includes four groups: type 1 diabetes, type 2 diabetes, other specific types (e.g., diabetes caused by genetic defects in β cell function or insulin action, disease or injury of the pancreas, or drug-induced diabetes), and gestational diabetes mellitus.

diastasis recti abdominis Separation of the two rectus muscles along the median line of the abdominal wall. This is often seen in women with repeated pregnancies or with a multiple gestation.

dietary reference intakes (DRIs) Nutritional recommendations for daily nutritional intakes that meet the needs of almost all of the healthy members of a population; divided into age, sex, and life-stage categories; can be used as goals in dietary planning.

dilation The enlargement or widening of the cervical opening and the cervical canal that occurs once labor has begun. The diameter of the cervix increases from being closed to full dilation (approximately 10 cm) to allow birth of a term fetus.

dilation and curettage (D&C) Surgical procedure in which the cervix is dilated if necessary and a curette is inserted to scrape the uterine walls and remove uterine contents. Uterine contents may also be removed by suction curettage, using a catheter attached to an electric-powered vacuum source.

diploid Containing two complete sets of chromosomes, one from each parent.

disenfranchised grief Occurs when a person's losses are not openly acknowledged or mourned publicly.

disseminated intravascular coagulation (DIC) Pathologic form of clotting that is diffuse and consumes large amounts of clotting factors, causing widespread external bleeding, internal bleeding, or both, and clotting. In obstetrics it is most often associated with placental abruption, amniotic fluid embolism, preeclampsia, HELLP syndrome (see entry later), and gram-negative sepsis. Also called consumptive coagulopathy.

dizygotic twins Twins developed from two separate ova fertilized by two separate sperm at the same time; fraternal twins.

dominant trait A trait or disorder expressed or phenotypically apparent when only one copy of an allele associated with the trait is present. Gene that is expressed whenever it is present in the heterozygous gene state (e.g., brown eyes are dominant over blue).

Doppler blood flow analysis Method for measuring blood flow noninvasively in the fetus and placenta using ultrasound to detect intrauterine growth restriction.

doula A specially trained, experienced female labor attendant. A doula is a professional or lay labor-support person who is present during labor to focus on the laboring woman and provide physical and emotional support.

Down syndrome (DS) Abnormality involving chromosome 21 that characteristically results in a typical picture of intellectual disability and altered physical appearance. This condition was formerly called mongolism.

dual diagnosis Coexistence of substance abuse and another psychiatric disorder. Mood and anxiety disorders are the psychiatric disorders most commonly seen along with substance abuse in women. The psychiatric illness usually occurs before substance use begins.

Dual process model An established theory of grief and bereavement; refers to the processes and strategies individuals use to manage grief and bereavement, as opposed to stages of grief.

DUB See dysfunctional uterine bleeding (DUB).

ductus arteriosus In fetal circulation an anatomic shunt between the pulmonary artery and arch of the aorta. It is obliterated after birth by a rising blood oxygen level and a change in intravascular pressures in the presence of normal pulmonary function. It normally becomes a ligament after birth but in some instances remains patent; this is called patent ductus arteriosus.

ductus venosus In fetal circulation a blood vessel carrying oxygenated blood between the umbilical vein and the inferior vena cava, bypassing the liver. It is obliterated and becomes a ligament after birth.

duration (of uterine contractions) Time (measured in seconds) from the beginning to the end of a contraction.

dysfunctional labor Long, difficult, or abnormal labor, caused by various conditions associated with the five factors affecting labor; also called dystocia.

dysfunctional uterine bleeding (DUB) Excessive uterine bleeding with no demonstrable organic cause, genital or extragenital; most frequently caused by anovulation. Subset of abnormal uterine bleeding.

dysmenorrhea Pain during or shortly before menstruation.

dysplasia Any abnormal development of tissues or organs; preinvasive lesions in cervical epithelium.

E

early deceleration (of the fetal heart rate) Visually apparent gradual (onset to lowest point ≥30 seconds) decrease in and return to baseline fetal heart rate associated with uterine contractions. It is thought to be caused by transient fetal head compression and is considered a normal and benign finding. In general, the onset, nadir (lowest point), and recovery of the deceleration correspond to the beginning, peak, and end of the contraction.

early neonatal death Death of a live-born infant less than 7 days old.

eclampsia Onset of seizure activity or coma in a woman with preeclampsia who has no history of preexisting pathology that can result in seizure activity.

ectopic pregnancy Pregnancy in which the fertilized ovum is implanted outside of its normal place in the uterine cavity. Locations include the abdomen, uterine tubes, and ovaries. Ectopic pregnancies are often called tubal pregnancies because at least 90% are located in the uterine tube.

EDB See estimated date of birth (EDB).

effacement The shortening and thinning of the cervix during the first stage of labor. Effacement generally progresses significantly in first-time term pregnancy before more than slight dilation occurs. In subsequent pregnancies, effacement and dilation of the cervix tend to progress together. Degree of effacement is expressed in percentages from 0% to 100%.

effleurage Light stroking, usually of the abdomen, in rhythm with breathing during contractions.

e-health literacy Ability to use information and communications technologies to improve health.

ELBW See extremely low birth weight (ELBW).

elective abortion Termination of pregnancy chosen by the woman that is not required for her physical safety.

elective cesarean birth A primary cesarean birth without medical or obstetric indication; sometimes referred to as cesarean on request or cesarean on demand.

ELSIs Ethical, legal, and social implications of genetics research.

embryo Conceptus from the second or third week of development until approximately the eighth week after conception, when mineralization (ossification) of the skeleton begins. This period is characterized by cellular differentiation and predominantly hyperplastic growth.

embryoblast Inner cell mass in blastocyst that gives rise to the embryo.

en face Face-to-face position in which the parent's and infant's faces are approximately 20 cm apart and on the same plane.

encephalocele A herniation of the brain and meninges through a skull defect.

endometrial cancer Most common malignancy of the reproductive system; slow-growing tumor that usually develops in the fundus of the uterus and can spread directly to the myometrium and cervix, as well as to the reproductive organs.

endometriosis Characterized by the presence and growth of endometrial glands and stroma outside of the uterus. Tissue closely resembling endometrial tissue but located outside the uterus in the pelvic cavity. Symptoms may include pelvic pain or pressure, dysmenorrhea, dyspareunia, abnormal bleeding from the uterus or rectum, and infertility.

endometritis Postpartum uterine infection, often beginning at the site of the placental implantation.

engagement Term used to indicate that the largest transverse diameter of the presenting part (usually the biparietal diameter) has passed through the maternal pelvic brim or inlet into the true pelvis and usually corresponds to station 0.

engorgement Painful overfilling of the breasts; occurs 3 to 5 days after birth with onset of lactogenesis II when milk production increases significantly; milk volume exceeds storage capacity of alveoli in breasts, resulting in tissue edema and compression of milk ducts; breasts and areolae are firm, tender, hot; nipples flatten.

engrossment A parent's absorption, preoccupation, and interest in his or her infant; term typically used to describe the father's intense involvement with his newborn.

entrainment Newborns move in time with the rhythms of adult speech but not to random noises or disconnected words or vowels. Entrainment is believed to be an essential factor in the process of maternal-infant bonding.

epidural block Type of regional anesthesia produced by injecting a local anesthetic alone or in combination with an opioid agonist analgesic into the epidural (peridural) space.

Epigenetics Epigenetics (which literally means over and above the genome) is "an emerging field of science that studies heritable changes caused by the activation and deactivation of genes without any change in the underlying DNA sequence of the organism."

episiotomy Surgical incision of the perineum at the end of the second stage of labor to enlarge the vaginal outlet, facilitate birth, and avoid laceration of the perineum.

episodic changes Changes from baseline patterns in the fetal heart rate that are not associated with uterine contractions.

epulis Red raised nodule on the gums that bleeds easily; tumorlike benign lesion of the gingiva seen in pregnant women. Also called gingival granuloma gravidarum.

erythema toxicum Transient rash of newborn, appearing within 24 to 48 hours after birth, lasting up to 3 weeks, and resolving spontaneously within a few days. Also called erythema neonatorum, newborn rash, or flea bite dermatitis.

erythroblastosis fetalis Hemolytic disease of the newborn usually caused by isoimmunization resulting from Rh incompatibility or ABO incompatibility.

esophageal atresia Congenital anomaly in which the esophagus ends in a blind pouch or narrows into a thin cord, thus failing to form a continuous passageway to the stomach.

estimated date of birth (EDB) Approximate date of birth. Usually determined by calculation using the Naegele rule; "due date."

ethnocentrism Belief in the rightness of one's culture's way of doing things.

euglycemia Normal blood glucose level.

euploid cell Cell with the correct or normal number of chromosomes within the cell.

evidence-based practice Providing care based on evidence gained through research and clinical trials.

exchange transfusion Replacing 75% to 85% of circulating blood by withdrawing the recipient's blood and injecting a donor's blood in equal amounts, the purposes of which are to prevent an accumulation of bilirubin in the blood greater than a dangerous level, to prevent the accumulation of other byproducts of hemolysis in hemolytic disease, and to correct anemia and acidosis.

exenteration, pelvic See pelvic exenteration.

exstrophy of the bladder Congenital abnormality in which the bladder, urethra, and ureteral orifices are exposed.

extended family Family form that includes the nuclear family and other blood-related persons.

external cephalic version (ECV) Turning the fetus to a vertex position by exertion of pressure on the fetus externally through the maternal abdomen.

extremely low birth weight (ELBW) A newborn birth weight of 1000 g (2.2 lb) or less.

F

FAB See fertility awareness–based (FAB) methods.

family planning See periodic abstinence.

FAS See fetal alcohol syndrome (FAS).

feeding-readiness cues Infant responses that indicate optimal times to begin a feeding; signs include sucking motions, hand-to-mouth or hand-to-hand movements, rooting reflex, or mouthing.

fertility awareness–based (FAB) methods Methods of contraception, also known as periodic abstinence or natural family planning, that depend on identifying the beginning and end of the fertile period of the menstrual cycle. These methods provide contraception by relying on avoidance of intercourse during fertile periods.

fertility rate Births per 1000 women from 15 to 44 years of age.

fertilization Union of an ovum and a sperm.

fetal alcohol spectrum disorder (FASD) Includes five conditions: fetal alcohol syndrome, partial fetal alcohol syndrome, alcohol-related neurodevelopmental disorder, alcohol-related birth defects, and neurobehavioral disorder associated with prenatal alcohol exposure.

fetal alcohol syndrome (FAS) The most severe fetal alcohol spectrum disorder; with specific dysmorphic facial features (short palpebral fissures, thin upper lip, smooth philtrum), growth deficiency, and central nervous system abnormalities (structural, neurologic, developmental, functional, or a combination of these).

fetal death Refers to any death prior to birth after 20 weeks of gestation. Fetal deaths are subdivided as early (20 to 27 weeks of gestation) or late (≥28 weeks of gestation).

fetal fibronectin (fFN) Glycoprotein "glue" found in plasma and produced during fetal life. It normally appears in cervical and vaginal secretions early in pregnancy and again in late pregnancy. Assessing for the presence or absence of fFN in vaginal secretions is used as a diagnostic test for preterm labor.

fetal heart rate (FHR) baseline The average rate during a 10-minute segment that excludes periodic or episodic changes, periods of marked variability, and segments of the baseline that differ by more than 25 beats/min. The normal range at term is 110 to 160 beats/min. In the preterm fetus the baseline rate is slightly higher.

fetal hydrops The most severe form of erythroblastosis fetalis, in which the fetus has marked anemia, cardiac decompensation, cardiomegaly, hepatosplenomegaly, and hypoxia.

fetus Unborn offspring in utero from approximately the eighth week after conception until birth.

fibroadenoma Benign condition of the breast; discrete, usually solitary lumps less than 3 cm in diameter.

fibrocystic change Characterized by lumpiness, with or without tenderness, in both breasts. Fibrocystic breast condition involves the glandular breast tissue.

first stage of labor Begins with the onset of regular uterine contractions and ends with full cervical effacement and dilation; consists of two phases: the latent phase and the active phase.

fistula Abnormal tubelike passage that forms between two normal cavities, possibly congenital or caused by trauma, abscesses, or inflammatory processes.

follicular cysts Develop most commonly in normal ovaries of young women as a result of the mature graafian follicle failing to rupture or when an immature follicle does not resorb fluid after ovulation.

foramen ovale Septal opening between the atria of the fetal heart. The opening normally closes shortly after birth, but if it remains patent, surgical repair usually is necessary.

forceps-assisted birth Birth in which forceps are used to assist in delivery of the fetal head.

fourth stage of labor Initial period of physical recovery from birth and the beginning of parent-infant bonding. It is usually considered to last for the first 1 to 2 hours after birth.

frequency (of uterine contractions) Time (measured in minutes) from the beginning of one contraction to the beginning of the next.

friability Easily broken. May refer to a fragile condition of the cervix, especially during pregnancy, that causes the cervix to bleed easily when touched.

funic souffle Soft, muffled, blowing sound produced by blood rushing through the umbilical vessels and synchronous with the fetal heart sounds.

G

galactorrhea Form of nipple discharge or lactation not associated with birth or breastfeeding; a bilaterally spontaneous, milky, sticky discharge. When associated with elevated prolactin levels, may be a symptom of a pituitary tumor.

galactogogue Medications or other substances that are believed to increase breast milk production.

galactosemia Inherited, autosomal recessive disorder of galactose metabolism, characterized by a deficiency of the enzyme galactose-1-phosphate uridyltransferase; resulting in the inability to convert galactose to glucose.

gamete Egg and sperm. Mature male or female germ cell; the mature sperm or ovum.

gastroschisis Abdominal wall defect at base of umbilical stalk; herniation of the bowel through a defect in the abdominal wall to the right of the umbilical cord.

gate-control theory of pain Helps explain the way hypnosis and the pain relief techniques taught in childbirth preparation classes work to relieve the pain of labor. According to this theory, pain sensations travel along sensory nerve pathways to the brain, but only a limited number of sensations, or messages, can travel through these nerve pathways at one time. Using distraction techniques such as massage or effleurage, stroking, music, focal points, and imagery reduces or completely blocks the capacity of nerve pathways to transmit pain. These distractions are thought to work by closing down a hypothetic gate in the spinal cord, thus preventing pain signals from reaching the brain.

gene Basic physical unit of inheritance passed from parents to offspring; contains the information needed to specify traits.

gene therapy Inserting a healthy copy of the defective gene into the somatic cells (of the affected individual).

general anesthesia Administration of several medications that combine to produce unconsciousness and pain relief (often referred to as being "put to sleep"). The major risks associated with general anesthesia are difficulty with or inability to intubate and aspiration of gastric contents.

genetics Study of individual genes and their effect on relatively rare single gene disorders.

genital self-examination (GSE) See vulvar self-examination (VSE).

genome Entire set of genetic instructions found in each cell.

genomics Study of all the genes in the human genome together, including their interactions with each other, the environment, and the influence of other psychosocial factors and cultural factors.

genotype An individual's collection of genes. Hereditary combinations in an individual determining physical and chemical characteristics. Some genotypes are not expressed until later in life (e.g., Huntington chorea); some hide recessive genes, which can be expressed in offspring, and others are expressed only under the proper environmental conditions (e.g., diabetes mellitus appearing under the stress of obesity or pregnancy).

germinal matrix hemorrhage-intraventricular hemorrhage The most common type of intracranial hemorrhage in preterm neonates; the germinal matrix is a vascular network of cells is beneath the lining of the lateral ventricles; hemorrhage extends from the germinal matrix into the ventricles; associated with high mortality.

gestational diabetes mellitus (GDM) Traditionally defined as carbohydrate intolerance with the onset or first recognition occurring during pregnancy. The American Diabetes Association defines GDM as diabetes diagnosed during pregnancy that is clearly not overt (pre-existing) diabetes.

gestational hypertension Onset of hypertension without proteinuria or other systemic findings diagnostic for preeclampsia after week 20 of pregnancy. Gestational hypertension does not persist longer than 12 weeks postpartum and usually resolves during the first postpartum week.

glycosylated hemoglobin A$_{1c}$ Test done to assess recent glycemic control. Hemoglobin A1c levels greater than 6 indicate elevated glucose levels during the previous 4 to 6 weeks.

Goodell sign Softening of the cervix, a probable sign of pregnancy, occurring during the second month.

gravida A woman who is pregnant.

gravidity Pregnancy.

grief The profound feelings of sadness and despair accompanying loss; recognized as a process through which bereaved persons work to make meaning of and come to terms with their loss.

growth spurts Times of increased infant growth that usually occur at approximately 6 to 10 days, 6 weeks, 3 months, and 5 to 6 months. The increased caloric needs necessitate more frequent feedings to increase the amount of milk needed.

H

habituation An acquired tolerance from repeated exposure to a particular stimulus. Also called negative adaptation; a decline and eventual elimination of a conditioned response by repetition of the conditioned stimulus.

haploid Cell that contains 23 chromosomes or half the number contained in a somatic cell; most gametes are haploid.

hCG See human chorionic gonadotropin (hCG).

health promotion Motivation to increase well-being and actualize health potential.

Hegar sign: Softening of the lower uterine segment; classified as a probable sign of pregnancy; may be present during the second and third months of pregnancy and is palpated during bimanual examination.

HELLP syndrome A laboratory diagnosis for a variant of preeclampsia that involves hepatic dysfunction, characterized by hemolysis (H), elevated liver enzymes (EL), and low platelet count (LP). HELLP syndrome can develop in women who do not have hypertension or proteinuria.

hematopoiesis Production of blood cells; formation of blood.

hemorrhage, subconjunctival See subconjunctival hemorrhage.

hemorrhage, subgaleal See subgaleal hemorrhage.

hemorrhagic shock Clinical condition in which the peripheral blood flow is inadequate to return sufficient blood to the heart for normal function, particularly oxygen transport to the organs or tissue. Also called hypovolemic shock.

heterozygous Having two dissimilar genes at the same site, or locus, on paired chromosomes (e.g., at the site for eye color, one chromosome carrying the gene for brown, the other for blue).

home birth Planned birth of the child at home, usually done under the supervision of a midwife.

homologous Similar in structure or origin but not necessarily in function.

homozygous Having two similar genes at the same locus, or site, on paired chromosomes.

hot flash Transient, sudden sensation of warmth in neck, head, and chest experienced by some women during or after menopause, resulting from autonomic vasomotor disturbances that accompany changes in the neurohormonal activity of the ovaries, hypothalamus, and pituitary gland.

hot flush Visible red flush of skin and perspiration experienced by some women during or after menopause; see also hot flash.

human chorionic gonadotropin (hCG) Hormone that is produced by chorionic villi; the biologic marker in pregnancy tests.

Human papillomavirus (HPV) Also known as condylomata acuminata, or genital warts, is the most common viral sexually transmitted infection seen in ambulatory health care settings. There are approximately 100 types of HPV, which is a double-stranded DNA virus, with approximately 40 of these types found to be causes of anogenital infections. There are several that can cause genital cancers, with two specific types (16 and 18) that are highly oncogenic, meaning they are highest risk for causing cancers of the cervix, vagina, vulva, penis, and oropharyngeal area. HPV is the primary cause of cervical neoplasia.

hydatidiform mole   See molar pregnancy.

hydramnios   See polyhydramnios.

hydrocele   Collection of fluid in a saclike cavity, especially in the sac that surrounds the testis, causing the scrotum to swell.

hydrocephalus   Accumulation of cerebrospinal fluid (CSF) in the subdural or subarachnoid spaces; caused by overproduction (rare) of CSF or a decrease in reabsorption.

hydrops fetalis   See fetal hydrops.

hyperbilirubinemia   Condition in which the total unconjugated serum bilirubin concentration in the blood is elevated. Values are evaluated based on gestational age, days of life, and the infant's general physical condition. See also jaundice.

hyperemesis gravidarum   Abnormal condition of pregnancy characterized by vomiting excessive enough to cause weight loss, electrolyte imbalance, nutritional deficiencies, and ketonuria.

hyperglycemia   Excess glucose in the blood.

hypermenorrhea   See menorrhagia.

hyperthermia   Body temperature greater than 37.5°C.

hyperthyroidism   Excessive functional activity of the thyroid gland.

hypoglycemia   Less than normal amount of glucose in the blood.

hypospadias   Anomalous positioning of urinary meatus on the undersurface of the penis.

hypothermia   Temperature that decreases to less than normal range, usually caused by exposure to cold.

hypothyroidism   Deficiency of thyroid gland activity with underproduction of thyroxine.

hypovolemic shock   See hemorrhagic shock.

hypoxemia   Deficiency of oxygen in the arterial blood.

hypoxia   Inadequate supply of oxygen at the cellular level that can cause metabolic acidosis.

hysterectomy   Surgical removal of the entire uterus.

I

icterus   See jaundice.

idiopathic thrombocytopenic purpura (ITP)   An autoimmune disorder in which antiplatelet antibodies decrease the life span of the platelets. Thrombocytopenia, capillary fragility, and increased bleeding time are diagnostic findings. Also called immune thrombocytopenic purpura.

illness prevention   Desire to avoid illness, detect it early, or maintain optimal functioning when illness is present.

immune thrombocytopenic purpura (ITP)   See idiopathic thrombocytopenic purpura.

imperforate anus   Congenital malformation in which the anus is absent or abnormally located.

implantation   Embedding of the fertilized ovum in the endometrium (uterine lining); nidation.

inborn error of metabolism   Hereditary deficiency of a specific enzyme needed for normal metabolism of specific chemicals (e.g., deficiency of phenylalanine hydroxylase results in phenylketonuria; a deficiency of hexosaminidase results in Tay-Sachs disease).

induced abortion   Purposeful interruption of a pregnancy before 20 weeks of gestation.

induction of labor   Chemical or mechanical initiation of uterine contractions before their spontaneous onset for the purpose of bringing about birth.

infant death   Death of a child during the first year of life.

infant mortality rate   Number of deaths per 1000 children 1 year of age or younger.

infantile hemangioma   Elevated lesion of immature capillaries and endothelial cells that usually regresses over a period of years. Also called nevus vascularis, strawberry hemangioma.

infertility   Decreased capacity to conceive. The term implies subfertility, a prolonged time to conceive, as opposed to sterility, which means inability to conceive.

insensible water loss (IWL)   Evaporative water loss that occurs mainly through the skin and respiratory tract.

intensity (of uterine contractions)   Strength of a contraction at its peak.

intermittent auscultation   Involves listening to fetal heart sounds at periodic intervals to assess the fetal heart rate.

interstitial deletion   Deletion anywhere in the chromosome except at the end.

intimate partner violence (IPV)   The actual or threatened physical, sexual, psychological, or emotional abuse by a spouse, ex-spouse, boyfriend, girlfriend, ex-boyfriend, ex-girlfriend, date, or cohabiting partner.

intraductal papilloma   A benign tumor that grows within the duct of the breast.

intrahepatic cholestasis of pregnancy (ICP)   Disorder unique to pregnancy that is characterized by generalized pruritus caused by elevated serum bile acids. The itching commonly affects the palms and soles but can occur on any part of the body and is usually worse at night. No skin lesions are present.

intrauterine growth restriction (IUGR)   Fetal undergrowth of any cause, such as deficient nutrient supply or intrauterine infection, or associated with congenital malformation; birth weight less than population 10th percentile corrected for gestational age.

intrauterine pressure catheter (IUPC)   Catheter inserted into uterine cavity to assess uterine activity and pressure by electronic means.

inversion of the uterus   Turning end for end, upside down, or inside out.

involution   Reduction in size of the uterus after birth and its return to its nonpregnant condition.

isoimmunization   Production of antibodies by one member of a species against something that is commonly found within that species (e.g., development of anti-Rh antibodies in an Rh-negative person; also called Rh incompatibility).

ITP   See idiopathic thrombocytopenic purpura (ITP). Note: The acronym ITP is also known as immune thrombocytopenic purpura.

IWL   See insensible water loss (IWL).

J

jaundice   Yellow discoloration of the body tissues caused by the deposit of bile pigments (unconjugated bilirubin); also called icterus. See also hyperbilirubinemia.

K

karyotype   Pictorial analysis of the number, form, and size of an individual's chromosomes. Schematic arrangement of the chromosomes within a cell to demonstrate their numbers and morphology.

Kegel exercises   Pelvic muscle exercises developed to strengthen the pubococcygeal muscles (supportive pelvic floor muscles) to control or reduce incontinent urine loss and to provide support for the pelvic organs and control of the muscles surrounding the vagina and urethra. Also beneficial during pregnancy and postpartum.

kernicterus   Irreversible, long-term consequences of bilirubin toxicity such as hypotonia, delayed motor skills, hearing loss, cerebral palsy, and gaze abnormalities.

ketoacidosis   The accumulation of ketone bodies in the blood as a consequence of hyperglycemia; leads to metabolic acidosis.

key informants   Individuals in specific positions who can provide information about a situation.

L

L/S ratio   See lecithin/sphingomyelin ratio.

labor   Series of processes by which the fetus is expelled from the uterus; parturition; birth.

Lactogenesis   Initiation of breast milk production. Stage I: initial synthesis of milk components beginning at approximately 16 to 18 weeks of pregnancy until approximately day 3 postpartum; the breasts prepare for milk production by producing colostrum. Stage II: begins with delivery of the placenta; progesterone levels drop and prolactin levels increase; onset of copious milk production on day 2 to 4 postpartum. Stage III: begins at approximately 10 days postpartum when mature milk is established and supply is maintained through autocrine control.

lactose intolerance   Inability to digest milk sugar (lactose) because of an inherited absence of the enzyme lactase in the small intestine.

lanugo   Downy, fine hair characteristic of the fetus between 20 weeks of gestation and birth that is most noticeable over the shoulders, forehead, and eyebrows.

LARC   Long-acting, reversible contraception.

large for gestational age (LGA)   Exhibiting excessive growth for gestational age; an infant whose birth weight falls above the 90th percentile on intrauterine growth curves.

latch   (1) Placement of the infant's mouth over the nipple, areola, and breast, making a seal between the mouth and breast to create adequate suction for milk removal. (2) Attachment of the infant to the breast for feeding.

late deceleration (of the fetal heart rate) Visually apparent gradual decrease in and return to baseline fetal heart rate associated with uterine contractions. It is thought to be caused by a disruption in oxygen transfer from the environment to the fetus. The deceleration begins after the contraction has started, and the nadir (lowest point) of the deceleration occurs after the peak of the contraction. The deceleration usually does not return to baseline until after the contraction is over.

late neonatal death Death of a newborn between 7 and 28 days after birth.

latent (early) phase of labor Phase in first stage of labor extending from the onset of labor, characterized by regular, painful uterine contractions that cause cervical change, to the beginning of the active phase.

latent ("laboring down") phase of labor Period of rest and relative calm at the beginning of second stage labor; sometimes referred to as delayed pushing, laboring down, or passive descent. During this phase the fetus continues to descend passively through the birth canal and rotate to an anterior position as a result of ongoing uterine contractions. The woman is quiet and often relaxes with her eyes closed between contractions. The urge to bear down is not strong, and some women do not experience it at all or only during the acme (peak) of a contraction.

LBW See low birth weight (LBW).

lecithin/sphingomyelin ratio Ratio of lecithin to sphingomyelin in the amniotic fluid. It is used to assess maturity of the fetal lung.

leiomyoma Slow-growing benign tumor arising from the muscle tissue of the uterus. Also known as fibroid tumor, fibroma, myoma, or fibromyoma.

letdown or let-down reflex See milk ejection reflex (MER).

leukorrhea White or slightly gray mucoid discharge from the cervical canal or the vagina with a faint musty odor, which may be normal physiologically or caused by pathologic states of the vagina and endocervix (e.g., *Trichomonas vaginalis* infections).

LGA See large for gestational age (LGA).

lie Relationship between the long axis (spine) of the fetus and the long axis (spine) of the mother. In a longitudinal lie, the fetus is lying lengthwise or vertically, whereas in a transverse lie, the fetus is lying crosswise or horizontally in the uterus.

lightening Sensation of decreased abdominal distention produced by uterine descent into the pelvic cavity as the fetal presenting part settles into the pelvis; it usually occurs 2 weeks before the onset of labor in nulliparas.

linea nigra Pigmented line extending from the symphysis pubis to the top of the fundus in the midline; common during pregnancy.

lithotomy position Position in which the woman lies on her back with her knees flexed and with abducted thighs drawn up toward her chest.

local perineal infiltration anesthesia Process by which a local anesthetic medication is injected into the skin and then subcutaneously to anesthetize a limited region of the body.

lochia Uterine/vaginal discharge after birth (during the puerperium) consisting of blood, tissue, and mucus.

lochia alba Thin, yellowish to white, vaginal discharge that follows lochia serosa approximately 10 to 14 days after birth and may last from 3 to 6 weeks postpartum; consists primarily of white blood cells and trophoblastic tissue debris.

lochia rubra Red, distinctly blood-tinged vaginal flow that follows birth and lasts 1 to 3 days; consists mainly of blood and decidual and trophoblastic debris.

lochia serosa Serous, pinkish brown, watery vaginal discharge that follows lochia rubra; from 4 to 10 days after birth; consists of old blood, serum, leukocytes, and tissue debris.

low birth weight (LBW) A newborn birth weight less than 2500 g (5.5 lb).

lumpectomy Removal of a small breast tumor and a small amount of surrounding healthy tissue to ensure there are clean margins.

M

macrosomia Birth weight more than 4000 to 4500 g or greater than the 90th percentile.

magnetic resonance imaging (MRI) Noninvasive nuclear procedure for imaging tissues with high fat and water content; in obstetrics, uses include evaluation of fetal structures, placenta, and amniotic fluid volume.

major depressive episode Disorder diagnosed in a person who has at least five of the following signs or symptoms nearly every day: depressed mood, often with spontaneous crying; markedly diminished interest in all activities; insomnia or hypersomnia; weight changes (increases or decreases); psychomotor retardation or agitation; fatigue or loss of energy; feelings of worthlessness or inappropriate guilt; diminished ability to concentrate; and suicidal ideation with or without a suicidal plan.

mammary duct ectasia An inflammation of the ducts behind the nipple.

mammography X-ray filming of the breast; examination technique used to screen for and evaluate breast lesions.

married-blended family Family formed as a result of divorce and remarriage, consisting of unrelated family members (stepparents, stepchildren, stepsiblings).

MAS See meconium aspiration syndrome (MAS).

mastectomy Removal of the breast including the nipple and areola; also called a simple or total mastectomy.

mastitis Infection in a breast, usually confined to a milk duct, characterized by influenza-like symptoms and redness and tenderness in the affected breast.

maternal mortality rate Number of maternal deaths per 100,000 births.

mechanical ventilation Technique used to provide predetermined amount of oxygen; requires intubation.

meconium First stools of infant: viscid, sticky; dark greenish brown, almost black; sterile; odorless.

meconium aspiration syndrome (MAS) Function of fetal hypoxia: with hypoxia, the anal sphincter relaxes and meconium is released; reflex gasping movements draw meconium and other particulate matter in the amniotic fluid into the infant's bronchial tree, obstructing the airflow after birth.

meconium-stained amniotic fluid Presence of green amniotic fluid that is either thin (light) or thick (heavy) in consistency; indicates that the fetus has passed meconium (first stool) before birth.

meiosis Process by which germ cells divide and decrease their chromosomal number by one-half; produces gametes (eggs and sperm).

melasma Blotchy, brownish hyperpigmentation of the skin over the cheeks, nose, and forehead, especially in dark-complexioned pregnant women and some women taking oral contraceptives; also known as chloasma, or mask of pregnancy.

MEN See minimal enteral nutrition (MEN).

menarche Onset, or beginning, of menstrual function; first menstruation.

menopausal hormone therapy (MHT) Hormonal therapy for menopausal symptoms; either as estrogen replacement therapy or estrogen therapy, in which a woman takes only estrogen, or hormonal replacement therapy or hormonal therapy, in which she takes both estrogen and progestins.

menopause From the Latin mensis (month) and Greek pausis (to cease); refers only to the last menstrual period; however, unlike menarche, menopause can be dated with certainty only 1 year after menstruation ceases.

menorrhagia Excessive menstrual bleeding, in either duration or amount; also known as hypermenorrhea.

menses (menstruation) (Latin plural of mensis [month].) Periodic uterine bleeding and vaginal discharge of bloody fluid from the nonpregnant uterus occurring approximately 14 days after ovulation. Menses begin at onset of puberty and cease with menopause.

menstruation See menses (menstruation).

MER See milk ejection reflex (MER).

metastasis Spread of cancer from its original site to other parts of the body. Results from seeding of cancer cells into the blood and lymph systems.

metrorrhagia Intermenstrual bleeding; refers to any episode of bleeding, whether spotting, menses, or hemorrhage, that occurs at a time other than the normal menses.

MHT See menopausal hormone therapy (MHT).

microcephaly Congenital abnormality in which the occipitofrontal head circumference is more than two standard deviations smaller than the mean for gestational age, weight, and sex; associated with cognitive impairment and developmental delays.

microdeletion Deletion too small to be detected by standard cytogenetic techniques.

milia Unopened sebaceous glands appearing as tiny, white, pinpoint papules on forehead, nose, cheeks, and chin of a neonate; disappear spontaneously in a few days or weeks.

milk ejection reflex (MER) Release of milk caused by the contraction of the myoepithelial cells within the milk glands in response to oxytocin; also called letdown or let-down reflex.

minimal enteral nutrition (MEN) Feeding small volumes of food to stimulate or prime the development of the immature gastrointestinal tract of the preterm infant, to achieve better absorption of nutrients when bolus or regular intermittent gavage feedings can be given. Also called trophic feeding.

miscarriage An in utero death prior to 20 weeks of gestation; also known as spontaneous abortion.

mitosis Process of somatic cell division in which a single cell divides, but both of the new cells have the same number of chromosomes as the first; body cells replicate to yield two cells with the same genetic makeup as the parent cell.

modified biophysical profile (mBPP) Combines the nonstress test with measurement of the quantity of amniotic fluid using ultrasound.

modified radical mastectomy Removal of breast tissue, skin, and axillary nodes.

molar pregnancy A benign proliferative growth of the placental trophoblast in which the chorionic villi develop into edematous, cystic, avascular transparent vesicles that hang in a grape-like cluster. Molar pregnancy is one of a group of pregnancy-related cancers without a viable fetus known as gestational trophoblastic neoplasia that are caused by abnormal fertilization. Also called hydatidiform mole.

mongolian spot Bluish gray or dark nonelevated pigmented area usually found over the lower back and buttocks; present at birth in some infants, primarily nonwhite; usually fades by school age.

monosomy Chromosomal aberration characterized by the absence of one chromosome from the normal diploid complement. Product of the union between a normal gamete and a gamete that is missing a chromosome.

monozygotic twins Twins developed from a single fertilized ovum; identical twins.

Montevideo units (MVUs) A method for evaluating the adequacy of uterine activity for achieving progress in labor. MVUs are calculated by subtracting the baseline uterine pressure from the peak contraction pressure for each contraction that occurs in a 10-minute window, and then adding together the pressures generated by each contraction that occurs during that period of time. MVUs can be calculated only using an intrauterine pressure catheter.

Montgomery glands Small, nodular prominences on the areolas around the nipples of the breasts that enlarge during pregnancy and lactation; hypertrophy of the sebaceous (oil) glands embedded in the primary areolae sebaceous glands. Also called Montgomery tubercles or tubercles of Montgomery.

morbidity (1) Condition of being diseased. (2) Number of cases of disease or of sick persons in relationship to a specific population; incidence.

morning sickness Nausea and vomiting that affect some women during the first few months of their pregnancy; can occur at any time of day.

morula Developmental stage of the fertilized ovum in which there is a solid mass of cells resembling a mulberry.

mosaicism Mixture of cells, some with a normal number of chromosomes and others entirely missing or having an extra chromosome.

mourning The process of finding the answers to the questions surrounding the loss, coping with grief responses, and determining how to live with the loss.

multifactorial inheritance Inheritance of phenotypic characteristics resulting from two or more genes on different chromosomes acting together. See also unifactorial inheritance.

multifetal pregnancy Pregnancy in which there is more than one fetus in the uterus at the same time; multiple pregnancy.

multigenerational family Family form consisting of three or more generations of relatives (grandparents, children, and grandchildren).

multigravida A woman who has had two or more pregnancies.

multipara A woman who has completed two or more pregnancies to 20 weeks of gestation or more.

mutation Spontaneous and permanent change in the normal gene structure in a gene or chromosome in gametes that may be transmitted to offspring.

mutuality Component of parent-infant attachment; the infant's behaviors and characteristics elicit a corresponding set of parental behaviors and characteristics.

myelomeningocele Congenital abnormality in which there is a herniation of spinal cord and neural elements through an opening in the spine with or without skin or vertebral covering.

myomectomy Removal of a tumor; specifically, removal of a benign tumor of the uterus leaving the uterine walls relatively intact.

N

Naegele rule Method for calculating the estimated date of birth or "due date."

NEC See necrotizing enterocolitis (NEC).

necrotizing enterocolitis (NEC) Acute inflammatory disease of the gastrointestinal mucosa that occurs primarily in preterm or low-birth-weight neonates; commonly complicated by bowel necrosis, perforation, and peritonitis.

neonatal abstinence syndrome Clinical signs in the newborn associated with withdrawal from opioids.

neonatal mortality rate (1) Number of neonatal deaths per 1000 births (or per live births). (2) Statistical rate of infant death during the first 28 days after live birth, expressed as the number of such deaths per 1000 live births in a specific geographic area or institution in a given period of time.

neural tube defect (NTD) Congenital abnormalities of the central nervous system resulting from defects in the closure of the neural tube during fetal development.

neurobehavioral disorder associated with prenatal alcohol exposure A relatively new term that reflects the teratogenic effects of alcohol on the developing fetus. Children affected this disorder lack the distinguishing physical features of fetal alcohol syndrome but have central nervous system damage that is manifested in functional impairments of neurocognition, self-regulation, and adaptive functioning.

neurofibroma: Benign, soft tumor.

neutral thermal environment (NTE) Environment that enables the neonate to maintain a body temperature of at least 36.5°C with minimum use of oxygen and energy.

nevus flammeus Port-wine stain; reddish, usually flat, discoloration of the face or neck; darkens with time; most often on the face and neck.

nitrazine A pH indicator dye.

nondirectiveness According to the principle of nondirectiveness, the individual who is providing genetic counseling respects the right of the individual or family being counseled to make autonomous decisions. Counselors using a nondirective approach avoid making recommendations and try to communicate genetic information in an unbiased manner.

nondisjunction Failure of two homologous chromosomes to separate during reduction division. One resulting cell contains both chromosomes, and the other contains none.

nonnutritive sucking Sucking opportunities not associated with feeding; most often using pacifier; useful for infant to calm, organize, or self-regulate.

nonphysiologic jaundice See jaundice, pathologic.

nonshivering thermogenesis Infant's method of producing heat through metabolism of brown fat.

nonstress test (NST) Evaluation of fetal response (fetal heart rate) to fetal movement, uterine contractions, or stimulation.

no-parent family Family form in which children live independently in foster or kinship care, such as living with a grandparent.

NTD See neural tube defect.

NTE See neutral thermal environment (NTE).

nuchal cord Encircling of fetal neck by one or more loops of umbilical cord.

nuclear family Traditional family in which male and female partners and their children live as an independent unit, sharing roles, responsibilities, and economic resources.

nullipara A woman who has not completed a pregnancy beyond 20 weeks of gestation.

nulligravida A woman who has never been pregnant and is not currently pregnant.

O

occurrence risk Estimated risk given to a couple who has not yet had children but are known to be at risk for having children with a genetic disease. See also recurrence risk.

oligohydramnios Decreased amount of amniotic fluid; indicated by an amniotic fluid index of less than 5 cm.

oligomenorrhea Infrequent menstrual periods characterized by intervals of 40 to 45 days or longer.

omphalocele Congenital abnormality resulting from failure of closure of the abdominal wall or muscles; a covered herniation abdominal contents into the base of the umbilical cord.

oogenesis Process of egg (ovum) formation; begins during fetal life in the female.

operculum Plug of mucus that fills the cervical canal during pregnancy; acts as a barrier against bacterial invasion.

ophthalmia neonatorum Infection in the neonate's eyes usually resulting from gonorrheal or other infection contracted when the fetus passes through the birth canal (vagina).

opioid (narcotic) agonist analgesics Medications that stimulate major opioid receptors, mu and kappa. They have no amnesic effect but create a feeling of well-being or euphoria and enhance a woman's ability to rest between contractions. Examples are meperidine (Demerol) and fentanyl (Sublimaze).

opioid (narcotic) agonist-antagonist analgesics Medications that are agonists at kappa opioid receptors and either antagonists or weak agonists at mu opioid receptors. In the doses used during labor, these mixed opioids provide adequate analgesia without causing significant respiratory depression in the mother or neonate. Examples are butorphanol (Stadol) and nalbuphine (Nubain).

opioid (narcotic) antagonist Medication that promptly reverses the central nervous system depressant effects, especially respiratory depression, of narcotics. An example is naloxone (Narcan).

osteoporosis Deossification of bone tissue resulting in structural weakness; generalized, metabolic disease characterized by decreased bone mass and increased incidence of bone fractures, especially after menopause.

outcomes-oriented care Measures effectiveness of care against benchmarks or standards.

ovarian cancer The second most frequently occurring reproductive cancer, which causes more deaths than any other female genital tract cancer. Also called cancer of the ovary.

ovulation Periodic ripening and discharge of the ovum from the ovary, usually 14 days before after the onset of menstrual flow; the release of a mature ovum from the ovary at intervals (usually monthly).

oxytocin Hormone produced by the posterior pituitary that stimulates uterine contractions and the release of milk in the mammary gland (milk-ejection reflex). Synthetic oxytocin (Pitocin) may be used to either induce or augment labor.

P

paced breathing techniques Various breathing methods used to control pain during labor. They include slow-paced, modified-paced, and pattern-paced breathing patterns.

palmar erythema Pinkish red, diffuse mottling or well-defined blotches seen over the palmar surfaces of the hands during pregnancy; related primarily to increased estrogen levels.

parity The number of pregnancies in which the fetus or fetuses have reached 20 weeks of gestation.

participant observation Assessment method in which the nurse actively participates in the community to understand the community more fully and to validate observations.

patent ductus arteriosus (PDA) Condition that occurs when the fetal ductus arteriosus fails to close after birth. Also see ductus arteriosus.

pathologic grief See complicated grief.

pathologic jaundice Jaundice usually first noticeable within 24 hours after birth; caused by some abnormal condition such as an Rh or ABO incompatibility and resulting in bilirubin toxicity (e.g., kernicterus); unconjugated hyperbilirubinemia that is either pathologic in origin or severe enough to warrant further evaluation and treatment. Also called nonphysiologic jaundice.

pathologic mourning See complicated grief.

PCOS See polycystic ovary syndrome (PCOS).

PDA See patent ductus arteriosus (PDA).

pelvic Pertaining or relating to the pelvis.

pelvic exenteration A total exenteration involves removal of the perineum, the pelvic floor, the levator muscles, and all reproductive organs. In addition, pelvic lymph nodes, rectum, sigmoid colon, urinary bladder, and distal ureters are removed, and a colostomy and ileal conduit are constructed.

pelvic inflammatory disease (PID) Infectious process that most commonly involves the uterine (fallopian) tubes (salpingitis), uterus (endometritis), and more rarely, the ovaries and peritoneal surfaces. Usually secondary to sexually transmitted infections.

pelvic relaxation Refers to the lengthening and weakening of the fascial supports of pelvic structures. Congenital or acquired weakness of the pelvic support structures.

percutaneous umbilical blood sampling (PUBS) Procedure during which a fetal umbilical vessel is accessed for blood sampling or for transfusions. Also called cordocentesis.

perimenopause Period of transition of changing ovarian activity before menopause and through first few years of amenorrhea; precedes menopause and lasts approximately 4 years. During this time, ovarian function declines. Ova slowly diminish, and menstrual cycles may be anovulatory, resulting in irregular bleeding. The ovary stops producing estrogen and eventually menses no longer occur.

perinatal bereavement The complex emotional responses experienced by women and their partners after the death of an expected child through miscarriage, stillbirth, neonatal death, or termination of pregnancy for fetal anomalies.

perinatal loss Loss associated with childbearing; particularly losses occurring after conception and after the woman has recognized that she is pregnant.

perinatal mood disorders Set of disorders that can occur any time during pregnancy as well as in the first year postpartum and can include depression, anxiety, obsessive-compulsive disorder, posttraumatic stress disorder, and postpartum psychosis.

perinatal mortality rate Combined fetal and neonatal mortality. See also death, perinatal.

perinatal palliative care A formalized end-of-life interprofessional care model specifically aimed at intervening when pregnancy is expected to end in stillbirth or neonatal death.

perineum A skin-covered muscular area that covers the pelvic structures. The perineum forms the base of the perineal body, a wedge-shaped mass that serves as an anchor for the muscles, fascia, and ligaments of the pelvis. Area between the vagina and rectum in the female and between the scrotum and rectum in the male.

periodic abstinence Contraceptive method in which a woman abstains from sexual intercourse during the fertile period of her menstrual cycle; also referred to as natural family planning because no other form of birth control is used during this period.

periodic changes Changes from baseline of the fetal heart rate that occur with uterine contractions.

persistent pulmonary hypertension of the newborn (PPHN) Combined findings of pulmonary hypertension, right-to-left shunting, and a structurally normal heart; formerly known as persistent fetal circulation.

phenotype An individual's observable traits. Refers to the observable expression of an individual's genotype, such as physical features, a biochemical or molecular trait, and even a psychological trait. Expression of certain physical or chemical characteristics in an individual resulting from interaction between genotype and environmental factors.

phenylketonuria (PKU) Inborn error of metabolism caused by a deficiency in the enzyme phenylalanine hydrolase. Absence of this enzyme impairs the body's ability to metabolize the amino acid phenylalanine found in all protein foods. Consequently, toxic accumulation of phenylalanine in the blood occurs, which interferes with brain development and function.

phototherapy Light therapy to reduce serum bilirubin levels by oxidating bilirubin into water-soluble compounds that are then processed in the liver and excreted into bile and urine.

physiologic anemia A modest decrease in the hemoglobin concentration and hematocrit in pregnancy, caused by the relative excess of plasma.

physiologic jaundice Yellow tinge to skin and mucous membranes in response to increased serum levels of unconjugated bilirubin; not usually apparent until after 24 hours; also called neonatal jaundice, physiologic hyperbilirubinemia, or nonpathologic unconjugated hyperbilirubinemia.

phytoestrogens Plant compounds that have a weak estrogenic effect in the human body; used in managing menopause as an alternative or complement to conventional hormone replacement therapy. Also known as isoflavones.

pica Unusual craving during pregnancy; the practice of consuming nonfood substances (e.g., clay, soil, and laundry starch) or excessive amounts of foodstuffs low in nutritional value (e.g., ice or freezer frost, baking powder or soda, and cornstarch) is often influenced by the woman's cultural background.

PID See pelvic inflammatory disease (PID).

placenta Latin, "flat cake"; afterbirth, specialized vascular disk-shaped organ for maternal-fetal gas and nutrient exchange. Normally it implants in the thick muscular wall of the upper uterine segment.

placenta accreta Abnormally firm placental attachment; accreta is a slight penetration of the myometrium. Sometimes referred to as a morbidly adherent placenta.

placenta increta Abnormally firm placental attachment; increta is deep penetration of the myometrium. Sometimes referred to as a morbidly adherent placenta.

placenta percreta Abnormally firm placental attachment; perceta is perforation of the myometrium. Sometimes referred to as a morbidly adherent placenta.

placenta previa Placenta is implanted in the lower uterine segment such that it completely or partially covers the cervix or is close enough to the cervix to cause bleeding when the cervix dilates or the lower uterine segment effaces. Placenta previa can be further classified as complete, marginal, or low-lying.

placental abruption See abruptio placentae.

plugged milk ducts Milk ducts blocked by small curds of dried milk.

PMDD See premenstrual dysphoric disorder (PMDD).

PMS See premenstrual syndrome (PMS).

polycystic ovary syndrome (PCOS) Occurs when an endocrine imbalance results in high levels of estrogen, testosterone, and luteinizing hormone and decreased secretion of follicle-stimulating hormone.

polyhydramnios Increased amount of amniotic fluid; indicated by an amniotic fluid index of more than 25 cm.

polyp Small tumorlike growth that projects from a mucous membrane surface.

polyploidy One of the two types of deviations from the correct number of chromosomes per cell, in which the deviation is an exact multiple of the haploid number of chromosomes or one chromosome set (23 chromosomes).

position Relationship of a reference point on the presenting part of the fetus to the front, back, or sides of the mother's pelvis.

positional plagiocephaly Asymmetry of an infant's skull; abnormally flattened shape and appearance, usually in the occipital region (the back of the head) as a result of lying consistently on the back.

positive signs of pregnancy Those signs attributed only to the presence of the fetus (e.g., hearing fetal hart tones, visualizing the fetus with ultrasound, palpating fetal movements).

postmenopause The time after menopause.

postpartum Occurring after birth; refers to the period after birth until maternal organs return to their nonpregnant state.

postpartum blues A let-down feeling, accompanied by irritability and anxiety, which usually begins 2 to 3 days after giving birth and disappears within a week or two. Sometimes called the baby blues.

postpartum depression (PPD) Major depressive episode with an onset in pregnancy or within the first year after birth; most often occurs 1 to 3 weeks after birth. (See major depressive episode.)

postpartum hemorrhage (PPH) Excessive bleeding after birth; traditionally defined as a loss of 500 mL or more after a vaginal birth and 1000 mL or more after a cesarean birth.

postpartum infection Any clinical infection of the genital canal that occurs within 28 days after miscarriage, induced abortion, or birth; in the United States, the presence of a fever of 38°C or more on 2 successive days of the first 10 postpartum days (not counting the first 24 hours after birth). Also called puerperal infection.

postpartum psychosis Postpartum depression with psychotic features, including auditory or visual hallucinations, paranoid or grandiose delusions, elements of delirium or disorientation, and extreme deficits in judgment accompanied by high levels of impulsivity that can contribute to increased risks of suicide or infanticide.

postterm pregnancy Pregnancy that extends past 42 completed weeks of gestation (294 days or more from the first day of the last menstrual period).

PPH See postpartum hemorrhage (PPH).

PPHN: See persistent pulmonary hypertension of the newborn (PPHN).

precipitous labor Labor that lasts less than 3 hours from the onset of contractions to the time of birth.

preconception care Care designed for health maintenance before pregnancy. Suggested components of preconception care are health promotion, risk assessment, and interventions.

predictive testing Genetic testing used to clarify the genetic status of asymptomatic family members.

predispositional testing Testing for a gene mutation that indicates susceptibility for developing a condition; a positive result does not indicate a 100% risk of developing the condition.

preeclampsia Pregnancy-specific condition in which hypertension and proteinuria develop after 20 weeks of gestation in a woman who previously had neither condition. In the absence of proteinuria, preeclampsia may be defined as hypertension along with either thrombocytopenia, impaired liver function, the new development of renal insufficiency, pulmonary edema, or new-onset cerebral or visual disturbances.

pregestational diabetes Type 1 or type 2 diabetes that existed before pregnancy.

prelabor rupture of membranes (PROM) Spontaneous rupture of the amniotic sac and leakage of amniotic fluid beginning before the onset of labor at any gestational age. Formerly termed premature rupture of membranes.

premenstrual dysphoric disorder (PMDD) A more severe variant of premenstrual syndrome in which 3% to 8% of women have marked irritability, dysphoria, mood lability, anxiety, fatigue, appetite changes, and a sense of feeling overwhelmed. The most common symptoms are those associated with mood disturbances.

premenstrual syndrome (PMS) Complex, poorly understood condition that includes one or more of a large number (more than 100) of physical and psychological symptoms beginning in the luteal phase of the menstrual cycle, occurring to such a degree that lifestyle or work is affected, and followed by a symptom-free period.

presentation The part of the fetus that enters the pelvic inlet first and leads through the birth canal during labor. The three main presentations are cephalic presentation, breech presentation, and shoulder presentation.

presenting part That part of the fetus that lies closest to the internal os of the cervix.

presumptive signs of pregnancy Those changes felt by the woman (e.g., amenorrhea, fatigue, breast changes).

presymptomatic testing Mutation analysis for a disorder in which symptoms are certain to appear if the individual lives long enough.

preterm birth Birth that occurs between 20 0/7 and 36 6/7 weeks of gestation. Preterm births are categorized as very preterm (<32 weeks of gestation), moderately preterm (32 to 34 weeks of gestation), and late preterm (34 to 36 weeks of gestation).

preterm labor Regular contractions along with a change in cervical effacement or dilation or both, or presentation with regular uterine contractions and cervical dilation of at least 2 cm before 37{0/7} weeks of gestation.

preterm prelabor rupture of membranes (preterm PROM) Premature rupture of membranes that occurs before 37{0/7} weeks of gestation. Formerly termed preterm premature rupture of membranes.

primigravida A woman who is pregnant for the first time.

primipara A woman who has completed one pregnancy with a fetus or fetuses who have reached at least 20 weeks of gestation.

primary dysmenorrhea Painful menstruation beginning 2 to 6 months after menarche, related to ovulation. Condition associated with abnormally increased uterine activity, due to myometrial contractions induced by prostaglandins in the second half of the menstrual cycle.

probable signs of pregnancy Those changes observed by an examiner (e.g., Hegar sign, ballottement, pregnancy tests).

prolapse of the umbilical cord Umbilical cord lies below the presenting part of the fetus; may be frank (visible) or occult (hidden, rather than visible).

prolonged deceleration (of the fetal heart rate) Visually apparent decrease (may be either gradual or abrupt) in fetal heart rate of at least 15 beats/min less than the baseline and lasting more than 2 minutes but less than 10 minutes.

prolonged grief See complicated grief.

PROM See premature rupture of membranes (PROM).

pruritic urticarial papules and plaques of pregnancy (PUPPP) The most common specific dermatosis in pregnancy. Lesions usually appear first on the abdomen but can spread to the arms, thighs, back, and buttocks. PUPPP classically appears in primigravidas during the third trimester. It almost always causes severe itching but is not associated with poor maternal or fetal outcomes.

pruritus Itching.

pruritus gravidarum Itching that occurs during pregnancy; usually occurs over the abdomen.

ptyalism Excessive salivation.

puberty Period in life in which the reproductive organs mature and one becomes functionally capable of reproduction; the entire transitional stage between childhood and sexual maturity.

pudendal nerve block Injection of a local anesthetic at the pudendal nerve root to produce numbness of the genital and perianal region.

puerperium The interval between the birth of the newborn and the return of the reproductive organs to their normal nonpregnant state; also called the fourth trimester of pregnancy or the postpartum period.

pyrosis A burning sensation in the epigastric and sternal region from stomach acid. Also called heartburn or acid indigestion.

Q

quickening Maternal perception of fetal movement ("feeling life"); usually occurs between weeks 16 and 20 of gestation but may be felt earlier by multiparous woman.

R

radical hysterectomy Surgical removal of the uterus, the tubes, the ovaries, the upper third of the vagina, the entire uterosacral and uterovesical ligaments, and all of the parametrium on each side, along with pelvic node dissection encompassing the four major pelvic lymph node chains: ureteral, obturator, hypogastric, and iliac.

rape Legal term that is defined differently by each state. Usually refers to forced sexual intercourse or penetration of the mouth, anus, or vagina by a body part or object without consent; it may or may not include the use of a weapon.

RDS See respiratory distress syndrome (RDS).

recessive trait A trait or disorder expressed or phenotypically, apparent only when two copies of the alleles associated with the trait are present. Genetically determined characteristic that is expressed only when present in the homozygotic state.

reciprocity Type of body movement or behavior that provides the observer with cues, such as the behavioral cues infants provide to parents and parents' responses to cues.

rectocele Herniation or protrusion of the anterior rectal wall through the relaxed or ruptured vaginal fascia and rectovaginal septum; it appears as a large bulge that may be seen through the relaxed introitus.

recurrence risk Estimated risk of a couple having a child with a specific genetic disease once they have produced one or more children with the same genetic disease.

regional analgesia Partial pain relief and motor block produced by a variety of local anesthetic agents.

regional anesthesia Complete pain relief and motor block produced by a variety of local anesthetic agents.

reproductive tract infection Encompasses both sexually transmitted infections and other common genital tract infections.

respiratory distress syndrome (RDS) Condition of the newborn resulting from decreased pulmonary gas exchange, leading to retention of carbon dioxide. Most common neonatal causes are prematurity, perinatal asphyxia, and maternal diabetes mellitus; also known as hyaline membrane disease.

retinopathy of prematurity (ROP) Associated with hyperoxemia, resulting in eye injury and blindness in premature infants.

Rh immune globulin A solution of gamma globulin that contains Rh antibodies; administered to prevent sensitization in an Rh negative woman who has had a fetomaternal transfusion of Rh positive fetal red blood cells.

ribonucleic acid (RNA) Element responsible for transferring genetic information within a cell; a template, or pattern.

rooming-in A family-centered care model in which the newborn stays in the room with the mother; in some facilities the newborn never leaves the mother's presence.

rooting reflex: Normal response of the newborn to move toward whatever touches the area around the mouth and to attempt to suck. This reflex usually disappears by 3 to 4 months of age.

ROP See retinopathy of prematurity (ROP).

S

second stage of labor Begins with full cervical dilation (10 cm) and complete effacement (100%) and ends with the baby's birth. It is composed of two phases: the latent phase and the active pushing (descent) phase.

secondary dysmenorrhea Acquired menstrual pain that develops later in life than primary dysmenorrhea, typically after age 25 years. This condition is associated with pelvic pathology, such as adenomyosis, endometriosis, pelvic inflammatory disease, endometrial polyps, or submucous or interstitial myomas (fibroids).

segmental mastectomy Includes tylectomy, wide excision, and quadrantectomy or segmental mastectomy and involves removal of the tumor, which may be larger, along with a rim of healthy tissue around it, to ensure clear margins.

selective reduction A procedure done during multifetal pregnancies to reduce the number of developing embryos to a number (usually one to three) that can be safely carried to near term.

semen analysis Basic test for male infertility; examination of semen specimen to determine liquefaction, volume, pH, sperm density, and normal morphology. Complete semen analysis includes the study of the effects of cervical mucus on sperm forward motility and survival and evaluation of the sperm's ability to penetrate an ovum.

sentinel event An unexpected occurrence involving death or serious physical or psychological injury or the risk thereof. Serious injury specifically includes loss of limb or function.

sepsis Bacterial infections of the bloodstream.

septic shock Caused by the toxins released into the bloodstream in septicemia. The most common sign is a decrease in blood pressure, a vital sign often not assessed in the care of the neonate. The infant often appears gray or mottled and can be noted to have cool extremities. Other signs are rapid, irregular respirations and pulse (similar to septicemia in general).

septicemia Generalized infection in the bloodstream.

sex chromosome Chromosome associated with determination of gender: the X (female) and Y (male) chromosomes. The normal female has two X chromosomes, and the normal male has one X and one Y chromosome.

sexual assault Intentional unwanted completed or attempted touching of the victim's genitals, anus, groin, or breasts, directly or through clothing as well as by voyeurism.

sexual response cycle The phases of physical changes that occur in response to sexual stimulation and sexual tension release. Divided into four phases: excitement phase, plateau phase, orgasmic phase, and resolution phase. The four phases occur progressively, with no sharp dividing line between any two phases. Specific body changes take place in sequence. The time, intensity, and duration for cyclic completion vary for individuals and situations.

sexual violence Broad term that encompasses a wide range of sexual victimization including sexual harassment, sexual assault, and rape.

sexually transmitted infections (STIs) Infections transmitted as a result of sexual activity with an infected individual; also called sexually transmitted diseases. Include more than 25 organisms that cause infections or infectious disease syndromes primarily transmitted by intimate contact.

SGA See small for gestational age (SGA).

shoulder dystocia Condition in which the head is born but the anterior shoulder cannot pass under the pubic arch to complete the birth of the entire fetus.

sibling rivalry Jealousy and other negative behaviors exhibited by siblings in response to the addition of a new baby in the family.

SIL See squamous intraepithelial lesion (SIL).

single-parent family Family form characterized by one parent (male or female) in the household. This may result from loss of spouse by death, divorce, separation, desertion, or birth of a child to a single woman.

sleep-wake states Variations in the state of consciousness of infants.

small for gestational age (SGA) Inadequate growth for gestational age; an infant whose rate of intrauterine growth was restricted and whose birth weight falls below the 10th percentile on intrauterine growth curves.

somatic cell Cell of the body of an individual that becomes differentiated and composes the tissues, organs, and parts of that individual. Diploid cell; not a gamete.

souffle: Soft, blowing sound or murmur heard by auscultation.

spermatogenesis Process by which mature spermatozoa are formed, during which the diploid chromosome number (46) is reduced by half (haploid, 23).

spina bifida The most common defect of the central nervous system; results from failure of the neural tube to close in early gestation; types are spina bifida occulta and spina bifida manifesta.

spinal anesthesia (block) Regional anesthesia induced by injection of a local anesthetic alone or in combination with an opioid agonist analgesic into the subarachnoid space at the level of the third, fourth, or fifth lumbar interspace.

spiral electrode A small electrode attached to the presenting fetal part (usually the head) to assess the fetal heart rate using the internal mode of monitoring.

spontaneous abortion Pregnancy that ends as a result of natural causes before fetal viability. A loss before 20 weeks of gestation or a fetal weight less than 500 g may be used to define an abortion. Also known as miscarriage.

spontaneous rupture of membranes (SROM) Rupture of membranes by natural means.

squamocolumnar junction Site in the endocervical canal where columnar epithelium and squamous epithelium meet, usually located just inside the cervical os; also called the transformation zone, the most common site for neoplastic changes; cells from this site are scraped for the Pap test.

squamous intraepithelial lesion (SIL) Term used to describe neoplastic changes of the cervix in abnormal cervical cytology reports.

standard of care Level of practice that a reasonable, prudent nurse would provide.

station Relationship of the presenting fetal part to an imaginary line drawn between the ischial spines of the pelvis. It is a measure of the degree of descent of the presenting part of the fetus through the birth canal.

sterilization Surgical procedure intended to render a person infertile or unable to produce children.

stillbirth A fetal death occurring at 20 weeks or later. Also referred to as an intrauterine fetal demise.

striae gravidarum Shining, slightly depressed reddish lines caused by stretching of the skin, often found on the abdomen, thighs, and breasts during pregnancy. These streaks turn to a fine pinkish white or silver tone in time in fair-skinned women and brownish in darker skinned women. Also called stretch marks.

subconjunctival hemorrhage Injuries resulting from rupture of subconjunctival capillaries, caused by increased intracranial pressure during birth.

subculture Group existing within a larger cultural system that retains its own characteristics.

subgaleal hemorrhage Bleeding into the subgaleal compartment, which is a potential space that contains loosely arranged connective tissue, located beneath the galea aponeurosis, the tendinous sheath that connects the frontal and occipital muscles and forms the inner surface of the scalp.

subinvolution Failure of a part (e.g., the uterus) to reduce to its normal size and condition after enlargement from functional activity (e.g., pregnancy).

substance abuse The continued use of substances despite related problems in physical, social, or interpersonal areas. Any use of alcohol or illicit drugs during pregnancy is considered abuse.

supine hypotension Fall in blood pressure caused by impaired venous return when gravid uterus presses on ascending vena cava, when woman is lying flat on her back; vena cava syndrome.

supply-meets-demand Physiologic basis for determining milk production. The volume of milk produced corresponds with the amount of milk removed from the breast.

surfactant Phosphoprotein necessary for normal respiratory function that prevents the alveolar collapse (atelectasis). See also lecithin and L/S ratio.

surgical menopause Occurs with hysterectomy and bilateral oophorectomy.

synchrony Fit between an infant's cues and the parent's response.

T

tachycardia Baseline fetal heart rate greater than 160 beats/min for 10 minutes or longer.

tandem nursing The practice of breastfeeding a newborn and an older child.

telephonic nursing Services such as warm lines, nurse advice lines, and telephonic nursing assessments using telephones, the internet, and Skype.

teratogens Nongenetic factors that cause malformations and disorders in utero.

term Birth after 37 weeks gestation; early term—37 0/7 through 38 6/7 weeks; full term—39 0/7 through 40 6/7 weeks; late term—41 0/7 through 41 6/7 weeks; postterm—42 weeks and beyond; postmature—born after completion of week 42 of gestation and showing the effects of progressive placental insufficiency.

terminal deletion Deletion at the end of a chromosome.

tetraploid Cell that has four times the normal number of chromosomes (4N); example of a polyploidy.

theca-lutein cysts Develop as a result of prolonged stimulation of the ovaries by human chorionic gonadotropin.

therapeutic abortion Pregnancy that has been intentionally terminated for medical reasons.

thermogenesis Creation or production of heat, especially in the body.

thermoregulation Control of temperature.

third stage of labor Stage of labor from the birth of the baby to the expulsion of the placenta.

thrombophlebitis Inflammation of a vein with secondary clot formation.

thrush Fungal infection of the mouth or throat that is characterized by the formation of white patches on a red, moist, inflamed mucous membrane and is caused by *Candida albicans*. Also called mycotic stomatitis.

tocolytics: Medications given to arrest labor after uterine contractions and cervical change have occurred. Also used to treat uterine tachysystole.

tocotransducer Electronic device for measuring uterine contractions using the external mode of monitoring. Also called a tocodynamometer.

TORCH infections Collective name for toxoplasmosis, other infections (e.g., hepatitis), rubella virus, cytomegalovirus, and herpes simplex virus, a group of organisms capable of crossing the placenta; these infections can affect a pregnant woman and her fetus.

tracheoesophageal fistula Congenital abnormality that is an abnormal connection between the esophagus and the trachea; often occurs with esophageal atresia.

transformation zone See squamocolumnar junction.

transition to parenthood The first months of having a child when parents define their parental roles and adjust to parenthood; it involves change and adaptation as the family adjusts to life with a new baby.

translocation Condition in which a chromosome breaks and there is an exchange of chromosomal material between two chromosomes; all or part of the broken chromosome is transferred to a different part of the same chromosome or to another chromosome.

trial of labor (TOL) Period of observation to determine if a laboring woman is likely to be successful in progressing to a vaginal birth.

trimester One of three periods of approximately 13 weeks each into which pregnancy is divided.

triploid Cell that has three times the normal number of chromosomes (3N); example of a polyploidy.

trisomy Product of the union of a normal gamete with a gamete containing an extra chromosome. Condition whereby any given chromosome exists in triplicate instead of the normal duplicate pattern.

trophoblast Outer layer of cells of the developing blastodermic vesicle (blastocyst) that develops the trophoderm or feeding layer, which will establish the nutrient relationships with the uterine endometrium.

tubercles of Montgomery See Montgomery glands.

twins Two neonates from the same impregnation developed within the same uterus at the same time.

U

UAE See uterine artery embolization (UAE).

UI See urinary incontinence (UI).

ultrasound transducer External signal source for monitoring fetal heart rate electronically.

unbalanced translocation Translocation in which part of a chromosome is transferred to a different chromosome; there is extra chromosomal material—extra of one chromosome but correct amount or deficient amount of other chromosome. The individual will be both genotypically and phenotypically abnormal.

unifactorial inheritance Inheritance of phenotypic characteristics controlled by a single gene. See also multifactorial inheritance.

urinary incontinence (UI) Disturbance in urinary control.

uterine Referring or pertaining to the uterus.

uterine artery embolization (UAE) Treatment during which polyvinyl alcohol pellets are injected into selected blood vessels to block the blood supply to the fibroid and cause shrinkage and resolution of symptoms.

uterine atony Relaxation of uterus; leads to postpartum hemorrhage. Failure of the uterine muscle to contract firmly.

uterine dehiscence Separation of a prior uterine scar. The potential for maternal or fetal complications as a result of uterine dehiscence is negligible because separation of a prior scar does not result in hemorrhage. Sometimes called incomplete uterine rupture.

uterine displacement Variation of the normal placement of the uterus, which is normally held in anteversion by the round ligaments, with the cervix pulled backward and upward by the uterosacral ligaments.

uterine polyps Tumors that are on pedicles (stalks) arising from the uterine mucosa; may be endometrial or cervical in origin.

uterine prolapse Falling, sinking, or sliding of the uterus from its normal location in the body. The degree of prolapse can vary from mild to complete. In complete prolapse the cervix and body of the uterus protrude through the vagina and the vagina is inverted.

uterine resting tone Degree of tension in the uterine muscle between contractions; relaxation of the uterus between contractions.

uterine rupture Rare but life-threatening obstetric injury in which there is complete nonsurgical disruption of all uterine layers. The major risk factor for uterine rupture is a scarred uterus as a result of previous cesarean birth or other uterine surgery.

uterine souffle A rushing or blowing sound of maternal blood flowing through uterine arteries; synchronous with the maternal pulse.

uterine tachysystole More than five contractions in 10 minutes, averaged over a 30-minute window, regardless of the presence of an abnormal fetal heart rate or pattern or the woman's perception of pain. The term applies to both spontaneous and stimulated labor.

uteroplacental insufficiency (UPI) Decline in placental function—exchange of gases, nutrients, and wastes—leading to fetal hypoxia and acidosis; evidenced by late fetal heart rate decelerations in response to uterine contractions.

V

vacuum-assisted birth Birth involving attachment of vacuum cup to fetal head and using negative pressure to assist in birth of the fetus. Also called vacuum extraction.

vaginal birth after cesarean (VBAC) Giving birth vaginally after having had a previous cesarean birth.

Valsalva maneuver Any forced expiratory effort against a closed airway such as holding one's breath and tightening the abdominal muscles (e.g., pushing during the second stage of labor).

variability (of the fetal heart rate) Irregular waves or fluctuations in the baseline fetal heart rate (FHR) of two cycles per minute or greater. It is a characteristic of the baseline FHR and does not include accelerations or decelerations of the FHR. Four possible categories of variability have been identified: absent, minimal, moderate, and marked.

variable deceleration (of the fetal heart rate) Visually abrupt (onset to nadir [lowest point] less than 30 seconds) decrease in fetal heart rate (FHR) to less than the baseline. The decrease is at least 15 beats/min or more below the baseline, lasts at least 15 seconds, and returns to baseline in less than 2 minutes from the time of onset. Variable decelerations are caused by compression of the umbilical cord.

vasa previa Occurs when fetal vessels lie over the cervical os and are implanted into the fetal membranes rather than into the placenta. There are two variations of vasa previa: velamentous insertion of the cord and succenturiate placenta.

vernix caseosa Protective gray-white fatty substance of cheesy consistency covering the fetal skin.

very low birth weight An infant whose birth weight is less than 1500 g (3.3 lb).

vestibular schwannoma Tumor on the eighth cranial nerves, the hearing and balance nerves.

viability The capacity to live outside the uterus; infants born at 22 to 25 weeks of gestation are considered to be on the threshold of viability.

vibroacoustic stimulation One of the methods of testing antepartum fetal heart rate response. Generally performed in conjunction with the nonstress test. Uses a combination of sound and vibration to stimulate the fetus. Also called the fetal acoustic stimulation test.

von Willebrand disease (vWD) A type of hemophilia; probably the most common of all hereditary bleeding disorders.

VSE See vulvar self-examination (VSE).

vulvar self-examination (VSE) Systematic examination of the vulva by the woman.

vulvectomy Surgical removal of all or parts of the vulva.

vulvodynia Complex condition thought to be a chronic pain disorder of the vulvar area; this term is used if pain is present with no visible abnormality or no identified neurologic diagnosis.

vWD See von Willebrand disease (vWD).

W

walking survey Using one's senses while traveling through a community to obtain information about sociocultural characteristics and the environment, housing, transportation, and local community agencies.

warm lines Telephone lines that are offered as a community service to provide new parents with support, encouragement, and basic parenting education.

X

X-linked dominant inheritance Mode of genetic inheritance by which a dominant gene is carried on the X chromosome.

X-linked recessive inheritance disorder Disorder for which the abnormal genes are carried on the X chromosome.

Z

Zika virus A virus spread by bites from the *Aedes* mosquito. It is also spread by sexual contact by semen. Women who become pregnant and are infected by the Zika virus have an increased risk of giving birth to an infant with microcephaly.

zygote Cell formed by the union of two reproductive cells or gametes; the fertilized ovum resulting from the union of a sperm and an ovum (egg).

INDEX

Note: Page numbers followed by "f" refer to illustrations; page numbers followed by "t" refer to tables; page numbers followed by "b" refer to boxes.

FEATURES

FEATURES — cont'd